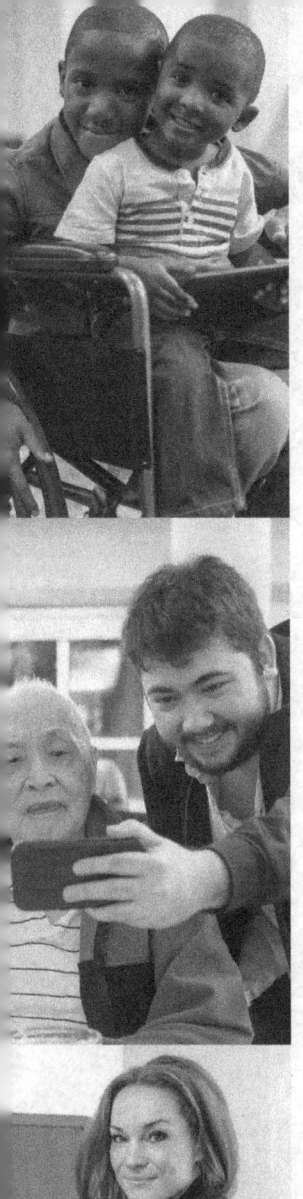

P9-BBP-740

THE
COMPLETE
DIRECTORY
FOR PEOPLE WITH
DISABILITIES

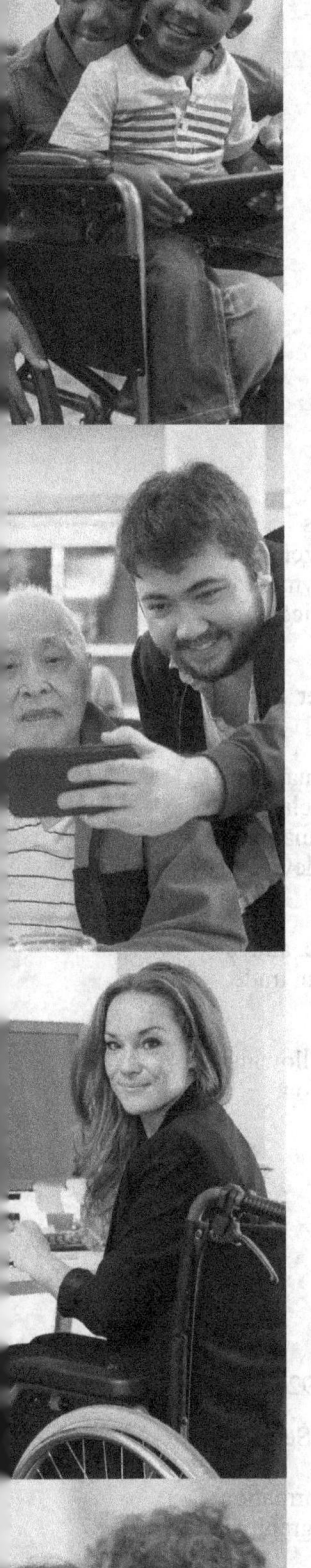

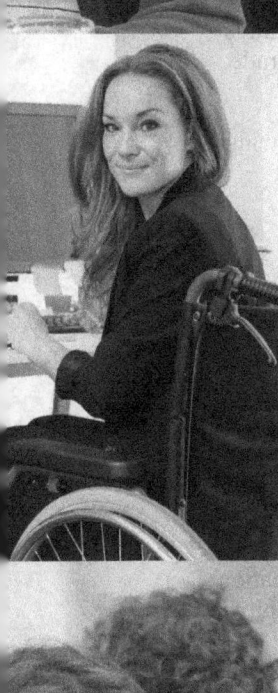

2018

TWENTY SIXTH EDITION

THE COMPLETE DIRECTORY FOR PEOPLE WITH DISABILITIES

A SEDGWICK PRESS BOOK

GREY HOUSE PUBLISHING

PUBLISHER: Leslie Mackenzie
EDITORIAL DIRECTOR: Laura Mars

PRODUCTION MANAGER & COMPOSITION: Kristen Hayes
MARKETING DIRECTOR: Jessica Moody

A Sedgwick Press Book
Grey House Publishing, Inc.
4919 Route 22
Amenia, NY 12501
518.789.8700
FAX 845.373.6390
www.greyhouse.com
e-mail: books@greyhouse.com

First edition published 1991
Twenty-sixth edition published 2017

The complete directory for people with disabilities : products, resources, books, services.-1992-2015

1. People with disabilities-Services for-United States-Directories. 2. People with disabilities-Services for-United States-Periodicals. 3. Disabled Persons-United States-Bibliography. 4. Disabled Persons-United States-Directory. 5. Information Services-United States-Bibliography. 6. Information Services-United States-Directory. 7. Mental Retardation-Rehabilitation-United States-Bibliography. 8. Mental Retardation-Rehabilitation-United States-Directory. 9. Rehabilitation-United States-Bibliography. 10. Rehabilitation-United States-Directory. I. Title: Directory for people with disabilities.

HV1553.C58
362.4/048/02573   92-658843

Printed in Canada
ISBN 13: 978-1-68217-377-0 Softcover

Table of Contents

General Resources for People with Disabilities

Arts & Entertainment

Assistive Devices

Associations

Camps

Table of Contents

Government Agencies

Table of Contents

Independent Living Centers

Law

Libraries & Research Centers

Rehabilitation Facilities, Acute

Table of Contents

Table of Contents

Table of Contents

Introduction

This 26th edition of the award-winning *Complete Directory for People with Disabilities* is an invaluable resource for all those living with a disability and all those committed to empowering these individuals. It offers thousands of ways for people with disabilities to succeed at work, in school, and in their community. Coverage includes Associations, Products, Camps, Living Facilities, Print and Electronic Resources and much more. The comprehensive Table of Contents guides you through the 31 chapters and more than 100 subchapters contained in this rich resource.

Careful research and compilation of the best data available maintains the reputation of *The Complete Directory for People with Disabilities* among educators, librarians and the disability community. This resource is a repeat recipient of the **National Mature Media Award** and the **National Health Information Award**.

Praise for previous editions:

> *"The strength of this source is in the information referral portion for each entry: the wide range of resources and organizations presented that can assist with additional information and support."*
>
> —ARBA

> *"...thousands of resources...covering a diverse range of services...separate section for specific disabilities...from aging to mobility and from the blind and deaf to speech and language disorders. Libraries...will want to consider..."*
>
> —Against the Grain

Sure to save hours of Internet research time, *The Complete Directory for People with Disabilities* provides comprehensive, critical and immediate information in one source that can be accessed quickly and easily. This edition provides **9,182 descriptive listings**, **24,348 key contacts**, **7,806 fax numbers**, **6,301 email addresses**, and **8,328 web sites**. Following this Introduction is a Glossary of Disability-Related terms.

Three indexes provide quick, easy access to the data:
- **Entry & Publisher Index** lists all directory listings alphabetically;
- **Geographic Index** organizes listings alphabetically by state;
- **Subject Index** alphabetically organizes directory listings by relevant topics, i.e. autism, language disorders.

In addition to the print directory, *The Complete Directory for People with Disabilities* is available for subscription on G.O.L.D., Grey House OnLine Databases. This gives you immediate access to the most valuable disability industry contacts in the United States, plus offers easy-to-use keyword searches, organization type and subject searches, hotlinks to web sites and emails, and so much more. Call 800-562-2139 for a free trial or visit http://gold.greyhouse.com for more information.

We welcome your comments, and look forward to another year of serving the disability community.

Glossary of Disability-Related Terms

Accessible: In the case of a facility, readily usable by a particular individual; in the case of a program or activity, presented or provided in such a way that a particular individual can participate, with or without auxiliary aids(s); in the case of electronic resources, accessible with or without the use of adaptive computer technology.

Access barrier: Any obstruction that prevents people with disabilities from using standard facilities, equipment and resources.

Accessible Web design: Creating World Wide Web pages according to universal design principles to eliminate or reduce barriers, including those that affect people with disabilities.

Accommodation: An adjustment to make a workstation, job, program, facility, or resource accessible to a person with a disability.

Adaptive technology: Hardware or software products that provide access to a computer that is otherwise inaccessible to an individual with a disability.

ALT attribute: HTML code that works in combination with graphical tags to provide alternative text for graphical elements.

Americans with Disabilities Act of 1990 (ADA): A comprehensive Federal law that prohibits discrimination on the basis of disability in employment, telecommunications, public services, public accommodations and services.

American Standard Code for Information Interchange (ASCII): Standard for unformatted text which enables transfer of data between platforms and computer systems.

Assistive technology: Technology used to assist a person with a disability (e.g., a handsplint or computer-related equipment).

Auxiliary aids and services: May include qualified interpreters or other effective methods of making aurally delivered materials available to individuals with hearing impairments; qualified readers, taped texts, or other effective methods of making visually delivered materials available to individuals with visual impairments; acquisition or modification of equipment or devices; and other similar services and actions.

Braille: A system of embossed characters formed by using a Braille cell, a combination of six dots consisting of two vertical columns of three dots each. Each simple Braille character is formed by one or more of these dots and occupies a full cell or space.

Browser: A program that runs on an Internet-connected computer and provides access to the World Wide Web. Web browsers may be text-only, such as Lynx, or graphical, such as Internet Explorer and Netscape Navigator.

Captioned film or videos: Transcription of the verbal portion of films or videos is displayed to make them accessible to people who have hearing impairments.

Closed Circuit TV Magnifier (CCTV): A camera used to magnify books or other materials on a monitor.

Cooperative education: Programs that work with students, faculty, staff, and employers to help students clarify career and academic goals, and expand classroom study by allowing students to participate in paid, practical work experiences.

Compensatory tools: Adaptive computing systems that allow people with disabilities to use computers to complete tasks that would be difficult without a computer (e.g., reading, writing, communicating, accessing information).

Disability: A physical or mental impairment that substantially limits one or more major life activities; a record of such an impairment; or being regarded as having such an impairment (Americans with Disabilities Act of 1990).

Discrimination: The act of treating a person differently in a negative manner based on factors other than individual merit.

Dymo Labeller: A device used to create raised print or Braille labels.

Electronic information: Any digital data for use with computers or computer networks, including disks, CD-ROMs, and World Wide Web resources.

Essential job functions: Those functions of a job or task which must be completed with or without an accommodation.

Facility: All or any portion of a physical complex, including buildings, structures, equipment, grounds, roads, and parking lots.

FM sound amplification system: An electronic amplification system consisting of three components: a microphone/transmitter, monaural FM receiver and a combination charger/carrying case. It provides wireless FM broadcasts from a speaker to a listener who has a hearing impairment.

Frame tags: A means of displaying Web pages. The browser reads the frame tags and produces an output that subdivides output within a browser into discrete windows.

Graphical user interface (GUI): Program interface that presents digital information and software programs in an image-based format as compared to a character-based format.

Hardware: Physical equipment related to computers.

Hearing impairment: Complete or partial loss of the ability to hear, caused by a variety of injuries or diseases, including congenital causes. Limitations, including difficulties in understanding language or other auditory messages and/or in production of understandable speech, are possible.

Independent study: A student works one-on-one with individual faculty members to develop projects for credit.

Informational interview: An activity where students meet with people working in careers to ask questions about their jobs and companies, allowing students to gain personal perspectives on career interests.

Input: Any method by which information is entered into a computer.

Internet: Computer network connecting governmental, educational, commercial, other organizations, and individual computer systems.

Internship: A time-limited, intensive learning experience outside of the typical classroom.

Interpreter: Professional person who assists a person who is deaf in communicating with hearing people.

Job shadowing: A short work-based learning experience where students visit businesses to observe one or more specific jobs to provide them with a realistic view of occupations in a variety of settings.

Keyboard emulation: Uses hardware and/or software in place of a standard keyboard.

Kinesthetic: Refers to touch-based feedback.

Large-print: Most ordinary print is six to ten points in height (about 1/16 to 1/8 of an inch). Large-print type is fourteen to eighteen points (about 1/8 to 1/4 of an inch) and sometimes larger.

Link: a connection between two electronic files or data items.

Lynx: A text-based World Wide Web browser.

Macro: A mini-program that, when run within an application, executes a series of predetermined keystrokes and commands to accomplish a specific task. Macros can automate tedious and often-repeated tasks or create special menus to speed data entry.

Mainstreaming: The inclusion of people with disabilities, with or without special accommodations, in programs, activities, and facilities with non-disabled people.

Major life activities: Functions such as caring for oneself, performing manual tasks, walking, seeing, hearing, speaking, breathing, learning, working, and participating in community activities (Americans with Disabilities Act of 1990).

Multimedia: A computer-based method of presenting information by using more than one medium of communication, such as text, graphics, and sound.

Optical Character Recognition (OCR): Machine recognition of printed or typed text. Using OCR software with a scanner, a printed page can be scanned and the characters converted into text in an electronic format.

Output: Any method of displaying or presenting electronic information to the user through a computer monitor or other device (e.g., speech synthesizer).

Portable Document Format (PDF): The file format for representing documents in a manner that is independent of the original application software, hardware and operating system used to create the documents.

Physical or mental impairment: Any physiological disorder or condition, cosmetic disfigurement, or anatomical loss affecting one or more, but not necessarily limited to, the following body systems: neurological; musculoskeletal; special sense organs; respiratory, including speech organs; cardiovascular; reproductive; digestive; genitourinary; hemic and lymphatic; skin and endocrine; or any mental or psychological disorder, such as mental retardation, organic brain syndrome, emotional or mental illness, and specific learning disabilities (Americans with Disabilities Act of 1990).

Plug-ins: Programs that work within a browser to alter, enhance, or extend the browser,s operation. They are often used for viewing video, animation or listening to audio files.

Proprietary software: Privately owned software based on trade secrets, privately developed technology, or specifications that the owner refuses to divulge, thus preventing others from duplicating a product or program unless an explicit license is purchased. The opposite of proprietary is open (publicly published and available for emulation by others).

Qualified individual with a disability: An individual with a disability who, with or without reasonable modification to rules, policies or practices, the removal of architectural, communication, or transportation barriers, or the provision of auxiliary aids and services, meets the essential eligibility requirements for the receipt of services or participation in programs or activities provided by a public entity (Americans with Disabilities Act of 1990).

Reader: Volunteer or employee of a blind or partially sighted individual who reads printed material in person or records to audiotape.

Relay service: A third-party service (usually free) that allows a hearing person without a TTY/TDD device to communicate over the telephone with a person who has a hearing impairment. The system also allows a person with a hearing impairment who has a TTY/TDD to communicate in voice through a third party, with a hearing person or business.

Screen reader: A text-to-speech system intended for use by computer users who are blind or have low vision that speaks the text content of a computer display using a speech synthesizer.

Service learning: A structured, volunteer work experience where students provide community service in non-paid, volunteer positions to give them opportunities to apply knowledge and skills learned in school while making a contribution to local communities.

Sign language: Manual communication commonly used by people who are deaf. Sign language is not universal; deaf people from different countries speak different sign languages. The gestures or symbols in sign language are organized in a linguistic way. Each individual gesture is called a sign. Each sign has three distinct parts: the hand shape, the position of the hands, and the movement of the hands. American Sign Language (ASL) is the most commonly used sign language in the United States.

Specific learning disability (SLD): A disorder of one or more of the basic psychological processes involved in understanding or in using language, spoken or written, which may manifest itself in difficulties listening, thinking, speaking, reading, writing, spelling, or doing mathematical calculations. Limitations may include hyperactivity, distractibility, emotional instability, visual and/or auditory perception difficulties and/or motor limitations, depending on the type(s) of learning disability.

Speech output system: A system that provides the user with a voice alternative to the text presented on the computer screen.

Speech impairment: A problem in communication and related areas, such as oral motor function, ranging from simple sound substitutions to the inability to understand or use language or use the oral-motor mechanism for functional speech and feeding. Some causes of speech and language disorders include hearing loss; neurological disorders; brain injury; mental retardation; drug abuse; physical impairments, such as cleft lip or palate; and vocal abuse or misuse.

Speech input system: A computer-based system that allows the operator to control the system using his/her voice.

Sticky keys: Enables a computer user to do multiple key combinations on a keyboard using only one finger at a time. The sticky keys function is usually used with the Ctrl, Alt, and Shift keys. Simultaneous keystrokes can be entered sequentially.

Telecommunications Device for the Deaf (TDD) or Teletypewriter (TTY): A device which enables someone who has a speech or hearing impairment to use a telephone when communicating with someone else who has a TDD/TTY. TDD/TTYs can be used with any telephone, and one needs only a basic typing ability to use them.

Trackball: A pointing device consisting of a ball housed in a socket containing sensors to detect the rotation of the ball " like an upside down mouse. The user rolls the ball with his thumb or the palm of his hand to move the pointer.

Traumatic Brain Injury (TBI): An open or closed head injury resulting in impairments in one or more areas, such as cognition; language; memory; attention; reasoning; abstract thinking; judgment; problem-solving; sensory, perceptual, and motor abilities; psychosocial behavior; physical functions; information processing; and speech. The term does not apply to brain injuries that are congenital or degenerative, or brain injuries induced by birth trauma.

Undue hardship: An action that requires significant difficulty or expense in relation to the size of the employer, the resources available, and the nature of the operation (Americans with Disabilities Act of 1990).

Universal design: Designing programs, services, tools, and facilities so that they are usable, without additional modification, by the widest range of users possible, taking into account a variety of abilities and disabilities.

Vocational Rehabilitation Act of 1973: An act prohibiting discrimination on the basis of disability which applies to any program that receives federal financial assistance. Section 504 of the act is aimed at making educational programs and facilities accessible to all people with disabilities. Section 508 of the act requires that electronic office equipment purchased through federal procurement meets disability access guidelines.

Voice input system: A computer-based system that allows the operator to control the system using his/her voice.

Vision impairments: A complete or partial loss of the ability to see, caused by a variety of injuries or diseases including congenital causes. Legal blindness is defined as visual acuity of 20/200 or less in the better eye with correcting lenses, on the widest diameter of the visual field subtending an angular distance no greater than 20 degrees.

World Wide Web (WWW, W3, or Web): Hypertext and multimedia gateway to the Internet.

DO-IT
University of Washington
Box 354842
Seattle, WA 98195-4842
doit@uw.edu
http://www.washington.edu/doit/
206-685-DOIT (3648) (voice/TTY)
888-972-DOIT (3648) (toll free voice/TTY)
206-221-4171 (FAX)
509-328-9331 (voice/TTY) Spokane

Director: Sheryl Burgstahler, Ph.D.

User Guide

Descriptive listings in *The Complete Directory for People with Disabilities* are organized into 31 chapters, by either resource type or disability category type. You will find the following types of listings throughout the book:

- National Agencies & Associations
- State Agencies & Associations
- Camps & Exchanges Programs
- Manufacturers of Assistive Devices, Clothing, Computer Equipment & Supplies
- Print & Electronic Media
- Living Centers & Facilities
- Libraries & Research Centers
- Conferences & Trade Shows

Below is a sample listing illustrating the kind of information that is or might be included in an Association entry. Each numbered item of information is described in the paragraphs on the following page.

---

1 ➡ 1234
2 ➡ **Advocacy Center for Seniors with Disabilities**
3 ➡ 1762 South Major Drive
New Orleans, LA 98087

4 ➡ **800-000-0000**

5 ➡ **058-884-0709**

6 ➡ **Fax: 058-884-0568**

7 ➡ **TDD: 800-000-0001**

8 ➡ **email: info@sadvoc.com**

9 ➡ **www.sadvoc.com**

10 ➡ Barbara Pierce, Executive Director
Diane Watkins, Marketing Director
Robert Goldfarb, Administrative Assistant

11 ➡ The mission of the Center is to advance the dignity, equality, self-determination and choices of senior citizens with disabilities. It provides referrals, publishes information, including a monthly newsletter, offers workshops and consultation on legal, social, travel, and medical issues. The Center works with various local organizations to help seniors with disabilities stay active in their community.

12 ➡ Founded 1964

13 ➡ 18 pages

14 ➡ Monthly

User Key

1 → **Record Number**: Entries are listed alphabetically within each category and numbered sequentially. The entry numbers, rather than page numbers, are used in the indexes to refer to listings.

2 → **Organization Name**: Formal name of company or organization. Where organization names are completely capitalized, the listing will appear at the beginning of the alphabetized section. In the case of publications, the title of the publication will appear first, followed by the publisher.

3 → **Address**: Location or permanent address of the organization.

4 → **Toll Free Number**: This is listed when provided by the organization.

5 → **Phone Number**: The listed phone number is usually for the main office of the organization, but may also be for the sales, marketing, or public relations office as provided by the organization.

6 → **Fax Number**: This is listed when provided by the organization.

7 → **TDD Number**: This is listed when provided. It refers to Telephone Device for the Deaf.

8 → **E-Mail**: This is listed when provided by the organization and is generally the main office e-mail.

9 → **Web Site**: This is also referred to as an URL address. These web sites are accessed through the Internet by typing *http://* before the URL address.

10 → **Key Personnel**: Name and titles of department heads of the organization.

11 → **Organization Description**: This paragraph contains a brief description of the organization and their services.

12 → **Year Founded:** The year in which the organization was established or founded. If the organization has changed its name, the founding date is usually for the earliest name under which it was known.

13 → **Number of Pages**: Number of pages if the listing is a publication.

14 → **Frequency:** The frequency of the listing if it is a publication.

Arts & Entertainment

Resources for the Disabled

1 AbleArts
P.O. Box 831
Bear, DE 19701
302-368-7477
AbleArts@AbleArts.org
ablearts.org

2 American Art Therapy Association (AATA)
4875 Eisenhower Avenue
Suite 240
Alexandria, VA 22304
703-548-5860
888-290-0878
Fax: 703-783-8468
info@arttherapy.org
arttherapy.org

Sarah P. Deaver, PhD, ATR-BC, President
Michele Basham, Director, Membership Information & Programs
Barbara Florence, Director, Communication, Education & Conference
Dean Sagar, Director of Public Policy
Organization of professionals who believe the art process is a beneficial and healing process.

3 American Council of the Blind
1703 N. Beauregard St.
Suite 420
Alexandria, VA 22311
202-467-5081
800-424-8666
Fax: 703-465-5085
info@acb.org
www.acb.org

Kim Charlson, President
Eric Bridges, Executive Director
Tony Stephens, Director of Advocacy and Governmental Affairs
The American Council of the Blind (ACB) is an association working to increase the independence, security, and opportunity for all blind or visually impaired individuals. The Council primarily focuses on developing and maintaining policies to implement the services needed for the blind or visually impaired.

4 American Dance Therapy Association (ADTA)
10632 Little Patuxent Pkwy
Ste 108
Columbia, MD 21044- 6258
410-997-4040
Fax: 410-997-4048
info@adta.org
www.adta.org/

Sharon Goodill, President
Jody Wager, MS, BC-DMT, Vice President
Gail Wood, Secretary
Meghan Dempsey, Treasurer
Dance-movement therapy is a psychotherapeutic use of movement as a process which furthers the emotional, cognitive and physical integration of the individual.

5 American Music Therapy Association (AMTA)
8455 Colesville Road
Suite 1000
Silver Spring, MD 20910-3392
301-589-3300
Fax: 301-589-5175
info@musictherapy.org
www.musictherapy.org

Andrea H. Farbman, Executive Director
Miss Angie K Elkins, Director of Membership Services & Information Systems
Al Bumanis, Director of Communications & Conferences
Jane P. Creagan, Director of Professional Programs
AMTA's purpose is the progressive development of the therapeutic use of music in rehabilitation, special education and community settings. Predecessors to the American Music Therapy Association included the National Association for Music Therapy founded in 1950 and the American Association for Music Therapy founded in 1971. AMTA is committed to the advancement of education, training, professional standards, credentials and research in support of the music therapy profession.

6 Arena Stage
The Mead Center for American Theater
1101 Sixth St. SW
Washington, DC 20024
202-554-9066
arenastage.org

Edgard Dobie, Executive Director
Molly Smith, Artistic Director
Anita Maynard Losh, Director, Community Engagement
Holly K. Oliver, Chief Development Officer
Arena Stage has played a pioneering role in providing access to all productions for people with disabilities. Access services and programs include wheelchair accessible seating; infrared assistive listening devices; Braille, large print, audio description and sign interpretation at designated performances.

7 Art Therapy SourceBook
McGraw-Hill Company
2 Penn Plaza
New York, NY 10121-101
212-904-2000
www.mhhe.com/hper/physed

Cathy Malchiodi, Author
An overview of the uses of art as a mentally therapeutic tool.
$18.00
272 pages
ISBN 1-565658-84-1

8 Art and Disabilities
Brookline Books
8 Trumbull Rd
Suite B-001
Northampton, MA 01060
413-584-0184
800-666-2665
Fax: 413-584-6184
brbooks@yahoo.com
www.brooklinebooks.com

Florence Ludins-Katz, Author
A step-by-step guide to establishing creative arts centers for people with disabilities. Includes philosophy and making creative arts centers happen.

9 Art and Healing: Using Expressive Art to Heal Your Body, Mind, and Soul
Three Rivers Press/Crown Publishing-Random House
1745 Broadway
New York, NY 10019
212-782-9000
crownpublicity@randomhouse.com
www.randomhouse.com/crown/trp.html

Barbara Ganim, Author
Markus Dohle, Chairman & CEO
Melanie Fallon-Houska, Dir., Corporate Contributions
The author believes creating a visual image through any medium can produce physical and emotional benefits for both the creator as well as those who view it. *$17.00*
256 pages
ISBN 0-609803-16-6

10 Art for All the Children: Approaches to Art Therapy for Children with Disabilities
Charles C. Thomas
2600 S First St
Springfield, IL 62704-4730
217-789-8980
800-258-8980
Fax: 217-789-9130
books@ccthomas.com
www.ccthomas.com

Frances E Anderson, Author
Sharon Moorman, Editorial Assistant
This second edition is for art therapists in training and for in-service professionals in art therapy, art education and special education who have children with disabilities as a part of their case/class load. *$56.95*
398 pages Paperback
ISBN 0-398060-07-7

11 **Arts Unbound**
542/544 Freeman Street
Orange, NJ   07050   973-675-2787
                                            Fax: 973-678-4408
                                          info@artsunbound.org
                                          www.artsunbound.org
Margaret Mikkelsen, Executive Director
Catherine Lazen, Founder and Board Chair
Alan Hirsh, Executive Vice President
Tashea Patterson Carless, Director of Agency Operations
Arts Unbound is a nonprofit organization dedicated to the artistic
achievement of youth, adults, and senior citizens with disabili-
ties.

12 **Association of Mouth and Foot Painting Artists (AMPFA)**
2070 Peachtree Court
Suite 101
Atlanta, GA   30341   770-986-7764
                                              877-637- 872
                                            Fax: 770-986-8563
                                          mfpausa@bellsouth.net
                                            www.mfpausa.com
Erich Stegmann, Founder
The AMPF is an international, for-profit association wholly
owned and run by disabled artists to help them meet their financial needs. Members paint with brushes held in their mouths or
feet as a result of a disability sustained at birth or through an accident or illness that prohibits them from using their hands.

13 **Awakenings Project, The**
PO Box 177
Wheaton, IL   60187   www.awakeningsproject.org
Robert Lundin, Co-Director
Irene O'Neill, President and Co-Director
Mary Lou Lowry, Secretary
John Rakow, Vice President
The Awakenings Project is an organization whose mission is to
assist those artists with psychiatric illnesses in developing their
talent and finding an outlet for their creative abilities through art
in all forms.

14 **Brookline Books**
8 Trumbull Rd
Suite B-001
Northampton, MA   01060   413-584-0184
                                              800-666-2665
                                            Fax: 413-584-6184
                                           brbooks@yahoo.com
                                          www.brooklinebooks.com

15 **Clinical Applications of Music Therapy in Developmental
Disability, Pediatrics and Neurolog**
Taylor & Francis
400 Market Street
Suite 400
Philadelphia, PA   19106-4738   215-922-1161
                                              866-416-1078
                                            Fax: 215-922-1474
                                           hello.usa@jkp.com
                                              www.jkp.com
Tony Wigram, Editor
Jessica Kingsley, Chairman, Managing Director
Jemima Kingsley, Director
Octavia Kingsley, Production Director
More and more, music therapy is being practiced as an interven-
tion in medical and special educational settings. This book de-
scribes and explains the planning and evaluation of music
therapy intervention and how it can be used for assessing com-
plex organic and emotional disabilities. *$34.95*
312 pages
ISBN 1-853027-34-0

16 **Contemporary Art Therapy with Adolescents**
Taylor & Francis
400 Market Street
Suite 400
Philadelphia, PA   19106-4738   215-922-1161
                                              866-416-1078
                                            Fax: 215-922-1474
                                           hello.usa@jkp.com
                                              www.jkp.com
Shirley Riley, Author
Jessica Kingsley, Chairman, Managing Director
Jemima Kingsley, Director
Octavia Kingsley, Production Director
Reviews contemporary theories on adolescent development and
therapy and offers solutions to the treatment of young people. *$
26.95*
285 pages
ISBN 1-853026-37-9

17 **Creative Arts Resources Catalog**
MMB Music
9051 Watson Road
Ste 161
St. Louis, MO   63126   314-531-9635
                                              80 -54 -377
                                            Fax: 314-531-8384
                                           info@mmbmusic.com
                                            www.mmbmusic.com
Norm Goldberg, Founder & Chair
Publisher and distributor of creative arts therapy materials in the
areas of music, dance, art, drama, and poetry. Free catalog con-
tains hundreds of books, recordings, and videos.

18 **Creative Growth Art Center**
355 - 24th St
Oakland, CA   94612   510-836-2340
                                            Fax: 510-836-0769
                                          info@creativegrowth.org
                                          www.creativegrowth.org
Becki Couch-Alvarado, Executive Director
Tom Di Maria, Director
Jennifer Strate O'Neal, Partnerships & Communications Manager
Creative Growth Art Center serves adult artists with developmen-
tal, mental and physical disabilities, providing a professional stu-
dio environment for artistic development, gallery exhibition and
representation and a social atmosphere among peers.

19 **Creativity Explored**
3245 16th Street
San Francisco, CA   94103   415-863-2108
                                            Fax: 415-863-1655
                                        info@creativityexplored.org
                                        www.creativityexplored.org
Jeff Spicer, President
Nina Sazevich, Vice President
Amy Taub, Executive Director
Ann Kappes, Marketing & Business Development Director
Creativity Explored is a nonprofit visual arts center for artists
with developmental disabilities.

20 **Dancing from the Inside Out**
Fanlight Productions
c/o Icarus Films
32 Court Street, 21st Floor
Brooklyn, NY 11201   718-488-8900
                                              800-876-1710
                                            Fax: 718-488-8642
                                           info@fanlight.com
                                            www.fanlight.com
Ben Achtenberg, Founder
This eloquent video looks at the lives and work of three talented
dancers who dance professionally with the acclaimed AXIS
Dance Troupe, which includes both disabled and non-disabled
dancers. They discuss the process they went through in adapting
to their disability and how they came to re-discover physical expression through dance.

21   Deaf West Theatre
5114 Lankershim Blvd.
Los Angeles, CA   91601
818-762-2998
Fax: 818-762-2981
info@deafwest.org
deafwest.org

Ed Waterstreet, Founding Artistic Director
David Kurs, Artistic Director
Mark Freund, President
Deaf West Theatre, Inc., was founded in 1991 to directly improve and enrich the cultural lives of the 1.2 million deaf and hard-of-hearing individuals who live in the Los Angeles area. DWT provides exposure and access to professional theatre, filling a void for deaf artists and audiences.

22   Dionysus Theatre
4930 W. Bellfort
Houston, TX   77035
713-728-0041
Fax: 713-779-7483
Deb@Dionysustheatre.org
www.dionysustheatre.net
Deborah E. Nowinski, Founder & Executive Director
Dionysus Theatre is a non profit organization bringing the theatre experience to actors with disabilities and those that are non-disabled together using the theatre as our creative venue.

23   Disability and Social Performance: Using Drama to Achieve Successful Acts
Brookline Books
8 Trumbull Rd
Suite B-001
Northampton, MA   01060
413-584-0184
800-666-2665
Fax: 413-584-6184
brbooks@yahoo.com
www.brooklinebooks.com
Bernie Warren, Author
This book makes a major contribution to the understanding of disability, people with disabilities and the creative power they possess which can be unleashed through performance. The books name is Disability and Social Performance: Using Drama to Achieve Successful Acts of Being. *$17.95*

24   Expressive Arts for the Very Disabled and Handicapped of All Ages
Charles C. Thomas
2600 S First St
Springfield, IL   62704-4730
217-789-8980
800-258-8980
Fax: 217-789-9130
books@ccthomas.com
www.ccthomas.com

Marilyn Wannamaker, Co-Author
Jane G. Cohen, Co-Author
The ideas presented are not only designed to hold the interest of the children and adults, but to meet the needs of professionals and volunteers working with the disabled artists. All crafts are rated on a sliding scale, are of a low difficulty rating, use inexpensive and safe materials, and include explicit instructions. *$ 49.95*
236 pages Spiral-Paper 1996
ISBN 0-398067-04-5

25   Fanlight Productions
c/o Icarus Films
32 Court Street, 21st Floor
Brooklyn, NY 11201
718-488-8900
800-876-1710
Fax: 718-488-8642
info@fanlight.com
www.fanlight.com
Ben Achtenberg, Founder
Fanlight Productions is a leading distributor of innovative film and video works on the social issues of our time, with a special focus on healthcare, mental health, professional ethics, aging and gerontology, disabilities, the workplace, and gender and family issues. Select titles include Acting Blind, Autism: A World Apart, Dancing from the Inside Out, and Able to Laugh.

26   Fountain House Gallery
702 Ninth Ave at 48th St
New York, NY   10019
212-262-2756
fountaingallerynyc.com
Ariel Wilmott, Director
Camille Tibaldeo, Communications Director
Fountain House Gallery provides an environment for artists living and working with mental illness to pursue their personal visions and to challenge the stigma that surrounds mental illness.

27   Friends In Art (FIA)
4317 Vermont Court
Columbia, MO   65203
573-445-5564
paltschul@centurytel.net
www.friendsinart.com

Peter Altschul, President
Lynn Hedl, Vice President
Don Horn, Corresponding Secretary
Arlo Monthei, Treasurer
Friends in Art is a national organization for blind, visually impaired, and deaf-blind artists, musicians and writers, and art enthusiasts. The organization is dedicated to enhancing the skills and broadening the opportunities of the individuals involved with the organization.

28   Future Horizons
721 West Abram Street
Arlington, TX   76013-6995
817-277-0727
800-489-0727
Fax: 817-277-2270
www.fhautism.com

R. Wayne Gilpin, President
Jennifer Gilpin, VP, Foreign Translations
Kelly Gilpin, Editorial Dir.
Teresa Corey, Conference Administration
Founded in 1996, Future Horizons is devoted to supporting and fostering works and programs for those who live and work with autism and asperger's syndrome.

29   Guide to the Selection of Musical Instruments
MMB Music
9051 Watson Road
Ste 161
St. Louis, MO   63126
314-531-9635
800-543-3771
Fax: 314-531-8384
info@mmbmusic.com
www.mmbmusic.com
Norm Goldberg, Founder & Chair
A marvelous resource book to aid therapists teaching those who are disabled to play musical instruments. *$7.75*

30   In-Definite Arts Society
8038 Fairmount Drive SE
Calgary, AB   T2H0Y
403-253-3174
Fax: 403-255-2234
ida@indefinitearts.com
www.indefinitearts.com

Darlene Murphy, Executive Director
Dijana Andric, Client Services Manager
Peter Kelsch, Accountant
Bernice Webb, Facility Coordinator
Promotes opportunities for people with developmental disabilities to express themselves and to grow and develop through their involvement in art.

31   Infinity Dance Theater
220 W 93rd St
New York, NY   10025
212-877-3490
info@infinitydance.com
infinitydance.com

Kitty Lunn, RDE, Founder/Artistic Director
Michael A. Fitch, Executive Director
Infinity Dance Theater is a non-traditional dance company committed to expanding the boundaries of dance by featuring dancers with and without disabilities. The company aims to inspire people with and without disabilities, encourage their artistic and other

professional aspirations, and empower them through the organization's educational and performance programs.

32 **Instrumental Music for Dyslexics: A Teaching Handbook**
Wiley & Sons
111 River Street
Hoboken, NJ 07030-5774 201-748-6000
Fax: 201-748-6088
info@wiley.com
www.wiley.com

Sheila Oglethorpe, Author
Stephen M. Smith, President and CEO
Ellis E. Cousens, Executive Vice President, Chief Operations Officer
MJ O'Leary, Senior Vice President, Human Resources
Describes dyslexia in layman's terms and explains how the various problems that a dyslexic may have can affect all aspects of learning to play a musical instrument. It alerts the music teacher with a problem pupil to the possibilities of that pupil having some form of dyslexia. It offers suggestions as to how to teach dyslexics, with particular reference to piano teaching, and it suggests ways in which the music teacher may contribute to the welfare of a dyslexic pupil. *$ 34.95*
200 pages
ISBN 1-861562-91-8

33 **Interact Center for the Visual and Performing Arts**
Interact Center
1860 Minnehaha Ave W
St. Paul, MN 55401 651-209-3575
Fax: 651-209-3579
info@interactcenter.com
interactcenter.com

Jeanne Calvit, Artistic & Executive Director
Shannon Forney, Managing Director
Beth Bowman, Director, Advancement
Creates art in a spirit of radical inclusion; Inspires artists and audiences to explore the full spectrum of human potential; Transforms lives by expanding ideas of what is possible.

34 **Kaleidoscope: Exploring the Experience of Disability through Literature & the Fine Arts**
United Disability Services
701 South Main St
Akron, OH 44311-1019 330-762-9755
Fax: 330-762-0912
kaleidoscope@udsakron.org
www.udsakron.org/services/kaleidoscope
Howard Taylor, President & CEO
Lisa Armstrong, Director of Community Relations & Managing Editor
Gail Willmott, Editor in Chief
Shelley Morris, Chief Financial Officer
Kaleidoscope is a magazine published by United Disability Services. Kaleidoscope challenges and transcends stereotypical, patronizing and sentimental attitudes about disability, looking at the experience of actually living with a disability from a more personal/individual perspective rather than a clinical, sociological or rehabilitative point of view. Included are a variety of articles, fiction, art and poetry relating to issues of disability, literature and the fine arts. *$10.00*
64 pages BiAnnually

35 **Keshet Dance and Center for the Arts**
4121 Cutler Ave NE
Albuquerque, NM 87110 505-224-9808
info@keshetarts.org
keshetarts.org

Shira Greenberg, Artistic Director
Adrian Moore Trask, Director of Business Advancement
Emily Dunkin, Events Director
Carolyn Tobias, Communications Director
Keshet offers youth and adult classes and workshops for individuals with varying levels of physical disabilities and dance experience. Within the Adaptive Dance programming, Keshet pairs dancers with disabilities with able-bodied dancers, which often include siblings, parents, and peers, to create professional-quality dance works.

36 **Learning Disabilities Sourcebook, 3rd Ed.**
Omnigraphics
Order Department
PO Box 8002
Aston, PA 19014-8002 610-461-3548
800-234-1340
Fax: 800-875-1340
contact@omnigraphics.com
www.omnigraphics.com

Joyce Brennfleck Shannon, Editor
Fred Ruffner, Founder
Peter Ruffner, Co-Founder
Learning Disabilities Sourcebook, Third Edition provides updated information about specific learning disabilities and other conditions that make learning difficult. These include dyscalculia, dysgraphia, dyslexia, auditory and visual processing, communication disorders, autism spectrum disorders, attention deficit/hyperactivity disorder, hearing and visual impairments, and brain injury. *$84.00*
600 pages Hard cover
ISBN 0-780810-39-6

37 **Manual of Sequential Art Activities for Classified Children and Adolescents**
Charles C. Thomas
2600 S First St
Springfield, IL 62704-4730 217-789-8980
800-258-8980
Fax: 217-789-9130
books@ccthomas.com
www.ccthomas.com

Rocco A L Fugaro, Author
Offers information to the special education professional on art therapy and management. *$41.95*
246 pages Softcover
ISBN 0-39805 -85-6

38 **Mozart Effect: Tapping the Power of Music to Heal the Body, Strengthen the Mind**
Harper Collins Publishers
10 E 53rd St
New York, NY 10022-5244 212-207-7000
www.harpercollins.com

Don Campbell, Author
Brian Murray, President and CEO
Michael Morrison, President and Publisher, U.S. General Books and Canada
Susan Katz, President and Publisher, HarperCollins Children's Books
Offers dramatic accounts of how doctors, shamans, musicians, and others use music to deal with everything from anxiety, cancer, and chronic pain, to dyslexia and mental illness. *$14.95*
352 pages
ISBN 0-060937-20-3

39 **Music Therapy**
Future Horizons, Inc.
721 West Abram St
Arlington, TX 76013-6995 817-277-0727
800-489-0727
Fax: 817-277-2270
www.fhautism.com

Betsey King Brunk, Author
R. Wayne Gilpin, President
Jennifer Gilpin, VP, Foreign Translations
Kelly Gilpin, Editorial Dir.
Music therapy is the use of music to address non-musical goals. Parents and professionals are finding that music can break down barriers for children with autism in areas such as cognition, socialization, and communication. *$19.95*
123 pages
ISBN 1-885477-53-8

40   Music Therapy and Leisure for Persons with Disabilities
Sagamore Publishing
1807 N Federal Drive
Urbana, IL 61801
217-359-5940
800-327-5557
Fax: 217-359-5975
books@sagamorepub.com
www.sagamorepub.com
Alicia L. Barksdale, Author
Joseph J. Bannon, Sr., Ph.D., Publisher & CEO
Peter L. Bannon, MBA, President
William Anderson, M.S., Director of Sales and Marketing
Explores the use of musical therapy in order to enhance the development of independent leisure skills with a variety of special populations. Suggestions are provided for alternative avenues through musical experiences enabling individuals to achieve their greatest potential for independence and a high quality of life. *$19.95*
ISBN 1-571675-11-6

41   Music Therapy for the Developmentally Disabled
Sage Publications
2455 Teller Road
Thousand Oaks, CA 91320
805-499-9774
800-818-7243
Fax: 800-583-2665
info@sagepub.com
www.sagepub.com
S. Venkatesan, Author
Included are practical guidelines, case samples and step-by-step instructions that enable a music therapist to bring about dramatic improvements in developmentally disabled adults and children. *$40.00*
269 pages Hardcover
ISBN 0-890791-90-2

42   Music Therapy in Dementia Care
Jessica Kingsley Publishers
400 Market Street
Suite 400
Philadelphia, PA 19106-4738
215-922-1161
866-416-1078
Fax: 215-922-1474
hello.usa@jkp.com
www.jkp.com
David Aldridge, Editor
Jessica Kingsley, Chairman, Managing Director
Jemima Kingsley, Director
Octavia Kingsley, Production Director
A comprehensive look at music therapy as a means of improving memory, health, and identity in those suffering from dementia, particularly Alzheimer's. For music therapists and those involved in psychogeriatry. *$29.95*
256 pages
ISBN 1-853027-76-6

43   Music Therapy, Sensory Integration and the Autistic Child
Jessica Kingsley Publishers
400 Market Street
Suite 400
Philadelphia, PA 19106-4738
215-922-1161
866-416-1078
Fax: 215-922-1474
hello.usa@jkp.com
www.jkp.com
Dorita S. Berger, Author
Jessica Kingsley, Chairman, Managing Director
Jemima Kingsley, Director
Octavia Kingsley, Production Director
Examines the human physiologic function, the brain, information processing, functional adaption, and how that might be affected by music interventions in persons with sensory integration difficulties. *$23.95*
256 pages
ISBN 1-843107-00-7

44   Music and Dyslexia: A Positive Approach
Wiley & Sons
111 River Street
Hoboken, NJ 07030-5774
201-748-6000
Fax: 201-748-6088
info@wiley.com
www.wiley.com
John Westcombe, Editor
Stephen M. Smith, President and CEO
Ellis E. Cousens, Executive Vice President, Chief Operations Officer
MJ O'Leary, Senior VP, Human Resources
This book shows how some people who have Dyslexia can be gifted musicians. The main point this books makes is that Dyslexic musicians can succeed provided only that they are given sufficient encouragement and understanding. *$34.95*
200 pages
ISBN 1-861562-05-5

45   Music for the Hearing Impaired
MMB Music
9051 Watson Road
Ste 161
St. Louis, MO 63126
314-531-9635
800-543-3771
Fax: 314-531-8384
info@mmbmusic.com
www.mmbmusic.com
Norm Goldberg, Founder & Chair
A resource manual and curriculum guide. It is the product of a four-year developmental music program, placing emphasis on the needs of those with severe and profound losses. *$29.95*

46   Music: Physician for Times to Come
Quest Books
P.O.Box 270
Wheaton, IL 60187-270
630-665-0130
800-669-9425
Fax: 630-665-8791
submissions@questbooks.net
www.questbooks.net
Don Campbell, Author
A resource guide for various types of music and their therapeutic outcome.
365 pages
ISBN 0-835607-88-7

47   NIAD Art Center (Nurturing Independence through Artistic Development)
551 23rd St.
Richmond, CA 94804-1626
510-620-0290
Fax: 510-620-0326
admin@niadart.org
www.niadart.org
Deborah Dyer, Executive Director
NIAD Art Center) promotes creativity, independence, dignity, and community integration for people with developmental and other disabilities. The visual arts studio supports artists with disabilities by providing materials, space to make art and facilitators to teach skills in drawing, painting, printmaking, ceramics, fiber arts and mixed media. The work that they make is exhibited in the Richmond gallery as well as in other galleries, on-line and other exhibition spaces.

48   National Arts and Disability Center (NADC)
Tarjan Center at UCLA
760 Westwood Plaza
Los Angeles, CA 90095-1759
310-825-5054
Fax: 310-794-1143
bstoffmacher@mednet.ucla.edu
www.semel.ucla.edu/nadc
Olivia Raynor, Director
Beth Stoffmacher, Center Coordinator
NADC has a database and website advocating for access to and participation in the arts by people with disabilities.

49   **National Association for Drama Therapy**
1450 Western Avenue
Suite 101
Albany, NY 12203   571-223-6440
     888-416-7167
     Fax: 518-463-8656
     office@nadta.org
     www.nadt.org

Nadya Trytan, MA, RDT/BCT, President
Jeremy Segall, MA, RDT, LCAT, Vice President
Jason Butler, RDT/BCT, LCAT, President-Elect
Whitney Sullivan, RDT, LCSW, Secretary
The National Association for Drama Therapy (NADT) was incorporated in 1979 to establish and uphold rigorous standards of professional competence for drama therapists. The NADT promotes drama therapy through information and advocacy.

50   **National Endowment for the Arts: Office for AccessAbility**
1100 Pennsylvania Ave NW
Washington, DC 20506-0001   202-682-5034
     Fax: 202-682-5666
     TTY:202-682-5496
     webmgr@arts.gov
     www.arts.gov/

Jane Chu, Chairman
Beth Bienvenu, Accessibility Director
Wendy Clark, Director of Museums, Visual Arts, and Indemnity
Ayanna N. Hudson, Arts Education Director
The National Endowment for the Arts Office for AccessAbility is the advocacy-technical assistance arm of the Arts Endowment to make the arts accessible for people with disabilities, older adults, veterans, and people living in institutions.

51   **National Library Service for the Blind And Physically Handicapped**
1291 Taylor St NW
Washington, DC 20011   202-707-5100
     Fax: 202-707-0712
     TTY:202-707-0744
     nls@loc.gov
     www.loc.gov/nls

Karen Keninger, Dir.
Erica Vaughns, Exec. Assistant to the Dir.
Michael Martys, Automation Officer
Neil Bernstein, R & D Officer
Administers a national library service that provides Braille and recorded books and magazines on free loan to anyone who cannot read standard print because of visual or physical disabilities.
Annual

52   **National Theatre Workshop of the Handicapped (NTWH)**
535 Greenwich Street
New York, NY 10013-1004   212-206-7789
     Fax: 212-206-0200
     www.ntwh.org

Jason Matthews, Director of Admissions
Rick Curry, President & CEO
John Spalla, General Manager
A non-profit organization that provides individuals within the disabled community with the communication skills and the artistic discipline necessary to pursue a life in professional theatre.

53   **National Theatre of the Deaf**
139 N Main St
West Hartford, CT 06107-1264   860-236-4193
     Fax: 860-574-9107
     Info@NTD.org
     www.ntd.org

Betty Beekman, Executive Director
William C. Martin, Marketing/PR Director
George Ghista, Accountant
Kathy Strauss, Company Interpreter
The mission of the National Theatre of the Deaf is to produce theatrically challenging work of the highest quality, drawing from as wide a range of the world's literature as possible and to perform these original works in a style that links American Sign Language with the spoken word.

54   **New Music Therapist's Handbook, 2nd Ed. Berklee School of Music**
Berklee Press Publications
1140 Boylston Street
Boston, MA 02215   617-747-2146
     866-237-5533
     www.berkleepress.com

Suzanne B. Hanser, Author
Dr. Hanser's well-respected Music Therapist's Handbook has been revised and thoroughly updated to reflect the latest developments in the field of music therapy. *$29.95*
256 pages
ISBN 0-634006-45-2

55   **No Limits**
9801 Washington Blvd
2nd Fl
Culver City, CA 90232   310-280-0878
     Fax: 310-280-0872
     michelle@nolimitsfordeafchildren.org
     nolimitsfordeafchildren.org

Michelle Christie, Founder & Executive Director
Juliana Scott, Director, Operations & Development
The mission of No Limits is to meet the auditory, speech and language needs of deaf children and enhance their confidence through the theatrical arts and individual therapy as well as provide family support and community awareness on the needs and talents of deaf children who are learning to speak.

56   **Non-Traditional Casting Project**
Ste 1600
1560 Broadway
New York, NY 10036-1518   212-730-4750
     Fax: 212-730-4820
     TTY:212-730-4913
     www.ntcp.org/

Nancy Kim, Manager
The Non-Traditional Casting Project (NTCP) is a not-for-profit advocacy organization whose purpose is to address and seek solutions to the problems of racism and exclusion in theatre, film and television. NTCP's principal concerns are those of artists of color, female artists, Deaf and hard of hearing artists, and artists with disabilities.

57   **Nuvisions For Disabled Artists, Inc.**
Kije Foschmann, Executive Director
1319 Magee Street
Philadelphia, PA 19111
Nuvisions was established to enable physically challenged artists to pursue professional and semi-professional artistic opportunities. Nuvisions supports these artists by sponsoring accessible exhibitions, special projects and educational opportunities in Southeastern Pennsylvania and Southern New Jersey.

58   **Open Circle Theatre**
102-500 King Farm Blvd
Rockville, MD 20850   240-683-8934
     info@opencircletheatre.org
     opencircletheatre.org

Suzanne Richard, Artistic Director
Ian Armstrong, Executive Producer
Open Circle Theatre is a professional theatre dedicated to producing productions that integrate the considerable talents of artists with disabilities. OCT was formed by a group of people with and without disabilities, who possess professional theater experience, love of the theater, and a commitment to full access for all persons in every opportunity our community has to offer.

59   Pied Piper: Musical Activities to Develop Basic Skills
Jessica Kingsley Publishers
400 Market Street
Suite 400
Philadelphia, PA   19106-4738   215-922-1161
                                                    866-416-1078
                                               Fax: 215-922-1474
                                               hello.usa@jkp.com
                                                    www.jkp.com

John Bean, Author
Jessica Kingsley, Chairman, Managing Director
Jemima Kingsley, Director
Octavia Kingsley, Production Director
Describes 78 enjoyable music activities for groups of children or
adults who may have learning difficulties. The emphasis is on using music, rather than learning songs or rhythms, so group members do not need any special skills to be able to participate. Full
details are given about any equipment required for the games, as
well as suggestions for variations or modifications. *$21.95*
96 pages
ISBN 1-853029-94-

60   Project Onward Gallery
Bridgeport Art Center
1200 W. 35th St
4th Fl
Chicago, IL   60609   773-940-2992
                                           info@projectonward.org
                                                  projectonward.org

61   Pure Vision Arts
The Shield Institute
114 W 17th St
3rd Fl
New York, NY   10011   212-366-4263
                                               Fax: 718-269-2059
                                                 progers@shield.org
                                                 purevisionarts.org

Pamala Rogers, Director
Pure Vision Arts mission is to provide people with autism and developmental disabilities opportunities for artistic expression and
to build public awareness of their important creative
contributions.

62   Reaching the Child with Autism Through Art
Future Horizons, Inc.
721 W Abram St
Arlington, TX   76013-6995   817-277-0727
                                                    800-489-0727
                                               Fax: 817-277-2270
                                                  www.fhautism.com
Toni Flowers, Author
R. Wayne Gilpin, President
Jennifer Gilpin Yacio, Vice President and Editorial Director
David Reasor, CPA and Administrative Director
This book uncovers how art encourages communication, positive
self-image, concept development, spatial relationships, fine-mo-
tor skills, and many more facets of health child development.
$19.95
130 pages

63   Survivors Art Foundation
PO Box 383
Westhampton, NY   11977   safe@survivorsartfoundation.com
                             www.survivorsartfoundation.org
Michael Herships, Ph.D, Project Leader & Board President
Candyce Brokaw, Art Director
Candyce M. Brokaw, Executive Director
Margaret Ashe Magistro, Secretary/Treasurer
Dedicated to encourage healing through the arts, committed to
empowering Trauma-Survivors with Effective Expressive Out-
lets via Internet Art Gallery, Outreach Programs, National Exhi-
bitions, Publications and Development of Employment Skills.

64   Teaching Asperger's Students Social Skills Through Acting
Future Horizons, Inc.
721 W Abram St
Arlington, TX   76013-6995   817-277-0727
                                                    800-489-0727
                                               Fax: 817-277-2270
                                                  www.fhautism.com
Amelia Davies, Author
R. Wayne Gilpin, President
Jennifer Gilpin Yacio, Vice President and Editorial Director
David Reasor, CPA and Administrative Director
This book provides the theories and activities needed for setting
up acting classes that double as social skills groups for individuals with Asperger's or high-functioning autism. Using these
skills, students will be able to develop social understanding
through repetition and generalization. *$19.95*
211 pages

65   Teaching Basic Guitar Skills to Special Learners
MMB Music
9051 Watson Road
Ste 161
St. Louis, MO   63126   314-531-9635
                                                    800-543-3771
                                               Fax: 314-531-8384
                                                 info@mmbmusic.com
                                                  www.mmbmusic.com
Norm Goldberg, Founder & Chair
The first-of-its-kind guitar book for use with persons who have
difficulty learning to play via traditional methods. *$16.00*

66   The Arts of Life
2010 W. Carroll Ave
Chicago, IL   60612   312-829-2787
                                                  info@artsoflife.org
                                                    artsoflife.org
Denise Fisher, Co-Founder & Executive Director
Sara Bemer, Development Coordinator
An organization comprised of people with and without disabili-
ties seeking to promote artistic expression, community building,
self-respect, and independence.

67   Theatre Without Limits
P.O.Box 4002
Portland, ME   04101   207-607-4016
                                               Fax: 207-761-4740
                                                  www.vsartsmaine.org
Kippy Rudy, Executive Director
VSA Maine is a 501(c)(3) non-profit organization providing edu-
cational, arts, and cultural opportunities to children and adults
with disabilities in Maine.

**68   VSA - The International Organization on Arts and
Disability**
2700 F Street, NW
Washington, DC   20566   202-467-4600
                                                    800-444-1324
                                               Fax: 202-429-0868
                                               TTY: 202-737-0645
                                                  info@vsarts.org
                                  www.kennedy-center.org/education/vsa/
Ambassador J Kennedy Smith, Founder
David M. Rubenstein, Chair
Michael M. Kaiser, President
Christoph Eschenbach, Music Director, NSO and Kennedy Center
VSA offers a large selection of guides, publications, and other re-
sources dealing with a wide variety of subject matter in educa-
tion, arts, and disabilities.

69   **VSA arts**
2700 F Street, NW
Washington, DC 20566
                                              202-467-4600
                                            800-444-1324
                                        Fax: 202-429-0868
                                        TTY: 202-737-0645
          www.kennedy-center.org/education/vsa/
Ambassador J Kennedy Smith, Founder
David M. Rubenstein, Chair
Michael M. Kaiser, President
Christoph Eschenbach, Music Director, NSO and Kennedy Center
VSA arts is an international, nonprofit organization founded in
1974 by Ambassador Jean Kennedy Smith whose mission is to
create a society where all people with disabilities learn through,
participate in, and enjoy the arts. Most states offer local programs, such as Arts in Action, that showcases the accomplishments of artists with disabilities and promotes increased access to
the arts for people with disabilities.

70   **We Are PHAMALY**
Fanlight Productions
c/o Icarus Films
32 Court Street, 21st Floor
Brooklyn, NY 11201
                                        718-488-8900
                                        800-876-1710
                                      Fax: 718-488-8642
                                      info@fanlight.com
                                      www.fanlight.com

Ben Achtenberg, Owner
Stands for Physically Handicapped Musical Actors League. This
dynamic troupe doesn't cut any corners or make any compromises. The musicals they perform are chosen for their appeal to
the audience, not because they are easy for the performers, who
have a variety of sensory and mobility handicaps. *$199.00*
ISBN 1-572954-08-6

Assistive Devices

Automobile

71   Ability Center
4797 Ruffner St.
San Diego, CA   92111   866-405-6806
info@abilitycenter.com
www.abilitycenter.com

Dan Monahan, Manager
Offers rear or side entry designed with painstaking craftsmanship using steel.

72   Acc-u-trol
Ace Mobility, LLC
9850 E 30th Street
Indianapolis, IN   46229   877-223-5301
info@acemobility.us
www.acemobility.us

73   Arcola Mobility
51 Kero Rd.
Carlstadt, NJ   07072-2601   201-507-8500
www.arcolasales.com

Andrew Rolfe, Executive Vice President
Jeff Krane, Sales Manager
John Akerlind, General Manager
Teresa Smeriglio, Commercial Bus Sales Coordinator
Arcola sells new and used accessible vehicles and adaptive driving equipment including hand controls, wheelchair lifts and securement systems. Daily, weekly and monthly vehicle rentals, stairway lift, porch elevators and ramps for the home are available.

74   Automobile Lifts for Scooters, Wheelchairs and Powerchairs
Bruno Independent Living Aids
1780 Executive Dr.
Oconomowoc, WI   53066   844-755-5546
888-832-6453
social@bruno.com
www.bruno.com

Michael R. Bruno, II, President and CEO
Over 18 different styles of automobile lifts for scooters, wheelchairs and power chairs for nearly any car, van, truck or sport utility vehicle that can raise most scooters or wheelchairs under 200 pounds and power chairs up to 300 pounds. All Bruno lifts are eligible for reimbursement of up to $1000.00 from GM, Saturn, Ford, and Chrysler under the terms of their Mobility Programs.

75   Blinker Buddy II Electronic Turn Signal
HARC Mercantile
5413 S Westnedge Ave.
Suite A
Portage, MI   49002-5317   269-324-1615
800-445-9968
TTY:800-445-9968
info@harc.com
www.harc.com

76   BraunAbility
631 W 11th St.
Winamac, IN   46996   800-488-0359
www.braunability.com

Ralph Braun, Founder
Manufactures wheelchair lifts and lowered floor minivans as well as many other mobility products.

77   Chevy Lowered Floor
Ace Mobility, LLC
9850 E 30th St.
Indianapolis, IN   46229   877-223-5301
info@acemobility.us
www.acemobility.us

78   Classic
Ricon
1135 Aviation Pl.
San Fernando, CA   91340   574-262-1239
800-322-2884
Fax: 800-962-1201
ripinsales@wabtec.com
www.riconcorp.com

79   DW Auto & Home Mobility
1208 N Garth Ave.
Columbia, MO   65203-4056   573-449-3859
800-568-2271
contactus@dwauto.com
www.dwauto.com

Shawn Bright, Owner
Angela Cornwell, Patient Service Representative
DW manufactures paratransit conversions and personalized conversions for the physically challenged including home elevators and lifts, scooter, wheelchairs and DME.
1967

80   Dodge Lowered Floor
Ace Mobility, LLC
9850 E 30th St.
Indianapolis, IN   46229   877-223-5301
info@acemobility.us
www.acemobility.us

81   Drive Master Company
37 Daniel Rd. W
Fairfield, NJ   07004-2521   973-808-9709
Fax: 973-808-9713
info@drivemastermobility.com
drivemastermobility.com

Peter B. Ruprecht, President
The Drive Master Company offers a full service mobility center, raised tops/doors, drop floors, custom driving equipment, distributor of name brand devices and systems for full sized and mini vans.

82   Driving Systems Inc.
16139 Runnymede St.
Van Nuys, CA   91406-2913   818-782-6793
www.drivingsystems.com

83   Dual Brake Control
Kroepke Kontrols
104 Hawkins St.
Bronx, NY   10464   718-885-1100

84   Entervan
BraunAbility
631 W 11th St.
Winamac, IN   46996   800-488-0359
www.braunability.com

Ralph Braun, Founder
The Entervan accessible features are designed to blend seamlessly into the original design of the Chrysler minivan with the only differences being the easily accessible qualities of the van.

85   Foot Pedal Extensions
Handicaps, Inc.
4335 S Santa Fe Dr.
Englewood, CO   80110-5417   303-781-2062
800-782-4335
info@handicapsinc.com
www.handicapsinc.com

86   Foot Steering
Drive Master Company
37 Daniel Rd. W
Fairfield, NJ   07004-2521   973-808-9709
                                Fax: 973-808-9713
                        info@drivemastermobility.com
                        drivemastermobility.com

Peter B. Ruprecht, President
This product is custom installed system to steer a vehicle with
your foot.

87   Foot Steering System
Ace Mobility, LLC
9850 E 30th St.
Indianapolis, IN   46229   877-223-5301
                              info@acemobility.us
                              www.acemobility.us

88   Ford Lowered Floor
Ace Mobility, LLc
9850 E 30th St.
Indianapolis, IN   46229   877-223-5301
                              info@acemobility.us
                              www.acemobility.us

89   Freedom Motors
Freedom Motors
740 Watkinds Rd.
Battle Creek, MI   49015   888-625-6335
                              www.freedommotors.com

90   Gear Shift Adaptor
Handicaps, Inc.
4335 S Santa Fe Dr.
Englewood, CO   80110-5417   303-781-2062
                                  800-782-4335
                          info@handicapsinc.com
                          www.handicapsinc.com

91   Gresham Driving Aids
30800 S Wixom Rd.
Wixom, MI   48393-2418   248-624-1533
                                800-521-8930
                            Fax: 248-624-6358
                        www.greshamdrivingaids.com

David Ohrt, General Manager
Craig Wigginton, Sales Consultant
Dexter Jackson, Service Manager
Joyce Martell, Customer Service
Gresham Driving Aids offers a full-service package to physically
challenged individuals including lowered floors, raised roofs and
doors and high-quad driver control systems. Dealer for Braun,
Ricon, Crow River and Bruno wheelchair lifts.

92   Hand Brake Control Only
Kroepke Kontrols
104 Hawkins St.
Bronx, NY   10464   718-885-2100

93   Hand Dimmer Switch
Gresham Driving Aids
30800 S Wixom Rd.
Wixom, MI   48393-2418   248-624-1533
                                800-521-8930
                            Fax: 248-624-6358
                        www.greshamdrivingaids.com

David Ohrt, General Manager
Craig Wigginton, Sales Consultant
Dexter Jackson, Service Manager
Joyce Martell, Customer Service
This switch is recommended for left leg handicaps or when a right
leg handicap uses a left foot throttle. *$36.25*

94   Hand Dimmer Switch with Horn Button
Gresham Driving Aids
30800 S Wixom Rd.
Wixom, MI   48393-2418   248-624-1533
                                800-521-8930
                            Fax: 248-624-6358
                        www.greshamdrivingaids.com

David Ohrt, General Manager
Craig Wigginton, Sales Consultant
Dexter Jackson, Service Manager
Joyce Martell, Customer Service
This decide attaches to the handle of control with a chrome plated
steel insulated switch box, giving an instant warning without re-
moving your hand from the steering wheel. *$28.75*

95   Hand Gas & Brake Control
Kroepke Kontrols
104 Hawkins St.
Bronx, NY   10464   718-885-2100

96   Hand Operated Parking Brake
Gresham Driving Aids
30800 S Wixom Rd.
Wixom, MI   48393-2418   248-624-1533
                                800-521-8930
                            Fax: 248-624-6358
                        www.greshamdrivingaids.com

David Ohrt, General Manager
Craig Wigginton, Sales Consultant
Dexter Jackson, Service Manager
Joyce Martell, Customer Service
This device converts foot parking brake to a hand operation for
easy access and manoeuvrability. *$30.20*

97   Hand Parking Brake
Kroepke Kontrols
104 Hawkins St.
Bronx, NY   10464   718-885-2100

98   Handicaps, Inc.
4335 S Santa Fe Dr.
Englewood, CO   80110-5417   303-781-2062
                                  800-782-4335
                          info@handicapsinc.com
                          www.handicapsinc.com

99   Handybar
Maxi Aids
42 Executive Blvd.
Farmingdale, NY   11735-4710   631-752-0521
                                    800-522-6294
                                Fax: 631-752-0689
                                TTY: 800-281-3555
                              sales@maxiaids.com
                              www.maxiaids.com

Elliot Zaretsky, Founder & President
This device is designed for those who have trouble getting in and
out of a car. Sturdy bar slides into door striker and allows you
better support to lift yourself out of the car. It stores easily under
the seats. *$39.95*

100   Headlight Dimmer Switch
Kroepke Kontrols
104 Hawkins St.
Bronx, NY   10464   718-885-2100

101   Horizontal Steering
Drive Master Company
37 Daniel Rd. W
Fairfield, NJ   07004-2521   973-808-9709
                                Fax: 973-808-9713
                          sales@drivemaster.net
                          www.drive-master.com

Peter B. Ruprecht, President
Horizontal Steering System is customized to meet the needs of the
high-level, spinally injured and all others who experience limited
arm strength and range of motion.

102   Horn Control Switch
Kroepke Kontrols
104 Hawkins St.
Bronx, NY   10464   718-885-2100

103   Joystick Driving Control
Ace Mobility, LLC
9850 E 30th St.
Indianapolis, IN   46229   877-223-5301
                                                info@acemobility.us
                                                www.acemobility.us

104   Kessler Institute for Rehabilitation
1199 Pleasant Valley Way
West Orange, NJ   07052   973-731-3600
                                                888-KES-SLER
                                                Fax: 973-243-6819
                                                www.kessler-rehab.com

Sue Kida, President

Driver evaluation training for the physically/mentally challenged offering state certified driving instructors. Door-to-door pickup at home, work or rehab centers are available.

105   Key Holders, Ignition & Door Keys
Gresham Driving Aids
30800 S Wixom Rd.
Wixom, MI   48393-2418   248-624-1533
                                                800-521-8930
                                                Fax: 248-624-6358
                                                www.greshamdrivingaids.com

David Ohrt, General Manager
Craig Wigginton, Sales Consultant
Dexter Jackson, Service Manager
Joyce Martell, Customer Service

These products offered by Gresham Driving Aids are designed for ease of accessibility for people with arthritist. *$18.70*

106   Latchloc Automatic Wheelchair Tiedown
Ace Mobility, LLC
9850 E 30th St.
Indianapolis, IN   46229   877-223-5301
                                                info@acemobility.us
                                                www.acemobility.us

107   Left Foot Accelerator
Gresham Driving Aids
30800 S Wixom Rd.
Wixom, MI   48393-2418   248-624-1533
                                                800-521-8930
                                                Fax: 248-624-6358
                                                www.greshamdrivingaids.com

David Ohrt, General Manager
Craig Wigginton, Sales Consultant
Dexter Jackson, Service Manager
Joyce Martell, Customer Service

A custom pedal designed for left-foot usage. Stainless steel cross bar attaches above the throttle pedal and leaves right pedal free for right foot use. *$80.50*

108   Left Foot Gas Pedal
Kroepke Kontrols
104 Hawkins St.
Bronx, NY   10464   718-885-2100

109   Left Foot Gas Pedal, The
Handicaps, Inc.
4335 S Santa Fe Dr.
Englewood, CO   80110-5417   303-781-2062
                                                800-782-4335
                                                info@handicapsinc.com
                                                www.handicapsinc.com

110   Left Hand Shift Lever
Gresham Driving Aids
30800 S Wixom Rd.
Wixom, MI   48393-2418   248-624-1533
                                                800-521-8930
                                                www.greshamdrivingaids.com

David Ohrt, General Manager
Craig Wigginton, Sales Consultant
Dexter Jackson, Service Manager
Joyce Martell, Customer Service

Converts steering wheel lever or automatic transmission selector lever to left hand usage for right arm handicaps. *$34.50*

111   Low Effort and No Effort Steering
Drive Master Company
37 Daniel Rd. W
Fairfield, NJ   07004-2521   973-808-9709
                                                Fax: 973-808-9713
                                                sales@drivemaster.net
                                                www.drive-master.com

Peter B. Ruprecht, President

Reduced effort steering modifications available for nearly all vehicles. Additional products are pedal extensions which are 1 inch to 4 inch clamp-on aluminum blocks and 6 inch to 12 inch adjustable fold-down pedals.

112   Mini-Bus and Mini-Vans
Arcola Mobility
51 Kero Rd.
Carlstadt, NJ   07072-2604   201-507-8500
                                                800-272-6521
                                                Fax: 201-507-5372
                                                JudyLongo@alliancebusgroup.com
                                                www.arcolasales.com

Andrew Rolfe, Executive Vice President
John Akerlind, General Manager
Sam Garcia, Parts Manager
Cory Mahady, Vehicle Service & Repair

Offers a virtually unlimited choice of chassis size, body style, floor plan and optional features. We provide transporters for almost every use, including school buses, vans, mini-coaches, medium-duty buses and personalized vans for the disabled.

113   Mini-Rider
Ricon
1135 Aviation Pl.
San Fernando, CA   91340   818-267-3000
                                                800-322-2884
                                                Fax: 818-962-1201
                                                ripinsales@wabtec.com
                                                www.riconcorp.com

114   Mobility Vehicle Stairlifts and Ramps
Arcola Mobility
51 Kero Rd.
Carlstadt, NJ   07072-2604   201-507-8500
                                                800-272-6521
                                                Fax: 201-507-5372
                                                JudyLongo@alliancebusgroup.com
                                                www.arcolasales.com

Andrew Rolfe, Executive Vice President
John Akerlind, General Manager
Sam Garcia, Parts Manager
Cory Mahady, Vehicle Service & Repair

Arcola Mobility is a leading dealer of personal, accessible mini and full-size vans with custom conversions and modifications available. Offers a complete line of adaptive driving equipment, including wheelchair lifts, ramps, hand controls, steering devices, scooter lifters, car top wheelchair carriers and power transfer seats.

115   Monarch Mark 1-A
Access Mobility Systems
7202 Evergreen Way
Everett, WA 98203

425-353-6563
800-854-4176
Fax: 425-355-6159
info@accessams.com
www.accessams.com

116   Monmouth Vans, Access and Mobility
Farmingdale, NJ 07727

877-275-4907
marketing@mobility.com
www.mobilityworks.com

117   PAC Unit
Ace Mobility, LLC
9850 E 30th St.
Indianapolis, IN 46229

877-223-5301
info@acemobility.us
www.acemobility.us

118   Park Brake Extension
Handicaps, Inc.
4335 S Santa Fe Dr.
Englewood, CO 80110-5417

303-781-2062
800-782-4335
info@handicapsinc.com
www.handicapsinc.com

119   Pedal Ease
Ace Mobility, LLC
9850 E 30th St.
Indianapolis, IN 46229

877-223-5301
info@acemobility.us
www.acemobility.us

120   Portable Hand Controls
Ace Mobility, LLC
9850 E 30th St.
Indianapolis, IN 46229

877-223-5301
info@acemobility.us
www.acemobility.us

121   Portable Hand Controls by Handicaps, Inc.
Handicaps, Inc.
4335 S Santa Fe Dr.
Englewood, CO 80110-5417

303-781-2062
800-782-4335
info@handicapsinc.com
www.handicapsinc.com

122   Power Seat Base (6-Way)
Ricon
1135 Aviation Pl.
San Fernando, CA 91340

818-267-3000
800-322-2884
Fax: 818-962-1201
ripinsales@wabtec.com
www.riconcorp.com

123   Rampvan
BraunAbility
631 W 11th St.
Winamac, IN 46996

800-488-0359
www.braunability.com

Ralph Braun, Founder
Fully accessible minivan conversions with automatic doors and
ramps, manufactured by Toyota, Chrysler, Dodge and Ford
minivans.

124   Reduced Effort Steering
Ace Mobility, LLC
9850 E 30th St.
Indianapolis, IN 46229

877-223-5301
info@acemobility.us
www.acemobility.us

125   Right Hand Turn Signal Switch Lever
Gresham Driving Aids
30800 S Wixom Rd.
Wixom, MI 48393-2418

248-624-1533
800-521-8930
Fax: 248-624-6358
www.greshamdrivingaids.com

David Ohrt, General Manager
Craig Wigginton, Sales Consultant
Dexter Jackson, Service Manager
Joyce Martell, Customer Service
This device converts signal switch to right hand usage for left arm
handicaps. *$34.50*

126   Slim Line Brake Only
Gresham Driving Aids
30800 S Wixom Rd.
Wixom, MI 48393-2418

248-624-1533
800-521-8930
Fax: 248-624-6358
www.greshamdrivingaids.com

David Ohrt, General Manager
Craig Wigginton, Sales Consultant
Dexter Jackson, Service Manager
Joyce Martell, Customer Service
A chrome plated steel handle, contour shaped, with a left hand or
right hand unit available. *$155.25*

127   Slim Line Control
Gresham Driving Aids
30800 S Wixom Rd.
Wixom, MI 48393-2418

248-624-1533
800-521-8930
Fax: 248-624-6358
www.greshamdrivingaids.com

David Ohrt, General Manager
Craig Wigginton, Sales Consultant
Dexter Jackson, Service Manager
Joyce Martell, Customer Service
A plated, strong, compact unit designed to be easily transferred
from car to car. Built of heavy steel tubing, welded and chrome
plated and contour-shaped for maximum driving room. *$201.25*

128   Slim Line Control: Brake and Throttle
Gresham Driving Aids
30800 S Wixom Rd.
Wixom, MI 48393-2418

248-624-1533
800-521-8930
Fax: 248-624-6358
www.greshamdrivingaids.com

David Ohrt, General Manager
Craig Wigginton, Sales Consultant
Dexter Jackson, Service Manager
Joyce Martell, Customer Service
Brake is actuated by pushing the control lever directly towards
the brake. Throttle is actuated by moving the lever at right angles
to the brake movement, toward the seat. The weight of the opera-
tor's hand is sufficient to hold the throttle at any designed speed.
$300.00

129   Steering Backup System
Ace Mobility, LLC
9850 E 30th St.
Indianapolis, IN 46229

877-223-5301
info@acemobility.us
www.acemobility.us

130   Steering Device
Handicaps, Inc.
4335 S Santa Fe Dr.
Englewood, CO 80110-5417

303-781-2062
800-782-4335
info@handicapsinc.com
www.handicapsinc.com

131   **Super Grade 4 Hand Controls**
Handicaps, Inc.
4335 S Santa Fe Dr.
Englewood, CO 80110-5417

303-781-2062
800-782-4335
info@handicapsinc.com
www.handicapsinc.com

132   **Super Grade IV Hand Controls**
Handicaps, Inc.
4335 S Santa Fe Dr.
Englewood, CO 80110-5417

303-781-2062
800-782-4335
info@handicapsinc.com
www.handicapsinc.com

133   **Tim's Trim**
25 Bermar Park
Rochester, NY 14624-1542

585-429-6270
888-468-6784
info@timstrim.com
www.timstrim.com

Tim Miller, Owner
Offers vehicle modifications, drop floors, raised tops/doors, driving equipment, touch pads and lifts.

134   **Transportation Equipment for People with Disabilities**
Gresham Driving Aids
30800 S Wixom Rd.
Wixom, MI 48393-2418

248-624-1533
800-521-8930
Fax: 248-624-6358
www.greshamdrivingaids.com

David Ohrt, General Manager
Craig Wigginton, Sales Consultant
Dexter Jackson, Service Manager
Joyce Martell, Customer Service
Wheelchair lifts and ramps, hand and foot controls, steering and braking modifications, complete van conversions, home modifications, wheelchairs and scooters and wheelchair accessible van rentals.

135   **Tri-Post Steering Wheel Spinner**
37 Daniel Rd. W
Fairfield, NJ 07004-2521

973-808-9709
Fax: 973-808-9713
sales@drivemaster.net
www.drive-master.com

Peter B. Ruprecht, President
Three nylon posts, adjustable for proper fit to drivers hand, to control the wheel, for use by persons with weak or limp wrists. *$40.25*

136   **Turn Signal Adapter**
Handicaps, Inc.
4335 S Santa Fe Dr.
Englewood, CO 80110-5417

303-781-2062
800-782-4335
info@handicapsinc.com
www.handicapsinc.com

137   **Ultra-Lite XL Hand Control**
Gresham Driving Aids
30800 S Wixom Rd.
Wixom, MI 48393-2418

248-624-1533
800-521-8930
Fax: 248-624-6358
www.greshamdrivingaids.com

David Ohrt, General Manager
Craig Wigginton, Sales Consultant
Dexter Jackson, Service Manager
Joyce Martell, Customer Service
This device allows the driver to operate gas and brake by hand (e.g., push for brake/pull for gas.) It can be installed in nearly every vehicle.

138   **United Access**
10232 Rahning Rd.
St. Louis, MO 63127

877-501-8267
www.unitedaccess.com

139   **Vantage Mini-Vans**
Vantage Mobility International
5202 S 28th Pl.
Phoenix, AZ 85040

855-864-8267
customeradvocate@vantafemobility.com
www.vantagemobility.com

140   **Wheelers Accessible Van Rentals**
6614 W Sweetwater
Glendale, AZ 85304

866-859-8880
info@wheelersvanrentals.com
www.wheelersvanrentals.com

141   **XL Steering**
Ace Mobility, LLC
9850 E 30th St.
Indianapolis, IN 46229

877-223-5301
info@acemobility.us
www.acemobility.us

Bath

142   **Adjustable Bath Seat**
AliMed, Inc.
297 High St.
Dedham, MA 02026-2852

781-329-2900
800-225-2610
Fax: 781-329-8392
info@alimed.com
www.alimed.com

Julian Cherubini, President
Bath seat that fits easily in any size tub. Easily adjustable to any height for easier maneuverability. *$44.00*

143   **Adjustable Raised Toilet Seat & Guard**
Invacare
1 Invacare Way
Elyria, OH 44035-4190

800-333-6900
Fax: 877-619-7996
www.invacare.com

Matthew E. Monaghan, Chairman, President & CEO
Dean Childers, Senior Vice President & General Manager
Patricia Stumpp, Senior Vice President of Human Resources
Robert K. Gudbranson, Senior Vice President and Chief Financial Officer
The seat features an exclusive pivot locking system so it won't slip or tip and the adjustable guard rail fits all toilets.

144   **ArjoHuntleigh**
2349 W Lake St.
Addison, IL 60101

800-323-1245
Fax: 888-389-2756
us.cc@arjohuntleigh.com
www.arjohuntleigh.us

145   **Bath Fixtures**
Fiat Products
41 Cairns Rd.
Mansfield, OH 44904

800-442-1902
www.fiatproducts.com

146   Bath Products
R82, Inc.
12801 E Independence Blvd.
P.O. Box 1739
Matthews, NC 28106   Fax: 704-882-0751
                                      information@R82.com
                                      www.r82.com

Kasper Lisby, Controller
Nanneke Dinklo, Marketing Director
Amy Wilson, Product Manager
Nancy Guzman, Product Specialist
Offers a wide range of products to meet the transportation, mobility, seating and bath aid needs for people of all ages. From car seats and standers for children with special needs to versatile wheelchairs that offer adults customized options and the freedom to go anywhere with confidence.

147   Bath Shower & Commode Chair
Clark Health Care Products
7830 Steubenville Pike
Oakdale, PA 15071-9226   724-695-2122
                                           888-347-4537
                                      Fax: 724-695-2922
                                      info@clarkehealthcare.com
                                      www.clarkehealthcare.com

148   Bath and Shower Bench 3301B
Mada Medical Products
625 Washington Ave.
Carlstadt, NJ 07072-2901   201-460-0454
                                             800-526-6370
                                        Fax: 201-460-3509
                                        saragannon@madamedical.com
                                        www.madamedical.com

149   Bathroom Transfer Systems
Inspired By Drive
11724 Willake St.
Santa Fe Springs, CA 90670-5032   800-454-6612
                                        info@inspiredbydrive.com
                                        www.inspiredbydrive.com

Matt Lawrence, Vice President & General Manager
Michael Gipson, Vice President of Sales
Brittany Commodore, Digital Media & Professional Relations Manager
Offers a complete line of bathroom transfer systems, bath lifts, reclining bath chairs, bath/shower/commode chairs, wrap-around bath supports, toilet supports, positioning commodes, premium air, foam and gel seat cushions, giant trainers and positioning restraint car seats that accommodate individuals from 20-130 pounds.

150   Bathtub Safety Rail
AliMed, Inc.
297 High St.
Dedham, MA 02026-2852   781-329-2900
                                          800-225-2610
                                     Fax: 781-329-8392
                                     info@alimed.com
                                     www.alimed.com

Julian Cherubini, President
Made of stainless steel, this safety rail fits in any size bathtub and offers safety and independence at bathing time. *$55.00*

151   BraunAbility
BraunAbility
631 W 11th St.
Winamac, IN 46996   800-488-0359
                                      www.braunability.com

Ralph Braun, Founder
Offers a variety of assistive devices for the bath and surrounding environment.

152   Can-Do Products Catalog
Independent Living Aids
137 Rano Rd.
Buffalo, NY 14207   716-332-2970
                                      800-537-2118
                                 Fax: 855-937-3906
                                 www.independentliving.com

84 pages Quarterly

153   Clarke Healthcare Products, Inc.
7830 Steubenville Pike
Oakdale, PA 15071-9226   724-695-2122
                                           888-347-4537
                                      Fax: 724-695-2922
                                      info@clarkehealthcare.com
                                      www.clarkehealthcare.com

154   Commode
Maxi Aids
42 Executive Blvd.
Farmingdale, NY 11735-4710   631-752-0521
                                               800-522-6294
                                          Fax: 631-752-0689
                                          TTY: 800-281-3555
                                          sales@maxiaids.com
                                          www.maxiaids.com

Elliot Zaretsky, Founder & President
Adjustable seat height for patient comfort. *$65.95*

155   Deluxe Bath Bench with Adjustable Legs
Maxi Aids
42 Executive Blvd.
Farmingdale, NY 11735-4710   631-752-0521
                                               800-522-6294
                                          Fax: 631-752-0689
                                          TTY: 800-281-3555
                                          sales@maxiaids.com
                                          www.maxiaids.com

Elliot Zaretsky, Founder & President
Bath bench with back support and adjustable legs. *$ 49.95*

156   Electric Leg Bag Emptier and Tub Slide Shower Chair
RD Equipment, Inc.
230 Percival Dr.
West Barnstable, MA 02668-1244   508-362-7498
                                              Fax: 508-362-7498
                                              info@rdequipment.com
                                              www.rdequipment.com

Richard Dagostino, Owner and Founder
Designed for independence, this small, lightweight, battery-operated valve attaches to the bottom of the leg bag. A simple flip of the switch empties the leg bag, allowing the user to take in unlimited amounts of fluids. Tub Slide Shower Chair is a complete bathroom care system. *$200.00*

157   Freedom Bath
ArjoHuntleigh
2349 W Lake St.
Addison, IL 60101   800-323-1245
                                 Fax: 888-389-2756
                                 us.cc@arjohuntleigh.com
                                 www.arjohuntleigh.us

158   Great Big Safety Tub Mat
Maxi Aids
42 Executive Blvd.
Farmingdale, NY 11735-4710   631-752-0521
                                               800-522-6294
                                          Fax: 631-752-0689
                                          TTY: 800-281-3555
                                          sales@maxiaids.com
                                          www.maxiaids.com

Elliot Zaretsky, Founder & President
Tub mat provides security against falls in the bath and shower. *$16.95*

159 Long Handled Bath Sponges
Therapro, Inc.
225 Arlington St
Framingham, MA   01702-8723

508-872-9494
800-257-5376
Fax: 508-268-6624
info@therapro.com
www.therapro.com

Karen Conrad, Owner
Plastic-handled, 18-inch bath sponge. Handle may be heated and bent for easy reach. *$2.50*

160 Mariner Shower and Commode Chair
Maxi Aids
42 Executive Blvd.
Farmingdale, NY   11735-4710

631-752-0521
800-522-6294
Fax: 631-752-0689
TTY: 800-281-3555
sales@maxiaids.com
www.maxiaids.com

Elliot Zaretsky, Founder & President
The all aluminum frame and stainless steel hardware provides optimum rust resistance making it ideal for use in the shower. Lightweight; folds easily for transport or storage. Padded 4-position seat with easy access, swing-away front riggings with tool-less adjustable height footrests. *$699.95*

161 Modular Wall Grab Bars
Invacare
1 Invacare Way
Elyria, OH   44035-4190

800-333-6900
Fax: 877-619-7996
www.invacare.com

Matthew E. Monaghan, Chairman, President & CEO
Dean Childers, Senior Vice President & General Manager
Patricia Stumpp, Senior Vice President of Human Resources
Robert K. Gudbranson, Senior Vice President and Chief Financial Officer
Engineered for strength and beauty, these bars can be assembled in various combinations to fit any bath or shower.

162 Portable Shampoo Bowl
JK Designs
4004 NE 4th St
Suite 107-456
Renton, WA   98059

206-999-8226
info@portableshampoobowl.com
www.portableshampoobowl.com

163 Prelude
Arjo Inc
2349 West Lake Street
Suite 250
Addison, IL   60101

630-785-4490
800-323-1245
Fax: 888-389-2756
usa.info@ArjoHuntleigh.com
www.arjohuntleigh.com

164 SLIDER Bathing System
Assistive Technology
21279 Protecta Dr
Elkhart, IN   46516-9539

574-522-7201
800-478-2363
Fax: 574-293-0202
info@pvcdme.com
www.pvcdme.com

165 Suregrip Bathtub Rail
Frohock-Stewart
1 Invacare Way
Elyria, OH   44035-4190

440-329-6000
800-333-6900
Fax: 877-619-7996
www.invacare.com

A Malachi Mixon III, Chairman
Gerald B. Blouch, President & CEO
Joseph B. Richey II, President, Invacare Technologies Division
Robert K. Gudbranson, Senior Vice President and Chief Financial Officer
Compact and versatile, the bars have a soft-touch, contoured, white vinyl gripping area for added safety.

166 Talking Bathroom Scale
Independent Living Aids
137 Rano Rd
Buffalo, NY   14207

516-937-1848
800-537-2118
855-746-7452
Fax: 516-937-3906
can-do@independentliving.com
www.independentliving.com

Irwin Schneidmill, President
Michael Gutierrez, Director of Operations
Pamela Strauss, Director of Marketing
Ursula Izurieta, Director of Merchandising
Talking scale. *$59.95*

167 Terry-Wash Mitt: Medium Size
Therapro, Inc.
225 Arlington St
Framingham, MA   01702-8723

508-872-9494
800-257-5376
Fax: 508-875-2062
info@therapro.com
www.therapro.com

Karen Conrad, Owner
Includes a thumb socket and a palm pocket to hold a bar of soap.
$8.00

168 Toilet Guard Rail
Maxi Aids
42 Executive Blvd.
Farmingdale, NY   11735-4710

631-752-0521
800-522-6294
Fax: 631-752-0689
TTY: 800-281-3555
sales@maxiaids.com
www.maxiaids.com

Elliot Zaretsky, Founder & President
Made of chrome-plated, heavy gauge steel. Fits securely to the toilet for maximum sturdiness. *$43.95*

169 Transfer Tub Bench
Arista Surgical Supply Company/AliMed
297 High St
Dedham, MA   02026-2852

781-329-2900
800-225-2610
Fax: 781-329-8392
info@alimed.com
www.alimed.com

Julian Cherubini, President
Curved padded backrest for comfortable support. Backrest also assists patient during lateral transfer. *$64.00*

170 Tri-Grip Bathtub Rail
Maxi Aids
42 Executive Blvd.
Farmingdale, NY   11735-4710

631-752-0521
800-522-6294
Fax: 631-752-0689
TTY: 800-281-3555
sales@maxiaids.com
www.maxiaids.com

Elliot Zaretsky, Founder & President

Two gripping heights for easy bathtub entrance or exit. *$36.95*

171   Tub Slide Shower Chair
RD Equipment
230 Percival Dr
West Barnstable, MA   02668-1244   508-362-7498
                                                Fax: 508-362-7498
                                            www.rdequipment.com
Richard Dagostino, Owner and Founder
The tub slide shower chair was designed for the elderly and disabled to make any bathroom (at home or when travelling) accessible with little or no renovations. Go from the bed, to the commode and over to the bathtub for a shower using one product. No transfers in the bathroom whatsoever. *$2000.00*

Bed

172   ASSISTECH Special Needs
4801 W Calle Don Miguel
Tucson, AZ   85757-1400   520-883-8600
                                                 866-674-3549
                                            Fax: 520-883-5926
                                            TTY: 520-883-5926
                                            www.assistech.com
Oliver Simoes, Owner
Sells hearing, visual and mobility aid devices. *$39.00*

173   Adjustable Bed
Golden Technologies
401 Bridge St
Old Forge, PA   18518-2323   570-451-7477
                                                 800-624-6374
                                            Fax: 800-628-5165
                                            www.goldentech.com
Richard Golden, CEO
Robert Golden, Co-Founder and Chairman
Fred Kiwak, Co-Founder and VP
Trouble-free gear motor, safety features, dual massage, variable speed timer and more, for the ultimate sleep experience.

174   Bye-Bye Decubiti Air Mattress Overlay
Ken McRight Supplies
401 Linden Center Drive
Fort Collins, CO   80524   970-484-7967
                                                 800-467-7967
                                            Fax: 970-484-3800
                                            info@randscot.com
                                            www.randscot.com
Joel Lerich, Co-Founder
Barbara , Co-Founder
Originally designed for hospital beds, converts any bed into an exceptionally therapeutic, flotation unit when used between the conventional mattress and pad. The complete overlay is comprised of five individually inflatable, 100 percent natural rubber, ventilated sections enclosed within separate pockets of a soft fleece cover. Conforms to any configuration of electric or manual beds. *$731.50*

175   Cervical Support Pillow
Wise Enterprises
5017 El Don Dr
Rocklin, CA   95677-4417   916-624-3848
                                                 888-947-3368
                                            sales@winsent.com
                                            www.wisent.com
Tom Wise, Owner
These hypoallergenic, antimicrobial fiber pillows support the neck in a natural position. Standard, midsize and petite pillows support the neck while sleeping on the back or side. The compact travel pillow offers support while sitting or lying down. The cervical roll has a gentle center and firm ends to ensure maximum comfort and proper support. Position the roll under the neck, back or knees. Standard and midsize fits adults, petite fits children and small adults.

176   Dual Security Bed Rail
Maxi Aids
42 Executive Blvd.
Farmingdale, NY   11735-4710   631-752-0521
                                                 800-522-6294
                                            Fax: 631-752-0689
                                            TTY: 800-281-3555
                                            sales@maxiaids.com
                                            www.maxiaids.com
Elliot Zaretsky, Founder & President
Sleep without worry! Dual rails for double the safety. Steel with Powder Coat. Rails adjust up and down.

177   Foam Decubitus Bed Pads
Profex Medical Products
P.O.Box 140188
Memphis, TN   38114   800-325-0196
                                            Fax: 901-454-9850
                                            customercare@ProfexMed.com
                                            www.profexmed.com
Robert Gates Watel, Founder
Convoluted foam provides extra back support and comfort for wheelchair users.

178   Global Assistive Devices, Inc.
1121 East Commercial Blvd. #39
Oakland Park, FL   33334-3920   954-776-1373
                                                 888-778-4237
                                            Fax: 954-776-8136
                                            TTY:954-776-1373
                                            sales@GlobalAssistive.com
                                            www.GlobalAssistive.com
Manufacturer of assistive devices designed to make life easier. Products include: vibrating watches/countdown timers, extra loud alarm clocks with adjustable tone and bed shaker option, door signalers, telephone ring signaler and caller identification for the television.

179   Hard Manufacturing Company
230 Grider St
Buffalo, NY   14215-3797   800-873-4273
                                            www.hardmfg.com

180   Jackson Cervipillo
Wise Enterprises
5017 El Don Dr
Rocklin, CA   95677-4417   916-624-3848
                                                 888-947-3368
                                            sales@winsent.com
                                            www.wisent.com
Tom Wise, Owner
The Jackson Cervipillo comfortably supports the neck vertebrae when sleeping on the side or on the back. Pillow measures 7 in diameter and is 17 long. A machine-washable cover is available separately.

181   NeckEase
Wise Enterprises
5017 El Don Dr
Rocklin, CA   95677-4417   916-624-3848
                                                 888-947-3368
                                            sales@winsent.com
                                            www.wisent.com
Tom Wise, Owner
Microwave NeckEase for penetrating heat that sooths stiff necks and shoulders, easing tension. NeckEase features a unique filling of organic, long grain rice and aromatic herbs and spices. When heated, this filling provides soothing, moist aromatherapy. Heat lasts about 30-45 minutes. Available in two sizes: small fits snugly around the neck, applying gentle pressure at the base of the skull; Large may be worn for a snug fit, or loosely for application on the shoulder and upper back.

182 Permaflex Home Care Mattress
BG Industries
8550 Balboa Blvd
Ste 214
Northridge, CA 91325-3564   818-894-0744
                                Fax: 818-894-7972
                                maxifloat@bgind.com

Larry Lankard, Director
Arnie Balonick, CEO/Director
Mattress with flame retardant upholstery material, water-repel-
lant, anti-microbial and tear-resistant cover, for extra comfort.

183 SleepSafe Beds
3629 Reed Creek Drive
Bassett, VA 24055   276-627-0088
                            866-852-2337
                            Fax: 276-627-0234
                    SleepSafeBed@SleepSafeBed.com
                            www.sleepsafebed.com

Gregg Weinschreider, President
Edward Hettig, Marketing
Casey Collins, Office Manager
Al Flora, Sales
Perfect for adult home or home care use. Offering twin or full size
bed frames in classic style, these beds offer an attractive alterna-
tive to a hospital bed. Keeps the user safe during rest and electri-
cally adjusts smoothly for user comfort and caregiver ease of use.

184 Sonic Alert Bed Shaker
ASSISTECH
4801 W Calle Don Miguel
Tucson, AZ 85757-1400   520-883-8600
                            866-674-3549
                            Fax: 520-883-5926
                            TTY: 520-883-5926
                            www.assistech.com

Oliver Simoes, Owner
Sells hearing, visual and mobility aid devices. *$49.00*

185 Vibes Bed Shaker
ASSISTECH
4801 W Calle Don Miguel
Tucson, AZ 85757-1400   520-883-8600
                            866-674-3549
                            Fax: 520-883-5926
                            TTY: 520-883-5926
                            www.assistech.com

Oliver Simoes, Owner
Sells hearing, visual and mobility aid devices.

186 Waterproof Sheet-Topper Mattress and Chair Pad
Pillow Talk
260 Madison Avenue
New York, NY 10016   732-780-9483
                            Fax: 732-780-0279
                    info@PTIproductmarketing.com
                            www.pillowtalkusa.com

Dorothy Fajerman, President
Jack Fajerman, Marketing Director
This soft pad lies on the top sheet, absorbing accidents from incontinence, pregnancy or medical problems. Waterproof barrier
locks out moisture, soiling and stains and eliminates midnight
linen changes and the resulting laundry. Available in bed sizes
W/4 Anchor, twin, full, queen, king, and crib.

Communication

187 ADA Hotel Built-In Alerting System
HARC Mercantile
5413 S. Westnedge Ave.
Suite A
Portage, MI 49002   269-324-1615
                            800-445-9968
                            Fax: 269-324-2387
                            TTY: 269-324-1615
                            info@harc.com
                            www.harc.com

188 Access Control Systems: NHX Nurse Call System
Aiphone Corporation
1700 130th Ave NE
Bellevue, WA 98005-2203   425-455-0510
                            800-692-0200
                            Fax: 425-455-0071
                            www.aiphone.com

Futoshi Tanaka, President/CEO
AIPHONE manufactures audio and video intercom systems for
home or business to help the physically disabled answer doors
and communicate through physical barriers; also ADA-compli-
ant emergency call intercom stations for use in public facilities
and an Environmental Control System for persons with limited
mobility.

189 Adaptek Systems
14224 Plank Street
Fort Wayne, IN 46818   260-637-8660
                            Fax: 260-637-8597
                            info@adapteksystems.com
                            www.adapteksystems.com

190 Akron Resources
20 La Porte St
Arcadia, CA 91006-2827   626-254-9005
                            800-841-0884
                            Fax: 626-254-9266
                            www.arkon.com

Paul Brassard, Owner
Aaron Roth, VP, Marketing & Sales
Benjamin Arana, Sr. Account Manager
Cleber Gandra, Account Manager
Manufacturers of infrared amplification systems for televisions
or stereos. $29-$69.00. The company name is Arkon Resources.

191 Amplified Handsets
HARC Mercantile
5413 S. Westnedge Ave.
Suite A
Portage, MI 49002   269-324-1615
                            800-445-9968
                            Fax: 269-324-2387
                            TTY: 269-324-1615
                            info@harc.com
                            www.harc.com

192 Amplified Phones
HARC Mercantile
5413 S. Westnedge Ave.
Suite A
Portage, MI 49002   269-324-1615
                            800-445-9968
                            Fax: 269-324-2387
                            TTY: 269-324-1615
                            info@harc.com
                            www.harc.com

193   Amplified Portable Phone
HARC Mercantile
5413 S. Westnedge Ave.
Suite A
Portage, MI 49002

269-324-1615
800-445-9968
Fax: 269-324-2387
TTY: 269-324-1615
info@harc.com
www.harc.com

194   Artificial Larynx
HARC Mercantile
5413 S. Westnedge Ave.
Suite A
Portage, MI 49002

269-324-1615
800-445-9968
Fax: 269-324-2387
TTY: 269-324-1615
info@harc.com
www.harc.com

195   Assistive Technology
333 Elm St
Dedham, MA 02026-4530

781-461-8200
800-793-9227
Fax: 781-461-8213
sales@tobiiATI.com
www.tobii.com/

Henrik Eskilsson, CEO
John Elvesjo, CTO and deputy CEO
Mårten Skogo, Chief Science Officer
Torbjorn Moller, Chief Operating Officer
A premiere developer of innovative technology solutions for people with physical and learning disabilities. Breakthrough products enable people of all ages and abilities to live and learn independently. Supportive material for teachers, clinicians and those with disabilities.

196   Big Red Switch
AbleNet
2625 Patton Road
Roseville, MN 55113-1308

651-294-2200
800-322-0956
Fax: 651-294-2222
customerservice@ablenetinc.com
www.ablenetinc.com

Bill Sproull, Chairman
Jennifer Thalhuber, CEO/President
William Mills, Board of Director
Five inches across the top and activates no matter where on its surface it is touched. It is made of shatterproof plastic and contains a cord storage compartment. Also available in green, yellow and blue. *$42.00*

197   Cornell Communications
7915 N 81st St
Milwaukee, WI 53223-3830

414-351-4660
800-558-8957
Fax: 414-351-4657
sales@cornell.com
www.cornell.com

George , Management Staff
Gary , Management Staff
Jim , Management Staff
Cornell's Rescue Assistance Systems allow personnel to request emergency assistance. Applications include handicapped evacuations, parking garages and elevators. Voice, intercom and visual only signaling systems are available.

198   Davis Center
110 Wesley St.
P.O. Box 508
Manlius, NY 13104

862-251-4637
Fax: 862-251-4642
ddavis@thedaviscenter.com
www.thedaviscenter.com

Dorinne S. Davis, MA, CCC-A, FAAA, President

The Davis Center's Sound Therapy Programs make positive changes for children and adults with autism, ADD/ADHD, auditory processing issues, Dyslexia, learning disabilities, and other learning and wellness challenges. Programs address issues such as phonics, spelling, writing, reading comprehension, hearing only parts of words, following directions, discriminating between sounds, sound sensitivity, behavioral responses, focus, attention, and more.

199   Flashing Lamp Telephone Ring Alerter
Independent Living Aids
137 Rano Rd
Buffalo, NY 14207

516-937-1848
800-537-2118
855-746-7452
Fax: 516-937-3906
can-do@independentliving.com
www.independentliving.com

Irwin Schneidmill, President
Michael Gutierrez, Director of Operations
Pamela Strauss, Director of Marketing
Ursula Izurieta, Director of Merchandising
Once your phone is plugged into the Telephone Ring Alerter, the lamp light will flash with each ring, alerting you that there is a phone call. *$62.00*

200   Harc Mercantile Ltd
HARC Mercantile
5413 S. Westnedge Ave.
Suite A
Portage, MI 49002

269-324-1615
800-445-9968
Fax: 269-324-2387
TTY: 269-324-1615
info@harc.com
www.harc.com

201   Ideal-Phone
IDEAMATICS
1364 Beverly Road
Suite 101
McLean, VA 22101-3617

703-903-4972
800-247-IDEA
Fax: 703-903-8949
ideamatics@ideamatics.net
www.ideamatics.com

David L Danner, President
Michael A. Schwartz, Vice President
Mark A. Moore, Vice President of Operations
John R. Kaplar, Director of Applications Development
Integrates the personal computer and the telephone into a single, efficient workstation. It is ideal for mobility-impaired persons and others who need a hands-free operation of the phone. The Ideal-Phone includes one PC Board, a Plantronics headset, software for access and logging and complete documentation. It can be integrated into programs or pops-up over any application. MS-DOS based, version 3.0 or higher are available. *$195.00*

202   IntelliKeys
IntelliTools
24 Prime Parkway
Natick, MA 01760

303-651-2829
800-547-6747
Fax: 720-382-7438
customerservice@cambiumlearning.com
www.intellitools.com

Arjan Khalsa, CEO
Card and cable to create keyboard port on Apple IIe computer to allow use of IntelliKeys alternative keyboard.

203   LPB Communications
960 Brook Rd
Norristown, PA 19401

856-365-8080
Fax: 856-365-8999

John Devecka, VP Sales
Limited area AM and FM broadcast systems for hearing assistance and language translation manufacturing since 1960. Sys-

tems for small conference halls, churches and Olympic stadiums. Components or complete system. *$400.00*

204 Language, Learning & Living
Prentke Romich Company
1022 Heyl Rd
Wooster, OH 44691-9786   330-262-1984
                                           800-262-1984
                                      Fax: 330-263-4829
                                      info@prentrom.com
                                      www.prentrom.com

David L Moffatt, President
Barry Romich, Co-Founder
Dave Moffatt, President & COO
A Minspeak application program designed for adolescent and adult individuals with developmental disabilities and associated learning difficulties. The software is used with Prentke Romich Company augmentative communication devices. *$355.00*

205 Large Button Speaker Phone
HARC Mercantile
5413 S. Westnedge Ave.
Suite A
Portage, MI 49002   269-324-1615
                                           800-445-9968
                                      Fax: 269-324-2387
                                      TTY: 269-324-1615
                                      info@harc.com
                                      www.harc.com

206 Large Print Telephone Dial
Maxi Aids
42 Executive Blvd
Farmingdale, NY 11735-4710   631-752-0521
                                           800-522-6294
                                      Fax: 631-752-0689
                                      TTY: 800-281-3555
                                      sales@maxiaids.com
                                      www.maxiaids.com

Elliot Zaretsky, Founder & President
Pressure sensitive dial with numbers that are easy to see for the disabled. *$69.00*

207 Large Print Touch-Telephone Overlays
Maxi Aids
42 Executive Blvd
Farmingdale, NY 11735-4710   631-752-0521
                                           800-522-6294
                                      Fax: 631-752-0689
                                      TTY: 800-281-3555
                                      sales@maxiaids.com
                                      www.maxiaids.com

Elliot Zaretsky, Founder & President
Pressure-sensitive and easy to apply overlays that make everyday phones accessible. *$49.00*

208 Liberator
Prentke Romich Company
1022 Heyl Rd
Wooster, OH 44691-9786   330-262-1984
                                           800-262-1984
                                      Fax: 330-263-4829
                                      info@prentrom.com
                                      www.prentrom.com

David L Moffatt, President
Barry Romich, Co-Founder
Dave Moffatt, President & COO
A portable electronic communication device that uses Minspeak so that symbols are used to represent words, sentences or phrases. Liberator can be accessed by pressing keys, optical headpointing and a wide variety of switch activated scans. It can be configured with 8, 32 or 128 locations. It offers a variety of unique features to permit the most effective communication possible. $7,345-$8,575.

209 Metropolitan Washington Ear
12061 Tech Rd.
Silver Spring, MD 20904-7826   301-681-6636
                                      Fax: 301-625-1986
                                      information@washear.org
                                      www.washear.org

Paul W. Schroeder, Chairman
Cornelia Oplinger, Executive Director
Multi-media reading service for blind and visually impaired. Offering 24 hour audio radio reading, dial-in newspapers and web casting, as well as audio description at theaters, museums and films.

210 Mini Teleloop
HARC Mercantile
5413 S. Westnedge Ave.
Suite A
Portage, MI 49002   269-324-1615
                                           800-445-9968
                                      Fax: 269-324-2387
                                      TTY: 269-324-1615
                                      info@harc.com
                                      www.harc.com

211 Multiple Phone/Device Switch
HARC Mercantile
5413 S. Westnedge Ave.
Suite A
Portage, MI 49002   269-324-1615
                                           800-445-9968
                                      Fax: 269-324-2387
                                      TTY: 269-324-1615
                                      info@harc.com
                                      www.harc.com

212 Personal FM Systems
HARC Mercantile
5413 S. Westnedge Ave.
Suite A
Portage, MI 49002   269-324-1615
                                           800-445-9968
                                      Fax: 269-324-2387
                                      TTY: 269-324-1615
                                      info@harc.com
                                      www.harc.com

213 Personal Infrared Listening System
HARC Mercantile
5413 S. Westnedge Ave.
Suite A
Portage, MI 49002   269-324-0301
                                           800-445-9968
                                      Fax: 269-324-2387
                                      TTY: 269-324-1615
                                      info@harc.com
                                      www.harc.com

214 Prentke Romich Company
1022 Heyl Rd
Wooster, OH 44691-9786   330-262-1984
                                           800-262-1984
                                      Fax: 330-263-4829
                                      info@prentrom.com
                                      www.prentrom.com

David L Moffatt, President
Barry Romich, Co-Founder
Dave Moffatt, President / COO
The Prentke Romich Company is a full service company offering easy, yet powerful communication aids. The company believes in supporting customers before and after the sale by offering funding assistance, distance learning training, extended warranty, service assistance and much more. Visit our website to view our full line catalog, read about our success stories and to sign up for our online newsletter.

215   Push to Talk Amplified Handset
HARC Mercantile
5413 S. Westnedge Ave.
Suite A
Portage, MI   49002

269-324-0301
800-445-9968
Fax: 269-324-2387
TTY: 269-324-1615
info@harc.com
www.harc.com

216   Room Valet Visual-Tactile Alerting System
HARC Mercantile
5413 S. Westnedge Ave.
Suite A
Portage, MI   49002

269-324-0301
800-445-9968
Fax: 269-324-2387
TTY: 269-324-1615
info@harc.com
www.harc.com

217   Silent Call Communications
5095 Williams Lake Rd
Waterford, MI   48329-3553

248-673-7353
800-572-5227
Fax: 248-673-7360
TTY: 800-572-5227
customerservice@silentcall.com
www.silentcall.com

George Elwell, President
Diana Elwell, President
Lisa DeLeuil, Director of Sales & Marketing
Alerting devices such as paging systems and smoke detectors for deaf and deaf-blind people.

218   Sonic Alert
Harris Communications
15155 Technology Dr
Eden Prairie, MN   55344-2273

952-906-1180
800-825-6758
Fax: 952-906-1099
TTY: 800-825-9187
info@harriscomm.com
www.harriscomm.com

Dr.Robert Harris, Owner
Lori Foss, Marketing Director
Offers visual alerting devices that provide safety and convenience by turning vital sound into flashing light: telephone ring signalers, doorbell signalers, baby cry signalers and wake up alarms. Free catalog available.

219   Sound Induction Receiver
HARC Mercantile
5413 S. Westnedge Ave.
Suite A
Portage, MI   49002

269-324-0301
800-445-9968
Fax: 269-324-2387
TTY: 269-324-1615
info@harc.com
www.harc.com

220   SpeakEasy Communication Aid
AbleNet
2625 Patton Road
Roseville, MN   55113-1308

651-294-2200
800-322-0956
Fax: 651-294-2259
customerservice@ablenetinc.com
www.ablenetinc.com

Bill Sproull, Chairman of the Board
Jennifer Thalhuber, President/CEO
William Mills, Board of Director
SpeakEasy is a digitalized voice output communication Aid that is ideal for anyone who is beginning to develop communication skills such as making choices and identifying symbols. It holds 12 messages totaling four minutes and 20 seconds of recording time.

It measures 7 1/2 inch by 1 3/4 inch and weighs only one pound. Activate messages using the built-in keyboard or via external switch. *$399.00*

221   Speech Discrimination Unit
HARC Mercantile
5413 S. Westnedge Ave.
Suite A
Portage, MI   49002

269-324-0301
800-445-9968
Fax: 269-324-2387
TTY: 269-324-1615
info@harc.com
www.harc.com

222   Speechmaker-Personal Speech Amplifier
HARC Mercantile
5413 S. Westnedge Ave.
Suite A
Portage, MI   49002

269-324-0301
800-445-9968
Fax: 269-324-2387
TTY: 269-324-1615
info@harc.com
www.harc.com

223   Standard Touch Turner Sip & Puff Switch
Access to Recreation
8 Sandra Ct
Newbury Park, CA   91320-4302

805-498-7535
800-634-4351
Fax: 805-498-8186
customerservice@accesstr.com
www.accesstr.com

Don Krebs, President /Founder
A page turning device.

224   Step-by-Step Communicator
AbleNet
2625 Patton Road
Roseville, MN   55113-1308

651-294-2200
800-322-0956
Fax: 651-294-2259
customerservice@ablenetinc.com
www.ablenetinc.com

Bill Sproull, Chairman of the Board
Jennifer Thalhuber, President/CEO
William Mills, Board of Director
Allows you to record a series of messages (as many as you want up to the 75 second limit). It has a 2 1/2 inches diameter switch surface and is 3 inches at its tallest point. Angled switch surface makes it easy to see and access. *$129.00*

225   Strobe Light Signalers
5413 S. Westnedge Ave.
Suite A
Portage, MI   49002

269-324-0301
800-445-9968
Fax: 269-324-2387
TTY: 269-324-1615
info@harc.com
www.harc.com

226   TTY's: Telephone Device for the Deaf
HARC Mercantile
5413 S. Westnedge Ave.
Suite A
Portage, MI   49002

269-324-0301
800-445-9968
Fax: 269-324-2387
TTY: 269-324-1615
info@harc.com
www.harc.com

227   TalkTrac Wearable Communicator
Ablenet
2625 Patton Road
Roseville, MN   55113-1308   651-294-2200
                                             800-322-0956
                                        Fax: 651-294-2259
                          customerservice@ablenetinc.com
                                        www.ablenetinc.com

Bill Sproull, Chairman of the Board
Jennifer Thalhuber, President/CEO
William Mills, Board of Director
The TalkTrac Wearable Communicator is a personal, portable
communication aid that is wearable on the wrist. TalkTrac features: simple to use, 75 seconds of recording time, four 3/4 x 1/2
message locations, rechargeable, water resistant, adjustable 9
inch band, Boardmaker compatible.

228   Talking Calculators
ASSISTECH
4801 W Calle Don Miguel
Tucson, AZ   85757-1400   520-883-8600
                                              866-674-3549
                                         Fax: 520-883-5926
                                          TTY: 520-883-5926
                                          www.assistech.com

Oliver Simoes, Owner
Marsha Neilson, Sales Representative
Carries a complete line of assistive products for the deaf and hard
of hearing, blind and visually impaired, speech impaired, and
physically challenged . They also feature products for everyone
such as medicine reminder watches and electronic language
translators.

229   Talking Clocks
HARC Mercantile
5413 S. Westnedge Ave.
Suite A
Portage, MI   49002   269-324-0301
                                              800-445-9968
                                         Fax: 269-324-2387
                                          TTY: 269-324-1615
                                             info@harc.com
                                              www.harc.com

230   Talking Watches
HARC Mercantile
5413 S. Westnedge Ave.
Suite A
Portage, MI   49002   269-324-0301
                                              800-445-9968
                                         Fax: 269-324-2387
                                          TTY: 269-324-1615
                                             info@harc.com
                                              www.harc.com

231   Telecaption Adapter
HARC Mercantile
5413 S. Westnedge Ave.
Suite A
Portage, MI   49002   269-324-0301
                                              800-445-9968
                                         Fax: 269-324-2387
                                          TTY: 269-324-1615
                                             info@harc.com
                                              www.harc.com

232   Touch Turner-Page Turning Devices
Touch Turner Company
13621 103rd Ave NE
Arlington, WA   98223-8827   360-651-1962
                                              888-811-1962
                                         Fax: 360-658-9380
                                        www.touchturner.com

233   Unity
Prentke Romich Company
1022 Heyl Rd
Wooster, OH   44691-9786   330-262-1984
                                              800-262-1984
                                         Fax: 330-263-4829
                                          info@prentrom.com
                                           www.prentrom.com

David L Moffatt, President
Barry Romich, Co-Founder
Dave Moffatt, President / COO
A Minspeak application program available for the Liberator and
Delta Talker communication devices. Provides single word vo-
cabulary to people of all ages at varying stages of language devel-
opment, who may be either cognitively intact or challenged.
$355.00

234   Vantage
Prentke Romich Company
1022 Heyl Rd
Wooster, OH   44691-9786   330-262-1984
                                              800-262-1984
                                         Fax: 330-263-4829
                                          info@prentrom.com
                                           www.prentrom.com

David L Moffatt, President
Barry Romich, Co-Founder
Dave Moffatt, President / COO
Vantage is a portable communication aid that features the Unity
Enhanced vocabulary software and a large high quality dynamic
display. Vantage also employs the recently upgraded 4.0 operating system that makes system settings quick and easy. Vantage
has synthesized speech powered by DECtalk Software, Spelling
and Word Protection software, built-in visor (flip-up protective
cover), digitized speech capability and built-in computer access
and ECU controls. 15 and 45 location keyguards available.
$6295.00

235   Vibrotactile Personal Alerting System
HARC Mercantile
5413 S. Westnedge Ave.
Suite A
Portage, MI   49002   269-324-0301
                                              800-445-9968
                                         Fax: 269-324-2387
                                          TTY: 269-324-1615
                                             info@harc.com
                                              www.harc.com

236   Voice Amplified Handsets
HARC Mercantile
5413 S. Westnedge Ave.
Suite A
Portage, MI   49002   269-324-0301
                                              800-445-9968
                                         Fax: 269-324-2387
                                          TTY: 269-324-1615
                                             info@harc.com
                                              www.harc.com

237   WalkerTalker
Prentke Romich Company
1022 Heyl Rd
Wooster, OH   44691-9786   330-262-1984
                                              800-262-1984
                                         Fax: 330-263-4829
                                          info@prentrom.com
                                           www.prentrom.com

David L Moffatt, President
Barry Romich, Co-Founder
Dave Moffatt, President / COO
A portable direct selection communication device for active persons. The 16 location keyboard and speakers are carried in a belt
that straps comfortably around the waist. The keyboard can be re-
moved from its pouch to use by activating keys. Two versions are
available, standard memory and expanded memory. *$1195.00*

Chairs

238 Adjustable Chair
Bailey Manufacturing Company
P.O.Box 130
Lodi, OH 44254-130
330-948-2655
800-321-8372
Fax: 800-224-5390
baileymfg@baileymfg.com
www.baileymfg.com

Larry Strimple, President
Sandy Mooney, Customer Service
Judie Butler, Dealer Contact
The seat and footboard of this versatile chair can be adjusted to accommodate children of various sizes. A classroom-suitable variation of this model is also available.

239 Adjustable Clear Acrylic Tray
Bailey Manufacturing Company
P.O.Box 130
Lodi, OH 44254-130
330-948-2655
800-321-8372
Fax: 800-224-5390
baileymfg@baileymfg.com
www.baileymfg.com

Larry Strimple, President
Sandy Mooney, Customer Service
Judie Butler, Dealer Contact
Adjusts for height and depth and is equipped with a spill rim for easy to clean edges.

240 Adjustable Rigid Chair
Kuschall North America
1811 Lefthand Cir
Ste B
Longmont, CO 80501-6785
303-682-2571
888-682-2571
Fax: 866-651-6973

Terry Mulkey, Owner
The Champion 3000 is a fully adjustable rigid frame chair weighing only 21 pounds with a new clamping system that adjusts seat height and angle without tools.

241 Adjustable Tee Stool
Bailey Manufacturing Company
P.O.Box 130
Lodi, OH 44254-130
330-948-2655
800-321-8372
Fax: 800-224-5390
baileymfg@baileymfg.com
www.baileymfg.com

Larry Strimple, President
Sandy Mooney, Customer Service
Judie Butler, Dealer Contact
May be used to encourage balance as well as develop integrative and perceptual motor skills.

242 BackSaver
BackSaver Products Company
53 Jeffrey Ave
Holliston, MA 01746-2084
508-893-6990
800-251-2225
Fax: 508-429-8698

Ed Foye, Owner
Eliminates slouching and extra pressure on your back and thighs which impairs circulation.

243 Better Back
Orthopedic Products Corporation
4100 1/2 Glencoe Ave
Marina Del Rey, CA 90292
323-584-6977
Fax: 310-306-0177

244 Carendo
Arjo Inc
2349 West Lake Street
Addison, IL 60101
630-785-4490
800-323-1245
Fax: 888-389-2756
usa.info@ArjoHuntleigh.com
www.arjo.com

Philip M. Croxford, President/ CEO
The Carendo hygiene chair has been designed for caregivers.

245 Century 50/60XR Sit
Arjo Inc
2349 West Lake Street
Addison, IL 60101
630-785-4490
800-323-1245
Fax: 888-389-2756
usa.info@ArjoHuntleigh.com
www.arjo.com

Philip M. Croxford, President/ CEO
This bathing system has a built-in cleaning/disinfectant injection system with adjustable flowmeter. The incorporation of an automatic hot water alarm/shut-off system, and digital temperature monitors, helps to assure resident safety and comfort.

246 Convert-Able Table
REAL Design
187 S Main St
Dolgeville, NY 13329-1455
315-429-3071
800-696-7041
Fax: 315-429-3071
rdesign@twcny.rr.com
www.realdesigninc.com

Sam Camardello, Owner
This table has push button height adjustment and interchangeable tops so it can become a desk, art easel or a sensory stimulation bowl.

247 Evac + Chair Emergency Evacuation Chair
Evac + Chair North America LLC
3000 Marcus Ave
Ste 3E6
Lake Success, NY 11042-1012
516-502-4240
Fax: 516-327-8220
sales@evac-chair.com
www.evac-chair.com

Richard Perl, VP Business Dev.
David Egen, Founder
Gravity driven evaluation chair allows one nondisabled person to smoothly glide a seated passenger down fire stairs and across landings to exit on a combination of wheels and track belts. Pivots in own width for tight landing turns. Aluminum; weight 19 pounds. Compactly stores on wall mount, 38 by 20 by 9 inches. Maximum capacity 330 pounds. Self braking features. No installation, works on all fire exit stairs. *$950.00*

248 Golden Technologies
401 Bridge St
Old Forge, PA 18518-2323
570-451-7477
800-624-6374
Fax: 800-628-5165
johngcei@excite.com
www.goldentech.com

Richard Golden, CEO
Robert Golden, Chairman of the Board
Fred Kiwak, VP of R & D
The largest facility in the world dedicated solely to the manufacture of lift chairs.

249 High-Low Chair
Rehab and Educational Aids for Living
NY
800-696-7041
rdesign@twcny.rr.com
www.realdesigninc.com/

Sam Camardello, President
Kris Wohnsen, Vice President

A high chair and mobile floor sitter in one. The high-low chair comes with colorful upholstered wipe clean seat and height adjustable tray. The chair has a single lever adjustment to change the seat height. Lateral and head supports are available as options. *$ 1199.00*

250 Ladybug Corner Chair
Rehab and Educational Aids for Living
NY   800-696-7041
                              rdesign@twcny.rr.com
                              www.realdesigninc.com/
Sam Camardello, President
Kris Wohnsen, Vice President
For children 0-3 years. This chair is adjustable for long legs for conventional sitting.

251 Lumex Recliner
Graham-Field Health Products
2935 Northeast Pkwy
Atlanta, GA 30360-2808   678-291-3207
                                        800-347-5678
                              Fax: 770-368-4702
                              cs@grahamfield.com
                              www.grahamfield.com
Kenneth Spett, President & Chief Executive Officer
Cherie Antoniazzi, SVP Quality, Regulatory and Risk Management
Ivan Bielik, Senior Vice President, Business Analyst
Marc Bernstein, Senior Vice President, Consumer Sales
Combines therapeutic benefits of position change with attractive appearance.

252 Modular QuadDesk
Gpk
535 Floyd Smith Dr
El Cajon, CA 92020-1228   619-593-7381
                                        800-468-8679
                              Fax: 888-755-5603
                              sales@gpk.com
                              www.gpk.com

253 Mulholland Positioning Systems
P.O.Box 70
839 Albion Avenue
Burley, ID 83318   208-878-3840
                                        800-543-4769
                              Fax: 208-878-3841
                              info@mulhollandinc.com
Larry Mulholland, Owner
Dick Stepan, Sales Manager
Provides a full line of standing aids, seating systems, adaptive components and bath aids.

254 Prime Engineering
Prime Engineering
4202 W Sierra Madre Ave
Fresno, CA 93722-3932   559-276-0991
                                        800-827-8263
                              Fax: 800-800-3355
                              info@primeengineering.com
                              www.primeengineering.com
Bruce Boegel, CFO
Mary Wilson Boegel, President
Mark Allen, Vice President
Dawn Smith Cobb, Customer Service
Prime Engineering is a leading manufacturer of adult and pediatric standing devices and patient transfer equipment. Products include the all-new Support Standing System, Granstand III MSS Standing System Kidstand III MSS Standing System Superstand Multi-Position Pediatric Stander, the Lift, the CindyLift and the Original Lift Walker.

255 Roll Chair
Bailey Manufacturing Company
P.O. Box 130
Lodi, OH 44254-130   330-948-2655
                                        800-321-8372
                              Fax: 800-224-5390
                              baileymfg@baileymfg.com
                              www.baileymfg.com
Larry Strimple, President
Sandy Mooney, Customer Service
Judie Butler, Dealer Contact
The padded roll helps maintain proper hip abduction and prevents scissoring of the legs.

256 Safari Tilt
Convaid Products
2830 California Street
Torrance, CA 90503   310-618-0111
                                        888-266-8243
                              Fax: 310-618-2166
                              www.convaid.com
Chris Braun, President
A semi-contour seat provides positioning with 5-45 degree tilt adjustment. One step design folds compactly into a lightweight chair.

257 Spatial Tilt Custom Chair
Redman Powerchair
Suite 107
1601 S Pantano Road
Tucson, AZ 85710-6791   520-546-6002
                                        800-727-6684
                              Fax: 520-546-5530
                              info@redmanpowerchair.com
                              www.redmanpowerchair.com
Don Redman, CEO
Paula Redman, CFO
Scott Evans, Regulatory affairs
Samuel Redman, General manager
Custom chair designed for comfort with a solid seat and back with modifications available for seat depth, height or width.

258 Transfer Bench with Back
Frohock-Stewart
1 Invacare Way
Elyria, OH 44035-4190   440-329-6000
                                        800-333-6900
                              Fax: 877-619-7996
                              www.invacare.com
A. Malachi Mixon III, Chairman of the Board
Gerald B. Blouch, President and Chief Executive Officer
Joseph B. Richey, II, President - Invacare Technologies Division
Robert K. Gudbranson, Senior Vice President and Chief Financial Officer
This bench with air-cushioned seat sections has a full, reversible backrest for safety and comfort.

Cushions & Wedges

259 Action Products
954 Sweeney Drive
Hagerstown, MD 21740-4910   301-797-1414
                                        800-228-7763
                              Fax: 301-733-2073
                              service@actionproducts.com
                              www.actionproducts.com
Mistie Witt, President
Janet Kaplan, Marketing Director
Wheelchair pads, mattress pads, positioning cushions and insoles that aid in the prevention and cure of pressure sores by reducing pressure. All products are made of Akton viscoelastic polymer that does not leak, flow or bottom out. Manufacturer of the Xact line of positioning cushions for patients with high risk of skin breakdown.

260 Adjustable Wedge
Bailey Manufacturing Company
P.O. Box 130
Lodi, OH 44254-130
800-321-8372
Fax: 800-224-5390
baileymfg@baileymfg.com
www.baileymfg.com

261 Back-Huggar Pillow
Bodyline Comfort Systems
3730 Kori Rd
Jacksonville, FL 32257-6036
904-262-4068
800-874-7715
Fax: 904-262-2225
info@bodyline.com
www.bodyline.com

Dr.John W. Fiore, Owner
Exclusive design makes almost any seat more comfortable by exerting soothing pressure against back muscles and discs.

262 Bye-Bye Decubiti (BBD)
Ken McRight Supplies
7456 S Oswego Ave
Tulsa, OK 74136-5903
918-492-9657
Fax: 918-492-9694

Ken McRight, President
The BBD therapeutic wheelchair cushions have been market-proven since 1951 — in the prevention and cure of pressure sores (decubiti). These natural rubber inflatable products have recently been expanded to include pediatric, sports and double-valve models. Moderately priced, they offer a viable and cost-effective alternative in the market. $84.00-$112.00.

263 Dynamic Systems, Inc.
104 Morrow Branch Rd.
Leicester, NC 28748-9635
828-683-3523
855-786-6283
Fax: 844-270-6478
dsi@sunmatecushions.com
www.sunmatecushions.com

Robin W. Yost, President/CEO
Melinda Garrett, Vice President/CFO
Andrew Biebinger, Plant Manager/COO
Susan Yost, Marketing Director
Systems, Inc. manufactures high-performance, medical-grade, orthopedic cushion materials for applications where pressure relief, body support, and skin health are critical. molding seat inserts. Sample packs and literature available upon request.

264 Econo-Float Water Flotation Cushion
Jefferson Industries
1985 Rutgers Blvd
Lakewood, NJ 08701-4569
732-905-9001
800-257-5145
Fax: 732-905-9899

Charles Landa, General Manager
An inexpensive, yet effective approach to the problem of pressure ulcers for patients confined to wheelchairs, geriatric chairs, etc. *$15.00*

265 Econo-Float Water Flotation Mattress
Jefferson Industries
1985 Rutgers Blvd
Lakewood, NJ 08701-4569
732-905-9001
800-257-5145
Fax: 732-905-9899

Charles Landa, General Manager
Helps prevent and treat pressure ulcers by reducing and distributing pressure over the patient's bony prominences while supporting the body evenly over a greater surface area. *$39.00*

266 Enhancer Cushion
ROHO Group
100 North Florida Avenue
Belleville, IL 62221-5429
618-277-9173
800-851-3449
Fax: 618-277-9561
tomb@therohogroup.com
www.therohogroup.com

Tom Borcherding, President
Bobby Graebe, CEO
Tim Richter, Vice President of Finance
Dave McCausland, Sr. VP of Planning & Gov Affairs
Uses AIR IN PLACE progressive positioning for enhanced midline channeling of the femurs, lateral stability and tissue protection.

267 Functional Forms
Consumer Care Products
1446 Pilgrim Rd
Plymouth, WI 53073-4969
920-893-4614
Fax: 800-977-2256
ccpi@consumercareinc.com

Terry Grall, Owner
These blocks, wedges, rolls, cervical pillows, head and leg supports and barrel rolls in resilient high density foam covered with durable antibacterial, antistatic, flame resistant, nonabsorbent vinyl are used to attain individualized support for the most difficult positioning needs for children and adults. Unique sizes allow fitting for almost any person. Use during exercise, feeding, therapy, recreation and rest at home, school and health care facilities. Packages available.

268 Gaymar Industries
Gaymar Industries
10 Centre Dr
Orchard Park, NY 14127-2295
716-662-2551
800-828-7341
Fax: 716-662-0748
webmaster@gaymar.com
www.gaymar.com

Dan Kormowicz, International Sales & Mktg
Cindy Sylvia, Educational Svcs Administrator
Heather Lindstrom, Medical Res
Brian McLaughlin, International Order Coordinator
Gaymar offers a complete line of support surfaces, including low-air-loss mattresses, specialty foam mattresses, turning mattresses, air overlays and fluid therapy beds. These products economically prevent and treat bedsores. Clinical and reimbursement professionals are available to answer any question related to bedsores (decubitus ulcers). Also offers a complete line of temperature control devices. The T-Pump delivers warm therapy to effectively dilate vessels and increase blood flow.

269 Geo-Matt for High Risk Patients
Span-America Medical Systems
70 Commerce Ctr
Greenville, SC 29615-5814
864-288-8877
800-888-6752
Fax: 864-288-8692
www.spanamerica.com

James D Ferguson, CEO
Helps prevent pressure sores in high risk patients.

270 High Profile Single Compartment Cushion
ROHO Group
100 North Florida Avenue
Belleville, IL 62221-5429
618-277-9173
800-851-3449
Fax: 618-277-9561
tomb@therohogroup.com
www.therohogroup.com

Tom Borcherding, President
Bobby Graebe, CEO
Tim Richter, Vice President of Finance
Dave McCausland, Sr. VP of Planning & Gov Affairs
With 4 inch cells, the HIGH PROFILE is the cushion of choice for individuals who suffer from ischemic ulcers (pressure sores) or who have a history of tissue breakdown.

271   Inflatable Back Pillow
Corflex
669 East Industrial Park Dr
Manchester, NH   03109-5625   603-623-3344
                                             800-426-7353
                                             Fax: 603-623-4111
                                             sales@corflex.com
                                             www.corflex.com

Paul Lorenzetti, CEO
Folds flat to fit into its own carrying case, this inflatable back pillow ensures comfort while at home or traveling.

272   Jobri
520 N Division St
Konawa, OK   74849-2223   580-925-3500
                                             800-432-2225
                                             Fax: 580-925-3501
                                             support@jobri.com
                                             www.jobri.com

Brian Gourley, CEO
Jobri manufactures ergonomic back supports, ergonomic chairs, orthopedic soft goods and sleep products.

273   Lumex Cushions and Mattresses
Graham-Field Health Products
2935 Northeast Pkwy
Atlanta, GA   30360-2808   678-291-3207
                                             800-347-5678
                                             Fax: 770-368-4702
                                             cs@grahamfield.com
                                             www.grahamfield.com

Kenneth Spett, President & Chief Executive Officer
Cherie Antoniazzi, SVP Quality, Regulatory and Risk Management
Ivan Bielik, Senior Vice President, Business Analyst
Marc Bernstein, Senior Vice President, Consumer Sales
Line of cushions and pillows give comfort and independence to the physically challenged.

274   Medpro Static Air Chair Cushion
Medpro
1950 Rutgers Blvd
Lakewood, NJ   08701-4537   800-257-5145
                                             Fax: 732-905-9899

Jody Gorran, President
Provides a protective layer of air beneath the patient helping prevent and treat pressure ulcers. $94.95

275   Medpro Static Air Mattress Overlay
Medpro
1950 Rutgers Blvd
Lakewood, NJ   08701-4537   800-257-5145
                                             Fax: 732-905-9899

Jody Gorran, President
Supports the patient on a cushioned network of air designed to redistribute the patient's weight reducing tissue interface pressure. Medpro's design incorporates a series of 65 air-breather vents that maintain air circulation. Medpro effectively reduces pressure and helps prevent and treat pressure ulcers. $164.95

276   Mini-Max Cushion
ROHO
100 North Florida Avenue
Belleville, IL   62221-5429   618-277-9173
                                             800-851-3449
                                             Fax: 618-277-9561
                                             tomb@therohogroup.com
                                             www.therohogroup.com

Tom Borcherding, President
Bobby Graebe, CEO
Tim Richter, Vice President of Finance
Dave McCausland, Sr. VP of Planning & Gov Affairs
Designed for the active individual with low risk of skin breakdown. The unique air cells of the MINI-MAX provide significant shock and impact absorption, skin protection and stability.

277   NEXUS Wheelchair Cushioning System
ROHO
100 North Florida Avenue
Belleville, IL   62221-5429   618-277-9173
                                             800-850-7646
                                             Fax: 618-277-9561
                                             tomb@therohogroup.com
                                             www.therohogroup.com

Tom Borcherding, President
Bobby Graebe, CEO
Tim Richter, Vice President of Finance
Dave McCausland, Sr. VP of Planning & Gov Affairs
A unique modular cushion that mates a contoured polyurethane foam base with a dry flotation support pad. It is designed to give the user positioning and stability, while offering maximum protection to the ischia, sacrum and coccyx.

278   Pediatric Seating System
ROHO
100 N Florida Ave
Belleville, IL   62221-5429   618-277-9173
                                             800-851-3449
                                             Fax: 618-277-9561
                                             tomb@therohogroup.com
                                             www.therohogroup.com

Tom Borcherding, President
Bobby Graebe, CEO
Tim Richter, Vice President of Finance
Dave McCausland, Sr. VP of Planning & Gov Affairs
ROHO Cushions for kids use individual air cells, creating the most versatile and dynamic cushioning products available. These cushions are designed to specifically fit pediatric wheelchairs.

279   Quadtro Cushion
ROHO
100 North Florida Avenue
Belleville, IL   62221-5429   618-277-9173
                                             800-851-3449
                                             Fax: 618-277-9561
                                             tomb@therohogroup.com
                                             www.therohogroup.com

Tom Borcherding, President
Bobby Graebe, CEO
Tim Richter, Vice President of Finance
Dave McCausland, Sr. VP of Planning & Gov Affairs
For individuals who require special positioning of the pelvis or thighs and are at risk of skin breakdown, the Quadtro, with 4 inch cell height and air in place, progressive positioning is the cushion of choice.

280   Silicone Padding
Spenco Medical Group
P.O. Box 2501
Waco, TX   76702-2501   254-772-6000
                                             800-877-3626
                                             spenco@spenco.com
                                             www.spenco.com

Jeff Antonioli, VP Sales
Ryan Cruthirds, Vice President
For the management of pressure sores, this padding provides a special support system which allows even distribution of pressure and cool, comfortable, well-ventilated support.

281   Soft-Touch Convertible Flotation Mattress
Medpro
1950 Rutgers Blvd
Lakewood, NJ   08701-4537   800-257-5145
                                             Fax: 732-905-9899

Jody Gorran, President
Gives the patient the option to choose between water and gel flotation depending on the needs of the patient. The mattress helps prevent and treat pressure ulcers by spreading the patient's weight over a greater surface area. $164.95-$239.95.

282   **Soft-Touch Gel Flotation Cushion**
Medpro
1940 Rutgers Blvd
Lakewood, NJ   08701-4537   732-905-9001
                                             800-257-5145
                                         Fax: 732-905-9899
Jody Gorran, President
Acts like an additional layer of fatty tissue beneath the patient to
help prevent and treat pressure sores. *$99.95*

283   **Spenco Medical Group**
P.O.Box 2501
Waco, TX   76702-2501   254-772-6000
                                              800-877-3626
                                          spenco@spenco.com
                                           www.spenco.com
Jeff Antonioli, VP Sales
Ryan Cruthirds, Vice President
Wheel chair cushions, silicone mattress pads, wound dressings,
second skin blister and burn pads, polysorb insoles, elbow, knee
and wrist supports and walking shoes.

284   **Stop-Leak Gel Flotation Mattress**
Jefferson Industries
1989 Rutgers Blvd
Lakewood, NJ   08701-4538   732-905-9001
                                             800-257-5145
                                         Fax: 732-905-9899
Charles Landa, General Manager
Protects persons from messy leaks while it protects from pressure
ulcers. *$54.00*

285   **Sun-Mate Seat Cushions**
Dynamic Systems
104 Morrow Branch Rd
Leicester, NC   28748-5710   828-683-3523
                                              855-786-6283
                                         Fax: 844-270-6478
                                    dsi@sunmatecushions.com
                                      www.sunmatecushions.com
Charles A Yost, CEO
Lewis McCrain, General Manager
Line of cushions, pads and accessory items for personal comfort
of the disabled. SunMate Orthopedic foam cushions and sheets
that contours slowly to give uniform pressure distribution and
soft spring back. Liquid SunMate for Foam-in-Place Seating
(FIPS) to make custom molded seat inserts.

286   **Twin-Rest Seat Cushion & Glamour Pillow**
Better Sleep
57 Industrial Rd
Berkeley Heights, NJ   07922-1501   908-464-6568
                                         Fax: 908-464-0058
William Emery Jr, President
Makes any seat more comfortable because it is ingeniously de-
signed to soothe sensitive areas while at work, in the car or at
home.

Dressing Aids

287   **Button Aid**
Maxi Aids
42 Executive Blvd
Farmingdale, NY   11735-4710   631-752-0521
                                              800-522-6294
                                         Fax: 631-752-0689
                                      TTY: 800-281-3555
                                      sales@maxiaids.com
                                       www.maxiaids.com
Elliot Zaretsky, Founder / President
Makes buttoning possible with the use of only one hand. *$9.95*

288   **Deluxe Sock and Stocking Aid**
Therapro, Inc.
225 Arlington St
Framingham, MA   01702-8723   508-872-9494
                                              800-257-5376
                                         Fax: 508-875-2062
                                      info@therapro.com
                                       www.therapro.com
Karen Conrad, ScD, OTR/L, Owner
Flexible plastic, lined with blue nylon to reduce friction and out-
side with beige terry cloth to hold sock firmly until it is on the
foot. *$12.95*

289   **Dressing Stick**
Maxi Aids
42 Executive Blvd
Farmingdale, NY   11735-4710   631-752-0521
                                              800-522-6294
                                         Fax: 631-752-0689
                                      TTY: 800-281-3555
                                       www.maxiaids.com
Elliot Zaretsky, Founder / President
Helps put on coats, sweaters and garments even when arm and
shoulder movement is limited. *$7.95*

290   **Elastic Shoelaces**
Therapro, Inc.
225 Arlington St
Framingham, MA   01702-8723   508-872-9494
                                              800-257-5376
                                         Fax: 508-875-2062
                                      info@therapro.com
                                       www.therapro.com
Karen Conrad, ScD, OTR/L, Owner
The elastic laces allow the wearer to slip tied shoes on and off.
$4.25

291   **Featherweight Reachers**
Therapro, Inc.
225 Arlington St
Framingham, MA   01702-8723   508-872-9494
                                              800-257-5376
                                         Fax: 508-875-2062
                                      info@therapro.com
                                       www.therapro.com
Karen Conrad, ScD, OTR/L, Owner
Useful in dressing or retrieving objects. *$17.95*

292   **Mirror Go Lightly**
AbleNet
2625 Patton Road
Roseville, MN   55113-1308   612-379-0956
                                              800-322-0956
                                         Fax: 612-379-9143
                                 customerservice@ablenetinc.com
                                       www.ablenetinc.com
Bill Sproull, Chairman of the Board
Jennifer Thalhuber, President/CEO
William Mills, Board of Director
Framed in plastic, the mirror can be tilted to provide either a nor-
mal or magnified image or to direct its lights at, or away from, the
user. *$22.00*

293   **Molded Sock and Stocking Aid**
Therapro, Inc.
225 Arlington St
Framingham, MA   01702-8723   508-872-9494
                                              800-257-5376
                                         Fax: 508-875-2062
                                      info@therapro.com
                                       www.therapro.com
Karen Conrad, ScD, OTR/L, Owner
Sock or stocking is pulled over the molded plastic and then can be
put on more easily. *$13.25*

294 **Say What**
Maxi Aids
42 Executive Blvd
Farmingdale, NY 11735-4710　　　　　　631-752-0521
　　　　　　　　　　　　　　　　　　　800-522-6294
　　　　　　　　　　　　　　　　　Fax: 631-752-0689
　　　　　　　　　　　　　　　　　TTY: 800-281-3555
　　　　　　　　　　　　　　　　　www.maxiaids.com

Elliot Zaretsky, Founder / President
Braille the tag with information that the wearer wants on the tag
and place the tag on a hanger. The custom-identification program
makes it easier for the user to remember and identify just the right
clothes. *$4.95*

295 **Shoe and Boot Valet: Decreased Mobility Aid**
Maxi Aids
42 Executive Blvd
Farmingdale, NY 11735-4710　　　　　　631-752-0521
　　　　　　　　　　　　　　　　　　　800-522-6294
　　　　　　　　　　　　　　　　　Fax: 631-752-0689
　　　　　　　　　　　　　　　　　TTY: 800-281-3555
　　　　　　　　　　　　　　　　　www.maxiaids.com

Elliot Zaretsky, Founder / President
This is the perfect device to alleviate and in many cases eliminate
the pain and embarrassment for millions of people who have a
problem doing the simple everyday task of putting on and taking
off their footwear. It works perfectly with shoes, boots, galoshes
and slippers. *$49.95*

Health Aids

296 **AMI**
P.O.Box 808
Groton, CT 06340-808　　　　　　　　860-536-3735
　　　　　　　　　　　　　　　　　　　800-248-4031
　　　　　　　　　　　　　　　　　Fax: 860-536-3735
　　　　　　　　　　　　　　　　　sales@aquamassage.com
　　　　　　　　　　　　　　　　　www.aquamassage.com

David M. Cote, President
Dow Cote, Vice President Sales
Hilaire Cote, Senior Vice President
Scott Gilbert, Customer Service Manager
The Aqua PT provides the major benefits of Hydrotherapy, Massage Therapy and Dry Heat Therapy. 36 water jets provide continuous full body or localized massage while the client remains
CLOTHED AND DRY! Adjustable water pressure, temperature
and pulsation frequency can massage in either a two direction
travel mode for musculoskeletal pain management or a one direction mode, flowing water from head to foot for a contrast mas-
sage-relax therapy. $25,000 to $30,000.

297 **American Medical Industries**
Ste 2
330 E 3rd St
Dell Rapids, SD 57022-1918　　　　　605-428-5501
　　　　　　　　　　　　　　　　　　　801-618-0444
　　　　　　　　　　　　　　　　　Fax: 605-428-5502
　　　　　　　　　　　　　　　　　www.ezhealthcare.com

Koby Jackson, Founder
Rick Martin, CEO
Kerina Blauer, VP Client Services
Jim Cannon, SVP Sales and Marketing
EZ-Swallow, EZ-Health, EZ-Home Care, Kleen-Handz,
Kleen-Scent, EZ-Irrigator, EZ-VU, Pureshark, Gobot and AMI
are all trademarks of American Medical Industries. Healthcare
products made easy.

298 **BIPAP S/T Ventilatory Support System**
Respironics
1010 Murry Ridge Ln
Murrysville, PA 15668-8517　　　　　724-387-5200
　　　　　　　　　　　　　　　　　Fax: 724-387-5010
　　　　　　　　　　　　　　　　　www.respironics.com

John L Miclot, CEO
Gerald McGinnis, Chairman
Daniel Bevevino, VP/CFO
Craig Reynolds, Executive VP/COO
Respironics, a recognized resource in the medical device market,
provides innovative products and unique designs to the health
care provider while helping them to grow and manage their busi-
ness efficiently.

299 **Bed Rails**
Mada Medical Products
625 Washington Ave
Carlstadt, NJ 07072-2901　　　　　　201-460-0454
　　　　　　　　　　　　　　　　　　　800-526-6370
　　　　　　　　　　　　　　　　　Fax: 201-460-3509
　　　　　　　　　　　　　dianelind@mail.madamedical.com
　　　　　　　　　　　　　　　　　www.madainternational.com

Jeffrey Adam, President
Chrome plated steel rails and crossbars, all welded construction,
telescopic side rail length adjustable, and a standard rail height of
16 inches.

300 **Coast to Coast Home Medical**
Ste 4d
3381 Fairlane Farms Rd
Wellington, FL 33414-8711　　　　　561-792-4009
　　　　　　　　　　　　　　　　　　　800-330-6316

Keri Suess, Owner
Home-delivered medical supplies for diabetes, respiratory, arthritis and impotence supplies.

301 **Drew Karol Industries**
P.O.Box 1066
Greenville, MS 38702-1066　　　　　662-378-2188
　　　　　　　　　　　　　　　　　Fax: 601-378-3188

Andrew K Hoszowski, Owner
Orally operated toothbrush and dental care system for persons
with limited or complete loss of hand or arm use - wheelchair accessible. *$600.00*

302 **Duraline Medical Products Inc.**
P.O.Box 67
324 Werner Street
Leipsic, OH 45856-1039　　　　　　419-943-2044
　　　　　　　　　　　　　　　　　　　800-654-3376
　　　　　　　　　　　　　　　　　Fax: 419-943-3637
　　　　　　　　　　　　　　　　　duraline@fairpoint.net
　　　　　　　　　　　　　　　　　www.dmponline.com

Kathy Peck, General Manager
An assortment of quality incontinence products for adults and
children.

303 **Duro-Med Industries**
1931 Norman Drive
Waukegan, IL 60085　　　　　　　　800-526-4753
　　　　　　　　　　　　　　　　　　　800-622-4714
　　　　　　　　　　　　　　　　　Fax: 800-479-7968
　　　　　　　　　　　　　　　　　www.mabisdmi.com

Mike Mazza, President
Tony D'Antonio, Senior VP of Sales
Alan Yefsky, Exec VP, Sales & Mktg
Manufacturers of a complete line of home health care products.
Featured products are patient gowns, back and seat cushions, pil-
lows and a complete line of aids for daily living.

304   Easy Ply
BioMedical Life Systems
P.O.Box 1360
Vista, CA 92085-1360   800-726-8367
                                               Fax: 760-727-4220
                                               information@bmls.com
                                               www.bmls.com

305   Electronic Stethoscopes
HARC Mercantile
5413 S. Westnedge Ave.
Suite A
Portage, MI 49002   269-324-0301
                                               800-445-9968
                                               Fax: 269-324-2387
                                               TTY: 269-324-1615
                                               info@harc.com
                                               www.harc.com

306   Fold-Down 3-in-1 Commode
Mada Medical Products
625 Washington Ave
Carlstadt, NJ 07072-2901   201-460-0454
                                               800-526-6370
                                               Fax: 201-460-3509
                                               dianelind@mail.madamedical.com
                                               www.madainternational.com
Jeffrey Adam, President
The Fold-Down commode is constructed of heavy duty, 1 inch diameter, steel tubing with X frame, has folding features convenient for storage and transport, easily removable back rest, and full length armrests.

307   Healing Dressing for Pressure Sores
Baxter Healthcare Corporation
1 Baxter Pkwy
Deerfield, IL 60015-4625   800-422-9837
                                               Fax: 800-568-5020
                                               www.baxter.com
Robert L Parkinson Jr, Chairman of the Board/CEO
Jean-Luc Butel, Corporate Vice President - President, International
Ludwig N. Hantson, Corporate Vice President - President, BioScience
Robert J. Hombach, Corporate VP/CFO
A dressing specifically designed to promote healing of pressure sores and other dermal ulcers.

308   Invacare Corporation
1 Invacare Way
Elyria, OH 44035-4190   440-329-6000
                                               800-333-6900
                                               Fax: 877-619-7996
                                               info@invacare.com
                                               www.invacare.com
A Malachi Mixon Iii, Chairman of the Board
Robert Gudbranson, Interim President & CEO; SVP & CFO
Joseph B. Richey, II, President - Invacare Technologies Division
Anthony C. LaPlaca, Senior Vice President /General Counsel
The world's leading manufacturer and distributor of innovative home and long-term care medical products which promote recovery and active lifestyles.

309   MADAMIST 50/50 PSI Air Compressor
Mada Medical Products
625 Washington Ave
Carlstadt, NJ 07072-2901   201-460-0454
                                               800-526-6370
                                               Fax: 201-460-3509
                                               dianelind@mail.madamedical.com
                                               www.madainternational.com
Jeffrey Adam, President
The new compressor rated at 50 PSI is designed to drive humidifiers, nebulizers, mist tents and is ideal to administer pentamidine aerosol therapy.

310   MedDev Corporation
730 N Pastoria Ave
Sunnyvale, CA 94085-3522   408-730-9702
                                               800-543-2789
                                               Fax: 408-730-9732
                                               info@meddev-corp.com
                                               www.meddev-corp.com

311   Medi-Grip
Therapro, Inc.
225 Arlington St
Framingham, MA 01702-8723   508-872-9494
                                               800-257-5376
                                               Fax: 508-875-2062
                                               info@therapro.com
                                               www.therapro.com
Karen Conrad, ScD, OTR/L, Owner
Reasonably priced, nonskid material. This nonslip material is available in marine blue, desert sand and burgundy rolls 12 inches x 144 inches. *$11.95*

312   Pocket Otoscope
HARC Mercantile
5413 S. Westnedge Ave.
Suite A
Portage, MI 49002   269-324-0301
                                               800-445-9968
                                               Fax: 269-324-2387
                                               TTY: 269-324-1615
                                               info@harc.com
                                               www.harc.com

313   Standard 3-in-1 Commode
Mada Medical Products
625 Washington Ave
Carlstadt, NJ 07072-2901   201-460-0454
                                               800-526-6370
                                               Fax: 201-460-3509
                                               dianelind@mail.madamedical.com
                                               www.madainternational.com
Jeffrey Adam, President
The standard commode is constructed of a heavy duty anodized aluminum frame, seat adjustment and an easily removable back rest.

314   Strider
Osborn Medical Corporation
7022 S. Revere Pkwy
Suite 240
Centennial, CO 80112   507-932-5028
                                               800-535-5865
                                               Fax: 507-932-5044
                                               info@osbornmedical.com
                                               www.osbornmedical.com
Bill Davis, President and CEO
Keith Walli-Ware, Vice President of Sales and Marketing
Ian MacDonald, COO
Strider allows you to exercise in most chairs found in your home. No more small, uncomfortable bicycle seats to sit on while exercising. With Strider, your hands are free to read the paper or your favorite book while you exercise.

315   Talking Clinical Thermometer
Maxi Aids
42 Executive Blvd
Farmingdale, NY 11735-4710   631-752-0521
                                               800-522-6294
                                               Fax: 631-752-0689
                                               TTY: 800-281-3555
                                               www.maxiaids.com
Elliot Zaretsky, Founder / President
Audible clinical thermometer. *$199.95*

316 Talking Thermometers
Maxi Aids
42 Executive Blvd
Farmingdale, NY 11735-4710   631-752-0521
                                                800-522-6294
                                        Fax: 631-752-0689
                                        TTY: 800-281-3555
                                        www.maxiaids.com

Elliot Zaretsky, Founder / President
Clearly announces temperature in Fahrenheit or Celcius. *$17.95*

317 Transfer Bench
Mada Medical Products
625 Washington Ave
Carlstadt, NJ 07072-2901   201-460-0454
                                                 800-526-6370
                                         Fax: 201-460-3509
                            dianelind@mail.madamedical.com
                                 www.madainternational.com

Jeffrey Adam, President
The transfer bench is a one piece bench with a wide base for stability, 1 inch diameter aluminum framework, corrosion resistant, and an adjustable seat.

Hearing Aids

318 Auditech: Personal PA Value Pack System
P.O.Box 821105
Vicksburg, MS 39182-1105   800-229-8293
                                         Fax: 800-221-8639
                                     info@auditechusa.com
                                     www.auditechusa.com

319 Auditech: Pocketalker Pro
P.O.Box 821105
Vicksburg, MS 39182-1105   800-229-8293
                                         Fax: 800-221-8639
                                     info@auditechusa.com
                                     www.auditechusa.com

320 Battery Device Adapter
AbleNet
2625 Patton Road
Roseville, MN 55113-1308   612-379-0956
                                                 800-322-0956
                                         Fax: 651-294-2259
                            customerservice@ablenetinc.com
                                     www.ablenetinc.com

Bill Sproull, Chairman of the Board
Jennifer Thalhuber, President/CEO
William Mills, Board of Director
A cable which connects to and adapts battery-operated devices for external switch control. Two sizes are available to adapt devices with either AA or C and D size batteries. *$8.00*

321 Custom Earmolds
Lloyd Hearing Aid Corporation
P.O.Box 1645
4435 Manchester Dr
Rockford, IL 61109-1645   815-964-4191
                                                 800-323-4212
                                         Fax: 815-964-8378
                                 info@lloydshearingaid.com
                                 www.lloydhearingaid.com

Andy PalmQuist, President
Hearing aid molds, custom built to the exact fit of the customer. *$29.95*

322 Digital Hearing Aids
Lloyd Hearing Aid Corporation
P.O.Box 1645
4435 Manchester Dr
Rockford, IL 61109-1645   815-964-4191
                                                 800-323-4212
                                         Fax: 815-964-8378
                                 www.lloydhearingaid.com

Andy PalmQuist, President
Latest hearing technology. *$7.50*

323 Doorbell Signalers
HARC Mercantile
5413 S. Westnedge Ave.
Suite A
Portage, MI 49002   269-324-0301
                                                 800-445-9968
                                         Fax: 269-324-2387
                                        TTY: 269-324-1615
                                             info@harc.com
                                             www.harc.com

324 Double Gong Indoor/Outdoor Ringer
HARC Mercantile
5413 S. Westnedge Ave.
Suite A
Portage, MI 49002   269-324-0301
                                                 800-445-9968
                                         Fax: 269-324-2387
                                        TTY: 269-324-1615
                                             info@harc.com
                                             www.harc.com

325 Duracell & Rayovac Hearing Aid Batteries
Lloyd Hearing Aid Corporation
P.O.Box 1645
4435 Manchester Dr
Rockford, IL 61109-1645   815-964-4191
                                                 800-323-4212
                                         Fax: 815-964-8378
                                 info@lloydhearingaid.com
                                 www.lloydhearingaid.com

Andy PalmQuist, President
Batteries for hearing aids at discounted prices. As low as 45 cents each.

326 Harris Communications
Harris Communications
15155 Technology Dr
Eden Prairie, MN 55344-2273   800-825-6758
                                         Fax: 952-906-1099
                                        TTY:800-825-9187
                                     info@harriscomm.com
                                     www.harriscomm.com

Dr.Robert Harris, Owner and President
A national distributor of assistive devices for the deaf and hard-of-hearing with many manufacturers represented. Catalog includes a wide range of assistive devices as well as a variety of books and video tapes related to deaf and hard-of-hearing issues. Products available for children, teachers, hearing professionals, interpreters and anyone interested in deaf culture, hearing loss and sign language.
180 pages Yearly

327 Hearing Aid Batteries
HARC Mercantile
5413 S. Westnedge Ave.
Suite A
Portage, MI 49002   269-324-0301
                                                 800-445-9968
                                         Fax: 269-324-2387
                                        TTY: 269-324-1615
                                             info@harc.com
                                             www.harc.com

328   Hearing Aid Battery Testers
HARC Mercantile
5413 S. Westnedge Ave.
Suite A
Portage, MI   49002
269-324-0301
800-445-9968
Fax: 269-324-2387
TTY: 269-324-1615
info@harc.com
www.harc.com

329   Hearing Aid Dehumidifier
HARC Mercantile
5413 S. Westnedge Ave.
Suite A
Portage, MI   49002
269-324-0301
800-445-9968
Fax: 269-324-2387
TTY: 269-324-1615
info@harc.com
www.harc.com

330   In the Ear Hearing Aid Battery Extractor
HARC Mercantile
5413 S. Westnedge Ave.
Suite A
Portage, MI   49002
269-324-0301
800-445-9968
Fax: 269-324-2387
TTY: 269-324-1615
info@harc.com
www.harc.com

331   Micro Audiometrics Corporation
655 Keller Rd
Murphy, NC   28906-5890
828-644-0771
800-729-9509
866-327-7226
Fax: 866-683-4447
sales@microaud.com
www.microaud.com
Jason Keller, President
Manufacturer and distributor of hearing testing instruments, including the complete line of Earscan.

332   Mushroom Inserts
Lloyd Hearing Aid Corporation
P.O.Box 1645
4435 Manchester Drive
Rockford, IL   61109- 1645
815-964-4191
800-323-4212
Fax: 815-964-8378
info@lloydhearingaid.com
www.lloydhearingaid.com
Andy PalmQuist, President
A universal earplug useful in wearing behind the ear type hearing instruments. *$2.50*

333   Oval Window Audio
33 Wildflower Ct
Nederland, CO   80466
303-447-3607
Fax: 303-447-3607
TTY:303-447-3607
info@ovalwindowaudio.com
www.ovalwindowaudio.com
Norman Lederman, Director of Research & Development
Paula Hendricks, Educational Director
Manufacturer of induction loop hearing assistance technologies compatible with telecoil-equipped hearing aids used by many hard of hearing people. The company also makes multisensory sound systems for use in speech and music therapy and science classes.

334   Starkey Hearing Foundation
6700 Washington Ave S
Eden Prairie, MN   55344
952-941-6401
866-354-3254
Fax: 952-828-6900
info@starkeyfoundation.org
www.starkeyhearingfoundation.org
Richard S Brown, President
Brady Forseth, Executive Director
Keith Becker, Senior Director of Operations
Bruce Schmaltz, Chief Financial Officer
The Starkey Hearing Foundation works to assist those with hearing impairments by offering hearing aids and aftercare services.
Quarterly

335   Ultratec
450 Science Dr
Madison, WI   53711
608-238-5400
800-482-2424
Fax: 608-238-3008
TTY: 800-482-2424
service@ultratec.com
www.ultratec.com
Jackie Morgan, Marketing Director
Amy Mueller, Marketing Communications Specialist
Ultratec works to make telephone access more convenient and reliable for people with hearing loss by providing assistive devices such as amplified phones and text phones.

Kitchen & Eating Aids

336   Bagel Holder
Maxi Aids
42 Executive Blvd
Farmingdale, NY   11735-4710
631-752-0521
800-522-6294
Fax: 631-752-0689
TTY: 800-281-3555
www.maxiaids.com
Elliot Zaretsky, Founder / President
Holds bagels in place for easy slicing. *$3.95*

337   Big Bold Timer Low Vision
Maxi Aids
42 Executive Blvd
Farmingdale, NY   11735-4710
631-752-0521
800-522-6294
Fax: 631-752-0689
TTY: 800-281-3555
www.maxiaids.com
Elliot Zaretsky, Founder / President
Sixty-minute mechanical timer with large, easy-to-read numbers for the vision impaired. *$9.95*

338   Box Top Opener
Sammons Preston Rolyan
W68 N158 Evergreen Blvd.
Cedarburg, WI   53012
630-378-6000
800-228-3693
Fax: 262-387-8748
sp@pattersonmedical.com
www.pattersonmedical.com
David P Sproat, President
Bruce Curtis, Sales Representative
This handy device exerts the pressure on those hard-to-open boxes of laundry/dishwasher soap, rice and prepared dinners. *$2.95*

339   Capscrew
Access with Ease
P.O.Box 1150
Chino Valley, AZ   86323-1150
928-636-9469
800-531-9479
Fax: 928-636-0292
KMJC@northlink.com

340 Cool Handle
Maxi Aids
42 Executive Blvd
Farmingdale, NY 11735-4710
631-752-0521
800-522-6294
Fax: 631-752-0689
TTY: 800-281-3555
www.maxiaids.com
Elliot Zaretsky, Founder / President
A specially designed, heat-resistant handle, available in three sizes which can be affixed to the handles of most fry, sauce and saute pans. *$7.95*

341 Cordless Receiver
AbleNet
2625 Patton Road
Roseville, MN 55113-1308
612-379-0956
800-322-0956
Fax: 651-294-2259
customerservice@ablenetinc.com
www.ablenetinc.com
Bill Sproull, Chairman of the Board
Jennifer Thalhuber, President/CEO
William Mills, Board of Director
The Cordless Receiver in conjunction with the Cordless Big Red Switch, can be used anywhere a switch is currently used to control battery or electrically-operated toys, games or appliances; augmentative communication systems; and computers (through a computer switch interface). *$79.00*

342 Deluxe Long Ring Low Vision Timer
Maxi Aids
42 Executive Blvd
Farmingdale, NY 11735-4710
631-752-0521
800-522-6294
Fax: 631-752-0689
TTY: 800-281-3555
www.maxiaids.com
Elliot Zaretsky, Founder / President
Bold black numerals on white background allows for easy reading at any distance. *$17.95*

343 Deluxe Roller Knife
Sammons Preston Rolyan
28100 Torch Parkway
Suite 700
Warrenville, IL 60555-3938
630-378-6000
800-323-5547
Fax: 630-393-7600
sp@pattersonmedical.com
www.pattersonmedical.com
David P Sproat, President
Bruce Curtis, Sales Representative
Stainless steel blade rolls smoothly, cutting food cleanly. *$10.95*

344 Dual Brush with Suction Base
Sammons Preston Rolyan
28100 Torch Parkway
Suite 700
Warrenville, IL 60555-3938
630-378-6000
800-323-5547
Fax: 630-393-7600
sp@pattersonmedical.com
www.pattersonmedical.com
David P Sproat, President
Bruce Curtis, Sales Representative
Two brushes clean the inside and outside of bottles and glasses at the same time using just one hand. *$14.50*

345 Easy Pour Locking Lid Pot
Maxi Aids
42 Executive Blvd
Farmingdale, NY 11735-4710
631-752-0521
800-522-6294
Fax: 631-752-0689
TTY: 800-281-3555
www.maxiaids.com
Elliot Zaretsky, Founder / President

Baked enamel and dishwasher safe, the pot comes with an easy lid that locks in place for extra safety. *$24.95*

346 Electric Can Opener & Knife Sharpener
Maxi Aids
42 Executive Blvd
Farmingdale, NY 11735-4710
631-752-0521
800-522-6294
Fax: 631-752-0689
TTY: 800-281-3555
www.maxiaids.com
Elliot Zaretsky, Founder / President
Features include a powerful magnetic lid holder, the ability to open odd-shaped cans, and easy operation for the physically challenged. *$19.95*

347 Evio Plastics
P.O.Box 2295
Sandusky, OH 44871-2295
419-621-1105
Fax: 419-626-2183
Doug Didion, Admininstrator Director
Danny Thomas, Owner
Handi Holder is a plastic holder for 1/2 gallon paper cartons of milk or juice. It is used to pour milk or juice without spills by using the handle.

348 Food Markers/Rubberbands
Maxi Aids
42 Executive Blvd
Farmingdale, NY 11735-4710
631-752-0521
800-522-6294
Fax: 631-752-0689
TTY: 800-281-3555
www.maxiaids.com
Elliot Zaretsky, Founder / President
These are durable plastic markers, easily identified by touch, texture, shape and form which help the visually impaired orient themselves to food location on the plate. *$11.95*

349 Good Grips Cutlery
Therapro, Inc.
225 Arlington St
Framingham, MA 01702-8723
508-872-9494
800-257-5376
Fax: 508-875-2062
info@therapro.com
www.therapro.com
Karen Conrad, ScD, OTR/L, Owner
Stainless steel utensils have a special twist built into the metal to facilitate bending of a spoon or fork at any angle for right or left handed people. *$7.50*

350 H.E.L.P. Knife
Maxi Aids
42 Executive Blvd
Farmingdale, NY 11735-4710
631-752-0521
800-522-6294
Fax: 631-752-0689
TTY: 800-281-3555
www.maxiaids.com
Elliot Zaretsky, Founder / President
Adjustable food slicing system guides the knife for even, uniform slices while protecting the user. *$11.95*

351 Handy-Helper Cutting Board
Maxi Aids
42 Executive Blvd
Farmingdale, NY 11735-4710
631-752-0521
800-522-6294
Fax: 631-752-0689
TTY: 800-281-3555
www.maxiaids.com
Elliot Zaretsky, Founder / President
Laminated cutting board with unique features to hold food in place with corner ledge for cutting and spreading. *$19.95*

352 **Innerlip Plates**
Therapro, Inc.
225 Arlington St
Framingham, MA   01702-8723

508-872-9494
800-257-5376
Fax: 508-875-2062
info@therapro.com
www.therapro.com

Karen Conrad, ScD, OTR/L, Owner
Food may be pushed to the side of the plate, then scooped up with
a fork and spoon. Available in beige or blue. *$5.00*

353 **Long Oven Mitts**
Sammons Preston Rolyan
28100 Torch Parkway
Suite 700
Warrenville, IL   60555-3938

630-378-6000
800-323-5547
Fax: 630-393-7600
sp@pattersonmedical.com
www.pattersonmedical.com

David P Sproat, President
Bruce Curtis, Sales Representative
Protect hands and forearms from heat, flames and oven grates
with these practical mitts that allow a longer reach and less bending. *$8.95*

354 **Magnetic Card Reader**
Maxi Aids
42 Executive Blvd
Farmingdale, NY   11735-4710

631-752-0521
800-522-6294
Fax: 631-752-0689
TTY: 800-281-3555
www.maxiaids.com

Elliot Zaretsky, Founder / President
Produces audible labels so a recorded card can be taped on cans of
food or a box of cake mix; even adding instructions for baking.
$159.95

355 **Maxi-Aids Braille Timer**
Maxi Aids
42 Executive Blvd
Farmingdale, NY   11735-4710

631-752-0521
800-522-6294
Fax: 631-752-0689
TTY: 800-281-3555
www.maxiaids.com

Elliot Zaretsky, Founder / President
Three raised dots at 15, 30 and 45, two raised dots at remaining
five minute intervals and one raised dot at remaining two and a
half minute intervals, offers ease of operation to make this a helpful aid for the visually impaired. *$12.95*

356 **Nosey Cup**
Therapro, Inc.
225 Arlington St
Framingham, MA   01702-8723

508-872-9494
800-257-5376
Fax: 508-875-2062
info@therapro.com
www.therapro.com

Karen Conrad, ScD, OTR/L, Owner
For those with a stiff neck or persons who can't tip their head back
while drinking. *$6.00*

357 **Paring Boards**
Therapro, Inc.
225 Arlington St
Framingham, MA   01702-8723

508-872-9494
800-257-5376
Fax: 508-875-2062
info@therapro.com
www.therapro.com

Karen Conrad, ScD, OTR/L, Owner
Suction feet stabilize board and stainless steel prongs hold food
in place for easy, one-handed cutting. *$32.50*

358 **PowerLink 2 Control Unit**
AbleNet
2625 Patton Road
Roseville, MN   55113-1308

612-379-0956
800-322-0956
Fax: 651-294-2259
customerservice@ablenetinc.com
www.ablenetinc.com

Bill Sproull, Chairman of the Board
Jennifer Thalhuber, President/CEO
William Mills, Board of Director
The PowerLink 2 Control Unit allows switch operation of electrical appliances. It can be used to activate 1 or 2 appliances (up to
1700 watts combined). If 2 appliances are used, they will activate
simultaneously. There are four modes of control on the
PowerLink 2; direct mode, timed (seconds) mode, timed (minutes) mode and latch mode. Meets safety standards from Under-
writers Laboratory (UL) and Canadian Standards Association
(CSA) for electrical appliances. *$159.00*

359 **Sammons Preston Rolyan**
28100 Torch Parkway
Suite 700
Warrenville, IL   60555-3938

630-378-6000
800-323-5547
Fax: 630-393-7600
sp@pattersonmedical.com
www.pattersonmedical.com

David P Sproat, President
Bruce Curtis, Sales Representative
Sammons Preston Rolyan is a leading provider of rehabilitation
and assistive devices to help those with disabilities meet daily
physical challenges and achieve their greatest level of independence. With one of the industry's largest catalogs, Sammons Preston Rolyan offers a wide range of products available.
Annually

360 **Slicing Aid**
Snug Seat
12801 E. Independence Blvd.
P.O.Box 1739
Matthews, NC 28106-1739

704-882-0666
800-336-7684
Fax: 704-882-0751
information@snugseat.com
www.snugseat.com

Scott Crosswhite, Vice President
Kirk Mackenzie, President
Greg Tilley, Controller
Angela Stegall, Purchasing
The design of these knives allows a better working posture and
makes optimal use of strength in the arms and hands.

361 **Small Appliance Receiver**
AbleNet
2625 Patton Road
Roseville, MN   55113-1308

612-379-0956
800-322-0956
Fax: 651-294-2259
customerservice@ablenetinc.com
www.ablenetinc.com

Bill Sproull, Chairman of the Board
Jennifer Thalhuber, President/CEO
William Mills, Board of Director
The Small Appliance Receiver, in conjunction with the Cordless
Big Red Switch, allows you to control small electrical appliances
in the environment without a cord. It should only be used with
low-wattage appliances (under 500 watts) which have two prong
plugs (i.e., radios, fans, lamps, blenders, etc.). It should not be
used with heat generating appliances. *$32.00*

362 Steel Food Guard
Maxi Aids
42 Executive Blvd
Farmingdale, NY 11735-4710
631-752-0521
800-522-6294
Fax: 631-752-0689
TTY: 800-281-3555
www.maxiaids.com

Elliot Zaretsky, Founder / President
Provides stable area to push against while eating. *$ 10.95*

363 Thick-n-Easy
Therapro, Inc.
225 Arlington St
Framingham, MA 01702-8723
508-872-9494
800-257-5376
Fax: 508-875-2062
info@therapro.com
www.therapro.com

Karen Conrad, ScD, OTR/L, Owner
Instant food thickener that sets in 30 seconds and will not become thicker even after refrigeration. *$6.50*

364 Thumbs Up Cup
Therapro, Inc.
225 Arlington St.
Framingham, MA 01702-8723
508-872-9494
800-257-5376
Fax: 508-875-2062
info@therapro.com
www.therapro.com

Karen Conrad, Owner
This cup is designed for those with limited strength or coordination or arthritis. The two backward-tilt handles and thumb rests allow finger joints to be used to their greatest mechanical advantage. *$9.50*

365 Undercounter Lid Opener
Sammons Preston Rolyan
28100 Torch Parkway
Suite 700
Warrenville, IL 60555-3938
630-378-6000
800-323-5547
Fax: 630-393-7600
sp@pattersonmedical.com
www.pattersonmedical.com

David P Sproat, President
Bruce Curtis, Sales Representative
The gripper of this unit which installs under the counter can help unscrew any cap. *$5.75*

366 Uni-Turner
Sammons Preston Rolyan
28100 Torch Parkway
Suite 700
Warrenville, IL 60555-3938
630-378-6000
800-323-5547
Fax: 630-393-7600
sp@pattersonmedical.com
www.pattersonmedical.com

David P Sproat, President
Bruce Curtis, Sales Representative
Odd shaped handles can be turned easily with one-handed, L-shaped Uni-Turner. *$16.50*

367 Universal Hand Cuff
Therapro, Inc.
225 Arlington St
Framingham, MA 01702-8723
508-872-9494
800-257-5376
Fax: 508-875-2062
info@therapro.com
www.therapro.com

Karen Conrad, ScD, OTR/L, Owner
Comfortable cuff with Velcro strap holds utensils, toothbrushes, etc. *$9.95*

Lifts, Ramps & Elevators

368 Accessibility Lift
Inclinator Company of America
601 Gibson Blvd
Harrisburg, PA 17104-3215
717-939-8420
800-343-9007
Fax: 717-939-8075
isales@inclinator.com
www.inclinator.com

Stephen Nock, President
An economical lift for restricted usage that provides barrier-free access that can be used by churches, schools, lodging halls and meeting halls to meet compliance requirements, with the dignified convenience and freedom they deserve.

369 Adjustable Incline Board
Bailey Manufacturing Company
P.O. Box 130
Lodi, OH 44254-130
800-321-8372
Fax: 800-224-5390
baileymfg@baileymfg.com
www.baileymfg.com

370 AlumiRamp
855 E Chicago Rd
Quincy, MI 49082-9450
800-800-3864
Fax: 517-639-4314
sales@alumiramp.com
www.alumiramp.com

Doug Cannon, General Manager
Complete line of modular, aluminum and portable ramps for both home and vehicle use. Welded construction and non-skid extruded surfaces are featured on all our ramps.

371 Area Access
7131 Gateway Court
Manassas, VA 20109-1015
703-396-4949
800-333-2732
Fax: 703-207-0446
www.areaaccess.com

372 Basement Motorhome Lift
Handicaps, Inc.
4335 S Santa Fe Dr.
Englewood, CO 80110
303-781-2062
800-782-4335
info@handicapsinc.com
www.handicapsinc.com

373 BraunAbility
631 W 11th St.
Winamac, IN 46996-310
800-488-0359
www.braunability.com

Ralph Braun, Founder/CEO
BraunAbility is the world's largest manufacturer of wheelchair-accessible vans, ramps and wheelchair lifts. Their products enable people with physical disabilities to regain their mobility and to lead active and independent lives.

374 Bruno Independent Living Aids
P.O.Box 84
1780 Executive Drive
Oconomowoc, WI 53066
262-567-4990
800-882-8183
Fax: 262-953-5510
www.bruno.com

Michael R. Bruno, II, President/CEO
Andrew Bayer, Product Mgr, Automotive Div.
Mike Krawczyk, Mktg Svcs Mgr
An ISO 9001 Certified Manufacturer of automotive lifts for scooter, wheelchairs, and power chairs, three and four wheel scooters, and straight and custom curve stairlifts.

375   Butlers Wheelchair Lifts
Flinchbaugh Company
629 Lowther Road #C
Lewisberry, PA 17339   717-938-4253
                                                888-847-0804
                                           Fax: 717-938-4238
                                           www.butlermobility.com

Hal Feinstein, VP Sales / Marketing
This wheelchair lift can be equipped with an end ramp and guard.
Automatically retractable, it locks firmly into place when the lift
is in operation.

376   Classique
Handi-Lift
730 Garden St
Carlstadt, NJ 07072-1625   201-933-0111
                                                800-432-5438
                                           Fax: 201-933-0050
                                           sales@handi-lift.com
                                           www.handi-lift.com

Douglas Boydston, President
The Classique elevator answers access problems in churches,
schools and small offices.

377   Columbus McKinnon Corporation
140 John James Audubon Pkwy
Amherst, NY 14228-1197   716-689-5400
                                                800-888-0985
                                           Fax: 716-689-5644
                                           www.cmworks.com

Timothy T. Tevens, President/CEO
Gregory P. Rustowicz, VP/CFO
Charles R. Giesige, VP, Corporate Dev.
Richard A. Steinberg, VP, Human Resources
Supplies various lift and transfer systems for independent or attended applications including ceiling mounted or freestanding
overhead track lifts and mobile floorbase units for homes,
schools and healthcare facilities. Lift Systems for transferring
between bed, chair, commode or bath are available with a variety
of slings, scales and accessories.

378   Curb-Sider
Bruno Independent Living Aids
PO Box 84
1780 Executive Drive
Oconomowoc, WI 53066   262-567-4990
                                                800-882-8183
                                           Fax: 262-953-5501
                                           www.bruno.com

Michael R. Bruno, II, President/CEO
Andrew Bayer, Product Mgr, Automotive Div.
Mike Krawczyk, Mktg Svcs Mgr
The lift of choice for storing your fully or partially assembled
scooter or power chair weighing up to 400 pounds in the rear of
your van or minivan, SUV, pickup truck or some station wagon
applications.

379   Curb-Sider Super XL
P.O.Box 84
1780 Executive Drive
Oconomowoc, WI 53066   262-567-4990
                                                800-882-8183
                                           Fax: 262-953-5510
                                           www.bruno.com

Michael R. Bruno, II, President/CEO
Andrew Bayer, Product Mgr, Automotive Div.
Mike Krawczyk, Mktg Svcs Mgr

380   Custom Lift Residential Elevators
Waupaca Elevator Company
1726 N Ballard Rd
Appleton, WI 54911-2444   920-991-9082
                                                800-238-8739
                                           Fax: 920-991-9087
                                           info@waupacaelevator.com
                                           waupacaelevator.com

Bill Mc Michael, Owner

Waupaca Elevator residential elevators and dumbwaiters add
value, convenience and reliability to today's homes.

381   Deluxe Convertible Exercise Staircase
Sammons Preston Rolyan
28100 Torch Parkway
Suite 700
Warrenville, IL 60555-3938   630-378-6000
                                                800-323-5547
                                           Fax: 630-393-7600
                                           sp@pattersonmedical.com
                                           www.pattersonmedical.com

David P Sproat, President
Bruce Curtis, Sales Representative
Here's an exercise staircase to fit any department configuration.
Just reposition a few nuts and bolts to change from a straight to a
corner type staircase.

382   E-Z Access Van Ramp
Maxi Aids
42 Executive Blvd
Farmingdale, NY 11735-4710   631-752-0521
                                                800-522-6294
                                           Fax: 631-752-0689
                                           TTY: 800-281-3555
                                           www.maxiaids.com

Elliot Zaretsky, Founder / President
Telescopic ramps for manual and electric wheel chairs. Bridges
gaps over steps and curbs and makes vans more accessible. Extends 7'ft. in length, locking securely in place with snap-button
catches. Easy to store. Holds up to 600lbs. *$299.95*

383   Easy Pivot Transfer Machine
Rand-Scot
401 Linden Center Dr
Fort Collins, CO 80524-2429   970-484-7967
                                                800-467-7967
                                           Fax: 970-484-3800
                                           info@randscot.com
                                           www.randscot.com

Joel Lerich, President
The Easy Pivot Patient Lifting System allows for strain-free,
one-caregiver transfers of the disabled individual.

384   Easy Stand
Altimate Medical
262 W. 1st St.
Morton, MN 56270-180   507-697-6393
                                                800-342-8968
                                           Fax: 507-697-6900
                                           info@easystand.com
                                           www.easystand.com

Andrew Gardeen, International Sales Manager
Designed to make standing fast and simple. The easy to operate,
hydraulic lift system provides a controlled lifting and lowering.
With the convenience of simply transferring to the chair and
reaching a standing position in seconds with no straps to struggle
with.

385   Economical Liberty
Handi-Lift
730 Garden St
Carlstadt, NJ 07072-1625   201-933-0111
                                                800-432-5438
                                           Fax: 201-933-0050
                                           sales@handi-lift.com
                                           www.handi-lift.com

Douglas Boydston, President
Installs quickly and easily on most straight stairways. It uses regular household current and mounts over the carpet or directly to
the stairs without marring.

386   Electra-Ride
Bruno Independent Living Aids
PO Box 84
1780 Executive Drive
Oconomowoc, WI   53066   262-567-4990
                                        800-882-8183
                                        Fax: 262-953-5501
                                        www.bruno.com
Michael R. Bruno, II, President/CEO
Andrew Bayer, Product Mgr, Automotive Div.
Mike Krawczyk, Mktg Svcs Mgr
Bruno stairlifts can fit almost any custom curve or straight rail application and require no structural modification to the stairway. Plus, battery power allows for uninterrupted operation even during a power outage.

387   Electra-Ride Elite
Bruno Independent Living Aids
P.O.Box 84
1780 Executive Drive
Oconomowoc, WI   53066   262-567-4990
                                        800-882-8183
                                        Fax: 262-953-5510
                                        www.bruno.com
Michael R. Bruno, II, President/CEO
Andrew Bayer, Product Mgr, Automotive Div.
Mike Krawczyk, Mktg Svcs Mgr
The new Electra-Ride Elite installs to within 5 inches of the wall and has a 350 pound weight capacity. Bruno stairlifts can fit almost any custom curve or straight rail application and require no structural modification to the stairway. Plus, battery power allows for uninterrupted operation even during a power outage.

388   Electra-Ride III
P.O.Box 84
1780 Executive Drive
Oconomowoc, WI   53066   262-567-4990
                                        800-882-8183
                                        Fax: 262-953-5510
                                        www.bruno.com
Michael R. Bruno, II, President/CEO
Andrew Bayer, Product Mgr, Automotive Div.
Mike Krawczyk, Mktg Svcs Mgr

389   Freedom Wheels
580 Tc Jester Blvd
Houston, TX   77007   713-864-1460
                                        888-422-5337
                                        Fax: 713-864-1469
                                        info@freedomwheels.com
                                        www.freedomwheels.com
Carlos Saez, Owner
An assistive technology and mobility equipment provider and is committed to people with disabilities and personal transportation options for an independent lifestyle.

390   Handi Home Lift
Handi-Lift
730 Garden St
Carlstadt, NJ   07072-1625   201-933-0111
                                        800-432-5438
                                        Fax: 201-933-0050
                                        sales@handi-lift.com
                                        www.handi-lift.com
Douglas Boydston, President
An outdoor lift designed to provide access over porch stairs or other steps that impede movement.

391   Handi Lift
730 Garden St
Carlstadt, NJ   07072-1625   201-933-0111
                                        800-432-5438
                                        Fax: 201-933-0050
                                        sales@handi-lift.com
                                        www.handi-lift.com
Douglas Boydston, President

Accessibility with Dignity. We create solutions that enable people with mobility impairments to live freely with products like wheelchair lifts and home elevators.

392   Handi Prolift
Handi-Lift
730 Garden St
Carlstadt, NJ   07072-1625   201-933-0111
                                        800-432-5438
                                        Fax: 201-933-0050
                                        sales@handi-lift.com
                                        www.handi-lift.com
Douglas Boydston, President
Provides dependable vertical transportation for multi-level buildings.

393   Handi-Ramp
Handi-Ramp
510 North Ave
Libertyville, IL   60048-2025   847-680-7700
                                        800-876-7267
                                        Fax: 847-816-7689
                                        info@handiramp.com
                                        www.handiramp.com
Thomas Disch, President/ CEO
Alicia C. Johns, Program Manager
Provides a complete line of economical, ADA Compliant access ramping products. Line includes van attachable and wheelchair tie downs; aluminum or expanded metal folding portables; aluminum channels; portable, sectional ramp systems; semi-permanent ramps, platforms and systems. All ramp series are available in varied lengths and widths in combination with platforms and optional hand railing, single or double bar construction with return ends. Special Order ramps and ramp systems.

394   Homewaiter
Inclinator Company of America
601 Gibson Blvd
Harrisburg, PA   17104-3215   717-939-8420
                                        800-343-9007
                                        Fax: 717-939-8075
                                        isales@inclinator.com
                                        www.inclinator.com
Stephen Nock, President
With its roller truck riding in a specially formed monorail, it is easy to install and highly adaptable to existing conditions. It can travel up to 35 feet, opening on any or all three sides at different stations, whether at counter level or floor level.

395   Horcher Lifting Systems
324 Cypress Rd
Ocala, FL   34472-3102   352-687-8020
                                        800-582-8732
                                        Fax: 866-378-3318
                                        us-office@horcher.com
                                        www.horcher.com
David Schultz, General Manager
Sharon Harbert, Administrative Assistant
Barrier Free Lifts by Horcher leads the industry for excellence in patient transfers and technology for over 18 years. They offer state of the art ceiling track systems, floor base lifts and bathing systems such as the Unilift, PC-2, Diana, Lexa, and Raisa to achieve greater mobility.

396   Inclinette
Inclinator Company of America
601 Gibson Blvd
Harrisburg, PA   17104-3215   717-939-8420
                                        800-343-9007
                                        Fax: 717-939-8075
                                        isales@inclinator.com
                                        www.inclinator.com
Stephen Nock, President
Inclinette provides comfort and convenience in providing multi-floor access to persons who have difficulty climbing stairs.

397   Independent Driving Systems
580 T.C. Jester
Houston, TX   77007   713-864-1460
                                                       888-422-5337
                                                  Fax: 713-864-1469
                                   www.independentdrivingsystems.com

Chad Donnelly, Owner
Provides adaptive driving systems for individuals with disabilities with more severe higher levels of injury that require more sophisticated types of assistive technology to enable them to drive safely.

398   Joey Interior Platform Lift
Bruno Independent Living Aids
PO Box 84
1780 Executive Drive
Oconomowoc, WI   53066   262-567-4990
                                                       800-882-8183
                                                  Fax: 262-953-5501
                                                       www.bruno.com

Michael R. Bruno, II, President/CEO
Andrew Bayer, Product Mgr, Automotive Div.
Mike Krawczyk, Mktg Svcs Mgr
Lifts and stores your unoccupied scooter or powerchair in the back of your minivan at the touch of a button.

399   Lectra-Lift
La-Z-Boy
1284 N Telegraph Rd
Monroe, MI   48162-5138   734-242-1444
                                                       800-375-6890
                                                  Fax: 734-457-2005
                                                      www.lazboy.com

Kurt L Darrow, CEO
David M Risley, SVP/CFO
Patrick H Norton, Chairman
Kurt Darrow, CEO
This power recliner has a single motor drive that operates three distinct cycles: lifting, leg elevation and full power recline.

400   Liberty LT
Handi-Lift
730 Garden St
Carlstadt, NJ   07072-1625   201-933-0111
                                                       800-432-5438
                                                  Fax: 201-933-0050
                                                 sales@handi-lift.com
                                                   www.handi-lift.com

Douglas Boydston, President
Stair lift with dual armrests that lock into position. The comfortable, contoured seat is designed to swivel and move forward at the bottom or top landings to facilitate transfer.

401   Lift-All
Amigo Mobility International
6693 Dixie Highway
Bridgeport, MI   48722-9725   989-777-0910
                                                       800-692-6446
                                                       800-248-9131
                                                  Fax: 800-334-7274
                                                  info@myamigo.com
                                                    www.myamigo.com

Al Thieme, Chairman and Founder
Beth Thieme, CEO
Tim Drumhiller, President
Sandy Humpert, Sales Rep
Leading manufacturer of electric mobility; Amigo's Lift-All transports your wheelchair easily into the trunk of an automobile and neatly stores it for easy access. Also available is the Lift-It. $965.00

402   Lifts for Swimming Pools and Spas
Aquatic Access
1921 Production Dr
Louisville, KY   40299-2110   502-425-5817
                                                       800-325-5438
                                                  Fax: 502-425-9607
                                                info@AquaticAccess.com
                                                 www.aquaticaccess.com

Linda Nolan, President
David Nolan, Vice President
Aquatic Access manufacturers and sells water-powered lifts providing access to in-ground and above-ground swimming pools, spas, boats and docks. *$2310.00*

403   Mac's Lift Gate
2801 South Street
Long Beach, CA   90805-3751   562-634-5962
                                                       800-795-6227
                                                  Fax: 562-529-3466
                                                sales@macsliftgate.com
                                                 www.macsliftgate.com

Randy Maner, Training Mgr
Sales and service of van and truck lifts. Sales and service of wheel chair lifts for vans and automobiles. Sales, installation and service of vertical home lifts, scooter lifts and pool lifts. Sales of scooters.

404   Mecalift Sling Lifter
Arjo Inc
2349 West Lake Street
Addison, IL   60101   630-785-4490
                                                       800-323-1245
                                                  Fax: 888-389-2756
                                               usa.info@ArjoHuntleigh.com
                                                        www.arjo.com

Philip M. Croxford, President/ CEO

405   Motorhome Lift
Handicaps, Inc.
4335 S Santa Fe Dr.
Englewood, CO   80110   303-781-2062
                                                       800-782-4335
                                                info@handicapsinc.com
                                                 www.handicapsinc.com

406   One for All Lift All
6693 Dixie Highway
Bridgeport, MI   48722-9725   989-777-0910
                                                       800-692-6446
                                                       800-248-9131
                                                  Fax: 800-334-7274
                                                  info@myamigo.com
                                                    www.myamigo.com

Al Thieme, Chairman and Founder
Beth Thieme, CEO
Tim Drumhiller, President
Amigo Mobility designs and manufactures a complete line of power operated vehicles/mobility scooters and accessories in Bridgeport, Mich.

407   Out-Sider III
P.O.Box 84
1780 Executive Drive
Oconomowoc, WI   53066   262-567-4990
                                                       800-882-8183
                                                  Fax: 262-953-5510
                                                       www.bruno.com

Michael R. Bruno, II, President/CEO
Andrew Bayer, Product Mgr, Automotive Div.
Mike Krawczyk, Mktg Svcs Mgr

408 Out-Sider Meridian
Bruno Independent Living Aids
P.O. Box 84
1780 Executive Drive
Oconomowoc, WI 53066   262-567-4990
                                         800-882-8183
                                    Fax: 262-953-5501
                                         www.bruno.com

Michael R. Bruno, II, President/CEO
Andrew Bayer, Product Mgr, Automotive Div.
Mike Krawczyk, Mktg Svcs Mgr
Lets you carry your scooter fully assembled and keeps your trunk
space available for other things.

409 Parker Bath
Arjo Inc
2349 West Lake Street
Addison, IL 60101   630-785-4490
                                         800-323-1245
                                    Fax: 888-389-2756
                              usa.info@ArjoHuntleigh.com
                                         www.arjo.com

Philip M. Croxford, President/ CEO
Ross Scavuzzo, President
This involves no manual lifting, strain or stress for the caregiver.

410 Patient Lifting & Injury Prevention
Arjo Inc
2349 West Lake Street
Addison, IL 60101   630-785-4490
                                         800-323-1245
                                    Fax: 888-389-2756
                              usa.info@ArjoHuntleigh.com
                                         www.arjo.com

Philip M. Croxford, President/ CEO
Aids in patient lifting while protecting the caregiver from the risk
of backstrain.

411 Ramplette Telescoping Ramp
Graham-Field Health Products
2935 Northeast Pkwy
Atlanta, GA 30360-2808   678-291-3207
                                         800-347-5678
                                    Fax: 770-368-4702
                                    cs@grahamfield.com
                                    www.grahamfield.com

Kenneth Spett, President & Chief Executive Officer
Cherie Antoniazzi, SVP Quality, Regulatory and Risk Management
Ivan Bielik, Senior Vice President, Business Analyst
Marc Bernstein, Senior Vice President, Consumer Sales
A multi-functional, easily moved, economical ramp weighing 25
pounds.

412 Rickshaw Exerciser
Access to Recreation
8 Sandra Ct
Newbury Park, CA 91320-4302   805-498-7535
                                         800-634-4351
                                    Fax: 805-498-8186
                              customerservice@accesstr.com
                                         www.accesstr.com

Don Krebs, President/ Founder
This Exerciser develops the muscle used most by those in wheelchairs. It develops the strength you need to lift yourself for pressure relief, doing transfers and pushing your wheelchair.

413 Ricon Corporation
1135 Aviation Pl.
San Fernando, CA 91340   818-267-3000
                                         800-322-2884
                                    Fax: 818-962-1201
                              ripinsales@wabtec.com
                                    www.riconcorp.com

414 Smart Leg
Invacare Corporation
1 Invacare Way
Elyria, OH 44035-4190   440-329-6000
                                         800-333-6900
                                    Fax: 877-619-7996
                                    info@invacare.com
                                         www.invacare.com

A Malachi Mixon Iii, Chairman of the Board
Gerald B. Blouch, President and Chief Executive Officer
Joseph B. Richey, II, President - Invacare Technologies Division
*Robert K. Gudbranson, Senior Vice President and Chief Financial
Officer*
An ingenious elevating leg rest that automatically extends to cor-
rectly fit every outstretched leg.

415 Smooth Mover
Dixie EMS
10101 Foster Ave
Brooklyn, NY 11236-3425   718-257-6400
                                         800-347-3494
                                    Fax: 718-257-6401
                              customerservice@dixieems.com
                                    www.dixieems.com

Eva Silverstein, President
Patient mover is a board designed to transfer patients from bed to
stretcher or table with one or two people. *$199.95*

416 SpectraLift
Inclinator Company of America
601 Gibson Blvd
Harrisburg, PA 17104-3215   717-939-8420
                                         800-343-9007
                                    Fax: 717-939-8075
                              isales@inclinator.com
                                    www.inclinator.com

Stephen Nock, President
A newly designed hydraulic wheelchair lift made of fiberglass
construction suitable for commercial and residential use.

417 Spectrum Aquatics
7100 Spectrum Ln
Missoula, MT 59808-8416   406-543-6823
                                         800-791-8056
                                    Fax: 800-791-8057
                              nkhaled@spectrumproducts.com
                                    www.spectrumproducts.com

Nabil Khaled, Director of Sales
Rob Nelson, Manager of Logistics and Customer Service
Philip Frandsen, Customer Service Representative
Josh Hartley, Business Development Specialist (Southeast Region)

418 Spectrum Products Catalog
Spectrum Products
982 County Route 1
Pine Island, NY 10969-1205   406-542-9781
                                         800-724-5305
                                    Fax: 800-791-8057
                              info@spectrumproducts.com
                                    www.spectrumproducts.com

Nabil Khaled, Dir. of Sales
Chris Rhyne, Business Dev. Specialist
Rob Nelson, Mgr of Logistics
Manufacturers of swimming pool disabled access products such
as lifts, ramps, railings, ladders, and stainless steel hydrotherapy
tanks for the swimming pool and medical therapy markets.

419 StairLIFT SC & SL
Inclinator Company of America
601 Gibson Blvd
Harrisburg, PA 17104-3215   717-939-8420
                                         800-343-9007
                                    Fax: 717-939-8075
                              isales@inclinator.com
                                    www.inclinator.com

Stephen Nock, President
Simple, self-contained and efficient stair units.

420 Stairway Elevators
Bruno Independent Living Aids
P.O. Box 84
1780 Executive Drive
Oconomowoc, WI 53066
262-567-4990
800-882-8183
Fax: 262-953-5510
www.bruno.com

Michael R. Bruno, II, President/CEO
Andrew Bayer, Product Mgr, Automotive Div.
Mike Krawczyk, Mktg Svcs Mgr
Bruno offers a full line of stairway elevators, including the Electra-Ride II featuring access during power interruptions, convenient installation, comfort and a powerful drive system. The Electra-Ride which features battery-powered technology, a rail width of 25 inches and seat rotation for easy transfers. The Comfort-Ride AC stair lift which is battery operated, has a rail width of 7.25 inches and folded width of less than 14.5 inches.

421 Straight and Custom Curved Stairlifts
Bruno Independent Living Aids
P.O.Box 84
1780 Executive Drive
Oconomowoc, WI 53066
262-567-4990
800-882-8183
Fax: 262-953-5501
www.bruno.com

Michael R. Bruno, II, President/CEO
Andrew Bayer, Product Mgr, Automotive Div.
Mike Krawczyk, Mktg Svcs Mgr
Bruno stairlifts can fit almost any curve or straight rail application and requires little or no structural modification to the stairway. Normal rail position for a Bruno inside turn is 7 to 8 inches from the wall or obstruction which is the tightest radius of any stairlift manufacturing company in the world. The Bruno inside turn is ideal for bi-level homes or staircases with mid-level doors. Bruno's unique battery power allows for uninterrupted operation even during a power outage.

422 Superarm Lift for Vans
Handicaps, Inc.
4335 S Santa Fe Dr.
Englewood, CO 80110
303-781-2062
800-782-4335
info@handicapsinc.com
www.handicapsinc.com

423 SureHands Lift & Care Systems
982 County Route 1
Pine Island, NY 10969-1205
845-258-6500
800-724-5305
Fax: 845-258-6634
info@surehands.com
www.surehands.com

Thomas Herceg, President
Joyce Moraczewski, Marketing Coordinator
Doug Siegel, General Sales Manager
SureHands specializes in lift & care systems for both homecare and professional settings where safety is most important, to assist an individual in overcoming physical and architectural barriers. Some of their products include lifting and body support systems, handi-slides, accessories and bathing equipment.

424 Thyssen Krupp Access
4001 E 138th St
Grandview, MO 64030-2837
816-200-1954
800-829-9760
Fax: 816-763-4467
dealerinfo@tkaccess.com
www.tkaccess.com

Jurrien van Akker, CEO
Scott Zoetewey, Vice President of Operations
Thomas Hance, President
Whether you want to open your facility or stay in the home you love, Thyssen Krupp Access has the perfect wheelchair lift, stair lift or elevator to suit your budget and needs. Our lifts have the best warranties. Our nationwide network of dealers are close by and ready to help.

425 Turning Automotive Seating (TAS)
Bruno Independent Living Aids
P.O.Box 84
Oconomowoc, WI 53066-84
262-567-4990
800-882-8183
Fax: 262-95- 550
info@bruno.com
www.bruno.com

Michael R. Bruno, II, President/CEO
Cindy Schmidt, Customer Relations
Steve Nelson, Service Manager
Thomas Jacobson, Senior Vice President
Transfer in and out of a car, minivan, pickup truck and full size van without any lifting!

426 Vangater, Vangater II, Mini-Vangater
BraunAbility
631 W 11th St.
Winamac, IN 46996
800-488-0359
www.braunability.com

Ralph Braun, Founder
Tri-fold and fold-in-half lifts represent a major innovation in the field of adapted van transportation.

427 Versatrainer
Pro- Max/ Division Of Bow- Flex Of America
2200 NE 65th Ave
Vancouver, WA 98661-6978
800-618-8853
800-952-7205
Fax: 360-993-3610
customerservice@bowflex.com
www.bowflex.com

428 Vestibular Board
Bailey Manufacturing Company
P.O. Box 130
Lodi, OH 44254-130
800-321-8372
Fax: 800-224-5390
baileymfg@baileymfg.com
www.baileymfg.com

429 Wheelchair Carrier
7325 Douglas Road
Lambertville, MI 48144-2624
734-568-6084
800-541-3213
Fax: 734-568-6705
admin@WheelChairCarrier.com
wheelchaircarrier.com

David Makulinsky, President
Mike Siler, Engineer
Christina Makulinski, Office Manager
Wheelchair, scooter and powerchair carriers for hitch mount on vehicles, priced from $199 to $999.

Major Catalogs

430 Access Store Products for Barrier Free Environments
Access Store.Com
820 W 7th St
Chico, CA 95928-5011
530-893-1596
800-497-2003
Fax: 530-893-1560
www.accessstore.com

Tim Vander Heiden, Owner
Lisa Bantum, Sales Administrator
One of the largest online ADA Compliance Catalogs available. Offers everything from innovative barrier removal products to survey equipment, to unique specialty products.

431   Access to Recreation
8 Sandra Ct
Newbury Park, CA 91320-4302   805-498-7535
800-634-4351
Fax: 805-498-8186
customerservice@accesstr.com
www.accesstr.com
Don Krebs, President
The Access to Recreation catalog is full of recreation and exercise equipment. One can find items such as electric fishing reels and other fishing and hunting equipment for the disabled sportsman. There are also adapted golf clubs, swimming pool lifts, wheelchair gloves and cuffs and bowling equipment. There are devices to help with embroidery, knitting and card playing, videos, books and practical aides such as wheelchair ramps and book.
64 pages Bi-Annually

432   Achievement Products
P.O. Box 6013
Carol Stream, IL 60197-6013   800-373-4699
Fax: 800-766-4303
Bids@achievement-products.com
www.specialkidszone.com
Teresa Cardon, VP
Offer a wide range of pediatric rehabilitation equipment and special education products including handwriting aids, weighted vests, positioning equipment, sensory integration products and adaptive furniture. Call for your free catalog.

433   Adaptive Clothing: Adults
Special Clothes
P.O.Box 333
E Harwich, MA 02645-333   508-430-2410
Fax: 508-430-2410
TTY:508-430-2410
SPECIALCLO@aol.com
www.special-clothes.com
Judith Sweeney, President
Special Clothes produces a catalogue of garments for adults with disabilities and/or incontinence. Offerings include: undergarments, snap-crotch tee shirts, sleepwear, jumpsuits, bibs and some footwear. The catalogue is available without charge. Comparable to department store prices. Special Clothes produces a catalog of adaptive clothing for children in sizes from toddler through young adults. A full line of clothing is included from undergarments through wheelchair jackets and ponchos.

434   Adaptive Technology Catalog
Synapse Adaptive
14 Lynn Ct
San Rafael, CA 94901-5114   415-455-9700
800-317-9611
Fax: 415-455-9801
info@synapse-ada.com
www.synapseadaptive.com
Martin Tibor, President
Adaptive technology for individuals with disabilities, ADA compliant workstations, and ergonomic furniture. Products accommodate blindness, low vision, mobility impairments or learning differences.

435   Adult Long Jumpsuit with Feet
Special Clothes
P.O.Box 333
E Harwich, MA 02645-333   508-896-7939
Fax: 508-896-7939
specialclo@aol.com
www.special-clothes.com
Judith Sweeney, President
Line of clothing for people with disabilities. Child and adult catalog available.

436   Adult Short Jumpsuit
Special Clothes
P.O.Box 333
E Harwich, MA 02645-333   508-896-7939
Fax: 508-896-7939
specialclo@aol.com
www.special-clothes.com
Judith Sweeney, President
This pull-on jumpsuit provides comfort and full coverage without bulk. Wide leg ribbing ends at mid-thigh, with snaps at the crotch. We use fine quality, comfortable cotton knit. 100% cotton knit. Made in USA. Option: long sleeves - add $3.00. Colors: white, navy, teal, light blue, light pink, red, burgundy, royal blue and black. Sm & Med: $36.50/3 for $104.00; L & XL: $39.00/3 for $111.25; and XXL: $42.00/3 for $119.25.

437   AliMed
297 High St
Dedham, MA 02026   781-329-2900
800-225-2610
Fax: 781-329-8392
customerservice@alimed.com
alimed.com

438   American Discount Medical
459 Main St
Ste 101-417
Trussville, AL 35173   205-467-6995
800-877-9100
Fax: 888-809-3029
Sales@AmericanDiscountMed.com
www.americandiscountmed.com
Tom Ruf, General Manager
Offers deep discounts for all major brands of medical products.

439   Apria Healthcare
26220 Enterprise Ct
Lake Forest, CA 92630-8405   949-639-2000
800-277-4288
contact_us@apria.com
www.apria.com
Dan Starck, Chief Executive Officer
Nichola Denney, Executive Vice President, Revenue Management
Lisa M. Getson, EVP, Government Relations, Investor Relations and Compliance
Bill Guidetti, Executive Vice President, East Zone
Lifts, chairs, bathroom aids, bedroom aids, eating utensils and independent living aids for the physically challenged.

440   Armstrong Medical
575 Knightsbridge Parkway
P.O. Box 700
Lincolnshire, IL 60069-700   847-913-0101
800-323-4220
Fax: 847-913-0138
csr@armstrongmedical.com
www.armstrongmedical.com
Armstrong, CEO
Diane Joseph, customer representative
Training aids, anatomical models, medical equipment, pediatrics equipment and rehabilitation equipment.

441   Assistive Technology Journal
1700 N Moore St
Suite 1905
Rosslyn, VA 22209-1905   703-243-1975
Fax: 703-524-6630
info@technologistsinc.com
www.technologistsinc.com
Bi-Annually

442   Assistive Technology Sourcebook
Special Needs Project
Ste H
324 State St
Santa Barbara, CA 93101-2364   805-962-8087
                                           818-718-9900
                                        Fax: 818-349-2027
                                    editor@specialneeds.com
                                    www.specialneeds.com

Hod Gray, Owner
Marian Hall, Editor
Provides you with 18 chapters of practical information on all aspects of assistive technology for individuals with functional limitations. *$60.00*
576 pages

443   Bailey
Bailey Manufacturing
P.O.Box 130
Lodi, OH 44254-130   800-321-8372
                                        Fax: 800-224-5390
                                    baileymfg@baileymfg.com
                                    www.baileymfg.com

70 pages

444   Best 25 Catalog Resources for Making Life Easier
Meeting Life's Challenges
9042 Aspen Grove Ln
Madison, WI 53717-2700   608-824-0402
                                        Fax: 608-824-0403
                                help@meetinglifeschallenges.com
                                www.meetinglifeschallenges.com
Shelley Peterman Schwarz, President
Deborah , Dir. of Mktg & Dev.
Unique reference guide to locate thousands of useful and hard-to-find adaptive devices to make dressing, eating, cooking, grooming, communicating, playing, exercising, etc. easier, safer and less frustrating for people of all ages and disabilities. A comprehensive, up-do-date reference for people with disabilities, caregivers and healthcare professionals. *$8.95*

36 pages
ISBN 1-891854-03-8

445   Body Suits
Special Clothes
P.O.Box 333
E Harwich, MA 02645-333   508-430-2410
                                        Fax: 508-430-2410
                                    specialclo@aol.com
                                    www.special-clothes.com

Judith Bari, President
Bodysuits, Jumpsuits, back opening garments, incontinence wear, bibs. Features include snap crotches and g-tube pockets.

446   Cambridge Career Products Catalog
Cambridge Educational
132 West 31st Street
17th Floor
New York, NY 10001   800-322-8755
                                           800-468-4227
                                        Fax: 609-679-0266
                                    custserv@films.com
                                    cambridge.films.com

Lisa Schmuclei, Marketing Director
A full color catalog featuring hundreds of products designed to aid people in career exploration, selecting specific occupations and obtaining these jobs through resume and interview preparation.
64 pages BiAnnual

447   Carex Health Brands
P.O. Box 2526
Sioux Falls, SD 57101-2526   800-328-2935
                                        Fax: 888-616-4297
                                customerservice@carex.com
                                carex.com

448   Carolyn's Low Vision Products
3938 S Tamiami Trl
Sarasota, FL 34231-3622   941-373-9100
                                           800-648-2266
                                        Fax: 941-739-5503
                                    info@carolynscatalog.com
                                    www.carolynscatalog.com

John Colton, Owner
Free mail-order catalog of items for visually impaired people. We also have a retail store.

449   Communication Aids for Children and Adults
Crestwood Communication Aids
6589 N
Crestwood Drive
Milwaukee, WI 53209   414-351-0311
                                        Fax: 414-351-0311
                                    crestcomm@aol.com
                                    www.communicationaids.com

Ruth B Leff, President
A free catalog of communication aids for children and adults with disabilities. Over 300 light and high tech switches and aids, and a large selection of adapted and voice-activated toys. Talking Pictures and Passports communication boards, easy to use and moderately priced talking aids.
32 pages Yearly

450   Danmar Products
221 Jackson Industrial Dr
Ann Arbor, MI 48103   734-761-1990
                                           800-783-1998
                                        Fax: 734-761-8977
                                    sales@danmarproducts.com
                                    www.danmarproducts.com

Dan Russo, President
Hidie Bowman, Chief Operating Officer
Manufactures adaptive equipment for persons with physical and mental disabilities. Products include seating and positioning equipment, flotation devices, toileting aids, and hard and soft shell helmets.

451   Dayspring Associates
2111 Foley Rd
Havre De Grace, MD 21078-1703   410-939-5900
                                        Fax: 410-939-6252
Benedict Schwartz, Manager
This publisher provides a directory of 1,000 rehabilitation aids.

452   Disabilities Sourcebook
Omnigraphics
155 West Congress
Suite 200
Detroit, MI 48226   313-961-1340
                                           800-234-1340
                                        Fax: 313-961-1383
                                    contact@omnigraphics.com
                                    www.omnigraphics.com

Paul Rogers, Publicity Associate
Georgiann Fratoni, Customer Service Manager
Peter Ruffner
$78.00
616 pages
ISBN 0-780803-89-2

453   Disability Bookshop Catalog
P.O.Box 129
Vancouver, WA 98666-129   360-694-2462
                                           800-637-2256
                                        Fax: 360-696-3210
                                    twinpeak@pacifier.com
                                    www.disabilitybookshop.virtualave.net/

40 pages

454 Dressing Tips and Clothing Resources for Making Life Easier
Attainment Company
504 Commerce Parkway
P.O.Box 930160
Verona, WI 53593-160   608-845-7880
                                                        800-327-4269
                                                   Fax: 608-845-8040
                                            info@attainmentcompany.com
                                            www.attainmentcompany.com
Don Bastian, Founder and CEO
Scott Meister, Director of Software Development
Sue Lockard, Director of Operations/Dealer Sales
Karen Riley, Shipping/Receiving Manager
Learn hundreds of simple tips and techniques to make dressing easier. Learn how to adapt/modify ready-to-wear garments to accommodate your special dressing needs. Find out how to locate more than 100 resources offering specially designed or easy-on/easy-off clothing for men, women, children and/or wheelchair users. You'll find everything you need to look your best. An invaluable resource for people with special dressing needs, people with disabilities, caregivers and healthcare professionals. *$19.00*
144 pages 2000
ISBN 1-578611-19-9

455 Enrichments Catalog
Sammons Preston Rolyan
28100 Torch Parkway
Suite 700
Warrenville, IL 60555-3938   630-378-6000
                                                        800-323-5547
                                                   Fax: 630-393-7600
                                            sp@pattersonmedical.com
                                            www.pattersonmedical.com
David P Sproat, President
Bruce Curtis, Sales Representative
Provides people with physical challenges with the products they need to help live their lives to the fullest. Includes items for everyday tasks and personal care; assistive products for home use; toileting and bathing aids; grooming and dressing devices; kitchen and dining aids. Also items for range of motion, mobility and exercise such as weights, therapy putty and exercise equipment; ergonomic gloves and supports; canes, crutches, walkers and wheelchair accessories. 36-page catalog.

456 Equipment Shop
34 Hartford Street
Bedford, MA 01730-33   781-275-7681
                                                        800-525-7681
                                                   Fax: 781-275-4094
                                            info@equipmentshop.com
                                            www.equipmentshop.com
Ken Larson, Owner
Barbara Johnston, General Manager
Specializing in oral motor therapy equipment including flexi cut cups, maroon spoons, chewy tubes, ARK grabbers and z-vibes. Also tricycle foot peal attachments and trike back supports as well as fat wheels.

457 Essential Medical Supply, Inc.
6420 Hazeltine National Dr
Orlando, FL 32822   407-770-0710
                                                        800-826-8423
                                                   Fax: 407-770-0624
                                            essentialmedicalsupply.com

458 Everest & Jennings
Division of Graham-Field
2935 Northeast Parkway
Atlanta, GA 30360   678-291-3207
                                                        800-347-5678
                                                   Fax: 770-368-2386
                                            cs@grahamfield.com
                                            www.grahamfield.com
Kenneth Spett, President & Chief Executive Officer
Cherie Antoniazzi, SVP Quality, Regulatory and Risk Management
Ivan Bielik, Senior Vice President, Business Analyst
Marc Bernstein, Senior Vice President, Consumer Sales
Manufactures more than 200 items for persons with physical disabilities, including wheelchairs, seat cushions, shower chairs, grab bars and more.

459 Express Medical Supply
218 Seebold Spur
Fenton, MO 63026   636-349-8448
                                                        800-633-2139
                                                   Fax: 800-633-9188
                                            sales@exmed.net
                                            www.exmed.net
Bill Nahm, President
Offers a full line of medical and ostomy supplies at discounted prices. Order by phone or online.

460 FlagHouse Rehab Resources
601 FLAGHOUSE DRIVE
Hasbrouck Heights, NJ 07604-3116   201-288-7600
                                                        800-793-7900
                                                   Fax: 800-793-7922
                                            www.flaghouse.com
George Carmel, President

461 FlagHouse Special Populations
601 FLAGHOUSE DRIVE
Hasbrouck Heights, NJ 07604-3116   201-288-7600
                                                        800-793-7900
                                                   Fax: 800-793-7922
                                            sales@flaghouse.com
                                            www.flaghouse.com
Brigid de Lime, Sr Brand Manager
Diana Hohman, Brand Manager
Contains over 2,000 products of interest to therapy professionals.
Bi-Annually

462 Freedom Rider
Freedom Rider
5225 Tudor Ct
Naples, FL 34112   603-540-0933
                                                        888-253-8811
                                                   Fax: 866-522-4708
                                            info@freedomrider.com
                                            www.freedomrider.com
Victoria Surr, President
A catalog of equipment for people with disabilities who ride and drive horses which includes instructional aids, vaulting equipment, and lots of hard to find items.

463 HAC Hearing Aid Centers of America: HARC Mercantile
Hearing Center
1111 W Centre Ave
Portage, MI 49024   269-324-0301
                                                        800-445-9968
                                                        888-426-6632
                                                   Fax: 269-324-2387
                                            info@harc.com
                                            www.hacofamerica.com

464   Health and Rehabilitation Products
Luminaud
8688 Tyler Blvd
Mentor, OH   44060   440-255-9082
                                                  800-255-3408
                                            Fax: 440-255-2250
                                            info@luminaud.com
                                            www.luminaud.com

Thomas M Lennox, President
Dorothy Lennox, VP
Switches for limited capability, stoma and trach covers, shower
protectors and thermo-stim oral motor stimulator. Personal voice
amplifiers for people with weak voices. Artificial larynges for
people with no voices. Small electronic communication boards.
Books for laryngectomies and speech pathologists.

465   HealthCare Solutions
Blue Chip II
3478 Hauck Rd
Cincinnati, OH   45241   513-271-5115
                                                  800-417-5115
                                            Fax: 513-527-3686
Michael Leabhart, Manager
Quality rehabilitation equipment sales and rental. Available
equipment includes manual and powered mobility, position-
ing/seating equipment, vehicle modification, environmental controls, augmentative and alternative communication devices,
adaptive computer access, ambulance aids and aids for daily living. Equipment provision is carried out through a total team
approach. .

466   Hear You Are
98 Us Highway 46
Budd Lake, NJ   07828-1818   973-347-7662
                                            Fax: 973-691-0611
Dorinne S Davis, President
A large catalog of various assistive and communication devices
for people who are hearing impaired. *$3.00*
42 pages

467   Hig's Manufacturing
8375 Sunset Rd Ne
Minneapolis, MN   55418-3238   763-795-9478
                                            Fax: 612-788-1926
Jim Murphy, Owner
Factory direct, lightweight aluminum, portable, 2 & 4-way folding, telescoping tracks, threshold, van, scooter and approach
ramps.

468   Huntleigh Healthcare
2349, W Lake Street
Suite 250
Addison, IL   60101   630-785-4490
                                                  800-323-1245
                                            Fax: 888-389-2756
                                        us.info@ArjoHuntleigh.com
                                        www.huntleigh-healthcare.com

469   Invacare Corporation
1 Invacare Way
Elyria, OH   44035-4190   800-333-6900
                                            Fax: 877-619-7996
                                            info@invacare.com
                                            invacare.com
Matthew E. Monaghan, Chair, President & CEO
*Dean Childers, Senior Vice President & General Manager, North
America*
The global leader in the manufacture and distribution of innova-
tive home and long-term care medical products that promote re-
covery and active lifestyles.

470   Kleinert's
433 Newton St
Elba, AL   36323   800-498-7051
                                            Fax: 305-937-0825
                                        customercare@kleinerts.com
                                            www.kleinerts.com
Michael Brier, President
Offers a complete line of sweat and odor protection products, incontinence products, and skin care products consisting of disposable and reusable panties for women and pants for men. Also
disposable liners, diapers and underpads.

471   LS&S
145 River Rock Drive
Buffalo, NY   14207   716-348-3500
                                                  800-468-4789
                                            Fax: 877-498-1482
                                            TTY: 800-317-8533
                                            www.LSSproducts.com
Melissa Balbach, President
John K Bace, Executive Vice President.
Specializes in products for the blind, visually impaired, hearing
impaired, and deaf. Free catalog upon request.

472   Lighthouse Low Vision Products
Lighthouse International
111 E 59th St
New York, NY   10022-1202   212-821-9200
                                                  800-829-0500
                                            Fax: 212-821-9707
                                            info@lighthouse.org
                                            www.lighthouse.org
Mark Ackermann, Chief Executive Officer
Joseph A Ripp, Chairman
Sarah Smith, Treasurer
This organization provides health care services related to vision
loss; Career and academic services for people with vision loss;
Music instruction and pre K curriculum for visually impaired
students.

473   Luminaud
8688 Tyler Blvd
Mentor, OH   44060-4348   440-255-9082
                                                  800-255-3408
                                            Fax: 440-255-2250
                                            info@luminaud.com
                                            www.luminaud.com
Thomas M Lennox, President
Dorothy Lennox, VP
Offers a line of artificial larynx, personal voice amplifiers, spe-
cial switches, stoma covers and other communication, health and
safety items.

474   MOMS Catalog
9385 Dielman Ind Dr
Saint Louis, MO   63132-2214   800-269-4663
                                            Fax: 314-997-0047
                                            custcare@hdis.com
                                            www.hdis.com
Bruce Grench, President
MOMS catalog features high quality, incontinence supplies, mobility products, bath safety products urological products, aids for
daily living products, ostomy supplies and many other adaptive
items. MOMS offers low prices, excellent customer service and
convenient home delivery to your doorstep.
52 pages

475   Maddak Inc.
661 Route 23 S
Wayne, NJ   07470   973-628-7600
                                                  800-443-4926
                                            Fax: 973-305-0841
                                        custservice@maddak.com
                                            maddak.com

476 Maxi Aids
42 Executive Blvd
Farmingdale, NY   11735-4710   631-752-0521
                                                800-522-6294
                                           Fax: 631-752-0689
                                           TTY: 800-281-3555
                                           sales@maxiaids.com
                                           www.maxiaids.com
Elliot Zaretsky, Founder/ President
Products specially designed for the blind, low vision, visually impaired, deaf, deaf-blind, hard of hearing, arthritic, diabetic and individuals with special needs.

477 New Vision Store
919 Walnut Street
Philadelphia, PA   19107   215-627-0600
                                           Fax: 215-922-0692
                                           asbinfo@asb.org
                                           www.asb.org
Patricia C. Johnson, President & Chief Executive Officer
Derby Ewing, Director, Human Services
Brian Rusk, Public Relations Officer
Richard Forsythe, Director, Braille Division and Custom Audio
Catalog for individuals with visual impairments, listing visual aids, magnifiers, large print books and more.
30 pages

478 Patterson Medical
28100 Torch Parkway
Ste 700
Warrenville, IL   60555-3938   630-393-6000
                                                800-323-5547
                                           Fax: 630-393-7600
                                           sp@pattersonmedical.com
                                           pattersonmedical.com

479 Pearson Performance Solutions
1 North Dearborn
Suite 1150
Chicago, IL   60602   800-922-7343
                                           Fax: 312-242-4403
                                           HCM.info@vangent.com
David Fabianski, Senior VP and General Mgr
Cindy Hotsky, finance Dir.
Julia McClung, VP, Talent Management Solutions
Publishes human resource assessment instruments for employment settings. The instruments include job analysis procedures to identify important characteristics for job success and objective assessment procedures to evaluate applicants and employees on these characteristics.

480 Pearson Reid London House
1 North Dearborn Street
Chicago, IL   60602-4335   *Fax:* 312-242-4403
                                           HCM.info@vangent.com
David Fabianski, Senior VP and General Mgr
Cindy Hotsky, finance Dir.
Julia McClung, VP, Talent Management Solutions

481 Potomac Technology
1500 Olympic Boulevard
Santa Monica, CA   90404   310-656-4924
                                                800-233-9130
                                           Fax: 310-450-9918
                                           TTY: 800-233-9130
                                           www.weitbrecht.com/
24 pages

482 Prentke Romich Company Product Catalog
1022 Heyl Rd
Wooster, OH   44691-9786   330-262-1984
                                                800-262-1984
                                           Fax: 330-263-4829
                                           info@prentrom.com
                                           www.prentrom.com
David L Moffatt, President
Dave Moffatt, President/ COO
Barry Romich, Co-Founder
A full line, product catalog containing information on speech-output communication devices, environmental controls and computer access products.

483 Products for People with Disabilities
LS&S
145 River Rock Drive
Buffalo, NY   14207   716-348-3500
                                                800-468-4789
                                           Fax: 877-498-1482
                                           TTY: 866-317-8533
                                           www.LSSproducts.com
John K Bace, Executive Vice President
LS&S, LLC has a free catalog of products for the blind, deaf, visually and hearing impaired including: TTYs, computer adaptive devices, CCTVs, talking blood pressure, blood glucose and talking scales.

484 Rehabilitation Engineering and Assistive Technology Society of North America (RESNA)
1700 North Moore Street
Suite 1540
Arlington, VA   22209- 1903   703-524-6686
                                           Fax: 703-524-6630
                                           TTY:703-524-6639
                                           membership@resna.org
                                           www.resna.org
Alex Mihailidis, PhD, P.Eng, President
Ray Grott, ATP, RET, President-Elect
Paul J. Schwartz, Treasurer
Jamie Arasz Prioli, ATP, Secretary
RESNA improves the potential of people with disabilities to achieve their goals through the use of technology. RESNA promotes research, development, education, advocacy and provision of technology; and by supporting the people engaged in these activities.

485 Sammons Preston Enrichments Catalog
Sammons Preston Rolyan
28100 Torch Parkway
Suite 700
Warrenville, IL   60555-3938   630-378-6000
                                                800-323-5547
                                           Fax: 630-393-7600
                                           sp@pattersonmedical.com
                                           www.pattersonmedical.com
David P Sproat, President
Bruce Curtis, Sales Representative
Our Enrichments Catalog offers products that make the tasks and challenges of living at home— bathing, getting dressed, getting around— a little easier. Choose from personal care items to kitchen and dining aids, household helpers to mobility devices, plus a complete selection of pain-reducing products, exercise items, health monitoring equipment and more.
40 pages Yearly

486 Sportaid
78 Bay Creek Rd
Loganville, GA   30052   770-554-5033
                                                800-743-7203
                                           Fax: 770-554-5944
                                           stuff@sportaid.com
                                           www.sportaid.com
Stacy Green, Owner
jimmy green, Owner

Offers an assortment of wheelchairs (everyday and racing), wheelchair sports equipment, replacement tires, hubs, spokes, pushrims, cushions and more. Call for free catalog.
68 pages Yearly

487 Store @ HDSC Product Catalog
Hearing, Speech & Deafness Center (HDSC)
1625 19th Ave.
Seattle, WA 98122-2848

206-323-5770
888-222-5036
Fax: 206-328-6871
seattlc@hsdc.org
www.hsdc.org

Lindsay Klarman, Executive Director
Michelle Coleman, Operations Director
Hearing, Speech & Deaf Center (HSDC) is a nonprofit for clients who are deaf, hard of hearing, or who face other communication barriers such as speech challenges. Their mission is to foster inclusive and accessible communities through communication, advocacy, and education.
32 pages Yearly

488 WCI/Weitbrecht Communications
1500 Olympic Boulevard
Santa Monica, CA 90405

310-656-4924
800-233-9130
Fax: 310-450-9918
TTY: 800-233-9130
www.weitbrecht.com

24 pages

489 Walgreens Home Medical Center
7173 Cermak Rd
Berwyn, IL 60402-2103

708-795-1295
800-323-2828
Fax: 708-795-1308

Stan Kozlowski, Manager
Hospital supplies and home medical equipment with nationwide direct mail delivery. .

490 Walton Way Medical
1225 Walton Way
Augusta, GA 30901-2141

706-722-0276
Fax: 706-722-0279

Michael Bower, President
Offers medical, therapeutic, urological, hygiene and skin care products for disabled persons.

Miscellaneous

491 Access-USA
242 James St
PO Box 160
Clayton, NY 13624-160

800-263-2750
Fax: 800-563-1687
info@access-usa.com
www.access-usa.com

Deborah Haight, PICOE
Access-USA provides one-stop alternate format transcription services for almost any type of document-reports, schedules, menus, monthly statements, brochures, reports, etc. Items may be submitted on computer disk, hard copy or email. Alternate formats include Braille, large print, Braille and print, audio recordings, adapted disks as well as video services-open/closed captioning and video descriptions. Accessible products also include Braille Business Cards and ADA signage.

492 Access-USA: Transcription Services
242 James St
PO Box 160
Clayton, NY 13624-160

800-263-2750
Fax: 800-563-1687
info@access-usa.com
www.access-usa.com

Deborah Haight, PICOE

Access-USA produces Braille business cards as well as offering alternate format services and products to enhance accessibility. Braille, large print, captioning, audio-descriptive forms are available. We help business, government, education, corporations by providing brochures, menus, manuals, books, collateral materials, videos, specialties and promotion items that can be more accessible to more people.

493 BeOK Key Lever
Sammons Preston Rolyan
28100 Torch Parkway
Suite 700
Warrenville, IL 60555-3938

630-378-6000
800-323-5547
Fax: 630-393-7600
www.pattersonmedical.com

David P Sproat, President
Bruce Curtis, Sales Representative
Handy accessory helps position key to provide maximum leverage enabling the user to work the most stubborn lock. *$11.50*

494 Big Lamp Switch
Maxi-Aids, Inc.
42 Executive Blvd.
Farmingdale, NY 11735-4710

631-752-0521
800-522-6294
Fax: 631-752-0689
TTY: 631-752-0738
www.maxiaids.com

Elliot Zaretsky, President
This big, three-spoke knob replaces small rotating knobs which are a problem for those with arthritis or other limitations of the fingers. *$6.75*

495 Bookholder: Roberts
Therapro, Inc.
225 Arlington St
Framingham, MA 01702-8723

508-872-9494
800-257-5376
Fax: 508-875-2062
info@therapro.com
www.therapro.com

Karen Conrad , ScD, OTR/L, Owner
Gray plastic, ideal for hand free reading, adjusts to all sizes of books and prevents pages from flipping for the physically challenged. *$27.50*

496 Brandt Industries
4461 Bronx Blvd
Bronx, NY 10470-1496

718-994-0800
800-221-8031
Fax: 718-325-7995
brandtequip@yahoo.com
www.brandtind.com

497 Bus and Taxi Sign
Maxi Aids
42 Executive Blvd
Farmingdale, NY 11735-4710

631-752-0521
800-522-6294
Fax: 631-752-0689
TTY: 800-281-3555
sales@maxiaids.com
www.maxiaids.com

498 Care Electronics
3301 W 151 Court
Broomfield, CO 8002

303-444-2273
888-444-8284
Fax: 303-447-3502
tmoody@careelectronics.com
www.medicalshoponline.com

Tom Moody, President
Care Electronics manufactures safety monitoring systems for caregivers, home-health care, and nursing homes. WanderCARE monitors loved ones who tend to wander away from home. Care Deluxe Occupancy systems monitor patients in bed and in wheel-

chairs to help prevent falls. WetSENSE provides incontinence monitors.

499   Child Convertible Balance Beam Set
Bailey Manufacturing Company
P.O. Box 130
Lodi, OH   44254-130

800-321-8372
Fax: 800-224-5390
baileymfg@baileymfg.com
www.baileymfg.com

500   Child Variable Balance Beam
Bailey Manufacturing Company
P.O. Box 130
Lodi, OH   44254-130

330-948-1080
800-321-8372
Fax: 330-948-4439
baileymfg@baileymfg.com
www.baileymfg.com

501   Child's Mobility Crawler
Bailey Manufacturing Company
P.O. Box 130
Lodi, OH   44254-130

800-321-8372
Fax: 800-224-5390
baileymfg@baileymfg.com
www.baileymfg.com

502   Choice Switch Latch and Timer
AbleNet
2625 Patton Road
Roseville, MN   55113-1308

651-294-2200
800-322-0956
Fax: 651-294-2259
customerservice@ablenetinc.com
www.ablenetinc.com

Bill Sproull, Chairman of the Board
Jennifer Thalhuber, President/CEO
William Mills, Board of Director
A Choice Switch Latch and Timer allows one user to learn to make choices. It has two switch inputs and can control two devices. Once one device has been activated, the other will not function until the first one is turned off or completes its timed cycle. *$83.00*

503   Cordless Big Red Switch
AbleNet
2625 Patton Road
Roseville, MN   55113-1308

651-294-2200
800-322-0956
Fax: 651-294-2259
customerservice@ablenetinc.com
www.ablenetinc.com

Bill Sproull, Chairman of the Board
Jennifer Thalhuber, President/CEO
William Mills, Board of Director
The Cordless Big Red Switch, when used in conjunction with either the Cordless Receiver or the Small Appliance Receiver, gives you cordless control of toys, games, and appliances in your environment. *$89.00*

504   DEUCE Environmental Control Unit
APT Technology
236a N Main St
Shreve, OH   44676

330-567-2001
888-549-2001
Fax: 330-567-3073
www.apt-technology.com

Grace Miller, Office Manager
Allows a severely disabled person to control a variety of useful devices via a dual switch. DEUCE controls phone, 4 AC powered devices such as a radio, 4 switch controlled devices such as a page turner and up to 16 lights and or appliances distributed around the environment. Starts at $1,500. .

505   Dazor Manufacturing Corporation
2079 Congressiona
Saint Louis, MO   63146

314-652-2400
800-345-9103
Fax: 314-652-2069
info@dazor.com
www.dazor.com

Kirk Cressey, Marketing Director
Bob Smith, National Sales Manager
Mark Hogrebe, President
Dazor is a US manufacturer of quality task lighting. Products include fluorescent, incandescent and halogen lighting fixtures. Illuminated magnifiers combine light and magnification to greatly enhance activities such as reading and make hobbies more enjoyable. All lamps come in a variety of mounting options to include desk bases, clamp on, floor stands and wall tracks. $95 - $450.

506   Digi-Flex
Therapro, Inc.
225 Arlington St
Framingham, MA   01702-8723

508-872-9494
800-257-5376
Fax: 508-875-2062
info@therapro.com
www.therapro.com

Karen Conrad , ScD, OTR/L, Owner
This is a unique hand and finger exercise unit. Recommended for use of individuation of fingers, web space and general strengthening of work hands. Available in a variety of resistances. *$ 17.50*

507   Dorma Architectural Hardware
DORMA Drive, Drawer AC
Reamstown, PA   17567-411

717-336-3881
866-401-6063
Fax: 717-336-2106
archdw@dorma-usa.com
www.dorma-usa.com

Larry O'Toole, CEO
Gary Phillips AHC, VP Regional Sales, East
Ken Theaker, VP Regional Sales West
DORMA provides a complete line of door controls, including barrier-free units that comply with the Americans with Disabilities Act. A wide variety of surface applied and concealed closers, low energy operators, exit devices and electronic access control systems are available to address these equipments.

508   Dual Switch Latch and Timer
AbleNet
2625 Patton Road
Roseville, MN   55113-1308

651-294-2200
800-322-0956
Fax: 651-294-2259
customerservice@ablenetinc.com
www.ablenetinc.com

Bill Sproull, Chairman of the Board
Jennifer Thalhuber, President/CEO
William Mills, Board of Director
A Dual Switch Latch and Timer allows two users to activate two devices at a time in the latch. Timed seconds or timed minutes mode of control. *$88.00*

509   Enabling Devices
50 Broadway
Hawthorne, CA   10532

914-747-3070
800-832-8697
Fax: 914-747-3480
customer_support@enablingdevices.com
www.enablingdevices.com

Elizabeth Bell, Marketing Manager
Karen O'Connor, VP Operations
Steven Kanor, Owner
For more than 25 years, Enabling Devices has been dedicated to providing affordable learning and assistive devices for the physically challenged. Products include augmentative communicators, adapted toys, capability switches, training and sensory devices and activity centers. Call for a free catalog.

510   Foot Inversion Tread
Bailey Manufacturing Company
P.O. Box 130
Lodi, OH 44254-130

800-321-8372
Fax: 800-224-5390
baileymfg@baileymfg.com
www.baileymfg.com

511   Foot Placement Ladder
Bailey Manufacturing Company
P.O. Box 130
Lodi, OH 44254-130

800-321-8372
Fax: 800-224-5390
baileymfg@baileymfg.com
www.baileymfg.com

512   HealthCraft SuperPole Traveller
Maxi Aids
42 Executive Blvd
Farmingdale, NY 11735-4710

631-752-0521
800-522-6294
Fax: 631-752-0689
TTY: 800-281-3555
sales@maxiaids.com
www.maxiaids.com

Elliot Zaretsky, President
Central to the system is a stylish floor-to-ceiling grab bar, which provides a secure structure that can be installed in minutes between a floor and ceiling. Use it beside a bed, bath, toilet or chair. *$193.00*

513   Home Bed Side Helper
Maxi Aids
42 Executive Blvd
Farmingdale, NY 11735-4710

631-752-0521
800-522-6294
Fax: 631-752-0689
TTY: 800-281-3555
sales@maxiaids.com
www.maxiaids.com

Elliot Zaretsky, President
The extra support you need getting in and out of bed is within your grasp with this easy to install Home Bed Side Helper. The rail itself features four easily accessible grasping points for the secure support you need when getting in or out of bed. *$126.75*

514   Hospital Environmental Control System
Prentke Romich Company
1022 Heyl Rd
Wooster, OH 44691-9786

330-262-1984
800-848-8008
800-262-1933
Fax: 330-263-4829
sales@prentrom.com
www.prentrom.com

David L Moffatt, President
Permits the non-ambulatory patient to operate a variety of electrical items in a single room. A large liquid crystal display is mounted in front of the user and they scan through the menu of operations and make a selection using a sip-puff switch. Options include nurse call, standard telephone functions, electric bed control, hospital television operation and electrical appliance on and off. *$3860.00*

515   Knock Light
HARC Mercantile
5413 S. Westnedge Ave.
Suite A
Portage, MI 49002

269-324-0301
800-445-9968
Fax: 269-324-2387
TTY: 269-324-1615
info@harc.com
www.harc.com

516   Leg Elevation Board
Bailey Manufacturing Company
P.O. Box 130
Lodi, OH 44254-130

800-321-8372
Fax: 800-224-5390
baileymfg@baileymfg.com
www.baileymfg.com

517   Leveron
Lindustries
21 Shady Hill Rd
Weston, MA 02193-1407

781-237-8177
877-794-9511
Fax: 651-989-2131
www.trademarkia.com/leveron-73486756.html

Willard H Lind, Owner
Louise T Lind, VP
Leveron is a doorknob lever handle for ease of operation. Leveron converts standard doorknobs to lever action without removing existing hardware. No gripping, twisting or pinching when hands are wet, arthritic or arms are full. Leveron provides convenience. Available in five colors: almond, satin brass, silver metallic, dark bronze and Hi-Glow (glows in the dark) at low cost to comply with ADA access requirements in public and private places. *$16.95*

518   Longreach Reacher
Therapro, Inc.
225 Arlington St
Framingham, MA 01702-8723

508-872-9494
800-257-5376
Fax: 508-875-2062
info@therapro.com
www.therapro.com

Karen Conrad , ScD, OTR/L, Owner
Reacher is useful when reaching, sitting or when standing. *$18.95*

519   Loop Scissors
Therapro, Inc.
225 Arlington St
Framingham, MA 01702-8723

508-872-9494
800-257-5376
Fax: 508-875-2062
info@therapro.com
www.therapro.com

Karen Conrad , ScD, OTR/L, Owner
Pliable, plastic handles that allow for easy and controlled cutting. *$14.25*

520   Pedal-in-Place Exerciser
Thoele Manufacturing
475 County Road 100 N
Montrose, IL 62445-3019

217-924-4553
Fax: 217-924-4553

521   Pet Partners
Delta Society National Service Dog Center
875 124th Ave NE
Ste 101
Bellevue, WA 98005-2531

425-679-5550
Fax: 425-379-5539
info@deltasociety.org
www.petpartners.org

Annie Peters Magnant, President & CEO
Mary Margaret Callahan, Senior National Director, Program Development
Evan Wight, National Director, Marketing
Linda Dicus, Executive Assistant
Pet Partners, formerly Delta Society, is a 501(c)(3) non-profit organization that helps people live healthier and happier lives by incorporating therapy, service and companion animals into their lives.

522 Plastic Card Holder
Therapro, Inc.
225 Arlington St
Framingham, MA 01702-8723
508-872-9494
800-257-5376
Fax: 508-875-2062
info@therapro.com
www.therapro.com

Karen Conrad , ScD, OTR/L, Owner
For those with reduced finger control. *$4.00*

523 Power Door
11240 Gemini Ln
Dallas, TX 75229-4710
800-688-1758
Fax: 972-620-9875
info@powerdoor.com

Jim Goldthwaite, National Sales Manager
Power door, low energy door operators.

524 ProtectaCap, ProtectaCap+PLUS, ProtectaChin Guard and ProtectaHip
Plum Enterprises
P.O.Box 85
Valley Forge, PA 19481-85
610-783-7377
800-321-PLUM
Fax: 610-783-7577
info@PlumEnt.com
www.plument.com

Janice Carrington, CEO
Plum Enterprises award winning, exquisite, ergonomic protective wear keeps you safe from the dangers of falls. ProtectCap+Plus and ProtectHips are engineered for superior shock-absorption and designed for exquisite simplicity and amazing lightweight comfort. The perfect blend of style and function.

525 Quad Commander
Gpk
535 Floyd Smith Dr
El Cajon, CA 92020-1228
619-593-7381
800-468-8679
Fax: 888-755-5603
info@gpk.com
www.gpk.com

526 Rocker Balance Square
Bailey Manufacturing Company
P.O. Box 130
Lodi, OH 44254-130
800-321-8372
Fax: 800-224-5390
baileymfg@baileymfg.com
www.baileymfg.com

527 Scott Sign Systems
7525 Pennsylvania Ave
Suite 101
Sarasota, FL 34243
941-355-5171
800-237-9447
Fax: 941-351-1787
info@scottsigns.com
www.scottsigns.com

Kathy Hannon, VP
Evelyn Brown, Sales
Call for a brochure.

528 Series Adapter
AbleNet
2625 Patton Road
Roseville, MN 55113-1308
651-294-2200
800-322-0956
Fax: 651-294-2259
customerservice@ablenetinc.com
www.ablenetinc.com

Bill Sproull, Chairman of the Board
Jennifer Thalhuber, President/CEO
William Mills, Board of Director

Allows two-switch operation of any battery-operated device or electrical devices. *$13.00*

529 Signaling Wake-Up Devices
HARC Mercantile
5413 S. Westnedge Ave.
Suite A
Portage, MI 49002
269-324-1615
800-445-9968
Fax: 269-324-2387
TTY: 269-324-1615
info@harc.com
www.harc.com

Ron Slager, Owner
Wake up devices. Vibrating alarm clocks, available with flashing lights, louder alarm noises and more. *$29.50*

530 Smoke Detector with Strobe
HARC Mercantile
5413 S. Westnedge Ave.
Suite A
Portage, MI 49002
269-324-1615
800-445-9968
Fax: 269-324-2387
TTY: 269-324-1615
info@harc.com
www.harc.com

Ron Slager, Owner
Most of the smoke alarms are twice as loud, and have a 120+ candela strobe that will wake a person from a sound sleep. Mounting hardware for ceiling or wall. *$165.95*

531 Spinal Network: The Total Wheelchair Resource Book
No Limits Communications & New Mobility
75-20 Astoria Blvd.
East Elmhurst, NY 11370
800-404-2898
888-850-0344
www.newmobility.com

Josie Byzek, Managing Editor
Jean Dobbs, Editorial Director
Tim Gilmer, Editor
Ian Ruder, Senior Editor
Nearly 600 pages of profiles, articles and resources on every topic of interest to wheelchair users. Subjects include health, coping, relationships, sexuality, parenthood, computers, sports, recreation, travel, personal assistance services, legal rights, financial strategies, employment, and media images. *$34.95*
400 pages

532 SteeleVest
Steele
P.O.Box 7304
Kingston, WA 98346-7304
360-297-4555
888-783-3538
Fax: 360-297-2816
www.steelevest.com

Sandra Steele, President
Vest developed by NASA provides an external cooling system.

533 TV & VCR Remote
AbleNet
2625 Patton Road
Roseville, MN 55113-1308
651-294-2200
800-322-0956
Fax: 651-294-2259
customerservice@ablenetinc.com
www.ablenetinc.com

Bill Sproull, Chairman of the Board
Jennifer Thalhuber, President/CEO
William Mills, Board of Director
Controls a TV, a VCR or a TV that is connected through a VCR tuner. It may be programmed to control functions such as on and off, channel up, preprogrammed TV channels and, if desired, other TV functions such as mute and pause. *$82.00*

534 Tactile Thermostat
Sense-Sations
919 Walnut Street
Philadelphia, PA 19107-5237   215-627-0600
Fax: 215-922-0692
asbinfo@asb.org
www.asb.org

Patricia C. Johnson, President & Chief Executive Officer
Derby Ewing, Director, Human Services
Brian Rusk, Public Relations Officer
Richard Forsythe, Director, Braille Division and Custom Audio
Large embossed numbers on cover ring and raised temperature
setting knob. *$31.50*

535 Therapy Putty
Therapro, Inc.
225 Arlington St
Framingham, MA 01702-8723   508-872-9494
800-257-5376
Fax: 508-875-2062
info@therapro.com
www.therapro.com

Karen Conrad , ScD, OTR/L, Owner
Designed to exercise and strengthen hands, ranging from soft to
firm for developing a stronger grasp. Available in two, four and
six ounce sizes. Three ounce putty in unique clear fist shaped con-
tainer.

536 Uppertone
535 Floyd Smith Dr
El Cajon, CA 92020-1228   619-593-7381
800-468-8679
Fax: 888-755-5603
info@gpk.com
www.gpk.com

537 Visual Alerting Guest Room Kit
HARC Mercantile
5413 S. Westnedge Ave.
Suite A
Portage, MI 49002   269-324-1615
800-445-9968
Fax: 269-324-2387
TTY: 269-324-1615
info@harc.com
www.harc.com

Ron Slager, Owner
ADA compliant visual alerting guest room kit for the hard of hearing and deaf. Includes visual smoke detector, phone alert, door
knock sensor, tactile alarm clock and telephone amplifier. Variations include TTY.

538 Window-Ease
A-Solution
5505 Barranca Oso Ct NE
Albuquerque, NM 87111   505-856-6632
Fax: 505-856-6652
info@windowease.com
www.windowease.com

Robert Gorrell, President
Jeff Dodd, Sales
Device adapts horizontally and vertically sliding windows to
ANSI A117.1 standards. 10:1 mechanical advantage at the crank
arm opens a 50lb window with 5lbs force. Price ranges from
$350.00-$450.00.

Office Devices & Workstations

539 Combination File/Reference Carousel
Center for Rehabilitation Technology
Ste 118
490 10th St NW
Atlanta, GA 30318-5754   404-712-5667
800-457-9555
Fax: 404-875-9409

TW Gannaway, Executive VP
Anthony Stringer PhD
Offers two reading platforms and file holders joined on one easily
rotated carousel. The carousel is easily rotated by head, mouth or
handstick. Page retainer adjusts to hold open a variety of books
and magazines. *$299.00*

540 Don Johnston
26799 W Commerce Dr
Volo, IL 60073-9675   847-740-0749
800-999-4660
800-889-5242
Fax: 847-740-7326
info@donjohnston.com
www.donjohnston.com

Don Johnston, President
A provider of quality products and services that enable people
with special needs to discover their potential and experience success. Products are developed for the areas of Physical Access,
Augmentative Communication and for those who struggle with
reading and writing.

541 Extensions for Independence
6100 Center Drive
Suite 1190
Los Angeles, CA 90045   757-416-6575
888-321-4678
Fax: 866-632-7149
support@inmotionhosting.com
www.mouthstick.net

Ted Sakis, Director of Operations
Develops, manufactures and markets special vocational equipment for the physically handicapped. Products: mouthsticks,
computer mechanical aids: key locks and diskette loaders. Also,
turntable desks, wheelchair portable desks, filing trays with
slanted sides, telephone adapters, and motorized artist easel. All
these products have been designed to solve the functional limitations of people with little or no use of hands and/or arms.

542 Fairway Spirit Adaptive Golf Car: Model4852
Fairway Golf Cars
Ste 300
3225 Gateway Rd
Brookfield, WI 53045-5139   262-790-9363
888-320-4850
888-320-4850
Fax: 262-790-9396
www.fairwaygolfcars.com

543 Freedom Ryder Handcycles
Brike International
20589 SW Elk Horn Ct
Tualatin, OR 97062-9518   503-692-1029
800-800-5828
Fax: 970-221-4308
Mike@Freedomryder.com
www.freedomryder.com

Mike Lofgren, Owner
Brian Stewart, VP
The finest handcycle in the world. The cycles incorporate body,
lean steering and the finest bicycle components to make this a
three-wheeled vehicle without equal. Suitable for both recreation
and competition. *$1995.00*

544 **Golf Xpress**
Emotorsports
4400 West M-61
Standish, MI 48658
989-846-6255
Fax: 989-846-6255
www.golfxpress.com

545 **Infogrip: AdjustaCart**
1899 E. Main Street
Ventura, CA 93001-3411
805-652-0770
800-397-0921
Fax: 805-652-0880
tech@infogrip.com
www.infogrip.com

546 **Infogrip: BAT Personal Keyboard**
1899 E. Main Street
Ventura, CA 93001-3411
805-652-0770
800-397-0921
Fax: 805-652-0880
tech@infogrip.com
www.infogrip.com

547 **Maxi Marks**
Maxi Aids
42 Executive Blvd
Farmingdale, NY 11735-4710
631-752-0521
800-522-6294
Fax: 631-752-0689
TTY: 800-281-3555
sales@maxiaids.com
www.maxiaids.com

Elliot Zaretsky, President
Braille writing and identification products. *$2.50*

548 **Pencil/Pen Weighted Holders**
Therapro, Inc.
225 Arlington St
Framingham, MA 01702-8723
508-872-9494
800-257-5376
Fax: 508-875-2062
info@therapro.com
www.therapro.com

Karen Conrad , ScD, OTR/L, Owner
Securely hold any pencil or pen. These weighted holders allow for more control along with proprioceptive feedback to encourage better writing skills.

549 **Perkins Brailler**
Maxi Aids
42 Executive Blvd
Farmingdale, NY 11735-4710
631-752-0521
800-522-6294
Fax: 631-752-0689
TTY: 800-281-3555
sales@maxiaids.com
www.maxiaids.com

Elliot Zaretsky, President
Can emboss 25 lines with 42 cells on an 11 x 11 1/2 sheet. *$495.00*

550 **PhoneMax Amplified Telephone**
Assistech
2738 N Campbell Ave
Tucson, AZ 85719-3141
520-883-8600
866-674-3549
Fax: 520-883-3172
www.assistivedevices.net

Oliver Simoes, Owner

551 **Raised Line Drawing Kit**
Maxi Aids
42 Executive Blvd
Farmingdale, NY 11735-4710
631-752-0521
800-522-6294
Fax: 631-752-0689
TTY: 800-281-3555
sales@maxiaids.com
www.maxiaids.com

Elliot Zaretsky, President
For writing script or drawing graphs by the use of special plastic paper. *$24.45*

552 **Reizen Braille Labeler**
Maxi Aids
42 Executive Blvd
Farmingdale, NY 11735-4710
631-752-0521
800-522-6294
Fax: 631-752-0689
TTY: 800-281-3555
sales@maxiaids.com
www.maxiaids.com

Elliot Zaretsky, President
Label everything in Braille with 3/8 or 1/2 wide labeling tape. *$47.95*

553 **Sharp Calculator with Illuminated Numbers**
Independent Living Aids
137 Rano Rd
Buffalo, NY 14207
516-937-1848
800-537-2118
855-746-7452
Fax: 516-937-3906
can-do@independentliving.com
www.independentliving.com

Irwin Schneidmill, President
Michael Gutierrez, Director of Operations
Pamela Strauss, Director of Marketing
Ursula Izurieta, Director of Merchandising
A trim desktop calculator with large illuminated numbers that can be carried anywhere. *$34.95*

554 **Signature and Address Self-Inking Stamps**
Independent Living Aids
137 Rano Rd
Buffalo, NY 14207
516-937-1848
800-537-2118
855-746-7452
Fax: 516-937-3906
can-do@independentliving.com
www.independentliving.com

Irwin Schneidmill, President
Michael Gutierrez, Director of Operations
Pamela Strauss, Director of Marketing
Ursula Izurieta, Director of Merchandising
Gives thousands of impressions before requiring re-inking. *$11.95*

555 **Steady Write**
Maxi Aids
42 Executive Blvd
Farmingdale, NY 11735-4710
631-752-0521
800-522-6294
Fax: 631-752-0689
TTY: 800-281-3555
sales@maxiaids.com
www.maxiaids.com

Elliot Zaretsky, President
Furnishes the writer with increased holding capacity and stabilizes the hand. *$6.95*

556 **Talking Desktop Calculators**
Maxi Aids
42 Executive Blvd
Farmingdale, NY 11735-4710   631-752-0521
800-522-6294
Fax: 631-752-0689
TTY: 800-281-3555
sales@maxiaids.com
www.maxiaids.com

Elliot Zaretsky, President
Unique voice synthesizers call out numerals and functions as they
are keyed in or read out data stored in memory. *$467.95*

557 **Talking Electronic Organizers**
Independent Living Aids
137 Rano Rd
Buffalo, NY 14207   516-937-1848
800-537-2118
855-746-7452
Fax: 516-937-3906
can-do@independentliving.com
www.independentliving.com

Irwin Schneidmill, President
Michael Gutierrez, Director of Operations
Pamela Strauss, Director of Marketing
Ursula Izurieta, Director of Merchandising
Electronic, portable, personal organizers that talk the user
through all the functions and are totally voice interactive.
$199.95 and up.

558 **Television Remote Controls with Large Numbers**
Independent Living Aids
137 Rano Rd
Buffalo, NY 14207   516-937-1848
800-537-2118
855-746-7452
Fax: 516-937-3906
can-do@independentliving.com
www.independentliving.com

Irwin Schneidmill, President
Michael Gutierrez, Director of Operations
Pamela Strauss, Director of Marketing
Ursula Izurieta, Director of Merchandising
Large 5 1/2 inch x 8 1/2 inch unit that has easy to see and use but-
tons. Can be used on nearly every TV, VCR and cable boxes.
$39.95

559 **Wheelchair Activity/Computer Table**
Maxi Aids
42 Executive Blvd
Farmingdale, NY 11735-4710   631-752-0521
800-522-6294
Fax: 631-752-0689
TTY: 800-281-3555
sales@maxiaids.com
www.maxiaids.com

Elliot Zaretsky, President
This powered height-adjustable table is a wheelchair accessible
activity table or computer workstation that's as stylish as it is
functional. Adjusts with the push of a button from 27-39 inches,
powered by an extremely quiet motor. ADA compliant computer
workstation for assistive technology and school computer labs.

Scooters

560 **Aerospace Compadre**
Aerospace America
900 Harry Truman Pkwy.
Bay City, MI 48706-4171   989-684-2121
800-237-6414
Fax: 989-684-4486
www.aerospaceamerica.com

Mike Alley, President
Fully customized golf cart type vehicle for the physically impaired person. Fully equipped with hand controls, wheelchair

rack, storage racks, head and tail lights and full safety belts.
$2500.00

561 **Alante**
Golden Technologies
401 Bridge St
Old Forge, PA 18518-2323   800-624-6374
Fax: 800-628-5165
www.goldentech.com

Robert Golden, Chairman
Richard Golden, CEO
Fred Kiwak, President
Rear-wheel-drive vehicle that represents the best in powered mo-
bility.

562 **Amigo Mobility International**
Amigo Mobility International
6693 Dixie Highway
Bridgeport, MI 48722   989-777-0910
800-248-9131
800-692-6446
Fax: 800-334-7274
info@myamigo.com
www.myamigo.com

Al Thieme, Chairman and Founder
Beth Thieme, CEO
Tim Drumhiller, President
An industry leader in power operated vehicles/scooters, Amigo
provides innovative, durable, and customized mobility solutions
for the disabled, injured, and seniors worldwide. Other services
include healthcare, travel and transportation services. *$1295.00*

563 **Amigo Mobility International Inc.**
6693 Dixie Hwy
Bridgeport, MI 48722-9725   989-777-0910
800-692-6446
888-892-2580
Fax: 800-334-7274
info@myamigo.com
myamigo.com

Al Thieme, Chairman & Founder
Beth Thieme, Chief Executive Officer
Amigo Mobility designs and manufactures a complete line of
power operated vehicles/mobility scooters and accessories in
Bridgeport, Michigan.

564 **Bravo! + Three-Wheel Scooter**
EZ-International
W194 N11301 McCormick Drive
Germantown, WI 53022   262-250-7740
800-824-1068
Fax: 262-250-7741
sales@ek-tech.com
www.ek-tech.com

565 **Cruiser Bus Buggy 4MB**
Convaid Products
2830 California Street
Torrance, CA 90503   310-618-0111
888-266-8243
Fax: 310-618-2166
www.convaid.com

rocio , Inside Sales Manager
In sizes from infant through young adult, this positioning buggy
is crash-tested.

566 **Cub, SuperCub and Special Edition Scooters**
1780 Executive Dr
Oconomowoc, WI 53066   262-567-4990
Fax: 262-953-5502
www.bruno.com

Michael R. Bruno, II, President/CEO
Michael R Bruno II, President/CEO
Steve Nelson, Service Manager

567   **Electric Mobility Corporation**
P.O.Box 156
Sewell, NJ 08080-156   856-468-0083
856-468-0083
800-257-7955
Fax: 856-468-3426
www.rascalscooters.com

Linda Autore, CEO
Manufactures Rascal Scooters.

568   **Explorer+ 4-Wheel Scooter**
EZ-International
W194 N11301 McCormick Drive
Germantown, WI 53022   262-250-7740
800-824-1068
Fax: 262-250-7741
sales@ek-tech.com
www.ek-tech.com/

569   **Featherlite**
No Boundaries
1 Monster Way
Corona, CA 92879   714-891-5899
800-426-7367
Fax: 714-891-0658
info@hansens.com
www.hansens.com

Hubert Hansen, Founder
Lightweight scooter folds in seconds without tools or bending down for hassle free travel on airplanes, cruise ships, trains, RVs, buses and more! Heaviest component weighs 27 pounds. Fits easily in almost any vehicle trunk.

570   **Invacare Fulfillment Center**
Invacare Corporation
1 Invacare Way
Elyria, OH 44035-4190   440-329-6000
800-333-6900
Fax: 877-619-7996
www.invacare.com

A Malachi Mixon Iii, Chairman of the Board
Gerald B. Blouch, President and Chief Executive Officer
Joseph B. Richey, II, President - Invacare Technologies Division
Robert K. Gudbranson, Senior Vice President and Chief Financial Officer
Invacare Corporation is the world's leading manufacturer and distributor of non-acute medical products which promote recovery and active lifestyles for people requiring home and other non-acute health care.

571   **Invacare Lynx L-3 Scooter**
Maxi Aids
42 Executive Blvd
Farmingdale, NY 11735-4710   631-752-0521
800-522-6294
Fax: 631-752-0689
TTY: 800-281-3555
sales@maxiaids.com
www.maxiaids.com

Elliot Zaretsky, President
The L-3 model conveniently disassembles into four compact pieces for easy transport. With an estimated seven miles of range, a plug-in battery charger and flat-free tires, consumers can plan their schedule around what they want to do, not around the limitations of their scooter. *$795.00*

572   **Leisure Lift**
Leisure Lift
1800 Merriam Ln
Kansas City, KS 66106-4714   913-722-5658
800-255-0285
Fax: 913-722-2614
Leisure-Lift@Leisure-Lift.com
www.pacesaver.com

Bill Burke, Founder
Leisure Lift offers light three wheel scooter models and seven power wheelchair models. *$2695.00*

573   **MVP+ 3-Wheel Scooter**
EZ-International
W194 N11301 McCormick Drive
Germantown, WI 53022   262-250-7740
800-824-1068
Fax: 262-250-7741
sales@ek-tech.com
www.ek-tech.com/contact.php

574   **Moxie**
No Boundaries
1 Monster Way
Corona, CA 92879   714-891-5899
800-426-7367
Fax: 714-891-0658
info@hansens.com
www.hansens.com

Hubert Hansen, Founder
Disassembles into three parts in less than a minute. Heaviest component weighs 41 pounds. Portable, affordable and downright snazzy!

575   **Outdoor Independence**
Palmer Industries
P.O.Box 5707
Endicott, NY 13763-5707   607-754-2957
800-847-1304
Fax: 607-754-1954
palmer@palmerind.com
www.palmerind.com

Jack Palmer, President
The futuristic, one, two and three seater, electric three-wheeler designed to take you almost anywhere.

576   **Pace Saver Plus II**
Leisure-Lift
1800 Merriam Ln
Kansas City, KS 66106-4714   913-722-5658
800-255-0285
Fax: 913-722-2614
www.pacesaver.com

Bill Burke, Founder
The scooter combines outdoor ruggedness with indoor maneuverability at a low price.

577   **Palmer Independence**
Palmer Industries
P.O.Box 5707
Endicott, NY 13763-5707   607-754-2957
800-847-1304
Fax: 607-754-1954
palmer@palmerind.com
www.palmerind.com

Jack Palmer, President
Futuristic electric outdoor three wheeler designed to take the rider almost anywhere.

578   **Palmer Twosome**
Palmer Industries
P.O.Box 5707
Endicott, NY 13763-5707   607-754-2957
800-847-1304
Fax: 607-754-1954
palmer@palmerind.com
www.palmerind.com

Jack Palmer, President
All electric two seat vehicle for those who can't pedal.

579   Phantom Compact Size Scooter
Maxi Aids
42 Executive Blvd
Farmingdale, NY   11735-4710   631-752-0521
                                      800-522-6294
                                 Fax: 631-752-0689
                                 TTY: 800-281-3555
                                 sales@maxiaids.com
                                 www.maxiaids.com

Elliot Zaretsky, President
Travel in style-ideal/affordable compact scooter. Great for both indoor and outdoor use. Three wheel design allows for small 32.3 turning radius. Top speed 4 miles per hour and a cruising range of 15 miles. Large carry basket.

580   Polaris Trail Blazer
Polaris Industries
2100 Highway 55
Medina, MN   55340-9770   763-542-0500
                                      888-704-5290
                                 Fax: 763-542-0599
                                 www.polarisindustries.com
Scott Wine, Chairman and Chief Executive Officer
Bennett J. Morgan, President and Chief Operating Officer
Michael W. Malone, Vice President - Finance and Chief Financial Officer
Todd-Michael Balan, Vice President - Corporate Development
A four-wheeler that has many engineered innovations, features such as: full floorboards for full comfort, single lever breaking with auxiliary foot brake, electronic throttle control, parking brake and adjustable handlebars.

581   Quickie 2
Sunrise Medical/Quickie Designs
2842 Business Park Avenue
Fresno, CA   93727   800-333-4000
                                      800-300-7502
                                 www.sunrisemedical.com

Pete Coburn, President
Randi Binstock, VP- Business Dev.
Peter Riley, Senior VP - Corporate CFO
Kevin Marshman, North American Controller
This custom, ultralight, folding, everyday scooter offers portability and performance plus modular flexibility.

582   Rascal 3-Wheeler
Electric Mobility Corporation
P.O.Box 156
Sewell, NJ   08080-156   856-468-1000
                                      800-257-7955
                                 Fax: 856-468-3426
                                 www.emobility.com

Scott Patrick, Manager
For primarily outdoor use, this three wheeler provides extra strength, durability and reliability.

583   Rascal ConvertAble
Electric Mobility Corporation
P.O.Box 156
Sewell, NJ   08080-156   856-468-1000
                                      800-257-7955
                                 Fax: 856-468-3426
                                 www.emobility.com
Scott Patrick, Manager
An electric vehicle that's a compact mobile chair one minute and a rugged outdoor scooter the next. Use both indoors and outdoors. Also available with joystick controls.

584   Regal Scooters
Bruno Independent Living Aids
Ste 84
1780 Executive Dr
Oconomowoc, WI   53066-4830   262-567-4990
                                      800-882-8183
                                 Fax: 262-953-5510
                                 webmaster@bruno.com
                                 www.bruno.com

Michael R. Bruno, II, President/CEO

This line includes the Regal Standard, the Regal Large Adult, the Regal Small Adult, the Regal Pediatric, The Regal Ten models 65 and 75, and The Regal Four. These scooters offer adjustable flip-up armrests, pneumatic tires front and rear, and more.

585   Regent
Golden Technologies
401 Bridge St
Old Forge, PA   18518-2323   570-451-7477
                                      800-624-6374
                                 Fax: 800-628-5165
                                 info@goldentech.com
                                 www.goldentech.com
Richard Golden, CEO
Lisa Miller, Senior Customer Service
Top-rated performance scooter, with extra features and economically priced.

586   Roadster 20
ATV Solutions
Unit 4
4700 W 60th Ave
Arvada, CO   80003-6928   303-450-2881
                                      866-777-9727
                                      888-867-1159
                                 Fax: 303-450-2880
                                 sales@atvsolutions.com
                                 www.atvsolutions.com
Andrew Miro, Owner
Great for indoor or outdoor use. The powerful, quiet drive system, independent front suspension and fully reclining high-back seat make for a smooth, quiet ride. The Roadster is loaded with great features at a bargain price.

587   Safari Scooter
Ranger All Seasons Corporation
P.O.Box 132
George, IA   51237-132   712-475-2811
                                      800-225-3811
                                 Fax: 712-475-2810
                                 www.rangerallseason.com

588   Scoota Bug
Golden Technologies
401 Bridge St
Old Forge, PA   18518-2323   570-451-7477
                                      800-624-6324
                                 Fax: 800-628-5165
                                 www.goldentech.com
Richard Golden, CEO
A lightweight, completely modular scooter, that disassembles and fits into most auto trunks.

589   Sierra 3000/4000
EZ-International
W194 N11301 McCormick Drive
Germantown, WI   53022   262-250-7740
                                      800-824-1068
                                 Fax: 262-250-7741
                                 Sales@EK-Tech.com
                                 www.ek-tech.com/

590   Solo Scooter
Ranger All Seasons Corporation
P.O.Box 132
George, IA   51237-132   712-475-2811
                                      800-225-3811
                                 Fax: 712-475-2810
                                 sales@rangerallseason.com
                                 www.rangerallseason.com

591   SoloRider Industries
Regal Research & Manufacturing Company
1200 East Plano Parkway
Plano, TX   75074   972-422-5324
                                       800-898-3353
                                  Fax: 972-422-8010
                                  info@solorider.com
                                  www.solorider.com

Roger Pretekin, Founder
Manufacturer and distributor of the Solorider Golf Cart. This revolutionary single rider adaptive cart is specifically designed to meet the needs of individuals with mobility impairments.

592   Sportster 10
ATV Solutions
Unit 4
4700 W 60th Ave
Arvada, CO   80003-6928   303-450-2881
                                       866-777-9727
                                       888-867-1159
                                  Fax: 303-450-2880
                                  sales@atvsolutions.com
                                  www.atvsolutions.com

Andrew Miro, Owner
Sportster 10 is our most maneuverable scooter, ideal for riders who must operate in tight spaces. Equipped with all of the great features of the Roadster 20, this three-wheeler is an exceptional buy.

593   Systems 2000
BioMedical Life Systems
P.O.Box 1360
Vista, CA   92085-1360   760-727-5600
                                       800-726-8367
                                  Fax: 760-727-4220
                                  information@bmls.com
                                  www.bmls.com

594   Terra-Jet: Utility Vehicle
TERRA-JET USA
P.O.Box 918
Junction Hwy. 417 & 419
Innis, LA   70747-918   225-492-2249
                                       800-864-5000
                                  Fax: 225-492-2226
                                  Terra-Jet@Terra-Jet.Com
                                  www.terra-jet.com

Larry Rabalais, President, General Manager and CEO
Shawn Oubre, Sales
TERRA-JET utility vehicles are unique in their ability to traverse many different types of terrain in remote areas otherwise inaccessible. It has a multitude of uses for industry, sportsmen or the whole family. Uniquely designed, industrial duty construction of low maintenance and low fuel consumption. $8,675-$21,995.

595   Terrier Tricycle
TRIAID
P.O.Box 1364
Cumberland, MD   21501-1364   301-759-3525
                                       800-306-6777
                                  Fax: 301-759-3525
                                  sales@triaid.com
                                  www.triaid.com

596   Trekker 40
ATV Solutions
Unit 4
4700 W 60th Ave
Arvada, CO   80003-6928   303-450-2881
                                       866-777-9727
                                       888-867-1159
                                  Fax: 303-450-2880
                                  www.atvsolutions.com

Andrew Miro, Owner
Our biggest, toughest scooter. With a huge 450 pound capacity and five inches of ground clearance, this machine is ideal for the daily outdoor user. The high top speed means you get there fast

and the four-wheel suspension makes the ride smooth and comfortable.

597   Tri-Lo's
TRIAID
P.O.Box 1364
Cumberland, MD   21501-1364   301-759-3525
                                       800-306-6777
                                  Fax: 301-759-3525
                                  sales@triaid.com
                                  www.triaid.com

598   Triumph 3000/4000
EZ-International
W194 N11301 McCormick Drive
Germantown, WI   53022   262-250-7740
                                       800-824-1068
                                  Fax: 262-250-7741
                                  Sales@EK-Tech.com
                                  www.ek-tech.com/

599   Triumph Scooter
EZ-International
W194 N11301 McCormick Drive
Germantown, WI   53022   262-250-7740
                                       800-824-1068
                                  Fax: 262-250-7741
                                  Sales@EK-Tech.com
                                  www.ek-tech.com/

Stationery

600   Access-USA
242 James St
PO Box 160
Clayton, NY   13624-160   800-263-2750
                                  Fax: 800-563-1687
                                  info@access-usa.com
                                  www.access-usa.com

Deborah Webster, PICOE
Access-USA provides one-stop alternate format transcription services for almost any type of document-reports, schedules, menus, monthly statements, brochures, reports, etc. Items may be submitted on computer disk, hard copy or email. Alternate formats include Braille, large print, Braille and print, audio recordings, adapted disks as well as video services-open/closed captioning and video descriptions. Accessible products also include Braille Business Cards and ADA signage.

601   Address Book
Sense-Sations
919 Walnut Street
Philadelphia, PA   19107-5237   215-627-0600
                                  Fax: 215-922-0692
                                  asbinfo@asb.org
                                  www.asb.org

Patricia C. Johnson, President & Chief Executive Officer
Derby Ewing, Director, Human Services
Brian Rusk, Public Relations Officer
Richard Forsythe, Director, Braille Division and Custom Audio
The big print address book is the first personal book to provide enlarged writing spaces, making it easier to write down and retrieve information. *$12.50*

602   Big Print Address Book
Maxi Aids
42 Executive Blvd
Farmingdale, NY   11735-4710   631-752-0521
                                       800-522-6294
                                  Fax: 631-752-0689
                                  TTY: 800-281-3555
                                  sales@maxiaids.com
                                  www.maxiaids.com

Elliott Zaretsky, Founder and President
Rods supported by two rubber blocks facilitate writing. *$16.95*

603 Bold Line Paper
Sense-Sations
919 Walnut Street
Philadelphia, PA 19107-5237   215-627-0600
Fax: 215-922-0692
asbinfo@asb.org
www.asb.org
Patricia C. Johnson, President & Chief Executive Officer
Derby Ewing, Director, Human Services
Brian Rusk, Public Relations Officer
Richard Forsythe, Director, Braille Division and Custom Audio
This pad consists of 100 sheets of paper with bold lines to help guide the writing of an individual with limited vision. *$2.50*

604 Braille Notebook
Maxi Aids
42 Executive Blvd
Farmingdale, NY 11735-4710   631-752-0521
800-522-6294
Fax: 631-752-0689
TTY: 800-281-3555
sales@maxiaids.com
www.maxiaids.com
Elliott Zaretsky, Founder and President
Made of heavy-duty board, covered with waterproof imitation leather and three rings for binding, including Braille paper and titles. *$12.95*

605 Braille: Desk Calendar
Maxi Aids
42 Executive Blvd
Farmingdale, NY 11735-4710   631-752-0521
800-522-6294
Fax: 631-752-0689
TTY: 800-281-3555
sales@maxiaids.com
www.maxiaids.com
Elliott Zaretsky, Founder and President
Schedule appointments, remember birthdays or write messages for a particular day. *$39.95*

606 Braille: Greeting Cards
Sense-Sations
919 Walnut Street
Philadelphia, PA 19107-5237   215-829-9997
Fax: 215-922-0692
asbinfo@asb.org
www.asb.org
Patricia C. Johnson, President & Chief Executive Officer
Derby Ewing, Director, Human Services
Brian Rusk, Public Relations Officer
Richard Forsythe, Director, Braille Division and Custom Audio
Birthday, anniversary, get well, sympathy and Christmas cards offering Braille print for the blind. *$.95*

607 Clip Board Notebook
Sense-Sations
919 Walnut Street
Philadelphia, PA 19107-5237   215-627-0600
Fax: 215-922-0692
asbinfo@asb.org
www.asb.org
Patricia C. Johnson, President & Chief Executive Officer
Derby Ewing, Director, Human Services
Brian Rusk, Public Relations Officer
Richard Forsythe, Director, Braille Division and Custom Audio
Kit includes a pack of Bold Line paper and black ink pen. *$5.95*

608 Deluxe Signature Guide
Maxi Aids
42 Executive Blvd
Farmingdale, NY 11735-4710   631-752-0521
800-522-6294
Fax: 631-752-0689
TTY: 800-281-3555
sales@maxiaids.com
www.maxiaids.com
Elliott Zaretsky, Founder and President

Rods supported by two rubber blocks facilitate writing. *$1.25*

609 Highlighter and Note Tape
Therapro, Inc.
225 Arlington St
Framingham, MA 01702-8723   508-872-9494
800-257-5376
Fax: 508-875-2062
info@therapro.com
www.therapro.com
Karen Conrad, Owner
A great way to highlight and draw attention to words without damaging original. Price ranges from $4.00-$7.00.

610 Letter Writing Guide
Independent Living Aids
137 Rano Rd
Buffalo, NY 14207   800-537-2118
855-746-7452
Fax: 516-937-3906
www.independentliving.com
Irwin Schneidmill, President
Michael Gutierrez, Director of Operations
Pamela Strauss, Director of Marketing
Ursula Izurieta, Director of Merchandising
Sturdy plastic sheet with 13 apertures corresponding to standard line spacing. *$3.49*

611 Lettering Guide Value Pack
Independent Living Aids
137 Rano Rd
Buffalo, NY 14207   800-537-2118
855-746-7452
Fax: 516-937-3906
www.independentliving.com
Irwin Schneidmill, President
Michael Gutierrez, Director of Operations
Pamela Strauss, Director of Marketing
Ursula Izurieta, Director of Merchandising
Included in this useful pack are four durable plastic lettering and number guides for tracing letters when the individual is unable to write letters unassisted. *$6.29*

Visual Aids

612 Aluminum Adjustable Support Canes for the Blind
Maxi Aids
42 Executive Blvd
Farmingdale, NY 11735-4710   631-752-0521
800-522-6294
Fax: 631-752-0689
TTY: 800-281-3555
sales@maxiaids.com
www.maxiaids.com
Elliott Zaretsky, Founder and President
Adjustable canes for the visually impaired. *$17.95*

613 Audio Book Contractors
P.O. Box 96
Riverdale, MD 20738-96   301-439-5830
Fax: 301-439-5830
info@audiobookcontractors.com
www.audiobookcontractors.com
Flo Gibson, President
Over 950 titles of unabridged classic books on audio cassettes in sturdy vinyl covers with picture and spine windows. Discounted prices for disabled patrons.

614 Beyond Sight
5650 S Windermere St
Littleton, CO 80120-1240   303-795-6455
Fax: 303-795-6425
jim@beyondsight.com
www.beyondsight.com
Scott Chaplick, Owner & President
Gina Whetzel, Sales & Merchandise Specialist

Products for the blind and visually impaired including talking clocks, watches and calculators, also carry a large selection of Braille products, magnifiers, reading machines and computer equipment.

615   Big Number Pocket Sized Calculator
Independent Living Aids
137 Rano Rd
Buffalo, NY   14207   516-937-1848
                                              800-537-2118
                                              855-746-7452
                                         Fax: 516-937-3906
                        can-do@independentliving.com
                              www.independentliving.com

Marvin Sandler, President
A handy pocket size calculator with big numbers that fits easily into purse or pocket. *$14.95*

616   Braille Compass
Maxi Aids
42 Executive Blvd
Farmingdale, NY   11735-4710   631-752-0521
                                               800-522-6294
                                          Fax: 631-752-0689
                                          TTY: 631-752-0738
                                      sales@maxiaids.com
                                         www.maxiaids.com

Elliott Zaretsky, Founder and President
The visually impaired can tell the direction by using this compass. *$42.95*

617   Braille Plates for Elevator
Maxi Aids
42 Executive Blvd
Farmingdale, NY   11735-4710   631-752-0521
                                               800-522-6294
                                          Fax: 631-752-0689
                                          TTY: 800-281-3555
                                      sales@maxiaids.com
                                         www.maxiaids.com

Elliott Zaretsky, Founder and President
The plates have curing type pressure sensitive material applied for metal to metal bonding. *$79.95*

618   Braille Touch-Time Watches
Independent Living Aids
137 Rano Rd
Buffalo, NY   14207   516-937-1848
                                              800-537-2118
                                              855-746-7452
                                         Fax: 516-937-3906
                        can-do@independentliving.com
                              www.independentliving.com

Marvin Sandler, President
White dial with black numerals and hands makes telling time possible quickly and easily for the visually impaired. *$44.95*

619   Circline Illuminated Magnifer
Dazor Manufacturing Corporation
2079 Congressional Dr.
St. Louis, MO   63146   314-652-2400
                                              800-345-9103
                                         Fax: 314-652-2069
                                        info@dazor.com
                                           www.dazor.com

Mark Hogrebe, Ph.D, Past President
Provides even, shadow free light under the magnifying lens with a 22-watt circline fluorescent. The magnifier is mounted on a floating arm that allows you to position the light source and lens with the touch of a finger.

620   Extra Loud Alarm with Lighter Plug
HARC Mercantile
5413 S. Westnedge Ave.
Suite A
Portage, MI   49002   269-324-1615
                                              800-445-9968
                                         Fax: 269-324-2387
                                         TTY: 269-324-1615
                                            info@harc.com
                                              www.harc.com

Ron Slager, Owner
Battery operated, easy to read, digital clock with extra loud alarm. *$45.00*

621   Low Vision Telephones
2738 N Campbell Ave
Tucson, AZ   85719-3141   520-883-8600
                                               866-674-3549
                                          Fax: 520-883-3172
                                 www.assistivedevices.net

Oliver Simoes, Owner

622   Magni-Cam & Primer
Innoventions
9593 Corsair Dr
Conifer, CO   80433-9317   303-797-6554
                                               800-854-6554
                                          Fax: 303-727-4940
                                        www.magnicam.com

Mark Freeman, President
Magni-Cam and Primer are hand-held, light weight, inexpensive auto-focus electronic magnification systems designed to meet the reading and writing needs of those with low vision. The systems present the image in black and white or in color with three different view modes. Connects to any TV monitor in minutes. Systems read any surface with no distortion. A battery powered system is available, providing total portability and flexibility.

623   Magnifier Bookweight
Levenger
420 S Congress Ave
Delray Beach, FL   33445-4693   901-566-5771
                                              800-544-0880
                                         Fax: 561-274-0263
                                   cservice@levenger.com
                                        www.levenger.com

Steve Leveen, CEO
The Magnifier Bookweight features an optical quality magnifier and is long enough to enlarge the full width of most book pages while holing the pages open. This magnifier is encased in embossed leather and enlarges approximately four lines of text at a time to twice the original size.

624   Man's Low-Vision Quartz Watches
Independent Living Aids
137 Rano Rd
Buffalo, NY   14207   516-937-1848
                                              800-537-2118
                                              855-746-7452
                                         Fax: 516-937-3906
                         can-do@independentliving.com
                               www.independentliving.com

Marvin Sandler, President
An inexpensive, easy-to-read watch with chrome case. *$27.95*

625   Men's/Women's Low Vision Watches & Clocks
Maxi Aids
42 Executive Blvd
Farmingdale, NY   11735-4710   631-752-0521
                                               800-522-6294
                                          Fax: 631-752-0689
                                          TTY: 800-281-3555
                                      sales@maxiaids.com
                                         www.maxiaids.com

Elliott Zaretsky, Founder and President
Choose from a wide range of watches from Braille automatic to quartz pocket watches.

626   **MonoMouse Electronic Magnifiers**
Maxi Aids
42 Executive Blvd
Farmingdale, NY 11735-4710   631-752-0521
                                          800-522-6294
                                       Fax: 631-752-0689
                                      TTY: 800-281-3555
                                     sales@maxiaids.com
                                       www.maxiaids.com

Elliott Zaretsky, Founder and President
Simple and affordable magnifier for people with Low Vision. Just about the size of a standard computer mouse. Allows you to read books, newspapers, product labels, etc. on either a computer or TV screen.

627   **Rigid Aluminum Cane with Golf Grip**
Maxi Aids
42 Executive Blvd
Farmingdale, NY 11735-4710   631-752-0521
                                          800-522-6294
                                       Fax: 631-752-0689
                                      TTY: 800-281-3555
                                     sales@maxiaids.com
                                       www.maxiaids.com

Elliott Zaretsky, Founder and President
A straight, tubular, heavy gauge aluminum rigid cane for blind and visually impaired persons. *$12.95*

628   **Stretch-View Wide-View Rectangular Illuminated Magnifier**
Dazor Manufacturing Corporation
2079 Congressional Dr.
St. Louis, MO 63146   314-652-2400
                                          800-345-9103
                                       Fax: 314-652-2069
                                        info@dazor.com
                                         www.dazor.com

Mark Hogrebe,Ph.D, Past President
Provides even, shadow free light under the magnifying lens with a 22-watt circline fluorescent. The magnifier is mounted on a floating arm that allows you to position the light source and lens with the touch of a finger.

629   **Timex Easy Reader**
Independent Living Aids
137 Rano Rd
Buffalo, NY 14207   516-937-1848
                                          800-537-2118
                                          855-746-7452
                                       Fax: 516-937-3906
                               can-do@independentliving.com
                                  www.independentliving.com

Marvin Sandler, President
An easy-to-read large face watch that's water resistant. *$29.95*

630   **Unisex Low Vision Watch**
Independent Living Aids
137 Rano Rd
Buffalo, NY 14207   516-937-1848
                                          800-537-2118
                                          855-746-7452
                                       Fax: 516-937-3906
                               can-do@independentliving.com
                                  www.independentliving.com

Marvin Sandler, President
Unisex watch with large numbers and wide hands. Gold-toned case with either expansion or leather band. *$31.95*

Walking Aids: Canes, Crutches & Walkers

631   **Air Lift Oxygen Carriers**
Air Lift Unlimited
1212 Kerr Gulch Rd
Evergreen, CO 80439-6397   800-776-6771
                                          888-343-3352
                                       Fax: 303-526-4700
                                        info@airlift.com
                               www.meridianmedicalusa.com

632   **Aluminum Crutches**
Arista Surgical Supply Company
297 High Street
Dedham, MA 02026-2852   781-329-2900
                                          800-225-2610
                                       Fax: 781-329-8392
                                        info@alimed.com
                                         www.alimed.com

Julian Cherubini, President
Lightweight aluminum crutches with wood underarms and handgrips. *$25.00*

633   **Aluminum Walking Canes**
Maxi Aids
42 Executive Blvd
Farmingdale, NY 11735-4710   631-752-0521
                                          800-522-6294
                                       Fax: 631-752-0689
                                      TTY: 800-281-3555
                                     sales@maxiaids.com
                                       www.maxiaids.com

Elliott Zaretsky, Founder and President
Lightweight but strong, these walking canes are made of a heavy gauge aluminum tube with safety locknuts and heavy-duty rubber tips. *$10.75*

634   **Compact Folding Travel Rollator**
Maxi Aids
42 Executive Blvd
Farmingdale, NY 11735-4710   631-752-0521
                                          800-522-6294
                                       Fax: 631-752-0689
                                      TTY: 631-752-0738
                                     sales@maxiaids.com
                                       www.maxiaids.com

Elliott Zaretsky, Founder and President
Is perfect for someone on the go. Pull strap for quick folding and disassembly. Folds down to half its assembled size in seconds, to a manageable 26 inch L x 22 inch W x 8 inch D for easy storage. *$149.95*

635   **Crutches**
Mada Medical Products
625 Washington Ave
Carlstadt, NJ 07072-2901   201-460-0454
                                          800-526-6370
                                       Fax: 201-460-3509
                              dianelind@mail.madamedical.com
                               www.madainternational.com

Jeffrey Adam, President
All aluminum construction, underarm crutch with double pushbutton height adjustment.

636   **Dapper Folding Adustable Cane**
Maxi Aids
42 Executive Blvd
Farmingdale, NY 11735-4710   631-752-0521
                                          800-522-6294
                                       Fax: 631-752-0689
                                      TTY: 631-752-0738
                                     sales@maxiaids.com
                                       www.maxiaids.com

Elliott Zaretsky, Founder and President
The Dapper walking stick can be folded and unfolded with only one hand and with minimum effort. The durable lanyard attached prevents loss and allows trailing of staff. Features a non-slip han-

dle, non-skid rubber tip and is made of high quality sturdy aluminum. $ 34.95

637   **Dapper Walking Stick**
Maxi Aids
42 Executive Blvd
Farmingdale, NY   11735-4710   631-752-0521
                                               800-522-6294
                                         Fax: 631-752-0689
                                         TTY: 631-752-0738
                                         sales@maxiaids.com
                                         www.maxiaids.com

Elliott Zaretsky, Founder and President
The Dapper walking stick is safe durable and sturdy allowing the user to conveniently store it when not in use. It can be folded and unfolded with only one hand and with minimum effort. The durable lanyard attached prevents loss and allows trailing of staff. Features a non-slip handle, non-skid rubber tip and is made of high quality sturdy aluminum construction. *$34.95*

638   **Deluxe Nova Wheeled Walker & Avant Wheeled Walker**
Sammons Preston Rolyan
W68n158 Evergreen Blvd
Cedarburg, WI   53012-2637   262-387-8720
                                               800-323-5547
                                         Fax: 800-547-4333
                    CustomerSupport@PattersonMedical.com
                              www.pattersonmedical.com/

Bruce Curtis, Sales Representative
David.P Sproat, President
Lightweight and simple to handle with an easy-to-operate braking system. *$425.40*

639   **Deluxe Standard Wood Cane**
Arista Surgical Supply Company/AliMed
297 High Street
Dedham, MA   02026-2852   781-329-2900
                                               800-225-2610
                                         Fax: 781-329-8392
                                         info@alimed.com
                                         www.alimed.com

Julian Cherubini, President
A standard old-fashioned wooden cane for the physically challenged. *$10.00*

640   **EasyStand 6000 Glider**
Access To Recreation
8 Sandra Ct
Newbury Park, CA   91320-4302   800-634-4351
                                         Fax: 805-498-8186
                    customerservice@accesstr.com
                              www.accesstr.com

Don Krebs, President
Provides dynamic leg motion for individuals who are unable to stand upright or walk on their own.

641   **Freedom Three Wheel Walker**
Mada Medical Products
625 Washington Ave
Carlstadt, NJ   07072-2901   201-460-0454
                                               800-526-6370
                                         Fax: 201-460-3509
                    dianelind@mail.madamedical.com
                              www.madainternational.com

Jeffrey Adam, President
The freedom walker has ultra light touch, locking loop brakes and sure grip hand grips.

642   **Liberty Lightweight Aluminum Stroll Walker**
Mada Medical Products
625 Washington Ave
Carlstadt, NJ   07072-2901   201-460-0454
                                               800-526-6370
                                         Fax: 201-460-3509
                    dianelind@mail.madamedical.com
                              www.madainternational.com

Jeffrey Adam, President

The Liberty walker has a spring loaded push down braking system, adjustable handle height with locking system, a 12in wide fully padded seat, and a removable shopping basket.

643   **Maxi Superior Cane**
Maxi Aids
42 Executive Blvd
Farmingdale, NY   11735-4710   631-752-0521
                                               800-522-6294
                                         Fax: 631-752-0689
                                         TTY: 800-281-3555
                                         sales@maxiaids.com
                                         www.maxiaids.com

Elliott Zaretsky, Founder and President
Convenient folding cane designed for optimum balance. Tapered joints provide rigidity when open, and are made of heavy gauge aluminum. *$17.50*

644   **Out-N-About American Walker**
742 Market St
Oregon, WI   53575-1059   608-835-9255
                                         Fax: 608-835-5234

Luann Smith, President
The lightweight Out-N-About is easy to handle. The four wheel design provides greater support and stability than any other walking aids. Its large rubber tires move effortlessly over most surfaces, indoors and out. The small turning radius makes it ideal for getting through confined spaces and narrow doorways. The attractive, burgundy colored, tubular steel frame is extremely durable. The Out-N-About folds flat and stands alone for easy storage. Made in USA.

645   **Patriot Extra Wide Folding Walkers**
Mada Medical Products
625 Washington Ave
Carlstadt, NJ   07072-2901   201-460-0454
                                               800-526-6370
                                         Fax: 201-460-3509
                    dianelind@mail.madamedical.com
                              www.madainternational.com

Jeffrey Adam, President
The extra wide walkers have padded foam hand grips, two-stage push button folding mechanism, dual width adjustment, height adjustment, and nonskid tips.

646   **Patriot Folding Walker Series**
Mada Medical Products
625 Washington Ave
Carlstadt, NJ   07072-2901   201-460-0454
                                               800-526-6370
                                         Fax: 201-460-3509
                    dianelind@mail.madamedical.com
                              www.madainternational.com

Jeffrey Adam, President
The patriot walker has high density, padded foam hand grips, high strength 1in lightweight, anodized, dull silver aluminum tube construction, adjustable height with push-button lock security, nonskid tips, and a single button folding mechanism.

647   **Patriot Reciprocal Folding Walkers**
Mada Medical Products
625 Washington Ave
Carlstadt, NJ   07072-2901   201-460-0454
                                               800-526-6370
                                         Fax: 201-460-3509
                    dianelind@mail.madamedical.com
                              www.madainternational.com

Jeffrey Adam, President
The reciprocal folding walkers have padded foam hand grips, adjustable height with snap-in security, double front cross brace, and nonskid tips.

648   Prone Support Walker
Consumer Care Products
W282 N7109 Main Street
Merton, WI   53056   262-820-2300
                                        info@consumercarellc.com
                                        www.consumercarellc.com

649   Push-Button Quad Cane
Arista Surgical Supply Company/AliMed
297 High Street
Dedham, MA   02026-2852   781-329-2900
                                            800-225-2610
                                       Fax: 781-329-8392
                                            info@alimed.com
                                            www.alimed.com
Julian Cherubini, President
A reliable walking cane offering independence to the physically
challenged user. *$25.00*

650   Quad Canes
Mada Medical Products
625 Washington Ave
Carlstadt, NJ   07072-2901   201-460-0454
                                            800-526-6370
                                       Fax: 201-460-3509
                            dianelind@mail.madamedical.com
                                    www.madainternational.com
Jeffrey Adam, President
There are large and small base quad canes with high density foam
grips.

651   Rand-Scot
401 Linden Center Dr
Fort Collins, CO   80524-2429   970-484-7967
                                            800-467-7967
                                       Fax: 970-484-3800
                                       TTY: 800-467-7967
                                            info@randscot.com
                                            www.randscot.com
Joel Lerich, President
Barbara Hoehn, President
Manufactures the Easy Pivot patient lift, the BBD wheelchair
cushion line and Saratoga Exercise products for the disabled. Offers a line of patient lifts and standers for the disabled. Rand-scot
products are designed to help the disabled achieve independence,
comfort, and stamina. A video or dvd is available at no charge for
potential users, $800-$3,000.

652   Secret Agent Walking Stick
Gold Violin
PO BOX 147
Jessup, PA   18434   877-648-8466
                                       Fax: 800-821-1282
Connie Hallquist, CEO
The Secret Agent Walking Stick features a built-in flashlight, a
red reflector and a built-in secret pill compartment. this folding
aluminum cane is height adjustable and has a derby-style handle
and a non-skid rubber tip. A nylon carrying case is included. The
walking stick comes in a choice of gold, bronze, or black shaft
with a faux burled walnut handle. . It has been taken over by
Orchard Brands.

653   StairClimber
Martin Technology
29 N Main St
Gloversville, NY   12078-3006   518-725-1837
                                            800-800-1410
                                       Fax: 518-725-9522
Michael Lewy, Owner
A walker-capable person can climb and descend stairs with this
walker-designed StairClimber.

654   Standing Aid Frame with Rear Entry
Consumer Care Products
W282 N7109 Main Street
Merton, WI   53056   262-820-2300
                                       Fax: 920-459-9070
                                            www.consumercarellc.com

655   Stick Canes
Mada Medical Products
625 Washington Ave
Carlstadt, NJ   07072-2901   201-460-0454
                                            800-526-6370
                                       Fax: 201-460-3509
                            dianelind@mail.madamedical.com
                                    www.madainternational.com
Jeffrey Adam, President
Mada's stick canes are adjustable with a locking security system.

656   Torso Support
Grandmar
5635 Peck Rd.
Arcadia, CA   91006-20   626-443-3143
                                            800-447-6739
                                       Fax: 800-767-3933
                                            info@posey.com
                                            www.posey.com
Ernest Posey, CEO
*Bob Kelleher, Senior Vice President of Supply Chain and Adminis-
tration*
Tracey Bertolina, CFO
Dale Clendon, President
An aid for people who are unable to maintain an upright position
in an automobile or a wheelchair.

657   U-Step Walking Stabilizer: Walker
Maxi Aids
42 Executive Blvd
Farmingdale, NY   11735-4710   631-752-0521
                                            800-522-6294
                                       Fax: 631-752-0689
                                       TTY: 631-752-0738
                                            sales@maxiaids.com
                                            www.maxiaids.com
Elliott Zaretsky, Founder and President
If you want to feel as stable as you would while holding onto another person's arm, the U-Step Walking Stabilizer is for you. The
innovative braking system is easy to use and puts you in complete
control; roll only when you want to. Plus, it easily folds for transport. *$ 539.95*

658   Ventura Enterprises
4431 S. Eastern Avenue
Las Vegas, NV   89119   702-457-7676
                                       Fax: 317-745-3179
                                            info@venturaenterprises.com
                                            www.venturaenterprises.com
Sam Ventura, President, CEO
Ron Ventura, Vice President of Development
Galit Rozen, Vice President of Acquisitions
Ofir Ventura, ESQ., In House General Council
Manufacturer of everyday living mobility aids. Products include
carrying aids for walkers and wheelchairs and also wheelchair
cushions.

659   WCIB Heavy-Duty Folding Cane
Maxi Aids
42 Executive Blvd
Farmingdale, NY   11735-4710   631-752-0521
                                            800-522-6294
                                       Fax: 631-752-0689
                                       TTY: 800-281-3555
                                            sales@maxiaids.com
                                            www.maxiaids.com
Elliott Zaretsky, Founder and President
A four section aluminum folding cane with a golf-type grip han-
dle and flexible wrist loop. Available in 34-60 lengths. *$17.95*

660 **Walker Leg Support**
Sammons Preston Rolyan
W68 N158 Evergreen Blvd
Cedarburg, WI 53012-2637   262-387-8720
                                         800-228-3693
                                         Fax: 262-387-8748
CustomerSupport@PattersonMedical.com
                                www.pattersonmedical.com/

Bruce Curtis, Sales Representative
David.P Sproat, President
For lower extremity trauma. An alternative to crutches that allows safe, stable ambulation and frees hands and arms for daily tasks. *$11.50*

Wheelchairs: Accessories

661 **Advantage Wheelchair & Walker Bags**
Laurel Designs
TORRANCE, CA 90505   800-556-6307
                                         Fax: 310-316-2561
                                    advantagebag@verizon.net
                                      www.advantagebag.com/

662 **Automatic Wheelchair Anti-Rollback Device**
Alzheimer's Store
3197 Trout Place Rd
Cumming, GA 30041-8260   678-947-4001
                                         800-752-3238
                                         Fax: 678-947-8411
                                          www.alzstore.com

Ellen Warner, President
As a wheelchair user transfers to and from the chair, a pair of brake arms grabs the tires to prevent the chair from rolling backwards. Once the individual is seated, the device switches to stand-by mode and the wheelchair returns to standard function.

663 **Battery Operated Cushion**
DA Schulman
3827 Creekside Lane
Holmen, WI 54636   608-782-0031
                                         866-782-9658
                                         Fax: 608-782-0488
                                      aquila@aquilacorp.com
                                        www.aquilacorp.com

664 **Dual-Mode Charger**
Lester Electrical
625 West A Street
Lincoln, NE 68522-1794   402-477-8988
                                         Fax: 402-474-1769
                                     sales@lesterelectrical.com
                                      www.lesterelectrical.com

665 **Equalizer 1000 Series**
Helm Distributing
P.O Box 25105 Deer Park P.O, Rd Dee
Alberta,   T4R 2   403-309-5551
                                         Fax: 403-342-5509
                                  james@equalizerexercise.com
                                     www.equalizerexercise.com

666 **Equalizer 5000 Home Gym**
Helm Distributing
P.O Box 25105
Deer Park P.O.
Red Deer, AB, Canada   T4R- 2M2   403-309-5551
                                         Fax: 403-342-5509
                                    info@equalizerexercise.com
                                     www.equalizerexercise.com

667 **Featherspring**
105 W Lincoln Hwy
DeKalb, IL 60115   800-628-4693
                                         Fax: 800-261-1164
                                   customerservice@luxis.com
                                          www.luxis.com

668 **Gem Wheelchair & Scooter Service: Mobility & Homecare**
176-39 Union Turnpike
Flushing, NY 11366-1515   718-969-8600
                                         800-943-3578
                                help@gemwheelchairservice.com
                                www.gemwheelchairservice.com/

669 **Lifestand**
Frank Mobility Systems
300 Duke Drive
Lebanon, TN 37090   800-736-0925
                                         Fax: 800-231-3256
                                     techsupport@permobil.com
                                       www.lifestandusa.com

Larry Jackson, President and CEO
Tom Rolick, VP Sales North America
Darin Lowery, VP of Operations
Rick Haynes, Senior HR Manager
Lifestand offers a full line of standing wheelchairs for manual operation. Power assisted are fully motorized. *$7000.00*

670 **Mat Factory**
6726 North Figueroa Street
Los Angeles, CA 90042   800-628-7626
                                         Fax: 323-254-4545
                                        www.matfactoryinc.com

671 **One Thousand FS**
Fortress
P.O.Box 489
Clovis, CA 93613-489   559-322-5437
                                         Fax: 559-323-0299

672 **Pac-All Wheelchair Carrier**
Pac-All Carriers
2321 Carolton Rd
Maitland, FL 32751-3624   407-830-6604
                                         800-628-6672
                                         Fax: 407-339-2847

LE Angel
No more lifting and no more pain wheelchair carrier. VA approved. Made in USA.
$158 - $226.40

673 **Safety Deck II**
Mat Factory
6726 North Figueroa Street
Los Angeles, CA 90042   800-628-7626
                                         Fax: 323-254-4545
                                        www.matfactoryinc.com

674 **Scooter & Wheelchair Battery Fuel Gauges and Motor Speed Controllers**
Curtis Instruments, Inc.
200 Kisco Ave
Mount Kisco, NY 10549-1407   914-666-2971
                                         Fax: 914-666-2188
                                        gomezj@curtisinst.com
                                         www.curtisinst.com

Stuart E Marwell, President and CEO
David Matthews, VP Sales Americas
Cheryl Leonaggeo, Customer Service Manager
Richard McFarlane, Customer Support Engineer
Provides a readable, accurate indication of battery in easy to read type of display. Innovative, efficient motor speed controllers for single or dual PM motor vehicles.

675 **Softfoot Ergomatta**
Mat Factory
6726 North Figueroa Street
Los Angelesa, CA 90042   949-645-3122
                                         800-628-7626
                                         Fax: 323-254-4545
                                        www.matfactoryinc.com

676 Tilt-N-Table
Osterguard Enterprises c/o Jim's Shop
3228 W Olive Ave
Fresno, CA 93722-5733   559-275-4695
Jim Ostergaard Ii, Owner
These are lightweight tables for wheelchairs that are angle and
height adjustable to your changing needs.

677 Wheel Life News
University of Virginia, Rehab Engineering Centers
3363 University Sta
Charlottesville, VA 22903   434-924-5118
                            www.medicine.virginia.edu
Kristine M. Garza, Ph.D., Executive Director of SACNAS
Steven T. DeKosky, Dean
Features tie downs and other adaptive technology for persons
with disabilities.

678 Wheelchair Accessories
Diestco Manufacturing Company
P.O.Box 6504
Chico, CA 95927-6504   800-795-2392
                                    info@diestco.com
                                    www.diestco.com

679 Wheelchair Aide
Graham-Field
400 Rabro Dr
Hauppauge, NY 11788-4258   631-348-1364

680 Wheelchair Back Pack and Tote Bag
Med Covers
320 Roebling Street
Suite 515
Brooklyn, NY 11211   718-302-1923
                                             800-320-7140
                                    Fax: 866-522-6967
                               info@1800wheelchair.com
                               www.1800wheelchair.com

681 Wheelchair Roller
Access To Recreation
8 Sandra Ct
Newbury Park, CA 91320-4302   800-634-4351
                                    Fax: 805-498-8186
                          customerservice@accesstr.com
                                    www.accesstr.com

Don Krebs, President
The McClain Wheelchair Roller allows you to build strength and
stamina in the comfort of your own home.

682 Wheelchair Work Table
Bailey Manufacturing Company
P.O. Box 130
Lodi, OH 44254-130   800-321-8372
                                    Fax: 800-224-5390
                             baileymfg@baileymfg.com
                                    www.baileymfg.com

Wheelchairs: General

683 21st Century Scientific, Inc. - Bounder Power Wheelchair
4931 N Manufacturing Way
Coeur D Alene, ID 83815-8931   208-667-8800
                                             800-448-3680
                                    Fax: 208-667-6600
                                    21st@wheelchairs.com
                                    wheelchairs.com

Ronald E. Prior, Ph.D., President and Founder
RD Davidson, Sales/Marketing Director
Susan Harris, CFO and Webmaster
High performance power chairs for active individuals. Very fast
(11+ MPH), OFF-ROAD and Bariatric options available. Power
seating options include tilt, recline, 13-inch seat elevator, reverse
tilt, leg rests, standing and front load (latitude). 6-drive program-

mable electronics standard; lights, horn, electric leg bag emptier
and many other options available. Customization is our specialty.

684 Arcoa Travel Chair
Maxi Aids
42 Executive Blvd
Farmingdale, NY 11735-4710   631-752-0521
                                             800-522-6294
                                    Fax: 631-752-0689
                                    TTY: 631-752-0738
                                    sales@maxiaids.com
                                    www.maxiaids.com
Elliott Zaretsky, Founder and President
The unique Comfort Travel Chair collapses into an easy to manage 25in x 26in x 11in and includes a strap for easy carrying. It
weighs just 16 lbs. but can hold up to 200 lbs., making it the perfect travel companion. You can rest assured that it will 'stay put'
with a dual wheel lock, while you enjoy the comfort and support
of the padded swing-back armrests and 16in seat. *$197.00*

685 Bariatric Wheelchairs Regency FL
Gendron
520 W. Mulberry St.
Suite 100
Bryan, OH 43506   800-537-2521
                                    Fax: 419-636-9261
                                    www.gendroninc.com

Roberta Jacobs, National Sales Manager
Bariatric wheelchairs, for users weighing up to seven hundred
pounds. Manual and power styles built to order for specific needs.

686 Breezy
Sunrise Medical/Quickie Designs
2842 Business Park Avenue
Fresno, CA 93727   800-333-4000
                                             800-300-7502
                                    webmaster@sunmed.com
                                    www.sunrisemedical.com

Pete Coburn, President
Randi Binstock, VP, Business Dev.
Peter Riley, Senior VP/Corporate CFO
Roxane Cromwell, SVP, Operations North America
This lightweight chair is durable, comfortable and flexible
enough to meet the needs of a wide range of wheelchair users.

687 Champion 1000
Kuschall of America
3601 Rider Trl S
Earth City, MO 63045-1116   314-512-7000
                                             800-654-4768
                                    Fax: 800-542-3567

688 Champion 2000
Kuschall of America
3601 Rider Trl S
Earth City, MO 63045-1116   314-512-7000
                                             800-654-4768
                                    Fax: 800-542-3567

689 Champion 3000
Kuschall of America
3601 Rider Trl S
Earth City, MO 63045-1116   314-512-7000
                                             800-654-4768
                                    Fax: 800-542-3567

690   Choosing a Wheelchair: A Guide for Optimal Independence
Patient-Centered Guides
1005 Gravenstein Hwy N
Sebastopol, CA   95472-3836   707-827-7019
                                            800-889-8969
                                       Fax: 707-824-8268
                                        order@oreilly.com
                                      www.patientcenters.com
Linda Lamb, Series Editor
Shawnde Paull, Marketing
Tim O'Reilly, Publisher
Gary Karp, Author
With the right wheelchair, quality of life increases dramatically
and even people with severe disabilities can have a considerable
degree of independence and activity. Choosing the wrong chair
can indeed the tantamount to confinement. This book describes
technology, options, and the selection process to help you identify the chair than can provide you with optimal independence.
$9.95
186 pages Paperback
ISBN 1-565924-11-8

691   Convaid
2830 California Street
Torrance, CA   90503   310-618-0111
                                            888-266-8243
                                       Fax: 310-618-2166
                                        www.convaid.com
Rocio , Sales Manager
Monica , National Account Representative
Veronica , Export Department
Five different styles of wheelchairs.

692   Custom
Fortress
P.O.Box 489
Clovis, CA   93613-489   559-322-5437
                                       Fax: 559-323-0299

693   Custom Durable
21279 Protecta Dr
Elkhart, IN   46516-9539   574-522-7201
                                            800-478-2363
                                       Fax: 574-293-0202
                                        info@pvcdme.com

694   Edge
Fortress
P.O.Box 489
Clovis, CA   93613-489   559-322-5437
                                       Fax: 559-323-0299

695   Etac USA: F3 Wheelchair
Ste J
2325 Parklawn Dr
Waukesha, WI   53186-2938   262-717-9910
                                            800-678-3822
                                       Fax: 262-796-4605
                                      etac1usa@execpc.com
Mark Samolyk, Manager
A Swedish wheelchair designed to provide function, comfort and
flexibility. Seat frame and upholstery are adjustable to fit each individual. Swing away, detachable footrests are standard. Available in frame widths from 14, 18 and 20 inch. Numerous
accessories are available in order to individualize each chair.
Lifetime warranty on frame for original user.

696   Evacu-Trac
Garaventa Canada
7505 - 134 A Street, Surrey, BC V3W
Blaine, WA   98231-1769   866-824-8314
                                      productinfo@evacutrac.com

697   Folding Chair with a Rigid Feel
Kuschall of America
3601 Rider Trl S
Earth City, MO   63045-1116   314-512-7000
                                            800-654-4768
                                       Fax: 800-542-3567

698   Formula Series Active Mobility Wheelchairs
Everest & Jennings
3233 Mission Oaks Blvd
Camarillo, CA   93012-5047   805-389-7450

699   Freestyle II
Fortress
P.O.Box 489
Clovis, CA   93613-489   559-322-5437
                                       Fax: 559-323-0299

700   Gadabout Wheelchairs
Gadabout Wheelchairs
1165 Portland Ave
Rochester, NY   14621-3945   585-338-2110
                                            800-828-4242
                                       Fax: 585-338-2696
Michael Fonte, Owner
Enjoy independence with the wheelchair that is lightweight, por-
table, convenient, comfortable and sturdy.

701   Gem Wheelchair & Scooter Service: Mobility & Homecare
176-39 Union Tpke
Flushing, NY   11366-1515   718-969-8600
                                            800-943-3578
                                       Fax: 718-969-8300
                                   help@gemwheelchairservice.com
                                   www.gemwheelchairservice.com/

702   Gendron
520 W. Mulberry St. Suite 100
Bryan, OH   43506   419-445-6060
                                            800-537-2521
                                       Fax: 419-636-9261
                                        www.gendroninc.com
Roberta Jacobs, National Sales Manager
Manufacturer of wheelchairs for a variety of other applications,
specializing in bariatric mobility products.

703   HiRider
Gaymar Industries
10 Centre Dr
Orchard Park, NY   14127-2280   716-662-2551
                                            800-828-7341
                                       Fax: 800-993-7890
                                          www.gaymar.com
Frank L Lumbar, CEO
John.K Whitney, Founder
Cindy Sylvia, Educational Svcs Administrator
Dan Kormowicz, International Sales Coordinator
A wheelchair that provides mobility in both sitting and standing
positions.

704   Innovative Products
4351 W College Ave
Appleton, WI   54914-3928   920-738-9090
                                            800-424-3369
                                       Fax: 920-738-9050
                                           www.att.com
Fritz H Heerdt, President
Wheelchairs; accessories.

705   Liberty
Fortress
P.O.Box 489
Clovis, CA   93613-489   559-322-5437
                                       Fax: 559-323-0299

706   Lightweight Breezy
Motion Design
2842 Business Park Avenue
Fresno, CA   93727
                                   800-333-4000
                            Fax: 800-300-7502
                            webmaster@sunmed.com
                            www.sunrisemedical.com

Pete Coburn, President
Randi Binstock, VP, Business Dev.
Peter · Riley, Senior VP/Corporate CFO
Roxane Cromwell, SVP, Operations North America
A lightweight wheelchair. $750.00

707   Majors Medical Equipment
415 W Wilshire Blvd., Suite A
Oklahoma City, OK   73116
                                   405-840-5272
                                   1 8-8 4-4 01
                            Fax: 405-840-5274
                            help@mmedsupply.com
                            www.majorsmedicalequipment.com

Pat Metz, Owner
America's largest selection of wheelchairs and homecare equipment.

708   Natural Access
PO Box 5729
Santa Monica, CA   90409
                                   310-392-9864
                                   800-411-7789
                            Fax: 310-392-3874
                            john_egan_2000@yahoo.com
                            www.landeez.com

John Egan, Owner
Provides the Landeez all-terrain wheelchair, that can roll easily on sand, gravel and snow for outdoor fun. The entire chair can fit inside a travel bag!

709   Patient Transport Chair
Mada Medical Products
625 Washington Ave
Carlstadt, NJ   07072-2901
                                   201-460-0454
                                   800-526-6370
                            Fax: 201-460-3509
                            dianelind@mail.madamedical.com
                            www.madainternational.com

Jeffrey Adam, President
Mada's lightweight design transport chair is constructed of heavy gauge chrome-plated, steel tubing with reinforced cross braces.

710   Posture-Glide Lounger
Graham-Field Health Products
2935 Northeast Pkwy
Atlanta, GA   30360-2808
                                   678-291-3207
                            Fax: 770-368-2386
                            cs@grahamfield.com
                            www.grahamfield.com

Kenneth Spett, President & CEO
Marc Bernstein, Senior Vice President, Consumer Sales
Cherie Antoniazzi, Senior Vice President, Quality, Regulatory & Risk Management
Ivan Bielik, Senior Vice President, Business Analyst
Provides all day comfort and safe, independent mobilization with feet or hands. The ergonomically engineered seat back provides correct support.

711   Prairie Cruiser
Wheelchairs of Kansas
204 West 2nd Street P.O.Box 32
Ellis, KS   67637-32
                                   785-726-4885
                                   800-537-6454
                            Fax: 800-337-2447
                            www.wheelchairsofkansas.com

712   Redman Apache
Redman Powerchair
1601 S Pantano Road Suite 107
Tucson, AZ   85710
                                   520-546-6002
                                   800-727-6684
                            Fax: 520-546-5530
                            info@redmanpowerchair.com
                            www.redmanpowerchair.com

Don Redman, CEO
Paula Redman, CFO
Scott Evans, Regulatory affairs
Samuel Redman, General Manager
These ultralight, active use wheelchairs offer quick release rear wheels, adjustable arm height and detachable arm swing-away.

713   Redman Crow Line
Redman Powerchair
1601 S Pantano Road Suite 107
Tucson, AZ   85710
                                   520-546-6002
                                   800-727-6684
                            Fax: 520-546-5530
                            info@redmanpowerchair.com
                            www.redmanpowerchair.com

Don Redman, CEO
Paula Redman, CFO
Scott Evans, Regulatory affairs
Samuel Redman, General Manager
Reclining wheelchair that reclines a full 90 degrees to flat and can be stopped anywhere on the axis.

714   Rolls 2000 Series
Invacare Corporation
1 Invacare Way
Elyria, OH   44035-4107
                                   440-329-6000
                                   800-333-6900
                            Fax: 877-619-7996
                            info@invacare.com
                            www.invacare.com

A. Malachi Mixon, III, Chairman of the Board
Gerald B. Blouch, President and Chief Executive Officer
Joseph B. Richey, II, President - Invacare Technologies Division & SVP
Robert K. Gudbranson, Senior Vice President and Chief Financial Officer
These wheelchairs are the first light-weight wheelchairs designed for rental use.

715   Skyway
Skyway Machine
4451 Caterpillar Rd
Redding, CA   96003-1496
                                   530-243-5151
                                   800-332-3357
                            Fax: 530-243-5104
                            sales@skywaywheels.com

Ken Coster, Sales Department
Parrey Cremeans, Sales Department
Rein Stolz, Engineering Department
Patrick McEachen, Customer Service
For over 20 years Skyway has been the world leader in composite wheels. Supplying over 650 different wheel combinations for wheelchairs, lawn and garden products, bicycles and a large assortment of wheeled devices. Wheel sizes range from 4 inch to 24 inch diameter.

716   Stand-Up Wheelchairs
Lifestand
P.O.Box 232171
Encinitas, CA   92023-2171
                                   800-782-6324
                            Fax: 610-586-0847
                            dallery@msn.com

Jacques A Dallery, President
Offers a complete line of manual, electric and stand-up wheelchairs for the disabled.

717 Standard Wheelchair
Mada Medical Products
625 Washington Ave
Carlstadt, NJ 07072-2901
201-460-0454
800-526-6370
Fax: 201-460-3509
www.madainternational.com

Jeffrey Adam, President
Mada's standard wheelchairs are designed and built for long-lasting, reliable operation. Each wheelchair is constructed of heavy gauge, chrome plated, steel framework and tube in tube construction at stress points. Mada's state-of-the art engineering uses the most modern components to provide the strength needed while keeping the chair's weight down.

718 Super Light Folding Transport Chair with Carry Bag
Maxi Aids
42 Executive Blvd
Farmingdale, NY 11735-4710
631-752-0521
800-522-6294
Fax: 631-752-0689
TTY: 631-752-0738
sales@maxiaids.com
www.maxiaids.com

Elliott Zaretsky, Founder and President
Folds like a conventional folding chair for added convenience and includes carry bag, fold-down footrests, padded flip back armrests, standard rear wheel locks and an attractive frame with durable lightweight nylon upholstery and limited lifetime warranty. Weighs only 18 pounds. Easy to push or transport. *$319.95*

719 Surf Chair
2052 S Peninsula Dr
Daytona Beach, FL 32118-5237
386-253-0986
800-841-6610
Fax: 386-253-7600

720 Vista Wheelchair
Arista Surgical Supply Company/AliMed
297 High Street
Dedham, MA 02026-2852
781-329-2900
800-225-2610
Fax: 781-329-8392
info@alimed.com
www.alimed.com

721 Wheelchair with Shock Absorbers
Iron Horse Productions
3114 Strawberry Ln
Port Huron, MI 48060-1727
810-987-6700
800-426-0354

Wheelchairs: Pediatric

722 Commuter & Kid's Commuter
Fortress
P.O.Box 489
Clovis, CA 93613-489
559-322-5437
Fax: 559-323-0299

723 Convaid
2830 California St
Torrance, CA 90503-3908
310-618-0111
888-266-8243
Fax: 310-618-2166
www.convaid.com

Rocio , Sales Manager
Monica , National Account Representative
Veronica
Convaid manufactures Mobile Positioning Systems for children. The Expedition, Safari Tilt, Cruiser, EZ Rider and Metro offer a non-institutional styling and are lightweight and compact-folding. The steel/aluminum structure is engineered for maximum comfort and durability. The mobile positioning lines come with more than 20 positioning features and a full range of positioning

adaptations. All chairs have been successfully crash-tested and offer a limited lifetime warranty (except the Metro).

724 Imp Tricycle
TRIAID
P.O.Box 1364
Cumberland, MD 21501-1364
301-759-3525
800-306-6777
Fax: 301-759-3525
sales@triaid.com
www.triaid.com

725 Kid's Custom
Fortress
P.O.Box 489
Clovis, CA 93613-489
559-322-5437
Fax: 559-323-0299

726 Kid's Edge
Fortress
P.O.Box 489
Clovis, CA 93613-489
559-322-5437
Fax: 559-323-0299

727 Kid's Liberty
Fortress
P.O.Box 489
Clovis, CA 93613-489
559-322-5437
Fax: 559-323-0299

728 Kid-Friendly Chairs
Vector Mobility
5030 E Jensen Ave
Fresno, CA 93725-4010
559-431-3334
800-441-0358
Fax: 559-431-5535

Dave Deatherage, Owner
Manual base offers the lowest available floor to seat height, growth capability, one-third the parts of a conventional chair and no welds to break. The power unit features standard shapes and personality designs from elephants to inch worms and autos to rainbows, lowest seat height, and smallest turning radius on the market.

729 Koala Miniflex
Permobil USA
300 Duke Dr
Lebanon, TN 37090
800-736-0925
Fax: 800-231-3256
info@permobilus.com
permobilus.com

730 Seven Fifty-Five FS
Fortress
P.O.Box 489
Clovis, CA 93613-489
559-322-5437
Fax: 559-323-0299

731 TMX Tricycle
TRIAID
P.O.Box 1364
Cumberland, MD 21501-1364
301-759-3525
800-306-6777
Fax: 301-759-3525
sales@triaid.com
www.triaid.com

Wheelchairs: Powered

732   Bounder Plus Power Wheelchair
21st Century Scientific
4931 N Manufacturing Way
Coeur D Alene, ID   83815-8931
208-667-8800
800-448-3680
Fax: 208-667-6600
21st@wheelchairs.com
wheelchairs.com

Ronald E. Prior, Ph.D., President and Founder
RD Davidson, Sales/Marketing Director
Susan Harris, CFO and Webmaster
Available in widths of 16 to 20 inches for users up to 500 pounds
with a 2 year warranty on the entire chair. It offers all the standard
features of a BOUNDER, plus reinforced rear wheel mounts, reinforced caster barrels, and super duty upholstery (with double
liner and web straps under every screw). The BOUNDER Plus
also features tandem cross struts, middle vertical support strut,
seat rails supported at five points and back upholstery attached
with machine screws.

733   Bounder Power Wheelchair
21st Century Scientific
4931 N Manufacturing Way
Coeur D Alene, ID   83815-8931
208-667-8800
800-448-3680
Fax: 208-667-6600
21st@wheelchairs.com
wheelchairs.com

Ronald E. Prior, Ph.D., President and Founder
RD Davidson, Sales/Marketing Director
Susan Harris, CFO and Webmaster
Available in a variety of widths from 16 to 18 inches for users up
to 250 pounds. The rugged frame is constructed with steel tubing.
The standard 12 position Adjustable Front Forks, made of 1/4
inch thick steel, provides impact dampening and seat tilt adjustment. A Dual Group 27 Sliding Battery Box provides extended
range and easy battery maintenance. *$8695.00*

734   Breez 1025
Electro Kinetic Technologies
W194 N11301 McCormick Dr
Germantown, WI   53022
262-250-7740
800-824-1068
Fax: 262-250-7741
info@ek-tech.com
ek-tech.com

735   Damaco D90
Damaco
28918 Hancock Parkway
Valencia, CA   91355
661-775-2020
877-528-2288
Fax: 661-775-2025
www.atbatt.com

736   Gem Wheelchair & Scooter Service: Mobility & Homecare
176-39 Union Turnpike
Flushing, NY   11366-1515
718-969-8600
800-943-3578
Fax: 718-969-8300
help@gemwheelchairservice.com
www.gemwheelchairservice.com/

737   Geronimo
Redman Powerchair
Ste 202
3840 S Palo Verde Rd
Tucson, AZ   85714-2076
520-294-1466
800-727-6684
Fax: 520-294-1460

Arnie Johnson, Owner
Wheelchair offering direct drive, two year electronic guarantee
and micro controls.

738   Invacare IVC Tracer EX2 Wheelchair with Legrest
Maxi Aids
42 Executive Blvd
Farmingdale, NY   11735-4710
631-752-0521
800-522-6294
Fax: 631-752-0689
TTY: 631-752-0738
sales@maxiaids.com
www.maxiaids.com

Elliott Zaretsky, Founder and President
Bob Messenger, Clinical Respiratory Specialist
The Tracer EX2 combines the design and technology of the
Invacare 9000 A true dual axle position allows for repositioning
the 24 inch rear wheels and 8 inch casters for adult and hemi
seat-to-floor heights. The new design also makes it possible to interchange components with the 9000 series chairs. *$189.95*

739   Jet 3 Ultra Power Wheelchair
Maxi Aids
42 Executive Blvd
Farmingdale, NY   11735-4710
631-752-0521
800-522-6294
Fax: 631-752-0689
TTY: 800-281-3555
sales@maxiaids.com
www.maxiaids.com

Elliott Zaretsky, Founder and President
Delivers a broad range of standard performance features like Ac-
tive-Trac Suspension and a powerful 50 amp PG VSI controller
on a very compact and maneuverable frame.

740   One Thousand FS
Fortress
P.O.Box 489
Clovis, CA   93613-489
559-322-5437
Fax: 559-323-0299

741   Permobil Max 90
Permobil
4020 Christopher Way
Plano, TX   75024
877-394-3941
mumu.moorthi@sigmabatteries.com
www.sigmabatteries.com

742   Permobil Super 90
Permobil
4020 Christopher Way
Plano, TX   75024
877-394-3941
mumu.moorthi@sigmabatteries.com
www.sigmabatteries.com

743   Power Wheelchairs
LaBac Systems
3845 Forest St
Denver, CO   80207-2516
800-370-6808
www.falconrehab.net

Power tilt and recline seating systems for wheelchairs, offering
more comfort and dependability for the physically challenged.

744   Power for Off-Pavement
Redman Powerchair
1601 S Pantano Road
Suite 107
Tucson, AZ   85710-2076
520-546-6002
800-727-6684
Fax: 520-546-5530
www.redmanpowerchair.com

Don Redman, CEO
Paula Redman, CFO
Scott Evans, Regulatory Affairs
Samuel Redman, General manager
Power-drive wheelchair has a solid seat and can handle safely and
securely knolls and off-pavement terrain.

Wheelchairs: Racing

745   Eagle Sportschairs, LLC
2351 Parkwood Rd
Snellville, GA   30039-4003

770-972-0763
800-932-9380
Fax: 770-985-4885
eaglesportschairs@gmail.com
www.eaglesportschairs.com

Barry Ewing, Owner
The Eagle line of custom lightweight performance chairs includes a range of options to fit all racing and sport needs including; track, baseball, quad-rugby, tennis, field events and waterskiing. Also popular for daily use. We are able to customize any chair to accommodate size and disability and all frames have a full five year warranty.

746   East Penn Manufacturing Company
East Penn Manufacturing Company
Deka Road P.O.Box 147
Lyon Station, PA   19536-147

610-682-6361
Fax: 610-682-4781
contactus@eastpenn-deka.com
www.eastpenn-deka.com

Harold DeLight, Breidegam
Chairman
Specially engineered for demanding deep-cycle applications Gelled electrolyte Deka Dominator Batteries provides maintenance-free operation, longer battery life and hours of reliable performance. Their excellent recharge characteristics provide quick turn around time.

747   Invacare Top End
1 Invacare Way
Elyria, OH   44035-4107

440-329-6000
800-333-6900
Fax: 877-619-7996
info@invacare.com
www.invacare.com

A. Malachi Mixon, III, Chairman of the Board
Gerald B. Blouch, President and Chief Executive Officer
Joseph B. Richey, II, President - Invacare Technologies Division & SVP
Robert K. Gudbranson, Senior Vice President and Chief Financial Officer
Manufacturers of light weight, rigid, sport-specific wheelchairs such as the Eliminator line of racing chairs, T-3 tennis and softball chairs, and the Terminator for quad rugby and basketball. The Excelerator, XLT three-wheel hand cycle for adults and juniors. Check out our full line of wheelchairs to fit every need. $1,895-$2,495

748   Invacare Top End Excelerator XLT Gold Handcyle
Maxi Aids
42 Executive Blvd
Farmingdale, NY   11735-4710

631-752-0521
800-522-6294
Fax: 631-752-0689
TTY: 631-752-0738
sales@maxiaids.com
www.maxiaids.com

Elliott Zaretsky, Founder and President
It's been completely re-designed to be light and faster with more control than ever before. The 27 speeds operated by Shimano Rapid fire hands-on-shifter/brake delivers smooth, responsive shifting and braking right at your fingertips. No foot pedaling! *$3036.00*

Associations

Associations

749 Indiana Association for Home and Hospice Care
6320-G Rucker Rd
Indianapolis, IN 46220   317-775-6675
                                      Fax: 317-775-6674
                                      savannah@iahhc.org
                                      www.iahhc.org

Gloria Horton, President & Co-Chair
Evan Reinhardt, Executive Director
Katie Ociepka, Director of Development
Tori Raderstorf, Communications & Event Coordinator
The Indiana Association for Home & Hospice Care (IAHHC) represents home nursing services and inpatient hospice care services. The association offers education and resources, advocacy and a career center to its members.

750 Volunteers of America
1660 Duke St
Alexandria, VA 22314   703-341-5000
                                            800-899-0089
                                            info@voa.org
                                            www.voa.org

Richard Cavanagh, Chair
Michael King, President & CEO
Joseph A Budzynski, Executive Vice President & Chief Financial Officer
Jatrice Martel Gaiter, Executive Vice President of External Affairs
Volunteers of America is a non-profit organization serving people with disabilities and behavioral health issues. Some services offered by them include housing and healthcare, community outreach, mental health services and senior care.

General Disabilities

751 A Loving Spoonful
1449 Powell St.
Vancouver, BC, Canada   V5L-1G8   604-682-6325
                                      Fax: 604-682-6327
                                      info@alovingspoonful.org
                                      alovingspoonful.org

Dean Malone, President
Christopher LaPrairie, Vice President
Ken Channon, Treasurer
Easter Armas, Secretary/Founder
A Loving Spoonful is a volunteer-driven, non-partisan Society that provides free, nutritious meals to people living with HIV/AIDS in Greater Vancouver. Every week volunteers deliver frozen meals and snack packs to men, women and children who are primarily homebound with AIDS.
1989

752 ACS Federal Healthcare
5270 Shawnee Rd.
Alexandria, VA 22312-2310   703-941-4387
Kimberly Brown, Executive Director
Project RSVP supports the SSA's initiative to expand operations vocational rehabilitation services through a national network of private providers. Rehabilitation companies interested in gaining access to a new client base, acquiring a new funding stream, and developing creative service delivery and entrepreneurial partnerships, may benefit from such a program.

753 AHEAD Association
107 Commerce Centre Dr.
Suite 204
Huntersville, NC   28078   704-947-7779
                                      Fax: 704-948-7779
                                      www.ahead.org

Jamie Axelrod, President
Stephan Smith, Executive Director
Gaeir Dietrich, Treasurer
Katy Washington, Secretary
AHEAD is a professional membership organization for individuals involved in the development of policy and in the provision of quality services to meet the needs of persons with disabilities involved in all areas of higher education, promoting full and equal participation.

754 AIDS Healthcare Foundation
6255 W. Sunset Blvd.
21st Fl.
Los Angeles, CA   90028   323-860-5200
                                            800-797-1717
                                            aidshealth.org

Michael Weinstein, President
Peter Reis, Senior Vice President
Rodney L. Wright, Secretary
Steve Carlton, Treasurer
The Los Angeles-based AIDS Healthcare Foundation (AHF) is a global nonprofit organization providing cutting-edge medicine and advocacy to people all around the world. AHF is currently the largest provider of HIV/AIDS medical care in the U.S.

755 AIDS Vancouver
803 East Hastings St.
Vancouver, BC, Canada   V6A-1R8   604-893-2201
                                      Fax: 604-893-2205
                                      contact@aidsvancouver.org
                                      aidsvancouver.org

Brian Chittock, Executive Director
Ilm Kassam, Program Manager & Clinical Supervisor
Michael Leclair, Chair
Shadi Mojtabavi, Vice Chair
AIDS Vancouver strives to create a community with no new HIV infections while ensuring support for those who are affected through case management services, financial assistance, grocery and nutrition support, and confidential helplines.
1983

756 APSE
416 Hungerford Dr.
Suite 224
Rockville, MD   20850   301-279-0060
                                      Fax: 301-279-0075
                                      membership@apse.org
                                      apse.org

Susie Rinne, President
Derek Nord, Vice President
Allison Wohl, Executive Director
Margaret T. Gilbride, Secretary
Through advocacy and education, the Association of People Supporting EmploymentFirst advances employment and self-sufficiency for all people with disabilities.

757 Abilities!
201 I.U. Willets Rd.
Albertson, NY   11507   516-465-1400
                                      info@viscardicenter.org
                                      www.viscardicenter.org

John D. Kemp, President
Sheryl P. Buchel, Executive Vice President & Chief Financial Officer
Gerard O'Connor, Chairperson
The Viscardi Center is a network of non-profit organizations that provides a lifespan of services for children and adults with disabilities.

758   Advocacy Center
1650 South Ave.
Suite 200
Rochester, NY   14620-1371   585-546-1700
                                     Fax: 585-224-7100
                                     www.starbridgeinc.org

Colin Garwood, President
Jason Blackwell, Vice President
Ida Jones, Vice President
Terry O'Hare, Vice President
A nonprofit organization dedicated to educating, supporting, and advocating people who have disabilities, their families and circles of support.

759   Advocacy Center of Louisiana
8325 Oak St.
New Orleans, LA   70118   800-960-7705
                                     Fax: 504-522-5507
                                advocacycenter@advocacyla.org
                                     advocacyla.org

Dale Higgins, President
Reagan Toledano, Vice President
Paget Bazile, Secretary
James Thompson, Treasurer
The Advocacy Center of Louisiana protects and advocates for the human and legal rights of people with disabilities and seniors living in Louisiana.

760   Advocacy Centre for the Elderly
2 Carlton St.
Suite 701
Toronto, ON, Canada   M5B-1J3   416-598-2656
                                          855-598-2656
                                     Fax: 416-598-7924
                                 advocacycentreelderly.org

Graham Webb, Executive Director
Lindsay O'Callaghan, Chair
Stacey Ferguson, Treasurer
Irene Carriere, Secretary
The Advocacy Centre for the Elderly (ACE) is a specialty community legal clinic that was established to provide a range of legal services to low-income seniors in Ontario. The legal services include advice and representation to individual and group clients, public legal education, law reform and community development activities.
1984

761   Advocates for Children of New York
151 West 30th St.
5th Floor
New York, NY   10001   212-947-9779
                                     Fax: 212-947-9790
                              info@advocatesforchildren.org
                              www.advocatesforchildren.org
Eric F. Grossman, President
Jamie A. Levitt, Vice President
Kim Sweet, Executive Director
Harriet Chan King, Secretary
AFC works on behalf of children from infancy to age 21 who are at risk for school-based discrimination and/or academic failure. These include children with disabilities, ethnic minorities, immigrants, homeless children, foster care children, limited English proficient children and those living in poverty.

762   Advocates for Developmental Disabilities
1225 Lincoln Ave. S
Owatonna, MN   55060   507-451-9769
                                 add_steele@hotmail.com
                        www.advocatesfordevelopmentaldisabilities.com
Laurie Running, Executive Director
Wendy Reller, President
Nancy Deetz, Secretary
Mary Butler-Fraser, Treasurer
The Advocates for Developmental Disabilities is a local agency that advocates the dissemination of information regarding developmental disabilities, the enhancement of existing services and develop new programs on behalf of individuals with developmental disabilities. Its goal is to develop a better understanding of developmental disabilities by families and others interested in the welfare of individuals with developmental disabilities.

763   Alliance for Technology Access
1119 Old Humboldt Rd.
Jackson, TN   38305   731-554-5282
                                          800-914-3017
                                     TTY:731-554-5284
                                 atainfo@ataccess.org
                                     www.ataccess.org
James Allison, President
Bob Van der Linde, Vice President
Margaret Doumitt, Executive Director
Mike Hewitt, Secretary/Treasurer
The ATA is a national network of technology resource centers, organizations, individuals and companies. ATA encourages and facilitates the empowerment of people with disabilities to participate fully in their communities. Through public education, information and referral, capacity building in community organizations, and advocacy/policy efforts, the ATA enables millions of people to live, learn, work, define their futures, and achieve their dreams.
1987

764   American Academy of Audiology
11480 Commerce Park Dr.
Suite 220
Reston, VA   20191   703-790-8466
                                          800-222-2336
                                     Fax: 703-790-8631
                                 infoaud@audiology.org
                                     audiology.org
Ian Windmill, President
Jackie Clark, President Elect
Holly Burrows, Secretary
Virginia Ramachandran, Treasurer
The American Academy of Audiology is the world's largest professional organization of, by, and for audiologists. The Academy is dedicated to providing quality hearing care services through professional development, education, research, and increased public awareness of hearing and balance disorders.

765   American Academy of Environmental Medicine
6505 E Central Ave
Suite 296
Wichita, KS   67206   316-684-5500
                                     Fax: 888-411-1206
                                 defox@aaemonline.org
                                     www.aaemonline.org
Gregg Govett, President
De Rodgers-Fox, Executive Director
Janette Hope, Secretary
James W Willoughby, Treasurer
The academy is an association of physicians and other professionals engaged in investigating and coming up with preventive strategies for medical care relating to environmentally triggered illnesses.

766   American Academy of Pain Medicine
8735 W. Higgins Rd.
Suite 300
Chicago, IL   60631-2738   847-375-4731
                                     Fax: 847-375-6477
                                 info@painmed.org
                                     painmed.org
Steven P. Stanos, President
Jianguo Cheng, President-Elect
Donna M. Bloodworth, Treasurer
Tim J. Lamer, Secretary
AAPM is an organization created for physicians practicing the specialty Of pain medicine in the United States. AAPM works provides the most up-to-date information available on the practice of Pain Medicine, advocate for its members and bring visibility and credibility to the specialty of pain medicine.

767   American Academy of Pain Medicine Foundation
American Academy of Pain Medicine
8735 W. Higgins Rd.
Suite 300
Chicago, IL   60631   847-375-4731
                                info@aapmfoundation.org
                                    aapmfoundation.org

Charles Argoff, President
Marsha Stanton, Treasurer & Secretary
Steven P. Stanos Jr., Liaison Director

The Foundation supports AAPM's core purpose to optimize the health of patients in pain and eliminate the major health problem of pain by advancing the practice and the specialty of pain medicine.
1911

768   American Academy of Pediatrics
141 NW Point Blvd.
Elk Grove Village, IL   60007-1098   800-433-9016
                                      Fax: 847-434-8000
                                         www.aap.org

Fernando Stein, President
Colleen A. Kraft, President Elect
Karen Remley, CEO/Executive Vice President

Organization of 60,000 pediatricians committed to the attainment of optimal physical, mental, and social health and well-being for all infants, children, adolescents and young adults.

769   American Association of Oriental Medicine
PO Box 96503
Suite 44114
Washington, DC   20090-6503   866-455-7999
                                      Fax: 866-455-7999
                                   admin@aaaomonline.org
                                    www.aaaomonline.org

Anne Biris, President
Amanda Gaitaud, Vice President
Aldo D'Aversa, Secretary
Carlos Chapa, Treasurer

Dedicated to the promotion and advancement of high ethical, educational, and professional standards in the practice of acupuncture and Oriental medicine (AOM) in the U.S.

770   American Association of People with Disabilities
2013 H St., NW
5th Floor
Washington, DC   20006   202-521-4316
                                         800-840-8844
                                     TTY:800-840-8844
                               communications@aapd.com
                                        www.aapd.com

Edward Kennedy, Chair
Joyce Bender, Vice Chair
Helena Berger, President/CEO
Jason Mida, Director of Development

The largest national nonprofit cross-disability member organization in the United States, dedicated to ensuring economic self-sufficiency and political empowerment for Americans with disabilities. AAPD works in coalition with other disability organizations for the full implimentation and enforcement of disability nondiscrimination laws, particularly the Americans With Disabilities Act (ADA) of 1990 and the Rehabilitation Act of 1973.

771   American Association on Health and Disability
110 N. Washington St.
Suite 328-J
Rockville, MD   20850   301-545-6140
                                      Fax: 301-545-6144
                                         contact@aahd.us
                                          www.aahd.us

Ronald G. Blankenbaker, President
Roberta Carlin, Executive Director
Charles E. Drum, Director

The American Association on Health and Disability (AAHD) is a cross-disability national non-profit organization committed to promoting health and wellness initiatives for children and adults with disabilities.

772   American Board of Professional Disability Consultants
4525 Harding Rd.
Second Floor
Nashville, TN   37205   615-327-2984
                                      Fax: 615-327-9235
                                    americanbd@aol.com
                                 www.americandisability.org

Kenneth Anchor, Executive Director

Certifies physicians, psychologists, attorneys, and counselors as specialists in disability and personal injury.

773   American Botanical Council
6200 Manor Rd.
Austin, TX   78723   512-926-4900
                                      Fax: 512-926-2345
                                     abc@herbalgram.org
                                    www.herbalgram.org

Neil Blomquist, Founder/President
Michael J. Balick, Vice President
Hannah Bauman, Assistant Editor
Janie Carter, Membership Coordinator

The American Botanical Council (ABC) is the leading independent, nonprofit, international member-based organization providing education using science-based ad traditional information to promote the responsible use of herbal medicine.

774   American Camp Association
5000 State Rd. 67 N.
Martinsville, IN   46151-7902   765-342-8456
                                         800-428-2267
                                      Fax: 765-342-2065
                                       www.acacamps.org

Ross Turner, Chair
Tony Oyenarte, Vice Chair
Tom Rosenberg, Chief Executive Officer
Craig Whiting, Treasurer

The American Camp Association is a community of camp professionals who have joined together to share their knowledge and experience and to ensure the quality of camp programs. Children and adults have the opportunity to engage with a community, developing character building and other skills.

775   American Chiropractic Association
1701 Clarendon Blvd.
Suite 200
Arlington, VA   22209   703-276-8800
                                      Fax: 703-243-2593
                                   memberinfo@acatoday.org
                                       www.acatoday.org

N. Ray Tuck, Chairman
David Herd, President
Karen Konarski, Vice President
Kelli Pearson, Director, Gov. District 1

The ACA is a professional organization representing Doctors of Chiropratic. Its mission is to preserve, protect, improve, and promote the chiropractic profession and the services of Doctors of Chiropratic for the benefit of the patients they serve. The purpose of the ACA is to provide leadership in health care and a positive vision for the chiropractic profession and its natural approach to health and wellness.

776   American College of Advancement in Medicine
380 Ice Center Ln.
Suite C
Bozeman, MT   59718   800-532-3688
                                      Fax: 406-587-2451
                                          info@acam.org
                                          www.acam.org

Michael Bauerschmidt, President
Lyn Patrick, Vice President/Secretary
Veronica Haynes, Executive Director
Allen Green, Treasurer

The American College for Advancement in Medicine (ACAM) is a nonprofit society dedicated to educating physicians and other health care professionals on the latest findings and emerging procedures in preventive/nutritional medicine. ACAM's goals are to improve skills, knowledge and diagnostic procedures as they relate to complimentary and alternative medicine; to support research; and to develop awareness of alternative methods of medical treatment.

777   **American College of Nurse Midwives**
8403 Colesville Rd.
Suite 1550
Silver Spring, MD   20910   240-485-1800
                                              Fax: 240-485-1818
                                               info@acnm.org
                                               www.midwife.org

Lisa Low, President
Carol Howe, Vice President
Stephanie Tillman, Secretary
Joan Slager, Treasurer
The American College of Nurse-Midwives (ACNM) is the oldest women's health care organization in the U.S. ACNM provides research, accredits midwifery education programs, administers and promotes continuing education programs, establishes clinical practice standards, creates liasons with state and federal agencies and members of Congress.

778   **American Counseling Association**
6101 Stevenson Ave.
Suite 600
Alexandria, VA   22304   703-823-9800
                                               800-347-6647
                                          Fax: 800-473-2329
                                        webmaster@counseling.org
                                              www.counseling.org

Gerard Lawson, President
Richard Yep, Chief Executive Officer
Simone Lambert, President-Elect
Brad Erford, Treasurer
The American Counseling Association is a not-for-profit, professional and educational organization that is dedicated to the growth and enhancement of the counseling profession.

779   **American Disability Association**
815 First Ave.
Suite 280
Seattle, WA   98104   205-328-9090
                                             freeman@adanet.org
                                              www.adanet.org

780   **American Disabled Golfers Association**
1295 SE Port St. Lucie Blvd.
Port St. Lucie, FL   34952   772-335-3216
                                               888-346-3290
                                          Fax: 772-335-3822
                                               info@usgtf.com
                                               www.usgtf.com

Geoff Bryant, President
The American Disabled Golfers Association helps to create handicapped accessibility to golf courses for disabled golfers.

781   **American Foundation for Suicide Prevention**
120 Wall St.
29th Fl.
New York, NY   10005   212-363-3500
                                               888-333-2377
                                          Fax: 212-363-6237
                                               info@afsp.org
                                               afsp.org

Robert Gebbia, Chief Executive Officer
Christine Moutier, Chief Medical Officer
Stephanie Coggin, Vice President of Communications and Marketing
the American Foundation for Suicide Prevention (AFSP) is a voluntary health organization that gives those affected by suicide a nationwide community empowered by research, education and advocacy to take action against this disease. AFSP achieves their goal by funding scientific research, educating th public about mental health and suicide prevention, and supporting survivors of suicide lose and all those affected by suicide.

782   **American Herbalists Guild**
67 Broadway
Asheville, NC   28801   617-520-4372
                                     office@americanherbalistsguild.com
                                       www.americanherbalistsguild.com

Bevin Clare, President
Phyllis D. Light, Vice President
Richard Mandelbaum, Secretary
David N. Harder, Treasurer
A non-profit, educational organization to represent the goals and voices of herbalists specializing in the medicinal use of plants. Their mission is to promote a high level of professionalism and education in the study and practice of theraputic herbalism.
1989

783   **American Holistic Medical Association**
6919 La Jolla Blvd.
San Diego, CA   92037   858-240-9033
                                               aihm.org

Mimi Guarneri, President
Brad Jacobs, Chair
Daniel M. Asimus, MD, MSEd, Vice President
Lucia Thorton, Secretary
The Academy of Integrative Health & Medicine unites healthcare professionals from family doctors to psychologists, acupuncturists to nurses, to build bridges between disciplines and offer credible educational and certification programs for licensed healthcare providers.

784   **American Massage Therapy Association**
500 Davis St.
Suite 900
Evanston, IL   60201-4695   877-905-0577
                                             info@amtamassage.org
                                              www.amtamassage.org

Dolly Wallace, President
Joan Nichols, Vice President
Nathan J. Nordstrom, Vice President
AMTA works to establish massage therapy as integral to the maintenance of good health and complementary to other therapeudic processes; to advance the profession through ethics and standards, certification, school accreditation, continuing education, professional publications, legislative efforts, public education, and fostering the development of members.

785   **American Occupational Therapy Association**
4720 Montgomery Ln.
Bethesda, MD   20814-3449   301-652-6611
                                               800-729-2682
                                               www.aota.org

Amy J. Lamb, President
Shawn Phipps, Vice President
Kathleen T. Foley, Secretary
Karen M. Sames, Treasurer
Advances the quality, availability, use and support of occupational therapy through standard setting, advocacy, education, and research on behalf of its members.

786   **American Organization for Bodywork Therapies of Asia**
PO Box 343
West Berlin, NJ   08091   856-809-2953
                                          Fax: 856-809-2958
                                             office@aobta.org
                                              www.aobta.org

Wayne Mylin, Managing Director
Lauren Paap, President
Andrea Sullivan, Vice President
Deborah Valentine Smith, Treasurer/Secretary
The American Organization for Bodywork Therapies of Asia (AOBTA) is a professional membership organizaton that promotes Asian Bodywork Therapy and its practitioners while honoring a diversity of disciplines. AOBTA serves its community of members by supporting appropriate credentialing; defining scope of practice and educational standards; and providing resources for training, professional development and networking. AOBTA advocates public policy to protect its members.

787 American Pain Society
American Academy of Pain Medicine
8735 W. Higgins Rd.
Suite 300
Chicago, IL 60631   847-675-4715
                          info@americanpainsociety.org
                          americanpainsociety.org

David A. Williams, President
William Maxiner, President Elect
Jennifer Haythornthwaite, Treasurer
Patrick M. Dougherty, Secretary
The American Pain Society is a multidisciplinary community that
brings together a diverse group of scientists, clinicians, and other
professionals to increase the knowledge of pain and transform
public policy and clinical practice to reduce pain-related
suffering.

788 American Public Health Association
800 I St., NW
Washington, DC 20001   202-777-2742
                               Fax: 202-777-2534
                               TTY:202-777-2500
                               www.apha.org

Jos, Ram¢n Fern ndez, Chair
Georges C. Benjamin, MD, Executive Director
Benjamin H. Hernandez, Treasurer
Thomas C. Quade, President
APHA is the oldest, largest and most diverse organization of public health professionals in the world. The association works to
protect all Americans and their communities from preventable,
seriuous health threats. APHA represents a broad array of health
officials, educators, environmentalists, policy-makers and health
providers at all levels working both within and outside governmental organizations and educational institutions.
1972

789 American Red Cross
431 18th Str., NW
Washington, DC 20006   202-303-4498
                                          800-733-2767
                                          www.redcross.org

Bonnie McElveen-Hunter, Chairman
Gail J. McGovern, President/CEO
Melissa B. Hurst, Chief Human Resources Officer
Jennifer L. Hawkins, Corporate Secretary & Chief of Staff
The American Red Cross offers services in five other areas: community services that help the needy; support and comfort for military members and their families; the collection, processing and
distribution of lifesaving blood and blood products; educational
programs that promote health and safety; and international relief
and development programs.

790 American Society for the Alexander Technique
11 W. Monument Ave.
Suite 510
Dayton, OH 45402-1233   937-586-3732
                                          800-473-0620
                               webteam@AmSATonline.org
                                          www.amsat.ws
Rick Carbaugh, Chair
Lisa Levinson, Treasurer
Holly Rocke, Secretary
Claire Creese, Member at Large
The Alexander Technique is a self-help method for improving
balance and coordination and increasing movement awareness by
eliminating habitual reactions of misuse in every day activities.
AmSats mission is to define, maintain and promote the Alexander
Technique at its highest standard of professional practice and
conduct.

791 American Society of Bariatric Physicians
101 University Blvd.
Suite 330
Denver, CO 80206   303-770-2526
                               Fax: 303-779-4834
                               info@obesitymedicine.org
                                          www.asbp.org

Deborah Bade Horn, President
Craig Primack, Vice President
Carly Crosby, Interim Executive Director
Rachel Nevers, Communication Manager
The American Society of Bariatric Physicians is an international
association and allied healthcare professionals with special inter-
est and experience in the comprehensive treatment of over-
weight, obesity and related disorders.

792 American Society of Clinical Hypnosis
140 N. Bloomingdale Rd.
Bloomingdale, IL 60108   630-980-4740
                               Fax: 630-351-8490
                                          info@asch.net
                                          www.asch.net

Milton H. Erickson, Founder
To provide and encourage education programs to further the
knowledge, understanding, and application of hypnosis in health
care; to encourage research and scientific publication in the field
of hypnosis; to promote the further recognition and acceptance of
hypnosis as an important tool in clinical health care and focus for
scientific research; to cooperate with other professional societies
that share mutual goals, ethics, and interests.

793 American Tinnitus Association
522 S.W. 5th Ave.
Suite 825
Portland, OR 97204-2143   503-248-9985
                                          800-634-8978
                               Fax: 503-248-0024
                                          tinnitus@ata.org
                                          ata.org

LaGuinn Sherlock, Chair
Randy E. Philips, Vice Chair
Scott C. Mitchell, Secretary
Gary P. Reul, Treasurer
ATA is the only patient-centered membership association that di-
rectly funds research related to tinnitus. ATA's research program
focuses on providing seed grants for the most new areas of
tinnitus scientific exploration.

794 Amputee Coalition
9303 Center St.
Suite 100
Manassas, VA 20110   865-524-8772
                                          888-267-5669
                                          amputee-coalition.org

Dan Berchinski, Chairman
John Kenney, Vice Chair
Thomas Coakley, Treasurer
David S. Sanders, Secretary
The Aputee Coalition is a nonprofit organization dedicated to as-
sisting and empowering people affected by limb loss through ed-
ucation, support groups and vocal advocacy.

795 Anxiety and Depression Association of America
8701 Georgia Ave.
Suite 412
Silver Spring, MD 20910   240-485-1001
                               Fax: 240-485-1035
                               information@adaa.org
                                          adaa.org

Karen Cassiday, President
Risa B. Weisberg, Treasurer
Cindy J. Aaronson, Secretary
The Anxiety and Depression Association of America (ADAA) is
an international nonprofit organization and a leader in education,
training, and research for anxiety, OCD, PTSD, depression, and
related disorders. ADAA encourages the advancement of scientific knowledge about the causes and treatment for mental health
issues.

796   Association for Applied Psychophysiology and Biofeedback
10200 W 44th Ave.
Suite 304
Wheat Ridge, CO   80033   303-422-8436
                                                 800-477-8892
                                                 info@aapb.org
                                                 www.aapb.org
Gabriel E. Sella, President
Patrick R. Steffen, President Elect
Mari Swingle, Board Member
Fred B. Shaffer, Treasurer
Provides names and phone numbers of local chapters. Mission is
to advance the development, dissemination and utilization of
knowledge about applied psychophysiology and biofeedback to
improve health and the quality of life through research, educa-
tion, and practice.

797   Association for Persons in Supported Employment
414 Hungerford Dr.
Suite 224
Rockville, MD   20850   301-279-0060
                                            Fax: 301-279-0075
                                                 cesp@apse.org
                                                 www.apse.org
Derek Nord, President
Allison Wohl, Executive Director
Jenny Stonemeier, Deputy Executive Director
Boshia McRoy, Administrative Associate
The Association of People Supporting Employment First (APSE)
is the only national organization with an exclusive focus on inte-
grated employment and career advancement opportunities for in-
dividuals with disabilities.
1988

798   Association for Persons with Severe Handicaps (TASH)
1875 Eye St. NW
Suite 582
Washington, DC   20006   202-429-2080
                                            Fax: 202-540-9019
                                                 info@tash.org
                                                 www.tash.org
Ruite-Marie Beckwith, Executive Director
Raquel Rosa, Special Projects Manager
Dawn Brown, Development Director
International association of people with disabilities, their family
members, other advocates and professionals, fighting for a soci-
ety in which inclusion of all people in all aspects of society is the
norm.

799   Association of Assistive Technology Act Programs
1020 S. Spring
Springfield, IL   62704   217-522-7985
                                             TTY:217-522-9966
                                                 www.ataporg.org
Alan Knue, Chair
Sachin Pavithran, Vice Chair
David Scherer, Treasurer
Wade Wingler, Secretary
The Association of Assistive Technology Act Programs (ATAP)
is a national, member-based organization, comprised of state
Assistive Technology Act Programs funded under the Assistive
Technology Act (AT Act).

800   Association of Children's Residential Centers
648 N. Plankinton Ave.
Suite 425
Milwaukee, WI   53203   877-332-2272
                                     ksisson@togetherthevoice.org
                                               togetherthevoice.org
Laurah Currey, President
Kari Sisson, Executive Director
Joe Ford, Vice President
Kerry Ann Goldsmith, Secretary
The Association of Children's Residential Centers believes that
children and adolescents, and their families, are entitled to treat-
ment which offers the maximum opportunity for growth and
change. They believe that clinically crafted residential treatment
options, ranging from community based homes through institu-

tional environments, are essential components in a
comprehensive system of behavioral health care.

801   Association of Educational Therapists
7044 S. 13th St.
Oak Creek, WI   53154   414-908-4949
                                       customercare@AETOnline.org
                                                 www.aetonline.org
Judith Brennan, President
Polly Brophy, Treasurer
Kaye Ragland, Secretary
Jose Chavez, Director
Educational Therapy offers children and adults with learning dis-
abilities and other learning challenges a wide range of intensive,
individualized interventions designed to remediate learning
problems.

**802   Association of Medical Professionals with Hearing Losses
         (Amphl)**
4850 Reliance Rd.
Front Royal, VA   22630   amphl.org
Jaime Wilson, President
Kyle DeCarlo, Vice President
Sarah Hein, Secretary
Keiko Kamiya, Treasurer
The Association of Medical Professionals With Hearing Losses
provides information, promote advocacy and mentorship, and
create a network for individuals with hearing loss interested in or
working in health care fields.

803   Association of University Centers on Disabilities
AUCD
1100 Wayne Ave.
Suite 1000
Silver Spring, MD   20910   301-588-8252
                                                 aucdinfo@aucd.org
                                                 www.aucd.org
Celia Feinstein, President
Andrew J. Imparato, Executive Director
Amy Hewitt, Treasurer
Philip Wilson, Secretary
The central office for the 61 University Centers for Excellence
programs and 21 Mental Retardation and Developmental Disabil-
ities Research Centers and is their representative to the federal
government. UCEDD's are located at major universities and
teaching hospitals. UCCED's target their activities to support the
independence, productivity and integration into the community
of individuals with developmental disabilities.

804   Bastyr University Natural Health Clinic
3670 Stone Way N.
Seattle, WA   98103   206-834-4100
                                            Fax: 206-834-4131
                                                 www.bastyrcenter.org

805   Beach Center on Families and Disability
University of Kansas
1200 Sunnyside Ave.
Rm 3134
Lawrence, KS   66045-7534   785-864-7600
                                                 866-783-3378
                                                 beachcenter@ku.edu
                                                 www.beachcenter.org
Michael Wehmeyer, Director
A federally funded center that conducts research and training in
the factors that contribute to the successful functioning of fami-
lies with members who have disabilities.

806   Beacon Tree
9201 Arboretum Pkwy
Suite 315
N. Chesterfield, VA 23236   800-414-6427
                                            info@beacontree.org
                                               beacontree.org

Anne Moss Rogers, President
Steven Genett, Vice President
Chris Demetrlus, Secretary/Treasurer
Lynette Brinkerhoff, Executive Director
Beacon Tree Foundation is dedicated to being an advocate for the family, providing education about treatment and financial resources to help heal children and teens struggling with mental health issues and to provide hope for the future.

807   Birth Defect Research for Children
976 Lake Baldwin Ln.
Suite 104
Orlando, FL 32814   407-895-0802
                                          staff@birthdefects.org
                                           www.birthdefects.org

Betty Mekdeci, Manager/Founder
A nonprofit organization that provides information about birth defects of all kinds to parents and professionals. Offers a library of medical books and files of information on less common categories of birth defects and is involved in research to discover possible links between environmental exposures and birth defects.

808   Bonnie Prudden Myotherapy
4330 E. Havasu Rd.
Tucson, AZ 85718   520-529-3979
                                          www.bonnieprudden.com

Enid Whittaker, Managing Director
Sandy Dirks, Treasurer
Lori Drummond, Secretary
Myotherapy is a method for relaxing muscle spasm, improving circulation and alleviating pain. Pressure is applied using elbows, knuckled or fingers, and held for several seconds to defuse trigger points. The success of this method depends upon the use of specific corrective exercises of the freed muscles.

809   Brain & Behavior Research Foundation
90 Park Ave.
16th Fl.
New York, NY 10016   646-681-4888
                                            800-829-8289
                                          info@bbrfoundation.org
                                            bbrfoundation.org

Jeffrey Borenstein, President & CEO
Anne Abramson, Vice President
John B. Hollister, Secretary
Arthur Radin, Treasurer
The Brain & Behavior Research Foundation is a nonprofit organization committed to alleviating the suffering caused by mental illness by awarding grants that will lead to advances and breakthroughs in scientific research.

810   Brain Injury Association of America
1608 Spring Hill Rd.
Suite 110
Vienna, VA 22812   703-761-0750
                                            800-444-6443
                                          Fax: 703-761-0755
                                          shconnors@biausa.org
                                            www.biausa.org

Bud Elkind, Chairman
Douglas L. Brewer, Vice Chairman
Susan H. Connors, President/CEO
Gregory W. Brickner, Treasurer
The Brain Injury Association of America (BIAA) is the leading national organization serving and representing individuals, families and professionals who are touched by a life-altering, often devistating, traumatic brain injury (TBI).
1980

811   CAPP National Parent Resource Center Federation for Children with Special Needs
15 Court Square
Suite 660
Boston, MA 02108   866-815-8122
                                          Fax: 617-542-7832
                                            info@ppal.net
                                            www.ppal.net

William O'Brien, Chair
Lisa Lambert, Executive Director
Joanna Allison, Clerk
Anne Metzger, Treasurer
A parent-run resource system designed to further the needs and goals of family-centered, community-based coordinated care for children with special health needs and their families. Offers written materials, training packages, workshops and presentations for parents and professionals on special education, health care financing and other topics.

812   CARF Rehabilitation Accreditation Commission
CARF International
6951 East Southpoint Rd.
Tucson, AZ 85756-9407   888-281-6531
                                          Fax: 520-318-1129
                                          TTY:520-495-7077
                                            info@carf.org
                                               carf.org

Brian J. Boon, President/CEO
An independent, nonprofit accreditor of human service providers in the areas of aging services, behavioral health, child and youth services, DMEPOS, employment and community services, medical rehabilitation, and opioid treatment programs.

813   Cambia Health Foundation
Portland, OR   503-225-4813
                                        cambiahealthfoundation.org

Peggy Maguire, President
Steve Lesky, Program Officer
Cambia Health Foundation is the corporate foundation of Cambia Health Solutions dedicated to transforming the way people experience health care to create a more person-focused and economically sustainable health care system.

814   Canadian Art Therapy Association
P.O. Box 658, Stn Main
Parksville, BC, Canada   V9P-2G7 cata.office.manager@gmail.com
                                          canadianarttherapy.org

Haley Toll, President
Michelle Winkel, Vice President
Sharona Bookdinder, Treasurer
CATA is a nonprofit organization that works in cooperation with other provincial art therapy associations to promote education and understanding of the value of art therapy, as well as provide ongoing education and professional standards for this field.
1977

815   Canine Companions for Independence
P.O.Box 446
Santa Rosa, CA 95402-0446   866-224-3647
                                            800-572-2275
                                          TTY:707-577-1756
                                             www.cci.org

John Miller, Chair
John McKinney, Vice Chair
Paul Mundell, Chief Executive Officer
Bob Street, Treasurer
A nonprofit organization that enhances the lives of people with disabilities by providing highly trained assistance dogs and ongoing support to ensure quality partnerships.

816   Canine Helpers for the Handicapped
Canine Helpers for the Handicapped, Inc.
5699 Ridge Rd.
Lockport, NY 14094   716-433-4035
                                          chhdogs@aol.com
                                          www.caninehelpers.org

Beverly D. Underwood, Executive Director

Canine Helpers for the Handicapped is a nonprofit organization dedicated to training dogs in order to assist people with disabilities and promote independence.

817   Cape Organization for Rights of the Disabled (CORD)
106 Bassett Ln.
Hyannis, MA   02601-3800   508-775-8300
                                          800-541-0282
                                    Fax: 508-775-7022
                                 cordinfo@cilcapecod.org
                                     www.cilcapecod.org

818   Case Management Society of America
6301 Ranch Dr
Little Rock, AR   72223   501-225-2229
                                          800-216-2672
                                    Fax: 501-221-9068
                                         cmsa@cmsa.org
                                           www.cmsa.org

Mary McLaughlin-Davis, President
Jose Santoro, Treasurer
Jody Luttrell, Secretary
Kathy Fraser, Executive Director
The Case Management Society of America is an international, non-profit organization dedicated to the support and development of the profession of case management through educational forums, networking opportunities and legislative involvement. Case management workers play a vital role in taking care of a patients' healthcare needs.

819   Center for Assistive Technology and Environmental Access
512 Means St., NW
Suite 300
Atlanta, GA   30318   404-894-4960
                                    Fax: 404-894-9320
                                 catea@design.gatech.edu
                                          www.catea.org

Jon Sanford, Director
Karen Milchus, Associate Director
Charlie Drummond, Administrative Assistant
Sarah Endicott, Research Scientist I
CATEA supports individuals with disabilities of any age within the State of Georgia and beyond through expert services, research, design and technological development, information dissemination, and educational programs.

820   Center for Creative Arts Therapy
4336 Saratoga Ave.
2nd Fl.
Downers Grove, IL   60515   847-477-8244
                            info@c4creativeartstherapy.com
                                 c4creativeartstherapy.com

Azizi Marshall, Founder & CEO
Jennifer Philips, Executive Administrator
The Center for Creative Arts Therapy offers arts-basd psychotherapy services to patients and their families as a healthy, proactive way to achieve wellness and balance in their lives. The Center provides creative therapeutic interventions, as well as professional counseling.

821   Center for Disability Resources
8301 Farrow Rd.
Columbia, SC   29208   803-935-5231
                                    Fax: 803-935-5059
                            David.Rotholz@uscmed.sc.edu
                                    uscm.med.sc.edu/cdrhome

822   Center for Mind-Body Studies
5225 Connecticut Ave., NW
Suite 414
Washington, DC   20015   202-966-7338
                                    Fax: 202-966-2589
                                         pcolina@cmbm.org
                                           www.cmbm.org

James S. Gordon. MD, President
Mark Hyman, MD, Director
Ann Hoopes, Director
Herman Bluestein, Secretary

The Center for Mind-Body Medicine is a non-profit educational organization dedicated to reviving the spirit and transforming the practice of medicine. The Center is working to create a more effective, comprehensive and compassionate model of healthcare and education. The Center's model combines the precision of modern science with the best of the world's healing traditions.

823   Center for Universal Design
NC State University
College of Design, NC State Uni
Campus Box 8613
Raleigh, NC   27695-8613   919-515-8359
                                            cud@ncsu.edu
                                 www.ncsu.edu/ncsu/design/cud

Sean Vance, Acting Director
Sharon Joines, Ergonomist
A federally funded resource center that works toward improving housing for people with disabilities. Provides technical assistance, training and publications on accessible housing and universal design.

824   Cerebral Palsy Foundation
3 Columbus Circle
15th Fl.
New York, NY   10019   212-520-1686
                                         info@yourcpf.org
                                              yourcpf.org

Lisa B. Baird, Chairman
Richard Ellenson, CEO
John Panagakis, Treasurer
James P. Volcker, Secretary
The Cerebral Palsy Foundation is dedicated to assisting and empowering people with celebral palsy through research in both medical breakthroughs and assitive technologies.

825   Challenged Athletes Foundation
9591 Waples St.
San Diego, CA   92121   858-866-0959
                                    Fax: 858-866-0958
                                 caf@challengedathletes.org
                                     challengedathletes.org

Virginia Tinley, Chief Executive Director
Dawna Callahan, Director of Programs
Lauren Ram, Programs Coordinator
James Sa, Communications Coordinator
The Challenged Athletes Foundation (CAF) provides opportunities and support to people with physical challenges so they can pursue active lifestyles through physical fitness and competitive athletics.

826   Change, Inc.
1413 Park Rd NW
Washington, DC   20010-2801   202-387-3725
                                    Fax: 202-387-3729
                                   changeinc@hotmail.com

Gracie Rolling, Executive Director
Offers counseling/assessment, emergency food and clothing referrals, rental assistance and job assistance to disabled persons in the District of Columbia area.

827   Child and Parent Resource Institute
600 Sanatorium Rd.
London, ON, Canada   N6H-3W7   519-858-2774
                                          877-494-2774
                                    Fax: 519-858-3913
                                    TTY: 519-858-0257
                                              www.cpri.ca

828   Children's Alliance
420 Capitol Ave.
Frankfort, KY   40601   502-875-3399
                                    Fax: 502-223-4200
                                 djchoate@windstream.net
                                 www.childrensallianceky.org

Jeff Choate, Chair
Jeff Hardin, Vice-Chair
Elizabeth Croney, Secretary
Chris Peck, Treasurer

An association of individuals and human services organizations committed to being a voice for at-risk children and families. Interacts with the legislative and executive branches of government and assists members in developing services that most effectively meet the needs of at-risk children and families.

829   Children's National Medical Center
111 Michigan Ave., NW
Washington, DC   20010   202-476-5000
                                                 888-884-BEAR
                                                 www.cnmc.org

Kurt Newman, President/CEO
Mark Batshaw, Executive Vice President
Denice Cora-Bramble, Chief Medical Officer
Vittorio Gallo, Chief Research Officer
The Children's National Medical Center provides healthcare services that enhance the health and well-being of children regionally, nationally and internationally. Through leadership and innovation, the organization will create solutions to pediatric healthcare problems.

830   Clay Tree Society
838 Old Victoria Rd.
Nanaimo, BC, Canada   V9R-6A1   250-753-5322
                                            Fax: 250-753-2749
                                            claytree@shaw.ca
                                            www.claytree.org

Kristopher Huberts, President
Dan Dube, Vice President
Glenys Patmor, Executive Director
Darlene Trinkwon, Secrtary
Non-profit society providing day programming for adults with various developmental disabilities governed by an elected Board of Directors and funded by Community Living British Columbia and BC Gaming.

831   Communitas Supportive Care Society
103-2776 Bourquin Cres. W
Abbotsford, BC, Canada   V2S-6A4   604-850-6608
                                                 800-622-5455
                                            Fax: 604-850-2634
                                            office@communitascare.com
                                            www.communitascare.com

Gary Falk, Board Chair
Karyn Santiago, CEO
Angelika Dawson, Communications Manager
Kelly Beaulieu, Chief Financial Officer
Communitas Supportive Care Society is a non-profit, faith-based organization providing care in communities across British Columbia to those living with disabilities, mental health challenges, and acquired brain injuries.

832   Community Enterprises
441 Pleasant St.
Northampton, MA   01060   413-584-1460
                                            Fax: 413-586-1121
                                            TTY:413-584-1460
                                            info@communityenterprises.com
                                            www.communityenterprises.com

William Donohue, Chair
Donald Miner, Vice-Chair
Brittney Kelleher, Treasurer
Joanne Carlisle, Clerk
Community Enterprise provides supported education services in a community college setting; supports employment including job training and placements; also offer transitional services from group homes and other setting to supported living within the community.

833   Council For Exceptional Children
2900 Crystal Dr.
Suite 1000
Arlington, VA   22202-3557   888-232-7733
                                            TTY:866-915-5000
                                            service@cec.sped.org
                                            www.cec.sped.org

Alexander T. Graham, Executive Director
Sharon Rodriguez, Senior Executive Assistant
Craig Evans, Director of Operations
The Council for Exceptional Children (CEC) is the largest international professional organization dedicated to improving the educational success of individuals with disabilities and/or gifts and talents.

834   DB-Link
National Consortium on Deaf-Blindness
345 N. Monmouth Ave.
Monmouth, OR   97361   503-838-8754
                                            Fax: 503-838-8150
                                            info@nationaldb.org
                                            www.nationaldb.org

Linda McDowell, Executive Director
Gail Leslie, Project Specialist
Jeff Denton, Lead Web Developer
Betsy McGinnity, Senior Advisor
Found at the National Consortium of Deaf-Blindness, DB-LINK is the largest collection of information related to deaf-blindness worldwide. A team of information specialists makes this extensive resource available in response to direct requests, via the NCDB website, through conferences, and via a variety of electronic medium.

835   Department of Physical Medicine & Rehabilitation at Sinai Hospital
2401 W Belvedere Ave.
Baltimore, MD   21215-5271   410-601-9000
                                            www.lifebridgehealth.org

Barry F. Levin, Esq., Chairman
Brian L. Moffet, Esq., Vice Chairman
Helen W. Whitehead, Treasurer
Harry W. Kaplan, Secretary
As one of largest, most comprehensive and most highly respected providers of health-related services to the people of the Northwest Baltimore region, LifeBridge heath advocates preventive services, wellness and fitness services and programs to educate and support the communities it serves. LifeBridge is dedicated to advancing the health of the community through a variety of health and wellness programs and services.

836   DisAbility LINK
1901 Montreal Rd.
Suite 102
Tucker, GA   30084   404-687-8890
                                            Fax: 404-687-8298
                                            TTY:404-711-8890
                                            info@disabilitylink.org
                                            www.disabilitylink.org

Dave Zilles, Chairman
Bill Nabors, Vice Chairman
Kim Gibson, Executive Director
Larry Brown, Finance Director
This center for rights and resources is committed to promoting the rights of all people with disabilities in allowing them to be independent, achieve goals, have access to their community and make decisions for themselves.

837   Disability Funders Network
14241 Midlothian Turnpike
Unit 151
Midlothian, VA   23113   703-795-9646
                                            disabilityfundingconsulting@yahoo.com
                                            www.cof.org

Javier Soto, Chair
Jamie Merisotis, Vice Chairman
Linda P. Evans, Secretary
Kenneth M. Jones II, Treasurer

Disability Funders Network is dedicated to the inclusion of the disability in grantmaking programs and organizations.

838   Disability Rights Bar Association
900 S. Crouse Ave.
Crouse-Hinds Hall, Suite 300
Syracuse, NY 13244-2130   *Fax:* 315-443-9725
                                  DRBA-Law@law.syr.edu
                                  disabilityrights-law.org

Scott LaBarre, Chair
Linda Dardarian, Vice Chair
William Myhill, Secretary
Amy Robertson, Treasurer
The DRBA is an online network of attorneys who specialize in disability civil rights law.

839   Disability Rights Florida
2473 Care Dr.
Suite 200
Tallahassee, FL 32308   850-488-9071
                                  800-342-0823
                                  Fax: 850-488-8640
                                  www.disabilityrightsflorida.org

Maryellen McDonald, Executive Director
Paige Morgan, Executive Assistant
Enrique Escallon, Chair
Stephanie Preshong Brown, Vice Chair
A non-profit organization providing protection and advocacy services in the State of Florida. The Center's mission is to advance the dignity, equality, self-determination and expressed choices of individuals with disabilities.

840   Disabled Athlete Sports Association
1236 Jungermann Rd.
Suite A
St. Peters, MO 63376   636-477-0716
                                  meghang@dasasports.org
                                  www.dasasports.org

Fred Schlichting, President
Bryan Krueger, Treasurer
Suzanne Bright, Secretary
Kelly Behlmann, Executive Director
The Disabled Athlete Sports Association (DASA) is a nonprofit organization specializing in adaptive sport and fitness opportunities. DASA relies heavily upon fundraising events, grants, and individual and corporate donations to sustain its mission.

841   Disabled Businesspersons Association
6367 Alvarado Crt.
Suite 350
San Diego, CA 92120   619-594-8805
                                  info@disabledbusiness.com
                                  disabledbusiness.org
1991

842   Disabled Children's Fund
P.O. Box 4712
Crofton, MD 21114   240-929-4281
                                  Fax: 240-929-4367
                                  helpsomechild@gmail.com
                                  disabled-child.org

Bill Collins, Co-Founder
Erma Collins, Co-Founder
Disabled Children's Fund (DCF) is a humanitarian organization committed to serving the indigent and oppressed children and their families worldwide.
1996

843   Disabled Drummers Association
18901 NW 19 Ave.
Miami Gardens, FL 33056   305-621-9022
                                  DDAFathertime@comcast.net
                                  www.disableddrummers.org

844   Disabled and Alone: Life Services for the Handicapped, Inc.
1440 Broadway
23rd Fl.
New York, NY 10018-2326   212-532-6740
                                  800-995-0066
                                  Fax: 212-532-6740
                                  info@disabledandalone.org
                                  www.disabledandalone.org

Leslie D. Park, Chairman
Rex L. Davidson, Vice President
Lee Alan Ackerman, Executive Director
William G. Shannon, Treasurer
A national nonprofit humanitarian organization whose primary concern is the well-being of handicapped persons, particularly when their families can no longer care for them. The organization helps families do sensible planning for and with their disabled children; provides advocacy and oversight when the parents cannot do so; and advises familieis, attorneys, and financial planners about life planning for a family with a member with a disability.
1988

845   Easterseal
141 W. Jackson Blvd.
Suite 1400A
Chicago, IL 60604   312-726-6200
                                  800-221-6827
                                  Fax: 312-726-1494
                                  info@easterseals.com
                                  www.easterseals.com

Rick Davidson, Chairman
Eileen Howard Boone, 1st Vice Chairman
Edward L. Wenzel, Treasurer
Nancy Goguen, Secretary
Easterseals provides services, education, outreach, and advocacy so that people living with autism and other disabilities can live, learn, work and play in our communities.

846   Easterseals
141 W. Jackson Dr.
Suite 1400A
Chicago, IL 60606   312-726-6200
                                  800-221-6827
                                  Fax: 312-726-1494
                                  info@easterseals.com
                                  easterseals.com

Joe Kern, Chair
Fred Maahs, First Vice Chairman
Eileen Howard Boone, Second Vice Chairman
Kathy Daly, Secretary
Easterseals provides exceptional services, education, outreach and advocacy so that people living with autism spectrum disorders and other disabilities can live, learn, work, and play in our communities.

847   Educational Accessibility Services
Wayne State University
5155 Gullen Mall
1600 Undergraduate Library
Detroit, MI 48202   313-577-1851
                                  Fax: 313-577-4898
                                  TTY:313-577-3365
                                  studentdisability@wayne.edu
                                  studentdisability.wayne.edu

848   Elwyn
111 Elwyn Rd.
Media, PA 19063   610-891-2000
                                  info@elwyn.org
                                  elwyn.org

Charles S. McLister, President
J. Richard Leaman, Jr., Chairman
H. Thomas Hollinger, Vice Chairman
Jared G. Culotta, Treasurer
A nonprofit organization developing programs for children and adults with disabilities and disadvantages.

849   Enable America Inc.
101 E. Kennedy Blvd.
Suite 3250
Tampa, FL   33602   877-362-2533
                                     Fax: 813-221-8811
                        richard.salem@enableamerica.org
                              www.enableamerica.org

Richard J. Salem, Founder/CEO
Chris Jadick, Executive Director
Sandy Moonert, Program Director
Enable America's objective is to increase employment among
people with disabilities in the United States.

850   Esalen Institute
55000 Highway One
Big Sur, CA   93920   831-667-3000
                                          888-837-2536
                                       info@esalen.org
                                       www.esalen.org

Gordon Wheeler, President
Cheryl Fraenzl, Director of Programs
Ben Tauber, Executive Director
Patrick Sheridan, Operations Director
An alternative education center devoted to East/West philoso-
phies, experiential/didactic workshops, and a steady influx of
philosophers, psychologists, artists, and religious thinkers.
1962

851   FOCUS Center for Autism
126 Dowd Ave.
P.O. Box 452
Canton, CT   06019   860-693-8809
                                     Fax: 860-693-0141
                        info@focuscenterforautism.org
                              www.focuscenterforautism.org

Patricia A. Cables, President
Timothy Grady, Secretary
Donna Swabson, Executive Director
Fred Evans, Associate Director
FOCUS Center for Autism is a nonprofit center to help children
and young adults with autism spectrum disorder, and other re-
lated disorders, achieve their full potential.

852   Family Resource Center on Disabilities
11 E. Adams St.
Suite 1002
Chicago, IL   60603   312-939-3513
                                     Fax: 312-854-8980
                                       info@frcd.org
                                       www.frcd.org

853   Family Voices
P.O. Box 37188
Albuquerque, NM   87176   505-872-4774
                                          888-835-5669
                                     Fax: 505-872-4780
                              nwells@familyvoices.org
                                 www.familyvoices.org

Nora Wells, Executive Director
Molly Cole, President
Leolinda Parlin, Treasurer
Grace P. Williams, Secretary
Not-for-profit organization dedicated to ensuring that children's
health issues are addressed as public and private healthcare systems undergo change in communities, states and the nation. National grassroots clearinghouse for information and education in
ways to assure and improve health care for children with disabilities and chronic conditions. Provides materials including pamphlets, a newsletter and one-page papers on important topics.

854   Favarh ARC
225 Commerce D.
Canton, CT   06019-2478   860-693-6662
                                     Fax: 860-693-8662
                                       favarh@favarh.org
                                       www.favarh.org

Augusto Russell, President
Fey Lenz, Vice President
Fran Traceski, Treasurer
Antoria D. Howard, Secretary
Provides a variety of programs and services to adults with devel-
opmental, physical or mental disabilities and their families
throughout the Farmington Valley communities of Avon,
Burlington and more. Favarh's programs are designed to enhance
the personal, social, emotional, vocational and living capabilities
of persons with disabilities.

855   Fedcap Rehabilitation Services
633 Third Ave.
6th Fl.
New York, NY   10017   212-727-4200
                                     Fax: 212-727-4374
                                   TTY:646-606-5905
                                       info@fedcap.org
                                       www.fedcap.org

Mark O'Donoghue, Chair
Laurence Ach, Vice Chair
Martha Sproule, Treasurer
Judy Bergtraum, Secretary
Fedcap helps people with barriers achieve economic independence through employment. Through evaluation, vocational and
soft-skills training, job placement, job creation and support programs, each year Fedcap helps thousands of Americans overcome
obstacles, rebuild their lives, and find and keep meaningful
employment.

856   Federation for Children with Special Needs
529 Main St.
Suite 1M3
Boston, MA   02129   617-236-7210
                                          800-331-0688
                                     Fax: 617-241-0330
                                       fcsninfo@fcsn.org
                                       www.fcsn.org

Anne Howard, President
Rich Robison, Executive Director
Maureen Jerz, Director of Development
Michael Weiner, Treasurer
The Federation for Children with Special Needs provides infor-
mation, support, and assistance to parents of children with dis-
abilities, their professional partners, and their communities.

857   Federation of Families for Children's Mental Health
12320 Parklawn Dr.
Rockville, MD   20855   240-403-1901
                                     Fax: 240-403-1909
                                       ffcmh@ffcmh.org
                                       www.ffcmh.org

Sherri Luthe, President
Terry Stevens, Vice President
Muriel Jones, Secretary
Larry English, Secretary
The FFCMH, a nationally family-run organization serves to provide advocacy at the national level for the rights of children and
youth with emotional, behavioral and mental health challenges
and their families. Provide leadership and technical assistance to
a nation-wide network of family run organizations. Collaborate
with family run and other child serving organizations to transform mental health care in America. The correct name is National
Federation of Families for Children's Mental Health.

858   Feingold Association of the US
11849 Suncatcher Dr.
Fishers, IN   46037   631-369-9340
                                       help@feingold.org
                                       www.feingold.org

859 Feldenkrais Guild of North America (FGNA)
401 Edgewater Pl.
Suite 600
Wakefield, MA 01880   781-876-8935
                                      Fax: 781-645-1322
                  executivedirector@feldenkrais.com
                              www.feldenkrais.com
Susan Marshall, Executive Director
This is the organization which sets the standards for and certifies all FELDENKRAIS practitioners in North America. In order to practice, a practitioner must be a graduate of an FGNA accredited program (a minimum of 800 instruction hours over a three to four year period), and agree to follow both the Code of Professional Conduct and the Standards of Practice. FGNA may be contacted for further information about the FELDENKRAIS METHOD or for a list of FELDENKRAIS practitioners sorted by region.

860 Freedom from Fear
308 Seaview Ave.
Staten Island, NY 10305   718-351-1717
                         help@freedomfromfear.org
                                  freedomfromfear.org
Mary Guardino, Founder/Executive Director
Freedom From Fear is a national non-profit mental health advocacy organization whose goal is to better the lives of all those affected by anxiety, depressive and related disorders through advocacy, education, research and community support.
1984

861 Geneva Centre for Autism
112 Merton St.
Toronto, ON, Canada M4S-2Z8   413-322-7877
                                      Fax: 416-322-5894
                                        info@autism.net
                                         www.autism.net
Judy Welikovitch, President
Sandra Fraser, Vice President
Alex Feness, Treasurer
Gabriella O'Rourke, Secretary
The Geneva Centre for Autism's mission is to empower individuals with Autism Spectrum Disorder, and their families, to fully participate in their communities.

862 Goodwill Industries International
15810 Indianola Dr.
Rockville, MD 20855   301-530-6500
                                           800-GOO-WILL
                                      Fax: 301-530-1516
                                      TTY: 301-530-9759
                                   contactus@goodwill.org
                                       www.goodwill.org
Jim Gibbons, President/CEO
Mohamed Alaoui, Regional Director of Operations
Strives to achieve the full participation in society of disabled persons and other individuals with special needs by expanding their opportunities and occupational capabilities through a network of autonomous, nonprofit, community-based organizations providing services throughout the world in response to local needs.

863 Grand Lodge of the International Association of Machinists and Aerospace Workers
9000 Machinists Pl.
Upper Marlboro, MD 20772-2687   301-967-4500
                                            www.goiam.org
Robert Martinez, President
Philip J. Gruber, General Vice President
Dora Cervantes, General Secretary-Treasurer
Offers placements, programs and resources for persons with disabilities.

864 HEATH Resource Center at the National Youth Transition Center
George Washington University
2134 G St., NW
Washington, DC 20052-0001   askheath@gwu.edu
                                           www.heath.gwu.edu
Carol Kochhar-Bryant, Chair
Julianna Taymans, Chair
Carol Hoare, Chair
Susan Wircenski, Chair
National clearinghouse for information about education after high school for people with disabilities. Also serves as an information exchange about educational support services, policies, procedures, adaptations and opportunities on American campuses, vocational-technical schools, adult education programs, independent living centers and other training entities after high school.

865 Haldimand-Norfolk Resource Education and Counseling
101 Nanticoke Creek Parkway
Townsend, ON, Canada N0A-1S0   519-587-2441
                                           800-265-8087
                                      Fax: 519-587-4798
                                       info@hnreach.on.ca
                                       www.hnreach.on.ca
Leo Massi, Executive Director
Ronelda Smith, President
Michelle Martin, Secretary/Treasurer
Stephanie Slaman, Member at Large
Haldimand-Norfolk REACH is a multi-service agency, providing children's mental health services, developmental services, Autism services, youth justice services, family services, a residential program for transitional-aged youth and several early learning and care services including licensed childcare, Ontario Early Years Centre(s) and Community Action Program for Children.

866 Hanger, Inc.
4534 Westgate Blvd.
Suite 114
Austin, TX 78745   512-614-4612
                                           877-442-6437
                                      Fax: 512-614-4615
                                           hangerclinic.com
Vinit K. Asar, CEO
Hanger Clinic specializes in orthotic and prosthetic services with clinic locations across the country.

867 Health Action
5276 Hollister Ave.
Suite 257
Santa Barbara, CA 93111   805-617-3390
                                          www.healthaction.net
Dr. Roger Jahnke, Co Founder and CEO
Rebecca Mclean, Co Founder
Health Action's mission is to foster innovation in healthcare that will increase health status, customer satisfaction, profitability, support provider efficiency and enhance clinical outcomes, and encourage consumer self-managed care.

868 Hearing Health Foundation
363 7th Ave.
10th Fl.
New York, NY 10001-3904   212-257-6140
                                           888-435-6104
                                             info@hhf.org
                                  hearinghealthfoundation.org
Elizabeth Keithley, Chair
Paul E. Orlin, Vice Chair
Robert Boucai, Treasurer
Michael Nolan, Secretary
Hearing Health Foundation's mission is to prevent and cure hearing loss and tinnitus through groundbreaking research and to promote hearing health.

869   High Technology Foundation
1000 Technology Dr.
Suite 1000
Fairmont, WV 26554   877-363-5482
                                       info@wvhtf.org
                                       www.wvhtf.org
James R. Haney, Chair
James L. Estep, President/CEO
Michael J. Basile, Director
Frank W. Blake, Director
High Technology Foundation performs cutting-edge research across a variety of scientific and engineering disciplines. Its members participate in world-class projects from concept through development, in some of today's most fascinating scientific fields.

870   Hogg Foundation for Mental Health
3001 Lake Austin Blvd.
Austin, TX 78703   512-471-5041
                                       haila.yates@austin.utexas.edu
                                       hogg.utexas.edu
Octavio N. Martinez Jr., Executive Director
Vicky Coffee, Program Manager
Haila Yates, Communications Manager
Bridget Lawrence, Assistant Director of Finance and Operations
The Hogg Foundation for Mental Health is a nonprofit organization is dedicated to the advancement of mental wellness for the people of Texas through out-reach programs, conferences, seminars, research grants and more.

871   Homeopathic Educational Services
812C Camelia St.
Berkeley, CA 94710   510-649-0294
                                       800-359-9051
                                       email@homeopathic.com
                                       www.homeopathic.com
Dana Ulman, Owner/Director
Resource center for homeopathic products and services including books, tapes, research, medicines, medicine kits, software for the general public and the health professional and correspondence courses.

872   Hope Network Neuro Rehabilitation
1490 E Beltline SE
Grand Rapids, MI 49506   616-940-0040
                                       855-407-7575
                                       Fax: 616-942-7130
                                       rehabreferral@hopenetwork.org
                                       www.hopenetworkrehab.org
Jeffrey Bennett, Chair
Phil Weaver, President & CEO
Richard Fabbrini, Chief Financial Officer
Jill Szyszko, Executive Administrator
Neuro Rehabilitation is a service line of Hope Network, helping those with brain or spinal cord injuries or other neurological conditions recover through treatment techniques and person-centered care.

873   Human Ecology Action League (HEAL)
P.O. Box 509
Stockbridge, GA 30281   770-389-4519
                                       Fax: 770-389-4520
                                       HEALNatnl@aol.com
                                       www.healnatl.org
1977

874   Immune Deficiency Foundation
110 West Rd.
Suite 300
Towson, MD 21204   800-296-4433
                                       Fax: 410-321-9165
                                       info@primaryimmune.org
                                       primaryimmune.org
Marcia Boyle, President/Founder
John Seymour, Chair
Steve Fietek, Vice Chair
Brian Rath, Secretary

The Immune Deficiency Foundation is the national patient organization dedicated to improving the diagnosis, treatment and quality of life of persons with primary immunodeficiency diseases through advocacy, education and research.

875   International Academy of Independent Medical Evaluators
PO Box 1537
Elk Grove Village, IL 60009-1537   312-663-1171
                                       Fax: 312-663-1175
                                       debbi@iaime.org
                                       www.iaime.org
Charles Xeller, President
James Williams, Vice President
Edward Dagher, Secretary/Treasurer
Sue O'Sullivan, Executive Director
IAIME is an organization serving physicians involved in disability management. Their courses and products cover disability management and evaluations for physicians, health care providers, attorneys, regulators, legislators, and others involved in the care of injured persons.

876   International Association of Yoga Therapists
PO Box 251563
Little Rock, AZ 72225   928-541-0004
                                       www.iayt.org
Dilip Sarkar, President
John Kepner, Executive Director
Amy Wheeler, Secretary
Eleanor Criswell, Treasurer
IAYT supports research and education in Yoga and serves Yoga practitioners, teachers, therapists, health care professionals, and researchers worldwide. Its mission is to establish Yoga as a recognised and respected therapy in the Western world. IAYT also serves members, the media, and the general public as a comprehensive source of information about contemporary Yoga education, research, and statistics.

877   International Child Amputee Network
P.O. Box 13812
Tuscon, AZ 85732   child-amputee.net
Sami Madden, President
Mike Holmes, Vice President
Pat Alexander, Secretary/Treasurer
Joyce Baughn, Director
I-CAN is an Internet mailing list to provide information and support contacts to children with absent or underdeveloped limbs and their parents. I-CAN is dedicated to promoting education, support, information, and empowerment to traumatic and congenital limb different children and their families.

878   International Chiropractors Association
6400 Arlington Blvd.
Suite 800
Falls Church, VA 22042   703-528-5000
                                       800-423-4690
                                       Fax: 703-528-5023
                                       chiro@chiropractic.org
                                       www.chiropractic.org
Huygo V. Gibson, DC, FICA, Chair
George B. Curry, DC, FICA, President
Stephen P. Welsh, DC, FIFA, Vice President
Selina Sigafoose-Jackson, Secretary-Treasurer
Established to empower humanity in the expression of maximum health, wellness and human potential through the universal chiropractic expression and utilization. Strives to advance chiropractics throughout the world as a distinct health care profession predicated upon its unique philosophy, science and art.
1926

879   International Clinic of Biological Regeneration
PO Box 509
Florissant, MO 63032   800-826-5366
                                       Fax: 314-921-8485
                                       icbr@aol.com
                                       www.icbr.com
Dr. C. Tom Smith, Medical Director
Judith A. Smith, Co Founder & Director
Dr. William Johnson, Director of Medical Services

The International Clinic of Biological Regeneration (ICBR) is a leading international cell therapy center dedicated to constantly improving theraputic results of the treatment by selecting newer, safer and more effective forumalations developed by European research centers.

880   International Expressive Arts Therapy Association
P.O. Box 40707
San Francisco, CA   94140-0707   415-489-0698
                                          info@ieata.org
                                          ieata.org

Yousef AlAjarma, Co-Chair
Anin Utigaard, Co-Chair
Fiona Chang, Co-Chair
Janet Raumussen, Secretary
The International Expressive Arts Therapy Association (IEATA) is a nonprofit organization dedicated to supporting expressive arts therapists, artists, educators, consultants, and others using intergrative, multimodal arts processes for personal and community growth and transformation.

881   International League Against Epilepsy
342 N. Main St.
Suite 301
West Hartford, CT   06117-2507   860-586-7547
                                          Fax: 860-586-7550
                                          pshisler@ilae.org
                                          ilae.org

Priscilla Shisler, Adaminsitrative Director
Emilio Perucca, President
Helen Cross, Secretary General
Sam Wiebe, Treasurer
ILAE is a nonprofit organization dedicated to the advancement and dissemination of knowledge about epilepsy, to promoting researcg, education and training to improve service and care for patients.

882   International Women's Health Coalition
333 7th Ave
6th Fl
New York, NY   10001   212-979-8500
                                          info@iwhc.org
                                          www.iwhc.org

Marlene Hess, Chair
Debora Diniz, Vice Chair
Catherine A. Gellert, Secretary
Francoise Girard, President
IWHC provides information and pamphlets on sexually transmitted diseases and other health concerns. The Coalition works to generate health and population policies, programs, and funding that promote and protect the rights and health of girls and women worldwide.

883   Invisible Disabilities Association
P.O. Box 4067
Parker, CO   80134   800-223-TALK
                                          invisibledisabilities.org

Wayne Connell, President/CEOr
Dirk Van Slyke, Chair
Brad Amman, Treasurer
Jim Calanni, JD, Secretary
The Invisible Disabilities Association (IDA) encourages, educates and connects people and organizations touched by illness, pain and disability around the globe.

884   JoanBorysenko.Com
PO Box 1300
Tesuque, NM   87574-9769   gilah@joanborysenko.com
                                  www.joanborysenko.com
Joan Borysenko, Founder
Publishes resources for credible information about the intersection of mind-body health, positive psychology, and spiritual exploration.

885   Job Accommodation Network
Office of Disability and Employment Policy
200 Constitution Ave. NW
Washington, DC   20210   800-526-7234
                                          TTY:877-781-9403
                                          www.jan.wvu.edu

Anne Hirsh, Co-Director
Louis Orslene, Co-Director
Linda Carter Batiste, Principal Consultants
Beth Loy, Principal Consultants
JAN's mission is to facilitate the employment and retention of workers with disabilities by providing employers, employment providers, people with disabilities, their family members and other interested parties with information on job accomodations, self-employment and small business opportunities and related subjects. JAN's efforts are in support of the employment, including self-employment and small business ownership, of people with disabilities.

886   Joni and Friends
30009 Ladyface Ct.
Agoura Hills, CA   91301   818-707-5664
                                          800-736-4177
                                          Fax: 818-707-2391
                                          TTY: 818-707-9707
                                          www.joniandfriends.org
Joni Eareckson-Tada, Founder/CEO
Doug Mazza, President/COO
Laura Pulido, Executive Vice President/CFO
Cate Given, Vice President of Human Resources
A nonprofit organization seeking to accelerate Christian ministry with people affected by disabilities. JAF educates churches and the community worldwide concerning the needs of the disabled and how those needs can be met. JAF sponsors family retreats for families with disabled members.

887   Juvenile Diabetes Research Foundation International
26 Broadway
14th Fl
New York, NY   10004   800-533-2873
                                          Fax: 212-785-9595
                                          info@jdrf.org
                                          www.jdrf.org
Mark Fischer-Colbrie, International Chairman
Ellen Leake, Vice Chairman
Grant Beard, Treasurer
Lisa F. Wallack, Secretary
A nonprofit, nongovernmental diabetes research organization. JDF's mission is to find a cure for diabetes and its complications through the support of research. JDF also sponsors international workshops and conferences for biomedical researchers, individual chapters offer support groups and other activities for families affected by diabetes. JDF has more than 110 chapters and affiliates worldwide. They publish a quarterly newsletter.
1970

888   Lambton County Developmental Services
339 Centre St.
P.O. Box 1210
Petrolia, ON, Canada   N0N- 1R0   519-882-0933
                                          Fax: 519-882-3386
                                          administration@lcds.on.ca
                                          www.lcds.on.ca

Kari Lupton, President
Frank Huybers, 1st Vice-President
Tony Hogervorst, 2nd Vice-President
Frank Backx, Treasurer
A network of experts and volunteers working together to provide services for people with developmental disabilities to facilitate the achievement of their life dreams.

889   Learning Disabilities Association of America
4156 Library Rd.
Pittsburgh, PA   15234-1349   412-341-1515
                                      Fax: 412-344-0224
                                      info@ldaamerica.org
                                      www.ldaamerica.org

Mary-Clare Reynolds, Executive Director
Stephanie Fedro-Byrom, Operations Manager
Joyce Kraemer, Conference Coordinator
Ericka Pardun, Communications Coordinator
LDA's mission is to create opportunities for success for all individuals affected by learning disabilities and to reduce the incidence of learning disabilities in future generations.

890   Learning Disabilities Association of New York State
Learning Disabilities Association of America
2555 Elmwood Ave.
Kenmore, NY   14217   518-608-8992
                                      Fax: 518-608-8993
                                      www.ldanys.org

Jeffrey Baker, President
Charles Giglio, Vice President
Helene Fallon, Treasurer
Martha Bernard, Secretary
The Learning Disabilities Association (LDA) is a non-profit organization advocating for children and adults with learning disabilities. LDA is a three-tiered organization comprised of a national organization, state affiliates and local chapters. In New York, LDA's state affiliate, the Learning Disabilities Association of New York State and its network of 8 local chapters serve as the conduit of information, advocacy and services for individuals with learning disabilities and their families.

891   Learning Disabilities Worldwide
179 Bear Hill Rd.
Suite 104
Waltham, MA   02451   978-897-5399
                                      Fax: 978-897-5355
                                      help@ldworldwide.org
                                      www.ldworldwide.org
Teresa Allissa Citro, Chief Executive Officer
Micheline Malow, Secretary
Learning Disabilities Worldwide, Inc. (LDWr), is an international professional organization dedicated to improving the educational, professional, and personal outcomes for individuals with learning disabilities (LD) and other related disorders.
1965

892   LoSeCa Foundation
215-1 Carnegie Dr.
St. Albert, AB, Canada   T8N-5B1   780-460-1400
                                      Fax: 780-459-1380
                                      chorpestad@loseca.ca
                                      www.loseca.ca

Carmen Horpestad, Executive Director
Jules Lefebvre, Director of Operations
Rebecca McLeod, Human Resources Manager
Practice Patterson, Administrative Coordinator
A non-profit organization that provides support services to adults with developmental disabilities.

893   Mainstream
300 S Rodney Parham Rd.
Suite 5
Little Rock, AR   72205- 4774   501-280-0012
                                      800-371-9026
                                      Fax: 501-280-9267
                                      TTY: 501-280-9262
                                      www.mainstreamilrc.com
1988

894   March of Dimes Birth Defects Foundation
1275 Mamaroneck Ave.
White Plains, NY   10605-5201   www.marchofdimes.com
Stacey D. Stewart, President
Jennifer L. Howse, CEO

The mission of the March of Dimes is to improve the health of babies by preventing birth defects and infant mortality.

895   McKinnon Body Therapy Center
2940 Webster St.
Oakland, CA   94609   510-465-3488
                                      info@mckinnonbtc.com
                                      mckinnonbtc.com
1973

896   Mental Health America
500 Montgomery St.
Suite 820
Alexandria, VA   22314   703-684-7722
                                      800-969-6642
                                      Fax: 703-684-5968
                                      info@mentalhealthamerica.net
                                      www.mentalhealthamerica.net
Reginald D. Williams II, Chair
Paul Gionfriddo, President/CEO
Michelle Hellebuyck, Program Manager
Jessica Kennedy, Chief of Staff/Vice President of Finance
Nonprofit organization addressing issues related to mental health and mental illness. NMHA works to improve the mental health of all Americans, especially the individuals with mental disorders, through advocacy, education, research and service.

897   Metametrix Clinical Laboratory
63 Zillicoa St.
Asheville, NC   28801-2552   828-253-0621
                                      800-522-4762
                                      info@gdx.net
                                      www.gdx.net
Chris Smith, President and CEO
Scott Madel, Vice President of Business Development
Darryl Landis, Chief Medical Officer
Ceco Ivanov, Chief Information Officer
Metametrix Clinical Laboratory is a pioneer and leader in the development of nutritional, metabolic, and toxicant analyses. Metametrix is committed to helping health care professionals identify nutritional influences on health and disease, and laboratory procedures in nutritional and biochemical testing.
1984

898   Muscular Dystrophy Association USA
222 S. Riverside Plaza
Suite 1500
Chicago, IL   60606   800-572-1717
                                      mda@mdausa.org
                                      www.mda.org
Kristine Welker, Interim President & CEO
Karen Lewis Alexander, Executive Vice President
Julie Faber, Chief Financial Officer
Eileen Timmins, Executive Vice President
MDA provides comprehensive medical services to people with neuromuscular diseases at hospital-affiliated clinics across the country. The Association's worldwide research program, which funds over 400 individual scientific investigations annually, represents the largest single effort to advance knowledge of neuromuscular diseases and to find cures and treatments for them. In addition, MDA conducts far-reaching educational programs for the public and professionals.

899   National Association for Holistic Aromatherapy
P.O. Box 27871
Raleigh, NC   27611-7871   919-894-0298
                                      Fax: 919-894-0271
                                      info@naha.org
                                      www.naha.org
Annette Davis, President
Jennifer Hochell, Vice President
Rose Chard, Secretary
Eric Davis, Treasurer
The NAHA is an educational, nonprofit organization dedicated to enhancing public awareness of the benefits of true aromatherapy. It offers aromatherapy Tele-classes & membership benefits, and acts as a referral service.

900   National Association of Blind Merchants
National Federation of the Blind
7450 Chapman Hwy #319
Knoxville, TN 37920   888-687-6226
                                    www.blindmerchants.org

Nicky Gacos, President
Harold Wilson, First Vice President
Ed Birmingham, Second Vice President
Pam Schnurr, Treasurer
Membership organization of blind persons employed in either self-employment work or the Randolph-Sheppard vending program. Provides information regarding rehabilitation, social security, tax and other issues which directly affect blind merchants. Serves as advocacy and support group.

901   National Association of Councils on Developmental Disabilities
1825 K Street NW
Suite 600
Washington, DC 20006   202-506-5813
                                    info@nacdd.org
                                    www.nacdd.org

Mat McCollough, President
Shannon Buller, Vice President
Steve Gieber, Secretary
Dan Shannon, Treasurer
NACDD is the national association for the 56 State and Territorial Councils on Developmental Disabilities (DD Councils) which receive federal funding to support programs that promote self-determination, integration, and inclusion for all Americans with developmental disabilities.

902   National Association of Disability Representatives
1305 W. 11th St.
Suite 222
Houston, TX 77008   202-822-2155
                                    800-747-6131
                             Fax: 972-245-6701
                                    www.nadr.org

Steven Skinner, President
Philip Litteral, Vice President
Barbara Manna, Secretary
Michael Wener, Treasurer
The NADR is an organization of Professional Social Security Claimants Representatives that focus on issues involving policies to protect the interest of people with disabilities. NADR conducts annual conventions open to members and non-members with educational seminars to keep practitioners up to date on Social Security rulings, regulatory changes and practice improvements.

903   National Association of State Directors of Developmental Disabilities Services (NASDDDS)
301 N Fairfax St.
Suite 101
Alexandria, VA 22314-2633   703-683-4202
                                    www.nasddds.org

Bernard Simons, President
John Martin, Vice President
Beverly A. Buscemi, Secretary/Treasurer
The association's goal is to promote and assist state agencies in developing effective, efficient service delivery systems that furnish high-quality supports to people with developmental disabilities.

904   National Business & Disability Council
201 I.U. Willets Rd.
Albertson, NY 11507-1516   516-465-1400
                                    info@viscardicenter.org
                             www.viscardicenter.org/services/nbdc
John D. Kemp, President/CEO
Sheryl P. Buchel, Executive Vice President
The NBDC is the leading resource for employers seeking to integrate people with disabilities into the workplace and companies seeking to reach them in the consumer marketplace.

905   National Center for Education in Maternal and Child Health
Georgetown University
PO Box 571272
Washington, DC 20057-1272   www.ncemch.org
Rochelle Mayer, Research Professor and Director
John Richards, Co-director
Jeanne Anastasi, Senior program specialist
Provides information on children with special health needs, child health and development, adolescent health, nutrition, violence and injury prevention and other issues of maternal and child health for health professionals and the public.

906   National Council on Disability
1331 F Street Northwest
Suite 850
Washington, DC 20004-1138   202-272-2004
                                    Fax: 202-272-2022
                                    TTY:202-272-2074
                                    ncd@ncd.gov
                                    www.ncd.gov
Clyde E. Terry, Chairperson
NCD is a small, independent federal agency charged with advising the President, Congress, and other federal agencies regarding policies, programs, practices, and procedures that affect people with disabilities.

907   National Council on Independent Living
2013 H St. NW
6th Fl
Washington, DC 20006   202-207-0334
                                    844-778-7961
                             Fax: 202-207-0341
                                    ncil@ncil.org
                                    www.ncil.org
Kelly Buckland, Executive Director
Lou Ann Kibbee, President
Sarah Launderville, Vice President
Derrel Christenson, Treasurer
NCIL advances independent living and the rights of people with disabilities through consumer-driven advocacy.

908   National Deaf Education Network and Clearinghouse
Oklahoma Department of Rehabilitation Services
800 Florida Ave NE
Gallaudet University
Washington, DC 20002-3695   202-651-5051
                                    Fax: 202-651-5054
                                    www.okdrs.org
Roberta Cordano, Chair
Paul Kelly, Vice Chair
Fred Weiner, Chief Executive Officer
Jean Cibuzar, Treasurer
The Clearinghouse disseminates information about deaf education and deaf and hard of hearing children ages 0-21, their families, and the professionals who serve them. All subjects related to the development of this population are addressed, including literacy, family involvement, transition, language development, sign language, hearing aids, cochlear implants, and other areas related to education of the deaf.

909   National Disability Rights Network
820 1st St. NE
Suite 740
Washington, DC 20002-3560   202-408-9514
                                    Fax: 202-408-9520
                                    TTY:202-408-9521
                                    info@ndrn.org
                                    www.ndrn.org
Kim Moody, President
Michae Kirkman, Vice President
Virgin K. Marcus, Secretary
Vicki Smith, Treasurer
Voluntary national membership association of protection and advocacy systems and client assistance programs. Promoting and strengthening the role and performance of its members in providing quality legally based advocacy services.

910   National Early Childhood Technical Assistance Center
CB 8040
Chapel Hill, NC   27599-8040   919-962-2001
                                                   Fax: 919-966-7463
                                                   ectacenter@unc.edu
                                                   ectacenter.org

Christina Kasprzak, Director
Betsy Ayankoya, Associate Director
Laura Curtis, Project Coordinator
Assists states and other designated governing jurisdictions as
they develop multidisciplinary, coordinated and comprehensive
services for children with special needs.

911   National Guild of Hypnotists
P.O. Box 308
Merrimack, NH   03054-0308   603-429-9438
                                                   Fax: 603-424-8066
                                                   ngh@ngh.net
                                                   www.ngh.net

Dr. Dwight Damon, President
Don Mottin, Vice President
Melody Damon-Bachand, Executive Director
Dawn Huard, Membership/Member Services
The National Guild of Hypnotists is a not-for-profit, educational
corporation in the State of New Hampshire committed to advanc-
ing the field of hypnotism.

912   National Institute on Disability and Rehabilitation Research
U.S. Department of Education
400 Maryland Ave. SW
Washington, DC   20202   800-872-5327
                                                   www.ed.gov

Charlie Lakin, Director
Conducts comprehensive and coordinated programs of research
and related activities to maximize the full inclusion, social integration, employment and independent living of individuals of all
ages with disabilities. NIDRR's focus includes research in areas
such as employment, health and function, technology for access
and function, independent living and community integration, and
other associated disability research areas.

913   National Organization on Disability
77 Water St.
Suite 204
New York, NY   10005   646-505-1191
                                                   Fax: 646-505-1184
                                                   info@nod.org
                                                   www.nod.org

Carol Glazer, President
Lindsay Beltzer, Chief of Staff
Amber Cecil, Communications Manager
Howard Green, Deputy Director
The National Organization on Disability promotes the full and
equal participation of men, women and children with disabilities
in all aspects of American life.
1982

914   National Rehabilitation Association (NRA)
P.O. Box 150235
Alexandria, VA   22315-4109   703-836-0850
                                                     888-258-4295
                                                   Fax: 703-836-0848
                                                   TTY: 703-836-0849
                                                   info@nationalrehab.org
                                                   www.nationalrehab.org

Fredric K. Schroeder, Executive Director
Sandra Mulliner, Administrative Assistant
Patricia Leahy, Governmental Affairs Director
Rachel Muchmore, Membership Director
NRA members work to eliminate barriers and increase employment opportunities for people with disabilities. They provide opportunities for advocacy and increased awareness of issues
through professional development and access to current research
topics.

915   National Rehabilitation Information Center (NARIC)
8400 Corporate Dr.
Suite 500
Landover, MD   20785-2245   800-346-2742
                                                   Fax: 301-459-4263
                                                   TTY:301-459-5984
                                                   naricinfo@heitechservices.com
                                                   www.naric.com

Mark Odum, Director
Mark X. Odum, Project Director
Jessica H. Chaiken, Information Services Manager
Natalie J. Collier, Library & Acquisitions Manager
NARIC is a federally-funded library and information center that
focuses on disability and rehabilitation information.

916   National University of Natural Medicine
049 SW Porter St.
Portland, OR   97201-4848   503-552-1555
                                                   rwright@nunm.edu
                                                   nunm.edu

David J. Schleich, President
Kathy Stanford, Vice President of Human Resources
NUNM offers two graduate professional degrees in accredited
and recognized programs that prepare you for licensed practice in
many states and provinces: Doctor of Naturopathic Medicine, a
four-year program of clinical sciences and holistic methods of
heal

917   National Vaccine Information Center
21525 Ridgetop Circle
Suite 100
Sterling, VA   20166-4737   703-938-0342
                                                   Fax: 571-313-1268
                                                   contactnvic@gmail.com
                                                   www.nvic.org

Barbara Loe Fisher, Co-Founder/President
Kathryn Williams, Co-Founder/VP
Theresa Wrangham, Executive Director
Paul Arthur, Director of Operations
A national nonprofit educational organization dedicated to preventing, through public education, vaccine injuries and deaths.
NVIC represents vaccine consumers and health care providers,
including parents whose children suffered illness or died following vaccination. NVIC supports the right of vaccine consumers to
have access to the safest and most effective vaccine as well as the
right to make informed, independent vaccination decisions.

918   National Women's Health Network
1413 K St., NW
4th Fl
Washington, DC   20005-3459   202-682-2640
                                                   Fax: 202-682-2648
                                                   nwhn@nwhn.org
                                                   www.nwhn.org

Cindy Pearson, Executive Director
Michelle M. Lockwood, Development Director
Erin Evans, Office Coordinator
Sarah Christophersan, Policy Advocacy Director
The National Women's Health Network improves the health of all
women by developing and promoting a critical analysis of health
issues in order to affect policy and support consumer decision-making. The Network aspires to a health care system that is
guided by social justice and reflects the needs of diverse women.

919   Native American Disability Law Center
3535 E. 30th St.
Suite 201
Farmington, NM   87402   505-566-5880
                                                     800-862-7271
                                                   Fax: 505-566-5889
                                                   info@nativedisabilitylaw.org
                                                   www.nativedisabilitylaw.org

Katie Toledo, President
Zacheree S. Kelin, President
The Native American Disability Law Center is a private nonprofit
organization that advocates for the legal rights of Native Americans with disabilities. Through advocacy and education, the cen-

ter empowers Native people with disabilities to lead independent lives in their own communities.

920   New York Therapeutic Riding Center-Equestria

212-535-3917
Fax: 212-535-3917
programinfo@equestria.nyc
www.equestria.org

Richard Brodie, Board Of Director
The Therapeutic Riding Center is a therapeutic horseback riding progams for children and adults with disabilites living in New York City. Its riding facility is located at the well-equipped Chateau Stables, and staffed by volunteers with experience in physical therapy, osteopathy, art therapy and other areas designed to deal with various aspects of disabled individuals.

921   North America Riding for the Handicapped Association
7475 Dakin St.
Denver, CO   80233   303-452-1212
                                          800-369-7433
                                   Fax: 303-252-4610
                                     pathintl@pathintl.org
                                        www.pathintl.org

Kathy Alm, CEO
Kaye Marks, Director of Marketing & Comunications
Kandis Branum, Executive Asistant & HR Specialist
National nonprofit equestrian organization dedicated to serving individuals with disability by giving disabled individuals the opportunity to ride horses. Establishes safety standards, provides continuing education and offers networking opportunities for both its individuals and center members. Produces educational materials including fact sheets, brochures, booklets, audio-visual tapes, a directory and NARHA's magazine Strides.

922   North Hastings Community Integration Association
2 Alice St.
P.O. Box 1580
Bancroft, ON, Canada   K0L-1C0   613-332-2090
                                   Fax: 613-332-4762
                               communityliving@nhcia.ca
                                           www.nhcia.ca

Sandy Phillips, Executive Director
Lloyd Churchill, President
Janice Stapley, Vice President
Stacy Masters, Treasurer
NHCIA offers daily living supports, life planning, community access, dual diagnosis supports, respite services, assistance with funding and resource referral information. The association works closely with many community services, groups, schools, and businesses to offer individualized supports to children, youth and adults with an intellectual disability and their families.

923   Nurse Healers: Professional Associates International
TTIA Box 130
Delmar, NY   12054   518-325-1185
                                   Fax: 509-693-3537
                               info@therapeutic-touch.org
                                   www.therapeutic-touch.org

Cindy Cole, President
Tama Recker, Communications
Marilyn Johnston-Svoboda, Education & Credentialing
Jennifer Browning, Membership
This international cooperative network of health care professionals is committed to excellence in healing through Therapeutic Touch. Its organization is a world-recognized resource for persons in the field of health care, laypersons and other organizations interested in information on Therapeutic Touch, and for therapists and teachers searching for teaching and learning materials related to Therapeutic Touch.

924   PACER Center (Parent Advocacy Coalition for Educational Rights)
8161 Normandale Blvd.
Bloomington, MN   55437-1044   952-838-9000
                                          800-537-2237
                                   Fax: 952-838-0199
                                        pacer@pacer.org
                                          www.pacer.org

Paula F. Goldberg, Executive Director
Alison Bakken, Secretary
Dan Levinson, Treasurer
Matthew Woodses, President
Mission is to expand opportunities and enhance the quality of life of children and young adults with disabilities and their families based on the concept of parents helping parents. Offers workshops, individual assistance and written information. Provides programs and materials that assist multicultural families, programs for students, schools and professionals with disability awareness puppet and child abuse prevention programs. Computer Resource Center/Software Lending Library available.

925   PEAK Parent Center
611 N Weber St.
Suite 200
Colorado Springs, CO   80903- 1072   719-531-9400
                                          800-284-0251
                                   Fax: 719-531-9452
                                       info@peakparent.org
                                        www.peakparent.org

Barbara Buswell, Executive Director
David Meeks, President
Vanessa Morrison, Vice President
Mark Cloer, Secretary
PEAK Parent Center is Colorado's federally-designated Parent Training and Information Center (PTI). As a PTI, PEAK supports and empowers parents, providing them with information and strategies to use when advocating for their children with disabilities. PEAK works one-on-one with families and educators helping them realize new possibilities for children with disabilities by expanding knowledge of special education and offering new strategies for success.

926   Pacific Institute of Aromatherapy
P.O. Box 6723
San Rafael, CA   94903   415-479-9120
                                   Fax: 415-479-0614
                                       contact@osapia.com
                         www.pacificinstituteofaromatherapy.com

927   Parent Professional Advocacy League
15 Court Sq.
Suite 660
Boston, MA   02108   866-815-8122
                                   Fax: 617-542-7832
                                           info@ppal.net
                                           www.ppal.net

Lisa Lambert, Executive Director
Anne Metzger, Treasurer
William O'Brien, Chair
Erin Edgecomb, Project Coordinator
An organization that promotes a strong voice for families of children and adolescents with mental health needs. PAL advocates for supports, treatment and policies that enable families to live in their communities in an environment of stability and respect.

928   Parents Helping Parents (PHP)
1400 Parkmoor Ave.
Suite 100
San Jose, CA   95126-3797   408-727-5775
                                   Fax: 408-286-1116
                                           info@php.com
                                           www.php.com

Maria Daane, Executive Director
Mark Fishler, Development Director
Jane Floethe Ford, Director of Education Services
Trudy Marsh Grable, Director of Community and Family Services
Dedicated to assisting children with any type of special need: mental, physical, emotional, or learning disability. Mission is to

help children with special needs receive love, hope, respect, and services needed to achieve their full potential by strengthening their families and the professionals who serve them. Developed and implemented numerous programs; produce a variety of educational and support materials, including information packets, brochures, database and a quarterly newletter.

929   People First of Canada
120 Maryland St.
Suite 5
Winnipeg, NB, Canada   R3G-1L1   204-784-7362
Fax: 204-784-7364
info@peoplefirstofcanada.ca
www.peoplefirstofcanada.ca
Kory Earle, President
Dewlyn Lobo, First Vice President
Donna Murphy, Second Vice President
Harold Barnes, Treasurer
People First of Canada is the national voice for people who have been labeled with an intellectual disability. People First is a movement of people who want all citizens to live equally in the country.

930   People-to-People Committee on Disability
2405 Grand Blvd.
Suite 500
Kansas City, MO   64108   816-531-4701
800-676-7874
Fax: 816-561-7502
ptpi@ptpi.org
www.ptpi.org
Mary Eisenhower, President and CEO
John Maloney, Director of Operations
Barbara Capozzi, Chair
Teresa Loar, Secretary
PTPI is dedicated to the advocacy of handicapped people and offer support through the dissemination of information, consultations, coordinating special assistance projects in developing countries and more.

931   Peter and Elizabeth C. Tower Foundation
2351 N Forest Rd.
Getzville, NY   14068-1225   716-689-0370
Fax: 716-689-3716
tas@thetowerfoundation.org
thetowerfoundation.org
Tracy A. Sawicki, Executive Director
Donald W. Matteson, Chief Program Officer
Charles E. Colston Jr., Program Officer
Megan T. MacDavey, Program Officer
The Peter and Elizabeth C. Tower Foundation supports community programming that results in children, adolescents, and young adults affected by substance use disorders, learning disabilities, mental illness, and intellectual disabilities achieving their full potential.

932   Postpartum Support International
6706 SW 54th Ave.
Portland, OR   97219   503-894-9453
800-944-4773
Fax: 503-894-9452
support@postpartum.net
postpartum.net
Ann Smith, President
Lita Simanis, Secretary
Lynn McFarland, Treasurer
Chris Raines, Chair
The mission of Postpartum Support International is to promote awareness, prevention and treatment of mental health issues related to childbearing in every country worldwide.

933   Project Inform
273 9th St.
San Francisco, CA   94103   415-558-8669
877-435-7443
Fax: 415-558-0684
projectinform.org
Dana Van Gorder, Executive Director
Ferdinand Garcia, President
Courtney Landis, Secretary
Andrew Bosco, Treasurer
Project Inform encourages the development of better treatments and cures for both HIV and hepatitis C. The project advocate for innovative, medically-based prevention strategies and provide up-to-date, life-saving information to help people living with HIV and hep C make the best choices regarding their treatment and care.

934   Raising Deaf Kids
3440 Market St.
4th Fl.
Philadelphia, PA   19104   215-590-7440
Fax: 215-590-1335
TTY:215-590-6817
raisingdeafkids.org
Annie Steinberg, Director
This website provides parents/guardians of children with hearing impairments with information and resources. The website is run and funded by the Deafness and Family Communication Center based at the Children's Hospital of Philadelphia.

935   Rehabilitation International
866 United Nations Plaza
Office 422
New York, NY   10017   212-420-1500
Fax: 212-505-0871
info@riglobal.org
www.riglobal.org
Venus Ilagan, Secretary General
Zhang Haidi, President
RI and its members develop and promote initiatives to protect the rights of people with disabilities and improve rehabilitation and other crucial services for disabled people and their families. RI also works toward increasing international collaboration and advocates for policies and legislation recognizing the rights of people with disabilities and their families, including the establishment of a UN Convention on the Rights and Dignity of Persons with Disabilities.

936   Rolf Institute
5055 Chaparral Ct.
Suite 103
Boulder, CO   80301-3326   303-449-5903
Fax: 303-449-5978
www.rolf.org
Christina Howe, Executive Director
Jessica Bystricky, Office Manager
Fahta Carter, Community Outreach Coordinator
Pat Heckman, Director of Education Services
The Rolf Institute is a nonprofit corporation, organized and existing under the laws of California and Colorado. It is recognized by the US Government as a tax-exempt educational and scientific research organization.
1971

937   Ronald McDonald House
1500 17th St.
Huntington, WV   25701-3956   304-529-1122
margaret@mchouse.org
www.mchouse.org
Wade Newell, President
Paul E. Smith, Vice President
Robert E. Yost, Secretary
Daniel Yon, Treasurer
A home-away-from-home, a temporary lodging facility for the families of seriously ill children being treated at nearby hospitals. Each house is run by a local nonprofit agency comprised of members of the medical community, McDonald's owners, businesses and civic organizations and parent volunteers.

938   Ryan White & Global HIV/AIDS Program
Health Resources & Services Administration
5600 Fishers Ln.
Rockville, MD 20857   301-443-1993
                                        877-974-2742
            hab.hrsa.gov/about-ryan-white-hivaids-program
Laura Cheever, Associate Administrator
Paul Belkin, Director of Operations & Executive Officer
Mahyar Mofidi, Director of Community HIV/AIDS Programs
The Ryan White HIV/AIDS Program provides a comprehensive system of care that includes primary medical care and essential support services for people living with HIV who are uninsured or underinsured. The Program works with cities, states, and local community-based organizations to provide HIV care and treatment services to more than half a million people each year.

939   Shirley Ryan Abilitylab
355 E. Erie
Chicago, IL 60611   312-238-1000
                                        800-354-7342
                                   Fax: 312-238-1369
                                        www.sralab.org
Jude Reyes, Chair
Thomas A. Reynolds III, Esq., Vice Chair
Mike P. Krasny, Vice Chair
Joanne C. Smith, MD, President/CEO
Shirley Ryan AbilityLab is the first-ever "translational" research hospital where clinicians, scientists, innovators and technologists work together in the same space, applying research real time to physical medicine and rehabilitation.

940   Society for Post-Acute and Long-Term Care Medicine
10500 Little Patuxent Pkw
Suite 210
Columbia, MD 21044   410-740-9743
                                        800-876-2632
                                   Fax: 410-740-4572
                                        info@paltc.org
                                        paltc.org
Heidi K. White, President
Cari R. Levy, Present Elect
Jeffery N. Nichols, Treasurer
Christopher Laxton, Executive Director
The Society for Post-Acute and Long-Term Care Medicine is the only medical specialty society representing the community of medical directors, physicians, nurse practitioners, physician assistants, and other practitioners working in the various post-acute and long-term care settings. The Society's members work in skilled nursing facilities, long-term care and assisted living communities, CCRCs, home care, hospice, PACE programs, and other settings.
1977

941   Sofia University
1069 E. Meadow Crl.
Palo Alto, CA 94303   650-493-4430
                                   Fax: 650-493-6835
                                        info@sofia.edu
                                        sofia.edu
Qiaoyun Li, Ph.D., President
Johan Vold, Managing Director
Marwan Jabri, CEO/Founder
Sofia University is a private, non-sectarian graduate school accredited by the Western Association of Schools and Colleges focusing on humanistic and transpersonal psychology.

942   St. Paul Abilities Network
4637-45 Ave.
St. Paul, AB, Canada T0A-3A3   780-645-3441
                                        866-645-3900
                                   Fax: 780-645-1885
                                   mail@spanet.ab.ca
                                   www.stpaulabilitiesnetwork.ca
Tom Melnyk, President
Trent Coulthard, Vice President
Amelia Harmse, Treasurer
Harpreet Chaggar, Director

Provides support and opportunities to encourage the development of an individual's full potential through education, advocacy and community partnerships.

943   Student Disability Services
Wayne State University
5155 Gullen Mall
1600 UGL
Detroit, MI 48202-3919   313-577-1851
                                   Fax: 313-577-4898
                                   studentdisability@wayne.edu
                                   www.studentdisability.wayne.edu
Randie Kruman, Director
Cherise Frost, Disability Specialist
Kelly Loftis, Disability Specialist
Kristen Swan, Disability Specialist
Their mission is to ensure a university experience in which individuals with disabilities have equitable access to programs and to empower students to self-advocate in order to fulfill their academic goals.

944   Stuttering Center of Western Pennsylvania
Children's Hospital of Pittsburgh of UPMC
One Children's Hospital Dr.
4401 Penn Ave.
Pittsburgh, PA 15224   412-383-6538
                                        jsyaruss@pitt.edu
                                        stutteringcenter.org
J. Scott Yaruss, Director
The Stuttering Center of Western Pennsylvania is a nonprofit organization that provides specialized assessment and treatment for children, adolescents, and adults who stutter and their families, to provide education, training, and support for speech-language pathologists who work with people who stutter, and conduct an active program of basic and clinical research on the nature and treatment of stuttering across age groups.

945   Technology and Media Division
Council For Exceptional Children
2900 Crystal Dr.
Suite 1000
Arlington, VA 22202-3557   888-232-7733
                                   TTY:866-915-5000
                                   service@cec.sped.org
                                   www.cec.sped.org
Alexander T. Graham, Executive Director
Sharon Rodriguez, Senior Executive Assistant
Craig Evans, Director of Operations
To support educational participation and improved results for individuals with disabilities and diverse learning needs through the selection, acquisition, and use of technology. The secondary purpose is to provide services to members and other units of CEC, to federal, state and local education agencies, and to business and industry regarding the current and future uses if technology and media with individuals with exceptionalities

946   The Advocacy Centre
521 Vernon St.
Nelson, BC, Canada V1L-4E9   250-352-5777
                                        877-352-5777
                                   Fax: 250-352-5723
                                   advocacycentre@nelsoncares.ca
                                   advocacycentre.org

947   The Cherab Foundation
P.O. Box 8524
Port St. Lucie, FL 34952-8524   772-335-5135
                                        cherabfoundation.org
Lisa Geng, Founder/President
Jolie Abreu, Vice President
The Cherab Foundation is a world-wide nonprofit organization working to improve the communication skills and education of all children with speech and language delays and disorders. The Cherab Foundation is committed to assisting with the development of new therapeutic approaches, preventions and cures to neurologically-based speech disorders.

948   The Davis Center
110 Wesley St.
P.O. Box 508
Manlius, NJ 13104   862-251-4637
                                          Fax: 862-251-4642
                                ddavis@thedaviscenter.com
                                www.thedaviscenter.com
Dorinne S Davis MA CCC-A FAAA, Director
Offers sound-based therapies supporting positive change in
learning, development, and wellness. All ages/all disabilities.
The Davis Model of Sound Intervention-an alternative approach.

949   The Hanen Centre
1075 Bay St.
Suite 515
Toronto, ON, Canada M5S-2B1   416-921-1073
                                              877-426-3655
                                          Fax: 416-921-1225
                                          info@hanen.org
                                          hanen.org
Elaine Weitzman, Executive Director
Cindy Earle, Program Director
The Hanen Centre's mission is to provide parents, caregivers,
early childhood educators and speech-language pathologists
with the knowledge and training they need to help young children
develop the best possible language, social and literacy skills.
This includes children with or at risk of language delays and those
with developmental challenges such as Autism Spectrum
Disorder.

950   The Steve Fund
P.O. Box 60923
Washington, DC 20039   202-723-0728
                                          info@stevefund.org
                                          stevefund.org
Terri Wright, Executive Director
Evan Rose, President
Jason Bell Rose, Co-Chair
Alfiee M. Breland-Noble, Senior Scientific Advisor
The Steve Fund is dedicated to the mental health and emotional
well-being of students of color. The fund offers programs and ser-
vices designed to assist both, institutions of higher education and
nonprofits, in improving their capacity to support the mental
health and emotional well-being of students of color. Programs
and services include workshops, webinars, expert speakers,
training and technology innovations.

951   Thresholds Psychiatric Rehabilitation Centers
4101 N. Ravenswood Ave.
Chicago, IL 60613-2196   773-572-5500
                                thresholds@thresholds.org
                                www.thresholds.org
Marianne Doan, President
Dan Klaff, Vice President
Harold E. D'Orazio, Treasurer
Kathy Graham, Secretary
A psychosocial rehabilitation agency serving persons with severe
and persistent mental illness. The agency offers its programming
at 22 service locations and more than 40 residential facilities
throughout Chicago and Northern Illinois. Also offers special-
ized programming for older adults, young adults, parents, the
homeless and the hearing impaired and mentally ill.
Sliding scale

952   United States Disabled Golf Association
598 Dixie Rd.
Clinton, NC 28328   910-214-5983
                                          info@usdga.net
                                          www.usdga.net
Jason Faircloth, Founder
Cheryl Stamp, Board Member
Patty George, Board Member
Vanessa Ward, Board Member
The US Disabled Golf Association provides people with physi-
cal, sensory, and mental disabilities an opportunity to play golf at
the highest level in the USA.

953   United States Trager Association
P.O. Box 1009
Burton, OH 44021-9005   440-834-0308
                                      Fax: 440-834-0365
                                          info@tragerus.org
                                          www.tragerus.org
Joe Rodin, President
Laura Lynn Giubardo, Vice President
Barbara Mason, Secretary
Anna Marie Bowers, Admininstration Director
The Trager approach is a pleasurable, gentle and effective ap-
proach to movement education and mind/body integration. The
Trager approach helps release deep-seated physical and mental
patterns and facilitates deep relaxation, increased physical mo-
bility, and mental clarity.

954   Universal Pediatric Services
6750 Westown Pkw.
Suite 115A
West Des Moines, IA 50266   515-280-2160
                                              800-383-0303
                                www.universalpediatrics.com
Tucker Anderson, President
Universal Pediatric Services provides high tech care to medically
fragile children and adults in the home setting. Emphasis is
placed on the provision of services in the rural areas, the ability to
service high tech needs and the promotion of primary nurse
concept.

955   Upledger Institute Clinic
11211 Prosperity Farms Rd.
Suite D325
Palm Beach Gardens, FL 33410-3487   561-622-4706
                                              800-311-9204
                                      Fax: 561-627-9231
                                          clinic@iahe.com
                                www.upledgerclinic.com
Kathy Woll, Chief Operating Officer
Dawn Langnes Shear, Chief Development Officer
Alex Jozefyk, Chief Financial Officer
JR Olson, Director of Sales & Community
A healthcare resource center recognized worldwide for its com-
prehensive education programs, advanced treatment options and
unique outreach initiatives. The Institute has trained more than
100,000 healthcare professionals throughout the globe in the
therapeutic approach.

956   Waban Projects
Waban Projects, Inc.
5 Dunaway Dr
Sanford, ME 04073   207-324-7955
                                      Fax: 207-324-6050
                                          connect@waban.org
                                          www.waban.org
Neal Meltzer, Executive Director
Gervaise Flynn, Deputy Director
Tim Hagelin, Chief Administrative Officer
Waban Projects is a nonprofit corporation working to create pro-
grams and services for individuals with autism, intellectual,
and/or developmental disabilities.

957   Women to Women
3 Marina Rd.
Yarmouth, ME 04096   888-303-8846
                                www.womentowomen.com
Marcelle Pick OB/GYN, NP, Co Founder/Director
Combination of alternative and conventional medicine in
women's health, bring science and disipline to natural and preventative methods. Publishes the Creating Health Guide, a quarterly collection of articles written by the health care professionals
at Women to Women.

958   World Federation for Mental Health
P.O. Box 807
Occoquan, VA   22125   info@wfmh.com
                                                www.wfmn.global

Gabriel Ivbijaro, President
Porsche Poh, Secretary
Janet Paleo, Treasurer
WFMH is an international membership organization founded to
advance the prevention of mental and emotional disorders, the
proper treatment and care of those with such disorders, and the
promotion of mental health.

959   World Institute on Disability
3075 Adeline Street
Suite 155
Berkeley, CA   94703   510-225-6400
                                     Fax: 510-225-0477
                                     TTY:510-225-0478
                                          wid@wid.org
                                          www.wid.org

Anita Shafer Aaron, Executive Director
Thomas Foley, Deputy Director/Access to Assets Program Director
Katherine Zigmont, Director of Strategy & Operations
Charity Peets, Project Coordinator
The mission of the World Institute on Disability (WID) is to elim-
inate barriers to full social integration and increase employment,
economic security and health care for persons with disabilities.
WID creates innovative programs and tools; conducts research,
public education, training and advocacy campaigns; and
provides technical assistance.

960   YAI: National Institute for People with Disabilities
460 W. 34th St.
11th Fl
New York, NY   10001-2382   212-273-6100
                                          www.yai.org

George Contos, Chief Executive Officer
Jeffery A. Mordos, Chairman
Kevin Hogan, Treasurer
YAI is dedicated to enhancing the lives of people with developmental disabilities and their families. The organization works
with individuals, families government, corporate partners, donors and foundations to ensure that people with disabilities are
recognized for their abilities, achieving the goals that are important to them, and integrated in the community.

Camps

Alabama

961 Camp Evoked Potential
Alabama's Special Camp for Children and Adults
PO Box 21
5278 Camp Ascca Dr.
Jacksons Gap, AL   36861   251-341-0170
                                     800-626-1582
                              info@campascca.org
                    www.efala.org/camp-evoked-potential
Matt Rickman, Camp Director
Amber Cotney, Program Director
Jocelyn Jones, Secretary
Camp Evoked Potential is held one week out of the year for children aged 6-18 with epilepsy at Camp ASCCA. Fully funded by The Epilepsy Foundation, persons wishing to attend the camp must apply. The camp provides a barrier free setting situated on 230 acres of wooded land at Lake Martin. The campe is staffed with medical personnel trained to care for children with all types of disabilities and provides a variety of camp activities.

962 Camp Rap-A-Hope
2701 Airport Blvd
Mobile, AL   36606   251-476-9880
                                Fax: 251-476-9495
                              info@camprapahope.org
                              www.camprapahope.org
Melissa McNichol, Executive Director
Roz Dorsett, Assistant Director
Camp Rap-A-Hope is an organization that offers a one week long summer camp for children who have, or who have had cancer. For children ages 7-17, the camp offers a wide range of summer camp activities, including but not limited to, swimming, kayaking, horseback riding, and arts. The camp is offered at no cost to campers or their families.

963 Camp Seale Harris
Southeastern Diabetes Education Services
500 Chase Park S.
Ste 104
Birmingham, AL   35244   205-402-0415
                                Fax: 205-402-0416
                              info@campsealeharris.org
                              www.campsealeharris.org
Tip McAlpin, Chair
David Jamieson, Vice Chairman
Rhonda McDavid, Executive Director
John Latimer, Camp & Community Programs Director
Offering overnight, family, day and community program camps, Camp Seale Harris is a nonprofit organization that offers residential camps for children and teens with diabetes. With multiple programs in Alabama, the volunteer camp counselors are trained adults living with diabetes, to better help the camp attendees gain independence in learning to manage their diabetes. Camp programs run all year round.

964 Camp Shocco for the Deaf
216 North St E.
PO Box 602
Talladega, AL   35161   800-264-1225
                              rvmilford23@charter.net
                    www.nchpad.org/Directories/Programs/9452
Ricky Milford, Rev.
Camp Shocco for the Deaf is a Christian Camp for children and teens with a hearing impairment, whose parents are deaf or are siblings of a person that are deaf. The camp runs for 1 week and offers a range of camp activities.

965 Camp Smile-A-Mile
Smile-A-Mile Place
1600 2nd Ave. S.
PO Box 550155
Birmingham, AL   35255   205-323-8427
                                     888-500-7920
                                Fax: 205-323-6220
                              info@campsam.org
                              www.campsam.org
Bruce Hooper, Executive Director
Jennifer Amundsen, Program Director
Savannah Lanier, Development Director
Madison Monday, Assitant Program Director
Camp Smile-A-Mile offers 7 different educational camp opportunities for children and their families who have been affected by childhood cancer in Alabama. The programs run all year long, in a variety of formats.

966 Camp Smile-A-Mile: Jr./Sr. Weekend Camp
Smile-A-Mile Place
1600 2nd Ave. S.
PO Box 550155
Birmingham, AL   35255   205-323-8427
                                     888-500-7920
                                Fax: 205-323-6220
                              info@campsam.org
                              www.campsam.org
Jennifer Amundsen, Program Director
Kellie Reece, Family Outreach Director
Camp Smile-A-Mile's Jr./Sr. Weekend Camp is for high school juniors, seniors, and new high school graduates that are both on and off therapy. The weekend camp works to instill independence and responsibility in regards to their diagnosis.

967 Camp Smile-A-Mile: Off Therapy Family Camp
Smile-A-Mile Place
1600 2nd Ave. S.
PO Box 550155
Birmingham, AL   35255   205-323-8427
                                     888-500-7920
                                Fax: 205-323-6220
                              info@campsam.org
                              www.campsam.org
Jennifer Amundsen, Program Director
Kellie Reece, Family Outreach Director
Camp Smile-A-Mile's Off Therapy Family Camp is a specialized camp for off-therapy patients and their families. Campers up to the age of 18 who are no longer receiving therapy are eligible to attend the camp.

968 Camp Smile-A-Mile: On Therapy Family Camp
Smile-A-Mile Place
1600 2nd Ave. S.
PO Box 550155
Birmingham, AL   35255   205-323-8427
                                     888-500-7920
                                Fax: 205-323-6220
                              info@campsam.org
                              www.campsam.org
Jennifer Amundsen, Program Director
Kellie Reece, Family Outreach Director
A program of Camp Smile-A-Mile, On Therapy Family Camp is for patients up to 18 years of age, who are currently receiving therapy. The Family Camp is designed to give patients and their immediate families the opportunity to connect outside of an hospital environment.

969 Camp Smile-A-Mile: Sibling Camp
Smile-A-Mile Place
1600 2nd Ave. S.
PO Box 550155
Birmingham, AL   35255   205-323-8427
                                     888-500-7920
                                Fax: 205-323-6220
                              info@campsam.org
                              www.campsam.org
Jennifer Amundsen, Program Director
Kellie Reece, Family Outreach Director

Camp Smile-A-Mile's Sibling Camp is a specialized camp for the siblings of children and teens with cancer. Campers attending the Sibling Camp range in age from 6-18 and no patients or parents attend the camp.

970　Camp Smile-A-Mile: Teen Camp
Smile-A-Mile Place
1600 2nd Ave. S.
PO Box 550155
Birmingham, AL　35255

205-323-8427
888-500-7920
Fax: 205-323-6220
info@campsam.org
www.campsam.org

Jennifer Amundsen, Program Director
Kellie Reece, Family Outreach Director
A weeklong summer camp session for children,13 through to the 10th grade, who have cancer. The session is open to those who are and aren't receiving therapy, with campers participating in activities such as swimming, snorkeling, and campfires.

971　Camp Smile-A-Mile: Young Adult Retreat
Smile-A-Mile Place
1600 2nd Ave. S.
PO Box 550155
Birmingham, AL　35255

205-323-8427
888-500-7920
Fax: 205-323-6220
info@campsam.org
www.campsam.org

Jennifer Amundsen, Program Director
Kellie Reece, Family Outreach Director
A program of Camp Smile-A-Mile, the Young Adult Retreat is for childhood cancer survivors ages 19-30. The retreat is held over a summer weekend and offers educational and camping activities for participants. Those wanting to attend the retreat do not have to be former campers of Camp Smile-A-Mile.

972　Camp Smile-A-Mile: Youth Weeklong Camp
Smile-A-Mile Place
1600 2nd Ave. S.
PO Box 550155
Birmingham, AL　35255

205-323-8427
888-500-7920
Fax: 205-323-6220
info@campsam.org
www.campsam.org

Jennifer Amundsen, Program Director
Kellie Reece, Family Outreach Director
A weeklong summer camp session for children, ages 6-12, who have cancer. The session is open to those who are and aren't receiving therapy, with campers participating in activities such as arts and crafts, fishing, boating, archery, and canoeing.

973　Camp WheezeAway
YMCA Camp Chandler
1240 Jordan Dam Rd
Wetumpka, AL　36092

334-229-0035
Fax: 334-649-7516
jreynolds@ymcamontgomery.org
ymcamontgomery.org/camp/wheezeaway

Jeff Reynolds, Executive Director
Matt Thomas, Camp Director
Art Mason, Operations Director
For children ages 8-12 with moderate to severe asthma, Camp WheezeAway offers week long summer camp programs that foster confidence building skills. The camp is free and managed by medical professionals. Those with children wishing to attend must apply to the camp and complete a selection process.

974　Easter Seals Camp ASCCA
PO Box 21
5278 Camp Ascca Dr.
Jacksons Gap, AL　36861

256-825-9226
800-843-2267
Fax: 256-269-0714
info@campascca.org
campascca.org

Matt Rickman, Camp Director
John Stephenson, Administrator
Jocelyn Jones, Secretary
Amber Cotney, Program Director
Easterseals Camp ASCCA is Alabama's Special Camp for Children and Adults, offering therapeutic recreation for children and adults with both physical and intellectual disabilities. The camp is located on 260 acres of barrier free woodland on Lake Martin and campers experience a wide variety of educational and recreational activities, including but not limited to: horseback riding, fishing, tubing, swimming, environmental education, arts, canoeing, and zip-lining.　1 week camp fees are $725.00.

975　Happy Camp
Merrimack Hall Performing Arts Center
3320 Triana Blvd SW.
Huntsville, AL　35805

256-534-6455
jsap@merrimackhall.com
www.merrimackhall.com/jsap/camp-merrimack

Alaska

976　Adam's Camp: Alaska
PO Box 242003
Anchorage, AK　99524

907-885-1758
alaska@adamscamp.org
www.adamscampalaska.org

977　Camp Abilities
Alpine Alternatives
2518 E. Tudor Road
Suite 105
Anchorage, AK　99507-1105

907-561-6655
Fax: 907-563-9232
alpinealternatives@arctic.net
www.alpinealternatives.org

Margaret Webber, Executive Director
Nancy Burnette, Bookkeeper/Program Administrator
LaVerne Lee, Director, Day Outing & Camp Alpine
A program of Alpine Alternatives, Camp Abilities is a 1 week developmental sports camp for children ages 9-19 who are blind or visually impaired.　The camp provides 1-on-1 instructional education, with campers participating in physical activities such as swimming, goalball, beep baseball, tandem biking, tack and field events, rock climbing, hiking, canoeing, and archery.

978　Camp Alpine
Alpine Alternatives
2518 E. Tudor Road
Suite 105
Anchorage, AK　99507-1105

907-561-6655
Fax: 907-563-9232
alpinealternatives@arctic.net
www.alpinealternatives.org

Margaret Webber, Executive Director
Nancy Burnette, Bookkeeper/Program Administrator
LaVerne Lee, Director, Day Outing & Camp Alpine
Operated by Alpine Alternatives, Camp Alpine offers a 4-5 day stay to Alaskans who experience some form of disability. Activities offered at the camp include but are not limited to, hiking, canoeing, outdoor games, sports, and nature identification.

Arizona

979 Arizona Camp Sunrise & Sidekicks
PO Box 27872
Tempe, AZ 85285   www.azcampsunrise.org

980 Camp AZDA
American Diabetes Association
5333 N 7th St.
Suite B212
Phoenix, AZ 85014   602-861-4731
                                          JGarcia@diabetes.org
                                          www.diabetes.org/adacampazda
Julie Garcia, Camp Director
Camp AZDA is the Arizona summer camp program of the American Diabetes Association for children with diabetes. The camp is held at Friendly Pines in Prescott, Arizona with children participating in traditional camp activities while receiving educational information on managing their diabetes.

981 Camp Abilities Tucson
PO Box 86838
Tucson, AZ 85754-6838   520-235-2582
                                          campabilitiestucson@gmail.com
                                          www.campabilitiestucson.org
Murry Everson, Camp Director
Maria Lepore-Stevens, Camp Director
Camp Abilities is a privately funded educational sport camp for children and young adults who are blind, deaf-blind or have multiple disabilities including visual impairment. The camp offers sports instruction, with a 1:1 camper to coach ratio, tailored to fit the needs of the individual. The location of camp sessions is the Arizona School for the Deaf and Blind and costs $300.00 per person.

982 Camp Candlelight
Epilepsy Foundation Arizona
3033A N. 7th Ave
Suite 104
Phoenix, AZ 85013   602-406-3581
                                          800-332-1000
                                          info@epilepsyaz.org
                                          epilepsyaz.org/programs/camp-candlelight/
Suzanne Matsumori, Executive Director
Min Skivington, Program Manager
Camp Candlelight provides children ages 8 to 15 a unique camp experience that mixes traditional summer camp with special sessions that teach campers about their seizures and gives them resources to manage the challenges that the seizures represent. Staff inclues a neurologist, several nurses, and a school psychologist, in addition to traditional camp staff who are given specialized training in responding appropriately to the needs of kids with epilepsy.

983 Camp Civitan
5008 N Civitan Rd
PO Box 457
Williams, AZ 56046   928-635-2944
                                          Fax: 928-635-2730
                                          camp@campcivitan.org
                                          www.civitanfoundationaz.com
Robert Adams, Camp Director
Dawn Trapp, Executive Director
Camp Civitan offers week long summer camp programs, and weekend programs throughout the year, to children with developmental disabilities. The camp is fully wheelchair accessible, is staffed by medical professionals and there is a 2:1 ratio of campers to staff. Camp Civitan offers campers the experience of traditional camp activities including, swimming, adaptive sports, fishing, music, arts and crafts, and talent shows.

984 Camp H.U.G
Arizona Hemophilia Association
826 North 5th Ave
Phoenix, AZ 85003   602-955-3947
                                          info@hemophiliaz.org
                                          www.arizonahemophilia.org/camp-programs
Cindy Komar, Chief Executive Officer
Chelsea Bolyard, Program Director
Yleana Highes, Director, Client Services
Camp H.U.G (Hemophilia Uniting Generations) is a weekend camp program of the Arizona Hemophilia Association. The camp is for families who have a member with hemophilia, WWD, and/or other bleeding disorders.

985 Camp Honor
Arizona Hemophilia Association
826 North 5th Ave
Phoenix, AZ 85003   602-955-3947
                                          info@hemophiliaz.org
                                          www.arizonahemophilia.org/camp-programs
Cindy Komar, Chief Executive Officer
Chelsea Bolyard, Program Director
Yleana Highes, Director, Client Services
Camp Honor offers a week long summer camp to children affected by an inherited bleeding disorders. The cost of the camp is $35 for a single camper and $50 dollars for a family (2 or more campers). Camp Honor offers children the chance to partcipate in outdoor activities and educational opportunities. In order to attend the camp there is an application process.

986 Camp Not-A-Wheeze
American Lung Association
Attn: Camp Director
102 W McDowell Rd.
Phoenix, AZ 85003   602-258-7505
                                          Fax: 877-276-2108
                                          PhoenixPrograms@Lungs.org
                                          www.lung.org

987 Camp Rainbow
Phoenix Childrens Hospital
1919 E Thomas Rd
Phoenix, AZ 85016-7710   602-933-0157
                                          ejarboe@phoenixchildrens.com
                                          ccbd.phoenixchildrens.org/support-services
Emilie Jarboe, Camp Director
Camp Rainbow is for children aged 7-17 who have or had cancer or a chronic blood disorder. The camp is offered for one week during the summer, held at camp Friendly Pines in Prescott, Arizona. Campers must be patients of Phoenix Children's Hospital's Center for Cancer and Blood Disorders, with the camp offering participants the opportunity to experience traditional camp activities including but not limited to, horseback riding, canoeing, fishing, swimming, and archery.

988 Lions Camp Tatiyee
5283 W White Mountain Blvd
Lakeside, AZ 85929   480-380-4254
                                          director@arizonalionscamp.org
                                          www.arizonalionscamp.com
Pamela Swanson, Executive Director
Lions Camp Tatiyee is the only organization in Arizona providing a week long summer camp for individuals with special needs. There is no cost for the camp and all of the programs are adaptable. Some activities that campers can participate in are, go-karting, fishing, art, games, cooking, rock wall, swimming, dances and campfires.

989 Nick & Kelly's Heart Camp
Nick & Kelly Children's Fund
1321 E Bayview Dr
Tempe, AZ 85283   480-838-1529
                                          contact@nickandkellyfund.org
                                          www.nickandkellyfund.org

Arkansas

990 **Camp Aldersgate**
2000 Aldersgate Road
Little Rock, AR 72205
  501-225-1444
  Fax: 501-225-2019
  info@campaldersgate.net
  www.campaldersgate.net
Sonya S. Murphy, Cheif Executive Officer
Ali Miller Berry, Director, Programs
Katie Jenkins, Program Coordinator
Kerri Daniels, Director, Development
Camp Aldersgate is a nonprofit organization, offering summer, weekend camps, and year-round social service programs to children, teens and adults with special needs. The camp promotes outdoor recreation and socialization in a completely accessible environment.

991 **Camp Laughter**
Arkansas Children's Neuroscience Center
1 Children's Way
2nd Floor
Little Rock, AR 72202
  501-364-5775
  Fax: 501-364-1649
  camplaughter@archildrens.org
  www.archildrens.org/programs-services

992 **Camp Quality Arkansas**
PO Box 9095
Jonesboro, AR 72403
  830-486-7106
  beth.cameron@campqualityusa.org
  www.campqualityusa.org/ar
Beth Cameron, Executive Director
Jordan Yoes, Camper Coordinator
Paige Parnell, Camp Coordinator Assistant
Betty Baureis, Treasurer
Camp Quality is an international camping program for children with cancer. The Arkansas Camp Quality is held at Camp Powderfork in Bald Knob, Arkansas and offers children and their siblings summer camps and year round camping opportunities. Volunteer doctors and nurses are at the camp 24 hours a day, and there is a 1:1 staff to camper ratio.

993 **Camp Sunshine**
Burn Program at Arkansas Children's
1 Children's Way
Slot 225
Little Rock, AR 72202
  501-364-1635
  wilkinsonge@archildrens.org
  www.archildrens.org/services/burn-progam
Gretta Wilkinson, RN, Camp Director
Camp Sunshine is a 4 day no cost summer camp for children and teens, 4-16, who have experienced burn injuries. Camp Sunshine works to assist campers in the transformation from burn victim to burn survivor. In order to attend the camp, campers must have survived a 10% or greater full thickness burn and/or may have significant scarring, disability or scarring to the hands or face.

994 **Kota Camp**
Junior League Of Little Rock
401 South Scott Street
Little Rock, AR 72201
  501-375-5557
  info@jllr.org
  www.jllr.org
Kimberly Logue, President
Dana Coburn, Vice President, Administrative
Kristen Bextermueller, Treasurer
Whitney Homan, Vice President, Community
Kota Camp is offered to children aged 6-16 with disabilities or medical conditions. "Kota" derived from a word used by the Quapaw Native American Tribe indigenous to Arkansas, means "friend", and reflects the goals of the camp. Children with a disability bring a sibling or friend without a disability, to create an environment of inclusion , participate in camp activities, and promote an understanding of those with special needs. The camp is held at Camp Aldersgate in Little Rock.

California

995 **Bearskin Meadow Camp**
Diabetic Youth Families
5167 Clayton Rd
Suite F
Concord, CA 94521
  925-680-4994
  Fax: 925-680-4863
  info@dyf.org
  www.dyf.org
Janet Kramschuster, Executive Director
Kaylor Glassman, Resident Camp Director
Christi Rossi, Development, Director
Patrick Mertes, Program Manager
Bearskin Meadow Camp, is a camp program offered by the Diabetes Youth Families organization to children (7-13), teens (14-17), and families who are affected by type 1 diabetes. The camp has traditional camp activities as well as educational opportunities for campers.

996 **Camp Beyond The Scars**
Burn Institute
8825 Aero Drive
Suite 200
San Diego, CA 92123-2269
  858-541-2277
  Fax: 858-541-7179
  ccoppenrath@burninstitute.org
  www.burninstitute.org/camp-beyond-the-scar s
Cat Coppenrath, MSW, Burn Survivor Support Coordinator
Susan Day, Executive Director
Benjamin Hemmings, Director, Operations
Camp Beyond the Scars, is a weeklong sleepaway summer camp for children aged 8-17 who have survived a burn injury. Staffed by adult burn survivors, healthcare professionals, and off-duty firefighters, the camp provides an inclusive environment for burn survivors to participate in activities including, swimming, basketball, volleyball, archery, golf, and arts and crafts. The camp is free of charge, and is hosted at a camp facility in Romano, California.

997 **Camp Bloomfield**
Junior Blind of America
35375 Mulholland Hwy
Malibu, CA 90265
  323-295-4555
  Fax: 310-321-3493
  jlucas@juniorblind.org
  www.juniorblind.org
Joshua Lucas, MS, Recreation Programs Manager
Miki Jordan, President & Chief Executive Officer
Corina Casco, LCSW, Chied Program Officer
Camp Bloomfield is a summer camp with week long sessions for children and youth who are blind, visually impaired or multi-disabled. The 45 acre campground offers campers a variety of activities, specifically designed to meet the needs of the children, with campers attending at no cost.

998 **Camp Christian Berets**
1317 Oakdale Rd.
Suite 340
Modesto, CA 95355
  209-524-7993
  Fax: 209-524-7979
  www.christianberets.org
James Woodhead, President
Karin Hoselton, Office Manager
Carletta Evans Steele, Secretary
Kelly Luth, Treasurer
Camp for children, students and adults with special needs.

999   Camp Conrad Chinnock
Diabetes Camping And Educational Services, Inc.
12045 E. Waterfront Dr.
Playa Vista, CA   90094   310-751-3057
                                           Fax: 888-800-4010
Rosie.DuBois@DiabetesCamping.org
www.diabetescamping.org
Rocky Wilson, Executive And Camp Director
Dale Lissy, Camp Manager
Ryan Martz, Program Director
McKenna Wilson, Program Director
Camp Conrad Chinnock offers year round recreational, social, and educational opportunities for children and families with type 1 diabetes.

1000   Camp Grizzly
NorCal Services For Deaf & Hard Of Hearing
4708 Roseville Rd
Suite 111
North Highlands, CA   95660   916-349-7500
                                           Fax: 916-349-7580
TTY:916-349-7500
campgrizzly@norcalcenter.org
www.campgrizzly.org
Molly Bowen, Program Leader
Cheryl Bella, Program Leader
A program of NorCal Services for Deaf & Hard of Hearing, Camp Grizzly is a coed camp for children aged 7-18 who have a hearing impairment. Camp Grizzly takes place at the Camp Lodestar campground facilities and offers sporting activities, performing and creative arts, hiking, swimming, playgrounds and campfires.

1001   Camp Hollywood HEART
One Heartland
2101 Hennepin Ave S
Suite 200
Minneapolis, MN   55405   888-216-2028
                                           Fax: 612-824-6303
helpkids@oneheartland.org
www.oneheartland.org
Patrick Kindler, Executive Director
Katie Donlin, Operations Manager
Allison Jones, Program Coordinator
Jill Rudolph, National Camp Director
A program of One Heartland, a nonprofit organization working to provide camping programs for children with serious illnesses or experiencing social isolation. Camp Hollywood HEART is a weeklong summer camp for youths, ages 15-20, who are infected or affected by HIV/AIDS. The camp is held in Malibu, California and is partnership camp between One Heartland and Hollywood Heart.

1002   Camp Kindle
Project Kindle
27203 Golden Willow Way
Santa Clarita, CA   91387   661-257-1901
877-800-2267
                                           Fax: 702-995-9186
info@projectkindle.org
www.projectkindle.org
Eva Payne, Founder & Executive Director
Mandy Nickolite, Vice President & PsychoSocial Lead
Kristen Nekovar, Program Coordinator
Camp Kindle provides year-round cost free recreational, educational and support services for children with special needs and life challenges.

1003   Camp Krem
Camping Unlimited
102 Brook Lane
Boulder Creek, CA   95006   831-338-3210
campkrem@gmail.com
campingunlimited.org
Katie Giampa, Program Director
Christina Krem, Program Director
Gail Zinegis, Intake Coordinator
Leon Wong, Head Counselor & Transportation Coordinator

Camp Krem - Camping Unlimited offers year-round and summer camping programs for children and adults with developmental disabilities. With a variety of different programs and many facilities on the campground such as a swimming pool, arts and crafts building, amphitheater, music pavilion, and archery range, Camp Krem provides its campers with recreation, education, and adventure opportunities.

1004   Camp No Limits California
No Limits Foundation
700 South Wren Drive
Big Bear Lake, CA   92315   207-240-5762
                                           Fax: 877-406-5106
campnolimits@gmail.com
www.nolimitsfoundation.org
Mary Leighton, Founder & Executive Director
Melanie Dash, Program Director
Pedro Pimenta, Director, Development
Missy Moreau, Project Coordinator
Camp No Limits California, a location of Camp No Limits, is a recreational and educational camp for youth who have experienced limb loss. Camp No Limits, is a program of the nonprofit organization No Limits Foundation. The California camp is held in Big Bear where campers have access to ropes courses, zip lines, and a swimming pool.

1005   Camp Okizu
Okizu Foundation
83 Hamilton Dr.
Suite 200
Novato, CA   94949-5755   415-382-9083
                                           Fax: 415-382-8384
info@okizu.org
www.okizu.org
Lori Sparrow, Executive Director
Suzie Randall, Executive Director, Operations
Kristen Hitchman, Camp Director
Camp Okizu offers a variety of medically supervised, residential camp programs for families who have a child diagnosed with cancer. Programs are offered throughout the year free of charge.

1006   Camp Okizu: Family Camp
Okizu Foundation
83 Hamilton Dr.
Suite 200
Novato, CA   94949-5755   415-382-9083
                                           Fax: 415-382-8384
enrollment@okizu.org
www.okizu.org
Lori Sparrow, Executive Director
Suzie Randall, Executive Director, Operations
Kristen Hitchman, Camp Director
Heather Ferrier, Director, Family Services
Camp Okizu's Family Camp is no cost camp designed for the families of children, and children who have been diagnosed with cancer. The Family Camp is offered as a weekend program, running on multiple weekends from April to September.

1007   Camp Okizu: Oncology Camp
Okizu Foundation
83 Hamilton Dr.
Suite 200
Novato, CA   94949-5755   415-382-9083
                                           Fax: 415-382-8384
enrollment@okizu.org
www.okizu.org
Lori Sparrow, Executive Director
Suzie Randall, Executive Director, Operations
Kristen Hitchman, Camp Director
Heather Ferrier, Director, Family Services
A program of Camp Okizu, the Oncology Camp is for children and teens, ages 6-17, who have or have had cancer. The camp is a residential summer camp program and is staffed by pediatric oncology departments from the participating hospitals.

1008 Camp Okizu: SIBS Camp
Okizu Foundation
83 Hamilton Dr.
Suite 200
Novato, CA 94949-5755   415-382-9083
                                  Fax: 415-382-8384
                                  enrollment@okizu.org
                                  www.okizu.org

Lori Sparrow, Executive Director
Suzie Randall, Executive Director, Operations
Kristen Hitchman, Camp Director
Heather Ferrier, Director, Family Services
SIBS (Special and Important Brothers and Sisters) Camp is for the sibling or siblings, ages 6-17, of a child who has, has had, or has died from cancer. The camp is a no charge, residential summer program, that provides campers the opportunity to learn new skills and get support from others who have experienced having a sibling with cancer.

1009 Camp Okizu: Teens-N-Twenties Camp
Okizu Foundation
83 Hamilton Dr.
Suite 200
Novato, CA 94949-5755   415-382-9083
                                  Fax: 415-382-8384
                                  enrollment@okizu.org
                                  www.okizu.org

Lori Sparrow, Executive Director
Suzie Randall, Executive Director, Operations
Kristen Hitchman, Camp Director
Heather Ferrier, Director, Family Services
Camp Okizu: Teens-N- Twenties Camp is a weekend recreation and support program that is offered 4 times a year for pediatric oncology patients and their siblings ages 18-25 .

1010 Camp Pacifica
California Lions Camp
45895 California Hwy 49
Ahwahnee, CA 93601
                                  559-683-4660
                                  www.camppacifica.org

Lisa Perez, Camp Director
Camp Pacifica provides a summer camp experience for children, boys and girls, aged 7-15 who have a hearing impairment. The camp is located in the foothills of Sierra on 52 acres of forested woodland. Activities include, but are not limited to, archery, canoeing, ropes course, swimming, horseback riding, and riflery. The camp costs $360.00 plus a registration fee.

1011 Camp Paivika
PO Box 3367
Crestline, CA 92325   909-338-1102
                                  Fax: 909-338-2502
                                  kkunsek@abilityfirst.org
                                  www.camppaivika.org

Kelly Kunsek, Camp Director
Lisa Duenas, Program Director
Tina Ronning-Fraynd, Coordinator, Camper Services
As a program of AbilityFirst, Camp Paivika offers overnight summer programs for children, teens and adults with developmental and physical disabilities. The camp is completely accessible and the staff is trained to provide any assistance or personal care a camper needs. Located in San Bernardino National Forest, Camp Paivika provides a traditional summer camp experience in a safe and fun environment.

1012 Camp ReCreation
2110 Broadway
Sacramento, CA 95818   916-733-0136
                                  Fax: 916-733-0195
                                  camprec@scd.org
                                  www.camprecreation.org

Kathi Barber, Camp Director
Chris Smrekar, Camp Ambassador
Michael Joyce, President
Marisa Bender, Vice President
Camp ReCreation offers residential summer camps and year round programs for children, teens, and adults with developmental disabilities. The summer camp is held at Camp Ronald Mc-

Donald in Lassen National Forest. With a 1:1 staff to camper ratio, Camp ReCreation offers wide variety of camp activities, and campers wishing to participate must fill out a camper application.

1013 Camp Reach for the Sky
The Seany Foundation
3530 Camino del Rio N
Suite 101
San Diego, CA 92108   858-551-0922
                                  info@theseanyfoundation.org
                                  www.theseanyfoundation.org/camp

Brian Bonert, Camp Advisory Chair
Claire Ellison, Sib Director
Steve Barbosa, Roc Camp Director
Pauline Kern, Day Camp Director
Previously run by the American Cancer Society, Camp Reach for the Sky (CR4TS) is now run by The Seany Foundation and provides an opportunity for children with cancer and their siblings to attend a free summer camp. Camp Reach for the Sky offers a multiple programs, including a Resident Oncology Camp, a Sibling Camp and Day Camps.

1014 Camp Ronald McDonald at Eagle Lake
2555 49th Street
Sacramento, CA 95817   916-734-4230
                                  Fax: 916-734-4238
                                  mdamos@RMHCNC.org
                                  www.campronald.org

Maria Damos, Camp Director
Camp Ronald McDonald at Eagle Lake collaborates with other nonprofit organizations to provide week long summer camp opportunities for children with special medical needs, financial hardship and/or emotional, developmental or physical disabilities. The camp is fully accessible.

1015 Camp Ronald McDonald for Good Times
1250 Lyman Place
Los Angeles, CA 90029   310-268-8488
                                  Fax: 310-473-3338
                                  www.rmhcsc.org/camp

Edward Lodgen, Esq., President
Jodie Lesh, Vice President
Sarah Orth, Executive Director
Chad Edwards, Program Director
Camp Ronald McDonald for Good Times, provides year round camping opportunities for children with cancer and their families. The Camp is a program of Ronald McDonald House Charities of Southern California.

1016 Camp Sunburst
Sunburst Projects United States Headquarters
2143 Hurley Way
Suite 240
Sacramento, CA 95825   916-440-0889
                                  Fax: 916-440-1208
                                  admin@sunburstprojects.org
                                  www.sunburstprojects.org

Geri DeLaRosa , PhD, Founder & Executive Director
Samantha Voelkel, Camp Director
Camp Sunburst is a youth oriented leadership camp that promotes and creates an environment to help youth learn self confidence to change negative social patterns and break cycles of HIV/AIDS infections. Activities campers will participate in include, boating, swimming, art, dance, and sports.

1017 Camp Sunshine Dreams
PO Box 28232
Fresno, CA 93729-8232   contact@campsunshinedreams.com
                                  www.campsunshinedreams.com

Anthony Aiello, Board of Directors
Pam Aiello, Board of Directors
Julie Bowen, Board of Directors
Jeff Clem, Board of Directors
Camp Sunshine Dreams provides a summer camp experience to children aged 8-15 with cancer and their siblings.

1018   Camp Taylor
Camp Taylor, Inc.
8224 West Grayson Rd.
Modesto, CA 95358-9094   209-581-0414
                                    Fax: 209-581-0421
                              kimberlie@kidsheartcamp.org
                                   www.kidsheartcamp.org
Kimberlie Gamino, Founder & Executive Director
With several programs, Camp Taylor provides youth, teens, and
the families of children with heart disease the opportunity to go to
a free medically supervised summer sleepaway camp. Campers
are able to enjoy activities such as, swimming, snorkeling, horseback riding, rock-wall, skits, archery, and heart education.

1019   Camp Taylor: Family Camp
Camp Taylor, Inc.
8224 West Grayson Rd.
Modesto, CA 95358-9094   209-581-0414
                                    Fax: 209-581-0421
                              Camp@KidsHeartCamp.org
                           www.kidsheartcamp.org/familycampca
Kimberlie Gamino, Founder & Executive Director
A program of Camp Taylor, Family Camp is for children of all
ages, with congenital heart disease and/or acquired heart disease,
and their family including parents and siblings. The camp offers
parental heart education and support programs for parents and
siblings. Family Camp is geared towards children too young to attend Youth or Teen Camp, or those who are not ready to attend a
residential camp.

1020   Camp Taylor: Leadership Camp
Camp Taylor, Inc.
8224 West Grayson Rd.
Modesto, CA 95358-9094   209-581-0414
                                    Fax: 209-581-0421
                          www.kidsheartcamp.org/leadershipcamp
Kimberlie Gamino, Founder & Executive Director
Leadership Camp is for teens and youth, ages 16-21, who have
previously attended a Camp Taylor California camp program,
wishing to be camp mentor for youth, teen, and family camps.
Campers wishing to attend this camp should make it known to either a camp counselor or camp director.

1021   Camp Taylor: Teen Camp
Camp Taylor, Inc.
8224 West Grayson Rd.
Modesto, CA 95358-9094   209-581-0414
                                    Fax: 209-581-0421
                              Camp@KidsHeartCamp.org
                             www.kidsheartcamp.org/teencamp
Kimberlie Gamino, Founder & Executive Director
The Teen Camp program at Camp Taylor is for teens ages 13-17,
with congenital heart disease and/or acquired heart disease.
Campers participate in heart education and traditional camp ac-
tivities. Campers wishing to attend the camp must apply, with
campers being accepted on a first come basis.

1022   Camp Taylor: Young Adult Program
Camp Taylor, Inc.
8224 West Grayson Rd.
Modesto, CA 95358-9094   209-581-0414
                                    Fax: 209-581-0421
                              YAP@KidsHeartCamp.org
                           www.kidsheartcamp.org/leadershipcamp
Kimberlie Gamino, Founder & Executive Director
The Young Adult Program at Camp Taylor is designed for previous heart campers ages 18-35 with congenital heart disease. The
program works to provide support, education, and the opportunities to participate in social events in order to help with the transition to adulthood.

1023   Camp Taylor: Youth Camp
Camp Taylor, Inc.
8224 West Grayson Rd.
Modesto, CA 95358-9094   209-581-0414
                                    Fax: 209-581-0421
                              Camp@KidsHeartCamp.org
                          www.kidsheartcamp.org/youthcamp
Kimberlie Gamino, Founder & Executive Director
A program of Camp Taylor, Youth Camp is designed for children,
ages 7-12, with congenital heart disease and/or acquired heart
disease. Campers participate in heart education and traditional
camp activities. Campers wishing to attend the camp must apply,
with campers being accepted on a first come basis.

1024   Camp Tuolumne Trails
22988 Ferretti Road
Groveland, CA 95321   209-962-7534
                                   info@tuolumnetrails.org
                                   www.tuolumnetrails.org
John Infelise, Camp & Operations Manager
Jessica Morrison, Program Director
Tuolumne Trails is a camp for individuals with special medical
needs. With week long summer camp options, Camp Tuolumne
Trails is a completely accessible camp, with a 3:1 staff to camper
ratio, that allows campers to participate in camping activities in a
safe environment. Campers wishing to attend must complete the
application and session assignment process.

1025   Camp del Corazon
11615 Hesby St
North Hollywood, CA 91601-3620   818-754-0312
                                         888-621-4800
                                    Fax: 818-754-0377
                                 info@campdelcorazon.org
                                 www.campdelcorazon.org
Samantha Lappin, Summer Camp Director
Lisa Knight, Executive Director & Co-Founder
Kevin Shannon, MD, President & Co-Founder & Medical Director
Kristina Wallace, Director, Development
Camp del Corazon, is a nonprofit corporation offering a no cost
summer camp and other programs to children aged 7-17 living
with heart disease. Campers or their guardians must fill out a
camp application, with acceptance into the camp dependant upon
a nurse review of the parent and cardiology portions of the
application.

1026   Camp-A-Lot and Camp-A-Little
The Arc of San Diego
3030 Market Street
San Diego, CA 92102   619-685-1175
                                    Fax: 619-234-3759
                                    info@arc-sd.com
                                    www.arc-sd.com
Lin Taylor, Camp Director
Programs of The Arc of San Diego, Camp - A - Lot (ages 18 and
up) and Camp - A - Little (ages 5-17) offer recreational summer
camp opportunities for individuals with physical and developmental disabilities. The cost of the camp program is $1,125.00
per camper.

1027   Coelho Epilepsy Youth Summer Camp
Epilepsy Foundation Of Northern California
1736 Franklin Street
Suite 450
Oakland, CA 94612   510-922-8687
                                         800-632-3532
                                    Fax: 510-922-8659
                                 camp@epilepsynorcal.org
                                 www.epilepsynorcal.org
Jody Eaton Iorns, Executive Director
Lauren Cotter, Program Coordinator
Tracie Ramsey, Event Coordinator
Carlos Quesada, Operations Manager
Offered to children aged 9-17, Coelho Epilepsy Youth Summer
Camp provides a week long sleepaway camp for children with ep-
ilepsy. Staffed by medical professional throughout the entire
week, campers participate in traditional camp activities. Parents

or guardians must fill out an application for a camper and the fee per camper is $650.00.

1028 Dream Street

Dream Street Foundation
324 S. Beverly Dr.
Suite 500
Beverly Hills, CA 90212
424-333-1371
Fax: 310-388-0302
dreamstreetca@gmail.com
www.dreamstreetfoundation.org

1029 Easterseals Camp

Easterseals Southern California
401 S Ivy St
Escondido, CA 92025
951-264-4855
Fax: 760-406-6048
amanda.showalter@essc.org
www.easterseals.com/southerncal
Amanda Showalter, Camp Director
Easterseals Camp is a week long summer camp for children and adults with disabilities. Held at Camp Oakes in the San Bernardino Mountains. Campers participate in activities including, crafts, hayrides, talent shows, dances, swimming, canoeing, archery, hiking, and rope courses. There is a 1:2 counselor to camper ratio and the cost of the camp is $775.00 per camper.

1030 Easterseals Camp Harmon

16403 Highway 9
Boulder Creek, CA 95006-9696
831-338-3383
Fax: 831-338-0200
campharmon@es-cc.org
www.campharmon.org
Scott Webb, Director, Camp Harmon
Cynthia Carman, Camp Registrar
Camp Harmon, the Easterseals Central California camp, offers residential summer camps programs to individuals ages 8-65 with disabilities. Each session at Camp Harmon is designed for a specific age group and offers campers the opportunity to experience traditional summer camp activities. There is a 3:1 counsellor to camper ratio, with camp fees are based on $140.00 a day base.

1031 Enchanted Hills Camp for the Blind

Lighthouse for the Blind
1155 Market St.
San Francisco, CA 94103
415-431-1481
ehc@lighthouse-sf.org
www.lighthouse-sf.org
Anthony Fletcher, Director, Enchanted Hills Camp and Retreat
Bryan Bashin, CEO
Enchanted Hills Camp for the Blind is located on 311 acres of land on Mt. Veeder, offering programs for children, teens, adults, deaf-blind, seniors, and families of the blind. The camp gives campers the experience of traditional summer camp but is adapted to meet the needs of the campers.

1032 Firefighters Kids Camp

Firefighters Burn Institute
3101 Stockton Blvd.
Sacramento, CA 95820
916-739-8525
marcos@ffburn.org
www.ffburn.org
Marco Reyes, Programs Coordinator
Mike Daw, Executive Director
Rachel Crowell, Assistant Director
Firefighters Kids Camp is a program run by the Firefighters Burn Institute for children ages 6-17, who are survivors of burns. With activities such as rocking climbing, bicycling, hiking, kayaking, swimming, and arts and crafts, the ratio of staff to campers is 3:1, with on site 24/7 nurse and physical therapist ensuring a safe and fun environment.

1033 Lions Wilderness Camp for Deaf Children, Inc.

Lions Wilderness Camp Headquarters
PO Box 8
Roseville, CA 95661-9998
campdirector@lionswildcamp.org
www.lionswildcamp.org
Kristina Frias, Camp Program Director
Lions Wilderness Camp gives deaf children aged 7-15 an outdoor camp experience helping children to learn outdoor skills and enjoy nature.

1034 Little Heroes Preschool Burn Camp

Firefighters Burn Institute
3101 Stockton Blvd.
Sacramento, CA 95820
916-739-8525
marcos@ffburn.org
www.ffburn.org
Marco Reyes, Programs Coordinator
Mike Daw, Executive Director
Rachel Crowell, Assistant Director
Little Heroes Preschool Burn Camp is a burn recovery program run by the Firefighters Burn Institute. The camp is for children ages 3-6, who are survivors of burns, and their families. The program runs for 3 days, providing support and education for those attending.

1035 New Horizons Summer Day Camp

CA
newhorizons@ymcaoc.org
www.ymcaoc.org/new-horizons

1036 Quest Camp

907 San Ramon Valley Blvd.
Suite 202
Danville, CA 94526
925-743-2900
800-313-9733
Fax: 925-820-9761
www.questcamps.com
Dr. Robert B Field, PhD., Founder & Executive Director
Debra Forrester-Field, MA, Administrative Director
Aprilyn Artz, MA, Clinical Director
Jodie Knott, Ph.D., Director
Quest Camps are designed using the Quest Camp Therapeutic System developed specifically to help and reduce a campers psychological disability. With locations in San Francisco East Bay, California, Huntington Beach, California, and Pittsburgh, Pennsylvania, camps have a 6:1 camper to staff ratio, with campers receiving sport instruction and participate in physical activity, arts, and games.

1037 Special Camp For Special Kids

31641 La Novia Ave
San Juan Capistrano, CA 92675
949-661-0108
Fax: 949-661-8637
lindsay.eres@smes.org
www.specialcamp.org
Lindsay Eres, Executive Director
Stefani Baker, Camp Operations Director
Elizabeth Stephens, Camper Coordinator
Sabine Scott, Development Coordinator
For youths with disabilities, Special Camps for Special Kids, offers day camps with a 1:1 volunteer counselor to camper.

1038 The Painted Turtle

1300 4th Street
Suite 300
Santa Monica, CA 90401
310-451-1353
866-451-5367
Fax: 310-451-1357
info@thepaintedturtle.org
www.thepaintedturtle.org
Chris Butler, Chief Executive Officer
Devon Page, Camper Admissions Manager
Allen McBroom, Chief Operations Officer
April Uyehara, Director, Camp Programs
The Painted Turtle provides year round camp programs for children, siblings, and families with children who have chronic and life threatening illnesses. The camp is located in Lake Hughes, California.

Colorado

1039 Adam's Camp
6767 South Spruce St.
Suite 102
Centennial, CO 80112 303-563-8290
Fax: 303-563-8291
Contact@AdamsCamp.org
www.adamscampcolorado.org
Jordan Ficke, Program Driector, Young Adults & Adventure Camp
Karel Horney, Founder
Anne Fiala, Volunteer & Operations Manager
Rob McIntire, Interim Executive Director & Finance Director
Adam's Camp is a nonprofit organization, with multiple locations across the United States, providing therapeutic programs and recreational camps for children, and the families of children with special needs and developmental delays.

1040 Adam's Camp: Colorado
Adam's Camp
6767 South Spruce St.
Suite 102
Centennial, CO 80112 303-563-8290
Fax: 303-563-8291
Contact@AdamsCamp.org
www.adamscampcolorado.org
Jordan Ficke, Program Driector, Young Adults & Adventure Camp
Karel Horney, Founder
Anne Fiala, Volunteer & Operations Manager
Rob McIntire, Interim Executive Director & Finance Director
Adam's Camp is a nonprofit organization providing therapeutic programs and recreational camps for children and the families of children with special needs. The Colorado location of Adam's Camp, offers both therapy and adventure camps. The adventure camp is held at the YMCA - Snow Mountain Ranch in Granby, Colorado.

1041 Aspen Camp
4862 Snowmass Creek Rd.
Snowmass, CO 81654 970-315-0513
Fax: 970-923-0643
TTY:970-315-0513
hi@aspencamp.org
www.aspencamp.org
Dr. Lesa Thomas, Executive Director
Zack Sisson, Facilities Director
Neal Matthews, Program Leader
Open to the deaf community, including family members and friends as well as those who are deaf, deaf blind, hard of hearing, and late deafened, Camp Aspen provides year round programs for youth and adults.
xxxx pages

1042 Breckenridge Outdoor Education Center
PO Box 697
Breckenridge, CO 80424 970-453-6422
800-383-2632
Fax: 970-453-4676
boec@boec.org
www.boec.org
Bruce Fitch, Executive Director
Marci Sloan, Development Director
Ella Greene, Associate Program Director, Operations
Breckenridge Outdoor Education Center (BOEC) provides year round educational outdoor experiences to individuals with physical and intellectual disabilities. Some programs BOEC offer include, Adaptive Ski and Ride School, Wilderness Programs and adaptive programs for individuals with brain injuries, multiple sclerosis, and Parkinson's Disease.

1043 CNI Cochlear Kids Camp
Colorado Neurological Institute
750 W Hampden Ave
Suite 400
Englewood, CO 80110 303-788-4010
Fax: 303-788-5469
cochlearcamp@thecni.org
www.thecni.org/cochlear-kids-camp
Tami Lack, MA, CFRE, Executive Director
Ellen Belle, MA, PT, MSSC, Director, Patient Services
Sheila Kutzer, MPS, Director, Development
Held at the YMCA Rockies Estes Park Center, the CNI Cochlear Kids Camp offers a wide range of activities for children from 3-17 years old with cochlear implants. The camp is 4 days and 3 nights, held during the summer and also offers programs for parents and families.

1044 Camp Rocky Mountain Village
Easterseals Colorado
5755 West Alameda Ave
Lakewood, CO 80226-3500 303-233-1666
Fax: 303-569-3857
campinfo@eastersealscolorado.org
www.easterseals.com/co
Lynn Robinson, President & CEO
Nancy Hanson, Vice President, Human Resources
A program of Easterseals Colorado, Rocky Mountain Village in Empire Colorado is a fully accessible camp, with summer camps sessions for children and adults with disabilities. Activities include but are not limited to swimming, fishing, overnight camping, outdoor cooking, day tips, arts and crafts, and a zip line.

1045 Camp Wapiyapi
191 University Boulevard
PO Box 294
Denver, CO 80206 303-534-0883
Fax: 303-534-0874
Wapiyapi@wapiyapi.org
www.campwapiyapi.org
Jeff Druck, President
Caryl Wojcik, Vice President
Chris Watts, Treasurer
Jason Elbot, Engineering Manager
Camp Wapiyapi is a nonprofit organization that offers free summer camps to children and families of children that have been affected by childhood cancer. The camp has a 1:1 staff or "companion" to camper ratio with onsite 24/7 volunteer medical staff.

1046 Challenge Aspen
PO Box 6639
Snowmass Village, CO 81615 970-923-0578
Fax: 970-923-7338
possibilities@challengeaspen.com
www.challengeaspen.org
Jeff Hauser, Chief Executive Officer
Anne Adams, Chief Operating Officer
Jenni Petersen, Chief Financial Officer
Challenge Aspen provides recreational, cultural experiences and summer camps for individuals who have cognitive or physical challenges. Programs are tailored to fit a diversity of needs and interests.

1047 Champ Camp
American Lung Association
CO 80481 303-847-0279
www.lung.org/
Bob Doyle, Director
Run by the American Lung Association, Champ Camp is an educational and recreational camp for children ages 7-14 with asthma. Children are able to participate in activities such as canoeing, hiking, and rock climbing. Volunteers and medical staff are on site 24/7 ensuring a safe environment for campers.

1048 Children's Hospital Burn Camps Program
13123 E 16th Ave.
PO Box 580
Aurora, CO 80045 720-777-8295
learnmore@noordinarycamps.org
www.noordinarycamps.org
Trudy Boulter, OTH CHT, Program Director
Brooke Cheley, Co-Director
The Children's Hospital Colorado Burn Camps Program provides rehabilitation and reintegration opportunities for children, teens, adults, and families who have been affected by burn injuries. The Camps Program has partnerships with 7 hospitals across the United States and offers year round programs.

1049 Children's Hospital Burn Camps Program: Cheley Children's Hospital Colorado Summer Burn Camp
13123 E 16th Ave.
PO Box 580
Aurora, CO 80045 720-777-8295
learnmore@noordinarycamps.org
www.noordinarycamps.org
Trudy Boulter, OTH CHT, Program Director
Brooke Cheley, Co-Director
The Cheley Children's Hospital Colorado Summer Burn Camp is part of the Children's Hospital Colorado Burn Camps Program, and offers a weeklong summer camp for children and teens, ages 8-18 who have been affected by burn injuries. The camp is held in Estes Park and activities include, hiking, mountain biking, challenge courses, horseback riding, mountain climbing, fishing, archery, crafts, riflery, and swimming.

1050 Children's Hospital Burn Camps Program: England Exchange Program Manchester Burn Camp
13123 E 16th Ave.
PO Box 580
Aurora, CO 80045 720-777-8295
learnmore@noordinarycamps.org
www.noordinarycamps.org
Trudy Boulter, OTH CHT, Program Director
Brooke Cheley, Co-Director
An international exchange program for campers ages, 13-15, between the Children's Hospital Burn Camps Program and The Manchester Children's Hospital Burns Camp in England. Campers are able to explore a new culture, food, and climate. The camp is located in the Lake District.

1051 Children's Hospital Burn Camps Program: Family Burn Camp
13123 E 16th Ave.
PO Box 580
Aurora, CO 80045 720-777-8295
learnmore@noordinarycamps.org
www.noordinarycamps.org
Trudy Boulter, OTH CHT, Program Director
Brooke Cheley, Co-Director
The Family Burn Camp is for families who have been affected by a burn injury. The camp is designed to give families the opportunity to interact and connect with other families who have had a similar experiences.

1052 Children's Hospital Burn Camps Program: Winter Burn Camp
13123 E 16th Ave.
PO Box 580
Aurora, CO 80045 720-777-8295
learnmore@noordinarycamps.org
www.noordinarycamps.org
Trudy Boulter, OTH CHT, Program Director
Brooke Cheley, Co-Director
The Winter Burn Camp is for older campers, ages 13-18, who have previously attended the Cheley Children's Hospital Colorado Summer Burn Camp. Held in Steamboat Springs, Colorado at the Steamboat Grand Lodge campers participate in a week of skiing and/or snowboarding.

1053 Children's Hospital Burn Camps Program: Young Adult Retreat
13123 E 16th Ave.
PO Box 580
Aurora, CO 80045 720-777-8295
learnmore@noordinarycamps.org
www.noordinarycamps.org
Trudy Boulter, OTH CHT, Program Director
Brooke Cheley, Co-Director
A program of the Children's Hospital Colorado Burn Camps Program, the Young Adult Retreat is designed to address the specific issues facing burn survivors ages 18-25. The retreat offers a variety of recreational and workshop opportunities working to address the topics of relationships, body image, and goal setting.

1054 City of Lakewood Recreation and Inclusion Services for Everyone (R.I.S.E.)
1555 Dover St
Lakewood, CO 80215 303-987-4869
Fax: 303-987-4802
TTY:303-987-7057
marsno@lakewood.org
www.lakewood.org/rise
Mark Snow, R.I.S.E Coordinator
Megan Cure, R.I.S.E. Program Specialist
Sasha Pietkiewicz, R.I.S.E. Program Specialist
The Recreation and Inclusion Services for Everyone (R.I.S.E.) of Lakewood is a therapeutic recreation program for individuals with disabilities, age 6 through senior adult. Some programs offered by R.I.S.E include field trips, social dances, sports and camping.

1055 Colorado Lions Camp
28541 Hwy 67 N
PO Box 9043
Woodland Park, CO 80863 719-687-2087
Fax: 719-687-7435
jodifranke@coloradolionscamp.org
www.coloradolionscamp.org
Jodi Franke, Executive Director
Michelle Werner, Executive Administrative Assistant
Colorado Lions Camp offers summer camp and weekend respite programs for individuals aged 8 and up with special needs. The camp is designed to promote independence and provide an opportunity for campers to discover their potential in a safe environment. The summer camp program costs $550.00 and weekend respite programs cost $200.00 .

1056 First Descents
3001 Brighton Blvd.
Suite 623
Denver, CO 80216 303-945-2490
Fax: 866-592-6911
info@firstdescents.org
www.firstdescents.org
Brad Ludden, Founder
Ryan O'Donoghue, Executive Director
Peta Sheridan, Director, Programs
Paul Kelly, Programs Manager
First Descents offers free outdoor adventure programs for young adults ages 18-39 who have, or who have had cancer. Activities include climbing, paddling and surfing, all offered in a safe environment.

1057 Roundup River Ranch
10 W Beaver Creek Blvd.
PO Box 8589
Avon, CO 81620-8589 970-748-9983
Fax: 970-748-9993
info@roundupriverranch.org
www.roundupriverranch.org
Ruth B. Johnson, JD, President & Chief Executive Officer
Sterling Nell Leija, Executive Camp Director
Kendra Perkins, Assustabt Camp Director
Alexis Klas, Program Coordinator
Roundup River Ranch provides traditional camp experiences for children and their families with chronic and serious illnesses. The

Ranch is located in Gypsum, Colorado, with all programs offered free of charge.

Connecticut

1058 Arthur C. Luf Children's Burn Camp
Connecticut Burns Care Foundation
601 Boston Post Rd.
Milford, CT 06460
203-878-6744
Fax: 203-878-4044
cbcf@ctburnsfoundation.org
www.ctburnsfoundation.org

Kathlene Gerrity, Executive Director
Armand J. Cantafio, President

The Arthur C. Luf Children's Burn Camp provides a free of charge camp experience for children and teens, ages 8-18, who have survived life altering burn injuries. Camp activities include hiking, fishing , archery, boating, ropes course, and campfires. The volunteer staff is composed of retired firefighters, medical personnel, and burn survivors.

1059 Camp Discovery
American Academy Of Dermatology
930 E Woodfield Rd.
PO Box 4014
Schaumburg, IL 60173
847-240-1280
866-503-7546
888-462-3376
Fax: 847-240-1859
www.campdiscovery.org

1060 Camp Horizons
127 Babcock Hill Rd.
PO Box 323
South Windham, CT 06266
860-456-1032
Fax: 860-456-4721
www.horizonsct.org

Adam Milne, Board Chairman
Chris McNaboe, President
Kathleen McNaboe, Board Vice President
L. Sanford (Sandy) Rice, Board Treasurer

Camp Horizons offers summer camp and weekend camps for children and adults with developmental disabilities.

1061 Camp Isola Bella
American School for the Deaf
139 N Main St.
West Hartford, CT 06107
860-570-2300
TTY:860-570-2222
IBDirector@asd-1817.org
www.campisolabella.org

Alyssa Pecorino, Director

Owned and operated by the American School for the Deaf, Camp Isola Bella provides summer camp opportunities for children who are deaf or hard of hearing. Staff is able to communicate with the campers regardless of the campers mode of communication including, sign language, oral, aural, lipreading or a mix, and activities include but are not limited to, swimming, ropes course, canoeing, water skiing, archery, hiking, sports, and sailing.

1062 Camp No Limits Connecticut
No Limits Foundation
Quinnipiac University
305 Sherman Avenue
Hamden, CT 06518
207-240-5762
Fax: 877-406-5106
campnolimits@gmail.com
www.nolimitsfoundation.org

Mary Leighton, Founder & Executive Director
Melanie Dash, Program Director
Pedro Pimenta, Director, Development
Missy Moreau, Project Coordinator

Camp No Limits Connecticut, a location of Camp No Limits, is a recreational and educational camp for youth who have experienced limb loss. Camp No Limits, is a program of the nonprofit organization No Limits Foundation. The Connecticut camp is

hosted at Quinnipiac's York Hill campus and provides campers the opportunity to participate in a variety of different sports, including ice and sled hockey.

1063 Easterseals Camp Hemlocks
Easterseals Coastal Fairfield County
733 Summer St.
Suite 104
Stamford, CT 6901
203-388-2192
Jillian.McCarthy@oakhillct.org
www.easterseals.com/cfc

Jillian McCarthy, Camp Contact

A summer camp program of Easterseals Coastal Fairfield County, Camp Hemlocks is a completely accessible camp for youth and adults with physical, sensory, intellectual, and developmental disabilities. Activities include, swimming, boating, fishing, arts and crafts, and climbing tower.

1064 SeriousFun Children's Network
SeriousFun Support Center Office
228 Saugatuck Ave.
Westport, CT 06880
203-562-1203
Fax: 203-341-8707
info@seriousfunnetwork.org
www.seriousfunnetwork.org

Blake Maher, Chief Executive Officer
Ingrid Milne, Chief Financial & Operations Officer
Mary Silvia, Associate Director, Global Partnerships & Programs

The SeriousFun Children's Network is an international organization of camps and programs for children and the families of children with serious illnesses. The Network has 9 camp locations in the United States and 21 international camp locations.

1065 Spina Bifida Association of Connecticut: Camp Harkness
PO Box 2545
Hartford, CT 06146-2545

1066 The Hole in the Wall Gang Camp
555 Long Wharf Dr.
New Haven, CT 06511
203-772-0522
info@holeinthewallgang.org
www.holeinthewallgang.org

James Canton, Chief Executive Officer
Pardraig Barry, Chief Program Officer
Hilary Gerson, Executive Camp Director
Ryan Thompson, Chief Communications Officer

The Hole in the Wall Gang Camp offers summer and weekend camp experiences for children, and the siblings of children with serious illnesses. Located in Ashford, Connecticut campers are able to participate in traditional camp activities in a medically safe environment.

1067 The Rainbow Club
The Barton Center for Diabetes Education, Inc.
30 Ennis Road
PO Box 356
North Oxford, MA 01537-0356
508-987-2056
Fax: 508-987-2002
info@bartoncenter.org
www.bartoncenter.org

Lynn Butler, Executive Director
Kenneth Follette, Clara Barton Camp Director
Lindsay Charest, Associate Director
Donna Joly, Facilities Director

A program of The Barton Center for Diabetes Education, The Rainbow Club is a day camp held in Greenwich, Connecticut for children and teens, ages 3-15, with diabetes. Campers receive diabetes education and participate in games, crafts, and water activities. An adult program designed for parents runs in conjunction with the day camp session.

Delaware

1068 Camp Manito & Camp Lenape
United Cerebral Palsy Of Delaware
700A River Road
Wilmington, DE 19809   302-764-2400
                                    Fax: 302-764-8713
                                    TTY:302-764-8708
                                    ucpde@ucpde.org
                                    www.ucpde.org/summer-camps
William J. McCool, III, Executive Director
Carma Carpenter, Camp Director
Camp Manito, located in New Castle County and Camp Lenape,
serving Kent and Sussex County, are summer camps run by the
United Cerebral Palsy of Delaware, Inc, for children and young
adults, ages 3-21, with orthopedic disabilities. Both campsites
are accessible and activities include, swimming, arts and crafts,
music, sports, computer education, and outings.

1069 Children's Beach House
100 W 10 Street
Suite 411
Wilmington, DE 19801-1674   302-655-4288
                                    Fax: 302-655-4216
                                    www.cbhinc.org
Richard T. Garrett, Executive Director
Stephanie Harmelin, Camp Director
Children's Beach House (CBH) is a nonprofit organization pro-
viding support and education for children with special needs.
CBH offers summer and weekend programs at the Lewes facility
on Delaware Bay. Activities are modified for each camper and in-
clude but are not limited to, swimming, sailing, kayaking, arts
and crafts, adventures, sports, and campfires.

1070 Easterseals Camp Fairlee
Easterseals Delaware & Maryland's Eastern Shore
22242 Bay Shore Rd.
Chestertown, MD 21620   410-778-0566
                                    Fax: 410-778-0567
                                    fairlee@esdel.org
                                    www.easterseals.com/de
Kenan J. Sklenar, CEO
Gary Cassedy, VP Programs
Sallie Price, Director of Camping and Recreation
Jeff Gosnear, Board Chair
Easterseals Camp Fairlee provides recreation and respite ser-
vices to children and adults with all types of disabilities. Best
known for traditional, residential, week long summer camp sessions. Summer activities include swimming, wall climbing, zip
line, horseback riding, canoeing, nature trails, arts/craft, outdoor
and indoor sports and games.

District of Columbia

1071 Camp Lighthouse
Columbia Lighthouse for the Blind
1825 K St. NW
Suite 1103
Washington, DC 20006   240-737-5136
                                    Fax: 202-955-6401
                                    plyman@clb.org
                                    www.clb.org
Patti Lyman, Camp Contact
Camp Lighthouse, is a 1 week day camp program run by the Co-
lumbia Lighthouse for the Blind. The camp is for children ages
6-12 with visual impairments.

Florida

1072 Camp Amigo
Children's Burn Camp Of North Florida, Inc.
PO Box 368
Tallahassee, FL 32302   850-509-6200
                                    www.campamigo.com
Rusty Roberts, President
Camp Amigo provides a 1 week summer camp experience for
children ages 6-18, living in North or Central Florida, who have
survived a burn injury.

1073 Camp Boggy Creek
30500 Brantley Branch Rd
Eustis, FL 32736   352-483-4200
                                    866-462-6449
                                    Fax: 352-483-0589
                                    info@campboggycreek.org
                                    www.boggycreek.org
June Clark, President & CEO
David Mann, Camp Director
Darren Dannelly, Chief Operating Officer
Kristin Cauraugh Youmans, Assitant Camp Director
Part of the SeriousFun Children's Network, Camp Boggy Creek
provides year round camping opportunities for children, and the
families of children with serious illnesses living in Florida. The
camp has week-long summer camp sessions and retreat
weekends.

1074 Camp No Limits Florida
No Limits Foundation
8411 25th Street
East Ellenton, FL 34219   207-240-5762
                                    Fax: 877-406-5106
                                    campnolimits@gmail.com
                                    dayspringfla.org
Mary Leighton, Founder & Executive Director
Melanie Dash, Program Director
Pedro Pimenta, Director, Development
Missy Moreau, Project Coordinator
Camp No Limits Florida, is a location of Camp No Limits, a recre-
ational and educational camp for youth who have experienced
limb loss. Camp No Limits is a program of the nonprofit organiza-
tion, No Limits Foundation. The 3 day camp is held at the Day
Spring Conference Center in Ellenton, Florida and includes a
visit to the Clearwater Marine Aquarium to visit Winter the dolphin. The camp takes place in February.

1075 Camp Thunderbird
Quest, Inc.
PO Box 531125
Orlando, FL 32853   407-218-4300
                                    888-807-8378
                                    Fax: 407-218-4301
                                    contact@questinc.org
                                    www.questinc.org/play.html
John Gill, President & Chief Executive Officer
Brooke Eakins, Chief Operating Officer
Kathy Lopus, Vice President, Development
A program of Quest, Inc. Camp Thunderbird provides recre-
ational programs for children and adults with developmental disabilities. The camp has 6 and 12 day overnight sessions with age
specific programming and typically have a 1:4 camper to staff
ratio.

1076 Center Academy at Pinellas Park
6710 86th Ave
Pinellas Park, FL 33782   727-541-5716
                                    Fax: 727-544-8186
                                    infopp@centeracademy.com
                                    www.centeracademy.com
Mack R Hicks PhD, Founder/Chairman of the Board
Eric V. Larson, Ph. D.,, President & COO
Andrew P Hicks PhD, CEO/Clinical Dir.
Lisa Hartmann, Dir. Education
Specifically designed for the learning disabled child and other
children with difficulties in concentration, strategy, social skills,

impulsivity, distractibility and study strategies. Programs offered include: attention training, visual-motor remediation, socialization skills training, relaxation training, horseback riding and more. The day camp meets weekdays from 9-3 for 3,4 or 5 week sessions.

1077 Dr. Moises Simpser VACC Camp
Nicklaus Children's Hospital
3200 S.W. 60 Ct.
Suite 203
Miami, FL 33155-4076
305-662-8222
Fax: 786-268-1765
bela.florentin@mch.com
www.vacccamp.com

Dr. Moises Simpser, Founder & Director
Ivette Hidalgo, Camp Clinical Coordinator
Bela Florentin, Camp Coordinator
VACC Camp gives families a fun opportunity to socialize with peers and enjoy activities not readily accessible to technology dependent children. The program includes sailing, swimming, field trips to local attractions, campsite entertainment, structured games, free play, and more - all to promote family growth and development while enhancing individual self-esteem and social skills. Parents have formal and informal opportunities to network among themselves.

1078 Dream Oaks Camp
Foundation For Dreams, Inc.
16110 Dream Oaks Pl.
Bradenton, FL 34212
941-746-5659
jfranke@foundationfordreams.org
www.foundationfordreams.org

1079 Easterseals Camp Challenge
Easterseals Of Florida
520 N Semoran Blvd
Suite 280
Orlando, FL 32807
407-306-9766
camp@fl.easterseals.com
www.easterseals.com/florida

Susan Ventura, President & Chief Executive Officer
Rob Porcaro, Chief Operating Officer
Jeff Lato, Chief Development Officer
Located in Sorrento, Florida, Easterseals Camp Challenge provides camp opportunities for children and adults with cognitive and physical disabilities.

1080 Florida Diabetes Camp
Florida Camp for Children & Adults w/Diabetes, Inc
PO Box 14136
Gainesville, FL 32604-2136
352-334-1321
Fax: 352-334-1326
fccyd@floridadiabetescamp.org
www.floridadiabetescamp.org

Gary Cornwell, Executive Director
Chris Stakely, Assistant Director
Amy Soileau, Outreach Director
Janet Silverstein, Medical Director
The Florida Diabetes Camp offers weekend and summer camps for children with type 1 diabetes. The camp combines traditional camp activities and diabetes related educational sessions for campers in order to provide a fun and safe environment.

1081 Florida Lions Camp
2819 Tiger Lake Rd
Lake Wales, FL 33898
863-696-1948
Fax: 863-696-2398
www.lionscampfl.org

Barbara Cage, Executive Director
Liz Cage, Program Director & Rentals
The Florida Lions Camp, is a nonprofit, inclusive camp dedicated to providing summer camp and weekend respite camp experiences for youth with physical and/or developmental disabilities. Campers can participate in activities including but not limited to, swimming, canoeing, fishing, hiking, camping, arts and crafts, and games.

1082 Hand Camp
Hands to Love
3450 Hull Rd.
PO Box 140572
Gainesville, FL 32614-0572
352-273-7382
Fax: 352-273-7388
info@handstolove.org
www.handstolove.org

Suzan Shaw, Executive Director
A program of Hands to Love, an organization for children and the families of children with upper limb differences, Hand Camp is annual networking event held in Starke, Florida at Camp Crystal Lake. Hand Camp has adapted camp activities, networking and support groups, and special guests.

1083 Kris' Camp
Kris' Camp/Therapy Intensive Programs, Inc.
1132 Green Hill Trace
Tallahassee, FL 32317
850-445-4821
kberger62@gmail.com
www.kriscamp.org

Kathy Berger, PT, Executive Director
Kris' Camp provides program for children with autism.

1084 Sertoma Camp Endeavor
1301 Camp Endeavor Blvd
PO Box 910
Dundee, FL 33838
miawilliams1965@gmail.com
www.sertomacampendeavor.net

Maria Williams, Camp Director
Charles Lake, President
Sertoma Camp Endeavor provides educational programs for deaf and hard of hearing youth. Programs are designed to promote social and personal growth, environmental awareness, and independence.

Georgia

1085 Aerie Experiences
GA
404-285-0467
mdweneta@aerieexperiences.com
aerieexperiences.com

Matthew Weneta, M.Ed., Owner & Director
Maggie Shay, BS, Program Director
Laurie Patrice, LPC, BCPC, Clinical Director
Located north of Atlanta, Georgia with summer camp expeditions taking place in Georgia, North Carolina, and Tennessee, Aerie Experiences provides programs for children, families and individuals with special needs. Aerie Experiences is focused on those affected by Aspergers, High Functioning Autism, Learning Disabilities, ADHD, and Neurobiological Disorders.

1086 Camp Breathe Easy
American Lung Association
2452 Spring Rd
Smyrna, GA 30080-3828
404-231-9887
LSchmitt@CampTwinLakes.org
www.campbreatheeasy.com

Lauren Schmitt, Camp Director
Operated by the Georgia Chapter of American Lung Association, Camp Breathe Easy, is a 1 week residential summer camp for children ages 7-13, with mild to severe asthma. Campers are able to participate in a wide variety of camp experiences such as, swimming, fishing, archery, and canoeing, with asthma education incorporated into the week.

1087 Camp Caglewood
Caglewood, Inc.
PO Box 158
Flowery Branch, GA 30542
678-405-9000
Fax: 770-441-3406
info@caglewood.org
www.caglewood.org

Paul Freeman, Co-Founder

A special needs camping program, Camp Caglewood provides active weekend programs for children and adults with developmental disabilities.

1088 Camp Dream
Camp Dream Foundation
4355 Cobb Pkwy
Suite J117
Atlanta, GA 30339   678-367-0040
                                         info@campdreamga.org
                                         www.campdreamga.org

Gary Marshall, Executive Director
Beverly Taylor, Program Director
JR Clark, President
Scott Little, Vice President
Camp Dream is a free camp where special needs children can camp and have fun regardless of their physical and/or mental condition. The camp offers many recreational activities and programs.

1089 Camp Firefly
The Firefly Foundation
5737 Kanan Road
Suite 180
Agoura Hills, CA 91301   CampFirefly89@gmail.com
                                         www.campfirefly.com

1090 Camp Hawkins
GA Baptist Childrens Homes & Family Ministries,Inc
PO Box 329
Palmetto, GA 30268   770-463-3344
                                         ksewell@gbchfm.org
                               www.gbchfm.org/Camp-Hawkins
Kendra Sewell, Camp Director
Camp Hawkins is a residential summer camp for youths ages 8-21 with developmental disabilities. Sessions are 5 days long with a staff to camper ratio of 1:1, activities include, swimming, canoeing, shows, arts and crafts, games, and bible study.

1091 Camp Independence
Camp Twin Lakes
1391 Keencheefoonee Rd
Rutledge, GA 30663   404-785-0631
                               campindependence@choa.org
                         www.choa.org/camps/camp-independence
Donna W. Hyland, President, Children's Healthcare Atlanta
Ruth Fowler, Chief Financial Officer
Danial Salinas, Chief Medical Officer
Camp Independence is Georgia's a overnight, week-long summer camp providing essential medical care, treatment & fun for kids with kidney disease and transplants. Camp Independence recognizes that campers are normal children but have special needs providing these children with opportunities for development & individual growth, peer support & normal life experiences. Activities include swimming, arts & crafts, fishing, horseback riding, and more. Ages 8-18.

1092 Camp Juliena
Georgia Center for the Deaf and Hard of Hearing
4151 Memorial Dr
Suite 103-B
Decatur, GA 30032   404-292-5312
                                         Fax: 404-299-3642
                                         TTY:800-541-0710
                                         gachiboard@gachi.org
                         www.gcdhh.org/gcdhh-programs/camp-juliena
Meredith Albert, President
Jimmy Peterson, Executive Director
LaQuanda Jackson, Executive Assistant
Kathy Keeter, Employment Support Coordinator
A weeklong residential summer camp for youths and teens who are deaf or hard of hearing. Through challenging, team-oriented activities, campers form lasting friendships and acquire valuable leadership, social and communication skills.

1093 Camp Kudzu
Camp Kudzu, Inc.
5885 Glenridge Drive
Suite 160
Atlanta, GA 30328   404-250-1811
                                         Fax: 404-250-1812
                                         info@campkudzu.org
                                         www.campkudzu.org

Alex Allen, Executive Director
Sandy Yates, Director, Development
Camp Kudzu is a nonprofit organization, offering overnight summer camp, day camp, family camps, and teen programs for individuals and the families of individuals with type 1 diabetes. Programs are held at various locations across Georgia and provide campers with traditional camp experiences and diabetes education.

1094 Camp Sunshine
1850 Clairmont Rd
Decatur, GA 30033-3405   404-325-7979
                                             866-786-2267
                                         Fax: 404-325-7929
                               info@mycampsunshine.com
                               www.mycampsunshine.com

Dorothy H. Jordan, Founder
Beth Abernathy, Chair
Randall Kirsch, Vice Chair
J. Preston Byers, Treasurer
Camp Sunshine provides children with cancer the opportunity partcipate in traditional camp activities such as horseback riding, swimming, and arts & crafts.

1095 Camp Twin Lakes
1100 Spring St.
Suite 260
Atlanta, GA 30309   404-231-9887
                                         Fax: 404-577-8854
                                         www.camptwinlakes.org

Jill Morrisey, Chief Executive Officer
Daniel C. Mathews, M.Ed., CTRS, Chief Operations Officer
Cheryl Belair, Director, Development
Camp Twin Lakes provides fully accessible, year round camp programs for children with serious illnesses, disabilities, and other life challenges. Camp Twin Lakes has 3 locations in Rutledge, Winder, and Warm Springs, Georgia with all locations working to deliver a fully adaptive, medically supported, and impactful experience for every camper.

1096 Camp Twin Lakes: Camp Dream
Roosevelt Warm Springs Institute for Rehab
6135 Roosevelt Hwy
Warm Springs, GA 31830   706-557-9070
                                         www.camptwinlakes.org
Jill Morrisey, Chief Executive Officer
Daniel C. Mathews, M.Ed., CTRS, Chief Operations Officer
Cheryl Belair, Director, Development

1097 Camp Twin Lakes: Rutledge
1391 Keencheefoonee Rd.
Rutledge, GA 30663   706-557-9070
                                         Fax: 706-557-9147
                                         www.camptwinlakes.org

Jill Morrisey, Chief Executive Officer
Daniel C. Mathews, M.Ed., CTRS, Chief Operations Officer
Cheryl Belair, Director, Development

1098 Camp Twin Lakes: Will-A-Way
210 S Broad St.
Unit 5
Winder, GA 30680   770-867-6123
                                         Fax: 770-867-6130
                                         www.camptwinlakes.org

Jill Morrisey, Chief Executive Officer
Daniel C. Mathews, M.Ed., CTRS, Chief Operations Officer
Cheryl Belair, Director, Development

1099 Squirrel Hollow Summer Camp
The Bedford School
5665 Milam Rd
Fairburn, GA 30213 770-774-8001
Fax: 770-774-8005
bbox@thebedfordschool.org
www.thebedfordschool.org
Betsy Box, Admissions Director
Jeff James, Head of School
Allison Day, Assistant Head of School
A program of The Bedford School, Squirrel Hollow Summer Camp, offers 2 summer sessions for students with academic needs due to a learning disability. Students receive academic instruction in reading, writing, and math through a variety of teaching techniques, with students grouped by age and skill level. The camp also incorporates recreational activities such as, swimming, games, and a challenge course.

Hawaii

1100 Camp Anuenue
Honolulu, HI 808-349-7325
campanuenue@gmail.com
www.campanuenue.com
B.K. Cannon, Director
Alison James, Director
Camp Anuenue is a nonprofit organization that offers a week long camping experience for children ages 7-18 who have, or have had cancer. The camp is held at Camp Mokule'ia on the North Shore of Oahu and accepts children from Hawaii (all the islands), and US territories in the Pacific including Guam, Saipan, Somoa, and Marshall Islands.

1101 Camp Taylor: Family Camp
Camp Taylor, Inc.
Hilton Hawaiian Village
2005 Kalia Road
Honolulu, HI 96815 209-581-0414
Fax: 209-581-0421
Camp@KidsHeartCamp.org
www.kidsheartcamp.org/familycamphi
Kimberlie Gamino, Founder & Executive Director
A program of Camp Taylor, Family Camp is for children of all ages, with congenital heart disease and/or acquired heart disease, and their family including parents and siblings. The camp offers parental heart education and support programs for parents and siblings. The camp is held at the Hilton Hawaiian Village and is open to families from all of the Hawaiian Islands.

Idaho

1102 Camp Hodia
Idaho Diabetes Youth Programs, Inc.
1701 N 12th St
Boise, ID 83702 208-891-1023
info@hodia.org
www.hodia.org
Lisa Gier, Programs Executive Director
Camp Hodia offers a variety of camp programs for children and teens in Idaho, Western Wyoming, and Eastern Oregon, ages 8-19, with type 1 diabetes.

1103 Camp No Limits Idaho
No Limits Foundation
Camp Cross Marine Rt.
Coeur d'Alene, ID 83814 207-240-5762
Fax: 877-406-5106
campnolimits@gmail.com
www.nolimitsfoundation.org
Mary Leighton, Founder & Executive Director
Melanie Dash, Program Director
Pedro Pimenta, Director, Development
Missy Moreau, Project Coordinator

Camp No Limits Idaho, a location of Camp No Limits, is a recreational and educational camp for youth who have experienced limb loss. Camp No Limits, is a program of the nonprofit organization No Limits Foundation. The camp is held at Camp Cross on Lake Coeur d'Alene.

1104 Camp Rainbow Gold
216 W Jefferson St.
Boise, ID 83702 208-350-6435
info@camprainbowgold.org
www.camprainbowgold.org
Elizabeth Lizberg, Executive Director
Tracy Bryan, Program Director
Jason Hosick, Program Manager
Christl Holzl, Development Director
Camp Rainbow Gold is a independent, nonprofit organization providing year round camp programs, support groups, and scholarships for children, siblings, and the family of children who have been diagnosed with cancer. All camp programs are offered free of charge, with campers participating in activities such as, fishing, hiking, campfires, and crafts. The camp is held in the the Sawtooth National Forest.

Illinois

1105 ADA Camp GrenADA
4-H Memorial Campground
499 Old Timber Rd.
Monticello, IL 61856 312-346-1805
illinoiscamps@diabetes.org
www.diabetes.org
Kalina Gurovski, Executive Director
Camp GranADA is an American Diabetes Association resident camp located in Monticello, Illinois at the 4H Memorial Camp owned by the University of Illinois. For children with diabetes, ages 8-16. Activities include swimming, canoeing, wall climbing, tie-dying shirts, arts & crafts and fun filled evening programs.

1106 ADA Teen Adventure Camp
YMCA Camp Duncan
32405 North Highway 12
Ingleside, IL 60041 312-346-1805
888-342-2383
SApsey@diabetes.org
www.nchpad.org/Directories/Programs/9566
Sue Apsey, Program Director
Camping for teenagers with diabetes. Coed, ages 14 to 18. Camp dates are early in August. Located at the YMCA Camp Duncan in Ingleside, Illinois. Featured activities include archery, boating, roller skating, ropes course, and swimming.

1107 ADA Triangle D Camp
Camp Duncan
32405 N Highway 12
Ingleside, IL 60041 888-342-2383
www.nchpad.org/Directories/Programs/9567
Sue Apsey, Program Director
Triangle D Camp is a resident camp program for children with diabetes. A coed camp for participants aged 9-13 years old, the camp ranges in price from $770 - $950, with swimming, row boating, canoeing, ropes course, camp games, archery, soccer, basketball, volleyball, and diabetes education as the camps features activities.

1108 Camp "I Am Me"
Illinois Fire Safety Alliance
426 W Northwest Hwy
Mount Prospect, IL 60056 847-390-0911
Fax: 847-390-0920
ifsa@ifsa.org
www.ifsa.org/programs/camp
Philip Zaleski, Executive Director
Stephanie Hiemer, Program Manager
Kim Mueller, Administrative Assistant

Camp "I Am Me" is a 1 week no cost summer camp for children and teens who have experienced burn injuries. The camp is held in Ingleside, Illinois at YMCA Camp Duncan. Activities include archery, games, canoes, kayaks, sailboats, campfires, fishing, ropes course, swimming, and specialized workshops related to burn injuries.

1109 Camp Callahan
Camp Callahan, Inc.
PO Box 5253
Quincy, IL 62305-5253　　　　　　217-833-2707
　　　　　　　　　　　www.campcallahan.com

1110 Camp Discovery
American Academy Of Dermatology
930 E Woodfield Rd.
PO Box 4014
Schaumburg, IL 60173　　　　　　847-240-1280
　　　　　　　　　　　　　　866-503-7546
　　　　　　　　　　　　　　888-462-3376
　　　　　　　　　　　　Fax: 847-240-1859
　　　　　　　　　　　www.campdiscovery.org

1111 Camp FRIENDship
Easterseals Chicagoland & Rockford
1939 W 13th Street
Suite 300
Chicago, IL 60608-1126　　　　　312-491-4110
　　　　　　　　　　www.easterseals.com/chicago
Cassie Wells, Director, Autism Services
A program of Easterseals, Camp FRIENDship is a summer camp program designed to help children ages 5-14 with autism, nonverbal learning disabilities, and intellectual disabilities. The camp promotes the acquiring of social skills in a safe and fun learning environment.

1112 Camp Little Giant
Touch of Nature Environmental Center
Camp Little Giant
SIU Mail Code 6888
Carbondale, IL 62901　　　　　　618-453-1121
　　　　　　　　　　　　　　Fax: 618-453-1188
　　　　　　　　　　　　　　tonec@siu.edu
　　　　　　　　　　　　　　www.ton.siu.edu

1113 Camp New Hope
PO Box 764
Mattoon, IL 61938-764　　　　　217-895-2341
　　　　　　　　　　　　　　Fax: 217-895-3658
officemanager@campnewhopeillinois.org
　　　　　　　　campnewhopeillinois.org
Carlissa Puckett, Executive Director
Jill Rohr, Program Director
Paul Semple, Office Assistant
Camp New Hope is a year round recreational experience for individuals 8 and up with developmental and physical disabilities. The camp offers summer, weekend respite, and bowling programs. Camp New Hope is situated on 41 acres of land on Lake Mattoon.

1114 Camp One Step
213 West Institute Place
Suite 306
Chicago, IL 60610　　　　　　　312-924-4220
　　　　　　　　　　　　　　Fax: 312-878-7374
　　　　　　　　　　　　　　info@camponestep.org
　　　　　　　　　　　　　　www.onestepcamp.org
Jeff Infusino, President
Darryl Winston Perkins, Jr., Director, Programs
Katie Weil, Development Officer
Lauren Kunkel, Program Coordinator
Camp One Step provides 11 different year round programs, including a 2 week overnight summer camp for children and teens aged 5-19, who have been diagnosed with cancer. Camp One Step is open to children and their families who live in Illinois, Wisconsin and throughout the Midwest.

1115 Camp Quality Illinois
PO Box 641
Lansing, IL 60438　　　　　　　708-895-8311
　　　　　　　　　　　　　　Fax: 708-895-8075
　　　　　　　　　　illinois@campqualityusa.org
　　　　　　　　　　www.campqualityusa.org/il
Mary Lockton, Executive Director
Dawn Winters, Treasurer
Linda Reece, Secretary/Staff Coordinator
Stacy Reynolds, Program Coordinator
Camp Quality is an international camping program for children with cancer. The Illinois Camp Quality is held in Frankfort, Illinois at Camp Manitoqua & Retreat Center and offers children and their siblings summer camps and year round support programs. Volunteer doctors and nurses are at the camp 24 hours a day, and there is a 1:1 staff to camper ratio.

1116 Camp Red Leaf
Jewish Council for Youth Services
26710 W Nippersink Rd
Ingleside, IL 60041　　　　　　　847-740-5010
　　　　　　　　　　　　　　enewport@jcys.org
　　　　jcys.org/locations/ingleside/camp-red-leaf
Erin Newport, Camp Red Leaf Director
Camp Red Leaf provides summer camp opportunities, weekend respite care, travel camp, and day camp for individuals 9 and up with special needs. The camp is a program of the Jewish Council for Youth Services and is located on 180 acres of land in Ingleside, Illinois.

1117 Illinois Wheelchair Sport Camps
University of Illinois
1207 S Oak St
Champaign, IL 61820-6901　　　　217-333-1970
　　　　　　　　　　　　　　Fax: 212-244-0014
　　　　　　　　　　　　　　sportscamp@illinois.edu
　　　　　　　　　　www.disability.illinois.edu/camps

1118 MDA Summer Camp
Muscular Dystrophy Association National Office
222 S Riverside Plaza
Suite 1500
Chicago, IL 60606　　　　　　　800-572-1717
　　　　　　　　　　　　　　mda@mdausa.org
　　　　　　　　www.mda.org/services-summer-camp
Kristine Welker, Interim President & CEO
Eileen Timmins, Ph.D, Executive Vice President, Chief People Officer
Steven G. Ford, Executive Vice President, Chief Communications & Marketing
MDA Summer Camp is a program of the Muscular Dystrophy Association providing a one week free summer camp for children with muscular dystrophy and related muscle-debilitating diseases.

1119 Nothern Suburban Special Recreation Association Day Camps
3105 MacArthur Blvd.
Northbrook, IL 60062　　　　　　847-509-9400
　　　　　　　　　　　　　　Fax: 847-509-1177
　　　　　　　　　　　　　　cbenson@nssra.org
　　　　　　　　　　www.nssra.org/programs/camps
Catherine Benson, Recreation Specialist, Camps
The Northern Suburban Special Recreation Association (NSSRA), offers year round day camps for children and youth 6-22 with disabilities. Summer day camps include: Afternoon Escapades, Awesome Post Camp, Camp Sunburst, Lake Forest Recreation Program, and NSSED/NSSRA Summer Program. Camp Igloo is the winter day camp which, is held over school winter break.

1120 **Rimland Services for Autistic Citizens**
1265 Hartrey Ave
Evanston, IL 60202 847-328-4090
Fax: 847-328-8364
TTY:847-328-4090
rimland.org/

Lorraine Ganz, President
Bernice Gryczan, VP
Barbara Cooper, Secretary
Wiliam Egan, Board Member

An accessible camp facility that can be utilized by groups for day use or overnight camping experiences. Six winterized cabins, a meeting facility, indoor pool, full food service, and an excellent staff are available. Educational programs can be arranged or you can utilize the facility to manage your own programs.

1121 **Shady Oaks Camp**
16300 Parker Rd
Homer Glen, IL 60491 708-301-0816
www.shadyoakscamp.org

Scott Steele, Executive Director
Amy Johnston, Associate Camp Director
Nikki Dunne, Associate Camp Director

Shady Oaks is a summer camp for people with disabilities. The camp provides a fun recreational camp experience, with a 1:1 camper to staff ratio.

1122 **Timber Pointe Outdoor Center**
Easterseals Central Illinois
507 E Armstrong Ave
Peoria, IL 61603-3201 309-686-1177
Fax: 309-687-2035
tpoc@ci.easterseals.com
www.easterseals.com/ci

Don Young, Chair
Jamoe Engstrom, Secretary

Timber Pointe Outdoor Center (TPOC) is a specialized outdoor recreational center for individuals with disabilities, which is owned and operated by Easterseals Central Illinois and is located on Lake Bloomington. TPOC offers year round programs, including summer and day camps, in a completely accessible environment.

Indiana

1123 **Anderson Woods**
4630 Adyeville Rd
Bristow, IN 47515 812-639-1079
www.andersonwoods.org

Judy Colby, Co-Founder
David Colby, Co-Founder
Isaac Gatwood, Executive Co-Director
Megan Gatwood, Executive Co-Director

Anderson Woods is a private, nonprofit organization providing summer camp experiences for children and adults with special needs.

1124 **CHAMP Camp**
704 S State Rd 135
Greenwood, IN 46143 317-679-1860
Fax: 317-245-2291
jenniferk@champcamp.org
www.champcamp.org

Jennifer Kobylarz, Executive Director
Dave Carter, Co-Camp Director & Founder
Jamie Mitchell, Co-Camp Director
Kristina Watkins, Program Coordinator

CHAMP Camp is a one week summer camp experience for children and youth, ages 6-18, who have tracheostomies or require respiratory assistance, including the use of ventilators and/or have physical challenges. The camp is held at Bradford Woods in Martinsville, Indiana, and activities include but are not limited to, fishing, boating, canoeing, arts, swimming, and a 50 foot alpine tower climb.

1125 **Camp About Face**
Heads Up!!! Foundation
PO Box 167
Medora, IN 47260 812-966-2761
Fax: 812-966-2927
headsupfoundation2012@gmail.com
www.headsupfoundation.org/camp_about_fac e.htm

1126 **Camp Brave Eagle**
Indiana Hemophilia & Thrombosis Center
8326 Naab Rd
Indianapolis, IN 46260 317-871-0000
www.campbraveeagle.org

Jennifer Maahs, MSN, PNP, Camp Director

Camp Brave Eagle is a summer camp for children and the siblings of children with bleeding disorders living in the state of Indiana. The camp is supervised by experienced medical staff.

1127 **Camp John Warvel**
American Diabetes Association
8604 Allisonville Rd.
Suite 140
Indianapolis, IN 46250 317-352-9226
Fax: 317-913-1592
cdixon@diabetes.org
www.diabetes.org/adacampjohnwarvel

Carol Dixon, Camp Director

A program of the American Diabetes Association, Camp John Warvel is a summer camp program for children with type 1 diabetes. The camp is designed to promote independence, confidence, and a healthy lifestyle through education, nutrition, and exercise. There is a 4:1 camper to staff ratio.

1128 **Camp Little Red Door**
Little Red Door Cancer Agency
1801 North Merideian St.
Indianapolis, IN 46202-1411 317-925-5595
Fax: 317-925-5597
mail@littlereddoor.org
www.littlereddoor.org

Fred Duncan, Director & CEO
Nick Duvall, Vice President, Development & Communications

Camp Little Red Door is a one week summer camp for children and teens, ages 8-18, who have, or have had cancer. The camp is held at Bradford Woods in Martinsville, Indiana with campers participating in traditional camp activities.

1129 **Camp Millhouse**
25600 Kelly Rd.
South Bend, IN 46614 574-233-2202
Fax: 574-233-2511
campmillhouse@gmail.com
www.campmillhouse.org

Diana Breden, Executive Director
Liz Richards, Camp Director

Camp Millhouse is a residential summer camp for children and adults with varying disabilities. Ages of campers range from 7 to 75+. They offer six one-week sessions and spring & fall camp weekends. Campers enjoy various daily activities including arts & crafts, recreation, music, and swimming in our in-ground, heated, fully accessible pool. They also have 24 hour on-site nursing and low camper to staff ratios.

1130 **Camp PossAbility**
Camp PossAbility, Inc.
Fort Wayne, IN 260-341-5732
info@camppossability.org
www.camppossability.org

Dr. Adam D. Keesling, Board President
Lauren E. Harmison, Founder & Board Vice President

Camp PossAbility is a 1 week summer camp designed for young adults ages 18-35 with physical disabilities. The camp is held at Bradford Woods in Martinsville, Indiana.

1131 Camp Quality Kentuckiana
PO Box 35474
Louisville, KY 40232 502-507-3235
charlie.obranowicz@campqualityusa.org
www.campqualityusa.org/ki

Charlie Obranowicz, Co-Director
Eddie Bobbitt, Co-Director
Meridith Nguyen, Camper Registrar
Linda Wickliffe, Companion Coordinator
Camp Quality is an international camping program for children with cancer. Camp Quality Kentuckiana, serves Kentucky and Indiana and offers children and their siblings summer camps and year round support programs. Volunteer doctors and nurses are at the camp 24 hours a day, and there is a 1:1 staff to camper ratio.

1132 Camp Red Cedar
3900 Hursh Road
Fort Wayne, IN 46845 260-637-3608
Fax: 260-637-5483
RedCedar@CampRedCedar.com
www.campredcedar.com

Carrie Perry, Director
Shelly Detcher, HR Recruiter & Program Manager
Camp Red Cedar is open to children and adults with or without disabilities. The camp offers summer residental, and summer day camps along with year round theraputic and conventional horseback riding. Other activities include, fishing, hiking, swimming and arts and crafts.

1133 Camp Riley
Riley's Children Foundation
30 S Meridian St.
Suite 200
Indianapolis, IN 46204-3509 317-634-4474
877-867-4539
Fax: 317-634-4478
riley@rileykids.org
www.rileykids.org/camp

Kevin O'Keefe, President & CEO
Katie Askey, Director, Development Operations
Viki Mech Hester, Chief Administrative Officer
Camp Riley is an annual summer camp program of the Riley Children's Foundation. The camp is designed to help children and teens ages 8-18 with physical disabilities, experience life without limits in a safe, fun, and accessible environment. The camp is held at Bradford Woods and campers can participate in activities such as, horseback riding, swimming, water skiing, climbing, and archery.

1134 Happiness Bag
Happiness Bag, Inc.
3833 Union Rd
Terre Haute, IN 47802 812-234-8867
Fax: 812-238-0728
www.happinessbag.org

Michelle , Service Coordinator
Happiness Bag provides adaptive education and recreational services, including summer day camps and respite care programs, for children and adults with disabilities.

1135 Hillcroft Services
Hillcroft Services: Isanogel
114 East Streeter Avenue
Muncie, IN 47304 765-284-4166
bwilliamson@hillcroft.org
www.hillcroft.org

Ted Baker, Chair
Brenda Llyod, Vice Chair
Bruce Baldwin, Director
Julie Bering, Secretary/ Treasurer
The camp is designed to improve the academic, social skills, and behaviors of children with autism spectrum disorders. The day camp is an 8-week intensive experience for children classified with autism spectrum disorders.

1136 Hoosier Burn Camp
PO BOX 233
Battle Ground, IN 47920 765-567-0115
Fax: 765-567-0195
markkoopman@hoosierburncamp.org
www.hoosierburncamp.org

Mark Koopman, Executive Director
Abby James, Program Manager
Kristin Burton, Administrative Assistant
Hossier Burn Camp is nonprofit organization that provides an annual summer camp and monthly events for children and teens, ages 8-18, who have suffered a burn injury. The camp is held at Camp Tecumseh in Brookston, Indiana.

1137 Indiana Deaf Camp
1434 S Wausau St
Warsaw, IN 46580 260-602-6758
TTY:5743063064
indeafcamp@hotmail.com
www.indeafcamps.org

Curtis Sigafoose, Director
Betty O'Hara, Program Corrdinator
Indiana Deaf Camp is for children ages 4-17 who have hearing loss or are related to individuals with hearing loss.

Iowa

1138 Camp Albrecht Acres
14837 Sherrill Rd
PO Box 50
Sherrill, IA 52073 563-552-1771
Fax: 563-552-2732
info@albrechtacres.org
www.albrechtacres.org

Eric Veltstra, Executive Director
Camp Albrecht Acres is a nonprofit organization offering a summer and winter programs for children and adults with special needs.

1139 Camp Courageous of Iowa
12007 190th St
PO Box 418
Monticello, IA 52310-0418 319-465-5916
Fax: 319-465-5919
info@campcourageous.org
www.campcourageous.org

Jeanne Muellerleile, Camp Director
Charlie Becker, Executive Director
Stephen Fasnacht, Assitant Program Director
A year round residential and respite care facility for individuals with special needs and their families. Campers range in age from 1-99 years old. Activities include traditional activities like canoeing, hiking, swimming, nature and crafts plus adventure activities like caving, and rock climbing.

1140 Camp Hertko Hollow
501 Grand Avenue
Des Moines, IA 50309 515-471-8523
855-502-8500
Fax: 515-288-2531
www.camphertkohollow.com

Jessica Thornton, Executive Director
Deb Holwegner, Camp Director
Camp Hertko Hollow is an education and recreational summer camping program for children and teens, ages 6-17 with diabetes. Campers participate in traditional camp activities and learn about living with diabetes.

1141 Camp Quality Heartland
PO Box 402
Council Bluffs, IA 51502 330-671-0167
Fax: 866-285-5208
angela.batson@campqualityusa.org
www.campqualityusa.org/htl

Angela Batson, Executive Director

Camp Quality is for children with cancer and their siblings. The camp offers a stress-free environment that offers exciting activities and fosters new friendships, while helping to give the children courage, motivation and emotional strength.

1142 Camp Sunnyside
Easter Seals Of Iowa
Attn: Camp Program
401 NE 66th Ave
Des Moines, IA 50313 515-289-1933
campandrespite@eastersealsia.org
www.easterseals.com/ia
Sherri Nielsen, President & Chief Executive Officer
Kristi Sterling, Chief Compliance Officer
Open to campers age 4 and up, with or without disabilities, Camp Sunnyside is owned and operated by Easterseals Iowa and offers week and day summer camps.

1143 Camp Tanager
1614 W Mount Vernon Rd
Mount Vernon, IA 52314 319-363-0681
Fax: 319-365-6411
campmail@tanagerplace.org
www.camptanager.org

Kansas

1144 CP Ranch
The Kansas Jaycees' Cerebral Palsy Foundation, Inc
PO Box 267
Augusta, KS 67207-267 316-775-2421
execdirector@cpranch.org
www.cpranch.cfsites.org
Cheryl Schmeidler, Executive Director
Sarah Walker, Camp Director
CP Ranch works to provide a camping experience and facility for children, teens, and adults with physical and intellectual disabilities. The ranch is located on 151 acres of land and included a lake, dorms, pool, and recreational pavilion.

1145 Camp Discovery Kansas
American Diabetes Association
608 W Douglas Ave.
Wichita, KS 67203 316-684-6091
Fax: 316-684-5675
lfurstner@diabetes.org
www.diabetes.org
Lora Furstner, Camp Contact
A program of the American Diabetes Association, Camp Discovery Kansas is for children and teens ages 8-16 with diabetes. Campers participate in traditional camp activities while receiving educational information on diabetes. The camp is held at Rock Springs 4-H Center in Junction City, Kansas and the cost is $400.00.

1146 Camp Planet D
American Diabetes Association
6900 College Blvd.
Suite 250
Leawood, KS 66211 913-383-8210
Fax: 913-383-2319
lfurstner@diabetes.org
Lora Furstner, Camp Contact
A program of the American Diabetes Association, Camp Planet D is for children and teens ages 7-15 with diabetes. Campers participate in traditional camp activities while receiving educational information on diabetes. The camp is held at the Tall Oaks Conference Center in Linwood, Kansas and the cost is $435.00.

1147 Camp Quality Kansas
2617 N 75th St.
Kansas City, KS 66109 913-424-8355
Fax: 913-334-2802
Susie.Mooney@CampQualityUSA.org
www.campqualityusa.org/ks
Susie Mooney, Executive Director

Camp Quality is an international camping program for children with cancer. Camp Quality Kansas offers children and their siblings summer camps and year round support programs. Volunteer doctors and nurses are at the camp 24 hours a day, and there is a 1:1 staff to camper ratio.

1148 Camp Sweet Betes
American Diabetes Association
608 W Douglas Ave.
Wichita, KS 67203 316-684-6091
Fax: 316-684-5675
lfurstner@diabetes.org
www.diabetes.org
Lora Furstner, Camp Contact
A program of the American Diabetes Association, Camp Sweet Betes is a day camp for children ages 5-8 with diabetes. Campers learn techniques for managing nutrition, exercise, and medication. The camp is held at Trinity Presbyterian Church in Wichita, Kansas and the cost is $100.00.

Kentucky

1149 Camp Quality Kentuckiana
PO Box 35474
Louisville, KY 40232 502-507-3235
charlie.obranowicz@campqualityusa.org
www.campqualityusa.org/ki
Charlie Obranowicz, Co-Director
Eddie Bobbitt, Co-Director
Meridith Nguyen, Camper Registrar
Linda Wickliffe, Companion Coordinator
Camp Quality is an international camping program for children with cancer. Camp Quality Kentuckiana, serves Kentucky and Indiana and offers children and their siblings summer camps and year round support programs. Volunteer doctors and nurses are at the camp 24 hours a day, and there is a 1:1 staff to camper ratio.

1150 Kids Cancer Alliance
607 W Main St, Suite 200
PO Box 24337
Louisville, KY 40224 502-365-1538
info@kidscanceralliance.org
www.kidscanceralliance.org
Shelby Russell, Executive Director
Leah McComb, Program Director
Brandon "Spot" Padgett, Program Coordinator
The Kids Cancer Alliance is a nonprofit organization that provides summer camps and support programs for children and the families of children with cancer. Camp programs include oncology and sibling camps, as well as teen and and family retreats.

1151 Lions Camp Crescendo
1480 Pine Tavern Rd
P.O. Box 607
Lebanon Junction, KY 40150 502-833-4427
888-879-8884
wibblesb@aol.com
www.lccky.org
Joe Westerman, Chairman
Cecil Warner, Vice Chairman
Kenneth Pierce, Secretary
Howard Cook, Treasurer
Organization dedicated to enhancing quality of life for youths, including those with disabilities, through the delivery of a traditional camping experience.

1152 The Center for Courageous Kids
1501 Burnley Rd
Scottsville, KY 42164 270-618-2900
Fax: 270-618-2902
info@courageouskids.org
www.courageouskids.org
Joanie O'Bryan, President & CEO
Emily Cosby, Camp Director
Elizabeth Chapman, Director, Development
Sarah Keltner, Director, Communications

The Center for Courageous Kids is a year round medical camp for children who have chronic or life threatening illnesses.

Louisiana

1153 Camp Bon Coeur
405 W. Main St.
Lafayette, LA 70501
337-233-8437
info@heartcamp.com
www.heartcamp.com

Susannah Craig, Executive Director
Camp Bon Coeur or Camp "Good Heart" is a nonprofit, one week overnight summer camp for children with cardiovascular issues. The camp is held annually in July and is based in South Louisiana.

1154 Camp Challenge
PO Box 10591
New Orleans, LA 70181
504-347-2267
Fax: 866-295-3803
campdirector@campchallenge.org
www.campchallenge.org

1155 Camp Pelican
PO Box 10235
New Orleans, LA 70181
888-617-1118
Fax: 866-295-3803
info@camppelican.org
www.camppelican.org

1156 Camp Quality Louisiana
1800 Forsythe Avenue
Suite 2, Box 307
Monroe, LA 71201
315-547-4319
alan.barth@CampQualityUSA.org
www.campqualityusa.org/la

Alan Barth, Executive Director & Camp Director
Gay Nell Barth, Camper Coordinator
Camp Quality is an international camping program for children with cancer. The Louisiana Camp is held at Jimmie Davis State Park in Chatham, Louisiana and offers children and their siblings summer camps and year round camping opportunities. Volunteer doctors and nurses are at the camp 24 hours a day, and there is a 1:1 staff to camper ratio.

1157 Camp Victory
American Diabetes Association
2424 Edenborn Ave.
Suite 600
Metairie, LA 70001
888-342-2383
Fax: 337-239-9975
www.lionscamp.org/html/diabetes-camp.html
Kasey Davis, Associate Director
Camp Victory is two one week residential summer camp sessions for children, ages 6-14, with Type 1 or Type II diabetes. The camp is run by the American Diabetes Association and the Lions Clubs of Louisiana and is held at the Lions Clubs location in Anacoco, Louisiana.

1158 Louisiana Lions Camp
292 L. Beauford Dr.
Anacoco, LA 71403
800-348-6567
Fax: 337-239-9975
www.lionscamp.org
Raymond E. Cecil, III, Executive Director & Camp Director
Owned and operated by the Louisiana Lions League, Inc. the Louisiana Lions Camp is a no cost residential summer camp for children with intellectual and physical disabilities. Campers are able to experience traditional summer camp activities in a medically safe and fun environment. The Camp is also host to the American Diabetes Association, Camp Victory, and to Camp Pelican, a camp for children with pulmonary disorders.

1159 MedCamps of Louisiana
102 Thomas Rd.
Suite 615
West Monroe, LA 71291
318-329-8405
info@medcamps.com
www.medcamps.com

Caleb Seney, Executive Director
Kacie Hobson, Camp Director
MedCamps of Louisiana offers free 1 week residential summer camp programs for children with chronic illnesses, physical and/or developmental disabilities. Each week during the summer a different camp is held specifically designed for a particular disability.

Maine

1160 Camp CaPella
PO Box 552
Holden, ME 04429
207-843-5104
www.campcapella.org

Dana Mosher, Executive Director
Deb Breindel, Camp Director
Camp CaPella provides recreational and educational opportunities for children and adults with disabilities. The camp is located on Phillips Lake in Dedham, Maine and offers a variety of programs including day camps, overnight camps, family vacation packages, and travel camp.

1161 Camp Lawroweld
228 West Side Rd
Weld, ME 04285
207-797-3760
tturcotte@nnec.org
www.lawroweld.org

1162 Camp No Limits Maine
No Limits Foundation
114 Pine Tree Camp Road
Rome, ME 04963
207-240-5762
Fax: 877-406-5106
campnolimits@gmail.com
www.nolimitsfoundation.org

Mary Leighton, Founder & Executive Director
Melanie Dash, Program Director
Pedro Pimenta, Director, Development
Missy Moreau, Project Coordinator
Camp No Limits Maine, a location of Camp No Limits, is a recreational and educational camp for youth who have experienced limb loss. Camp No Limits, is a program of the nonprofit organization No Limits Foundation. The camp is held at Pine Tree Camp in Rome, Maine and is supported by Maine Adaptive Sports & Recreation.

1163 Camp Snow Maine
No Limits Foundation
15 South Ridge Road
Newry, ME 04261
207-240-5762
Fax: 877-406-5106
campnolimits@gmail.com
www.nolimitsfoundation.org

Mary Leighton, Founder & Executive Director
Melanie Dash, Program Director
Pedro Pimenta, Director, Development
Missy Moreau, Project Coordinator
A program of the nonprofit organization No Limits Foundation, Camp No Limits provides recreational and educational camp opportunities for youth who have experienced limb loss. With locations across the United States, camps offer therapeutic programs with specialized professionals, support programs, and recreational activities. The camp costs $500.00.

1164 Camp Sunshine
35 Acadia Rd
Casco, ME 04015
                                    207-655-3800
                                    Fax: 207-655-3825
                                    info@campsunshine.org
                                    www.campsunshine.org
Michael Katz, Executive Director
Maureen McAllister, Director, Operations
Michael Smith, Development Director
Camp Sunshine is a free, year round camp for children and families of children with cancer, hematologic conditions, renal disease, systemic lupus, and solid organ transplantation. The camp also has bereavement programs for families.

1165 Camp Winnebago
19708 Camp Winnebago Rd
Caledonia, MN 55921
                                    507-724-2351
                                    Fax: 507-724-3786
                                    campwinnebagodirector@gmail.com
                                    www.campwinnebago.org

1166 Camp sNOw Maine
No Limits Foundation
265 Centre Rd
Wales, ME 04280
                                    207-240-5762
                                    Fax: 877-406-5106
                                    campnolimits@gmail.com
                                    www.nolimitsfoundation.org
Mary Leighton, Founder & Executive Director
Melanie Dash, Program Director
Pedro Pimenta, Director, Development
Missy Moreau, Project Coordinator
Camp sNOw Maine, is a location of Camp No Limits, a recreational and educational camp for youth who have experienced limb loss. Camp No Limits is a program of the nonprofit organization, No Limits Foundation. Partnered with Maine Adaptive Sports & Recreation, the camp is weekend of winter activities including, skiing and snowboarding. The camp takes place in March.

1167 Pine Tree Camp
Pine Tree Society
149 Front Street
Bath, ME 04530
                                    207-386-5990
                                    Fax: 207-443-1070
                                    TTY:207-443-3341
                                    ptcamp@pinetreesociety.org
                                    www.pinetreesociety.org
Dawn Willard-Robinson, Camp Director
Offering day camps, overnight camps, retreats, and specialized programs, Pine Tree Camp is run by the Pine Tree Society, and provides children and adults with disabilities the opportunity to participate in recreational activities, such as swimming, fishing, kayak, hiking, and boating. The camp is located in North Pond in Rome, Maine.

Maryland

1168 Camp Fairlee
Easterseals Delaware & Maryland's Eastern Shore
61 Corporate Circle
New Castle, DE 19720
                                    302-324-4444
                                    contact@esdel.org
                                    www.easterseals.com/de
Kenan J. Sklenar, President & CEO
David Dougherty, Secretary
Christine Sauers, Treasurer
Easterseals Camp Fairlee provides accessible summer camp and year round respite weekends to individuals with physical and intellectual disabilities. Activities include but are not limited to, swimming, wall climbing, zip lining, horseback riding, arts and crafts, and games.

1169 Camp Great Rock
Epilepsy Foundation Metropolitan Washington
8301 Professional Place
Suite 200
Landover, MD 20785-2353
                                    301-459-3700
                                    800-332-1000
                                    Fax: 301-459-1569
                                    www.brainycamps.com/camps/camp-great-rock

1170 Camp Littlefoot
The Treatment and Learning Centers
2092 Gaither Rd
Suite 100
Rockville, MD 20850
                                    301-424-5200
                                    Fax: 301-424-8063
                                    TTY:301-424-5203
                                    LTorvik@ttlc.org
Lisa Torvik, Camp Contact
Camp Littlefoot offers a variety of programs for children requiring speech-language and/or occupational therapy.

1171 Camp No Limits Maryland
No Limits Foundation
11 Horseshoe Point Lane
North East, MD 21901
                                    207-240-5762
                                    Fax: 877-406-5106
                                    campnolimits@gmail.com
                                    www.nolimitsfoundation.org
Mary Leighton, Founder & Executive Director
Melanie Dash, Program Director
Pedro Pimenta, Director, Development
Missy Moreau, Project Coordinator
Camp No Limits Maryland, a location of Camp No Limits, is a recreational and educational camp for youth who have experienced limb loss. Camp No Limits, is a program of the nonprofit organization No Limits Foundation.

1172 Camp Sunrise
John Hopkins Kimmel Cancer Center
750 E Pratt St
Suite 1700
Baltimore, MD 21201   campsunriseappliations@gmail.com
                                    www.hopkinsmedicine.org/kimmel_cancer_center/
Marilyn Scalf, Staffing Director
Jennifer Seiler, Camper Coordinator
Ashley Richards, Programs
Michelle Ruff, Programs
Camp Sunshine is a free 1 week summer camp open to children and teens, ages 4-18 who are currently being treated for cancer or who have undergone bone marrow transplants at John Hopkins Hospital. Camp Sunshine offers a day camp for children ages 4 and 5, a residential camp for children and teens ages 6-16, and a leadership in training program for campers ages 17-18.

1173 Camp Superkids
John Hopkins Bayview Medical Center
4940 Eastern Ave
Baltimore, MD 21224
                                    717-578-0465
                                    campsuperkids@gmail.com
                                    www.hopkinsbayview.org/campsuperkids
Heather Dougherty, Camp Administrator
Camp Superkids is an overnight camp for children between the ages of 7.5-12 with asthma. Campers partcipate in a wide range of traditional camp activities and learn how to manage their asthma. Camp Superkids costs $400.00.

1174 Deaf Camps
MD   deafcampsinc@gmail.com
                                    deafcampsinc.wordpress.com
Kathy MacMillan, President
Louise Rollins, Treasurer
David Shepard, Secretary
Deaf Camps, Inc. is a nonprofit organization dedicated to providing a fun, safe, and communication-rich 1 week summer camps for deaf, and hard of hearing children and children learning American Sign Language.

1175 League at Camp Greentop
The League for People with Disabilities, Inc.
1111 E. Cold Spring Lane
Baltimore, MD 21239   410-323-0500
info@leagueforpeople.org
www.leagueforpeople.org
David Greenberg, President & Chief Executive Officer
Marsha Legg, Vice President, Workforce & Youth Development
Bill Morgan, Vice President, Recreation & Fitness
A traditional sleepaway summer camp for youth and adults with
disabilities. The League at Camp Greentop is located in
Thurmont, Maryland, and has youth and all ages sessions, with
campers participating in activities such as swimming, arts and
crafts, sports, and games.

1176 Lions Camp Merrick
PO Box 56
Nanjemoy, MD 20662   301-870-5858
Fax: 301-246-9108
info@LionsCampMerrick.org
www.lionscampmerrick.org
Heidi A. Fick, Executive Director
Donna Wadsworth, Office Administrator
A recreational camp for children, ages 6-16 who are deaf, hard of
hearing, and/or blind or visually impaired. Camp activities in-
clude but are not limited to, archery, canoeing, ropes courses,
swimming, fishing, and games.

Massachusetts

1177 Adam's Camp: Nantucket
Adam's Camp
6767 South Spruce St.
Suite 102
Centennial, CO 80112   603-715-2298
newhampshire@adamscamp.org
www.adamscampnewengland.org
Adrienne Evans, Executive Director
Ann Poyant, Nantucket Program Coordinator
A program of Adam's Camp, Adam's Camp Nantucket is held on
Nantucket Island, offering a variety of programs for children and
the families of children with special needs and developmental delays. The Nantucket camp has 2 therapy programs, Pathfinder
(ages 4 and up) and Trailblazer (ages 8 and up), and 1 transition
program, Discovery, for ages 13 and up.

1178 Camp Howe
557 East St.
PO Box 326
Goshen, MA 01032   413-268-7635
office@camphowe.com
www.camphowe.com
Terrie Campbell, Executive Director
The Echo Program at Camp Howe is designed for youth ages 7-17
with physical or developmental disabilities. The program is offered in 1 or 2 week sessions with campers experiencing every aspect of a traditional summer camp program and camping
community. The program is not a specialized therapeutic program
and the camper to staff ratio is 2:1.

1179 Camp Jabberwocky
200 Greenwood Ave Ext.
PO Box 1357
Vineyard Haven, MA 02568   508-687-0967
info@campjabberwocky.org
www.campjabberwocky.org
Liza Gallagher, Executive Director
Jack Knower, Session Director
Nora Olsen, Session Director
Kristen 'Sully' St. Amour, Session Director
Camp Jabberwocky offers summer camp and family camp pro-
grams for individuals with physical and intellectual disabilities.
The camp is located in Martha's Vineyard with campers usually
staying between 1 and 4 weeks. Camp activities include day trips,
horseback riding, barbeques, boating, biking, and spending time
at the beach.

1180 Camp Starfish
636 Great Rd
Suite 2
Stow, MA 01775   978-637-2617
Fax: 978-637-2617
info@campstarfish.org
www.campstarfish.org
Emily Golinsky, Executive Director
Adam Sparks, Camp Director
Matt Nalley, Program Director
Camp Starfish provides summer camps, day camps, and year
round respite programs for children with emotional, behavioral,
and learning disabilities. Camp Starfish has a 1:1 staff to camper
ratio at all times, promoting an individualized camping experience, the building of social skills, and the teaching coping
mechanisms.

1181 Eagle Hill School: Summer Program
Eagle Hill School
242 Old Petersham Road
PO Box 116
Hardwick, MA 01037- 0116   413-477-6000
Fax: 413-477-6837
www.eaglehill.school
Frederick Macdonald, Director, Development
Peter McDonald, Headmaster
Eric Stone, Dean of Education
A program of Eagle Hill School, a school for students diagnosed
with learning disabilities including ADHA. The Eagle Hill Sum-
mer session is a 5 week camp, for students 10-16 who has been di-
agnosed with a learning disability and/or ADHD. The summer
session incorporates education and recreation to address the specific academic and social skills of the student.

1182 Kamp for Kids at Camp Togowauk
Carson Center for Human Services
754 Russell Rd
Westfield, MA 01085   413-562-5678
TTY:800-764-0200
abenoit@carsoncenter.org
www.carsoncenter.org/programs
Anne Benoit, Director
Kamp for Kids at Camp Togowauk is an integrated summer camp
for youth with or without disabilities.

1183 Open Hearts Camp
The Edward J. Madden Open Hearts Camp
250 Monument Valley Rd
Great Barrington, MA 01230   413-528-2229
hearts@openheartscamp.org
www.openheartscamp.org
David Zaleon, Executive Director
The Open Hearts Camp is a eight week summer camp program divided into four age specific sessions for children and teens who
have had open heart surgery. Campers must be in stable health and
the program blends sports, recreation, arts and crafts and rest periods into a campers day.

1184 Summer@Carroll
Carroll School
25 Baker Bridge Rd
Lincoln, MA 01773-3199   781-259-8342
gsummers@carrollschool.org
www.carrollschool.org
Greely Summers, Director
Donna Brown, Assistant Director
A program of the Carroll School, an independent day school for
elementary and high school students diagnosed with learning disabilities, Summer@Carroll is a 5 week day camp incorporating
education and recreation for children with learning disabilities.
Students participate in academic classes in the morning, splitting
into smaller groups during the afternoon for recreational activities. Campers attending the day camp do not have to be students
of the school during the regular school year.

1185 The Barton Center
The Barton Center for Diabetes Education, Inc.
30 Ennis Road
PO Box 356
North Oxford, MA   01537-0356   508-987-2056
                                        Fax: 508-987-2002
                                        info@bartoncenter.org
                                        www.bartoncenter.org

Lynn Butler, Executive Director
Kenneth Follette, Clara Barton Camp Director
Lindsay Charest, Associate Director
Donna Joly, Facilities Director
The Barton Center for Diabetes Education, is year round camp, retreat, and conference center; offering education, recreation, and support programs for the families of children, and children and teens with insulin dependent diabetes. The center offers a variety of programs in Massachusetts, Connecticut, and New York.

1186 The Barton Center Camp Joslin
The Barton Center for Diabetes Education, Inc.
30 Ennis Rd
PO Box 356
North Oxford, MA   01537-0356   508-987-2056
                                        Fax: 508-987-2002
                                        info@bartoncenter.org
                                        www.bartoncenter.org

Lynn Butler, Executive Director
Kyler Jesanis, Camp Joslin Director
Lindsay Charest, Associate Director
Donna Joly, Facilities Director
A summer camp program of The Barton Center for Diabetes Education, Camp Joslin provides boys ages 6-16, with insulin-dependent diabetes a traditional summer camp experience combined with diabetes education. Activities include sports, swimming, kayaking, canoeing, fishing, hiking, arts and crafts, and campfires.

1187 The Barton Center Clara Barton Camp
The Barton Center for Diabetes Education, Inc.
30 Ennis Road
PO Box 356
North Oxford, MA   01537-0356   508-987-2056
                                        Fax: 508-987-2002
                                        info@bartoncenter.org
                                        www.bartoncenter.org

Lynn Butler, Executive Director
Kenneth Follette, Clara Barton Camp Director
Lindsay Charest, Associate Director
Donna Joly, Facilities Director
A summer camp program of the Barton Center for Diabetes Education, Clara Barton Camp provides girls ages 6-16, with insulin-dependent diabetes a traditional summer camp experience combined with diabetes education. Activities include sports, swimming, kayaking, canoeing, fishing, hiking, arts and crafts, and campfires.

1188 The Barton Center Danvers Day Camp
The Barton Center for Diabetes Education, Inc.
30 Ennis Road
PO Box 356
North Oxford, MA   01537-0356   508-987-2056
                                        Fax: 508-987-2002
                                        info@bartoncenter.org
                                        www.bartoncenter.org

Lynn Butler, Executive Director
Kenneth Follette, Clara Barton Camp Director
Lindsay Charest, Associate Director
Donna Joly, Facilities Director
A coed day camp for children and teens, ages 6-15, with type 1 diabetes. The camp is held in Danvers, Massachusetts at the St. John's Preparatory School. Campers get the opportunity to explore the 175-acre facility, play games, and construct art pieces.

1189 The Barton Center Family Camp
The Barton Center for Diabetes Education, Inc.
30 Ennis Road
PO Box 356
North Oxford, MA   01537-0356   508-987-2056
                                        Fax: 508-987-2002
                                        info@bartoncenter.org
                                        www.bartoncenter.org

Lynn Butler, Executive Director
Kenneth Follette, Clara Barton Camp Director
Lindsay Charest, Associate Director
Donna Joly, Facilities Director
The Barton Center Family Camp is offered twice a year for the families of youth with diabetes. Families participate in traditional camp activities and diabetes education sessions.

1190 The Barton Center Worcester Day Camp
The Barton Center for Diabetes Education, Inc.
30 Ennis Road
PO Box 356
North Oxford, MA   01537-0356   508-987-2056
                                        Fax: 508-987-2002
                                        info@bartoncenter.org
                                        www.bartoncenter.org

Lynn Butler, Executive Director
Kenneth Follette, Clara Barton Camp Director
Lindsay Charest, Associate Director
Donna Joly, Facilities Director
A coed day camp for children and teens, ages 6-15, with diabetes. The camp is held in North Oxford, Massachusetts at the Clara Barton Birthplace Museum, campers experience boating, canoeing, arts and crafts, and camp games.

1191 The Bridge Center
470 Pine St
Bridgewater, MA   02324-2112   508-697-7557
                                        info@TheBridgeCtr.org
                                        www.thebridgectr.org

Jackie Ross, Interim Executive Director
Abby Ross, Year Round & Summer Camp Program Coordinator
A therapeutic recreational facility in Bridgewater, Massachusetts offering after-school programs, special events, school vacation full-week and summer day camp programs for individuals with disabilities.

Michigan

1192 Camp Barefoot
The Fowler Center for Outdoor Learning
2315 Harmon Lake Rd
Mayville, MI   48744   989-673-2050
                                        Fax: 989-673-6355
                                        info@thefowlercenter.org
                                        www.thefowlercenter.org

Kyle L Middleton, Executive Director
Lynn M. Seeloff, Assistant Director
Offered to adults 18 or older with traumatic brain injuries/closed head injuries. A wide variety of activities are offered. The participants in Camp Barefoot request their week's activities, allowing each participant to design their own activity schedule.

1193 Camp Catch-A-Rainbow
YMCA Storer Camps
6941 Stony Lake Rd
Jackson, MI   49201   517-536-8607
                                        Fax: 517-536-4922
                                        storer@ymcastorercamps.org
                                        www.ymcastorercamps.org

Katie Wilson, Camp Catch-A-Rainbow Coordinator
Brian Frawley, Associate Executive Director
Madeline Lombardo, Program Executive
Camp Catch-A-Rainbow is a free camp for cancer survivors ages 4-15. The camp is held at YMCA Storer Camps in Jackson, Michigan.

1194 Camp Chris Williams
MI Coalition for Deaf & Hard of Hearing People
PO Box 16234
Lansing, MI 48901-6234   586-718-0344
                                        campchris@michdhh.org
                    michdhh.weebly.com/camp-chris-williams.html

1195 Camp Grace Bentley
8250 Lakeshore Rd
Burtchville Township, MI 48059   313-962-8242
                                campgracebentley@gmail.com
                                        campgracebentley.org
Jim Ellis, President
Camp Grace Bentley offers 9 day summer camp programs for
children and teens ages 7-16, with physical and mental disabilities. Each camper is screened before attending the camp to ensure
the camp can meet the needs of the camper. Activities include
swimming, campfires, movie nights, team sports, arts and crafts,
karaoke night, and dances.

1196 Camp Midicha
American Diabetes Association
300 Galleria Officentre #111
Southfield, MI 48034   248-433-3830
                                    campmidicha@diabetes.org
                                        www.diabetes.org/camp
Krista Lang, Camp Director
Camp Midicha is the Michigan summer camp program of the
American Diabetes Association for children with diabetes. The
camp is hosted at YMCA Camp Copneconic in Fenton, Michigan.

1197 Camp Quality Michigan
PO Box 345
Boyne City, MI 49712   231-582-2471
                                        Fax: 866-564-7637
                                    mioffice@campqualityusa.org
                                    www.campqualityusa.org/MI
Kristyn Balog, Executive Director
Tom Fasca, North Camp Director
Camp Quality is an international camping program for children
with cancer. The Michigan Camp Quality is held in Lake Ann,
Michigan and offers children and their siblings summer camps
and year round camping opportunities. Volunteer doctors and
nurses are at the camp 24 hours a day, and there is a 1:1 staff to
camper ratio.

1198 Camp Quality South Michigan
PO Box 345
Boyne City, MI 49712   231-582-2471
                                        Fax: 866-564-7637
                                    mioffice@campqualityusa.org
                                    www.campqualityusa.org/MI
Kristyn Balog, Executive Director
Jeff Cram, South Camp Director
Camp Quality is an international camping program for children
with cancer. The South Michigan Camp Quality is held in Fenton,
Michigan and offers children and their siblings summer camps
and year round camping opportunities. Volunteer doctors and
nurses are at the camp 24 hours a day, and there is a 1:1 staff to
camper ratio.

1199 Echo Grove Camp
Salvation Army
1101 Camp Rd
Leonard, MI 48367-2812   248-628-3108
                                        Fax: 248-628-7055
                            vicky_purkey@usc.salvationarmy.org
                                        www.echogrove.org
Mark Mc Clenaghan, Camp Director
Sharon McClenaghan, Associate Camp Director
Jeanie Engle, Program Director
Martin Soffran, Site & Facility Manager
Since 1921, the Army's Echo Grove Camp has offered a struc-
tured camping program for children, adults and seniors referred
through Corps Community Centers. During the course of Echo
Grove's 12 week season, the camp includes programs geared for

every need and interest. In addition to outdoor recreation, camps
may include religious, musical and skill-building instruction.

1200 Indian Trails Camp
IKUS Life Enrichment Services
O-1859 Lake Michigan Dr NW
Grand Rapids, MI 49534   616-677-5251
                                        Fax: 616-677-2955
                                        info@ikuslife.org
                                        www.ikuslife.org
Tim Hileman, Executive Director
Mary Allis, Camp Director & Respite Coordinator
Amy DeMott, Director, Programs & Services
The Indian Trails Camp is a program of IKUS Life Enrichment
Services. The camp offers summer, day, and weekend respite pro-
grams for individuals of all ages with disabilities. Campers are
able to participate in adaptive recreation opportunities in a
barrier-free environment.

1201 St. Francis Camp On The Lake
10120 Murrey Rd
Jerome, MI 49249   517-688-9212
                                        Fax: 517-688-9298
                                    info@saintfranciscamp.org
                                    www.saintfranciscamp.org
Michelle L. Hatfield, Camp Director
St. Francis Camp on the Lake offers residential summer camps,
day camps, and respite care for children and adults with developmental disabilities.

1202 Trail's Edge Camp
Trail's Edge Camp
c/o Mott Respiratory Care, 8-714
1540 E Hospital Dr. SPC 4208
Ann Arbor, MI 48109-4208   734-764-1817
                            director.trailsedgecamp@gmail.com
                                        www.trailsedgecamp.org
Jeff Cain, RRT, Director
Betsy Howell, Activities Coordinator
Trail's Edge Camp is a free, 1 week summer camp for children and
teens ages 5-18, who are ventilator dependent. Campers are able
to participate in camp activities such as games, horseback riding,
and fishing. The camp is limited to 32 campers and they must be
able to interact and communicate with other children through
speech or sign language.

Minnesota

1203 AuSM Summer Camp
Autism Society of Minnesota
2380 Wycliff St.
#102
St. Paul, MN 55114   651-647-1083
                                        camp@ausm.org
                                        www.ausm.org
Jean Bender, President
Paul D'Arco, Vice President
Katie Knutson, Secretary
Paul Schmidt, Treasurer
A program of the Autism Society of Minnesota (AuSM), the Sum-
mer Camps are offered to children, teens, and adults with autism,
ages 6 and up, in a variety of formats including day and residen-
tial summer camp. Camp Hand in Hand is held at Camp Knutson
in Crosslake, Minnesota, Camp Discovery is held at True
Friends/Courage North in Lake George, Minnesota, and Wahode
Day Camps are held at Camp Butwin. Campers wishing to attend
the summer camp programs must be members of the AuSM

1204 Camp Buckskin
PO Box 389
Ely, MN 55731   763-432-9177
                                    info@campbuckskin.com
                                    www.campbuckskin.com
Tom Bauer, Camp Co-Director
Mary Bauer, Camp Co-Director
David Williamson, Program Director

Camp Buckskin is for campers ages 6-18 with underdeveloped social skills who may struggle to interact with others and make friends. The camp is also open to children who have been diagnosed with AD/HD, Aspergers, and/or a learning disability.

1205 Camp Confidence
Confidence Learning Center
1620 Mary Fawcett Drive W
East Gull Lake, MN 56401   218-828-2344
                                        info@campconfidence.com
                                        www.campconfidence.com

Jeff Olson, Executive Director
Bob Slaybaugh, Program Director
Camp Confidence works to promote self-confidence and self-esteem for individuals with developmental and cognitive disabilities. Programs run year round with campers participating in hands on activities and outdoor recreation experiences .

1206 Camp Discovery
American Academy Of Dermatology
930 E Woodfield Rd.
PO Box 4014
Schaumburg, IL 60173   847-240-1280
                                                    866-503-7546
                                                    888-462-3376
                                        Fax: 847-240-1859
                                        www.campdiscovery.org

1207 Camp Heartland
One Heartland
2101 Hennepin Ave S
Suite 200
Minneapolis, MN 55405   888-216-2028
                                        Fax: 612-824-6303
                                        helpkids@oneheartland.org
                                        www.oneheartland.org

Patrick Kindler, Executive Director
Katie Donlin, Operations Manager
Allison Jones, Program Coordinator
Jill Rudolph, National Camp Director
A program of One Heartland, a nonprofit organization working to provide camping programs for children with serious illnesses or experiencing social isolation, Camp Heartland is a weeklong summer camp for children, ages 7-15, who are infected or affected by HIV/AIDS. The camp is held in Willow River, Minnesota.

1208 Camp Knutson
11148 Manhattan Pt. Blvd.
Crosslake, MN 56442   218-543-4232
                                        campknutson@lssmn.org
                                        www.lssmn.org/camp

Jared Griffin, Camp Director
Caitlin Malin, Program Director
Camp Knutson is an accessible camp that hosts a variety of different programs for children with special needs such as skin disease, autism, down syndrome, heart diseases, and children who are infected or affected with HIV/AIDS.

1209 Camp Odayin
275 3rd St S, Suite 104
PO Box 2068
Stillwater, MN 55082   651-351-9185
                                        Fax: 651-351-9187
                                        info@campodayin.org
                                        www.campodayin.org
Sara Meslow, Executive Director
Alison Boerner, Assistant Director
Camp Odayin provides camping experiences for youth and the families of youth with heart disease. Camp Odayin offers a variety of programs including residential, day, family, and winter camps as well as retreats.

1210 Camp Odayin Day Camp
Camp Odayin
275 3rd St S, Suite 104
PO Box 2068
Stillwater, MN 55082   651-351-9185
                                        Fax: 651-351-9187
                                        info@campodayin.org
                                        www.campodayin.org

Sara Meslow, Executive Director
Alison Boerner, Assistant Director
A program of Camp Odayin, the Day Camp is geared for children in kindergarten to grade 3 with heart disease. Located at the Dodge Nature Center in West St. Paul, Minnesota , Camp Odayin's Day Camp offers campers recreational experiences in a safe and fun environment.

1211 Camp Odayin Summer Camp
Camp Odayin
275 3rd St S, Suite 104
PO Box 2068
Stillwater, MN 55082   651-351-9185
                                        Fax: 651-351-9187
                                        info@campodayin.org
                                        www.campodayin.org

Sara Meslow, Executive Director
Alison Boerner, Assistant Director
Camp Odayin offers a variety of summer camp programs for children in grades 1 - 11 with heart disease. Camper eligibility is determined upon the recommendation of a pediatric cardiologist and the camps medical director. The camp is held at 2 locations, with campers able to attend Camp Lutherdale in Elkhorn, Wisconsin or Camp Knutson in Crosslake, Minnesota.

1212 Camp Odayin Winter Camp
Camp Odayin
275 3rd St S, Suite 104
PO Box 2068
Stillwater, MN 55082   651-351-9185
                                        Fax: 651-351-9187
                                        info@campodayin.org
                                        www.campodayin.org

Sara Meslow, Executive Director
Alison Boerner, Assistant Director
Offered to campes who attended either Camp Odayin's Summer or Day Camps, the Winter Camp is for children and teens who have heart disease. The camp is held in Amery, Wisconsin at Camp Wapogasset.

1213 Camp Odayin Young Adult Retreat
Camp Odayin
275 3rd St S, Suite 104
PO Box 2068
Stillwater, MN 55082   651-351-9185
                                        Fax: 651-351-9187
                                        info@campodayin.org
                                        www.campodayin.org

Sara Meslow, Executive Director
Alison Boerner, Assistant Director
Camp Odayin's Young Adult Retreat is a weekend program for adults 18-22 who previously attended Camp Odayin. The retreat is designed to help with the transition to adulthood and give retreat goers a chance to share their experiences.

1214 Courage Center Camps
Courage Center
3915 Golden Valley Road
Minneapolis, MN 55422   763-588-0811
                                                    866-734-3273
                                        Fax: 320-963-3698
                                        TTY: 763-520-0245
                                        couragekenny@allina.com
                                        www.couragecenter.org/camps

Jan Malcolm, CEO
Pamela J. Lindemoen, Exec VP of Operations
Stephen Bariteau, Chief Dev. Officer
Alice Johnson, Chief Financial Officer

Camp is located in Maple Lake, Minnesota. Summer sessions for campers with a variety of disabilities. Coed, ages 6-99, families, seniors.

1215 Down Syndrome Camp
Down Syndrome Foundation
MN   651-321-2267
www.downsyndromefoundation.org
Angie Kniss, President & Founder
Nick Engbloom, Secretary
Ellie Wilson, Counselor Coordinator
A weeklong summer, coed camp for youths, ages 10-21 who have Down Syndrome. The camp is held at Camp Knutson in Cross Lake, Minnesota . The camp is fully accessible and activities include swimming, boating, fishing, tubing, paddleboarding, horseback riding, arts and crafts, and campfires. The camp staff is trained to work with children and adults with special needs.

1216 True Friends
10509 108th St NW
Annandale, MN   55302   952-852-0101
800-450-8376
Fax: 320-852-0123
news@truefriends.org
Conor McGrath, Director, Camp & Operations
Jon Salmon, Associate Camp Director & Customer Relations
True Friends provides camp experiences for children and adults with disabilities. 5 locations make up True Friends including Camp Courage in Maple Lake, Minnesota, Camp Friendship on Clearwater Lake, Camp Eden Wood, a fully accessible camp in Eden Prairie, Minnesota, Camp Courage North in Paul Bunyan State Forest, and Camp New Hope near McGregor, Minnesota in Savannah State Forest and Park.

Mississippi

1217 Camp Dream Street
3863 Morrison Rd.
Utica, MS   39175   225-229-6277
info@dreamstreetms.org
www.dreamstreetms.org
Kyle Goldich, Advisory Board Chair
David Zapletal, Advisory Board Finance Vice Chair
Kimberly Evans, Advisory Board Marketing Vice Chair
Ellie Streiffer, Advisory Board Programming Vice Chair
Dream Street is a 5 day, 4 night camp for children ages 8-14 with physical and sometimes related cognitive disabilities. The camp offers activities such as swimming, arts and crafts, horseback riding and more.

Missouri

1218 Camp Barnabas
PO Box 3200
Springfield, MO   65808   417-476-2565
info@campbarnabas.org
www.campbarnabas.org
Jason Brawner, Chief Operations Officer
Mike Mrosko, Director, Operations
Camp Barnabas is a Christian camp for children, the siblings of children, and adults with special needs. The camp has two locations in Purdy and Shell Knob, Missouri serving children and adults, ages 7-45. The camp costs $750.00.

1219 Camp Encourage
4025 Central St.
Kansas City, MO   64111   816-830-7171
info@campencourage.org
www.campencourage.org
Jenny Hines, President
Kaye Otten, President Elect
Kelly Lee, Executive Director
Elizabeth Boresow, Secretary

Encourages social growth, independence and self esteem in children and young adults with autism spectrum disorder through a quality, overnight camp experience located in the greater Kansas City area.

1220 Camp Hickory Hill
PO Box 1942
Columbia, MO   65205   573-445-9146
CampHickoryHill@gmail.com
www.camphickoryhill.com
David Bernhardt, CPA, Executive Director
Jessica Bernhardt, Camp Director
Christina Barron, Program Director
Frank La Mantia, Development Director
Camp Hickory Hill is a residential summer camp for children, ages 7-17, with diabetes. Campers participate in traditional summer camp activities as well as educational programs.

1221 Camp MITIOG
Share, Inc.
7615 N. Platte Purchase Dr
Suite 116
Kansas City, MO 64118   www.campmitiog.org

1222 Camp No Limits Missouri
No Limits Foundation
13528 State Route AA
Potosi, MO   63664   207-240-5762
Fax: 877-406-5106
campnolimits@gmail.com
www.nolimitsfoundation.org
Mary Leighton, Founder & Executive Director
Melanie Dash, Program Director
Pedro Pimenta, Director, Development
Missy Moreau, Project Coordinator
Camp No Limits Missouri, is a location of Camp No Limits, a recreational and educational camp for youth who have experienced limb loss. Camp No Limits, is a program of the nonprofit organization No Limits Foundation.

1223 Camp Quality Central Missouri
PO Box 953
Jefferson City, MO   65012-0953   636-795-7229
cmo@campqualityusa.org
www.campqualityusa.org/cmo
Casey Bucher, Co-Director
Erin Carl, Co-Director
Camp Quality is an international camping program for children with cancer. The Central Missouri Camp is held in St.Clair, Missouri and offers children and their siblings summer camps and year round camping opportunities. Volunteer doctors and nurses are at the camp 24 hours a day, and there is a 1:1 staff to camper ratio.

1224 Camp Quality Greater Kansas City
3111 SE 3rd Terr.
Lee's Summit, MO   64086   816-809-8600
Fax: 888-456-1611
crystal.davison@campqualityusa.org
www.campqualityusa.org/gkc
Crystal Davison, Executive Director
Camp Quality is an international camping program for children with cancer. The Greater Kansas City Camp is held in Excelsior Springs, Missouri and offers children and their siblings summer camps and year round camping opportunities. Volunteer doctors and nurses are at the camp 24 hours a day, and there is a 1:1 staff to camper ratio.

1225 Camp Quality Northwest Missouri
PO Box 9044
St. Joseph, MO   64508   816-232-2267
Fax: 816-232-2920
nwmo@campqualityusa.org
www.campqualityusa.org/nwmo
Adam Nelson, Co-Director
Gabe Bailey, Co-Director

Camp Quality is an international camping program for children with cancer. The Northwest Missouri Camp is held in Stewartsville, Missouri and offers children and their siblings summer camps and year round camping opportunities. Volunteer doctors and nurses are at the camp 24 hours a day, and there is a 1:1 staff to camper ratio.

1226 Camp Quality Ozarks
PO Box 302
Joplin, MO 64802

ozarks@campqualityusa.org
www.campqualityusa.org/oz

1227 Wonderland Camp
18591 Miller Circle
Rocky Mount, MO 65072

573-392-1000
info@wonderlandcamp.org
www.wonderlandcamp.org

Cory Polk, Executive Director
Dustin Baker, Interim Camp Director
Linda Fiers, Office Manager
Wonderland Camp provides residential summer camps and year round weekend camps for children, teens, and adults with disabilities.

Montana

1228 Big Sky Kids Cancer Camps
Eagle Mount-Bozeman
6901 Goldenstein Lane
Bozeman, MT 59715

406-586-1781
Fax: 406-586-5794
bigskykids@eaglemount.org
www.eaglemount.org

Mary Peterson, Executive Director
Maggee Harrison, Equestrian Program Director
Chad Biggerstaff, Big Sky Program Director
Tracey Wheeler, Finance Director
Provides recreational opportunities for kids and young adults ages 5-23 with cancer. Big Sky offers skiing, swimming, fishing, ice-skating, golf, cycling, and other outdoor activities.

1229 Camp Mak-A-Dream
2110 Johnson Street
Missoula, MT 59801

406-549-5987
Fax: 406-549-5933
info@campdream.org
www.campdream.org

Kim McKearnan, Executive Director
Beth Jones, Camp Director
Jennifer Bentoon, Program Manager
Jake Wood, Property Manager
Camp Mak-A-Dream provides a cost-free summer camp experience to children, teens, young adults, women and families affected by cancer. Participants can expect to experience regular camp activities such as swimming and zip lining, as well as the chance to interact with ranch staff.

1230 Camp Montana
Beartooth Mountain Christian Camp
130 Trinity Trail
Fishtail, MT 59028

720-855-1102
Fax: 720-855-1302
emfay@diabetes.org
www.diabetes.org

Emily Fay, Camp Director
Camp Montana is an American Diabetes Association summer camp for children with diabetes, ages 8-17. The goal of Camp Montana is to provide a safe and fun camping experience, while also educating campers about managing their diabetes.

1231 Charles Campbell Childrens Camp
The Billings Lions Club
PO Box 23342
Billings, MT 59104

406-670-2496
campbellcamp@msn.com

Doug Hanson, Director
Sue Hanson, Director
Camp is open to young adults with physical disabilities that include sight or hearing impairment, spina bifida, cerebral palsy, gross motor skill impairments and other disabilities. Campers enjoy hiking, swimming, fishing, dances, campfires and much more.

Nebraska

1232 Camp Floyd Rogers
Floyd Rogers Foundation
PO BOX 541058
Omaha, NE 68154

402-885-9022
director@campfloydrogers.com
www.campfloydrogers.com

Erin Hoffman, President
Greg Penny, Vice President
Ashley Moore, Treasurer
Mike German, Secretary
A camp for children, ages 8-18, with Type 1 diabetes. While at the camp, children will enjoy activities, participate in special events, engage in innovative evening programs, and meet other children their own age with diabetes. Camp Floyd Rogers offers young people an opportunity to share some of life's adventures with others who also happen to have diabetes.

1233 Camp Kindle
Project Kindle/Camp Kindle
PO BOX 81147
Lincoln, NE 68501

661-257-1901
877-800-2267
Fax: 702-995-9186
info@projectkindle.org
www.campkindle.org

Eva Payne, Founder and President
Mandy Nickolite, Vice President
Erin FitzGerald, Program Coordinator
Nikki Wiener, Medical Director
The camp offers children with HIV and AIDS a safe environment where they can go to strengthen their self esteem through interactive participation in educational and recreational programming.
Held in June each year

1234 Easter Seals Nebraska
Easter Seals Nebraska
12565 West Center Road
Suite 100
Omaha, NE 68144-8144

402-345-2200
Fax: 402-345-2500
ahowell@ne.easterseals.com
www.ne.easterseals.com

James C. Summerfelt, President & CEO
Angela Howell, Vice President Easter Seals Nebr
Lily Sughroue, Director of Camp, Respite & Recr
Offers a variety of services to help people with disabilities address life's challenges and achieve personal goals. Terrific fun for campers and a much needed respite for families and caregivers from the daily challenges of caring for special needs individuals.

1235 Kamp Kaleo
46872 Willow Springs Rd
Burwell, NE 68823

308-346-5083
kampkaleo@gmail.com
www.kampkaleo.com

Gaylene O'Brien, Facilities Administrator
Sandy Denton, Minister of Faith Development
An overnight summer camp for individuals who are blind/visually impaired or have developmental disabilities. Coed, ages 9-18 and families, seniors, single adults. Participants can expect to experience outdoor recreational activities such as canoeing, fish-

ing, and swimming, and there is a strong focus on religous education.

1236 National Camps for Blind Children
Christian Record Services
5900 S 58th St
Suite M
Lincoln, NE 68516
402-488-0981
Fax: 402-488-7582
services@christianrecord.org
www.christianrecord.org

Diane Thurber, President
Andrea Ahrens, Development Director
Jeri Lyn Rogge, Communication Director
Kalvin Follett, Studio & Library Services Director

Provides free Christian publications and programs to people who are legally blind or physically incapable of holding reading material. Free services include subscription magazines in braille, large-print and audio; lending library on digital cartridge and on-line download; Full-Vision books, combining braille, audio and print; gift Bibles and study guides; camping for people age 9-65 through National Camps for Blind Children; and scholarship assistance.

Nevada

1237 Camp Buck
Nevada Diabetes Association
18 Stewart Street
Reno, NV 89501
775-856-3839
800-379-3839
Fax: 775-348-7591
camp@diabetesnv.org
www.diabetesnv.org

Sarah Gleich, Executive Director
Mylan Hawkins, Founder
Diana Kern, Dirctor of Development
Lynn Wexler, Southern Nevada Dir. Of dev.

Co-ed summer camp for children with diabetes ages 8-17. While at the camp, the children develop a better understanding of their diabetes while enjoying a week filled with recreational and athletic activities such as swimming, kayaking, fishing and arts & crafts.

1238 Camp Lotsafun
Amplify Life
164 Hubbard Way
Suite D
Reno, NV 89502
775-827-3866
Fax: 775-827-0334
www.camplotsafun.com

Gayla Ouellette, Director
Stephanie Rice, Chairwoman
Linda Barnes, Director
Alan Herak, Treasurer

Provides therapeutic, educational, and recreational opportunities for individuals with developmental disabilities, while providing respite care for their families. Children, teens and adults with autism, down syndrome, traumatic brain injury, cerebral palsy and attention deficit hyperactive disorder are among some of the individuals who attend camp for fun and recreational activities such as swimming, kayaking, pet therapy, arts & crafts, drama and music.

1239 Camp SignShine
Deaf Centers of Nevada
6490 S McCarran Blvd.
Bldg. F, Suit 46 & 47
Reno, NV 89509
775-473-9452
888-240-4684
Fax: 702-685-0324
info@dcnv.org
www.dhharc.org

J. Farrell Cafferata Jenkins, President

Week long camp for children ages 7-19 who are deaf or hard of hearing and their siblings. Campers enjoy recreational and educational activities in a safe and comfortable environment.

1240 CampCare
P.O. Box 12155
Reno, NV 89510-2155
775-323-3737
cmoore@campcarenevada.org
www.campcarenevada.org

1241 Discovery Day Camp
Nevada Blind Children's Foundation
9330 West Martin Ave.
Las Vegas, NV 89148
702-735-6226
info@nvblindchildren.org
nvblindchildren.org/programs/day-camp/

Emily Smith, Executive Director
Veronica Atkins, Development Director
Briana Myers, Program Director

A summer day camp program for children in grades K through 8 who are blind/visually impaired. Disocvery Day camp provides traditional camp activities that have been adapted to meet the needs of children with visual impairments.

New Hampshire

1242 Adam's Camp: New Hampshire
Adam's Camp
60 Loon Mountain Road
Lincoln, NH 03251
603-715-2298
newhampshire@adamscamp.org
www.adamscampnewengland.org

Adrienne Evans, Executive Director

The New Hampshire location of Adam's Camp, offers both therapy and adventure camps for children and the families of children with special needs and developmental delays. The New Hampshire Camp is located in Loon Mountain at the Loon Mountain Resort.

1243 Camp Allen
56 Camp Allen Road
Bedford, NH 03110-6606
603-622-8471
Fax: 603-626-4295
michael@campallennh.org
www.campallennh.org

Michael Constance, Executive Director
Deb Shulte, Camp Allen Office Manager
Stephen Daley, Camp Director
Deaglan O'Rourke

A residential summer camp for individuals with disabilities. All of the activities are conducted by individual coordinators under the supervision of the Program Director. Some of the activities include, aquatics, arts, crafts, games and nature programs. All camp events, special events, evening programs, and field trips are scheduled throughout the summer and are structured to meet the individual abilities and needs of each camper.

1244 Camp Connect
Easter Seals New Hampshire
555 Auburn Street
Manchester, NH 03103
603-621-3407
Fax: 603-625-1148
www.easterseals.com/nh

Andrew MacWilliam, Chariman
Charles Goodwin, Vice Chairman
Tom Sullivan, Vice Chairman
Matthew Boucher, Treasurer

A summer day camp for children in grades K-12 with Asperger Syndrome, High Functioning Autism, Nonverbal Learning Disorder, and other social communication disorders. The camp has a large focus on continuing to address academic needs of the campers, but also incorporates music, drama, and arts & crafts.

1245 Camp Inter-Actions
Inter-Actions
170 West Rd.
Suite 6-B
Portsmouth, NH   03801

603-319-6120
campinfo@inter-actions.org
inter-actions.org/

Debbie Gross, Camp Director
Duy Bui, Music Director
Camp Inter-Actions is a summer camp for children, ages 8-15, who are blind or visually impaired. The camp is located in Kingston, New Hampshire, and runs one, two, and three week sessions. Activities include swimming, fishing, adapted sports/games, woodworking, pottery, and more.

1246 Camp Sno Mo
Easter Seals: New Hampshire
555 Auburn St
Manchester, NH   03103

603-623-8863
Fax: 603-625-1148
rkelly@eastersealsnh.org
www.easterseals.com/nh/

Andrew MacWilliam, Chairman
Charles Goodwin, Vice Chairman
Matthew Boucher, Treasurer
Charles Panasis, Secretary
Camp Slo Mo is is a residential camp program where children and young adults, ages 11-21, with disabilities and special needs participate alongside Boy Scouts in a variety of outdoor recreational activities.

1247 Camp Yavneh: Yedidut Program
Summer Address
18 Lucas Pond Rd.
Northwood, NH   03261

603-942-5593
info@campyavneh.org
www.campyavneh.org/yedidut/

Nanette Fridman, President
Bil Zarch, Camp Director
Jeff Weener, Associate Director
Miriam Loren, Inclusion Coordinator/Yedidut Director
A residential Jewish summer camp program for 4-5 campers ages 9-12 at Camp Yevnah. Traditional camp activities with a strong focus on Judaism and Jewish education.

1248 Wediko Summer Program
New Hampshire Campus
11 Bobcat Blvd.
Windsor, NH   03244

603-478-5236
Fax: 603-478-2049
www.wediko.org/

Miklos Oyler, Director
Jennifer Walsh, Program Operations Manager
Ed Zadravec, Clinical Director
This program is a 45 day residential program for children, teens, and young adults, ages 9-19 with social, emotional, and behaviour challenges. This program serves children with disabilities such as ADD/ADHD, Asperger's, Ausitsm, and others.

New Jersey

1249 Camp Carefree
1846 West Seventh St.
Piscataway, NJ   08854

603-483-3803
director@campcarefreekids.org
www.campcarefreekids.org

Phyllis Woestemeyer, Camp Director
The camp is located at Lions Camp Pride in New Durham, New Hampshire. Camp Carefree is a American Diabetes Association summer camp for children with diabetes.

1250 Camp Chatterbox
Children's Specialized Hospital
150 New Providence Rd.
Mountainside, NJ   07092

908-301-5548
campchatterbox@childrens-specialized.org
www.childrens-specialized.org

Sara Barnhill, MS, CCC-SLP, Clinical Coordinator
Camp Chatterbox is an overnight camp for people ages 5-22 who use augmentative communication devices. The camp offers recreational activities such as swimming, arts, sports and exploring nature.

1251 Camp Deeny Riback
208 Flanders-Netcong Rd.
Flanders, NJ   07836

973-929-2901
Fax: 973-463-3998
camps@jccmetrowest.org
cdr.jccmetrowest.org/

Julie Perlow, Director
Ben Gilbert, Assistant Director
Debra Scher, Registrar
A Jewish summer camp for children of all ages. The camp integrates children with special needs through their Camp Friends program. The camp provide traditional outdoor camp activities.

1252 Camp Dream Street
Kaplen JCC On The Palisades
411 East Clinton Ave.
Tenafly, NJ   07670

201-569-7900
Fax: 201-569-7448
info@jccotp.org
www.jccotp.org

Kyle Goldich, Advisory Board Chair
David Zapletal, Advisory Board Finance Vice Chair
Kimberly Evans, Advisory Board Marketing Vice Chair
Ellie Streiffer, Advisory Board Programming Vice Chair
Dream Street is a 5 day, 4 night camp for children ages 8-14 with physical and sometimes related cognitive disabilities. The camp offers activities such as swimming, arts and crafts, horseback riding and more.

1253 Camp Jotoni
ARC of Somerset County
141 S Main St
Manville, NJ   08835-1803

908-725-8544
lauraz@thearcofsomerset.org
www.thearcofsomerset.org

Josh Burke, Director
Chris Reagan, Director, Travel Camp
Vicky Thornton, Program Coordinator
Kristin Wells, Program Coordinator
Sponsored by the Arc of Somerset County, Camp Jotoni is a day and residential camp for children and adults with developmental disabilities. Campers are ages five to adult. Set on 15 acres in Somerset County, the camp features a junior Olympic size pool, cabins, dining hall, playgrounds, open air pavilions, unspoiled woods, and wildlife.

1254 Camp Merry Heart
Easter Seals: New Jersey
25 Kennedy Blvd
Suite 600
East Brunswick, NJ   08816

732-257-6662
Fax: 732-257-7373
camp@nj.easterseals.com
www.easterseals.com/nj/

Brian Fitzgerald, President
Helen Drobnis, Chied Advancement Officer
Shelley Samuels, Chief Program Officer
Judy Fellenz, Executive Assistant
An organized program of swimming, arts and crafts, boating, nature study and travel offered to campers with a variety of disabilities. Coed, ages 5-80, families, seniors. Fall and spring travel programs for adults.

1255   Camp Nejeda
Camp Nejeda Foundation
910 Saddlebrook Rd
P.O. Box 156
Stillwater, NJ   07875   973-383-2611
                                      Fax: 973-383-9891
                                  info@campnejeda.org
                                   www.nejeda.convio.net
Ernest Post, MD, Secretary
Scott Ross, President
Bill Vierbuchen, Executive Director
Jim Daschbach, Camp Director
For children with diabetes, ages 7-15. Provides an active and safe
camping experience which enables the children to learn about
and understand diabetes. Activities include boating, swimming,
fishing, archery, as well as camping skills.

1256   Camp Oakhurst
New York Service for the Handicapped
111 Monmouth Rd
Oakhurst, NJ   07755   732-531-0215
                                      Fax: 732-531-0292
                                         info@nysh.org
                                         www.nysh.org/
Robert Pacenza, Executive Director
Charles Sutherland, Camp Director
Andy Arno, Board Member
Hope Bach, Board Member
A summer and day camp for adults and children with with special
needs, including autism and physical and intellectual disabilities.
Campers will experience all the traditional camp activities while
gaining skills for greater independence.

1257   Camp Quality New Jersey
PO Box 264
Adelphia, NJ   07710   330-671-0167
                                      Fax: 866-285-5208
                                  info@campqualityusa.com
                                  www.campqualityusa.org/nj
Vicki Irey, President
Anneliese Kulakofsky, Vice President
Dennis Hart, Secretary
Lois Hartje, Treasurer
Camp Quality is for children with cancer and their siblings. The
camp offers a stress-free environment that offers exciting activi-
ties and fosters new friendships, while helping to give the chil-
dren courage, motivation and emotional strength.

1258   Camp Sun'N Fun
ARC of Gloucester
1555 Gateway Blvd.
West Deptford, NJ   08096   856-848-8648
                                  camp@thearcgloucester.org
                                   www.thearcgloucester.org
William Gordon, Assistant Executive Director
Ana Rivera, Executive Director
Camp is located in Williamstown, New Jersey. Summer sessions
for campers with developmental disabilities. Coed, ages 8-88.
Activities include swimming, arts & crafts, nature, sports, games,
music, dance and drama.

1259   Explorer's Club Camp
New Behavioural Network
2 Pin Oak Lane
Suite 250
Cherry Hill, NJ   08003   856-874-1616
                                      Fax: 856-424-7660
                                   nbh@nbngroup.com
                    www.newbehavioralnetwork.com/summer-camp/

1260   Happiness Is Camping
62 Sunset Lake Rd
Hardwick, NJ   07825   908-362-6733
                                      Fax: 908-362-5197
                                  rich@happinessiscamping.org
                                   www.happinessiscamping.org
Laura San Miguel, RN, PNP, President
Julie McMahon, RN, Secretary
Alexander Chou, MD, Medical Director
Paulette Kelly, RN, Nursing Director
Located in Hardwick, New Jersey, Happiness is Camping is a
week-long camp for kids with cancer and their siblings, ages
6-15. The camp is free for all attendees, and campers will partici-
pate in a variety of traditional outdoor activities, including
canoeing, fishing, swimming, archery, and more.

1261   Harbor Haven Summer Program
470 Prospect Ave.
Suite 203B
West Orange, NJ   07052   908-964-5411
                                      Fax: 908-964-0511
                                   info@harborhaven.com
                                   www.harborhaven.com/
Robyn Tanne, Director/Owner
Brad Haimowitz, Assistant Director
Kristie Thomas, Program Coordinator
A 7-week summer day program for children, ages 3-15, with mild
special needs. Harbor Haven offers traditional outdoor recreation
activities, and a daily academic period which reinforces math,
reading, and language arts.

1262   Mane Stream
83 Old Turnpike Rd.
P.O. Box 305
Oldwick, NJ   08858   908-439-9636
                                      Fax: 908-439-2338
                                   info@manestreamnj.org
                                   www.manestreamnj.org/
Holland Kochanski, Camp Director
Trish Hegeman, Executive Director
Linda Dietz, President
Karen Mikita Kaufhold, Vice President
A summer day camp for children with physical and cognitive
challenges, their siblings, and non-disabled children. The camp is
primarily focused on horsemanship lessons, with activities such
as riding lessons, grooming, tacking, leading, basic horse care,
and more. Eight week-long sessions available.

1263   New Jersey Camp Jaycee
Camp Jaycee Administrative Office
985 Livingston Ave
North Brunswick, NJ   08902   732-737-8279
                                      Fax: 732-737-8279
                                   info@campjaycee.org
                                   www.campjaycee.org
Frank Pirrello, President
John O'Brien, Vice President
Patricia Rhein, Secretary
James Sandham, Treasurer
Camp Jaycee is located on 185 acres of forests, fields and streams
in the Pocono Mountains, a short distance from the New Jersey
border. Sessions for children and adults, ages 7-85, with autism
and developmental disabilities. Goals of Camp Jaycee are centered around developing social skills, improving self esteem, increasing confidence, learning in a fun environment, developing
physical fitness, and establishing meaningful relationships with
new friends.

1264   Round Lake Camp
New Jersey YMHA/YWHA
21 Plymouth Street
Fairfield, NJ   07004   973-575-3333
                                      Fax: 973-575-4188
                                   info@njycamps.org
                                   www.roundlakecamp.org
Aryn Barer, Director

Round Lake Camp is for children, ages 7-18, with learning differences and social communication disorders. Campers can enjoy swimming, boating, sailing, mountain biking, and arts and crafts.

1265   Summit Camp
322 Route 46 West
Suite 210
Parisppany, NJ   07054   973-732-3230
                                       Fax: 973-732-3226
                                    info@summitcamp.com
                                     www.summitcamp.com

Eugene Bell, Senior Director
Leah Love, Assistant Director
Thea Mullis, Travel Director
Maryann Santora, Clinical Social Worker/Admission
The camp is located in Honesdale, Pennsylvania, and is for children, ages 8-19, who have a variety of developmental, social, or learning issues. In addition to regular camp activities like swimming, sports, and arts and crafts, Summit Camp has a strong focus on social skills development and interpersonal growth.

New Mexico

1266   Camp Enchantment
Monzano Mountain Retreat
201A Los Pinetos
Torreon, NM   87061   505-384-4467
                               info@campenchantment.org
                                   campenchantment.org/

Jessica Lin, Board of Directors
Cameron Rodger, Board of Directors
Berdel Boulenger, Board of Directors
Melissa O'neill, Board of Directors
A pediatric summer camp for kids and teens, ages 7-17, diagnosed with cancer. The camp is held at the Monzano Mountain Retreat in Torreon, New Mexico. Activities include swimming, kayaking, dancing, archery, and more. The camping session is 7 days. Camp Enchantment also runs Camp Superstars, a summer camp for siblings of cancer patients.

1267   Camp Rising Sun
Center for Development and Disability
2300 Menaul Blvd. NE
Albuquerque, NM   87107   505-272-3000
                                          800-270-1861
                                       Fax: 505-272-2014
                                   PBrouse@salud.unm.edu
                            www.cdd.unm.edu/camprisingsun/

Paul Brouse, Camp Director
Maia Wynn, Program Coordinator
Natalie Kossar, Administrative Assistant
Held at the Manzano Mountain Retreat southeast of Albuquerque, Camp Rising sun is a summer camp designed specifially for children and teens with Autism Spectrum Disorder and their peers, ages 8-17. Activities include hiking, sports, photography, kayaking, campouts, and other nature activities.

1268   Camp for Kids With Diabetes: Camp 180
American Diabetes Association
Manzano Mountain Retreat
County Road AO03, Post 210
Torreon, NM   87061   602-861-4731
                                       Fax: 602-995-1344
                                     jgarcia@diabetes.org
                                        www.diabetes.org

Julie Garcia, Director
The main goal of the program at American Diabetes Association Camp for Kids is to allow the campers the ability to feel at ease and accepted in a community where having diabetes is the rule, not the exception. The campers learn to understand diabetes and the process of self-management, under skilled and continuous medical supervision. It is the hope of the staff that these children go home feeling more self-confident, self-reliant and having gained the invaluable knowledge.

New York

1269   ADA Camp Aspire
Sunshine Campus
809 Five Points Rd
Rush, NY   14543   585-533-2080
                                     esmythe@diabetes.org
                                        www.diabetes.org/

Amanda Capizzi, Co-Director
Alicia Harper, Co-Director
The American Diabetes Association New York Area's Camp is a residential camp for children with diabetes. The program is held on the Rotary Sunshine Campus in Rush, only 15 miles from Rochester. The camp is located on 133 acres of land in a rural setting including modern year round cabins, an Olympic-sized swimming pool, nature trails, athletic fields and a fishing pond. Ages 8-16; held during July.

1270   Autism Summer Respite Program
Samuel Field Y
58-20 Little Neck Parkway
Little Neck, NY   11362   718-225-6750
                                       Fax: 718-225-3910
                                  Sfysummercamps@sfy.org
                                  www.sfysummercamps.org/

Gerrie Mayerhoff, Director, Special Services
Amanda Smith, Camp Dirctor, Autism Summer Respite
An afternoon camping program for children, teens, and young adults, ages 5-21 with Autism and similar disabilities. Located at the Samuel Field Y.

1271   AutismUp: YMCA Summer Social Skills Program
AutismUp Headquarters
855 Publishers Prkwy
Webster, NY   14580   585-248-9011
                                       Fax: 585-248-9159
                                    contact@autismup.org
                                         autismup.org

Lisa Fetkenhour, President, AutismUp
Betsy Brugg, Vice President
Dawn Vogler-Elias, Secretary
This program is a collaboration between AutismUp and the Greater Rochester YMCA. The Summer Social Skills Program is a day camp held at Camp Arrowhead and Camp Bay View for children, 4-16, with Autism Spectrum Disorders. Half day and full day sessions available, and campers are integrated into regular camp activities.

1272   Barton Day Camp Long Island
The Barton Center for Diabetes Education, Inc.
30 Ennis Road
PO Box 356
North Oxford, MA   01537-0356   508-987-2056
                                       Fax: 508-987-2002
                                    info@bartoncenter.org
                                      www.bartoncenter.org

Lynn Butler, Executive Director
Kenneth Follette, Clara Barton Camp Director
Lindsay Charest, Associate Director
Donna Joly, Facilities Director
A program of The Barton Center for Diabetes Education, The Barton Day Camp Long Island is held in Long Island, New York for children and teens, ages 5-15, with diabetes. The camp offers a 1 week or 2 week session, with campers receiving diabetes education and participating in activities such as swimming, arts and crafts, and games.

1273   Camp Abilities Brockport
The College at Brockport, State Univ of New York
350 New Campus Drive
Brockport, NY   14420   585-395-5361
                           campabilitiesbrockport01@gmail.com
                             www.campabilitiesbrockport.org

Dr. Lauren Lieberman, PhD, Camp Director
Tiffany Mitrakos, MEd, Assistant Director
Emily Gilbert, Aquatic and Boating Director
Maria Lepore-Stevens, Aquatic and Boating Director

A one-week sports camp for children who are visually impaired, blind or deaf blind. Children learn to be more physically active, which in turn improves their health and well being.

1274   Camp Adventure
KiDS NEED MoRE
P.O. Box 305
Copiague, NY   11726   631-608-3135
                                          Fax: 631-532-4944
                                          info@kidsneedmore.org
                                          kidsneedmore.org/

Melissa Firmes, President
Kim Bjorklund, Vice President
John Ray, Treasurer
Jaqueline Lorenz, Secretary
Camp Adventure is a one-week sleep away camp for children and teens ages 6-18 dealing with cancer and other life threatening illnesses. The camp takes place on Shelter Island at Quinipet Camp and Retreat Center.

1275   Camp Anne
AHRC New York
228 Four Corners Rd.
Ancramdale, NY   12503   518-329-5649
                                          Michael.Rose@ahrcnyc.org
                                          camping.ahrcnyc.org/

Michael Rose, Camp Director
Angelo Aponte, President
Edward J. Leahy, 1st Vice President
A day summer camp program for children and adults with intellectual and developmental disabilities. The camp offers activities such as cooking, crafts, nature, sports, swimming, and more. Camp Anne offers three 11-day sessions for adults ages 21-59, and two 11-day sessions for childres ages 5-20. Each session can accomodate 100 campers.

1276   Camp EAGR
YMCA of Greater Buffalo
301 Cayuga Rd
Suite 100
Buffalo, NY   14225   716-565-6000
                                          Fax: 716-565-6007
                                          www.ymcabuffaloniagara.org
Scott Weigley, Executive Director, Camp Weona
Carolyn Blaine, Program Director, Camp Weona
Nick Reid, Assistant Program Director, Camp Weona
April Williams, Office Manager, Camp Weona
Camp EAGR is held at YMCA's Camp Weona, located in Gainesville, New York. Camping sessions for children and adults with epilepsy. Coed, ages 7-16, families and single adults. Nestled in 1,000 acres of hardwood and pine forests, Weona has miles of hiking trails, brooks, a heated outdoor pool and a world class adventure ropes course. Indoor facilities include arts and crafts studios, environmental classrooms and a challenging rock climbing wall.

1277   Camp Good Days and Special Times
1332 Pitsford-Mendon Rd
PO Box 665
Mendon, NY   14506   585-624-5555
                                             800-785-2135
                                          Fax: 585-624-5799
                                          www.campgooddays.org
J. Robert Bleier, Board President
Eric Foster, Board Vice President
Michael Mercier, Board Treasurer
Patricia Stevens, Board Secretary
The camp is dedicated to improving the quality of life for children, adults and their families whose lives have been touched by cancer and/or other life challenges. The camp offers week-long sessions that are free of charge.

1278   Camp High Hopes
P.O. Box 165
Afton, NY   13730   607-644-6969
                                          badlands056@gmail.com
                                          www.camphighhopes.org/
Matt Palmeri, Camp Director
Joe Brennan, President of the Board
Hope Woodcock-Ross, Health Director
During the six-day camp boys with Hemophilia and their brothers participate in individual and group activities designed for fun and fitness. The camp held each year in mid-June has a 24-hour physician and nursing staff. Ages 7-17, boys only.

1279   Camp Huntington
56 Bruceville Road
High Falls, NY   12440   845-687-7840
                                             855-707-2267
                                          Fax: 855-707-2267
                                          www.camphuntington.com

Alex Mellor, Camp Director
Daniel Falk, Camp Owner
Margaret Short, Health Director
Cathy Crowley, Program Supervisor
A co-ed residential summer camp specifically designed to focus on Adaptive and Therapeutic Recreation. Campers include those with learning and developmental disabilities, ADD/HD, Autism Spectrum Disorders, Asperger's, PDD, and other special needs. Three programs are offered that focus on: recreation and social skills; independence; and participation. Campers may attend for a week at a time with a full summer lasting nine weeks.

1280   Camp Kehilla
Henry Kaufmann Campgrounds
75 Colonial Spring Rd.
Wheatley Heights, NY   11798   516-484-1545
                                          mcaira@sjjcc.org
                                          www.campkehilla.org/
Pam Zimmer, Director
Marissa Caira, Assistant Director
A year-round camp for children, teens, and young adults with a variety of disabilities. Ages 4-21.

1281   Camp Little Oak
Aldersgate Camp & Retreat Center
7955 Brantingham Rd.
Greig, NY   13345   425-770-1801
                                          hannahbanana90@juno.com
                                          camplittleoak.org/
Hannah Russell, Camp Director
Hope Woodcock-Ross, Health Director
A non-profit, week-long summer camp for girls diagnosed with a bleeding disorder. The camp is held at Aldersgate Camp in Greig, New York. Camp Little Oak runs traditional summer camp activities, such as swimming, canoeing, and archery, as well as provides education about blood disorders and conducts community service projects.

1282   Camp Mark Seven
Mark Seven Deaf Foundation
144 Mohawk Hotel Rd
Old Forge, NY   13420   315-207-5706
                                          TTY:315-357-6089
                                          registrar@campmark7.org
                                          www.campmark7.org
Dave Staehle, Camp Director
Adirondack Mountain camp for hard-of-hearing, deaf and hearing people. Coed, ages 1-99, families, seniors and single adults.

1283   Camp Northwood
132 State Route 365
Remsen, NY   13438-5700   315-831-3621
                                          northwoodprograms@hotmail.com
                                          www.nwood.com
Gordon W Felt, Director
Donna Felt, Director
Camp Northwood is an overnight camp for children with non-agressive learning issues such as Asperger's Syndrome, At-

tention Deficits, HFA, and other learning issues. The camp is co-ed and accepts children ages 8-18. The camp has a strong focus on developing age appropriate skills, as well as traditional camping activities.

1284 Camp Pa-Qua-Tuck
2 Chet Swezey Rd.
Center Moriches, NY   11934   631-878-1070
www.camppaquatuck.com/
Steve Kronman, Board Member
Barbara Caldwell, Board Member
Newton Homan, Board Member
Marcella Weiss, Board Member
Camp Pa-Qua-Tuck is a residential camp for children ages 6-21 with physical and developmental disabilities. 50 campers are accepted per weekly session. The camp also offers Respite Camp, a weekend camp program for ages 6-21.

1285 Camp Ramapo
22 Camp Ramapo Rd
Rhinebeck, NY   12572   845-876-8403
Fax: 845-876-8414
office@ramapoforchildren.org
www.ramapoforchildren.org
Adam Weiss, CEO
Teri Goldberg Horowitz, President
David Ross, VP
Bob Dean, Treasurer
Ramapo's specific focus is adventure-based, experiential learning programs that promote positive character values in children and teens with special needs.

1286 Camp Reece
Summer Address
815 North Broadway
Saratoga Springs, NY   12866   212-289-4872
info@campreece.org
www.campreece.org/
Duncan Lester, Executive Director
Octavia Man, Camp Director
Lisa Howles, Administrative Associate
A sleep-away camp for children, ages 10-16, with special needs. The camp is located at Skidmore College, and offers activities such as photography, rafting, biking, sports, and more. The camp serves boys and girls with disabilities such as ADD/ADHD, learning disabilities, and High-functioning Autism. There are two 3-week sessions or the full 6-week session available.

1287 Camp Sisol
Jewish Community Center of Greater Rochester/JCC
1200 Edgewood Ave
Rochester, NY   14618   585-461-2000
Fax: 585-461-0805
www.jccrochester.org
Richard Gray, President
Daniel Goldstein, Vice President
Arnie Sohinki, Executive Director
Howard Cohen, Treasurer
Camp is located in Honeoye Falls, New York. Coed, ages 5-16. Camp Sisol accomodates children with special needs.

1288 Camp Tova
92nd Street Y
1395 Lexington Ave
New York, NY   10128   212-415-5500
www.92y.org
Marc S. Lipschultz, President
Henry Timms, Executive Director
Laurence D. Belfer, Vice President
Lori A. Kasowitz, Vice President
Children with learning and developmental disabilities thrive in Camp Tova's small group setting. Making friends and developing a wide variety of creative, social, and physical skills are the goals for Tova campers.

1289 Camp Venture, Inc.
25 Smith Street
Suite 510
Nanuet, NY   10954   845-624-3860
www.campventure.org
John Murphy, President
Celia Solomita, Chief Financial Officer
Debra Archambault, Associate Executive Director
Lisa Kirrane, Associate Executive Director
Camp Venture is a day camp for children, ages 5-12, with and without developmental disabilities. Located in Stony Point, the camp also offers a young adult group for teens, ages 13-21, with developmental disabilities. Children will experience the fun of regular camp activities, while benefitting from group engagement.

1290 Camp Whitman on Seneca Lake
Presbyterian Church USA
150 Whitman Road
Penn Yan, NY   14527   315-536-7753
Fax: 315-531-4002
camp@campwhitman.org
www.campwhitman.org
Lea Kone, Camp Director
Aline Trombley, Office Manager
Taylor Eike, Coordinator
Courtney Ormsby, Coordinator
To give the developmentally disabled youth/adult, ages 10-60, the opportunity to enjoy him/herself in a camping program. Campers are encouraged to participate in a full range of activities including games, sports, swimming, singing, and dancing.

1291 Clover Patch Camp
Center for Disability Services
55 Helping Hand Ln
Glenville, NY   12302   518-384-3042
Fax: 518-384-3001
cloverpatchcamp@cfdsny.org
www.cloverpatchcamp.org
Laura Taylor, Camp Director
Christopher Schelin, Program Administrator
Clover Patch Camp is operated by the Center for Disability Services, and is located in Glenville, New York. The camp is for individuals with a variety of disabilities between the ages of 5-18.

1292 Double H Ranch
97 Hidden Valley Road
Lake Luzerne, NY   12846   518-696-5676
Fax: 518-696-4528
myurenda@doublehranch.org
www.doublehranch.org
Vincent T. Riggi, Chairman
Ed Mitzen, Vice Chairman
Max Yurenda, CEO/Executive Director
Jacqui Royael, Director Of Operations
Summer residential camp and winter sports programs for children and young adults ages 6-16 who have cancer and other life threatening illnesses. The programs are free of charge and some of the recreational activities include bead making, arts & crafts, kickball, tennis, soccer, and volleyball.

1293 Friendship Circle Summer Camp
121 West 19th Street
New York, NY   10011   646-820-1066
www.friendshipnyc.com

1294 Gow School Summer Programs
2491 Emery Road
South Wales, NY   14139   716-652-3450
Fax: 716-652-3457
summer@gow.org
www.gow.org

Douglas B. Cotter, Director of Admissions
Bradley Rogers Jr., Headmaster
Jon Chafin, Assistant Summer Program Director
Joseph Cendrowski, Summer Program Administrator

Co-ed summer programs for students ages 8-16 with dyslexia or similar learning disabilities offer a balanced blend of morning academics, afternoon/evening traditional camp activities and weekend overnights. The primary purpose of these programs is to provide a positive experience. Committed to the creation of a positive and enjoyable experience for each participant by defining and merging the goals of the camp and the school with those of camper students.

1295 Kamp Kiwanis
New York District Kiwanis Foundation
9020 Kiwanis Rd
Taberg, NY 13471   315-336-4568
                                                  Fax: 315-336-3845
                                           kamp@kampkiwanis.org
                                           www.kamp-kiwanis.org

Rebecca L. Clemence, Executive Director
Sal Anelli, Foundation President
Kamp Kiwanis is a mainstream camp for underprivileged youth with and without special needs. 20 campers with disabilities are integrated into weekly sessions. Coed, ages 8-14, seniors and single adults.

1296 Katy Isaacson Elaine Gordon Lodge
AHRC New York
653 Colgate Rd.
Box 37
East Jewett, NY 12424   518-589-6000
                                     Matthew.Hatcher@ahrcnyc.org
                                           camping.ahrcnyc.org/

Matt Hatcher, Camp Director
Angelo Aponte, President
Edward J. Leahy, 1st Vice President
An alternative and traditional summer day camp for adults and teens with intellectual and developmental disabilities. The lodge offers fice 11-day sessions for adults ages 18-29, and one session for teens ages 13-17. Activities include boating, swimming, pony rides, sports, and more.

1297 Lisa Beth Gerstman Camp
Samuel Field Y
58-20 Little Neck Parkway
Little Neck, NY 11362   718-225-6750
                                                  Fax: 718-225-3910
                                          Sfysummercamps@sfy.org
                                          www.sfysummercamps.org/

Gerrie Mayerhoff, Director, Special Services
Shari Rebhun, Director, Lisa Beth Gerstman Camp
A summer day camp for children ages 6-13 who are hard of hearing or deaf. Activities include simming, sports, and arts and crafts. The program is held at the Bay Terrace Pool Club.

1298 Maplebrook School
5142 Route 22
Amenia, NY 12501   845-373-9511
                                                  Fax: 845-373-7029
                                     admissions@maplebrookschool.org
                                          www.maplebrookschool.org

Donna Konkolics, Head of School
Roger Fazzone, President
Jennifer Scully, Assistant Head, Postsecondary Studies
Lori Hale, Executive Director
A coeducational boarding school which offers a six week camp for children with learning differences and ADD.

1299 Marist Brothers Mid-Hudson Valley Camp
P.O.Box 197
Esopus, NY 12429   845-384-6620
                                     info@maristbrotherscenter.org
                                     www.maristbrotherscenter.org/

Amy Reinwald-Earle, Camp Director, Special Children
Brother Owen Ormsby, Executive Director
Scott Kuhner, Director of Operations
Mike Trainor, Facilities Director
The camp provides week-long summer sessions for children who have a variety of special needs/illnesses, such as cancer, HIV, deaf or mental disabilities. Each session is specific to the special need/illness.

1300 Mosholu Day Camp
Mosholu Montefiore Community Center
3450 Dekalb Ave.
Bronx, NY 10467   718-882-4000
                                                  contact@mmcc.org
                                           www.mosholudaycamp.com

Rita Santelia, Cheif Executive Officer
Laurie Meltzer Bandremer, Director of Development
Ivan Diaz, Facilities Director
A day camp program for children in 1st-10th grade. The day camp offers specific programs for children and teens who are developmentally disabled. Camp Sunshine is for children ages 5-12, and Camp Elan is for children who are ages 12-16.

1301 Samuel Field Y Day Camp
58-20 Little Neck Parkway
Little Neck, NY 11362   718-225-6750
                                                  Fax: 718-225-3910
                                          Sfysummercamps@sfy.org
                                          www.sfysummercamps.org/

Gerrie Mayerhoff, Director, Special Services
Samuel Field Y offers a day camp for children, ages 5-21, with developmental disabilities. Activities include dancing, swimming, arts and crafts, and community-based field trips. Older campers are offered a Campsite program, which allows them to attend activities at the Henry Kaufmann Campgrounds.

1302 Southampton Fresh Air Home
36 Barkers Island Rd.
Southampton, NY 11968   631-283-1594
                                                  Fax: 631-283-7596
                                                  www.sfah.org/

Michaela Kezler, Chairman
Catherine Kuehn Price, Chariman
Susan Nappa Cocke, Vice Chairman
Kirsten Solsvig Galef, President
A residential camp facility that accomodates physically challenged children. The Special Needs Summer Camp is for children and teens ages 8-18. one or three week sessions available, as well as day camp. The SFAH provides adapted programs and activities that allow campers to develop physically, emotionally, and psychologically.

1303 Sunshine Campus
Rochester Rotary Club
180 Linden Oaks
Suite 200
Rochester, NY 14625   585-546-7435
                                     brandi@rochesterrotary.org
                                          www.sunshinecampus.org

Laura Speers, Camp Director
James Allessi, Camp Director
Brandi Koch, Sunshine Campus Partner Director
Seth Sykes, Sunshine Campus Facilities Manager
The camp is located in Rush, New York. Camping sessions for children and young adults with a variety of disabilities. Ages 7-21. Campers experience a variety of traditional summer camp activities, including climbing wall, swimming, boating, hiking, and sports.

1304 VISIONS Vacation Camp for the Blind
VISIONS Center on Blindness
500 Greenwich St
3rd Floor
New York, NY 10013-1354   212-625-1616
                                                  888-245-8333
                                                  Fax: 212-219-4078
                                                  info@visionsvcb.org
                                                  www.visionsvcb.org

Nancy T. Jones, President
Steve E. Kent, Vice President
Burton M. Strauss, Jr., Treasurer
Jasmine M. Campirides, Secretary
Is a non profit agency that promotes the independence of people of all ages who are blind or visually impaired. Camp offers Braille classes, computers with large print and voice output, support groups, discussions, mobility lesions, cooking classes, personal and home management training, large print and Braille books.

1305 Wagon Road Camp
Children's Aid Society
711 Third Ave
Suit 700
New York, NY 10017   212-949-4800
webmaster@childrensaidsociety.org
www.childrensaidsociety.org

Iris Abrons, Chair
Richard Edelman, Vice Chair
Kevin J. Watson, Treasurer
Amy Engel Scharf, Secretary
Wagon Road Day Camp is a co-ed program for children ages 6-13 with a variety of disabilities held within Chappaqua, New York. Uniquely qualified specialists in Project Adventure activities, athletics, horsemanship, theater arts, nature/ecology studies and arts/crafts complement the day camp staff. Special events including Carnival, Olympics, Crazy Hat Day, Western Day, and optional sleepovers add to the summer excitement providing children with an enriching multicultural experience.

1306 West Hills Day Camp: Gersh Academy
West Hills Day Camp
21 Sweet Hollow Rd.
Huntington, NY 11743   631-427-6700
Fax: 631-427-6504
info@westhillscamp.com
westhillsdaycamp.com/

Kevin Gersh, Owner/President
Scott Zlochower, Director, Gersh Academy
A summer day camp program for children with Autism Spectrum disorders an other related neurobiological disorders. Located on Long Island, activities include swimming, climbing/ropes course, photography, arts & crafts, and more.

1307 YMCA Camp Chingachgook on Lake George
Capital District YMCA
1872 Pilot Knob Rd
Kattskill Bay, NY 12844   518-656-9462
Fax: 518-656-9362
chingachgook@cdymca.org
camp.cdymca.org/

John Lefner, Executive Director
Carol Lewis, Office Manager
Jin, Andreozzi, Summer Camp Program Director
Tricia Biles, Groups Services Director
Sailing programs for people with disabilities. Coed, ages 7-16, families, seniors and single adults.

North Carolina

1308 Camp Carefree
275 Carefree Lane
Stokesdale, NC 27357   336-427-0966
directors@campcarefree.org
www.campcarefree.org

Lynn Tuttle, Executive Director
Tony McCallum, Program Director
JeNai Davis, Program Director
Grace Turner, Program Director
A free, one-week camp for youngsters with serious health problems. The camp gives the children a chance to have the freedom to play, learn and enjoy all the recreational and craft activities the camp has to offer.

1309 Camp Carolina Trails
American Diabetes Association
YMCA Camp Hanes
1225 Camp Hanes Road
King, NC 27021   919-743-5400
888-342-2383
Fax: 919-783-7838
btonkin@diabetes.org
www.diabetes.org

Brooke Tonkin, Director
The camp is for children aged 7-17 years of age who have diabetes. The camp is held on the YMCA's Camp Hanes campground,

next to Hanging Rock State Park. Activities include swimming, hiking, and field games. The camp employs a complete medical staff consisting of registered nurses, dieticians, and pediatric endocrinologists.

1310 Camp Dogwood
7050 Camp Dogwood Dr.
Sherrills Ford, NC 28673   800-662-7401
susan@nclionsinc.org
nclionscampdogwood.org/

Susan King, Camp Director
Keisha Ramseur, Camp Secretary
A recreational facility on Lake Norman, offering 10 week-long sessions for adults who are blind and visually impaired. Ages 18 and up. Activities include swimming, tubing, local field trips, bowling, and more. Service dogs welcome.

1311 Camp New Hope
P.O. Box 154
Glendale Springs, NC 28629   336-982-3797
campnewhopenc.com/

Randy S. Brown, Camp Director
Camp New Hope is a privately owned facility where children with life threatening conditions and their families can go to relax and enjoy the joys of the outdoors. There are no scheduled events/activities, but families are able to enjoy fishing, canoeing, tubing, swimming, and more entirely at their leisure. Attendance is completely free.

1312 Camp Royall
250 Bill Ash Rd
Moncure, NC 27559   919-542-1033
Fax: 919-542-6343
camproyall@autismsociety-nc.org
www.autismsociety-nc.org/camp-royall/

Lesley Fraser, Program Director, Camp Royall
Cindy Lodestro, Administrative Assisstant
Sara Gage, Director, Social Recreation Services
Curtis Sobie, Fellow
A week-long overnight and day camp for children and adults with autism. Campers will participate in traditional camp activities in a structured environment that helps them develop confidence, independence, and a willingness to try new things.

1313 Camp Sertoma
Millstone 4-H Center
1296 Mallard Dr
Ellerbe, NC 28338   336-593-8057
SertomaDeafCamp@gmail.com
www.campsertomaclub.org/

Sandy Waterman, Camp Setoma
Keith Russell, Camp Director, Millstone 4-H Center
Erehn N. Frye, Program Director, Millstone 4-H Center
Camp Sertoma is a place where deaf and hard of hearing children can come to meet people just like them, with out communication barriers. Activities include swimming, canoeing, fishing, hiking, hayrides, campfires, games, astronomy, and nature crafts. Ages 8-16, co-ed.

1314 Camp Tekoa UMC
United Methodist Camp Tekoa
P.O. Box 160
Hendersonville, NC 28793-0160   828-692-6516
Fax: 828-697-3288
ecampbell@camptekoa.org
www.camptekoa.org

James Johnson, Executive Director
John Isley, Assistant Director
Karen Rohrer, Business Manager
Melisa Coates, Administrative Assistant
Camping for children with developmental disabilities. Day camps available for children aged 8-12, and overnight programs for adults aged 18 and up.

1315 SOAR Summer Adventures
NC Base Camp
226 SOAR Lane
P.O.Box 388
Balsam, NC 28707
828-456-3435
Fax: 801-820-3050
admissions@soarnc.org
www.soarnc.org

John Wilson, Executive Director
Laura Pate, Director of Operations
Catey Terry, Chief Financial Officer
Lynne Neaves, Admissions Director
A nonprofit adventure program working with disadvantaged youth diagnosed with learning disabilities in an outdoor, challenge based environment. Focuses on esteem building and social skills development through rock climbing, backpacking, whitewater rafting, mountaineering, sailing, snorkeling, and much more. Offers two week, one month, and semester programs. SOAR programs utilize North Carolina, Florida, Colorado, American Southwest, Alaska, and Jamaica as program areas.

1316 Talisman Summer Camp
64 Gap Creek Rd
Zirconia, NC 28790
828-697-6313
info@talismancamps.com
talismancamps.com

Douglas Smathers, Camp Director & Owner
Linda Tatsapaugh, Operations Director & Owner
Robyn Mims, Admissions Director
Lee Kisselburg, Facilities Manager
Talisman Summer Camp is located 40 minutes south of Asheville, North Carolina. Offers a program of hiking, rafting, climbing, and caving for learning disabled ADD/ADHD and autistic young people. Coed, ages 6-22.

1317 Victory Junction Gang Camp
4500 Adam's Way
Randleman, NC 27317
336-498-9055
info@victoryjunction.org
www.victoryjunction.org

Chad Coltrane, President/CEO
Kyle Petty, Founder/Chairman
Brian Flynn, Executive Board Member
Carolyn Bechtel, Executive Board Member
The camp serves children with a variety of chronic medical conditions or serious illnesses, including Autism, Cancer, Craniofacial Anomalies, Diabetes, Sickle Cell, Spina Bifida and more. Victory Junction provides all the regular camp activities, but also includes a NASCAR themed area where kids can play wii, dress up in a racing suit, and sit in an authentic NASCAR racecar.

North Dakota

1318 Camp Sioux
American Diabetes Association
106 Solid Rock Circle
Park River, ND 58270
763-593-5333
Fax: 952-582-9000
rbarnett@diabetes.org
www.diabetes.org

Becky Barnett, Camp Director
Carol Holten, Associate Manager
Camp Sioux, located in Park River, ND, is a week-long residential summer camp for children ages 8-15 who are living with diabetes. Programs encourage independence and self management with appropriate medical supervision to ensure the best possible experience for every camper. Nutrition activities, blood glucose monitoring, and injections/medications are integrated into the camp program.

Ohio

1319 CYO Camp Happiness Day Camp
Catholic Charities Disability Services
7911 Detroit Ave
Cleveland, OH 44102
216-334-2963
contactus@clevelandcatholiccharities.org
ccdocle.org/disability

Dennis McNulty, Director, Disability Services
Marilyn Scott, Program Director, Disability Services
Camp Happiness welcomes children and young adults ages 6-21 with cognitive and other developmental disabilities. In addition to recreational services, Camp Happiness also provides educational and social services to help participants continue to practice and develop skills throughout the year.

1320 Camp Arye
Jewish Community Center of Greater Columbus
1125 College Ave
Columbus, OH 43209
614-231-2731
Fax: 614-231-8222
arardain@columbusjcc.org
www.columbusjcc.org

Austen Rardain, Director, Camp Arye
Karen Causey, Site Director, Camp Hoover
A Jewish summer camp for children and young adults with developmental, physical, emotional, mental and learning disabilities. Camp Arye is co-ed and for ages 5-22.

1321 Camp Cheerful
Achievement Centers For Children
15000 Cheerful Ln
Strongsville, OH 44136-5420
440-238-6200
Fax: 440-238-1858
jennie.amodio@achievementctrs.org
www.achievementcenters.org

Julie Boland, Chairwoman
James Kacic, Vice Chairman
Nicole Hilbert, Treasurer
Jennifer Vergilli, Secretary
Camp Cheerful provides a number of day and overnight camping options for children and adults who have disabilities. The camp hosts traditional camp activities, as well as year-round Therapeutic Horseback Riding sessions and a handicap-accessible High Ropes challenge course during the summer. The focus of activities is to increase the quality of life while encouraging confidence and independence.

1322 Camp Christopher: SumFun Day Camp
Camp Christopher
1930 N Hametown Rd.
Akron, OH 44333
330-726-2961
800-296-2267
campchristopher@ccdocle.org
ccdocle.org/program/sumfun

Tess Flannery, Program Contact
A multi-week summer day camp for children, teens, and young adults, ages 5-21, with developmental disabilities. Campers participate in regular camp activities, while building confidence and social skills.

1323 Camp Courageous
12701 Waterville-Swanton Rd
Whitehouse, OH 43571
419-875-6828
Fax: 419-875-5598
camping@campcourageous.com
www.campcourageous.com

1324 Camp Echoing Hills
36272 County Road 79
Warsaw, OH 43844   800-419-6513
                                Fax: 740-327-2333
                        info@echoinghillsvillage.org
                        www.campechoinghills.org/

Lauren Unger, Camp Administrator
Emily Smith, Program Director
Dan Peterson, Camp Nurse
Donald Smith, Operations & Activities Coordinator

Summer camp for children and adults with physical and intellectual disabilities. There is a strong focus on religion, social interaction, and development of skills.

1325 Camp Emanuel
P.O. Box 752343
Dayton, OH 45475   937-477-5504
                        crawford@campenamuel.org
                        www.campemanuel.weebly.com

Brian Demarke, President
Stephanie Ackner, Vice President
Mary Foreman, Secretary
Nan Crawford, Executive Director

Camp Emanuel is a camp for hearing impaired and normal hearing youth. There are day sessions for children 5-14, and overnight resident sessions for children and teens 9-17. The camp aims to promote descision making, self-esteem, and acceptance by integrating non-hearing children with hearing children.

1326 Camp Hamwi
Central Ohio Diabetes Association
1100 Dennison Ave.
Columbus, OH 43201   614-884-4400
                                Fax: 614-884-4484
                        coda@diabetesohio.org
                        www.diabetesohio.org/

Tim Cotter, President
Jay Meglich, Treasurer
Jon Yoon, Secretary

A summer camp for kids with diabetes, ages 7-18. Sessions are divided by age group, with a Junior Challenge Week for ages 7-12, and a Senior Challenged week for ages 13-17. Activities include horseback riding, sports, swimming, and other outdoor activities.

1327 Camp Ho Mita Koda
14040 Auburn Rd
Newbury, OH 44065   info@chmkfoundation.org
                        www.chmkfoundation.org/

Julia Blanchette, Health Director
Ted Rusinoff, Board Member
Kristin Warzocha, Board Member

Camp Ho Mita Koda is a summer camp for children with type 1 diabetes. The camp aims to provide fun outdoor activties, while also educating and building life skills for children with diabetes. Day camp available for ages 5-11, and two overnight sessions for children ages 8-11 and 12-15.

1328 Camp Joy
10117 Old 3C Hwy.
P.O. Box 157
Clarksville, OH 45113   937-289-2031
                        camp-joy.org/

Dave Palm, President
Jeff Yancey, Secretary
John Kramer, Treasurer

A summer camp organization for children and teens with a variety of disabilities. Sessions for children, teens and young adults with asthma, HIV/AIDS, spina bifidia, limb loss, cancer, blood diseases, and immune disorers.

1329 Camp Ko-Man-She
Diabetes Dayton
2555 S Dixie Drive
Suite 112
Dayton, OH 45409   937-220-6611
                                Fax: 937-224-0240
                        dada@diabetesdayton.org
                        www.diabetesdayton.org

Tyler Starline, President
Michael Martens, Vice President
Becky Roberts, Secretary
Sheila DeWeese, Treasurer

Camp Ko-Man-She is located in Bellefontaine, Ohio, and is held annually for children with type 1 diabetes. The camp's goal is for children to socialize with other children who also have diabetes and to have fun outdoors in a medically supervised setting. Co-ed, ages 8-17.

1330 Camp Korelitz
Camp Joy
10117 Old 3C Hwy.
Clarksville, OH 45113   513-759-9330
                                Fax: 513-421-2203
                        jloving@diabetes.org
                        www.diabetes.org

Jen Loving, Camp Director

A week-long residential camp for children, ages 8-15, with type 1 or type 2 diabetes. Camp Korelitz is a camping program of the American Diabetes Association, and is held at Camp Joy in Clarksville, Ohio. Activities include climbing walls, archery, and canoeing, as well as discussions and education about nutrition and diabetes.

1331 Camp Nuhop
Nuhop Corporate Office
404 Hillcrest Dr
Ashland, OH 44805   419-289-2227
                        www.nuhop.org

Trevor Dunlap, CEO
Nate Holton, Summer Camp Director
Chris Clyde, Associate Director
Ben King, Director of Outdoor Education

A summer residential program for any youngster from 6 to 18 with a learning disability, behavior disorder or Attention Deficit Disorder. Campers and staff members live on site in groups of to seven campers to every three counselors. Activities focus on positive self-concept and behaviors and teaches children to learn how to find their strengths, abilities and talents from a positive, yet realistic viewpoint. Each program is around 6 weeks long.

1332 Camp Oty'Okwa
24799 Purcell Rd.
South Bloomingville, OH 43152-9740   614-839-2447
                        mbayes@bbbscentralohio.org
                        campotyokwa.org/

David Schirner, Director
Megan Bayes

Owned and operated by Big Brothers and Sisters of Central Ohio, this summer camp accommodates children with disabilities such as ADD/ADHD, Autism, learning disabilities, or beahviour/mood disorders.

1333 Camp Paradise
SHC, The ARC of Medina County
4283 Paradise Rd.
Seville, OH 44273   330-722-1900
                        shc@shc-medina.org
                        shc-medina.org/camp-paradise/

Melanie Kasten-Krause, Executive Director
Michael Beh, Director of Finance
Lynn Emmons, Director of Human Resources
Melissa Hart, Comminuty Operations Manager

Camp Paradise is a summer camp for adults with developmental disabilities. The camp offers 5 weeks of themed summer camp, day and overnight sessions available. Activities include music, art therapy, sports, swimming, bonfires, and more.

1334 Camp Quality Ohio
PO Box 358
Uniontown, OH 44685 216-236-2400
Fax: 216-236-2409
Sandra.Kelly@campqualityusa.org
www.campqualityusa.org/oh
Sandra Kelly, Executive Director
Brian Krebs, Summer Camp Director
Kelly Krebs, Camper Registrar
Allison Whoroski, Companion Coordinator
Camp Quality is for children with cancer and their siblings. The camp offers a stress-free environment that offers exciting activities and fosters new friendships, while helping to give the children courage, motivation and emotional strength.

1335 Camp Stepping Stone
Stepping Stones Center
5650 Given Rd
Cincinnati, OH 45243 513-831-4660
Fax: 513-831-5918
steppingstonesohio.org/
Chris Adams, Executive Director
Sam Browne Allen, Programs Director
Chris Brockman, Facilities Director
Kelly Crow, Director of Development
Day and overnight camps for children ages 5-22, serving persons with autism, cognitive deficits, Down Syndrome, cerebral palsy, brain injury, and multiple disabilities. This non-profit organization has four camp locations in Ohio: Camp Given, Camp Allyn, Camp BeauVita West and Camp UCP.

1336 Camp Tiponi
Camp Willson
2732 County Road 11
Bellefontaine, OH 43311 800-423-0427
www.diabetesdaytoncamp.com/camp-tiponi
Tyler Starline, President, Diabetes Dayton
Michael Martens, Vice President, Diabetes Dayton
Becky Roberts, Secretary, Diabetes Dayton
Sheila DeWeese, Treasurer, Diabetes Dayton
A summer camp for children, ages 8-17, for children and teens who have Insulin Resistance, prediabetes, or type 2 diabetes. Campers will participate in activities such as swimming, tennis, archery, and hiking, as well as gaining education and skills needed to maintain a healthy lifestyle.

1337 Champ Camp
Achievement Centers for Children
4255 Northfield Rd.
Highland Hills, OH 44128 216-292-9700
Fax: 216-292-9721
www.achievementcenters.org/
Julie Boland, Chairwoman
James Kacic, Vice Chairman
Nicole Hilbert, Treasurer
Jennifer Vergilii, Secretary
A day camp for children with and without special needs, ages 5-18. Activities include nature study, arts & crafts, music, and special guest performers. Camp is offered in one-week sessions from mid-June through mid-August.

1338 Flying Horse Farms
5260 State Route 95
Mt. Gilead, OH 43338 419-751-7077
Fax: 419-751-7010
info@flyinghorsefarms.org
flyinghorsefarms.org/
Mimi Dane, CEO/President
Kathleen Starkoff, Chair
Tony Garrison, Vice Chair
Robin Grant, Secretary
Flying Horse Farms is a camp for children with serious illnesses, ages 8-15, and their families. The camp serves campers diagnosed with cancer, heart conditions, asthma, blood disorders, and more. Activities include swimming, fishing, and other traditional camp activities.

1339 Highbrook Lodge
Cleveland Sight Center
1909 East 101st St
Cleveland, OH 44106 216-791-8118
877-776-9563
Fax: 216-791-1101
TTY: 216-791-8119
info@clevelandsightcenter.org
www.clevelandsightcenter.org
Lawrence Benders, President/Executive Director
Kevin R. Krencisz, Chief Financial Officer
Karen Bain Hiller, Director of Development
Michael McManamon, Chief Information Officer
Camp is located in Chardon, Ohio. Summer sessions for children, adults and families who are blind or have low vision. Sessions include a wide range of outdoor camp activities. Camp activities focus on gaining independent skills, mobility, orientation and self confidence in an accessible and traditional camp setting.

1340 Insight Horse Camp
Marmon Valley
7754 State Route 292 S.
Zanesfield, OH 43360 937-593-8000
Fax: 937-593-6900
mwiley@marmonvalley.com
marmonvalley.com/
Matt Wiley, Executive Director
Steve Olsen, Operations Manager
Natalie Frueh, Program Director
A coed resident camp program for children, ages 7-17, who are blind/visually impaired. The main focus of camp is on learning basic horsemanship skills, however, campers also particiapte in traditional camp activities and Bible study discussions.

1341 Recreation Unlimited: Day Camp
Recreation Unlimited Foundation
7700 Piper Rd
Ashley, OH 43003 740-548-7006
Fax: 740-747-2640
info@recreationunlimited.org
www.recreationunlimited.org
Paul L. Huttlin, Executive Director & CEO
Chris Link, Operations Manager
Sarah Kelley, Program Manager
Zane Clouse, Program Coordinator
Camping sessions for children and teens, ages 5-22, with physical or developmental disabilities and their siblings. Day camps provide a full day of traditional camp activities and aims to create an inclusive experience for all participants to have fun and grow.

1342 Recreation Unlimited: Residential Camp
Recreation Unlimited Foundation
7700 Piper Rd
Ashley, OH 43003 740-548-7006
Fax: 740-747-2640
info@recreationunlimited.org
www.recreationunlimited.org
Paul L. Huttlin, Executive Director & CEO
Chris Link, Operations Manager
Sarah Kelley, Program Manager
Zane Clouse, Program Coordinator
Camping sessions for children and adults with a variety of physical and developmental disabilities. Two week long sessions for ages 8-22, one week long session for ages 18-35, and four week long sessions for ages 23 and up. The camp provides traditional outdoor recreation such as fishing, archery, exploration, campfires and more.

1343 Recreation Unlimited: Respite Weekend Camp
Recreation Unlimited Foundation
7700 Piper Rd
Ashley, OH 43003
740-548-7006
Fax: 740-747-2640
info@recreationunlimited.org
www.recreationunlimited.org
Paul L. Huttlin, Executive Director & CEO
Chris Link, Operations Manager
Sarah Kelley, Program Manager
Zane Clouse, Program Coordinator
Camping sessions for children and adults with a variety of physical and developmental disabilities. There are seven weekends for youths ages 8-22, and eight weekend camps for adults ages 23 and up. Traditional outdoor activities are provided, along with lodging, meals, site nursing, and more.

1344 Recreation Unlimited: Specialty Camp
Recreation Unlimited Foundation
7700 Piper Rd
Ashley, OH 43003
740-548-7006
Fax: 740-747-2640
info@recreationunlimited.org
www.recreationunlimited.org
Paul L. Huttlin, Executive Director & CEO
Chris Link, Operations Manager
Sarah Kelley, Program Manager
Zane Clouse, Program Coordinator
Weekend and weeklong camping sessions for youth and adults dedicated to a specific disability or health concern. The camp runs traditional outdoor activities that have been created to meet the needs of specific disabilities.

1345 Rotary Camp
4460 Rex Lake Dr
Akron, OH 44319
330-644-4512
Fax: 330-644-1013
rotarycamp@akronymca.org
www.akronymca.com
Grady P. Appleton, President/CEO
Laura Bennett, Board Member
Robert R. Beiswenger, President
Cindy Dormo, Vice President
Offers camping experiences for children and adults with disabilities. Rotary Camp is American Camping Association (ACA) accredited and provides a nurturing and enriching atmosphere where campers develop friendships, skills and memories that will last a lifetime. Coed, ages 6-17.

1346 St. Augustine Rainbow Camp
Disability Ministries at St. Augustine Parish
2486 W 14th St
Cleveland, OH 44113
216-781-5530
Fax: 216-781-1124
www.staugustine-west14.org
Sr. Corita Ambro, Program Director
Fr. Joseph D McNulty, Director, All Ministries
Day camp for all disabled children, and operated by the St. Augustine Church.

1347 Stepping Stones: Camp Allyn
Stepping Stones Center
5650 Given Rd
Cincinnati, OH 45243
513-831-4660
Fax: 513-831-5918
steppingstonesohio.org/
Chris Adams, Executive Director
Sam Browne Allen, Programs Director
Chris Brockman, Facilities Director
Kelly Crow, Director of Development
A residential camp in Batavia, Ohio for children and adults with disabilities. Coed, ages 7-60. Campers participate in crafts, swimming, hiking, nature, sports and motor activities. Camp sessions range from 3 to 10 days, are theme oriented, and geared to individual abilities and interests. Also offers day camps for children ages 5-22.

1348 YMCA Outdoor Center Campbell Gard
4803 Augspurger Rd
Hamilton, OH 45011
513-887-0600
Fax: 513-867-0127
camp@gmvymca.org
www.gmvymca.org
Pete Fasano, Executive Director
Katie Depew, Summer Camp Director
Wendi Moore, Office Manager
Tom Andrews, Properties & Facilities Manager
The camp is located in Hamilton, Ohio. The camp is for children and young adults with developmental disabilities. Runs overnight and day sessions for ages 7-22 and families.

Oklahoma

1349 Camp CANOE
Camp Fire: Camp DaKaNi
3309 E. Hefner Rd.
Oklahoma City, OK 73131
405-254-2080
info@campfireusa-ok.org
campdakani.org/
Penn Henthorn, Camp Director
Elizabeth Logan, Assistant Director
Abbie Dedmon, Camp Office Manager
Camp CANOE is a summer day camp for children with autism in grades K-12. Held at Camp DeKaNi, Camp CANOE focuses on skills such as self-reliance, confidence, communication & social skills, problem-solving, and more.

1350 Camp ClapHans
J.D. McCarty Center
2002 E Robinson St.
Norman, OK 73071
405-307-2865
800-777-1272
Fax: 405-307-2801
camp@jdmc.org
www.campclaphans.com
Bobbie Hunter, Camp Director
Vicki Kuestersteffen, Director/CEO, J.D. McCarty Center
A summer camp for children, teens, and young adults, ages 8-18 with developmental disabilities. Activities include archery, arts & crafts, scavenger hunts, stargazing, and more. Sessions are four days and three nights, and are limited to 12 campers per session (6 boys and 6 girls).

1351 Camp Endres
Diabetes Solutions of Oklahoma, Inc.
3333 NW 63rd
Suite 100
Oklahoma City, OK 73116
405-843-4386
Fax: 888-665-2741
kim@dsok.net
dsok.net/programs/camp-endres/
Kim Boaz-Wilson, RN, Executive Director/Camping Director
Tracy Pappas, Administrative Assistant
Camp Endres is a summer camp for children and teens, ages 8-18, diagnosed with diabetes. The camp is divided into Junior, ages 8-12, and Senior, ages 13-18, sessions. Activities include capture the flag, swimming, horseback riding, and more.

1352 Camp Loughridge
4900 W. 71st St.
Tulsa, OK 74131
918-446-4194
registrar@camploughridge.org
camploughridge.org
Don Skillern, Executive Director
Michael Staires, Summer Camp Program Director
Bart Boatright, Chair
Jeff McMains, Vice Chair
Camp Loughridge is a Christian summer day camp for children ages 6-12. The camp runs for 8 weeks, and has an Autism Inclusion program for children diagnosed with Austism. Space is limited to 4 campers with Autism per session.

1353 Camp Perfect Wings
Crosstimbers Conference Center
5039 Hwy 77 South
Davis, OK 73030 405-942-3800
campperfectwings@bgco.org
www.bgco.org/campperfectwings
Becka Johnson, Camp Director
Keith Burkhart, Family & Men's Ministry Specialist
Sara Pruegert, Family & Men's Ministry Assistant
Pat Jones, Childhood Ministry Assistant
Specifically for children ages 8-17 with special needs. Campers enjoy supervised activities such as canoeing, pool games, low ropes challenges, and crafts. Held in spring/early summer.

1354 Easter Seals Oklahoma
701 NE 13th St
Oklahoma City, OK 73104 405-239-2525
info@eastersealsoklahoma.org
eastersealsok.org/
Keith McCombs, Chairman
Krista Massad, Chairman-Elect
Cassie Wilson, Secretary
Matt Vance, Treasurer
A nationally accredited, full-day program welcoming all children, including those with disabilities and those at risk of disability. The center offers developmentally appropriate learning activities and services to meet the unique needs of each child. Our Adult Day Health Center provides solutions to meet the physical, social and emotional needs of adults from the ages of 21 to 100+.

Oregon

1355 Adventures Without Limits
1341 Pacific Ave
Forest Grove, OR 97116 503-359-2568
Fax: 503-359-4671
info@awloutdoors.org
awloutdoors.com
Brad Bafaro, Founder/Executive Director
Ashley Borman, Program Director
Lartz Stewart, Assistant Executive Director
Laura Stallard, Office Manager
Adventures Without Limits facilitates inclusive, outdoor adventure for people of all ages and ability levels. Trip activities include hiking, rafting, caving, rock climbing, kayaking, snowshoeing, and more.

1356 B'nai B'rith Camp: Kehila Program
9400 SW Beaverton Hillsdale Hwy
Suite 200
Beaverton, OR 97005 503-452-3443
Fax: 503-452-0750
info@bbcamp.org
bbcamp.org/
Michelle Koplan, Executive Director
Ben Charlton, Camp Director
Barb Gordon, Executive Assistant
Shayna Sigman, Inclusion Coordinator
The Kehila Program at B'nai B'rith Camp is a Jewish summer camp program for children with special needs. This program is run during the camp's Maccabee session.

1357 Camp Magruder
Oregon-Idaho Conference Center
17450 Old Pacific Hwy
Rockaway Beach, OR 97136 503-355-2310
Fax: 503-355-8701
office@campmagruder.org
www.campmagruder.org
Troy Taylor, Camp Director
Rik Gutzke, Facilities Manager
Angie Nebeker, Guest Services Manager
Hope Montgomery, Program Director
Camp is located in Rockaway Beach, Oregon. Sessions for teens and adults with developmental disabilities through Camp Hope.

1358 Camp Meadowood Springs
Camp Meadowood Office
122 SE Court Ave
P.O. Box 1025
Pendleton, OR 97801 541-276-2752
Fax: 541-276-7227
info@meadowoodsprings.org
www.meadowoodsprings.org

1359 Camp Millennium
2726 NE Diamond Lake Blvd.
Roseburg, OR 97470 541-677-0600
campmoregon@gmail.com
campmillennium.com/
Sherry Fromdahl, Dirctor
Ryan Boles, Camp Contact
A week-long residential summer camp for children diagnosed with cancer, ages 5-16. The camp is free to attent, and activities include hiking, archery, horeseback riding, and more.

1360 Camp Starlight
P.O. Box 13107
Portland, OR 97213 503-964-1516
info@camp-starlight.org
camp-starlight.org
Melanie Smith-Wilusz, Camp Director
Kit Noble, Operations Director
Spike Huntington-Kline, Program Director
Christy Alger-Williams, Mental Health Director
Camp Starlight is a week-long sleep-away summer camp for children in Oregon and Washington whose lives are affected by HIV/AIDS. There is no charge to attend, and Camp Starlight aims to give children the ability to forget about their illness and enjoy the outdoors.

1361 Camp Taloali
15934 N Santiam Hwy SE
P.O. Box 32
Stayton, OR 97383 503-877-3864
camp@taloali.org
www.taloali.org

1362 Camp Ukandu
601 SW 2nd Ave.
Suite 2300
Portland, OR 97204 503-276-2178
campukandu.org/
Jason Hickox, Executive Director
Susan Lindemulder, Chair
Cindy Geiger, Vice Chair
Julie Desimone, Treasurer
Camp Ukandu is a summer camp for children and teens with cancer, ages 8-18, and their siblings. Activities include campfires, horseback riding, rock walls, and more. The camp is free to attend.

1363 Creating Memories
Creating Memories for Disabled Children
P.O. Box 586
Enterprise, OR 97828 541-426-6538
creating-memories.com/
Ken Coreson, Founder
Jack Burgoyne, Board Member
Enoch Stallcup, Board Member
Creating Memories for Disabled Children is a camp for children and adults with disabilities. The camp's goal is to connect individuals with diabilities to nature. The camp offers a variety of outdoor activities, including hunting, camping, fishing, and more. Attendance is free of charge.

1364   Gales Creek Diabetes Camp
Gales Creek Camp Foundation
1100 NE 28th Ave
Suit 106
Portland, OR   97232   503-968-2267
                                    Fax: 971-255-1575
                              rob@galescreekcamp.org
                              www.galescreekcamp.org

Angie Evans, President
Tom Talbot, Vice President
Scott Sloan, Secretary
Alex Stephens, Treasurer
Camp is located in Gales Creek, Oregon. Summer sessions for
children with Type 1 diabetes. Coed and family and pre-school
family camps also available. Gales Creek also helps teach campers about testing themselves, giving injections, and how to manage their own bodies.

1365   Hull Park
43233 SE Oral Hull Rd
Sandy, OR   97055   503-668-6195
                                    oralhull@gmail.com
                                          oralhull.org

Steve Butler, President
Tom Ciesielski, Vice President
Edwina Swart, Secretary
Don Jageman, Treasurer
The Oral Hull Foundation for the Blind is dedicated to providing
a special place for persons with blindness or low vision by pro-
viding recreational, educational and social activities programs
specially designed to fit the needs of guests with vision loss.

1366   Mt Hood Kiwanis Camp
Kiwanis Club of Montavilla
10725 SW Barbur Blvd.
Suite 50
Portland, OR   97219   503-452-7416
                                       info@mhkc.org
                                         www.mhkc.org

Kaleen Deatherage, Executive Director
Kayla Johnson, Camp Director
Allan Cushing, Director of Programs
Byron Rose, Campsite & Facilities Director
Camp is located in Government Camp, Oregon. Summer sessions
for children and adults with a variety of disabilities. Coed, ages
11 and up. Family and off-site adventure programs available.

1367   Strength for the Journey
Oregon-Idaho Conference Center
1505 SW 18th Ave
Portland, OR   97201-2524   503-226-7931
                                          800-593-7539
                              suttlelake@gocamping.org
                              suttlelake.gocamping.org/

Jane Petke, Suttle Lake Camp Director
Geneva Cook, Registrar
Camp is located near Sisters, Oregon at Suttle Lake Camp.
Strength for the Journey is a program for adults living with
HIV/AIDS.

1368   Suttle Lake Camp
29551 Suttle Lake Rd
Sisters, OR   97759   541-595-6663
                              suttlelake@gocamping.org
                              suttlelake.gocamping.org/

Jane Petke, Co-Director
Daniel Petke, Co-Director
Camp is located in Sisters, Oregon. Camping sessions for children and adults with AIDS/HIV. Coed, ages 6-18, families, seniors and single adults.

1369   Upward Bound Camp
P.O.Box C
Stayton, OR   97383   503-897-2447
                                    Fax: 503-897-4116
                              Fun@UpwardBoundCamp.org
                              www.upwardboundcamp.org

Pennsylvania

1370   Aces Adventure Weekend
Camp Hebron
957 Camp Hebron Rd.
Halifax, PA   17032   412-281-7244
                              www.easterseals.com/wcpenna

James G. Bennett, President/CEO
Ronald Palmer, Chairman
Pete Licastro, 1st Vice President
A weekend respite program for teens and you adults with
high-functioning Austism, ages 11-22. Activities include canoe-
ing, rock climbing, and cooking. The camp takes place at Camp
Hebron in Halifax, Pennsylvania.

1371   Achieva
711 Bingham St
Pittsburgh, PA   15203   412-995-5000
                                          888-272-7229
                                    Fax: 412-995-5001
                                         www.achieva.info

Marsha S. Blanco, President and CEO
Gary K. Horner, Executive Vice President
Reid Wolfe, Senior Vice President
Nancy J. Murray, President, The ARC of Greater Pittsburg
Achieva provides life-long services such as early intervention
therapies, in-home support, older adult protective services, and
more, to individuals with disabilities. Offers camp weekends
September through June for all ages.

1372   Camp AIM
YMCA of Greater Pittsburgh
420 Fort Duquesne Blvd.
Suit 625
Pittsburgh, PA   15222   412-227-3800
                              campaiminfo@gmail.com
                              www.ycamps.org/camp-aim/

Kevin Bolding, President & CEO
Stephan Davis, Senior Vice President, Human Resources
Carolyn Grady, Senior Vice President/Chief Development Officer
Greg Swetoha, Vice President, Operations
Camp AIM is a 6-week summer program for children, teens, and
young adults with physical, cognitive, social/communication,
and emotional/behavioral disabilities. The program combines
life skills, social and recreational activities with music, art, physical education, and more. Ages 3-21.

1373   Camp Akeela
Camp Akeela Winter Address
314 Bryn Mawr Ave
Bala Cynwyd, PA   19004   802-866-0380
                                    Fax: 866-462-2828
                                      www.campakeela.com

Eric Sasson, Camp Director
Debbie Sasson, Camp Director
Kevin Trimble, Assistant Director
Nicole Frederick, Head Counselor
Camp Akeela Vermont is a co-ed, overnight camp for children
and young adults ages 9-17 who have been diagnosed with
Asperger's Syndrome or a non verbal learning disability.

1374   Camp Amp
Easter Seals Western & Central Pennsylvania, York
2550 Kingston Rd.
Suite 219
York, PA   17402   717-741-3891
                                    Fax: 717-741-5359
                                  www.veryspecialcamps.com

James G. Bennett, President/CEO
Ronald Palmer, Chairman
Pete Licastro, 1st Vice Chairman
Bill Warfel, Treasurer
Camp Amp is an overnight summer camp for children, ages 7-17,
with any disability or special need. The camp offers a mini session and a full week session. Activities include talent shows,
sports, swimming, ropes course, hiking, and more. Camp Amp's
goal is to foster independenge and encourage socialization.

1375 Camp Can Do
Administrative Office
3 Unami Trail
Chalfont, PA 18914
717-273-6525
info@campcandoforever.com
campcandoforever.org

Tom Prader, Board
Karen MacAinsh, Board
Stephanie Cole, Board
Amy McGonigal, Board
Camp Can Do is for children, ages 8-17, who have been diagnosed with cancer in the last 5 years. The camp also offers a session for siblings of children with cancer.

1376 Camp Courage
YMCA Camp Soles
134 Camp Soles Ln.
Rockwood, PA 15557
412-824-1181
Fax: 412-471-1315
rmitchell@diabetes.org
www.diabetes.org/

Robert Mitchell, Camp Director
A summer camp program of the American Diabetes Association. The camp is held at the YMCA Camp Soles, and is for children ages 8-16 with diabetes. The camp runs traditional outdoor activities, and employs on-site medical staff and dieticians.

1377 Camp Discovery
American Academy Of Dermatology
930 E Woodfield Rd.
PO Box 4014
Schaumburg, IL 60173
847-240-1280
866-503-7546
888-462-3376
Fax: 847-240-1859
www.campdiscovery.org

1378 Camp Freedom
157 Game Farm Rd
Schwenksville, PA 19473
610-828-5003
mfoster@diabetes.org
www.diabetes.org

Les Weiser, Director, Camp Kweebec
Maddy Weiser, Director
Michelle Foster, Director, Camp Freedom
Camp Freedom is a resident summer camp, located in Schwenksville, Pennsylvania at Camp Kweebec. Sessions for children and teens with diabetes. Coed, ages 6-16.

1379 Camp Hot-to-Clot
Camp Kon-O-Kwee
126 Nagel Rd.
Fombell, PA 16123
724-758-6238
877-962-2565
www.hemophilia.org

Nathan Rost, President, National Hemophilia Foundation Western PA
Matthew Suarez Pace, Vice President, National Hemophilia Foundation Western PA
Mike Covert, Secretary
Camp Hot-to-Clot is a summer camp for children, ages 7-17, diagnosed with a bleeding disorder and their siblings. The camp is held at the YMCA Camp Kon-O-Kwee, and activities include rock wall climbing, arts & crafts, field games, and more.

1380 Camp Lee Mar
Winter Address
805 Redgate Rd
Dresher, PA 19025
215-658-1708
Fax: 215-658-1710
ari@leemar.com
www.leemar.com

Ari Segal, Executive Director
Laura Leibowitz, Assistant Director
Lynsey Trohoske, Admisstions Director
Seven week summer camp for children and young adults, ages 7-21, with mild to moderate developmental disabilities. Camp

Lee Mar incorporates an Academic and Speech program with traditional camp activities.

1381 Camp Lily Lehigh Valley
Easter Seals: Eastern Pennsylvania
1501 Lehigh St
Suit 201
Allentown, PA 18103
610-289-0114
www.easterseals.com/esep/

Dolores Bertoti, Chairperson
William Blumer, Vice Chairperson
Lisa Lavender, Treasurer
Nancy Knoebel, Secretary
Camp Lily is a week-long day camp for children and young adults with a variety of disabilities. Coed, ages 8-21. The camp offers a variety of traditional camp activities and field trips so that campers can enhance their social skills and increase their independence.

1382 Camp Orchard Hill
640 Orange Rd.
Dallas, PA 18612
570-333-4098
Fax: 570-333-4058
office@camporchardhill.com
www.camporchardhill.com/

Jim Payne, Executive Director
Derek Hodne, Program Director
Kacey Poe, Program Manager
Colin Kirby, Program Manager
Camp Orchard Hill provides day and overnight summer camps for ages 4-17. The camp is inclusive to children with mild to moderate special needs. Special needs campers participate alongside non-disabled campers in a multitude of outdoor activities.

1383 Camp Ramah in the Poconos Education, Inc.
2100 Arch St
Philadelphia, PA 19103
215-885-8556
Fax: 215-885-8905
info@ramahpoconos.org
www.ramahpoconos.org

Rabbi Joel Seltzer, Executive Director
Michelle Sugarman, Associate Director
Bruce Lipton, Director of Finance & Operation
Missy Stein, Development Director
Camp Ramah is a Jewish summer camp that runs three separate programs for children with various disabilities and their families. There are two residential programs and one family program, the Tikvah Family Camp.

1384 Camp STAR
2504 Atlas St.
Pittsburgh, PA 15235
412-370-5481
cindymcq1@gmail.com
www.chp.edu/

Cindy McCue, Camp Director
A week-long summer camp for children and teens, ages 8-18, who are amputees. The camp is held at the YMCA Camp Kon-O-Kwee in Zelienople, Pennsylvania. Activities include arts & crafts, zip lining, campfires, high ropes course, and more. Campers are also able to learn about their prosthetic, physical/recreation therapy, and limb care.

1385 Camp Setebaid
Setebaid Services, Inc.
P.O.Box 196
Winfield, PA 17889-0196
570-524-9090
866-738-3224
Fax: 570-523-0769
info@setebaidservices.org
www.setebaidservices.org

Mark Moyer, Executive Director
Camping sessions for children with diabetes. Coed, ages 3-18 years. The camp also hosts a family day for children with diabetes and their families.

1386 Camp Spencer Superstars
YMCA Camp Kon-O-Kwee
126 Nagel Rd.
Fombell, PA 16123   724-758-6238
                                         877-962-2565
                               campkon-o-kwee@ymcapgh.org
                                        www.ycampkok.org

Tim Murphy, Executive Director
Charlie Deer, Camp Spencer Director
Adam Stevenson, Program Director
An overnight respite camp for adults, ages 18 and up, with special
needs. The camp is fully inclusive, and aims to encourage campers to develop social and life skills. Campers have access to all activities and programs, such as canoeing, bonfires, swimming, and
more.

1387 Camp Victory
58 Camp Victory Rd
P.O. Box 810
Millville, PA 17846   570-458-6530
                                        www.campvictory.org

Dennis Wolff, President
Paul Kettlewell, Vice President
Art Girio, Vice President
Tara Holdren, Secretary
At Camp Victory, partner groups with specialized knowledge and
training provide camping opportunities for children with chronic
health problems or physical or mental challenges.

1388 Camp Wesley Woods: Exceptional Persons Camp
Western PA United Methodist Church
1001 Fiddlersgreen Rd
Grand Valley, PA 16420   814-436-7802
                                   info@wesleywoods.com
                                      www.wesleywoods.com

Nate Greenway, Executive Director
Kira Argot, Program & Marketing Director
Penny Boehme, Office Manager
The Exceptional Person's Camp is for children with emotional
and intellectual handicaps. Ages 13 and up.

1389 Camp Woodlands
The Woodlands Foundation
134 Shenot Rd
Wexford, PA 15090   724-935-6533
                               www.woodlandsfoundation.org

Douglas A. Clark, Chairman
Andrew J. Morrison, Vice Chairman
William P. Rydell, Treasurer
Edward A. Vargo, Secretary
Camp Woodlands is a one-of-a-kind camp for youth, teens, and
adults with varying disabilities and chronic illness where the em-
phasis is on the campers abilities rather than their disabilities.
The camp runs a number of programs for kids, teens, adults, and
seniors.

1390 Dragonfly Forest Summer Camp
YMCA Camp Speers
143 Nichecronk Rd
Dingmans Ferry, PA 18328   570-828-2329
                                    Fax: 570-828-2984
                                 campspeers@philaymca.org
                                   www.dragonflyforest.org

John E. Colburn, Chairman
Chris Wilson, Board Member
Chavis Patterson, Board Member
Jeff Daly, Board Member
Dragonfly Forest Summer Camp program, provides children with
Autism and medical needs such as asthma, sickle cell anemia and
hemophilia the opportunity to enjoy an overnight camp experi-
ence in an environment that is safe and equipped to meet a variety
of physical, medical, and psychological needs.

1391 Handi Camp
Handi Vangelism Ministries International
P.O.Box 122
Akron, PA 17501-0122   717-859-4777
                                    Fax: 717-721-7662
                                         info@hvmi.org
                                         www.hvmi.org

Tim Sheetz, Executive Director
Mark Amey, Assistant Director, Handi Camp
Kathy Sheetz, Executive Secretary
Brian Robinson, Office Manager, Handi Camp
Christian, overnight camping program for people with disabili-
ties, ages 7-50, in Eastern Pennsylvania. Sponsored by Handi
Vangelism Ministries International.

1392 Innabah Camps
United Methodist Church: Eastern Pennsylvania
712 Pughtown Rd
Spring City, PA 19475   610-469-6111
                                    Fax: 610-469-0330
                                         www.innabah.org

Michael Hyde, Director
Kelly Nelson, Program Coordinator
Gina James, Office Manager
Erin Slye, Summer Camp Registrar
Innabah Camps runs a number of sessions for children, teens, and
adults with developmental disabilities. The Challenge camps are
for ages 4-18, families and seniors.

1393 Lions Camp Kirby
1735 Narrows Hill Rd
Upper Black Eddy, PA 18972   610-982-5731
                                  info@lionscampkirby.org
                                   www.lionscampkirby.org

Alice Breon, Camp Director
Offers 2-week camps for deaf and hearing impaired children and
their siblings in eastern Pennsylvania.

1394 Mainstay Life Services Summer Program
Mainstay Life Services
200 Roessler Road
Pittsburgh, PA 15220   412-344-3640
                                    Fax: 412-344-5486
                               info@mainstaylifeservices.org
                                  mainstaylifeservices.org

James R. Kirk, CEO
Brian Cox, Chair
Rebekah Herman, Vice Chair
Steven Dobis, Treasurer
Mainstay Life Services' Summer program is a unique, urban
camping experience. The program runs for one or two week sessions on a college campus in Pittsburgh, Pennsylvania. The program is open to adults age 18 and over who live with families and
caregivers.

1395 Outside In School Of Experiential Education, Inc.
P.O.Box 639
Greensburg, PA 15601   724-837-1518
                                    Fax: 724-837-0801
                                      www.myoutsidein.org

Michael C. Henkel, Executive Director
Camp programs primarily focus on substance abuse, but some
services are available for special needs related to school/work.
Programs are for boys ages 13-18.

1396 Phelps School Academic Support Program
583 Sugartown Rd
Malvern, PA 19355   610-644-1754
                                    Fax: 610-540-0156
                                 admis@thephelpsschool.org
                                   www.thephelpsschool.org

Dan Knopp, Head of School
Stephany Phelps Fahey, President
Gerald D. Fahey, Treasurer
Andrew Wilmerding, Secretary
The Phelps School is a day and boarding school for grades 6-12.
They run an Academic Support Program for English, Reading,

Mathematics, and Study Skills for students who have diagnosed learning differences.

1397 Sequanota Lutheran Conference Center and Camp
P.O. Box 245
Jennerstown, PA 15547 814-629-6627
contact@sequanota.com
www.sequanota.com/
Rev. Carol Custead, President
David Shoemaker, Vice President
Chris Brant, Treasurer
Megan Will, Secretary
Runs Camp Bethesda, a summer camp for adults with developmental disabilities and speech/communication impairment. For ages 18 and up.

1398 Variety Club Camp & Development Center
2950 Potshop Rd
P.O.Box 609
Worcester, PA 19490 610-584-4366
Fax: 610-584-5586
www.varietyphila.org
Douglas I. Zeiders, President
Maribeth Roman Schmidt, Vice President
Donald F. Faul, Treasurer
Mark Tierney, Secretary
Year-round camping and recreation facility for children with special needs and their families. Includes summer camping, aquatics, weekend retreats and other specialty programs. Coed, ages 5-21.

1399 West Penn Burn Camp
Camp Kon-O-Kwee
126 Nagel Rd.
Fombell, PA 16123 412-578-5295
www.ahn.org/
Christine Perlick, Outreach Coordinator
Founded in 1986, West Penn Burn camp is a week-long overnight camp for children and teens, ages 7-17, who have burn injuries. Campers are able to participate in a fun, stress free week of regular camp activities. The camp also provides therapeutic services through the support and guidance of camp counselors. The camp is held at the YMCA Camp Kon-O-Kwee in Fombell, Pennsylvania.

1400 YMCA Camp Fitch
The YMCA's Camp Fitch On Lake Erie
12600 Abels Rd
North Springfield, PA 16430 814-922-3219
877-863-4824
Fax: 814-922-7000
hannahkight@campfitchymca.org
campfitchymca.org
Matt Pose, Executive Director
Tom Parker, Associate Executive Director
Hannah Kight, Office Manager
Jon Tully, Program Director
Camp is located in North Springfield, Pennsylvania. Camping sessions for children and adults with diabetes or epilepsy. Ages 8-16, families and seniors.

Rhode Island

1401 Camp Mauchatea
Rhode Island Lions Sight Foundation, Inc.
PO Box 19671
Johnston, RI 02919-0671 401-769-7000
domgbranco@msn.com
www.lions4sight.org
Francine Murphy-Brillon, First Vice President
Linda Hughes, Secretary
Domingos Branco, President
Michael Haws, Treasurer
Camp serving those who are blind/visually impaired. Campers enjoy developing and maintaining friendships with fellow campers. Some of the activities include boating and other water sports, as well as hiking and nature studies.

1402 Camp Ruggles
PO Box 353
Chepachet, RI 02814 401-567-8914
campruggles@gmail.com
www.campruggles.org
Gregory Gauthier, President
Brandon Ruotolo, Vice President
Jim Field, Camp Director
Ethan Roe, Assistant Director
Camp Ruggles is located in Glocester, RI, and is a summer day camp for emotionally and behaviourally handicapped children. The camp offers a 6 week co-ed summer session for 60 children ages 6-12.

1403 Canonicus Camp
Canonicas Camp and Conference Center
54 Exeter Road
Exeter, RI 02822 401-294-6318
Fax: 401-294-7780
colleen@abcori.org
www.hasbrochildrenshospital.org/
Colleen Tolhurst, Office Manager
Linda Moore, Camp Registrar
Jason Clark, Food Service Manager
Matt Black, Facilities Manager
Canonicus Camp hosts Asthma Camp, an initiative of the Community Asthma Programs at Hasbro Children's Hospital. This camp program is for children with asthma/respiratory ailments. Coed, ages 9-13.

1404 Hasbro Children's Hospital Asthma Camp
593 Eddy Street
Providence, RI 02903 401-444-7409
malsina@lifespan.org
www.hasbrochildrenshospital.org/
Timothy J. Babineau,MD, President & CEO
Lisa Abbott, Senior Vice President
Mamie Wakefield, Executive Vice President
Paul Adler, Senior Vice President
Camp for children with asthma, hosted by Canonicus Camp and Conference Center. Children learn about asthma and asthma management through interactive, educational and fun activities. The camp also offers activities such as swimming, canoeing and arts & crafts. Coed, ages 9-13.

South Carolina

1405 Burnt Gin Camp
SC Department of Health and Environmental Control
2600 Bull St
Columbia, SC 29201 803-898-3432
Fax: 803-898-0613
aimonemi@dhec.sc.gov
www.scdhec.gov
Marie I Aimone, Camp Director
David Wilson, Acting Director, Deparment of Health & Environment Control
Jennifer Read, Chief of Staff, DHEC
A residential camp for children who have physical disabilities and/or chronic illnesses. Camp Burnt Gun runs four seven-day sessions for 7-15 year olds, two six-day session for 16-19 year olds, and one four-day session for 21-25 year olds. Limited to residents of South Carolina.

1406 Camp Adam Fisher
P.O. Box 5226
Columbia, SC 29250 campadamfisher@gmail.com
www.campadamfisher.com
Maria McGregor, Board of Directors
Scott McFarland, Board of Directors
Bryan Epps, Board of Directors
Erin Massengale, Board of Directors
A week-long overnight camp for children with diabetes and their siblings, ages 6-17. Campers enjoy swimming, horseback riding, tubing, basketball, volleyball and arts & crafts, while also learn-

ing how to manage their diabetes so they can live longer, healthier lives.

1407   Camp Courage
Greenvile Health Services Children's Hospital
701 Grove Rd.
Greenville, SC   29605   864-455-8741
                          www.ghschildrens.org/camp-courage.php
Marguerite R Wyche, Chair
Charles E. Dalton, Board Member
David Lominack, Board Member
Robert T. Nitto, Board Member
Camp Courage is a non-profit organization that provides a summer camp experience for children and teens with cancer or blood disorders. Activities include horseback riding, riflery, climbing wall, and more. The camp is held at the Pleasant Ridge Camp & Retreat Center.

1408   Camp Debbie Lou
726 Lucky Run
Latta, SC   29565   843-752-5416
                                   info@campdebbielou.com
                                   www.campdebbielou.com
Judy Richardson, Chairwoman
John Rayne, Vice Chair
Rita Isenhour, Secretary
Robyn Queen, Treasurer
For children between the ages of 4-14, that have been diagnosed with cancer and their families.

1409   Camp Luv-A-Lung
Pleasant Ridge Camp & Retreat Center
4232 Highway 11
Marietta, SC   29661   864-546-1567
              www.ghschildrens.org/camp-luv-a-lung.php
Marguerite R Wyche, Chair
Charles E. Dalton, Board Member
David Lominack, Board Member
Robert T. Nitto, Board Member
A summer camp for children in grades 1-8 who have respiratory problems. The camp takes place at Pleasant Ridge Camp & Retreat Center in Marietta, South Carolina. Activities include swimming, archery, campfires, and more.

1410   Camp Spearhead
Greenville County Recreation District
4806 Old Spartanburg Rd
Taylors, SC   29687   864-288-6470
                                   Fax: 864-288-6499
                           rmurr@greenvillecounty.org
                                   www.campspearhead.org
Gene Smith, Executive Director
Chanell Moore, Deputy Director
Peggy Baxter, President
Jeff Dezen, Vice President
Camp for children with disabilities age 8 years and up. The mission of Camp Spearhead is to provide an environment of unconditional acceptance for children and adults with disabilities. A caring staff, creative programming, and a state-of-the-art campsite all combine to offer a safe and nurturing camp experience for every camper.

South Dakota

1411   Camp Friendship
P.O. Box 1986
Rapid City, SD   57709   campfriendshipdirector@hotmail.com
                                   www.campfriendship.org

1412   Camp Gilbert
Camp Gilbert, Inc.
P.O. Box 89406
Sioux Falls, SD   57109-9406   605-212-6027
                                   campgilbertinfo@gmail.com
                                   www.campgilbert.com
Cindy Matthes, Pediatric Dietician
Nancy Hartung, Staffing
For children ages 8-18 with diabetes. Campers can enjoy a week of canoeing, swimming, sing-a-longs, crafts, and games, while also attending educational programs covering nutrition, exercise and lifestyle management.

1413   NeSoDak
Lutherans Outdoors in South Dakota
3285 Camp Dakota Dr.
Waubay, SD   57273   605-947-4440
                                                800-888-1464
                                   nesodak@losd.org
                                   www.losd.org/
Jake Hanson, Director, NeSoDak
Sharon Oliver, Officer Manager, NeSoDak
Kris Mueller, Hospitality Director, NeSoDak
Camp is located in Waubay, South Dakota. Hosts Camp Gilbert, a summer camp program for children with diabetes. Coed, ages 8-18.

Tennessee

1414   ACM Lifting Lives Music Camp
Vanderbilt Kennedy Center
110 Magnolia Circle
Nashville, TN   37203   615-322-8240
                           vkc.mc.vanderbilt.edu/vkc/
Donna Eskind, Chair
Honey Alexander, Leaderchip Council Member
Jean Ann Banker, Leadership Council Member
Melissa Beasley, Leadership Council Member
A camp for individuals with developmental disabilities where they can come to celebrate music by participating in songwriting workshops, recording sessions and live performances. For ages 16 and up. The program is specifically designed for people with Williams syndrome.

1415   All Days Are Happy Days Summer Camp
Boling Center
711 Jefferson Ave
Memphis, TN   38105   901-448-6511
                                                888-572-2249
                                   Fax: 901-448-7097
                                   TTY:901-448-4677
                                   www.uthsc.edu/bcdd/
Jenness Roth, MEd, Family Faculty Coordinator
Bruce Keisling, PhD, Executive Director
Zach DeBerry, MS, RDN, LEND Training Coordinator
Vanessa Baker, Business Manager
Week long camp for children ages 6-11 years of age who have been diagnosed with ADHD. The goal of the camp is to provide activities specifically designed for children with ADHD and to educate children and their parents on the treatment and management of ADHD and related behaviours.

1416   Bill Rice Ranch
627 Bill Rice Ranch Road
Murfreesboro, TN   37128   615-893-2767
                                                800-253-7423
                                   Fax: 615-898-0656
                                   info@billriceranch.org
                                   www.billriceranch.org
Wil Rice IV, President
Troy Carlson, Director
Nathan McConnell, Deaf Ministries Director
Matt Downs, Camp Director
Camping for hearing impaired children and youths ages 9-19. Also runs camps and retreats for deaf/hearing impaired adults.

1417   Camp Agape
Lakeshore Camp & Retreat Center
1458 Pilot Knob Rd.
Eva, TN 38333   731-584-6102
                                      Fax: 731-584-2267
                          office@lakeshorecamp.org
                          lakeshorecamp.org/summer-camp
Rev. Gary D. Lawson, Sr., Executive Director
Vicki Lawson, Office Manager
Tiffany Dowdy, Program Director
A summer camp for children and teens, ages 8-17, with disabilities. The camp takes place at Lakeshore Camp & Retreat Center. Activities include swimming, crafts, games, pontoon boat rides, and more traditional camp activities.

1418   Camp Conquest
4100 Raleigh Millington Rd.
Memphis, TN 38128   901-490-7164
                          markp@campconquest.com
                          www.campconquest.com/
Mark Price, Co-Founder
Amanda Price, Co-Founder
Becca Bryant, Camp Director
JT Dick, Camp Director
Camp Conquest is a week-long overnight Christian summer camp for children and adults with special needs, disabilities, and chronic illnesses. Ages 6-16 for session 1 and ages 17 and up for session 2. Activities include horseback riding, canoeing, ropes course, climbing wall, and more.

1419   Camp Discovery
Tennessee Jaycees and Tennessee Jaycee Foundation
400 Camp Discovery Ln
Gainesboro, TN 38562   931-704-0107
                          director@jayceecamp.org
                          www.jayceecamp.org
Chester Lowe, Vice President of Camp Operation
Faith Henshaw, Camp Director
Millie Dawkins, Camp Off Season Rentals
Serves children, teens, and adults between teh ages of 7 and 90 with disabilities. The camp is a project of the Tennessee Jaycees and the Tennessee Jaycee Foundation.

1420   Camp Joy
Lakeshore Camp & Retreat Center
1458 Pilot Knob Rd.
Eva, TN 38333   731-584-6102
                                      Fax: 731-584-2267
                          office@lakeshorecamp.org
                          lakeshorecamp.org/summer-camp/
Rev. Gary D. Lawson, Sr., Executive Director
Tiffany Dowdy, Program Director
Vicki Lawson, Office Manager
A summer camp for teens and adults, ages 14 and up, with disabilities. The camp takes place at Lakeshore Camp & Retreat Center. The camp runs regular camp activities such as swimming, arts & crafts, and other outdoor activities.

1421   Camp Koinonia
University Of Tennessee
1914 Andy Holt Ave
HPER Building 362
Knoxville, TN 37996   865-974-4363
                          thecampkoinonia@gmail.com
                          www.kftn.org/campkoinonia/
Lindsay Willis, Chair
Robbie Proffitt, Vice Chair
Carlene LeCompte, Treasurer
Helen Porter, Secretary
Outdoor education program for children and young adults ages 7-22 who have multiple disabilities. The camp offers recreational activities such as canoeing, music and games.

1422   Camp Oginali
The Camp Koinonia
1914 Andy Holt Ave.
HPER Building 362
Knoxville, TN 37996   865-974-4363
                          thecampkoinonia@gmail.com
                          www.kftn.org/campkoinonia/
Lindsay Willis, Chair
Robbie Proffitt, Vice Chair
Carlene LeCompte, Treasurer
Helen Porter, Secretary
A weekend retreat in October for individuals, aged 7 and older, with Down syndrome. The retreat is held at Camp Montvale. Activities include fishing, low ropes courses, cooking, outdoor adventure, and more.

1423   Camp Okawehna
Dialysis Clinic, Inc.
1633 Church Street
Suite 500
Nashville, TN 37203   615-327-3061
                                            877-326-1109
                          www.dciinc.org/campo/
Andy Parker, Camp Director
Week-long summer camp for critically ill children ages 6-18 years suffering from kidney disease. Children who have had kidney transplants as well as children on hemodialysis and peritoneal dialysis are welcome. The camp focuses on the critically ill child who needs to have fun and be in the company of other children who suffer from the same disease.

1424   Camp Sugar Falls
Camp Widjiwagan
3088 Smith Springs Rd
Antioch, TN 37013   615-298-3066
                                      Fax: 615-271-2151
                          mwilson@diabetes.org
                          www.diabetes.org
Melissa Wilson, Camp Director
Camp Sugar Falls is a day camp for children, ages 6-17, who have type 1 or type 2 diabetes and their siblings. Activities include education sessions, athletics and exercise.

1425   Easter Seals Tennessee Camping Program
Easter Seals Tennessee
750 Old Hickory Blvd
#2-260
Brentwood, TN 37027   615-292-6640
                                      Fax: 615-251-0994
                          www.easterseals.com/tennessee/
John Pfeiffer, Chairman
Chuck Mataya, Vice Chairman
Jeff Bridges, Treasurer
Jeff Bridges, Treasurer
Offers overnight, day, and weekend programs for youths ages 7-16 and adults ages 16 and up with diabilities or traumatic brain injuries. The camps are held at the YMCA's Camp Widjiwagan.

1426   LeBonheur Cardiac Kids Camp
LeBonheur Children's Hospital
848 Adams Ave.
Memphis, TN 38103   901-287-5437
                          info@lebonheur.org
                          www.lebonheur.org
Christopher Knott-Craig, MD, Co-Director, Heart Institute
Jeffrey Towbin, MD, Co-Director, Heart Institute
Camp for children and young adults ages 9-17 with cardiac-related diagnoses. Children enjoy a fun-filled week at camp where they learn about their heart conditions and meet other children just like them.

1427 Paddy Rossbach Youth Camp
Amputee Coalition Of America
900 East Hill Ave.
Suite 390
Knoxville, TN 37915
888-267-5669
Camp@amputee-coalition.org
www.amputee-coalition.org

Dan Berschinski, Chairman
John Kenney, Vice Chair
Jack Richmond, President/CEO
Carole Folta, Chief Financial Officer

A 6-day camp for youths ages 10-17 years of age who have limb loss or limb difference. Activities include sports, swimming, fishing, arts and crafts.

Texas

1428 Adam's Camp: Texas
Adam's Camp
6767 South Spruce St.
Suite 102
Centennial, CO 80112
303-552-4418
adamscamptexas@gmail.com
www.adamscamptexas.org

Heath Remedies, President
Lulu Jones, Program Director

The Texas location of Adam's Camp, offers 3 therapy programs, for children and the families of children with special needs and developmental delays. Early Start (ages 1-preschool), Pathfinder (ages 4 and up) and Trailblazer (ages 8 and up).

1429 Camp Ailihpomeh
National Hemophilia Foundation: Lone Star Chapter
5600 Northwest Central Dr.
Suite 140
Houston, TX 77092
713-686-6100
Fax: 832-383-4601
info@camp-ailihpomeh.org
www.camp-ailihpomeh.org/
Melissa Compton, Executive Director, NHF Lone Star Chapter
Dan Bond, President, NHF Lone Star Chapter
Allison Pohl, 1st Vice President, NHF Lone Star Chapter
James Setliff, 2nd Vice President, NHF Lone Star Chapter

A six-day overnight camp for boys, ages 7-17, who have a bleeding disorder. The camp takes place at Camp John Marc, and provides recreational and educational activities.

1430 Camp Aranzazu
5420 Loop 1781
Rockport, TX 78382
361-727-0800
Fax: 361-727-0818
info@camparanzazu.org
www.camparanzazu.org/

Virginia C. Ballard, President
Amanda Praet, Program Manager
Alexa Rosenblat, Program Manager
Mark White, Facilities Manager

A summer camp program for children with a variety of special needs and chronic illnesses, such as cancer, autism, asthma, cerebral palsy, Down Syndrome, epilepsy, and more. Activities center around emphasizing spiritual awareness, environmental awareness, team building and sports, the arts, and social skills.

1431 Camp Aurora
YMCA Camp Carter
6200 Sand Springs Rd.
Fort Worth, TX 76114
972-392-1181
Fax: 972-392-1366
shill@diabetes.org
www.diabetes.org

Sherry Hill, Camp Director

A week-long summer camp program of the American Diabetes Association, for children ages 6-12 with diabetes. The camp is held at the YMCA Camp Carter, and is dedicated to providing children with a fun and safe camp experience. Activities include swimming, fishing, horseback riding, and more.

1432 Camp Be An Angel
2003 Aldine-Bender Rd.
Houston, TX 77032
281-219-3313
angel@beanangel.org
www.beanangel.org/prog_camp.html#.VZAxuvmqqko
Robbie Schilhab, Chairman
Marti Boone, Executive Director
Russ Massey, Program Director
Larry Blanton, Office Manager

Camp Be An Angel is designed to be a retreat for special needs children under the age of 22 and their immediate families.

1433 Camp Blessing
Administrative Office
P.O. Box 2268
Tomball, TX 77377
281-259-5789
Fax: 823-203-4417
office@campblessing.org
campblessing.org/

Brad DeLoach, Bussiness Director
Caleb Elder, Program Coordinator
Dan Taylor, Board Chairman

A residential summer camp for children and young adults with special needs and their siblings. The camp serves kids ages 7-13 with a physical, developmental, or intellectual disability. The camp provides specialized programs that allow for participation for all levels of abilities.

1434 Camp CAMP
Children's Association for Maximum Potential
P.O. Box 27086
San Antonio, TX 78227
210-671-5411
Fax: 210-671-5225
campmail@campcamp.org
www.campcamp.org

Ken McConnell, Chairman
Julie Allen, Vice Chair
Susan Osborne, Executive Director
Brandon G. Briery, Ph.D, Executive Camping Director

Camping for children, teens, and adults ages 5-50 with a variety of disabilities and their siblings. The camp offer a series of sessions that run for 6 days, and is held at Camp CAMP in Center Point, Texas. Activities are modified to include everyone, no matter the severity of physical or developmental needs.

1435 Camp CPals
5501A Balcones
Suite 160
Austin, TX 78731
866-74C-PATH
info@cpathtexas.com
www.cpathtexas.com

Victoria Polega, President
Marielle Deckard, Secretary
Ilona McCauley, Public Relations
Jamie L. Eppele, Development

Camp CPals is an overnight weekend camp for campers of all ages with cerebral palsy. The camp's goal is to allow campers to gain confidence, independence, learn new skills, and meet other kids suffering from cerebral palsy.

1436 Camp Can-Do
YMCA Camp Carter
6200 Sand Springs Rd.
Fort Worth, TX 76114
817-738-9241
camper@ymcafw.org
campcarter.org/other-camps/camp-can-do/

Andy Hockenbrock, Executive Director
Jessica Wilmoth, Business Operations Director
Stephanie Williams, Program Operation Director
David Hagel, Camp Program Director

A week-long summer camp designed specifically for blind/visually impaired children, ages 6-12. The camp is held at the YMCA Camp Carter, and activities include hiking, canoeing, skeet shooting, and more.

1437 Camp Discovery
American Academy Of Dermatology
930 E Woodfield Rd.
PO Box 4014
Schaumburg, IL   60173

847-240-1280
866-503-7546
888-462-3376
Fax: 847-240-1859
www.campdiscovery.org

1438 Camp John Marc
Special Camps for Special Kids
2929 Carlisle Street
Suite 355
Dallas, TX   75204

214-360-0056
mail@campjohnmarc.org
www.campjohnmarc.org

Kevin Randles, Executive Director
Megan White, Camp Director
Kyle Lamb, Associate Camp Director
Bre Loveless, Assistant Camp Director
Year-round camping for children with a variety of chronic medical and physical challenges. Campers can participate in a number of traditional camp activities.

1439 Camp Neuron
Epilepsy Foundation Texas
2401 Fountain View Dr.
Suite 900
Houston, TX   77057

713-789-6295
888-548-9716
Fax: 713-789-5628
info@eftx.org
eftx.org

Donna Stahlhut, Founder/ CEO
Rebecca Moreau, Programs Director
Shannon Robbins, Assistant Director
Jeanette Hartshorn, Clinic Services Director
Camp Neuron offers an overnight camping experience for children and teens, ages 8-14, with epilepsy or a diagnosed seizure disorder. There is no cost to attend the camp, and the camp is located at the Texas Lions Camp in Kerrville, Texas.

1440 Camp New Horizons North
Cross Creek Ranch
3406 Dublin Rd.
Parker, TX   75002

972-392-1181
Fax: 972-392-1366
shill@diabetes.org
www.diabetes.org

Sherry Hill, Camp Director
A week-long summer camp program of the American Diabetes Association, for children ages 4-12 with diabetes. The camp is held at Cross Creek Ranch in Parker, Texas. Activities include games, sports, swimming, and more. The camp aims to allow kids a fun camp experience alongside others with diabetes, and to educate both children and parents on how to manage diabetes.

1441 Camp New Horizons South
The Southern Cross Ranch
1800 W. Dowdy Ferry Rd.
Dallas, TX   75217

972-392-1181
Fax: 972-392-1366
shill@diabetes.org
www.diabetes.org/

Sherry Hill, Camp Director
A summer camp program of the American Diabetes Association, for children ages 4-12 with diabetes. The camp is held at the Southern Cross Ranch, and traditional outdoor camp activities are provided. The camp aims to educate children and parents on diabetes and how to manage it.

1442 Camp No Limits Texas
No Limits Foundation
6301 Rehburg Rd
Burton, TX   77835

207-240-5762
Fax: 877-406-5106
campnolimits@gmail.com
www.nolimitsfoundation.org

Mary Leighton, Founder & Executive Director
Melanie Dash, Program Director
Pedro Pimenta, Director, Development
Missy Moreau, Project Coordinator
Camp No Limits Texas, is a location of Camp No Limits, a recreational and educational camp for youth who have experienced limb loss. Camp No Limits, is a program of the nonprofit organization No Limits Foundation. The weeklong camp is for children ages 5 and up, with campers participating in a variety of activities such as archery, kayaking, and fishing. The camp is held at Camp For All in Burton, Texas.

1443 Camp Quality Texas
3801 Spring Run Ln.
Melissa, TX   75454

214-578-3054
texas@campqualityusa.org
www.campqualityusa.org/TX

Stephanie Weber, Camp Director
Anneliese Kulakofsky, Executive Director
Camp Quality is for children with cancer and their siblings. The camp offers a stress-free environment that offers exciting activities and fosters new friendships, while helping to give the children courage, motivation and emotional strength.

1444 Camp Rainbow
Circle Lake Retreat Center
P.O. Box 1410
Pinehurst, TX   77362-1408

713-977-7706
eanadu@diabetes.org
www.diabetes.org/

Edith Anadu, Camp Director
A 4-day summer day camp for children with diabetes. A program of the American Diabetes Association, the camp is held at the Circle Lake Retreat Center. Activities will include regular outdoor camp activities. Siblings are allowed to attend as space allows.

1445 Camp Sandcastle
Camp Aranzazu
5420 FM 1781
Rockport, TX   78382

361-850-8778
Fax: 361-885-0051
karodriguez@diabetes.org
www.diabetes.org/

Kassandra Rodriguez, Camp Director
A week long day camp for children, ages 5-17, with type 1 diabetes. This camp is a program of the American Diabetes Association, and provides kids with fun outdoor activities while educating children and teens about positive diabetes management.

1446 Camp Spike 'n' Wave
Epilepsy Foundation Texas
2401 Fountain View Dr.
Suite 900
Houston, TX   77057

713-789-6295
888-548-9716
Fax: 713-789-5628
info@eftx.org
eftx.org

Donna Stahlhut, Founder/ CEO
Rebecca Moreau, Programs Director
Shannon Robbins, Assistant Director
Jeanette Hartshorn, Clinic Services Director
Camp Spike 'n' Wave is a residential camp for children and teens, ages 8-14, with epilepsy or a seizure disorder. The camp is located at Camp For All in Burton, Texas, and runs activities such as swimming, boating, and sports. There is no cost to attend the camp.

1447 Camp Summit
17210 Campbell Rd
Suite 180-W
Dallas, TX   75252   972-484-8900
                                        Fax: 972-620-1945
                              camp@campsummittx.com
                              www.campsummittx.org

Carla R Weiland, President & CEO
Lisa Braziel, Camp Director
Megan Attwood, Marketing Manager
Pam Chicol, Director of Development
Camp Summit offers camping for children and adults with a variety of disabilities. The program is coed, for ages 6-99.

1448 Camp Sweeney
Camp Sweeney
P.O.Box 918
Gainesville, TX   76241   940-665-2011
                                        Fax: 940-665-9467
                              info@campsweeney.org
                              www.campsweeney.org

T. Milton Dickson, Jr. DDS, Chair
Robert D. Vandermeer, MD, Vice Chair
Ernie Fernandez, M.D., Camp Director
Skip Rigsby, Program Director
Camp Sweeney teaches self-care and self-reliance to children ages 5-18 with type 1 diabetes. Campers participate in activities such as swimming, fishing, horseback riding and arts and crafts while learning about how to self manage their diabetes.

1449 Camp for All
Camp for All Foundation
6301 Rehburg Rd
Burton, TX   77835   979-289-3752
                                        Fax: 979-289-5046
                              bdeans@campforall.org
                              www.campforall.org

Rogers Crain, Chairman
Belinda Munsell, Development Director
Pat Prior Sorrells, President and CEO
Kurt R. Podeszwa, Camp Director
Camp For All is a fully-accessible year round camp facility located in Burton, Texas. The camp is for children and adults with a variety of disabilities. Coed, ages 5-35 and up and families. Some disabilities that the camp serves are cancer, autism, muscular dystrophy, spinal cord injuries, and more.

1450 Charis Hills Camp
498 Faulkner Rd.
Sunset, TX   76270   940-964-2145
                                        Fax: 940-964-2147
                              info@charishills.org
                              www.charishills.org/

Rand Southard, President/Foudner
Colleen Southard, Founder
Molly Southard, Assistant Program Director
Cara Krueger, Assistant Program Director
A Christian summer camp for children with learning disabilities, such as ADD/ADHD, Austism, Asperger's, and more. Campers will participate in traditional camp activities, while also learning about Christ and improving social skills, self esteem and confidence.

1451 Dallas Academy
950 Tiffany Way
Dallas, TX   75218   214-324-1481
                                        Fax: 214-327-8537
                              www.dallas-academy.com

Terrence S. Welch, Chair
Jim Lucius, Vice Chair
Chris Bellew, Secretary
Redonna Higgins, Treasurer
Dallas Academy is a school for children with diagnosed learning differences such as autism, ADD/ADHD, dyslexia, and more. The academy offers a number of academic or athletic summer school programs.

1452 Hill School of Fort Worth
4817 Odessa Ave.
Fort Worth, TX   76133   817-923-9482
                                        Fax: 817-923-4894
                              hillschool@hillschool.org
                              www.hillschool.org

John W. Wright, Chairman
Randall Connelly, Vice Chair
Joanna Gant, Business Manager
Roxann Breyer, Head of School
Provides an alternative learning environment for students who have average or above-average intelligence with learning differences. Hill School caters to individuals with disabilities by offering smaller class sizes and individualized learning programs. Offers and academic summer program during the month of June.

1453 Kamp Kaleidoscope
Epilepsy Foundation Texas
2401 Fountain View Dr.
Suite 900
Houston, TX   77057   713-789-6295
                                            888-548-9716
                                        Fax: 713-789-5628
                              info@eftx.org
                              eftx.org

Donna Stahlhut, Founder/ CEO
Rebecca Moreau, Programs Director
Shannon Robbins, Assistant Director
Jeanette Hartshorn, Clinic Services Director
Kamp Kaleidoscope is a residential camp for teens, ages 15-19, with epilepsy or a seizure disorder. The camp takes place at the YMCA Collin County Adventure Camp in Anna, Texas, and is provided at no cost.

1454 Texas Lions Camp
Lions Club of Texas
P.O.Box 290247
Kerrville, TX   78029   830-896-8500
                                        Fax: 830-896-3666
                              www.lionscamp.com

Stephen Mabry, Executive Director
Steven King, Director of Operations
Patty Rodriguez, Program Supervisor
Bailey Carter, Program Supervisor
Texas Lions Camp is a camp dedicated to seving children in Texas with physical diabilities, ages 7-16. While at camp, campers will participate in a variety of acitivties and they will be encouraged to become more independent and self-confident.

Utah

1455 Action Camp
National Ability Center
P.O. Box 682799
Park City, UT   84068   435-649-3991
                                        Fax: 435-658-3992
                              info@DiscoverNAC.org
                              www.discovernac.org

Michael Kerby, President
Sean Carroll, Vice Presiednt, People
Andy Dahmen, Vice President, Facilities & Capital
Steve Ward, Vice President, Programs
Winter and Summer camps designed for youths, ages 9-16, who have amputations or spinal cord injuries. Campers are challenged with Paralymic activities and sports training. Some activities at that can be expected at camp are paddle sports, cycling, skiing/snowboarding, adaptive horseback riding, and more.

1456 Camp Giddy-Up
National Ability Center
PO Box 682799
Park City, UT 84068   435-649-3991
                                 Fax: 435-658-3992
                              info@DiscoverNAC.org
                              www.discovernac.org

Michael Kerby, President
Sean Carroll, Vice President, People
Andy Dahmen, Vice President, Facilities & Capital
Steve Ward, Vice President, Programs
Camp Giddy Up is a horsemanship camp, ages 8-18, for campers
with and without disabilities. Campers will be participating in all
activities related to horseback riding, including grooming, rid-
ing, and barn activities.

1457 Camp Hobe
P.O. Box 520755
Salt Lake City, UT 84152-0755   801-631-2742
                              wapitimama@camphobekids.org
                              www.camphobekids.org
Christina Beckwith, PharmD, President, Executive Director
Phillip Barnette, MD, Medical Director, Vice President
Bruce LeBaron, Secretary
Jamie Seale, Medical Co-Director
A summer camp for children with cancer and their siblings. The
camp's goal is to allow kids to take part in a normal aspect of
childhood in a safe and medically supervised environment. Camp
Hobe offers a two-day Day Camp sessions for ages 4-7, one
five-day session for ages 6-12, and one five-day session for ages
12-19.

1458 Camp ICANDO
Grace Lutheran School
1815 E. 9800 S.
Sandy, UT 84092   801-363-3024
                              bbartel@diabetes.org
                              www.diabetes.org/
Beverly Bartel, Camp Director
A summer camp program of the American Diabetes Association.
Camp ICANDO is for children ages 4-8 who have been diagnosed
with diabetes. The camp runs traditional camp activities and combines them with informal diabetes education. Children are encouraged to build self-esteem and learn how to take age
appropriate responsibility for their diabetes management.

1459 Camp Kostopulos
Kostopulos Dream Foundation
4180 E. Emigration Canyon Road
Salt Lake City, UT 84108   801-582-0700
                                 Fax: 801-583-5176
                              kdf@campk.org
                              www.campk.org

Rick Lifferth, Chairman
Andrea Moss, Vice Chair
Layne Smith, Vice Chair, Legal
Mircea Divricean, President & CEO
Summer camping for children and adults ages 7-65 with a variety
of disabilities. There are 4 types of summer camp programs offered: Day Camp, Residential Camp, Travel Trip Camp, and Partner Day Camps. There is also year round recreation on site and
community based activities. Programs are designed to foster independence, confidence, physical fitness, and social and
communication skills.

1460 Camp Nah-Nah-Mah
University Health Care Burn Camp Programs
50 N. Medical Drive
Salt Lake City, UT 84132   801-581-2700
                              healthcare.utah.edu/burncenter/
Mark Davis, Board Member, University of Utah Health
David Burton, Board Member, University of Utah Health
Phil Clinger, Board Member, University of Utah Health
For children ages 6-12 years of age that are burn survivors. Some
of the activities include canoeing, rock climbing and archery. The
camp takes place in Millcreek Canyon, and is a five-day over-
night camp.

1461 Camp Vision
National Ability Center
PO Box 682799
Park City, UT 84068   435-649-3991
                                 Fax: 435-658-3992
                              info@DiscoverNAC.org
                              www.discovernac.org

Michael Kerby, President
Sean Carroll, Vice President, People
Andy Dahmen, Vice President, Facilities & Capital
Steve Ward, Vice President, Programs
Camp Vision is an overnight summer camp designed for teens and
young adults with visual impairments. Activities include horse-
back riding, cycling, and more. The camp provides experienced
guides for all activities.

1462 Camp X-Treme
National Ability Center
PO Box 682799
Park City, UT 84068   435-649-3991
                                 Fax: 435-658-3992
                              info@DiscoverNAC.org
                              www.discovernac.org

Michael Kerby, President
Sean Carroll, Vice President, People
Andy Dahmen, Vice President, Facilities & Capital
Steve Ward, Vice President, Programs
Camp X-Treme is a week-long outdoor overnight camp for teens
with physical disabilities. Activities include zip lining, alpine
slide, skiing, snowboarding, and more. Programs are available in
the summer and winter.

1463 Discovery Camps
National Ability Center
PO Box 682799
Park City, UT 84068   435-649-3991
                                 Fax: 435-658-3992
                              info@DiscoverNAC.org
                              www.discovernac.org

Michael Kerby, President
Sean Carroll, Vice President, People
Andy Dahmen, Vice President, Facilities & Capital
Steve Ward, Vice President, Programs
Discovery Camps are summer camps for kids, ages 8-18, with
physical disabilities, intellectual disabilities, and Autism Spectrum Disorders. The camp is divided into various ses-
sions-Pathfinders, Crusaders, and Adventurers- depending on
the disability. Primarily day camps, with a few overnight activities. Discovery Camps also offers a session for siblings.

1464 FCYD Camp Utada
Foundation for Children and Youth with Diabetes
1995 West 9000 South
West Jordan, UT 84084   801-566-6913
                              www.fcydcamp.org

David Okubo, MD, Co-Founder, Trustee
Elizabeth Elmer, Co-Founder, Trustee
Nathan Gedge, Co-Founder, Trustee
Camp Utada is a summer camp for children with diabetes. Coed,
ages 1-18 and families.

1465 Overnight Camps
National Ability Center
PO Box 682799
Park City, UT 84068   435-649-3991
                                 Fax: 435-658-3992
                              info@DiscoverNAC.org
                              www.discovernac.org
Michael Kerby, President
Sean Carroll, Vice President, People
Andy Dahmen, Vice President, Facilities & Capital
Steve Ward, Vice President, Programs
Overnight Camps are available for teens and young adults, ages
15-24, depending on the specific camp. Campers participate in
traditional camp activities during the day. During the evenings,
campers may attend campfires and sometimes sleep in tents.

Vermont

1466 Camp Thorpe
680 Capen Hill Rd.
Goshen, VT 05733
802-247-6611
kathy@campthorpe.org
www.campthorpe.org

Ruth I. Durkee, Board of Trustee
Elizabeth Giard, Board of Trustee
Richard Giard, Board of Trustee
Ralph O. Hathaway, Board of Trustee
Camp Thorpe is a residential summer camp for children, teens and adults with a range of social, behavioural, mental, and developmental disabilities. Two separate campus' are available, the Mountain Reach Campus for ages 10-21, and the Pine Haven Campus for ages 21 and up.

1467 Silver Towers Camp
56 Silver Towers Rd
Ripton, VT 05766
802-388-6446
Fax: 802-388-0219
cdravenna@comcast.net
www.vtelks.org/programs/silver-towers/
Brian Guara, President
Henry Diemer, 1st Vice President
Carolyn Ravenna, Camp Director
Carol Sylvia, Secretary
Two-week residential camp for ages 6-75 who are physically or mentally challenged. Campers gain the social skills and personal enrichment they seek. Activities include swimming, horseback riding, music, sing-a-longs, dancing, nature studies and more.

1468 Vermont Overnight Camp
The Barton Center for Diabetes Education, Inc.
30 Ennis Rd
PO Box 356
North Oxford, MA 01537-0356
508-987-2056
Fax: 508-987-2002
info@bartoncenter.org
www.bartoncenter.org
Lynn Butler, Executive Director
Kyler Jesanis, Camp Joslin Director
Lindsay Charest, Associate Director
Donna Joly, Facilities Director
A summer camp program of the Barton Center for Diabetes Education and SLAMDiabetes, the Vermont Overnight Camp provides children and teens, ages 6-16, with insulin-dependent diabetes a traditional summer camp experience combined with diabetes education. Activities include sports, swimming, kayaking, canoeing, fishing, hiking, arts and crafts, and campfires. The camp is held in South Hero, Vermont.

Virginia

1469 Camp Dickenson
Holston Conference of United Methodist Church
801 Camp Dickson Ln
P.O. Box 232
Fries, VA 24330
276-744-7241
campdickenson@centurylink.net
www.campdickenson.com
Michael Snow, Camp Director
Kory Tomlinson, Program Director
Wayne Roberts, Facilities Manager
Camp Dickenson offers camping sessions for children and adults with developmental disabilities. Coed, ages 5-18 and 18 and up, families, seniors and single adults.

1470 Camp Easter Seals Virginia
Easter Seals: Virginia
900 Camp Easter Seals Rd.
New Castle, VA 24127
540-777-7325
camp@eastersealsucp.com
www.easterseals.com

Alex Barge, Camp Director
Luanne Welch, President & CEO
Rick Anicetti, Chair
Dave Sweyer, 1st Vice Chair
Summer camp sessions for children and adults ages 5-99 with physical disabilities, cognitive disabilities and sensory impairments. Therapeutic recreation activities including swimming, fishing, sports, horseback riding, rock climbing, and more.

1471 Camp Holiday Trails
400 Holiday Trails Ln.
Charlottesville, VA 22903
434-977-3781
Fax: 434-977-8814
info@campholidaytrails.org
Ann Wicks, President
Kurt A. Friesen, Vice President
Tina La Roche, Executive Director
Ana Baggiano, Program Director
Private, nonprofit camp for children with special health needs and various chronic illnesses. Coed 5-17, nationwide and international. Activities include canoeing, swimming, horseback riding, arts and crafts, drama, ropes course, etc. 24-hour medical supervision by doctor and nursing staff.

1472 Camp Jordan
Camp Hanover
3163 Parsleys Mill Rd.
Mechanicsville, VA 23111
804-779-2811
info@camphanover.org
www.camphanover.org/
Doug Walters, Executive Director
Lisa VanderPloeg, Office Manager
Harry Zweckbronner, Program Director
Camp Jordan is a sleepover camp session for children with diabetes in grades 6-12. The camp is a part of Camp Hanover, and activities include hiking, archery, campfires, paddle boards, and more.

1473 Camp Loud And Clear
Holiday Lake 4-H Educational Center
1267 4-H Camp Rd.
Appomattox, VA 24522
434-248-5444
Fax: 434-248-6749
bgoin@vt.edu
holidaylake4h.com/camploud.php
Preston Willson, President/ CEO
Heather Benningrove, Program Director
Chris Hawn, Center Director
Rich Hilbers, Facilities Manager
Camp Lound And Clear is a summer camp for children, ages 8-13, who are deaf or suffer from hearing loss. Activities include swimming, archery, bible study, and more.

1474 Camp Virginia Jaycee
Camp Jaycee Rd.
P.O. Box 648
Blue Ridge, VA 24064
540-947-2972
info@campvajc.org
www.campvajc.org

William B. Robertson, Founder
Summer camping for children and adults with developmental disabilities. Coed, ages 7-70. Weekend respite camps for children and adults with mental retardation.

1475 Camps for Children & Teens with Diabetes
American Diabetes Association
2451 Crystal Dr.
Suite 900
Arlington, VA   22202   800-342-2383
                                                     www.diabetes.org/

David A. DeMarco, PhD, Chair
Brenda Montgomery, President, Health Care & Education
Alvin Powers, President, Medicine & Science
Umesh Verma, Secretary/Treasurer
The American Diabetes Association sponsors day camps, family camps and resident camps for children and teens. These camps provide an opportunity for children with diabetes to go to camp, meet other children and gain a better understanding of their diabetes. The total experience can help campers develop more confidence in their abilities to control their diabetes effectively while enjoying the traditional camp experience. Camps are located all across the country.

1476 Civitan Acres for the Disabled
Civitan Acres
2210 Cedar Rd.
Chesapeake, VA   23323-6303   757-487-6062
                                                Fax: 757-487-4143
                                          info@egglestonservices.org
                                          www.egglestonservices.org
Paul Atkinson, President and CEO
Dennis Bailey, Chief Financial Officer
Thomas L. Redmond, Vice President, Marketing
Chris Hoagland, Vice President, Government Contracts
Offers a summer camp for adults and children with disabilities. Sessions run for one week, and aims to help campers improve their emotional, intellectual, and physical dimensions of life.

1477 Loudoun County Adaptive Recreation Camps
Loudoun County Local Government
P.O. Box 7000
Leesburg, VA   20177   703-777-0100
                                                Fax: 703-771-5354
                                                   prcs@loudoun.gov
                                                   www.loudoun.gov
Phyllis J. Randall, Chair
Ralph M. Buona, Vice Chairman
Suzanne M. Volpe, Board Member
Ron A. Meyer, Board Member
Loudoun County's Adaptive Recreation Camps offers and promotes integration opportunities for individuals with disabilities. All camps are designed to meet the individual needs of the participants, and aim to provide traditional summer camp experiences.

1478 Oakland School & Camp
128 Oakland Farm Way
Troy, VA   22974   434-293-9059
                                                Fax: 434-296-8930
                                       information@oaklandschool.net
                                             www.oaklandschool.net
Carol Williams, Head of School
Abby Sprague, Admissions Director
Amanda Baber, Admissions Director
Pete Cormons, Operations Director
A highly individualized program that stresses improving reading ability. Subjects taught are reading, English composition, math and word analysis. Recreational activities include horseback riding, sports, swimming, tennis, crafts, archery and camping. For girls and boys, ages 8-14. Students who attend the summer camp often have a variety of learning disabilities, such as ADHD, dyslexia, visual/auditory processing disorders, and more.

Washington

1479 Camp Goodtimes
The Goodtimes Project
7400 Sand Point Way NE
#101S
Seattle, WA   98115   206-940-0062
                                                Fax: 206-877-4437
                                        tanya@thegoodtimesproject.org
                                         www.thegoodtimesproject.org/
Tanya Khron, Camp Director
Zac Johnson, Executive Director
A week-long residential summer camp for children ages 7-25 diagnosed with cancer and their siblings. The Goodtimes Project also runs Kayak Adventure Camp for childhood cancer survivors, aged 18-25.

1480 Camp Killoqua
Camp Fire Snohomish County
4312 Rucker Ave
Everett, WA   98203   425-258-KIDS
                                                Fax: 425-252-2267
                                         killoqua@campfiresnoco.org
                                       www.campfireusasnohomish.org
Elizabeth Johnson, President
Rebekah Couper-Noles, Vice President
Dave Surface, Executive Director
Carol Johnson, Assistant Executive Director
Camp Killoqua offers Inclusion Programs for all of its traditional camp programs. The inclusion program allows campers, ages 7-21, with mild to moderate developmental disabilities the chance to participate in any Camp Killoqua session.

1481 Camp Korey
19301 33rd Ave W.
Suite 211
Lynnwood, WA   98036   425-440-0850
                                                Fax: 425-404-2158
                                                   info@campkorey.org
                                                       campkorey.org/
Chris McReynolds, President
Kenneth G. Smith, Treasurer
Claudia Campanile, Secretary
A summer camp for children with life threatening illnesses and their families. Camp Korey is completely free, and aims to allow kids to experience a normal childhood experience in a safe, and fun camp environment with specialized medical support.

1482 Camp Prime Time
6 S. 2nd Street
Suite 815
Yakima, WA   98901   509-248-2854
                                                Fax: 509-248-5505
                                         families@campprimetime.org
                                            www.campprimetime.org
Ralph Berthon, Co-Founder
Dave Berthon, Co-Founder
Dick Haapala, President
Mike Burnam, Vice President
Prime Time serves children and adults with disabilities or have terminal or serious illnesses.

1483 Camp Sealth
14500 SW Camp Sealth Rd.
Vashon, WA   98070-8222   206-463-3174
                                                Fax: 206-463-6936
                                                 campfireseattle.org/
Hillary U, President
Lisa Luchau, Vice President
Patrick Hayes, Secretary
Jodi Colligan, Treasurer
With support from the American Diabetes Association, Camp Sealth runs a overnight summer camp session for children ages 5-17 during session 5. The ADA provides a team of medical staff and dieticians to ensure that campers are safe and health during their stay at camp.

1484   Camp Stix
Camp STIX Diabetes Programs
P.O. Box 8308
Spokane, WA 99203   509-484-1366
                                Fax: 888-958-5730
                        campstix@campstix.org
                        www.campstix.org/Default.aspx

Bill Martin, Medical Director
Lynn Sander, Education Director
Camp Stix is an independent summer camp for children and teens with diabetes. Coed, ages 9-18. The camp is help for one week at the Riverview Bible Camp on the Pend Oreille River.

1485   Easter Seals Camp Stand by Me
Easter Seal Society of Washington
17809 S. Vaughn Rd KPN
PO Box 289
Vaughn, WA 98394   253-884-2722
                        jmayer@wa.easterseals.com
                        www.wa.easterseals.com

Jeff Pavey, Board Chair
Carol Basile, Vice Chair
Ellen Briggs, Treasurer
Joshua Mayer, Camp Director
Camp Stand by Me is a summer camp for adults and children with any disability. Coed, ages 7-65, seniors. Respite weekends offered throughout the year. Activities include campfires, fishing, swimming, sports, archery, and more.

1486   Northwest Kiwanis Camp
Camp Beausite NW
P.O.Box 1227
Port Hadlock, WA 98339   360-732-7222
                        campbeausitenw.org

Dr. Claudia Edmondson, Director
Cheryl Smith, Director of Programs
Northwest Kiwanis Camp is also known as Camp Beausite NW, and is located in Chimacum, Washington. Campers range from 6-65 in age, and includes those with developmental disabilities, cerebral palsy, autism, downs syndrome, and other physical and/or mental handicaps. The camp currently offers five week-long overnight summer camp sessions for adults and children.

West Virginia

1487   Mountaineer Spina Bifida Camp
534 New Goff Mountain Rd
Charleston, WV 25313   304-776-7513
                        info@drewsday.org
                        www.drewsday.org/

Suzie Humphreys
A summer camp for individuals with spina bifida. Campers can participate in activities such as swimming, wheelchair hockey, baseball, and more.

Wisconsin

1488   Camp Daypoint
YMCA Camp St. Croix
532 County Road F
Hudson, WI 54016   763-593-5333
                        Fax: 952-582-9000
                        rbarnett@diabetes.org
                        www.diabetes.org

Becky Barnett, Camp Director
Camp Daypoint is a day camp for children, ages 5-9, who have been diagnosed with diabetes. Activities include swimming, crafts, hikes, games, and more. Camp runs from 9am to 3:30pm, and buses return campers to Minneapolis and St. Paul locations.

1489   Camp Kee-B-Waw
Easter Seals Wisconsin
8001 Excelsior Dr.
Suite 200
Madison, WI 53717   608-277-8288
                                     800-422-2324
                                Fax: 608-277-8333
                                TTY: 608-277-8031
                camp@eastersealswisconsin.com
                camp.eastersealswisconsin.com

Christine Fessler, President/CEO
Sandee Horn, Executive Assistant
Stevie Thomas, Summer Director, Camp Wawbeek
Located at Camp Wawbeek, Camp Kee-B-Waw is a day camp for children ages 6-13 from Wisconsin Dells and surrounding communities.

1490   Camp Klotty Pine
Great Lakes Hemophilia Foundation
638 North 18th St.
Milwaukee, WI 53233   414-937-6782
                                     888-797-GLHF
                                info@glhf.org
                                glhf.org

Pete Fisher, President, Great Lakes Hemophilia Foundation
Andy Barragry, Secretary
Jeff Koopmeiners, Vice President
Robin Grehn, Treasurer
An overnight summer camp for children, ages 7-15, who have been diagnosed with a bleeding disorder. The camp is held at Camp Lakotah in Wautoma, Wisconsin. The Camp runs recreational camp activities such as archery, canoeing, and campfires, as well as education about their disorder and self-infusion instruction.

1491   Camp Lakota
Wisconsin Lions Camp
3834 County Road A
Rosholt, WI 54473   608-222-7785
                                Fax: 608-222-7795
                        jjoswiak@diabetes.org
                        www.diabetes.org

Jenna Joswiak, Camp Director
A program of the American Diabetes Association, Camp Lakota is a summer camp for children, ages 9-16, who have been diagnosed with diabetes. The camp is held at the Wisconsin Lions Camp, and is only open to Wisconsin residents. Activities include hiking, climbing walls, sailing, and more.

1492   Camp Needlepoint
American Diabetes Association
YMCA Camp St. Croix
532 County Road F
Hudson, WI 54016   763-593-5333
                                Fax: 952-582-9000
                        rbarnett@diabetes.org
                        www.diabetes.org

Becky Barnett, Camp Director
Carol Holton, Associate Manager
Camp Needlepoint is a summer camp for children who have type 1 diabetes. Coed, ages 8-16. The Camp takes place at the YMCA Camp St. Croix. The aim of Camp Needlepoint is to provide a safe camping expeience where children with diabetes can meet others with type 1 diabetes.

1493 Easter Seal Camp Wawbeek
Easter Seals: Wisconsin
8001 Excelsior Dr.
Suite 200
Madison, WI 53717   608-277-8288
                                  800-422-2324
                             Fax: 608-277-8333
                             TTY: 608-277-8031
                camp@eastersealswisconsin.com
                camp.eastersealswisconsin.com

Christine Fessler, President/CEO
Sandee Horn, Executive Assistant
Stevie Thomas, Summer Director, Camp Wawbeek
Alex Peters, Assistant Director, Camp Wawbeek
Camp Wawbeek is a summer camp for children and adults with physical disabilities. Coed, ages 7 and up. During the summer, the camp runs six-day youth and teen sessions; a six-day adult, young adult, and transition sessions; as well as weekend sessions from September to May.

1494 Lutherdale Bible Camp
Lutherdale Ministries
N7891 US Highway 12
Elkhorn, WI 53121   262-742-2352
                             Fax: 888-248-4551
                                info@lutherdale.org
                                www.lutherdale.org

Jeff Bluhm, Executive Director
David Box, Program Director
Robert Couden, Operations/Facilities Manager
Jeff Thompson, Program Director
Lutherdale Bible Camp currently offers Team USA, a summer camp program for adults with developmental disabilities. Activities include talent show, parade, and campfire worships.

1495 Phantom Lake YMCA Camp
S110W30240 YMCA Camp Road
Mukwonago, WI 53149   262-363-4386
                office@phantomlakeymca.org
                www.phantomlakeymca.org

James Scharine, Chair of the Board
Jay Wall, Vice Chair
Dr. Karin Mulrooney, Secretary
Jodi Jacobsen, Treasurer
Phantom Lake Camp offers day and residential camping sessions for boys, girls, and a coed session. All programs are open to individuals with disabilities as the camp welcomes any child, ages 3-17, regardless of race, religon, disability, etc.

1496 Timbertop Nature Adventure Camp
YMCA Camp Glacier Hollow
1000 Division St.
Stevens Point, WI 54481   715-342-2980
                             Fax: 715-342-2987
                             pmatthai@spymca.org
            www.glacierhollow.com/timbertop-camp/
Pete Matthai, Camp Director
Tiffany Praeger, Summer Camp Program Director
For children who can benefit from an individualized program of learning in a non-competitive outdoor setting under the skilled leadership of people who understand the environment and the unique potential of these children. Timbertop combines traditional camp programs with extra reading practice and special group activities. The camp lasts 7 days, and activties include stargazing, canoeing, archery, and more.

1497 Wisconsin Badger Camp
Wisconsin Badger Camp
P.O. Box 723
Platteville, WI 53818   608-348-9689
                             Fax: 608-348-9737
            wiscbadgercamp@centurytel.net
                    www.badgercamp.org

Carol Beals, Chair
Bruce Rathe, Vice Chair
Michelle Eno, Treasurer
Kim Martens, Board Member

Wisconsin Badger Camp, established in 1966, is a summer camp that serves individuals with developmental disabilities. Badger camp offers eight one-week camps and one two-week camp for ages 3-93. One week is for ages 14-25, one week for ages 3-13 and all other weeks for ages 18 and older.

1498 Wisconsin Elks/Easter Seals Respite Camp
1550 Waubeek Road
Wisconsin Dells, WI 53965   608-254-2502
                                  800-422-2324
                             Fax: 608-277-8333
                             TTY: 608-277-8031
                camp@eastersealswisconsin.com
                camp.eastersealswisconsin.com

Cyndi Hemmer, Director, Respite Camp
Christine Fessler, President/CEO
Sandee Horn, Executive Assistant
The Wisconsin Elks/Easter Seals Respite Camp is a year-round camp for individuals with disabilities, including those with severe or multiple disabilities. Activities include arts and crafts, sports, games, high ropes course, and local field trips.

1499 Wisconsin Lions Camp
Wisconsin Lions Foundation
3834 County Road A
Rosholt, WI 54473   715-677-4969
                                  877-463-6953
                             Fax: 715-677-4527
            info@wisconsinlionscamp.com
            www.wisconsinlionscamp.com

Evett J. Hartvig, Executive Director
Andrea Yenter, Camp Director
Summer Allen, Program Supervisor
Dale Schroeder, Facility Director
Serves children who have either a visual, hearing or mild cognitive disability, as well as diabetes types I and II. Program activities include sailing, ropes course, hiking and canoe trips, environmental education, swimming, camping, canoeing, outdoor living skills and handicrafts. ACA accredited, located in central Wisconsin, near Stevens Point.

Wyoming

1500 Camp Hope
3920 West 45th St.
Casper, WY 82604   307-265-5865
                             Fax: 307-472-5008
                             sjohnrph1@gmail.com

Steve Johnson, Director
Nancy Johnson, Director
Camp Hope is a camp for children and young adults with diabetes. Some of the activities include hiking, swimming, sports and games.

1501 Eagle View Ranch
SOAR
184 Uphill Rd.
P.O. Box 584
Dubois, WY 82513   307-455-3084
                             Fax: 801-820-3050
                             admissions@soarnc.org
                                www.soarnc.org

John Willson, M.S., Executive Director
Jonathan Jones, Founder
Laura Pate, Operations Director
Jeremy Neidens, Director, Eagle View Ranch
Camp for youths with learning disabilities and attention deficit disorder. Campers enjoy a broad range of wilderness adventure experiences that help to empower them to overcome challenges, while helping them to learn how to develop problem solving skills, effective communication strategies and social skills.

Clothing

Dresses & Skirts

1502 Budget Cotton/Poly Open Back Gown
Buck & Buck
3111 27th Ave S
Seattle, WA 98144-6502
206-722-4196
800-458-0600
Fax: 800-317-2182
info@buckandbuck.com
www.buckandbuck.com

Julie Buck, Owner
Short raglan sleeves, lace at neck and bodice over lapping
snapback closure. *$14.00*

1503 Budget Flannel Open Back Gown
Buck & Buck
3111 27th Ave S
Seattle, WA 98144-6502
206-722-4196
800-458-0600
info@buckandbuck.com
www.buckandbuck.com

Julie Buck, Owner
3/4 raglan sleeve, lace at neck and bodice. *$17.00*

1504 Cotton/Poly House Dress
Buck & Buck
3111 27th Ave S
Seattle, WA 98144-6502
206-722-4196
800-458-0600
info@buckandbuck.com
www.buckandbuck.com

Julie Buck, Owner
Comes in short and long sleeves, assorted florals and plaids.
$36.00

1505 Dusters
Buck & Buck
3111 27th Ave S
Seattle, WA 98144-6502
206-722-4196
800-458-0600
info@buckandbuck.com
www.buckandbuck.com

Julie Buck, Owner
Three types: Floral, Budget Better. Snap front styles and gathered
yokes, flannel $16.00-$24.00. *$36.00*

1506 Flannel Gowns
Buck & Buck
3111 27th Ave S
Seattle, WA 98144-6502
206-722-4196
800-458-0600
info@buckandbuck.com
www.buckandbuck.com

Julie Buck, Owner
Comes in long or short with a deep button-front opening for ease
of slipping on. Shorter long length. *$21.00*

1507 Float Dress
Buck & Buck
3111 27th Ave S
Seattle, WA 98144-6502
206-722-4196
800-458-0600
info@buckandbuck.com
www.buckandbuck.com

Julie Buck, Owner
A safe bet for everyone from a size medium to a 3X. Gathered
yoke front and back and literally yards of fabric for fullness. Comes in cotton or polyester. *$32.00*

1508 Muu Muu
Buck & Buck
3111 27th Ave S
Seattle, WA 98144-6502
206-722-4196
800-458-0600
info@buckandbuck.com
www.buckandbuck.com

Julie Buck, Owner
Comes in long and short styles, assorted bright floral prints.
$20.00-$22.00. *$31.00*

1509 Polyester House Dress
Buck & Buck
3111 27th Ave S
Seattle, WA 98144-6502
206-722-4196
800-458-0600
info@buckandbuck.com
www.buckandbuck.com

Julie Buck, Owner
Comes in short and long sleeves, assorted florals. *$ 36.00*

Footwear

1510 Booties with Non-Skid Soles
Buck & Buck
3111 27th Ave S
Seattle, WA 98144-6502
206-722-4196
800-458-0600
Fax: 800-317-2182
info@buckandbuck.com
www.buckandbuck.com

Julie Buck, Owner
Acrylic knit or quilted cotton/poly and shearling inner. *$17.00*

1511 Foot Snugglers
Buck & Buck
3111 27th Ave S
Seattle, WA 98144-6502
206-722-4196
800-458-0600
Fax: 800-317-2182
info@buckandbuck.com
www.buckandbuck.com

Julie Buck, Owner
Quilted poly/cotton outers lined with plush shearling pile, provide a thick, comfortable cushion which helps minimize the pressure points on tender areas. *$.30*

1512 Propet Leather Walking Shoes
Buck & Buck
3111 27th Ave S
Seattle, WA 98144-6502
206-722-4196
800-458-0600
Fax: 800-317-2182
info@buckandbuck.com
www.buckandbuck.com

Julie Buck, Owner
Two velcro straps, leather upper, shock-absorbing sole. *$58.00*

1513 TRU-Mold Shoes
42 Breckenridge St
Buffalo, NY 14213-1555
716-881-4484
800-843-6653
Fax: 716-881-0406
www.trumold.com

Husain Syed, Production Manager
Custom made, fully molded shoes, relieve pressure in sensitive
areas by taking all of the weight off the painful areas.

1514 Velcro Booties
Buck & Buck
3111 27th Ave S
Seattle, WA 98144-6502
206-722-4196
800-458-0600
Fax: 800-317-2182
info@buckandbuck.com
www.buckandbuck.com
Julie Buck, Owner
The high-domed toe, and extra-wide, non-skid sole design accommodates virtually every foot related problem. *$20.00*

1515 Washable Shoes
Buck & Buck
3111 27th Ave S
Seattle, WA 98144-6502
206-722-4196
800-458-0600
Fax: 800-317-2182
info@buckandbuck.com
www.buckandbuck.com
Julie Buck, Owner
Vinyl upper with velcro closure, nonskid sole. *$20.00*

Miscellaneous & Catalogs

1516 Adaptations by Adrian
PO Box 7
San Marcos, CA 92079-0007
760-744-3565
888-214-8372
Fax: 760-471-7560
adrians1@sbcglobal.net
www.adaptationsbyadrian.com

1517 Adaptive Clothing: Adults
Special Clothes
P.O.Box 333
E Harwich, MA 02645-333
508-430-2410
Fax: 508-430-2410
specialclo@aol.com
www.special-clothes.com
Judith Sweeney, President
Special Clothes produces a catalogue of garments for adults with disabilities and/or incontinence. Offerings include: undergarments, snap-crotch tee shirts, jumpsuits, and denim travel cath. The catalogue is available without charge. Comparable to department store prices. Special Clothes produces a catalog of adaptive clothing for children in sizes from toddler through young adults. A full line of clothing is included from undergarments through wheelchair jackets and ponchos.

1518 Adult Short Jumpsuit
Special Clothes
P.O.Box 333
E Harwich, MA 02645-333
508-430-2410
Fax: 508-430-2410
specialclo@aol.com
www.special-clothes.com
Judith Sweeney, President
This pull-on jumpsuit provides comfort and full coverage without bulk. Wide leg ribbing ends at mid-thigh, with snaps at the crotch. We use fine quality, comfortable cotton knit. 100% cotton knit. Made in USA. Option: long sleeves - add $3.00. Colors: white, navy, teal, light blue, light pink, red, royal blue, black, khaki and juvenile print. S,M & L $43.00; XL & XXL $45.00

1519 Body Suits
Special Clothes
P.O.Box 333
E Harwich, MA 02645-333
508-430-2410
Fax: 508-430-2410
specialclo@aol.com
www.special-clothes.com
Judith Sweeney, President
These are one piece garments that can be used to protect skin under braces, to add warmth and to shield incisions. S,M & L $42.00; XL & XXL $44.00.

1520 Buck and Buck Clothing
3111 27th Ave S
Seattle, WA 98144-6502
206-722-4196
800-458-0600
Fax: 800-317-2182
info@buckandbuck.com
www.buckandbuck.com
Julie Buck, Owner
Clothing for the disabled and elderly.
88 pages Yearly

1521 Carolyn's Catalog
3938 S Tamiami Trl
Sarasota, FL 34231-3622
941-373-9100
800-648-2266
Fax: 941-739-5503
www.carolynscatalog.com
John Colton, Owner
Free, mail-order catalog of items for visually impaired people.

1522 Exquisite Egronomic Protective Wear
Plum Enterprises
P.O.Box 85
Valley Forge, PA 19481-85
610-783-7377
800-321-7586
Fax: 610-783-7577
info@plument.com
www.plument.com
Janice Carrington, President/CEO
Egronomic Protective Wear; ProtectaCap custom-fitting headgear has earned an unparalleled reputation for quality, safety, and comfort. ProtectaCap+Plus technologically-advanced protective headgear closes the gap between hard and soft helmets. Comes with optional ProtectaChin Guard and new sporty design. Protectahip protective undergarment is the intelligent, innovative solution to the problem of hip injuries for both men and women. Ladies' styles are covered with attractive stretch lace.

1523 Headliner Hats
Designs for Comfort
PO Box 671044
Marietta, GA 30066-2429
770-565-8246
800-443-9226
Fax: 770-565-8425
headliner@mindspring.com
www.headlinerhats.com
Curt Maurer, President
A patented cap and hairpiece combination, the Headliner is both a quick, stylish coverup and an upbeat wig alternative for women experiencing hair care problems or hair loss. Ideal for social gatherings and outdoor activities as well as for sleeping and hospital stays. *$ 25.00*

1524 Knee Socks
Buck & Buck
3111 27th Ave S
Seattle, WA 98144-6502
206-722-4196
800-458-0600
Fax: 800-317-2182
info@buckandbuck.com
www.buckandbuck.com
Julie Buck, Owner
Comes in regular and large size. $3.00 - $8.00

1525 M&M Health Care Apparel Company
Fashion Collection
1541 60th St
Brooklyn, NY 11219-5023
718-871-8188
800-221-8929
Fax: 718-436-2067
info@fashionease.com
www.fashionease.com
Abraham Klein, Owner
Specialized clothing for disabled people.

1526 Professional Fit Clothing
Ste 1
831 N Lake St
Burbank, CA 91502-1600   818-563-1975
                                         800-422-2348
                                  Fax: 818-563-1834
                      sales@professionalfit.com
                      www.professionalfit.com

Kurt Rieback, Owner
Professional fit clothing caters to homes that care for people with
developmental disabilities and individuals who are physically
challenged. Our clothing is fashionable, affordable and can be
adapted to each person's special needs.

1527 Spec-L Clothing Solutions
849 Performance Drive
Stockton, CA 95206   714-427-0781
                                         800-445-1981
                                  Fax: 800-683-6510
                      www.clothingsolutions.com

Jim Lechner, Owner
The nation's leading designer and manufacturer of assistive
clothing for men and women. Free 56 page catalog available.

1528 Special Clothes Adult Catalogue
Special Clothes
P.O.Box 333
E Harwich, MA 02645-333   508-430-2410
                                  Fax: 508-430-2410
                      specialclo@aol.com
                      www.special-clothes.com

Judith Sweeney, President
Produces a catalogue of adaptive clothing for adults with disabilities. Offers include undergarments, casual bottoms, jumpsuits,
swimwear, footwear and bibs. Prices are comparable to
deparment store prices. The catalogue is free.

1529 Special Clothes for Special Children
Special Clothes
P.O.Box 333
E Harwich, MA 02645-333   508-430-2410
                                  Fax: 508-430-2410
                      specialclo@aol.com
                      www.special-clothes.com

Judith Sweeney, President
All special adaptations, such as velcro closures, snap crotches,
bib fronts and G-tube access openings. Every item is fully washable. Offering optional features to customize each item to meet
the needs of your child.

1530 Specialty Care Shoppe
16126 E 161st St S
Bixby, OK 74008-7325   918-366-2901
                                  Fax: 918-366-9445
                      www.specialtycareshoppe.com

K J Marshall, Owner
Catalog of attractive, affordable clothing and accessories for
adults with special needs. Includes items for edema, incontinence, alzheimers, limited mobility, and hand impairment.

1531 Super Stretch Socks
Buck & Buck
3111 27th Ave S
Seattle, WA 98144-6502   206-722-4196
                                         800-458-0600
                                  Fax: 800-317-2182
                      info@buckandbuck.com
                      www.buckandbuck.com

Julie Buck, Owner
This sock has been improved to stretch laterally throughout the
foot area as well as at the top. *$3.75*

1532 Thigh-Hi Nylon Stockings
Buck & Buck
3111 27th Ave S
Seattle, WA 98144-6502   206-722-4196
                                         800-458-0600
                                  Fax: 800-317-2182
                      info@buckandbuck.com
                      www.buckandbuck.com

Julie Buck, Owner
A sheer, full length stocking. *$4.50*

1533 Waterproof Bib
Buck & Buck
3111 27th Ave S
Seattle, WA 98144-6502   206-722-4196
                                         800-458-0600
                                  Fax: 800-317-2182
                      info@buckandbuck.com
                      www.buckandbuck.com

Julie Buck, Owner
Made with 3 layers of fabric including waterproof backing, these
attractive bibs will not soak through like most others, protecting
clothing from stains. *$18.00*

1534 Wishing Wells Collection
Ste 965
11684 Ventura Blvd
Studio City, CA 91604-2699   818-840-6919
                                  Fax: 818-760-3878
                      wishingwells@dawn-wells.com
                      www.dawnwells.com

Dawn Wells, Owner
Lorraine Parker, General Manager
Features designs full of back overlap construction and all velcro
closures clothing.

Robes & Sleepwear

1535 Creative Designs
3704 Carlisle Ct
Modesto, CA 95356-924   209-523-3166
                                         800-335-4852
                      robes4you@aol.com
                      www.robes4you.com

Barbara Arnold, Owner
Designer of the original Change-A-Robe and the new
Handi-Robe, which allows the wearer to put it on without having
to stand up. Robes are designed especially for physically challenged, disabled individuals, and wheelchair users. *$69.95*

1536 Flannel Pajamas
Buck & Buck
3111 27th Ave S
Seattle, WA 98144-6502   206-722-4196
                                         800-458-0600
                                  Fax: 800-317-2182
                      info@buckandbuck.com
                      www.buckandbuck.com

Julie Buck, Owner
$25.00

1537 His & Hers
Wishing Wells Collection
Ste 965
11684 Ventura Blvd
Studio City, CA 91604-2699   818-840-6919
                                  Fax: 818-760-3878
                      www.dawnwells.com

Dawn Wells, Owner
This sleep shirt is designed for him or her. *$21.99*

1538   Nightshirts
Buck & Buck
3111 27th Ave S
Seattle, WA 98144-6502   206-722-4196
                                           800-458-0600
                                      Fax: 800-317-2182
                                   info@buckandbuck.com
                                   www.buckandbuck.com
Julie Buck, Owner
Come in flannel or cotton patterns and prints in sizes S/M, 4XL,
2XL/3XL *$29.00*

1539   Open Back Nightgowns
Buck & Buck
3111 27th Ave S
Seattle, WA 98144-6502   206-722-4196
                                           800-458-0600
                                      Fax: 800-317-2182
                                   info@buckandbuck.com
                                   www.buckandbuck.com
Julie Buck, Owner
Come in cotton (sizes S-4X) or flannel (sizes S-3X). *$20.00*

1540   Seersucker Shower Robe
Buck & Buck
3111 27th Ave S
Seattle, WA 98144-6502   206-722-4196
                                           800-458-0600
                                      Fax: 800-317-2182
                                   info@buckandbuck.com
                                   www.buckandbuck.com
Julie Buck, Owner
Totally covers a man or woman being wheeled to and from the
shower or bath. A crisp, light weight shower robe. *$34.00*

Shirts & Tops

1541   Basic Rear Closure Sweat Top
Buck & Buck
3111 27th Ave S
Seattle, WA 98144-6502   206-722-4196
                                           800-458-0600
                                      Fax: 800-317-2182
                                   info@buckandbuck.com
                                   www.buckandbuck.com
Julie Buck, Owner
Top opens completely down the back for ease of dressing with
snaps. *$19.00*

1542   Cotton Full-Back Vest
Buck & Buck
3111 27th Ave S
Seattle, WA 98144-6502   206-722-4196
                                           800-458-0600
                                      Fax: 800-317-2182
                                   info@buckandbuck.com
                                   www.buckandbuck.com
Julie Buck, Owner
Wide shoulder straps that don't slide off shoulders. *$5.00*

1543   Dutch Neck T-Shirt
Buck & Buck
3111 27th Ave S
Seattle, WA 98144-6502   206-722-4196
                                           800-458-0600
                                      Fax: 800-317-2182
                                   info@buckandbuck.com
                                   www.buckandbuck.com
Julie Buck, Owner
Stretchy neck makes it easy to get over the head. *$ 5.50*

1544   Printed Rear Closure Sweat Top
Buck & Buck
3111 27th Ave S
Seattle, WA 98144-6502   206-722-4196
                                           800-458-0600
                                      Fax: 800-317-2182
                                   info@buckandbuck.com
                                   www.buckandbuck.com
Julie Buck, Owner
Comes in assorted colors, plain or with animal motifs and snaps
all the way down the back. *$28.00*

1545   Rear Closure Shirts
Buck & Buck
3111 27th Ave S
Seattle, WA 98144-6502   206-722-4196
                                           800-458-0600
                                      Fax: 206-722-1144
                                   info@buckandbuck.com
                                   www.buckandbuck.com
Julie Buck, Owner
Snaps down the back on T-shirts and dress shirts. *$ 33.00*

1546   Rear Closure T-Shirt
Buck & Buck
3111 27th Ave S
Seattle, WA 98144-6502   206-722-4196
                                           800-458-0600
                                      Fax: 800-317-2182
                                   info@buckandbuck.com
                                   www.buckandbuck.com
Julie Buck, Owner
Closes down the back with velcro snaps. *$10.00*

Slacks & Pants

1547   Jumpsuits
Special Clothes
PO Box 333
E Harwich, MA   02645-333   508-430-2410
                                      Fax: 508-430-2410
                                       lou@lnrmusic.com
                                   www.special-clothes.com
Judith Sweeney, President
Several styles of one-piece garments are available for dressing
ease. Front opening styles are designed for easy access. Prices
range from $32.20-$44.00. *$55.00*

1548   Side Velcro Slacks
Buck & Buck
3111 27th Ave S
Seattle, WA 98144-6502   206-722-4196
                                           800-458-0600
                                      Fax: 800-317-2182
                                   info@buckandbuck.com
                                   www.buckandbuck.com
Julie Buck, Owner
Slacks open down both sides from waist to hip with snap closures
at sides. *$36.00*

1549   Side-Zip Sweat Pants
Buck & Buck
3111 27th Ave S
Seattle, WA 98144-6502   206-722-4196
                                           800-458-0600
                                      Fax: 800-317-2182
                                   info@buckandbuck.com
                                   www.buckandbuck.com
Julie Buck, Owner
Out-seam zippers un-zip 22-inch zippers down both sides to en-
able dressing a resident with severe leg contractures. *$25.00*

1550 Trunks
Buck & Buck
3111 27th Ave S
Seattle, WA 98144-6502
206-722-4196
800-458-0600
Fax: 800-317-2118
info@buckandbuck.com
www.buckandbuck.com

Julie Buck, Owner
Come in cotton or nylon, flare leg, full cut. *$5.00*

Undergarments

1551 Adult Absorbent Briefs
Special Clothes
PO Box 333
E Harwich, MA 02645-333
508-430-2410
Fax: 508-430-2410
lou@lnrmusic.com
www.special-clothes.com

Judith Sweeney, President
Soft, comfortable, 100% cotton knit brief is seven layers thick at the crotch. Sides of the brief are a non-bulky single layer. The waistband elastic is enclosed in a soft cotton knit casing and does not touch the skin. Comfortable cotton rib knit bands circle the leg. This brief will not replace a diaper, but provides absorbency for light incontinence. *$18.50*

1552 Adult Lap Shoulder Bodysuit
Special Clothes
PO Box 334
E Harwich, MA 02645-333
508-430-2410
Fax: 508-430-2410
TTY:508-430-2410
lou@lnrmusic.com
www.special-clothes.com

1553 Adult Sleeveless Bodysuit
Special Clothes
PO Box 335
E Harwich, MA 02645-333
508-430-2410
Fax: 508-430-2410
lou@lnrmusic.com
www.special-clothes.com

Judith Sweeney, President
Bodysuit styles fasten at the crotch with sturdy snaps to stay neatly tucked. All are made of soft, absorbent 100% cotton knit for maximum comfort. They are cut wide at the hip and seat for full coverage, and will accomodate a diaper if necessary. Soft knit rib circles the neck and leg. This cool tank style slips on easily. Deep armholes are banded with rib knit. All styles: S,M,L $42, XL,XXL $44. A choice of 12 colors.

1554 Adult Swim Diaper
Special Clothes
PO Box 336
E Harwich, MA 02645-333
508-430-2410
Fax: 508-430-2410
lou@lnrmusic.com
www.special-clothes.com

Judith Sweeney, President
This pant is made of soft, silent, light-weight, impermeable fabric- waterproof and secure. It is a containment brief, designed to be used in the pool in place of cloth or disposable diapers, which can become waterlogged or disintegrate in the water. Waist and legbands should be snug for proper fit, so please consult sizing chart before ordering. Darlex with lining of 100% cotton knit. Lycra waist and legbands. Made in USA. *$40.00*

1555 Adult Tee Shoulder Bodysuit
Special Clothes
PO Box 337
E Harwich, MA 02645-333
508-430-2410
Fax: 508-430-2410
TTY:508-430-2410
lou@lnrmusic.com
www.special-clothes.com

1556 Adult Waterproof Overpant
Special Clothes
PO Box 338
E Harwich, MA 02645-333
508-430-2410
Fax: 508-430-2410
lou@lnrmusic.com
www.special-clothes.com

Judith Sweeney, President
Overpants are made of a soft, silent, lightweight fabric which is waterproof and very secure. It is designed to be used over our Adult Absorbent Brief, or cloth diapers. It is completely latex-free and is an excellent non-allergenic substitute for rubber or vinyl pants. Waist and legbands should be snug to minimize leakage, so please consult the sizing chart before ordering. Lycra waist and legbands. Made in USA. *$40.00*

1557 Briefs
Special Clothes
P.O.Box 333
E Harwich, MA 02645
508-430-2410
Fax: 508-430-2410
specialclo@aol.com
www.special-clothes.com

Judith Sweeney, President
A variety of unique brief styles available for easy access and practicality.

1558 Panties
Buck & Buck
3111 27th Ave S
Seattle, WA 98144-6502
206-722-4196
800-458-0600
Fax: 800-317-2182
info@buckandbuck.com
www.buckandbuck.com

Julie Buck, Owner
Come in nylon or cotton, band leg for comfort. *$5.00*

1559 Support Plus
5581 Hudson Industrial Parkway
PO Box 2599
Hudson, OH 44236-0099
508-359-2910
866-229-2910
Fax: 800-950-9569
www.supportplus.com

Ed Janos, President
Offers a selection of support undergarments, braces and shoes for the physically challenged and medical professionals.

Computers

Assistive Devices

1560 Ability Research
PO Box 1721
Minnetonka, MN 55345-721   952-939-0121
Fax: 952-227-5809
info@abilityresearch.net
www.abilityresearch.net
Suzanne Severson, Administrator
Manufacturers and marketers of assistive technology equipment.

1561 Academic Software Inc
3504 Tates Creek Rd
Lexington, KY 40517-2601   859-552-1020
Fax: 253-799-4012
asistaff@acsw.com
www.acsw.com
Warren E Lacefield PhD, President
Penelope Ellis, Marketing Director
Sylvia P Lacefield, Graphic Artist
Employs a unique, goal-oriented approach to aid individuals in identifying adaptive devices with potential to support various physical limitations. Devices are categorized in seven databases: Existence, Travel, In-situ Motion, Environmental Adaptation, Communication, and Sports & recreation. ADLS provides its users with device descriptions, pictures and lists of sources for locating products and product information.

1562 Adaptivation
Ste 100
2225 W 50th St
Sioux Falls, SD 57105-6536   605-335-4445
800-723-2783
Fax: 605-335-4446
info@adaptivation.com
www.adaptivation.com
Jonathan Eckrich, President
Manufacturers of switches, voice output devices and enviromental controls.

1563 Analog Switch Pad
Academic Software
331 W 2nd St
Lexington, KY 40507-1113   859-233-2332
800-842-2357
Fax: 859-231-0725
Warren E Lacefield PhD, President
Penelope Ellis, Marketing Director
A touch-activated, force-adjustable, low-voltage DC, electronic switch designed to control battery-operated toys, environmental controls, and computer access interfaces. This device features a large activation area that is soft and compliant to the touch. Force sensitivity is adjusted by a small dial from approximately 1 ounce to 32 ounces activation pressure, applied over an area ranging from the size of a fingertip to the size of the entire switch surface.

1564 Arkenstone: The Benetech Initiative
480 S California Ave
Palo Alto, CA 94306-1609   650-644-3400
Fax: 650-475-1066
www.hrdag.org
Jim Fruthterman, CEO
Roberta G Brosnaha, General Manager/VP
Patrick Ball, Executive Director
Offers various models of ready-to-read personal computers for the disabled.

1565 Augmentative Communication Systems (AAC)
ZYGO-USA
48834 Kato Road
Suite 101A
Freemont, CA 94538   510-249-9660
800-234-6006
Fax: 510-770-4930
zygo@zygo-usa.com
www.zygo-usa.com
Lawrence Weiss, President
Full range of AAC systems and assistive technology including computer-based systems and computer access programs and devices.

1566 Away We Ride IntelliKeys Overlay
Soft Touch Inc
12301 Central Ave NE
Ste 205
Blaine, NE 55434   763-755-1402
888-755-1402
sales@marblesoft.com
www.softtouch.com
Joyce Meyer, President
Four full color preprinted overlays to use with Away We Ride. Just put them on an IntelliKeys keyboard and you are ready to go.

1567 BIGmack Communication Aid
AbleNet
2625 Patton Road
Roseville, MN 55113   651-294-2200
800-322-0956
Fax: 651-294-2222
customerservice@ablenetinc.com
www.ablenetinc.com
Jen Thalhuber, CEO
A single message communication aid, BIGmack has 2 minutes of memory and has a 5 inches in diameter switch surface. *$86.00*

1568 Close-Up 6.5
Norton- Lambert Corporation
PO Box 4085
Santa Barbara, CA 93140-4085   805-964-6767
sales@norton-lambert.com
www.norton-lambert.com
Jeannie Vesely, Marketing Coordinator
Remotely controls PC's via modem. Telecommute from your home or laptop PC to your office PC. Run applications, update spreadsheets, print documents remotely and access networks on remote PCs. Features: fast screen and file transfers, synchronize files, unattended transfers, multi-level security, transaction logs, automated installation. *$99.95*

1569 Concepts on the Move Advanced Overlay CD
Soft Touch Inc
12301 Central Ave NE
Ste 205
Blaine, MN 55434   763-755-1402
888-755-1402
Fax: 763-862-2920
sales@marblesoft.com
www.softtouch.com
Joyce Myer, President
Use this overlay CD with Concepts on the Move Advanced Preacademics. Overlays match the concepts and graphics in the program. Includes standard overlays with all the choices and SoftTouch's changeable format overlays. Print and laminate the blank templates. Then print and laminate the picture keys in all three sizes - small, medium and large. Includes Overlay Printer by IntelliTools for easy printing. *$115.00*

1570 Concepts on the Move Basic Overlay CD
Soft Touch Inc
12301 Central Ave NE
Ste 205
Blaine, MN 55434   763-755-1402
                                            888-755-1403
                                    Fax: 763-862-2920
                                    sales@marblesoft.com
                                    www.softtouch.com

Joyce Meyer, President
Use this Overlay CD with Concepts on the Move Basic
Preacademics. Overlays match the concepts and graphics in the
program. Includes standard overlays with all the choices and
SoftTouch's changeable format overlays. Print and laminate the
blank templates. Then print and laminate the picture keys in all
three sizes - small, medium and large. It is easy and fast to place
the images on the blank templates. *$115.00*

1571 Darci Too
WesTest Engineering Corporation
810 Shepard Ln
Farmington, UT 84025-3846   801-451-9191
                                    Fax: 801-451-9393
                                    larryk@westest.com
                                            westest.com

Robert Lessmann, President
A universal device which allows people with physical disabilities
to replace the keyboard and mouse on a personal computer with a
device that matches their physical capabilities. DARCI TOO
works with almost any personal computer and provides access to
all computer functions. *$995.00*

1572 Eyegaze Computer System
LC Technologies Inc
10363A Democracy Lane
Fairfax, VA 22030   703-385-7133
                                            800-393-4293
                                    Fax: 703-385-7137
                                    info0309@eyegaze.com
                                            www.eyegaze.com

Nancy Cleveland, Medical Coordinator
Enables people with physical disabilities to do many things with
their eyes that they would otherwise do with their hands.

1573 Five Green & Speckled Frogs IntelliKeys Overlay
Soft Touch Inc
12301 Central Ave NE
Ste 205
Blaine, MN 55434   763-755-1402
                                            888-755-1403
                                    Fax: 763-862-2920
                                    sales@marblesoft.com
                                    www.softtouch.com

Joyce Meyer, President
Seven full color preprinted overlays to use with Five Green and
Speckled Frogs. Just put them on an IntelliKeys keyboard and
you are ready to go. *$49.00*

1574 GW Micro
725 Airport North Office Park
Fort Wayne, IN 46825-6707   260-489-3671
                                    Fax: 260-489-2608
                                    sales@gwmicro.com
                                    www.gwmicro.com

Dan Weirich, Sales Executive
Marty Hord, Sales Manager
Computer hardware and software products for people with dis-
abilities.

1575 InvoTek, Inc.
1026 Riverview Dr
Alma, AR 72921   479-632-4166
                                    Fax: 479-632-6457
                                            invotek.org

Thomas Jakobs, President
Diane Jakobs, Vice President, Operations
John Riggins, Chief Marketing Officer

InvoTek, Inc. is a research and development company that improves the quality of life for people who find it difficult or impossible to use their hands by giving them new, efficient ways to
access computers.

1576 Jelly Bean Switch
AbleNet
2625 Patton Road
Roseville, MN 55113-1308   651-294-2200
                                            800-322-0956
                                    Fax: 651-294-2259
                                    customerservice@ablenetinc.com
                                    www.ablenetinc.com

Jen Thalhuber, CEO
A momentary touch switch made of shatterproof plastic, small
and sensitive to 2-3 ounces of pressure, this switch is provided
audible feedback when activated and is a compact version of the
Big Red Switch. Choice of colors: red, blue, green and yellow.

1577 Large Print Keyboard Labels
Hooleon Corp
P.O.Box 589
Melrose, NM 88124-589   575-253-4503
                                            800-937-1337
                                    Fax: 928-634-4620
                                    sales@hooleon.com
                                    www.hooleon.com

Shannen Aikman, Admin Manager/Sales
Joan Crozier, President/Sales
Pressure sensitive labels for computer keyboards.

1578 MessageMate
Words+ Inc
42505 10th Street W
Lancaster, CA 93534-7059   661-723-6523
                                            800-869-8521
                                    Fax: 661-723-2114
                                    www.words-plus.com

Jeff Dahlan, President
Ginger Woltosz, General Manager
Lightweight, hand-held communicator providing high-quality
analog recording capability using either direct select keyboards
or 1 to 2 switch access. Price ranges from $549.00 to $999.00.
$1550.00

1579 Mouthsticks
Sammons Preston Rolyan
1000 Remington Blvd
Suite 210
Bolingbrook, IL 60440-5117   630-378-6000
                                            800-323-5547
                                    Fax: 630-378-6010
                                    www.pattersonmedical.com

Sandra Brown, Customer Service Director
Wide offering of mouthsticks featuring various functions (BK
5380, 5381, 5383, 5385, 6002, or BK 5370 series).

1580 Old MacDonald's Farm IntelliKeys Overlay
Soft Touch Inc
12301 Central Ave NE
Ste 205
Blaine, MN 55434   763-755-1402
                                            888-755-1403
                                    Fax: 763-862-2920
                                    sales@marblesoft.com
                                    www.softtouch.com

Joyce Meyer, President
Extend your students' learning with more than 45 pre-made overlays that support all of the skills learned at the farm. Use with the
IntelliKeys keyboard. Simply print and use. Print an extra set to
make off computer activities, too. Note: Requires Overlay Maker
or Overlay Printer by IntelliTools.

1581 **Origin Instruments Corporation**
854 Greenview Dr
Grand Prairie, TX 75050   972-606-8740
                                            Fax: 972-606-8741
                                            support@orin.com
                                            www.orin.com

1582 **Perfect Solutions**
2685 Treanor Ter
Wellington, FL 33414-6460   561-790-1070
                                             800-726-7086
                                             Fax: 561-790-0108
                                             perfect@gate.net
                                             www.perfectsolutions.com
Andrew Kramer, President
A computer for every student and it speaks! Wireless laptop computers starting at $299.00 are ideal for students to carry with them all day. Text-to-speech and web browsing are available. *$299.00*

1583 **Phillip Roy**
13064 Indian Rocks Road
PO Box 130
Indian Rocks Beach, FL 33785-130   727-593-2700
                                           800-255-9085
                                           Fax: 877-595-2685
                                           info@philliproy.com
                                           www.philliproy.com
Ruth Bragman PhD, President
Phil Padol, VP
Offers multimedia materials appropriate for use with individuals with disabilities. Programs range from preschool through the adult level. Many of the programs are high interest topics/low vocabulary, ideal for transition and employability skills. Materials are also available which focus on social and personal development. Call for a free catalog.

1584 **SS-Access Single Switch Interface for PC'swith MS-DOS**
Academic Software
3504 Tates Creek Road
Lexington, KY 40517-2601   859-552-1020
                                            800-842-2357
                                            Fax: 253-799-4012
                                            asistaff@acsw.com
                                            www.acsw.com
Warren E Lacefield PhD, President
Penelope Ellis, Marketing Director
A general purpose single switch hardware and software interface for DOS and the IBM and compatible PC family. It is designed to be easy to install, simple to use, and compatible with the widest possible range of computers and application software programs. SS-ACCESS! connects to one of the PC serial ports and provides a jack to connect an external switch. The DOS version of the software works by sending a user defined keystroke to the PC keyboard buffer whenever the switch is pressed. *$ 90.00*

1585 **Simplicity**
Words+
42505 10th Street W
Lancaster, CA 93534-7059   661-723-6523
                                            800-869-8521
                                            Fax: 661-723-2114
                                            info@words-plus.com
                                            www.words-plus.com
Jeff Dahlan, President
Ginger Wolosz, General Manager
Swing-down mount for portable computers and other devices is made from high-quality aircraft aluminum. Simplicity contains very few moving parts and installs in minutes, providing a positive, secure support for computer/device in both the stored and overlap position. *$1199.00*

1586 **Slim Armstrong Mounting System**
AbleNet
2625 Patton Road
Roseville, MN 55113-1308   612-379-0956
                                            800-322-0956
                                            Fax: 651-294-2259
                                            customerservice@ablenetinc.com
                                            www.ablenetinc.com
Jen Thalhuber, CEO
Slim Armstrong is a mounting system strong enough to hold up to five pounds in any position. Mix and match parts to create the system length you desire. *$188.00*

1587 **Songs I Sing at Preschool IntelliKeys Overlay**
Soft Touch
12301 Central Ave NE
Ste 205
Blaine, MN 55434   763-755-1402
                                            888-755-1403
                                            Fax: 763-862-2920
                                            sales@marblesoft.com
                                            www.softtouch.com
Joyce Meyer, President
Pre-made overlays for use with Songs I Sing at Preschool. Simply print and use with an IntelliKeys keyboard. Print an extra set to make off computer activities, too.

1588 **Switch Basics IntelliKeys Overlay**
Soft Touch
12301 Central Ave NE
Ste 205
Blaine, MN 55434   763-755-1402
                                            888-755-1403
                                            Fax: 763-862-2920
                                            sales@marblesoft.com
                                            www.softtouch.com
Joyce Meyer, President
Four preprinted overlays to use with Switch Basics. Just put them on an IntelliKeys keyboard and you're ready to go.

1589 **Teach Me Phonemics Blends Overlay CD**
SoftTouch Inc.
12301 Central Ave NE
Ste 205
Blaine, MN 55434   763-755-1402
                                            888-755-1403
                                            Fax: 763-862-2920
                                            sales@marblesoft.com
                                            wwww.softtouch.com
Roxanne Butterfield, Marketing
Joyce Meyer, President
Teach Me Phonemics Blends Overlay CD contains over 40 IntelliKeys overlays for use with Teach Me Phonemics - Blends program. Choose either 4-item or 9-item layout to match the presentation you use in the program. Print extra copies of the overlays for off computer activites, too.

1590 **Teach Me Phonemics Medial Overlay CD**
SoftTouch Incorporated
Ste C
17117 Oak Dr
Omaha, NE 68130-2193   402-330-1301
                                             877-763-8868
                                             Fax: 402-334-8478
                                             support@softtouch.com
                                             www.softtouch.com
Kip Fisher, Manager
Roxanne Butterfield, Marketing
Teach Me Phonemics Medial Overlay CD contains over 40 IntelliKeys overlays for use with Teach Me Phonemics - Medial program. Choose either 4-item or 9-item layout to match the presentation you use in the program. Print extra copies of the overlays for off computer activites, too.

1591 Teach Me Phonemics Overlay Series Bundle
SoftTouch
Ste 401
4300 Stine Rd
Bakersfield, CA 93313-2352
661-396-8676
877-763-8868
Fax: 661-396-8760
softtouch@funsoftware.com
www.softtouch.com

Roxanne Butterfield, Marketing
Joyce Meyer, President
Teach Me Phonemics Overlay Series Bundle includes one copy of
each Teach Me Phonemics Overlay CD - Initial, Medial, Final and
- four CD's in all.

1592 Teach Me to Talk Overlay CD
Soft Touch
12301 Central Ave NE
Ste 205
Blaine, MN 55434
763-755-1402
888-755-1403
Fax: 763-862-2920
sales@marblesoft.com
www.softtouch.com

Joyce Meyer, President
For older version of Teach Me to Talk. Mac only version with red
label and PC only version with yellow label. More than 48
pre-made overlays that match the activities on Teach Me to Talk.
Simply print and use with an IntelliKeys keyboard. Print an extra
set to make off computer activities, too.

1593 Teach Me to Talk: USB-Overlay CD
Soft Touch
12301 Central Ave NE
Ste 205
Blaine, MN 55434
763-755-1402
888-755-1403
Fax: 763-862-2920
sales@marblesoft.com
www.softtouch.com

Joyce Meyer, President
Revised version of Teach Me to Talk Overlays for the newest version that is USB IntelliKeys compatible. This CD contains more
than 48 overlays that match the activities and updated graphics of
Teach Me to Talk. Includes Overlay Printer by IntelliTools for
easy printing.

1594 Teen Tunes Plus IntelliKeys Overlay
Soft Touch
12301 Central Ave NE
Ste 205
Blaine, MN 55434
763-755-1402
888-755-1403
Fax: 763-862-2920
sales@marblesoft.com
www.softtouch.com

Joyce Meyer, President
Seven full color, preprinted overlays to use with Teen Tunes Plus.
Just put them on an IntelliKeys keyboard and you're ready to go.
$49.00

1595 U-Control III
Words+
42505 10th St W
Lancaster, CA 93534-7059
575-253-4503
800-869-8521
Fax: 661-723-2114
www.words-plus.com

Jeff Dahlen, President
Ginger Wolosz, General Manager
Works with the Words+ system (EX Keys, Morse WSKE, Scan-
ning WSKE, Talking Screen) to provide wireless, portable con-
trol of items which are already infrared-controlled such as a TV,
VCR, CD player, etc. *$499.00*

1596 Universal Switch Mounting System
AbleNet
2625 Patton Road
Roseville, MN 55113-1308
612-379-0956
800-322-0956
Fax: 651-294-2259
customerservice@ablenetinc.com
www.ablenetinc.com

Jen Thalhuber, CEO
Mounting system that allows switch placement in any position. A
single lever locks all joints securely in place. Extends to 20 1/2
inches and holds up to five pounds. A mounting system for quick
and easy positioning. *$210.00*

**1597 WinSCAN: The Single Switch Interface for PC's with
Windows**
Academic Software
3504 Tates Creek Rd
Lexington, KY 40517-2601
859-522-1020
Fax: 253-799-4012
asistaff@acsw.com
www.acsw.com

Warren E Lacefield, President
Penelope Ellis, Marketing Director/COO
A general purpose single-switch control interface for Windows.
It provides single-switch users independent control access to educational and productivity software, multimedia programs, and
recreational activities that run under Windows 3.1 and higher versions on IBM and compatible PC's. The user can navigate
through Windows; choose program icons and run programs,
games, and CD's; even surf the Internet with WinSCAN and his or
her adaptive switch. *$349.00*

1598 Words+ IST (Infrared, Sound, Touch)
Words+
42505 10th St W
Lancaster, CA 93534-7059
575-253-4503
800-869-8521
Fax: 661-723-2114
www.words-plus.com

Jeff Dahlan, President
Ginger Wolosz, General Manager
A unique switch that is activated by slight movement or faint
sound. The switch provides user control when connected to a device driven by a single switch. Individuals are currently accessing a wide variety of communication and computer systems with
movement using the IST switch. *$395.00*

Braille Products

1599 Braille Keyboard Labels
Hooleon Corporation
PO Box 589
Melrose, NM 88124-589
928-634-7515
800-937-1337
Fax: 928-634-4620
sales@hooleon.com
www.hooleon.com

Barry Green, Sales Manager
Joan Crozier, President/Sales
Also large print keyboard labels and large print with Braille.

1600 Brailon Thermoform Duplicator
American Thermoform Corporation
1758 Brackett St
La Verne, CA 91750-5855
909-593-6711
800-331-3676
Fax: 909-593-8001
pnunnelly@americanthermoform.com
www.americanthermoform.com

Patrick Nunnelly, VP
Gary Nunnelly, Owner
This copy machine, for producing tactile images, copies any
brailled or embossed original, by a vacuum forming process. This
model is for the reproduction of teaching aids and mobility maps.

1601   Computer Paper for Brailling
Maxi Aids
42 Executive Blvd
Farmingdale, NY   11735-4710   631-752-0521
                                                800-522-6294
                                           Fax: 631-752-0689
                                           TTY: 631-752-0738
                                           sales@maxiaids.com
                                           www.maxiaids.com

Elliot Zaretsky, President
Specially made paper for braille printing. 1,500 sheets/case
$85.99

1602   Duxbury Braille Translator
Duxbury Systems
Ste 6
270 Littleton Rd
Westford, MA   01886-3523   978-692-3000
                                           Fax: 978-692-7912
                                           info@duxsys.com
                                           www.duxburysystems.com

Joe Sullivan, President
A complete line of easy to use word processing and Braille translation software available for Windows (including 64 bit windows. Applications for anyone wanting to produce or
communicate with Braille; signs, note cards, textbooks, business
communications and forms, telephone bills, etc. Simple to use,
FREE technical support. Free one year upgrades. DBT is for producing Braille in English, Spanish, French, Portuguese, Italian,
Latin, Greek, German and 125 other languages. *$600.00*

1603   Enabling Technologies Company
1601 NE Braille Pl
Jensen Beach, FL   34957-5345   772-225-3687
                                                800-777-3687
                                           Fax: 772-225-3299
                                           info@brailler.com
                                           www.brailler.com

Tony Schenk, President
Kate Schenk, Product Manager Western US
Greg Schenk, Sales & Marketing
Manufactures the most complete line of American made Braille
embossers, including desktop or portable models capable of producing high quality single sided or interpoint Braille. Also carries a complete line of adaptive technology aids for the blind
community at affordable prices.

1604   Freedom Scientific Blind/Low Vision Group
11800 31st Ct N
St Petersburg, FL   33716-1805   727-803-8000
                                                800-444-4443
                                           Fax: 727-803-8001
                                           info@freedomscientific.com
                                           www.freedomscientific.com

Brad Davis, VP Hardware Product Management
Dr Lee Hamilton, President/CEO
Developer and manufacturer of assistive technology products for
people who are blind or who have low vision. Innovative blindness products include: JAWS® screen reading software; the PAC
Mate Omni™, an accessible Pocket PC; the SARA™ scanning
and reading appliance; OpenBook™ scanning and reading software; FSReader™ DAISY player; FaceToFace™ deaf-blind
communications solution; and PAC Mate and Focus Braille Displays. *$16.95*

1605   Hooleon Corporation
PO Box 589
Melrose, NM   88124-589   928-634-7515
                                                800-937-1337
                                           Fax: 928-634-4620
                                           sales@hooleon.com
                                           www.hooleon.com

Kim Green, Manager
Joan Crozier, President/Sales
Large print and combination Braille adhesive keytop labels for
computer keyboards. Helps visually impaired computer users access correct key strokes either by sight or by touch. Raised Braille
meets ADA specifications and large print fills key top surface.

1606   Humanware
1 UPS Way
P.O. Box 800
Champlain, NY   12919   800-722-3393
                                           Fax: 888-871-4828
                                           info@humanware.com
                                           humanware.com

Gilles Pepin, CEO
Humanware manufactures electronics to provide solutions that
empower the visually impaired.

1607   Infogrip: Large Print/Braille Keyboard Labels
1899 E. Main Street
Ventura, CA   93001   805-652-0770
                                                800-397-0921
                                           Fax: 805-652-0880
                                           sales@infogrip.com
                                           www.infogrip.com

Liza Jacobs, President
Aaron Gaston, VP
Makes a standard keyboard more accessible for visually impaired
individuals with large print or Braille keyboard labels. Characters on the large print labels are .5 by .25 inches, about 3 times
larger than standard keyboard characters. Braille labels are available as clear labels with Braille dots or large print with Braille.
Each set includes all the keys used on a standard Windows keyboard. *$29.00*

1608   Raised Dot Computing
Duxbury Systems Incorporated
270 Littleton Rd.
Unit 6
Westford, MA   01886-3523   978-692-3000
                                           Fax: 978-692-7912
                                           info@duxsys.com
                                           www.duxburysystems.com

Joe Sullivan, President
Peter Sullivan, VP of Software Development
Genevieve Sullivan, Treasurer
Dana Winikates, Software Engineer
Software for the visually impaired.

1609   Touchdown Keytop/Keyfront Kits
Hooleon Corporation
P.O.Box 589
304 West Denby Ave
Melrose, NM   88124   575-253-4503
                                                800-937-1337
                                           Fax: 575-253-4299
                                           Sales@Hooleon.com
                                           www.hooleon.com

Bob Crozier, Founder
Joan Crozier, President
Barry Green, Sales Manager
These kits enlarge the key legends of a computer and include
Braille for easy recognition.

Information Centers & Databases

1610   ATTAIN
Division of Disability Aging & Rehab Services
Ste 1400
32 E Washington St
Indianapolis, IN   46204-3552   317-232-1147
                                                800-528-8246
                                           Fax: 317-486-8809
                                           www.attaininc.org

Gary R Hand, Executive Director
Peter Bisbecos, Manager
Nonprofit organization that creates system change by expanding
the availability of community-based technology-related activities, outreach services, empowerment and advocacy activities
through the development of a comprehensive, consumer-responsive, statewide program to serve individuals with disabilities, of
all ages and all disabilities, their families, caregivers, educators

and service providers. Provides training, information and referrals, system change and assessments for equipment needs.

1611 AbleData
103 W Broad St
Suite 400
Falls Church, VA 22046   301-608-8998
                                        800-227-0216
                                        Fax: 301-608-8958
                                        TTY: 301-608-8912
                                        abledata@neweditions.net
                                        www.abledata.com

Katherine Belknap, Director
David Johnson, Publications Director
AbleData is an electronic database containing information on assistive technology and rehabilitation equipment products for children and adults with physical, cognitive and sensory disabilities. AbleData staff can perform database searches or the database can be searched via the website, informed consumer guides or fact sheets.

1612 Aloha Special Technology Access Center
710 Green St
Honolulu, HI 96813-2119   808-523-5547
                                        Fax: 808-536-3765
                                        astachi@yahoo.com
                                        www.alohastac.org

Ali Silvert, President
Ms. Jacquely Brand, Founder
Computer technology center.

1613 Audiogram/Clinical Records Manager
The Davis Center
110 Wesley St.
P.O. Box 508
Manlius, NY 13104   862-251-4637
                                        Fax: 862-251-4642
                                        ddavis@thedaviscenter.com
                                        www.thedaviscenter.com

Dorinne S. Davis, Director
Sound-based therapy uses sound vibration with special equipment, specific programs, modified music, and/or specific tones/beats, the need for which is identified with appropriate testing. *$414.75*

1614 Birmingham Alliance for Technology Access Center
Birmingham Independent Living Center
206 13th St S.
Birmingham, AL 35233-1317   205-251-2223
                                        Fax: 205-251-0605
                                        TTY: 205-251-2223
                                        judy.roy@drradvocates.org
                                        www.drradvocates.org

Kathy Lovell, President
Phil Klebine, Vice President
Daniel Kessler, Executive Director
Judy Roy, Programs Coordinator
Computer technology center.

1615 Bluegrass Technology Center
409 Southland Drive
Lexington, KY 40503   859-294-4343
                                        800-209-7767
                                        Fax: 866-576-9625

Debbie Sharon, Acting Executive Director
Linnie Lee, Assistive Technology Specialist
Jean Isaacs, Assistive Technology Consultant
Linda Gassaway, PhD, Assistive Technology Consultant
Provides assistive technology information, consulting and training for education, health professionals, consumers and parents of consumers. Maintains extensive lending library of assistive devices and adapted toys. Statewide training such as; AAC, how to obtain funding for assistive technology, augmentative and alternate communication, equipment implementation strategies, specific to hardware and software, etc.

1616 CITE: Lighthouse for Central Florida
215 East New Hampshire Street
Orlando, FL 32804   407-898-2483
                                        Fax: 407-898-0236
                                        csacca@lcf-fl.org
                                        www.lighthousecentralflorida.org/Default.asp
Lee Nasehi, MSW, President/CEO
Donna Esbensen CPA,MBA, VP/CFO
Jeff Whitehead, MPA, MS, Director of Program Services
Casey Mathews, Access Technology Specialist
CITE promotes the independence of adults and children with blindness, low vision and other disabilities through technology, education, support and advocacy.

1617 Carolina Computer Access Center
P.O.Box 247
Cramerton, NC 28032   704-342-3004
                                        Fax: 704-342-1513

Linda Schilling, Executive Director
Nonprofit, community-based technology resource center for people with disabilities, providing information about and demonstration of the technology tools that enable individuals with disabilities to control and direct their own lives. Services and programs include: assessments, demonstrations, resource information, lending library, workshops and outreach.

1618 Center for Accessible Technology
3075 Adeline
Suite 220
Berkeley, CA 94703   510-841-3224
                                        Fax: 510-841-7956
                                        info@cforat.org
                                        www.cforat.org

Dmitri Belser, Executive Director
Eric Smith, Associate Director
A consumer-based technology resource and demonstration center for adults and children with disabilities, families, teachers, and professionals. The primary focus is on assistive technology for computer access. Seen by appointment only.

1619 Center for Applied Special Technology
40 Harvard Mills Square
Suite 3
Wakefield, MA 01880-3233   781-245-2212
                                        Fax: 781-245-5212
                                        cast@cast.org
                                        www.cast.org/

Anne Meyer, Founder
David H. Rose, Founder
Lisa Poller, Co-President
Gabrielle Rappolt-Schlichtmann, Co-President
Expands opportunities for individuals with special needs through innovative use of computers and related technology. We pursue this mission through research and product development that further universal design for learning.

1620 Center for Assistive Technology & Inclusive Education Studies
2000 Pennington Rd.
P.O.Box 7718
Ewing, NJ 08628-0718   609-771-3016
                                        Fax: 609-637-5179
                                        caties@tcnj.edu
                                        caties.pages.tcnj.edu

Amanda Norvell, President
Matt Bender, VP
Regina Morin, Parliamentarian
Laurie Wanat, Secretary
Computer technology center offering resource time, workshops, technology, training and evaluations.

1621   Center on Evaluation of Assistive Technology
National Rehabilitation Hospital
102 Irving St NW
Washington, DC   20010   202-877-1000
                                            TTY:202-726-3996
                                   justin.m.carter@medstar.net
                                      www.medstarhealth.org
Kenneth A. Samet, FACHE, President, CEO
Michael J. Curran, EVP, Chief Administrative and Financial Officer
Christine Swearingen, EVP, Planning, Marketing and Community Relations
Stephen R.T. Evans, MD, EVP, Medical Affairs and Chief Medical Officer
The center develops ways of collecting, producing and distributing information to help users, prescribers and third-party payers make intelligent selections of devices.

1622   Compuserve: Handicapped Users' Database
5000 Arlington Centre Blvd
Columbus, OH   43220-2913   614-326-1002
                                                 800-848-8990
                                            Fax: 614-538-4023
                                webcenters.netscape.compuserve.com

1623   Computer & Web Resources for People With Disabilities
Alliance for Technology Access
Ste 240
1304 Southpoint Blvd
Petaluma, CA   94954-7464   707-778-3011
                                            Fax: 707-765-2080
                                            TTY:707-778-3015
                                               www.ataccess.org
Sharon Hall, Manager
A guide to maneuvering the growing world of computers, both the mainstream and the assistive technology.
ISBN 0-897933-00-1

1624   Computer Access Center
P.O. Box 12464
Albuquerque, NM   87195   505-242-9588
                                                  info@cac.org
                                                   www.cac.org
Richard Barlow, Board of Director
Richard Rohr, Board of Director
Michael Poffenberger, Board of Director
Damien Faughnan, Board of Director
Computer technology center.

1625   Computer Center for Visually Impaired People: Division of Continuing Studies
Baruch College
1 Bernard Baruch Way
Box H-648
New York, NY   10010   646-312-1420
                                            Fax: 646-312-5101
                                   judith.gerber@baruch.cuny.edu
                                      www.baruch.cuny.edu/ccvip
Karen Gourgey, Director
Judith Gerber, Operations Manager
Lynette Tatum, Training Specialist
William Reed, Assistant Director
Offers courses, tutors, equipment and assistance.

1626   Computer Resources for People with Disabilities
Hunter House Publishers, Inc
424 Church Street
Suite 2240
Nashville, TN   37219   615-255-BOOK
                                   info@turnerpublishing.com
                                       www.hunterhouse.com
Kiran Rana, Publisher
Chris Alexander, Author
Sheila Alson, Author
Peter Axt, Author
Part One describes conventional and assistive technologies and gives strategies for accessing the Internet. Part Two features

easy-to-use charts organized by key access concerns, and provides detailed descriptions of software, hardware, and communication aids. Part Three is a gold mine of Web resources, publications, support organizations, government programs, and technology vendors.

1627   Computer-Enabling Drafting for People with Physical Disabilities
County College of Morris
214 Center Grove Road
Randolph, NJ   07869-2086   973-328-5000
                                                 888-226-8001
                                            Fax: 973-328-5067
                                                   www.ccm.edu
Edward J Yaw, President
Dr. Dwight Smith, Vice President of Academic Affairs
Karen VanDerhoof, Vice President for Business and Finance
Dr. Bette M. Simmons, VP of Student Development & Enrollment Management
Since they opened in 1968, more than 40,000 graduates have passed through their halls. Many have become teachers, nurses, police officers, doctors and engineers. CCM has also been a community resource for those seeking to enhance their careers through additional education. They drafted a newsletter on Computer-Enabling Drafting for People with Physical Disabilities

1628   DIRLINE
National Library of Medicine
8600 Rockville Pike
Bethesda, MD   20894   301-594-5983
                                                 888-346-3656
                                            Fax: 301-402-1384
                                            TTY:800-735-2258
                                               www.nlm.nih.gov/
Dr. Donald A B. Lindberg, Director
Milton Corn, Deputy Director
Betsy Humphreys, Deputy Director
Todd Danielson, Office of Administration
18,000 listings of organizations that serve as information resources, including libraries, professional associations and government agencies.

1629   Developmental Disabilities Council
626 Main Street, Suite A
P.O.Box 3455
Baton Rouge, LA 70821-3455   225-342-6804
                                                 800-450-8108
                                            Fax: 225-342-1970
                                      shawn.fleming@la.gov
                                               www.laddc.org
Sandee Winchell, Executive Director
Shawn Fleming, Deputy Director
Derek White, Program Manager
Robbie Gray, Program Monitor
The Louisiana Developmental Disabilities Council is made up of people from every region of the state who are appointed by the governor to develop and implement a five year plan to address the needs of persons with disabilities. Membership includes persons with developmental disabilities, parents, advocates, professionals, and representatives from public and private agencies.

1630   Employment Resources Program
330 South Grand Avenue West
Springfield, IL   62704   217-523-2587
                                                 800-447-4221
                                            Fax: 217-523-0427
                                            TTY: 217-523-2587
                                                 scil@scil.org
                                                  www.scil.org
Pete Roberts, Executive Director
Susanne Cooper, Program Director
Robin Ashton- Hale, Reintegration Coordinator
Kathryn Cline, Business Manager
An information and referral service that encourages inquiries from professionals, individuals with disabilities, family members, organizations or anyone requesting information pertaining to disabilities. The staff at DRN uses both computer listings and in-house library files to provide the programs services. The DRN

program is funded by a grant from the Illinois Department of Rehabilitation Services.

1631   Functional Skills Screening Inventory
Functional Resources
3905 Huntington Dr
Amarillo, TX   79019-4047   806-353-1114
                                        Fax: 806-353-1114
                                        info@winfssi.com
                                        www.winfssi.com

Ed Hammer, Owner
Heather Becker PhD, Owner
Assesses the individual's level of functional skills and identifies supports needed by educational, rehabilitation and residential programs serving moderately and severely disabled persons. Includes environmental assessments as well as profiles of jobs and training sites.

1632   High Tech Center
Sacremento State
6000 J Street
Sacramento, CA   95819   916-278-6011
                                        sswd@csus.edu
                                        www.csus.edu

Alexander Gonzalez, President
Judy Dean, Co-Director
Melissa Repa, Co-Director
Terry Gomez, Office Manager
The Center offers assessment and training in adaptive hardware/software for eligible students with disabilities at Sacramento State upon referral from the Office of Services to Students with Disabilities.

1633   Idaho Assistive Technology Project
121 W 3rd St
Moscow, ID   83843-2268   208-885-3557
                                        Fax: 208-885-3628
                                        www.idahoat.org
Ron Seiler, Project Director
Sue House, Information Specialist
A federally funded program managed by the center on disabilities and human development at the university of Idaho. The goal of the IATP is to increase the availability of assistive technology devices and services for Idahoans with disabilities. The IATP offers free trainings and technical assistance, a low-interest loan program, assistive technology assessments for children and agriculture workers, and free informational materials.

1634   Increasing Capabilities Access Network
525 W.Capitol
Little Rock, AR   72201   501-666-8868
                                        800-828-2799
                                        Fax: 501-666-5319
                                        TTY: 501-666-8868
                                        nfo@ar-ican.org
                                        www.arkansas-ican.org
Bryen Ayres, Member of Advisory Council
Billy Altom, Member of Advisory Council
Adrienne Brown, Member of Advisory Council
Carolyn Boyles, Member of Advisory Council
A consumer responsive statewide systems change program promoting assistive technology for persons of all ages with disabilities. The program provides information on new and existing technology and maintains an equipment exchange free of charge. Training on assistive technology is also provided.

1635   International Center for the Disabled
340 E 24th St
New York, NY   10010-4019   212-585-6000
                                        Fax: 212-585-6161
                                        info@icdnyc.org
                                        www.icdnyc.org
Jill Bowman, Manager
Les Halpert, CEO
The ICD is a comprehensive outpatient rehabilitation facility, providing medical rehabilitation, behavioral health and vocational services to children and adults with a broad range of physical, communication, emotional and cognitive disabilities.

1636   Kentucky Assistive Technology Service Network
200 Juneau Dr.
Suite 200
Louisville, KY   40243   502-429-4484
                                        800-327-5287
                                        Fax: 502-429-7114
                                        www.katsnet.org
Derrick Cox, Manager
Statewide network of four regional assistive technology centers with a central coordinating office in Louisville and two regional centers in eastern Kentucky. Network services include but are not limited to assistive technology of services, loan of assistive devices, funding information and referral, assessment and evaluations, consultations on appropriate technologies, training, and technical assistance.

1637   Learning Independence Through Computers
2301 Argonne Drive
Baltimore, MD   21218   410-554-9134
                                        Fax: 410-261-2907
                                        info@linc.org
                                        www.linc.org
Theo Pinette, Executive Director
Sandy Fishman, Office and Computer Center Coordinator
Angela Tyler, Volunteer Services Manager
Christy Wooden, AT Learning Specialist
V-LINC creates technological solutions to improve the independence and quality of life for individuals of all ages with disabilities in Maryland. We do this through a mix of off-the-shelf computer software and equipment, and one-of-a-kind, customized assistive technology.

1638   MEDLINE
Dialog Corporation
2250 Perimeter Park Drive
Suite 300
Morrisville, NC 27560   800-334-2564
                                        919-804-6400
                                        Fax: 919-804-6410
                                        www.dialog.com
Tim Wahlberg, Genral Manager
Morten Nicholaisen, VP Global Sales and Account Mana
Libby Trudell, VP Strategic Initiatives
Tim Hall, Director Integration and Busines
Bibliographic citations to biomedical literature.

1639   Maine CITE
University of Maine at Augusta
46 University Avenue
Augusta, ME   04330   207-621-3195
                                        Fax: 207-629-5429
                                        TTY:877-475-4800
                                        iweb@mainecite.org
                                        www.mainecite.org
Robert McPhee, Member of Advisory Council
Deborah Gardner, Member of Advisory Council
Anita Dunham, Member of Advisory Council
Sandra Jaeger, Member of Advisory Council
Computer technology center.

1640   Maryland Technology Assistance Program
Maryland Department of Disabilities
2301 Argonne Drive
Rm T-17
Baltimore, MD   21218   410-554-9361
                                        800-832-4827
                                        Fax: 410-554-9237
                                        TTY: 866-881-7488
                                        www.mdtap.org
James McCarthy, Executive Director
Denise Schuler, Assistive Technology Specialist
Tanya Goodman, Loan Program Assistant Director
Lori Markland, Director of Communications, Outreach &Program Development
Assistive technology center. Information and referral, equipment display loans and demonstration, funding sources, alternative media, training, workshops and seminars. Rural outreach for individuals with disability in Maryland.

1641 **Minnesota STAR Program**
358 Centennial Office Building 658
Saint Paul, MN   55155- 1402   651-201-2640
                                               800-627-3529
                                               888-234-1267
                                        Fax: 651-282-6671
                                  star.program@state.mn.us
                    www.admin.state.mn.us/assistivetechnology
Chuck Rassbach, Program Director
Jennis Delisi, Program Staff
Jaoan Gillum, Program Staff
Kim Moccia, Program Staff
STAR's mission is to help all Minnesotans with disabilities gain
access to and acquire the assistive technology they need to live,
learn, work and lay. The Minnesota STAR program is federally
funded by the Rehabilitation Services Administration.

1642 **Mississippi Project START**
2550 Peachtree Street
Jackson, MS 39216   601-987-4872
                                              800-852-8328
                                       Fax: 601-364-2349
                                     pgaltelli@mdrs.ms.gov
                                      www.msprojectstart.org
Patsy Galtelli, Executive Director
Dorothy Young, Project Director
Nekeba Simmons, Administrative Assistant
Jason Mac McMaster, Repair Specialist
Project START is a Tech Act project established to bring about
systems change in the field of assistive technology in the State of
Mississippi. Activities include providing training opportunities
for consumers and service providers on subjects such as
state-of-the-art AT devices, their application and funding resources; referral information on AT evaluation centers; technical
assistance to AT users; establishment of an AT equipment loan
program and an Information and Referral Service.

1643 **National Technology Database**
American Foundation for the Blind/ AF B Press
2 Penn Plaza
Suite 1102
New York, NY 10121   212-502-7600
                                              800-232-5463
                                       Fax: 888-545-8331
                                         afbinfo@afb.net
                                             www.afb.org
Carl.R Augusto, President and CEO
Robin Vogel, Vice President, Resource Development
Kelly Bleach, Chief Administrative Officer
Rick Bozeman, Chief Financial Officer
This database includes resources for visually impaired persons.
$99.00

1644 **New Jersey Department of Labor & Workforce
Development**
Office of the Commissioner
1 John Fitch Plaza
P.O.Box 110
Trenton, NJ 08625-0110   609-292-7060
                                       Fax: 609-633-1359
                                   cmycoff@dol.state.nj.us
                                       www.state.nj.us/labor
Harold J. Wirths, Commissioner
Aaron R. Fichtner, Ph.D., Deputy Commissioner
Frederick J. Zavaglia, Chief of Staff
David Ramsay, Director
Oversees various federal and state vocational rehabilitation ser-
vices including sheltered workshops and independent living cen-
ters; adjudication of permanent disability claims filed with the
Social Security Administration; oversees New Jersey's tempo-
rary disability program covering non-work related illnesses and
injuries

1645 **New Mexico Technology Assistance Program**
435 Saint Michaels Drive
Ste D
Santa Fe, NM 87505-7679   505-827-8535
                                              800-866-2253
                                       Fax: 505-954-8608
                                             www.nmtap.com
Julie Martinez, Program Director
Examines and works to eliminate barriers to obtaining assistive
technology in New Mexico. Has established a statewide program
for coordinating assistive technology services; is designed to assist people with disabilities to locate, secure, and maintain
assistive technology.

1646 **Northern Illinois Center for Adaptive Technology**
3615 Louisiana Rd
Rockford, IL 61108   815-229-2163
Dave Grass, President
Computer technology center.

1647 **OCCK**
1710 W. Schilling Road
Salina, KS 67402-1160   785-827-9383
                                              800-526-9731
                                       Fax: 785-823-2015
                                        TTY: 785-827-9383
                                           occk@occk.com
                                             www.occk.com
Shelia Nelson Stout, President, CEO
Carolee Miner, CEO
Computer technology center; training center for employment and
independent living for people with disabilities; family support
center. Kansas AgrAbility program coordinator, Kansas
equipment exchange site.

1648 **Options, Resource Center for Independent Living**
318 3rd St. NW
East Grand Forks, MN 56721   218-773-6100
                                              800-726-3692
                                       Fax: 218-773-7119
                                      options@myoptions.info
                                             www.rcil.com
Burt Danovitz, Executive Director
The RCIL aggressively advocates for and defends the rights of
persons with disabilities. RCIL believes in integration adn assisting people to reach their full potential, encouraging a culture of
risk-taking, creativity and innovation through our programs and
services. They monitor and assess the current legal climate
around rights for persons with disabilities on an ongoing bases
and are committed and deliberate in speaking about the problems
and obstacles faced by persons with disabilities.

1649 **Parents, Let's Unite for Kids**
516 N 32nd St
Billings, MT 59101-6003   406-255-0540
                                              800-222-7585
                                       Fax: 406-255-0523
                                        TTY: 406-657-2055
                                             info@pluk.org
                                             www.pluk.org
Roger Holt, Executive Director
Computer technology center. Parents, Let's Unite for Kids offers
an assistive technology lab that is open to people of all ages. The
lab is a computer and assistive technology demonstration site.
There is no charge for services.

1650 **Pennsylvania's Initiative on Assistive Technology**
Temple University
1755 N. 13th St.
Student Center, Room 411 South
Philadelphia, PA 19122-6024   215-204-1356
                                              800-204-7428
                                       Fax: 215-204-6336
                                        TTY: 866-268-0579
                                          ATinfo@temple.edu
                                     www.disabilities.temple.edu
Kim Singleton, Director

Pennsylvania's Initiative on Assistive Technology (PIAT) offers information and referral about assistive Technology (AT), device demonstrations, and awareness-level presentations. PIAT also operates Pennsylvania's AT Lending Library, a free, state-supported program that loans AT devices to Pennsylvanians of all ages.

1651 Rehabilitation Engineering & Assistive Technology Society of North America (RESNA)
1700 North Moore Street
Suite 1540
Arlington, VA 22209
703-524-6686
Fax: 703-524-6630
TTY:703-524-6639
membership@resna.org
www.resna.org

Alex Mihailidis, PhD, P.Eng, President
Ray Grott, ATP, RET, President-Elect
Paul J. Schwartz, Treasurer
Michael J. Brogioli, Executive Director
Improves the potential of people with disabilities to achieve their goals through the use of technology and disability. Promotes research, development, education, advocacy and provision of technology, and by supporting the people engaged in theses activities.

1652 SACC Assistive Technoloy Center
P.O.Box 1325
Simi Valley, CA 93062-1325
805-582-1881
www.semel.ucla.edu

Debi Schultze, CEO
SACC connects children, adults and seniors with special needs to computers, technologies and resources. We provide information and referral, assessments, tutoring, presentations and outreach awareness.

1653 South Dakota Department of Human Services: Computer Technology Services
Properties Plaza
500 East Capitol Avenue
Pierre, SD 57501
605-773-5990
800-265-9684
Fax: 605-773-5483
TTY: 605-773-6412
infodhs@state.sd.us
dhs.sd.gov

Dan Lusk, Division Director
Ted Williams, Director
Eric Weiss, Director
Gaye Mattke, Director
Computer technology center.

1654 Star Center
1119 Old Humboldt Rd
Jackson, TN 38305-1752
731-668-3888
888-398-5619
Fax: 731-668-1666
TTY: 731-668-9664
information@starcenter.tn.org
www.starcenter.tn.org

John Borden, CEO
Nation's largest assistive technology center dedicated to helping children and adults with disabilities achieve their goals for competitive employment, effective learning, returning to or starting school and independent living. Programs include: high-tech training, music therapy, art therapy, low vision evaluation, orientation and mobility evaluation and training, augmentative communication evaluation, vocational evaluations, assistive technology, job placement services and job skills training.

1655 Students with Disabilities Office
University of Texas at Austin
100 West Dean Keeton A5800
Austin, TX 78712-1100
512-471-5017
Fax: 512-471-7833
deanofstudents@austin.utexas.edu
deanofstudents.utexas.edu

Soncia Reagins-Lilly, Ed.D., Senior Associate VP for Student Affairs & Dean of Students
Douglas Garrard, Ed.D., Senior Associate Dean of Students
Wanda Brune, Administrative Associate
Sara LeStrange, Manager of Communications

1656 TASK Team of Advocates for Special Kids
100 W Cerritos Ave
Anaheim, CA 92805
714-533-8275
866-828-8275
Fax: 714-533-2533
task@taskca.org
www.taskca.org

Marta Anchondo, Executive Director
Tom Bratkovich, Treasurer
Leana Way, Director
Computer technology center.

1657 Tech Connection
35 Haddon Avenue
Shrewsbury, NJ 07702
732-747-5310
Fax: 732-747-1896
info@frainc.org
www.frainc.org

Bill Sheeser, President
Nancy Phalanukom, Executive Director
Sue Levine, Program Administrator
Vicky Butler, EI Program Coordinator
Offers a noncommercial center to examine and try computers, adapted equipment, alternative input devices, and a variety of software. Program of Family Resource Associates and a member of the Alliance for Technology Access (ATA), a growing national coalition of computer resource centers, professionals, technology developers and vendors, interacting with new technology to enrich the lives of people with disabilities. Tech Connection offers evaluations, for computer technology.

1658 Tech-Able
1451 Klondike Road, Suite D
Conyers, GA 30094
770-922-6768
Fax: 770-922-6769
www.techable.org

Cassandra Baker, Executive Director
Pat Hanus, Program Assistant
Erika Ruffin-Mosley, Assistive Technology Trainer
Jason Chadwell, AT & Blind / Low Vision Trainer
Provide assistive technology to individuals with disabilities, toy-lending and software libraries, product demonstration, access to technology devices and fabrication of keyguards for keyboards. Low vision consultant on Thursdays; computer training for persons with disabilities.

1659 Technology Access Center of Tucson
P.O.Box 13178
Tucson, AZ 85732-3178
520-638-2733
Fax: 520-519-7954
tact1@qwestoffice.net
http://www.uacoe.arizona.edu/tact/

1660 Technology Assistance for Special Consumers
1856 Keats Dr NW.
Huntsville, AL 35810
256-859-8300
Fax: 256-859-4332
tasc@ucphuntsville.org
ucphuntsville.org/what-we-do/t-a-s-c/

Cheryl Smith, Chief Executive Officer
T.A.S.C. is a computer resource center with 10 computers, which are equipped with special adaptations for those who are blind, visually impaired, or severely physically disabled. The staff demonstrates and trains individuals on this equipment so that they can become more independent at home, school, and work. Over 2,500

pieces of educational software are available for individuals who are learning disabled, mentally retarded or who have developmental delays.

1661 Tidewater Center for Technology Access Special Education Annex
1415 Laskin Rd
Virginia Beach, VA 23451
757-424-2672
Fax: 757-263-2801
www.tcta.access.org

Pat Mc Gee, Manager
Myra Jessie Flint, Designee
Nonprofit organization providing persons with disabilities access, support, and knowledge—re: technology; organization contracts for consultations, workshops and training, or conventional and assistive technologies including computers, augmented communication devices and software; resources: extensive lending library of educational software; books and videotape library; yearly individual membership and corporate membership fees; working/presentation and evaluation fees available upon request.

1662 Vermont Assistive Technology Project: Department of Aging & Disabilities
Agency of Human Services
103 South Main Street
Weeks Building
Waterbury, VT 05671-2305
802-871-3353
800-750-6355
Fax: 802-871-3048
TTY: 802-241-1464
amber.fulcher@state.vt.us
atp.vermont.gov

Amber Fulcher, Program Director
Sharon Alderman, Assistive Technology Reuse Coordinator
Emma Cobb, Assistive Technology Services Coordinator
Increase the awareness and change policies to insure assistive technology is available to all Vermonters with disabilities.

Keyboards, Mouses & Joysticks

1663 A4 Tech (USA) Corporation
5585 Brooks St
Montclair, CA 91763-4547
909-988-9633
info@a4tech.com
www.a4tech.com
Robert C
Manufacturers of a cordless mouse, trackballs and joysticks that emulate mouse controls, flatbed scanners, modified keyboards, and other specialty mouses.

1664 Abacus
3150 Patterson Ave SE
Grand Rapids, MI 49512
616-698-0330
800-451-4319
Fax: 616-698-0325
www.abacuspub.com

Arnie Lee, President
Designs a mouse software program that permits programs written for one computer to be run on another computer.

1665 Ability Center of Greater Toledo
5605 Monroe Street
Sylvania, OH 43560
419-885-5733
Fax: 419-882-4813
www.abilitycenter.org

Tim Harrington, Executive Director
Dale Abell, Director of Program Development
Debbie Andriette, Director of Human Resources
Kimberley Arnett, Director of Community Services
Manufactures keyboard wrist supports to help prevent repetitive motion disorders.

1666 Dreamer
TS Micro Tech
17109 Gale Ave
City of Industry, CA 91745-1810
626-939-8998
Fax: 626-839-8516

Steve Heung, Owner
An intelligent, add-on function keyboard providing single-keystroke access to multiple-keystroke functions.

1667 FlexShield Keyboard Protectors
Hooleon Corporation
P.O.Box 589
Melrose, NM 88124-589
928-634-7515
800-937-1337
Fax: 928-634-4620
sales@hooleon.com
www.hooleon.com

Barry Green, Sales Manager
Joan Crozier, President
Transparent keyboard protectors allowing instant recognition of keytop legends. They have a matte finish to reduce glare. Also available are large print and braille keyboard labels and large print/braille combo labels.

1668 Infogrip: King Keyboard
1899 E. Main Street
Ventura, CA 93001
805-652-0770
800-397-0921
Fax: 805-652-0880
support@infogrip.com
www.infogrip.com

Lisa Jacobs, President
Giant alternative keyboard that plugs directly into a computer—no special interface is required. The keys are 1.25 inches in diameter, slightly recessed, and provide both tactile and auditory feedback. The King has a built-in keyboard so that you can rest on its surface without activating keys. This keyboard allows you to control both keyboard and mouse functions, so it's great for people who have difficulty maneuvering a standard mouse. *$130.00*

1669 Infogrip: Large Print Keyboard
1899 E. Main Street
Ventura, CA 93001
805-652-0770
800-397-0921
Fax: 805-652-0880
support@infogrip.com
www.infogrip.com

Lisa Jacobs, President
Standard Windows keyboard with large print keys. The keyboard and its keys are the same size as a standard keyboard; however, the print has been enhanced. The characters measure .5 by .25 inches, about 3 times larger than standard keyboard characters. *$130.00*

1670 Infogrip: OnScreen
1899 E. Main Street
Ventura, CA 93001
805-652-0770
800-397-0921
Fax: 805-652-0880
support@infogrip.com
www.infogrip.com

Lisa Jacobs, President
OnScreen features word prediction/completion (with an editable dictionary), Key Dwell Timer (a timer that selects a key under the cursor), integrated Verbal Keys Feedback, Show and Hide Keys (turns on/off keys to prevent access and minimize confusion) a Smart Window (automatically re-positions the keyboard or panels off of the area in use). On Screen also offers edit, numeric, macro, calculator and Windows enhancement capabilities. *$200.00*

1671 IntelliKeys
Intelli Tools
1720 Corporate Circle
Petaluma, CA 94954
707-773-2000
800-899-6687
Fax: 707-773-2001
info@intellitools.com
www.intellitools.com

Dayton Johnson, VP, Sales
Arjan Khalsa, CEO
Alternative, touch-sensitive keyboards; plugs into any Macintosh or Windows computer. *$395.00*

1672 IntelliKeys USB
Intelli Tools
1720 Corporate Circle
Petaluma, CA 94954
707-773-2000
800-899-6687
Fax: 707-773-2001
info@intellitools.com
www.intellitools.com

Dayton Johnson, VP, Sales
Arjan Khalsa, CEO
IntelliKeys alternative keyboard for USB computers and Windows 2000, Mac OSX. *$69.95*

1673 Key Tronic KB 5153 Touch Pad Keyboard
KeyTronic
N. 4424 Sullivan Road
Spokane Valley, WA 99216
509-928-8000
Fax: 509-927-5555
EMSsales@keytronicems.com
www.keytronic.com

Craig.D Gates, President/CEO
Ronald.F Klawitter, EVP of Administration and Chief Financial Officer
Douglas G. Burkhardt, Executive Vice President of Worldwide Operations
Philip S. Hochberg, Executive Vice President of Business Development
Integrates a regular full-function keyboard, a numeric keypad with a cursor key capability and a touch pad into one unit.

1674 Magic Wand Keyboard
In Touch Systems
11 Westview Road
Spring Valley, NY 10977
845-354-7431
800-332-6244
sc@magicwandkeyboard.com
www.magicwandkeyboard.com

Jerry Crouch, President
Susan Crouch, VP
The magic wand keyboard allows your child to use a keyboard and mouse easily-no light beams, microphones, or sensors to wear of position. This miniature computer keyboard has zero-force keys that work with the slightest touch of a wand (hand-held of mouthstick). No strength required.

1675 McKey Mouse
In Touch Systems
11 Westview Road
Spring Valley, NY 10977
845-354-7431
800-332-6244
sc@magicwandkeyboard.com
www.magicwandkeyboard.com

Jerry Crouch, President
Susan Crouch, VP
Microsoft compatible mouse for persons with little or no hand/arm movement; it's an option for the Magic Wand Keyboard and adds full mouse function without adding any extra devices.

1676 PortaPower Plus
Words+
42505 10th Street West
Lancaster, CA 93534-7059
661-723-7723
800-869-8521
Fax: 661-723-5524
info@simulations-plus.com
www.simulations-plus.com

Walter S Woltosz, M.S., M.A.S., President, CEO
John A. DiBella, Vice President, Marketing & Sales
John R. Kneisel, Chief Financial Officer
Robert D. Clark, Ph.D., Director, Life Sciences
Rechargeable battery pack designed to give longer life and remote usage time to laptop computers and other portable battery-operated devices and accessories. Requires a 12 volt auto adapter. *$149.00*

1677 Unicorn Keyboards
Intelli Tools
1720 Corporate Circle
Petaluma, CA 94954
707-773-2000
800-899-6687
Fax: 707-773-2001
info@intellitools.com
www.intellitools.com

Dayton Johnson, VP, Sales
Arjan Khalsa, CEO
Alternative keyboards with membrane surface and large, user-defined keys. Large and small sizes are available. *$250.00*

Scanners

1678 Scanning WSKE
Words+
42505 10th Street West
Lancaster, CA 93534-7059
661-723-7723
888-266-9294
Fax: 661-723-5524
info@simulations-plus.com
www.simulations-plus.com

Walter S Woltosz, M.S., M.A.S., President, CEO
John A. DiBella, Vice President, Marketing & Sales
John R. Kneisel, Chief Financial Officer
Robert D. Clark, Ph.D., Director, Life Sciences
A software and a hardware product designed to operate on an IBM compatible PC. The software provides dual word prediction, abbreviation expansion, five different methods of voice output, and access to commercial software applications.

1679 System 2000/Versa
Words+
42505 10th Street West
Lancaster, CA 93534-7059
661-723-7723
800-869-8521
Fax: 661-723-5524
info@simulations-plus.com
www.simulations-plus.com

Walter S Woltosz, M.S., M.A.S., President, CEO
John A. DiBella, Vice President, Marketing & Sales
John R. Kneisel, Chief Financial Officer
Robert D. Clark, Ph.D., Director, Life Sciences
Provides all of the strategies currently being used in AAC, from dynamic display color pictographic language, to dual-word prediction text language, in a single system.

1680 Zygo-Usa
SVC Corporation
48834 Kato Road Suite 101-A
Fremont, CA 94538
510-249-9660
800-234-6006
Fax: 510-770-4930
zygo@zygo-usa.com
www.zygo-usa.com

Adam Weiss, Vp Sales & Marketing
ZYGO-USA has been involved in manufacturing and distributing assistive technologies since 1974. They specialize in

augmentative and alternative computer access. They offer a wide range of technology products to our clients so they can achieve a greater independence and to enhance the quality of their lives. These soloutins improve and individual's ability to learn, work, and interact with family and friends.

Screen Enhancement

1681 Boxlight
Boxlight Corporation
151 State Highway 300, Suite A
P.O. Box 2609
Belfair, WA 98528

360-464-2119
866-972-1549
sales@boxlight.com
www.boxlight.com

Herb Myers, CEO/Founder
Sloan Myers, Founder
Hank Nance, President
BOXLIGHT is a global presentation solutions partner for trainers, educators and professional speakers. Solutions include projector sales, national rental service, technical support, repair, and presentation peripherals. For more information visit us online.

1682 FDR Series of Low Vision Reading Aids
Optelec U S
Breslau 4
Barendrecht, LT 92081-8358

886-783-444
800-826-4200
Fax: 886-783-400
info@optelec.com
in.optelec.com

Stephan Terwolbeck, President
Michiel van Schaik, VP
Janet Lennex, Director of Customer Excellence
Jade Arbelo, Director of Human Resources
The Low Vision Reading Aids features; high resolution, positive and negative display, a high-quality zoom lens, versatile swivel and a 12 inch or 19 inch high-resolution monitor, color or black and white, computer compatible, or portable.

1683 InFocus
AI Squared
130 Taconic Business Park Road
Manchester Center, VT 05255

802-362-3612
800-859-0270
Fax: 802-362-1670
sales@aisquared.com
www.aisquared.com

David Wu, CEO
Jost Eckhardt, VP of Engineering
Scott Moore, VP of Marketing
Shawn Warren, VP of Product Support
A memory-resident program that magnifies text and graphics - the entire screen, a single line or a portion of the screen.

1684 Portable Large Print Computer
Human Ware
1800, Michaud street
Drummondville, CA 94520-1213

819-471-4818
888-723-7273
Fax: 925-681-4630
ca.info@humanware.com
www.humanware.com/en-australia/home

Real Goulet, Chairman
Gilles Pepin, CEO
Michel Cote, Corporate Director
Georges Morin, Corporate Director
A portable large print computer which magnifies up to 64 times. It is linked to a PC and has a hand-held camera.

1685 ZoomText
A I Squared
130 Taconic Business Park Road
Manchester Center, VT 05255

802-362-3612
800-859-0270
Fax: 802-362-1670
sales@aisquared.com
www.aisquared.com

David Wu, CEO
Jost Eckhardt, VP of Engineering
Scott Moore, VP of Marketing
Shawn Warren, VP of Product Support
A RAM-resident program that enlarges screen characters up to eight times. It runs on IBM PC, XT, AT and PS/2.

Speech Synthesizers

1686 Artic Business Vision (for DOS) and Artic WinVision (for Windows 95)
Artic Technologies
3456 Rodchester Road
Troy, MI 48083

248-689-9883
Fax: 248-588-2650
info@ablezone.com

Dale McDaniel, Founder
Kathy Gargagliano, Founder
A speech processor for blind computer users featuring true interactive speech with spread sheets, word processors, database managers, etc. Now available with both Windows 3.1 and Windows 95 access. *$ 495.00*

1687 Computerized Speech Lab
Kay Elemetrics Corporation
3 Paragon Drive
Montvalle, NJ 07645

973-628-6200
800-289-5297
Fax: 201-391-2063
www.kaypentax.com

John Crump, President
Hardware/software for the acquisition, analysis/display, playback and storage of speech signals.

1688 DynaVox Technologies Speech Communication Devices
Dyna Vox Technologies
2100 Wharton St
Suite 400
Pittsburgh, PA 15203-1945

412-381-4883
866-396-2869
Fax: 412-381-5241
Ray.Merk@dynavoxtech.com
www.dynavoxtech.com

Ed Donnelly, CEO
Michelle Heying, President and COO
Kenneth Misch, CFO
Ray Merk, VP Finance
Develops and manufactures speech communication devices that help individuals who are unable to speak due to speech, language and/or learning disabilities to communicate quickly and easily.

1689 Electronic Speech Assistance Devices
Luminaud
8688 Tyler Blvd
Mentor, OH 44060-4348

440-255-9082
800-255-3408
Fax: 440-255-2250
info@luminaud.com
www.luminaud.com

Thomas M Lennox, President
Dorothy Lennox, VP
Offers a full line of speech aids, voice amplifiers, mini-vox amplifiers, laryngectomec products.

1690 Keywi
Hoffmann + Krippner Inc.
200 Westpark Drive
Suite 270
Peachtree City, GA 30269 770-487-1950
Fax: 770-487-1945
www.keywi-usa.com

1691 Little Mack Communicator
AbleNet
2625 Patton Road
Roseville, MN 55113-1308 651-294-2200
800-322-0956
Fax: 651-294-2259
customerservice@ablenetinc.com
www.ablenetinc.com

Bill Sproull, Chairman
Jennifer Thalhuber, President/CEO
Paul Sugden, Former Vice President of Finance
William Mills, Board of Directors
The Little Mack Communicator has 2 minutes of memory and has an angled switch surface making it easy to see and access. The switch surface is 2 1/2 inches in diameter. Detachable mounting base makes it easy to position a single unit in a variety of locations. *$129.00*

1692 Mega Wolf Communication Device
Wayne County Regional Educational Service Agency
33500 Van Born Rd
Wayne, MI 48184-2474 734-334-1300
Fax: 734-334-1620
www.resa.net

Lynda S. Jackson, President
Kenneth E. Berlinn, Vice President
James Petrie, Secretary
Mary E. Blackmon, Treasurer
A low cost voice output communication device which is primarily intended to provide the power of speech to those individuals who are most severely challenged mentally and/or physically. The WOLF device is User programmable and uses the Texas Instruments' Touch and Tell case and touch panel; ADAMLAB electronics with synthesized (robotic) voice. For users able to point with approximately 6 ounces of pressure. *$400.00*

1693 Talking Screen
Words+
42505 10th St W
Lancaster, CA 93534-7059 661-723-7723
888-266-9294
Fax: 661-723-5524
info@simulations-plus.com
www.simulations-plus.com
Walter S Woltosz, M.S., M.A.S., Chairman, President and Chief Ex
John R. Kneisel, Chief Financial Officer
John DiBella, Vice President, Marketing and Sales
Robert D. Clark, Ph.D, Director, Life Sciences
An augmentative communication program that allows the user to select graphic symbols on the display to produce speech output. Symbols can be used either singly or in sequence as picture abbreviations. *$ 1395.00*

1694 Turnkey Computer Systems for the Visually, Physically, and Hearing Impaired
E V A S
39 Canal St P.O. Box 371
Westerly, RI 02891-1511 401-596-3155
800-872-3827
Fax: 401-596-3979
TTY: 401-596-3500
contact@evas.com
www.evas.com

Gerald Swerdlick, Owner
Jerry Swerdlick, CEO
Offers clear speech with pleasant inflection and tonal quality as well as variable pitch, intonation and voices.

1695 Voice-It
V XI Corporation Incorporated
271 Locust Street
Denver, NH 03820 603-742-2888
800-742-8588
Fax: 603-742-5065
info@vxicorp.com
www.vxicorp.com

Michael Ferguson, President
Tom Manero, Chief Financial Officer
Phil Pane, Vice President Operations
Brian Cole, Vice President Engineering
Adds voice to popular spreadsheet and word processing applications on IBM PCs and compatibles, turning spreadsheets and word processing documents into talking documents.

1696 Window-Eyes
G W Micro
725 Airport North Office Park
Fort Wayne, IN 46825 260-489-3671
Fax: 260-489-2608
sales@gwmicro.com
www.gwmicro.com

Dan Weirich, Owner/Vice President of Sales an
Doug Geoffray, Owner
Provides access to available software automatically reading information important to the user while ignoring the rest. A screen reader for the windows operative system.

Software: Math

1697 AIMS Multimedia
Discovery Education
8145 Holton Dr
Florence, KY 41042-3009 859-342-7200
Fax: 877-324-6830

Mike Wright, Director
Lynn Fassett, Administrative Assistant
Cindy Vogt, Human Resources Executive
AIMS Multimedia is a leader in the production and distribution of training and educational programs for the business and K-12 communities via YHS, interactive CD-ROM, DVD and Internet streaming video.

1698 Basic Math: Detecting Special Needs
Allyn & Bacon
One Liberty Square
Suite 1200
Boston, MA 02109-3988 617-261-0040
800-852-8024
Fax: 617-944-7273
samplingdept@pearson.com
www.greenellp.com

Thomas M Greene, Attorney at Law
Michael Tabb, Attorney at Law
Describes special mathematics needs of special learners.
180 pages
ISBN 0-205116-35-3

1699 Campaign Math
Mindplay
4400 E. Broadway Blvd
Suite 400
Tucson, AZ 85711-1726 520-888-1800
800-221-7911
Fax: 520-888-7904
mail@mindplay.com
www.mindplay.com

Judith Bliss, CEO
Brian Williams, Development Manager
Lisa Garcia, Director of Educational Services
Chris Coleman, Vice President of Business Development
A complete program on the electoral process as well as a math package which teaches ratios, fractions and percentages.

1700 Educational Activities Software
5600 W 83rd Street
Suite 300, 8200 Tower
Bloomington, MN 55437 866-243-8464
Fax: 239-225-9299
jwest@orchardlng.com
www.edmentum.com

Vin Riera, President & Chief Executive Officer
Rob Rueckl, Chief Financial Officer
Dave Adams, Chief Academic Officer
Paul Johansen, Chief Technology Officer
Comprehensive MATH SKILLS software tutorials teach concepts ranging from rounding and tables to measuring area. MAC/WIN compatible. *$369.00*
Per Unit

1701 Fraction Factory
Queue
80 Hathaway Drive
Stratford, CT 06615 800-232-2224
Fax: 800-775-2729
jdk@queueinc.com
qworkbooks.com

Anna Christopoulos, General Manager
Peter Uhrynowski, Comptroller
Steve Pernett, Director of Printing and Graphic
Ann Pleszko, Shipping Manager
In 1980, Jonathan Kantrowitz started Queue, Inc. as an educational software company. After twenty thriving years publishing and distributing high-quality software to educators, Queue began transitioning from software to workbooks, focusing on state-specific test preparation.

1702 Information & Referral Services
Information + Referral Services
2590 N. Alvernon Way
Tucson, AZ 85712 520-323-1708
Fax: 520-325-8841
inform@azinfo.org
www.azinfo.org

Patti Caldwell, Executive Director
Chuck Palm, Treasurer
Ben Rensvold, Vice President
Tom DeSollar, President
Provides information about health and human services for people in Arizona over the telephone. Information specialists help callers clarify their needs, and provide referrals to the appropriate service agency.

1703 King's Rule
WINGS for Learning
1600 Green Hills Rd
Scotts Valley, CA 95066-4981 831-426-2228
Fax: 831-464-3600

Ani Stocks, Owner
A software mathematical problem solving game. Students discover mathematical rules as they work their way through a castle and generate and test a working hypothesis by asking questions.

1704 Learning About Numbers
C&C Software
5713 Kentford Cir
Wichita, KS 67220-3131 316-683-6056
800-752-2086
Carol Clark, President
Three programs use the power of computer graphics to provide young children with a variety of experiences in working with numbers. *$50.00*

1705 Math Rabbit
Learning Company
Ste 1900
100 Pine St
San Francisco, CA 94111-5205 415-659-2000
800-825-4420
Fax: 415-659-2020
thelearningco@hmhpub.com
www.hmhco.com

Linda K. Zecher, President, Chief Executive Officer and Director
Eric Shuman, Chief Financial Officer
William Bayers, Executive Vice President and General Counsel
Dr. Tim Cannon, Executive Vice President,
Teaches early math concepts by matching objects to numbers, then adding and subtracting up to 18.

1706 Math for Everyday Living
Educational Activities Software
5600 W 83rd Street
Suite 300, 8200 Tower
Bloomington, MN 55437 866-243-8464
Fax: 239-225-9299
jwest@orchardlng.com
www.edmentum.com

Vin Riera, President & Chief Executive Officer
Rob Rueckl, Chief Financial Officer
Dave Adams, Chief Academic Officer
Paul Johansen, Chief Technology Officer
Real life math skills are taught with this tutorial and practice software program. Examples include Paying for a Meal (addition and subtraction), Working with Sales Slips (multiplication), Unit Pricing (division), Sales Tax (percent), Earning with Overtime (fractions) plus more. Software: CD-ROM, Windows, MAC, and DOS. *$159.00*

1707 Math for Successful Living
Siboney Learning Group
5600 W 83rd Street
Suite 300, 8200 Tower
Bloomington, MN 55437 866-243-8464
Fax: 239-225-9299
jwest@orchardlng.com
www.edmentum.com

Vin Riera, President & Chief Executive Officer
Rob Rueckl, Chief Financial Officer
Dave Adams, Chief Academic Officer
Paul Johansen, Chief Technology Officer
These programs include managing a checking account, budgeting, shopping strategies and buying on credit.

1708 Piece of Cake Math
Queue Inc
80 Hathaway Drive
Stratford, CT 06615 800-232-2224
Fax: 800-775-2729
jdk@queueinc.com
www.qworkbooks.com

Anna Christopoulos, General Manager
Peter Uhrynowski, Comptroller
Steve Pernett, Director of Printing and Graphic
Ann Pleszko, Shipping Manager
In 1980, Jonathan Kantrowitz started Queue, Inc. as an educational software company. After twenty thriving years publishing and distributing high-quality software to educators, Queue began transitioning from software to workbooks, focusing on state-specific test preparation.

1709 Puzzle Tanks
WINGS for Learning
1600 Green Hills Rd
Scotts Valley, CA 95066-4981 831-426-2228
Fax: 831-464-3600

Ani Stocks, Owner
A mathematical problem solving game that involves multi-step problems.

1710 Right Turn
WINGS for Learning
1600 Green Hills Rd
Scotts Valley, CA 95066-4981   831-426-2228
                                       Fax: 831-464-3600

Ani Stocks, Owner
Requires students to predict, experiment and learn about the mathematical concepts of rotation and transformation.

1711 RoboMath
4400 E. Broadway Blvd
Suite 400
Tucson, AZ 85711-1726   520-888-1800
                                800-221-7911
                           Fax: 520-888-7904
                           mail@mindplay.com
                           www.mindplay.com

Judith Bliss, CEO
Brian Williams, Development Manager
Lisa Garcia, Director of Educational Services
Chris Coleman, Vice President of Business Development
A complete program on the electoral process as well as a math package which teaches ratios, fractions and percentages.

1712 Stickybear Math I Deluxe
Optimum Resource
1 Mathews Drive
Suite 107
Hilton Head Island, SC 29926- 3689   843-689-8000
                                        Fax: 843-689-8008
                                        info@stickybear.com
                                        www.stickybear.com

Richard Hefter, President
Sharpen basic addition and subtraction skills with this captivating series of math exercises. Grades Pre-K to 2. Available in as single edition with sizing up to 30 users at a site. English/Spanish. *$59.95*

1713 Stickybear Math II Deluxe
Optimum Resource
1 Mathews Drive
Suite 107
Hilton Head Island, SC 29926- 3689   843-689-8000
                                        Fax: 843-689-8008
                                        info@stickybear.com
                                        www.stickybear.com

Richard Hefter, President
Multiplication and division, beginning with the elementary problems and developing into the more complex problems with regrouping. Grades 2-4. Available for single user through the 30 user site package. English/Spanish. *$59.95*

1714 Stickybear Math Splash
Optimum Resource
1 Mathews Drive
Suite 107
Hilton Head Island, SC 29926- 3689   843-689-8000
                                        Fax: 843-689-8008
                                        info@stickybear.com
                                        www.stickybear.com

Richard Hefter, President
Unique multiple activities keep the learning level high while children acquire skills in addition, subtraction, multiplication and division. K-5th grade. Available as single edition up to 30 user site package. English/Spanish. *$59.95*

1715 Stickybear Math Word Problems
Optimum Resource
1 Mathews Drive
Suite 107
Hilton Head Island, SC 29926- 3689   843-689-8000
                                        Fax: 843-689-8008
                                        info@stickybear.com
                                        www.stickybear.com

Richard Hefter, President
Hundreds of different word problems make it easy for students to practice basic math skills around analyzing and solving word problems. Grades 1-5. Available as single edition up to 30 user site package. English/Spanish. *$59.95*

1716 Stickybear Money
Optimum Resource
1 Mathews Drive
Suite 107
Hilton Head Island, SC 29926- 3667   843-689-8000
                                        Fax: 843-689-8008
                                        info@stickybear.com
                                        www.stickybear.com

Chris Gintz, President
Teaches children to recognize US coins and paper money and introduces simple counting. K to 3rd grade. Bilingual. *$59.95*

1717 Stickybear Numbers Deluxe
Optimum Resource
1 Mathews Drive
Suite 107
Hilton Head Island, SC 29926- 3689   843-689-8000
                                        Fax: 843-689-8008
                                        info@stickybear.com
                                        www.stickybear.com

Richard Hefter, President
Counting and number recognition are as easy as 1-2-3 with this award-winning program. Teaches number recognition of numbers 0-9 and 0-30. Pre-K to 2nd grade. Available as single edition up to 30 user site package. *$59.95*

1718 Tomorrow's Promise: Mathematics
Compass Learning
203 Colorado Street
Austin, TX 78701   512-478-9600
                           800-678-1412
                           866-586-7387
                           www.compasslearning.com

Eric Loeffel, President
Trey Chambers, Chief Financial Officer
ARTHUR VANDERVEEN, Vice President, Business Strategy and Development
CHIPP WALTERS, Chief Designer Officer
By integrating interdisciplinary content and real-world application of skills, this product emphasizes the practical value of fundamental math skills. It helps your students develop a problem-solving aptitude for ongoing mathematics achievement.

Software: Miscellaneous

1719 Adventures in Musicland
Electronic Courseware Systems
1713 S State St
Champaign, IL 61820-7258   217-359-7099
                                    800-832-4965
                               Fax: 217-359-6578
                               support@ecsmedia.com
                               http://ecsmedia.com.np/

G Peters, President
Jodie Varner, Marketing Manager
This unique set of music games features characters from Lewis Carroll's, Alice in Wonderland. Players learn through pictures, sounds, and animation which help develop understanding of musical tones, composers, and musical symbols. Games include MusicMatch, Melody Mixup, Picture Perfect and Sound Concentration. *$49.95*

1720 Ai Squared
130 Taconic Business Park Road
Manchester Center, VT 05255-669   802-362-3612
                                          800-859-0270
                                     Fax: 802-362-1670
                                     sales@aisquared.com
                                     http://www.aisquared.com

David Wu, CEO
Jost Eckhardt, VP of Engineering
Scott Moore, VP of Marketing
Shawn Warren, VP of Product Support

Developers of software for the visually impaired.

1721 All About You: Appropriate Special Interactions and Self-Esteem
P CI Educational Publishing
P.O.Box 34270
San Antonio, TX   78265-4270
210-377-1999
800-594-4263
800-471-3000
Fax: 888-259-8284
submissions@pcieducation.com

Lee Wilson, President and CEO
Randy Pennington, Executive VP
Jeff McLane, Founder
David Keith, Vice President of IT
This game offers parents and game players a new line of communication when discussing various issues such as learning to be thoughtful, respecting the rights and feelings of others, how to make and keep friends and more. *$49.95*

1722 All Star Review
Tom Snyder Productions
100 Talcott Ave
Watertown, MA   02472-5703
800-342-0236
www.tomsnyder.com

Rick Abrams, Manager
Tom Synder, Founder
Bridget Dalton, Ed.D., Author
Peggy Healy Stearns, Ph.D., Author
This package turns group review into a baseball game for small and large groups.

1723 Attainment Company
I ET Resources
P.O.Box 930160
Verona, WI   53593-160
608-845-7880
800-327-4269
Fax: 608-845-8040
info@attainmentcompany.com
www.attainmentcompany.com

Don Bastian, President
Julie Denu, Technical Support
Theresa O'Connor, Office Manager
Augmentative/alternative communication, software, videos, print and hands-on functional life skills and basic acdemics materials for developmental and cognitive disabilities.

1724 Attention Getter
Soft Touch
12301 Central Ave NE Ste 205
4300 Stine Rd
Blaine, MN 55434
763-755-1402
888-755-1402
Fax: 763-862-2920
support@marblesoft.com
www.softtouch.com

Joyce Meyer, President
The whimsical photos morph to another photo and then to a third photo in categories. Paired with interesting sounds and music, the photo animations are so engaging that the student is motivated to activate the computer to see and hear the next one. This is a perfect vehicle to achieve goals aimed at attention getting, activating a switch or intentionally. Compatible with USB IntelliKeys keyboards.

1725 Attention Teens
Soft Touch
12301 Central Ave NE Ste 205
Blaine, MN   55434
763-755-1403
888-755-1403
Fax: 763-862-2921
support@marblesoft.com
www.softtouch.com

Joyce Meyer, President
Attention Teens (formerly known as Loony Teens) is a program for teens with disabilities who need powerful input to get their attention. Attention Teens is a computer program to do just this. Paired with interesting sounds and music, the photo animations

are so engaging that the student is motivated to activate the computer to see and hear the next one. Compatible with USB IntelliKeys keyboards.

1726 Away We Ride
Soft Touch
12301 Central Ave NE Ste 205
4300 Stine Rd
Blaine, MN 55434
763-755-1404
888-755-1404
Fax: 763-862-2922
support@marblesoft.com
www.softtouch.com

Joyce Meyer, President
Software for children and teens. For Macintosh and PC.

1727 Battenberg & Associates
11135 Rolling Springs Dr
Carmel, IN   46033-3629
317-843-2208
Jan Battenberg, Owner
Offers various software programs that develop the user's visual memory, sequencing skills, word recognition, hand-eye coordination and more.

1728 Behavior Skills: Learning How People Should Act
PCI Education Publishing
P.O.Box 34270
San Antonio, TX   78265-4270
210-377-1999
800-471-3000
Fax: 888-828-
www.pcieducation.com

Jeff Clain, CEO
Erin Kinard, VP Product Development/Publisher
Helps players learn what behavior is acceptable and what behavior is not acceptable in the real world. *$49.95*

1729 Blocks in Motion
Don Johnston
26799 W Commerce Dr
Volo, IL   60073-9675
847-740-0749
800-999-4660
Fax: 847-740-7326
info@donjohnston.com
www.donjohnston.com

Ruth Ziolkowski, President
Don Jhonson, Founder
This unique art and motion program makes drawing, creating and animating fun and educational for all users. Based on the Piagetian Theory for motor-sensory development, this program promotes the concept that the process is as educational and as much fun as the end result. *$79.00*

1730 Car Builder Deluxe
Optimum Resource
1 Mathews Drive
Suite 107
Hilton Head Island, SC   29926- 3689
843-689-8000
Fax: 843-689-8008
info@stickybear.com
www.stickybear.com

Richard Hefter, President
As design engineers, users build cars on screen, specifying chassis length, wheelbase, engine type, transmission, fuel tank size, suspension, steering, tires and brakes. All functional choices are interrelated and will affect the performance of the final design. Grades 3 & up. *$59.99*

1731 Center for Best Practices in Early Childhood
Horrabin Hall 32
Macomb, IL   61455
309-298-1634
Fax: 309-298-2305
jk-johanson@wiu.edu
www.wiu.edu/thecenter/

Linda Robinson, Assistant Director
The Center, part of the College of Education and Human Services at Western Illinois University, provides products, training mate-

rials, and information related to best practices for educators and families of young children with disabilities.

1732   Clock
Compass Learning
203 Colorado Street
Austin, TX   78701-3922

512-478-9600
800-678-1412
866-586-7387
www.compasslearning.com

Eric Loeffel, President
Trey Chambers, Chief Financial Officer
Arthur Vanderveen, Vice President, Business Strategy and Development
Chipp Walters, Chief Designer Officer
An extremely simple, easy-to-use program for children who are learning how to read the time of day from clocks and digital displays. Apple and MS-DOS and Mac available. *$39.95*

1733   Community Skills: Learning to Function in Your Neighborhood
Programming Concepts
8700 Shoal Creek Boulevard
Austin, TX   78757-6897

210-377-1999
800-594-4263
800-471-3000
Fax: 888-259-8284
www.proedinc.com

Lee Wilson, President and CEO
Randy Pennington, Executive VP
Jeff McLane, Founder
David Keith, Vice President of IT
Offers parents and educators a functional way to teach community life skills. *$49.95*

1734   Companion Activities
Soft Touch
12301 Central Ave NE Ste 205
4300 Stine Rd
Blaine, MN 55434

763-755-1404
888-755-1404
Fax: 763-862-2922
support@marblesoft.com
www.softouch.com

Joyce Meyer, President
Print your own books, worksheets, flash cards, board games, matching games, bingo games, card games and many more. This CD offers numerous companion activities to different SoftTouch software titles. Activities range from very easy to difficult. Companion activities are great tools to reinforce learning. Use the work sheets - black and white and color - in the inclusion class for students with special needs.

1735   Concepts on the Move Advanced Preacademics
Soft Touch
12301 Central Ave NE Ste 205
P.O.Box 490215
Blaine, MN 55449

763-862-2920
888-755-1402
Fax: 763-862-2922
support@marblesoft.com
www.marblesoft.com

Joyce Meyer, President
Choose from five concepts groups: categories, occupations, functions, goes with and prepositions. Use our Steps to Learning Design to choose how many concepts to present at one time and where to place each one in the scan array, on screen keyboard or IntelliKeys keyboard. Watch and listen as the concept morphs or changes and music plays. The words are also shown to reinforce emerging literacy skills. Compatible with USB IntelliKeys.

1736   Cooking Class: Learning About Food Preparation
Programming Concepts
8700 Shoal Creek Boulevard
Austin, TX   78757-6897

512-451-3246
800-897-3202
800-471-3000
Fax: 800-397-7633
general@proedinc.com
www.proedinc.com

Jeff McLane, Founder
Lee Wilson, President and CEO
Randy Pennington, Executive VP
David Keith, Vice President of IT
This game offers parents and educators a new way to teach basic preparation skills. Kitchen safety and sanitation are stressed throughout the game. *$49.95*

1737   Dilemma
Educational Activities Software
5600 West 83rd Street
Suite 300, 8200 Tower
Bloomington, MN   55437

800-447-5286
Fax: 239-225-9299
info@edmentum.com
www.edmentum.com

Vin Riera, President/CEO
Dan Juckniess, SVP, Sales & Professional Services
Stacey Herteux, VP, Human Resources
Rob Rueckl, Chief Financial Officer
Realistic stories with a choice of different gripping endings, color graphics, a built-in dictionary and a user controlled reading rate make these computer programs compelling enough to interest all students. Comprehension and vocabulary questions follow each story. *$159.00*

1738   Dino-Games
Academic Software
3504 Tates Creek Road
Lexington, KY   40517-2601

859-552-1020
859-552-1040
Fax: 253-799-4012
asistaff@acsw.com
www.acsw.com

Dr. Warren E Lacefield PhD, President
Penelope D. Ellis, COO, Sales & Marketing Director
Sylvia B. Lacefield, Graphic Artist
Cindy L George, Author
Dino-Games are single switch software programs for early switch practice. Dinosaur games provide practice in pattern recognition, cause and effect demonstration, directionality training, number concepts and problem solving. They are compatible with most popular switch interfaces and alternate keyboards. For Macintosh, IBM and compatibles. DINO-LINK is a matching game; DINO-MAZE is a series of maze games; DINO-FIND is a game of concentration; and DINO-DOT is a collection of dot-to-dot games.
$39.95 per game

1739   Directions: Technology in Special Education
DREAMMS for Kids
273 Ringwood Road
Freeville, NY   13068-5606

607-539-3027
Fax: 607-539-9930
janet@dreamms.org
www.dreamms.org

Janet P. Hosmer, Editor/Publisher
Chester D. Hosmer, Jr., Technical Editor
Susan Lait, Regular Contributor
Lorianne Hoenninger, Regular Contributor
A CD containing all of 'Directions' past articles and information gathered from their newsletter which lists resources for assistive and adaptive computer ethnologies in the home, school and community. *$24.95*

1740 ESI Master Resource Guide
Educational Software Institute
4213 S 94th St
Omaha, NE 68127-1223
402-592-3300
800-955-5570
Fax: 402-592-2017

Lee Myers, President
Kathy Cavanaugh, Catalog Manager
Educational Software Institute (ESI) provides a one-stop shop to purchase software titles by all of the best publishers. The ESI Master Gold Book catalog and CD-ROM represents more than 400 software publishers, with information on more than 8,000 software titles. Take the confusion out of software selection by calling ESI for all of your software needs - including competitive prices, software previews, knowledgeable assistance, and the largest selection available all in one place.
Yearly

1741 EZ Keys
Words+
42505 10th Street West
Suite 109
Lancaster, CA 93534- 7059
661-723-7723
888-266-9294
Fax: 661-723-5524
info@simulations-plus.com
www.simulations-plus.com
Walter S Woltosz, M.S., M.A.S., Chairman, President and Chief Executive Officer
John A. Dibella, VP, Marketing & Sales
Virginia E. Woltosz. M.B.A., Secretary & Treasurer
John R. Kneisel, Chief Financial Officer
A software and hardware product designed to operate on an IBM compatible PC. The software provides dual word prediction, abbreviation expansion, five different methods of voice output and access to commercial software applications. *$1395.00*

1742 Early Games for Young Children
Queue Incorporated
80 Hathaway Drive
Stratford, CT 06615
800-232-2224
Fax: 800-775-2729
jdk@queueinc.com
www.qworkbooks.com
Anna Christopoulos, General Manager
Peter Uhrynowski, Comptroller
Steve Perrett, Director of Printing and Graphics
Ann Pleszko, Shipping Manager
Software that includes nine activities that entertain preschoolers in honing basic math and language skills.

1743 Early Music Skills
Electronic Courseware Systems
1713 S State St
Champaign, IL 61820-7258
217-359-7099
800-832-4965
Fax: 217-359-6578
support@ecsmedia.com
www.ecsmedia.com
G Peters, President
Jodie Varner, Marketing Manager
A tutorial and drill program designed for the beginning music student. It covers four basic music reading skills: recognition of line and space notes; comprehension of the numbering system for the musical staff; visual and aural identification of notes moving up and down; and recognition of notes stepping and skipping up and down. *$ 39.95*

1744 Eating Skills: Learning Basic Table Manners
PCI Education Publishing
P.O.Box 34270
San Antonio, TX 78265-4270
210-377-1999
800-594-4263
Fax: 210-377-1121
www.pcieducation.com
Erin Kinard, VP Product Development/Publisher
Jeff Clain, CEO

Offers parents and educators a functional way to teach and reinforce basic table manners. *$49.95*

1745 Electronic Courseware Systems
1713 S State St
Champaign, IL 61820-7258
217-359-7099
800-832-4965
Fax: 217-359-6578
support@ecsmedia.com
www.ecsmedia.com
Jodie Varner, Manager
G Peters, President
Offers a complete library of instructional software for music, math, science and social studies.

1746 Fall Fun
Soft Touch
12301 Central Ave NE Ste 205
P.O.Box 490215
Blaine, MN 55449
763-862-2920
888-755-1402
Fax: 763-862-2922
support@marblesoft.com
www.marblesoft.com
Joyce Meyer, President
Your students can begin their day with the Pledge of Allegiance, Pumpkins, Owls, and Cats. Witches adorn Five Pumpkins Sitting on the Gate. Five Fat Turkeys out smart the pilgrims with song and antics. The owl and cat have songs of their own. A variety of activities reinforce concepts such as short, tall, first, second, third, same and different. Fall Fun includes cause and effect and easy to more difficult levels. Eight songs in all.

1747 Five Green & Speckled Frogs
Soft Touch
12301 Central Ave NE Ste 205
P.O.Box 490215
Blaine, MN 55449
763-862-2920
888-755-1402
Fax: 763-862-2922
support@marblesoft.com
www.marblesoft.com
Joyce Meyer, President
Laugh, learn and sing with Five Humorous Frogs. Activities start with cause and effect and progress to teach directionality and simple subtraction. This classic song makes learning numbers and number worlds easy. Selections can be set to 2, 3, 4, 5, or 6 on-screen choices. Two games are included. One teaches direction on a number line. If the child moves the frog in the correct direction, the frog gets a point. The other game teaches beginning subtraction.

1748 Free and User Supported Software for the IBM PC: A Resource Guide
McFarland & Company
960 NC Highway 88 W
P.O.Box 611
Jefferson, NC 28640-8813
336-246-4460
800-253-2187
Fax: 336-246-5018
info@mcfarlandpub.com
www.mcfarlandpub.com
Robert McFarland Franklin, Founder
Kenneth.J Ansley, Author
Victor.D Lopez, Author
A selection of word processing, database management, spreadsheets, and graphics programs are described and evaluated. Describes how the program works and its strengths and weaknesses. Rating charts cover such aspects as ease of use, ease of learning, documentation, and general utility. *$27.50*
224 pages Paperback
ISBN 0-89950 -99-0

1749 GoalView: Special Education and RTI Student Management Information System
Learning Tools International
2391 Circadian Way
Santa Rosa, CA 95407-5439 707-521-3530
800-333-9954
info@goalview.com
www.ltools.com

Cathy Zier, President/CEO
Natalie Sipes, VP
Michael R. Paul, Director of IT/Senior Web Engine
A Web Based information system for students, educators and parents that enables accountability and achievement tracking; prepares IDEA compliant IEP's in minutes; provides over 250,000 education standards and special education goals and objectives in English and Spanish; generates Federal compliance reports; and creates IDEA GoalCard progress reports for students, schools and districts for every reporting period.

1750 HELP
V OR T Corporation
P.O.Box G (George)
Menlo Park, CA 94026 650-322-8282
888-757-8678
Fax: 650-327-0747
custserv@vort.com
vort.com

Tom Holt, Owner
A software version of HELP, covers over 650 skills in 6 developmental areas; cognitive, motor skills, language, gross motor, social and self-help.

1751 Handbook of Adaptive Switches and Augmentative Communication Devices
Academic Software
3504 Tates Creek Road
Lexington, KY 40517-2601 859-552-1020
859-552-1040
Fax: 253-799-4012
asistaff@acsw.com
www.acsw.com

Dr. Warren E Lacefield PhD, President
Penelope D. Ellis, COO, Sales & Marketing Director
Cindy L George, Author
Sylvia B. Lacefield, Graphic Artist
This second edition contains physical descriptions and laboratory test data for a variety of commercially available pressure switches and augmentative communication devices and chapters on physical interaction, seating and positioning, and control access. It is an essential tool for assistive technology professionals and therapists who make decisions concerning physical access.
$60.00
300 pages Hardcover

1752 HandiWARE
Microsystems Software
600 Worcester Rd
Framingham, MA 01702-5303 508-626-8511
800-828-2600
Fax: 508-879-1069
infor@microsys.com
www.handiware.com

Terri McGrath, Sales/Marketing
Bill Kilroy, Product Manager
Adapted access software, assists persons with physical, hearing and visual impairments in accessing computers running DOS and Windows. HandiWARE is a suite of 8 software programs which provide users with screen magnification, alternate keyboard access, word prediction, augmentative communication, hands free telephone access, a visual beep. $20.00-$595.00.

1753 How to Write for Everyday Living
Educational Activities Software
5600 West 83rd Street
Suite 300, 8200 Tower
Bloomington, MN 55437-585 800-447-5286
Fax: 239-225-9299
info@edmentum.com
www.edmentum.com

Vin Riera, President/CEO
Dan Juckniess, SVP, Sales & Professional Services
Stacey Herteux, VP, Human Resources
Rob Rueckl, Chief Financial Officer
An individualized Life Skills WRITING Software program emphasizing the reading, writing, communication and reference skills needed for real-life tasks: preparing a resume, an employment form, a business letter and envelope, a learner's permit, a social security application and banking forms. *$159.00*

1754 I KNOW American History
Soft Touch
12301 Central Ave NE Ste 205
P.O.Box 490215
Blaine, MN 55449-2352 763-862-2920
888-755-1402
Fax: 763-862-2922
support@marblesoft.com
www.marblesoft.com

Joyce Meyer, President
The new I KNOW programs is the way students practice attending, choice making and turn-taking while uncovering learning puzzles. Each press reveals more of the image while the narrator reads the text on the screen. Offers three levels of language: short phrases, short sentences and longer sentences to match the student's learning level. Choose from the five topic areas: American Symbols, Westward Movement, Early Colonial Americans, Industrial Revolution and Biographies.

1755 I KNOW American History Overlay CD
Soft Touch
12301 Central Ave NE Ste 205
P.O.Box 490215
Blaine, MN 55449-2352 763-862-2920
888-755-1402
Fax: 763-862-2922
support@marblesoft.com
www.marblesoft.com

Joyce Meyer, President
Use this Overlay CD with I KNOW American History program. Includes standard overlays and SoftTouch's changeable overlays. Includes Overlay Printer by IntelliTools. Use Overlay Maker by IntelliTools (not included) to modify the overlays or to make additional learning materials.

1756 Incite Learning Series
Don Johnston
26799 West Commerce Drive
Volo, IL 60073 847-740-0749
800-999-4660
Fax: 847-740-7326
info@donjohnston.com
www.donjohnston.com

Don Johnston, Founder
Ruth Ziolkowski, President
A collection of original short films and a thought-provoking instruction model to engage every student in the critical thinking and feeling process. This research-based program was developed around the science of how students learn best using the theory of 'anchored instruction' and 'front-loading' standards-based curriculum. *$79.00*

1757 Innovation Management Group
179 Niblick Rd
Ste 454
Paso Robles, CA 93446   818-701-1579
                                        800-889-0987
                                    Fax: 818-936-0200
                                    cs@imgpresents.com
                                    www.imgpresents.com
Jerry Hussong, VP of Marketing
Publisher of the Assistive Technology Suite. The ultimate set of
general purpose, adaptive computer access available today. Site
License includes ALL computers and ALL active students and
teachers at a single or multi-site location.

1758 IntelliPics Studio 3
Intelli Tools
1720 Corporate Cir
Petaluma, CA 94954-6924   707-773-2000
                                        800-547-6747
                                    Fax: 707-773-2001
                                    info@intellitools.com
                                    www.intellitools.com
Arjan Khalsa, CEO
Multimedia authoring tool for both students and teachers to cre-
ate activities, games, quizzes, slide shows, reports and presenta-
tions. *$395.00*

1759 KIDS (Keyboard Introductory Development Series)
Electronic Courseware Systems
1713 S State St
Champaign, IL 61820-7258   217-359-7099
                                        800-832-4965
                                    Fax: 217-359-6578
                                    support@ecsmedia.com
                                    www.ecsmedia.com
G Peters, President
Jodie Varner, Marketing Manager
A four disk series for the very young. Zoo Puppet Theater rein-
forces learning correct finger numbers for piano playing; Race
Car Keys teaches keyboard geography by recognizing syllables
or note names; Dinosaurs Lunch teaches placement of the notes
on the treble staff; and Follow Me asks the student to play notes
that have been presented aurally. *$49.95*

1760 Keyboard Tutor, Music Software
Electronic Courseware Systems
1713 S State St
Champaign, IL 61820-7258   217-359-7099
                                        800-832-4965
                                    Fax: 217-359-6578
                                    support@ecsmedia.com
                                    www.ecsmedia.com
G Peters, President
Jodie Varner, Marketing Manager
Presents exercises for learning elementary keyboard skills in-
cluding knowledge of names of the keys, piano keys matched to
notes, notes matched to piano keys, whole steps and half steps.
Each lesson allows unlimited practice of the skills. The program
may be used with or without a midi keyboard attached to the computer. *$39.95*

1761 Keyboarding by Ability
Teachers Institute for Special Education
9933 NW 45th St
Sunrise, FL 33351-4744   954-235-7940
                                    Fax: 866-843-0765
                            Support@Special-Education-Soft.com
                                www.special-education-soft.com
Gary Byowitz, President
Allows the learning disabled or dyslexic student to acquire
keyboarding skills through visually cued alphabetical approach
designed and tested to meet the specific learning style needs of
this unique population at every grade level. Package contains:
IBM software, a set of lesson plans and instructional goals; supplemental graded data input exercises. *$369.00*

1762 Keyboarding for the Physically Handicapped
Teachers Institute for Special Education
9933 NW 45th Street
Sunrise, FL 33351   954-235-7940
                                    Fax: 866-843-0765
                            Support@Special-Education-Soft.com
                                www.special-education-soft.com
Jack Heller, Director/Owner
Gary Byowitz, President
Custom designed touch typing programs for any student. A person needs order by the number of usable fingers on each hand (not
counting the thumb), and whether or not a one finger or a
head-pointer edition is wanted. Package includes IBM software;
a complete set of lesson plans and instructional goals. *$149.95*

1763 Keyboarding with One Hand
Teachers Institute for Special Education
P.O.Box 2300
Wantagh, NY 11793-140   *Fax:* 516-781-4070
                                    jackheller@aol.com
Jack Heller, Director
This 22 lesson tutorial developed through 25 years of research,
testing and teaching allows a student with one hand to acquire em-
ployable keyboarding skills using a touch system designed for
the standard IBM PC keyboard. *$79.95*

1764 LPDOS Deluxe
Optelec U S
3030 Enterprise Court
STE C
Vista, CA 92081-8358   800-826-4200
                                    Fax: 800-368-4111
                                    info@optelec.com
                                    us.optelec.com
Stephan Terwolbeck, President
Michiel van Schaik, VP
Janet Lennex, Director of Customer Excellence
Jade Arbelo, Director of Human Resources
Large print software programs. *$595.00*

1765 Large Print DOS
Optelec U S
3030 Enterprise Court
STE C
Vista, CA 92081-8358   800-826-4200
                                    Fax: 800-368-4111
                                    info@optelec.com
                                    us.optelec.com
Stephan Terwolbeck, President
Michiel van Schaik, VP
Janet Lennex, Director of Customer Excellence
Jade Arbelo, Director of Human Resources

1766 Laureate Learning Systems
110 E Spring St
Winooski, VT 05404-1898   802-655-4755
                                        800-562-6801
                                    Fax: 802-655-4757
                                    info@llsys.com
                                    www.laureatelearning.com
Mary Wilson, Owner
Kathy Hollandsworth, Office Manager
Laureate publishes award-winning talking software for children
and adults with disabilities. Programs cover cause and effect, language development, cognitive processing, and reading.
High-quality speech, colorful graphics and amusing animation
make learning fun. Accessible with touchscreen, single switch,
keyboard and mouse. No reading required. Available on a hybrid
CD-ROM for Windows and Macintosh. Visit our website for
more information or call for a free catalog.

1767 Learning Company
Ste 400
222 3rd Ave SE
Cedar Rapids, IA 52401-1542
319-395-9626
888-242-6747
Fax: 319-395-0217
info@riverdeep.net
http://web.riverdeep.net
Barry O'Callaghan, Executive Chairman & Chief Executive Officer
Tony Mulderry, Executive Vice President, Corporate Development
Ciara Smyth, Executive Vice President, Global Business Operations
Scott Campbell, Executive Vice President, Strategic Sales
Software for children. For Macintosh or Windows (3.1 DOS or Windows 95, Windows 98 required). The Learning Company has been added to Riverdeep.

1768 Little Red Hen
Compass Learning
203 Colorado Street
Austin, TX 78701
512-478-9600
800-678-1412
866-586-7387
Fax: 619-622-7873
support@compasslearning.com
www.compasslearning.com
Eric Loeffel, President, CEO
Tammy Deal, VP, Human Resources
Eric Wasser, VP, Sales
Eileen Shihadeh, VP, Marketing
Children learn about the rewards of hard work when they discover who the Little Red Hen's friends miss out on freshly baked bread. Puzzles, rhymes, story writing and other interactive exercises enhance the creative learning process. *$34.95*

1769 Looking Good: Learning to Improve Your Appearance
Programming Concepts
8700 Shoal Creek Boulevard
Austin, TX 78757-6897
512-451-3246
800-897-3202
800-471-3000
Fax: 800-397-7633
general@proedinc.com
www.proedinc.com
Jeff McLane, Founder
Lee Wilson, President and CEO
Randy Pennington, Executive VP
David Keith, Vice President of IT
This game offers a creative way to discuss all areas of grooming. *$49.95*

1770 Monkeys Jumping on the Bed
Soft Touch
12301 Central Ave NE Ste 205
P.O.Box 490215
Blaine, MN 55449-2352
763-862-2920
888-755-1402
Fax: 763-862-2922
support@marblesoft.com
www.marblesoft.com
Joyce Meyer, President
This program combines a favorite preschool song with number and color activities. Children and adults will enjoy engaging music and delightful animation. Students with cognitive delays respond to upbeat music and interesting sounds. Large graphics help learners focus on the action. Several important concepts are presented in enjoyable activity formats. Students learn cause and effect in Let's Play and Just for Fun.

1771 Morse Code WSKE
Words+
42505 10th Street West
Suite 109
Lancaster, CA 93534- 7059
661-723-7723
888-266-9294
Fax: 661-723-5524
info@simulations-plus.com
www.simulations-plus.com
Walter S Woltosz, M.S., M.A.S., Chairman, President and Chief Executive Officer
John A. Dibella, VP, Marketing & Sales
Virginia E. Woltosz. M.B.A., Secretary & Treasurer
John R. Kneisel, Chief Financial Officer
A software and hardware product designed to operate on an IBM compatible PC.

1772 Multi-Scan Single Switch Activity Center
Academic Software
3504 Tates Creek Road
Lexington, KY 40517-2601
859-552-1020
859-552-1040
Fax: 253-799-4012
asistaff@acsw.com
www.acsw.com
Dr. Warren E Lacefield PhD, President
Penelope D. Ellis, COO, Sales & Marketing Director
Cindy L George, Author
Sylvia B. Lacefield, Graphic Artist
A single switch activity center containing four educational games: Match, Maze, Dot-to-Dot, and Concentration, along with six graphics libraries; Dinosaurs, Sports, Animals, Independent Living, Vocations, and Cosmetology. MULTI-SCAN allows you to select a graphic library, choose games for each user, and adjust the difficulty level and other settings for each game. Other features allow you to save the game setups under each user's name and print out individual performance reports after sessions. *$154.00*

1773 Muppet Learning Keys
WINGS for Learning
1600 Green Hills Rd
Scotts Valley, CA 95066-4981
831-426-2228
Fax: 831-464-3600
Ani Stocks, Owner
Designed to introduce children to the world of the computer as they become familiar with letters, numbers and colors.

1774 My Own Pain
Soft Touch
12301 Central Ave NE Ste 205
P.O.Box 490215
Blaine, MN 55449-2352
763-862-2920
888-755-1402
Fax: 763-862-2922
support@marblesoft.com
www.marblesoft.com
Joyce Meyer, President
Three activities - three levels. Press the switch and the paint brush chooses the color and paints the vehicle. Music reinforces the sounds when the picture is complete. A second activity allows the student to choose the color and paint the vehicle parts any color he or she wants. The third activity is a blueprint. Print the color that matches the one in the wire drawing. Color the drawing to complete the picture.

1775 NanoPac
4823 S Sheridan Rd
Suite 302
Tulsa, OK 74145-5717
918-665-0329
800-580-6086
Fax: 918-665-0361
TTY: 918-665-2310
info@nanopac.com
www.nanopac.com
Silvio Cianfrone, President
NanoPac offers assistive technology for those with low vision, blindness and reading disabilities. Some of their products include

voice recognition, environmental controls, text to speech, magnifiers and door openers.

1776 Old MacDonald's Farm Deluxe
Soft Touch
12301 Central Ave NE Ste 205
P.O.Box 490215
Blaine, MN 55449-2352   763-862-2920
                                                     888-755-1402
                                                Fax: 763-862-2922
                                        support@marblesoft.com
                                               www.marblesoft.com

Joyce Meyer, President
Toddlers, preschoolers and early elementary students will be entertained and captivated by the six major activities and animations in the delightful program. Includes 18 real animation images or 9 cartoon like characters. The teacher or child can choose which animals they want to sing about. Some activities are designed for children within the normal population, others are designed for students with moderate and severe disabilities.

1777 Optimum Resource Educational Software
Optimum Resource
1 Mathews Drive
Suite 107
Hilton Head Island, SC 29926   843-689-8000
                                   Fax: 843-689-8008
                                   info@stickybear.com
                                     www.stickybear.com

Richard Hefter, President
A complete topical curriculum of reading, math, keyboard skills and science programs that are age and skill specific. Programs include: Early Learning for Pre-K to 1st grade with introductions to numbers, language, shapes, and time; Language Arts from Pre-K to 12; Math for Pre-K to 12; two distinct Science programs; Tools for Educators provides Spelling and Math generators; and Bilingual programs for Pre-K through 9th grade. All are available as single user up to 30 user site packages.

1778 Optimum Resources/Stickybear Software
1 Mathews Drive
Suite 107
Hilton Head Island, SC 29926   843-689-8000
                                   Fax: 843-689-8008
                                   info@stickybear.com
                                     www.stickybear.com

Richard Hefter, President
Publisher of award-winning educational software for thirty years. Programs in use by millions of students nationwide.
$59.95

1779 Please Understand Me: Software Program and Books
Cambridge Educational
132 West 31st Street
17th Floor
New York, NY 10001   800-322-8755
                                   Fax: 800-678-3633
                                   custserv@films.com
                                        www.films.com

209 pages BiAnnual
ISBN 0-927368-56-x

1780 Pond
WINGS for Learning
1600 Green Hills Rd
Scotts Valley, CA 95066-4981   831-426-2228
                                   Fax: 831-464-3600
Ani Stocks, Owner
Software game that teaches pattern recognition and encourages observation, trial and error and the interpretation of data.

1781 Print, Play & Learn #1 Old Mac's Farm
Soft Touch Incorporated
12301 Central Ave NE Ste 205
P.O.Box 490215
Blaine, MN 55449-2352   763-862-2920
                                                     888-755-1402
                                                Fax: 763-862-2922
                                        support@marblesoft.com
                                               www.marblesoft.com

Joyce Meyer, President
Once your students have completed Old Mac's Farm, let them use the fun off-computer activities to continue learning. Over 25 activities with 250 sheets you print. Board games, dot-to-dot drawings, word puzzles, make a scene, flash cards. Concentration, sentence strips, worksheets and much more are available for teachers to expand their teaching goals. This CD is full of activities to print and use.

1782 Print, Play & Learn #7: Sampler
Soft Touch
12301 Central Ave NE Ste 205
P.O.Box 490215
Blaine, MN 55449-2352   763-862-2920
                                                     888-755-1402
                                                Fax: 763-862-2922
                                        support@marblesoft.com
                                               www.marblesoft.com

Joyce Meyer, President
Print, Play and Learn Sampler gives you over 200 activities organized by training, easy, medium and hard levels so you can ready to help your student advance. Activities cover a wide range of basic knowledge, including colors, shapes, numbers, letters and much, much more. Note: Requires Overlay Maker or Overlay Printer by IntelliTools and a color printer.

1783 Puzzle Power: Sampler
Soft Touch
12301 Central Ave NE Ste 205
P.O.Box 490215
Blaine, MN 55449-2352   763-862-2920
                                                     888-755-1402
                                                Fax: 763-862-2922
                                        support@marblesoft.com
                                               www.marblesoft.com

Joyce Meyer, President
Puzzle Power - Sampler offers a variety of puzzles in different themes. Each theme puzzle is followed by a puzzle of one item in this category. For example, first solve a puzzle for occupations. Then, solve a puzzle that is a baker. The pictures are large, clear and easily identifiable.

1784 Puzzle Power: Zoo & School Days
Soft Touch
12301 Central Ave NE Ste 205
P.O.Box 490215
Blaine, MN 55449-2352   763-862-2920
                                                     888-755-1402
                                                Fax: 763-862-2922
                                        support@marblesoft.com
                                               www.marblesoft.com

Joyce Meyer, President
Here is a program for all of our students who need puzzle skills, but cannot access commercial puzzles. Puzzle Power puzzles start with just two pieces and progress to 16 pieces. The pictures are large, clear and easily identifiable. Four different activities enable all students to be successful. Automatic Placement: the student just presses the switch or keyboard to place the pieces. Magnet Mouse: all the student needs to do is move the mouse and it drops into place.

1785 Rodeo
Soft Touch
12301 Central Ave NE Ste 205
P.O.Box 490215
Blaine, MN 55449-2352   763-862-2920
                                       888-755-1402
                                 Fax: 763-862-2922
                             support@marblesoft.com
                                 www.marblesoft.com
Joyce Meyer, President
Rodeo action and familiar tunes for teens and preteens. Four activities invite students to learn, laugh, and sing as they go to the rodeo with up to six age-peer friends. Age-appropriate graphics with surprising animations reinforce the learning. The graphics are large and colorful, the melodies familiar, and the words descriptive of the action on the screen.

1786 Shop Til You Drop
Soft Touch
12301 Central Ave NE Ste 205
P.O.Box 490215
Blaine, MN 55449-2352   763-862-2920
                                       888-755-1402
                                 Fax: 763-862-2922
                             support@marblesoft.com
                                 www.marblesoft.com
Joyce Meyer, President
Designed specifically for preteens and teens with moderate and severe disabilities, this program will become a staple for the classroom. The student goes shopping and can choose which outfits to put together. They may choose to purchase the outfit - of course, with mom's credit card. Another activity is a video arcade game about money. Shop 'Til You Drop can be adjusted from a single switch cause-and-effect program to row-and-column scanning to direct choice.

1787 Songs I Sing at Preschool
Soft Touch
12301 Central Ave NE Ste 205
P.O.Box 490215
Blaine, MN 55449-2352   763-862-2920
                                       888-755-1402
                                 Fax: 763-862-2922
                             support@marblesoft.com
                                 www.marblesoft.com
Joyce Meyer, President
Songs I Sing at Preschool offers many options for the teacher and the student. Over the years, our software has used music because our students really respond to the sounds and rhythms of songs. Teachers select which songs to present, how many to present at one time and where to place each song on the overlay, keyboard or scan array.

1788 Stickybear Early Learning Activities
Optimum Resource
1 Mathews Drive
Suite 107
Hilton Head Island, SC 29926   843-689-8000
                                 Fax: 843-689-8008
                               info@stickybear.com
                                 www.stickybear.com
Richard Hefter, President
Two modes of play allow youngsters to learn through prompted direction or by the discovery method. Lively animation and sound keep attention levels high as children learn writing, counting, shapes, opposites and colors. Stickybear Early Learning Activities is bilingual, so youngsters can build skills in both English and Spanish. Pre-K to 1st grade. *$59.95*

1789 Stickybear Kindergarden Activities
Optimum Resource
1 Mathews Drive
Suite 107
Hilton Head Island, SC 29926   843-689-8000
                                 Fax: 843-689-8008
                               info@stickybear.com
                                 www.stickybear.com
Richard Hefter, President
This dynamic new multifaceted program covers a wide range of preschool skills that go far beyond the strictly academic. At Stickybear's house, children discover the alphabet, numbers, shapes, colors, plus - social skills, important safety messages and delightful off-screen activities that foster creativity. Over three hours of original music can be composed by a child and saved for future use. *$59.95*

1790 Stickybear Science Fair Light
Optimum Resource
1 Mathews Drive
Suite 107
Hilton Head Island, SC 29926   843-689-8000
                                 Fax: 843-689-8008
                               info@stickybear.com
                                 www.stickybear.com
Richard Hefter, President
The first in the new series of science-based programs Stickybear Science Fair Light presents a content rich environment which allows students in grades 7-12 to explore, experiment with and understand light and it's properties. The program presents experiments, both structured and free-form, which allow users to work with prisms, lenses, color mixing, optical illusions and more. *$59.95*

1791 Stickybear Town Builder
Optimum Resource
1 Mathews Drive
Suite 107
Hilton Head Island, SC 29926   843-689-8000
                                 Fax: 843-689-8008
                               info@stickybear.com
                                 www.stickybear.com
Richard Hefter, President
Children learn to read maps, build towns, take trips and use a compass in this simulation program. *$59.95*

1792 Stickybear Typing
Optimum Resource
1 Mathews Drive
Suite 107
Hilton Head Island, SC 29926   843-689-8000
                                 Fax: 843-689-8008
                               info@stickybear.com
                                 www.stickybear.com
Richard Hefter, President
Sharpen typing skills with three challenging activities: Stickybear Keypress, Stickybear Thump and Stickybear Stories. Pre-K to 5th. *$59.95*

1793 Storybook Maker Deluxe
Compass Learning
203 Colorado Street
Austin, TX 78701   512-478-9600
                                       800-678-1412
                                       866-586-7387
                                 Fax: 619-622-7873
                      support@compasslearning.com
                          www.compasslearning.com
Eric Loeffel, President, CEO
Tammy Deal, VP, Human Resources
Eric Wasser, VP, Sales
Eileen Shihadeh, VP, Marketing
Using Storybook Maker Deluxe and their imaginations, students can create and publish stories filled with exciting graphics. Students can write stories and watch as the text appears in the setting they've chosen. Engaging sounds and music, plus lively animations, provide positive learning reinforcement throughout the program. *$44.95*

1794   Super Challenger
Electronic Courseware Systems
1713 S State St
Champaign, IL   61820-7258   217-359-7099
                                              800-832-4965
                                          Fax: 217-359-6578
                                          www.ecsmedia.com

Jodie Varner, Manager
G Peters, President
An aural-visual musical game that increases the player's ability
to remember a series of pitches as they are played by the computer. The game is based on a 12-note chromatic scale, a major
scale, and a minor scale. Each pitch is reinforced visually with a
color representation of a keyboard on the display screen. Com-
puter/software. *$39.95*

1795   Switch Basics
Soft Touch
12301 Central Ave NE Ste 205
P.O.Box 490215
Blaine, MN 55449-2352   763-862-2920
                                              888-755-1402
                                          Fax: 763-862-2922
                                          support@marblesoft.com
                                          www.marblesoft.com

Joyce Meyer, President
Discover whimsical animations and real life pictures while learning switch operations. Intriguing and humorous, nine different
programs offer a multitude of learning experiences for all ages.
Program options include: cause and effect, scanning, step scanning, row and column activities for one or two players. Watch the
clouds roll away revealing African animals; visit the beauty salon
or barber shop; work two to sixteen piece puzzles; or add
swimming fish to a huge aquarium.

1796   Switch Interface Pro 5.0
Don Johnston
26799 West Commerce Drive
Volo, IL   60073   847-740-0749
                                              800-999-4660
                                          Fax: 847-740-7326
                                          info@donjohnston.com
                                          www.donjohnston.com

Don Johnston, Founder
Ruth Ziolkowski, President
Allows individuals with physical disabilities to access the computer. Five ports accommodate multiple switches and emulate everything from a single-click to a return. Consequently,
individuals gain access to the widest variety of switch-accessible
software available. It requires no software and can be used with
both Windows and Macintosh computers. *$79.00*

1797   Teach Me Phonemics Series Bundle
SoftTouch
Ste 401
4300 Stine Rd
Bakersfield, CA   93313-2352   661-396-8676
                                              877-763-8868
                                          Fax: 661-396-8760
                                          support@softtouch.com
                                          www.funsoftware.com

Joyce Meyer, President
Roxanne Butterfield, Marketing
The Teach Me Phonemics Series Bundle includes one copy of
each Teach Me Phonemics program - Initial, Medial, Final and
Blends - four CD's in all.

1798   Teach Me Phonemics Super Bundle
SoftTouch
Ste 401
4300 Stine Rd
Bakersfield, CA   93313-2352   661-396-8676
                                              877-763-8868
                                          Fax: 661-396-8760
                                          softtouch@funsoftware.com
                                          www.funsoftware.com

Roxanne Butterfield, Marketing
Joyce Meyer, President

Teach Me Phonemics Super Bundle includes all 4 Teach Me Phonemics programs and all 4 Teach Me Phonemics overlay CD's -
eight CD's in all.

1799   Teach Me Phonemics: Blends
SoftTouch
Ste 401
4300 Stine Rd
Bakersfield, CA   93313-2352   661-396-8676
                                              877-763-8868
                                          Fax: 661-396-8760
                                          softtouch@funsoftware.com
                                          www.funsoftware.com

Roxanne Butterfield, Marketing
Joyce Meyer, President
Teach Me Phonemics - Blends helps students explore words and
hear the initial blend sounds. It features musical interludes and
movement to engage the student. Teachers select the best combination options to motivate and engage the student. Options turn
off and on the fly so you can quickly make changes to keep the
student engaged.

1800   Teach Me Phonemics: Final
SoftTouch
Ste 401
4300 Stine Rd
Bakersfield, CA   93313-2352   661-396-8676
                                              877-763-8868
                                          Fax: 661-396-8760
                                          www.funsoftware.com

Roxanne Butterfield
Joyce Meyer, President
Teach me Phonemics - Final helps students explore words and
hear the final sounds. It features musical interludes and movement to engage the student. Options turn off and on the fly so you
can quickly make changes to keep the student engaged.

1801   Teach Me Phonemics: Initial
SoftTouch
12301 Central Ave NE
Ste 205
Blaine, MN   55434   763-755-1402
                                              888-755-1403
                                          Fax: 763-862-2920
                                          sales@marblesoft.com
                                          www.softtouch.com

Roxanne Butterfield, Marketing
Joyce Meyer, President
Teach Me Phonemics - Initial helps students explore the words
and hear the initial sounds. It features musical interludes and
movement to engage the student. Teachers select the best combination options to motivate and engage the student. Options turn
off and on the fly so you can quickly make changes to keep the
student engaged.

1802   Teach Me Phonemics: Medial
SoftTouch
12301 Central Ave NE
Ste 205
Blaine, MN   55434   763-755-1402
                                              888-755-1403
                                          Fax: 763-862-2920
                                          sales@marblesoft.com
                                          www.softtouch.com

Roxanne Butterfield, Marketing
Joyce Meyer, President
Teach Me Phonemics - Medial helps students explore the words
and hear the medial sounds. It features musical interludes and
movement to engage the student. Teachers select the best combination options to motivate and engage the student. Options turn
off and on the fly so you can quickly make changes to keep the
student engaged.

1803 Teach Me to Talk
Soft Touch
12301 Central Ave NE Ste 205
P.O.Box 490215
Blaine, MN 55449-2352 763-862-2920
888-755-1402
Fax: 763-862-2922
support@marblesoft.com
www.marblesoft.com

Joyce Meyer, President
The first activity Teach Me to Talk is used as a springboard for the student to learn to speak the word. There are 150 real pictures. When a picture is chosen, it appears on a clear background with musical interludes, movement, written word and spoken word. It culminates by morphing to the corresponding black and white Mayer-Johnson symbol. The second activity Story Time, takes some of these nouns and puts them in four line poetry. This helps students hear the word in the midst of a sentence.

1804 Teen Tunes Plus
Soft Touch
12301 Central Ave NE Ste 205
P.O.Box 490215
Blaine, MN 55449-2352 763-862-2920
888-755-1402
Fax: 763-862-2922
support@marblesoft.com
www.marblesoft.com

Joyce Meyer, President
Introduce switch use to older students with disabilities. Large interesting graphics, a variety of musical interludes, and surprising animations are combined with calm soothing music and beautiful pictures in the software specifically designed for preteens and teens with severe cognitive delays and/or physical disabilities, and older students learning to use a switch.

1805 There are Tyrannosaurs Trying on Pants in My Bedroom
Compass Learning
203 Colorado Street
Austin, TX 78701-3922 512-478-9600
800-678-1412
866-586-7387
Fax: 619-622-7873
support@compasslearning.com
www.compasslearning.com

Eric Loeffel, President, CEO
Tammy Deal, VP, Human Resources
Eric Wasser, VP, Sales
Eileen Shihadeh, VP, Marketing
In this popular story, Saturday chores turn into fun-filled frolicking when dinosaurs come for a visit. Sounds, music and animation make learning about phonics and vocabulary dyno-mite. *$34.95*

1806 Three Billy Goats Gruff
Compass Learning
203 Colorado Street
Austin, TX 78701-3922 512-478-9600
800-678-1412
866-586-7387
Fax: 619-622-7873
support@compasslearning.com
www.compasslearning.com

Eric Loeffel, President, CEO
Tammy Deal, VP, Human Resources
Eric Wasser, VP, Sales
Eileen Shihadeh, VP, Marketing
Motivating exercises and creative activities provide hours of learning fun while young students follow the adventure of The Three Billy Goats Gruff in this animated version of the timeless tale. *$ 34.95*

1807 Three Little Pigs
Compass Learning
203 Colorado Street
Austin, TX 78701-3922 512-478-9600
800-678-1412
866-586-7387
Fax: 619-622-7873
support@compasslearning.com
www.compasslearning.com

Eric Loeffel, President, CEO
Tammy Deal, VP, Human Resources
Eric Wasser, VP, Sales
Eileen Shihadeh, VP, Marketing
Help young students build reading comprehension and writing skills with this interactive version of the children's classic, The Three Little Pigs. Animated storytelling and creative activities inspire children to read, write and rhyme. *$34.95*

1808 TouchCorders
Soft Touch
12301 Central Ave NE Ste 205
P.O.Box 490215
Blaine, MN 55449-2352 763-862-2920
888-755-1402
Fax: 763-862-2922
support@marblesoft.com
www.marblesoft.com

Joyce Meyer, President
TouchCorders are the flexible and easy-to-use communicator designed by Jo Meyer and Linda Bidabe for reach classroom use. TouchCorders are sensitive to touch at every angle and give the student kinesthetic feedback. With the unique Add 'n Touch system, Jo connects the puzzles bases of 2 or more TouchCorders on the fly to present vocabulary, sequencing, story telling, social stories, concepts and other curriculum and communication opportunities.

1809 TouchWindow Touch Screen
Riverdeep Incorporated
100 Pine Street
Suite 1900
San Francisco, CA 94111 415-659-2000
800-542-4222
Fax: 415-659-2020
info@riverdeep.net
www.riverdeep.net

Barry O'Callaghan, Executive Chairman & Chief Executive Officer
Tony Mulderry, Executive Vice President, Corporate Development
Ciara Smyth, Executive Vice President, Global Business Operations
Scott Campbell, Executive Vice President, Strategic Sales
Software for children. *$335.00*

1810 Turtle Teasers
Soft Touch
12301 Central Ave NE Ste 205
P.O.Box 490215
Blaine, MN 55449-2352 763-862-2920
888-755-1402
Fax: 763-862-2922
support@marblesoft.com
www.marblesoft.com

Joyce Meyer, President
Three Games, Three Levels from Easy, Medium to Hard. The Shell Game - easy: Watch one of the three turtles get the tomato. Then watch carefully as they switch positions and pop shut. Choose incorrectly and the frog disappears until the correct one is displayed. The Pond - medium: Watch the tomato disappear somewhere in the pond scene. Tomato Dump - hard: Hit the shell and it turns into the tomato, giving a score. There are different difficulty levels to equalize all students.

1811 What Was That!
Compass Learning
203 Colorado Street
Austin, TX 78701-3922

512-478-9600
800-678-1412
866-586-7387
Fax: 619-622-7873
support@compasslearning.com
www.compasslearning.com

Eric Loeffel, President, CEO
Tammy Deal, VP, Human Resources
Eric Wasser, VP, Sales
Eileen Shihadeh, VP, Marketing
In this bedtime story, noises in the night send three brother bears scurrying out of bed. Thoughtful questions test young readers' comprehension, while games, voice recording, writing practice and other playful activities stimulate their creativity.

1812 Wivik 3
Prentke Romich Company
1022 Heyl Road
Wooster, OH 44691

330-262-1984
800-262-1984
Fax: 330-263-4829
info@prentrom.com
www.prentrom.com

David L Moffatt, President
On-screen keyboard provides access to any application in the latest Windows operating systems. Selections are made by clicking, dwelling or switch scanning. Enhancements include word prediction and abbreviation expansion.

1813 WordMaker
Don Johnston
26799 West Commerce Drive
Volo, IL 60073

847-740-0749
800-999-4660
Fax: 847-740-7326
info@donjohnston.com
www.donjohnston.com

Don Johnston, Founder
Ruth Ziolkowski, President
The computer version of Dr Patricia Cunningham's book 'Systematic Sequential Phonics They Use.' The program systematically builds spelling and word decoding skills for struggling readers and writers. *$79.00*

1814 Write: Out Loud
Don Johnston
26799 West Commerce Drive
Volo, IL 60073

847-740-0749
800-999-4660
Fax: 847-740-7326
info@donjohnston.com
www.donjohnston.com

Don Johnston, Founder
Ruth Ziolkowski, President
Write: Out Loud is an easy-to-use talking word processor that uses text-to-speech and revision and editing supports to help students write more effectively, more often and with more enthusiasm as they share creative thoughts on paper. *$79.00*

1815 You Tell Me: Learning Basic Information
Programming Concepts
8700 Shoal Creek Boulevard
Austin, TX 78757-6897

512-451-3246
800-897-3202
800-471-3000
Fax: 800-397-7633
general@proedinc.com
www.proedinc.com

Jeff McLane, Founder
Lee Wilson, President and CEO
Randy Pennington, Executive VP
David Keith, Vice President of IT
This game teaches and reinforces basic information all individuals need to know. Questions asked in this game help prepare peo-

ple to communicate personal identification information important to community survival. *$49.95*

Software: Professional

1816 Acrontech International
5500 Main St
Williamsville, NY 14221-6755

Fax: 716-854-4014

1817 DPS with BCP
V OR T Corporation
P.O.Box G (George)
Menlo Park, CA 94026

650-322-8282
888-757-8678
Fax: 650-327-0747
custserv@vort.com
vort.com

Tom Holt, Owner
This program uses unique DPS branching techniques to access goals and objectives.

1818 Diagnostic Report Writer
Parrot Software
P.O. Box 250755
West Bloomfield, MI 48325

248-788-3223
800-727-7681
Fax: 248-788-3224
support@parrotsoftware.com
www.parrotsoftware.com

Dr. Frederic Weiner, Ph. D., CCC-SP, President, Owner
Creates a three page single-spaced diagnostic report for a child with a communication disorder from a list of questions; sections of the report include developmental and background history, oral peripheral exam, speech and language analysis, summary and recommendations.

1819 Discriptive Language Arts Development
Educational Activities Software
5600 West 83rd Street
Suite 300, 8200 Tower
Bloomington, MN 55437

888-351-4199
800-447-5286
Fax: 239-225-9299
info@edmentum.com
www.edmentum.com

Vin Riera, President/CEO
Dan Juckniess, SVP, Sales & Professional Services
Stacey Herteux, VP, Human Resources
Rob Rueckl, Chief Financial Officer
This multimedia language arts development program provides instruction and application of fundamental English skills and concepts. *$395.00*

1820 Draft: Builder
Don Johnston
26799 West Commerce Drive
Volo, IL 60073

847-740-0749
800-999-4660
Fax: 847-740-7326
info@donjohnston.com
www.donjohnston.com

Don Johnston, Founder
Ruth Ziolkowski, President
A software-based graphic organizer that breaks down the writing process into manageable chunks to structure planning, organizing, and draft-writing. *$79.00*

1821 EZ Dot
CAPCO Capability Corporation
3910 S. Union Court
Spokane Valley, WA 99206-6345

509-927-8195
800-827-2182
Fax: 800-827-2182
info@skilltran.com
www.skilltran.com

Jeff Truthan, President

A critical software tool used in vocational counseling, job restructuring, recruitment and placement, better utilization of workers, and safety issues. This software offers occupational data by title, code, industry, GEO, DPT, or OGA. *$295.00*

1822   EZ Keys for Windows
Words+
Ste 109
42505 10th St W
Lancaster, CA   93534-7059   661-723-6523
                                          800-869-8521
                                     Fax: 661-723-2114
                                     info@words-plus.com
                                     www.words-plus.com

Jean Dobbs, Editorial Director
Tim Gilmer, Editor
Josie Byzek, Managing Editor
Doug Lathrop, Senior Correspondent
A software and hardware product designed to operate on an IBM compatible PC. The software provides dual word prediction, abbreviation expansion, five different methods of voice output and access to commercial software applications. *$1395.00*

1823   Goals and Objectives
JE Stewart Teaching Tools
P.O.Box 15308
Seattle, WA   98115-308   206-262-9538
                                     Fax: 206-262-9538

Jeff Stewart, Owner
Goals and Objectives software helps teachers make student plans including IEP's, IPP's and IHP's. The system provides curricula for all students and programs to develop and evaluate plans, print reports and make data forms. Systems are available for Windows and Macintosh for $139.

1824   Goals and Objectives IEP Program Curriculum Associates LLC
153 Rangeway Road
P.O.Box 2001
North Billerica, MA 01862-0901   978-667-8000
                                          800-225-0248
                                     Fax: 800-366-1158
                                     www.curriculumassociates.com

Frank E. Ferguson, Chairman
Renee Foster, President & Publisher
Woody Palk, Senior Vice President, Sales
Robert Waldron, CEO
BRIGANCE CIBS-R standardized scoring conversion software, is a teacher's tool that prints goal and objective pages of the IEP. In less than two minutes per student, a teacher types student data into the computer.

1825   Nasometer
Kay Elemetrics Corporation
3 Paragon Drive
Montvale, NJ   07645   973-628-6200
                                          800-289-5297
                                     Fax: 201-391-2063
                                     sales@kaypentax.com
                                     www.kaypentax.com

John Crump, President
Steve Crump, Direct Sales
Measures the ratio of acoustic energy for the nasal and real-time visual cueing during therapy. Used clinically in the areas of cleft palate, motor speech disorders, hearing impairment and palatal prosthetic fittings.

1826   PSS CogRehab Software
Psychological Software Services
3304 W 75th St
Indianapolis, IN   46268-1664   317-257-9672
                                     Fax: 317-257-9674
                                     nsc@neuroscience.cnter.com
                                     www.neuroscience.cnter.com

Odie L Bracy, Executive Director
PSS CogRehab Software is a comprehensive and easy-to-use multimedia cognitive rehabilitation software available, for clinical and educational use with head injury, stroke LD/ADD and

other brain compromises. The packages include 64 computerized therapy tasks which contain modifiable parameters that will accommodate most requirements. Exercises include attention and executive skills, multiple modalities of visuosatial and memory skills, simple, complex, problem-solving skills.
$260 - $2500

1827   Parrot Easy Language Simple Anaylsis
Parrot Software
P.O.Box 250755
West Bloomfield, MI   48325   248-788-3223
                                          800-727-7681
                                     Fax: 248-788-3224
                                     support@parrotsoftware.com
                                     www.parrotsoftware.com

Dr. Frederic Weiner, Ph. D., CCC-SP, President, Owner
Designed for grammatical analysis of language samples. The user types and translates language samples of up to 100 utterances.

1828   SOLO Literacy Suite
Don Johnston
26799 West Commerce Drive
Volo, IL   60073   847-740-0749
                                          800-999-4660
                                     Fax: 847-740-7326
                                     info@donjohnston.com
                                     www.donjohnston.com

Don Johnston, Founder
Ruth Ziolkowski, President
Places all of the right tools, and a wide-range of embedded learning supports, at their fingertips. SOLO includes word prediction, a text reader, graphic organizer and talking word processor, putting students in charge of their own learning and accommodations. Students of varying ages and abilities have access to, and make progress in, the general education curriculum. *$79.00*

1829   TOVA
Universal Attention Disorders
3321 Cerritos Avenue
Los Alamitos, CA   90720   562-594-7700
                                          800-729-2886
                                     Fax: 800-452-6919
                                     info@tovatest.com
                                     www.tovatest.com

Lawrence M. Greenberg, MD
A computerized assessment which, in conjunction with classroom behavior ratings, is a highly effective screening tool for ADD. TOVA includes software, complete instructions, and supporting data including norms.

1830   Visi-Pitch III
Kayelemetrics Corporation
3 Paragon Drive
Montvale, NJ   07645   973-628-6200
                                          800-289-5297
                                     Fax: 201-391-2063
                                     sales@kaypentax.com

John Crump, President
Steve Crump, Direct Sales
Assists the speech/voice clinician in assessment and treatment tasks across an expansive range of disorders.

Software: Reading & Language Arts

1831   Choices, Choices 5.0
Tom Snyder Productions
100 Talcott Avenue
Watertown, MA   02472-5703   800-342-0236
                                     Ask@tomsnyder.com
                                     www.tomsnyder.com

Tom Snyder, Founder
Bridget Dalton, Ed.D, Author
Peggy Healy Stearns, Ph.D., Author
David Dockterman, Ed.D., Author

Teaches students to take responsibility for their behavior. Helps students develop the skills and awareness they need to make wise choices and to think through the consequences of their actions.

1832 Co: Writer
Don Johnston
26799 West Commerce Drive
Volo, IL 60073
847-740-0749
800-999-4660
Fax: 847-740-7326
info@donjohnston.com
www.donjohnston.com

Don Johnston, Founder
Ruth Ziolkowski, President

A software-based writing assistant that uses word prediction to cut through writing barriers and improve written expression. It is intended for students who struggle to write because of difficulty with spelling, syntax, and translating thoughts into writing. As students type, Co: Writer learns the context of the sentence and accurately 'predicts' words even when spelled phonetically or inventively. *$79.00*

1833 Community Exploration
Compass Learning
203 Colorado Street
Austin, TX 78701-3922
512-478-9600
800-678-1412
866-586-7387
Fax: 619-622-7873
support@compasslearning.com
www.compasslearning.com

Eric Loeffel, President, CEO
Tammy Deal, VP, Human Resources
Eric Wasser, VP, Sales
Eileen Shihadeh, VP, Marketing

An award-winning learning adventure takes students who are learning English as a second language on a field trip to the make-believe town of Cornerstone. More than 50 community locations come to life with sound and animation. While exploring places in this typical American community where people live, work and play, students also enhance important English language skills. Offers an exciting approach for any age student who needs to improve their English language proficiency. 4-12. *$19.95*

1834 Conversations
Educational Activities Software
5600 West 83rd Street
Suite 300, 8200 Tower
Bloomington, MN 55437
888-351-4199
800-447-5286
Fax: 239-225-9299
info@edmentum.com
www.edmentum.com

Vin Riera, President/CEO
Dan Juckniess, SVP, Sales & Professional Services
Stacey Herteux, VP, Human Resources
Rob Rueckl, Chief Financial Officer

Using American digitized voices, CONVERSATIONS provides 14 different dialogues in which the student can participate. The topics offer learners important information about American culture and the workplace. Available for DOS. *$195.00*

1835 Core-Reading and Vocabulary Development
Educational Activities
P.O.Box 87
Baldwin, NY 11510
516-223-4666
800-797-3223
Fax: 516-623-9282
www.edact.com

Alfred Harris, President
Carol Stern, VP

Students begin with 36 basic words and progress to more than 200. Reading and writing activities are coordinated and integrated throughout the program for more substantial permanent learning. Five units covering readability levels from pre-primer to grade three.

Full Program

1836 Friday Afternoon
203 Colorado Street
Austin, TX 78701-3922
512-478-9600
800-678-1412
866-586-7387
Fax: 619-622-7873
support@compasslearning.com
www.compasslearning.com

Eric Loeffel, President, CEO
Tammy Deal, VP, Human Resources
Eric Wasser, VP, Sales
Eileen Shihadeh, VP, Marketing

Save hours of preparation time and dazzle your students with interesting new activities to supplement their classroom learning. With Friday afternoon, you'll produce flash cards, word puzzles, even customized bingo cards and more, all at the click of a mouse. MacIntosh diskette. *$99.95*

1837 How to Read for Everyday Living
Educational Activities Software
5600 West 83rd Street
Suite 300, 8200 Tower
Bloomington, MN 55437
888-351-4199
800-447-5286
Fax: 239-225-9299
info@edmentum.com
www.edmentum.com

Vin Riera, President/CEO
Dan Juckniess, SVP, Sales & Professional Services
Stacey Herteux, VP, Human Resources
Rob Rueckl, Chief Financial Officer

Basic vocabulary and key words are taught and, when need, retaught using alternative teaching strategies. Passages that students read help put the vocabulary into context. Each lesson is followed by crossword and other puzzles check comprehension.

1838 Learning English: Primary
203 Colorado Street
Austin, TX 78701-3922
512-478-9600
800-678-1412
866-586-7387
Fax: 619-622-7873
support@compasslearning.com
www.compasslearning.com

Eric Loeffel, President, CEO
Tammy Deal, VP, Human Resources
Eric Wasser, VP, Sales
Eileen Shihadeh, VP, Marketing

Four stories and rhymes help students familiarize themselves with essential English language concepts, recognize patterns in language and associate words with objects. *$49.95*

1839 Learning English: Rhyme Time
Compass Learning
203 Colorado Street
Austin, TX 78701-3922
512-478-9600
800-678-1412
866-586-7387
Fax: 619-622-7873
support@compasslearning.com
www.compasslearning.com

Eric Loeffel, President, CEO
Tammy Deal, VP, Human Resources
Eric Wasser, VP, Sales
Eileen Shihadeh, VP, Marketing

Using classic children's rhymes in an animated multimedia program, students work on language skills, vocabulary and comprehension.

1840   Lexia I, II and III Reading Series
Lexia Learning Systems
200 Baker Ave Ext.
Concord, MA   01742   978-405-6200
                                       800-435-3942
                                       800-507-2772
                                    Fax: 978-287-0062
                                  info@lexialearning.com
                                  www.lexialearning.com

Nick Gaehde, President and CEO
Paul More, Vice President, Finance
Collin Earnst, Vice President of Marketing
Peter Koso, Vice President of Operations
Lexia's software helps children and adults with learning disabilities master their core reading skills. Based on the Orton Gillingham method, Lexia Early Reading, Phonics Based Reading and SOS (Strategies for Older Students) apply phonics principles to help students learn essential sound-symbol correspondence and decoding skills. The Quick Reading Tests generate detailed skill reports in only 5-8 minutes per student to provide data for further instruction. Price: $40-400 per workstation.

1841   Memory Castle
WINGS for Learning
1600 Green Hills Rd
Scotts Valley, CA   95066-4981   831-426-2228
                                    Fax: 831-464-3600

Ani Stocks, Owner
Introduces a strategy to increase memory skills via an adventure Q198game. Set in a castle, the game requires memory, reading, spelling skills and more to win.

1842   On a Green Bus: A UKanDu Little Book
Don Johnston
26799 West Commerce Drive
Volo, IL   60073   847-740-0749
                                       800-999-4660
                                    Fax: 847-740-7326
                                  info@donjohnston.com
                                  www.donjohnston.com

Don Johnston, Founder
Ruth Ziolkowski, President
This early literacy program that consists of several create-your-own 4-page animated stories that help build language experience on each page and then watch the page come alive with animation and sound. After completing the story, students can print it out to make a book which can be read over and over again. Because there are no wrong answers, all children can have a successful literacy experience. *$ 45.00*

1843   Open Book
Freedom Scientific
11800 31st Court North
St Petersburg, FL   33716   727-803-8000
                                       800-444-4443
                                    Fax: 727-803-8001
                                 info@freedomscientific.com
                                 www.freedomscientific.com

Lee Hamilton, President, CEO, and Chairman of
Mike Self, Sales Representative (Alabama)
Joseph McDaniel, Sales Representative (Alaska and
Bobby Lakey, Sales Representative (Arkansas)
Software that reads scanned text allowed and includes other features that aid the vision-impaired. *$995.00*

1844   Optimum Resource Software
1 Mathews Drive
Suite 107
Hilton Head Island, SC   29926   843-689-8000
                                    Fax: 843-689-8008
                                   info@stickybear.com
                                   www.stickybear.com

Richard Hefter, President
Optimum Resource publishes over 100 K-12 education curriculum software titles under its varietal brands, StickyBear, MiddleWare, High School and Tools for Teachers. Most pro-

grams are available in Bilingual English/Spanish, and are offered with options for the single user through 30 users.

1845   Parts of Speech
Optimum Resource
1 Mathews Drive
Suite 107
Hilton Head Island, SC   29926   843-689-8000
                                    Fax: 843-689-8008
                                   info@stickybear.com
                                   www.stickybear.com

Richard Hefter, President
Designed to help students build grammar and vocabulary as they strengthen reading and writing ability. Grades 3 to 9. *$59.95*

1846   Programs for Aphasia and Cognitive Disorders
Parrot Software
P.O.Box 250755
West Bloomfield, MI   48325   248-788-3223
                                       800-727-7681
                                    Fax: 248-788-3224
                                 support@parrotsoftware.com
                                 www.parrotsoftware.com

Dr. Frederic Weiner, Ph. D., CCC-SP, President, Owner
Over 50 different computer programs that facilitate language, memory and attention training. Programs are available for MS DOS, WINDOWS and Apple II.

1847   Punctuation Rules
Optimum Resource
1 Mathews Drive
Suite 107
Hilton Head Island, SC   29926   843-689-8000
                                    Fax: 843-689-8008
                                   info@stickybear.com
                                   www.stickybear.com

Richard Hefter, President
Punctuation Rules is designed to help students improve their punctuation skills. Students work with appropriate level sentences which follow common rules of punctuation. The program covers material ranging from categories of sentences to forming possessives and allows students to gain strength in their ability to correctly use periods, commas, apostrophes, question marks, colons, hyphens, quotation marks, exclamation points and more. Grades 3-9. Bilingual. *$59.95*

1848   Quick Reading Test, Phonics Based Reading, Reading SOS (Strategies for Older Students)
Lexia Learning Systems
200 Baker Ave Ext.
Concord, MA   01742   978-405-6200
                                       800-435-3942
                                       800-507-2772
                                    Fax: 978-287-0062
                                  info@lexialearning.com
                                  www.lexialearning.com

Nick Gaehde, President and CEO
Paul More, Vice President, Finance
Collin Earnst, Vice President of Marketing
Peter Koso, Vice President of Operations
Lexia's software helps children and adults with learning disabilities master their core reading skills. Based on the Orton Gillingham method, Phonics Based Reading and S.O.S. (Strategies for the Older Student) apply phonics principles to help students learn essential sound-symbol correspondence and decoding skills. The Quick Reading Tests generate detailed phonemic skills reports in only 5-8 minutes per student to provide teachers with accurate data to focus their instruction. Price: $67-$500.

1849 Quick Talk
Educational Activities Software
5600 West 83rd Street
Suite 300, 8200 Tower
Bloomington, MN 55437
888-351-4199
800-447-5286
Fax: 239-225-9299
info@edmentum.com
www.edmentum.com

Vin Riera, President/CEO
Dan Juckniess, SVP, Sales & Professional Services
Stacey Herteux, VP, Human Resources
Rob Rueckl, Chief Financial Officer
Students will learn and use new vocabulary immediately: high-frequency, everyday vocabulary words are introduced and used contextually using human speech, graphics and text. Voice-interactive program (MS-DOS). *$65.00*

1850 Race the Clock
Mindplay
4400 E. Broadway Blvd
Suite 400
Tucson, AZ 85711
520-888-1800
800-221-7911
Fax: 520-888-7904
mail@mindplay.com
www.mindplay.com

Dan Figurski, Senior Vice President of Business
Chris Coleman, VP, Business Development
Judith Bliss, CEO
Brian Williams, Development Manager
A matching game, uses the animation capabilities to teach verbs. The player chooses a matching game from a menu.

1851 Read: Out Loud
Don Johnston
26799 West Commerce Drive
Volo, IL 60073
847-740-0749
800-999-4660
Fax: 847-740-7326
info@donjohnston.com
www.donjohnston.com

Don Johnston, Founder
Ruth Ziolkowski, President
An accessible text reader that provides access to the curriculum. It features high-quality text to speech and study tools that help students read with comprehension. *$79.00*

1852 Reader Rabbit
Learning Company
Ste 1900
100 Pine St
San Francisco, CA 94111-5205
415-659-2000
800-825-4420
Fax: 415-659-2020
thelearningco@hmhpub.com
www.thelearningcompany.com

Linda K. Zecher, President and CEO
Eric Shuman, Chief Financial Officer
John K. Dragoon, Executive Vice President and Chi
William Bayers, Executive Vice President and Gen
Supports young students in building fundamental reading readiness skills in a playful, multi-sensory environment.

1853 Reading Comprehension Series
Optimum Resource
1 Mathews Drive
Suite 107
Hilton Head Island, SC 29926- 3765
843-689-8000
Fax: 843-689-8008
info@stickybear.com
www.stickybear.com

Richard Hefter, President
The Reading Comprehension Series, includes seven volumes packed with intriguing multi-level stories. Each volume will capture the interest of children ages 8-14 while teaching them crucial reading comprehension skills. These open-ended programs are versatile and easy to use, and Bilingual. *$59.95*

1854 Simon SIO
Don Johnston
26799 West Commerce Drive
Volo, IL 60073
847-740-0749
800-999-4660
Fax: 847-740-7326
info@donjohnston.com
www.donjohnston.com

Don Johnston, Founder
Ruth Ziolkowski, President
A researched and widely field-tested phonics program for beginning readers, developed in collaboration with Dr. Ted Hasselbring of Vanderbilt University. The program uses a personal tutor to deliver individualized instruction and corrective feedback. *$79.00*

1855 Sound Sentences
Educational Activities Software
5600 West 83rd Street
Suite 300, 8200 Tower
Bloomington, MN 55437
888-351-4199
800-447-5286
Fax: 239-225-9299
info@edmentum.com
www.edmentum.com

Vin Riera, President/CEO
Dan Juckniess, SVP, Sales & Professional Services
Stacey Herteux, VP, Human Resources
Rob Rueckl, Chief Financial Officer
This sound-interactive program breaks away from traditional language instruction. Instead of formal concentration on verb and basic vocabulary, students meet everyday English with colloquialisms they will hear in real life situations. They reinforce their knowledge of sentence structure while acquiring the ability to communicate in daily settings. (For MAC, MS-DOS and Windows). *$65.00*

1856 Spelling Rules
Optimum Resource
1 Mathews Drive
Suite 107
Hilton Head Island, SC 29926- 3765
843-689-8000
Fax: 843-689-8008
info@stickybear.com
www.stickybear.com

Richard Hefter, President
A curriculum based, easy-to-use program that provides students with the practice they need to build strong spelling skills. Concepts discussed include plurals, compounds, i-before-e, capitalization, and more. Grades 3 to 9. Bilingual. *$59.95*

1857 Start-to-Finish Library
Don Johnston
26799 West Commerce Drive
Volo, IL 60073
847-740-0749
800-999-4660
Fax: 847-740-7326
info@donjohnston.com
www.donjohnston.com

Don Johnston, Founder
Ruth Ziolkowski, President
Offers struggling readers a wide selection of engaging narrative chapter books written at two readability levels (2-3rd and 4-5th grade) and delivered in three media formats. Professionally-narrated audio and computer supports help scaffold reading to ensure success. *$79.00*

1858 Start-to-Finish Literacy Starters
Don Johnston
26799 West Commerce Drive
Volo, IL 60073
847-740-0749
800-999-4660
Fax: 847-740-7326
info@donjohnston.com
www.donjohnston.com

Don Johnston, Founder
Ruth Ziolkowski, President

A reading series intended for students with multiple disabilities who are in 3-12th grade, but reading at a beginning level. Dr. Karen Erickson developed this series, which combines switch-accessible software with three types of text. *$79.00*

1859 Stickybear Reading Comprehension
Optimum Resource
1 Mathews Drive
Suite 107
Hilton Head Island, SC 29926- 3765   843-689-8000
                                        Fax: 843-689-8008
                                        info@stickybear.com
                                        www.stickybear.com

Richard Hefter, President

This multi-level reading comprehension program helps children improve reading skills with 30 high-interest stories and question sets created by the Weekly Reader editors. Children learn to recognize main ideas, define sequence, using context to identify words, and more. Grades 2 to 4. Bilingual. *$59.95*

1860 Stickybear Reading Fun Park
Optimum Resource
1 Mathews Drive
Suite 107
Hilton Head Island, SC 29926- 3765   843-689-8000
                                        Fax: 843-689-8008
                                        info@stickybear.com
                                        www.stickybear.com

Richard Hefter, President

Children discover and practice critical reading skills as the Stickybear family guides users through unique, action-packed activities, each with multiple levels of difficulty and skills that address both the auditory and visual needs of budding readers. Pre-K through 3rd grade. *$59.95*

1861 Stickybear Reading Room Deluxe
Optimum Resource
1 Mathews Drive
Suite 107
Hilton Head Island, SC 29926- 3765   843-689-8000
                                        Fax: 843-689-8008
                                        info@stickybear.com
                                        www.stickybear.com

Richard Hefter, President

Children build vocabulary and reading comprehension skills using hundreds of word/picture sets and thousands of put-together sentence parts. K-3rd grade. Bilingual, English/Spanish. *$59.95*

1862 Stickybear Spelling
Optimum Resource
1 Mathews Drive
Suite 107
Hilton Head Island, SC 29926- 3765   843-689-8000
                                        Fax: 843-689-8008
                                        info@stickybear.com
                                        www.stickybear.com

Richard Hefter, President

Children discover and practice critical spelling skills as they work with three unique action-packed activities, each with four graded levels of difficulty. The program is open-ended and teachers may add, change and modify the word lists for each individual. Stickybear Spelling contains more than 2000 recorded words. Levels may be set to allow students of different ages or abilities to compete effectively. Grades 2 through 4. *$59.95*

1863 Tomorrow's Promise: Language Arts
Compass Learning
13500 Evening Creek Drive North
Suite 600
San Diego, CA 92128   858-668-2586
                          866-475-0317
                          Fax: 858-408-2903
                          info@bridgepointeducation.com
                          www.bridgepointeducation.com

Andrew S. Clark, Founder, Chief Executive Officer
Diane Thompson, SVP, General Counsel
Charlene Dackerman, SVP, Human Resources
Daniel J. Devine, Executive Vice President & CFO

You'll strengthen students' grammar, usage and vocabulary skills and promote higher order thinking skills with this comprehensive Language Arts curriculum. It utilizes cross-curricular, thematic instruction engaging multimedia learning exercises that encourage writing, speaking and listening proficiency. Promotes higher order thinking skills. *$279.95*

1864 Tomorrow's Promise: Reading
Compass Learning
203 Colorado Street
Austin, TX 78701-3922   512-478-9600
                            800-678-1412
                            866-586-7387
                            Fax: 619-622-7873
                            support@compasslearning.com
                            www.compasslearning.com

Eric Loeffel, President, CEO
Tammy Deal, VP, Human Resources
Eric Wasser, VP, Sales
Eileen Shihadeh, VP, Marketing

This multimedia curriculum balances thematic, interactive exploration with core skills development, increasing your students' early reading proficiency, building a solid literacy foundation and fostering a lifelong love for reading. *$279.95*

1865 Tomorrow's Promise: Spelling
Compass Learning
203 Colorado Street
Austin, TX 78701-3922   512-478-9600
                            800-678-1412
                            866-586-7387
                            Fax: 619-622-7873
                            support@compasslearning.com
                            www.compasslearning.com

Eric Loeffel, President, CEO
Tammy Deal, VP, Human Resources
Eric Wasser, VP, Sales
Eileen Shihadeh, VP, Marketing

Lovable characters and engaging multimedia effects put young students on a fast-track to early spelling proficiency with fourteen activities and three games. A full year's instruction on each CD includes 30 world lists per grade, in story context, or create word lists to suit your needs. This program addresses students' multiple learning styles and rewards students as they progress through each stage of spelling skill acquisition. *$99.95*

1866 Vocabulary Development
Optimum Resource
1 Mathews Drive
Suite 107
Hilton Head Island, SC 29926- 3765   843-689-8000
                                        Fax: 843-689-8008
                                        info@stickybear.com
                                        www.stickybear.com

Richard Hefter, President

A featured program in the middle school series. Vocabulary Development is designed to help students increase vocabulary as they strengthen reading skills. Students relate their current knowledge of vocabulary to the context in which they discover an unfamiliar word. Utilizing a variety of contextual aids, this program illustrates synonyms, antonyms, prefixes, suffixes, homophones, multiple meanings and context clues, allowing students to apply experience and context. *$59.95*

1867 Whoops
Cornucopia Software
P.O.Box 6111
Albany, CA 94706   510-528-7000
                        supportstaff@practicemagic.com
                        www.practicemagic.com

Christina Morua, Manager

Checks spelling three ways. It checks words as they are typed, it checks an entire screen and highlights the errors and it reads ASCII text files from a disk and lists errors.

Software: Vocational

1868 Films Media Group
Infobase Publishing
132 W 31st St, 17th Floor
New York, NY 10001
800-322-8755
Fax: 800-678-3633
custserv@factsonfile.com
www.infobaselearning.com

Melinda Gallo, Senior Account Executive
Educational publisher of DVD programming for schools and libraries. *$64.86*
ISBN 0-927368-59-5

1869 Functional Literacy System
Conover Company
4 Brookwood Court
Appleton, WI 54914
920-231-4667
800-933-1933
Fax: 800-933-1943
support@conovercompany.com
www.conovercompany.com

Terry Schmitz, Founder and Owner
Mike , Vice President of Operations
Art Janowiak, Vice President of Sales
Assessment and skill building for basic functional literacy. This multimedia software program is adult in format and uses live action video taken in actual community settings to help learners become more capable of functioning independently. Twenty different programs are currently available. *$99.00*

1870 Learning Activity Packets
4 Brookwood Court
Appleton, WI 54914
920-231-4667
800-933-1933
Fax: 800-933-1943
support@conovercompany.com
www.conovercompany.com

Terry Schmitz, Founder and Owner
Mike , Vice President of Operations
Art Janowiak, Vice President of Sales
Demonstrates how basic academic skills relate to 30 major career areas. LAPs provide valuable diagnostics in applied academic applications and demonstrates to users the importance of academics as they relate to the workplace. Software. *$99.00*

1871 Microcomputer Evaluation of Careers & Academics (MECA)
Conover Company
4 Brookwood Court
Appleton, WI 54914
920-231-4667
800-933-1933
Fax: 800-933-1943
support@conovercompany.com
www.conovercompany.com

Terry Schmitz, Founder and Owner
Mike , Vice President of Operations
Art Janowiak, Vice President of Sales
A cost-effective, technology-based, career development system which provides users with opportunities to get their hands dirty. The MECA system utilizes work simulations and is built around common occupational clusters. Each cluster, or career area, consists of hands-on WORK SAMPLES which provide a variety of career exploration and assessment experiences, linked to LEARNING ACTIVITY PACKETS, which integrate basic academic skills into the career planning and placement process. $580-$1,070.

1872 OASYS
Vertek
12835 Bellevue-Redmond Road
Suite 310
Bellevue, WA 98005
425-455-9921
800-220-4409
Fax: 425-454-7264
sales@vertekinc.com
www.vertekinc.com

Debra Callahan, Sales Representative, Northern California
Tim Whitney, Sales Representative, Ohio, Michigan
Beverly Duncan, Sales Representative, Florida
Debbie Gordon, Sales Representative, Illinois
A software system that matches a person's skills and abilities to occupations and employers.

1873 Reading in the Workplace
Educational Activities Software
5600 West 83rd Street
Suite 300, 8200 Tower
Bloomington, MN 55437-585
888-351-4199
800-447-5286
Fax: 239-225-9299
info@edmentum.com
www.edmentum.com

Vin Riera, President/CEO
Dan Juckniess, SVP, Sales & Professional Services
Stacey Herteux, VP, Human Resources
Rob Rueckl, Chief Financial Officer
A job-based, reading software program using real-life problems and solutions to capture students' attention and improve their vocabulary and comprehension skills. Units include: automotive, clerical, health care and construction. *$295.00*

1874 Stickybear Typing
Optimum Resource
1 Mathews Drive
Suite 107
Hilton Head Island, SC 29926- 3765
843-689-8000
Fax: 843-689-8008
www.stickybear.com

Richard Hefter, President
The award winning Stickybear Typing program allows users to sharpen typing skills and achieve keyboard mastery with three engaging and amusing multi-level activities. *$59.95*

1875 Work-Related Vocational Assessment Systems: Computer Based
Valpar International
P.O.Box 5767
Tucson, AZ 85703-767
262-797-0840
800-633-3321
Fax: 262-797-8488
sales@valparint.com
www.valparint.com

Neal Gunderson, President
Criterion-referenced to Department of Labor standards. Evaluate academic levels for reading, spelling, math and language, interests, personalities, cognitive and physical aptitudes.

1876 Workplace Skills: Learning How to Function on the Job
Programming Concepts
8700 Shoal Creek Boulevard
Austin, TX 78757-6897
512-451-3246
800-897-3202
Fax: 800-397-7633
general@proedinc.com
www.proedinc.com

Jeff McLane, Founder
Lee Wilson, President and CEO
Randy Pennington, Executive VP
David Keith, Vice President of IT
Offers parents and educators a functional means by which to discuss all aspects of finding and keeping a job. *$49.95*

Word Processors

1877   DARCI
Wes Test Engineering Corporation
810 Shepard Lane
Farmington, UT 84025

801-451-9191
Fax: 801-451-9393
webmail@westest.com
westest.com

Robert Lessmann, President
James Lynds
Provides transparent access to all computer functions by replacing the computer's keyboard with a smart joystick. *$975.00*

1878   Eye Relief Word Processing Software
SkiSoft Publishing Corporation
P.O.Box 364
Lexington, MA 02420-4

781-863-1876
www.skisoft.com

Ken Skier, President
Cynthia Skier, CFO
Large-type word processing program for visually-impaired PC users. *$295.00*

1879   IntelliTalk
Intelli Tools
24 Prime Parkway
Natick, MA 01760

707-773-2000
800-547-6747
Fax: 707-773-2001
customerservice@cambiumtech.com
www.intellitools.com

Beth Davis, Director Sales Operations
Lori Castle, Supervisor
Arjan Khalsa, CEO
Talking word-processing program available for MacIntosh, Apple IIe, IBM compatible and Windows computers. *$39.95*

1880   Large Type
P.O.Box T
Hewitt, NJ 07421-2088

973-853-6585
800-736-2216
Fax: 928-832-2894
http://www.angelfire.com

Don Selwyn, Vice President
Rev. Tom Schwanda, President & Chairman
Robt. Fondiller, Ph.D., P.E, Vice President
Everett G. Ball, Treasurer
Display enlargement programs for visually impaired users. Consist of a variety of programs for different needs, ranging from basic to full-featured.

1881   Pegasus LITE
Words+
Ste 109
42505 10th St W
Lancaster, CA 93534-7059

661-723-6523
800-869-8521
Fax: 661-723-2114
info@words-plus.com
www.words-plus.com

Phil Lawrence, VP
Provides all of the strategies currently being used in AAC, from dynamic display color pictographic language, to dual-word prediction text language, in a single system. *$6995.00*

1882   Up and Running
Intelli Tools
24 Prime Parkway
Natick, MA 01760

707-773-2000
800-547-6747
Fax: 707-773-2001
customerservice@cambiumtech.com

Beth Davis, Director Sales Operations
Lori Castle, Supervisor
Arjan Khalsa, CEO

Instantly use hundreds of popular commercial software programs with this custom collection of setups and overlays. *$69.95*

1883   Write: OutLoud
Don Johnston
26799 West Commerce Drive
Volo, IL 60073-9675

847-740-0749
800-999-4660
Fax: 847-740-7326
info@donjohnston.com
www.donjohnston.com

Don Johnston, Founder
Ruth Ziolkowski, President
The award-winning feasible and user friendly talking word processor with talking spell checker. Text-to-speech technology provides multi-sensory learning and positive reinforcements for writers of all ages and ability levels. *$99.00*

Conferences & Shows

General

1884   AACRC Annual Meeting
American Assn. of Children's Residential Centers
648 N. Plankinton Ave.
Suite 425
Milwaukee, WI   53203   877-332-2272
                                ksisson@togetherthevoice.org
                                    togetherthevoice.org

Kari Sisson, Executive Director
Laurah Currey, President
Joe Ford, Vice President
Kerry Ann Goldsmith, Secretary
One-day program that addresses accreditation as it relates to current behavioral health care challenges held in Pasadena, CA.
October

1885   AADB National Conference
American Association of the Deaf-Blind
3825 LaVista Rd. W-2
Tucker, GA   30084   aadb-info@aadb.org
                                        www.aadb.org

Jen,e Alleman-Goodman, President
Ren, Pellerin, Vice President
Chris Woodfill, Secretary
Mark Gasaway, Treasurer
A week of general meetings, workshops, tours and evening recreational activities.

1886   AAIDD Annual Meeting
American Association on Mental Retardation
501 3rd St. NW
Suite 200
Washington, DC   20001   202-387-1968
                                    Fax: 202-387-2193
                                        maria@aaidd.org
                                        www.aamr.org

Susan Havercamp, President
Elizabeth Perkins, President Elect
Laura Lee McIntyre, Vice President
Alexandra Bonardi, Secretary/Treasurer
This annual meeting offers a full compliment of workshops, symposia, and multiperspective sessions that fill four days including social events.
May/June

1887   AAO Annual Meeting
American Academy Of Opthamology
655 Beach St.
San Francisco, CA   94109-1336   415-561-8500
                                    Fax: 415-561-8533
                                        faao@aao.org
                                        www.faao.org

Cynthia Ann Bradford, President
David W. Parke II, Chief Executive Officer
Maria M. Aaron, Secretry for Annual Meeting
Matthew W. MacCumber, Chair
Offers the most comprehensive program with more than 2000 scientific presentations and six subspecialty day programs.
October

1888   ABD Winter Conference
American Board of Disability Analysts
4525 Harding Rd.
Second Floor
Nashville, TN   37205   americanbd@aol.com
                                    www.americandisability.org

Kenneth Anchor, Executive Director
A bi-annual event hosted by the American Board of Disability Analysts cover topics including: case studies, applied research, polemical/ideological talks, ethics, innovative techniques, evaluation strategies, forensic experiences, customized software, economic issues, private practice insights, earnings loss projec-

tions, life care plans, hedonic assessments, and labor market surveys.
october

1889   ACA Annual Conference
American Counseling Association
6101 Stevenson Ave.
Alexandria, VA   22304   703-823-9800
                                        800-347-6647
                                    Fax: 800-473-2329
                                    webmaster@counseling.org
                                        www.counseling.org

Gerard Lawson, President
Simone Lambert, President Elect
Julie Beaver, Executive Assistant
Richard Yep, CEO
Promotes the development of professional counselors, advancing the counseling profession, and using the profession and practice of counseling to promote respect for human dignity and diversity.
March/April

1890   ADA Annual Scientific Sessions
American Diabetes Association
2451 Crystal Dr.
Suite 900
Arlington, VA   22201   703-549-1500
                                        800-342-2383
                                    Fax: 703-836-7439
                                    webmaster@diabetes.org
                                        www.diabetes.org

David A. DeMarco, Chairman
Brenda Montgomery, President
Alvin C. Powers, President
Umesh Verma, Secretary/Treasurer
Brings together physicians, scientists and other health care professionals from around the world to learn about the latest advances in basic and clinical science for diabetes.

1891   AER Annual International Conference
Assoc. for Educ. & Rehab of the Blind/Vis. Imp.
1703 N. Beauregard St.
Suite 440
Alexandria, VA   22311- 1744   703-671-4500
                                    Fax: 703-671-6391
                                        aer@aerbvi.org
                                        www.aerbvi.org

Jim Adams, President
Louis Tutt, Executive Director
Ginger Croce, Deputy Executive Director & Chief Marketing Officer
Angela Smith, Director of Prefessional Development & Internal Relations
Dedicated to rendering support and assistance to the professionals who work in all phases of education and rehabilitation of blind and visually impaired children and adults.
July

1892   AG Bell Convention
Alexander Graham Bell Association
3417 Volta Pl., NW
Washington, DC   20007   202-337-5220
                                    Fax: 202-337-8314
                                    TTY:202-337-5221
                                        info@agbell.org
                                        www.agbell.org

Ted A. Meyer, Chair
Catharine McNally, Chair-Elect
Susan Lenihan, Secretary
Emilio Alonso Mendoza, Chief Executive Officer
Over 60 booths offering information on resources and technology for the deaf and hard of hearing.
June

1893 APSE National Conference
Association for Persons in Supported Employment
414 Hungerford Dr.
Suite 224
Rockville, MD 20850

301-279-0060
Fax: 301-279-0075
cesp@apse.org
www.apse.org

Derek Nord, President
Allison Wohl, Executive Director
Jenny Stonemeier, Deputy Executive Director
Boshia McRoy, Administrative Associate

A major conference on Supported Employment. The conference includes 130 sessions presented by nationally recognized leaders in the field. Conference attendees come from all 50 states, Canada and several foreign countries and include professionals in supported employment, occupational therapy, rehabilitation technology and other related fields.
July

1894 ASHA Convention
American Speech-Language-Hearing Association
2200 Research Blvd.
Rockville, MD 20850-3289

301-296-5700
800-638-8255
convention@asha.org
www.asha.org

Gail J. Richard, President
Elise Davis-Mcfarland, President-Elect
Margot L. Beckerman, Chair
Arlene A. Pietranton, Chief Executive Officer

Exhibits by companies specializing in alternative and augmentative communication products, publishers, software and hardware companies, and hearing aid testing equipment manufacturers. Speech-Language Pathologists are professionals who identify, assess, and treat speech and language problems. Audiologists are hearing health care professionals who specialize in preventing, identifying and assessing hearing disorders as well as providing audiologic treatment including hearing aids and more.
November

1895 ASIA Annual Scientific Meeting
American Spinal Injury Association
2209 Dickens Rd.
Richmond, VA 23230-2005

804-565-6396
Fax: 804-282-0090
asia.office@asia-spinalinjury.org
www.asia-spinalinjury.org

Patty Duncan, Executive Director
Carolyn Moffatt, Association Manager
Cynthia Bolden, Administrative Assistant

Professional association for physicans and other health professionals working in all aspects of spinal cord injury. Also holds an annual scientific that surveys the latest advancements in the field.
May

1896 ATIA Conference
Assistive Technology Industry Association
330 N. Wabash Ave.
Suite 2000
Chicago, IL 60611-4267

312-321-5172
877-687-2842
Fax: 312-673-6659
info@atia.org
atia.org

Tara Rudnicki, Board President
Bruce Miles, Treasurer
Dave Hershberger, Secretary

The ATIA Conference is the largest international conference showcasing excellence in assistive technology.

1897 Abilities Expo
16501 Ventura Blvd.
Suite 510
Encino, CA 91436

310-405-1317
Fax: 424-238-6358
abilities.com/expos

David Korse, President & CEO
Caryn Bates, Director of Operations

Abilities Expo is a national event for people with disabilities, their families, caregivers, and healthcare professionals. Meets in Chicago, Houston, Boston, Bay Area, Los Angeles, New York, and Toronto.

1898 American Academy for Cerebral Palsy and Developmental Medicine Annual Conference
555 East Wells
Suite 1100
Milwaukee, WI 53202

414-918-3014
Fax: 414-276-2146
info@aacpdm.org
www.aacpdm.org

Unni Narayanan, President
Sarah Winter, First Vice President
Uri Givon, Secretary
Sylvia Ounpuu, Treasurer

The Annual Meeting is a 3-day event, held in the Fall, designed to provide targeted opportunities for dissemination of information in the basic sciences, prevention, diagnosis, treatment, and technical advances as applied to persons with cerebral palsy and development disorders.
September

1899 American Academy of Environmental Medicine: Annual Conference
6505 E. Central Ave.
Suite 296
Wichita, KS 67206

316-684-5500
defox@aaemonline.org
aaemonline.org

Gregg Govett, President
Derek Lang, President Elect
Janette Hope, Secretary
James W. Willoughby, Treasurer

AAEM is dedicated to the education of health care professionals from all traditional and alternative disciplines, the public, government, industry, and health insurance officials, and are looking for more efficacious and cost effective ways to understand, diagnose, treat, and prevent these disorders. Annual Meeting of the Academy is an open forum addressing aspects of Environmental Medicine as well as related topics, such as mental health.

1900 American Board of Disability Analysts Annual Conference
Disability Analyst
4525 Harding Rd.
Second Floor
Nashville, TN 37205

americanbd@aol.com
www.americandisability.org

Kenneth Anchor, Executive Director

Annual conference held for members to meet and discuss current events and attend seminars.

1901 Annual Conference on Dyslexia and Related Learning Disabilities
New York Branch International Dyslexia Association
1550 Deer Park Ave.
Suite C
Long Island, NY 11729

631-261-7441
info@lidyslexia.org
www.lidyslexia.org

Concetta Russo, President
Glenna Rubin, Vice President
Carolyn McIntyre, Secretary
Julia Bunyatov, Treasurer

The International Dyslexia Association (IDA) is an organization focused on the complex issues of dyslexia and related lan-

guage-based learning disabilities which make it difficult to learn to read and write.
March

1902   Annual TASH Conference
TASH
1875 Eye St. NW
Suite 582
Washington, DC   20006
                                        202-429-2080
                                        Fax: 202-540-9019
                                        info@tash.org
                                        tash.org/conferences-events
Ruthie-Marie Beckwith, Executive Director
Dawn Brown, Development Director
Ralph Edwards, President
Ruby Moore, Vice President
Each year, the TASH Conference strengthens the disability field by connecting attendees to innovative information and resources, facilitating connections between stakeholders within the disability movement, and helping attendees reignite their passion for an inclusive world.

1903   Arc National Convention, The
The Arc
1825 K St., NW
Suite 1200
Washington, DC   20006
                                        202-955-6148
                                        info@thearc.org
                                        convention.thearc.org
Elise McMillan, President
Frederick Misilo, Vice President
Carol Wheeler, Secretary
Doug Church, Treasurer
Experts and professionals gather from all over the world share best practices, struggles, successes and hopes for the future, and continue the conversation about protecting and promoting the human and civil rights for individuals with intellectual and developmental disabilities.

1904   Association on Higher Education and Disability
107 Commerce Centre Dr.
Suite 204
Huntersville, NC   28078
                                        704-947-7779
                                        Fax: 704-948-7779
                                        www.ahead.org
Jamie Axelrod, President
Gaeir Dietrich, Treasurer
Jstephan Smith, Executive Director
Katy Washington, Secretary
AHEAD is a professional membership organization for individuals involved in the development of policy and in the provision of quality services to meet the needs of persons with disabilities involved in all areas of higher education, promoting full and equal participation.
July

1905   Attention Deficit Disorders Association, Southern Region: Annual Conference
12345 Jones Rd.
Suite 287-7
Houston, TX   77070
                                        281-897-0982
                                        Fax: 281-894-6883
                                        addaoffice@sbcglobal.net
                                        www.adda-sr.org
Carlye Read, President
Barbara Beard, Vice President
Judy German, Treasurer
The Attention Deficit Disorders Association provides a resource network, supports individuals impacted by ADHHD and related condition and to advocate for the development of community resources.
February

1906   Blind Children's Center Annual Meeting
Blind Children's Center
4120 Marathon St.
Los Angeles, CA   90029-3584
                                        323-664-2153
                                        www.blindchildrenscenter.org
Sarah E. Orth, CEO
Dannett M. Beck, President
Lawrence F. Meyer, Treasurer
Lisa D. Hansen, Secretary
A family-centered agency which serves children with visual impairments from birth to school-age. The center-based and home-based services help the children to acquire skills and build their independence. The Center utilizes its expertise and experience to serve families and professionals worldwide through support services, education and research.
September

1907   Blinded Veterans Association National Convention
Blinded Veterans Association
125 N West St
Suite 300
Alexandria, VA   22314
                                        202-371-8880
                                        800-669-7079
                                        Fax: 202-371-8258
                                        bva@bva.org
                                        www.bva.org
Dale Stamper, National President
Joe Parker, National Vice President
Albert Avina, Executive Director
Stuart Nelson, Manager of Communications
The convention has three functions: to serve as a platform for Association business, to educate blinded veterans about the resources available to them, and to provide a means whereby blinded veterans can support one another.
August

1908   CQL Accreditation
Council on Quality and Leadership
100 West Rd.
Suite 300
Towson, MD   21204
                                        410-583-0060
                                        info@thecouncil.org
                                        www.c-q-l.org
Gayle DiCesare, President and CEO
Gary Edwards, Executive Director
William Beattie, Board Chairperson
Jennifer Becher, Vice Chairperson
CQL Accreditation is a leader in working with human service organizations and systems to continuously define, measure and improve quality of life and quality of services.

1909   Centers of Excellence Leadership Conference
National Parkinson Foundation
200 SE 1st St.
Suite 800
Miami, FL   33131
                                        800-473-4636
                                        Fax: 305-537-9901
                                        contact@parkinson.com
                                        parkinson.org
John L. Lehr, CEO
James Beck, Vice President
Yashnahia Cortorreal, Vice President
Curt DeGreff, Senior Vice President
The mission of the National Parkinson Foundation is to make life better for people affected by Parkinson's through expert care, research, and education. The goal of the conference is to convene the medical directors, center coordinators and other leaders from the Centers of Excellence to discuss the latest research and best practices in care delivery and to highlight NPF's programs.
July/August

1910   Closing the Gap's Annual Conference
P.O. Box 68
Henderson, MN   56044
                                        507-248-3294
                                        Fax: 507-248-3810
                                        www.closingthegap.com
Dolores Hagen, Co-Founder
Budd Hagen, Co-Founder

Topics cover a broad spectrum of technology as it is being applied to all disabilities and age groups in education, rehabilitation, vocation and independent living. People with disabilities, special educators, rehabilitation professionals, administrators, service/care providers, personnel managers, government officials, and hardware/software developers share their experiences and insights at this significant networking experience.
October

1911   Council for Exceptional Children Annual Convention and Expo
2900 Crystal Drive
Suite 1000
Arlington, VA 22202-3557   888-232-7733
                                             TTY:866-915-5000
                                        service@cec.sped.org
                                             www.cec.sped.org

Alexander T. Graham, Executive Director
Sharon Rodriguez, Senior Executive Assistant
Craig Evans, Director of Operations
Works to improve the educational success of children with disabilities and/or gifts and talents.
April

1912   Disability Matters
Springboard Consulting
14 Glenbrook Dr.
Mendham, NJ 07945   973-813-7260
                                        Fax: 973-813-7261
                                   info@consultspringboard.com
                                   www.consultspringboard.com

James C. Barrood, Executive Director
Steve Cody, Managing Partner & Co-founder
Meryle Mahrer Kaplan, Vice President
Bill Dueease, President
Features outstanding content as delivered by leading disability experts from corporations, academia, national non-profits and governments across North America. Conferences also take place in Europe and Asia-Pacific.

1913   Eye Bank Association of America Annual Meeting
Eye Bank Association of America
1101 17th St., NW
Suite 400
Washington, DC 20036   202-775-4999
                                        Fax: 202-429-6036
                                     malene@restoresight.org
                                         www.restoresight.org

Kevin Corcoran, CAE, President & CEO
Molly Georgakis, Vice-President of Member Services
Bernie Dellario, Director of Finance
Jennifer DeMatteo, Director of Regulations and Standards
A four day program, which includes a series of presentations in administrative, hospital development, scientific and technical fields that are relative to eye banking.
June

1914   IDF National Conference
Immune Deficiency Foundation
110 West Rd.
Suite 300
Towson, MD 21204   800-296-4433
                                        Fax: 410-321-9165
                                           www.primaryimmune.org

Marcia Boyle, President & Founder
Katherine Antilla, Vice President, Education & Volunteers
Christine Belser, Vice President, Programs & Communications
Lawrence A. LaMotte, Vice President, Public Policy
The Immune Deficiency Foundation (IDF) brings together the community every other year for a three-day conference, the world's largest gathering of people living with primary immunodeficiency diseases. From physicians to nurses to specialized life management experts, individuals and families are presented with an opportunity to network with those involved in research and treatment.
June

1915   Joint Conference with ABMPP Annual Conference
American Board of Disability Analysts
4525 Harding Rd.
Second Floor
Nashville, TN 37205   americanbd@aol.com
                                        www.americandisability.org

Kenneth Anchor, Executive Director
Joint Conference with ABMPP Annual Conference Charleston, South Carolina.
May

1916   Lowe Syndrome Conference
Lowe Syndrome Association
P.O. Box 417
Chicago Ridge, IL 60415   216-630-7723
                                          www.lowesyndrome.org

Lisa Waldbaum, President
Jane Gallery, Treasurer
Fiona Fisher, Secretary
Jessica Hanson, Board Member
An international conference held approximately every two years where family, friends, medical and other professionals gather to exchange ideas and information.
June

1917   NACDD Annual Conference
1825 K St., NW
Suite 600
Washington, DC 20006   202-506-5813
                                             info@nacdd.org
                                             www.nacdd.org

Mat McCollough, Executive Director/President
Shannon Buller, Vice President
Steve Gieber, Secretary
Dan Shannon, Treasurer
NACDD is the national association for the 56 State and Territorial Councils on Developmental Disabilities (DD Councils) which receive federal funding to support programs that promote self-determination, integration, and inclusion for all Americans with developmental disabilities.

1918   NADD
National Association for the Dually Diagnosed
132 Fair St.
Kingston, NY 12401   845-331-4336
                                             800-331-5362
                                        Fax: 845-331-4569
                                             info@thenadd.org
                                             www.thenadd.org

Robert Fletcher, CEO
Donna McNelis, President
Julia Pearce, Secretary
Terrence McNelis, Treasurer
NADD is a non-for-profit membership organization designed to promote awareness of, and services for, individuals who have co-occuring intellectual disability and mental illness. NADD provides training, consultation services, and publishes journals and books.
November

1919   NADR Conference
National Association of Disability Representatives
1305 W 11th St.
Suite 222
Houston, TX 77008   202-822-2155
                                             800-747-6131
                                        Fax: 972-245-6701
                                             www.nadr.org

Steven Skinner, President
Philip Litteral, Vice President
Barbara Manna, Secretary
Michael Wener, Treasurer
The NADR is an organization of Professional Social Security Claimants Representatives that focus on issues involving policies to protect the interest of people with disabilities. NADR conducts annual conventions open to members and non-members with educational seminars to keep practitioners up to date on So-

cial Security rulings, regulatory changes and practice improvements.

1920   NASW-NYS Chapter
NASW
188 Washington Ave.
Albany, NY 12210
518-463-4741
800-724-6279
Fax: 518-463-6446
info@naswnys.org
www.naswnys.org

Mark Buttiglieri, President
N. Lael Telfeyan, Vice President
Jessica Russo, Secretary
Workshops, keynote speakers, and presentations offered at this event will develop and enhance practice skills and knowledge in the provision of quality mental health and community services.
March

1921   National Council on the Aging Conference
251 18th St. S.
Suite 500
Arlington, VA 22202
571-527-3900
membership@ncoa.org
www.ncoa.org

James Firman, President and CEO
Donna Whitt, Senior Vice President, Chief Financial Officer
Rina Pennacchia, Vice President, Human Resources & Talent Management
Howard Bedlin, Vice President, Public Policy & Advocacy
Offers ideas and programs to increase program and administrative skills through NCOA's professional development tracks and offering of continuing education units.
May

1922   PVA Summit & Expo
Paralyzed Veterans Of America
801 18th St. NW
Washington, DC 20006-3517
800-424-8200
summit@pva.org
summitpva.org

David Zurfluh, President
Sherman Gillums, Executive Director
Ken Weas, Senior Vice President
James Thomas Wheaton Jr., Treasurer
The annual 3-day medical conference will bring together renowned leaders from medicine, health care, policy, and government to explore and implement holistic strategies to strengthen the continuum of care for patients with spinal cord injuries or related diseases.

1923   PWSA (USA) Conference
Prader-Willi Alliance Of New York
244 5th Ave.
Suite D-110
New York, NY 10001
800-442-1655
alliance@prader-willi.org
www.prader-willi.org

Amy McDougall, President
Barbara McManus, Treasurer
Brian Burgin, Secretary
Nina Roberto, Executive Director
Through conferences, publications, electronic communication and networking (parent-to-parent, parent-to professional, and professional-to-professional), the Prader-Willi Alliance provides a valuable resource for individuals and families sharing the same concerns.
July

1924   Pacific Rim International Conference on Disability And Diversity
1410 Lower Campus Rd.
Unit 171F
Honolulu, HI 96822
808-956-7539
Fax: 808-956-4437
cccrocke@hawaii.edu
www.pacrim.hawaii.edu

Charmaine Crockett, Conference Organizer
Patricia Morrissey, Director of the Center on Disability
The Pacific Rim International Conference on Disability and Diversity encourages and respects voices from diverse perspective across numerous areas including voices from persons representing all disability areas, and experiences of family members and supporters across all disability and diversity areas.

1925   RESNA Annual Conference
Rehab Engineering & Assistive Tech. North America
1560 Wilson Blvd.
Suite 850
Arlington, VA 22209
703-524-6686
Fax: 703-524-6630
conference@resna.org
www.resna.org

Roger O. Smith, President
Maureen Linden, Treasurer
Meghan Donahue, Secretary
Carmen DiGiovine, Board Member
Sponsored by a multidisciplinary association for the advancement of rehabilitation and assistive technologies, this annual conference brings together a large number of rehabilitation professionals, products and services from around the world and has something to offer for both professionals and consumers. The conference provides an informative and thought provoking forum for anyone with interests in rehabilitation technology.
June

1926   Rehabilitation International
866 United Nation Plaza
Office 422
New York, NY 10017
212-420-1500
Fax: 212-505-0871
info@riglobal.org
riglobal.org

Zhang Haidi, President
Susan Parker, Treasurer
Venus Ilagan, Secretary General
RI is a global network of people with disabilities, service providers, researchers, government agencies, and advocates protecting and promoting the rights and inclusion of people with disabilities.

1927   Source-APTA Audio Conference
American Physical Therapy Association
1111 North Fairfax St.
Alexandria, VA 22314-1488
703-684-2782
800-999-2782
Fax: 703-706-8536
consumer@apta.org
apta.org

Sharon L. Dunn, President
Lisa K. Saladin, Vice President
Roger A. Herr, Secretary
Jeanine Gunn, Treasurer
The American Physical Therapy Association is a national professional organization sponsors this annual conference. The goal is to foster advancements in physical therapy practice, research, and education.

1928   Southwest Conference On Disability
University of New Mexico
2300 Menaul Blvd., NE
Albuquerque, NM 87107
505-272-3000
Fax: 505-272-9594
acahill@salud.unm.edu
cdd.unm.edu/swconf

Dr. Anthony Cahill, Conference Director
Heidi Fredine, Disability & the Arts Program

The Center for Development and Disability (CDD), is New Mexico's University Center for Excellence in Developmental Disabilities Education, Research and Service that respond to the needs of individuals with developmental disabilities and their families.

1929   TSA National Conference
Tourette Syndrome Association
42-40 Bell Blvd.
Suite 205
Bayside, NY   11361   800-237-0717
                                               Fax: 718-279-9596
                                               support@tourett.org
                                               taoa.convio.net
John Miller, President & CEO
Diana Felner, Executive VP
This is a biannual conference that includes members of the TS community and their families, educators, TS advocates, physicians, researchers, allied professionals, and TSA staff members. Attendees interact, socialize, share ideas, discuss issues of concern, and learn from experts.
Spring 1972

1930   Young Onset Parkinson Conference
National Parkinson Foundation & ADPF
200 SE 1st St.
Suite 800
Miami, FL   33131   800-473-4636
                                               Fax: 305-537-9901
                                               contact@parkinson.org
                                               www.parkinson.org
John L. Lehr, President and CEO
James Beck, Vice President, Chief Scientific Officer
Yasnahia Cortorreal, Vice President, Human Resources & Administration
Curt DeGreff, Vice President, Chief Development Officer
Purpose is to find the cause and cure for Parkinson's Disease and related neurodegenerative disorders through research, education and dissemination of current information to patients, care-givers and families.
Annual

Construction & Architecture

Associations

1931 Adaptive Environments Center
200 Portland Street
Suite 1
Boston, MA 02114 617-695-1225
Fax: 617-482-8099
info@HumanCenteredDesign.org
www.humancentereddesign.org
Ralph Jackson, FAIA, President
Chris Pilkington, Vice President
Nancy Jenner, Treasurer
Valerie Fletcher, Executive Director
Develops educational programs and materials on universal design, Americans with Disabilities Act, home adaptation, and more. Central Adaptive Environments publication list also available.

1932 Building Owners and Managers Association International
1101 15th St., NW
Suite 800
Washington, DC 20005 202-408-2662
Fax: 202-326-6377
info@boma.org
www.boma.org
John G. Oliver, Chair and Chief Elected Officer
Kent C. Gibson, CPM, Chair-Elect
Henry H. Chamberlain, President, COO
Brian Harnetiaux, Vice Chair
Conducts seminars nationwide and publishes resource guidebooks for building owners and managers on ADA requirements for commercial facilities and places of public accommodation.

1933 Institute for Human Centered Design
Formerly Adaptive Environments
200 Portland St
Ste 1
Boston, MA 02214 617-695-1225
Fax: 617-482-8099
TTY:617-695-1225
info@humancentereddesign.org
humancentereddesign.org
Valerie Fletcher, Executive Director
Gabriela Bonome-Sims, Director, Administration
Insititute focused on collaborating and working with citizens to design communal places to be accessible for all, including those with disabilities.

1934 Mark Elmore Associates Architects
Ste 104
42 East St
Crystal Lake, IL 60014-4400 815-455-7260
800-801-7766
Fax: 815-455-2238
mark@elmore-architects.com
www.elmore-architects.com
Mark A Elmore, Owner
Architectural designs for accessible residential and commercial buildings. ADA compliance reviews.

1935 National Conference on Building Codes and Standards
505 Huntmar Park Drive
Suite 210
Herndon, VA 20170 703-437-0100
Fax: 703-481-3596
membership@ncsbcs.org
www.ncsbcs.org
Cynthia Wilk, President
Robert C. Wible, Executive Director
Debbie Becker, Administrative Assistant
Kevin Egilmez, Project Manager
Serves as a forum in the interchange of information and provides technical services, education and training to our members to enhance the public's social and economic well being through safe, durable, affordable, accessible and efficient buildings.

1936 National Council of Architectural Registration Boards (NCARB)
1801 K Street NW
Suite 700K
Washington, DC 20006 202-879-0520
ncarb.org
Gregory L. Erny, President
David L. Hoffman, First Vice President
Terry L. Allers, Second Vice President
Robert M. Calvani, Treasurer
Research service in print and online information. Large collection of books and periodicals on the building/architectural environments.

1937 Overcoming Mobility Barriers International
1022 S 4st St
Omaha, NE 68105 402-342-5731
Fax: 402-342-5731
Kay Neil, Executive Director
Members are government officials, service consumers and providers, and other persons interested in removing mobility barriers for elderly, handicapped and disadvantaged persons. Advises and works in conjunction with other groups and government agencies to establish safety standards for special equipment used in retrofitting vehicles and works to retrain drivers in the use of nonconventional driving controls.

1938 Paradigm Design Group
Paralyzed Veterans of America
801 Eighteenth Street, NW
Washington, DC 20006-3517 202-872-1300
800-424-8200
Fax: 202-785-4432
info@pva.org
www.pva.org
Bill Lawson, National President
Homer S. Townsend Jr., Executive Director
Al F. Kovach Jr., National Senior Vice Presedent
Craig F. Enenbach, National Treasurer
Specialized firm providing architectural consulting services related to accessible designs. Experience includes product design and building codes and standards.

1939 United States Access Board
Ste 1000
1331 F St NW
Washington, DC 20004-1111 202-272-0080
800-872-2253
Fax: 202-272-0081
TTY: 800-993-2822
info@access-board.gov
www.access-board.gov
Dave Yanchulis, Public Affairs Specialist
Offers information and technical assistance to the public on accessible design under the Americans with Disabilities Act and other laws. Guidance and publications are available free that address access to facilities, transit vehicles and information technology.

Publications & Videos

1940 Access Currents
United States Access Board
1331 F Street, NW
Suite 1000
Washington, DC 20004-1111 202-272-0080
800-872-2253
Fax: 202-272-0081
TTY: 800-993-2822
info@access-board.gov
www.access-board.gov
Michael K. Yudin, Chair, Department of Education
Sachin Dev Pavithran, Vice Chair, Logan, Utah
Regina Blye, Public Member
Patrick D. Cannon, Public Member
Offers information and referrals on architectural accessibility for architects, designers, government agencies, building owners and consumers. A list of free publications is available on request.
bi-monthly

1941 Access Equals Opportunity
Council of B BB s Foundation
3033 Wilson Blvd
Suite 600
Arlington, VA 22201 703-276-0100
media@cbbb.bbb.org
www.bbb.org
Beverly Baskin, Senior VP, Chief Mission Officer
Genie Barton, Vice President and Director, Onl
Rodney L. Davis, Senior VP Enterprise Programs
Joseph E. Dillon, VP and CFO
These six Title III compliance guides for existing small businesses offer creative cheap and easy suggestions for complying with the public accommodations section of the ADA. Each guide is industry specific for: retail stores, car sales/service, restaurants/bars, medical offices and fun/fitness centers. They include suggestions for readily achievable removal of architectural barriers; effective communication; and guidance for nondiscriminatory policies or procedures. *$2.50*

1942 Access for All
Hospital Audiences
548 Broadway
3rd Floor
New York, NY 10012 212-575-7676
Fax: 212-575-7669
David Sweeny, Executive Director
Jane Kleinsinger, Director of Operations
Jill Bernard, Marketing & Outreach Manager
JoAnne Brockways, Chief Financial Officer
Provides physical and program accessibility information for people with disabilities to New York City cultural institutions including theaters, museums, galleries, etc.

1943 Accessible Home of Your Own
Accent Special Publications
Bloomington, IL 61702-700
Raymond C Cheever, Publisher
Betty Garee, Editor
This guide includes 14 articles on the popular subject of how to make a disabled persons home more accessible. *$7.99*
52 pages Paperback 1990
ISBN 0-915708-29-9

1944 Adaptable Housing: A Technical Manual for Implementing Adaptable Dwelling
H UD U SE R
P.O.Box 23268
Washington, DC 20026-3268 202-708-3178
800-245-2691
Fax: 202-708-9981
TTY: 800-927-7589
helpdesk@huduser.org
www.huduser.org
Patrick J. Tewey, Director, Budget, Contracts, and Program Control Division
Jacqueline D Buford, Director, Management and Administrative Services Division
Jean Lin Pao, General Deputy Assistant Secretary
Katherine M. O'Regan, Assistant Secretary for Policy Development and Research
An illustrated manual describing methods for implementing adaptability in housing. *$3.00*

1945 Consumer's Guide to Home Adaptation
Adaptive Environments Center
200 Portland Street
Suite 1
Boston, MA 02114 617-695-1225
Fax: 617-482-8099
info@HumanCenteredDesign.org
www.humancentereddesign.org
Ralph Jackson, FAIA, President
Chris Pilkington, Vice President
Nancy Jenner, Treasurer
Valerie Fletcher, Executive Director
A workbook that enables people with disabilities to plan the modifications necessary to adapt their homes. Describes how to widen doorways, lower countertops, etc. *$12.00*
52 pages Paperback

1946 Design for Acessibility
National Endowment for the Arts Office
400 7th Street, SW
Washington, DC 20506-0001 202-682-5400
Fax: 202-682-5715
webmgr@arts.gov
arts.gov
Jane Chu, Chairman
Joan Shigekawa, Senior Deputy Chairman
Mike Burke, Chief Information Officer
Joseph Smith, Deputy Chief Information Officer
A handbook for compliance with Section 504 of the Rehabilitation Act of 1973 and the Americans with Disabilities Act of 1990 including technical assistance on making arts programs accessible to staff, performers and audience.
101 pages
ISBN 0-160042-83-6

1947 Directory of Accessible Building Products
N AH B Research Center
400 Prince George's Blvd
Upper Marlboro, MD 20774 301-249-4000
800-638-8556
Fax: 301-430-6180
www.homeinnovation.com
Michael Luzier, CEO & President
Michelle Desiderio, Vice President of Innovation Services
Tom Kenney, P.E, Vice President of Engineering & Research
Phil Davis, Senior Economist & Analyst
Contains descriptions of more than 200 commercially available products designed for use by people with disabilities and age-related limitations. Paperback. *$5.00*
104 pages Yearly

1948 Do-Able Renewable Home
A AR P Fulfillment
601 E Street NW
Washington, DC   20049   202-434-3525
                                       888-687-2277
                                       877-342-2277
                                  Fax: 202-434-3443
                                  member@aarp.org
                                  www.aarp.org
John Wider, President, CEO, AARP Services Inc.
Lisa M. Ryerson, President, AARP Foundation
Robert R. Hagans, Jr., Executive Vice President & Chief Financial
Officer
Hollis Terry Bradwell III, Executive Vice President & Chief
Information Officer
Describes how individuals with disabilities can modify their
homes for independent living. Room-by-room modifications are
accompanied by illustrations.

**1949 ECHO Housing: Recommended Construction and
Installation Standards**
601 E Street NW
Washington, DC   20049   202-434-3525
                                       888-687-2277
                                       877-342-2277
                                  Fax: 202-434-3443
                                  member@aarp.org
                                  www.aarp.org
John Wider, President, CEO, AARP Services Inc.
Lisa M. Ryerson, President, AARP Foundation
Robert R. Hagans, Jr., Executive Vice President & Chief Financial
Officer
Hollis Terry Bradwell III, Executive Vice President & Chief
Information Officer
Illustrated design, construction, and installation standards for
temporary dwelling units for elderly people on single family resi-
dential property.

1950 Electronic House: Enhanced Lifestyles with Electronics
Electronic House
111 Speen Street, Suite 200
P.O. Box 989
Framingham, MA 01701-2000   508-663-1500
                                       800-375-8015
                                  Fax: 508-663-1599
                                  cheditorial@ehpub.com
                                  electronichouse.com
Kenneth D. Moyes, President
Karen Bligh, Marketing Director
John Brillon, Web Creative Director
Guy Caiola, Director of Internet Operations
Dedicated to home automation. Featuring both extravagant and
affordable smart homes that can be controlled with one touch. EH
covers electronic systems that give homeowners more security,
entertainment, convenience, and fun. Articles cover whole house
control and subsystems like residential lighting, security, home
theater, energy management and telecommunications. *$23.95*
84 pages BiMonthly
ISSN 0886-66 3

1951 Fair Housing Design Guide for Accessibility
National Council on Multifamily Housing Industry
1201 15th Street NW
Washington, DC   20005   202-266-8200
                                       800-368-5242
                                  Fax: 202-266-8400
                                  www.nahb.com
Kevin Kelly, Chairman of the Board
Tom Woods, First Vice Chairman of the Board
Ed Brady, Second Vice Chairman of the Board
Gerald M. Howard, CEO
Specifically tailored to address the needs of architects and build-
ers. The book includes a detailed technical analysis of the legisla-
tion's impact on multifamily design, highlights potential
construction problems, and identifies possible solutions. *$29.95*

1952 Ideas for Making Your Home Accessible
Accent Books & Products
P.O.Box 700
Bloomington, IL   61702-0700   309-378-2961
                                       800-787-8444
                                  Fax: 309-378-4420
                                  acmtlvng@aol.com
                                  www.accentonliving.com
Raymond C Cheever, Publisher
Betty Garee, Editor
Offers over 100 pages of tips and ideas to help build or remodel a
home. Includes many special devices and where to get them.
$7.50
94 pages Paperback
ISBN 0-91570 -08-6

1953 North Carolina Accessibility Code
North Carolina Department of Insurance
325 N. Salisbury St.
Raleigh, NC   27603   919-647-0014
                                  Fax: 919-715-0067
                                  laurel.wright@ncdoi.gov
Laurel W. Wright, Chief Accessibility Code Consultant
Making buildings and facilities accessible to and usable by the
physically disabled. *$20.00*
678 pages Triannually

**1954 Removing the Barriers: Accessibility Guidelines and
Specifications**
A PP A
1643 Prince Street
Alexandria, VA   22314   703-684-1446
                                  Fax: 703-549-2772
                                  webmaster@appa.org
                                  www.appa.org
John F. Bernhards, Associate Vice President
E. Lander Medlin, Executive VP
Steve Glazner, Director of Knowledge Management
Suzanne M. Healy, Director of Professional Development
Offers site accessibility, building entrances, doors, interior circu-
lation, restrooms and bathing facilities, drinking fountains and
additional resources. *$45.00*
125 pages
ISBN 0-91335 -59-9

**1955 Smart Kitchen/How to Design a Comfortable, Safe &
Friendly Workplace**
Ceres Press
P.O.Box 87
Woodstock, NY   12498-87   845-679-5573
                                  Fax: 845-679-5573
                                  cem620@aol.com
                                  healthyhighways.com
David Goldbeck, Owner
This book provides information about designing kitchens that
may be helpful to people with disabilities as well as safe and en-
ergy efficient. *$16.95*
132 pages Paperback

1956 United Spinal Association
75-20 Astoria Blvd
Suite 120
East Elmhurst, NY   11370- 1177   718-803-3782
                                       800-444-0120
                                  Fax: 718-803-0414
                                  mkurtz@unitedspinal.org
                                  www.unitedspinal.org
Paul Tobin, President
Maria Kurtz, Executive Assistant
Information on spinal cord injury and laws and regulations con-
cerning people with disabilities, including veterans.
Monthly

Education

Aids for the Classroom

1957   AEPS Child Progress Record: For Children Ages Three to Six
Brookes Publishing
PO Box 10624
Baltimore, MD   21285-624
410-337-9580
800-638-3775
Fax: 800-638-3775
custserv@brookespublishing.com
www.brookespublishing.com

Paul Brooks, President
Melissa Behm, Executive VP
George Stamathis, VP and Publisher
This chart helps monitor change by visually displaying current abilities, intervention targets, and child progress. In packages of 30. *$21.00*
8 pages Gate-fold
ISBN 1-557662-51-7

1958   AEPS Curriculum for Three to Six Years
Brookes Publishing
PO Box 10624
Baltimore, MD   21285-0624
410-337-9580
800-638-3775
Fax: 410-337-8539
webmaster@brookespublishing.com
www.brookespublishing.com

Paul H. Brookes, Chairman of the Board
Jeffrey D. Brookes, President
George S. Stamathis, VP/Publisher
Melissa A. Behn, Executive Vice President
Used after the AEPS® Test is completed and scored, this developmentally sequenced curriculum allows professionals to match the child's IFSP/IEP goals and objectives with activity-based interventions — beginning with simple skills and moving on to more advanced skills. *$ 65.00*
304 pages Spiral-bound
ISBN 1-557665-65-6

1959   AEPS Data Recording Forms: For Children Ages Three to Six
Brookes Publishing
PO Box 10624
Baltimore, MD   21285-624
410-337-9580
800-638-3775
Fax: 800-638-3775
custserv@brookespublishing.com
www.readplaylearn.com

Paul Brooks, President
These forms can be used by child development professionals on four separate occasions to pinpoint and then monitor a child's strengths and needs in the six key areas of skill development measured by the AEPS Test. Packages of 10. *$24.00*
36 pages Saddle-stiched
ISBN 1-557662-49-5

1960   AEPS Family Interest Survey
Brookes Publishing
PO Box 10624
Baltimore, MD   21285-624
410-337-9580
800-638-3775
Fax: 800-638-3775
custserv@brookespublishing.com
www.brookespublishing.com

Paul Brooks, President
Tracy Gracy, Educational Sales Manager
This is a 30-item checklist that helps families to identify interests and concerns to address in a child's IEP/IFSP. Comes in packages of 30. *$15.00*
8 pages Saddle-stiched
ISBN 1-557660-98-0

1961   Adaptivemall.com
15 South Second Street
Dolgeville, NY   13329
315-429-7112
800-371-2778
Fax: 315-429-8862
info@adaptivemall.com
www.adaptivemall.com

Katie Bergeron Peglow,PT,MS, COO
Adaptivemall.comr help families find the best equipment to support their children at their highest functioning level.

1962   Advanced Language Tool Kit
School Specialty
625 Mt. Auburn Street, 3rd Floor
PO Box 9031
Cambridge, MA 02139-9031
617-547-6706
800-225-5750
Fax: 888-440-2665
Feedback.EPS@schoolspecialty.com
eps.schoolspecialty.com

Rick Holden, President, EPS
Jean S Osman, Co-Author
Paula D Rome, Author
Provides an overview o the structure, organization, and sound units that are needed to develop skills for advanced reading and spelling. The kit contains a teacher's manual and 3 pack of cards, with features similar to the cards in the Language Tool Kit. *$60.00*
ISBN 0-838885-48-9

1963   All Kinds of Minds
School Specialty
625 Mt. Auburn Street, 3rd Floor
PO Box 9031
Cambridge, MA 02139-9031
617-547-6706
800-225-5750
Fax: 888-440-2665
Feedback.EPS@schoolspecialty.com
eps.schoolspecialty.com

Rick Holden, President, EPS
Melvin D Levine, Author
A fictitious account of five different students who have learning disabilities. *$33.00*
296 pages
ISBN 0-838820-90-5

1964   American Sign Language Handshape Cards
T J Publishers, Distributor
Ste 206
817 Silver Spring Ave
Silver Spring, MD   20910- 4617
301-585-4440
800-999-1168
Fax: 301-585-5930
tjpubinc@aol.com

Angela K Thames, President
Jerald A Murphy, VP
Durable flashcards illustrate basic handshapes, classifiers and the American manual alphabet. An instructional booklet describes games for differing skill levels to improve vocabulary, increase hand and eye coordination, sign recognition and usage. *$16.95*

1965   Asthma Action Cards: Child Care Asthma/Allergy Action Card
Asthma and Allergy Foundation of America
8201 Corporate Drive
Suite 1000
Landover, MD   20785
202-466-7643
800-727-8462
Fax: 202-466-8940
info@aafa.org
www.aafa.org

Tom Flanigan, Chariman
William Mclin, President and CEO
Yolanda Miller, VP and CFO
Includes necessary information a provider needs to care for a young child who has asthma and allergies. The card includes a

medication plan, a list of the child's specific signs and symptoms that indicate the child is having trouble breathing, and steps on how to handle an emergency situation.

1966 Asthma Action Cards: Student Asthma Action Card
Asthma and Allergy Foundation of America
1233 20th St NW
Suite 610
Washington, DC 20036-2330   202-833-1700
800-727-8462
Fax: 202-833-2351
info@aafa.org
www.swmlaw.com
Bill Mc Lin, Executive Director
Ben C Hadden, VP Finance & Treasurer
Bill Lin, Executive Director
Tool for communicating school aged children's and teen's asthma managment plan to school personnel. Includes sections for asthma triggers, daily medications, and emergency directions.

1967 Auditech: Classroom Amplification System Focus CFM802
PO Box 821105
Vicksburg, MS 39182-1105   800-229-8293
Fax: 800-221-8639
info@auditechusa.com
www.auditechusa.com

1968 Auditech: Personal FM Educational System
PO Box 821105
Vicksburg, MS 39182-1105   800-229-8293
Fax: 800-221-8639
info@auditechusa.com
www.auditechusa.com

1969 Auditory-Verbal Therapy for Parents and Professionals
Alexander Graham Bell Association
3417 Volta Place, NW
Washington, DC 20007   202-337-5220
Fax: 202-337-8314
TTY:202-337-5221
info@agbell.org
www.listeningandspokenlanguage.org
Meredith K. Sugar, Esq. (OH), President
Donald M. Goldberg, Immediate Past President
Ted A. Meyer, M.D., Ph.D. (SC, President-Elect, Secretary, Treasurer
Emilio Alonso Mendoza (DC), Chief Executive Officer
A must-have for hearing health professionals, students entering hearing health fields and parents who want to explore the theory and practices of auditory-verbal therapy. *$54.95*
313 pages Paperback

1970 Autism Community Store
7800 E. Iliff Ave.
Suite J
Denver, CO 80231   303-309-3647
866-709-4344
Fax: 303-756-2311
support@autismcommunitystore.com
www.autismcommunitystore.com
Shannon Sullivan, Co-Founder
The Autism Community Store is a parent-owned autism and special needs resource, a special little shop helping families, teachers and therapists get hard-to-find products for kids with ASD, PDD-NOS, Aspergers, SPD, ADHD and other special needs at reasonable prices.

1971 Autism-Products.com
8776 E. Shea Blvd.
Suite 106-552
Scottsdale, AZ 85260   *Fax:* 815-550-1819
Kelly@Autism-Products.com
www.autism-products.com

1972 Barrier Free Education
Center for Assistive Technology & Env Access
490 10th St NW
Atlanta, GA 30332-156   404-894-4960
800-726-9119
Fax: 404-894-9320
catea@coa.gatech.edu
www.catea.org
Elizabeth Bryant, Project Director
Math and science activities pose unique accommodation challenges for students with disabilities. The Barrier Free Education resource on accessible science experiments was developed for high school chemistry and physics students with physical or visual disabilities under the National Science Foundation's Program for Persons with Disabilities.

1973 Beginning Reasoning and Reading
School Specialty
625 Mt. Auburn Street, 3rd Floor
PO Box 9031
Cambridge, MA 02139-9031   617-547-6706
800-225-5750
Fax: 888-440-2665
Feedback.EPS@schoolspecialty.com
eps.schoolspecialty.com
Rick Holden, President, EPS
Joanne Carlisle, Author
This workbook develops basic language and thinking skills that build the foundation for reading comprehension. Workbook exercises reinforce reading as a critical reasoning activity. *$10.45*
ISBN 0-838830-01-3

1974 Buy!
JE Stewart Teaching Tools
PO Box 15308
Seattle, WA 98115-308   206-262-9538
Fax: 206-262-9538
Jeff Stewart, Owner
Teaches 50 words as they appear in commercial and community situations such as clinic, sale, receipt, price and cleaner. These words are functional at school, on the job and shopping. *$32.50*
116 pages
ISBN 1-877866-05-9

1975 Catalog for Teaching Life Skills to Persons with Development Disability
PCI Education Publishing
PO Box 34270
San Antonio, TX 78265-4270   210-377-1999
800-594-4263
Fax: 888-259-8284
www.pcieducation.com
Lee Wilson, President/CEO
Erin Kinard, VP Product Development/Publisher
Randy Pennington, VP, Sales & Marketing
Over 200 educational products that help individuals learn and maintain the life skills they need to succeed in an inclusive society.

1976 Classroom GOAL: Guide for Optimizing Auditory Learning Skills
Alexander Graham Bell Association
3417 Volta Pl., NW
Washington, DC 20007   202-337-5220
Fax: 202-337-8314
info@agbell.org
www.agbell.org
Ted A. Meyer, Chair
Catharine McNally, Chair-Elect
Susan Lenihan, Secretary
Emilio Alonso Mendoza, Chief Executive Officer
This reader-friendly teacher's guide filled with tips, source materials and sample charts and plans is designed for educators who have yearned for a resource that explains how to incorporate auditory goals into academic learning for students with different degrees of hearing loss. *$34.95*
Paperback

1977 Classroom Notetaker: How to Organize a Program Serving Students with Hearing Impairments
Alexander Graham Bell Association
3417 Volta Pl. NW
Washington, DC 20007 202-337-5220
Fax: 202-337-8314
info@agbell.org
www.agbell.org

Ted A. Meyer, Chair
Catharine McNally, Chair-Elect
Susan Lenihan, Secretary
Emilio Alonso Mendoza, Chief Executive Director

This detailed manual for instructors, administrators and staff notetakers promotes classroom notetaking within long-term educational programs as absolutely vital for students who are deaf and hard of hearing from elementary school to college. *$24.95*
127 pages Paperback

1978 Community Services for the Blind and Partially Sighted
Store: Sight Connection
9709 Third Ave NE
Ste 100
Seattle, WA 98115-2027 206-525-5556
800-458-4888
Fax: 206-525-0422
info@sightconnection.org
www.sightconnection.org

Miles Otoupal, Chair
Jonathan Avedovech, Vice Chair
David McBride, Treasurer
Mary Lewis, Secretary

Over 400 products specifically designed to make life easier for people with vision loss.

1979 Community Signs
JE Stewart Teaching Tools
P.O.Box 15308
Seattle, WA 98115-308 206-262-9538
Fax: 206-262-9538

Jeff Stewart, Owner

Teaches 50 words like go, fire, rest room, men, women, danger and walk needed to successfully navigate our environment. *$ 32.50*

1980 Comprehensive Assessment of Spoken Language (CASL)
AGS
PO Box 99
Circle Pines, MN 55014-99 800-328-2560
Fax: 800-471-8457
agsmail@agsnet.com
www.agsnet.com

Kevin Brueggeman, President
Robert Zaske, Market Manager

CASL is an individually and orally administered research-based, theory-drive oral language assessment battery for ages 3 through 21. Fifteen tests measure language processing skills - comprehension, expression, and retrieval - in four language structure categories: lexical/semantic, syntactic, supralinguistic and pragmatic. *$299.95*

1981 Creative Arts Therapy Catalogs
MMB Music
9051 Watson Road
Suite 161
Saint Louis, MO 63126-1019 314-531-9635
800-543-3771
Fax: 314-531-8384
info@mmbmusic.com
www.mmbmusic.com

Marcia Goldberg, President

Catalogs of books, videos, recordings for the creative arts and wellness (music, art, dance, poetry, drama, therapies, photography).

1982 Cursive Writing Skills
School Specialty
625 Mt. Auburn Street, 3rd Floor
PO Box 9031
Cambridge, MA 02139-9031 617-547-6706
800-225-5750
Fax: 888-440-2665
Feedback.EPS@schoolspecialty.com
eps.schoolspecialty.com

Rick Holden, President, EPS
Diana Hanbury King, Author

Boosts writing achievement through handwriting skills. Handwriting instruction helps students become fluent writers, allowing them to focus on their thoughts and ideas rather than on letter and word formation. *$12.00*

1983 Different Roads to Learning
37 East 18th Street
10th Floor
New York, NY 10003 212-604-9637
800-853-1057
Fax: 212-206-9329
info@difflearn.com
www.difflearn.com

Julie Azuma, Founder

Its product line supports the social, academic and communicative development of children on the autism spectrum through Applied Behavior Analysis (ABA) and Verbal Behavior interventions

1984 Discount School Supply
PO Box 6013
Carol Stream, IL 60197-6013 800-627-2829
Fax: 800-879-3753
customerservice@discountschoolsupply.com
www.discountschoolsupply.com

Ron Elliott, Founder
Kelly Crampton, Chief Executive Officer

Discount School Supply offers the highest quality educational products at the lowest possible prices, supported by an extraordinary level of service.

1985 Do2learn
3204 Churchill Road
Raleigh, NC 27607 919-755-1809
Fax: 919-420-1978
www.do2learn.com

1986 Don Johnston
26799 West Commerce Drive
Volo, IL 60073-9675 847-740-0749
800-999-4660
Fax: 847-740-7326
info@donjohnston.com
www.donjohnston.com

Don Johnston, Founder
Ruth Ziolkowski, President
Kevin Johnston, Director of Product Design
Ben Johnston, Director of Marketing

A provider of quality products and services that enable people with special needs to discover their potential and experience success. Products are developed for the areas of Physical Access, Augmentative Communication and for those who struggle with reading and writing.

1987 Dyslexia Training Program
School Specialty
625 Mt. Auburn Street, 3rd Floor
PO Box 9031
Cambridge, MA 02139-9031 617-547-6706
800-225-5750
Fax: 888-440-2665
Feedback.EPS@schoolspecialty.com
eps.schoolspecialty.com

Rick Holden, President, EPS

This 2-year, cumulative series of daily 1-hour video lessons and accompanying Student's Books and Teacher's Guides is a structured, multisensory sequence of alphabet, reading, spelling, cursive handwriting, listening, language history, and review activities. Written by the Texas Scottish Rite Hospital for Children.

1988 ESpecial Needs
11704 Lackland Industrial Drive
St. Louis, MO   63146   314-692-2424
                                               877-664-4565
                                          Fax: 314-692-2428
                                        www.especialneeds.com

1989 Encyclopedia of Basic Employment and Daily Living Skills
Phillip Roy, Inc.
13064 Indian Rocks Road
P.O. Box 130
Indian Rocks Beach, FL   33785   727-593-2700
                                               800-255-9085
                                          Fax: 727-595-2685
                                          info@philliproy.com

Ruth Bragman PhD, President
Phil Padol, Consultant
Contains developmental skills for special education students. Contains lessons in 6 curriculum areas covering 80 objects with 541 lessons. Also includes objectives, instructional strategies, and assessment tasks.

1990 Exceptional Teaching Inc
Exceptional Teaching Inc
3994 Oleander Way
PO Box 2330
Castro Valley, CA   94546   510-889-7282
                                               800-549-6999
                                          Fax: 510-889-7382
                                 info@exceptionalteaching.com
                                 www.exceptionalteaching.com

Helene Holman, Owner/manager
Providing educational products for those with special needs via catalog and online store.

1991 Explode the Code
School Specialty
625 Mt. Auburn Street, 3rd Floor
PO Box 9031
Cambridge, MA   02139-9031   617-547-6706
                                               800-225-5750
                                          Fax: 888-440-2665
                              Feedback.EPS@schoolspecialty.com
                                      eps.schoolspecialty.com

Rick Holden, President, EPS
Nancy M Hall, Author
Helps students build the essential literacy skills needed for reading success: phonological awareness, decoding, vocabulary, comprehension, fluency and spelling. *$6.20*
Grades K-4, 1-3

1992 Food!
JE Stewart Teaching Tools
PO Box 15308
Seattle, WA   98115-308   206-262-9538
                                          Fax: 206-262-9538

Jeff Stewart, Owner
Teaches 50 words like salt, pepper, hamburger, fruit, milk and soup, seen commonly on menus, packages and in directions used at home and at play. *$32.50*

1993 Fun for Everyone
AbleNet
2625 Patton Road
Roseville, MN   55113-1308   651-294-2200
                                               800-322-0956
                                          Fax: 651-294-2259
                              customerservice@ablenetinc.com
                                          www.ablenetinc.com

Jen Thalhuber, CEO
Ann Meyer, Vice President
Paul Sugden, VP Finance
Jason Voiovich, VP Marketing

Today, simple technology allows children and adults with disabilities to participate in leisure activities they were limited or excluded from in the past. *$20.00*

1994 Fundamentals of Autism
Slosson Educational Publications Inc.
538 Buffalo Road
East Aurora, NY   14052-280   716-652-0930
                                               800-655-3840
                                               888-756-7760
                                          Fax: 716-655-3840
                                     slossonprep@gmail.com
                                          www.slosson.com

Steven Slosson, President
John Slosson, VP
David Slosson, VP
The Fundamentals of Autism handbook provides a quick, user friendly, effective and accurate approach to help in identifying and developing educationally related program objectives for children diagnosed as autistic. These materials have been designed to be easily and functionally used by teachers, therapists, special education/learning disability resource specialists, psychologists and others who work with children diagnosed as autistic. *$56.00*
72 pages

1995 GO-MO Articulation Cards- Second Edition
Sage Publications
2455 Teller Road
Thousand Oaks, CA   91320   805-499-9774
                                               800-818-7243
                                          Fax: 800-583-2665
                                          info@sagepub.com
                                          www.sagepub.com

Blaise R Simqu, President & CEO
Tracey Ozmina, VP and COO
Chris Hickok, Senior VP and CFO
Stephen Barr, Managing Director
The most popular system used for remedying defective speech articulation in children and adults. This popular card set was the first and is still the best therapy tool of its kind, as it continues to produce results and maintains the interest of students of all ages.

1996 Gillingham Manaual
School Specialty
625 Mt. Auburn Street, 3rd Floor
PO Box 9031
Cambridge, MA   02139-9031   617-547-6706
                                               800-225-5750
                                          Fax: 888-440-2665
                              Feedback.EPS@schoolspecialty.com
                                      eps.schoolspecialty.com

Rick Holden, President, EPS
Anna Gillingham, Author
Bessie W Stillman, Co-Author
Remedial training for children with specific disability in reading, spelling, and penmanship.
352 pages 69.95
ISBN 0-83880 -00-

1997 Guide to Teaching Phonics
School Specialty
625 Mt. Auburn Street, 3rd Floor
PO Box 9031
Cambridge, MA   02139-9031   617-547-6706
                                               800-225-5750
                                          Fax: 888-440-2665
                              Feedback.EPS@schoolspecialty.com
                                      eps.schoolspecialty.com

Rick Holden, President, EPS
June Lyday Orton, Author
This flexible teacher's guide presents multisensory procedures developed in association with the late Dr. Samuel Orton. They consist of 100 phonograms for teaching phonetic elements and their sequences in words for reading, writing and spelling. Also contains coordinated Phonics Cards. *$19.25*
96 pages
ISBN 0-838802-41-9

1998   **Homemade Battery-Powered Toys**
Special Needs Project
Ste H
324 State St
Santa Barbara, CA   93101-2364   818-718-9900
                                                 800-333-6867
                                            Fax: 818-349-2027
                                        editor@specialneeds.com
                                        www.specialneeds.com

Hod Gray, Owner
Laraine Gray, Coordinator
Describes how to make simple switches and educational devices
for severely handicapped children. *$7.50*

1999   **Idaho Assistive Technology Project**
University of Idaho
PO Box 444061
Moscow, ID   83844-4061   208-885-6097
                                                 800-432-8324
                                            Fax: 208-885-6145
                                          janicec@uidaho.edu
                                             www.idahoat.org

Janice Carson, Project Director
Sue House, Information/Referral Specialst
A federally funded program managed by the Center on Disabilities and Human Development at the University of Idaho. The goal
is to increase the availability of assistive technology devices and
services for Idahoans with disabilities. *$15.00*

2000   **If It Is To Be, It Is Up To Me To Do It!**
AVKO Educational Research Foundation
3084 Willard Road
Birch Run, MI   48415-9404   810-686-9283
                                                 866-285-6612
                                            Fax: 810-686-1101
                                          webmaster@avko.org
                                              www.avko.org

Don McCabe, President, Research Director Emeritus, Birch Run,
Michigan
Linda Heck, VP, Clio, Michigan
Michael Lane, Treasurer, Clio, Michigan
Amy Messer, Board Member, Flint, Michigan
A student and tutor's text, for use on dyslexics and non-dyslexics,
by parents, spouses, or friends. *$29.95*
206 pages
ISBN 1-564007-42-1

2001   **Inclusive Play People**
Educational Equity Concepts
Fl 8
100 5th Ave
New York, NY   10011-6903   212-243-1110
                                            Fax: 212-627-0407
                                           TTY:212-725-1803
                                           www.iconcapital.com

Jacqueline Johnson, Manager
Six sturdy multiracial wooden figures that provide a unique variety of nonstereotyped work and family roles and are inclusive of
disabled and nondisabled people of various ages. For block building and dramatic play. *$25.00*

2002   **Individualized Keyboarding**
AVKO Educational Research Foundation
3084 Willard Road
Birch Run, MI   48415-9404   810-686-9283
                                                 866-285-6612
                                            Fax: 810-686-1101
                                          webmaster@avko.org
                                              www.avko.org

Don McCabe, President, Research Director Emeritus, Birch Run,
Michigan
Linda Heck, VP, Clio, Michigan
Michael Lane, Treasurer, Clio, Michigan
Amy Messer, Board Member, Flint, Michigan

Utilizes a multi-sensory approach to teach typing skills. It not
only teaches typing skills, it also reinforces the reading patterns
that are necessary for typing proficiency. *$14.95*
96 pages
ISBN 1-654004-01-5

2003   **Instruction of Persons with Severe Handicaps**
McGraw-Hill School Publishing
PO Box 182604
Columbus, OH   43272   877-833-5524
                                            Fax: 614-759-3749
                                  customer.service@mcgraw-hill.com
                                        www.mcgraw-hill.com

Harold McGraw, President and CEO
Jack Callahan, Executive VP
John Berisford, Executive VP of HR
A complete introduction to the status of education as it pertains to
people with severe handicaps.

2004   **Kaplan Early Learning Company**
1310 Lewisville Clemmons Rd
Lewisville, NC   27023   336-766-7374
                                                 800-334-2014
                                            Fax: 800-452-7526
                                           info@kaplanco.com
                                             www.kaplanco.com

Hal Kaplan, President & CEO
Kaplan Early Learning Company is a international provider of
products and services that enhance children's learning.

2005   **Keeping Ahead in School**
Educators Publishing Service
PO Box 9031
Cambridge, MA   2139-9031   617-547-6706
                                                 800-225-5750
                                            Fax: 888-440-2665
                                        feedback@epsbooks.com
                                             www.epsbooks.com

Charles H Heinle, VP
Alexandra S Bigelow, Author
Gunnar Voltz, President
This book helps students not only understand their own strengths
and weaknesses but also more fully appreciate their individuality.
He suggests specific ways to approach work, bypass or overcome
learning disorders, and manage other struggles that may beset
students in school. *$24.75*
320 pages Paperback
ISBN 0-838820-69-7

2006   **KeyMath Teach and Practice**
AGS
P.O.Box 99
Circle Pines, MN   55014-99   800-328-2560
                                            Fax: 800-471-8457
                                          agsmail@agsnet.com
                                               www.agsnet.com

Kevin Brueggeman, President
Robert Zaske, Market Manager
This set of materials provides all the tools needed to assess stu-
dents' math skills...and the strategies to deal with problem areas.
Three sets are available: Basic Concepts Package; Operations
Package; and Applications Package. $219.95 each or $599.95 for
whole set.

2007   **Lakeshore Learning Materials**
2695 E. Dominguez Street
Carson, CA   90895   310-537-8600
                                                 800-421-5354
                                            Fax: 800-537-5403
                                    lakeshore@lakeshorelearning.com
                                      www.lakeshorelearning.com

Bo Kaplan, President/CEO
Josh Kaplan, VP Merchandising
Mat , Vice President of Operations

Offers books, resources, testing materials, assessment information and special education materials for the professional in the field of special education.
190 pages

2008 Language Parts Catalog
School Specialty
625 Mt. Auburn Street, 3rd Floor
PO Box 9031
Cambridge, MA 02139-9031
617-547-6706
800-225-5750
Fax: 888-440-2665
Feedback.EPS@schoolspecialty.com
eps.schoolspecialty.com

Rick Holden, President, EPS
Melvin D Levine, Author
Offers a humorous and informative explanation of the various aspects of language and how they operate. Laid out in the form of a catalog, the book presents various parts that can help students improve their language abilities. *$12.65*
ISBN 0-838819-80-X

2009 Language Tool Kit
School Specialty
625 Mt. Auburn Street, 3rd Floor
PO Box 9031
Cambridge, MA 02139-9031
617-547-6706
800-225-5750
Fax: 888-440-2665
Feedback.EPS@schoolspecialty.com
eps.schoolspecialty.com

Rick Holden, President, EPS
Paula D Rome, Author
Jean S Osman, Co-Author
Designed for use by a teacher or parents, teaches reading and spelling to students with specific language disability. *$43.25*
32 pages English Edition
ISBN 0-838885-20-3

2010 Language, Speech and Hearing Services in School
American Speech-Language-Hearing Association
10801 Rockville Pike
Rockville, MD 20852-3226
301-296-5700
800-638-8255
Fax: 301-296-8580
actioncenter@asha.org
www.asha.org

Paul Rao, President
Robert Augustine, VP of Finance
Arlene Pietranton, Executive Director
Professional journal for clinicians, audiologists and speech-language pathologists. *$30.00*

2011 Learning American Sign Language
Harris Communications
15155 Technology Dr
Eden Prairie, MN 55344-2273
952-906-1180
800-825-6758
Fax: 952-906-1099
info@harriscomm.com
www.harriscomm.com

Robert Harris, President
Kevin Horsky, Business Director
Offers over 700 titles on ASL including books, videotapes, CDs & DVDs. Free catalog available. *$78.95*
350 pages Video & Book

2012 Learning Resources
380 N. Fairway Drive
Vernon Hills, IL 60061
800-333-8281
Fax: 888-892-8731
info@learningresources.com
www.learningresources.com

2013 Learning to Sign in My Neighborhood
T J Publishers
2544 Tarpley Rd
Suite 108
Carrollton, TX 75006-2288
972-416-0800
800-999-1168
Fax: 301-585-5930
tjpubinc@aol.com

Angela K Thames, President
Jerald A Murphy, VP
Beautifully illustrated coloring book lets children learn signs from kids just like themselves! Recommended for ages 4 and up, let children have fun while they learn signs for words typically used in day-to-day activities. *$3.50*
32 pages Softcover
ISBN 0-93266 -36-1

2014 Literacy Program
School Specialty
625 Mt. Auburn Street, 3rd Floor
PO Box 9031
Cambridge, MA 02139-9031
617-547-6706
800-225-5750
Fax: 888-440-2665
Feedback.EPS@schoolspecialty.com
eps.schoolspecialty.com

Rick Holden, President, EPS
Paula D Rome, Author
Jean S Osman, Co-Author
Written by the Texas Scottish Rite Hospital for Children. A one-year course that consists of 160 one-hour videotaped lessons accompanied by student workbooks, designed for high school students and adults who read below sixth grade level.

2015 Literature Based Reading
Oryx Press
4041 N Central Ave
Phoenix, AZ 85012-3330
602-265-2651
800-279-6799
Fax: 800-279-4663

2016 Living an Idea: Empowerment and the Evolution of an Alternative School
Brookline Books
8 Trumbull Rd, Suite B-001
Northampton, MA 1060-4533
413-584-0184
800-666-2665
Fax: 413-584-6184
brbooks@yahoo.com
www.brooklinebooks.com

William H Walters, Author
Esther Wilder, Co-Author
This book is about the creation and 14 year evolution of a public alternative inner-city high school. The school lived an idea - empowerment. Students were encouraged to participate in shaping many aspects of their education, teachers were responsible for running the school, and parents invited to help govern. *$27.95*
ISBN 0-91479 -68-9

2017 Low Tech Assistive Devices: A Handbook for the School Setting
Therapro, Inc.
225 Arlington Street
Framingham, MA 02139-8723
508-872-9494
800-257-5376
800-268-6624
Fax: 508-875-2062
info@therapro.com
www.therapro.com

Karen Conrad, Owner
A how-to book with step by step directions and detailed illustrations for fabrication of frequently requested low-tech assistive devices. *$45.00*
320 pages Paperback

2018 MTA Readers
Educators Publishing Service
625 Mt. Auburn Street, 3rd Floor
PO Box 9031
Cambridge, MA 02139-9031   617-547-6706
                                         800-225-5750
                                    Fax: 888-440-2665
                         Feedback.EPS@schoolspecialty.com
                                         www.epsbooks.com

Rick Holden, President, EPS
Illustrated readers for grades 1-3 that accompany the MTA Reading and Spelling Program (Multisensory Teaching Approach). Phonetic elements in a structured, but entertaining context.
48+ pages $4.65 - $11.65
ISBN 0-83882 -33-3

2019 Making School Inclusion Work: A Guide to Everyday Practice
Brookline Books
8 Trumbull Rd, Suite B-001
Northampton, MA 2445-4533   413-584-0184
                                         800-666-2665
                                    Fax: 413-584-6184
                               brbooks@yahoo.com
                               www.brooklinebooks.com

William H Walters, Author
Esther Wilder, Co-Author
This book tells the reader how to conduct a truly inclusive program, regardless of ethnic or racial background, economic level and physical or cognitive ability. *$24.95*
254 pages
ISBN 0-914791-96-4

2020 Making the Writing Process Work: Strategies for Composition and Self-Regulation
Brookline Books
8 Trumbull Rd, Suite B-001
Northampton, MA 2445-4533   413-584-0184
                                         800-666-2665
                                    Fax: 413-584-6184
                               brbooks@yahoo.com
                               www.brooklinebooks.com

William H Walters, Author
Esther Wilder, Co-Author
This book is geared toward students who have difficulty organizing their thoughts and developing their writing. The specific stategies teach students how to approach, organize, and produce a final written product.. *$24.95*
240 pages Paperback
ISBN 1-571290-10-9

2021 Manual Alphabet Poster
TJ Publishers
Ste 108
2544 Tarpley Rd
Carrollton, TX 75006-2288   972-416-0800
                                         800-999-1168
                                    Fax: 972-416-0944
                               TJPubinc@aol.com
                               www.TJpublishers.com

Pat O'Rourke, President
Poster presents the manual alphabet. *$4.50*

2022 Many Faces of Dyslexia
40 York Rd.
4th Floor
Baltimore, MD 21204-5243   410-296-0232
                                    Fax: 410-321-5069
                               info@interdys.org
                               www.interdys.org

Rick Smith, Chief Executive Officer
Jennifer Topple, Chair
Elsa Cardenas-Hagan, Vice Chair
Provides information on the teaching and rehabilitation techniques for people with dyslexia. *$16.50*
Paperback

2023 Match-Sort-Assemble Job Cards
Exceptional Education
PO Box 15308
Seattle, WA 98115-308   206-262-9538
Jeff Stewart, Owner
Teaches workers to use a series of symbolic cues to control their own production cycles. *$565.00*
Class Set

2024 Match-Sort-Assemble Pictures
Exceptional Education
PO Box 15308
Seattle, WA 98115-308   206-262-9538
Jeff Stewart, Owner
People with profound, severe and moderate mental retardation have immediate access with MSA Pictures. Students work with pictures (and if necessary a template) to match, sort, assemble and disassemble parts that vary in shape, length and diameter. *$426.00*
Class Set

2025 Match-Sort-Assemble SCHEMATICS
Exceptional Education
PO Box 15308
Seattle, WA 98115-308   206-262-9538
Jeff Stewart, Owner
Students with moderate and mild mental retardation and those who have completed MSA Pictures are ready for MSA Schematics. It increases abstraction and displacement of instruction from the work clearly and simply. *$495.00*
Class Set

2026 Match-Sort-Assemble TOOLS
Exceptional Education
PO Box 15308
Seattle, WA 98115-308   206-262-9538
                                    Fax: 475-486-4510
Jeff Stewart, Owner
Students and clients learn to use the tools required for many jobs in light industry. Mastery of the production cycle with independence, endurance and the ability to learn new tasks through pictures and schematics and basic hand functions will help clients acquire and maintain employment in a competitive field. *$595.00*
Class Set

2027 Meeting-in-a-Box
Asthma and Allergy Foundation of America
1233 20th St NW
Suite 610
Washington, DC 20036-7322   202-833-1700
                                         800-7AS-THMA
                                    Fax: 202-833-2351
                               info@aafa.org
                               www.swmlaw.com

Bill Mc Lin, Executive Director
Bill Mclin, Executive Director
A series of self-contained, comprehensive kits that contain all the necessary components for a successful asthma presentation.

2028 More Food!
JE Stewart Teaching Tools
PO Box 15308
Seattle, WA 98115-308   206-262-9538
                                    Fax: 206-262-9538
Jeff Stewart, Owner
Teaches 50 more words found in restaurants, grocery stores, cookbooks such as pizza, carrot, tacos, oysters and pineapple. These words are functional at home, going shopping and during leisure. *$32.50*

2029 More Work!
J E Stewart Teaching Tools
PO Box 15308
Seattle, WA 98115-308   206-262-9538
                                    Fax: 206-262-9538
Jeff Stewart, Owner

Teaches 50 words as they appear on parts, tools, job instructions, signs and labels, such as fill, grasp, release, lock, search, position and select. These words are functional in school and on-the-job. *$32.50*

2030   Multisensory Teaching Approach
Educators Publishing Service
PO Box 9031
Cambridge, MA   2139-9031   617-367-2700
                                             800-225-5750
                                        Fax: 617-547-0412
                                           www.epsbooks.com

$110 - $140
ISBN 0-83888 -10-9

2031   National Autism Resources
6240 Goodyear Rd.
Benicia, CA   94510   707-745-3308
                                             877-249-2393
                                        Fax: 877-259-9419
customerservice@nationalautismresources.com
              www.nationalautismresources. com

2032   Peabody Articulation Decks
AGS
PO Box 99
Circle Pines, MN   55014-99   651-287-7220
                                             800-328-2560
                                        Fax: 763-786-9007
                                          agsmail@agsnet.com
                                             www.agsnet.com

Keith Powel, Special Education Transition Coo
Robert Zaske, Marketing Manager
Complete kit of playing-card sized PAD decks let students focus on the 18 most commonly misarticulated English consonants and blends. *$115.95*
ISBN 0-88671 -75-4

2033   Phonemic Awareness in Young Children: A Classroom Curriculum
Brookes Publishing
PO Box 10624
Baltimore, MD   21285-624   410-337-9580
                          custserv@brookespublishing.com
                             www.brookespublishing.com
Clary Creighton, Exhibits Coordinator
Tracy Gray, Educational Sales Manager
Paul Brooks, Owner

This is a supplemental, whole-class curriculum for improving pre-literacy listening skills. It contains activities that are fun, easy to use, and proven to work in any kindergarten classroom - general, bilingual, inclusive, or special education. This program takes only 15-20 minutes a day. *$24.95*
208 pages Spiral-bound
ISBN 1-557663-21-1

2034   Phonics for Thought
Educators Publishing Service
PO Box 9031
Cambridge, MA   2139-9031   617-367-2700
                                             800-225-5750
                                        Fax: 617-547-0412
                                           www.epsbooks.com
Paperback

2035   Phonological Awareness Training for Reading
Sage Publications
2455 Teller Road
Thousand Oaks, CA   91320   805-499-9774
                                             800-818-7243
                                        Fax: 800-583-2665
                                           info@sagepub.com
                                             www.sagepub.com

Blaise R Simqu, President & CEO
Tracey Ozmina, Executive VP
Chris Hickok, Executive VP and CFO
Stephen Barr, Managing Director

Designed to increase the level of phonological awareness in young children. Can be taught individually or in small groups and takes about 12 to 14 weeks to complete if children are taught in short sessions three or four times a week. *$129.00*

2036   Play!
JE Stewart Teaching Tools
PO Box 15308
Seattle, WA   98115-308   206-262-9538
                                        Fax: 206-262-9538

Jeff Stewart, Owner
Teaches 50 more words as they appear at recreation sites, on signs and labels and in newspapers and magazines, such as movie, visitor, ticket, gallery and zoo. These words are functional in school and at leisure. *$32.50*

2037   Power Breathing Program
Asthma and Allergy Foundation of America
8201 Corporate Drive
Suite 1000
Landover, MD   20785   202-466-7643
                                             800-727-8462
                                        Fax: 202-466-8940
                                              info@aafa.org
                                               www.aafa.org
Bill McLin, Executive Director
Devoloped the only asthma education program specifically designed for and pre-tested with teens. Teens with asthma have special challenges. This interactive program covers everything from the basics of asthma to dealing with their asthma in social situations, in college, and on the job. Includes everything you need to present this three-four session program. *$295.00*

2038   Primary Phonics
School Specialty
625 Mt. Auburn Street, 3rd Floor
PO Box 9031
Cambridge, MA   02139-9031   617-547-6706
                                             800-225-5750
                                        Fax: 888-440-2665
                        Feedback.EPS@schoolspecialty.com
                               eps.schoolspecialty.com
Rick Holden, President, EPS
Barbara W Makar, Author
A program of storybooks and coordinated workbooks that teaches reading for grades K-2. A structured phonetic approach. Contains 8 student workbooks, with 8 sets of 10 coordinated storybooks; consonant workbooks; initial consonant blend workbooks; picture dictionary, and coloring book.
ISSN 0838-83 0

2039   Reading for Content
School Specialty
625 Mt. Auburn Street, 3rd Floor
PO Box 9031
Cambridge, MA   02139-9031   617-547-6706
                                             800-225-5750
                                        Fax: 888-440-2665
                        Feedback.EPS@schoolspecialty.com
                               eps.schoolspecialty.com
Rick Holden, President, EPS
Carol Einstein, Author
A series of 4 books designed to help students improve their reading comprehension skills. Each book contains 43 reading passages followed by 4 questions. Two questions as for a recall of main ideas, and two ask the student to draw conclusions from what they have read. *$ 11.45*
96 pages

2040 Reading from Scratch
Educators Publishing Service
P.O.Box 9031
Cambridge, MA   2139-9031

617-367-2700
800-225-5750
Fax: 617-547-0412
www.epsbooks.com

$6.25 - $49.30
ISBN 0-83888 -75-5

2041 Recipe for Reading
School Specialty
625 Mt. Auburn Street, 3rd Floor
PO Box 9031
Cambridge, MA 02139-9031

617-367-2700
800-225-5750
Fax: 888-440-2665
Feedback.EPS@schoolspecialty.com
eps.schoolspecialty.com

Rick Holden, President, EPS
Nina Traub, Author
Frances Bloom, Co-Author
Contains comprehensive, multisensory, phonics-based reading program presents a skill sequence and lesson structured designed for beginning, at-risk, or struggling readers.

2042 Rewarding Speech
Speech Bin
PO Box 1579
Appleton, WI 54912-1579

772-770-0007
888-388-3224
Fax: 888-388-6344
customercare@schoolspecialty.com
www.speechbin.com

Jan J Binney, Senior Editor
Reproducible reward certificates for children. *$12.95*
32 pages

2043 SAYdee Posters
Speech Bin
PO Box 1579
Appleton, WI 54912-1579

772-770-0007
888-388-3224
Fax: 888-388-6344
customercare@schoolspecialty.com
www.speechbin.com

Jan J Binney, Senior Editor
Colorful speech and language posters. *$20.00*
24 pages
ISBN 0-93785 -47-5

2044 Sensation Products
74 Cotton Mill Hill
Unit A-350
Brattleboro, VT 5301

802-254-4480
Fax: 802-254-4481
www.sensationproducts.com

2045 Sensory University Toy Company, The
4992 Bristol Industrial Hwy
Buford, GA 30518

888-831-4701
Fax: 770-904-6418
sales@sensoryuniversity.com
sensoryuniversity.com

2046 Sequential Spelling: 1-7 with 7 Student Response Books
AVKO Educational Research Foundation
3084 Willard Rd
Birch Run, MI 48415-9404

810-686-9283
866-285-6612
Fax: 810-686-1101
webmaster@avko.org
www.avko.org

Deborah Wolf, President
Aaron Miller, Vice President
Sequential Spelling uses immediate student self-correction. It builds from easier words of a word family such as all and then builds on them to teach; all, tall, stall, install, call, fall, ball, and their inflected forms such as: stalls, stalled, stalling, installing, installment. *$89.95*
72 pages $8.95 each
ISBN 1-56400 -11-6

2047 Signing Naturally Curriculum
Harris Communications
15155 Technology Dr
Eden Prairie, MN   55344-2273

952-906-1180
800-825-6758
Fax: 952-906-1099
info@harriscomm.com
www.harriscomm.com

Robert Harris, President
Kevin Horsky, Business Director
A series based on the functional approach that is the most popular and widely used sign language curriculum designed for teaching American Sign Language. Book and videotape set for level 1 & 2. Teacher's curriculum is also available. *$59.95*

2048 Small Wonder
AGS
PO Box 99
Circle Pines, MN   55014-99

651-287-7220
800-328-2560
Fax: 763-786-9007
agsmail@agsnet.com
www.agsnet.com

Kevin Brueggeman, President
Robert Zaske, Marketing Manager
This infant through toddler program offers a delightful array of activities to teach babies about themselves, others, their surroundings and the world outside. Level One - zero to 18 months; Level Two 18-36 months. Discount price of $389.95 when both levels ordered. *$229.95*
ISBN 0-91347 -62-5

2049 Solving Language Difficulties
School Specialty
625 Mt. Auburn Street, 3rd Floor
PO Box 9031
Cambridge, MA 02139-9031

617-547-6706
800-225-5750
Fax: 888-440-2665
Feedback.EPS@schoolspecialty.com
eps.schoolspecialty.com

Rick Holden, President, EPS
Amey Steere, Author
Caroline Z Peck, Co-Author
This basic workbook can be used in any corrective reading program. It deals extensively with syllables, syllable division, prefixes, suffixes and accent. *$9.75*
176 pages
ISBN 0-838803-26-1

2050 Speech Bin
Abilitations
PO Box 1579
Appleton, WI 54912-1579

772-770-0007
800-513-2465
onlinehelp@schoolspecialty.com
www.speechbin.com

Jan J Binney, Senior Editor
Activities, worksheets and games to encourage practice of speech and language skills. *$25.00*
128 pages
ISBN 0-93785 -42-4

2051 Speech-Language Delights
1965 25th Ave
Vero Beach, FL 32960-3062

772-770-0007

2052 **Spell of Words**
School Specialty
625 Mt. Auburn Street, 3rd Floor
PO Box 9031
Cambridge, MA 02139-9031 617-547-6706
800-225-5750
Fax: 888-440-2665
Feedback.EPS@schoolspecialty.com
eps.schoolspecialty.com

Rick Holden, President, EPS
Elsie T Rak, Author
Covers syllabication, word building along with prefixes, phonograms, word patterns, suffixes, plurals, and possessives. *$14.70*
128 pages Grades 7-Adult

2053 **Spellbound**
School Specialty
625 Mt. Auburn Street, 3rd Floor
PO Box 9031
Cambridge, MA 02139-9031 617-547-6706
800-225-5750
Fax: 888-440-2665
Feedback.EPS@schoolspecialty.com
eps.schoolspecialty.com

Rick Holden, President, EPS
Elsie T Rak, Author
This workbook begins with teaching simple, consistent rules and
then moves on to those that are more difficult. By an inductive
process, students use their own observations to confirm the spelling rules they learn. Each portion of the text is followed by exercises for drill and kinesthetic reinforcement. *$12.85*
144 pages Grades 7-Adult
ISBN 0-838801-65-X

2054 **Spelling Dictionary**
School Specialty
625 Mt. Auburn Street, 3rd Floor
PO Box 9031
Cambridge, MA 02139-9031 617-547-6706
800-225-5750
Fax: 888-440-2665
Feedback.EPS@schoolspecialty.com
eps.schoolspecialty.com

Rick Holden, President, EPS
Gregory Hurray, Author
Contains the most frequently used and misspelled words for students at these grade levels. Designed to be useable and reliable, to
build research and writing skills, and to help teachers promote independent learning in a classroom setting *$6.35*
ISBN 0-838820-56-5

2055 **Starting Over**
School Specialty
625 Mt. Auburn Street, 3rd Floor
PO Box 9031
Cambridge, MA 02139-9031 617-547-6706
800-225-5750
Fax: 888-440-2665
Feedback.EPS@schoolspecialty.com
eps.schoolspecialty.com

Rick Holden, President, EPS
Joan Knight, Author
For students who are ready to try to learn to read again, or for
those who are learning English as a second language. *$38.40*
ISBN 0-838881-65-5

2056 **Studio 49 Catalog**
MMB Music
9051 Watson Road
Suite 161
Saint Louis, MO 63126-1019 314-531-9635
800-543-3771
Fax: 314-531-8384
info@mmbmusic.com
www.mmbmusic.com

Marcia Goldberg, President
Michelle Greenlaw, VP

Percussion instruments for school, therapy, church and family.

2057 **Syracuse Community-Referenced Curriculum Guide for
Students with Disabilties**
Brookes Publishing
PO Box 10624
Baltimore, MD 21285-624 410-337-9580
800-638-3775
Fax: 410-337-8539
custserv@brookespublishing.com
www.readplaylearn.com

Paul Brooks, President
Serving learners from kindergarten through age 21, this
field-tested curriculum is a for professionals and parents devoted
to directly preparing a student to function in the world. it examines the role of community living domains, functional academics,
and embedded skills and includes practical implementation strategies and information for preparing students whose learning
needs go beyond the scope of traditional academic programs.
$54.95
416 pages Spiral-bound
ISBN 1-557660-27-1

2058 **Teaching Individuals with Physical and Multiple Disabilities**
McGraw-Hill, School Publishing
PO Box 182604
Columbus, OH 43272 877-833-5524
Fax: 614-759-3749
customer.service@mcgraw-hill.com
www.mcgraw-hill.com

Harold McGraw, President and CEO
Jack Callahan, Executive VP
John Berisford, Executive VP of HR
Focuses on the functional needs of the handicapped and the teaching skills of background teachers that they need to help them
reach the highest possible level of self-sufficiency.
410 pages

2059 **Teaching Students Ways to Remember**
Brookline Books
8 Trumbull Rd, Suite B-001
Northampton, MA 1060 800-666-2665
Fax: 413-584-6184
brbooks@yahoo.com
www.brooklinebooks.com

ISBN 0-914797-67-0

2060 **Teaching Test-Taking Skills: Helping Students Show What
They Know**
Brookline Books
8 Trumbull Rd, Suite B-001
Northampton, MA 1060 60- 66- 703
800-666-2665
Fax: 414-584-6184
brbooks@yahoo.com
www.brooklinebooks.com

ISBN 0-914797-76-X

2061 **Therapy Shoppe**
PO Box 8875
Grand Rapids, MI 49518 616-696-7441
800-261-5590
Fax: 616-696-7471
info@therapyshoppe.com
www.therapyshoppe.com

2062 **To Teach a Dyslexic**
AVKO Educational Research Foundation
3084 Willard Rd
Birch Run, MI 48415-9404 810-686-9283
866-686-9283
Fax: 810-686-1101
webmaster@avko.org
www.avko.org

Deborah Wolf, President
Aaron Miller, Vice President

A video available in DVD or video CD that shows Don McCabe working with a dyslexic teenager. The video helps teachers learn more about dyslexia and how to go about teaching a dyslexic student using the AVKO methodology and philosophy. This is a free video.

288 pages Paperback

2063   Tools for Transition
AGS
PO Box 99
Circle Pines, MN   55014-99
651-287-7220
800-328-2560
Fax: 763-786-9007
agsmail@agsnet.com
www.agsnet.com

Kevin Brueggeman, President
Robert Zaske, Marketing Manager
This program prepares students with learning disabilities for postsecondary education. *$129.95*

2064   United Art and Education
PO Box 9219
Fort Wayne, IN   46899-9219
260-478-1121
800-322-3247
Fax: 800-858-3247
www.unitednow.com

2065   VAK Tasks Workbook: Visual, Auditory and Kinesthetic
Educational Tutorial Consortium
4400 S 44th St
Lincoln, NE   68516-1109
402-489-8133
Fax: 402-489-8160

T Elli Cross, Owner
A workbook emphasizing the multisensory approach to teaching vocabulary and spelling. It is intended for middle-grade and older students working with prefixes, roots, suffixes, homonyms, and the spelling of easily confused endings. Includes spelling posters. *$7.00*

96 pages Paperback

2066   Volunteer Transcribing Services
Ste 200
205 E 3rd Ave
San Mateo, CA   94401-4028
650-357-1571
Fax: 650-632-3510

Alanah Hoffman, Coordinator
VTS is a nonprofit California corporation that produces large print school books for visually impaired students in grades K-12.

2067   Wordly Wise 3000
School Specialty
625 Mt. Auburn Street, 3rd Floor
PO Box 9031
Cambridge, MA   02139-9031
617-547-6706
800-225-5750
Fax: 888-440-2665
Feedback.EPS@schoolspecialty.com
eps.schoolspecialty.com

Rick Holden, President, EPS
Kenneth Hodkinson, Author
Sandra Adams, Co-Author
Cheryl Dressler, Co-Author
Begins with a word list of 8-12 words, followed by clear, brief definitions and sentences that illustrate the meaning of the word. Books B and C often present more than one meaning of a word. Throughout all three books, drawings illustrate the meanings.
ISSN 0838-84 8

2068   Work!
JE Stewart Teaching Tools
PO Box 15308
Seattle, WA   98115-308
206-328-7664
Fax: 206-262-9538

Jan Gleason, Executive Director
Teaches 50 words as they appear on parts, tools, job instructions, signs, labels such as: hard hat, assembly, clamp, cut, drill, pack-

age and schedule. These words are functional in school and on-the-job. *$32.50*

2069   Working Together & Taking Part
A GS
PO Box 99
Circle Pines, MN   55014-99
651-287-7220
800-328-2560
Fax: 763-786-9007
agsmail@agsnet.com
www.agsnet.com

Kevin Brueggeman, President
Robert Zaske, Market Manager
Two programs to build children's social skills in grades 3-6 through folk literature. Has 31 activity-rich lessons, teaching skills like: following rules, accepting differences, speaking assertively and helping others. Discount price of $279.00 when ordering both. *$149.95*

Associations

2070   AVKO Educational Research Foundation
3084 Willard Rd
Birch Run, MI   48415-9404
810-686-9283
Fax: 810-686-1101
webmaster@avko.org
www.avko.org

Don McCabe, President
Linda Heck, Vice President
Comprised of individuals interested in helping others learn to read and spell. Develops and sells materials for teaching dyslexics or others with learning disabilities using a method involving audio, visual, kinesthetic and oral (multi-sensory) techniques.

2071   Academy of Rehabilitative Audiology
PO Box 2323
Albany, NY   12220-0323
952-920-0484
ara@audrehab.org
www.audrehab.org

Claire Bernstein, Ph.D, President
Sherri Smith, Ph.D, Treasurer
Kristin Vasil-Dilaj, Ph.D, Secretary
Sheila Pratt, Ph.D, JARA Editor
The Academy of Rehabilitative Audiology provides professional education, research and programs for hearing handicapped persons. The primary purpose of the ARA is to promote excellence in hearing care through the provision of comprehensive rehabilitative and habilitative services.

2072   Alternative Work Concepts
PO Box 11452
Eugene, OR   97440
541-345-3043
Fax: 541-345-9669
www.alternativeworkconcepts.org

Liz Fox, Executive Director
To promote individualized, integrated, and meaningful employment opportunities in the community for adults with multiple disabilities; to improve the quality of life and provide continuous opportunities for personal growth for these individuals; and to assist businesses with workforce diversification.

2073   American Council for Headache Education(ACHE)
19 Mantua Rd.
Mount Royal, NJ   08061
856-423-0043
Fax: 856-423-0082
amf@talley.com
www.achenet.org

David W. Dodick, Chairman
Nonprofit, patient-health, professional partnership dedicated to advancing the treatment and management of headaches and to raising the public awareness of headache as valid, biologically based illness.

2074 American School Counselor Association
American Counselling Association
1101 King St.
Suite 310
Alexandria, VA   22314-2957   703-683-2722
                                             800-306-4722
                                        Fax: 703-997-7572
                                     asca@schoolcounselor.org
                                     www.schoolcounselor.org
Richard Wong, Executive Director
Kathleen Rakestraw, Director of Communications
Jennifer Walsh, Director of Education and Training
ASCA focuses on providing professional devleopment, enhancing school counseling programs, and research effective school counseling practices. Mission is to promote excellence in professional school counseling and the development of all students.

2075 Association for Driver Rehabilitation Specialists
200 First Ave. NW
Suite 505
Hickory, NC   28601   866-672-9466
                                        Fax: 828-855-1672
                                             info@aded.net
                                             www.aded.net
Dan Allison, President
Elizabeth Green, Executive Director
Beth Gibson, Secretary
Robert Dan, Office Manager
The Association for Driver Rehabilitation Specialists was established to support professionals working in the field of driver education and driver training and transportation equipment modifications for persons with disabilities through education and information dissemination.

2076 Association on Higher Education and Disability
107 Commerce Centre Dr.
Suite 204
Huntersville, NC 28078-5870   704-947-7779
                                        Fax: 704-948-7779
                                             www.ahead.org
Jamie Axelrod, President
Gaeir Dietrich, Treasurer
Stephan Smith, Executive Director
Katy Washington, Secretary
AHEAD is a professional membership organization for individuals involved in the development of policy and in the provision of quality services to meet the needs of persons with disabilities involved in all areas of higher education, promiting full and equal participation.

2077 CARF International (Commission on Accreditation of Rehabilitation Facilities)
CARF International
6951East Southpoint Rd.
Tucson, AZ 85756-9407   888-281-6531
                                        Fax: 520-318-1129
                                        TTY:520-495-7077
                                             info@carf.org
                                                  carf.org
Brian J. Boon, President/CEO
An independent, nonprofit accreditor of human service providers in the areas of aging services, behavioral health, child and youth services, DMEPOS, employment and community services, medical rehabilitation, and opioid treatment programs.

2078 Council for Exceptional Children
2900 Crystal Dr.
Suite 1000
Arlington, VA 22202-3557   888-232-7733
                                        TTY:866-915-5000
                                        service@cec.sped.org
                                             www.cec.sped.org
Alexander T. Graham, Executive Director
Sharon Rodriguez, Senior Executive Assistant
Craig Evans, Director of Operations
The largest international professional organization dedicated to improving the educational success of individuals with disabilities and/or gifts and talents. Advocates for appropriate govern-

mental policies, sets professional standards, provides professional development, advocates for individuals with exceptionalities, and helps professionals obtain conditions and resources necessary for effective professional practice.

2079 Division for Early Childhood of the Council for Exceptional Children
Council for Exceptional Children
2900 Crystal Dr.
Suite 100
Arlington, VA   22202-3557   310-428-7209
                                             888-232-7733
                                        Fax: 855-678-1989
                                        TTY:866-912-5000
                                             dec@dec-sped.org
                                             www.dec-sped.org
Peggy Kemp, Executive Director
Ben Rogers, Associate Director
Brittany Clark, Operations Coordinator
Promotes policies and advances evidence-based practices that support families and enhance the optimal development of young children who have or are at risk for developmental delays and disabilities.

2080 Division for Physical, Health & Multiple Disabilities
Council for Exceptional Children (CEC)
2900 Crystal Dr.
Suite 1000
Arlington, VA   22202   888-232-7733
                                        TTY:866-915-5000
                                        service@cec.sped.org
                                             www.cec.sped.org
Alexander T. Graham, Executive Director
Sharon Rodriguez, Senior Executive Assistant
Craig Evans, Director of Operations
The DPHD is the official division of the CEC that advocates for quality education for all individuals with physical disabilities, multiple disabilities, and special health care needs served in schools, hospitals, or home settings. The goals of DPHD include: promoting the continued development adequate resources and programs; disseminating relevant and timely information on issues, instructional strategies, and research through meetings and publications; and many more services and activities.

2081 Filomen M. D'Agostino Greenberg Music School
Lighthouse Guild
250 West 64th St.
New York, NY   10023   646-874-8660
                                             800-284-4422
                                     musicschool@lighthouseguild.org
                                             lighthouseguild.org
Leslie Jones, Executive Director
The Filomen M. D'Agostino Greenberg Music School is the only community music school in the US for people who are blind or visually impaired, offering instruction and an accessible music technology center.

2082 HEAL: Health Education AIDS Liaison
New York, NY   347-867-4497
                                     michaelellner2@gmail.com
                                             www.healaids.com
Michael Ellner, President
Barnett J. Weiss, Board Member
Roberto Giraldo, Board Member
Nonprofit, community-based educational organization providing information, hope, and support to people who are HIV positive or living with AIDS. The men and women at HEAL are health professionals, people living with life threatening diseases, and volunteers.

2083 Incight
111 SW Columbia St
Suite 1170
Portland, OR 97201   971-244-0305
                                             info@incight.org
                                                  incight.org
Scott Hatley, Development & Community Relations Officer

Incight in a non-profit organization that supports people with disabilities in the areas of education, employment, and independent living. Incight offers programs that address workplace descrimination, college application process and recreational needs of those they serve.

2084 International Childbirth Education Association
110 Horizon Dr.
Suite 210
Raleigh, NC 27615   919-674-4183
    800-624-4934
    Fax: 919-459-2075
    www.icea.org

Debra Tolson, President
Bonita Katz, President Elect
Michaelle Hardy, Treasurer
Vonda Gates, Secretary

The Association offers teaching certificates, seminars, continuing education workshops, and mail order center.

2085 International Dyslexia Association
40 York Rd.
4th Floor
Baltimore, MD 21204-5243   410-296-0232
    Fax: 410-321-5069
    info@interdys.org
    www.interdys.org

Rick Smith, Chief Executive Officer
Jennifer Topple, Chair
Elsa Cardenas-Hagan, Vice Chair
Lisa Goldstein, President

Provides free information and referral services for diagnosis and tutoring for parents, educators, physicians, and individuals with dyslexia. Membership includes yearly journal and quarterly newsletter, and Pennsylvania newsletter; discounts to conferences and events.

2086 Job Accommodation Network
Office of Disability and Employment Policy
200 Constitution Ave. NW
Washington, DC 20210   800-526-7234
    TTY:877-781-9403
    www.jan.wvu.edu

Anne Hirsh, Co-Director
Louis Orslene, Co-Director

International toll-free consulting service that provides information about job accommodations and the employability of people with disabilities. Also provides information regarding the Americans with Disabilities Act (ADA).

2087 LD Online
2775 S. Quincy St.
Arlington, VA 22206   *Fax:* 703-998-2060
    ldonline.org

Noel Gunther, Executive Director
Christian Lindstrom, Director
Lydia Breiseth, Manager
Tina Chovanec, Director

LD OnLine seeks to help children and adults reach their full potential by providing accurate and up-to-date information and advice about learning disabilities and ADHD. The site features hundreds of helpful articles, multimedia, monthly columns by noted experts, first person essays, children's writing and artwork, a comprehensive resource guide, very active forums, and a Yellow Pages referral directory of professionals, schools, and products.

2088 Lighthouse Guild
250 W 64th St.
New York, NY 10023-6601   800-284-4422
    TTY:TTY 711
    www.lighthouseguild.org

James M. Dubin, Chairman
Alan R. Morse, President
Sarah E. Smith, Treasurer
Robert B. Okun, Secretary

Lighthouse Guild is a not-for-profit vision & healthcare organization, addressing the needs of people who are blind or visually impaired, including those with multiple disabilities or chronic medical conditions.

2089 Michigan Psychological Association
124 W Allegan St.
Suite 1900
Lansing, MI 48933-1768   517-347-1885
    Fax: 517-484-4442
    office@michiganpsychologicalassociation.org
    www.michiganpsychologicalass ociation.org

Kristin Sheridan, President
LaVone Swanson, Executive Director
Debra Smith, Treasurer
Cynthia S. Rodriguez, Secretary

Nonprofit organization of over 1000 psychologists, working to advance psychology as a science and a profession and to promote the public welfare by encouraging the highest professional standards, offering public education and providing a public service, and by participating in the public policy process on behalf of the profession and health care consumers.

2090 National Association for Adults with Special Learning Needs
PO Box 716
Bryn Mawr, PA 19010   naasln.org

Richard Cooper, President
Frances A. Holthaus, Vice President
Jeanne Brunette-Tregoning, Treasurer

NAASLN is an association for those who serve adults with special learning needs. NAASLN members include educators, trainers, employers and human service providers.

2091 National Association of Colleges and Employers
62 Highland Ave.
Bethlehem, PA 18017-9481   610-868-1421
    cnader@naceweb.org
    naceweb.org

Glen Fowler, President
Norma Guerra Gaier, President Elect
Cecelia M. Nader, Administration

A national association with services for career planning, placement and recruitment professionals.

2092 National Association of Parents with Children in Special Education
3642 E Sunnydale Dr.
Chandler Heights, AZ 85142   800-754-4421
    Fax: 800-424-0371
    contact@napcse.org
    www.napcse.org

Dr. George Giuliani, President

(NAPCSE)is a national membership organization dedicated to rendering all possible support and assistance to parents whose children receive special education services, both in and outside of school.

2093 National Association of State Directors of Special Education
225 Reinekers Ln.
Suite 420
Alexandria, VA 22314   703-519-3800
    Fax: 703-519-3808
    www.nasdse.org

Glenna Gallo, President
Bill East, Executive Director
Nancy Reder, Deputy Executive Director
Bill Hussey, Secretary/Treasurer

NASDSE focuses on improving educational services and outcomes for children and youth with disabilities throughout the United States, the Department of Defense, the federated territories and the Freely Associated States of Palau, Micronesia and the Marshall Islands.

2094   National Center for Homeopathy
1120 Route 73
Suite 200
Mount Laurel, NJ   08054   856-437-4752
                                     Fax: 856-439-0525
                          nationalcenterforhomeopathy.org

Abby Beale, President
Lauri Grossman, Secretary
Glenna Tinney, Treasurer
Alison Teitelbaum, Executive Director
The National Center for Homeopathy (NCH) is a non-profit organization dedicated to promoting health through homeopathy by advancing the use and practice of homeopathy.

2095   National Council on Rehabilitation Education (NCRE)
1099 E. Champlain Dr.
Suite A-137
Fresno, CA   93720   559-906-0787
                                        info@ncre.org
                                             ncre.org

Michael Accordino, President
Denise Catalano, First Vice President
Matt Bruinekool, Second Vice President
Members include academic institutions and organizations, professional educators, researchers, and students. Assists in the documentation of the effect of education in improving services to persons with disabilities; determines the skills and training necessary for effective rehabilitation services; develops role models, standards and uniform licensure and certification requirements for rehabilitation personnel.

2096   National Education Association of the United States
1201 16th St. NW
Washington, DC   20036-3290   202-833-4000
                                     Fax: 202-822-7974
                                           www.nea.org

Lily Eskelsen Garcia, President
Becky Pringle, Vice President
Princess R. Moss, Secretary/Treasurer
John C. Stocks, Executive Director
The National Education Association (NEA) is committed to advancing the cause of public education.

2097   National Society for Experiential Education
19 Mantua Rd.
Mount Royal, NJ   08061   856-423-3427
                                     Fax: 856-423-3420
                                        nsee@talley.com
                                           www.nsee.org

Stephanie Thomason, President
Marianna Savoca, Vice President
Bath Odahlen, Executive Director
Alan Grose, Treasurer
National nonprofit organization which advocates experiential learning and works with college administrators and high school and college internship programs.

2098   SSD (Services for Students with Disabilities)
College Board
P.O. Box 7504
London, KY   40742-7504   212-713-8333
                                          844-255-7728
                                     Fax: 866-360-0114
                                       TTY: 609-882-4118
                             ssd@info.collegeboard.org
                                  www.collegeboard.com

David Coleman, President
Jeremy Singer, Chief Operating Officer
John McGrath, Senior Vice President
National, nonprofit association dedicated to preparing, inspiring and connecting students to college and opportunity. Provide the accomodations students with disabilities need to complete test and other evaluations.

2099   Society for Disability Studies
P.O. Box 5570
Eureka, CA   95502   510-206-5767
                                        sds@disstudies.org
                                          www.disstudies.org

Phil Smith, President
Carol Goldin, Treasurer
Joanne Woiak, Vice President
SDS is a scholarly association of more than 400 artists, scholars and activists who promote Disability Studies, recognizing disability as a complex and valuable aspect of human experience.

2100   The AG Academy for Listening and Spoken Language
Alexander Graham Bell Association
3417 Volta Pl. NW
Washington, DC   20007-2737   202-337-5220
                                     Fax: 202-337-8314
                                       academy@agbell.org
                                          www.agbell.org

Ted A. Meyer, Chair
Catharine McNally, Chair-Elect
Emilio Alonso Mendoza, Chief Executive Officer
Listening and Spoken Language Specialsts (LSLST) work with infants and children who are deaf or hard of hearing and their families seeking a listening and spoken language outcome in a variety of settings: home-based intervention, public schools, independent schools, private therapy, clinical centers for the deaf and hard of hearing, audiological and cochlear implant centers.

2101   United Cerebral Palsy
1825 K St. NW
Suite 600
Washington, DC   20006-5638   202-776-0406
                                          800-872-5827
                                            www.ucp.org

Armando Contreras, President/CEO
Diane Wilush, Chair
Christobel Selecky, Vice Chair
Melvin Hurley, Treasurer
United Cerebral Palsy (UCP) educates, advocates and provides support services to ensure a life without limits for people with a spectrum of disabilities. UCP and its nearly 68+ affiliates have a mission to advance the independence, productivity and full citizenship of people with a broad range of disabilities by providing services and support to children and adults.

Directories

2102   ADDitude Directory
108 West 39th St.
Suite 805
New York, NY   10018   646-366-0830
                                     Fax: 646-366-0842
                          customerservice@additudemag.com
                               directory.additudemag.com

2103   BOSC: Directory of Facilities for People with Learning Disabilities
Books on Special Children
PO Box 3378
Amherst, MA   1004-3378   413-256-8164
                                     Fax: 413-256-8896
                                      irene@boscbooks.com
                                         www.boscbooks.com

Michael Young, President
Directory of schools, independent living programs, clinics and centers, colleges and vocational programs, agencies and commercial products. Five sections in special post binder that can be updated annually. Hardcover. *$70.00*
300+ pages Yearly
ISSN 0961-3888

2104 Community Resource Directory
5300 Hiatus Road
Sunrise, FL 33351 954-745-9779
800-963-5337
webmaster@adrcbroward.org
www.adrcbroward.org

2105 Complete Directory for Pediatric Disorders
Sedgwick Press/Grey House Publishing
4919 Route 22
P.O. Box 56
Amenia, NY 12501 518-789-8700
800-562-2139
Fax: 518-789-0556
books@greyhouse.com
www.greyhouse.com

Leslie Mackenzie, Publisher
Laura Mars, Editorial Director
Jessica Moody, Marketing Director
Diana Delgado, Editorial Assistant
An annual directory for professionals, parents and caregivers.
Provides valuable information on more than 200 pediatric conditions, disorders, diseases and disabilities, including informative descriptions and a wide variety of resources, from associations to publications. *$165.00*
1000 pages Annual
ISBN 1-592374-30-1

2106 Complete Directory for People with Chronic Illness
Sedgwick Press/Grey House Publishing
4919 Route 22
P.O. Box 56
Amenia, NY 12501 518-789-8700
800-562-2139
Fax: 518-789-0556
books@greyhouse.com
www.greyhouse.com

Leslie Mackenzie, Publisher
Laura Mars, Editorial Director
Jessica Moody, Marketing Director
Diana Delgado, Editorial Assistant
This directory is structured around the ninety most prevalent chronic illnesses. Each chronic illness chapter includes an informative description, plus a comprehensive listing of resources and support services available for people diagnosed with chronic illness and their network of supportive individuals. *$165.00*
1000 pages Annual
ISBN 1-592374-15-8

2107 Complete Learning Disabilities Directory
Sedgwick Press/Grey House Publishing
4919 Route 22
P.O. Box 56
Amenia, NY 12501 518-789-8700
800-562-2139
Fax: 518-789-0556
books@greyhouse.com
www.greyhouse.com

Leslie Mackenzie, Publisher
Laura Mars, Editorial Director
Jessica Moody, Marketing Director
Diana Delgado, Editorial Assistant
A comprehensive educational guide offering over 6,500 listings on associations and organizations, schools, government agencies, testing materials, camps, products, books, newsletters, legal information, classroom materials and more. Includes separate chapters on ADD and Literacy, as well as informative articles.
$150.00
800 pages Annual
ISBN 1-592375-86-3

2108 Complete Mental Health Directory
Sedgwick Press/Grey House Publishing
4919 Route 22
P.O. Box 56
Amenia, NY 12501 518-789-8700
800-562-2139
Fax: 518-789-0556
books@greyhouse.com
www.greyhouse.com

Leslie Mackenzie, Publisher
Laura Mars, Editorial Director
Jessica Moody, Marketing Director
Diana Delgado, Editorial Assistant
This directory offers comprehensive information covering the field of behavioral health, with critical information for both the layman and the mental health professional. It covers, in depth, 25 specific mental disorders, and includes informative descriptions and a complete list of resources. *$165.00*
800 pages Annual
ISBN 1-592375-44-8

2109 Directory Of Services For People With Disabilities
117 W. Duval St.
Suite 205
Jacksonville, FL 32202-4111 904-630-4940
Fax: 904-630-3476
TTY:904-630-4933
disabledservices@coj.net
www.coj.net

2110 Directory for Exceptional Children
Prorter Sargent
2 LAN Drive
Suite 100
Westford, MA 01886 978-692-5092
800-342-7470
Fax: 978-692-4714
info@carnegiecomm.com
www.carnegiecomm.com

Joe Moore, President, CEO
Mark Cunningham, SVP, Enrollment Marketing
Melissa Rekos, SVP, Digital Services
Gary Allen Williams, VP, Special Projects
Supports parents and professionals seeking the optimal educational, therapeutic or clinical environment for special-needs youth. *$75.00*
1120 pages Trienniel
ISBN 0-875581-50-1

2111 Educators Resource Directory
Sedgwick Press/Grey House Publishing
4919 Route 22
PO Box 55
Amenia, NY 12501 518-789-8700
800-562-2139
Fax: 845-373-6390
books@greyhouse.com
www.greyhouse.com

Leslie Mackenzie, Publisher
Laura Mars, Editorial Director
Jessica Moody, Marketing Director
Kristen Thatcher, Production Manager
Gives education professionals immediate access to Associations and Organizations, Conferences and Trade Shows, Educational Research Centers, Employment Opportunities and Teaching Abroad, School Library Services, Scholarships, Financial Resources and much more. *$145.00*
650 pages Annual
ISBN 1-592377-43-5

2112   Greater Milwaukee Area Health Care Guide for Older Adults
PO Box 285
Germantown, WI   53022   262-253-0901
Fax: 262-253-0903
info@seniorresourcesonline.com
www.seniorresourcesonline.com

Gary Knippen, President
This directory is designed for older adults, family members and professionals looking for health care options in Milwaukee, Ozaukee, Washington and Waukesha counties. The directory is comprehensive with all providers included at no charge.

2113   Greater Milwaukee Area Senior Housing Options
PO Box 285
Germantown, WI   53022   262-253-0901
Fax: 262-253-0903
info@seniorresourcesonline.com
www.seniorresourcesonline.com

Gary Knippen, President
This directory is designed for older adults, family members and professionals looking for senior housing options in Milwaukee, Ozaukee, Washington and Waukesha counties. The directory is comprehensive with all providers included at no charge.

2114   Increasing and Decreasing Behaviors of Persons with Severe Retardation and Autism
Research Press
P.O. Box 7886
Champaign, IL   61826   217-352-3273
800-519-2707
Fax: 217-352-1221
orders@researchpress.com
www.researchpress.com

Robert W. Parkinson, Founder
Dr Richard M Foxx, Author
Shows how to increase desirable behaviors by using techniques such as shaping, prompting, fading, modeling, backward chaining and graduated guidance. Offers specific guidelines for arranging and managing the learning environment as well as standards for evaluating and maintaining success. *$21.95*
230 pages
ISBN 0-878222-65-0

2115   Indiana Directory of Disability Resources
225 S. University Street
ABE Bldg.
West Lafayette, IN 47907-2093   765-494-5013
800-825-4264
bng@ecn.purdue.edu
engineering.purdue.edu/~bng/IDDR/

2116   Nevada's Care Connection
3416 Goni Road
Suite D-132
Carson City, NV   89706   702-486-3600
cpasquale@adsd.nv.gov
www.nevadaadrc.com

Cheyenne Pasquale, ADRC Project Manager
Nevada's Care Connection: Aging and Disability Resource Center (ADRC) program provides information and access to programs and services that benefit Nevada's seniors, people with disabilities and caregivers.

2117   Northeast Wisconsin Directory of Servicesfor Older Adults
PO Box 285
Germantown, WI   53022   262-253-0901
Fax: 262-253-0903
info@seniorresourcesonline.com
www.seniorresourcesonline.com

Gary Knippen, President
This directory is designed for older adults, family members and professionals looking for housing and health care options in Brown, Calumet, Door, Fond du Lac, Green Lake, Kewaunee, Manitowoc, Marinette, Marquette, Oconto, Outagamie, Shawano, Sheboygan, Waupaca, Waushara and Winnebago counties.

2118   ODHH Directory of Resources and Services
1521 N. 6th Street
Harrisburg, PA   17102   717-783-4912
TTY:717-783-4912
RA-LI-OVR-ODHH@pa.gov

2119   Responding to Crime Victims with Disabilities
2000 M Street NW
Suite 480
Washington, DC   20036   202-467-8700
Fax: 202-467-8701
webmaster@ncvc.org
www.victimsofcrime.org

Philip M. Gerson, Chair
G. Morris Gurley, Vice-Chair
Mai Fernandez, Executive Director
Jeffrey R. Dion, Deputy Executive Director
The mission of the National Center for Victims of Crime is to forge a national commitment to help victims of crime rebuild their lives. It is dedicated to serving individuals, families, and communities harmed by crime.

2120   Selective Placement Program Coordinator Directory
1900 E Street, NW
Washington, DC   20415-1000   202-606-1800
www.opm.gov

2121   South Central Wisconsin Directory of Services for Older Adults
PO Box 285
Germantown, WI   53022   262-253-0901
www.seniorresourcesonline.com

Gary Knippen, President
This directory is designed for older adults, family members and professionals looking for housing and health care options in Columbia, Dane, Dodge, Grant, Green, Iowa, Jefferson, Juneau, Lafayette, Richland, Rock, Sauk, and Walworth counties.

2122   Southeast Wisconsin Directory of Servicesfor Older Adults
PO Box 285
Germantown, WI   53022   262-253-0901
www.seniorresourcesonline.com

Gary Knippen, President
This directory is designed for older adults, family members and professionals looking for housing and health care options in Kenosha, Racine and Walworth counties.

2123   Teaching Special Students in Mainstream
Books on Special Children
P.O.Box 305
Congers, NY   10920-305   845-638-1236
Fax: 845-638-0847
irene@boscbooks.com

515 pages Softcover

Educational Publishers

2124   AFB Press
American Foundation for the Blind / AFB Press
2 Penn Plaza
Suite 1102
New York, NY   10121   212-502-7600
Fax: 888-545-8331
afbinfo@afb.net
www.afb.org

Carl R. Augusto, President and CEO
Paul Schroeder, Vice President, Programs and Policy
Rick Bozeman, Chief Financial Officer
Kelly Bleach, Chief Administrative Officer
Develops, publishes, and sells a wide variety of informative books, pamphlets, periodicals, and videos for students, professionals, and researchers in the blindness and visual impairment fields, for people professionally involved in making the mainstream community accessible, and for blind and visually impaired people and their families; publication and video orders.

2125 Academic Therapy Publications
Academic Therapy Publications / High Noon Books
20 Leveroni Ct
Novato, CA 94949-5746   415-883-3314
                                            800-422-7249
                                            888-287-9975
                           sales@academictherapy.com
                           www.academictherapy.com

Jim Arena, President
Stacy Frauwirth, Assessment Project Manager
Holly Melton, Head Writer & Senior Project Manager
Academic Therapy Publications produces and distributes psychological and educational tests used by professionals involved in special education and learning differences in the K-12 school system as well as adult services.

2126 AccessText Network
512 Means Street NW
Suite 250
Atlanta, GA 30318   866-271-4968
                                       Fax: 404-894-7565
                           membership@accesstext.org
                           www.accesstext.org

2127 American Association of University Affiliated Programs for Persons with Dev Disabilities
1100 Wayne Ave.
Suite 1000
Silver Spring, MD 20910   301-588-8252
                                       Fax: 301-588-2842
                           aucdinfo@aucd.org
                           www.aucd.org/

Andrew J. Imparato, JD, Executive Director
Abigail Alberico, MPH, Project Manager
Leon Barnett, MSEd, Program Specialist
Anna Costalas, MPA, Program Specialist
The Association of University Centers on Disabilities (AUCD) is a membership organization that supports and promotes a national network of university-based interdisciplinary programs

2128 American Counseling Association
5999 Stevenson Ave
Alexandria, VA 22304   703-823-0252
                                            800-347-6647
                                       Fax: 800-473-2329
                           webmaster@counseling.org
                           www.counseling.org

Robert L. Smith, President
Thelma Duffey, President Elect
Brian Canfield, Treasurer
Richard Yep, CEO
Offers tools and books for the professional.

2129 Brookes Publishing Company
PO Box 10624
Baltimore, MD 21285-0624   410-337-9580
                                            800-638-3775
                                       Fax: 410-337-8539
                           webmaster@brookespublishing.com
                           www.brookespublishing.com

Paul H. Brookes, Chairman of the Board
Jeffrey D. Brookes, President
George S. Stamathis, VP/Publisher
Melissa A. Behn, Executive Vice President
Publishes highly respected resources in early childhood, early intervention, inclusive and special education, developmental disabilities, learning disabilities, communication and language, behavior and mental health.

2130 Brookline Books
8 Trumbull Rd
B-001
Northampton, MA 01060   413-584-0184
                                            800-666-2665
                                       Fax: 413-584-6184
                           brbooks@yahoo.com
                           www.brooklinebks.com

2131 Brooks/Cole Publishing Company
511 Forest Lodge Rd
Pacific Grove, CA 93950-5040   831-373-0728
                                            800-354-9706
                                       Fax: 831-375-6414

2132 BurnsBooks Publishing
680 Ridge Road
Middletown, CT 6457   860-344-0233
                                       Fax: 860-344-0233
                           burnsbookspub@aol.com
                           www.burnsbookspublishing.com

2133 Charles C Thomas Publisher LTD
2600 S 1st Street
Springfield, IL 62704-4730   217-789-8980
                                            800-258-8980
                                       Fax: 217-789-9130
                           books@ccthomas.com
                           www.ccthomas.com

Michael P. Thomas, President
Publishes specialty titles and textbooks in medicine, dentistry, nursing, and veterinary medicine, as well as a complete line in the behavioral sciences, criminal justice, education, special education, and rehabilitation. Aims to accommodate the current needs for information.

2134 DisabilityAdvisor.com
37 North Orange Ave.
Suite 500
Orlando, FL 32801   321-332-7800
                                            888-393-1010
                                       Fax: 888-985-6060
                           joeram@disabilityadvisor.com
                           www.disabilityadvisor.com

Joseph E. Ram, Publisher
Kay Derochie, Editor
Jackie Booth, Ph.D., Editor
Lisa Nuss, Writer
DisabilityAdvisor.com provides free information on federal and state disability benefits programs and other resources for readers and their families. This includes disabled children and students, military veterans, injured workers and disabled seniors. Readers are encouraged to submit their questions and comments online. The website also offers information on managing finances, education, parenting, relationships and other issues of interest to the disabled and their friends and families.

2135 Dolphin Computer Access
231 Clarksville Road
Suite 7
Princeton Junction, NJ 8550   866-797-5921
                                       Fax: 609-799-0475
                           info@dolphinusa.com
                           www.yourdolphin.com

Noel Duffy, Managing Director
Dolphin helps vision and print impairments

2136 Eric Clearinghouse on Disabilities and Gifted Education
Council for Exceptional Children
2900 Crystal Dr.
Suite 1000
Arlington, VA 22202-3557   888-232-7733
                                       TTY:866-915-5000
                           service@cec.sped.org
                           www.cec.sped.org

Alexander T. Graham, Executive Director
Sharon Rodriguez, Senior Executive Assistant
Craig Evans, Director of Operations
Provides information on special and gifted education. Provides referrals, offers patient networking services and provides information on current research programs. Focuses its efforts on prevention, identification, assessment, intervention and enrichment both in special settings and within mainstream communities. Offers a variety of materials including brochures and Spanish language matereials.

2137 Gallaudet University Press
800 Florida Avenue, NE
Washington, DC 20002-3695   202-651-5488
                                Fax: 202-651-5489
                                gupress@gallaudet.edu
                                gupress.gallaudet.edu
David F Armstrong, Executive Director
Publishes scholarly trade books and journals about deaf people
and their language, history, and culture for deaf people, parents of
deaf children, professionals, educators and the general public.
Produces spring and fall catalogs.

2138 Greenwood Publishing Group
88 Post Rd W
Westport, CT 06880-4208   203-226-3571
                                Fax: 203-222-1502
                                webmaster@greenwood.com
                                greenwood.com

Wayne Smith, President
Kirstin Olsen, Author
ABC-CLIO and Greenwood Press are recognized as indus-
try-leading providers of the highest-quality reference materials.
These imprints offer authoritative reference scholarship and innovative coverage of history and humanities topics across the
secondary and higher education curriculum.

2139 Grey House Publishing
4919 Route 22
P.O. Box 56
Amenia, NY 12501   518-789-8700
                                800-562-2139
                                Fax: 518-789-0556
                                books@greyhouse.com
                                www.greyhouse.com

Leslie Mackenzie, Publisher
Laura Mars, Editorial Director
Jessica Moody, Marketing Director
Kristen Thatcher, Production Manager
Grey House Publishing publishes directories, handbooks and ref-
erence works for public, high school and academic libraries and
the business and health communities. Most titles are available as
online databases.

2140 Hammill Institute on Disabilities
8700 Shoal Creek Blvd.
Austin, TX 78757-6897   512-451-3521
                                Fax: 512-451-3728
                                info@hammill-institute.org
                                hammill-institute.org

2141 Harbor House Law Press
PO Box 480
Hartfield, VA 23071   804-758-8400
                                Fax: 202-318-3239
                                webmaster@wrightslaw.com
                                www.harborhouselaw.com

2142 High Noon Books
Academic Therapy Publications / High Noon Books
20 Leveroni Ct
Novato, CA 94949-5746   800-422-7249
                                888-287-9975
                                products@academictherapy.com
                                www.highnoonbooks.com

Jim Arena, President
Holly Melton, Head Writer & Senior Project Manager
High Noon Books produces and distributes a variety of pho-
nic-based and high-interest/low level chapter books, ebooks, and
audio for beginning, at-risk, and struggling readers.

2143 Information from HEATH Resource Center
National Clearinghouse on Postsecondary Education
2134 G Street, N.W.
Washington, DC 20052   202-939-9320
                                800-544-3284
                                Fax: 202-833-5696
                                heath@ace.nche.edu
                                www.HEATH-resource-center.org

2144 Lynne Rienner Publishers
1800 30th St.
Ste. 314
Boulder, CO 80301   303-444-6684
                                Fax: 303-444-0824
                                questions@rienner.com
                                www.rienner.com

2145 MAPCON Technologies
8191 Birchwood Court
Suite A
Johnston, IA 50131-2930   515-331-3358
                                800-223-4791
                                Fax: 515-331-3373
                                www.mapcon.com

Joel Tesdall, President/CEO
Diane Wiand, Client Solutions Advocate
Lora Whicker, Accounting
Bailey Merritt, Administrative Assistant
MAPCON is a computerized maintainance management soft-
ware.

2146 McGraw-Hill Company
PO Box 182605
Columbus, OH 43218   800-338-3987
                                Fax: 609-308-4480
                                customer.service@mheducation.com
                                www.mcgraw-hill.com

David Levin, President, CEO
Ellen Haley, President, CTB
Peter Cohen, President, School Education
Mark Dorman, President, International
Offers a catalog of testing resources and materials for the special
educator.

2147 National Association of School Psychologists
4340 East West Highway
Suite 402
Bethesda, MD 20814   301-657-0270
                                866-311-6277
                                Fax: 301-657-0275
                                TTY: 301-657-4155
                                webmaster@naspweb.org
                                www.nasponline.org

Stephen E. Brock, President
Todd A. Savage, President-Elect
Laura Benson, Chief Operating Officer
Susan Gorin, Executive Director
Represents over 22,500 school psychologists and related professionals. It serves its members and society by advancing the profession of school psychology and advocating for the rights,
welfare, education and mental health of children, youth and their
families.

2148 National Center for Learning Disabilities
32 Laight St
2nd Floor
New York, NY 10013   212-545-7510
                                888-575-7373
                                Fax: 212-545-9665
                                info@ncld.org
                                www.ncld.org

Frederic M Poses, Chairman
Mimi Corcoran, President & CEO
Rashonda Ambrose, Director of Strategic Partnerships
Michele Aweeky, Manager of Communications & Content
Contains features, articles, human interest news and other practi-
cal material to benefit children and adults with learning disabili-
ties and their families, as well as educators and other helping

professionals. The center also offers online forums and other resources on their website.
Quarterly

2149 PEAK Parent Center
611 N Weber
Suite 200
Colorado Springs, CO 80903-1072   719-531-9400
                                          800-284-0251
                                      Fax: 719-531-9452
                                      info@peakparent.org
                                      www.peakparent.org
Barbara Buswell, Executive Director
PEAK Parent Center is a federally-designated Parent Training and Information Center (PTI). As a PTI, PEAK supports and empowers parents, providing them with information and strategies to use when advocating for their children with disabilities. PEAK works one-on-one with families and educators helping them realize new possibilities for children with disabilities by expanding knowledge of special education and offering new strategies for success.

2150 PRO-ED
8700 Shoal Creek Boulevard
Austin, TX 78757-6897   512-451-3246
                                          800-897-3202
                                      Fax: 512-451-8542
                                      info@proedinc.com
                                      www.proedinc.com

2151 Peytral Publications
P.O. Box 1162
Minnetonka, MN 55345   952-949-8707
                                      TTY:952-906-9777
                                      www.peytral.com

2152 Prufrock Press
PO Box 8813
Waco, TX 76714-8813   254-756-3337
                                          800-998-2208
                                      Fax: 800-240-0333
                                      jmcintosh@prufrock.com
                                      www.prufrock.com
Joel McIntosh, Publisher & Marketing Director
Lacy Compton, Senior Editor
Rachel Taliaferro, Editor
Raquel Trevino, Graphic Designer and Production Coordinator
Publishes books, textbooks, teaching aids, journals, and magazines supporting gifted education and gifted children.

2153 Research Press
P.O. Box 7886
Champaign, IL 61826   217-352-3273
                                          800-519-2707
                                      Fax: 217-352-1221
                                      orders@researchpress.com
                                      www.researchpress.com
Robert W. Parkinson, Founder
Dr Richard M Foxx, Author
Jeffrey S. Allen, Author
Bryce Alvord, Author
Research Press is an independent, family-owned business founded in 1968 by Robert W. Parkinson (1920-2001). During the past 40 years, the company has earned a solid reputation for publishing practical and effective educational and mental health resources. Authors from the early years include well-known names in the field of psychology, such as B.F. Skinner, Albert Ellis, Gerald Patterson, Wesley Becker, John Guttmann, Richard Foxx, Arnold Lazarus, and Joseph Cautela.

2154 Research Press Company
2612 N. Mattis Ave.
Champaign, IL 61822   217-352-3273
                                          800-519-2707
                                      Fax: 217-352-1221
                                      www.researchpress.com

2155 Sage Publications
2455 Teller Road
Thousand Oaks, CA 91320   805-499-0721
                                          800-818-7243
                                      Fax: 800-583-2665
                                      info@sagepub.com
                                      www.sagepub.com
Sara Miller McCune, Founder, Publisher & Executive Chairman
Blaise R Simqu, President/CEO
Chris Hickok, Senior Vice President & Chief Financial Officer
Stephen Barr, Managing Director/SAGE London, President of SAGE Internation
Publishes books, text books, journals, reference books, and databases mainly related to psychology, special education and speech, language and hearing.

2156 Special Needs Project
324 State St
Ste H
Santa Barbara, CA 93101   818-718-9900
                                      Fax: 818-349-2027
                                      hgray@specialneeds.com
                                      www.specialneeds.com
Hod Gray, Owner
Publishes child development textbooks, books about aspergers syndrome, autism, and other disabilities.

2157 Supporting Success for Children with Hearing Loss
15619 Premiere Drive
Suite 101
Tampa, FL 33624   850-363-9909
                                      Fax: 480-393-4331
                                      accounting@successforkidswithhearingloss.com
                                      successforkidswithhearinglo ss.com
Karen Anderson, PhD, Director
Improving the Outcomes of Children with Hearing Loss

2158 Woodbine House
6510 Bells Mill Road
Bethesda, MD 20817   800-843-7323
                                      info@woodbinehouse.com
                                      www.woodbinehouse.com

State Agencies: Alabama

2159 Alabama Department of Education: Division of Special Education Services
50 North Ripley St
P.O. Box 302101
Montgomery, AL 36104   334-242-9700
                                      Fax: 334-262-2677
                                      www.alsde.edu
Crystal Richardson, Program Coordinator
Provides technical assistance to all education agencies serving Alabama's gifted children as well as children with disabilities.

State Agencies: Alaska

2160 Alaska Department of Education: Special Education
State of Alaska
801 West 10th St
Ste 200, P.O.Box 110500
Juneau, AK 99811-0500   907-465-8693
                                      Fax: 907-465-2806
                                      TTY:907-465-2815
                                      sped@alaska.gov
                                      www.education.alaska.gov/TLS/SPED
Dr. Susan McCauley, Division Director
Paul Prussing, Deputy Director
Cassidy Jones, Special Education Programs Manager
Administers special educational programs to the disabled residents of Alaska, through the Division of Teaching & Learning Support.

State Agencies: Arkansas

2161   Arkansas Department of Special Education
1401 West Capitol Ave, Victory Bldg
Suite 450
Little Rock, AR   72201   501-682-4221
                                      Fax: 501-682-3456
                                       TTY:501-682-4222
                                  spedsupport@arkansas.gov
                                       arksped.k12.ar.us

Tom Hicks, Interim Associate Director
Ella Albert, Management Project Analyst
Howie Knoff, Director
Tony Boaz, Director
Provides oversight of all educational programs for children and
youth with disabilities, ages 3 to 21. Provides technical assis-
tance to all public agencies providing educational services to this
population.

State Agencies: California

**2162   California Department of Education: Special Education
Division**
1430 N Street
Sacramento, CA   95814-5901   916-319-0800
                                      Fax: 916-327-3516
                                    scheduler@cde.ca.gov
                                         www.cde.ca.gov

*Tom Torlakson, State Superintendent of Public Instruction and Di-
rector of E*
Fred Balcom, Director
Gordon Jackson, Director
Phyllis Bramson, Director
Information and resources to serve the unique needs of persons
with disabilities so that each person will meet or exceed high stan-
dards of achievement in academic and nonacademic skills.

State Agencies: Colorado

**2163   Colorado Department of Education: Special Education
Service Unit**
Colorado Department of Education
201 E Colfax Ave
Denver, CO   80203-1704   303-866-6600
                                      Fax: 303-830-0793
                                  steinberg_e@cde.state.co.us
                                      www.cde.state.co.us

Ed Steinberg, Commissioner
Provides consultation on materials and educational services for
visually handicapped children, supervises volunteer services,
transcribes textbooks for visually handicapped students.

State Agencies: Connecticut

**2164   Connecticut Department of Education: Bureau of Special
Education**
165 Capitol Avenue
Hartford, CT   06106   860-713-6543
                                      Fax: 860-713-7014
                                  annelouise.thompson@ct.gov
                                          www.sde.ct.gov

Anne Louise Thompson, Bureau Chief
Lisa Spooner, Administrative Assistant
Regina Gaunichaux, Secretary
Carol Leddy, Secretary, Due Process Unit
The State Board of Education believes each student is unique and
needs an educational environment that provides for, and accom-
modates, his or her strengths and areas of needed improvement.

**2165   Department of Rehabilitation Services & Bureau of
Education And Services for the Blind**
State of Connecticut Agency
184 Windsor Ave
Windsor, CT   06095-4536   860-602-4000
                                           800-842-4510
                                      Fax: 860-602-4020
                                       TTY: 860-602-4221
                                     brian.sigman@ct.gov
                                       www.ct.gov/besb

State Agencies: Delaware

**2166   Department of Public Instruction: Exceptional Children &
Special Programs Division**
Department of Education
Ste 2
401 Federal St
Dover, DE   19901-3639   302-739-5471
                                      Fax: 302-739-2388
                                       www.doe.k12.de.us

Martha Toomey, Executive Director

State Agencies: DC

2167   Administration for Community Living
One Massachusetts Avenue NW
Washington, DC   20001   202-401-4634
                                           800-677-1116
                                      Fax: 202-357-3555
                                     aclinfo@acl.hhs.gov
                                           www.acl.gov

Kathy Greenlee, Administrator
Sharon Lewis, Principal Deputy Administrator
Edwin Walker, Deputy Assis Secretary for Aging
Aaron Bishop, Comm., Admin on Disabilities
ACL brings together the efforts and achievements of the Administration on Aging, the Administration on Intellectual and Developmental Disabilities, and the HHS Office on Disability to serve
as the Federal agency responsible for increasing access to community supports, while focusing attention and resources on the
unique needs of older Americans and people with disabilities
across the lifespan.

**2168   District of Columbia Public Schools: Special Education
Division**
1200 First Street, NE
Washington, DC   20002-4210   202-442-5885
                                           202-442-5517
                                      Fax: 202-442-5026
                                          www.dcps.dc.gov

Paul L Vance MD, Superintendent
Committed to providing a continuum of services that offers students with disabilities the opportunity to actively participate in
the learning environment of their neighborhood school.

2169   Federal Emergency Management Agency
500 C Street S.W.
Washington, DC   20472   202-646-2500
                                           800-621-3362
                                       TTY:800-427-5593
                                           www.fema.gov

W. Craig Fugate, Administrator
Michael Coen, Jr., Chief of Staff
Joseph Nimmich, Deputy Administrator
Alyson Vert, Director
FEMA's mission is to support the citizens and first responders to
ensure that as a nation we work together to build, sustain and im-
prove our capability to prepare for, protect against, respond to, re-
cover from and mitigate all hazards.

2170 Lab School of Washington
4759 Reservoir Rd NW
Washington, DC 20007-1921   202-965-6600
                                    labschool@webmail.org
                                       www.labschool.org

Mimi W. Dawson, Chair
Mac Bernstein, Vice Chair
Mike Tongour, Secretary
Bill Tennis, Treasurer

The Lab School six week summer session includes individualized reading, spelling, writing, study skills and math programs. A multisensory approach addresses the needs of bright learning disabled children. Related services such as speech/language therapy and occupational therapy are integrated into the curriculum. Elementary/Intermediate; Junior High/High School.

2171 National Clearinghouse on Family Support and Children's Mental Health
Ste 800
1 Dupont Cir NW
Washington, DC 20036-1149   202-939-9320
                                             800-544-3284
                                       Fax: 202-833-4760
                                       heatah@ace.nche.edu
                                        ncfy.acf.hhs.gov/

State Agencies: Florida

2172 Florida Department of Education: Bureau of Exceptional Education And Student Services
325 West Gaines Street
Turlington Building, Suite 1514
Tallahassee, FL 32399   850-245-0505
                                       Fax: 850-245-9667
                                 Monica.Verra-Tirado@fldoe.org
                                        www.fldoe.org/ese

Monica Verra-Tirado, Ed.D., Bureau Chief
Gerard Robinson, Commissioner
Randy Hanna, Chancellor
Pam Stewart, Chancellor

Administers programs for students with disabilities and for gifted students. Coordinates student services throughout the state and participates in multiple inter-agency efforts designed to strengthen the quality and variety of services to students with special needs.

2173 Florida State College at Jacksonville Services for Students with Disabilities
501 W State St
Jacksonville, FL 32202   904-633-8100
                                             888-873-1145
                                       Fax: 904-633-5955
                                           info@fscj.edu
                                              fscj.edu

Randle P DeFoor, Chair
Cynthia A Bioteau, President
Richard Turner, Associate Vice President of Enrollment Management
Sarah Ashbrook, Project Coordinator

Florida State College ensures acessibility of its services, activities, facilities and academic programs to students with disabilities. Special accmmodations are provided to anyone with a physical, mental or learning disability.

State Agencies: Hawaii

2174 Hawaii Department of Education: Special Needs
Hawaii Department of Education
3430 Leahi Ave
Honolulu, HI 96815-4246   808-941-3894
                                       Fax: 808-941-3894

Margaret Donovan MD, State Administrator

Provides consultation on educational services for local schools, offers psychological testing and evaluation, maintains resource rooms in district schools and more for the blind and handicapped throughout the state.

State Agencies: Illinois

2175 Illinois State Board of Education: Department of Special Education
100 N 1st St
Springfield, IL 62777   217-782-5589
                                       Fax: 217-782-0372
                                           www.isbe.net

Elizabeth Hanselman, Asst Superintendent Special Ed.

Mission is to advance the human and civil rights of people with disabilities in Illinois. Statewide advocacy organization providing self-advocacy assistance, legal services, education and public policy initiatives. Designated to implement the federal protection and advocacy system; has broad statutory power to enforce the rights of people with physical and mental disabilities, including developmental disabilities and mental illnesses.

State Agencies: Indiana

2176 Indiana Department of Education: Special Education Division
Indiana Department of Education
South Tower, Suite 600
115 W. Washington Street
Indianapolis, IN 46204-2731   317- 23- 661
                                             877-851-4106
                                       Fax: 317- 23- 800
                                      webmaster@doe.in.gov
                                         www.doe.in.gov/

Robert A Marra, Manager
Tony Bennett, Chair

Provides consultation on educational services for local schools, offers psychological testing and evaluation, maintains resource rooms in district schools and more for the blind and handicapped throughout the state.

State Agencies: Iowa

2177 Iowa Department of Public Instruction: Bureau of Special Education
400 E 14th St
Des Moines, IA 50319-9000   515-457-2000
                                       Fax: 515-242-6019
                                        www.educateiowa.gov/

Tom Kuehl, CEO
Jason Glass, Director
Jeff Berger, Administrative Services

State Agencies: Kansas

2178 Kansas State Board of Education: Special Education Services
900 SW Jackson Street
Topeka, KS 66612-1212   785-296-3201
                                             800-203-9462
                                       Fax: 785-296-7933
                                       TTY: 785-296-6338
                                          contact@ksde.org
                                            www.ksde.org

Ethan Erickson, Director
Kathy Gosa, Director
Denise Kahler, Director
Scott Myers, Director

Provides leadership and support for exceptional learners receiving special education services throughout Kansas schools and communities.

State Agencies: Kentucky

2179 **Kentucky Department of Education: Divisionof Exceptional Children's Services**
500 Mero St
Capital Tower Plaza
Frankfort, KY   40601   502-564-4770
Fax: 502-564-7749
www.education.ky.gov

Darlene Jesse, Director
Provides consultation on educational services for local schools, offers psychological testing and evaluation, maintains resource rooms in district schools and more for the blind and handicapped throughout the state.

State Agencies: Louisiana

2180 **Louisiana Department of Education: Office of Special Education Services**
Louisiana Department of Education
1201 North Third Street
Baton Rouge, LA   70802   225-342-0090
877-453-2721
Fax: 225-342-0193
www.doe.state.la.us

David Elder, Manager
Kim Fitch, Director Human Resources
George Nelson, President

State Agencies: Massachusetts

2181 **Getting Ready for the Outside World (G.R.O.W.)**
Riverview School
551 Route 6A East Sandwich
Cape Cod, MA   2537-1448   508-888-0489
Fax: 508-833-7001
admissions@riverviewschool.org
www.riverviewschool.org

Janice James, Vice Chairman
Deborah Cowan, Vice Chair
James Shallcross, Treasurer
Kathleen Yazbak, Secretary
Riverview School's G.R.O.W. Program is a unique ten month transitional prgoram (1-3 years) for young adults with complex language, learning and cognitive disabilities. This post secondary program is designed to further develop academic, vocational and independent living skills, to enable students to function as independently as possible.

2182 **Massachusetts Department of Education: Program Quality Assurance**
Massachusetts Department of Education
75 Pleasant Street
Malden, MA   2148-4906   781-388-3300
Fax: 617-388-3476
boe@doe.mass.edu
www.doe.mass.edu/pqa/
Pamela Kaufamann, Administrator

State Agencies: Maryland

2183 **Agency for Healthcare Research and Quality**
540 Gaither Road
Rockville, MD   20850   301-427-1364
www.ahrq.gov

Richard G. Kronick, PhD, Director, Director
Sharon B. Arnold, PhD, Deputy Director
The Agency for Healthcare Research and Quality's (AHRQ) mission is to produce evidence to make health care safer, higher quality, more accessible, equitable, and affordable, and to work

within the U.S. Department of Health and Human Services and with other partners to make sure that the evidence is understood and used.

2184 **Center for Mental Health Services**
Room 6-1057
1 Choke Cherry Road
Rockville, MD   20857   240-276-1310
Fax: 240-276-1320
www.samhsa.gov

Paolo del Vecchio, M.S.W., Director
Elizabeth Lopez, Ph.D., Deputy Director
Elizabeth Lopez, Ph.D., Acting Director
Anne Mathews-Younes, Ed.D., Director
The Center for Mental Health Services leads federal efforts to promote the prevention and treatment of mental disorders. Congress created CMHS to bring new hope to adults who have serious mental illness and children with emotional disorders.

2185 **Centers for Medicare & Medicaid Services**
7500 Security Boulevard
Baltimore, MD   21244   410-786-3000
877-267-2323
TTY:866-226-1819
Mandy.Cohen@cms.hhs.gov
www.cms.gov

Dr. Mandy Cohen, M.D., MPH, Chief of Staff
Deborah Taylor, Acting Chief Operating Officer
Andy Slavitt, Acting Administrator
Patrick Conway, MD, MSc, Acting Principal Deputy Admin
US federal agency which administers Medicare, Medicaid, and the State Children's Health Insurance Program.

2186 **Maryland State Department of Education: Division of Special Education**
200 West Baltimore Street
Baltimore, MD   21201-2595   410-767-0100
888-246-0016
Fax: 410-333-8165
www.marylandpublicschools.org

Nancy S Grasmick, State Superintendent
Dr. Lillian Lowery, Superintendent of Schools
James V. Foran, Assistant State Superintendent
Katharine Oliver, Assistant State Superintendent
Collaborates with families, local early intervention systems, and local school systems to ensure that all children and youth with disabilities have access to appropriate services and educational opportunities to which they are entitled under federal and state laws.

2187 **National Human Genome Research Institute**
National Institutes of Health
Building 31, Room 4B09
31 Center Drive, MSC 2152
Bethesda, MD   20892-2152   301-402-0911
Fax: 301-402-2218
lbrody@mail.nih.gov
www.genome.gov

Eric D. Green, M.D., Ph.D., Director
Lawrence Brody, Ph.D., Director
Bettie Graham, Ph.D., Director
Ellen Rolfes, M.A., Director, Division of Management
The National Human Genome Research Institute began as the National Center for Human Genome Research (NCHGR), which was established in 1989 to carry out the role of the National Institutes of Health (NIH) in the International Human Genome Project (HGP).

2188 **National Institute of General Medical Sciences**
45 Center Drive MSC 6200
Bethesda, MD   20892-6200   301-496-7301
info@nigms.nih.gov
www.nigms.nih.gov

Jon R. Lorsch, Ph.D., Director
Judith H. Greenberg, Ph.D., Deputy Director
Ann Hagan, Ph.D., Associate Director
Sally Lee, Executive Officer

The National Institute of General Medical Sciences (NIGMS) supports basic research that increases understanding of biological processes and lays the foundation for advances in disease diagnosis, treatment and prevention.

State Agencies: Michigan

2189 **Michigan Department of Education: Special Education Services**
608 W. Allegan Street
PO Box 30008
Lansing, MI 48909
517-373-3324
Fax: 517-373-7504
DHS-OCS-PEP@michigan.gov
www.michigan.gov/mde
John C. Austin, President
Kathleen N. Straus, President of the State Board
Michelle Fecteau, Executive Director
Daniel Varner, Chief Executive Officer of Excellent Schools Detroit
Oversees the administrative funding of education and early intervention programs and services for young children and students with disabilities.

2190 **Services for Students with Disabilities**
University of Michigan
G-664 Haven Hall
505 South State St.
Ann Arbor, MI 48109-1045
734-763-3000
Fax: 734-936-3947
TTY:734-615-4461
ssdoffice@umich.edu
www.ssd.umich.edu
Stuart Segal, Director
Offers information to students of the University of Michigan and their parents.

State Agencies: Minnesota

2191 **Community Supports for People with Disabilities (CSP)**
South Central Technical College (SCTC)
1920 Lee Blvd
North Mankato, MN 56003-2504
507-389-7200
800-722-9359
online@southcentral.edu
www.southcentral.edu
Christensen Tami, Executive Director
Keith Stover, President
Human services program available as a physical or online program, designed for those wanting to earn a certificate, diploma or associate degree as a Direct Support Professional for use in the health and human services industries. The program comprises eight courses relating to professional services and support for people with disabilities.

2192 **Professional Development Programs**
6303 Osgood Ave. N.
Ste 104
Stillwater, MN 55082
651-439-8865
877-439-8865
Fax: 877-259-5906
www.pdppro.com
Cindy Lacosse, VP
Lori Lacrosse, President
Sponsors cutting edge and popular continuing education workshops and symposia of interest to professionals who provide services to children and adults with special needs.

State Agencies: Missouri

2193 **Missouri Department of Elementary and Secondary Education: Special Education Programs**
205 Jefferson St
PO Box 480
Jefferson City, MO 65102
573-751-5739
Fax: 573-526-4404
TTY:800-735-2966
Stephen Barr, Assistant Commissioner
The Office of Special Education administers state and federal funds to support services for students and adults with disabilities.

State Agencies: Mississippi

2194 **Mississippi Department of Education: Office of Special Services**
359 North West Street
P.O. Box 771
Jackson, MS 39201
601-359-3513
Fax: 601-987-3892
www.mde.k12.ms.us
Dr Tom Burnham, Superintendent
Key priorities are: reading, early literacy, student achievement, teachers/teaching, leadership/principals, safe and orderly schools, parent relations/community involvement, and technology.

State Agencies: Montana

2195 **Department of Public Health Human Services**
PO Box 4210
Helena, MT 59604-4210
406-444-5622
Fax: 406-444-1970
hhsea@mt.gov
www.dphhs.mt.gov
Anna Whitin Sorrell, Director
Bernie Jacobs, Chief Legal Counsel
Deb Sloat, Human Resources Office
Jon Ebelt, Public Information Office
Provides consultation on educational services for local schools, offers psychological testing and evaluation, maintains resource rooms in district schools and more for the blind and handicapped throughout the state.

State Agencies: North Carolina

2196 **National Institute of Environmental Health Sciences**
111 T.W. Alexander Drive
Research Triangle Park, NC 27709
919-541-4580
birnbaumls@niehs.nih.gov
www.niehs.nih.gov
Linda S. Birnbaum, Ph.D., Director
Richard Woychik, Ph.D., Deputy Director
Sheila A. Newton, Ph.D., Policy, Planning, and Evaluation
Ericka Reid, Ph.D., Science Education & Diversity
The mission of the NIEHS is to discover how the environment affects people in order to promote healthier lives.

2197   **North Carolina Department of Public Instruction: Exceptional Children Division**
301 N Wilmington St
Raleigh, NC   27601   919-807-3300
Fax: 919-715-1569
lharris@dpi.state.nc.us
www.ncpublicschools.org
June St. Clair Atkinson, Ed.D, State Superintendent of Public Instruction
Mike McLaughlin, Senior Policy Advisor to the State Superintendent
Rachel Beaulieu, Legislative & Community Affairs Director
Jeani Allen, Director of Internal Auditing
The mission is to assure that students with disabilities develop mentally, physically, emotionally, and vocationally through the provision of an appropriate individualized education in the least restrictive environment.

State Agencies: North Dakota

2198   **North Dakota Department of Education: Special Education**
600 E. Boulevard Avenue, Dept. 201
Floors 9, 10, and 11
Bismarck, ND   58505-0440   701-328-2260
866-741-3519
Fax: 701-328-2461
TTY: 701-328-4920
mdanderson@nd.gov
www.dpi.state.nd.us
Kirsten Baesler, State Superintendent
Jerry Coleman, Director, School Finance & Organization
Linda Schloer, Child Nutrition & Food Distribution, Director
Gerry Teevens, Director, Special Education
Provides consultation on educational services for local schools, offers psychological testing and evaluation, maintains resource rooms in district schools and more for the blind and handicapped throughout the state.

State Agencies: Nebraska

2199   **Nebraska Department of Education: Special Populations Office**
1200 N Street, Suite 400
PO Box 98922
Lincoln, NE   68509   402-471-2186
877-253-2603
Fax: 402-471-2909
NDEQ.moreinfo@Nebraska.gov
deq.ne.gov
Rod Gangwish Shelton, Council Member
Douglas Anderson Aurora, Council Member
Mark Whitehead Lincoln, Council Member
Mark Czaplewski Grand Islan, Council Member
Assists school districts in establishing and maintaining effective special education programs for children with disabilities (date of diagnosis through the school year when a child reaches 21). Major function: provide technical assistance to school districts and to parents of children with disabilities, assist programs in meeting state and federal special education regulations. Also responsible for assuring that the rights of children with disabilities and their parents are protected.

State Agencies: New Hampshire

2200   **Institute on Disability**
University of New Hampshire
10 West Edge Drive
Suite 101
Durham, NH   03824   603-862-4320
Fax: 603-862-0555
contact.iod@unh.edu
www.iod.unh.edu
Charles E. Drum, Director & Professor
Andrew Houtenville, Director of Research
Matthew Gianino, Director of Communications
Mary Schuh, Director of Development and Consumer Affairs
Provides coherent university-based focus for the improvement of knowledge, policies, and practices related to the lives of persons with disabilities and their families.

2201   **New Hampshire Department of Education: Bureau for Special Education Services**
101 Pleasant Street
Concord, NH   03301-3860   603-271-3494
Fax: 603-271-1953
Lori.Temple@doe.nh.gov
www.education.nh.gov
Santina Thibedeau, Administrator
Virginia Barry, Commissioner
Linda Breden, Secretary
Traci Biron, Secretary
The mission of Special Education is to improve educational outcomes for children and youth with disabilities by providing and promoting leadership, technical assistance and collaboration statewide. Provides oversight and implementation of federal and state laws that ensure a free appropriate public education for all children and youth with disabilities in New Hampshire.

State Agencies: New Jersey

2202   **New Jersey Department of Education: Office of Special Education Program**
New Jersey Department of Education
PO Box 500
Trenton, NJ   8625-500   609-292-0147
Fax: 609-984-8422
www.nj.gov/education/specialed/info/
Barbara Gantwerk, Director
Alfred Murray, Executive Director

2203   **New Jersey Speech-Language-Hearing Association**
174 Nassau St
Suite 337
Princeton, NJ   08542   888-906-5742
Fax: 888-729-3489
info@njsha.org
njsha.org
Mary Faella, President
Robynne Kratchman, Vice President
Joan Warner, Treasurer
Kristie Soriano, Secretary
The New Jersey Speech-Language-Hearing Association offers services to audiologists, speech-language pathologists, and scientists studying in these fields. Services include resources, advocacy, information and programs to help foster professional development.

2204   **The Arc of New Jersey**
985 Livingston Ave
North Brunswick, NJ   08902   732-246-2525
Fax: 732-214-1834
info@arcnj.org
arcnj.org
Joanne Bergin, President
Thomas Baffuto, Executive Director
Celine Fortin, Associate Executive Director
Anna Scruggs, Coordinator, Financial Services

The Arc of New Jersey is committed to enhancing the quality of life of children and adults with intellectual and developmental disabilities and their families, through advocacy, empowerment, education and prevention.

State Agencies: New Mexico

2205 New Mexico State Department of Education
300 Don Gaspar Ave
Santa Fe, NM 87501-2744
505-827-6508
Fax: 505-827-6696
www.sde.state.nm.us

Bill Trant, Assistant Director
Judy Parks, Assistant Director
Provides consultation on educational services for local schools, offers psychological testing and evaluation, maintains resource rooms in district schools and more for the blind and handicapped throughout the state.

State Agencies: Nevada

2206 Nevada Department of Education: Special Eduction Branch
700 E Fifth St
Carson City, NV 89701-5096
775-687-9800
Fax: 775-687-9101
www.doe.nv.gov

Nick Gakalatos, Manager
The Office of Special Ed and School Improvement Program of the Nevada State Department of Education is responsible for management of state and federal programs providing educational opportunities for students with diverse learning needs. Included are such programs as: special education/disabled (IDEA); disadvantaged/at-risk programs (Title I/IASA); early childhood programs (Title I/ESEA); early childhood programs; migrant education; English language learners; NRS 395 student placement program.

State Agencies: New York

2207 New York State Education Department
1606 One Commerce Plz
Albany, NY 12234
518-474-5930
Fax: 518-486-6880
www.nysed.gov

Bernard Margolis, Manager
Provides vocational rehabilitation and educational services for eligible individuals with disabilities throughout New York State. Services include evaluation, counseling, job placement, and referral to other agencies.

State Agencies: Ohio

2208 Ohio Department of Education: Division of Special Education
Ohio Department of Education
25 S Front St
Columbus, OH 43215-4183
614-995-1545
877-644-6338
Fax: 614-728-1097
TTY: 888-886-0181
www.ode.state.oh.us

Mike Armstrong, Manager
Provides technical assistance to educational agencies for the development and implementation of educational services to meet the needs of students with disabilities and/or those who are gifted. Provides information to parents. Administers state and federal funds allocated to educational agencies for the provision of services to students with disabilities and/or those who are gifted.

2209 The Arc of Allen County
546 S Collett St
Lima, OH 45805
419-225-6285
Fax: 419-228-7770
info@thearcofohio.org
www.arcallencounty.org

Brad Perrott, Executive Director
Vicki Alves, Day Service Manager
Lisa Hengstler, Office Assistant
Elaine Copeland, Day Care Aide
Offers services to people with intellectual and developmental disabilities. Some programs include day care, educational training, human rights advocacy, and information and referral.

State Agencies: Oklahoma

2210 Oklahoma State Department of Education
2500 N Lincoln Blvd
Oklahoma City, OK 73105-4599
405-521-3301
Fax: 405-521-6205

Misty Kimbrough, Manager
Sandy Garrett, Administrator
Janet Barresi, State Superintendent
Provides consultation on educational services for local schools, offers psychological testing and evaluation, maintains resource rooms in district schools and more for the blind and handicapped throughout the state.

State Agencies: Oregon

2211 Oregon Department of Education: Office of Special Education
Oregon Department of Education:
255 Capitol St NE
Salem, OR 97310-1300
503-945-5600
Fax: 503-378-2897
www.dpeducation.com

Bruce Goldberg, Manager
Heidi Cockrell, Executive Assistant
Katy Coba, Executive Director
State agency ensuring provision of special education services to children with disabilities from birth to age 21.

State Agencies: Pennsylvania

2212 Pennsylvania Department of Education: Bureau of Special Education
333 Market St
Harrisburg, PA 17126-333
717-783-6788
Fax: 717-783-6139
TTY: 717-783-8445
00specialed@psupen.psu.edu
www.pde.state.pa.us

Linda Rhen, Administrator
John Tommasini, Assistant Director
Provides effective and efficient administration of the Commonwealth of Pennsylvania's resources dedicated to enabling school districts to maintain high standards in the delivery of special education services and programs for all exceptional students.

State Agencies: Rhode Island

2213 Rhode Island Department of Education: Office of Special Needs
255 Westminster St
Providence, RI 2903
401-222-4600
Fax: 401-784-9513
www.ride.ri.gov

Al Moscola, Manager
Alfred Moscola, Manager

Provides consultation on educational services for local schools, offers psychological testing and evaluation, maintains resource rooms in district schools and more for the blind and handicapped throughout the state.

State Agencies: South Carolina

2214 **South Carolina Assistive Technology Program (SCATP)**
Center for Disability Resources
8301 Farrow Rd
Columbia, SC 29208-3245 803-935-5263
800-915-4522
Fax: 800-935-5342
www.sc.edu/scatp

Carol Page, Program Director
Mary Bechter, Program Coordinator
SCATP is a federally funded project concerned with getting technology into th hands of people with disabilities so that they might live, work, learn and be a more independent part of the community.

2215 **South Carolina Department of Education: Office of Exceptional Children**
1429 Senate St
Suite 808
Columbia, SC 29201-3730 803-734-8224
Fax: 803-734-4824
sdeservicedesk@sde.ok.gov
www.scschools.com

Susan Durant, State Director
Provides consultation on educational services for local schools, offers psychological testing and evaluation, maintains resource rooms in district schools and more for the blind and handicapped throughout the state.

State Agencies: South Dakota

2216 **South Dakota Department of Education & Cultural Affairs: Office of Special Education**
700 Governors Dr
Pierre, SD 57501-2291 605-773-3804
Fax: 605-773-6041

Chelle Somsen, Manager
Dorothy Liegl, Manager

State Agencies: Tennessee

2217 **Tennessee Department of Education**
710 James Robertson Pkwy
Nashville, TN 37243-1219 615-741-2731
888-212-3162
Fax: 615-741-1791
www.state.tn.us/education

Ruth S Letson, Manager
Kevin Huffman, Commissioner
Provides consultation on educational services for local schools, offers psychological testing and evaluation, maintains resource rooms in district schools and more for the blind and handicapped throughout the state.

State Agencies: Texas

2218 **Texas Education Agency**
1701 N Congress Ave
Austin, TX 78701-1494 512-463-8532
Fax: 512-463-8057
www.tealighthouse.org

Shirley J Neeley, Commissioner of Education
Provides consultation on educational services for local schools, offers psychological testing and evaluation, maintains resource

rooms in district schools and more for the blind and handicapped throughout the state.

2219 **Texas Education Agency: Special Education Unit**
1701 Congress Ave
PO Box 420637
Austin, TX 77242-637 512-463-8532
Fax: 512-463-8057
info@tdea.org
www.tdea.org

Gene Lenz, Deputy Associate Commissioner
Shirley Neeley, Administrator

2220 **Texas School of the Deaf**
1102 S Congress Ave
Austin, TX 78704-1791 512-462-5353
800-332-3873
Fax: 512-462-5424
ercod@tsd.state.tx.us
tsd.state.tx.us

Claire Bugen, Superintendent
Russell West, Residential Services Director
Gary Bego, Business and Operations Director
Brenda Fraenkel, Special Education Director
Ensures that students excel in an environment where they learn, grow and belong. Supports deaf students, families and professionals in Texas by providing resources through outreach services.

State Agencies: Utah

2221 **Utah State Office of Education: At-Risk and Special Education Service Unit**
Utah State Office of Education
250 East 500 South
P.O.Box 144200
Salt Lake City, UT 84114-4200 801-538-7500
Fax: 801-538-7521
webmaster@schools.utah.gov
schools.utah.gov

Sandra Cox, Financial Analyst
Mark Peterson, Director
Glenna Gallo, State Director of Special Educat
Rebecca Donovan, Administrative Secretary
Provides consultation on educational services for local schools, offers psychological testing and evaluation, maintains resource rooms in district schools and more for the blind and handicapped throughout the state.

State Agencies: Virginia

2222 **National Science Foundation**
4201 Wilson Blvd
Arlington, VA 22230 703-292-5111
TTY:703-292-5090
info@nsf.gov
www.nsf.gov

France A. Cerdova, Director
Richard O. Buckius, Chief Operating Officer
Michael Van Woert, Executive Officer/Director
Dr. James L. Olds, Assistant Director
NSF is the only federal agency whose mission includes support for all fields of fundamental science and engineering, except for medical sciences.

2223   Virginia Department of Education: Divisionof Pre & Early Adolescent Education
Virginia Department Of Education
James Monroe Building, 101, N. 14th
P.O.Box 2120
Richmond, VA   23219
                              804-236-3631
                         Fax: 804-236-3635
                    webmaster@doe.virginia.gov
                         www.pen.k12.va.us
Dr. Steven R Staples, Superintendent of Public Instruction
Kent Dickey, Deputy Superintendent, Finance & Operations
Chris Sorensen, Director, Budget
Becky Marable, Director, Human Resources
Provides consultation on educational services for local schools, offers psychological testing and evaluation, maintains resource rooms in district schools and more for the blind and handicapped throughout the state.

State Agencies: Washington

2224   Superintendent of Public Instruction: Special Education Section
Old Capitol Building, 600 Washingto
P.O. Box 47200
Olympia, WA 98504-7200
                              360-725-6000
                         Fax: 360-586-0247
                         TTY:360-664-3631
                       webmaster@k12.wa.us
                         www.k12.wa.us
Randy I. Dorn, State Superintendent of Public I
Alan Burke, Deputy Superintendent
Robert Butts, Assistant Superintendent
Bob Harmon, Assistant Superintendent
Provides leadership, service and support for the development and implementation of research-based curriculum to assure that all learners achieve at all levels.

State Agencies: West Virginia

2225   West Virginia Department of Education: Office of Special Education
Rm 6
1900 Kanawha Blvd E
Charleston, WV 25305-0001
                              304-558-3660
                         Fax: 304-558-3741
                         wvde.state.wv.us
Liza Cordeiro, Executive Director
Mary Nunn, Assistant Director
Marshall Patton, Executive Director
Brenda Williams, Executive Director
Provides consultation on educational services for local schools, offers psychological testing and evaluation, maintains resource rooms in district schools and more for the blind and handicapped throughout the state.

State Agencies: Wyoming

2226   Wyoming Department of Education
2300 Capitol Avenue
Hathaway Building, 2nd Floor
Cheyenne, WY 82002-2060
                              307-777-7690
                         Fax: 307-777-6234
                         edu.wyoming.gov
Cindy Hill, WDE Superintendent
Deb Lindsey, Division Administrator, Assessment
Teri Wigert, Division Administrator, Support Systems & Resources
Dianne Bailey, Division Administrator, Finance & Data
Mission is to lead, model, and support continuous improvement of education for everyone in Wyoming.

Magazines & Journals

2227   Adapted Physical Activity Programs
Human Kinetics
1607 N. Market Street
P.O.Box 5076
Champaign, IL   61820
                              800-747-4457
                         Fax: 217-351-1549
                         info@hkusa.com
                         www.humankinetics.com
Patty Lehn, Publicity Manager
Lori Cooper, Marketing Manager
Bill Dobrik, Sales Associate
Dan Stebel, Sales Associate
Human Kinetics produces a variety of resources for adapted physical education practitioners, including books on activities, a research journal and higher education references. *$24.00*
Quarterly
ISSN 0736-58 9

2228   Advance for Providers of Post-Acute Care
Merion Publications
2900 Horizon Drive
King of Prussia, PA   19406
                              610-278-1400
                              800-355-5627
                         Fax: 610-278-1421
                    webmaster@advanceweb.com
                         advanceweb.com
Timothy Baum, MS, CRNP, Author
A free magazine for providers of post-acute care.

2229   American Journal on Intellectual and Developmental Disabilities
501 3rd Street, NW
Suite 200
Washington, DC   20001
                              202-387-1968
                         Fax: 202-387-2193
                         mnygren@aaidd.org
                         aaidd.org
Deborah Fidler,PhD, Editor
Glenn T. Fujiura, PhD, Editor
Michael L. Wehmeyer, PhD, Co-Editor
Karrie A. Shogren, PhD, Co-Editor
American Journal on Intellectual and Developmental Disabilities (AJIDD)is a scientific, scholarly, and archival multidisciplinary journal for reporting original contributions of the highest quality to knowledge of intellectual disability, its causes, treatment, and prevention.

2230   CEC Catalog
Council for Exceptional Children
2900 Crystal Dr.
Suite 1000
Arlington, VA   22202-3557
                              888-232-7733
                         TTY:866-915-5000
                         service@cec.sped.org
                         www.cec.sped.org
Alexander T. Graham, Executive Director
Sharon Rodriguez, Senior Executive Assistant
Craig Evans, Director of Operations
Semi-annual catalog from the Council for Exceptional Children offering books, guides, materials, products and services for the special educator.
18 pages

2231   Career Development and Transition for Exceptional Individuals
2455 Teller Road
Thousand Oaks, CA   91320
                              800-818-7243
                         Fax: 800-583-2665
                         journals@sagepub.com
                         cde.sagepub.com
Blaise R. Simqu, President/ CEO
Tracey A. Ozmina, EVP/ COO
Chris Hickok, SVP/ CFO
Phil Denvir, Global Chief Information Officer

Career Development and Transition for Exceptional Individuals (CDTEI) specializes in the fields of secondary education, transition, and career development for persons with documented disabilities and special needs.

2232   Case Manager Magazine
Elsevier Health
3251 Riverport Lane
Maryland Heights, MO   63043   314-447-8070
                                      800-222-9570
                             textbook@elsevier.com
                             journals.elsevierhealth.com
Thomas Reller, Vice President Global Corporate
Harald Boersma, Senior Manager Corporate Relatio
Ylann Schemm, Corporate Relations Manager
Sacha Boucherie, Press Officer
This national magazine is for medical case managers, social workers, counselors and home health professionals who work with people with serious injury or illness. It is a membership benefit of CMSA, the national association for case managers. *$55.00*
84 pages BiMonthly

2233   Catalyst
The Catalyst
Ste 275
1259 El Camino Real
Menlo Park, CA   94025-4208   800-647-0314
Sue Swezey, Editor
Digest of news and information on the use of computers in special education. *$15.00*
20 pages Quarterly

2234   Challenge Magazine
451 Hungerford Drive
Suite 100
Rockville, MD   20850   301-217-0960
                       Fax: 301-217-0968
                          Info@dsusa.org
                          www.disabledsportsusa.org

Kirk Bauer, Executive Director
Claire Duffy, Program Coordinator
Orlando Gill, Field Representative
Huarya Gomez-Garcia, Program Manager
Challenge Magazine is a publication of Disabled Sports USA, providing adaptive sports information to adults and children with disabilities, including those who are visually impaired, amputees, spinal cord injured (paraplegic and quadriplegic), and those who have multiple sclerosis, head injury, cerebral palsy, autism and other related intellectual disabilities.

2235   Clinical Connection
American Advertising Dist of Northern Virginia
708 Pendleton St
Alexandria, VA   22314-1819   703-549-5126
                          Fax: 703-548-5563
Kathie Harrington, M.A., CCC, Author
Covers speech language pathology.

2236   College and University
AACRAO
One Dupont Circle NW
Suite 520
Washington, DC   20036   202-293-9161
                          Fax: 202-872-8857
                          reillym@aacrao.org
                          aacrao.org

Brad Myers, President
Dan Garcia, President Elect
Adrienne McDay, Past President
Stan DeMerritt, VP, Finance
Scholarly research journal. American Association of Collegiate Registrars and Admissions Offers (AACRAO) is a nonprofit, voluntary, professional, educational association of degree-granting, postsecondary institutions, government agencies, private educational organizations and education-oriented businesses in the

United States and abroad. $80 per year US; $90 per year international.
30 pages Quarterly
ISSN 0010-0889

2237   Communication Disorders Quarterly
2455 Teller Road
Thousand Oaks, CA   91320   800-818-7243
                          Fax: 800-583-2665
                          journals@sagepub.com
                          cde.sagepub.com

Blaise R. Simqu, President/ CEO
Tracey A. Ozmina, EVP/ COO
Chris Hickok, SVP/ CFO
Phil Denvir, Global Chief Information Officer
Communication Disorders Quarterly (CDQ) presents cutting edge information on typical and atypical communication — from oral language development to literacy.

2238   Continuing Care
Stevens Publishing Corporation
14901 Quorum Dr,
Suite 425
Dallas, TX   75254   972-687-6700
                          Fax: 972-687-6750
                          info@1105media.com
                          1105media.com

Neal Vitale, President & Chief Executive Officer
Richard Vitale, Senior Vice President & Chief Financial Officer
Mike Valenti, Executive Vice President
Jeff Klein, Non-Executive Chairman of the Board
A national magazine for case management and discharge planning professionals published monthly except for December. *$119.00*
34 pages Monthly

2239   Counseling Psychologist
American Psychological Association
2455 Teller Road
Thousand Oaks, CA   91320   805-499-0721
                                      800-818-7243
                          Fax: 800-583-2665
                          info@sagepub.com
                          www.sagepub.com

Sara Miller McCune, Founder, Publisher & Executive Chairman
Blaise R Simqu, President/CEO
Chris Hickok, Senior Vice President & Chief Financial Officer
Stephen Barr, Managing Director/SAGE London
Thematic issues in the theory, research and practice of counseling psychology. *$78.00*
Bi-Monthly

2240   Counseling and Values
American Counseling Association
5999 Stevenson Ave
Alexandria, VA   22304   703-823-0252
                                      800-347-6647
                          Fax: 800-473-2329
                          webmaster@counseling.org
                          counseling.org

Robert L. Smith, President
Thelma Duffey, President Elect
Brian Canfield, Treasurer
Richard Yep, CEO
Counseling and Values is the official journal of the Association for Spiritual, Ethical, and Religious Values in Counseling (ASERVIC), a member association of the American Counseling Association. Counseling and Values s a professional journal of theory, research, and informed opinion concerned with the relationships among psychology, philosophy, religion, social values, and counseling. *$12.00*
TriAnnual

2241 Disability & Society
711 3rd Avenue
8th Floor
New York, NY   10017   212-216-7800
                                                        800-634-7064
                                                    Fax: 212-564-7854
                                                    www.routledge.com

Len Barton, Author
The study of disability has traditionally been influenced mainly
by medical and psychological models. The aim of this new text,
Disability and Society, is to open up the debate by introducing alternative perspectives reflecting the increasing sociological
interest in this important topic.

2242 Disability Studies Quarterly
552 Park Hall
Buffalo, NY   14260-4130   marembis@buffalo.edu
                                              dsq-sds.org
Michael Rembis, Interim Editor-in-Chief
Tanja Aho, Interim Managing Editor
Disability Studies Quarterly (DSQ) is the journal of the Society
for Disability Studies (SDS). It is a multidisciplinary and international journal of interest to social scientists, scholars in the humanities, disability rights advocates, creative writers, and others
concerned with the issues of people with disabilities.

2243 Disability and Health Journal
110 N. Washington Street
Suite 328-J
Rockville, MD   20850   301-545-6140
                                                   Fax: 301-545-6144
                                                        www.aahd.us
Ronald G. Blankenbaker, President
Roberta Carlin, Executive Director
E. Clarke Ross, Public Policy Director
Wanda C. Smith, Program Associate
Disability and Health Journal is a scientific, scholarly and
multidisciplinary journal for reporting original contributions
that advance knowledge in disability and health.

2244 Early Intervention
Early Childhood Intervention Clearinghouse
51 Gerty Drive
Room 20
Champaign, IL   61820-7469   217-333-1386
                                                       877-275-3227
                                                   Fax: 217-244-7732
                                           Illinois-eic@illinois.edu
                                             www.eicclearinghouse.org
Susan Fowler, Director
Features articles, conference calendar, material reviews and
news concerning early childhood intervention and disability.
4 pages Quarterly

2245 Emerging Horizon
PO Box 278
Ripon, CA   95366-0278   209-599-9409
                                               emerginghorizons.com

2246 Exceptional Children
Council for Exceptional Children
2900 Crystal Drive
Suite 1000
Arlington, VA   22202-3557   703-620-3660
                                                       866-509-0218
                                                       888-232-7733
                                                   Fax: 703-264-9494
                                                   TTY:866-915-5000
                                                  service@cec.sped.org
                                                       cec.sped.org
Robin D. Brewer, President
James P. Heiden, President Elect
Christy A. Chambers, Immediate Past President
Mikki Garcia, Executive Director

Articles include research, literature surveys and position papers
concerning exceptional children, special education and
mainstreaming. *$58.00*
96 pages BiMonthly

2247 Focus on Autism and Other Developmental Disabilities
Sage Publications
2455 Teller Road
Thousand Oaks, CA   91320   805-499-0721
                                                       800-818-7243
                                                   Fax: 800-583-2665
                                                    info@sagepub.com
                                                    www.sagepub.com
Sara Miller McCune, Founder, Publisher & Executive Chairman
Blaise R. Simqu, President & CEO
Chris Hickok, Senior Vice President & Chief Financial Officer
Stephen Barr, Managing Director/SAGE London
Practical management, treatment and planning strategies; a must
for persons working with individuals with autism and other de-
velopmental disabilities. *$43.00*
64 pages Quarterly

2248 Focus on Exceptional Children
Love Publishing Company
9101 East Kenyon Avenue
Suite 2200
Denver, CO   80237   303-221-7333
                                                   Fax: 303-221-7444
                                               lpc@lovepublishing.com
                                               www.lovepublishing.com
Steve Graham, Consulting Editor
Ron Nelson, Consulting Editor
Eva Horn, Consulting Editor
Contains research and theory-based articles on special education
topics, with an emphasis on application and intervention, of inter-
est to teachers, professors and administrators. *$36.00*
Monthly

2249 HomeCare Magazine
Cahaba Media Group
1900-28th Ave S.
Ste 200
Birmingham, AL   35209   205-212-9402
                                                     cahabamedia.com
Wally Evans, Publisher
Greg Meineke, Vice President, Sales
Stephanie Gibson Lepore, Editor
The business magazine of the home medical equipment industry
offering information on legislation and regulations affecting the
homecare industry, monthly profiles of suppliers, operational
tips, newest products in the industry, advice on sales, government
regulations. *$ 65.00*
120 pages Monthly

2250 I Wonder Who Else Can Help
AARP
601 E Street NW
Washington, DC   20049   202-434-3525
                                                       888-687-2277
                                                       877-342-2277
                                                   Fax: 202-434-3443
                                                    member@aarp.org
                                                        www.aarp.org
John Wider, President, CEO, AARP Services Inc.
Lisa M. Ryerson, President, AARP Foundation
*Robert R. Hagans, Jr., Executive Vice President & Chief Financial
Officer*
*Hollis Terry Bradwell III, Executive Vice President & Chief
Information Officer*
Contains information about crisis counseling, needs and re-
sources, written in lay terms.

2251 Inclusion
501 3rd Street, NW
Suite 200
Washington, DC 20001   202-387-1968
                          Fax: 202-387-2193
                          mnygren@aaidd.org
                          aaidd.org
Deborah Fidler, PhD, Editor
Glenn T. Fujiura, PhD, Editor
Michael L. Wehmeyer, PhD, Co-Editor
Karrie A. Shogren, PhD, Co-Editor
Inclusion is an open submission ejournal. Inclusion is published quarterly in an online-only format, enabling timely dissemination of emerging and promising research, policy, and practices.

2252 Intellectual and Developmental Disabilities
501 3rd Street, NW
Suite 200
Washington, DC 20001   202-387-1968
                          Fax: 202-387-2193
                          mnygren@aaidd.org
                          aaidd.org
Deborah Fidler, PhD, Editor
Glenn T. Fujiura, PhD, Editor
Michael L. Wehmeyer, PhD, Co-Editor
Karrie A. Shogren, PhD, Co-Editor
Intellectual and Developmental Disabilities (IDD) is a peer reviewed multidisciplinary journal of policy, practices, and perspectives.

2253 International Rehabilitation Review
Rehabilitation International
41 Madison Avenue
Office 3141
New York, NY 10010   212-420-1500
                          Fax: 212-505-0871
                          info@riglobal.org
                          riglobal.org
Anne Hawker, President
Patric Fougeyrollas, Deputy Vice President for the No
Marca Bristo, Vice President for the North Ame
Martin Grabois, Treasurer
International overview of activities and programs in vocational and medical rehabilitation, prosthesis and orthotics and special education. *$30.00*
TriAnnual

2254 Intervention in School and Clinic
Sage Publications
2455 Teller Road
Thousand Oaks, CA 91320   805-499-0721
                          800-818-7243
                          Fax: 800-583-2665
                          info@sagepub.com
                          www.sagepub.com
Sara Miller McCune, Founder, Publisher & Executive Chairman
Blaise R. Simqu, President & CEO
Chris Hickok, Senior Vice President & Chief Financial Officer
Stephen Barr, Managing Director/SAGE London
A hands-on, how-to resource for teachers and clinicians working with students for whom minor curriculum and environmental modifications are ineffective. *$35.00*
64 pages

2255 Journal of Applied School Psychology
Haworth Press
711 Third Avenue
New York, NY 10017   212-216-7800
                          800-354-1420
                          Fax: 212-244-1563
                          subscriptions@tandf.co.uk
                          www.haworthpress.com
BiAnnually

2256 Journal of Counseling & Development
American Counseling Association
5999 Stevenson Ave
Alexandria, VA 22304-3304   703-823-0252
                          800-347-6647
                          Fax: 800-473-2329
                          webmaster@counseling.org
                          counseling.org
Robert L. Smith, President
Thelma Duffey, President Elect
Brian Canfield, Treasurer
Richard Yep, CEO
Publishes archival material, also publishes articles that have broad interest for a readership composed mostly of counselors and other mental health professionals who work in private practice, schools, colleges, community agencies, hospitals, and government. An appropriate outlet for articles that: critically integrate published research; examine current professional and scientific issues; report research, new techniques, innovative programs and practices; and examine ACA as an organization. *$140.00*
128 pages Quarterly

2257 Journal of Disability Policy Studies
2455 Teller Road
Thousand Oaks, CA 91320   800-818-7243
                          Fax: 800-583-2665
                          journals@sagepub.com
                          cde.sagepub.com
Blaise R. Simqu, President/ CEO
Tracey A. Ozmina, EVP/ COO
Chris Hickok, SVP/ CFO
Phil Denvir, Global Chief Information Officer
Journal of Disability Policy Studies (DPS) addresses compelling variable issues in ethics, policy and law related to individuals with disabilities.

2258 Journal of Emotional and Behavioral Disorders
Sage Publications
2455 Teller Road
Thousand Oaks, CA 91320   805-499-0721
                          800-818-7243
                          Fax: 800-583-2665
                          info@sagepub.com
                          www.sagepub.com
Sara Miller McCune, Founder, Publisher & Executive Chairman
Blaise R. Simqu, President & CEO
Chris Hickok, Senior Vice President & Chief Financial Officer
Stephen Barr, Managing Director/SAGE London
An international, multidisciplinary journal featuring articles on research, practice and theory related to individuals with emotional and behavioral disorders and to the professionals who serve them. *$39.00*
64 pages Quarterly

2259 Journal of Learning Disabilities
Sage Publications
2455 Teller Road
Thousand Oaks, CA 91320   805-499-0721
                          800-818-7243
                          Fax: 800-583-2665
                          info@sagepub.com
                          www.sagepub.com
Sara Miller McCune, Founder, Publisher & Executive Chairman
Blaise R. Simqu, President & CEO
Chris Hickok, Senior Vice President & Chief Financial Officer
Stephen Barr, Managing Director/SAGE London
An international, multidisciplinary publication containing articles on practice, research and theory related to learning disabilities. Published bi-monthly. *$49.00*
Magazine

2260 Journal of Motor Behavior
Heldref Publications
325 Chestnut Street
Suite 800
Philadelphia, PA 19106

215-625-8900
800-354-1420
Fax: 215-625-2940
customer.service@taylorandfrancis.com
www.heldref.org

Emilli Pawlowsky, Marketing Manager
Laura Rosse, Assistant Marketing Manager
Douglas Kirkpatrick, Publisher
A professional journal aimed at psychologists, therapists and educators who work in the areas of motor behavior, psychology, neurophysiology, kinesiology, and biomechanics. Offers up-to-date information on the latest techniques, theories and developments concerning motor control. Titles previously published by Heldref Publications will be joining the T&F portfolio. *$77.00*
115 pages Quarterly

2261 Journal of Musculoskeletal Pain
Haworth Press
711 Third Avenue
New York, NY 10017

212-216-7800
800-354-1420
Fax: 212-244-1563
subscriptions@tandf.co.uk
www.haworthpress.com

110 pages Quarterly

2262 Journal of Positive Behavior Interventions
2455 Teller Road
Thousand Oaks, CA 91320

800-818-7243
Fax: 800-583-2665
journals@sagepub.com
cde.sagepub.com

Blaise R. Simqu, President/ CEO
Tracey A. Ozmina, EVP/ COO
Chris Hickok, SVP/ CFO
Phil Denvir, Global Chief Information Officer
Journal of Positive Behavior Interventions (PBI) offers sound, research-based principles of positive behavior support for use in school, home and community settings with people with challenges in behavioral adaptation.

2263 Journal of Postsecondary Education & Disability
AHEAD
107 Commerce Centre Dr.
Suite 204
Huntersville, NC 28078

704-947-7779
Fax: 704-948-7779
rwessel@bsu.edu
www.ahead.org/publications/jped

Roger Wessel, Executive Editor
Jamie Axelrod, President
Stephan Smith, Executive Director
An annual publication dedicated to the advancement of full participation in higher education for persons with disabilities. The journal focuses on a variety of related topics that emphasize research, issues, and trends relatedto the theory and practice of postsecondary disability services.

2264 Journal of Prosthetics and Orthotics
330 John Carlyle Street
Suite 210
Alexandria, VA 22314

703-836-7114
Fax: 703-836-0838
info@abcop.org
www.abcop.org

Catherine Carter, Executive Director
Debbie Ayres, Director, Marketing & Public Relations
Stephen Fletcher, CPO, LPO, Director, Clinical Resources
Heather Harris, Director, Continuing Education Programs
Provides the latest research and clinical thinking in orthotics and prosthetics, including information on new devices, fitting techniques and patient management experiences. Each issue contains research-based information and articles reviewed and approved by a highly qualified editorial board. *$60.00*
64 pages Quarterly
ISSN 1040-88 0

2265 Journal of Reading, Writing and Learning Disabled International
Hemisphere Publishing Corporation
7625 Empire Drive
Florence, KY 41042-2919

800-634-7064
Fax: 800-248-4724
orders@taylorandfrancis.com
www.taylorandfrancis.com

2266 Journal of School Health Association
Suite 403
4340 East West Highway
Bethesda, MD 20814

301-652-8072
Fax: 301-652-8077
info@ashaweb.org
ashaweb.org

Jeffrey K. Clark, President
Stephen Conley, Executive Director
Julie Greenfield, Marketing and Conferences Direct
Beverly Samek, Chair of Advocacy
This is a monthly journal which offers information to professionals and parents on school health. Membership dues, $95.00.

2267 Journal of Special Education
Sage Publications
2455 Teller Road
Thousand Oaks, CA 91320

805-499-0721
800-818-7243
Fax: 800-583-2665
info@sagepub.com
www.sagepub.com

Sara Miller McCune, Founder, Publisher & Executive Chairman
Blaise R. Simqu, President & CEO
Chris Hickok, Senior Vice President & Chief Financial Officer
Stephen Barr, Managing Director/SAGE London
Internationally known as the prime research journal in special education. JSE provides research articles of special education for individuals with disabilities, ranging from mild to severe. Published quarterly. *$39.00*
Magazine

2268 Journal of Vocational Behavior
Academic Press, Journals Division

www.academicpress.com/jvb

2269 Learning Disabilities: A Contemporary Journal
179 Bear Hill Rd.
Suite 104
Waltham, MA 02451

978-897-5399
Fax: 978-897-5355
help@ldworldwide.org
www.ldw-ldcj.org

Matthias Grunke, Editor
Teresa Allissa Citro, Editor
Marco G. P. Hessels, Associate Editor
Erin K. Washburn, Associate Editor
Learning Disabilities: A Contemporary Journal (LDCJ) is a peer-reviewed forum for research, practice, and opinion regarding learning disabilities (LD) and associated disorders.

2270 Learning Disabilities: A Multidisciplinary Journal
Learning Disabilities Association of America
4156 Library Road
Pittsburgh, PA 15234-1349

412-341-1515
Fax: 412-344-0224
info@ldaamerica.org
ldaamerica.org

Nancie Payne, President
Allen Broyles, First Vice President
Evalynne W. Lindberg, Secretary
Myrna Soule, Treasurer

The journal is a vehicle for disseminating the most current thinking on learning disabilities and to provide information on research, practice, theory, issues, and trends regarding learning disabilities from the perspectives of varied disciplines involved in broadening the understanding of learning disabilities.

2271   Learning Disability Quarterly
2455 Teller Road
Thousand Oaks, CA 91320   800-818-7243
                                            Fax: 800-583-2665
                                            journals@sagepub.com
                                            ldq.sagepub.com

Blaise R. Simqu, President/ CEO
Tracey A. Ozmina, EVP/ COO
Chris Hickok, SVP/ CFO
Phil Denvir, Global Chief Information Officer
Learning Disability Quarterly (LDQ) publishes high-quality research and scholarship concerning children, youth, and adults with learning disabilities.

2272   MDA Newsmagazine
Muscular Dystrophy Association
3300 E. Sunrise Drive
Tucson, AZ 85718   520-529-2000
                                            800-572-1717
                                            Fax: 520-795-3989
                                            tusconservices@mdausa.org
                                            alsn.mda.org
Danielle Trzyna, Manager
Presents news related to muscular dystrophy and other neuromuscular diseases including research, personal profiles, fundraising activities and patient services.

2273   Measurement and Evaluation in Counseling
5999 Stevenson Ave
Alexandria, VA 22304-3304   703-823-0252
                                            800-347-6647
                                            Fax: 800-473-2329
                                            webmaster@counseling.org
                                            www.counseling.org
Robert L. Smith, President
Thelma Duffey, President Elect
Brian Canfield, Treasurer
Richard Yep, CEO
The American Counseling Association is a not-for-profit, professional and educational organization that is dedicated to the growth and enhancement of the counseling profession

2274   Movement Disorders
555 East Wells Street
Suite 1100
Milwaukee, WI 53202- 3823   414-276-2145
                                            Fax: 414-276-3349
                                            info@movementdisorders.org
                                            www.movementdisorders.org
Matthew B. Stern, President
Oscar S. Gershanik, President-Elect
Francisco Cardoso, Secretary
Christopher Goetz, Treasurer
Movement Disorders, the official Journal of the International Parkinson and Movement Disorder Society (MDS), is a highly read and referenced journal covering all topics of the field - both clinical and basic science.

2275   People & Families
PO Box 700
Trenton, NJ 8625-700   609-292-345
                                            800-792-8858
                                            Fax: 609-292-7114
                                            TTY: 609-777-3238
                                            njcdd@njcdd.org
                                            www.njcdd.org
Kevin T. Jonathan, Waller
Editor
People & Families, the NJCDD's nationally recognized magazine, focuses on issues of importance to the developmental disabilities community in New Jersey.

2276   Psychiatric Staffing Crisis in Community Mental Health
Nat l Council for Community Behavioral Healthcare
76 Ninth Avenue
New York, NY 10011   201-559-3882
                                            800-THE-BOOK
                                            amilevoj@bn.com
                                            www.barnesandnoble.com
Andy Milevoj, Vice President, Investor Relations
Mary Ellen Keating, SVP, Corporate Communications & Public Affairs
Carolyn Brown, Director of Corporate Communications
Find out some of the simple, low-cost ways you can increase workplace satisfaction among staff psychiatrists and compete successfully for their talents. $20.00

2277   Readings: A Journal of Reviews and Commentary in Mental Health
American Orthopsychiatric Association
3524 Washington Avenue
P.O. Box 1048
Sheboygan, WI 53081-1048   920-457-5051
                                            800-558-7687
                                            Fax: 920-457-1485
                                            info@americanortho.com
                                            www.americanortho.com
Michael Bogenschuetz, President
Randy Benz, Chief Executive Officer
Charles Achter, Assistant Controller
Deb Schmidt, Administrative Manager
Reviews of recent books in mental health and allied disciplines. Includes essay reviews and brief reviews. $25.00
32 pages Quarterly

2278   Rehab Pro
1926 Waukegan Rd
Suite 1
Glenview, IL 60025-1770   847-657-6964
                                            Fax: 847-657-6963
                                            carlw@tcag.com
                                            www.rehabpro.org
Carl Wangman, Executive Director
The magazine is to promote the profession and to inform the public about the activities of the national organization, its state chapter affiliates, and the work of its special interest sections.
38 pages BiMonthly

2279   Remedial and Special Education
Sage Publications
2455 Teller Road
Thousand Oaks, CA 91320   805-499-0721
                                            800-818-7243
                                            Fax: 800-583-2665
                                            info@sagepub.com
                                            www.sagepub.com
Sara Miller McCune, Founder, Publisher & Executive Chairman
Blaise R. Simqu, President & CEO
Chris Hickok, Senior Vice President & Chief Financial Officer
Stephen Barr, Managing Director/SAGE London
A professional journal that bridges the gap between theory and practice. Emphasis is on topical reviews, syntheses of research, field evaluation studies and recommendations for the practice of remedial and special education. Published six times a year. $39.00
64 pages

2280   Teaching Exceptional Children
Council for Exceptional Children
2900 Crystal Dr.
Suite 1000
Arlington, VA 22202-3557   888-232-7733
                                            TTY:866-915-5000
                                            service@cec.sped.org
                                            www.cec.sped.org
Alexander T. Graham, Executive Director
Sharon Rodriguez, Senior Executive Assistant
Craig Evans, Director of Operations

Journal designed for teachers of gifted students and students with disabilities, featuring practical methods and materials for classroom use. *$58.00*
96 pages BiMonthly

Newsletters

2281 APA Access
750 First Street, NE
Washington, DC 20002-4242
202-336-5500
800-374-2721
rllowman@gmail.com
www.apa.org

Rodney L. Lowman, PhD, Chair
Barry Anton, PhD, President
Bonnie Markham, PhD, PsyD, Treasurer
Norman Anderson, PhD, CEO, EVP
Exclusively for APA members, APA Access provides a helpful insider's view of the latest APA news. Each monthly issue highlights an array of current topics, such as advocacy updates, continuing education opportunities, press releases, previews of Monitor on Psychology articles, APA publishing news, new APA products and a calendar of events.

2282 Alert
Association on Handicapped Student Service Program
P.O.Box 21192
Columbus, OH 43221
614-365-5216
Fax: 614-365-6718

2283 Camp Virginia Jaycee Newsletter
Dare Care Charity
2494 Camp Jaycee Rd
P.O. Box 648
Blue Ridge, VA 24064
540-947-2972
info@campvajc.org
www.campvajc.org

Tom King, Chairman
Kathleen King, Vice Chair
Lisa Parrish, Treasurer
William Hartz, Past Chair
Summer camping for children and adults with developmental disabilities. Coed, ages 7-70. Weekend respite camps for children and adults with mental retardation.
8 pages quarterly

2284 Children's Mental Health and EBD E-news
8161 Normandale Blvd.
Bloomington, MN 55437
952-838-9000
800-537-2237
888-248-0822
Fax: 952-838-0199
www.pacer.org

Paula F. Goldberg, Executive Director
It can be quite difficult to address children's mental health and emotional or behavioral issues. From multiple diagnoses and co-occurring conditions to the confusion of navigating often overlapping systems of care, it is often overwhelming for parents. PACER's goal is to provide family friendly, culturally competent resources to help parents be effective advocates for their child.

2285 Counseling Today
American Counseling Association
5999 Stevenson Ave
Alexandria, VA 22304-3304
703-823-0252
800-347-6647
Fax: 800-473-2329
webmaster@counseling.org
counseling.org

Robert L. Smith, President
Thelma Duffey, President Elect
Brian Canfield, Treasurer
Richard Yep, CEO
Aims to serve individuals active in professional counseling, in the school and university, in the workplace and the marketplace, as well as other citizens, community leaders and policy makers

who appreciate the importance of the role of professional counselors in today's society.
Monthly

2286 Counselor Education and Supervision
American Counseling Association
5999 Stevenson Ave
Alexandria, VA 22304-3304
703-823-0252
800-347-6647
Fax: 800-473-2329
webmaster@counseling.org
www.counseling.org

Robert L. Smith, President
Thelma Duffey, President Elect
Brian Canfield, Treasurer
Richard Yep, CEO
Dedicated to the growth and development of the counseling profession and those who are served. *$18.00*
Quarterly

2287 Disability Compliance for Higher Education
LRP Publications
P.O. Box 24668
West Palm Beach, FL 33416-4668
561-622-2423
800-341-7874
Fax: 561-622-1375
custserve@lrp.com
lrp.com

Kenneth F. Kahn, Owner and President
Ed Chase, Vice President
The only newsletter that is dedicated to the exclusive coverage of disability issues that affect colleges and universities. *$195.00*
8 pages Monthly

2288 Disability Pride Newsletter
900 Rebecca Avenue
Pittsburgh, PA 15221
800-633-4588
Fax: 412-371-9430
lgray@trcil.org
trcil.myfastsite.net

Rachel Rogan, CEO
Gregory Daigle, Chief Financial Officer
Lisa Wilson, HR Program Manager
Victoria Johnson, Human Resources Assistant
Three Rivers Center for Independent Living (TRCIL) is a non-residential, non-profit, community-based human service organization. There purpose is to assist people with disabilities to lead self-directed and productive lives within the community.

2289 Disability Resources Monthly
Disability Resources
4 Glatter Ln
South Setauket, NY 11720-1032
631-585-0290
Fax: 631-585-0290

Avery Klauber, Executive Director
A newsletter that monitors, reviews and reports on resources for independent living. A monthly newsletter that features short topical articles, news items and reviews of books, pamphlets, periodicals, videotapes, on-line services, organizations and other resources for and about people with disabilities. It is intended primarily for librarians, social workers, educators, rehabilitation specialists, disability advocates, ADA coordinators and other health and social service professionals. *$33.00*
4 pages Monthly
ISSN 1070-72 0

2290 Early Childhood Connection
8161 Normandale Blvd.
Bloomington, MN 55437
952-838-9000
800-537-2237
888-248-0822
Fax: 952-838-0199
www.pacer.org

Paula F. Goldberg, Executive Director
PACER's Early Childhood Family Information and Resources Project gives parents of children ages birth through 5 years the

confidence, knowledge, and skills they need to help their children obtain the education, health care, and other services they deserve.

2291   Early Childhood E-News
8161 Normandale Blvd.
Bloomington, MN 55437   952-838-9000
                                                      800-537-2237
                                                      888-248-0822
                                          Fax: 952-838-0199
                                                      www.pacer.org
Paula F. Goldberg, Executive Director
Highlights early childhood news and information. Published quarterly.

2292   Early Childhood Reporter
LRP Publications
P.O. Box 24668
West Palm Beach, FL 33416-4668   561-622-2423
                                                      800-341-7874
                                          Fax: 561-622-1375
                                            custserve@lrp.com
                                                      www.lrp.com
Kenneth F. Kahn, Owner and President
Ed Chase, Vice President
Monthly reports with information on federal, state, and local legislation affecting the implementation of early intervention and preschool programs for children with disabilities. *$145.00*
12-16 pages $10 shipping

2293   FYI
501 3rd Street, NW
Suite 200
Washington, DC 20001   202-387-1968
                                          Fax: 202-387-2193
                                            mnygren@aaidd.org
                                                      aaidd.org
Deborah Fidler, PhD, Editor
Glenn T. Fujiura, PhD, Editor
Michael L. Wehmeyer, PhD, Co-Editor
Karrie A. Shogren, PhD, Co-Editor
This monthly eblast provides news and information about AAIDD resources, educational opportunities, and other activities.

2294   Fellow Insider
501 3rd Street, NW
Suite 200
Washington, DC 20001   202-387-1968
                                          Fax: 202-387-2193
                                            mnygren@aaidd.org
                                                      aaidd.org
Deborah Fidler, PhD, Editor
Glenn T. Fujiura, PhD, Editor
Michael L. Wehmeyer, PhD, Co-Editor
Karrie A. Shogren, PhD, Co-Editor
Published quarterly.

2295   Field Notes
501 3rd Street, NW
Suite 200
Washington, DC 20001   202-387-1968
                                          Fax: 202-387-2193
                                            mnygren@aaidd.org
                                                      aaidd.org
Deborah Fidler, PhD, Editor
Glenn T. Fujiura, PhD, Editor
Michael L. Wehmeyer, PhD, Co-Editor
Karrie A. Shogren, PhD, Co-Editor
This monthly eblast promotes the translation of research to practice by providing a brief summary of approximately 10 studies recently published in peer reviewed journals with links to the original articles.

2296   Gram Newsletter, The
PO Box 1114
Claremont, CA 91711   909-621-1494
                                            contact@ldaca.org
                                                      www.ldaca.org
Arline Krieger, President
Pam Hamilton, 1st Vice-President
EunMi Cho, 3rd Vice-President
William McKinley, Treasurer
The Learning Disabilities Association of California's (LDA-CA's) quarterly newsletter, The GRAM, provides LDA-CA members with timely information.

2297   Growing Readers
2775 S. Quincy St.
Arlington, VA   *Fax:* 703-998-2060
                                                      www.ldonline.org
Noel Gunther, Executive Director
Bridget Brady, Web Assistant
Lydia Breiseth, Manager
Tina Chovanec, Director
Monthly tips for raising strong readers and writers, written especially for parents. Used by schools and PTAs in parent newsletters, and by libraries and community literacy organizations.

2298   HEALTH E-News
8161 Normandale Blvd.
Bloomington, MN 55437   952-838-9000
                                                      800-537-2237
                                                      888-248-0822
                                          Fax: 952-838-0199
                                                      www.pacer.org
Paula F. Goldberg, Executive Director
If you need information or individual assistance about navigating the health care system, PACER's F2F HICcan help. It provides a central source for Minnesota families of children and youth with special health care needs and/or disabilities and the professionals who serve them to obtain support, advocacy, and information about the health care system.

2299   Healthline
CV Mosby Company
1600 John F. Kennedy Boulevard
Suite 1800
Philadelphia, PA 19103-2822   215-239-3900
                                                      800-523-1649
                                          Fax: 215-239-3990
                                            www.us.elsevierhealth.com
Monthly

2300   Help Newsletter
Learning Disabilities Association of Arkansas
P.O. Box 23514
Little Rock, AR 72221   501-666-8777
                                          Fax: 501-666-8777
                                                      www.ldaarkansas.org
Nathan Green, President
Rebecca Walker, VP
Becca Green, Past President, Treasurer
Doris Pierce, Secretary
Information on how to overcome obstacles and to achieve in spite of learning disabilities. *$30.00*
8 pages Quarterly

2301   Insights
135 Parkinson Avenue
Staten Island, NY 10305   800-223-2732
                                          Fax: 718-981-4399
                                            apda@apdaparkinson.org
                                                      www.apdaparkinson.org
Fred Greene, Chairman
Patrick McDermott, 1st Vice Chairman
Jerry Wells, Esq., Secretary
Elena Imperato, Treasurer
APDA was founded in 1961 with the dual purpose to Ease the Burden - Find the Cure for Parkinson's disease.

2302 International Rolf Institute
5055 Chaparral Ct.
Suite 103
Boulder, CO 80301 303-449-5903
800-530-8875
Fax: 303-449-5978
dyourell@rolf.org
rolf.org

Kevin McCoy, Chairperson
Diana Yourell, Executive Director
Jim Jones, Director of Education
Carah Wertheimer, Admissions Advisor
Information, practitioner training and certification.

2303 LD Monthly Report
2775 S. Quincy St.
Arlington, VA *Fax:* 703-998-2060
www.ldonline.org

Noel Gunther, Executive Director
Bridget Brady, Web Assistant
Lydia Breiseth, Manager
Tina Chovanec, Director
LD OnLine seeks to help children and adults reach their full potential by providing accurate and up-to-date information and advice about learning disabilities and ADHD.

2304 Learning Disabilities Consultants Newsletter
Learning Disabilities Consultants
P.O.Box 716
Bryn Mawr, PA 19010 610-446-6126
800-869-8336
Fax: 610-446-6129
rcooper-ldr@comcast.net
www.thebrookhospitals.com/Resources
Richard Cooper, Director
Newsletter providing information about learning disabilities and differences. It contains both local and national news items and includes in each issue articles about various aspects of learning problems encountered in both children and adults. *$10.00*
6 pages 5x Year

2305 MA Report
National Allergy and Asthma Network
Ste 200
3554 Chain Bridge Rd
Fairfax, VA 22030-2709 703-385-4403
Fax: 703-352-4354
Monthly

2306 Member Update
501 3rd Street, NW
Suite 200
Washington, DC 20001 202-387-1968
Fax: 202-387-2193
mnygren@aaidd.org
aaidd.org

Deborah Fidler,PhD, Editor
Glenn T. Fujiura, PhD, Editor
Michael L. Wehmeyer, PhD, Co-Editor
Karrie A. Shogren, PhD, Co-Editor
This weekly eblast updates readers on time-sensitive professional development opportunities, such as conferences and webinars, job postings, calls for papers, and opportunities to join advisory committees and provide comments on federal initiatives.

2307 O&P Almanac
American Orthotic & Prosthetic Association
330 John Carlyle Street
Suite 200
Alexandria, VA 22314 571-431-0876
Fax: 571-431-0899
info@aopanet.org
www.aopanet.org

Anita Liberman-Lampear, MA, President
Charles H. Dankmeyer, Jr, CPO, President-Elect
James Campbell, CO, Ph.D., Vice President
Jim Weber, MBA, Treasurer
Offers in-depth coverage on orthotics and prosthetics to current professional, government, business and reimbursement activities affecting the orthotics and prosthetics industry. *$59.00*
80 pages Monthly

2308 Occupational Therapy in Health Care
Haworth Press
711 Third Avenue
New York, NY 10017 212-216-7800
800-354-1420
Fax: 212-244-1563
subscriptions@tandf.co.uk
www.haworthpress.com

2309 Ohio Coalition for the Education of Children with Disabilities
165 W Center St, 3rd Floor, Chase B
Suite 302
Marion, OH 43302 740-382-5452
800-374-2806
Fax: 740-383-6421
ocecd@ocecd.org
www.ocecd.org

Martha Lause, Manager
Lee Ann Derugen, Co-Director
Margaret Burley, Executive Director
Lee Ann Derugen, Co-Director
Forum is a newsletter reporting on educational, legislative and other developments affecting persons with disabilities.
8 pages

2310 PACER E-News
8161 Normandale Blvd.
Bloomington, MN 55437 952-838-9000
800-537-2237
888-248-0822
Fax: 952-838-0199
www.pacer.org

Paula F. Goldberg, Executive Director
Published monthly, it provides resources and information for children with disabilities and their families.

2311 PACER Partners
8161 Normandale Blvd.
Bloomington, MN 55437 952-838-9000
800-537-2237
888-248-0822
Fax: 952-838-0199
www.pacer.org

Paula F. Goldberg, Executive Director
Connecting families, friends, donors, and staff of PACER. Published by the Development Office at PACER.

2312 PACESETTER
8161 Normandale Blvd.
Bloomington, MN 55437 952-838-9000
800-537-2237
888-248-0822
Fax: 952-838-0199
www.pacer.org

Paula F. Goldberg, Executive Director
PACER's main newsletter; information on special education, PACER programs, and resources.

2313 SAMHSA News
U S Department of Health and Human Services
1 Choke Cherry Road
Rockville, MD   20857   202-690-7650
                                             877-SAM-SA 7
                                       TTY:800-487-4889
                                          www.samhsa.gov
Pamela S. Hyde, J.D., Administrator
Kana Enomoto, M.A., Principal Deputy Administrator
Daryl W. Kade, M.A., Chief Financial Officer and Director,OFR
Marla Hendriksson, M.P.M., Director, Office of Communications
This quarterly agency newsletter reports on information on substance abuse, mental health treatment and prevention programs of the Substance Abuse and Mental Health Services Administration.
Quarterly

2314 Sibling Information Network Newsletter
AJ Pappanikou Center
270 Farmington Avenue
Suite 181
Farmington, CT   06030   860-679-1500
                                             866-623-1315
                                        Fax: 860-679-1571
                                       TTY: 860-679-1502
                              contact.us.ucedd@uchc.edu
                                        www.uconnucedd.org
Mary Beth Bruder, PhD, UCEDD/LEND Director
Gerarda Hanna, J.D., M.Ed., Associate UCEDD Director
Gabriela Freyre-Calish, MSW, Coordinator, Director, Cultural Diversity
Linda Procko, Program Coordinator
Contains information aimed at the varying interested of our membership. Program descriptions, requests for assistance, conference announcements, literature summaries and research reports.
$8.50

2315 Sibpage
AJ Pappanikou Center
270 Farmington Avenue
Suite 181
Farmington, CT   06030   860-679-1500
                                             866-623-1315
                                        Fax: 860-679-1571
                                       TTY: 860-679-1502
                              contact.us.ucedd@uchc.edu
                                        www.uconnucedd.org
Mary Beth Bruder, PhD, UCEDD/LEND Director
Gerarda Hanna, J.D., M.Ed., Associate UCEDD Director
Gabriela Freyre-Calish, MSW, Coordinator, Director, Cultural Diversity
Linda Procko, Program Coordinator
Developed specifically for children containing games, recipes, pen pals, and articles written by siblings relating to developmental disabilities.
4 pages

2316 Special Edge
Resources in Special Education
Fl 4
1107 9th St
Sacramento, CA 95814-3616   916-492-9999
                                             877-493-7833
                                        Fax: 916-492-4004
                                          rise@wested.org
Virigina Reynolds, President
Provides education news, collaborative programs, amendments to the laws, tools for accommodations, resource information, a calendar of events, and more.
BiMonthly

2317 Special Education Report
LRP Publications
360 Hiatt Dr
Dept. 150F
Palm BeachGardens, FL 33418   800-341-7874
                                        Fax: 561-622-2423
                                       custserve@lrp.com
                                                  lrp.com

Current, pertinent information about federal legislation, regulations, programs and funding for educating children with disabilities. Covers federal and state litigation on the Individuals with Disabilities Education Act and other relevant laws. Looks at innovations and research in the field.

2318 Tech Notes
8161 Normandale Blvd.
Bloomington, MN   55437   952-838-9000
                                             800-537-2237
                                             888-248-0822
                                        Fax: 952-838-0199
                                            www.pacer.org
Paula F. Goldberg, Executive Director
Events, resources and more for families and professionals interested in assistive technology, published quarterly.

2319 Tiny Tech
8161 Normandale Blvd.
Bloomington, MN   55437   952-838-9000
                                             800-537-2237
                                             888-248-0822
                                        Fax: 952-838-0199
                                            www.pacer.org
Paula F. Goldberg, Executive Director
Highlights technology and resources of interest to parents and professionals of children age 0 - 5, published monthly.

2320 Topics in Early Childhood Special Education
Sage Publications
2455 Teller Road
Thousand Oaks, CA   91320   805-499-0721
                                             800-818-7243
                                        Fax: 800-583-2665
                                        info@sagepub.com
                                           www.sagepub.com
Sara Miller McCune, Founder, Publisher & Executive Chairman
Blaise R. Simqu, President & CEO
Chris Hickok, Senior Vice President & Chief Financial Officer
Stephen Barr, Managing Director/SAGE London
Designed for professionals helping young children with special needs in areas such as assessment, special programs, social policies and developmental aids. *$43.00*
Quarterly

2321 Treatment Review
AIDS Treatment Data Network
57 Willoughby St.
2nd Floor
Brooklyn, NY 11201   347-473-7400
                                             800-734-7104
                                       TTY:212-925-9560
                              info@housingworks.org
                                     www.housingworks.org
Charles King, Chair
Linney Smith, Vice Chair
Earl Ward, Vice Chair
Andrew Coarney, Secretary
Individual members receive treatment education, counseling, referrals and case management support. Services are available in both English and Spanish. The Treatment Review newsletter includes descriptions of approved, alternative and experimental treatments, as well as announcements of seminars and forums on treatments and clinical trials.
Quarterly

2322 VIP Newsletter
Blind Children's Fund
6761 West US 12
P.O. Box 363
Three Oaks, MI 49128   989-779-9966
                                        Fax: 269-756-3133
                         BCF@blindchildrensfund.org
                             www.blindchildrensfund.org
Karla B. Kwast, Executive Director
Jeremy Murphy, President
Robert R. Storrer Jr., Vice President
Carrie L. Owens, Director

Provides parents and professionals with information, materials and resources that help them successfully teach and nurture blind, visually and multi-impaired infants and preschoolers. *$10.00*

Professional Texts

2323   7 Steps for Success
Council for Exceptional Children
2900 Crystal Dr.
Suite 1000
Arlington, VA   22202-3557   888-232-7733
                                    TTY:866-915-5000
                                    service@cec.sped.org
                                    www.cec.sped.org

Elizabeth C. Hamblet, Author
A book helping young adults with disabilities transitioning from high school.

2324   A Guide to Teaching Students With Autism Spectrum Disorders
Council for Exceptional Children
2900 Crystal Dr.
Suite 1000
Arlington, VA   22202-3557   888-232-7733
                                    TTY:866-915-5000
                                    service@cec.sped.org
                                    www.cec.sped.org

Monica E. Delano, Co-Author
Darlene E. Perner, Co-Author
This book is a resource for all special educators and general educators who work with students with autism spectrum disorders (ASD). The underlying premise is that students with ASD should be explicitly taught a full range of social, self-help, language, reading, writing and math skills, as are their typically developing classmates.

2325   A Teacher's Guide to Isovaleric Acidemia
150 North 18th Avenue
Phoenix, AZ   85007   602-542-1025
                                    Fax: 602-542-0883
                                    www.azdhs.gov

Will Humble, Director
Thomas Salow, Manager
Resource book for preschool teachers and school staff on isovaleric academia basics and classroom activities. *$2.50*

2326   A Teacher's Guide to Methylmalonic Acidemia
Arizona State Department of Health Services
150 North 18th Avenue
Phoenix, AZ   85007   602-542-1025
                                    Fax: 602-542-0883
                                    www.azdhs.gov

Will Humble, Director
Thomas Salow, Manager
Resource book for preschool teachers and school staff on methylmalonic academia basics and classroom activities. *$2.50*

2327   A Teacher's Guide to PKU
Arizona Department of Health Services
150 North 18th Avenue
Phoenix, AZ   85007   602-542-1025
                                    Fax: 602-542-0883
                                    www.azdhs.gov

Will Humble, Director
Thomas Salow, Manager
Resource book for preschool teachers and school staff on PKU basics, NutraSweet warning, and classroom activities. *$2.50*
13 pages

2328   AD/HD and the College Student: The Everything Guide to Your Most Urgent Questions
750 First Street, NE
Washington, DC   20002-4242   202-336-5500
                                    800-374-2721
                                    rllowman@gmail.com
                                    www.apa.org

Patricia O. Quinn, MD, Author
Whether you are looking for information or facing an urgent situation,AD/HD and the College Studentprovides answers to your most pressing questions. Organized in a question-and-answer format, this guide is loaded with helpful information, practical tips, and resources.

2329   ADD Challenge: A Practical Guide for Teachers
2612 N. Mattis Ave.
P.O. Box 7886
Champaign, IL   61822   217-352-3273
                                    800-519-2707
                                    Fax: 217-352-1221
                                    orders@researchpress.com
                                    www.researchpress.com

Robert W. Parkinson, Founder
Steven B. Gordon, Author
Dr Richard M Foxx, Author
Michael J. Asher, Author
Research Press is an independent, family-owned business founded in 1968 by Robert W. Parkinson (1920-2001).

2330   ADHD Coaching: A Guide for Mental Health Professionals
750 First Street, NE
Washington, DC   20002-4242   202-336-5500
                                    800-374-2721
                                    rllowman@gmail.com
                                    www.apa.org

Frances Prevatt, PhD, Co-Author
Abigail Levrini, PhD, Co-Author
This book describes the underlying principles as well as the nuts and bolts of ADHD coaching. Step-by-step details for gathering information, conducting the intake, establishing goals and objectives, and working through all stages of coaching are included, along with helpful forms and a detailed list of additional resources.

2331   ADHD in the Classroom: Strategies for Teachers
Guilford Publication
72 Spring Street
New York, NY   10012   212-431-9800
                                    800-365-7006
                                    Fax: 212-966-6708
                                    info@guilford.com
                                    www.guilford.com

Bob Matloff, President
Seymour Weingarten, Editor-in-Chief
Russell A. Barkley, Author
Gary Stoner, Author
Designed specifically to help teachers with their ADHD students, thereby providing a better learning environment for the entire class. *$95.00*
ISBN 0-898629-85-3

2332   ADHD in the Schools: Assessment and Intervention Strategies
72 Spring Street
New York, NY   10012   212-431-9800
                                    800-365-7006
                                    Fax: 212-966-6708
                                    info@guilford.com
                                    www.guilford.com

Bob Matloff, President
Seymour Weingarten, Editor-in-Chief
George J. DuPaul, Author
Gary Stoner, Author
The landmark volume emphasizes the need for a team effort among parents, community-based professionals, and educators. Provides practical information for educators that is based on empirical findings. Chapters Focus on how to identify and assess students who might have ADHD, the relationship between

ADHD and learning disabilities; how to develop and supplement classroom-based programs. Communication strategies to assist physicians and the need for community-based treatments *$36.00*
269 pages Paperback
ISBN 0-898622-45-X

2333 AEPS Curriculum for Birth to Three Years
Brookes Publishing
P.O.Box 10624
Baltimore, MD 21285-0624 410-337-9580
800-638-3775
Fax: 410-337-8539
custserv@brookespublishing.com
readplaylearn.com
496 pages
ISBN 1-557660-96-4

2334 Access to Health Care: Number 3&4
World Institute on Disability
3075 Adeline Street
Suite 155
Berkeley, CA 94703 510-225-6400
Fax: 510-225-0477
TTY:510-225-0478
wid@wid.org
www.wid.org
Paul W. Schroeder, Chairman
Linda M. Dardarian, Vice Chairman
Anita Shafer Aaron, Executive Director
Mary Brooner, Treasurer
These policy bulletins focus on the capacity of the private and public health insurance systems to respond to the health care needs of persons with disabilities or chronic illness. *$6.50*
91 pages Paperback

2335 Activity-Based Approach to Early Intervention, 2nd Edition
Brookes Publishing
P.O.Box 10624
Baltimore, MD 21285-0624 410-337-9580
800-638-3775
Fax: 410-337-8539
webmaster@brookespublishing.com
www.brookespublishing.com
Paul H. Brookes, Chairman of the Board
Jeffrey D. Brookes, President
George S. Stamathis, VP/Publisher
Melissa A. Behn, Executive Vice President
Activity-based intervention shows how to use natural and relevant events to teach infants and young children, of all abilities, effectively and efficiently. *$24.00*
240 pages
ISBN 1-55766-87-5

2336 Adapted Physical Education for Students with Autism
Charles C. Thomas
2600 S First St
Springfield, IL 62704-4730 217-789-8980
800-258-8980
Fax: 217-789-9130
books@ccthomas.com
www.ccthomas.com
Kimberly Davis, Author
Focuses on the physical education needs and curriculum for autistic children. Available in cloth, paperback and hardcover. *$27.95*
142 pages Paper
ISBN 0-398060-85-1

2337 Adapting Early Childhood Curricula for Children with Special Needs (9th Edition)
Pearson Higher Education
330 Hudson St
New York, NY 10013 212-641-2400
www.pearsonhighered.com
Ruth E. Cook, Author
M. Diane Klein, Author
Deborah Chen, Author

This highly readable, well researched, and current resource uses a developmental focus, rather than a disability orientation, to discuss typical and atypical child development and curricular adaptations, and encourage the treatment of students as children first, without regard to their learning differences. *$102.67*
528 pages Loose-Leaf or Access Code Card 1915
ISBN 0-134019-41-3

2338 Adapting Instruction for the Mainstream: A Sequential Approach to Teaching
McGraw-Hill School Publishing
P.O. Box 182605
Columbus, OH 43218 800-338-3987
Fax: 609-308-4480
customer.service@mheducation.com
mcgraw-hill.com
David Levin, President, CEO
Ellen Haley, President, CTB
Peter Cohen, President, School Education
Mark Dorman, President, International
This text gives both regular and special education teachers everything they need to help mildly handicapped students succeed in the mainstream.
226 pages

2339 Adaptive Education Strategies Building on Diversity
Brookes Publishing Company
P.O.Box 10624
Baltimore, MD 21285-0624 410-337-9580
800-638-3775
Fax: 410-337-8539
webmaster@brookespublishing.com
www.brookespublishing.com
Paul H. Brookes, Chairman of the Board
Jeffrey D. Brookes, President
George S. Stamathis, VP/Publisher
Melissa A. Behn, Executive Vice President
Based on more than two decades of systematic research, this comprehensive manual provides a road map to the effective implementation of adaptive education. *$35.00*
304 pages Paperback
ISBN 1-557880-84-0

2340 Adolescents and Adults with Learning Disabilities and ADHD
370 Seventh Avenue
Suite 1200
New York, NY 10001-1020 800-365-7006
Fax: 212-966-6708
info@guilford.com
www.guilford.com
No%ol Gregg, PhD, Author
Most of the literature on learning disabilities and attention-deficit/hyperactivity disorder (ADHD) focuses on the needs of elementary school-age children, but older students with these conditions also require significant support.

2341 Advanced Sign Language Vocabulary: A Resource Text for Educators
Charles C. Thomas
2600 S First St
Springfield, IL 62704-4730 217-789-8980
800-258-8980
Fax: 217-789-9130
books@ccthomas.com
www.ccthomas.com
Elizabeth E. Wolf, Author
Janet R. Coleman, Author
This book is a collection of advanced sign language vocabulary for use by educators, interpreters, parents or anyone wishing to enlarge their sign vocabulary. *$53.95*
202 pages Spiralbound
ISBN 0-398057-22-2

2342 Advances in Cardiac and Pulmonary Rehabilitation
Haworth Press
711 Third Avenue
New York, NY   10017   212-216-7800
                                            800-354-1420
                                        Fax: 212-244-1563
                                    subscriptions@tandf.co.uk
                                        www.haworthpress.com

74 pages Hardcover
ISBN 0-866869-86-3

2343 Aging Brain
Taylor & Francis Group
Ste 800
325 Chestnut St
Philadelphia, PA   19106-2608   215-625-8900
                                           800-354-1420
                                       Fax: 215-625-2940
                                 www.taylorandfrancisgroup.com

225 pages Paperback
ISBN 0-85066-78-0

2344 Aging and Disability: Crossing Network Lines
Springer Publishing
11 West 42nd Street
15th Floor
New York, NY   10036   212-431-4370
                                           877-687-7476
                                       Fax: 212-941-7842
                                  marketing@springerpub.com
                                            springerpub.com

Theodore C. Nardin, CEO/Publisher
Jason Roth, VP/Marketing Director
Annette Imperati, Marketing/Sales Director
Stephanie Drew, Acquisitions Editor,Social Work
Michelle Putnam has set forth this volume to reflect the current
research, facilitate collaboration across service networks, and
encourage movement toward more effective service policies.
Professional stakeholders evaluate the bridges and barriers to
crossing network lines, and chapter on current websites, agencies, and coalitions provides the much needed tools to bring
collaboration into practice.

2345 Aging and Rehabilitation II: The State ofthe Practice
Springer Publishing Company
11 W 42nd St
15th Fl
New York, NY   10036-8002   212-431-4370
                                           877-687-7476
                                       Fax: 212-941-7842
                                       cs@springerpub.com
                                        www.springerpub.com

Ted Nardin, chief Executive Officer
Jason Roth, Vice President, Marketing & Sales
Kathy Weiss, Senior Sales Director
Annette Imperati, Sales Director, Corporate, Government, &
Associations
Current, multidisciplinary investigations of various practice issues. Leading experts in the field use a practical perspective to
provide specific comments on interventions. The scope of this
work encompasses the autonomy of elderly disabled, mobility,
mental health and value issues, as well as basic aspects in rehabilitation of the elderly. *$8.95*
348 pages Hardcover 1990
ISBN 0-826170-80-3

2346 Alphabetic Phonics Curriculum
Educators Publishing Service
625 Mount Auburn Street
3rd Floor
Cambridge, MA   02138- 3039   617-547-6706
                                           800-225-5750
                                Feedback.EPS@schoolspecialty.com
                                          www.cpsbooks.com

Rick Holden, President, EPS
Ungraded multisensory curriculum for teaching phonics and the
structure of language. Uses Orton-Gillingham approach to teach
handwriting, spelling, reading, reading comprehension, and oral

and written expression. program includes basic manual, workbooks, tests, teachers' guides, drill cards and all cards. *$28.15*
ISSN 8388-42

2347 Alternative Educational Delivery Systems
National Association of School Psychologists
4340 East West Highway
Suite 402
Bethesda, MD   20814   301-657-0270
                                           866-331-NASP
                                       Fax: 301-657-0275
                                       TTY: 301-657-4155
                                   webmaster@naspweb.org
                                           nasponline.org

Stephen E. Brock, President
Todd A. Savage, President-Elect
Laura Benson, Chief Operating Officer
Susan Gorin, Executive Director
A book offering information to the professional on how to en-
hance educational options for all students.

2348 Alternative Teaching Strategies
Special Needs Project
324 State St
Ste H
Santa Barbara, CA   93101   818-718-9900
                                       Fax: 818-349-2027
                                    hgray@specialneeds.com
                                      www.specialneeds.com

Hod Gray, Owner
Offers help for teachers who teach behaviorally troubled students.

**2349 Antecedent Control: Innovative Approaches to Behavioral
Support**
Brookes Publishing
P.O.Box 10624
Baltimore, MD   21285-0624   410-337-9580
                                           800-638-3775
                                       Fax: 410-337-8539
                              webmaster@brookespublishing.com
                                  www.brookespublishing.com

Paul H. Brookes, Chairman of the Board
Jeffrey D. Brookes, President
George S. Stamathis, VP/Publisher
Melissa A. Behn, Executive Vice President
This book explains the theory and methodology of antecedent
control. The treatment techniques in this book are effective for
both children and adults.
416 pages Paperback
ISBN 1-55766-34-3

**2350 Anxiety-Free Kids: An Interactive Guide for Parents and
Children**
Prufrock Press
PO Box 8813
Waco, TX   76714-8813   800-998-2208
                                       Fax: 800-240-0333
                                       info@prufrock.com
                                         www.prufrock.com

Joel McIntosh, Publisher & Marketing Director
Lacy Compton, Senior Editor
Rachel Taliaferro, Editor
Raquel Trevino, Graphic Designer and Production Coordinator
Offers parents strategies that help children happy and worry-free,
methods that relieve a child's excessive anxieties and phobias,
and tools for fostering interaction and family-oriented solutions.
$19.95
280 pages Paperback
ISBN 1-593633-43-1

2351 Applied Rehabilitation Counseling (Springer Series on Rehabilitation)
Springer Publishing Company
11 W 42nd St
15th Fl
New York, NY   10036-8002
212-431-4370
877-687-7476
Fax: 212-941-7842
cs@springerpub.com
www.springerpub.com

Ted Nardin, Chief Executive Officer
Jason Roth, Vice President, Marketing & Sales
Kathy Weiss, Senior Sales Director
Annette Imperati, Sales Director, Corporate, Government, & Associations

This comprehensive text describes current theories, techniques, and their applications to specific disabled populations. Perspectives on varying counseling approaches such as psychodynamic, existential, gestalt, behavioral and psychoeducational orientations are systematically outlined in an easy-to-follow format. Practical applications for counseling are emphasized with attention given to strategies, goal-setting and on-going evaluations. *$43.95*
404 pages Paperback 1986
ISBN 0-826153-71-2

2352 Art-Centered Education and Therapy for Children with Disabilities
Charles C. Thomas
2600 S First St
Springfield, IL   62704-4730
217-789-8980
800-258-8980
Fax: 217-789-9130
books@ccthomas.com
www.ccthomas.com

Frances E. Anderson, Author

This book has been written to help both the regular education, and art and special education teachers, both pre- and in-service, better understand some of the issues and realities of providing education and remediation to children with disabilities. The book is also offered as model concept that has govern the author's personal and professional career of over thirty years. *$41.95*
284 pages Paperback
ISBN 0-398060-06-1

2353 Assessing the Handicaps/Needs of Children
Books on Special Children
P.O.Box 3378
Amherst, MA   01004-3378
413-256-8164
Fax: 413-256-8896
irene@boscbooks.com

260 pages Hardcover
ISBN 0-12218 -02-0

2354 Assessment & Management of Mainstreamed Hearing-Impaired Children
Sage Publications
2455 Teller Road
Thousand Oaks, CA   91320
805-499-0721
800-818-7243
Fax: 800-583-2665
info@sagepub.com
www.sagepub.com

Sara Miller McCune, Founder, Publisher & Executive Chairman
Blaise R. Simqu, President & CEO
Chris Hickok, Senior Vice President & Chief Financial Officer
Stephen Barr, Managing Director/SAGE London

The theoretical and practical considerations of developing appropriate programming for hearing-impaired children who are being educated in mainstream educational settings are presented in this book.

2355 Assessment Log & Developmental Progress Charts for the Carolina Curriculum
Brookes Publishing
P.O.Box 10624
Baltimore, MD   21285-0624
410-337-9580
800-638-3775
Fax: 410-337-8539
webmaster@brookespublishing.com
www.brookespublishing.com

Paul H. Brookes, Chairman of the Board
Jeffrey D. Brookes, President
George S. Stamathis, VP/Publisher
Melissa A. Behn, Executive Vice President

This 28-page booklet allows the progress of children with skills in the 12-36 month development range to be easily recorded. Available in packages of 10. *$23.00*
28 pages Saddle-stiched
ISBN 1-557662-21-5

2356 Assessment and Remediation of Articulatoryand Phonological Disorders
McGraw-Hill School Publishing
PO Box 182604
Columbus, OH   43218
877-833-5524
800-338-3987
Fax: 609-308-4480
customer.service@mheducation.com
www.mcgraw-hill.com

David Levin, President/Chief Executive Officer
David Stafford, Senior Vice President/General Counsel
Maryellen Valaitis, Senior Vice President Human Resources
Patrick Milano, Chief Financial Officer/Chief Administrative Officer

Offers comprehensive coverage of articulation disorders.

2357 Assessment in Mental Handicap: A Guide to Assessment Practices & Tests
Brookline Books
8 Trumbull Rd
Suite B-001
Northampton, MA   01060
413-584-0184
800-666-2665
Fax: 413-584-6184
brbooks@yahoo.com
www.brooklinebooks.com

Esther Wilder, Co-Author

Helps professionals understand the rationale and uses for assessment practices, and provides details of appropriate instruments within each type: adaptive behavior scales, assessment of behavioral disturbances, early development and Plagetian tests. *$20.00*
Hardcover
ISBN 0-91479 -31-X

2358 Assessment of Children and Youth
Longman Education/Addison Wesley
1185 Avenue of the Americas
New York, NY   10036-2601
212-997-8500
866-203-6215
TTY:800-231-5469
www.hess.com

Dr. Mark R. Williams, Chairman of the Board
Gregory P. Hill, President/COO
John B. Hess, Chief Executive Officer
Gary Boubel, Senior Vice President-Developments

Introductory text for preservice and in-service special educators on assessment, based on the principle that every child is unique. Comprehensive coverage of both formal and informal assessment instruments. *$50.00*
640 pages Paperback
ISBN 0-80131 -02-5

2359 Assessment of Individuals with Severe Disabilities
Brookes Publishing Company
PO Box 10624
Baltimore, MD 21285-0624   410-337-9580
                                             800-638-3775
                                        Fax: 410-337-8539
                           custserv@brookespublishing.com
                               www.brookespublishing.com
Paul H. Brookes, Chairman
Jeffrey D. Brookes, President
Melissa A. Behm, ExecutiveVice President
George S. Stamathis, Vice President & Publisher
This expanded text offers instructors guidelines to design a comprehensive educational assessment for individuals with severe disabilities. *$34.00*
432 pages Paperback
ISBN 1-557660-67-0

2360 Assessment of the Technology Needs of Vending Facilitiy Managers In Tennessee
Mississippi State University
108 Herbert - South
Room 150/PO Drawer 6189
Mississippi State Univers, MS 39762-6189   662-325-2001
                                             800-675-7782
                                        Fax: 662-325-8989
                                        TTY: 662-325-2694
                                   nrtc@colled.msstate.edu
                                     www.blind.msstate.edu
Jacqui Bybee, Research and Training Coordinato
Michele Capella McDonnall, Ph.D., Research Professor/Interim Director
Jessica Thornton, Business Manager
Marty Giesen, Ph.D., Senior Research Scientist
This report summarizes the results and recommendations of a survey conducted of vending facility managers throughout the state of Tennessee who participate in the Randolph-Sheppard program. *$15.00*
39 pages Paperback

2361 Assessment: The Special Educator's Role
Brookes Publishing Company
PO Box 10624
Baltimore, MD 21285-0624   410-337-9580
                                             800-638-3775
                                        Fax: 410-337-8539
                           custserv@brookespublishing.com
                               www.brookespublishing.com
Paul H. Brookes, Chairman
Jeffrey D. Brookes, President
Melissa A. Behm, ExecutiveVice President
George S. Stamathis, Vice President & Publisher
Aimed at students with little or no classroom experience in assessment, the book focuses on the integration of dynamic, curriculum-based and norm-referenced data for diagnostic decisions and program planning.
580 pages Casebound
ISBN 0-53421-32-1

2362 Assistive Technology in the Schools: A Guide for Idaho Educators
Idaho Assistive Technology Project
University of Idaho
1187 Alturas Dr.
Moscow, ID 83843- 8331   205-885-3557
                                             800-432-8324
                                        Fax: 208-885-6102
                                       idahoat@uidaho.edu
                                           www.idahoat.org
LaRhae Rhoads, Author
Ron Seiler, Author
Michelle Doty, Author
This manual is designed to provide educators, parents, students with disabilities and related service providers with assistance in identifying, selecting, and acquiring assistive technology (AT) devices and services.

2363 Asthma Management and Education
Asthma and Allergy Foundation of America
8201 Corporate Drive
Suite 1000
Landover, MD   20785   202-466-7643
                                             800-727-8462
                                            info@aafa.org
                                             www.aafa.org
Lynn Hanessian, Chair
Mitchell Grayson, MD, Chair, Research
Barbara Corn, Chair, Governance
Calvin Anderson, Chair/Finance/Treasurer
One session, two hour program developed to educate allied health professionals about up-to-date asthma care and patient education, information and materials. Includes hands on experience with peak flow meters and demonstrations of medical devices.

2364 Aston-Patterning
PO Box 3568
Incline Village, NV 89450-3568   775-831-8228
                                       Fax: 775-831-8955
                                  office@astonkinetics.com
                                    www.astonkinetics.com
J Aston, Owner
Angelina Calafiore, Office Manager
Integrated system of movement education, body assessment, environmental modification and fitness training.

2365 Attention Deficit Disorder in Children
Charles C. Thomas
2600 S First St
Springfield, IL 62704-4730   217-789-8980
                                             800-258-8980
                                        Fax: 217-789-9130
                                     books@ccthomas.com
                                      www.ccthomas.com

2366 Aural Habilitation
Alexander Graham Bell Association
3417 Volta Pl NW
Washington, DC 20007-2737   202-337-5220
                                        Fax: 202-337-8314
                                        TTY:202-337-5221
                                         info@agbell.org
                           www.listeningandspokenlanguage.org
Meredith K. Sugar, Esq. (OH), President
Ted A. Meyer, M.D., Ph.D, President-Elect/Secretary-Treasurer
Emilio Alonso-Mendoza, Chief Executive Officer
Susan Boswell, Director of Communications and Marketing
This classic text for professionals, educators and parents discusses verbal learning and aural habilitation of young children with hearing losses to ensure that each child is educated in the best setting. It discusses communication, normal development of spoken language, speech audiologic assessment, hearing aids and use of residual hearing, and program designs for individualized needs, including the assessment and planning of IEPs. *$26.95*
324 pages

2367 Behavior Analysis in Education: Focus on Measurably Superior Instruction
Brookes Publishing Company
PO Box 10624
Baltimore, MD 21285-0624   410-337-9580
                                             800-638-3775
                                        Fax: 410-337-8539
                           custserv@brookespublishing.com
                               www.brookespublishing.com
Paul H. Brookes, Chairman
Jeffrey D. Brookes, President
Melissa A. Behm, ExecutiveVice President
George S. Stamathis, Vice President & Publisher
Designed to disseminate measurably superior instructional strategies to those interested in advancing sound, pedagogically effective, field-tested educational practices, this book is intended for graduate-level courses and seminars in special education and/or psychology focusing on behavior analysis and instruction.
512 pages Casebound
ISBN 0-53422 -60-9

2368   Behavior Modification
Sage Publications
2455 Teller Rd
Thousand Oaks, CA   91320-2218   805-499-0721
                                        800-818-7243
                                        Fax: 800-583-2665
                                        info@sagepub.com
                                        www.sagepub.com
Sara Miller McCune, Founder, Publisher and Executive Chairman
Blaise R. Simqu, President & CEO
Chris Hickok, Senior Vice President & Chief Financial Officer
Stephen Barr, Managing Director/SAGE London
Describes in detail for replication purposes assessment and modi-
fication techniques for problems in psychiatric, clinical, educa-
tional and rehabilitation settings. *$53.00*
640 pages Quarterly

2369   Behavioral Disorders
Council for Exceptional Children
2900 Crystal Dr.
Suite 1000
Arlington, VA   22202-3557   888-232-7733
                                    TTY:866-915-5000
                                    services@cec.sped.org
                                    www.cec.sped.org
Alexander T. Graham, Executive Director
Sharon Rodriguez, Senior Executive Assistant
Craig Evans, Director of Operations
Provides professionals with a means to exchange information and
share ideas related to research, empirically tested educational in-
novations and issues and concerns relevant to students with
behavioral disorders.
Quarterly

2370   Behind Special Education
Love Publishing Company
9101 E Kenyon Ave
Suite 2200
Denver, CO   80237-1854   303-221-7333
                                 Fax: 303-221-7444
                                 lpc@lovepublishing.com
                                 www.lovepublishing.com

ISBN 0-89108-17-4

2371   Biomedical Concerns in Persons with Down's Syndrome
Paul H Brookes Publishing Company
PO Box 10624
Baltimore, MD   21285-0624   410-337-9580
                                    800-638-3775
                                    Fax: 410-337-8539
                                    custserv@brookespublishing.com
                                    www.brookespublishing.com
Paul H. Brookes, Chairman
Jeffrey D. Brookes, President
Melissa A. Behm, ExecutiveVice President
George S. Stamathis, Vice President & Publisher
Written by leading authorities and spanning many disciplines and
specialties, this comprehensive resource provides vital informa-
tion on biomedical issues concerning individuals with Down's
Syndrome. *$45.00*
336 pages Hardcover
ISBN 1-557660-89-1

2372   Breaking Barriers
AbleNet
2625 Patton Road
Roseville, MN   55113-5423   651-294-2200
                                    800-322-0956
                                    Fax: 651-294-2259
                                    customerservice@ablenetinc.com
                                    www.ablenetinc.com
Bill Sproull, Chairman of the Board
William Mills, Board of Directors, Chair
Jennifer Thalhuber, President/CEO
Paul Sugden, Vice President of Finance, IT & CFO, Trustee
A practical resource for parents, caregivers, teachers and thera-
pists. *$15.00*

2373   Building Skills for Independence in the Mainstream
15619 Premiere Drive
Suite 101
Tampa, FL   33624   850-363-9909
                           Fax: 480-393-4331
                           accounting@successforkidswithhearingloss.com
                           successforkidswithhearinglo ss.com
Karen L. Anderson, Director/ Co-Author
Gale Wright, Co-Author
Building Skills for Independence in the Mainstream was devel-
oped as a Guide for DHH professionals to support their work with
classroom teachers and with students to develop the skills needed
for independence with hearing aids and self-advocacy.

2374   Building Skills for Success in the Fast-Paced Classroom
15619 Premiere Drive
Suite 101
Tampa, FL   33624   850-363-9909
                           Fax: 480-393-4331
                           accounting@successforkidswithhearingloss.com
                           successforkidswithhearinglo ss.com
Karen L. Anderson, PhD, Co-Author
Kathleen A. Arnoldi, MA
The purpose of this book is to provide resources that will assist
these students in optimizing their achievement through improved
access and self-advocacy. The information contained in this book
targets the expanded core curriculum, or those skills that must be
mastered in order to benefit from the core curriculum. This book
is meant to be a practical ready-to-go resource for professionals
who work with school-age children with hearing loss.

**2375   Building the Healing Partnership: Parents, Professionals
and Children with Chronic Illnesses**
Brookline Books
8 Trumbull Rd
Ste B-001
Northampton, MA   01060   413-584-0184
                                 800-666-2665
                                 Fax: 413-584-6184
                                 brbooks@yahoo.com
                                 www.brooklinebks.com
Patricia Tanner Leff, Author
Elaine H. Walizer, Author
Successful programs understand that the disabled child's needs
must be considered in the context of a family. This book was specifically written for practitioner's who must work with families
but who have insufficient training in family systems assessment
and intervention. It is a valuable blend of theory and practice with
pointers for applying the principles. *$24.95*
312 pages Paperback 1992
ISBN 0-914797-60-3

**2376   CAI, Career Assessment Inventories for the Learning
Disabled**
Academic Therapy Publications
20 Leveroni Crt
Novato, CA   94949-5746   415-883-3314
                                 800-422-7249
                                 Fax: 888-287-9975
                                 sales@academictherapy.com
                                 www.academictherapy.com
Carol Weller, Author
Mary Buchanan, Author
Takes personality, ability and interest into account in pointing
learning disabled students of all ages toward intelligent and real-
istic career choices. Contains binder with paperback teaching
guide plus 50 interest inventories and 50 abilities inventories.
64 pages 1983
ISBN 0-878793-50-X

2377 Caring for Children with Chronic Illness
11 W 42nd St
15th Floor
New York, NY   10036-8002   212-431-4370
                                    877-687-7476
                                 Fax: 212-941-7842
                              cs@springerpub.com
                              www.springerpub.com

Ursula Springer, President
Theodore C. Nardin, CEO/Publisher
Jason Roth, VP/Marketing Director
James C. Costello, Vice President, Journal Publishing

A critical look at the current medical, social, and psychological framework for providing care to children with chronic illnesses. Emphasizing the need to create integrated, interdisciplinary approaches, it discusses issues such as the roles of families, professionals, and institutions in providing health care, the impact of a child's illness on various family structures, financing care, the special problems of chronically ill children as they become adolescents and more. *$36.95*
320 pages Hardcover
ISBN 0-82615 -00-1

2378 Carolina Curriculum for Infants and Toddlers with Special Needs (3rd Edition)
Brookes Publishing
P.O. Box 10624
Baltimore, MD   21285-0624   410-337-9580
                                    800-638-3775
                                 Fax: 410-337-8539
                           custserv@brookespublishing.com
                              www.brookespublishing.com

Nancy M. Johnson-Martin, Author
Susan M. Attermeier, Author
Bonnie J. Hacker, Author

This book includes detailed assessment and intervention sequences, daily routine integration strategies, sensorimotor adaptations, and a sample 24-page assessment log that shows readers how to chart a child's individual progress.
504 pages Spiral-bound

2379 Carolina Curriculum for Preschoolers with Special Needs
Brookes Publishing
PO Box 10624
Baltimore, MD   21285-0624   410-337-9580
                                    800-638-3775
                                 Fax: 410-337-8539
                           custserv@brookespublishing.com
                              www.brookespublishing.com

Paul H. Brookes, Chairman
Jeffrey D. Brookes, President
Melissa A. Behm, ExecutiveVice President
George S. Stamathis, Vice President & Publisher

This curriculum provides detailed teaching and assessment techniques, plus a sample 28-page assessment log that shows readers how to chart a child's individual progress. This guide is for children between 2 and 5 in their developmental stages who are considered at risk for developmental delay or who exhibit special needs. *$34.00*
352 pages Spiral-bound
ISBN 1-55766 -32-8

2380 Challenge of Educating Together Deaf and Hearing Youth: Making Manistreaming Work
Charles C. Thomas
2600 S First St
Springfield, IL   62704-4730   217-789-8980
                                      800-258-8980
                                   Fax: 217-789-9130
                                books@ccthomas.com
                                   www.ccthomas.com

198 pages Hardcover
ISBN 0-398063-91-5

2381 Challenged Scientists: Disabilities and the Triumph of Excellence
Greenwood Publishing Group
130 Cremona Drive
Santa Barbara, CA   93117   805-968-1911
                                    800-368-6868
                                 Fax: 866-270-3856
                           CustomerService@abc-clio.com
                                www.abc-clio.com

208 pages
ISBN 0-275938-73-5

2382 Child Care and the ADA: A Handbook for Inclusive Programs
Brookes Publishing
PO Box 10624
Baltimore, MD   21285-0624   410-337-9580
                                    800-638-3775
                                 Fax: 410-337-8539
                           custserv@brookespublishing.com
                              www.brookespublishing.com

Paul H. Brookes, Chairman
Jeffrey D. Brookes, President
Melissa A. Behm, ExecutiveVice President
George S. Stamathis, Vice President & Publisher

This book is designed for educators and administrators in child care settings. It offers a straightforward discussion of the Americans with Disabilities Act including children with disabilities in community programs. *$25.95*
240 pages Paperback
ISBN 1-55766 -85-5

2383 Child with Disabling Illness
Lippincott, Williams & Wilkins
16522 Hunters Green Pkwy
Hagerstown, MD   21740   301-223-2300
                                 800-638-3030
                              Fax: 301-223-2400
                              orders@lww.com
                                 www.lww.com

700 pages

2384 Childhood Behavior Disorders: Applied Research & Educational Practice
Sage Publications
2455 Teller Road
Thousand Oaks, CA   91320-2218   805-499-0721
                                         800-818-7243
                                      Fax: 800-583-2665
                                    info@sagepub.com
                                       www.sagepub.com

Sara Miller McCune, Founder, Publisher, Chairperson
Blaise R. Simqu, President/CEO
Chris Hickok, Senior Vice President & Chief Fi
Stephen Barr, Managing Director/SAGE London, P

The only comprehensive overview of childhood behavior disorders. This book gives you the how and why for helping children with behavior disorders.

2385 Childhood Disablity and Family Systems(Routledge Library Editions) (Volume 5)
Routledge (Taylor & Francis Group)
711 Third Ave
New York, NY   10017   212-216-7800
                               800-634-7064
                            Fax: 202-564-7854
                       enquiries@taylorandfrancis.com
                            www.routledge.com

Michael Ferrari, Editor
Marvin B. Sussman, Editor

Focuses on what the presence of a disabled child means to a family. Those professionals involved in teaching, research, and direct care with families having disabled children will value the coverage of such topics as the contemporary context of disability, ethical issues, family effects, and care systems. First published in

1987 by Haworth Press, the book is now published under Routledge. *$140.00*
256 pages Hardcover 1916
ISBN 1-138101-55-9

2386 Children and Youth Assisted by Medical Technology in Educational Settings, 2nd Edition
Brookes Publishing
PO Box 10624
Baltimore, MD   21285-0624   410-337-9580
800-638-3775
Fax: 410-337-8539
custserv@brookespublishing.com
www.brookespublishing.com
Paul H. Brookes, Chairman
Jeffrey D. Brookes, President
Melissa A. Behm, ExecutiveVice President
George S. Stamathis, Vice President & Publisher
Contains detailed daily care guidelines and emergency-response techniques, including information on working with a range of students who have the HIV infection, that rely on ventilators, that utilize tube feeding, or require catheterization. Also covers every aspect of planning for inclusive classrooms, including information on personnel training, entrance planning and transition, legal requirements, and transportation issues. *$52.00*
432 pages Spiral-bound
ISBN 1-55766 -36-3

2387 Children's Needs Psychological Perspective
National Association of School Psychologists
8455 Colesville Rd
Suite 1000
Silver Spring, MD   20910- 3392   301-589-3300
Fax: 301-589-5175
www.musictherapy.org
637 pages

2388 Choices: A Guide to Sex Counseling with Physically Disabled Adults
Krieger Publishing Company
1725 Krieger Dr
Malabar, FL   32950   321-724-9542
800-724-0025
Fax: 321-951-3671
info@krieger-publishing.com
www.krieger-publishing.com
Maureen E. Neistadt, Author
Provides rehabilitation professionals with the basic information necessary for limited sexuality counseling of physically disabled adults. *$20.90*
132 pages
ISBN 0-898749-03-4

2389 Choosing Options and Accommodations for Children
Brookes Publishing
PO Box 10624
Baltimore, MD   21285-0624   410-337-9580
800-638-3775
Fax: 410-337-8539
custserv@brookespublishing.com
www.brookespublishing.com
192 pages
ISBN 1-55766 -06-5

2390 Cirriculum Development for Students with Mild Disabilities
Charles C. Thomas
2600 S First St
Springfield, IL   62704-4730   217-789-8980
800-258-8980
Fax: 217-789-9130
books@ccthomas.com
www.ccthomas.com
Carroll J. Jones, Author

This book was designed to provide the foundation from which to write cirrocumuli that will provide academic and social skills for Individual Education Programs (IEPs). *$38.95*
258 pages Spiral-Paper
ISBN 0-398070-18-2

2391 Classroom Success for the LD and ADHD Child
John F. Blair Publishing
1406 Plaza Dr
Winston Salem, NC   27103-1470   336-768-1374
800-222-9796
Fax: 336-768-9194
sparrow@blairpub.com
www.blairpub.com
Steve Kirk, Editor-In-Chief
Anna Sutton, Vice President, Sales & Marketing
Artie Sparrow, Office Manager & Customer Service
Suzanne H. Stevens, Author
This book offers suggestions on teaching techniques, adapting texts, recognition of children with disabilities and testing, grading and mainstreaming the learning disabled and ADHD child. *$13.95*
333 pages Paperback 1997
ISBN 0-895871-59-9

2392 Clinical Alzheimer Rehabilitation
Springer Publishing
11 W 42nd St
15th Floor
New York, NY   10036-8002   212-431-4370
877-687-7476
Fax: 212-941-7842
cs@springerpub.com
www.springerpub.com
Theodore C. Nardin, CEO/Publisher
Jason Roth, VP/Marketing Director
Annette Imperati, Marketing/Sales Director
James C. Costello, Vice President, Journal Publishing
This comprehensive and easy-to-read guidebook contains the latest research on dementia and AD in the elderly population, including the causes and risk factors of AD, diagnosis information, and symptoms and progressions of the disease. Significant emphasis is given to the physical, mental, and verbal rehabilitation challenges of patients with AD. The authors outline specific rehabilitation goals for the physical therapist, speech-language pathologist, and general caregiver.

2393 Clinical Management of Childhood Stuttering, 2nd Edition
Sage Publications
2455 Teller Road
Thousand Oaks, CA   91320-2218   805-499-0721
800-818-7243
Fax: 800-583-2665
info@sagepub.com
www.sagepub.com
Sara Miller McCune, Founder, Publisher, Chairperson
Blaise R. Simqu, President/CEO
Chris Hickok, Senior Vice President/CFO
Stephen Barr, Managing Director/SAGE London
Updates and integrates recent findings in childhood stuttering into a broad range of therapeutic strategies for assessing and treating the young dysfluent child. *$38.00*
336 pages

2394 Cognitive Approaches to Learning Disabilities
Sage Publications
2455 Teller Road
Thousand Oaks, CA   91320-2218   805-499-0721
800-818-7243
Fax: 800-583-2665
info@sagepub.com
www.sagepub.com
Sara Miller McCune, Founder, Publisher, Chairperson
Blaise R. Simqu, President/CEO
Chris Hickok, Senior Vice President/CFO
Stephen Barr, Managing Director/SAGE London

The first to bridge the gap between cognitive psychology and information processing theory in understanding learning disabilities. *$39.00*
495 pages Hardcover

2395   Cognitive Strategy Instruction That Really Improves Children's Academic Skills
Brookline Books
8 Trumbull Rd
Suite B-001
Northampton, MA   01060   413-584-0184
                                           800-666-2665
                                   Fax: 413-584-6184
                                   brbooks@yahoo.com
                                   www.brooklinebooks.com
Esther Isabe Wilder, Author
A concise and focused work that summarily presents the few procedures for teaching strategies that aid academic subject matter learning: decoding reading comprehension, vocabulary, math, spelling and writing. Learning unrelated facts and science. Completely revised in 1995. *$27.95*
Paperback
ISBN 1-571290-07-9

2396   Collaborating for Comprehensive Services for Young Children and Families
Brookes Publishing Company
PO Box 10624
Baltimore, MD   21285-0624   410-337-9580
                                           800-638-3775
                                   Fax: 410-337-8539
                                   custserv@brookespublishing.com
                                   www.brookespublishing.com
Paul H. Brookes, Chairman
Jeffrey D. Brookes, President
Melissa A. Behm, ExecutiveVice President
George S. Stamathis, Vice President & Publisher
Taking collaboration a step beyond basic implementation, this useful book shows agency and school leaders how to coordinate their efforts to stretch human services dollars while still providing quality programs. Provides the building blocks needed to establish a local interagency coordinating council. *$37.00*
272 pages
ISBN 1-557661-03-0

2397   Collaborative Teams for Students with Severe Disabilities
Brookes Publishing
PO Box 10624
Baltimore, MD   21285-0624   410-337-9580
                                           800-638-3775
                                   Fax: 410-337-8539
                                   custserv@brookespublishing.com
                                   www.brookespublishing.com
Paul H. Brookes, Chairman
Jeffrey D. Brookes, President
Melissa A. Behm, ExecutiveVice President
George S. Stamathis, Vice President & Publisher
How can educators, parents and therapists work together to ensure the best possible educational experience for students with severe disabilities? This resource describes how a collaborative team can successfully create exciting learning opportunities for students, while teaching them to participate fully at home, school, work and play. *$ 30.00*
304 pages
ISBN 1-55766 -88-3

2398   Communicating with Parents of Exceptional Children
Love Publishing Company
9101 E Kenyon Ave
Suite 2200
Denver, CO   80237-1854   303-221-7333
                                   Fax: 303-221-7444
                                   lpc@lovepublishing.com
                                   www.lovepublishing.com
Roger L. Kroth, Author
Denzil Denzil Edge, Author

This book shows how teachers can facilitate parent involvement with children's education. It presents the mirror model of parent involvement, family, dynamics, how to listen actively to parents, values and perceptions, problem-solving, parent conferences and training groups. *$19.95*
ISBN 0-89108 -67-4

2399   Communication & Language Acquisition: Discoveries from Atypical Development
Brookes Publishing
PO Box 10624
Baltimore, MD   21285-0624   410-337-9580
                                           800-638-3775
                                   Fax: 410-337-8539
                                   custserv@brookespublishing.com
                                   www.brookespublishing.com
Paul H. Brookes, Chairman
Jeffrey D. Brookes, President
Melissa A. Behm, ExecutiveVice President
George S. Stamathis, Vice President & Publisher
This text demonstrates how the study of language acquisition in children with atypical development promotes advances in basic theory. *$44.00*
352 pages Hardcover
ISBN 1-557662-79-7

2400   Communication Skills for Working with Elders
Springer Publishing Company
11 W 42nd St
15th Floor
New York, NY   10036-8002   212-431-4370
                                           877-687-7476
                                   Fax: 212-941-7842
                                   cs@springerpub.com
                                   www.springerpub.com
Ursula Springer, President
Theodore C. Nardin, CEO/Publisher
Jason Roth, VP/Marketing Director
James C. Costello, Vice President, Journal Publishing
How aging and illness affects communication. *$17.95*
160 pages Softcover
ISBN 0-82615 -20-7

2401   Communication Unbound
Teachers College Press
Ste 2115
14781 Memorial Dr
Houston, TX   77079-5210   415-738-4323
                                   Fax: 415-738-4329
                                   tcc.orders@aidcvt.com
                                   www.pearsonhighered.com
240 pages Paperback
ISBN 0-087737-21-4

2402   Complete Handbook of Children's Reading Disorders: You Can Prevent or Correct LDs
Gallery Bookshop
319 Kasten Street
PO Box 270
Mendocino, CA 95460-270   707-937-2215
                                   Fax: 707-937-3737
                                   info@gallerybookshop.com
                                   www.gallerybooks.com
Tony Miksak, Owner
The complete handbook of children's reading disorders. *$34.95*
732 pages Paperback
ISBN 0-80772 -83-3

2403   Computer Access/Computer Learning
Special Needs Project
324 State St
Suite H
Santa Barbara, CA   93101-2364   805-962-8087
                                                  800-333-6867
                                             Fax: 805-962-5087
                                        editor@specialneeds.com
                                          www.specialneeds.com
Mark Darrow, Founder, The Prolotherapy Institu
A resource manual in adaptive technology and computer training.
$22.50

2404   Consulting Psychologists Press
1055 Joaquin Rd
Suite. 200
Mountain View, CA   94043-1243   650-969-8901
                                                  800-624-1765
                                             Fax: 650-969-8608
                                            custserv@cpp.com
Carl E. Thoresen, Chairman
Jeffrey Hayes, President and Chief Executive Officer
Andrew Bell, Vice President of International
Catey DeBalko, Vice President of Marketing
Catalog offering job assessment software, career development
reports, educational assessment information and books for the
professional.

**2405   Counseling Persons with Communication Disorders and
           Their Families**
Sage Publications
2455 Teller Road
Thousand Oaks, CA   91320-2218   805-499-0721
                                                   800-818-7243
                                             Fax: 800-583-2665
                                              info@sagepub.com
                                               www.sagepub.com
Sara Miller McCune, Founder, Publisher, Chairperson
Blaise R. Simqu, President & CEO
Chris Hickok, Senior Vice President & Chief Fi
Stephen Barr, Managing Director/SAGE London, P
A learning manual for speech-language pathologists and audiolo-
gists on how to deal with the emotional issues facing them in their
work with clients with communication disorders and their fami-
lies. *$ 29.00*
187 pages

2406   Counseling in the Rehabilitation Process
Charles C. Thomas
2600 S First St
Springfield, IL   62704-4730   217-789-8980
                                                   800-258-8980
                                             Fax: 217-789-9130
                                            books@ccthomas.com
                                              www.ccthomas.com
Gerald L. Gandy, Author
E. Davis Martin Jr, Author
Richard E. Hardy, Author
This text provides the reader with a comprehensive overview and
introduction to the field of rehabilitation counseling and ser-
vices, and also has applicability in the growing field of commu-
nity counseling. *$51.95*
358 pages paper 1999
ISBN 0-398069-70-4

**2407   Creating Positive Classroom Environments: Strategies for
           Behavior Management**
Brooks / Cole Publishing Company
511 Forest Lodge Rd
Pacific Grove, CA   93950-5040   831-373-0728
                                                   800-354-9706
                                             Fax: 831-375-6414
                                          bc-info@brookscole.com
                                              www.cengage.com
448 pages Paperbound
ISBN 0-53422-54-4

2408   Cristine M. Trahms Program for Phenylketonuria
University of Washington
PO Box 357920
Seattle, WA   98195   206-598-1800
                                                   877-685-3015
                                             Fax: 206-598-1915
                                          pku@u.washington.edu
                                       www.depts.washington.edu/pku
C. Ronald Scott, MD, Professor, Pediatrics, Division
Clinical program for children and adults with phenylketonuria.

**2409   Critical Voices on Special Education: Problems & Progress
           Concerning the Mildly Handicapped**
State University of New York Press
22 Corporate Woods Boulevard
3rd Floor
Albany, NY   12211-2504   518-472-5000
                                                   866-430-7869
                                             Fax: 518-472-5038
                                             info@sunypress.edu
                                              www.sunypress.edu
James Peltz, Associate Director
Janice Vunk, Assistant to the Director
Scott B Sigmon, Editor
Problems and progress concerning the mildly handicapped.
$24.95
265 pages Paperback 1990
ISBN 0-79140 -20-3

**2410   Cultural Diversity, Families and the Special Education
           System**
Teachers College Press
1234 Amsterdam Ave
New York, NY   10027-6602   212-678-3929
                                                   800-575-6566
                                             Fax: 212-678-4149
                                          tcpress@tc.columbia.edu
                                       www.teacherscollegepress.com
Beth Harry, Author
This timely and thought-provoking book explores the quadruple
disadvantage faced by the parents of poor, minority, handicapped
children whose first language is not that of the school they attend.
$22.95
296 pages Paperback
ISBN 0-807731-19-6

**2411   Curriculum Decision Making for Students with Severe
           Handicaps**
Teachers College Press
1234 Amsterdam Ave
New York, NY   10027-6602   212-678-3929
                                                   800-575-6566
                                             Fax: 212-678-4149
                                       www.teacherscollegepress.com
192 pages Paperback
ISBN 0-807728-61-6

**2412   Deciphering the System: A Guide for Families of Young
           Disabled Children**
Brookline Books
8 Trumbull Rd
Ste B-001
Northampton, MA   01060   413-584-0184
                                                   800-666-2665
                                             Fax: 413-584-6184
                                           brbooks@yahoo.com
                                            www.brooklinebks.com
Paula Beckman, Author
This book informs parents of disabled children (0-5) of their
rights and the service system, e.g., ways to manage the cumulat-
ing information, tips on IEP and IFSP meetings and the educational assessment process, and how parents can work with
multiple service providers. It includes contributions from both
parents and professionals who have experience with the service
system. *$21.95*
208 pages Paperback 1999
ISBN 0-914797-87-5

2413 Defining Rehabilitation Agency Types
Mississippi State University
108 Herbert - South
Room 150 Industrial Education Depar
Mississippi State, MS 39762-6189

662-325-2001
800-675-7782
Fax: 662-325-8989
TTY: 662-325-2694
nrtc@colled.msstate.edu
www.blind.msstate.edu

Jacqui Bybee, Research Associate II
Michele Capella McDonnall, Ph.D., Research Professor/Interim Director
Jessica Thornton, Business Manager
Marty Giesen, Ph.D., Senior Research Scientist
Relationships of participant selection and cost factors of service delivery across rehabilitation agency types. A national survey of state agencies for the blind was conducted to examine factors that define the characteristics of different agencies; similar programs were grouped together. Classification criteria were developed to distinguish agencies into logical groups based on line of authority, funding and operating procedures. *$10.00*
15 pages Paperback

2414 Designing and Using Assistive Technology: The Human Perspective
Brookes Publishing
PO Box 10624
Baltimore, MD 21285-0624

410-337-9580
800-638-3775
Fax: 410-337-8539
custserv@brookespublishing.com
www.brookespublishing.com

Paul H. Brookes, Chairman
Jeffrey D. Brookes, President
Melissa A. Behm, ExecutiveVice President
George S. Stamathis, Vice President & Publisher
Presented here is a holistic perspective on how and why people choose and use AT. Features personal insights and the latest research on design and development. *$31.00*
352 pages Paperback
ISBN 1-55766 -14-9

2415 Developing Cross-Cultural Competence:Guideto Working with Young Children & Their Families
Brookes Publishing
PO Box 10624
Baltimore, MD 21285-0624

410-337-9580
800-638-3775
Fax: 410-337-8539
custserv@brookespublishing.com
www.brookespublishing.com

Paul H. Brookes, Chairman
Jeffrey D. Brookes, President
Melissa A. Behm, ExecutiveVice President
George S. Stamathis, Vice President & Publisher
This enlightening book perceptively and sensitively explores cultural, ethnic, and language diversity in human services. For those who work with families whose infants and young children may have or be at risk for a disability or chronic illness. (Second Edition) *$ 32.00*
448 pages Paperback
ISBN 1-55766 -31-9

2416 Developing Individualized Family Support Plans: A Training Manual
Brookline Books
Suite B-001
8 Trumbull Rd
Northampton, MA 01060

413-584-0184
800-666-2665
Fax: 413-584-6184
brbooks@yahoo.com
www.brooklinebooks.com

Esther Wilder, Co-Author
This manual provides in-service training coordinators, administrators, supervisors and university personnel with a compact package of functional and practical methods to train profession-

als about implementing family-centered individualized family support plans (IFSP'S). Also, case studies provide concrete examples to aid in learning to write IFSP's. *$24.95*
ISBN 0-914797-69-7

2417 Developing Staff Competencies for Supporting People with Disabilities
Brookes Publishing
PO Box 10624
Baltimore, MD 21285-0624

410-337-9580
800-638-3775
Fax: 410-337-8539
custserv@brookespublishing.com
www.brookespublishing.com

Paul H. Brookes, Chairman
Jeffrey D. Brookes, President
Melissa A. Behm, ExecutiveVice President
George S. Stamathis, Vice President & Publisher
This timely second edition, now in a new easier to read format, gives service providers helpful strategies for increasing effectiveness and maintaining well-being while working in the rewarding yet challenging field of human services. *$34.00*
480 pages Paperback
ISBN 1-55766 -07-3

2418 Development of Language
McGraw-Hill, School Publishing
220 E Danieldale Rd
Desoto, TX 75115-2490

800-648-2970
Fax: 800-593-4418
www.mhschool.com

464 pages

2419 Developmental Disabilities of Learning
Gallery Bookshop
319 Kasten Street
PO Box 270
Mendocino, CA 95460-270

707-937-2215
Fax: 707-937-3737
info@gallerybookshop.com
www.gallerybooks.com

Tony Miksak, Owner
Manual for professionals on developmental and learning disabilities in the growing child. *$25.00*
224 pages Illustrated

2420 Developmental Disabilities: A Handbook for Occupational Therapists
Haworth Press
711 Third Avenue
New York, NY 10017

212-216-7800
800-354-1420
Fax: 212-244-1563
subscriptions@tandf.co.uk
www.haworthpress.com

268 pages Hardcover
ISBN 0-866569-59-6

2421 Developmental Disabilities: A Handbook for Interdisciplinary Practice
Brookline Books
8 Trumbull Rd
Suite B-001
Northampton, MA 01060

413-584-0184
800-666-2665
Fax: 413-584-6184
brbooks@yahoo.com
www.brooklinebooks.com

Esther Wilder, Co-Author
Successful interdisciplinary team practice for persons with developmental disabilities that require each team member to understand and respect the contributions of the others. This handbook explains the professions most often represented on interdisciplinary teams: their natures, concerns and roles in the interdisciplinary context. *$29.95*
256 pages
ISBN 1-571290-03-6

2422 Developmental Variation and Learning Disorders
Educators Publishing Service
PO Box 9031
Cambridge, MA 02139-9031   617-367-2700
                                             800-225-5750
                                        Fax: 617-547-0412
                                     eps@schoolspecialty.com
                                          www.epsbooks.com

Rick Holden, President
Discusses seven major areas of development and four major areas
of academic proficiency and then ties this information together
by examining factors that predispose a child to dysfunction and
disability, offering guidelines to assessment and management,
and analyzing long-range outcomes and factors that promote re-
siliency for parents, educators and clinicians. *$69.00*
640 pages Cloth
ISBN 0-838819-92-3

2423 Digest of Neurology and Psychiatry
Institute of Living: Hartford Hospital
80 Seymour Street
Hartford, CT 06106-3309   860-545-5000
                                             800-673-2411
                                        Fax: 860-545-5066
                                            www.harthosp.org

Douglas Elliot, Chair of the Board
Stuart K. Markowitz, MD, FACR, President/SVP
*Gerald J. Boisvert, HHC Regional Vice President / Chief Financial
Officer,*
Peter Q. Fraser, Regional Vice President Human Resources
Abstracts and reviews of selected current literature in psychiatry,
neurology and related fields.

2424 Disability Funding News
8204 Fenton St
Silver Spring, MD 20910-4502   301-588-6380
                                             800-666-6380
                                        Fax: 301-588-6385
                                      www.cdpublications.com
Mike Gerecht, Publisher

2425 Disability Studies and the Inclusive Classroom
711 3rd Avenue
8th Floor
New York, NY 10017   212-216-7800
                                             800-634-7064
                                        Fax: 212-564-7854
                                           www.routledge.com

Susan Baglieri, Co-Author
Arthur Shapiro, Co-Author
This book's mission is to integrate knowledge and practice from
the fields of disability studies and special education. Parts I & II
focus on the broad, foundational topics that comprise disability
studies (culture, language, and history) and Parts III & IV move
into practical topics (curriculum, co-teaching, collaboration,
classroom organization, disability-specific teaching strategies,
etc.) associated with inclusive education.

2426 Disability and Rehabilitation
Taylor & Francis
7625 Empire Dr
Florence, KY 41042-2919   800-634-7064
                                        Fax: 800-248-4724
                                   orders@taylorandfrancis.com
                                     www.taylorandfrancis.com
Monthly
ISSN 0963-82 8

2427 Disability, Sport and Society
711 3rd Avenue
8th Floor
New York, NY 10017   212-216-7800
                                             800-634-7064
                                        Fax: 212-564-7854
                                           www.routledge.com

Nigel Thomas, Co-Author
Andy Smith, Co-Author

Disability sport is a relatively recent phenomenon, yet it is also
one that, particularly in the context of social inclusion, is attracting increasing political and academic interest. The purpose of
this important new text - the first of its kind - is to introduce the
reader to key concepts in disability and disability sport and to examine the complex relationships between modern sport, disability and other aspects of wider society.

**2428 Disabled Rights: American Disability Policy and the Fight
for Equality**
3240 Prospect Street, NW
Suite 250
Washington, DC 20007   202-687-5889
                                        Fax: 202-687-6340
                                     gupress@georgetown.edu
                                       press.georgetown.edu/

Jacqueline Vaughn Switzer, Author
Disabled Rights explains how people with disabilities have been
treated from a social, legal, and political perspective in the
United States.

**2429 Divided Legacy: A History of the Schism in Medical
Thought, The Bacteriological Era**
North Atlantic Books
2526 Martin Luther King Jr. Way
Berkeley, CA 94704   510-549-4270
                                             800-337-2665
                                        Fax: 510-549-4276
                                  orders@northatlanticbooks.com
                                     www.northatlanticbooks.com
Alla Spector, Director of Finance & Office Operations
Doug Reil, Executive Director/Associate Publisher
Ed Angel, Director of Office Administration
Janet Levin, Senior Director of Sales & Distribution
Concluding volume of Coulter's history of medical philosophy,
from ancient times to today. Covers the origins of bacteriology
and immunology in world medicine; describes the clash between
orthodox and alternative medicine.

2430 Dual Relationships in Counseling
5999 Stevenson Ave
Alexandria, VA 22304-3304   703-823-0252
                                             800-347-6647
                                        Fax: 800-473-2329
                                    webmaster@counseling.org
                                          www.counseling.org

Robert L. Smith, President
Thelma Duffey, President-Elect
Brian Canfield, Treasurer
Catherine Roland, Representative
Publishes archival material, also publishes articles that have
broad interest for a readership composed mostly of counselors
and other mental health professionals who work in private practice, schools, colleges, community agencies, hospitals, and government. An appropriate outlet for articles that: critically
integrate published research; examine current professional and
scientific issues; report research, new techniques, innovative
programs and practices; and examine ACA as an organization.

**2431 Early Communication Skills for Children with Down
Syndrome**
Woodbine House
6510 Bells Mill Rd
Bethesda, MD 20817-1636   301-897-3570
                                             800-843-7323
                                        Fax: 301-897-5838
                                       info@woodbinehouse.com
                                       www.woodbinehouse.com

Nancy Gray Paul, Acquisitions Editor
Libby Kumin, Author
An expert shares her knowledge of speech and language development in young children with Down syndrome. Intelligibility,
hearing loss, apraxia and other factors that affect communications are discussed. It also covers speech-language assessments
and alternative communication options and literacy. *$19.95*
368 pages
ISBN 1-890627-27-5

2432 Early Intervention: Implementing Child & Family Services for At-Risk Infants and Toddlers
PRO-ED Inc.
8700 Shoal Creek Blvd
Austin, TX 78757-6897   512-451-3246
                                        800-897-3202
                                    Fax: 800-397-7633
                                    general@proedinc.com
                                    www.proedinc.com

Marci J. Hanson, Author
Eleanor W. Lynch, Author
New directions and recent legislation have produced a need for this guide which is designed for professionals facing the challenge of program development for disabled and at-risk infants, toddlers and their families. *$68.20*
394 pages Paperback 1995
ISBN 0-890796-21-1

2433 Ecology of Troubled Children
Brookline Books Publications
8 Trumbull Rd
Suite B-001
Northampton, MA 01060   413-584-0184
                                        800-666-2665
                                    Fax: 413-584-6184
                                    brbooks@yahoo.com
                                    www.brooklinebooks.com

Esther Isabe Wilder, Author
Designed for frontline mental health clinicians working with children with serious emotional disturbances; shows how to make children's' worlds more supportive by changing the places, activities and people in their lives. *$15.95*
256 pages
ISBN 1-571290-57-5

2434 Educating Children with Disabilities: A Transdisciplinary Approach
Brookes Publishing
PO Box 10624
Baltimore, MD 21285-0624   410-337-9580
                                        800-638-3775
                                    Fax: 410-337-8539
                                    custserv@brookespublishing.com
                                    www.brookespublishing.com

Paul H. Brookes, Chairman
Jeffrey D. Brookes, President
Melissa A. Behm, ExecutiveVice President
George S. Stamathis, Vice President & Publisher
Widely respected textbook presents you with the strategies you need for developing an inclusive curriculum, integrating health care and educational programs and addressing needs and concerns. *$38.00*
512 pages
ISBN 1-557662-46-0

2435 Educating Children with Multiple Disabilities: A Transdisciplinary Approach
Brookes Publishing
PO Box 10624
Baltimore, MD 21285-0624   410-337-9580
                                        800-638-3775
                                    Fax: 410-337-8539
                                    custserv@brookespublishing.com
                                    www.brookespublishing.com

Paul H. Brookes, Chairman
Jeffrey D. Brookes, President
Melissa A. Behm, ExecutiveVice President
George S. Stamathis, Vice President & Publisher
Emphasizing transdisciplinary cooperation between teachers, therapists, nurses and parents, this book describes a general model and specific techniques for effectively educating children with multiple disabilities. *$29.00*
496 pages Paperback
ISBN 1-557662-46-0

2436 Educating Individuals with Disabilities: IDEIA 2004 and Beyond (1st Edition)
Springer Publishing Company
11 W 42nd St
15th Fl
New York, NY 10036-8002   212-431-4370
                                        877-687-7476
                                    Fax: 212-941-7842
                                    cs@springerpub.com
                                    www.springerpub.com

Ted Nardin, Chief Executive Officer
Jason Roth, Vice President, Marketing & Sales
Kathy Weiss, Director, Sales
Elena L. Grigorenko, Editor
Discusses how learning-disabled students are identified and assessed today, in light of the 2004 Individuals with Disabilities Education Improvement Act. Grigorenko's interdisciplinary collection is the first to comprehensively review the IDEIA 2004 Act and distill the changes professionals working with learning-disabled students face. The text takes an overarching perspective, first discussing the IDEIA in its historical, political, and legal context. *$100.00*
512 pages Hardcover 1908
ISBN 0-826103-56-1

2437 Educating Students Who Have Visual Impairments with Other Disabilities
Brookes Publishing
PO Box 10624
Baltimore, MD 21285-0624   410-337-9580
                                        800-638-3775
                                    Fax: 410-337-8539
                                    custserv@brookespublishing.com
                                    www.brookespublishing.com

Paul H. Brookes, Chairman
Jeffrey D. Brookes, President
Melissa A. Behm, ExecutiveVice President
George S. Stamathis, Vice President & Publisher
This introductory text provides techniques for facilitating functional learning in students with a wide range of visual impairments and multiple disabilities. With a concentration on educational needs and learning styles, the authors of this multidisciplinary volume demonstrate functional assessment and teaching adaptations that will improve students' inclusive learning experiences. *$49.95*
552 pages Paperback
ISBN 1-557662-80-0

2438 Educating all Students in the Mainstream
Brookes Publishing Company
PO Box 10624
Baltimore, MD 21285-0624   410-337-9580
                                        800-638-3775
                                    Fax: 410-337-8539
                                    custserv@brookespublishing.com

Paul H. Brookes, Chairman
Jeff Brookes, President
Melissa A. Behm, ExecutiveVice President
Cary Gold, Educational Sales Representative
Incorporating the research and viewpoints of both regular and special educators, this textbook provides an effective approach for modifying, expanding, and adjusting regular education to meet the needs of all students. *$34.00*
304 pages
ISBN 1-557660-22-0

2439 Educational Audiology for the Limited Hearing Infant and Preschooler
Charles C. Thomas
2600 S First St
Springfield, IL 62704-4730   217-789-8980
                                        800-258-8980
                                    Fax: 217-789-9130
                                    books@ccthomas.com
                                    www.ccthomas.com

Donald Goldberg, Author
Nancy Coleffe-Schenck, Author
Doreen Pollack, Author

Offers information on current concepts and practices in audio-logic screening and evaluation, development of the listening function, development of speech, development of language, the role of parents, parent education, mainstreaming of the limited-hearing child, and program modifications for the severely learning disabled child. Also includes information on auditory assessment, sensory aides, cochlear implants, acoupedics and auditory verbal programs. *$79.95*
430 pages Paperback
ISBN 0-398067-51-1

2440   Educational Care
Educators Publishing Service
625 Mount Auburn St
3rd Floor
Cambridge, MA   02138-3039   617-547-6706
                                       800-225-5750
                         Feedback.EPS@schoolspecialty.com
                              www.eps.schoolspecialty.com

Paula Fabbro, Sales Consultant
Leo Micale, Sales Consultant
Kristen Colson, Sales Consultant
Flora Francis, Sales Consultant
This book, written for both parents and teachers, is based on the view that education should be a system of care that is able to look after the specific needs of individual students. Using case studies, it analyzes various types of learning disorders and then suggests ways to help students with these problems. *$31.50*
325 pages
ISBN 0-838819-87-7

2441   Educational Intervention for the Student
Charles C. Thomas
2600 S First St
Springfield, IL   62704-4730   217-789-8980
                                       800-258-8980
                                  Fax: 217-789-9130
                                  books@ccthomas.com
                                  www.ccthomas.com

2442   Educational Prescriptions
Educators Publishing Service
625 Mount Auburn St
3RD Floor
Cambridge, MA   02138-3039   617-547-6706
                                       800-225-5750
                         Feedback.EPS@schoolspecialty.com
                              www.eps.schoolspecialty.com

Paula Fabbro, Sales Consultant
Leo Micale, Sales Consultant
Kristen Colson, Sales Consultant
Flora Francis, Sales Consultant
This book provides specific recommendations for the classroom management of students who are experiencing subtle developmental and/or learning difficulties. Intended for regular classroom teachers, specific examples of accommodations teachers can make are provided for grades 1-3 and 4-6. *$13.50*
64 pages
ISBN 0-838819-90-7

2443   Effective Instruction for Special Education
Sage Publications
2455 Teller Road
Thousand Oaks, CA   91320-2218   805-499-0721
                                       800-818-7243
                                  Fax: 800-583-2665
                                  info@sagepub.com
                                  www.sagepub.com

Sara Miller McCune, Founder, Publisher, Chairperson
Blaise R. Simqu, President/CEO
Chris Hickok, Senior Vice President/CFO
Stephen Barr, Managing Director/SAGE London, P
This exciting and wide-ranging book provides special educators with effective methods for teaching students with mild and moderate learning and behavioral problems, as well as for teaching remedial students in general. *$37.00*
419 pages Paperback

2444   Effectively Educating Handicapped Students
Longman Publishing Group
9th Fl
Upper Saddle River, NJ   07458-1813   201-236-3281
                                       800-922-0579
                                  Fax: 201-236-3290
                                  www.pearsoned.com
468 pages Paperback
ISBN 0-801303-17-6

2445   Emotional Problems of Childhood and Adolescence
McGraw-Hill School Publishing
PO Box 182604
Columbus, OH   43218   877-833-5524
                                       800-338-3987
                                  Fax: 609-308-4480
                         customer.service@mheducation.com
                              www.mcgraw-hill.com

David Levin, President/Chief Ex
David Stafford, Senior Vice President/General Counsel
Maryellen Valaitis, Senior Vice President Human Resources
Patrick Milano, Chief Financial Officer Chief Administrative Officer
For future special educators, psychologists and others who work with emotionally disturbed children and adolescents.

2446   Enabling & Empowering Families: Principles & Guidelines for Practice
Brookline Books
8 Trumbull Rd
Suite B-001
Northampton, MA   01060   413-584-0184
                                       800-666-2665
                                  Fax: 413-584-6184
                                  brbooks@yahoo.com
                                  www.brooklinebooks.com

Esther Wilder, Co-Author
This book was written for practitioners who must work with families but who have insufficient training in family systems assessment and intervention. The authors' system enables professionals to help the family identify its needs, locate the formal and informal resources to meet these needs and develop the abilities to effectively access these resources. *$24.95*
220 pages
ISBN 0-914797-59-X

2447   Evaluation and Educational Programming of Students with Deafblindness & Severe Disabilities
Charles C. Thomas
2600 S First St
Springfield, IL   62704-4730   217-789-8980
                                       800-258-8980
                                  Fax: 217-789-9130
                                  books@ccthomas.com
                                  www.ccthomas.com

Carroll J. Jones, Author
Subtitle: Sensorimotor Stage. This second edition offers a very complete package of information on the special education of deaf-blind students; including detailed diagnostic information to assist the instructor in evaluating the physical, social, mental status of the student, as well as the educational progress. *$50.95*
265 pages Spiral-Paper 2001
ISBN 0-398072-16-2

2448   Evaluation and Treatment of the Psychogeriatric Patient
Haworth Press
711 Third Avenue
New York, NY   10017   212-216-7800
                                       800-354-1420
                                  Fax: 212-244-1563
                         subscriptions@tandf.co.uk
                              www.haworthpress.com

111 pages Hardcover
ISBN 1-560240-52-0

2449   Exceptional Children in Focus
McGraw-Hill School Publishing
PO Box 182604
Columbus, OH   43218   877-833-5524
                                              800-338-3987
                                         Fax: 609-308-4480
                              customer.service@mheducation.com
                                          www.mcgraw-hill.com

David Levin, President/Chief Ex
David Stafford, Senior Vice President/General Counsel
Maryellen Valaitis, Senior Vice President Human Resources
Patrick Milano, Chief Financial Officer Chief Administrative
Officer
Combines a light, personal look at the problems of special educators experiences with the basic facts of exceptionality.
288 pages

2450   Exceptional Lives: Special Education in Today's Schools, 4th Edition
Pearson Education
1 Lake St
Upper Saddle River, NJ   07458-1813   201-236-3281
                                              800-922-0579
                                         Fax: 201-236-3290
                                           www.pearsoned.com

592 pages
ISBN 0-131126-00-8

2451   Facilitating Self-Care Practices in the Elderly
Haworth Press
711 Third Avenue
New York, NY   10017   212-216-7800
                                              800-354-1420
                                         Fax: 212-244-1563
                               subscriptions@tandf.co.uk
                                          www.haworthpress.com

185 pages Hardcover
ISBN 1-560240-13-X

2452   Family-Centered Early Intervention with Infants and Toddlers
Brookes Publishing
PO Box 10624
Baltimore, MD   21285-0624   410-337-9580
                                              800-638-3775
                                         Fax: 410-337-8539
                               custserv@brookespublishing.com
                                       www.brookespublishing.com

Paul H. Brookes, Chairman
Jeffrey D. Brookes, President
Melissa A. Behm, ExecutiveVice President
George S. Stamathis, Vice President & Publisher
This informative text provides professionals with insight and practical guidelines to help fulfill the federal requirements for provision of early intervention services. *$37.00*
368 pages Hardcover
ISBN 1-557661-24-3

2453   Feeding Children with Special Needs
Arizona Department of Health Services
150 North 18th Avenue
Phoenix, AZ   85007-2607   602-542-1025
                                         Fax: 602-542-0883
                                              www.azdhs.gov

Will Humble, Director
Jeff Bloomberg, J.D., Manager
Robert Lane, Esq., Administrative Counsel
Lynn Golder, Esq., Administrative Counsel & HIPAA Privacy
Officer
Guide designed to help develop a greater awareness of the special challenges involved in the nutrition and feeding concerns for children with special health care needs, and ways to approach the issues. *$5.00*

2454   Focal Group Psychotherapy
New Harbinger Publications
5674 Shattuck Ave
Oakland, CA   94609-1662   510-652-0215
                                              800-748-6273
                                         Fax: 800-652-1613
                               customerservice@newharbinger.com
                                          www.newharbinger.com

Matthew McKay, Founder
Patrick Fanning, Co-Founder/Writer
Guide to leading brief, theme-based groups. This book offers an extensive week-by-week description of the basic concepts and interventions for 14 theme or focal groups for: codependency, rape victims, shyness, survivors of incest, agoraphobia, survivors of toxic parents, depression, child molesters, anger control, domestic violence offenders, assertiveness, alcohol and drug abuse, eating disorders, and parent training. *$59.95*
544 pages Cloth
ISBN 1-879237-18-0

2455   Free Hand: Enfranchising the Education of Deaf Children
TJ Publishers
Margaret Walworth, Author
Donald F. Moores, Author
Terrence J. O'Rourke, Author
A select group of nationally prominent educators, linguists and researchers met at Hofstra University to consider the most vital and controversial question in education of the deaf: what role should ASL play in the classroom? Become part of that discussion with A Free Hand. *$16.95*
204 pages Softcover
ISBN 0-93266-40-X

2456   Friendship 101
Council for Exceptional Children
2900 Crystal Dr.
Suite 1000
Arlington, VA   22202-3557   888-232-7733
                                          TTY:866-915-5000
                                         service@cec.sped.org
                                            www.cec.sped.org

Juliet E. Hart Barnett, Co-Author/Editor
Kelly J. Whalon, Co-Author/Editor
An essential characteristic of autism spectrum disorder (ASD) is difficulty acquiring the social skills needed to develop social competence, including the ability to form and maintain friendships and relationships with others. This webinar, designed for general and special educators who work with children with ASD, presents evidence-based practices shown to enhance social competence in children and youth with ASD.

2457   Functional Assessment Inventory Manual
Stout Vocational Rehab Institute
655 15th St. NW
Suite 800
Washington, DC   20005   715-232-1411
                                              800-538-3742
                                         Fax: 715-232-2356
                               botterbuschd@uwstout.edu
                                              www2.epa.gov

Gina McCarthy, Administrator
Gwen Keyes Fleming, Chief of Staff
Bob Perciasepe, Deputy Administrator
Craig E. Hooks, Office of Administration and Resource Management (OARM)
The Functional Assessment is a systematic enumeration of a client's vocationally relevant strengths and limitations. *$12.00*
96 pages Paperback
ISBN 0-916671-53-4

2458   Get Ready for Jetty!: My Journal About ADHD and Me
750 First Street, NE
Washington, DC   20002-4242   202-336-5500
                                              800-374-2721
                                         rllowman@gmail.com
                                              www.apa.org

Jeanne Kraus, Author

Jetty writes about these things as well as her recent ADHD diagnosis in her journal.

2459 Getting Around Town
Council for Exceptional Children
2900 Crystal Dr.
Suite 1000
Arlington, VA 22202-3557 888-232-7733
TTY:866-915-5000
service@cec.sped.org
www.cec.sped.org

M. Sherril Moon, Co-Author
Emily M. Luedtke, Co-Author
Elizabeth Halloran-Tornquist, Co-Author
This book provides examples of possible IEP goals and field-tested lesson plans for individual students or entire classes across all age and grade levels.

2460 Global Perspectives on Disability: A Curriculum
Mobility International U SA
132 E Broadway
Suite 343
Eugene, OR 97401-3155 541-343-1284
Fax: 541-343-6812
TTY:541-343-1284
info@miusa.org
www.miusa.org

Susan Sygall, CEO/Founder
Cerise Roth-Vinson, Chief Operating Officer
Cindy Lewis, Director of Programs
Stephanie Gray, Program Managers
Designed for secondary and higher education instructors. Includes five lesson plans covering disability awareness, disability rights and international perspectives on disability. Available in alternative formats. *$40.00*

2461 Glossary of Terminology for Vocational Assessment/Evaluation/Work
Rehabilitation Resource University
University of Wisconsin-Stou
Menomonie, WI 54751 715-232-2236
Fax: 715-232-2356
gundlachj@uwstout.edu
Ronald Fry, Manager
Jennifer Gundlach Klatt, Program Assistant
This glossary contains 254 terms and their definitions. Primary focus is on the terminology related to the practice and professionals of vocational assessment, vocational evaluation and work adjustment. *$9.50*
40 pages Softcover

2462 Graduate Technological Education and the Human Experience of Disability
Haworth Press
711 Third Avenue
New York, NY 10017 212-216-7800
800-354-1420
Fax: 212-244-1563
subscriptions@tandf.co.uk
www.haworthpress.com

115 pages Hardcover
ISBN 0-789060-08-6

2463 HIV Infection and Developmental Disabilities
Brookes Publishing
PO Box 10624
Baltimore, MD 21285-0624 410-337-9580
800-638-3775
Fax: 410-337-8539
custserv@brookespublishing.com
www.brookespublishing.com

Paul H. Brookes, Chairman
Jeffrey D. Brookes, President
Melissa A. Behm, Executive Vice President
George S. Stamathis, Vice President & Publisher

A resource for service providers pinpointing the most crucial medical, legal and educational issues to control HIV infection. *$47.00*
320 pages
ISBN 1-557660-83-2

2464 Handbook for Implementing Workshops for Siblings of Special Children
Special Needs Project
324 State St
Suite H
Santa Barbara, CA 93101-2364 805-962-8087
800-333-6867
Fax: 805-962-5087
editor@specialneeds.com
www.specialneeds.com

Mark Darrow, Founder, The Prolotherapy Institu
Based on three years of professional experience, this handbook provides guidelines and techniques for those who wish to start and conduct workshops for siblings. *$40.00*

2465 Handbook for Speech Therapy
Psychological & Educational Publications
PO Box 520
Hydesville, CA 95547 800-523-5775
Fax: 800-447-0907
psych-edpublications@suddenlink.net
www.psych-edpublications.com

143 pages paperback

2466 Handbook for the Special Education Administrator
Edwin Mellen Press
PO Box 450
Lewiston, NY 14092-1205 716-754-2266
Fax: 716-754-4056
jrupnow@mellenpress.com
www.mellenpress.com

Arthur R. Crowell, Author
Bonnie Crogan, Marketing
Irene Miller, Accounting
Patricia Schultz, Production
Organization and procedures for special education. *$ 49.95*
96 pages Hardcover
ISBN 0-88946 -22-9

2467 Handbook of Acoustic Accessibility
15619 Premiere Drive
Suite 101
Tampa, FL 33624 850-363-9909
Fax: 480-393-4331
accounting@successforkidswithhearingloss.com
successforkidswithhearinglo ss.com

Joseph J. Smaldino, Co-Author
Carol Flexer, Co-Author
Most students with hearing loss are educated in mainstream education classrooms the majority of each school day. Communication - between peers and with teachers - is the coin of education and upon which a wealth of knowledge is built. Unfortunately for students with hearing loss, the typical classroom environment is hazardous for listening and interferes with access to all classroom communication.

2468 Handbook of Developmental Education
Greenwood Publishing Group
130 Cremona Drive
Santa Barbara, CA 93117 805-968-1911
800-368-6868
Fax: 866-270-3856
CustomerService@abc-clio.com
www.abc-clio.com

This comprehensive handbook has brought together the leading practitioners and researchers in the field of developmental education to focus on the developmental learning agenda. Hardcover.
400 pages $65 - $75
ISBN 0-275932-97-4

2469 Handbook on Supported Education for Peoplewith Mental Illness
Brookes Publishing
PO Box 10624
Baltimore, MD 21285-0624   410-337-9580
                                             800-638-3775
                                        Fax: 410-337-8539
                          custserv@brookespublishing.com
                               www.brookespublishing.com

Paul H. Brookes, Chairman
Jeffrey D. Brookes, President
Melissa A. Behm, ExecutiveVice President
George S. Stamathis, Vice President & Publisher
Here you will find all necessary information that mental health professionals need in order to provide supported education services. There are specific suggestions on how to help people with mental illness return to or remain in college, trade school, or GED programs. Also addressed are funding and legal issues, accommodations, and specific interventions.
208 pages Paperback
ISBN 1-55766 -52-1

2470 Head Injury Rehabilitation: Children
Taylor & Francis
47 Runway Dr
Ste G
Levittown, PA 19057-4738   267-580-2622
                                        Fax: 215-785-5515
460 pages Cloth
ISBN 0-85066 -67-1

2471 Health Care Management in Physical Therapy
Charles C. Thomas
2600 S First St
Springfield, IL 62704-4730   217-789-8980
                                             800-258-8980
                                        Fax: 217-789-9130
                                  books@ccthomas.com
                                     www.ccthomas.com

2472 Health Care for Students with Disabilities
Brookes Publishing Company
PO Box 10624
Baltimore, MD 21285-0624   410-337-9580
                                             800-638-3775
                                        Fax: 410-337-8539
                          custserv@brookespublishing.com
                               www.brookespublishing.com

Paul H. Brookes, Chairman
Jeffrey D. Brookes, President
Melissa A. Behm, ExecutiveVice President
George S. Stamathis, Vice President & Publisher
This practical guidebook provides detailed descriptions of the 16 health-related procedures most likely to be needed in the classroom by students with disabilities. *$25.00*
304 pages Paperback
ISBN 1-557660-37-9

2473 Helping Learning- Disabled Gifted Children Learn Through Compensatory Active Play
Charles C. Thomas
2600 S First St
Springfield, IL 62704-4730   217-789-8980
                                             800-258-8980
                                        Fax: 217-789-9130
                                  books@ccthomas.com
                                     www.ccthomas.com

James Harry Humphrey, Author
$36.95
156 pages Hardcover 1990
ISBN 0-398056-95-1

2474 Helping Students Grow
American College Testing Program
500 ACT Drive
PO Box 168
Iowa City, IA 52243-0168   319-337-1000
                                     info@keytrain.com
                                         www.act.org

Jon Whitmore, Chief Executive Officer
Tom J. Goedken, Chief Financial Officer/Senior Vice President
Patricia C. Steinbrech, Chief Information Officer
Janet E. Godwin, Chief of Staff/Accountability Officer
Designed to assist counselors in using the wealth of information generated by the ACT Assessment.

2475 Home Health Care Provider: A Guide to Essential Skills
Springer Publishing
11 W 42nd St
15th Floor
New York, NY 10036-8002   212-431-4370
                                             877-687-7476
                                        Fax: 212-941-7842
                                   cs@springerpub.com
                                    www.springerpub.com

Theodore C. Nardin, CEO/Publisher
Jason Roth, VP/Marketing Director
Annette Imperati, Marketing/Sales Director
James C. Costello, Vice President, Journal Publishing
This book is designed to foster quality care to home care recipients. Prieto provides information, tips, and techniques on personal care routines as well as additional responsibilities, including home safety and maintenance, meal planning, errand running, caring for couples, and making use of recreational time. The book focuses on the psycho-social needs of home care recipients, stressing the need to maintainthe house as a home, and sustaining the recipient's way of life throughout caregiving.

2476 How to Teach Spelling/How to Spell
Educators Publishing Service
625 Mount Auburn St
3rd Floor
Cambridge, MA 02138-3039   617-547-6706
                                             800-225-5750
                       Feedback.EPS@schoolspecialty.com
                            www.eps.schoolspecialty.com

Paula Fabbro, Sales Consultant
Leo Micale, Sales Consultant
Kristen Colson, Sales Consultant
Flora Francis, Sales Consultant
This is a comprehensive resource manual based on the Orton-Gillingham approach to reading and spelling. It recommends what and how much to teach at each grade level at the beginning of each lesson or section. There are four student manuals that accompany this. *$22.50*
Teachers Manual
ISBN 0-838818-47-1

2477 Human Exceptionality: School, Community,and Family (12th Edition)
Cengage Learning
20 Channel Center St
Boston, MA 02210   617-289-7700
                                             617-289-7844
                                      www.cengage.com/us

Michael L. Hardman, Author
M. Winston Egan, Author
Clifford J. Drew, Author
An evidence-based testament to the critical role of cross-professional collaboration in enhancing the lives of exceptional individuals and their families. This text's unique lifespan approach combines powerful research, evidence-based practices, and inspiring stories, engendering passion and empathy and enhancing the lives of individuals with exceptionalities.
544 pages Hardcover

2478   I Can't Hear You in the Dark: How to Lean and Teach Lipreading
Charles C. Thomas
2600 S First St
Springfield, IL 62704-4730   217-789-8980
                                           800-258-8980
                                      Fax: 217-789-9130
                                     books@ccthomas.com
                                        www.ccthomas.com

Betty Woerner Carter, Author
The goal of this text is to improve communication and strengthen relationships with others. *$40.95*
226 pages Spiral-Paper 1997
ISBN 0-398067-89-2

2479   I Heard That!
3417 Volta Pl NW
Washington, DC 20007-2737   202-337-5220
                                      Fax: 202-337-8314
                                      TTY:202-337-5221
                                        info@agbell.org
                           www.listeningandspokenlanguage.org
Meredith K. Sugar, Esq. (OH), President
Ted A. Meyer, M.D., Ph.D, President-Elect/Secretary-Treasurer
Emilio Alonso-Mendoza, Chief Executive Officer
Susan Boswell, Director of Communications and Marketing
Provides a framework for teachers, clinicians and parents when writing objectives and designing activities to develop listening skills in children with hearing loss from newborn to 3 years.
$7.95
36 pages

2480   I Heard That!2
Alexander Graham Bell Association
3417 Volta Pl NW
Washington, DC 20007-2737   202-337-5220
                                      Fax: 202-337-8314
                                      TTY:202-337-5221
                                        info@agbell.org
                           www.listeningandspokenlanguage.org
Meredith K. Sugar, Esq. (OH), President
Ted A. Meyer, M.D., Ph.D, President-Elect/Secretary-Treasurer
Emilio Alonso-Mendoza, Chief Executive Officer
Susan Boswell, Director of Communications and Marketing
Provides a framework for teachers, clinicians and parents when writing objectives and designing activities to develop listening skills in children who are deaf or hard of hearing. *$7.95*
36 pages

2481   If It Is To Be, It Is Up To Us To Help!
AVKO Educational Research Foundation
3084 Willard Rd
Ste W
Birch Run, MI 48415-9404   810-686-9283
                                           866-285-6612
                                      Fax: 810-686-1101
                                     webmaster@avko.org
                                         www.avko.org

Don Mc Cabe, President
Ted A. Meyer, M.D., Ph.D, Vice-President
Michael Lane, Treasurer
Birch Run, Research Director Emeritus
A book of lesson plans for an Adult Community Education Course for Volunteer Tutors. Contains information on how to go about establishing such a course and how to secure cooperation from local and national organizations. Free as an e-book for Foundation members. *$ 14.95*
ISBN 1-56400 -42-1

2482   Images of the Disabled, Disabling Images
ABC-CLIO
130 Cremona Dr
Santa Barbara, CA 93117   805-968-1911
                                           800-368-6868
                                      Fax: 866-270-3856
                                  customerservice@abc-clio.com
                                        www.abc-clio.com

Alan Gartner, Author
Combines an examination of the presentation of persons with disabilities in literature, film and the media with an analysis of the ways in which these images are expressed in public policy concerning the disabled. *$84.00*
227 pages Hardcover 1986
ISBN 0-275921-78-6

2483   Implementing Family-Centered Services in Early Intervention
Brookline Books
8 Trumbull Rd
Suite B-001
Northampton, MA 01060   413-584-0184
                                           800-666-2665
                                      Fax: 413-584-6184
                                       brbooks@yahoo.com
                                     www.brooklinebooks.com

180 pages Paperback
ISBN 0-91479 -62-

2484   Including All of Us: An Early Childhood Curriculum About Disability
Educational Equity Concepts
71 Fifth Avenue
6th Floor
New York, NY 10003   212-243-1110
                                      Fax: 212-627-0407
                                       lcolon@fhi360.org
                                        www.edequity.org

Frank Schneiger, President
Antonia Cottrell Martin, Founder and President
Merle Froschl, Co-director
Barbara Sprung, Co-director
The first nonsexist, multicultural, mainstreamed curriculum. Step-by-step activities incorporate disability into three curriculum areas: Same/Different (hearing impairment), Body Parts (visual impairment), and Transportation (mobility impairment). *$14.95*
144 pages
ISBN 0-93162 -00-4

2485   Including Students with Severe and Multiple Disabilites in Typical Classrooms
Brookes Publishing
PO Box 10624
Baltimore, MD 21285-0624   410-337-9580
                                           800-638-3775
                                      Fax: 410-337-8539
                                  custserv@brookespublishing.com
                                    www.brookespublishing.com

Paul H. Brookes, Chairman
Jeffrey D. Brookes, President
Melissa A. Behm, ExecutiveVice President
George S. Stamathis, Vice President & Publisher
This straightforward and jargon free resource gives instructors the guidance needed to educate learners who have one or more sensory impairments in addition to cognitive and physical disabilities. *$32.95*
224 pages Paperback
ISBN 1-55766 -39-8

2486 Including Students with Special Needs: A Practical Guide for Classroom Teachers
Allyn & Bacon
75 Arlington St
Suite 300
Boston, MA   02116-3988   ab_webmaster@abacon.com
www.pearson.com/us/higher-education.html
544 pages
ISBN 0-20528 -85-4

2487 Inclusive & Heterogeneous Schooling: Assessment, Curriculum, and Instruction
Brookes Publishing
PO Box 10624
Baltimore, MD   21285-0624   410-337-9580
800-638-3775
Fax: 410-337-8539
custserv@brookespublishing.com
www.brookespublishing.com

Paul H. Brookes, Chairman
Jeff Brookes, President
Melissa A. Behm, ExecutiveVice President
Cary Gold, Educational Sales Representative
Presents methods for successfully restructuring classrooms to enable all students, particularly those with disabilities, to flourish. Provides specific strategies for assessment, collaboration, classroom management, and age-specific instruction. *$34.95*
448 pages Paperback
ISBN 1-55766 -02-9

2488 Independent Living Approach to Disability Policy Studies
World Institute on Disability
3075 Adeline Street
Suite 155
Berkeley, CA   94703   510-225-6400
Fax: 510-225-0477
TTY:510-225-0478
wid@wid.org
www.wid.org

Paul W. Schroeder, Chairman
Linda M. Dardarian, Vice Chairman
Mary Brooner, Treasurer
Cassandra Malry, Secretary
This collection of essays and bibliographies attempts to build a framework for understanding how the relationship between public policy, disability studies and disability policy studies will impact us in the future. *$17.50*
240 pages Paperback

2489 Information & Referral Center
Mississippi State University
108 Herbert - South
Room 150/PO Drawer 6189
Mississippi State Univers, MS   39762-6189   662-325-2001
800-675-7782
Fax: 662-325-8989
TTY: 662-325-2694
nrtc@colled.msstate.edu
www.blind.msstate.edu

Jacqui Bybee, Research and Training Coordinato
Michele Capella McDonnall, Ph.D., Research Professor/Interim Director
Jessica Thornton, Business Manager
Marty Giesen, Ph.D., Senior Research Scientist
A comprehensive website that includes information about client assistance programs, vocational rehabilitation agencies, low vision clinics and information about blindness and low vision. *$25.00*
150 pages

2490 Instructional Methods for Students
Allyn & Bacon
75 Arlington St
Suite 300
Boston, MA   02116-3988   ab_webmaster@abacon.com
www.home.pearsonhighered.com
450 pages
ISBN 0-205087-35-3

2491 Interactions: Collaboration Skills for School Professionals
Longman Education/Addison Wesley
75 Arlington St
Suite 300
Boston, MA   02116-3988   ab_webmaster@abacon.com
270 pages Paperback
ISBN 0-80131 -21-2

2492 International Journal of Arts Medicine
MMB Music
9051 Watson Road
Suite 161
Saint Louis, MO   63126   314-531-9635
800-543-3771
Fax: 314-531-8384
info@mmbmusic.com
www.mmbmusic.com

Norm Goldberg, Founder/chairman
Exploration of the creative arts and healing. Presents peer-reviewed articles clearly written by educators in the creative arts, as well as internationally prominent physicians, therapists and health care professionals.

2493 Interpreting Disability: A Qualitative Reader
Teachers College Press
1234 Amsterdam Avenue
New York, NY   10027   212-678-3929
800-575-6566
Fax: 212-678-4149
tcpress@tc.columbia.edu
www.tcpress.com

Brian Ellerbeck, Executive Acquisitions Editor
Marie Ellen Larcada, Senior Acquisitions Editor
Emily Spangler, Acquisitions Editor
Meg Hartmann, Acquisitions Assistant
This book offers a collection of exemplary qualitative research affecting people with disabilities and their families. Instead of focusing upon methodological details, the chapters illustrate the variety of styles and formats that interpretive research can adopt in reporting its results. *$24.95*
328 pages Paperback
ISBN 0-807731-21-8

2494 Intervention Research in Learning Disabilities
Gallery Bookshop
319 Kasten Street
PO Box 270
Mendocino, CA   95460-270   707-937-2215
Fax: 707-937-3737
info@gallerybookshop.com
www.gallerybooks.com

Tony Miksak, Owner
Based on the Symposium on Intervention Research, this volume presents 12 papers addressing issues in intervention research, academic interventions, social and behavioral interventions, and postsecondary interventions. *$30.00*
347 pages

2495 Introduction to Learning Disabilities
Allyn & Bacon
75 Arlington St
Suite 300
Boston, MA   02116-3988   ab_webmaster@abacon.com
www.pearsonhighered.com

608 pages
ISBN 0-20529 -43-4

2496   Introduction to Mental Retardation
Allyn & Bacon
75 Arlington St
Suite 300
Boston, MA   02116-3988   ab_webmaster@abacon.com
                                 www.pearsonhighered.com
350 pages Casebound
ISBN 0-134879-27-9

2497   Introduction to Special Education: Teaching in an Age of Challenge, 4th Edition
Allyn & Bacon
75 Arlington St
Suite 300
Boston, MA   02116-3988   www.pearsonhighered.com
640 pages cloth
ISBN 0-20526-94-4

2498   Introduction to the Profession of Counseling
McGraw-Hill School Publishing
PO Box 182604
Columbus, OH   43218   877-833-5524
                                       800-338-3987
                                  Fax: 609-308-4480
                      customer.service@mheducation.com
                                   www.mcgraw-hill.com
David Levin, President/Chief Executive Officer
David Stafford, Senior Vice President/General Counsel
Maryellen Valaitis, Senior Vice President Human Resources
Patrick Milano, Chief Financial Officer/Chief Administrative Officer
Offers information, theories and techniques for counseling numerous cases from drug addiction to special populations.
464 pages

2499   Issues and Research in Special Education
Teachers College Press
PO Box 20
Williston, VT   05495-0020   800-575-6566
                                  Fax: 802-664-7626
                            tcp.orders@aidcvt.com
                          www.teacherscollegepress.com
264 pages Hardcover
ISBN 0-807731-95-1

2500   Kendall Demonstration Elementary School Curriculum Guides
Gallaudet University Bookstore
800 Florida Ave NE
Washington, DC   20002-3695   202-651-5488
                                       800-621-2736
                                  Fax: 202-651-5489
                                  TTY: 888-630-9347
                              gupress@gallaudet.edu
                            www.gupress.gallaudet.edu
Dr. T Alan Hurwitz, President
Edward Bosso, Vice President for Administration
Dr. Lynne Murray, Vice President for Development
Donald Beil, Chief of Staff
KDES is a day school serving students from birth through age 15, beginning with the Parent-Infant Program and ending in grade 8. Students come from the Washington, D.C., metropolitan area.

2501   Language Arts: Detecting Special Needs
Allyn & Bacon
75 Arlington St
Suite 300
Boston, MA   02116-3988   617-848-7500
                                       800-852-8024
                                  Fax: 617-944-7273
                           www.home.pearsonhighered.com
Bill Barke, Chairman/CEO
Nancy Forfyth, President
Kevin Stone, Vice President, National Sales M
Thomas A. Rakes, Author

Describes special language arts needs of special learners.
180 pages paperback
ISBN 0-205116-36-1

2502   Language Learning Practices with Deaf Children
Sage Publications
2455 Teller Road
Thousand Oaks, CA   91320   805-499-9774
                                       800-818-7243
                                  Fax: 800-583-2665
                             books.claim@sagepub.com
                                    www.sagepub.com
Sara Miller McCune, Founder, Publisher, Chairperson
Stephen P. Quigley, Co-Author
Susan Rose, Co-Author
Patricia L. McAnally, Co-Author
This new edition describes the variety of language-development theories and practices used with deaf children without advocating anyone. $38.00
321 pages Hardcover

2503   Language and Communication Disorders in Children
McGraw-Hill School Publishn
PO Box 182604
Columbus, OH   43218   877-833-5524
                                       800-338-3987
                                  Fax: 609-308-4480
                      customer.service@mheducation.com
                                   www.mcgraw-hill.com
David Levin, President/Chief Executive Officer
David Stafford, Senior Vice President/General Counsel
Maryellen Valaitis, Senior Vice President Human Resources
Patrick Milano, Chief Financial Officer/Chief Administrative Officer
Comprehensive coverage encompassing all aspects of children's language disorders.
512 pages

2504   Learning Disabilities, Literacy, and Adult Education
Brookes Publishing
PO Box 10624
Baltimore, MD   21285-0624   410-337-9580
                                       800-638-3775
                                  Fax: 410-337-8539
                        custserv@brookespublishing.com
                            www.brookespublishing.com
Paul H. Brookes, Chairman
Jeffrey D. Brookes, President
Melissa A. Behm, ExecutiveVice President
George S. Stamathis, Vice President & Publisher
This book focuses on adults with severe learning disabilities and the educators who work with them. Described are the characteristics, demographics, and educational and employment status of adults with LD and the laws that protect them in the workplace and in educational settings.
450 pages Paperback
ISBN 1-55766-47-5

2505   Learning Disabilities: Concepts and Characteristics
McGraw-Hill School Publishing
220 E Danieldale Rd
Desoto, TX   75115-2490   972-224-4772
                                       800-442-9685
                                  Fax: 972-228-1982
Harold McGraw III, Chairman/ President/ Chief Ex
Jack F. Callahan, Executive Vice President, Chief
James A. McLoughlin, Co-Author
Gerald Wallace, Co-Author
Covers the conceptual basis of learning disabilities, identification, etiology and diagnosis.
448 pages

2506 Learning Disability: Social Class and the Cons of Inequality In American Education
Greenwood Publishing Group
130 Cremona Drive
Santa Barbara, CA 93117

805-968-1911
800-368-6868
Fax: 866-270-3856
CustomerService@abc-clio.com
www.abc-clio.com

James Carrier, Author
Presents a detailed historical description of the social and educational assumptions integral to the idea of learning disability.
167 pages $43.95 - $47.95
ISBN 0-313253-96-X

2507 Learning and Individual Differences
National Association of School Psychologists
8455 Colesville Rd
Suite 1000
Silver Spring, MD 20910- 3392

301-589-3300
Fax: 301-589-5175
info@musictherapy.org
www.musictherapy.org

Andrea Farbman, EdD, Executive Director
Judy Simpson, MT-BC, Director of Government Relations
Jane Creagan, MME, MT-BC, Director of Professional Program
E.L. Grigorenko, Editor
A multidisciplinary journal in education.

2508 Learning to Feel Good and Stay Cool: Emotional Regulation Tools for Kids With AD/HD
750 First Street, NE
Washington, DC 20002-4242

202-336-5500
800-374-2721
rllowman@gmail.com
www.apa.org

Judith M. Glasser, PhD, Co-Author
Kathleen G. Nadeau, PhD, Co-Author
Packed with practical advice and fun activities, this book will show you how to Understand your emotions, Practice healthy habits to stay in your Feel Good Zone, Feel better when you get upset, Know the warning signs that you are heading into your Upset Zone, Problem-solve so upsets come less often

2509 Learning to See: American Sign Language asa Second Language
Gallaudet University Press
800 Florida Ave NE
Washington, DC 20002-3695

202-651-5206
800-621-2736
Fax: 800-621-8476
TTY: 888-630-9347
clerc.center@gallaudet.edu
www.gupress.gallaudet.edu

Dr. T Alan Hurwitz, President
Edward Bosso, Vice President for Administration
Phyliss Wilcox, Co-Author
Sherman Wilcox, Co-Author
This important book has been updated to help teachers teach American Sign Language as a second language, including information on Deaf culture, the history and structure of ASL, teaching methods and issues facing educators. *$19.95*
160 pages Softcover

2510 Let's Write Right: Teacher's Edition
AVKO Educational Research Foundation
3084 Willard Rd
Ste W
Birch Run, MI 48415-9404

810-686-9283
866-285-6612
Fax: 810-686-1101
webmaster@avko.org
www.avko.org

Barry Chute, President
Julie Guyette, Vice President
Don Mc Cabe, Research Director
Clifford Schroeder, Treasurer

A manuscript and cursive writing program designed not only to teach handwriting but help with reading and spelling patterns as well. Teaches students to learn to read cursive as manuscript is being taught and ease the transition to cursive by using a D'Nealian-like script. Exercises involve phoically consistent patterns to help reinforce fluency with spelling and handwriting. *$39.95*
164 pages

2511 Library Manager's Guide to Hiring and Serving Disabled Persons
McFarland & Company
960 NC Hwy 88 W
Jefferson, NC 28640

336-246-4460
800-253-2187
Fax: 336-246-5018
infoinso@mcfarlandpub.com
www.mcfarlandbooks.com

Kieth C. Wright, Author
Judith F. Davie, Author
Information for library staff on hiring and serving disabled persons. *$27.50*
171 pages Library binding 1990
ISBN 0-899505-16-3

2512 Life-Span Approach to Nursing Care for Individuals with Developmental Disabilities
Brookes Publishing
PO Box 10624
Baltimore, MD 21285-0624

410-337-9580
800-638-3775
Fax: 410-337-8539
custserv@brookespublishing.com
www.brookespublishing.com

Paul H. Brookes, Chairman
Jeffrey D. Brookes, President
Melissa A. Behm, ExecutiveVice President
George S. Stamathis, Vice President & Publisher
This reference book was written by and for nurses. This guide addresses fundamental nursing issues such as health promotion, infection control, seizure management, adaptive and assistive technology, and sexuality. Also offered are in-depth case studies, helpful charts and tables, and problem-solving strategies. *$49.95*
464 pages Hardcover
ISBN 1-557661-51-0

2513 Mainstreaming Deaf and Hard of Hearing Students: Questions and Answers
Gallaudet University Bookstore
800 Florida Ave NE
Washington, DC 20002-3600

202-651-5000
800-451-1073
Fax: 202-651-5489
TTY: 888-630-9347
clerc.center@gallaudet.edu
www.gupress.gallaudet.edu

Dr. T Alan Hurwitz, President
Debra S. Lipkey, University Budget Director
Donald Beil, Chief of Staff
Edward Bosso, Vice President for Administratio
This booklet presents mainstreaming as one educational option and suggests some considerations for parents, teachers and administrators. *$6.00*
40 pages

2514 Mainstreaming Exceptional Students: A Guide for Classroom Teachers
Allyn & Bacon
75 Arlington St
Suite 300
Boston, MA 02116-3988 617-848-7500
800-852-8024
Fax: 617-944-7273
www.home.pearsonhighered.com
Nancy Forfyth, President
Bill Barke, CEO
Jane B. Schulz, Co-Author
C. Dale Carpenter, Co-Author
Covers the various categories of exceptional students and discusses educational strategies and classroom management.
464 pages paperback
ISBN 0-20515-24-6

2515 Mainstreaming: A Practical Approach for Teachers
McGraw-Hill School Publishing
PO Box 182604
Columbus, OH 43218 877-833-5524
800-338-3987
Fax: 609-308-4480
customer.service@mheducation.com
www.mcgraw-hill.com
David Levin, President/Chief Executive Officer
David Stafford, Senior Vice President/General Counsel
Maryellen Valaitis, Senior Vice President Human Resources
Patrick Milano, Chief Financial Officer/Chief Administrative Officer
Provides teachers, administrators and school psychologists with the background, techniques and strategies they need to offer appropriate services for mildly handicapped students in the mainstream classroom.

2516 Managing Diagnostic Tool of Visual Perception
Gallery Bookshop
319 Kasten Street
PO Box 270
Mendocino, CA 95460-270 707-937-2215
Fax: 707-937-3737
info@gallerybookshop.com
www.gallerybooks.com
Constantine Mangina, Author
For diagnosing specific perceptual learning abilities and disabilities. *$14.00*
ISBN 0-80580-83-4

2517 Medical Rehabilitation
Lippincott, Williams & Wilkins
227 S 6th St
Suite 227
Philadelphia, PA 19106-3713 215-545-5630
800-777-2295
Fax: 215-732-9988
www.lpub.com
Cheryl Murkey, Manager
Information for the professional on new techniques and treatments in the medical rehabilitation fields. *$80.50*
368 pages Illustrated
ISBN 0-88167-85-5

2518 Meeting the ADD Challenge: A Practical Guide for Teachers
Research Press
PO Box 7886
Champaign, IL 61826-9177 217-352-3273
800-519-2707
Fax: 217-352-1221
rp@researchpress.com
www.researchpress.com
Robert W. Parkinson, Founder
Dr. Michael Asher, Co-Author
Dr. Steven B Gordon, Co-Author
  $24.95
ISBN 0-878223-45-9

2519 Mental & Physical Disability Law Digest
A BA Commission on Mental and Physical Disability
1050 Connecticut Ave. N.W.
Suite 400
Washington, DC 20036-1019 202-662-1000
800-285-2221
Fax: 202-442-3439
cmpdl@abanet.org
www.americanbar.org
Robert M. Carlson, Chair, House of Delegates:
James R. Silkenat, President
William C. Hubbard, President-Elect
Cara Lee, Secretary
Provides comprehensive, summary and analysis of federal and state disability and state disability laws from mental disability law and disability discrimination law perspectives. *$60.00*
376 pages
ISBN 1-590310-05-5

2520 Mental Health Concepts and Techniques for the Occupational Therapy Assistant
Lippincott, Williams & Wilkins
227 S 6th St
Suite 227
Philadelphia, PA 19106-3713 215-521-8300
800-777-2295
Fax: 301-824-7390
www.lpub.com
J Lippincott, CEO
This text offers clear and easily understood explanations of the various theoretical and practiced health models. *$36.00*
344 pages
ISBN 0-88167-53-X

2521 Mental Health and Mental Illness
Lippincott, Williams & Wilkins
227 S 6th St
Suite 227
Philadelphia, PA 19106-3713 215-592-5400
800-777-2295
Fax: 301-824-7390
www.lpub.com
Kathy Sykes, Manager
Concise, comprehensive and completely up to date, this book presents the most current theory in mental health nursing for the student and the new practitioner. *$28.95*
480 pages
ISBN 0-39755-73-7

2522 Mentally Ill Individuals
Mainstream
Ste 830
3 Bethesda Metro Ctr
Bethesda, MD 20814-6301 301-961-9299
800-247-1380
Fax: 301-654-6714
info@mainstreaminc.org
Charles Moster
Mainstreaming mentally ill individuals into the workplace. *$2.50*
12 pages

2523 Midland Treatment Furniture
Sammons Preston Rolyan
W68 N158 Evergreen Blvd
Cedarburg, WI 53012-2637 262-387-8720
800-228-3693
Fax: 262-387-8748
CustomerSupport@PattersonMedical.com
www.pattersonmedical.com
Free

2524 Multidisciplinary Assessment of Children With Learning Disabilities and Mental Retardation
Gallery Bookshop
319 Kasten Street
PO Box 270
Mendocino, CA 95460-270
707-937-2215
Fax: 707-937-3737
info@gallerybookshop.com
www.gallerybooks.com

David L. Wodrich, Author
James E. Joy, Editor
Assessment of children with learning disabilities and mental retardation. $24.00
346 pages Illustrated
ISBN 0-93371-62-1

2525 Multisensory Teaching of Basic Language Skills: Theory and Practice
Brookes Publishing
PO Box 10624
Baltimore, MD 21285-0624
410-337-9580
800-638-3775
Fax: 410-337-8539
custserv@brookespublishing.com
www.brookespublishing.com

Paul H. Brookes, Chairman
Jeffrey D. Brookes, President
Melissa A. Behm, ExecutiveVice President
George S. Stamathis, Vice President & Publisher
This book presents specific multisensory methods for helping students who are having trouble learning to read due to dyslexia or other learning disabilities. Recommended techniques are offered for teaching alphabet skills, composition, comprehension, handwriting, math, organization and study skills, phonological awareness, reading and spelling. $59.00
608 pages Hardcover
ISBN 1-557663-49-1

2526 Music, Disability, and Society
1852 North 10th Street
Philadelphia, PA 19122
215-926-2140
800-621-2736
www.temple.edu/tempress

Alex Lubet, Author
In Music, Disability, and Society, Alex Lubet challenges the rigid view of technical skill and writes about music in relation to disability studies. He addresses the ways in which people with disabilities are denied the opportunity to participate in music.

2527 No Longer Immune: A Counselor's Guide to AIDS
American Counceling Association
5999 Stevenson Ave
Alexandria, VA 22304-3304
703-823-9800
800-347-6647
Fax: 703-823-0252
membership@counseling.org
www.counseling.org

Robert L. Smith, President
Thelma Duffey, President-Elect
Cirecie A. West-Olatunji, Past-President
Brian Canfield, Treasurer
Covers a broad range of issues such as working with specific populations, handling pre and post testing situations, coping with fear, grief and survivor guilt, struggling with spiritual issues and dealing with counter transference. $26.95
295 pages
ISBN 1-55620-64-1

2528 Occupational Therapy Across Cultural Boundaries
Haworth Press
711 Third Avenue
New York, NY 10017
212-216-7800
800-354-1420
Fax: 212-244-1563
subscriptions@tandf.co.uk
www.taylorandfrancisgroup.com

Derek Mapp, Non-Executive Chairman
Roger Horton, CEO
Emma Blaney, Group HR Director - Head of Corporate Responsibility
Isobel Peck, Group Chief Marketing Officer
Examines the concept of culture from a unique perspective, that of individual occupational therapists who have worked in environments very different from those in which they were educated or had worked previously. Journal publications formerly published by Haworth Press are now listed on the Taylor & Francis Journals website. $74.95
107 pages Hardcover
ISBN 1-560242-23-X

2529 Occupational Therapy Approaches to Traumatic Brain Injury
Routledge (Taylor & Francis Group)
711 Third Ave
New York, NY 10017
212-216-7800
800-634-7064
Fax: 212-564-7854
enquiries@taylorandfrancis.com
www.routledge.com

Laura H. Krefting, Author
Jerry A. Johnson, Author
Focusing on the disabled individual, the family, and the societal responses to the injured, this comprehensive book covers the spectrum of available services from intensive care to transitional and community living. Formerly published by Haworth Press, titles are now listed on Routledge/Taylor Francis Group. $140.00
137 pages Hardcover
ISBN 1-560240-64-4

2530 Overcoming Dyslexia in Children, Adolescents and Adults
Sage Publications
2455 Teller Road
Thousand Oaks, CA 91320
805-499-9774
800-818-7243
Fax: 800-583-2665
books.claim@sagepub.com
www.sagepub.com

Sara Miller McCune, Founder, Publisher, Chairperson
Blaise R Simqu, President/CEO
Tracey A. Ozmina, Executive Vice President & Chief
Dale R. Jordan, Author
This book describes some forms of dyslexia in detail and then relates those problems to the social, emotional and personal development of dyslexic individuals. $34.00
350 pages Paperback

2531 Oxford Textbook of Geriatric Medicine
Oxford University Press
198 Madison Ave
New York, NY 10016-4308
212-726-6000
800-445-9714
Fax: 919-677-1303
custserv.us@oup.com
global.oup.com

Rebecca Seger, Director, Institutional Sales, Americas
Lesa Moran Owen, Library Sales Operations Manager
Lenny Allen, Director, Institutional Accounts
Nancy Roy, Library Sales Manager
This comprehensive text brings together extensive experience in clinical geriatrics with a strong scientific base in research. $125.00
784 pages

2532 Pain Centers: A Revolution in Health Care
Lippincott Williams And Wilkins
227
227 S 6th St
Philadelphia, PA   19106-3713   215-521-8300
                                        800-777-2295
                                   Fax: 301-824-7390
                                        www.lpub.com

J Lippincott, CEO
   $103.00
   280 pages

2533 Parental Concerns in College Student Mental Health
Haworth Press
711 Third Avenue
New York, NY   10017   212-216-7800
                                        800-354-1420
                                   Fax: 212-244-1563
                              subscriptions@tandf.co.uk
                           www.taylorandfrancisgroup.com
Derek Mapp, Non-Executive Chairman
Roger Horton, CEO
Emma Blaney, Group HR Director - Head of Corporate Responsibility
Isobel Peck, Group Chief Marketing Officer
An instructive guide for parents and mental health professionals regarding the most important issues about psychological development in college students. Journal publications formerly published by Haworth Press are now listed on the Taylor & Francis Journals website. *$74.95*
204 pages Hardcover
ISBN 0-866567-20-8

2534 Parents and Teachers
Alexander Graham Bell Association
3417 Volta Pl NW
Washington, DC   20007-2737   202-337-5220
                                        866-337-5220
                                   Fax: 202-337-8314
                                   TTY: 202-337-5221
                                        info@agbell.org
                         www.listeningandspokenlanguage.org
Kathleen S. Treni, M.Ed., M.A., President
Meredith K. Knueve, Esq., Secretary-Treasurer
Alexander T. Graham, Executive Director/CEO
Corrine Altman, Director
This excellent book offers in-depth guidance to parents and teachers whose partnership can foster language in school-aged children with hearing impairments. The first section examines roles of parents, teachers, professionals and children in language acquisition, residual hearing and audiological management, language development stages and readying children for preschool. The second portion of the book presents specific objectives and teaching strategies to use at school and at home. *$27.95*
386 pages

2535 Patient and Family Education
Springer Publishing Company
11 W 42nd St
15th Floor
New York, NY   10036-8002   212-431-4370
                                        877-687-7476
                                   Fax: 212-941-7842
                                      cs@springerpub.com
                                       www.springerpub.com
Dr. Ursula Springer, President
Ted Nardin, CEO
James C. Costello, Vice President, Journal Publishi
James C. Costello, Vice President, Journal Publishing
This guide outlines the actual clinical content needed to develop, implement and maintain patient education programs. Conveniently arranged in one-hour long lesson plans, each disease or condition is organized in an easy-to-follow format. *$26.95*
272 pages Softcover
ISBN 0-82615 -41-7

2536 Person to Person: Guide for Professionals Working with the Disabled
Paul H Brookes Publishing Company
PO Box 10624
Baltimore, MD   21285-0624   410-337-9580
                                        800-638-3775
                                   Fax: 410-337-8539
                             custserv@brookespublishing.com
                               www.brookespublishing.com
Paul H. Brookes, Chairman
Jeffrey D. Brookes, President
Melissa A. Behm, ExecutiveVice President
George S. Stamathis, Vice President & Publisher
This second edition of an already-popular book helps professionals approach interactions with a people-first, disability second attitude. *$29.00*
288 pages Paperback
ISBN 1-557661-00-6

2537 Personality and Emotional Disturbance
Taylor & Francis
Ste G
47 Runway Dr
Levittown, PA   19057-4738   267-580-2622
                                   Fax: 215-785-5515
Richard Roberts, CEO
The brain injured person has unique needs. Recent findings have highlighted that it is the personality, behavioral and emotional problems which most prohibit a return to work, create the greatest burden for the long-term care and rehabilitation of physical and cognitive functions. *$72.00*
260 pages Cloth
ISBN 0-85066 -71-3

2538 Phenomenology of Depressive Illness
Human Sciences Press
233 Spring St
New York, NY   10013-1522   212-229-2859
                                        877-283-3229
                                   Fax: 212-463-0742
                                        ainy@aveda.com
                                        www.aveda.edu

263 pages Cloth
ISBN 0-89885 -69-9

2539 Physical Disabilities and Health Impairments: An Introduction
McGraw-Hill School Publishing
PO Box 182604
Columbus, OH   43218   877-833-5524
                                        800-338-3987
                                   Fax: 609-308-4480
                           customer.service@mheducation.com
                                     www.mcgraw-hill.com
David Levin, President/Chief Executive Officer
David Stafford, Senior Vice President/General Counsel
Maryellen Valaitis, Senior Vice President Human Resources
Patrick Milano, Chief Financial Officer/Chief Administrative Officer
A comprehensive text which presents a wealth of up-to-date medical information for teachers.

2540 Physical Education and Sports for Exceptional Students
McGraw-Hill Company
2460 Kerper Blvd
Dubuque, IA   52001-2224   800-338-3987
                                   Fax: 614-755-5654
                           customer.service@mcgraw-hill.com
                                   www.mhhe.com/hper/physed
Michael Horvat, Author
Harold McGraw III, Chairman, President and Chief Ex
Jack F. Callahan, Executive Vice President, Chief
John Berisford, Executive Vice President, Human
Physical education for exceptional students and teaching students with learning and behavior exceptionalities.
Cloth

2541 Physical Management of Multiple Handicaps: A Professional's Guide
Brookes Publishing Company
PO Box 10624
Baltimore, MD   21285-0624   410-337-9580
                                     800-638-3775
                                Fax: 410-337-8539
                         custserv@brookespublishing.com
                         www.brookespublishing.com
Paul H. Brookes, Chairman
Jeffrey D. Brookes, President
Melissa A. Behm, ExecutiveVice President
George S. Stamathis, Vice President & Publisher
Comprehensive guide, takes a transdisciplinary approach to therapeutic/technological management of persons with multiple handicaps. *$36.00*
352 pages Hardcover
ISBN 1-557660-47-6

2542 Physically Handicapped in Society
Ayer Company Publishers
Ste 322
400 Bedford St
Manchester, NH   03101-1195   603-669-9307
                                     888-267-7323
                                Fax: 603-669-7945
                                     stg@ncia.net
                                     www.ayerpub.com
Kathy Train, Office Manager
Ellie Phipps, Customer Service
A group of 39 books. Biographies that offer studies on attitudes, sociological and psychological. Please write or call for catalog. *$965.00*
Hardcover
ISBN 0-40513 -00-3

2543 Practicing Rehabilitation with Geriatric Clients
Springer Publishing Company
11 W 42nd St
15th Floor
New York, NY   10036-8002   212-431-4370
                                     877-687-7476
                                Fax: 212-941-7842
                                     cs@springerpub.com
                                     www.springerpub.com
Dr. Ursula Springer, President
Ted Nardin, CEO
James C. Costello, Vice President, Journal Publishi
James C. Costello, Vice President, Journal Publishing
Physical therapy in the geriatric client, psychological and psychiatric considerations in the rehabilitation of the elderly. *$32.95*
256 pages Hardcover
ISBN 0-82616 -80-5

2544 Pragmatic Approach
Educators Publishing Service
625 Mount Auburn St
3RD Floor
Cambridge, MA   02138-3039   617-547-6706
                                     800-225-5750
                                Fax: 617-547-0285
Paula Fabbro, Sales Consultant
Leo Micale, Sales Consultant
Kristen Colson, Sales Consultant
Flora Francis, Sales Consultant
Monograph on evaluation of children's performances on Slingerland Pre-Reading Screening Procedures to Identify First Grade Academic Needs. *$6.00*
56 pages
ISBN 0-838816-85-1

2545 Preschoolers with Special Needs: Children At-Risk, Children with Disabilities
Allyn & Bacon
75 Arlington St
Suite 300
Boston, MA   02116-3988   617-848-7500
                                  800-852-8024
                             Fax: 617-944-7273
                         www.home.pearsonhighered.com
Bill Barke, CEO
Janet W. Lerner, Co-Author
Barbara Lowenthal, Co-Author
Rosemary W. Egan, Co-Author
Explores ways of providing preschool children with special needs and their families with a learning environment that will help them develop and learn. Emphasizes the needs of preschoolers age three to six and provides information to teachers and others who work with young children in all settings. Current models of curricula, which incorporate new features from research and practical expreiences with children who have special needs, are described and discussed. *$59.00*
336 pages cloth
ISBN 0-205358-79-9

2546 Preventing Academic Failure - Teachers Handbook
Educators Publishing Service
625 Mount Auburn St
3rd Fl
Cambridge, MA   02138-3039   617-547-6706
                                     800-225-5750
                                Fax: 617-547-0285
                                     eps.schoolspecialty.com
Paperback
ISBN 0-838852-71-8

2547 Preventing School Dropouts
Sage Publications
2455 Teller Road
Thousand Oaks, CA   91320   805-499-9774
                                     800-818-7243
                                Fax: 800-583-2665
                         books.claim@sagepub.com
                                     www.sagepub.com
Sara Miller McCune, Founder, Publisher, Chairperson
Blaise R Simqu, President/ CEO
Tracey A. Ozmina, Executive Vice President & Chief
Thomas C. Lovitt, Author
For secondary teachers, special education and regular, who have difficulty teaching youth in their classes. Presented are 120 tactics, specific instructional techniques, for helping adolescents to stay in school. Each tactic is written in a format that includes five sections. *$38.00*
509 pages

2548 Prevocational Assessment
Exceptional Education
P.O.Box 15308
Seattle, WA   98115-308   206-262-9538
                             Fax: 475-486-4510
Jeff Stewart, Owner
Use the PACG to assess your students in nine areas (attendance and endurance, learning and behavior, communication skills, social skills, grooming and eating and toileting) covering 46 specific workshop experiences. *$12.00*
16 pages Complete Set
ISBN 1-87786 -23-7

2549 Primary Special Needs and the National Curriculum
7625 Empire Drive
Florence, KN   41042-2919   800-634-4724
                         orders@taylorandfrancis.com
                                     www.psypress.com
Ann Lewis, Author
This new edition of Ann Lewis's widely acclaimed text has been substantially revised and updated to take into account the recent revisions to the National Curriculum and the guidance of the Code of Practice.

2550 Progress Without Punishment: Approaches for Learners with Behavior Problems
Teachers College Press
1234 Amsterdam Ave
New York, NY 10027-6602 212-678-3929
800-575-6566
Fax: 212-678-4149
tcpress@tc.columbia.edu
www.teacherscollegepress.com
Anne M. Donnellan, Author
In this volume, the authors argue against the use of punishment, and instead advocate the use of alternative intervention procedures. *$17.95*
184 pages Paperback
ISBN 0-807729-11-6

2551 Promoting Postsecondary Education for Students with Learning Disabilities
Sage Publications
2455 Teller Road
Thousand Oaks, CA 91320 805-499-9774
800-818-7243
Fax: 800-583-2665
books.claim@sagepub.com
www.sagepub.com
Sara Miller McCune, Founder, Publisher, Chairperson
Stan F. Shaw, Co-Author
Joan M. McGuire, Co-Author
Loring Cowles Brinckerhoff, Co-Author
Primarily designed for postsecondary service providers who are responsible for serving college students with learning disabilities. *$41.00*
440 pages

2552 Psychiatric Mental Health Nursing
Lippincott, Williams & Wilkins
227 S 6th St
Suite 227
Philadelphia, PA 19106-3713 215-521-8300
800-777-2295
Fax: 301-824-7390
www.lpub.com
J Lippincott, CEO
This text emphasizes and contrasts the roles of the generalist nurse and the psychiatric nurse specialist. *$52.00*
1120 pages Illustrated

2553 Psychoeducational Assessment of Visually Impaired and Blind Students
Sage Publications
2455 Teller Road
Thousand Oaks, CA 91320 805-499-9774
800-818-7243
Fax: 800-583-2665
books.claim@sagepub.com
www.sagepub.com
Sara Miller McCune, Founder, Publisher, Chairperson
Blaise R Simqu, President/CEO
Tracey A. Ozmina, Executive Vice President & Chief
Sharon Bradley-Johnson, Author
Professional reference book that addresses the problems specific to assessment of visually impaired and blind children. Of particular value to the practitioner are the extensive reviews of available tests, including ways to adapt those not designed for use with the visually handicapped. *$29.00*
140 pages Paperback
ISBN 0-890791-08-2

2554 Psychological and Social Impact of Illness and Disability
Springer Publishing
11 W 42nd St
15th Floor
New York, NY 10036-8002 212-431-4370
877-687-7476
Fax: 212-941-7842
cs@springerpub.com
www.springerpub.com
Dr. Ursula Springer, President
Ted Nardin, CEO
Ph.D. Orto Arthur E. Dell, Editor
James C. Costello, Vice President, Journal Publishing
The newest edition of Psychological and Social Impact of Illness and Disability continues the tradition of presenting a realistic perspective on life with disabilities and then improves upon its predecessors with the inclusion of illness as a major influence on client care needs. Further broadening the scope of this edition is the inclusion of personal perspectives and stories from those living with illness or disabilities. These stories offer a look into what it is like to cope with these issues.

2555 Reading and Deafness
Sage Publications
2455 Teller Road
Thousand Oaks, CA 91320 805-499-9774
800-818-7243
Fax: 800-583-2665
books.claim@sagepub.com
www.sagepub.com
Sara Miller McCune, Founder, Publisher, Chairperson
Beverly J Trezek, Co-Author
Peter V. Paul, Co-Author
Ye Wang, Co-Author
Three areas are looked at in this book: deaf children's prereading development of real-world knowledge, cognitive abilities and linguistic skills. *$39.00*
422 pages

2556 Readings on Research in Stuttering
Longman Publishing Group
1 Penn Plaza
Suite 2222
New York, NY 10119 646-556-8401
Fax: 646-556-8415
coffee@rothfos.com
www.rothfos.com
Dan Dwyer, CEO
Thomas Minogue, CFO
Maria Tanpinco-Queyquep, Traffic Manager
Joseph P. Thomas, Traffic Coordinator
Collection of the key journal articles published on stuttering over the past decade, addressing trends in recent research in the field.
231 pages Paperback
ISBN 0-801304-10-5

2557 Recreation Activities for the Elderly
Springer Publishing Company
11 W 42nd St
15th Floor
New York, NY 10036-8002 212-431-4370
877-687-7476
Fax: 212-941-7842
cs@springerpub.com
www.springerpub.com
Dr. Ursula Springer, President
Ted Nardin, CEO
James C. Costello, Vice President, Journal Publishi
James C. Costello, Vice President, Journal Publishing
Included in this volume are simple crafts that utilize easily obtainable, inexpensive materials, hobbies focusing on collections, nature, and the arts' and games emphasizing both mental and physical activity. *$23.95*
240 pages Softcover
ISBN 0-82616 -30-1

2558 Reference Manual for Communicative Sciences and Disorders
Pro- Ed Publications
8700 Shoal Creek Blvd
Austin, TX 78757-6897
512-451-3246
800-897-3202
Fax: 512-451-8542
info@proedinc.com
www.proedinc.com

Raymond D. Kent, Author
An indispensable guide to standards and values essential in the assessment of communication disorders. *$54.00*
393 pages

2559 Rehabilitation Interventions for the Institutionalized Elderly
Haworth Press
711 Third Avenue
Floor 8th
New York, NY 10017
212-216-7800
800-354-1420
Fax: 212-564-7854
subscriptions@tandf.co.uk
www.taylorandfrancisgroup.com

Derek Mapp, Non-Executive Chairman
Roger Horton, CEO
Emma Blaney, Group HR Director - Head of Corporate Responsibility
Isobel Peck, Group Chief Marketing Officer
Gerontology professionals offer suggestions to enrich the quality of rehabilitation services offered to the institutionalized elderly. This volume examines up to the minute ideas, some that would have been unlikely even a few years ago, that focus exclusively on rehabilitation services for the institutionalized elderly. Journal publications formerly published by Haworth Press are now listed on the Taylor & Franc *$44.95*
77 pages Hardcover
ISBN 0-866568-33-6

2560 Rehabilitation Nursing for the Neurological Patient
Springer Publishing Company
11 W 42nd St
15th Fl
New York, NY 10036-8002
212-431-4370
877-687-7476
Fax: 212-941-7842
cs@springerpub.com
www.springerpub.com

Ted Nardin, Chief Executive Officer
Jason Roth, Vice President, Sales & Marketing
Kathy Weiss, Director, Sales
Marcia Hanak, Author
Reviews the physiology, pathophysiology, & nursing management of problems frequently encountered in neuro- rehabilitation and reviews the pathphysiology of specific disabilities & the related nursing interventions. *$32.95*
229 pages Hardcover 1992
ISBN 0-826176-60-7

2561 Rehabilitation Resource Manual: VISION
Resources for Rehabilitation
22 Bonad Rd
Winchester, MA 01890-1302
781-368-9094
Fax: 781-368-9096
info@rfr.org
www.rfr.org

Marshall E. Flax, MS, Author
A desk reference that enables service providers, librarians and others to make effective referrals. Includes guidelines on establishing self-help groups, information on research and service organizations, and chapters on assistive technology, for special population groups and by eye condition. *$44.95*
Biennial

2562 Rehabilitation Technology
CRC Press
6000 Broken Sound Pkwy NW
Ste 300
Boca Raton, FL 33487
800-634-7064
Fax: 800-374-3401
orders@crcpress.com
www.crcpress.com

Glenn E. Hedman, Author
Learn how the use of technological devices can enhance the lives of disabled children. Informs physical therapists, occupational therapists, and rehabilitation technologists about the devices that are available today and provides important background information on these devices. CRC Press is part of the Taylor & Francis Group. *$39.95*
173 pages Hardcover 1990
ISBN 1-560240-33-4

2563 Report Writing in Assessment and Evaluation
Stout Vocational Rehab Institute
University of Wisconsin-Stout
712 South Broadway
Menomonie, WI 54751
715-232-1478
Fax: 715-232-2356
giffordj@uwstout.edu
www.uwstout.edu

Charles W. Sorensen, Chancellor
Judy Gifford, Director
Stephen W. Thomas, Author
Linda Vanderloop, CFSC Office
This examines questions of who are you writing for and what does the referral source want. Defines characteristics of good reports, common problems, writing in different settings, types of reports, getting ready to write, and writing prescriptive recommendations. *$ 17.75*
188 pages Softcover

2564 Resource Room, The
State University of New York Press
22 Corporate Woods Boulevard
3rd Floor
Albany, NY 12210-2314
518-472-5000
866-430-7869
Fax: 518-472-5038
info@sunypress.edu
www.sunypress.edu

Barry Edwards McNamara, Author
Provides teachers and administrators with helpful, practical information and explores the role of the resource room teacher as it relates to three major functions: assessment, instruction and consultation. It will also assist supervisors and administrators in evaluating their resource programs. *$28.95*
148 pages Paperback
ISBN 0-887069-84-0

2565 Resources for Rehabilitation
22 Bonad Rd
Winchester, MA 01890-1302
781-368-9094
Fax: 781-368-9096
info@rfr.org
www.rfr.org

2566 Restructuring High Schools for All Students: Taking Inclusion to the Next Level
Brookes Publishing
PO Box 10624
Baltimore, MD 21285-0624
410-337-9580
800-638-3775
Fax: 410-337-8539
custserv@brookespublishing.com
www.brookespublishing.com

Paul H. Brookes, Chairman
Jeffrey D. Brookes, President
Melissa A. Behm, ExecutiveVice President
George S. Stamathis, Vice President & Publisher

Details the process of creating an inclusive, collaborate community of learners and teachers at the secondary level. *$29.95*
304 pages Paperback
ISBN 1-557663-13-0

2567 Restructuring for Caring and Effective Education: Administrative Guide
Brookes Publishing
PO Box 10624
Baltimore, MD   21285-0624   410-337-9580
                                            800-638-3775
                                        Fax: 410-337-8539
                        custserv@brookespublishing.com
                        www.brookespublishing.com
Paul H. Brookes, Chairman
Jeffrey D. Brookes, President
Melissa A. Behm, ExecutiveVice President
George S. Stamathis, Vice President & Publisher
In this empowering book, leading general and special education schools reform experts synthesize the major school restructuring initiatives and describe the processes and rationale for changing the organizational structure and instructional practices of schools. *$ 29.00*
384 pages Paperback
ISBN 1-55766 -91-3

2568 Scoffolding Student Learning
Brookline Books
8 Trumbull Rd
Suite B-001
Northampton, MA   01060   413-584-0184
                                         800-666-2665
                                     Fax: 413-584-6184
                        brbooks@yahoo.com
                        www.brooklinebooks.com
Paul H. Brookes, Chairman
Jeffrey D. Brookes, President
Melissa A. Behm, ExecutiveVice President
George S. Stamathis, Vice President & Publisher
Collection of papers on the theory and practice of scoffolding—an interactive style of instructions that helps students develop more powerful thinking tools. *$21.95*
180 pages Paperback
ISBN 1-571290-36-2

2569 Selective Nontreatment of Handicapped
Oxford University Press
2001 Evans Rd
Cary, NC   27513-2009   919-677-0977
                                       800-445-9714
                                   Fax: 919-677-1303
                        custserv.us@oup.com
                        www.global.oup.com
Lesa Moran Owen, Library Sales Operations Manager
Rebecca Seger, Director, Institutional Sales, Americas
Lenny Allen, Director, Institutional Accounts
Nancy Roy, Library Sales Manager
Information on selective nontreatment of handicapped newborns, moral dilemmas in neonatal medicine. *$17.95*
304 pages Paperback

2570 Semiotics and Dis/ability: Interogating Categories of Difference
State University of New York Press
22 Corporate Woods Boulevard
3rd Floor
Albany, NY 12210-2314   518-472-5000
                                       866-430-7869
                                   Fax: 518-472-5038
                        info@sunypress.edu
                        www.sunypress.edu
James Peltz, Associate Director
Linda Rogers, Editor
Beth Blue Swadener, Editor

Examines the ways the words disability and difference and socially and culturally constructed. *$25.95*
265 pages Paperback 1990
ISBN 0-791449-06-6

2571 Service Coordination for Early Intervention: Parents and Friends
Brookline Books
8 Trumbull Rd
Suite B-001
Northampton, MA   01060   413-584-0184
                                         800-666-2665
                                     Fax: 413-584-6184
                        brbooks@yahoo.com
                        www.brooklinebooks.com
Deborah D. Hatton, Co-Author
R. A. McWilliam, Co-Author
P. J. Winton, Co-Author
This book helps administrators and professionals to structure early intervention and ongoing services so that professionals work collaboratively with parents to promote the health, well being and development of children with special needs. *$19.95*
110 pages Paperback
ISBN 0-91479 -91-3

2572 Services for the Seriously Mentally Ill: A Survey of Mental Health Centers
Nat'l Council for Community Behavioral Healthcare
12300 Twinbrook Pkwy
Ste 320
Rockville, MD   20852-1606   301-984-6200
                                        Fax: 301-881-7159
Linda Rosenberg, CEO
Dale K Klatzker, Board Chair
This ground-breaking report documents what administrators and practitioners have maintained for many years: community mental health organizations devote a significant percentage of the human and financial resources to serving the seriously mentally ill. *$30.00*

2573 Sexuality and Disability
Springer Publishing
11 W 42nd St
15th Fl
New York, NY   10036-8002   212-431-4370
                                        Fax: 212-460-1575
                        www.springer.com
Sigmund Hough, Editor-in-Chief
A journal devoted to the psychological and medical aspects of sexuality in rehabilitation and community settings. The journal features original scholarly articles that address the psychological and medical aspects of sexuality in the field of rehabilitation, case studies, clinical practice reports, and guidelines for clinical practice.
Quarterly

2574 Shop Talk
PO Box 7886
Champaign, IL   61826-9177   217-352-3273
                                           800-519-2707
                                       Fax: 217-352-1221
                        rp@researchpress.com
                        www.researchpress.com
Robert W. Parkinson, Founder
Philip Roth, Author

2575 Signed English Schoolbook
Gallaudet University Press
800 Florida Ave NE
Washington, DC 20002-3600
202-651-5488
800-451-1073
Fax: 202-651-5489
TTY: 888-630-9347
clerc.center@gallaudet.edu
www.gupress.gallaudet.edu

Harry Bornstein, Co-Author
Karen L. Saulnier, Co-Author
Dr. T Alan Hurwitz, President
Edward Bosso, Vice President for Administratio
The Signed English Schoolbook provides vocabulary for teachers and others who serve school-age children and adolescents and covers the full range of school activities. *$13.95*
184 pages Softcover

2576 Social Skills for Students With Autism Spectrum Disorders and Other Dev Disabilities
Council for Exceptional Children
2900 Crystal Dr.
Suite 1000
Arlington, VA 22202-3557
888-232-7733
TTY:866-915-5000
service@cec.sped.org
www.cec.sped.org

Laurence R. Sargent, Co-Author
Toni Cook, Co-Author
Darlene E. Perner, Co-Author
A book teaching children to understand their own behaviours and when step away from a situation.

2577 Social Studies: Detecting and Correcting Special Needs
Allyn & Bacon
75 Arlington St
Suite 300
Boston, MA 02116-3988
617-848-7500
800-852-8024
Fax: 617-944-7273
www.home.pearsonhighered.com

Harry Bornst Barke, CEO
Nancy Forfyth, President
Lana J. Smith, Co-Author
Dennie L. Smith, Co-Author
Describes social studies and special needs for special learners.
180 pages
ISBN 0-205121-51-9

2578 Social and Emotional Development of Exceptional Students: Handicapped
Charles C. Thomas
2600 S First St
Springfield, IL 62704-4730
217-789-8980
800-258-8980
Fax: 217-789-9130
books@ccthomas.com
www.ccthomas.com

Michael P. Thomas, President
Carroll J. Jones, Author
Sixteen years after the passage of P.L. 94-142, the dream of special educators to educate the handicapped and nonhandicapped children and youth together resulting in increased academic gains and age-appropriate school skills for handicapped children and youth has not yet materialized. This book helps eliminate an existing void by providing teachers with understandable information regarding the social and emotional development of exceptional students. Also in cloth at $41.95 (ISBN# 0-398-05781-8) *$29.95*
218 pages Softcover
ISBN 0-398061-94-7

2579 Special Education Today
LifeWay Christian Resources Southern Baptist Conv.
One LifeWay Plaza
Nashville, TN 37234
615-251-2000
800-458-2772
Fax: 615-532-9412
specialed@lifeway.com
www.lifeway.com

Thom S. Rainer, President/CEO
Brad Waggoner, Executive Vice President
Eric Geiger, Vice President, Church Resources Division
Tim Hill, Vice President/Chief Information Officer
This unique quarterly publications ministers to people with special education needs and to their families, the church, and other caregivers. It offers a variety of helps and encouragement, including: What's working in churches, Suggestions for adapting teaching techniques, inspirational stories about people who have disabilities, Parenting and family issues, Ideas for reaching, witnessing, worship, and recreation. *$4.25*
36 pages Quarterly

2580 Special Education for Today
Allyn & Bacon
75 Arlington St
Suite 300
Boston, MA 02116-3988
617-848-7500
800-852-8024
Fax: 617-944-7273
www.home.pearsonhighered.com

See search r Barke, CEO
Michael S. Rosenberg, Co-Author
David L. Westling, Co-Author
James McLeskey, Co-Author
An undergraduate introduction to special education covering all major areas of exceptionality. Contains pedagogical features designed to make the book accessible to the undergraduate.
576 pages hardcover
ISBN 0-138264-53-8

2581 Speech and the Hearing-Impaired Child
Alexander Graham Bell Association
3417 Volta Pl NW
Washington, DC 20007-2737
202-337-5220
866-337-5220
Fax: 202-337-8314
TTY: 202-337-5221
info@agbell.org
www.listeningandspokenlanguage.org
Meredith K. Sugar, Esq. (OH), President
Ted A. Meyer, M.D., Ph.D, President-Elect/Secretary-Treasurer
Emilio Alonso-Mendoza, Chief Executive Officer
Susan Boswell, Director of Communications and Marketing
This textbook for professionals deals with basic theoretical issues in the acquisition of speech and the form of language (phonetics and phonology) in children with hearing losses. It provides a systematic framework to develop and evaluate speech target behaviors and their underlying subskills. *$29.95*
402 pages Paperback

2582 Speech-Language Pathology and Audiology: An Introduction
McGraw-Hill School Publishing
PO Box 182604
Columbus, OH 43218
877-833-5524
800-338-3987
Fax: 609-308-4480
customer.service@mheducation.com
www.mcgraw-hill.com

David Levin, President/Chief Executive Officer
David Stafford, Senior Vice President/General Counsel
Maryellen Valaitis, Senior Vice President Human Resources
Patrick Milano, Chief Financial Officer & Chief Administrative Officer
Offers classroom-tested coverage of clinical objectives and functioning.
301 pages

2583 Spinal Cord Dysfunction
Oxford University Press
2001 Evans Rd
Cary, NC 27513-2009 919-677-0977
800-451-7556
Fax: 919-677-1303
humanres@oup-usa.org
www.global.oup.com
Lesa Moran Owen, Library Sales Operations Manager
Rebecca Seger, Director, Institutional Sales, Americas
Lenny Allen, Director, Institutional Accounts
Nancy Roy, Library Sales Manager
Offers information on restoration of function after spinal cord damage as seen from the point of view of identification of impaired or absent function in the nerve cells and processes which survive after the initial insult, intact but with impaired functions.
$95.00
368 pages

2584 Steps to Success: Scope & Sequence for Skill Development
15619 Premiere Drive
Suite 101
Tampa, FL 33624 850-363-9909
Fax: 480-393-4331
accounting@successforkidswithhearingloss.com
successforkidswithhearinglo ss.com
Lynne H. Price, Author
Steps to Success is a curriculum for students who are deaf or hard of hearing in grades kindergarten through 12.

2585 Strategies for Teaching Learners with Special Needs
McGraw-Hill School Publishing
PO Box 182604
Columbus, OH 43218 877-833-5524
800-338-3987
Fax: 609-308-4480
customer.service@mheducation.com
www.mcgraw-hill.com
David Levin, President/Chief Executive Officer
David Stafford, Senior Vice President/General Counsel
Maryellen Valaitis, Senior Vice President Human Resources
Patrick Milano, Chief Financial Officer & Chief Administrative Officer
This is a text that helps special educators develop the full range of teaching competencies needed to be effective.
560 pages

2586 Strategies for Teaching Students with Learning and Behavior Problems
Allyn & Bacon
75 Arlington St
Suite 300
Boston, MA 02116-3988 617-848-7500
800-852-8024
Fax: 617-944-7273
www.home.pearsonhighered.com
Bill Barke, CEO
Nancy Forfyth, President
Sharon R. Vaughn, Co-Author
Candace S. Bos, Co-Author
Provides descriptions of methods and strategies for teaching students with learning and behvior problems, managing professional roles, and collaborating with families, professionals, and paraprofessionals.
544 pages
ISBN 0-205113-89-3

2587 Students with Acquired Brain Injury: The School's Response
Brookes Publishing
PO Box 10624
Baltimore, MD 21285-0624 410-337-9580
800-638-3775
Fax: 410-337-8539
custserv@brookespublishing.com
www.brookespublishing.com
Ann Glang, Editor
Bonnie Todis, Editor
Paul H. Brooks, Chairman of the Board
Cary Gold, Educational Sales Representative
This book is designed for school professionals and describes a range of issues that this population faces and presents proven means of addressing them in ways that benefit all students. Included topics are hospital-to-school transitions, effective assessment strategies, model programs in public schools, interventions to assist classroom teachers, and ways to involve family members in the educational program. *$29.95*
424 pages Paperback
ISBN 1-55766 -85-1

2588 Students with Mild Disabilities in the Secondary School
Longman Group
75 Arlington St
Suite 300
New York, NY 10036-2601 212-782-3300
800-852-8024
www.home.pearsonhighered.com
William Hitchings, Co-Author
Michael Horvath, Co-Author
Bonnie Schmalle, Co-Author
Paul Retish, Co-Author, Editor
Provides methods and strategies for curriculum delivery to students with mild disabilities at the secondary school level.
2313G pages Paperback
ISBN 0-801301-66-1

2589 Supporting and Strengthening Families
Brookline Books
8 Trumbull Rd
Suite B-001
Northampton, MA 01060 413-584-0184
800-666-2665
Fax: 413-584-6184
brbooks@yahoo.com
www.brooklinebooks.com
Carl J Dunst, Author
A collection of papers addressing the theory, methods, strategies, and practices involved in adopting an empowerment and family-centered resources approach to supporting families and strengthening individual and family functioning. *$30.00*
252 pages Paperback
ISBN 0-91479 -94-8

2590 TESTS
Slosson Educational Publications
538 Buffalo rd
PO Box 280
East Aurora, NY 14052 716-652-0930
888-756-7766
Fax: 800-665-3840
slossonprep@gmail.com
www.slosson.com
Steven W. Slosson, President
Dr. Georgina Moynihan, Office Personnel
Slosson Educational Publications, Inc. offers educators an extensive selection of testing products, along with books on autism. ADED and other special needs materials. Our catalog includes 30 pages of speech-language testing and language rehabilitation products. The behavioral conduct. Special needs section includes checklist and scales on aberrant/disruptive behavior, tapes on ADD, as well as products for dyslexia and remediation of reversals.

2591 Teacher's Guide to Including Students with Disabilities in Regular Physical Education
Brookes Publishing
PO Box 10624
Baltimore, MD 21285-0624   410-337-9580
                                            800-638-3775
                                      Fax: 410-337-8539
                            custserv@brookespublishing.com
                               www.brookespublishing.com
Martin E. Block, Author
Melissa A. Behm, Executive Vice President
Paul H. Brooks, Chairman of the Board
Cary Gold, Educational Sales Representative
Provides simple and creative strategies for meaningfully including children with disabilities in regular physical education programs. *$39.00*
288 pages Paperback
ISBN 1-557661-56-1

2592 Teachers Working Together
Brookline Books
8 Trumbull Rd
Suite B-001
Northampton, MA 01060   413-584-0184
                                         800-666-2665
                                   Fax: 413-584-6184
                                 brbooks@yahoo.com
                                www.brooklinebooks.com
Carol Davis, Co-Author
Alice Yang, Co-Author
This collection of papers describes collaborabative efforts for such classroom settings as preschools, elementary, middle and high schools, for content area teaching and into the transition to work. Each chapter describes actual practice and analyzes what is required to accomplish this collaboration. *$19.95*
Paperback
ISBN 1-57139 -66-4

2593 Teachig Students with Special Needs in Inclusive Classrooms
SAGE Publications
2455 Teller Rd
Thousand Oaks, CA 91320   800-818-7243
                                      Fax: 800-583-2665
                                 orders@sagepub.com
                                   us.sagepub.com
Diane P. Bryant, Author
Brian P. Bryant, Author
Deborah D. Smith, Author
Using the research-validated ADAPT framework, Teaching Students with Special Needs in Inclusive Classrooms helps future teachers determine how, when, and with whom to use proven academic and behavioral interventions to obtain the best outcomes for students with disabilities. This book will provide the skills and inspiration that teachers need to make a positive difference in the educational lives of struggling learners.

2594 Teaching Adults with Learning Disabilities
Krieger Publishing Company
1725 Krieger Drive
Malabar, FL 32902   321-724-9542
                                     800-724-0025
                               Fax: 321-951-3671
                          info@krieger-publishing.com
                             www.krieger-publishing.com
Dale R. Jordan, Author
R Krieger, Owner
Designed to teach literacy providers and classroom instructors how to recognize specific learning disability (LD) patterns and block reading, spelling, writing and arithmetic skills in students of all ages. One of the major problems faced by literary providers is keeping low-skill adults involved in basic education programs long enough to increase their literacy skills to the level of success. Shows instructors in adult education how to modify teaching strategies. *$25.50*
160 pages
ISBN 0-894649-10-8

2595 Teaching Children With Autism in the General Classroom
Prufrock Press
PO Box 8813
Waco, TX 76714-8813   254-756-3337
                                         800-998-2208
                                   Fax: 254-756-3339
                                 gbates@prufrock.com
                                   www.prufrock.com
Joel McIntosh, Publisher & Marketing Director
Ginny Bates, Customer Service and Office Manager
Lacy Compton, Senior Editor
Rachel Taliaferro, Editor
Provides an introduction to inclusionary practices that serve children with autism, giving teachers the practical advice they need to ensure each students receives the quality education he or she deserves. *$39.95*
350 pages Paperback
ISBN 1-593633-64-6

2596 Teaching Disturbed and Disturbing Students: An Integrative Approach
Sage Publications
2455 Teller Road
Thousand Oaks, CA 91320   805-499-9774
                                         800-818-7243
                                   Fax: 800-583-2665
                               books.claim@sagepub.com
                                   www.sagepub.com
Sara Miller McCune, Founder, Publisher, Chairperson
Blaise R Simqu, President & CEO
Tracey A. Ozmina, Executive Vice President & Chief
Paul Zionts, Author
Using an integrative approach, this text provides teachers with step-by-step details of how to implement and use the methods and theories discussed in each chapter. *$37.00*
465 pages

2597 Teaching Every Child Every Day: Integrated Learning in Diverse Classrooms
Brookline Books
8 Trumbull Rd
Suite B-001
Northampton, MA 01060   413-584-0184
                                         800-666-2665
                                   Fax: 413-584-6184
                                 brbooks@yahoo.com
                                www.brooklinebooks.com
Karen R. Harris, Editor
Steve Graham, Editor
Don Deshler, Editor
Collection of articles addressing various issues in teaching to diverse classrooms—varied in need for special educational services, English proficiency, and socioeconomic and racial backgrounds. *$19.95*
224 pages Paperback
ISBN 0-57129 -40-0

2598 Teaching Infants and Preschoolers with Handicaps
Mc Graw- Hill, School Publishing
PO Box 182604
Columbus, OH 43218   877-833-5524
                                     800-338-3987
                               Fax: 609-308-4480
                        customer.service@mheducation.com
                               www.mcgraw-hill.com
David Levin, President/Chief Executive Officer
David Stafford, Senior Vice President/General Counsel
Maryellen Valaitis, Senior Vice President Human Resources
Patrick Milano, Chief Financial Officer & Chief Administrative Officer
Builds a solid background in early childhood special education.
380 pages

2599 Teaching Language-Disabled Children: A Communication/Games Intervention
Brookline Books
8 Trumbull Rd
Ste B-001
Northampton, MA 01060

413-584-0184
800-666-2665
Fax: 413-584-6184
brbooks@yahoo.com
www.brooklinebks.com

Susan Conant, Author
Offers practitioners specific teaching methods for helping students play communication games. *$22.95*
185 pages Hardcover 1983
ISBN 0-914797-38-7

2600 Teaching Learners with Mild Disabilities: Integrating Research and Practice
Brooke Publishing
PO Box 10624
Baltimore, MD 21285-0624

410-337-9580
800-638-3775
Fax: 410-337-8539
custserv@brookespublishing.com
www.brookespublishing.com

Ruth Lyn Meese, Author
Melissa A. Behm, Executive Vice President
Paul H. Brooks, Chairman of the Board
Cary Gold, Educational Sales Representative
The authors illustrate interactions among regular teachers, special education teachers and students with mild disabilities through the use of hypothetical case studies of students and teachers.
496 pages Paperbound
ISBN 0-53421 -02-0

2601 Teaching Mathematics to Students with Learning Disabilities
Sage Publications
2455 Teller Road
Thousand Oaks, CA 91320

805-499-9774
800-818-7243
Fax: 800-583-2665
books.claim@sagepub.com
www.sagepub.com

Sara Miller McCune, Founder, Publisher, Chairperson
Blaise R Simqu, President & CEO
Nancy S. Bley, Co-Author
Carol A. Thornton, Co-Author
New trends in school mathematics have surfaced in the teaching world. Problem-solving, estimation and the use of computers are receiving considerably greater emphasis than in the past and these areas are included in the new text. *$38.00*
486 pages Paperback

2602 Teaching Mildly and Moderately Handicapped Students
Allyn & Bacon
75 Arlington St
Suite 300
Boston, MA 02116-3988

617-848-7500
800-852-8024
Fax: 617-944-7273
www.home.pearsonhighered.com

Bill Barke, CEO
Nancy Forfyth, President
B. R. Gearheart, Author
Kevin Stone, Vice President, National Sales M
A cross-categorical text providing teaching ideas and techniques. Focuses on the theme of learning as a constructive process in which the learner interacts with the environment, constructing new systems of knowledge, Behavioral techniques and research are also presented.
hardcover
ISBN 0-138939-00-4

2603 Teaching Reading to Children with Down Syndrome: A Guide for Parents and Teachers
Woodbine House
6510 Bells Mill Rd
Bethesda, MD 20817-1636

301-897-3570
800-843-7323
Fax: 301-897-5838
info@woodbinehouse.com
www.woodbinehouse.com

Irvin Shapell, Publisher
Patricia Logan Oelwein, Author
Beth Binns, Special Marketing Manage
Fran Marinaccio, Marketing Manager
Guide includes lessons customized to meet the unique interests and learning style of each child. *$16.95*
371 pages Paperback
ISBN 0-933149-55-7

2604 Teaching Reading to Disabled and Handicapped Learners
Charles C. Thomas
2600 S First St
Springfield, IL 62704-4730

217-789-8980
800-258-8980
Fax: 217-789-9130
books@ccthomas.com
www.ccthomas.com

Michael P. Thomas, President
Freddie W. Litton, Author
Harold D. Love, Author
Designed as a text for undergraduate and graduate students, this resource aims to help the many children, adolescents, and adults who encounter difficulty with reading. It guides prospective and present special education teachers in assisting and teaching handicapped learners to read. The text integrates traditional methods with newer perspectives to provide and effective reading program in special education. *$43.95*
252 pages Paperback 1996
ISBN 0-398062-48-X

2605 Teaching Reading to Handicapped Children
Love Publishing Company
9101 E Kenyon Ave
Suite 2200
Denver, CO 80237-1854

303-221-7333
Fax: 303-221-7444
lpc@lovepublishing.com
www.lovepublishing.com

Charles H. Hargis, Author
The author covers skills teaching through letter sound association, word identification, synthetic and analytic methods and others, plus testing and assessment. *$24.95*
ISBN 0-89108 -13-5

2606 Teaching Self-Determination to Students with Disabilities
Brookes Publishing
PO Box 10624
Baltimore, MD 21285-0624

410-337-9580
800-638-3775
Fax: 410-337-8539
custserv@brookespublishing.com
www.brookespublishing.com

Michael L. Wehmeyer, Co-Author
Martin Agran, Co-Author
Paul H. Brooks, Chairman of the Board
Cary Gold, Educational Sales Representative
Basic skills for successful transition. This teacher-friendly source will help educators prepare students with disabilities with the specific skills they need for a satisfactory, self-directed life once they leave school. *$34.95*
384 pages Paperback
ISBN 1-55766 -02-5

2607 **Teaching Students with Learning Problems**
McGraw-Hill School Publishing
PO Box 182604
Columbus, OH 43218 877-833-5524
800-338-3987
Fax: 609-308-4480
customer.service@mheducation.com
www.mcgraw-hill.com
David Levin, President/Chief Executive Officer
David Stafford, Senior Vice President/General Counsel
Maryellen Valaitis, Senior Vice President Human Resources
Patrick Milano, Chief Financial Officer & Chief Administrative Officer
Expanded coverage of learning strategies, generalization training, self-monitoring techniques, and techniques for increasing the time students spend on academic tasks.
608 pages

2608 **Teaching Students with Learning and Behavior Problems**
Sage Publications
2455 Teller Road
Thousand Oaks, CA 91320 805-499-9774
800-818-7243
Fax: 800-583-2665
books.claim@sagepub.com
www.sagepub.com
Sara Miller McCune, Founder, Publisher, Chairperson
Blaise R Simqu, President & CEO
Sharon R. Vaughn, Co-Author
Candace S. Bos, Co-Author
$65.00
444 pages Paperback
ISBN 0-890799-28-4

2609 **Teaching Students with Mild and Moderate Learning Problems**
Allyn & Bacon Longman College Faculty
75 Arlington St
Suite 300
Boston, MA 02116-3988 617-367-0025
800-852-8024
Fax: 617-367-2155
www.home.pearsonhighered.com
Bill Barke, CEO
John Langone, Author
Kevin Stone, Vice President, National Sales M
Kevin Stone, Vice President, National Sales M
Provides teachers with skills for assisting students with mild to moderate handicaps in making successful transitions in school and community environments.
496 pages
ISBN 0-205123-62-7

2610 **Teaching Students with Moderate/Severe Disabilities, Including Autism**
Charles C. Thomas
2600 S First St
Springfield, IL 62704-4730 217-789-8980
800-258-8980
Fax: 217-789-9130
books@ccthomas.com
www.ccthomas.com
Michael P. Thomas, President
Elva Duran, Author
This resource and guide was written to help teachers, parents, and other caregivers provide the best educational opportunities for their students with moderate and severe disabilities. The author addresses functional language and other language intervention strategies, vocational training, community based instruction, transition and postsecondary programming, the adolescent student with autism, students with multiple disabilities, parent and family issues, and legal concerns. *$58.95*
416 pages Paperback
ISBN 0-398067-01-5

2611 **Teaching Students with Special Needs in Inclusive Settings**
Allyn & Bacon
75 Arlington St
Suite 300
Boston, MA 02116-3988 617-848-7500
800-852-8024
Fax: 617-944-7273
www.home.pearsonhighered.com
Tom E.C. Smith, Co-Author
Edward A. Polloway, Co-Author
James Patton, Co-Author
Carol A. Dowdy, Co-Author
This text is intended to be a survey text providing practical guidance to general education teachers. It will help them to meet the diverse needs of students with disabilities.
544 pages
ISBN 0-20527-16-6

2612 **Teaching Young Children to Read**
Brookline Books
8 Trumbull Rd
Suite B-001
Northampton, MA 01060 413-584-0184
800-666-2665
Fax: 413-584-6184
brbooks@yahoo.com
www.brooklinebooks.com
Dolores Durkin, Author
John P.
Detailed instructions on teaching reading to preschoolers. Gradually develops full fluency. *$16.95*
192 pages Paperback
ISBN 0-57129-48-6

2613 **Teaching the Bilingual Special Education Student**
Ablex Publishing Corporation
P.O.Box 811
Stamford, CT 06904-811 *Fax:* 201-767-6717
ISBN 0-89391-23-4

2614 **Teaching the Learning Disabled Adolescent: Strategies and Methods**
Love Publishing Company
9101 E Kenyon Ave
Ste 2200
Denver, CO 80237-1813 303-221-7333
Fax: 303-221-7444
lpc@lovepublishing.com
www.lovepublishing.com
Gordon R. Alley, Author
This book gives expert strategies and methods for teaching learning disabled adolescents how, rather than what, to learn. *$39.95*
360 pages Hardcover 1979
ISBN 0-891080-94-5

2615 **Teaching the Mentally Retarded Student: Curriculum, Methods, and Strategies**
Allyn & Bacon
75 Arlington St
Suite 300
Boston, MA 02116-3988 617-367-0025
800-852-8024
Fax: 617-367-2155
www.home.pearsonhighered.com
Bill Barke, CEO
Richard L. Luftig, Author
Nancy Forfyth, President
Kevin Stone, Vice President, National Sales M
Represents a comprehensive approach to curriculum, methods and strategies for teaching the mildly mentally retarded student.
640 pages hardcover
ISBN 0-205102-62-X

2616   Technology and Handicapped People
Springer Publishing Company
11 W 42nd St
15th Floor
New York, NY   10036-8002   212-431-4370
                                   877-687-7476
                              Fax: 212-941-7842
                              cs@springerpub.com
                              www.springerpub.com
Dr. Ursula Springer, President
Ted Nardin, CEO
James C. Costello, Vice President, Journal Publishi
James C. Costello, Vice President, Journal Publishing
Important information for concerned professionals about new re-
habilitation techniques and treatments for handicapped people.
$29.95
224 pages Hardcover
ISBN 0-82614-10-8

**2617   Textbooks and the Student Who Can't Read Them: A Guide
for Teaching Content**
Brookline Books
8 Trumbull Rd
Suite B-001
Northampton, MA   01060   413-584-0184
                                 800-666-2665
                            Fax: 413-584-6184
                            brbooks@yahoo.com
                            www.brooklinebooks.com
Paperback
ISBN 0-91479-57-3

2618   The Education of Children with Acquired Brain Injury
David Fulton Publishers (Routledge)
711 Third Ave
New York, NY   10017   212-216-7800
                         Fax: 212-564-7854
                         orders@taylorandfrancis.com
                         www.routledge.com
Sue Walker, Author
Beth Wicks, Author
Teachers have to be aware of their pupils' special educational
needs. Find out what an acquired brain injury is and how to maximize learning opportunities for those with the condition with this
book.
128 pages

**2619   The Fundamentals of Special Education: A Practical Guide
for Every Teacher**
Corwin Press Inc.
2455 Teller Rd
Thousand Oaks, CA   91320   805-499-9734
                                   800-233-9936
                              Fax: 805-499-5323
                              order@corwin.com
                              us.corwin.com
Bob Algozzine, Author
Jim Ysseldyke, Author
This guide highlights major concepts in special education-from
disability categories, identification issues, and IEPs to appropriate learning environments and the roles general and special
educators play.
104 pages

**2620   The K&W Guide to Colleges for Studentswith Learning
Disabilties (13th Edition)**
The Princeton Review - Penguin Random House
1745 Broadway
New York, NY   10019   212-782-9000
                         customerservice@penguinrandomhouse.com
                         www.penguinrandomhouse.com
848 pages Paperback 1916
ISBN 1-101920-38-6

2621   There's a Hearing Impaired Child in My Class
Gallaudet University Bookstore
800 Florida Ave NE
Washington, DC   20002-3600   202-651-5000
                                     800-451-1073
                                Fax: 202-651-5489
                                TTY: 888-630-9347
                                clerc.center@gallaudet.edu
Debra Nussbaum, Author
Dr. T Alan Hurwitz, President
Edward Bosso, Vice President for Administratio
Donald Beil, Chief of Staff
This complete package provides basic facts about deafness, prac-
tical strategies for teaching hearing impaired children, and the
question-and-answer information for all students. *$16.95*
44 pages

2622   Toward Effective Public School Program for Deaf Students
Teachers College Press
525 W 120th St
New York, NY   10027-6605   212-678-3000
                                   800-575-6566
                              Fax: 212-678-4149
                              webcomments@tc.columbia.edu
                              www.tc.columbia.edu
Susan H. Fuhrman, Ph.D., President of the College
Harvey Spector, Vice President for Finance and Administration
*Suzanne M. Murphy, Vice President for Development and External
Affairs*
*Janice S. Robinson, Vice President for Diversity and Community
Affairs*
This book translates research and data into useable recommenda-
tions and possible courses of action for organizing effective pub-
lic school programs for deaf students. *$22.95*
272 pages Paperback
ISBN 0-807731-59-5

**2623   Treating Adults with Disabilities: Access and
Communication**
World Institute on Disability
3075 Adeline Street
Suite 155
Berkeley, CA   94703   510-225-6400
                         Fax: 510-225-0477
                         TTY:510-225-0478
                         wid@wid.org
                         www.wid.org
Paul W. Schroeder, Chairman
Linda M. Dardarian, Vice Chairman
Mary Brooner, Treasurer
Cassandra Malry, Secretary
This training curriculum is for medical professionals who want to
improve the quality of care for people with disabilities and
chronic illnesses. Also covers architectural, communication, attitudinal and economic policy barriers to quality health care and
specific skills to increase good communication and rapport.
$6.50
63 pages Paperback

2624   Treating Cerebral Palsy for Clinicians by Clinicians
Sage Publications
2455 Teller Road
Thousand Oaks, CA   91320   805-499-9774
                                   800-818-7243
                              Fax: 800-583-2665
                              books.claim@sagepub.com
                              www.sagepub.com
Sara Miller McCune, Founder, Publisher, Chairperson
Blaise R Simqu, President & CEO
Tracey A. Ozmina, Executive Vice President & Chief
Eugene T. McDonald, Editor
A clinical manual for professionals beginning to work with per-
sons who have cerebral palsy. *$31.00*
312 pages

2625 Treating Disordered Speech Motor Control
Sage Publications
2455 Teller Road
Thousand Oaks, CA 91320　　　805-499-9774
　　　　　　　　　　　　　　　800-818-7243
　　　　　　　　　　　　Fax: 800-583-2665
　　　　　　　　　　　books.claim@sagepub.com
　　　　　　　　　　　　　www.sagepub.com
Sara Miller McCune, Founder, Publisher, Chairperson
Blaise R Simqu, President & CEO
Deanie Vogel, Author
Michael Cannito, Editor
This book about neuromotor disturbances of speech production is
aimed at practicing professionals and advanced graduate stu-
dents interested in the neuropathologies of communication.
$36.00
410 pages

2626 Treating Families of Brain Injury Survivors
Springer Publishing Company
11 W 42nd St
15th Floor
New York, NY 10036-8002　　　212-431-4370
　　　　　　　　　　　　　　　877-687-7476
　　　　　　　　　　　　Fax: 212-941-7842
　　　　　　　　　　　cs@springerpub.com
　　　　　　　　　　　　www.springerpub.com
Dr. Ursula Springer, President
Ted Nardin, CEO
James C. Costello, Vice President, Journal Publishi
James C. Costello, Vice President, Journal Publishing
Provides the mental health practitioner with a comprehensive
program for helping families of head injury survivors cope with
the change in their lives. Includes background on medical aspects
of head injury, family structure functioning and special needs of
various family members.
220 pages
ISBN 0-82616 -20-1

**2627 Understanding and Teaching Emotionally Disturbed
Children & Adolescents**
Sage Publications
2455 Teller Road
Thousand Oaks, CA 91320　　　805-499-9774
　　　　　　　　　　　　　　　800-818-7243
　　　　　　　　　　　　Fax: 800-583-2665
　　　　　　　　　　　　　www.sagepub.com
Sara Miller McCune, Founder, Publisher, Chairperson
Blaise R Simqu, President & CEO
Tracey A. Ozmina, Executive Vice President & Chief
Phyllis L. Newcomer, Author
The teacher's handbook provides information that will change
misconceptions about children who are frequently labeled as
emotionally disturbed. It also gives information about a wide variety of intervention methods and approaches for use in educational settings. *$41.00*
620 pages Hardover

**2628 Using the Dictionary of Occupational Titles in Career
Decision Making**
Stout Vocational Rehab Institute
University of Wisconsin Stou
Menomonie, WI 54751　　　715-232-2470
　　　　　　　　　　　　Fax: 715-232-5008
　　　　　　　　　　　　luij@uwstout.edu
　　　　　　　　　　　　www.svri.uwstout.edu
John Lui, Contact Person
This is a self-study manual for learning how to use the 1991 U.S.
Department of Labor's Dictionary of Occupational Titles. It
gives the DOT user a tool to understand the DOT and then put its
information to work. Shows how to quickly obtain information
about the work performed in 12,741 occupations listed and described in the DOT and the worker requirements for those occupations. *$24.00*
142 pages Softcover

2629 VBS Special Education Teaching Guide
Life Way Christian Resources Southern Baptist Conv
1 Lifeway Plz
Nashville, TN 37234-1001　　　615-251-2000
　　　　　　　　　　　　　　　www.lifeway.com
Tom Hellam, VP of Executive Communications a
Thom Rainer, President & CEO
This book contains teaching plans for five bible study sessions
with reproducible handouts for learners. The plans use
multisensory, experiential-based learning activities designed for
adults and older youth who have mental retardation. Suggestions
for Bible learning, crafts, recreation, snacks and theme interpretation are included. Designed primarily for Vacation Bible
School, but may be used in camp/retreat settings. *$9.95*
56 pages Yearly

2630 Vermont Interdependent Services Team Approach (VISTA)
Brookes Publishing
PO Box 10624
Baltimore, MD 21285-624　　　410-337-9580
　　　　　　　　　　　　　　　800-638-3775
　　　　　　　　　　　　Fax: 410-337-8539
　　　　　　　　　custserv@brookespublishing.com
　　　　　　　　　　　www.brookespublishing.com
Paul Kelly, National Textbook Sales Manager
Tracy Gray, Educational Sales Manager
Paul Brooks, President
A guide to coordinating educational support services. This man-
ual enables IEP team members to fulfill the related services provi-
sions of IDEA as they make effective support services decisions
using a collaborative team approach. *$27.95*
176 pages Spiral bound
ISBN 1-55766 -30-4

2631 What School Counselors Need to Know
Council for Exceptional Children
2900 Crystal Dr.
Suite 1000
Arlington, VA 22202-3557　　　888-232-7733
　　　　　　　　　　　　　　TTY:866-915-5000
　　　　　　　　　　　　service@cec.sped.org
　　　　　　　　　　　　　www.cec.sped.org
Barbara E. Baditoi, Co-Author
Pamelia E. Brott, Co-Author
This book provides counselors (and school administrators) with
essential information to make the most of their participation in
providing special education services.

**2632 When You Have a Visually Impaired Student in Your
Classroom: A Guide for Teachers**
American Foundation for the Blind
2 Penn Plaza
Suite1102
New York, NY 10121　　　212-502-7600
　　　　　　　　　　　　　800-232-5463
　　　　　　　　　　Fax: 888-545-8331
　　　　　　　　　　　afbinfo@afb.net
　　　　　　　　　　　　afb.org
Carl Augusto, President
This guide provides information on students' abilities and needs,
resources and educational team members, federal special educa-
tion requirements, and technology materials used by students.
$9.95
84 pages
ISBN 0-891283-93-5

**2633 Working Bibliography on Behavioral and Emotional
Disorders**
Natl. Clearinghouse for Alcohol & Drug Information
1 Choke Cherry Road
Rockville, MD 20857　　　301-468-2600
　　　　　　　　　　　　877-SAM-SA 7
　　　　　　　　　　Fax: 301-468-6433
Lizabeth J Foster, Librarian/Info. Resource Manager
Pamela S. Hyde, Administrator
NCADI is a service of the U.S. Substance Abuse and Mental
Health Services Administration. As the national focal point for

information on alcohol and other drugs, NCADI collects, prepares, classifies, and distributes information about alcohol, tobacco and other drugs, prevention strategies and materials, research, treatment, etc.
40 pages

2634 Working Together with Children and Families: Case Studies
Brookes Publishing Company
PO Box 10624
Baltimore, MD 21285-624

410-337-9580
800-638-3775
Fax: 410-337-8539
custerv@brookespublishing.com
www.brookespublishing.com

Paul Kelly, National Textbook Sales Manager
Tracy Gray, Educational Sales Manager
Paul Brooks, Owner
Early interventionists will be able to bridge the gap between theory and practice with this edited collection of case studies.
$23.00
336 pages
ISBN 1-557661-23-5

2635 Working with Visually Impaired Young Students: A Curriculum Guide for 3 to 5 Year Olds
Charles C. Thomas
2600 S First St
Springfield, IL 62704-4730

217-789-8980
800-258-8980
Fax: 217-789-9130
books@ccthomas.com
www.ccthomas.com

Michael P. Thomas, President
Ellen Trief, Editor
The first step in the education process of a visually impaired child is the early identification and treatment by an eye care specialist. This book is geared to the age of birth through 3-years. Available in cloth, paperback and hardcover. *$42.95*
194 pages Paperback
ISBN 0-398068-75-2

Testing Resources

2636 ADD-SOI Center, The
2007 Cedar Avenue
Manhattan Beach, CA 90266

310-546-6500
Fax: 310-546-9068
ADDSOI@aol.com
www.addsoi.com

2637 AEPS Child Progress Report: For Children Ages Birth to Three
Brookes Publishing
PO Box 10624
Baltimore, MD 21285-624

410-337-9580
800-638-3775
Fax: 410-337-8539
custserv@brookespublishing.com
www.brookespublishing.com

Paul Kelly, National Textbook Sales Manager
Tracy Gray, Educational Sales Manager
Paul Brooks, Owner
This chart helps monitor change by visually displaying current abilities, intervention targets, and child progress. In packages of 30. *$18.00*
6 pages Gate-fold
ISBN 1-55766-65-0

2638 AEPS Data Recording Forms: For Children Ages Birth to Three
Brookes Publishing
PO Box 10624
Baltimore, MD 21285-624

410-337-9580
800-638-3775
Fax: 410-337-8539
custserv@brookespublishing.com
readplaylearn.com

Paul Brooks, Owner
Melissa Behm, Executive Vice President
These forms can be used by child development professionals on four separate occasions to pinpoint and then monitor a child's strengths and needs in the six key areas of skill development measured by the AEPS Test. Packages of 10. *$23.00*
36 pages Saddle-stiched
ISBN 1-55766 -97-2

2639 AEPS Measurement for Birth to Three Years
Brookes Publishing
PO Box 10624
Baltimore, MD 21285-624

410-337-9580
800-638-3775
Fax: 410-337-8539
custserv@brookespublishing.com
www.brookespublishing.com

Paul Kelly, National Textbook Sales Manager
Tracy Gray, Educational Sales Manager
Paul Brooks, Owner
This dynamic volume explains the Assessment, Evaluation and Programming System, provides the complete AEPS Test and parallel assessment/evaluation tools for families and includes the forms and plans needed for implementation. *$39.00*
352 pages

2640 AEPS Measurement for Three to Six Years
Brookes Publishing
PO Box 10624
Baltimore, MD 21285-624

410-337-9580
800-638-3775
Fax: 410-337-8539
custserv@brookespublishing.com
www.brookespublishing.com

Paul Kelly, National Textbook Sales Manager
Tracy Gray, Educational Sales Manager
Paul Brooks, Owner
Resources in early childhood, early intervention, inclusive and special education, developmental disabilities, learning disabilities, communication and language, behavior, and mental health.
$57.00
400 pages Spiral-bound
ISBN 1-55766 -87-1

2641 AIR: Assessment of Interpersonal Relations
Sage Publications
2455 Teller Road
Thousand Oaks, CA 91320

805-499-0721
800-818-7243
Fax: 800-583-2665
info@sagepub.com
www.sagepub.com

Sara Miller McCune, Founder, Publisher, Chairperson
Blaise R Simqu, President & CEO
A thoroughly researched and standardized clinical instrument assessing the quality of adolescents' interpersonal relationships in a hierarchical fashion, including global relationship quality and relationship quality with three domains: Family, Social and Academic. *$89.00*

2642 ALST: Adolescent Language Screening Test
Sage Publications
2455 Teller Road
Thousand Oaks, CA 91320
805-499-0721
800-818-7243
Fax: 800-583-2665
info@sagepub.com
www.sagepub.com

Sara Miller McCune, Founder, Publisher, Chairperson
Blaise R Simqu, President & CEO
Provides speech/language pathologists and other interested professionals with a rapid thorough method for screening adolescents (ages 11-17). *$119.00*

2643 Adaptive Mainstreaming: A Primer for Teachers and Principals, 3rd Edition
Longman Publishing Group
1330 Avenue of the Americas
New York, NY 10019
212-641-2400
800-745-8489
wendy.spiegel@pearsoned.com
www.pearson.com

Glen Moreno, Chairman
Marjorie Scardino, Chief Executive Officer
An introduction to education for handicapped and gifted students. Presents research-based rationales for teaching exceptional students in the least restrictive environment. Provides historical perspectives, offers realistic descriptions of prevailing practices in the field, and reviews trends and new directions.
366 pages Paperback
ISBN 0-582285-04-6

2644 Ages & Stages Questionnaires
Brookes Publishing
PO Box 10624
Baltimore, MD 21285-624
410-337-9580
800-638-3775
Fax: 410-337-8539
custserv@brookespublishing.com
www.brookespublishing.com

Paul Kelly, National Textbook Sales Manager
Tracy Gray, Educational Sales Manager
Paul Brooks, Owner
ASQ is an economical and field-tested system for identifying whether infants and young children may require further developmental evaluation and offers a screening and tracking program that helps early intervention professionals, service coordinators, and administrators maximize financial resources while promoting the health and growth of the children they serve. Set includes 11 color-coded, reproducible questionnaires, 11 reproducible, age appropriate scoring sheets. *$135.00*

2645 American College Testing Program
500 Act Drive
PO Box 168
Iowa City, IA 52243-168
319-337-1000
Fax: 319-339-3021
act.org

John Whitmore, CEO
Mark D Musik, President Emeritus
An independent, nonprofit organization that provides a variety of educational services to students and their parents, to high schools and colleges, and to professional associations and government agencies.

2646 Assessing Students with Special Needs
Longman Publishing Group
10 Bank Street
9th Floor
White Plains, NY 10606-1933
914-993-5000
www.ablongman.com

Joanne Dresner, President
Step-by-step guide to informal, classroom assessment of students with special needs.
174 pages Paperback
ISBN 0-801301-77-7

2647 Assessment Log & Developmental Progress Charts for the CCPSN
Brookes Publishing
P.O.Box 10624
Baltimore, MD 21285-624
410-337-9580
800-638-3775
Fax: 410-337-8539
custserv@brookespublishing.com
www.brookespublishing.com

Paul Kelly, National Textbook Sales Manager
Tracy Gray, Educational Sales Manager
Paul Brooks, Owner
This 28-page booklet allows readers to actually chart the ongoing progress of each preschool child. Available in packages of 10.
$22.00
28 pages Saddle-stiched
ISBN 1-55766 -39-5

2648 Assessment of Learners with Special Needs
Allyn & Bacon
75 Arlinton Street
Ste 300
Boston, MA 2116-3988
617-848-7500
800-852-8024
Fax: 617-944-7273
www.ablongman.com

Bill Barke, CEO
Thomas Longman, Founder
The central goal of this book is to help teachers become sophisticated, informed test consumers in terms of choosing, using and interpreting commercially prepared tests for their special needs students.
508 pages Casebound
ISBN 0-205227-33-3

2649 Benchmark Measures
Educators Publishing Service
PO Box 9031
Cambridge, MA 2139
617-547-6706
800-225-5750
Fax: 888-440-2665
feedback@epsbooks.com
www.epsbooks.com

Charles H Heinle, VP
Alexandra S Bigelow, Author
Gunnar Voltz, President
Ungraded test containing three sequential levels that assess alphabet and dictionary skills, reading, handwriting and spelling, and correspond to the first three schedules of the Alphabetic Phonics curriculum. The tests can be used at any level to measure a student's general knowledge of phonics. *$64.40*
Kit

2650 Brain Clinic, The
19 West 34th Street
Penthouse
New York, NY 10001
212-268-8900
nurosvcs@aol.com
thebrainclinic.com

Dr. James Lawrence Thomas, Director
The brain clinic offers diagnosis and Treatment of ADD, Learning Disabilities, Migraines, and Traumatic Brain Injury.

2651 CREVT: Comprehensive Receptive and Expressive Vocabulary Test
Sage Publications
2455 Teller Road
Thousand Oaks, CA 91320
805-499-0721
800-818-7243
Fax: 800-583-2665
info@sagepub.com
www.sagepub.com

Sara Miller McCune, Founder, Publisher, Chairperson
Blaise R Simqu, President & CEO
A new, innovative, efficient measure of both receptive and expressive oral vocabulary. The CREVT has two subtests and is

based on the most current theories of vocabulary development, suitable for ages 4 through 17. *$174.00*
Complete Kit

2652   Carolina Curriculum for Preschoolers with Special Needs
Brookes Publishing
P.O.Box 10624
Baltimore, MD 21285-624   410-337-9580
                                            800-638-3775
                                        Fax: 410-337-8539
                        custserv@brookespublishing.com
                            www.brookespublishing.com
Paul Kelly, National Textbook Sales Manager
Tracy Gray, Educational Sales Manager
Paul Brooks, Owner
This curriculum provides detailed teaching and assessment techniques, plus a sample 28-page Assessment Log that shows readers how to chart a child's individual progress. This guide is for children between 2 and 5 in their developmental stages who are considered at risk for developmental delay or who exhibit special needs. *$35.95*
352 pages Spiral-bound
ISBN 1-557660-32-8

2653   Center For Personal Development
405 North Wabash Ave.
Suite 208 & 1114
Chicago, IL 60611   312-755-7000
                                        Fax: 312-755-7001
                            info@chicagotherapist.com
                            www.chicagotherapist.com
Steven Nakisher, Licensed Clinical Psychologist
Cara McCanse, Licensed Clinical Psychologist
Sarah Kremarik, Staff Psychotherapist
Amy Zurawic, Staff Psychotherapist
The Center for Personal Development was founded in 1998 to provide a diverse range of high-quality mental health services.

2654   Center for Human Potential
525 East 100 South
Suite 120
Salt Lake City, UT 84102   801-483-2447
                                             801-486-8705
                                            www.c4hp.com
C. Brendan Hallett Psy.D., Clinical Director
Michael DeCaria, Ph.D., Licensed Clinical Psychologist
Annice Julian, Psy.D., Licensed Clinical Psychologist
Stephanie Voigt, Psy.D., Licensed Clinical Psychologist
Center for Human Potentialis a human services company that helps individuals, businesses and organizations reach their potential by achieving balance in the fundamental areas of life: Emotional, Physical, Mental, Spiritual and Financial. We offer individual, couples, and family counseling to help with a number of issues.

2655   Center for Neuropsychology, Learning & Development
1955 Pauline Blvd
Suite 100A
Ann Arbor, MI 48103   734-994-9466
                                        Fax: 734-994-9465
                                            www.cnld.org
Roger E. Lauer, Clinical Director
Jodene Goldenring Fine, Ph.D., Licensed Psychologist
CNLD was founded over 20 years ago to serve Southeast Michigan and the greater Ann Arbor community by providing quality mental health care for children, adolescents, adults and families.

2656   Center for Student Health and Counseling
1825 SW Broadway
Portland, OR 97201   503-725-3000
                                             800-547-8887
                                        Fax: 503-725-4882
                                    askadm@pdx.edu
                            www.pdx.edu/shac/ldadhd

2657   Children's Assessment Center, The
2500 Bolsover St.
Houston, TX 77005   713-986-3300
                                        Fax: 713-986-3553
                                    info@cac.hctx.net
                                    cachouston.org
Brady E. Crosswell, Chairman
Gail Prather, President
Elaine Stolte, Executive Director
Mark Anderson, Treasurer
The Children's Assessment Center (CAC)provides a safe haven to sexually abused children and their families.

2658   Cognitive Solutions Learning Center
2409 N. Clybourn Ave.
Chicago, IL 60614   773-755-1775
                                        Fax: 773-439-5499
                                    info@helpforld.com
                        www.helpforld.com/index.php/about-us/
Dr. Ari Goldstein, Founder
Jason Almodovar, M.S.Ed., Office Manager
Cognitive Solution offers a broad range of services, including learning disability and attention deficit disorder assessment and remediation, executive functions training, and the latest neurofeedback technologies.

2659   DAYS: Depression and Anxiety in Youth Scale
Sage Publications
2455 Teller Road
Thousand Oaks, CA 91320   805-499-0721
                                             800-818-7243
                                        Fax: 805-376-9443
                                    info@sagepub.com
                                    www.sagepub.com
Sara Miller McCune, Founder, Publisher, Chairperson
Blaise R Simqu, President & CEO
A unique battery of three norm-references scales useful in identifying major depressive disorder and overanxious disorders in children and adolescents. *$129.00*
Complete Kit

2660   DOCS: Developmental Observation Checklist System
Pro- Ed Publications
8700 Shoal Creek Blvd
Austin, TX 78757-6897   512-451-3246
                                             800-897-3202
                                        Fax: 800-397-7633
                                    general@proedinc.com
                                    www.proedinc.com
Donald D Hammill, Owner
Courtney King, Marketing Coordinator
A three-part system for the assessment of very young children with respect to general development, adjustment behavior and parent stress and support. *$124.00*

2661   Dennis Developmental Center
1 Children's Way
Little Rock, AR 72202-3591   501-364-1100
                                        TTY:501-364-1184
                                    www.archildrens.org

2662   Developmental Services Center
Therapeutic Nursery Program
4525 Lee St NE
Washington, DC 20019   202-388-3216
                                        Fax: 202-576-8799
Alice Anderson
Offers assessment information and evaluation for developmentally delayed students.

2663 Frames of Reference for the Assessment of Learning Disabilities
Brookes Publishing
P.O.Box 10624
Baltimore, MD 21285-624   410-337-9580
                                  800-638-3775
                            Fax: 410-337-8539
                    custserv@brookespublishing.com
                       www.brookespublishing.com
Paul Kelly, National Textbook Sales Manager
Tracy Gray, Educational Sales Manager
Paul Brooks, Owner
New views on measurement issues. Here you'll find an in=depth look at the fundamental concerns facing those who work with children with learning disabilities - assessment and identification. *$55.00*
672 pages Hardcover
ISBN 1-55766 -38-3

2664 How to Conduct an Assessment
FSSI
3905 Huntington Dr
Amarillo, TX 79109-4047   806-353-1114
                            Fax: 806-353-1114
                        webmaster@winfssi.com
                           www.winfssi.com
Ed Hammer, Owner
The Functional Skills Screening Inventory,this behavioral check-list allows for parents and professionals to observe critical behaviors in individuals with multiple disabilities (7 years to adult years).

2665 Inclusive & Heterogeneous Schooling: Assessment, Curriculum, and Instruction
Brookes Publishing
P.O.Box 10624
Baltimore, MD 21285-624   410-337-9580
                                  800-638-3775
                            Fax: 410-337-8539
                    custserv@brookespublishing.com
                       www.brookespublishing.com
Paul Kelly, National Textbook Sales Manager
Tracy Gray, Educational Sales Manager
Paul Brooks, Owner
Presents methods for successfully restructuring classrooms to enable all students, particularly those with disabilities, to flourish. Provides specific strategies for assessment, collaboration, classroom management, and age-specific instruction. *$34.95*
448 pages Paperback
ISBN 1-557662-02-9

2666 Infant & Toddler Convection of Fairfield: Falls Church
Joseph Willard Health Center
3750 Old Lee Hwy
Fairfax, VA 22030-1806   703-246-7180
                            Fax: 703-246-7307
Susan Sigler, Program Coordinator
Allan Phillips, Director Early Intervention
Offers assessments, evaluations and educational/therapeutic infant programs for parents infants and toddlers birth to age 3.
Sliding Scale

2667 K-BIT: Kaufman Brief Intelligence Test
AGS
Ste 1000
5910 Rice Creek Pkwy
Shoreview, MN 55126-5023   651-287-7220
                                  800-328-2560
                            Fax: 800-471-8457
                         agsmail@agsnet.com
                           www.agsnet.com
Kevin Brueggeman, President
Robert Zaske, Market Manager
Quick and easy-to-use, KBIT assesses verbal and non-verbal abilities through two reliable subtests - vocabulary and matricies.
$ 124.95
Ages 4-90

2668 K-FAST: Kaufman Functional Academic Skills Test
AGS
Ste 1000
5910 Rice Creek Pkwy
Shoreview, MN 55126-5023   651-287-7220
                                  800-328-2560
                            Fax: 800-471-8457
                         agsmail@agsnet.com
                           www.agsnet.com
Robert Zaske, Market Manager
Helps assess a person's capacity to function effectively in society regarding functional reading and math skills. *$99.95*
Ages 15-85+

2669 K-SEALS: Kaufman Survey of Early Academic and Language Skills
AGS
5910 Rice Creek Pkwy
Shoreview, MN 55126-5025   651-287-7220
                                  800-328-2560
                            Fax: 800-471-8457
                         agsmail@agsnet.com
                           www.agsnet.com
Kevin Brueggeman, President
Robert Zaske, Market Manager
An individually administered test of children's of both expressive and receptive skills, pre-academic skills and articulation. K-SEALS offers reliable scores usually in less than 25 minutes. *$ 179.95*
Ages 3-0; 6-11

2670 KLST-2: Kindergarten Language Screening Test Edition, 2nd Edition
Sage Publications
2455 Teller Road
Thousand Oaks, CA 91320   805-499-9774
                                  800-818-7243
                            Fax: 800-583-2665
                          info@sagepub.com
                           www.sagepub.com
Paul Kelly, National Textbook Sales Manager
Blaise R Simqu, President & CEO
Identifies children who need further diagnostic testing to determine whether or not they have language deficits that will accelerate academic failure. *$94.00*

2671 Kaufman Test of Educational Achievement(K-TEA)
AGS
PO Box 99
Circle Pines, MN 55014-99   800-328-2560
                            Fax: 800-471-8457
                         agsmail@agsnet.com
                           www.agsnet.com
Robert Zaske, Marketing Manager
Kevin Brueggeman, President
K-TEA is an individually administered diagnostic battery that measures reading, mathematics, and spelling skills. Setting the standards in achievement testing today, K-TEA Comprehensive provides the complete diagnostic information you need for educational assessment and program planning. The Brief Forum is indispensable for school and clinical psychologists, special education teachers when a quick a measure of achievement is needed. *$249.95*

2672 Learning House
264 Church Street
Guilford, CT 6437   203-453-3691
                     www.learninghouse-ct.com
Susan Santora, Founder and Director
Learning House is a professional community committed to enhancing the lives of individuals with dyslexia and other learning disabilities in safe and supportive surroundings.

2673   LearningRx
5085 List Drive
Suite 200
Colorado Springs, CO   80919   719-264-8808
                                                www.learningrx.com
Dr. Ken Gibson, Founder
LearningRx is a brain training program.

**2674   Life Centered Career Education: A Contemporary Based
Approach**
Council for Exceptional Children
2900 Crystal Dr.
Suite 1000
Arlington, VA   22202-3557   888-232-7733
                                                TTY:866-915-5000
                                                service@cec.sped.org
                                                www.cec.sped.org
Alexander T. Graham, Executive Director
Sharon Rodriguez, Senior Executive Assistant
Craig Evans, Director of Operations
Provides a framework for building 97 functional skill competencies appropriate for preparing for adult life and special education students. *$28.00*
175 pages

2675   Measure of Cognitive-Linguistic Abilities(MCLA)
Speech Bin
PO Box 1579
Appleton, VA   54912-1579   772-770-0007
                                                888-388-3224
                                                Fax: 888-388-6344
                                                onlinehelp@schoolspecialty.com
                                                www.speechbin.com
Jan J Binney, Senior Editor
A diagnostic test of cognitive-linguistic abilities of adolescents and adults with traumatically induced brain injuries. High level. Normed. *$89.00*
100 pages
ISBN 0-93785-72-

2676   Miriam
501 Bacon Avenue
St. Louis, MO   63119-1512   314-968-3893
                                                Fax: 314-962-0482
                                                athorp@miriamstl.org
                                                www.miriamstl.org/learning-center
Andrew Thorp, Executive Director
Sarah Scott, Development Director
Carol Faust, Business Manager
Tam Nguyen, Facilities Manager
Miriam improves the quality of life for children with learning disabilities and their families through innovative and comprehensive programs.

2677   Neuropsychology Assessment Center
One University Place
Chester, PA   19013   610-499-4273
                                                www.widenernac.org
Mary F. Lazar, PsyD, Director
Wendy M. Sarkisian, PsyD, Assistant Director
Located in the Philadelphia area, the Neuropsychology Assessment Center (NAC) specializes in neuropsychological evaluations for the investigation of a variety of psychological conditions.

2678   ONLINE
West Virginia Research and Training Center
P.O.Box 1004
Institute, WV   25112-1004   304-766-9495
                                                800-624-8284
                                                Fax: 304-766-2689
                                                www.icdi.wvu.edu
Clifford Lantz, President
A quarterly newsletter offering information about hardware technology, software (commercial and home grown); applications that work and bonuses such as an exchange program for copyright-free software. *$25.00*
Quarterly

2679   OWLS: Oral and Written Language Scales LC/OE & WE
AGS
P.O.Box 99
Circle Pines, MN   55014-99   800-328-2560
                                                Fax: 800-471-8457
                                                agsmail@agsnet.com
                                                www.agsnet.com
Kevin Brueggeman, President
Robert Zaske, Market Manager
One kit provides an assessment of listening comprehension while the other assesses oral expression tasks: semantic, syntactic, pragmatic, and supralinguistic aspects of language. Written Expression may be administered individually or in small groups. *$249.95*

2680   PAT-3: Photo Articulation Test
Sage Publications
2455 Teller Road
Thousand Oaks, CA   91320   805-499-9774
                                                800-818-7243
                                                Fax: 800-583-2665
                                                info@sagepub.com
                                                www.sagepub.com
Paul Kelly, National Textbook Sales Manager
Blaise R Simqu, President & CEO
This test consists of 72 color photographs. The first 69 photos test consonants and all but one vowel and one diphthong. The remaining pictures test connected speech and the remaining vowel and diphthong. *$144.00*
Complete Kit

2681   Peabody Early Experiences Kit (PEEK)
AGS
P.O.Box 99
Circle Pines, MN   55014-99   800-328-2560
                                                Fax: 800-471-8457
                                                agsmail@agsnet.com
                                                www.agsnet.com
Kevin Brueggeman, President
Robert Zaske, Market Manager
1,000 activities and all the materials you need to build youngsters' cognitive, social and language skills. Manuals, puppets, manipulatives, picture card deck, picture mini decks and more to teach early development concepts. *$789.95*

**2682   Peabody Individual Achievement Test-Revised Normative
Update (PIAT-R-NU)**
AGS
P.O.Box 99
Circle Pines, MN   55014-99   800-328-2560
                                                Fax: 800-471-8457
                                                agsmail@agsnet.com
                                                www.agsnet.com
Kevin Brueggeman, President
Robert Zaske, Market Manager
PIAT-R-NU is an efficient individual measure of academic achievement. Reading, mathematics, and spelling are assessed in a simple, non-threatening format that requires only a pointing response for most items. This multiple choice format makes the PIAT-R ideal for assessing individuals who hesitate to give a spoken response, or have limited expressive abilities. *$289.98*

2683   Peabody Language Development Kits (PLDK)
AGS
P.O.Box 99
Circle Pines, MN   55014-99   800-328-2560
                                                Fax: 800-471-8457
                                                agsmail@agsnet.com
                                                www.agsnet.com
Kevin Brueggeman, President
Robert Zaske, Market Manager
The main goals of the Peabody Kit language program are to stimulate overall language skills in Standard English and, for each

level of the program, advance children's cognitive skills about a year. $ 649.95
Level P
ISBN 0-88671 -25-1

2684 Pediatric Early Elementary (PEEX II) Examination
Educators Publishing Service
625 Mount Auburn Street
3rd Floor
Cambridge, MA 2138- 3039   617-547-6706
     800-225-5750
Fax: 888-440-2665
feedback@epsbooks.com
www.epsbooks.com

Charles H Heinle, VP
Alexandra S Bigelow, Author
Gunnar Voltz, President
Assesses the second-fourth grade child's performance on thirty-two tasks in six specific areas of development: fine-motor function, language, gross-motor function, memory, visual processing, and delayed recall. At three points during the exam, the child is rated on selective attention and behavior and effect.
$15.40 - $93
ISBN 0-83888 -80-6

2685 Pediatric Exam of Educational-PEERAMID Readiness at Middle Childhood
Educators Publishing Service
625 Mount Auburn Street
3rd Floor
Cambridge, MA 2138- 3039   617-547-6706
     800-225-5750
Fax: 888-440-2665
feedback@epsbooks.com
www.epsbooks.com

Charles H Heinle, VP
Alexandra S Bigelow, Author
Gunnar Voltz, President
Assesses the 4th-10th grade child's performance on thirty-one tasks in six specific areas: minor neurological indicators, fine-motor function, language, gross-motor function, temporal-sequential organization, and visual processing. Complete set.
$15.40 - $109
ISBN 0-83888 -99-3

2686 Pediatric Examination of Educational Readiness
Educators Publishing Service
625 Mount Auburn Street
3rd Floor
Cambridge, MA 2139- 3039   617-547-6706
     800-225-5750
Fax: 888-440-2665
feedback@epsbooks.com
www.epsbooks.com

Charles H Heinle, VP
Alexandra S Bigelow, Author
Gunnar Voltz, President
Assesses the Pre-1st grade child's performance on twenty-nine tasks in six specific areas of development: orientation, gross-motor, visual-fine motor, sequential, linguistic and preacademic learning. The child is rated on ten dimensions of selective attention/activity processing efficiency and adaptation. Complete set.
$12.85 - $86.40
ISBN 0-83888 -80-1

2687 Pediatric Extended Examination at-PEET Three
Educators Publishing Service
625 Mount Auburn Street
3rd Floor
Cambridge, MA 2138- 3039   617-547-6706
     800-225-5750
Fax: 888-440-2665
feedback@epsbooks.com
www.epsbooks.com

Charles H Heinle, VP
Alexandra S Bigelow, Author
Gunnar Volta, President

Assesses the preschool-age child's performance on twenty-eight tasks in five basic areas of development: gross-motor, language, visual-fine motor, memory, and intersensory integration. Complete set.
$13.75 - $126
ISBN 0-83888 -79-4

2688 Pre-Reading Screening Procedures
Educators Publishing Service
625 Mount Auburn Street
3rd Floor
Cambridge, MA 2138- 3039   617-547-6706
     800-225-5750
Fax: 888-440-2665
feedback@epsbooks.com
www.epsbooks.com

Charles H Heinle, VP
Alexandra S Bigelow, Author
Gunnar Voltz, President
This revised group test, for grades K-1, evaluates auditory, visual and kinesthetic strengths in order to identify children who may have some form of dyslexia or specific language disability. $ 18.00
Grades K-1
ISBN 0-83885 -23-4

2689 Preparing for ACT Assessment
American College Testing Program
500 Act Drive
PO Box 168
Iowa City, IA 52243-168   319-337-1000
Fax: 319-339-3021
act.org

Richard L Ferguson, CEO
Designed to help high school students ready themselves for the ACT Assessment's subject area tests, explains the purposes of the four tests, describes their content and format, provides tips and exercises to improve student's test-taking skills and includes a complete sample text with scoring key.

2690 Psycho-Educational Assessment of Preschool Children
National Association of School Psychologists
Ste 105
4340 East West Hwy
Bethesda, MD 20814-4468   301-657-0270
     866-331-NASP
Fax: 301-657-0275
ADMIN@SOELIN.COM
soelin.com

Susan Gorin, Executive Director
This is a contributed text on assessing specific skills of preschool children.
592 pages

2691 RULES: Revised
Speech Bin
PO Box 1579
Appleton, VA 54912-1579   772-770-0007
     888-388-3224
Fax: 888-388-6344
customercare@schoolspecialty.com
www.speechbin.com

Jan J Binney, Senior Editor
Treatment program for young children who have phonological disorders. $43.95
280 pages
ISBN 0-93785 -51-3

2692 Receptive-Expressive Emergent-REEL-2 Language Test, 2nd Edition
Sage Publications
2455 Teller Road
Thousand Oaks, CA 91320   805-499-9774
                                 800-818-7243
                                 Fax: 800-583-2665
                                 info@sagepub.com
                                 www.sagepub.com
Paul Kelly, National Textbook Sales Manager
Blaise R Simqu, President & CEO
A revision of the popular scale used for the multidimensional analysis of emergent language. The REEL-2 is specifically designed for use with a broad range of at risk infants and toddlers in the new multidisciplinary programs developing under P.L. 99-457. *$79.00*

2693 Regents' Center for Learning Disorders
103 Hooper Street
Athens, GA 30602   706-542-4589
                          Fax: 706-583-0001
                          rcld@uga.edu
                          rcld.uga.edu
Tasha Falkingham, Office Manage
Karen Myers, Budget Analyst
Trish Foels, Staff Clinician, Psychologist
Lisa McLain, Staff Clinician
Provide assessment, training, research, andresources related to students who have learning disorders (e.g., Attention-Deficit/Hyperactivity Disorder, Autism Spectrum Disorders, Learning Disabilities, Emotional Disorders, and Traumatic Brain Injury) that impact their functioning in the academic environment.

2694 Schmieding Developmental Center
519 Latham Drive
Lowell, AR 72745   479-750-0125
                          Fax: 479-750-0323
                          www.archildrens.org
Mary Ann Scott, PhD, Program Director
Damon Lipinski, PhD, Program Director
Jerie Beth Karkos, MD, Medical Director
Arkansas Children's Hospital (ACH) is the a pediatric medical center in Arkansas.

2695 Slingerland Screening Tests
Educators Publishing Service
625 Mount Auburn Street
3rd Floor
Cambridge, MA 2138- 3039   617-547-6706
                                   800-435-7728
                                   Fax: 888-440-2665
                                   feedback@epsbooks.com
                                   www.epsbooks.com
Charles H Heinle, VP
Alexandra S Bigelow, Author
Gunnar Voltz, President
These tests, by Beth Slingerland, for individuals or groups of children, grades 1-6, identify children who show indications of having specific language disability in reading, handwriting, spelling or speaking. Form D evaluates personal orientation in time and space as well as the ability to express ideas in writing. *$14.80 - $27.45*
ISBN 0-83882 -02-2

2696 Special Needs Advocacy Resource Book
Prufrock Press
PO Box 8813
Waco, TX 76714-8813   800-998-2208
                             Fax: 800-240-0333
                             info@prufrock.com
                             www.prufrock.com
Joel McIntosh, Publisher & Marketing Director
Rich Weinfield, Author
Michelle Davis, Author
Subtitle: What You Can Do Now to Advocate for Your Exceptional Child's Education. This is a unique hadnbook that teaches parents how to work with schools to achieve optimal learning situations and accommodations for their child's needs. *$19.95*
328 pages
ISBN 1-593633-09-7

2697 Speech Bin
PO Box 1579
Appleton, VA 54912-1579   772-770-0007
                                  888-388-3224
                                  Fax: 888-388-6344
                                  customercare@schoolspecialty.com
                                  www.speechbin.com
Jan J Binney, Senior Editor
Catalog offering test materials, assessment information, books and special education resources for speech-language pathologists, occupational and physical therapists, audiologists, and other rehabilitation professionals in schools, hospitals, clinics and private practices.
ISSN 4773-324

2698 Stuttering Severity Instrument for Children and Adults
Psychological & Educational Publications
P.O.Box 520
Hydesville, CA 95547-520   707-768-1807
                                   800-523-5775
                                   Fax: 800-447-0907
                                   www.psych-edpublications.com
Morrison Gardner, President
With this tool teachers can determine whether to schedule a child for therapy or to evaluate the effects of treatment.

2699 Taking Part: Introducing Social Skills to Young Children
AGS
P.O.Box 99
Circle Pines, MN 55014-99   800-328-2560
                                    Fax: 800-471-8457
                                    www.agsnet.com
Kevin Brueggeman, President
Robert Zaske, Market Manager
The first social skills curriculum to be linked directly to an assessment tool. More than 30 lessons correlate with the skills assessed by the Social Skills Rating System, a multirater approach to assessing prosocial and problem behaviors. *$149.95*

2700 Teaching of Reading: A Continuum from Kindergarten through College, The
AVKO Educational Research Foundation
3084 Willard Rd
Birch Run, MI 48415-9404   810-686-9283
                                   866-285-6612
                                   Fax: 810-686-1101
                                   webmaster@avko.org
                                   avko.org
Don Mc Cabe, Executive Director
A textbook for teaching teachers how to teach language arts with lessons about dyslexia, phonics, learning to write, the connection between reading and spelling, and diagnostic and prescriptive tests. Free as an e-book for Foundation members. *$49.95*
364 pages

2701 Test Critiques: Volumes I-X
Sage Publications
2455 Teller Road
Thousand Oaks, CA 91320   805-499-9774
                                  800-818-7243
                                  Fax: 800-583-2665
                                  info@sagepub.com
                                  www.sagepub.com
Paul Kelly, National Textbook Sales Manager
Blaise R Simqu, President & CEO
Provides the professional and nonprofessional with in-depth, evaluative studies of more than 800 of the most widely used of these assessment instruments. *$649.00*

2702 Test of Early Reading Ability Deaf or Hard of Hearing
Pro- Ed Publications
8700 Shoal Creek Blvd
Austin, TX 78757-6816

512-451-3246
800-897-3202
Fax: 800-397-7633
general@proedinc.com
www.proedinc.com

Donald D Hammill, Owner
Courtney King, Marketing Coordinator
This adaptation of the TERA-2 for simultaneous communication of American Sign Language is the ONLY individually administered test of reading designed for children with moderate to profound sensory hearing loss. *$169.00*
Complete Kit

2703 Test of Language Development: Primary
Sage Publications
2455 Teller Road
Thousand Oaks, CA 91320

805-499-9774
800-818-7243
Fax: 800-583-2665
info@sagepub.com
www.sagepub.com

Paul Kelly, National Textbook Sales Manager
Blaise R Simqu, President & CEO
TOLD P:2 and TOLD 1:2 are the most popular tests of spoken language used by clinicians today. They are used to identify children who have language disorders and to isolate the particular types of disorders they have. Primary Edition for ages 1-4 to 8-11: Intermediate Edition for ages 8-6 to 12-11.

2704 Test of Mathematical Abilities, 2nd Edition
Sage Publications
2455 Teller Road
Thousand Oaks, CA 91320

805-499-9774
800-818-7243
Fax: 800-583-2665
info@sagepub.com
www.sagepub.com

Paul Kelly, National Textbook Sales Manager
Blaise R Simqu, President & CEO
The latest version was developed for use in grades 3 through 12. It measures math performance on the two traditional major skill areas in math as well as attitude, vocabulary and general application of math concepts in real life. *$84.00*

2705 Test of Nonverbal Intelligence, 3rd Edition
Sage Publications
2455 Teller Road
Thousand Oaks, CA 91320

805-499-9774
800-818-7243
Fax: 800-583-2665
info@sagepub.com
www.sagepub.com

Paul Kelly, National Textbook Sales Manager
Blaise R Simqu, President & CEO
A language-free measure of intelligence, aptitude and reasoning. The administration of the test requires no reading, writing, speaking or listening on the part of the test subject. The items included in this test are problem-solving tasks that increase in difficulty. Each item presents a set of figures in which one or more components is missing. The test items include one or more of the characteristics of shape, position, direction, rotation, contiguity, shading, size, movement or pattern. *$229.00*
Complete Kit

2706 Test of Phonological Awareness
Sage Publications
2455 Teller Road
Thousand Oaks, CA 91320

805-499-9774
800-818-7243
Fax: 800-583-2665
info@sagepub.com
www.sagepub.com

Paul Kelly, National Textbook Sales Manager
Blaise R Simqu, President & CEO

Measures young children's awareness of the individual sounds in words. Children who are sensitive to the phonological structure of words in oral language have a much easier time learning to read than children who are not. *$143.00*

2707 Test of Written Spelling, 3rd Edition
Pro- Ed Publications
8700 Shoal Creek Blvd
Austin, TX 78757-6897

512-451-3246
800-897-3202
Fax: 800-397-7633
general@proedinc.com
www.proedinc.com

Donald D Hammill, Owner
Courtney King, Marketing Coordinator
This revised edition assesses the student's ability to spell words whose spellings are readily predictable in sound-letter patterns, words whose spellings are less predictable and both types of words considered together. *$74.00*

2708 Texas Scottish Rite Hospital for Children
2222 Welborn Street
Dallas, TX 75219

214-559-5000
Fax: 800-421-1121
tsrhdv@tsrh.org
www.tsrhc.org

Robert L. Walker, President/ CEO
Mark G. Bateman, SVP, Public Relations
Leslie A. Clonch, Jr., Vice President/ CIO
Stephanie Brigger, Vice President, Development
TSRHC treats children with orthopedic conditions, such as scoliosis, clubfoot, hand disorders, hip disorders and limb length differences, as well as certain related neurological disorders and learning disorders, such as dyslexia.

2709 Treatment and Learning Centers
2092 Gaither Road
Suite 100
Rockville, MD 20850

301-424-5200
Fax: 301-424-8063
TTY:301-424-5203
info@ttlc.org
www.ttlc.org

Dr Lisa Lenhart, Tutoring/Testing Services Dir
Diagnostic evaluations are provided on an individual basis to identify the learning differences and needs of students who may have learning disabilities, or who are struggling with the academic environment.

2710 Woodcock Reading Mastery Tests
Pearson
5601 Green Valley Dr
Bloomington, MN 55437-1099

800-627-7271
Fax: 800-232-1223
pearsonassessments@pearson.com
www.pearsonassessments.com

Christine Carlson, Product Manager
Doug Kubach, President & CEO
The Woodcock Reading Mastery Tests - Revised provides an interpretive system and age range to help you assess reading skills of children and adults. Two forms, G and II, make it easy to test and retest, or you can combine the results of both forms for a more comprehensive assessment. Revised with recent updates. *$329.95*

2711 Young Children with Special Needs: A Developmentally Appropriate Approach
Allyn & Bacon
75 Arlington Street
Ste 300
Boston, MA 2116-3988

617-848-7500
800-852-8024
Fax: 617-944-7273
www.ablongman.com

Bill Barke, CEO
Thomas Longman, Founder

This book is designed to prepare students in making curriculum decisions in order to care for and foster the development of young children with special needs in normal early childhood settings.
270 pages
ISBN 0-20518-94-X

Treatment & Training

2712   ABLE Program MCC-Longview
3200 Broadway
Kansas City, MO   64111-2105   816-604-1000
                                        Fax: 816-672-2719
                                        joan.bergstrom@mcckc.edu
                                        mcckc.edu/ABLE

Joan Bergstrom, Director
Kay Owens, Administrative Assistant
Intensive support services program for post secondary students with neurological disabilities. The ABLE Program can be reached at http://mcckc.edu/ABLE

2713   Academy for Guided Imagery
30765 Pacific Coast Hwy
Ste 355
Malibu, CA   90265-3643   800-726-2070
                                        Fax: 800-727-2070
                                        info@acadgi.com
                                        www.acadgi.com

David E Bresler, President
The Academy aims to teach people to access and use the power of the mind/body connection for healing, and to further understanding of the imagery process in human life and development. They provide systematic training and guidance to health professionals who are interested in the use of Guided Imagery in their practice. The Academy's Imagery Store offers guided imagery CDs, DVDs and books for self-healing.

2714   Adventist HealthCare
820 West Diamond Avenue
Suite 600
Gaithersburg, MD   20878   301-315-3030
                                        Fax: 301-315-3000
                                        www.adventisthealthcare.com

David E. Weigley, M.B.A., Chairman
Robert T. Vandeman, Vice-Chair
Terry Forde, Secretary
dventist HealthCare, based in Gaithersburg, Md., is a not-for-profit organization of dedicated professionals who work together to provide excellent wellness, disease management and health-care services to the community.

2715   Asthma & Allergy Education for Worksite Clinicians
Asthma and Allergy Foundation of America
8201 Corporate Drive
Suite 1000
Landover, VA   20785   202-466-7643
                                        800-727-8462
                                        Fax: 202-466-8940
                                        info@aafa.org
                                        aafa.org

Bill Mc Lin, President & CEO
Helen Taylor, Information Specialist
Developed to teach health professionals in the worksite about asthma and allergies and ultimately improve the health of the employees who have theses de\iseases. The program gives worksite clinicians the knowledge and tools they need to give employees guidance on how to control environmental factors both in the home and in the workplace, self-manage thier asthma and/or allergies and to determaine if ti is necessary for employees to see an allergist if symptoms persist.

2716   Asthma & Allergy Essentials for Children's Care Provider
Asthma and Allergy Foundation of America
8201 Corporate Drive
Suite 1000
Landover, VA   20785   202-466-7643
                                        800-727-8462
                                        Fax: 202-466-8940
                                        info@aafa.org
                                        aafa.org

Bill Mc Lin, President & CEO
Helen Taylor, Information Specialist
Course gives child care providers the tools and knowledge they need to care for children with asthma and allergies. During the interactive, three hour program, a trained health professional teaches providers how to recognize the signs and symptoms of an asthma or allergy episode, how to institute environmental control measures to prevent these episodes, and how to properly use medication and the tools for asthma management. In areas of the country serviced by AAFA's 14 chapters.

2717   Asthma Care Training for Kids (ACT)
Asthma and Allergy Foundation of America
8201 Corporate Drive
Suite 1000
Landover, VA   20785   202-466-7643
                                        Fax: 202-466-8940
                                        info@aafa.org
                                        www.aafa.org

Bill Mc Lin, President & CEO
Helen Taylor, Information Specialist
Interactive program for children ages seven to 12 and their families. Children and their families attend three group sessions seperately to learn their own unique styles and then come together at the end of each session to share their knowledge.

2718   Ayurvedic Institute
PO Box 23445
Albuquerque, NM   87292-1445   505-291-9698
                                        800-863-7721
                                        Fax: 505-294-7572
                                        ayurveda.com

Wynn Werner, Administrator
Directed by Dr. Vasant Lad, trains people in Ayurveda.

2719   Brooks Rehabilitation Hospital
3599 University Blvd S
Jacksonville, FL   32216   904-345-7600
                                        Fax: 904-345-7619
                                        www.brookshealth.org

Gary W. Sneed, Chairman
Michael Spigel, President/ COO
Douglas M. Baer, Chief Executive Officer
Bruce M. Johnson, Vice-Chair
Brooks Rehabilitation provides the most advanced therapy and medical care.

2720   Center for Parent Information and Resources
35 Halsey St
4th Floor
Newark, NJ   07102   973-642-8100
                                        malizo@spannj.org
                                        www.parentcenterhub.org

Debra A. Jennings, Director
Myriam Alizo, Project Assistant
Lisa K☐pper, Product Development Coordinator
Jessica Wilson, Communications Director
The Center for Parent Information and Resources (CPIR) serves as a central resource of information and products to the community of Parent Training Information (PTI) Centers and the Community Parent Resource Centers (CPRCs), so that they can focus their efforts on serving families of children with disabilities.

2721 Center for Spinal Cord Injury Recovery
261 Mack
Detroit, MI 48201 866-724-2368
Fax: 313-745-9064
krodgers@dmc.org
www.centerforscirecovery.org
Krystal Rodgers, Administrative Assistant
The Center for SCI Recoveryr (CSCIR)provides long-term, high intensity, non-traditional, activity based therapy to maximize recovery.

2722 Cottage Rehabilitation Hospital
400 W. Pueblo Street
Santa Barbara, CA 93105 805-682-7111
mzate@sbch.org
www.cottagehealth.org

2723 Courage Kenny Rehabilitation Institute
800 E. 28th St.
Minneapolis, MN 55407 612-863-4200
866-880-3550
couragekenny@allina.com
www.couragecenter.org

2724 Harriet & Robert Heilbrunn Guild School
JGB Audio Library for the Blind
15 W 65th St
New York, NY 10023-6601 212-769-6200
800-284-4422
Fax: 212-769-6266
info@JGB.org
www.JGB.org
Allen R Morse, JD, PhD, President & CEO
Ken Stanley, Manager
A Jewish Guild for the blind.

2725 Howard School, The
1192 Foster St NW
Atlanta, GA 30318-4329 404-377-7436
Fax: 404-377-0884
admissions@howardschool.org
howardschool.org
Marifred Cilella, Head Of School
The Howard School educates students 5 years old through 12th grade with language learning disabilities and learning differences. Small student/teacher ratios allow for instruction that is personalized to complement the individual learning styles and to help each student understand his/her learning process. Students gain the tools and strategies needed to become independent, life-long learners.

2726 Kennedy Krieger Institute
707 North Broadway
Baltimore, MD 21205 443-923-9200
800-873-3377
888-554-2080
www.kennedykrieger.org
Jennifer Accardo, M.D., Neurologist
Adrianna Amari, Ph.D., Training & Research Coordinator
Roberta L. Babbitt, Ph.D, Program Director
Amy J. Bastian, Ph.D., P.T., Chief Science Officer
Kennedy Krieger Institute is an internationally recognized institution dedicated to improving the lives of children and young adults with pediatric developmental disabilities and disorders of the brain, spinal cord and musculoskeletal system, through patient care, special education, research, and professional training.

2727 Kessler Rehabilitation Corporation
1199 Pleasant Valley Way
West Orange, NJ 7052 973-731-3600
Fax: 973-243-6819
www.kessler-rehab.com
Robert Brehm, President
Bruce M. Gans, MD, Executive VP and CMO
Sue Kida, PT, MHA, VP and COO
Steven Kirshblum, MD, Medical Director

Provides physical medicine and rehabilitation by delivering an exceptional patient experience through the integration of quality care, technology, education, research, and advocacy.

2728 Lake Michigan Academy
West Michigan Learning Disabilities Foundation
2428 Burton St SE
Grand Rapids, MI 49546-4806 616-464-3330
Fax: 616-285-1935
www.wmldf.org
Amy Barto, Executive Director
Is a private day school for children with learning disabilities.

2729 Levinson Medical Center
98 Cutter Mill Road
Suite 90
Great Neck, NY 11021 516-482-2888
800-334-7323
Fax: 516-482-2480
drlevinson@aol.com
www.dyslexiaonline.com
Dr. Harold Levinson, Psychiatrist, Neurologist
Carolyn Malman, Office Manager
Lisa Danziger, Patient Coordinator
Dr. Margaret , Neurological Test & Evaluations
Medical center groundbreaking medical treatment offers rapid and often dramatic help to suffering dyslexic/ADHD children and adults

2730 Mad Hatters: Theatre That Makes a World of Difference
P.O.Box 50002
Kalamazoo, MI 49005-2 *Fax:* 269-385-5868
Bobbe A Luce, Executive Director
A nationally-known theater which has presented effective and innovative programs to more than 175,000 people in over 1,150 performances in the past 15 years. Our presentations and training programs are a proven method of changing attitudes and behaviors. The Mad Hatters is a leader in the field of sensitivity training to build community and foster the inclusion of all people in society. Fees: $500-$4000 per program, depending on topic and audience.

2731 MedStar National Rehabilitation Network
102 Irving Street NW
Washington, DC 20010 202-877-1000
www.medstarnrh.org

2732 Missouri Rehabilitation Center
One Hospital Drive
Columbia, MO 65212 573-882-4141
www.muhealth.org

2733 Neuroxcel
401 Northlake Blvd.
North Palm Beach, FL 33048 866-391-6247
www.neuroxcel.com

2734 Ramapo Training
Ramapo for Children
Route 52/Salisbury Turnpike
PO Box 266
Rhinebeck, NY 12572 845-876-8403
Fax: 845-876-8414
office@ramapoforchildren.org
www.ramapoforchildren.org
Richard Rosenthal, President
Teri Goldberg Horowitz, First Vice President
Claude Ann Mellins, Ph.D., Vice President
Deusdedi Merced, Esq., Vice President
Ramapo Training was established to provide staff training and program support for educational and recreational programs, especially those that serve children-at-risk and those with special needs.

2735 Sandhills School
1500 Hallbrook Dr
Columbia, SC 29209-4021   803-695-1400
Fax: 803-695-1214
info@sandhillsschool.org
www.sandhillsschool.org
Anne Vickers, Head of School
Erika Senneseth, Asst Head of School
Angela Daniel, Director of Development
Carmen Kennedy, Business Manager
Exists to provide educational programs and intellectual development for average to above average students, six to 15, who learn differently and to promote the development of self-awareness, joy in learning and a vision of themselves as life-long learners.

2736 Senior Program for Teens and Young Adults with Special Needs
Camp J CC
6125 Montrose Rd
Rockville, MD 20852-4860   301-881-0100
Fax: 301-881-6549
jcccamp@jccgw.org
www.jccgw.org
Scott Cohen, President
Mindy Burger, Vice President for Development
The senior Program is a transitional program for teens and young adults with mental retardation, severe learning disabilities and multiple disabilities. Socialization, recreation and independent living skills are enhanced ina fun enviroment. Activities include art, music, recreational swim and more.

2737 Spinal Cord Injury Center
132 S. 10th Street
375 Main Building
Philadelphia, PA 19107   215-955-6579
Fax: 215-955-5152
www.spinalcordcenter.org
Marilyn P. Owens, RN, BSN, Project Coordinator
Brittany Hayes, Research Coordinator
Jacqueline Robinson, Administrative Assistant
Susan Sakers Sammartino, BS, Data Coordinator
SCI provides medical care for their injuries, along with emotional, social, vocational and psychological rehabilitation to cope with the changes in their bodies and in their lifestyles that often result from the injury.

2738 Stanford Health Care
300 Pasteur Drive
Stanford, CA 94304   650-498-3333
800-756-9000
stanfordhealthcare.org
Amir Dan Rubin, President and CEO
Raj Behal, MD, Chief Quality Officer
James Hereford, Chief Operating Officer
Daniel J. Morissette, Chief Financial Officer
Stanford Health Care provides patients with the very best in diagnosis and treatment.

2739 Teacher of Students with Visual Impairments
3635 Coal Mountain Rd.
Cumming, GA 30028 c.willings@teachingvisuallyimpaired.com
www.teachingvisuallyimpaired.com

2740 The Glenholme School
Devereux Advanced Behavioral Health Connecticut
81 Sabbaday Ln.
Washington, CT 06793   860-868-7377
Fax: 860-868-7894
info@theglenholmeschool.org
www.theglenholmeschool.org

2741 UAB Spain Rehabilitation Center
1720 2nd Ave South
Birmingham, AL 35294   205-934-4011
TTY:205-934-4642
www.uab.edu
Ray L. Watts, M.D., President
G. Allen Bolton Jr., VP, Financial Affairs
UAB's missionis to be a research university and academic health center that discovers, teaches and applies knowledge for the intellectual, cultural, social and economic benefit of Birmingham, the state and beyond.

2742 University of Maryland Rehabilitation and Orthopaedic Institute
Uni of MD Rehab & Ortho Institute
2200 Kernan Drive
Baltimore, MD 21207   410-448-2500
888-453-7626
TTY:800-735-2258
www.umrehabortho.org
Cynthia A. Kelleher, MPH, MBA, Interim President and CEO
John P. Straumanis, VP, Medical Affairs
W. Walter Augustin, III, CPA, VP of Financial Services
Cheryl D. Lee, RN, MSN, CRRN, VP, Patient Care Services
University of Maryland Rehabilitation & Orthopaedic Institute (formerly Kernan Hospital), a committed provider of orthopaedic surgery and the largest inpatient rehabilitation hospital and provider of rehabilitation services in the state of Maryland, has been serving the Baltimore community for over 100 years.

2743 Vanguard School, The
Valley Forge Specialized Educational Services
1777 N Valley Rd
Paoli, PA 19301   610-296-6700
Fax: 610-640-0132
www.vanguardschool-pa.org
Tim Lanshe, Director of Education
James Kirkpatrick, CFO
Peg Osborne, Admissions Director
An Approved Private School (APS) for students aged 4-21 years with exceptionalities including autism spectrum disorder, mild emotional disturbances and/or neurological impairments.

2744 Worthmore Academy
3535 Kessler Boulevard East Dr
Indianapolis, IN 46220-5154   317-902-9896
877-700-6516
Fax: 317-251-6516
bjackson@worthmoreacademy.org
www.worthmoreacademy.org
Brenda Jackson, Director
Alyssa Blaire Cook, Assistant Director
A place where children with learning disabilities receive individualized instruction to help remediate his or her condition. The most common learning disabilities we work with are Dyslexic, A.D.D, A.D.H.D, Autism Spectrum (including Asperger's Syndrome), and communication disorders.

Exchange Programs

General

2745 A Guide to International Educational Exchange
Mobility International USA
132 E. Broadway
Suite 343
Eugene, OR   97401-2767

541-343-1284
Fax: 541-343-6812
info@miusa.org
www.miusa.org

Susan Sygall, CEO
A Guide to International Educational Exchange, Community Service and Travel for People with Disabilities includes information travel and international programs, as well as personal experience stories from people with disabilities who have had successful international experiences. *$45.00*
600 pages
ISBN 1-880034-24-7

2746 American Institute for Foreign Study
River Plaza 9 W Broad St
Stamford, CT   6902-3788

203-399-5000
866-906-2437
Fax: 203-399-5590
info@aifs.com
www.aifs.com

William L Gertz, CEO
Organizes cultural exchange programs throughout the world for more than 50,000 students each year and arranges insurance coverage for our own participants as well as participants of other organizations. Also provides summer travel programs overseas and in the US ranging from one week to a full academic year.

2747 American Universities International Programs
307 S College Ave
Fort Collins, CO   80524-2801

970-495-0084
888-730-2847
Fax: 970-495-0114
info@auip.com
www.auip.com

Laurie Klith, Executive Director
Study abroad organization sending students to universities in Australia and New Zealand.

2748 American-Scandinavian Foundation
58 Park Ave
38 Street
New York, NY   10016-3007

212-779-3587
Fax: 212-686-1157
info@amscan.org
scandinaviahouse.org

Edward Gallagher, President
Promotes international understanding through educational and cultural exchange between the United States and Denmark, Finland, Iceland, Norway and Sweden.

2749 Antioch College
One Morgan Place
Yellow Springs, OH   45387-1635

937-319-6082
Fax: 937-319-6085

Mark Roosevelt, President
Thomas Brookley, CFO & COO
Gariot Louima, Chief Communications Officer
Education abroad offers numerous programs which can be included in undergraduate and graduate study programs.

2750 Army and Air Force Exchange Services
PO Box 660202
Dallas, TX   75266-202

214-312-2011
800-527-2345
Fax: 800-446-0163
TTY: 800-423-2011
www.aafes.com

James Moore, Senior VP
MG Bruce Casella, Commander/CEO
Brings a tradition of value, service, and support to its 11.5 million authorized customers at military installations in the United States, Europe and in the Pacific.

2751 Association for International Practical Training
10400 Little Patuxent Pkwy
Suite 250
Columbia, MD 21044-3519

410-997-2200
Fax: 410-992-3924
aipt@aipt.org
aipt.org

Elizabeth Chazottes, CEO
Nonprofit organization dedicated to encouraging and facilitating the exchange of qualified individuals between the US and other countries so they may gain practical work experience and improve international understanding.

2752 Basic Facts on Study Abroad
International Education
809 United Nations Plz
New York, NY   10017-3503

212-883-8200
Fax: 212-984-5452
publications@un.org
iie.org

Allen E Goodman, CEO
Peggy Blumenthal, Executive Vice President
Information book including foreign study planning, educational choices, finances and study abroad programs. *$35.00*
30 pages

2753 Beaver College
Arcadia University
450 S Easton Rd
Glenside, PA   19038-3215

215-572-2901
888-232-8379
Fax: 215-572-2174

Lorna Stern, Deputy Director
One of the largest college-based study abroad programs in the country. Prices from $8000.00 semester to $22000.00 a year.

2754 Buffalo State (SUNY)
1300 Elmwood Ave
South Wing 410
Buffalo, NY   14222-1095

716-878-4620
Fax: 716-878-3054
intleduc@buffalostate.edu
www.buffalostate.edu/studyabroad

Lee Ann Grace, Asst Dean Int'l/Exchange Program
Provides international educational exchange opportunities for students of university age and older through its Office of International Education.

2755 Building Bridges: Including People with Disabilities in International Programs
Mobility International USA
132 E Broadway
Suite 343
Eugene, OR   97401-3155

541-343-1284
Fax: 541-343-6812
info@miusa.org
miusa.org

Susan Sygall, CEO
Michele Scheib, Project Specialist
Melissa Mitchell, Public Relations Coordinator
Empowers people with disabilities around the world through international exhange and international development to achieve their human rights. The international exchange programs usually last two-four weeks and are held throughout the year in the US

and abroad. Activities include living with homestay families, leadership seminars, disability rights workshops, cross cultural learning and teambuilding activities such as river rafting and challenging courses.

2756   Davidson College, Office of Study Abroad
Davidson College
PO Box 7171
Davidson, NC   28035-7171   704-894-2000
                                      Fax: 704-894-2005
                                 kocampbell@davidson.edu
                                      www3.davidson.edu

Carol Quillen, President
Recognizes the value of study abroad for both the devlopment of worl understanding and the development of the student as a broadminded, objective and mature individual.

2757   High School Students Guide to Study, Travel, and Adventure Abroad
300 Fore Street
Portland, ME   4101   207-553-4000
                                      Fax: 207-553-4299
                                        contact@ciee.org
                                          www.ciee.org

Robert E. Fallon, CEO & President
Kenton Keith, Senior Vice President for Progra
This guide provides high school students with all the information they need for a successful trip abroad. Included are sections to help students find out if they're ready for a trip abroad, make the necessary preparations and get the most from their experience. Over 200 programs are described including language study, summer camps, homestays, study tours and work camps. The program descriptions include information for people with disabilities.
ISSN 0312-11

2758   International Christian Youth Exchange
134 W 26th St
New York, NY   10001-6803   212-206-7307
                                      Fax: 212-633-9085
Ed Gragert
Offers participants a unique experience to learn about another culture and make friends from different countries.

2759   International Partnership for Service-Learning and Leadership
1515 SW 5th Avenue
Suite 606
Portland, OR   97201   503-954-1812
                                      Fax: 503-954-1881
                                          info@ipsl.org
                                             ipsl.org

Nevin Brown, President
A not for profit educational organization incorporated in New York State serving students, colleges, universities, service agenices and related organizations around the world by fostering programs that link volunteer service to the community and academic study.

2760   International Student Exchange Programs (I SEP)
1655 N Fort Myer Drive
Suite 400
Arlington, VA   22209   703-504-9960
                                      Fax: 703-243-8070
                                          info@isep.org
                                          www.isep.org

Dr. Thomas Hochstettler, Chair
Dr. Tony Atwater, President
ISEP is a network of 275 post-secondary institutions in the United States and 38 other countries cooperating to provide affordable international educational experiences for a diverse student population.

2761   International University Partnerships
University of Pennsylvania
1011 South Dr
Indiana, PA   15705-1046   724-357-2100
                                      Fax: 724-357-6213
                                             iup.edu

David Werner, President
Offers a variety of international educational exchange programs to students who wish to study overseas.

2762   Lake Erie College
391 W. Washington St.
Painesville, OH   44077   440-296-1856
                                          800-533-4996
                                      Fax: 440-375-7005
                                       admissions@lec.edu
                                           www.lec.edu

Michael Victor, President
Michael Keresman lll, Director
Sends students abroad for a term or longer to develop intellectual awareness and individual maturity.

2763   Lane Community College
4000 E 30th Ave
Eugene, OR   97405   541-463-3100
                                      Fax: 541-463-5201
                                       asklane@lanecc.edu
                                          www.lanecc.edu

Margaret Hamilton, Ph.D, President
Lane Community College offers a wide variety of instructional programs including transfer credit programs, career and technical degree and certificate programs, continuing education noncredit courses, ESL, GED programs, and customized training for local businesses. The college offers support services for those with disabilities through their Center for Accessible Resources.

2764   Lions Clubs International
300 W 22nd St
Oak Brook, IL   60523-8842   630-571-5466
                                      Fax: 630-571-8890
                                       www.lionsclubs.org

Joe Preston, International President
Jitsuhiro Yamada, First Vice President
Robert E. Corlew, Second Vice President
Eric R. Carter, First Year Directors
Over 46,000 individual clubs in over 194 countries and geographical areas which provide community service and promote better international relations. Clubs work with local communities to provide needed and useful programs for sight, diabetes and hearing, and aid in study abroad.

2765   Lisle
900 County Road 269
Leander, TX   78641-1633   512-259-4404
                                          lisle2@io.com

Barbara E Bratton, Owner
Educational organization which works toward world peace and better quality of human life through increased understanding between persons of similar and different cultures.

2766   National 4-H Council
7100 Connecticut Ave
Chevy Chase, MD   20815-4934   301-961-2800
                                      Fax: 301-961-2894
                                           www.4-h.org

Donald Floyd, President
Jennifer Sirangelo, Executive Vice President
4-H opened the door for young people to learn leadership skills and explore ways to give back. 4-H revolutionized how youth connected to practical, hands-on learning experiences while outside of the classroom.

2767 New Directions for People with Disabilities
5276 Hollister Avenue
Suite 207
Santa Barbara, CA 93111-3068   805-967-2841
                                       888-967-2841
                                  Fax: 805-964-7344
                       hello@newdirectionstravel.org
                       www.newdirectionstravel.org

Dee Duncan, Executive Director
Jeanne Mohle, Director of Operations
Danna Mead, Program Director
Colette Piacentini, Business Manager
Provides high quality local, national, and international travel vacations and holiday programs for people with mild to moderate developmental disabilities. Through these programs, people with disabilities are increasingly understood, appreciated and more accepted as important and contributing members of our world.

2768 People to People International
911 Main Street
Suite 2110
Kansas City, MO   64105-2246   816-531-4701
                                  Fax: 816-561-7502
                                       ptpi@ptpi.org
                                       www.ptpi.org

Mary Eisenhower, CEO
Roseanne Rosen, Senior Vice President of Operati
Brian Hueben, Senior Director, Administration
Stacey Chance, Director, Publications
Exchanges international understanding and friendship through educational, cultural and humanitarian activities involving the exchange of ideas and experiences directly among people of different countries and diverse cultures. Is also dedicated to enhancing cross cultural communication within each community and across communities and nations.

2769 Rotary Youth Exchange
Rotary International
1560 Sherman Ave
Evanston, IL   60201-4818   847-866-3000
                                   866-976-8279
                              Fax: 847-328-4101
                       youthexchange@rotary.org
                              www.rotary.org

Kalyan Banerjee, International President
Noel A Bajat, Vice President
Kenneth R Boyd, Director
Elizabeth Demaray, Director
This worldwide organization of business and professional leaders provides humanitarian service, encourages high ethical standards in all vocations, and helps build goodwill and peace in the world. Approximately 1.2 million Rotarians belong to more than 31,000 Rotary clubs located in 167 countries for exchange opportunities.

2770 Scandinavian Exchange
24 Dickinson Street
Amherst, MA   1002   413-253-9737
                       Fax: 413-253-5282
             howery@scandinavianseminar.org
             www.scandinavianseminar.org

Jacqueline D Waldman, CEO
William Kaufmann, Chair
Student exchange program founded in 1949.

2771 Sister Cities International
915 15th Street, NW
4th Floor
Washington, DC   20005   202-347-8630
                           Fax: 202-393-6524
                           info@sister-cities.org
                           sister-cities.org

Patrick Madden, President
Jim Doumas, Executive Vice President, & Inte
A non profit citizen diplomacy network creating and strengthening partnerships between US and international communities in an effort to increase global cooperation at the municipal level, to promote cultural understnading and to stimulate economic devel-

opment. Encourages local community development and volunteer action by motivating and empowering private citizens, municipal officials and business leaders to conduct long term programs of mutual benefits including exchange situations.

2772 State University of New York
1400 Washington Ave
Albany, NY   12222-100   518-442-3300
                           Fax: 518-442-5383
                           ugadmissions@albany.edu
                           www.albany.edu

George Philip, President
Alain Kaloyeros, Senior Vice President & CEO
Susan Phillips, Provost & VP for Academic Affai
James Dias, VP for Research
Offers over 150 international educational exchange programs in 37 different countries. Broad mission of excellence in undergraduate and graduate education, research and public service engages 17,000 diverse students in nine schools and colleges across three campuses.

2773 University of Minnesota at Crookston
2900 University Ave
Crookston, MN   56716-5000   218-281-6510
                                    800-862-6466
                               Fax: 218-281-8050
                               UMCinfo@umn.edu
                               www.crk.umn.edu

Charles Casey, CEO
Eric Kaler, President
The University of Minnesota, Crookston (UMC) is a public, baccalaureate, coeducational institution and a coordinate campus of the University of Minnesota

2774 University of Oregon
5000 N Willamette Blvd
Portland, OR   97203-5798   503-943-8000
                              Fax: 503-725-3067
                              webmaster@up.edu
                              up.edu

Patricia Esley, Manager
Rev.E.Willia Beauchamp, President
James Lyons, VP University Relations
Jim Ravelli, VP for University Research
Study/cultural experience is available in Tokyo and other Japanese cities as part of the Japan Studies Program at the University.

2775 Western Washington University
516 High St
Bellingham, WA   98225-5996   360-650-3000
                                Fax: 360-650-3022
                                www.wwu.edu

Bruce Shepard, President
Paul Dunn, Senior Executive Asst. to the Pr
Barbara Stoneberg, Assistant to the President
Mary Lacher, Receptionist, President & Provis

2776 World Experience Teenage Exchange Program
2440 S Hacienda Blvd
Suite 116
Hacienda Heights, CA 91745-4763   626-330-5719
                                        800-633-6653
                                   Fax: 626-333-4914

Kerry Gonzales, President
Marge Archaumbault, President
Offers a quality and affordable program for over two decades and continues to provide students and host families a youth exchange program based on individual attention, with the help of an international network of overseas directors and USA coordinators.

2777 **World of Options**
Mobility International USA
132 E Broadway
Suite 343
Eugene, OR 97401-3155

541-343-1284
Fax: 541-343-6812
info@miusa.org
miusa.org

Susan Sygall, CEO
Cerise Roth-Vinson, COO
Susan Dunn, Executive Asst. to the CEO
Alison Eker, Project Assistant
Empowering people with disabilities around the world through
international exchange and international development to achieve
their human rights. *$16.00*
338 pages
ISBN 1-880034-01-8

2778 **Youth for Understanding International Exchange**
6400 Goldsboro Road
Suite 100
Bethesda, MD 20817-5841

240-235-2100
800-833-6243
Fax: 240-352-2104
admissions@yfu.org
yfu.org

Rachel Andreson, Founder
Samantha Brizzolara, Chair
Youth for Understanding (YFU) International Exchange, an educational, nonprofit organization, prepares young people for the
opportunities and responsabilities in a changing, independent
world. With YFU, students can choose a year, semenster, or summer program in one or more than 35 countries worldwide. More
than 200,000 young people from more than 50 nations in Asia,
Europe, North and South America, Africa and the Pacific have
participated in YFU exchanges.

Foundations & Funding Resources

Alabama

2779 Alabama Power Foundation
PO Box 2641
Birmingham, AL 35291-11
205-257-2508
800-245-2244
Fax: 205-257-1860
rsking@southernco.com
powerofgood.com

John O. Hudson III, President
Richard King, Director of Charitable Giving
Alisa Summerville, Manager of Charitable Giving
Kim Thrift, Program Manager

Honoring its mission to strengthen the communities the company serves, the foundation focuses its efforts on organizations that support education, civic activities, health services, the environment and the arts. By supporting the state's educational system □ from pre-K to universities □ the foundation is investing in Alabama's future and the well-being of its residents.

2780 Andalusia Health Services
700 River Falls Street
PO Box 667
Andalusia, AL 36420
334-222-2030
Fax: 334-222-7844
chrissie@andalusiachamber.com
www.andalusiachamber.com

Janna McGlamory, President
Debbie Marcum, Vice President
Ashley Eiland, Executive Vice President
Gail Hayes, Treasurer

Only offers grants to the residents of Covington County in Alabama who are pursuing a degree in a medical field.

2781 Arc Of Alabama, The
557 S Lawrence St
Montgomery, AL 36104-4611
334-262-7688
866-243-9557
Fax: 334-834-9737
info@thearcofAl.org
www.thearcofal.org/#!contact/c1d94

Larry Bailey, President
Sherron Culpepper, 1st Vice President
Bruce Koppenhoeffer, 2nd Vice President
Jack Knight, Treasurer

The Arc of Alabama, Inc. is a volunteer-based membership organization made up of individuals with intellectual (such as mental retardation, an old and outdated term seldom used anymore), developmental and other disabilities, their families, friends, interested citizens, and professionals in the disability field.

Alaska

2782 Arc of Alaska
The Arc of Anchorage
2211 Arca Dr
Anchorage, AK 99508-3462
907-277-6677
800-258-2232
Fax: 907-272-2161
TTY: 907-277-0735
info@thearcofanchorage.org

Rod Shipley, President
Dave Falsey, Vice President
Meredith Parham, Secretary
Sharon Purkis, Treasurer

The Arc helps Alaskans who experience developmental disabilities, behavioral health concerns or deafness achieve lives of dignity and independence as valued members of our community.

2783 Rasmuson Foundation
301 West Northern Lights Blvd.
Suite 400
Anchorage, AK 99503
907-297-2700
877-366-2700
Fax: 907-297-2770
rasmusonfdn@rasmuson.org
www.rasmuson.org

Edward B. Rasmuson, Chairman
Cathryn Rasmuson, Vice Chair
Diane Kaplan, President & CEO
Chris Perez, Program Officer

The Rasmuson Foundation invests both in individuals and well managed organizations dedicated to improving the quality of life for Alaskans.

Arizona

2784 American Foundation Corporation
4518 North 32nd Street
Phoenix, AZ 85018
602-955-4770
Fax: 602-955-4700
info@americanfoundation.org
www.americanfoundation.org

Ben L. Schaub, Founder and CEO

The American Foundation can be your sponsor, and help your company set up a corporate foundation in a public charity or support organization format.

2785 Arizona Autism Resources
The Arc of Arizona
PO Box 90714
Phoenix, AZ 85066
602-234-2721
800-433-5255
Fax: 602-234-5959
arc@arcarizona.org
www.arcarizona.org

Robert Snyder, President
Michael Leyva, Vice President
Jon Meyers, Executive Director
Kim Dorshaw, Secretary

The Arc, a national organization on mental retardaion, is committed to securing for all people with developmental disabilities the opportunity to choose and realize their goals in regard to where they live, learn, work and play.

2786 Arizona Community Foundation
2201 E Camelback Road
Suite 405B
Phoenix, AZ 85016
602-381-1400
800-222-8221
Fax: 602-381-1575
info@azfoundation.org
www.azfoundation.org

Ron Butler, Chair
Shelly Cohn, Vice Chair
Steven G. Seleznow, President & CEO
John Gogolak, Treasurer

The mission of the Arizona Community Foundation is to empower and align philanthropic interests with community needs and build a legacy of living.

2787 Arizona Instructional Resource Center for Students who are Blind or Visually Impaired, The
Foundation For Blind Children
1235 E. Harmont Drive
Phoenix, AZ 85020
602-678-5800
800-322-4870
Fax: 602-678-5819
mashton@SeeItOurWay.org
www.seeitourway.org

Dee Nortman, CFO
Marc Ashton, Chief Executive Officer
Barbra Smith, Chief of Staff
Alexander Pushman, Director, Mark & Dev

The Foundation for Blind Children contracts with the Arizona Department of Education to provide statewide media services for students between pre-kindergarten and 12th grade who have a visual impairment or are blind andEneed their instructional materials in a specialized medium such as braille, large print, or electronic files as well as adaptive equipment.

2788 Margaret T Morris Foundation
PO Box 592
Prescott, AZ 86302-592   928-445-6633
                                        Fax: 928-445-6633

Susan Rheem, Executive Director

Arkansas

2789 Arc of Arkansas
2004 Main St
Little Rock, AR 72206-1526   501-375-7770
                                        Fax: 501-372-4621
                                        www.arcark.org

Willie Jones, President
Steve Hitt, Chief Executive Officer
Roger Williams, Chief Financial Officer
Cynthia Stone, Chief Operating Officer
Serving people with disabilites and their families for over fourty years.

2790 Winthrop Rockefeller Foundation
225 East Markham Street
Suite 200
Little Rock, AR 72201   501-376-6854
                                        Fax: 501-374-4797
                                        webfeedback@wrfoundation.org
                                        www.wrfoundation.org

Phillip N. Baldwin, Chair
David Rainey, Ed.D., Vice chair
Sherece Y. West-Scantlebury, Ph.D, President & CEO
Andrea M. Dobson, CPA, COO & CFO
Mission is to improve the quality of life in Arkansas. It focuses its grantmaking efforts in three areas: education, economic development and civic affairs. Education projects funded in the past have included grants to schools that are working to involve teachers and parents in making decisions about what happens at their schools, projects that work to remove prejudice from the educational process and more. Major grants are made to support the development of new programs.

California

2791 Ahmanson Foundation
9215 Wilshire Blvd
Beverly Hills, CA 90210   310-278-0770
                                        info@theahmansonfoundation.org
                                        www.theahmansonfoundation.org

William H. Ahmanson, President
Karen Ahmanson Hoffman, Managing Director & Secretary
Kristen K. O'Connor, CFO & Treasurer
Jennie H. Chin, Senior Accountant
The Foundation primarily gives in Southern California with major emphasis in Los Angeles County. The Foundation focuses on the arts and humanities, education, mental health and support for a broad range of social welfare programs.

2792 Alice Tweed Touhy Foundation
205 E Carrillo Street
Suite 219
Santa Barbara, CA 93101-7186   805-962-6430
Jeanne Mc Kay, Manager
Rehabilitation, recreation and building funds are given to organizations only within the Santa Barbara area.

2793 Alternating Hemiplegia of Childhood Foundation
2000 Town Center
Suite 1900
Southfield, MI 48075   313-663-7772
                                        Fax: 313-733-8987
                                        sharon@ahckids.org
                                        ahckids.org

Lynn Egan, President
Joshua Marszalek, Vice President
Gene M Andrasco, Treasurer
Vicky Platt, Secretary
Non-profit organization dedicated to promoting professional and public awareness of Alternating Hemiplegia of Childhood (AHC) and providing current information to affected individuals and their families. The foundation also supports ongoing medical research into the cause, treatment and potential cure of AHC and maintains a registry of families, affected chidren and physicians who are familiar with AHC.

2794 Arc of California
1225 8th Street
Suite 350
Sacramento, CA 95815   916-552-6619
                                        800-698-6619
                                        Fax: 916-441-3494
                                        www.thearcca.org

Tony Anderson, Executive Director
Richard Fitzmaurice, President
Betsy Katz, Secretary
Bruce MacKenzie, Treasurer
Advocates for people with intellectual and all developmental disabilities since 1953. The ARC of California is committed to securing for all people with developmental disabilities, in partnership with thier families, legal guardians or conservators the opportunity to choose and realize their goals of where and how they learn, live, work and play.

2795 Atkinson Foundation
1660 Bush Street
Suite 300
San Mateo, CA 94109   415-561-6540
                                        Fax: 650-357-1101
                                        sangeles@pfs-llc.net
                                        www.atkinsonfdn.org

Elizabeth Curtis, Administrator
Stacey Angels, Grants Manager
The Foundation focuses and awards grants to community service and civic organizations serving the residents of San Mateo County, California through programs that benefit children, youth, seniors, the disadvantaged and those in need of rehabilitation. Grants are also made to local churches and schools, and overseas for sustainable development, health education and family planning. No grants to individuals or for research, travel, special events, annual campaigns, media and publications.

2796 Baker Commodities Corporate Giving Program
4020 Bandini Blvd
Vernon, CA 90058   323-268-2801
                                        Fax: 323-268-5166
                                        info@bakercommodities.com
                                        www.bakercommodities.com

Jim Andreoli, President
Baker Commodities has been one of the nation's leading providers of rendering, and grease removal services. Baker Commodities, Inc. is a completely sustainable company, recycling animal by-products and kitchen waste into valuable products that can be used to feed livestock, power vehicles, and act as a base for everyday items.

2797 Bank of America Foundation
315 Montgomery St
Fl 8
San Francisco, CA 94104-1803   415-622-8248
                                        888-488-9802
                                        Fax: 704-386-6444
                                        www.bankamerica.com/foundation

Ilana Orin, Manager

The Foundation will consider grants in four categories including: Health & Human Services, which provides support to health & human service organizations primarily through grants to the United Way campaigns; Education, with the focus on preparing people to become productive employees and participating citizens; Conservation & Environment, the improvement of California communities for the benefit of their citizens; and Culture & The Arts, supporting the leading performing and visual arts groups.

2798 Blind Babies Foundation
1814 Franklin Street
Suite 300
Oakland, CA 94612 510-446-2229
Fax: 510-446-2262
bbfinfo@blindbabies.org
www.blindbabies.org

Dottie Bridge, President
Sharon Sacks, PhD, 1st Vice President
Clare Friedman, PhD, 2nd Vice President
Deborah Orel-Bixler, PhD, OD, Secretary
Founded in 1949, the foundation provides home-based early intervention services to families with young children with vision impairment in the Northern and Central regions of California.

2799 Bothin Foundation
1660 Bush Street
Suite 300
San Francisco, CA 94109 415-561-6540
Fax: 415-561-6477
ccasey@pfs-llc.net

Lyman H. Casey, President
A. Michael Casey, Vice President & Treasurer
Devon Laycox, Vice President
Charlie Casey, Program Officer
The Bothin Foundation makes grants for capital, building, and equipment needs to organizations providing direct services to low-income, at risk children, youth and families, the elderly, and the disabled in San Francisco, Marin, Sonoma, and San Mateo counties.

2800 Briggs Foundation
1969 Lancewood Ln
Carlsbad, CA 92009-6826 760-704-6481
Fax: 760-704-6483

Blaine A Briggs, President
Private non-operating foundation.

2801 Burns-Dunphy Foundation
5 3rd Street
Suite 528
San Francisco, CA 94103-3213 415-421-6995
Fax: 415-882-7774

Walter Gleason
Cressey Nakagawa
Grants are given to promote wellness for the visually impaired, physically and mentally disabled and to promote research in these areas.

2802 California Community Foundation
221 S. Figueroa Street
Suite 400
Los Angeles, CA 90012 213-413-4130
Fax: 213-383-2046
info@ccf-la.org
www.calfund.org

Cynthia A. Telles, Chairman
Antonia Hernandez, President & CEO
John E. Kobara, EVP & COO
Stephen J. Cobb, VP & CFO
Areas of funding priority include grants for the disabled, child welfare, rehabilitation, developmentally disabled, employment projects, research and computer projects. Giving is limited to the greater Los Angeles area.

2803 California Endowment
1000 N Alameda St
Los Angeles, CA 90012 213-628-1001
800-449-4149
Fax: 213-703-4193
questions@calendow.org

Zac Guevara, Vice Chair
Robert Ross, President & CEO
Martha Jimenez, EVP/ Counsel
Anthony Iton, SVP
California Endowment's mission is to expand access to affordable, quality health care for underserved individuals and communities, and to promote fundamental improvements in the health status of all Californians.

2804 Carrie Estelle Doheny Foundation
707 Wilshire Boulevard
Suite 4960
Los Angeles, CA 90017 213-488-1122
Fax: 213-488-1544
doheny@dohenyfoundation.org
www.dohenyfoundation.org

Robert A. Smith,III, President
Nina Shepherd, CAO/ CFO
Pam Thomas, Grants Administrator
Lisa Rogers, Grants Administrator
The Foundation primarily funds local, not-for-profit organizations endeavoring to advance education, medicine and religion, to improve the health and welfare of the sick, aged, incapacitated, and to aid the needy.

2805 Coeta and Donald Barker Foundation
3740 Cahuenga Blvd
Studio City, CA 91604 760-340-1162
818-980-3630
Fax: 818-980-2709
info@scga.org
www.scga.org

Nancy Harris, President
Kevin Heaney, Executive Director
Andrea Fredlin, Admin Asst., Club Services
Evan Belfi, Asst. Director, Marketing
It is an independent organization that gives its attention to organizations that are charitable or nonprofit under the laws of the state of Oregon or California.

2806 Conrad N Hilton Foundation
30440 Agoura Road
Agoura Hills, CA 91301 818-851-3700
Fax: 310-694-9051
cnhf@hiltonfoundation.org
hiltonfoundation.org

Steven M. Hilton, Chairman, President & CEO
Barron Hilton, Chairman Emeritus
Donald H Hubbs, Director Emeritus
Katherine Miller, Facilities and Office Services M
Our grant-making style is to initiate and develop major long-term projects and then seek out the organizations to implement them. As a consequence of this proactive approach, the Foundation does not generally consider unsolicited proposals. Our major projects currently include: blindness prevention and treatment, support the work of the Catholic Sisters, drug abuse prevention among youth, support of the Conrad N. Hilton College of Hotel and Restaurant Management, and much more.

2807 Crescent Porter Hale Foundation
1660 Bush Street
Suite 300
San Francisco, CA 94109 415-561-6540
Fax: 415-561-5477
evalentine@pfs-llc.net
www.crescentporterhale.org

E. William Swanson, President
Sr. Estela Morales, MSW, Vice President
Eunice Valentine, Executive Director
Patricia Fata, Secretary/Treasurer
Serves organizations in the San Francisco Bay Area who are involved in the following areas of concern: education in the fields

of art and music; private elementary, high school and university education; capital funding; and other worthwhile programs which can be demonstrated as serving broad community purposes, leading toward the improvement of the quality of life.

2808   David and Lucile Packard Foundation
343 Second Street
Los Altos, CA   94022   650-917-7142
                                                      Fax: 650-948-5793
                                              communications@packard.org
                                                        www.packard.org

Susan Packard Orr, Chairman
Julie E. Packard, Vice Chairman
Nancy Packard Burnett, Vice Chairman
Carol S Larson, President & CEO
This foundation provides grants to nonprofit organizations in the following areas: conservation; population; science; children, familes, and communities; arts and organizational effectiveness; and philanthropy. It provides national and international grants and also has a special focus on the Northern California Counties.

2809   Deutsch Foundation
5454 Beethoven St
Los Angeles, CA   90066   310-862-3000
                                                           877-340-7700
                                                      Fax: 310-862-3100
                                                          deutschinc.com

Linda Sawyer, Chairman
Kim Getty, President, North America
Val Difebo, CEO, Deutsch NY
Mike Sheldon, CEO, North America
Learning disabled, visually impaired, mental health, eye research, child welfare, speech and hearing impaired, physically disabled and independence projects are funded through this Foundation. Giving is limited to California.

2810   East Bay Community Foundation
De Domenico Building
200 Frank H Ogawa Plaza
Oakland, CA 94612   510-836-3223
                                                      Fax: 510-836-7418
                                                     jwhead@eastbaycf.org
                                                           www.ebcf.org

Sherry M. Hirota, Chair
Ingrid Lamirault, Vice Chair
Peter Garcia, Vice Chair
James W. Head, President & CEO
A collection of funds created by many people, organizations and businesses, the Foundation helps those people and groups to support effective nonprofit organizations to the East Bay and beyond.

2811   Evelyn and Walter Hans Jr
114 Sansome Street
Suite 600
San Francisco, CA   94104   415-856-1400
                                                      Fax: 415-856-1500
                                                           www.haasjr.org

Walter J. Haas, Chair
Ira S. Hirschfield, President & Trustee
Michael Blake, VP of Finance
Robert D. Haas, Treasurer
A private foundation interested in programs which assist people who are hungry, homeless, or at risk of homelessness; enable older adults to maintain independent lives in the community and support Hispanic community development in San Francisco's Mission District. The Foundation also encourages proposals for corporate social responsibility efforts within the business community.

2812   Family Caregiver Alliance
785 Market St.
Suite 750
San Francisco, CA   94103   415-434-3388
                                                           800-445-8106
                                                      Fax: 415-434-3508
                                                       info@caregiver.org
                                                        www.caregiver.org

Ping Hao, MBA, President
Jacquelyn Kung, Vice President
Kathleen Kelly,MPA, Executive Director
Deborah Wolter, Secetary
To improve the quality of life for caregivers and those they care for through information, services, and advocacy.

2813   Financial Aid for the Disabled and Their Families
Reference Service Press
2310 Homestead Rd.
Suite C1 #219
Los Altos, CA   94024   650-861-3170
                                                      Fax: 650-861-3171
                                                      info@rspfunding.com
                                                       www.rspfunding.com

Gail Schlachter, President
R David Weber, Editor-in-Chief
Mike Fields, Database and Website Manager
Sandy Perez, Online and Print Sales
This directory, which Children's Bookwatch calls invaluable describes more than 1,100 financial aid opportunities available to support persons with disabilities and members of their families. Updated ever 2 years. *$39.50*
300 pages
ISBN 1-588410-31-5

2814   Firemans Fund Foundation
Firemans Fund Insurance Companies
777 San Marin Dr
Novato, CA   94998   415-899-2000
                                                           800-227-1700
                                                      Fax: 415-899-3600
                                                  customerrelations@ffic.com
                                                        www.firemansfund.com

Lori Dickerson Fouche, President & CEO
Jill Paterson, Chief Financial Officer
Eleanor Barnard, Chief Distribution & Sales
Sally Narey, Chief Counsel, Corp. Secretary
Provides discretionary grants to the disabled only in Marin and Sonoma counties in the San Francisco Bay area.

2815   Fred Gellert Foundation
1038 Redwood Highway
Building B, Suite 2
Mill Valley, CA 94941   415-381-7575
                                                      Fax: 415-381-8526
                                                     patty@fgffoundation.com
                                          foundationcenter.org/grantmaker/fredgellert/
Fred Gellert, Founder
Patty Oday, Administrator
Focuses on organizations and programs serving residents of San Mateo and San Francisco and Marin counties in California, with the exception of environmentally concerned organizations.

2816   Gallo Foundation
P.O. Box 1130
Modesto, CA   95353-1130   209-579-3204
                                                           877-687-9463
                                                      Fax: 209-341-3307
                                                         www.ejgallo.com

John Gallo, Senior VP Operations
Physically and mentally disabled, child welfare, Special Olympics, United Cerebral Palsy and Easter Seal Society are among the grants provided by this foundation.

2817 Glaucoma Research Foundation
251 Post Street
Suite 600
San Francisco, CA 94108   415-986-3162
                                         800-826-6693
                                    Fax: 415-986-3763
                                 question@glaucoma.org
                                      www.glaucoma.org
Andrew Iwach, MD, Board Chair
Robert L. Stamper, MD, Vice Chair
Thomas M. Brunner, President/CEO
Fred H. Brinkmann, Treasurer
A national organization dedicated to protecting the sight of people with glaucoma through research and education. The Foundation conducts and supports research that contributes to improved patient care and a better understanding of the disease process. Provides education, advocacy and emotional support to patients and their families.

2818 Harden Foundation
1636 Ercia Street
Salinas, CA 93906   831-442-3005
                                    Fax: 831-443-1429
                                  joe@hardenfoundation.org
                                  www.hardenfoundation.org
Patricia Tynan Chapman, President
C. Bill Elliott, Vice President/Treasurer
Joseph C. Grainger, Executive Director
Linda Taylor, Secretary
Founded to assist charitable organizations in the Salinas Valley.

2819 Henry J Kaiser Family Foundation
2400 Sand Hill Rd
Menlo Park, CA 94025-6941   650-854-9400
                                    Fax: 650-854-4800
                                         www.kff.org
Drew Altman, President/CEO
Gary Claxton, Vice President
Esther Dicks, Vice President
Mollyann Brodie, SVP for Executive Operations
A non-profit, private operating foundation focusing on the major health care issues facing the US, with a growing role in global health. Kaiser develops and runs its own research and communications programs, sometimes in partnership with other non-profit research organizations or major media companies.

2820 Henry W Bull Foundation
Santa Barbara Bank & Trust
P.O. Box 2340
Santa Barbara, CA 93120   202-720-7871
                                    Fax: 805-884-1404
                                  info@coreprojects.com
                              www.activistfacts.com/about/
Janice Gibbons, VP/Senior Trust Officer
Grant given to a wide range of organizations that include those which provide services for the disabled; arts, education, services for elderly and youth grants awarded two times a year. Grant size ranges from $500 to $5,000. Proposal deadlines April 1, Sept 1.

2821 Irvine Health Foundation
18301 Von Karman Avenue
Suite 440
Irvine, CA 92612-0120   949-253-2959
                                    Fax: 949-253-2962
                                         info@ihf.org
                                         www.ihf.org
Timothy L. Strader, Sr., Chairman
Carol Mentor McDermott, Vice Chairman
Edward B. Kacic, President
Ptricia A. Meredith, VP, Administration & Programs
Mission is to improve the physical, mental and emotional well-being of all Orange County residents.

2822 Joseph Drown Foundation
1999 Avenue of the Stars
Suite 2330
Los Angeles, CA 90067   310-277-4488
                                    Fax: 310-277-4573
                                      staff@jdrown.org
                                       www.jdrown.org
Norman C Obrow, President
Giving is focused primarily in California. No support for religious purposes or to individuals. Goal is to assist individuals in becoming successful, self-sustaining, contributing citizens.

2823 Junior Blind of America
5300 Angeles Vista Blvd
Los Angeles, CA 90043   323-295-4555
                                         800-352-2290
                                    Fax: 323-296-0424
                                    info@juniorblind.org
                                     www.juniorblind.org
Harold A. Davidson, DBA, Chair
Robert D. Held, Vice Chair
Miki Jordan, President/CEO
Scott Farkas, Treasurer
Junior Blind provides programs and services for children and adults who are blind or visually impaired and their families to achieve independence and self-esteem. Programs include; Camp Bloomfield, Visions: Adventures in Learning, Infant-Family Program, Early Childhood Program, Special Education School, Children's Residential Program, Davidson Program for Independence, and Student Transition and Enrichment Program, Vision Screening and After School enrichment.

2824 Kenneth T and Eileen L Norris Foundation
11 Golden Shore
Suite 450
Long Beach, CA 90802   562-435-8444
                                    Fax: 562-436-0584
                                      grants@ktn.org
                                  www.norrisfoundation.org
Lisa D Hanson, Chairman
Ronald R Barnes, Executive Director & Trustee
Walter J Zanino, Controller
William G Corey, Medical Advisor
The Foundation is primarily focused on medicine and education. To a lesser extent the foundation contributes to community programs including visually impaired, autism, mentally and physically disabled, deaf and mental health in the Southern California area. Average grant size in this area is $5,000-$10,000. Grants are also given in the area of culture and youth.

2825 Koret Foundation
33 New Montgomery Street
Suite 1090
San Francisco, CA 94105-4526   415-882-7740
                                    Fax: 415-882-7775
                                   info@koretfoundation.org
                                    www.koretfoundation.org
Susan Koret, Board Chair
Anita L. Friedman, President
Michael J. Boskin, President
Jeffery A. Farber, CEO
Koret seeks to fund outstanding examples of innovative approaches to community challenges and opportunities.

2826 LA84 Foundation
2141 W Adams Blvd
Los Angeles, CA 90018   323-730-4600
                                    Fax: 323-730-9637
                                        info@la84.org
                                        www.la84.org
Frank M. Sanchez, Chair
Anita L. DeFrantz, President
F. Patrick Escobar, VP, Grants & Programs
Robert Wagner, Vice President, Partnerships
The LA84 Foundation was established to manage Southern California's share of the surplus from the highly successful 1984 Olympic Games in Los Angeles and offers sports programs, a premier sports library and meeting facilities. The foundation cur-

rently serves two million youth in eight Southern California counties.

2827 LJ Skaggs and Mary C Skaggs Foundation
1221 Broadway
21st Floor
Oakland, CA 94612-1837   510-451-3300
                                 Fax: 510-451-1527
                                 skaggs@fablaw.com

Philip M Jelley, President
Jayne C Davis, Vice President
Robert N Janopaul, Director
Joseph W Martin, Jr., Secretary, Treasurer
The Foundation presently makes grants under four program categories: performing arts, social concerns, projects of historic interest and special projects.

2828 Legler Benbough Foundation
2550 Fifth Avenue
Suite 132
San Diego, CA 92103   619-235-8099
                                 Fax: 619-235-8077
                                 peter@benboughfoundation.org
                                 www.benbough.org

Peter K. Elsworth, President
John G. Rebelo, Jr., Treasurer
Nbob Kelly, Director
Peter K. Ellsworth, Director
The mission of the foundation is to improve the quality of life of the people of San Diego. The foundation focuses on three target areas for funding, one in the area of providing economic opportunity, one in the area of enhancing cultural opportunity, and one that provides focus for health, education and welfare funding.

2829 Levi Strauss Foundation
1155 Battery St
San Francisco, CA 94111-1264   415-501-7208
                                 800-872-5384
                                 Fax: 415-544-3490
                                 www.levistrauss.com/levi-strauss-foundation

Chip Bergh, President & CEO
Roy Bagattini, EVP/President
Lisa Collier, EVP/President
James Curleigh, EVP/President
Has a funding initiative to support organizations which provide services for people with AIDS, and/or educational programs which help prevent the further spread of the HIV virus. The Foundation will assist in the development and enhancement of such services only in those communities where Levi Strauss & Co. has plants and distribution centers.

2830 Louis R Lurie Foundation
555 California Street
Suite 5100
San Francisco, CA 94104-1707   415-392-2470
                                 Fax: 415-421-8669
                                 www.foundationcenter.org/grantmaker/lurie
Nancy Terry, Foundation Administrator
Visually impaired, hard-of-hearing and physically disabled in the San Francisco Bay Area and Metropolitan Chicago areas only.

2831 Luke B Hancock Foundation
360 Bryant St
Palo Alto, CA 94301-1409   650-321-5536
                                 Fax: 650-321-0697
Ruth Ramel, Director
Has concentrated its resources over the past year on programs which provide job training and employment for at-risk youth. Consortium funding with other foundations in areas where there is unmet need; emergency and transitional funding; and selected funding for music education. .

2832 Marin Community Foundation
5 Hamilton Landing
Suite 200
Novato, CA 94949   415-464-2500
                                 Fax: 415-464-2555
                                 info@marincf.org
                                 www.marincf.org

Cleveland Justis, Chair
Thomas Peters, Ph.D., President & CEO
Sid Hartman, CFO/COO
Aileen Sweeney, VP Of Finance
Mission is to encourage and apply philanthropic contributions to help improve the human condition, embrace diversity, promote a humane and democratic society, and enhance the communities quality of life, now and for future generations.

2833 Mary A Crocker Trust
57 Post Street
Suite 610
San Francisco, CA 94104-5023   650-576-3384
                                 Fax: 415-982-0141
                                 staff@mactrust.org
                                 www.mactrust.org

2834 MedicAlert Foundation International
5226 Pirrone Crt
Salida, CA 95368   800-432-5378
                                 customer_service@medicalert.org
                                 www.medicalert.org
Barton G. Tretheway, CAE, Chairt
David Leslie, President & CEO
Melody Howard, Vice President Of Call Center Operations
A trusted emergency support network dedicated to educating emergency responders and medical personnel for facing everyday emergency situations, as well as providing emergency care services for members.

2835 National Center on Caregiving at Family Caregiver Alliance (FCA)
785 Market Street
Suite 750
San Francisco, CA 94103   415-434-3388
                                 800-445-8106
                                 Fax: 415-434-3508
                                 info@caregiver.org
                                 www.caregiver.org

Ping Hao, MBA, President
Jacquelyn Kung, Vice President
Kathleen Kelly, MPA, Executive Director
Jeff Kumataka, CPA, MBA, Treasurer
FCA offers programs at national, state and local levels to support and sustain caregivers. The National Center on Caregiving (NCC) program works to advance the development of high-quality, cost-effective policies and programs for caregivers in every state of the country. Uniting research, public policy and services, the NCC serves as a central source of information on caregiving and long term care issues for policy makers, service providers, media, funders and family caregivers.

2836 National Foundation of Wheelchair Tennis
940 Calle Amanecer
Suite B
San Clemente, CA 92673-6218   714-361-3663
                                 Fax: 714-361-6603
                                 www.nfwt.org

Bill Butler
Founded in January of 1980, the intention of this foundation is to assist the newly physically disabled individual to realize his full potential in society by enhancing his esteem, independence productivity and physical capabilities regardless of age, sex, creed or disability extent.

2837 Parker Foundation
2604-B El Camino Real
Suite 244
Carlsbad, CA 92008   760-720-0630
                                    Fax: 760-720-1239
                              mail@theparkerfoundation.org
                              www.theparkerfoundation.org
Judy McDonald, President
Gordon Swanson, Vice President
Ann Davies, Secretary
Raymond Ellis, Treasurer
The assets are directed to projects which will contribute to the
betterment of any aspect of the people of San Diego County, Cali-
fornia and solely to entities which, among other things, are orga-
nized exclusively for charitable purposes and are operating in
San Diego County, California.

2838 Pasadena Foundation
301 East Colorado Boulevard
Suite 810
Pasadena, CA 91101-2824   626-796-2097
                                    Fax: 626-583-4738
                              pcfstaff@pasadenacf.org
                              www.pasadenacf.org
David M. Davis, Chair
Judy Gain, Vice Chair
Jennifer Fleming DeVoll, Executive Director
Mariver Copeland, Director of Finance
The mission of the Pasadena Foundation is to improve the quality
of life for citizens of the Pasadena area through support of non-
profit organizations that provide services beneficial to the
community.

2839 RC Baker Foundation
P.O. Box 6150
Orange, CA 92863-6150   714-750-8987
F L Scott, Manager
Established in 1952, for general philanthropic purposes. The
bulk of assistance and support has been to religious, scientific,
educational institutions and youth organizations.

2840 Ralph M Parsons Foundation
888 West Sixth Street
Suite 700
Los Angeles, CA 90017   213-362-7600
                                    Fax: 213-482-8878
                              www.rmpf.org
James A. Thomas, Chairman
Elizabeth Lowe, Vice Chairman
Wendy Garen, President & CEO
Astra Anderson Galang, CFO
The Foundation is concerned with the encouragement and sup-
port of projects and programs deemed beneficial to mankind in
several major areas of interest such as: education; social impact;
civic and cultural; health and special products. Only funds in Los
Angeles County.

2841 Robert Ellis Simon Foundation
312 S Canyon View Drive
Los Angeles, CA 90049-3812   310-275-7335
Joan Willens
Mental health and visually impaired grants are the main concerns
of this organization.

2842 San Francisco Foundation
One Embarcadero Cente
Suite 1400
San Francisco, CA 94111   415-733-8500
                                    Fax: 415-477-2783
                              info@sff.org
                              www.sff.org
Sandra R Hernandez, CEO
Nick Hodges, VP for Philanthropic Services
Bobbie Chapman, Director of Business Development
Shona Carter, Donor Relations Officer
The Foundation's purpose is to improve life, promote greater
equality of opportunity and assist those in need or at risk in the
San Francisco Bay Area. The Foundation strives to protect and
enhance the unique resources of the Bay Area, committed to
equality of opportunity for all and the elimination of any injus-
tice, seeks to enhance human dignity and seeks to establish mutual trust, respect and communication among the Foundation.

2843 Santa Barbara Foundation
1111 Chapala Street
Suite 200
Santa Barbara, CA   93101   805-963-1873
                                    Fax: 805-966-2345
                              info@sbfoundation.org
                              www.sbfoundation.org
Eileen Sheridan, Chair
James Morouse, Vice Chair
Ronald Gallo, President & CEO
Maria Caudillo, Exec. Asst. to President & CEO
The Foundations mission is to enrich the lives of the people of
Santa Barbara County through philanthropy. The Foundation
awards grants to nonprofits within the County in the areas of edu-
cation, health, human services, personal development, cluture,
recreation, community enhancement and environment. No sup-
port is given to individuals except through student aid.

2844 Sidney Stern Memorial Trust
860 Via de la Paz
PO Box 457
Pacific Palisades, CA   90272   310-459-2117
                              info@sidneysternmemorialtrust.org
                              www.sidneysternmemorialtrust.org
Betty Hoffenberg, Director
A Southern California-based foundation providing grants to non-
profit organizations for various projects. The foundation gives
priority to the following areas of interest: education, health and
science, community service projects, youth, services to the mentally and emotionally disabled, the arts, organizations and activities serving California. The Board prefers to make contributions
to organizations that use the funds directly in the furtherance of
their charitable and public purposes.

2845 Sierra Health Foundation
1321 Garden Hwy
Sacramento, CA 95833   916-922-4755
                                    Fax: 916-922-4024
                              info@sierrahealth.org
                              www.sierrahealth.org
Jose Hermocillo, Chair
David W. Gordon, Vice Chair
Chet P. Hewitt, President & CEO
Gil Alvarado, VP of Administration/CFO
The Foundation strives to establish a collaborative relationship
with its grantees, and with other funders and foundations,
through an open dialogue. The Foundation approaches each grant
as a partnership, with opportunities for the grantee and grantor to
work cooperatively to enhance the effectiveness of the grant
project.

2846 Silicon Valley Community Foundation
2400 West El Camino Real
Suite 300
Mountain View, CA 94040-1498   650-450-5400
                                    Fax: 650-450-5401
                              info@siliconvalleycf.org
                              www.siliconvalleycf.org
C.S. Parker, Chair
Samuel Johnson,Jr., Vice Chair
Emmitt D. Carson, Ph.D, President & CEO
George Dallas, Administrative Asst.
Serving all of San Mateo & Santa Clara counties, Silicon Valley
Foundation has more than $1.5B in assets under management and
1500 philanthropic funds. The community provides grants
through donor advised and corporate funds in addition to its own
Community Endowment Fund. In addition, the community foun-
dation serves as a regional center for philanthropy, providing do-
nors simple and effective ways to give locally & globally.

2847 Sonora Area Foundation
362 S Stewart Street
Sonora, CA 95370
209-533-2596
Fax: 209-533-2412
edwyllie@sonora-area.org
www.sonora-area.org

Jim Johnson, President SAF
Roger Francis, Vice President
Edward B. Wyllie, Executive Director
Lin Freer, Program Manager
The Sonora Area Foundation strengthens its community through
assisting donors, making grants, and providing leadership.

**2848 Stella B Gross Charitable Trust C/O Bank of The West Trust
Department**
PO Box 1121
San Jose, CA 95108-1121
408-947-5203
Gabe Padilla, Trust Admin
Organization must be federal and state tax-exempt and reside
within the bounds of Santa Clara County, California to be eligi-
ble.

2849 Teichert Foundation
3500 American River Dr
Sacramento, CA 95864
916-484-3011
Fax: 916-484-6506
www.teichert.com

Frederick Teichert, LHD, Executive Director
Awards grants to community organizations and provides employee matching grants. Teichert Foundation expresses the
companie's commitment to build and preserve a healthy and pros-
perous region.

2850 WM Keck Foundation
550 South Hope Street
Suite 2500
Los Angeles, CA 90071- 2617
213-680-3833
Fax: 213-614-0934
info@wmkeck.org
www.wmkeck.org

Allison Keller, Executive Director & CFO
Maria Pellegrini, Ph.D, Executive Director of Programs
Thomas Everhart, Ph.D, Senior Scientific Advisor
Matesh Varma, Ph.D, Senior Program Director
Created to support accredited colleges and universities with par-
ticular emphasis on the sciences, engineering and medical re-
search. The Foundation also maintains a Southern California
Grant Program that provides support for non-profit organizations
in the field of civic and community services, health care,
precollegiate education and the arts.

2851 Whittier Trust
Whittier Trust Company
1600 Huntington Dr
South Pasadena, CA 91030
626-441-5111
Fax: 626-441-0420
hrdept@whittiertrust.com
www.whittiertrust.com

Michael J Casey, Chairman
David A Dahl, President & CEO
Brian H Flynn, Senior Vice President, Business Development
Sandip A Bhagat, Chief Investment Officer
Whittier Trust offers financial services and expertise in the area
of family wealth management. Some of their other areas of con-
sultation include philanthropic advising, investment manage-
ment, legal services and real estate.

2852 Willam G Gilmore Foundation
1660 Bush Street
Suite 300
San Francisco, CA 94109
415-561-0650
Fax: 415-561-5477

William N Hancock, Owner

Colorado

2853 AV Hunter Trust
650 South Cherry Street
Suite 535
Glendale, CO 80246- 1897
303-399-5450
Fax: 303-399-5499
afreeman@pfs-llc.net
www.avhuntertrust.org

Mary K. Anstine, President
George C. Gibson, Vice President
Barbara L. Howie, Executive Director
Jessica Sutton, Grants Manager
Donated nearly $50 million to nonprofit organizations serving
those who captured Mr. Hunter's attention and sparked his com-
passion. Trust gives aid, comfort, support, or assistance to chil-
dren or aged people or indigent adults.

2854 Adolph Coors Foundation
215 St. Paul Street
Suite 300
Denver, CO 80206
303-388-1636
Fax: 303-388-1684
www.coorsfoundation.org

John W. Jackson, Executive Director
Jeanne L. Bistranin, Senior Program Officer
Carrie C. Tynan, Program Officer
Carol S. Strathman, Financial/Special Projects Coord
Applicant organizations must be classified as 501 and must oper-
ate within the United States. The areas covered by the Foundation
are health, education, youth, community services, civic and cul-
tural and public affairs.

2855 Arc of Colorado
1580 Logan Street
Suite 730
Denver, CO 80203
303-864-9334
800-333-7690
Fax: 303-864-9330
mrymer@thearcofco.org
www.thearcofco.org

Randy Patrick, President
Tonna Kelly, Vice President
Marijo Rymer, Executive Director
Lynnelle Zackroff, Secretary
A private not-for-profit, membership-based, grassroots associa-
tion. The Arc of Colorado is the state office whith local units lo-
cated in various areas throughout the state.

2856 Bonfils-Stanton Foundation
Daniels and Fisher Tower
1601 Arapahoe Street
Suite 500
Denver, CO 80202
303-825-3774
Fax: 303-825-0802
webinfo@bonfils-stanton.org
bonfils-stantonfoundation.org

Gary P. Steuer, President & CEO
Gina A. Ferrari, Director, Grants Program
Ann M. Hovland, CFO/Treasurer
Monique M. Loseke, Executive Asst.
Grants limited to Colorado 501 (c) (3) organizations. Grants are
for general, charitable philanthropic activities within the State.
Major categories include education, scientific (including hospi-
tal and health services), civic and cultural, community and human
services. Organizations should request foundation guidelines
before submitting a proposal.

2857 Comprecare Foundation
PO Box 740610
Arvada, CO 80006
303-432-2808
Fax: 303-432-2808
www.comprecarefoundation.org

Milton W. Bollman, Chairman of the Board
Dr. Ellen Mangione, MD, MPH, Vice Chairman
James R. Gilsdorf, Executive Director
Dennis E. Baldwin, Secretar/Treasurer

The purpose of the Comprecare Foundation is to encourage, aid or assist specific health related programs and to make grants to support the activities of organizations which are designed to advance and promote health care education, the delivery of health care services, and the improvement of community health and welfare.

2858 Denver Foundation
55 Madison Street
8th Floor
Denver, CO 80206

303-300-1790
Fax: 303-300-6547
information@denverfoundation.org
www.denverfoundation.org

Sandra Shreve, Chair
Ginny Bayless, Vice Chair and Chair-Elect
David M Miller, President & CEO
Sarah Bock, Secretary
Neighbors helping neighbors, that's what the foundation is for. As Denver's only community foundation we've been accepting charitable donations since 1925. Those funds have been given back to the community in ongoing grants to nonprofit organizations - organizations that touch nearly every meaningful artistic, cultural, civic, health and human services interest of metro Denver's citizens.

2859 El Pomar Foundation
10 Lake Circle
Colorado Springs, CO 80906

719-633-7733
800-554-7711
Fax: 719-577-5702
grants@elpomar.org
www.elpomar.org

William J. Hybl, Chairman/CEO
William Ward, Vice Chair
R. Thayer Tutt, Jr., President/CIO
Kyle Hybl, COO/General Counsel
Mission of El Pomar is to enhance, encourage and promote the current and future well being of the people of Colorado through grantmaking and community stewardship.

2860 Helen K and Arthur E Johnson Foundation
1700 Broadway
Suite 1100
Denver, CO 80290-1718

303-861-4127
800-232-9931
Fax: 303-861-0607
www.johnsonfoundation.org

Ms. Lynn H. Campion, Chairman
Ms. Berit K. Campion, Vice Chair
John H Alexander Jr, President
Jacque Beaty, Finance Director
A nonprofit, grantmaking private foundation incorporated under the laws of the State of Colorado in 1948. The Foundation is a general purpose foundation whose grant program consists of a wide variety of creative efforts to solve problems and to enrich the quality of life. The areas of interest are: education, youth, health, community services, civic and culture and senior citizens. Grants limited to the state of Colorado.

Connecticut

2861 Aetna Foundation
151 Farmington Ave
Hartford, CT 06156

860-273-0123
800-872-3862
www.aetnahealthinsurance.com

Mark T Bertolini, Chairman/CEO
Karen S. Rohan, President
William J. Casazza, EVP & General Counsel
Richard di Benedetto, EVP, Aetna International
The Aetna Foundation is the independent charitable and philanthropic arm of Aetna Inc. The Foundation helps build healthy communities by promoting volunteerism, forming partnerships and funding initiatives that improve the quality of life where our employees and customers live and work.

2862 Arc of Connecticut
43 Woodland Street
Suite 260
Hartford, CT 6105-2300

860-246-6400
Fax: 860-246-6406
arcct@aol.com
www.arcct.com

Leslie Simoes, Interim Executive Director
The Arc of Connecticut is an advocacy organization committed to protecting the rights of people with intellectual, cognitive, and developmental disabilities and to promoting opportunities for their full inclusion in the life of thier communities.

2863 Community Foundation of Southeastern Connecticut
68 FederalStreet
PO Box 769
New London, CT 06320

860-442-3572
877-442-3572
Fax: 860-442-0584
maryam@cfect.org
www.cfect.org

Susan Pochal, Chair
Dianne E. Williams, Vice Chair
Maryam Elahi, President & CEO
Alison Woods, Vice President & COO
Provides donors with an easy and convenient way to give back to our community with joy and impact. We make grants to nonprofit organizations and support their efforts to strengthen our community.

2864 Connecticut Mutual Life Foundation
140 Garden St
Hartford, CT 6154

860-727-3000
Astrida Olds, Executive Director
Distinguished throughout its long history by unusual commitment to high principles of corporate purpose and business ethics. That commitment has been reflected not only in the firm belief that normal business functions must be carried out with a sense of responsibility beyond that required by the marketplace. Maintains an ongoing program of corporate contributions, a nationwide matching gifts plan for all employees on behalf of private and public education, skills training programs, and more.

2865 Cornelia de Lange Syndrome Foundation
302 West Main Street
#100
Avon, CT 06001

860-676-8166
800-753-2357
Fax: 860-676-8337
info@cdlsusa.org
www.cdlsusa.org

Robert Boneberg, Esq., President
Richard Haaland, Ph.D., Vice President
David Harvey, Vice President
Wendy Miller, Esq., Secretary
Provides information about birth defects caused by Cornelia de Lange Syndrome.

2866 Fidelco Guide Dog Foundation
103 Vision Way
Bloomfield, CT 06002

860-243-5200
Fax: 860-769-0567
admissions@fidelco.org
www.fidelco.org

Karen C. Tripp, Chair
G. Kenneth Bernhard, Esq., Vice Chair
Gregg Barratt, Chief of Staff
Julie Unwin, Chief Operating Officer
The Fidelco Guide Dog Foundation creates increased freedom and independence for men and women who are blind by providing them with guide dogs.

2867 GE Foundation
General Electric Company
3135 Easton Tpke
Fairfield, CT 6828
203-373-3216
Fax: 203-373-3029
gefoundation@ge.com
www.ge.com
Jeffrey R. Immelt, Chairman/ CEO
Daniel C. Heintzelman, Vice Chair
Jeffrey S. Bornstein, SVP & CFO, GE
Shane Fitzsimons, SVP Global Operations
Believes that our greatest national resource is the work force. If we are to successfully compete in the global arena, then we become involved in improving the education of all of our citizens. The Foundation sets examples for others to emulate helping people with their international grant program to higher education and to health care for children in developing countries.

2868 Hartford Foundation for Public Giving
10 Columbus Blvd
8th Floor
Hartford, CT 06106
860-548-1888
Fax: 860-524-8346
lindakelly@hfpg.org
www.hfpg.org
Yvette Melendez, Chair
Bonnie J. Malley, Vice Chair
Linda J. Kelly, President
Julie Feidner, Exec. Asst. to the President
Developmentally disabled, housing, deaf, recreation and education grants.

2869 Hartford Insurance Group
1 Hartford Plz
Hartford, CT 6155-1708
860-547-5000
www.thehartford.com
Christopher Swift, Chairman/ CEO
Doug Elliot, President
Beth Bombara, Chief Financial Officer
Kathy Bromage, Chief Marketing Officer
Giving is primarily in the Hartford, CT area and in communities where the company has a regional office. No support is available for political or religious purposes. Grants are given in the areas of education, health and United Way organizations.

2870 Henry Nias Foundation
20 Carmen Rd
Milford, CT 6460-7508
203-874-2787
Charles D Fleischman, President
Giving limited to NY metropolitan area. Arts, cultural programs, medical school/education, and children and youth.

2871 Jane Coffin Childs Memorial Fund for Medical Research
333 Cedar St, SHM
L300
New Haven, CT 6510-3206
203-785-4612
Fax: 203-785-3301
www.jccfund.org
Dr Randy Schekman, Director
The Fund awards fellowships to suitably qualified individuals for full time postdoctoral studies in the medical and related sciences bearing on cancer.

2872 John H and Ethel G Nobel Charitable Trust
Bankers Trust Company
1 Fawcett Pl
PO Box 1297
New York, NY 1008-1297
203-629-7120
Fax: 203-629-7170
Paul J Bisset, VP

2873 Scheuer Associates Foundation
960 Lake Ave
Greenwich, CT 6831-3032
203-622-5002
Fax: 203-622-5002
Thomas Scheuer, President

2874 Swindells Charitable Foundation Trust
Shawmut Bank
1221SW YamhillStreet
Suite 100
Portland, OR 97205-2303
503-222-0689
Fax: 503-222-0726
dwecker@swindellstrust.org
www.swindellstrust.org
Maggie Willard, President
Grants made to charitable organizations or societies incorporated for the relief of sick and suffering poor children and/or the relief of sick suffering and indigent aged men and women and/or the support of public charitable hospitals. Geographic area includes Hartford, CT area primarily. Application is required, deadlines are Feb. 1 and Aug. 1.

Delaware

2875 Arc of Delaware
2 S Augustine Street
Suite B
Wilmington, DE 19804-2504
302-996-9400
Fax: 302-996-0683
TTY:800-232-5460
eraign@arcde.org
www.thearcofdelaware.org
Bill Seufert, President
Becky Hill, Vice President
Merry Jones, Vice President
Barbara Robeleto, Vice President
The Arc of Delaware is a non-profit organization of volunteers and staff who work together to improve the quality of life for people with disabilitiesand their families. We strive to include all children and adults with cognitive, intellectual and developmental disabilities in every community.

2876 Longwood Foundation
100 W 10th St
Suite 1109
Wilmington, DE 19801-1694
302-683-8200
Fax: 302-654-2323
www.longwoodfoundation.com
ThŠre du Pont, President
Peter Morrow, Executive Director
Offers grants to the mentally and physically disabled - capital, program, education and housing grants in the state of Delaware.

District of Columbia

2877 Alexander and Margaret Stewart Trust
Brawner Building
888 17th Street NW
Suite 1250
Washington, DC 20006-3321
202-333-1277
Fax: 202-333-3128
aplatt@projectsinternational.com
www.projectsinternational.com
Chas W. Freeman, Chairman
Peter J.C, Young, President
Imtiaz T. Ladak, Chief Financial Officer
Landon K. Thorne, Managing Director
Grants are given only to the Washington, DC area organizations providing care or treatment to cancer patients or those with childhood afflictions.

2878 Arc of the District of Columbia
415 Michigan Avenue, NE
Suite 150
Washington, DC 20017- 2144 202-636-2950
Fax: 202-635-7086
arcdc@arcdc.net
www.arcdc.net

Robert A. Anderson, President
Mary Lou Meccariello, Executive Director
Michael Gonzales, Chief Operating Officer
Ed Cabatic, Director of Finance
Advocating for and providing services to persons with mental retardation. Mission is to improve the quality of life of all persons with mental retardation and their families through supports and advocacy.

2879 Eugene and Agnes E Meyer Foundation
The Meyer Foundation
1250 Connecticut Ave NW
Suite 800
Washington, DC 20036- 2620 202-483-8294
Fax: 202-328-6850
meyer@meyerfdn.org
www.meyerfoundation.org

Joshua Bernstein, Chair
Deborah Ratner Salzberg, Vice Chair
Nicky Goren, President & CEO
Barbara Lang, Secretary-Treasurer
Awards grants to projects dealing with the learning disabled, blind, mental health and vocational training in the Washington metropolitan area.

2880 Federal Student Aid Information Center
US Department of Education
400 Maryland Ave SW
Washington, DC 20202 202-275-5446
800-872-5327
www.ed.gov

Arne Duncan, Secretary of Education
Tony Miller, Deputy Secretary
Martha Kanter, Under Secretary
Answers questions about Federal student aid from students, parents and Members of Congress, as well as financial aid administrators.

2881 GEICO Philanthropic Foundation
1 Geico Plz
Washington, DC 20076 301-986-3000
800-841-3000
Fax: 301-986-2851
www.geico.com

Tony M Nicely, CEO
Hospitals, physically disabled and Special Olympics.

2882 Jacob and Charlotte Lehrman Foundation
1836 Columbia Rd NW
Washington, DC 20009-2002 202-328-8400
Fax: 202-338-8405
www.lehrmanfoundation.org

Elizabeth Berry, Director
Robert Lehrman, Trustee
Samuel Lehrman, Trustee
Barbara Ferguson, Administrative/Program assistant
The Jacob & Charlotte Lehrman Foundation supports and seeks to enrich Jewish life in Washington DC, Israel and around the world. It is committed to making Washington a better place for all people and supports the arts, education and undeserved children, the environment, and healthcare.

2883 John Edward Fowler Memorial Foundation
79 Fifth Avenue
16th Street
New York, NY 10003-3076 212-620-4230
800-424-9836
Fax: 212-807-3677
www.foundationcenter.org

Bradforth K. Smith, President
Lisa Philp, Vice President
Lawrence T. McGill, Vice President
Jen Bokoff, Director
Although not a program priority, the foundation does offer grants to the physically disabled in the Washington, DC area only.

2884 Joseph P Kennedy Jr Foundation
1133 19th Street NW
12th Floor
Washington, DC 20036-3604 202-393-1250
Fax: 202-824-0351
jpkf@jpkf.org
www.jpkf.org

Rebecca Salon, President
Steven Eidelman, Executive Director
Has two firm objectives: to seek the prevention of mental retardation, and to improve the way society deals with its citizens who are already mentally retarded. The Foundation uses its funds in areas where a multiplier effect can be achieved through development of innovative models for the prevention and amelioration of mental retardation, through provision of seed money that encourages new researchers, and thorough use of the Foundation's influence to promote public awareness.

2885 Kiplinger Foundation
1100 13th Street, NW
Suite 750
Washington, DC 20005-3938 202-887-6400
800-544-0155
Fax: 202-778-8976
foundation@kiplinger.com
www.kiplinger.com

Knight Kiplinger, VP
Limited to the greater Washington, DC area, the grants focus primarily on education, social welfare, cultural activities and community programs. Matching grants to eligible secondary or higher education institutions are provided on behalf of employees and retirees of Kiplinger Washington Editors, Inc. The Foundation does not fund scholarships.

2886 Morris and Gwendolyn Cafritz Foundation
1825 K St NW
Ste 1400
Washington, DC 20006-1271 202-223-3100
800-544-0155
Fax: 202-296-7567
info@cafritzfoundation.org
www.cafritzfoundation.org

Calvin Cafritz, Chairman/President/ CEO
John E. Chapoton, Vice Chairman and Treasurer
Ed McGeogh, Vice President - Asset Managemen
Rohan Rodrigo, Vice President - Finance
Grants are awarded to only 501(c)(3) organizations that are in the DC area. Grants are not awarded for capitol purposes, special events, endowments, or to individuals.

2887 Paul and Annetta Himmelfarb Foundation
4545 42nd St NW
Ste 203
Washington, DC 20016-4623 202-966-3796
M Preston, Executive Director
Primary areas of interest include health, children, human need, and Israel.

2888 Public Welfare Foundation
1200 U St NW
Washington, DC 20009-4443   202-965-1800
info@publicwelfare.org
www.publicwelfare.org

Lydia M. Marshall, Chair
Mary E. McClymont, President
Phillipa Taylor, Chief Financial and Administrati
Alyssa Piccirilli, Manager of Administration
The foundation's funding is specifically targeted to economically disadvantaged populations. Proposals must fall within one of the following categories: criminal justice, disadvantaged elderly, disadvantaged youth, environment, health and population and reproductive health, human rights and global security, and community economic developmental and participation. Proposals should be addressed to the Review Committee.

Florida

2889 Able Trust
3320 Thomasville Road
Suite 200
Tallahassee, FL 32308   850-224-4493
Fax: 850-224-4496
TTY:850-224-4493
info@abletrust.org
www.abletrust.org

Susanne Homant, President
Guenevere Crum, Senior Vice President
Kathryn McManus, MA, Chief Development Director
Allison Chase, MS, State Director, Florida High Sch
The Able Trust is a non-profit, public/private partnership that supports non-profit vocational rehabilitation programs throughout Florida with fundraising, grant making and public awareness of disability issues.

2890 Arc of Florida
2898 Mahan Dr
Ste 1
Tallahassee, FL 32308-5462   850-921-0460
800-226-1155
info@arcflorida.org
www.arcflorida.org

Pat Young, President
Dick Bradley, Vice President Administration
Linda Bloom, Vice President Advocacy
Greg Roe, Treasurer
Promotes, for all people with mental retardation and other developmental disablilities, through education, awareness, research, advocacy and the support of families, friends and community.

2891 Bank of America Client Foundation
50 Central Avenue
Suite 750
Sarasota, FL 34236-5900   941-951-4103
maryann.l.smith@ustrust.com
www.fdnweb.org/boacf/
Maryann L. Smith, Vice President, Senior Trust Off
Committed to creating meaningful change in the communities we serve through our philanthropic efforts, associate volunteerism, community development activities and investing, support of arts and culture programming and environmental initiatives.

2892 Barron Collier Jr Foundation
2600 Golden Gate Pkwy
Naples, FL 34105-3227   239-262-2600
Fax: 239-262-1840
ContactUs@BarronCollier.com
www.barroncollier.com
Karen V. Triplett, Director of Property Management
Jose Medina, Facilities Manager
Barron Collier Companies - dedicated to the responsible development, management and stewardship of its extensive land holdings and other assets in the businesses of agriculture, real estate, and mineral management.

2893 Camiccia-Arnautou Charitable Foundation
Ste 402
980 N Federal Hwy
Boca Raton, FL 33432-2712   561-368-5757
Fax: 561-368-8505
Ronda Gluck, President

2894 Chatlos Foundation
PO Box 915048
Longwood, FL 32791-5048   407-862-5077
info@chatlos.org
www.chatlos.org
Bill Chatlos, Trustee
Funds nonprofit organizations in the USA and around the globe. Funding is provided in the following areas of giving: Bible Colleges/Seminaries, Religious Causes, Medical Concerns, Liberal Arts Colleges and Social Concerns. Category of placement is determined by the organizations overall mission rather than the project under consideration. The Foundation does not make scholarship grants directly to individuals but rather to educational institutions which in turn select recipients.

2895 Edyth Bush Charitable Foundation
199 E Welbourne Ave
Ste 100
Winter Park, FL 32789-4365   407-647-4322
888-647-4322
Fax: 407-647-7716
dodahowski@edythbush.org
www.edythbush.org
Gerald F. Hilbrich, Chairman
Herbert W. Holm, Vice Chairman
David A. Odahowski, President/CEO
Mary Ellen Hutcheson, Vice-President/Treasurer
Funding is resrticted to 501c3 nonprofit organizations located and operating in Orange, Osceola, Seminole and Lake Counties, Florida. Visit www.edythbush.org for a list of funding policies.

2896 FPL Group Foundation
700 Universe Blvd
Juno Beach, FL 33408-2657   561-694-4000
888-488-7703
Fax: 561-694-4620
PoweringFlorida@FPL.com
www.fpl.com
Maria V. Fogarty, Senior Vice President, Internal
James L. Robo, President and Chief Operating Of
Joseph T. Kelliher, Executive Vice President, Federa
Antonio Rodriguez, Executive Vice President, Power
The company consistently outperforms national averages for service reliability while customer bills are below the national average. A clean energy leader, FPL has one of the lowest emissions profiles and one of the leading energy efficiency programs among utilities nationwide. FPL is a subsidiary of Juno Beach, Fla.-based NextEra Energy, Inc.

2897 Jefferson Lee Ford III Memorial Foundation
9600 Collins Ave
Bal Harbour, FL 33154-2202   305-868-2609
Fax: 305-868-2640
Sanford L King, Director
Yvonne Quatrale, President
Disabled children, hearing and speech center. Grants are only given to tax exempt organizations, no individual grants are offered.

2898 Jessie Ball duPont Fund
40 East Adams Street
Ste 300
Jacksonville, FL 32202-3302   904-353-0890
800-252-3452
Fax: 904-353-3870
contactus@dupontfund.org
www.dupontfund.org
Sherry P. Magill, President
Mark D. Constantine, Vice President for Strategy, Pol
Barbara Roole, Senior Program Officer
Katie Ensign, Senior Program Officer

Established under the terms of the will of the late Jessie Ball duPont. The fund is a national foundation having a special though not exclusive interest in issues affecting the South. The Fund works with the approximately 325 individual institutions to which Mrs. duPont personally contributed during the five-year period, 1960 through 1964.

2899   Lost Tree Village Charitable Foundation
8 Church Lane
North Palm Beach, FL   33408-2908   561-622-3780
Fax: 561-841-6773
info@losttreefoundation.org
www.losttreefoundation.org
Pam Rue, Executive Director
Teresa Elu, Executive Assistant
Bob Heon, Controller
The Lost Tree Village Charitable Foundation is dedicated to building a stronger community and improving the quality of life for all local residents. Grants are awarded annually to local non-profit health and human service organizations providing information, expertise and assistance to those in need. Applications are only accepted from organizations located in Palm Beach and Southern Martin Counties. Visit the website for guidelines and further information.

2900   Miami Foundation, The
40 NW 3rd Street
Suite 405
Miami, FL   33128   305-371-2711
Fax: 305-371-5342
info@miamifoundation.org
www.miamifoundation.com
Javier Alberto Soto, President and CEO
Rebecca Mandelman, VP for Strategy and Engagement
The Foundation approaches all of its program activities with a focus on building the community. We conduct acticvities and support efforts that build community assets and relationships among individuals, organizations, and communities that connect people with resources and opportunities to improve their quality of life.

2901   Mount Sinai Medical Center
4300 Alton Road
Miami Beach, FL   33140-6574   305-674-2121
305-674-2777
www.msmc.com/foundation
Wayne Chaplin, Chairman
Steven D. Sonenreich, President & CEO
Jason Loeb, Foundation President
Kenneth L. Davis, MD, Chief Executive Officer and Pres
Autism Research

2902   National Parkinson Foundation
200 SE 1st Street
Suite 800
Miami, FL   33131-1494   305-243-6666
800-473-4636
Fax: 305-537-9901
contact@parkinson.org
www.parkinson.org
John W. Kozyak, Chairman
Joyce Oberdorf, President/CEO
Amy Gray, Vice President, Chapter and Comm
Peter Schmidt, PhD, Vice President, Programs, Chief
The mission of the NPF is to improve the quality of care for people with Parkinson's disease through research, education, and outreach.

2903   Publix Super Markets Charities
Publix Super Market Corporation Office
PO Box 407
Lakeland, FL   33802-0407   800-242-1227
www.publix.com
Gino DiGrazia, Vice President of Finance
Maria Brous, Director of Media & Community R
Kimberly Reynolds, Media & Community Relations
In addition to giving to thousands of local projects, Publix annually supports five organizations in companywide campaigns:

Special Olympics, March of Dimes, Children's Miracle Network, United Way and Food for All

Georgia

2904   Arc Of Georgia
100 Edgewood Ave NE
Ste 1675
Atlanta, GA   30303-3068   678-733-8969
888-401-1581
Fax: 678-733-8970
info@thearcofgeorgia.org
www.thearcofgeorgia.org
Torin Togut, President
David Glass, Vice President
Julie Lee, Secretary
Will Hudson, Treasurer
The Arc of Georgia advocates for the rights and full participation of all children and adults with intellectual and developmental disabilities. Together with our network of members and other local Chapters, we improve systems of supports and services, connect families, inspire communities, and influence public policy.

2905   Community Foundation for Greater Atlanta
50 Hurt Plz SE
Ste 449
Atlanta, GA   30303-2915   404-688-5525
Fax: 404-688-3060
info@cfgreateratlanta.org
www.cfgreateratlanta.org
Suzanne Boas, Board Chair
Alicia Philipp, President
Robert Smulian, Vice President of Philanthropic
Lesley Grady, Senior Vice President of Communi
The Community Foundation for Greater Atlanta is a creative, cost-effective and tax-efficient way for people to invest in our community. We help donors and their families meet their charitable goals by educating them or critical issues and by matching them with organizations that serve their interests. By working with donors and the community, we improve the quality of life for residents in our region.

2906   Florence C and Harry L English Memorial Fund
Sun Trust Bank Atlanta
PO Box 4418
Mail Code 041
Atlanta, GA   30302   404-588-8250
Fax: 404-724-3082
raymond.king@suntrust.com
www.suntrustatlantafoundation.org
Anil T. Cheriyan, Chief Information Officer
Kenneth J. Carrig, Chief Human Resources Officer
Rilla S. Delorier, Chief Marketing and Client Exper
Thomas E. Freeman, Chief Risk Officer
Grants only made to Metro Atlanta non-profit organizations; no grants to churches or individuals.

2907   Georgia Power
96 Annex
Atlanta, GA   30308-3374   404-506-6526
888-655-5888
www.georgiapower.com
W. Paul Bowers, Chairman/ President/ CEO
John L. Pemberton, Senior VP/SPO
Georgia Power is an investor-owned, tax-paying utility that serves 2.25 million customers in all but four of Georgia's 159 counties.

2908 Grayson Foundation
1701 Willa Place Drive
Kernersville, NC 2728   336-650-9914
graysonfoundation@gmail.com
www.graysonfoundation.net
Donna Sherrell, Finance- Public Relations
Tricia Gladstone, Behavior Analyst-Finance Public
Roger Sherrell, Information Technology-Web Manag
Bob Sherrell, Finance
Grayson Foundation enhances the quality of public educationfor the students of the Grayson cluster of schools by providing funds which enrich and extend educational oppurtunities.

2909 Harriet McDaniel Marshall Trust in Memory of Sanders McDaniel
Sun Trust Bank Atlanta
96 Annex
PO Box 4418
Atlanta, GA 30396   404-588-8250
888-891-0938
Fax: 404-724-3082
raymond.king@suntrust.com
Anil T. Cheriyan, Chief Information Officer
Kenneth J. Carrig, Chief Human Resources Officer
Rilla S. Delorier, Chief Marketing and Client Exper
Thomas E. Freeman, Chief Risk Officer
Grants only made to Metro Atlanta non-profit organizations, no grants to churches or individuals.

2910 IBM Corporation
1 New Orchard Rd
Armonk, NY 10504-1772   914-499-1900
800-425-3333
TTY:804-068-4225
response@in.ibm.com
www.ibm.com
Samuel J Palmisano, Chairman
Virginia M. Rometty, President and Chief Executive Of
Rodney C. Adkins, Senior Vice President
Michael E. Daniels, Senior Vice President and Group
Manages disability programs (which leverage IBM resources through partnerships) designed to train persons with disabilities and assist them in gaining employment. Also, disseminates information regarding products and resources for persons with disabilities with those of other companies and organizations.

2911 John H and Wilhelmina D Harland Charitable Foundation
3565 Piedmont Road, NE
Two Piedmont Center, Suite 710
Atlanta, GA 30305-1502   404-264-9912
Fax: 404-266-8834
info@harlandfoundation.org
www.harlandfoundation.org
Margaret C. Reiser, President
Winifred S. Davis, Vice President/Treasurer
Robert E. Reiser, Secretary
Jane G. Hardesty, Executive Director
The Harland Charitable Foundation was established in 1972 by John H. and Wilhelmina D. Harland to support worthy local causes in Atlanta, with a particular interest in improving the welfare of children and youth as well as support of community services and arts and culture.

2912 Lettie Pate Whitehead Foundation
191 Peachtree Street NE
Suite 3540
Atlanta, GA 30303- 2951   404-522-6755
Fax: 404-522-7026
fdns@woodruff.org
www.woodruff.org
James B. Williams, Chairman
James M. Sibley, Vice Chairman
Lawrence L. Gellerstedt, President /CEO
J. Lee Tribble, Treasurer
Non-profit organization dedicated to the support of needy women in nine southeastern states.

2913 Rich Foundation
222 Summer Street
Stamford, CT 06901   203-359-2900
Fax: 203-328-7980
info@fdrich.com
www.fdrich.com

2914 SunTrust Bank, Atlanta Foundation
Sun Trust Bank Atlanta
PO Box 4418
Mail Code 041
Atlanta, GA 30302   404-588-8250
Fax: 404-724-3082
www.suntrust.com
Anil T. Cheriyan, Chief Information Officer
Kenneth J. Carrig, Chief Human Resources Officer
Rilla S. Delorier, Chief Marketing and Client Exper
Thomas E. Freeman, Chief Risk Officer

Hawaii

2915 Arc of Hawaii
3989 Diamond Head Rd
Honolulu, HI 96816-4413   808-737-7995
Fax: 808-732-9531
info@thearcinhawaii.org
www.thearcinhawaii.org
Thomas Huber, President
Lee Moriwaki, Vice President
Duane Bartholomew, Secretary
Kevin Dooley, Treasurer
The Arc is a national, grassroots organization of and for people with intellectual and related developmental disabilities. With more then 140,000 members in 1000 local and state chapters. The Arc is the largest volunteer organization devoted soley to working on behalf of people with intellectual disabilities.

2916 Atherton Family Foundation
827 Fort Street Mall
Honolulu, HI 96813-2817   808-566-5524
888-731-3863
Fax: 808-521-6286
foundations@hcf-hawaii.org
Patricia R. Giles, Vice President
Judith M. Dawson, President
Frank C. Atherton, Vice President and Treasurer
Paul F. Morgan, Vice President
Supports educational projects, programs and institutions as the highest priority, with the enterprises of a religious nature and those concerned with health and social services given careful attention. The Foundation is one of the largest private resources in the State devoted exclusively to the support of activities of a charitable nature.

2917 GN Wilcox Trust
Bank of Hawaii
PO Box 3170
Honolulu, HI 96802-3170   808-649-8580
800-272-7262
Fax: 808-538-4006
stafford.kiguchi@boh.com
www.boh.com
Paul Boyce, AVP and Grants Administrator
Elaine Moniz, Trust Specialist
William L. Carpenter, Senior Vice President
Diane W. Murakami, Senior Vice President
Benefits the people of Hawaii by funding programs that support social services, education, culture, the arts, youth services, religion, health and rehabilitation.

2918 Hawaii Community Foundation
827 Fort Street Mall
Honolulu, HI 96813-2817   808-537-6333
                               888-731-3863
                          Fax: 808-521-6286
                          info@hcf-hawaii.org
                www.hawaiicommunityfoundation.org

Kelvin Taketa, President/CEO
Chris van Bergeijk, Vice President/Chief Operating O
Joseph Martyak, Vice President of Communications
Tom Kelly, Vice President for Knowledge, Ev
The Hawaii Community Foundation is a public, statewide, charitable services and grantmaking organization supported by donor contributions for the benefit of Hawaii's people.

2919 McInerny Foundation Bank Of Hawaii, Corporate Trustee
PO Box 3170
Honolulu, HI 96802-3170   808-649-8580
                               800-272-7262
                          Fax: 808-538-4006
                          stafford.kiguchi@boh.com
                          www.boh.com

Paula Boyce, Avp And Grants Administrator
Elaine Moniz, Trust Specialist
William L. Carpenter, Senior Vice President
Diane W. Murakami, Senior Vice President
Although the Trust is broad-purposed, it does not make grants to churches or individuals, nor for endowments, reserve purposes, deficit financing, or for the purchase of real estate.

2920 Sophie Russell Testamentary Trust Bank Of Hawaii
PO Box 3170
Honolulu, HI 96802-3170   808-649-8580
                               800-272-7262
                          Fax: 808-538-4006
                          stafford.kiguchi@boh.com
                          www.boh.com

Paula Boyce, Asst. Vice President
Elaine Moniz, Trust Specialist
William L. Carpenter, Senior Vice President
Diane W. Murakami, Senior Vice President
Supports qualified tax-exempt charitable organizations, in the State of Hawaii only. Offers grants to the Humane Society and institutions giving nursing care and serving the physically and mentally handicapped.

Illinois

2921 Alzheimer's Association
225 N Michigan Ave
Fl 17
Chicago, IL 60601-7633   312-335-8700
                               800-272-3900
                          Fax: 866-699-1246
                          TTY: 312-335-5886
                          info@alz.org
                          www.alz.org

Stewart Putnam, Chair
Christopher Binkley, Vice Chair
Harry Johns, President /CEO
Deborah Jones, Secretary
Mission is to eliminate Alzheimer's disease through the advancement of research, to provide and enhance care and support for all affected, and to reduce the risk of dementia through the promotion of brain health.

2922 American National Bank and Trust Company
33 N La Salle St
PO Box 191
Danville, VA 24543-0191   312-661-6000
                               800-240-8190
                          Fax: 815-961-7745
                          www.amnb.com

Charles H. Majors, Chairman/ CEO
Jeffrey V. Haley, President
Charles T. Canaday, Jr., Senior Vice President
R. Helm Dobbins, Senior Vice President
Supports the endeavors of organizations working to meet the critical needs of the city and its surrounding communities. Success is greatly affected by the well-being of the communities the company serves, thus the foundation seeks to fulfill the social obligations both through financial funding and human resources. The Foundation funding categories include organizations and programs involved in economic development, education, community and social services, healthcare and culture and the arts.

2923 Amerock Corporation
P.O.Box 7018
Rockford, IL 61125-7018   815-963-9631
                               800-435-6959
                          Fax: 800-618-6733
                          www.amerock.com

Robert Bailey, President
Grants are given to organizations promoting wellness, health and rehabilitation of the visually impaired and physically disabled.

2924 Arc of Illinois
The Illinois Life Span Project
20901 S La Grange Rd
Ste 209
Frankfort, IL 60423-3213   815-464-1832
                               800-588-7002
                          Fax: 815-464-5292
                          www.thearcofil.org

Brain Rubin, President
Therese Devine, Vice President
Tony Paulauski, Executive Director
Janet Donahue, Director of Development
The Arc of Illinois is committed to empowering persons with disabilities to achieve full participation in community life thru informed choices.

2925 Benjamin Benedict Green-Field Foundation
18313 Greenleaf Ct
Tinley Park, IL 60487-2176   708-444-4241
                          Fax: 708-614-0496
                          kathy@greenfieldfoundation.org
                          www.greenfieldfoundation.org

Colin Fisher, Chairman of the Board
Kathryn Groenendal, President
Dan Jarke, Vice President
Sheldon K. Rachman, Secretary
A privately endowed grantmaking organization trying to improve the qaulity of life for children and the elderly in the city of chicago.

2926 Blowitz-Ridgeway Foundation
1701 E Woodfield Rd
Suite 201
Schaumburg, IL 60173-5127   847-330-1020
                          Fax: 847-330-1028
                          laura@blowitzridgeway.org
                          www.blowitzridgeway.org

Daniel L Kline, President
Pierre R. LeBreton, Ph.D., Vice-President
Thomas P. Fitzgibbon, Treasurer
Sandra Swantek, M.D., Secretary
Provides limited program, capital and research grants to organizations aiding the physically and mentally disabled, and agencies serving children and youth. Grants generally limited to Illinois.

2927 Chaddick Institute for Metropolitan Development
2352 N. Clifton Ave.
Suite 130
Chicago, IL 60614-2302   773-325-7310
Fax: 312-362-5506
lasadvising@depaul.edu
las.depaul.edu

Joseph P Scwieterman PhD, Director
Marisa Schulz, LEED AP, Assistant Director
Justin Kohls, Program Manager
Susan Aaron, Civic Program Design
Advances the principals of effective land use, transportation, and community planning. Offers planners, attorneys, developers, and entrepreneurs a forum to share expertise on difficult land-use issues through workshops, conferences, and policy studies.

2928 Chicago Community Trust
225 North Michigan Avenue
Suite 2200
Chicago, IL 60601- 4501   312-616-8000
Fax: 312-616-7955
alla@cct.org
www.cct.org

Frank M. Clark, Chairman
Terry Mazany, President /CEO
Jamie Phillippe, Vice President-Development and D
Chae Dawning, Sr. Director of Human Resources
A community foundation established in 1915, which receives gifts and bequests from individuals, families or organizations interested in providing through the community foundation, financial support for the charitable agencies or institutions which serve the residents of metropolitan Chicago.

2929 Chicago Community Trust and Affiliates
225 North Michigan Avenue
Suite 2200
Chicago, IL 60601- 4501   312-616-8000
Fax: 312-616-7955
TTY:312-853-0394
www.cct.org

Frank M. Clark, Chairman
Terry Mazany, President /CEO
Jamie Phillippe, Vice President-Development and D
Chae Dawning, Sr. Director of Human Resources
Provides critical charitable resources in the arts, community and economic development, education, health and wellness, hunger and homeless alleviation, legal services, programs for youth, the elderly, and people with disabilities, and services to assure that basic human needs are met for all members of our community.

2930 Community Foundation of Champaign County
307 W University Ave
Champaign, IL 61820-3411   217-359-0125
Fax: 217-352-6494
cfcc@soltec.net
www.cfeci.org

Brooke Didier Starks, Chair
Tom Costello, Vice-Chair
Joan M. Dixon, President /CEO
Bradley Uken, Treasurer
A network of cultural resource providers and educational organizations who collaborate in the creation, coordination, and promotion of cultural resource programs for Champaign County Schools.

2931 Dr Scholl Foundation
1033 Skokie Blvd
Ste 230
Northbrook, IL 60062-4109   847-559-7430
www.drschollfoundation.com

Pamela Scholl, President
The Foundation is dedicated to providing financial assistance to organizations committed to improving our world. Grants are made annually after an executive review by the staff and all the directors.

2932 Duchossois Foundation
Chamberlain Group
845 N Larch Ave
Elmhurst, IL 60126-1114   630-279-3600
Fax: 630-530-6091
employment@duch.com
www.duch.com

Richard L. Duchossois, Chairman
Robert L. Fealy, President /COO
Craig J. Duchossois, Chief Executive Officer
Michael E. Flannery, Executive Vice President/Chief F
Established in 1984, the foundation returns dollars to the communities supporting its facilities and employees. Within these following areas, organizations are carefully selected on the basis of community needs and the organization's value and performance. Areas aimed at include: medical research, children/youth programs and cultural institutions.

2933 Evenston Community Foundation
1560 Sherman Ave
Suite 535
Evanston, IL 60201-5910   847-492-0990
Fax: 847-492-0904
info@evanstonforever.org
www.evanstonforever.org

Sara Schastok, Phd., President and CEO
Gwen Jessen, Vice President for Philanthropy
Marybeth Schroeder, Vice President for Programs
Jan Fischer, Chief Financial Officer
The Foundation is a publicly supported plilanthropic organization dedicated to enriching Evanston and the lives of its people, now and in the future. The Foundation builds and manages its own and other community endowments, addresses Evanston's changing needs through grant making, and provides leadership on important community needs.

2934 Field Foundation of Illinois
200 S Wacker Dr
Ste 3860
Chicago, IL 60606-5848   312-831-0910
Fax: 312-831-0961
byoung@fieldfoundation.org
www.fieldfoundation.org

Lyle Logan, Board Chair
Aurie A. Pennick, Executive Director and Treasurer
Sarah M. Linsley, Secretary
Mark C. Murray, Program Director
The Field Foundation seeks to provide support for community, civic and cultural organizations in the Chicago area, enabling both new and established programs to test innovations, to expand proven strengths or to address specific, time-limited operational needs.

2935 Francis Beidler Charitable Trust
53 W Jackson Blvd
Ste 530
Chicago, IL 60604-3422   312-922-3792
Fax: 312-922-3799

Francis Beidler, Owner
Children/youth, services. Community development, business promotion, crime and violence prevention. Federated giving programs, higher education, human services and family planning.

2936 Fred J Brunner Foundation
9300 King St
Franklin Park, IL 60131-2114   847-678-3232
Fax: 847-678-0642

Fred J Brunner, CEO
General disability grants.

2937 George M Eisenberg Foundation for Charities
Ste 480
2340 S Arlington Heights Rd
Arlington Heights, IL 60005-4507   847-981-0545
Fax: 847-941-0548

James Marousis, Manager

2938 Grover Hermann Foundation
233 S Wacker Dr
Suite 6600
Chicago, IL 60606-6473 312-258-5500
Fax: 312-258-5600
rsafer@schiffhardin.com
www.schiffhardin.com

Ronald S. Safer, Managing Partner, Executive Comm
Provides funds for educational, health, public policy, community and religious organizations throughout the United States. Its major interests are in higher education and health.

2939 John D and Catherine T MacArthur Foundation
Office of Grants Management
140 S Dearborn St
Chicago, IL 60603-5285 312-726-8000
Fax: 312-920-6258
TTY:312-920-6285
4answers@macfound.org
www.macfound.org

Marjorie M. Scardino, Chair
Julia Statch, Interim President
Cecilia A. Conrad, Vice President-MacArthur Fellows
Susan E. Manske, Vice President/Chief Investment
The Foundation supports creative people and effective institutions committed to building a more just, verdant, and peaceful world. In addition, we work to defend human rights, advance global conservation, & security, make cities better places, and understand how technology is affecting children and society.

2940 Les Turne Amyotrophic Laterial Sclerosis Foundation
5550 Touhy Ave
Ste 302
Skokie, IL 60077-3254 847-679-3311
888-257-1107
Fax: 847-679-9109
info@lesturnerals.org
www.lesturnerals.org

Ken Hoffman, President
Andrea Paul Backman, Executive Director
Shari Diamond, RN, BSN, Director of Patient Services
Kim McIver, Director
Voluntary health organization dedicated to raising funds for ALS research, patient services and public awareness. Provides educational materials for affected individuals and family members, health care professionals, and the general public. Program services include referrals and counseling; audio-visual aids and periodic newsletters. Offers support groups and patient networking to affected individuals, family members, and caregivers.

2941 Little City Foundation
1760 W Algonquin Rd
Palatine, IL 60067-4799 847-358-5510
Fax: 847-358-3291
info@littlecity.org
www.littlecity.org

Matthew B. Schubert, President
B. Timothy Desmond, Executive Vice President
David Rose, Vice President
Douglas A. Wilson, Vice President
We offer innovative and personalized programs to fully assist and empower children & adults with autism and other intellectual and developmental disabilities. With a commitment to attaining a greater quality of life for Illinois most vulnerable citizens, we actively promote choice, person-centered planning and a holistic approach to health and wellness. 'ChildBridge' services include in-home personal & family supports, clinical behavior intervention, 24/7 residential services and much more.

2942 MAGIC Foundation for Children's Growth
6645 North Ave
Oak Park, IL 60302-1057 708-383-0808
800-362-4423
Fax: 708-383-0899
ContactUs@magicfoundation.org
www.magicfoundation.org

Rich Buckley, Chairman
Ken Dickard, Vice Chairman
Mary Andrews, CEO and Co-Founder
Dianne Kremidas, Executive Director
This is a national nonprofit organization providing support and education regarding growth disorders in children and related adult disorders, including adult GHD. Dedicated to helping children whose physical growth is affected by a medical problem by assisting families of afflicted children through local support groups, public education/awareness, newsletters, specialty divisions and programs for the children.

2943 McDonald's Corporation Contributions Program
2111 McDonalds Dr
Oak Brook, IL 60523-5500 630-623-3000
800-244-6227
Fax: 630-623-5700
www.mcdonalds.com

Don Thompson, President and Chief Executive Of
Tim Fenton, Chief Operating Officer
Peter J. Bensen, Executive Vice President and Chi
Jose Armario, Corporate Executive Vice Preside

2944 Michael Reese Health Trust
150 N Wacker Dr
Ste 2320
Chicago, IL 60606-1608 312-726-1008
Fax: 312-726-2797
wpalmer@healthtrust.net
www.healthtrust.net

Herbert S. Wander, Chairman
The Hon. How Carroll, Vice Chairman
Walter R. Nathan, Secretary
Gregory S. Gross, EdD, President
The trust seeks to improve the health of people in Chicago's metropolitan communities through effective grantmaking in health care, health education, and health research.

2945 National Eye Research Foundation
910 Skokie Blvd
Ste 207a
Northbrook, IL 60062-4033 847-564-9400
800-621-2258
Fax: 847-564-0807
info@nerf.org
www.subway.com

Joel Tenner, Manager
Dedicated to improving eye care for the public and meeting the professional needs of eye care practitioners; sponsors eye research projects on contact lens applications and eye care problems. Special study sections in such fields as orthokertology, primary eyecare, pediatrics, and through continuing education programs. Provides eye care information for the public and professionals. Educational materials including pamphlets. Program activities include education and referrals.

2946 National Foundation for Ectodermal Dysplasias
6 Executive Dr
Suite 2
Fairview Heights, IL 62208-1360 618-566-2020
Fax: 618-566-4718
info@nfed.org
www.nfed.org

Anil Vora, President
George Barbar, Vice President
Mary Fete, Executive Director
Kelley Atchison, Director
To empower and connect people touched by ectodermal dysplasias through education, support, and research.

2947   National Headache Foundation
820 N Orleans St
Ste 411
Chicago, IL   60610-3131   312-274-2650
                                            888-643-5552
                                            Fax: 312-640-9049
                                            info@headaches.org
                                            www.headaches.org
Seymour Diamond, M.D., Executive Chairman
Roger K. Cady, M.D., Associate Executive Chairman
Arthur H. Elkind, M.D., President
Vincent Martin, M.D., Vice President
Foundation exists to enhance the healthcare of headache sufferers. It is a source of help to sufferers' families, physicians who treat headache sufferers, allied healthcare professionals and to the public.

2948   OMRON Foundation OMRON Electronics
1 Commerce Dr
Schaumburg, IL   60173-5330   847-843-7900
                                            800-556-6766
                                            Fax: 847-884-1866
                                            aoisales@omron.com
                                            www.omron247.com
Tastu Goto, CEO
Supports local community projects through direct donations and matching employee-directed contributions.

2949   Parkinson's Disease Foundation
1359 Broadway
Suite 1509
New York, NY   10018-2331   212-923-4700
                                            800-457-667
                                            Fax: 212-923-4778
                                            info@pdf.org
                                            www.pdf.org
Howard D. Morgan, Chair
Constance Woodruff Atwell, Ph.D., Vice Chair
Robin Anthony Elliott, President
James Beck, Ph.D., Vice President
International voluntary not-for-profit organization dedicated to patient services; education of affected individuals, family members, and healthcare professionals; and promotion and support of research for Parkinson's Disease and related disorders. Offers an extensive referral service to guide affected individuals to proper diagnosis and clinical care. Provides referrals to genetic counseling and support groups; promotes patient advocacy; and offers a variety of educational and support materials
Quarterly

2950   Peoria Area Community Foundation
331 Fulton St
Ste 310
Peoria, IL   61602-1449   309-674-8730
                                            Fax: 309-674-8754
                                            jim@communityfoundationci.org
                                            www.communityfoundationci.org
Donna Maracci, Chair
David Wynn, Vice Chair
Mark Roberts, CEO
Jessica Dillon, Program Manager
Established to meet a wide variety of social, cultural, educational and other charitable needs throughout Central Illinois.

2951   Polk Brothers Foundation
20 W Kinzie St
Ste 1110
Chicago, IL   60654-5815   312-527-4684
                                            Fax: 312-527-4681
                                            questions@polkbrosfdn.org
                                            www.polkbrosfdn.org
Sandra P. Guthman, Chair
Raymond F. Simon, Vice Chair
Gordon S. Prussian, Secretary
Gillian Darlow, CEO
The Polk Brothers Foundation seeks to improve the quality of life for the people of Chicago. We partner with local nonprofit organizations that work to reduce the impact of poverty and provide area

residents with better access to quality education, preventive health care and basic human services.

2952   Retirement Research Foundation
8765 W Higgins Rd
Ste 430
Chicago, IL   60631-4170   773-714-8080
                                            Fax: 773-714-8089
                                            info@rrf.org
                                            www.rrf.org
Nathaniel P. McParland, M.D., Chairman
Ruth Ann Watkins, Secretary
Downey R. Varey, Treasurer
Irene Frye, Executive Director
A private philanthropy with primary interest in improving the quality of life of older persons in the United States.

2953   Sears-Roebuck Foundation
3333 Beverly Rd
Hoffman Estates, IL   60179   847-286-2500
                                            800-932-3188
                                            Fax: 800-326-0485
                                            www.sears.com
W Bruce Johnson, CEO
Has a special interest in projects that address women, families, and diversity, but awards most of its funding to disease-specific charities and United Way in the Chicago area.

2954   Siragusa Foundation
1 E Wacker Dr
Ste 2910
Chicago, IL   60601-1912   312-755-0064
                                            Fax: 312-755-0069
                                            www.siragusa.org
John E. Hicks, Chair & President
Ross D. Siragusa, Vice Chair
John R. Siragusa, Treasurer
Sharmila Rao Thakkar, Executive Director
The Siragusa Foundation, is a private family foundation that is committed to honoring its founder by sustaining and developing Chicago's extraordinary nonprofit resources.

2955   Square D Foundation
1415 S Roselle Rd
Palatine, IL   60067-7337   847-397-2600
                                            Fax: 847-925-7500
                                            www.schneider-electric.com

2956   WP and HB White Foundation
540 W Frontage Rd
Ste 3240
Northfield, IL   60093-1232   847-446-1441
Margaret Blandford, Executive Director
The Foundation's funds are allocated on a continuing basis within the metropolitan area of Chicago where our founder's business prospered. The Foundation helps organizations specializing in the visually impaired, mental health, youth and recreation.

2957   Washington Square Health Foundation
875 N Michigan Ave
Ste 3516
Chicago, IL   60611-1957   312-664-6488
                                            Fax: 312-664-7787
                                            washington@wshf.org
                                            www.wshf.org
William N. Werner, MD, MPH, Board Chair
Howard Nochumson, Executive Director/President
William B. Friedeman, Secretary
James M. Snyder, Treasurer
Grants funds in order to promote and maintain access to adequate healthcare for all people in the Chicagoland area regardless of race, sex, creed or financial need.

2958 Wheat Ridge Ministries
1 Pierce Pl
Ste 250 E
Itasca, IL   60143-2634   630-766-9066
                                            800-762-6748
                                       Fax: 630-766-9622
                                          www.wheatridge.org

Kevin Boettcher, Chair
Richard Herman, President
Brain Becker, Senior Vice President
Holly Harrison Fiala, Vice President of Advancement
Weat Ridge supports more then 100 new health-related ministries
each year through a variety of grant programs

Indiana

2959 Arc of Indiana
107 N Pennsylvania St
Suite 800
Indianapolis, IN   46204- 2423   317-977-2375
                                            800-382-9100
                                       Fax: 317-977-2385
                                          thearc@arcind.org
                                             www.arcind.org

Kerry Fletcher, President
Marlene Lu, Vice President
Mike Foddrill, Treasurer
Erika Steuterman, Secretary
Arc of Indiana is commited to people with cognitive and develop-
mental disabilities realizing their goals of learning, living, work-
ing, and playing in the community.

2960 Ball Brothers Foundation
222 S Mulberry St
Muncie, IN   47305-2802   765-741-5500
                                       Fax: 765-741-5518
                                            info@ballfdn.org
                                             www.ballfdn.org

James A. Fisher, Chairman/ CEO
Jud Fisher, President/Chief Operating Office
Frank B. Petty, Vice Chairman
Tammy Phillips, Treasurer, ex-officio
The Ball Brothers Foundation is dedicated to the stewardship leg-
acy of the Ball brothers and to the pursuit of improving the quality
of the Muncie, Delaware County, east Central Indiana and Indi-
ana, through philanthropy and leadership.

2961 Community Foundation of Boone County
102 N. Lebanon
Suite 200
Lebanon, IN   46052   317-873-0210
                                       Fax: 317-873-0219
                                 info@communityfoundationbc.org
                                   www.communityfoundationbc.org

Marc Applegate, Chairman of the Board
Ray Ingham, Vice Chair
Mike Harlos, Treasurer
Suzy Rich, Secretary
The Community Foundation of Boone County provides pathways
for connecting people who care with causes that matter for now
and in the future.

2962 John W Anderson Foundation
402 Wall St
Valparaiso, IN   46383-2562   219-462-4611
                                       Fax: 219-531-8954
                                         andersonfnd@aol.com

Bruce Wargo, Manager
Physically and mentally disabled, recreation and youth agencies
in Northwest Indiana area.

Iowa

2963 Arc of Iowa
114 S. 11th Street
Ste 302
West Des Moines, IA   50265- 3259   515-402-1618
                                            800-362-2927
                                       Fax: 515-330-2195
                                         casey@thearcofiowa.org
                                          www.thearcofiowa.org

Casey Westhoff, Executive Director
The Arc of Iowa exists to ensure that people with intellectual disabilities and developmental disabilities receive the services, supports and opportunities necessary to fully realize their right to
live, work and enjoy life in the community without
discrimination.

2964 Hall-Perrine Foundation
115 3rd St SE
Ste 803
Cedar Rapids, IA   52401-1222   319-362-9079
                                       Fax: 319-362-7220
                                        kristin@hallperrine.org
                                          www.hallperrine.org

William Whipple, Chairman
Jack Evans, President
Darrel Morf, Vice President
Iris Muchmore, Secretary
This foundation is dedicated tio improving the quality of life for
peole in Linn County, IA by responding to the changing social,
economic, and cultural needs of the community.

2965 Mid-Iowa Health Foundation
3900 Ingersoll Ave
Ste 104
Des Moines, IA   50312-3535   515-277-6411
                                       Fax: 515-271-7579
                                        info@midiowahealth.org
                                          www.midiowahealth.org

Becky Miles-Polka, Chairman
Rob Hayes, Vice Chair
Suzanne Mineck, President
Cheryl Harding, Secretary/Treasurer
Mission is to serve as a partner and catalyst for improving the
health of vulnerable people in greater Des Moines.

2966 Principal Financial Group Foundation
711 High St
Des Moines, IA   50392   515-247-5111
                                            800-986-3343
                                       Fax: 515-235-5724

Larry Zimpleman, Chairman/ President/ CEO
Daniel J. Houston, President - Retirement, Insuranc
James P. McCaughan, President - Principal Global Inv
Luis Valdes, President - Principal Internatio
The Principal Financial Group is a leading global financial com-
pany offering businesses, individuals and industrial clients a
wide range of financial products and services.

2967 Siouxland Community Foundation
505 5th St
Suite 412
Sioux City, IA   51101-1507   712-293-3303
                                       Fax: 712-293-3303
                                 office@siouxlandcommunityfoundation.org
                                  www.siouxlandcommunityfoundation .org

Richard J. Dehner, President
Robert F. Meis, Vice President
Marilyn J. Hagberg, Secretary
Mary E. Anderson, Treasurer
The Siouxland Community Foundation strives to enhance the
quality of life in the greater Siouxland tri-state area by seeking
charitable gifts to build permanent endowments as charitable
capital for the community, providing a flexable vehicle to receive
and distribute gifts of any size, making grants in response to community needs, and providing services that will help shape the
well-being of Siouxland.

Kansas

2968   Arc of Kansas
2701 SW Randolph Ave
Topeka, KS   66611-1536
785-232-0597
Fax: 785-232-3770
info@tarcinc.org
www.tarcinc.org

Barbara Duncan, President
Matthew Bergman, Vice President
Travis Stryker, Secretary
Kim Savage, Treasurer
Organzation works to ensure that the estimated 7.2 million Americans with intellectual and developmental disabilities have the services and supports they need to grow, develop, and live in communities across the nation.

2969   Hutchinson Community Foundation
1 North Main, Suite 501
PO Box 298
Hutchinson, KS 67504-0298
620-663-5293
Fax: 620-663-9277
info@hutchcf.org
www.hutchcf.org

Aubrey Abbot Patterson, President and Executive Director
Terri L. Eisiminger, Vice President of Administration
Janet Hamilton, Community Investment Officer
Maria G. Kicklighter, Finance Assistant
Connects donors to community needs and opportunities, increases philanthropy and provides community leadership.

2970   Richard W Higgins Charitable Foundation
Marshall & Ilsley Trust of Florida
2520 South Iowa
Ste 100
Lawrence, KS   66046-2713
877-202-9234
www.applebees.com

Ken Krei, President
Jessica James, Executive Chef
Patrick Humphrey, Executive Chef
Michael Slavin, Executive Chef
Gives primarily for medical research with geographical focus on New York and Florida.

Kentucky

2971   Arc of Kentucky
706 E. Main Street
Suite A
Frankfort, KY   40601-2408
502-875-5225
800-281-1272
Fax: 502-875-5226
arcofky@aol.com
arcofky.org

James Cheely, President
Patty Dempsey, Executive Director
Ellen Nicholson, Secretary
Bob Gray, Treasurer
The Arc of Kentucky works to ensure a quality of life for children and adults with intellectual and developmental disabilities to help in securing a positive future. The Arc values services and supports that enhance the quality of life through independence, friendship, choice and respect for individuals with intellectual and developmental disabilities.

Louisiana

2972   Arc of Louisiana
606 Colonial Dr
Ste G
Baton Rouge, LA   70714-6535
225-383-1033
866-966-6260
Fax: 225-383-1092
info@thearcla.org
www.thearcla.org

Larry Pete, President
Henry Friloux, Vice President
Kelly Serrett, Executive Director
Ashley Courville, Project Director
The Arc of Louisiana advocates for and with individuals with intellectual and developmental disabilities and their families that they shall live to their fullest potential.

2973   Baton Rouge Area Foundation
402 N 4th St
Baton Rouge, LA   70802-5506
225-387-6126
877-387-6126
Fax: 225-387-6153
mverma@braf.org
www.braf.org

C. Kris Kirkpatrick, Chair
S. Dennis Blunt, Vice Chair
John G. Davies, President/CEO
Annette D. Barton, Secretary
The Foundation provides grants to nonprofits to make lives better in the region. It also takes on projects, often with parters, to remake Baton Rouge.

2974   Community Foundation of Shreveport-Bossier
401 Edwards St
Ste 105
Shreveport, LA   71101-5551
318-221-0582
Fax: 318-221-7463
info@cfnla.org
www.cfnla.org

Janie D. Richardson, Chairman
Thomas H. Murphy, Vice Chairman
Terry C. Davis, Ph.D, Secretary
Rand Falbaum, Treasurer
Provides a variety of charitable funds and gift options to help our partners achieve their vision for a stronger, more vibrant community. By bringing together fund donors, their financial advisors and non profit agencies, the Foundation is a powerful catalyst for building charitable giving and effecting positive change in our area

Maine

2975   BCR Foundation
83 Mussey Rd.
Scarborough, ME   04074
207-883-8000
800-227-6111
Fax: 207-883-0100
solutions@bcr.net
www.bcr.net

2976   UNUM Charitable Foundation
Maine Association of Non Profits
565 Congress St
Ste 301
Portland, ME   04101-3308
207-871-1885
Fax: 207-780-0346
Manp@NonprofitMaine.org
www.nonprofitmaine.org

Doug Woodbury, Board President
Ted Scontras, Board Vice President
Joan Smith, Board Treasurer
Stephanie Eglinton, Board Secretary
The Foundation encourages projects that: stimulate others in the private or public sector to participate in problem solving; ad-

vance innovative and cost-effective approaches for addressing defined, recognized needs; and demonstrate ability to obtain future project funding, if needed. The foundation generally limits its consideration of capital campaign requests to the Greater Portland, Maine area.

Maryland

2977 American Health Assistance Foundation
22512 Gateway Center Dr
Clarksburg, MD 20871-2005
301-948-3244
800-437-2423
Fax: 301-258-9454
info@brightfocus.org
www.brightfocus.org

Stacy Pagos Haller, President / CEO
Donna Callison, Vice President of Development
Michael Buckley, Vice President of Public Affairs
Guy Eakin, Ph.D., Vice President of Scientific Aff

The American Health Assistance Foundation (AHAF) is a registered non-profit organization that funds research into cures for Alzheimer's disease, macular degeneration and glaucoma, and provides the public with informantion about risk factors, preventative lifestyles, availiable treatments and coping strategies.

2978 American Occupational Therapy Foundation
4720 Montgomery Lane
Suite 202
Bethesda, MD 20814-3449
240-292-1079
Fax: 240-396-6188
aotf@aotf.org
aotf.org

Diana L. Ramsay, Chair
Wendy J. Coster, Vice Chair
Scott Campbell, CEO
Emily Kringle, President

AOFT provides advanced research, education and public awareness for occupational therapy, so that all people may participate fully in life regardless of their physical, social, mental or developmental circumstances.

2979 Arc of Maryland
121 Cathedral St, 2B
PO Box 1747
Annapolis, MD 21401- 1747
410-571-9320
888-272-3449
Fax: 410-974-6021
info@thearcmd.org
www.thearcmd.org

Richard Dean, President
Aileen O'Hare, Vice President
Annette Hinkle, Treasurer
Adam Vanderhook, Secretary

The Arc of Maryland works to create a world where children and adults with cognitive and developmental disabilities have and enjoy equal rights and opportunities.

2980 Baltimore Community Foundation
2 E Read Street
Floor 9
Baltimore, MD 21202-6903
410-332-4171
Fax: 410-837-4701
questions@bcf.org
www.bcf.org

Raymond L. Bank, Chair
Tedd Alexander, Vice Chair
Laura L. Gamble, Vice Chair
Thomas E. Wilcox, President

Makes grants in Baltimore City and Baltimore County; see website for how to apply. BCF is governed by a 30-member board of trustees, made up of a cross section of Baltimore.

2981 Candlelighters Childhood Cancer Foundation
10920 Connecticut Ave.
PO Box 498
Kensington, MD 20895- 0498
301-962-3520
855-858-2226
Fax: 301-962-3521
staff@acco.org
www.acco.org

Naomi Bartley, President
Janine Lynne, Vice President
Ken Phillips, Treasurer
Judy Mendoza, Secretary

An international organization providing information and support, and advocacy to parents of children with cancer and survivors of childhood cancer.Health and Education professionals also welcome as members.Network of local support groups. Information on disabilities related to treatment of childhood cancer. Publications.

2982 Children's Fresh Air Society Fund
Baltimore Community Foundation
2 E Read St
Baltimore, MD 21202-2470
410-332-4171
Fax: 410-837-4701
grants@bcf.org
bcf.org

Tom E. Wilcox, President
Danista Hunte, Vice President, Community Invest
Ralph M. Serpe, CFRE, Vice President, Development
Amy T. Seto, CPA, Vice President, Finance and Admi

Makes grants to nonprofit camps to provide tuition for disadvantaged and disabled Maryland children to attend summer camp. See website for how to apply.

2983 Clark-Winchcole Foundation
3 Bethesda Metro Ctr
Suite 550
Bethesda, MD 20814-5358
301-654-3607
Laura Phillips, President

Supported tax-exempt charitable organizations operating in the metropolitan area of Washington, DC in the following areas: deaf, higher education and physically disabled.

2984 Columbia Foundation
10630 Little Patuxent Parkway
Century Plaza, Suite 315
Columbia, MD 21044
410-730-7840
Fax: 410-997-6021
info@columbiafoundation.org
www.cfhoco.org

Bruce Harvey, Chair
Joseph Maranto, Vice Chair
Barb Van Winkle, Secretary
Lynne Schaefer, Treasurer

The Columbia Foundation serves as a catalyst for building a more caring, creative and effective community in Howard County by promoting and creating opportunities for personal and corporate philanthropy, managing endowments, anticipating and responding to community needs, and strategically granting funds.

2985 Corporate Giving Program
Ryland Group
11000 Broken Land Pkwy
Columbia, MD 21044
410-715-7022
800-267-0998
Fax: 410-715-7909
Bruce N Haas, President

Contributions of equipment, volunteers and financial support to organizations working to meet the challenges and needs of modern society.

2986 Cystic Fibrosis Foundation
6931 Arlington Rd
2nd floor
Bethesda, MD 20814-5200   301-951-4422
                                            800-344-4823
                                     Fax: 301-951-6378
                                            info@cff.org
                                            www.cff.org
Catherine C. McLoud, Board Chair
Robert J. Beall, Ph.D., President/Chief Executive Office
C. Richard Mattingly, Executive Vice President/Chief O
Preston W. Campbell, III, M.D., Executive Vice President for Med
The mission of the Cystic Fibrosis Foundation, a nonprofit donor-supported organization is to assure the development of the means to cure and control cystic fibrosis and to improve the quality of life for those with the disease.

2987 Foundation Fighting Blindness
7168 Columbia Gateway Dr.
Suite 100
Columbia, MD 21046   410-423-0600
                                            800-683-5555
                                     TTY:410363713951
                                     info@FightBlindness.org
                                            www.blindness.org
William T. Schmidt, Chief Executive Officer
Valerie Navy-Daniels, Chief Development Officer
Stephen M. Rose, PhD, Chief Research Officer
The Foundation Fighting Blindness (FFB) works to promote research in order to prevent, treat and restore vision. FFB is currently the world's leading private funder of retinal disease research, funding over 100 research grants and 150 researchers.

2988 George Wasserman Family Foundation
Grossberg Company
6707 Democracy Blvd
Suite 300
Bethesda, MD 20817-1176   301-571-4977
                                     Fax: 301-571-6250
Helen Salud, Manager
Anthony Cpa, Partner

2989 Giant Food Foundation
8301 Professional Pl
Ste 115
Landover, MD 20785-2351   301-341-4100
                                            888-469-4426
                                     jmiller@giantfood.com
                                            www.giantfood.com
Anthony Hucker, President
Brian Beatty, Md. Director of Marketing and Ex
Stefanie Cain, Md. District Director
Bob Haas, Md. District Director
Offers grants in the areas of mental health, recreation, community and cultural programs, art, and educational programs for the health and prosperity of the greater Washington area.

2990 Harry and Jeanette Weinberg Foundation
7 Park Center Ct
Owings Mills, MD 21117-4200   410-654-8500
                                     Fax: 410-654-4900
                                     cdemchak@hjweinberg.org
                                            hjweinbergfoundation.org
Ellen M. Heller, Chair
Barry I. Schloss, Treasurer
Alvin Awaya, Vice-President
Rachel Garbow Monroe, President and Chief Executive Of
The Harry & Jeanette Weinberg Foundation, Inc. is dedicated to assisting the poor, primarily through operating and capital grants to direct service organizations located in Baltimore, Hawaii, Northeastern Pennsylvania, New York, Israel and the Former Soviet Union. These grants are focused on meeting basic needs such as shelter, nutrition, health & socialization & on enhancing an individual's ability to meet those needs. Within that focus, emphasis is placed on the elderly & Jewish community.

2991 Kennedy Krieger Institute
707 North Broadway
Baltimore, MD 21205   443-923-9200
                                            800-873-3377
                                            888-554-9400
                                     TTY:443-923-2645
                                     findaspecialist@kennedykrieger.org
                                            www.kennedykrieger.org
Gary W. Goldstein, MD
Internationally recognized for improving the lives of children and adolescents with disorders and injuries of the brain, spinal cord and musculoskeletal system, the Kennedy Krieger Institute serves more than 20,000 individuals each year through inpatient and outpatient clincs, home and community services and school-based programs. Kennedy Krieger provides a wide range of services for children and young adults with developmental concerns mid to severe, and is home to a team of investigators.

2992 Miracle-Ear Children's Foundation
5000 Cheshire Ln N
Minneapolis, MN 55446-3706   763-268-4000
                                            800-464-8002
                                     Fax: 763-268-4365
                                     www.miracle-ear.com/en-us/

2993 National Federation of the Blind
200 E. Wells St.
at Jernigan Place
Baltimore, MD 21230- 4998   410-659-9314
                                     Fax: 410-685-5653
                                            nfb@nfb.org
                                            nfb.org
John Berggren, Executive Director, Operations
John G. Par, Jr., Executive Director, Advocacy & Policy
Anil Lewis, Executive Director, NFB Jernigan Institute
The National Federation of the Blind (NFB) is the largest organization of the blind in the world. The Federation's purpose is to help blind people achieve self-confidence, self-respect, and self-determination. Their goal is the complete integration of the blind into society on a basis of equality.

2994 Optometric Extension Program Foundation
2300 York Road
Suite 113
Timonium, MD 21093   410-561-3791
                                     Fax: 949-250-8157
                                     Kelin.Kushin@oep.org
                                            www.oepf.org
Paul A. Harris, OD, President
Robin Lewis, OD, Vice President
Kelin Kushin, Executive Director
Eric Ikeda, Secretary-Treasurer
Vision care for learning disabilities and head trauma patients.

2995 Sjogren's Syndrome Foundation
6707 Democracy Blvd
Suite 325
Bethesda, MD 20817-1164   301-530-4420
                                            800-475-6473
                                     Fax: 301-530-4415
                                            tms@sjogrens.org
                                            www.sjogrens.org
Kenneth Economou, Chairman of the Board
Stephen Cohen, OD, Chairman-Elect
Vidya Sankar, DMD, MHS, Treasurer
Janet Ee. Church, Secretary
Provides patients practical information and coping strategies that minimize the effects of Sjogren's syndrome. In addition, the Foundation is the clearinghouse for medical information and is the recognized national advocate for Sjogren's syndrome.
$25.00
Monthly

Massachusetts

2996   Abbot and Dorothy H Stevens Foundation
P.O. Box 111
North Andover, MA   01845   978-688-7211
                                        Fax: 978-686-1620

Josh Miner, Executive Director
Established in 1953, Purpose is giving primarily to the arts, education, conservation, and health and human services.

2997   Arc of Massachusetts, The
217 South St
Waltham, MA   02453-2710   781-891-6270
                                        Fax: 781-891-6271
                                        arcmass@arcmass.org
                                        www.arcmass.org

Leo Sarkissian, Executive Director
Joshua Komyerox, Government Affairs Director
Brenda Asis, Development Director
Quarterly newsletter for The Arc of Massachusetts is Advocate.

2998   Arc of Northern Bristol County
141 Park St
Attleboro, MA   02703-3020   508-226-1445
                                             888-343-3301
                                        Fax: 508-226-1476
                                        info@arcnbc.org
                                        arcnbc.org

Richard Harwood, Chairperson
Valerie Zagami, Vice Chairperson
Paul Oliveira, Treasurer
D. Randall Hays, III, Secretary/Clerk
Mission is to strive for the right of all people with developmental disabilities to be valued as individuals, to experience choice, and to be fully included in all aspects of community life

2999   Boston Foundation
75 Arlington St
10th Fl
Boston, MA   02116-3992   617-338-1700
                                        Fax: 617-338-1604
                                        info@tbf.org
                                        tbf.org

Michael Keating, Esq., Chair
Catherine D'Amato, Vice Chair
Paul S. Grogan, President & CEO
Alfred F. Van Ranst, Jr., CFO and Treasurer
The Foundation's grantmaking, special initiatives and civic leadership promote innovation across a broad range of compelling community issues, from educational excellence to affordable housing to workforce development and the arts.

3000   Boston Globe Foundation
P.O. Box 55819
Boston, MA   02205-5819   617-929-2000
                                        bostonglobe.com

Mary Jacobus, President
The mission of the Boston Globe Foundation is to empower community-based organizations to effect real change in the ares of greatest need, where the Globe is uniquely postioned to add the most value. Priority focus areas: strengthen the reading, writing and critical thinking of young people, while fostering their inherent love of learning. Strengthen the roads that link people to culture. Strengthen the civic fabric of the city. Be responsive to the needs of our immediate community.

3001   Bushrod H Campbell and Ada F Hall Charity Fund
Palmer & Dodge
111 Huntington Ave
Boston, MA   02199-7610   617-239-0540
                                        Fax: 617-227-4420

Brenda Taylor, Foundation Administrator
The fund's areas of interest include organizations and/or their projects supporting aid to the elderly, healthcare and population control. Medical research grants are administered through the Medical Foundation. No grants are awarded to individuals and the geographical area of support is limited to organizations located in Massachusetts within the area of Boston and Route 128.

3002   Clipper Ship Foundation
77 Summer St
8th Floor
Boston, MA   02110-1006   617-391-3088
                                        Fax: 617-426-7087
                                        hblaisdell@gmafoundations.com
                                        clippershipfoundation.org

Ron Ancrum, President
Makes grants to federally tax-qualified non-profit organizations offering human services to individuals living in Greater Boston and the cities of Lawrence and Brockton.

3003   Community Foundation of Western Massachusetts
1500 Main Street, Suite 2300
P.O. Box 15769
Springfield, MA   01115-5769   413-732-2858
                                        Fax: 413-733-8565
                                        wmass@communityfoundation.org
                                        www.communityfoundation.org

Katie Allan Zobel, President and CEO
Nancy Reiche, M.S.W., Vice President for Programs
Donna Roseman David, Chief Financial Officer/Chief Ad
Kristin Leutz, Vice President of Philanthropic
Provides a simple way to achieve the charitable objectives of donors most effectively; supports nonprofit organizations that offer programs in the arts, education, human services, healthcare, housing, and the environment; and works to improve the quality of life in our region.

3004   Frank R and Elizabeth Simoni Foundation
1401 Boston Providence Tpke
Norwood, MA   02062-5053   781-762-3449
                                        Fax: 781-769-6166

Matthew Mac Donald, President
Ann Mac Donald, Secretary
Robert Mac Donald, Clerk

3005   Frank Stanley Beveridge Foundation
3 Upland Lane
West Newbury, MA   01985   800-229-9667
                                        administrator@beveridge.org
                                        www.beveridge.org

Ward Slocum Caswell, President
Philip Caswell, Chairman and Vice President
Ruth S. DuPont, Treasurer
Leah Beveridge Richardson, Clerk
The mission of The Frank Stanley Beveridge Foundation, Inc. is to preserve and enhance the quality of life by embracing and perpetuating Frank Stanley Beveridge's philanthropic vision through grantmaking initiatives in support of The Stanley Park of Westfield, Inc. and programs in youth development, health, education, religion, art and environment primarily in Hampden and Hampshire Counties, Massachusetts.

3006   Friendly Ice Cream Corp Contributions Program
1855 Boston Rd
Wilbraham, MA   01095-1002   413-543-3544
                                             800-966-9970
                                        Fax: 413-731-4467
                                        friendlys.com

John Maguire, Chief Financial Officer
Steve Weigel, EVP, Chief Operating Officer
Pat Hickey, EVP, Chief Financial Officer
Tim Hopkins, EVP, Retail and Manufacturing

3007 Greater Worcester Community Foundation
370 Main St
Ste 650
Worcester, MA 01608-1738   508-755-0980
                                     Fax: 508-755-3406
                               info@greaterworcester.org
                                     greaterworcester.org

Gerald Gaudette III, Chair
Warner S. Fletcher, Vice Chair
Thomas J. Bartholomew, Treasurer
Carolyn Stempler, Clerk
By focusing on the entire community rather then on any specific
issue, the community foundation is able to address matters of
greater importance to the people of the region. The Foundation
has built a permanent, flexable endowment and has distributed
grants and awards to a broad range of organizations and people
throughout the region.

3008 Hyams Foundation
50 Federal St
9th Floor
Boston, MA 02110   617-426-5600
                                     Fax: 617-426-5696
                               info@hyamsfoundation.org
                                     hyamsfoundation.org

Martella Wilson-Taylor, Chair
Angela Brown, Director of Programs
Mike Givens, Communications Manager
Jocelyn V Sargent, Executive Director
The mission of the foundation is to increase economic and social
stregnth within low-income communities in Boston and Chelsea,
Massachusetts. Some areas they provide funding to include com-
munity identified issues, racial justice and transitional funding.

3009 Raytheon Company Contributions Program
870 Winter St
Waltham, MA 02451-1449   781-522-3000
                                     Fax: 781-860-2172
                                          raytheon.com

Thomas A. Kennedy, Chief Financial Officer
David C. Wajsgras, Senior Vice President and Chief
Keith J. Peden, Senior Vice President - Human Re
Jay B. Stephens, Senior Vice President - General
Industry leader in defense and government electronics, space, in-
formation technology, technical services, and business aviation
and special mission aircraft.

3010 TJX Foundation
TJX Companies
770 Cochituate Rd
Framingham, MA 01701-4666   508-390-1000
                                     Fax: 508-390-2091
                                          www.tjx.com

Carol Meyrowitz, CEO
The purpose of the TJX Foundation's Giving Program is to support qualified, tax-exempt nonprofit organizations that provide
services which promote and improve the quality of life for children, women and families in need.

3011 Vision Foundation
8901 Strafford Cir
Knoxville, TN 37923-1500   865-357-4603
                                     Fax: 865-690-9322
                               gordon@visionfoundation.net
                                     www.visionfoundation.net

Gordon Adams, President
Offers counseling, support groups, seminars and transportation
for the blind providing 600 members.

Michigan

3012 Ann Arbor Area Community Foundation
301 N Main St
Ste 300
Ann Arbor, MI 48104-1296   734-663-0401
                                     Fax: 734-663-3514
                                          info@aaacf.org
                                          aaacf.org

Michelle Crumm, Chair
Tim Wadhams, Vice Chair
Neel Hajra, President & CEO
Shelley Strickland, Vice President
Interested in funding projects which will improve the quality of
life for citizens of the Ann Arbor area. Eligible projects generally
fall within these categories: education, culture, social service,
community development, environmental awareness and health
and wellness. The Foundation aims to support creative approaches to community needs and problems by making grants
which will benefit the widest possible range of people.

3013 Arc of Michigan
State of Michigan
1325 S Washington Ave
Lansing, MI 48910-1652   517-487-5426
                                          800-292-7851
                                     Fax: 517-487-0303
                                          dhoyle@arcmi.org
                                          arcmi.org

Shari Fitzpatrick, President
Kim Brown, Vice President
Bob Altizer, Secretary
Laurel Robb, Treasurer
The Arc Michigan empowers local chapters to assure that citizens
with disabilities are valued and that they and their families partic-
ipate fully in and contribute to the life of their community.

3014 Berrien Community Foundation
2900 S State St
Ste 2e
Saint Joseph, MI 49085-2467   269-983-3304
                                     Fax: 269-983-4939
                               bcf@BerrienCommunity.org
                                     berriencommunity.org

Hillary Bubb, Chair
Mabel Mayfield, Vice Chair
Lisa Cripps-Downey, President
Sandra Tardi, Finance Director
The Foundation is a union of numerous gifts, bequests and other
contributions that form permanent endowments and other funds.

3015 Blind Children's Fund
P.O. Box 187
Grand Ledge, MI 48837   517-488-4887
                               info@blindchildrensfund.org
                                     www.blindchildrensfund.org

Carrie L Owens, Board President
Diana Popp, Executive Director
Provides parents and professionals information materials and resources to help them teach and nurture blind and visually impaired children so they may reach their potential.

3016 Community Foundation of Monroe County
P.O. Box 627
28 S. Macomb St.
Monroe, MI 48161-627   734-242-1976
                                     Fax: 734-242-1234
                                          info@cfmonroe.org
                                          cfmonroe.org

Kathleen Russeau, MBA, Executive Director
Michele Sandiefer, Office Manager
Julie Rhinehart, YAC Coordinator
Doug Redding, Project Manager
The mission of the Community Foundation of Monroe County is
to encourage and facilitate philanthropy in Monroe County.

3017 Cowan Slavin Foundation
7881 Dell Rd
Saline, MI 48176-9744   734-944-1439
                                      Fax: 734-944-3529

David Bovee, Owner

3018 Daimler Chrysler
Automobility Program
P.O. Box 5080
Troy, MI 48007-5080   800-255-9877
                                      Fax: 855-409-0475
                              rebates@chrysler.com
                              www.chryslerautomobility.com

3019 Frank & Mollie S VanDervoort Memorial Foundation
4646 Okemos Rd
Okemos, MI 48864-1795   517-349-7232
Ann L Gessert, Secretary

3020 Fremont Area Community Foundation
4424 W. 48th Street
PO Box B
Fremont, MI 49412-176   231-924-5350
                                      Fax: 231-924-5351
                                             tfacf.org

Robert Zeldenrust, Chair
William Johnson, Vice Chair
Carla Roberts, President & CEO
Cathy Kissinger, Secretary
A local nonprofit organization serving the residence of Newaygo County. We connect the needs of the community with those who have the conviction to make a lasting impact. Our mission is to improve the quality of life for the people of Newaygo County.Zeldenrust

3021 Grand Rapids Foundation
185 Oakes St SW
Grand Rapids, MI 49503-4008   616-454-1751
                                      Fax: 616-454-6455
                              grfound@grfoundation.org
                                      grfoundation.org

Paul M. Keep, Chair
Laurie Finney Beard, Vice Chair
Diana R. Sieger, President
Ren Guttrich, Executive Assistant
Grand Rapids Community Foundation leads the community in making positive, sustainable change. Through our grantmaking and leadership initiatives we help foster academic achievement, build economic prosperity, achieve healthy ecosystems, encourage healthy people, support social enrichment, and create vibrant neighborhoods.

3022 Granger Foundation
6267 Aurelius Rd
Lansing, MI 48911-2187   517-393-1670
                                      Fax: 517-393-1382
                              grangerconstruction.com

Alton Granger, Chairman
Glenn D. Granger, President & CEO
The primary purpose of the Granger Foundation is to enhance the quality of life within the Greater Lansing, Michigan Area. Our mission is to support Christ-centered activities. We also support efforts that enhance the lives of youth in our community.

3023 Harvey Randall Wickes Foundation
4800 Fashion Square Blvd
Suite 472
Saginaw, MI 48604- 2677   989-799-1850
                                      Fax: 989-799-3327
                                             www.tgci.com

James Finkbeiner
Grants for rehabilitation.

3024 Havirmill Foundation
3505 Greenleaf Blvd
Ste 203
Kalamazoo, MI 49008-2580   269-375-1193
                              millenniumrestaurants.com

Ken Miller, CEO, Principal Partner
Matthew Burian, President
Bob Lewis, Operating Partner
Shelly Pastor, Operating Partner

3025 Kelly Services Foundation
999 W Big Beaver Rd
Troy, MI 48084-4782   248-362-4444
                                      Fax: 248-244-4588
                              kfirst@kellyservices.com
                                      kellyservices.com

George S. Corona, Chief Operating Officer
Carl T. Camden, President & CEO
Terence E. Adderley, Executive Chairman
Olivier Thirot, Acting Chief Financial Officer

3026 Kent County Arc
2922 Fuller Ave. NE
Ste 201
Grand Rapids, MI 49505   616-459-3339
                                      Fax: 401-737-8907
                                      info@arckent.org
                                      www.arckent.org

Pam Cross, President
Tim Lundgren, Vice-President
Tammy Finn, Executive Director
Maggie Kolk, Advocate/WIPA Benefits Counselor
Providing individuals with disabilties meaningful opportunities throughout their communities.

3027 Kresge Foundation
3215 W Big Beaver Rd
Troy, MI 48084-2818   248-643-9630
                                      Fax: 248-643-0588
                                      info@kresge.org
                                             kresge.org

Rip Rapson, President and CEO
Amy B. Coleman, VP/ CFO
Ariel H. Simon, Vice President, Chief Program
Marcus L. McGrew, Director of Grants Management
This foundation offers challenge grants for capital projects, most often for construction or renovation of buildings, but also for the purchase of major equipment and real estate. As challenge grants, they are intended to stimulate new, private gifts in the midst of an organized fund raising effort. Offers special opportunities to build capacity, both in providing enhanced facilities in which to present programs and in generating private support. Only charitable organizations may apply.

3028 Lanting Foundation
1575 S Shore Dr
Holland, MI 49423-4436   616-335-2033
Arlyn Lanting, Partner

3029 Rollin M Gerstacker Foundation
PO Box 1945
Midland, MI 48641-1945   989-631-6097
                              www.gerstackerfoundation.org

Gail E. Lanphear, Chairperson
Lisa J. Gerstacker, President
E. N. Brandt, Vice President /Secretary
Alan W Ott, Vice President /Treasurer
The Rollin M. Gerstacker Foundation was founded by Mrs. Eda U. Gerstacker in 1957, in memory of her husband. Its primary purpose is to carry on, indefinitely, financial aid to charities of all types supported by Mr. and Mrs. R.M. Gerstacker during their lifetimes. These charities are concentrated in the states of Michigan and Ohio.

3030 Steelcase Foundation
PO Box 1967
GH-4E
Grand Rapids, MI 49501-1967
616-246-4695
Fax: 616-475-2200
foundation@Steelcase.com
steelcase.com

Julie Ridenour, President
The Foundation focuses on the areas of human service, health, education, community development, the arts and the environment; giving particular concern to people who are disadvantaged, disabled, young and elderly as they attempt to improve the quality of their lives.
1951

Minnesota

3031 Arc of Minnesota
800 Transfer Road
Suite 7A
St. Paul, MN 55114
651-523-0823
800-582-5256
Fax: 651-523-0829
mail@arcmn.org
www.arcmn.org

John Rentschler, President
Lisa Schoneman, Vice President
Amy Hewitt, Secretary
Rob Wolf, Treasurer
Your membership in The Arc of Minnesotta benefits persons with developmental disabilities and their families as they live, learn, work and play. Please join today!

3032 Deluxe Corporation Foundation
Deluxe Corporation
3680 Victoria St N
Shoreview, MN 55126-2966
651-483-7111
800-328-0304
Fax: 651-483-7270
feedback@deluxe.com
ww.deluxe.com

Lee J Schram, CEO
Terry D. Peterson, CFO /Senior VP
Malcolm J. McRoberts, Senior Vice President, Small Bus
John D. Filby, Senior Vice President, Financial
Funds programs such as schools, museums, programs for the disadvantaged. We believe programs and services like these represent the heart and soul of our communities.

3033 General Mills Foundation
P.O. Box 9452
Minneapolis, MN 55440-9452
800-248-7310
Fax: 763-764-8330
corporate.response@genmills.com
generalmills.com

Kendall J. Powell, Chairman / CEO
Ann W.H. Simonds, Senior Vice President/ Chief Mar
Keith A Woodward, Vice President, Treasurer
Gary Chu, Senior Vice President

3034 Hugh J Andersen Foundation
342 5th Ave N
Suite 200
Bayport, MN 55003-4502
651-439-1557
888-439-9508
Fax: 651-439-9480
contact@srinc.biz
www.srinc.biz

Brad Kruse, Program Director
Established in 1962, this fund is a nonprofit charitable corporation classified as a private foundation. The Foundation was established as a general charitable fund, but now identifies projects that build individual and community capacity to be a priority. Giving is focused primarily in the counties of Washington, Minnesota, & St, Croix, Polk and Pierce of Wl. Grants are given in the areas of human services, health, education, arts and culture, community services and the environment.

3035 James R Thorpe Foundation
5866 Oakland Avenue
Minneapolis, MN 55417-5418
763-250-9304
info@jamesrthorpefoundation.org
www.jamesrthorpefoundation.org

Tim Thorpe, President
Robert C. Cote, Treasurer
Kerrie Blevins, Foundation Manager
S. Ruggles Cote, Board Member
Foundation based on values of respect and compassion, and is dedicated to making the greater Minneapolis area better for all its citizens.

3036 Jay and Rose Phillips Family Foundation
615 First Ave. NE
Ste. 330
Minneapolis, MN 55413
612-623-1654
Fax: 612-623-1653
info@phillipsfamilyfoundationmn.org

Patrick Troska, Executive Director
Joel Luedtke, Senior Program Officer
Tracy Lamparty, Grants and Operations Manager
Salena Acox, Vista Program Manager

3037 Minneapolis Foundation
80 S 8th St
800 IDS Center
Minneapolis, MN 55402-2100
612-672-3878
866-305-0543
Fax: 612-672-3846
email@mplsfoundation.org
www.mplsfoundation.org

Sandra L. Vargus, President and CEO
Jean M. Adams, Chief Operating Officer/Chief Fi
Teresa Morrow, Vice President, External Relatio
Luz Maria Frias, Vice President, Community Impact
Provides a variety of charitable fund and gift options to help Minnesotans make a difference.

3038 Ordean Foundation
424 W Superior St
Duluth, MN 55802-1591
218-726-4785
Steve Mangan, Executive Director
Grants are given for a variety of purposes including: treatment and rehabilitation for persons who are chronically or temporarily mentally ill, persons whose physical capacity is impaired by injury or illness, promotes mental and physical health of the elderly, provides for youth guidance programs designed to avoid delinquency, and provides relief, aid and charity to people with no or low incomes. Grants are only offered to certain cities and townships near and around St. Louis County/Duluth.

3039 Otto Bremer Foundation
445 Minnesota St
Ste 2250
Saint Paul, MN 55101-2161
651-227-8036
888-291-1123
Fax: 651-312-3665
obf@ottobremer.org
www.ottobremer.org

Kari Suzuki, Director of Operations
Diane Benjamin, Executive Director
Danielle Cheslog, Grants Manager
Rose Carr, Program Officer
Mission is to assist people in achieving full economic, civic and social participation in and for the betterment of their communities.

3040 Rochester Area Foundation
400 South Broadway
Suite 300
Rochester, MN 55904 507-282-0203
Fax: 507-282-4938
info@rochesterarea.org
rochesterarea.org

JoAnn Stormer, President
Max Evans, Administration/Communications
Ann Fahy-Gust, Grants and Impact Officer
Paul Harkess, Development Officer
The mission of the Rochester Area Foundation is to strengthen community philanthropy by promoting responsible and informed giving and to assist donors in meeting their charitable objectives.

Mississippi

3041 Arc of Mississippi
704 North President Street
Jackson, MS 39202 601-355-0220
800-717-1180
Fax: 601-355-0221
info@arcms.org
www.arcms.org

Kim Duffy, President
Ronnie Raggio, Senior Vice-President
Shirley Miller, Secretary
Cherri Hedglin, Treasurer
The Arc is Committed to securing for all people with developmental disabilities the opportunity to choose and realize their goals of where and how they learn live work and play.

Missouri

3042 Allen P & Josephine B Green Foundation
1055 Broadway
Suite 130
Kansas City, MO 64105 816-627-3420
Fax: 816-268-3420
greenfoundation@gkccf.org
www.greenfdn.org
Matthew Fuller, Manager of Community Investment
While the Foundation makes grants in a variety of fields, in the past its major support was in the field of medical research. During a 20-year period, 1951-71, it contributed over $900,000 to research in Parkinson's and related diseases of the nervous system; $600,000 for research in pediatric neurology and lesser amounts in other areas of medical research, but the board is now trending in other directions. Grants are limited to Missouri and none are offered to individuals.

3043 Anheuser-Busch
1 Busch Pl
Saint Louis, MO 63118-1852 314-577-2000
800-342-5283
Fax: 314-577-2900
anheuser-busch.com

August A Busch Iv, President
Supports education, helped fund health and human services organizations, provided disaster relief, and worked to preserve the environment.

3044 Arc of the US Missouri Chapter
PO Box 7823
Columbia, MO 65205 573-552-7648
arcmoinfo@arcofmissouri.org
www.arcofmissouri.org

3045 Greater Kansas City Community Foundation & Affiliated Trusts
1055 Broadway Blvd
Suite 130
Kansas City, MO 64105-1595 816-842-0944
866-719-7886
Fax: 816-842-8079
info@gkccf.org
www.growyourgiving.org
William S. Berkley, Past Chair
Dr. Jim Hinson, Vice Chair
William H. Coughlin, President
Mary Bloch, Community Volunteer
Mission is to improve the quality of life in Greater Kansas City by increasing charitable giving, connecting donors to community needs they care about, and providing leadership on critical community issues.

3046 Greater St Louis Community Foundation
319 N 4th St
Ste 300
Saint Louis, MO 63102-1906 314-588-8200
Fax: 314-588-8088
dluckes@gstlcf.org
gstlcf.org
Stephen J. Rafferty, Chair
Thomas R. Collins, Vice Chair & Secretary
Amelia A.J. Bond, President & CEO
Mara Mitch Meyers, Treasurer
To improve the quality of life across the region by helping individuals, families and businesses make a difference through charitable giving.

3047 H&R Block Foundation
1 H and R Block Way
Kansas City, MO 64105-1905 816-854-4363
Fax: 816-854-8025
foundation@hrblock.com
www.blockfoundation.org
Henry W. Bloch, Chairman/ Treasurer/ Director
Thomas M. Bloch, Vice Chairman & Director
David P. Miles, President
Carey Wilker Looney, Vice President and Secretary
A charitable organization under the not-for-profit corporation law of the state of Missouri. Grants are made only to organizations which are tax exempt from Federal Income taxation and which are not classified as private foundations. Major emphasis is placed in the metropolitan areas of Kansas City, Missouri: and Columbus, Ohio. The goal is to provide proportionately significant support of relatively few activities, as opposed to minor support for a great many.

3048 James S McDonnell Foundation
1034 S Brentwood Blvd
Suite 1850
Saint Louis, MO 63117- 1284 314-721-1532
Fax: 314-721-7421
info@jsmf.org
jsmf.org
Susan M Fitzpatrick, President
John T. Bruer, President Emeritus
Cheryl A. Washington, Grants Manager
M. Brent Dolezalek, Senior Program Associate
The Foundation supports scientific, educational, and charitable causes locally, nationally and internationally.

3049 Lutheran Charities Foundation of St Louis
8860 Ladue Road
Suite 200
Saint Louis, MO 63124 314-231-2244
Fax: 314-727-7688
info@lutheranfoundation.org
www.lutheranfoundation.org
Karl A. Dunajcik, Chairperson of the Board
Ann L. Vazquez, President/ CEO
Melinda K. McAliney, Program Director
Donna Luker, Office/Grants Manager

Seeks the improved care of people in the greater St. Louis metropolitan region. Lutheran Foundation of St. Louis manages the endowment established upon the sale of the Lutheran Medical Center and provides grant awards for health, human care, Lutheran congregations' community service programs, and Lutheran education.

3050 **RA Bloch Cancer Foundation**
1 H and R Block Way
Kansas City, MO   64105-1905   816-854-5050
                                     800-433-0464
                               Fax: 816-854-8024
                          hotline@blochcancer.org
                               www.blochcancer.org
Vangie Rich, Executive Director
Rosanne Wickman, Hotline Director
Provides a hotline that matches newly diagnosed cancer patients with someone who has survived the same kind of cancer. Offers free infomration, resources and support groups, and distributes lists of multidisciplinary second opinion centers. Also supplies three books at no charge: Fighting Cancer; Cancer... There's Hope; and A Guide for Cancer Supporters. All services and books are free of charge.

3051 **Victor E Speas Foundation**
10434 Indiana Ave
Kansas City, MO   64137-1532   816-868-9300
                          mo.grantmaking@ustrust.com
                             www.bankofamerica.com
Latricia Scott Adams, President
VCC is a membership-based organization that brings together area volunteer managers and others interested in volunteerism for mutual support, exchange of ideas and information, and educational programs of timely interest.

Nebraska

3052 **Arc of Nebraska**
215 Centennial Mall South
Suite 508
Lincoln, NE   68508   402-475-4407
                                     888-519-6524
                               Fax: 402-475-0214
                           info@arc-nebraska.org
                             www.arc-nebraska.org
Debbie Salomon, President
David Rowe, 1st Vice President
Kadi Holmberg, 2nd Vice President
Michael Chittenden, Executive Director
Arc of Nebraska is commited to helping children and adults with disabilities secure the oppurtunity to choose and realize their goals of where and how they learn, live, work, and play.

3053 **Cooper Foundation**
1248 O St
Suite 870
Lincoln, NE   68508-1493   402-476-7571
                               Fax: 402-476-2356
                         info@cooperfoundation.org
                               cooperfoundation.org
Jack Campbell, Chair
Brad Korell, VP Business Development
Art Thompson, President
Robert Nefsky, Attorney & Partner
Serves only Nebraska with the primary interest in education, arts and humanities and the human services area.

3054 **Mosaic**
4980 S 118th St
Omaha, NE   68137-2200   402-896-9988
                                     877-366-7242
                               Fax: 402-896-1511
                              info@mosaicinfo.org
                               www.mosaicinfo.org
Linda Timmons, President / CEO
Cindy Schroeder, Chief Financial Officer
Raul Saldivar, Chief Operating Officer
Scott Hoffman, Senior Vice President of Finance
Headquarters for the faith-based organization providing services to people with disabilities in communities nationwide, and in conjunction with international partners. Mosaic was born of a merger of these two Lutheran organizations: Bethpage and Martin Luther Homes Society.

3055 **Slosburg Family Charitable Trust**
10040 Regency Cir
Ste 200
Omaha, NE   68114-3734   402-391-7900
                               Fax: 402-391-2991
                                     richdale.com
David Slosburg, Owner

3056 **Union Pacific Foundation**
1400 Douglas Street
Omaha, NE   68179   402-544-5000
                                     888-870-8777
                                     888-877-7267
                               Fax: 402-501-0021
                                     www.up.com
John J. Koraleski, Executive Chairman
Lance M. Fritz, President & COO of Union Pacific
Eric L. Butler, EVP, Marketing and Sales
Diane K. Duren, EVP/ Corporate Secretary
The Union Pacific Foundation is the philanthropic arm of the Union Pacific Corporation and Union Pacific Railroad. Union Pacific believes that the quality of life in the commuinities in which its employees live and work is an integral part of its own success.

Nevada

3057 **EL Wiegand Foundation**
165 W Liberty St
Suite 200
Reno, NV   89501-1955   775-333-0310
                               Fax: 775-333-0314
                      www.thewiegandfoundationinc.com
Kristen A Avansino, President/Executive Director

3058 **Nell J Redfield Foundation**
PO Box 61
Reno, NV   89504-0061   775-323-1373
                               Fax: 775-323-4476
                       redfieldfoundation@yahoo.com
Jerry Smith, Manager
Gerald C. Smith, V.P. and Secy

3059 **William N Pennington Foundation**
441 W Plumb Ln
Reno, NV   89509-3766   775-333-9100
                               Fax: 775-333-9111
William Pennington, Owner

New Hampshire

3060   Agnes M Lindsay Trust
660 Chestnut St
Manchester, NH   03104-3550   603-669-1366
                                              866-669-1366
                                        Fax: 603-665-8114
                                      admin@lindsaytrust.org
                                            lindsaytrust.org

Susan E. Bouchard, Administrative Director
Ernest E. Dion, CPA, Trustee
Alan G. Lampert, Esq., Trustee
Michael S. Delucia, Esq., Trustee
Funding for health and wefare organizations, special needs, mental health, blind, deaf and cultural programs to organizations, specifically for capital needs, not operating funds, located in the New England states of Maine, Massachusetts, New Hampshire and Vermont. We highly recommend you visit our web site.

3061   Foundation for Seacoast Health
100 Campus Dr
Ste 1
Portsmouth, NH   03801-5892   603-422-8200
                                        Fax: 603-422-8206
                                   ffsh@communitycampus.org
                                                  ffsh.org

Debra S. Grabowski, Executive Director
Kathleen Taylor, Finance Director
Eligio Santana, Facility Manager
Noreen Hodgdon, Executive Assistant
Giving limited to Portsmouth, Rye, New Castle, Greenland, Newington, North Hampton, NH; and Kittery, Eliot, and York, ME.

New Jersey

3062   Arc of New Jersey
985 Livingston Ave
N Brunswick, NJ   08902-1843   732-246-2525
                                        Fax: 732-214-1834
                                                  arcnj.org

Robert Hage, President
Joanne Bergin, First Vice President
Kevin Sturges, Second Vice President
Elspeth Moore, Secretary
The Arc of New Jersey is committed to enhancing the quality of life of children and adults with intellectual and developmental disabilities and their families, through advocacy, empowerment, education and prevention.

3063   Arnold A Schwartz Foundation
15 Mountain Blvd
Warren, NJ   7059-5611   908-757-7800
                                        Fax: 908-757-8039

Steven A Kunzman, President

3064   Campbell Soup Foundation
1 Campbell Pl
Camden, NJ   08103-1701   800-257-8443
                                    media@campbellsoup.com
                                            campbellsoup.com

Denise M. Morrison, President/ CEO
Anthony P. DiSilvestro, Senior Vice President and Chief
Mark Alexander, President
Carlos J. Barraso, Senior Vice President - Global R
Goal of this foundation is to match the company's assets with community needs in order to help forge solutions to community challenges. The Foundation believes that involvement at the community level can play a catalytic role in improving the quality of life. Giving is located in the areas of education, nutrition and health, cultural and youth related programs. The major focus of the foundation is on nutrition and health related matters, and places a high priority on Camden, New Jersey areas.

3065   Children's Hopes & Dreams Wish Fulfillment Foundation
280 US Highway 46
Dover, NJ   07801-2084   706-482-2248
                                        Fax: 706-482-2289
                                            www.helpingnow.org

3066   Community Foundation of New Jersey
35 Knox Hill Road Morristown
PO Box 338
Morristown, NJ 07963-0388   973-267-5533
                                              800-659-5533
                                        Fax: 973-267-2903
                                                info@cfnj.org
                                                www.cfnj.org

Hans Dekker, President
Madeline Rivera, Program Officer
Susan I. Soldivieri, Chief Financial Officer
Faith Krueger, Chief Operating Officer
The Community Foundation of New Jersey is an alliance of families, businesses, and foundations that work together to create lasting differences in lives and communities today and tomorrow.

3067   FM Kirby Foundation
17 DeHart Street
PO Box 151
Morristown, NJ   07963-0151   973-538-4800
                            www.fdncenter.org/grantmaker/kirby

S. Dillard Kirby, President and Director
Jefferson W Kirby, Vice President and Director
Alice Kirby Horton, Assistant Secretary and Director
Walker D. Kirby, Director
Family foundation, grants made to a wide range of nonprofit organizations in education, health and medicine, the arts and humanities, civic and public affairs, as well as religious, welfare and youth organizations.

3068   Fannie E Rippel Foundation
14 Maple Avenue
Suite 200
Morristown, NJ   07960   973-540-0101
                                        Fax: 973-540-0404
                                    info@rippelfoundation.org
                                    www.rippelfoundation.org

Laura K Landy, President/ CEO
Chana Fitton, Chief Operating Officer
John D. Campbell, Chairman
Elizabeth G. Christopherson, Secretary
Core purposes: research and treatment related to cancer and heart disease, the health of women and the elderly, and the quality of our nation's hospitals.

3069   Fund for New Jersey
One Palmer Square East
Suite 303
Princeton, NJ   08542   609-356-0421
                                      lmandell@fundfornj.org
                                                fundfornj.org

Kiki Jamieson, President
Lucy Vandenberg, Senior Program Officer
Laura Mandell, Office Manager
Ami Kachalia, Program Associate
Our grants promote projects that share a high purpose of furthering effective democracy through a range of methods encompassing education, advocacy, public policy analysis, and community problem-solving.

3070   Merck Company Foundation
2000 Galloping Hill Road
Kenilworth, NJ   07033   908-740-4000
                                                  merck.com

Kenneth C. Frazier, Chairman
Robert M. Davis, Executive Vice President and Chi
Willie A. Deese, EVP and President, Merck Manufac
Clark Golestani, Executive Vice President and Chi
Mission of the foundation is to support organizations and innovative programs in alignment with four strategic profiles: Improving access to quality health care and the appropriate use of

medicines and vaccines,building capacity in the biomedical and health sciences, promoting environments that support innovation, economic growth and development in and ethical and fair context, and supporting communities where Merck employees work and live.

3071 Nabisco Foundation
7 Campus Dr
Parsippany, NJ 07054-4413   973-682-7096
                                     Fax: 973-503-3018

Henry Sandbach, Director

3072 Ostberg Foundation
PO Box 1098
Alpine, NJ 07620-1098   201-569-6800
                                     Fax: 201-767-8006

3073 Prudential Foundation
Prudential Financial
751 Broad St
15th Floor
Newark, NJ 07102-3714   973-802-6000
                                     Fax: 973-802-7486
                         community.resources@prudential.com
                                          prudential.com

John R Strangfeld, Chairman and CEO
Mark B. Grier, Vice Chairman
Charles Lowrey, Executive Vice President, Chief
Sharon C. Taylor, Senior Vice President, Corporate
Gives priority to national programs that further our objectives and programs serving areas where The Prudential has a substantial employee presence. Places special emphasis on the home state of New Jersey and the headquarters city, Newark.

3074 Robert Wood Johnson Foundation
Route 1 and College Road East
P.O. Box 2316
Princeton, NJ 08543-2316   609-452-8701
                                             877-843-7953
                                     Fax: 888-727-1966
                                           mail@rwjf.org
                                              rwjf.org

Roger S. Fine, Chairman
Risa Lavizzo-Mourey, President and CEO
Robin E. Mockenhaupt, Chief of Staff
Joan F. McKay, Executive Assistant, Executive O
Our mission is to assure that all Americans have access to basic health care at reasonable cost, improve care and support for people with chronic health conditions, promote healthy communities and lifestyles and also, reduce the personal, social and economic harm caused by substance abuse.

3075 Victoria Foundation
31 Mulberry Street
5th Floor
Newark, NJ 07102-1397   973-792-9200
                                     Fax: 973-792-1300
                               info@victoriafoundation.org
                               www.victoriafoundation.org

Frank Alvarez, President
Margaret H. Parker, Vice President
Gary M. Wingens, Treasurer
Irene Cooper-Basch, Executive Officer
Desire is to help individuals in need reach their potential remains. Provides emergency coal for needy families and treated rheumatic fever in children.

New Mexico

3076 Arc of New Mexico
3655 Carlisle NE
Albuquerque, NM 87110-1644   505-883-4630
                                             800-358-6493
                                     Fax: 505-883-5564
                                         rcostales@arcnm.org
                                              arcnm.org

John Hall, President
Dolores Harden, Senior Vice President
Elaine Palma, Secretary
Randy Costales, Executive Director
Our mission is to improve the quality of life for individuals with developmental disabilities of all ages by advocating for equal opportunities and choices in where and how they learn, live, work, play and socialize. The Arc of New Mexico promotes self-determination, healthy families, effective community support systems and partnerships.

3077 Frost Foundation
511 Armijo St
Suite A
Santa Fe, NM 87501-2899   505-986-0208
                                         info@frostfound.org
                                            frostfound.org

Mary Amelia Whited-Howell, President
Philip B. Howell, Executive Vice President
Taylor F. Moore, Secretary/Treasurer
Ann Rogers Gerber, Board Member
The Frost Foundation was created to be operated excusively for educational, charitable, and religious purposes.

3078 McCune Charitable Foundation
345 E Alameda St
Santa Fe, NM 87501-2229   505-983-8300
                                     Fax: 505-983-7887
                                        mccune@nmmccune.org
                                            nmmccune.org

Sarah McCune Losinger, Chair
Wendy Lewis, Executive Director
Henry Rael, Program Officer
Carla Romero, Administrative Director
Dedicated to enriching the health, education, environment, and cultural and spiritual life of New Mexicans.

3079 Santa Fe Community Foundation
501 Halona Street
Santa Fe, NM 87505   505-988-9715
                                     Fax: 505-988-1829
                               foundation@santafecf.org
                                      www.santafecf.org

Suzanne Ortega Cisneros, Chair
Barry Herskowitz, Vice Chair
Kenneth Romero, Secretary
Stephen G. Gaber, Treasurer

New York

3080 AFB Center on Vision Loss
American Foundation for the Blind
2 Penn Plaza
Suite 1102
New York, NY 10121-4524   212-502-7600
                                     Fax: 888-545-8331
                                           afbinfo@afb.net
                                               afb.org

Carl R Augusto, President & CEO
Kelly Bleach, Chief Administrative Officer
Rick Bozeman, Chief Financial Officer
Paul Schroeder, Vice President
National nonprofit organization that expands possibilities for people with vision loss.

3081   AT&T Foundation
32 Avenue of the Americas
24th Floor
New York, NY 10013-2473   212-226-2216
                                    Fax: 212-387-5097
                                        info@att.com
                                         www.att.com
Randall L Stephenson, Chairman, Chief Executive Office
John T. Stanky, Group President and Chief Strate
Wayne Watts, Senior Executive Vice President
John Stephens, Senior Executive Vice President
Committed to advancing education, strengthening communities
and improving lives.

3082   Altman Foundation
521 5th Ave
Fl 35
New York, NY 10175-3500   212-682-0970
                                    Fax: 212-682-1648
                                        info@altman.org
                                     altmanfoundation.org
Karen L. Rosa, President
Jeremy Tennenbaum, Chief Financial Officer
Ann E. Maldonado, Office Manager
Megan McAllister, Program Officer
For the benefit of such charitable and educational institutions in
the City of New York as said directors shall approve. Foundation
grants support programs and institutions that enrich the quality of
life in the city, with a particular focus on initiatives that help individuals, families and communities benefit from the services and
opportunities that will enable them to achieve their full potential.

3083   Ambrose Monell Foundation
1 Rockefeller Plz
Suite 301
New York, NY 10020-2002   212-586-0700
                                    Fax: 212-245-1863
                                    info@monellvetlesen.org
                                     www.monellvetlesen.org
Ambrose K. Monell,, President and Treasurer
Eugene P. Grisanti, Vice-President
George Rowe, Vice-President
Kristen G. Pemberton, Secretary
Voluntary aiding and contributing to religious, charitable, scien-
tific, literary, and educational uses and purposes, in New York,
elsewhere in the US and throughout the world.

3084   American Chai Trust
41 Madison Ave
Suite 400
New York, NY 10010-2202   212-889-0575
                                    Fax: 212-743-8120
                                 info@perlmanandperlman.com
                                  www.perlmanandperlman.com

3085   American Foundation for the Blind
2 Penn Plaza
Suite 1102
New York, NY 10121   800-232-5463
                                        info@afb.org
                                         www.afb.org
Kirk Adams, President & CEO
Darren M. Davis, Executive Administrator Executive Office
The American Foundation for the Blind (AFB) is a national non-
profit that is dedicated to removing barriers, creating solutions,
and expanding possibilities for the blind and visually impaired.
The AFB is focused on spreading access to technology, elevating
the quality of information and tools for professional who serve
people with vision loss, and the promotion of independent living
for those with vision loss.

3086   Arthur Ross Foundation
20 E 74th St
Ste 4c
New York, NY 10021-2654   212-737-7311
                                    Fax: 212-650-0332
Arthur Ross, President

3087   Artists Fellowship
47 5th Ave
New York, NY 10003-4303   212-255-7740
                                    info@artistsfellowship.org
                                     www.artistsfellowship.org
Babette Bloch, President
Private, charitable foundation that assists professional fine arts
and their families in times of emergency, disability, or
bereavement.

3088   Bodman Foundation
767 3rd Ave
4th Floor
New York, NY 10017-2023   212-644-0322
                                    Fax: 212-759-6510
                                  www.achelis-bodman-fnds.org
John N. Irwin III, Chairman
Russell P. Pennoyer, President
Peter Frelinghuysen, Vice President
John B. Krieger, Executive Director
Foundation concentrates their grant programs in New York City,
but foundation also makes some grants in Northern New Jersey.
Funding is concentrated in six program areas: Arts & Culture, Ed-
ucation, Employment, Health, Public Policy and Youth and
Families.

3089   Brooklyn Home for Aged Men
P.O.Box 280062
Brooklyn, NY 11228   718-745-1638
                                    Fax: 718-745-0813
                                     www.brooklynhome.org
Catherine M. Birdseye, Co-President
William E. Spaulding, Co-President
Andelusia Wheeler, Co-President
Edwin A. Ames, Co-President
The Brooklyn Home For Aged Men has served the community for
more than one hundred years. Although originally set up as a resi-
dence for men, it later accepted women and couples as well.

3090   Cancer Care
275 7th Avenue
22nd Floor
New York, NY 10001-6754   212-712-8400
                                        800-813-4673
                                    Fax: 212-712-8495
                                     info@cancercare.org
                                      www.cancercare.org
Patricia J. Goldsmith, Chief Executive Officer
John Rutigliano, Chief Operating Officer
Sue Lee, Senior Director of Development
Ann Navarria, Director of Human Resources
A national non-profit organization that provides free, profes-
sional support services to anyone affected by cancer: people with
cancer, caregivers, children, loved ones, and the bereaved.

3091   Children's Tumor Foundation
120 Wall Street
16th Floor
New York, NY 10005-3904   212-344-6633
                                        800-323-7938
                                    Fax: 212-747-0004
                                        info@ctf.org
                                          ctf.org
Linda Halliday Martin, Chairperson
Colin Bryar, Vice Chairperson
Annette Bakker, PhD, President and Chief Scientific Officer
Tracy Galloway, Secretary
A nonprofit 501 (c)(3) medical foundation, dedicated to improving the health and well-being of individuals and families affected
by neurofibromatosis. The Foundation sponsors medical research, clinical services, public education programs and patient
support services. It is the central source for up-to-date and accurate information about NF. It also assists patients and families
with referrals to NF clinics and healthcare professionals specializing in NF. The goal is to find a cure for NF.

3092   Commonwealth Fund
1 E 75th St
New York, NY   10021-2692   212-606-3800
                                        Fax: 212-606-3500
                                          info@cmwf.org
                                    www.commonwealthfund.org

Benjamin K. Chu, Chairman
Cristine Russell, Vice Chairman
Donald Moulds, Executive Vice President for Pro
Barry Scholl, Senior Vice President for Commun
A private foundation with the broad charge to enhance the common good. Carries out this mandate by supporting efforts that help people live healthy and productive lives, and by assisting certain groups with serious and neglected problems. Supports independent research on health and social issues and makes grants to improve heathcare practice and policy.

3093   Community Foundation for Greater Buffalo
726 Exchange Street,
Suite 525
Buffalo, NY   14210   716-852-2857
                                        Fax: 716-852-2861
                                           mail@cfgb.org
                                                cfgb.org

Marsha Joy Sullivan, Chair
William Joyce, Vice Chair
Gary L. Mucci,, Secretary
Ross Eckert, Treasurer
Mission is connecting people, ideas, and resources to improve lives in Western New York

3094   Community Foundation of Herkimer & Oneida Counties
2608 Genesee Street
Utica, NY   13502-4728   315-735-8212
                                        Fax: 315-735-9363
                                     info@foundationhoc.org
                                        foundationhoc.org

Alicia Dicks, President/CEO
Gilles Lauzon, Director of Finance
Elayne Johnson, Director of Fund Administration
Laura Cohen, Program Officer
Mission of the foundation is to improve the lives of the residents of Herkimer and Oneida Counties.

3095   Community Foundation of the Capitol Region
Six Tower Place
Albany, NY   12203-3749   518-446-9638
                                        Fax: 518-446-9708
                                          info@cfgcr.org
                                           www.cfgcr.org

Karen Bilowith, President/CEO
Mindy Derosia, Development Officer
Shelly Connolly, Program Assistant
Jackie Mahoney, Vice President of Programs
Mission is to strengthen our community by attracting charitable endowments both large and small, maximizing benefits to donors, making effective gtants, and providing leadership to address community needs.

3096   Comsearch: Broad Topics
Foundation Center
79 5th Ave
New York, NY   10003-3034   212-620-4230
                                             800-424-9836
                                        Fax: 212-807-3677
                             communications@foundationcenter.org
                                        www.fdncenter.org

Bradford K. Smith, President
Lisa Philip, Vice President for Strategic Phi
Jen Bokoff, Director of GrantCraft
Steven Lawrence, Director of Research
Subset publications of The Foundation Grants Index, are printouts of actual foundation grants, covering 26 key areas of grantmaking. This tool is designed for fundraisers who wish to examine grantmaking activities in a broad field of interest.
$55.00

3097   DE French Foundation
Ste 503
120 Genesee St
Auburn, NY   13021-3672   315-252-3634
Walter Lowe, Owner

3098   Dana Foundation
Dana Alliance for Brain Initiatives
505 Fifth Avenue
6th floor
New York, NY   10017   212-223-4040
                                        Fax: 212-317-8721
                                         danainfo@dana.org
                                           www.dana.org

Edward F Rover, President /Chairman
Burton M. Mirsky, Executive Vice President, Financ
Barbara Rich, Ed.D., EVP, Communications; Assistant S
Barbara E Gill, Executive Vice President
A private philanthropy with principal interests in brain science, immunology, and arts education.

3099   David J Green Foundation
Ste 12
599 Lexington Ave
New York, NY   10022-6030   212-317-8820
                                        Fax: 212-371-5099
                                         www.djgreene.com

Valerie Ventolora, Manager
Michael Greene, Manager

3100   Easter Seals New York
40 W 37th St
Suite 503
New York, NY   10018-7907   212-220-2290
                                             800-727-8785
                                        Fax: 212-695-4807
                                    www.easterseals.com/newyork

John W. McGrath, MPA, Chief Executive Director
Aris Pavlides, Senior Vice President Developmen
Thomas Renart, M.A., M.S., Senior Vice-President Program Se
Kevin Carey, Director of Finance
Offers resources and expertise that allow children and adults with disabilities to live with dignity and independence. A long standing commitment to serve those for whom no other resources exist. Statewide, provides innovative solutions that enhance the lives of people with disabilities, while heightening community awareness and acceptance.

3101   Edna McConnel Clark Foundation
415 Madison Ave
Tenth Floor
New York, NY   10017-7949   212-551-9100
                                        Fax: 212-421-9325
                                          info@emcf.org
                                               emcf.org

Nancy Roob, President
Woodrow C. McCutchen, Vice President, Senior Portfolio
Kelly Fitzsimmons, Vice President, Chief Program an
Charles Harris, Portfolio Manager
Helps young people, ages 9-24, from low-income backgrounds become independent, productive adults.

3102   Edward John Noble Foundation
Fl 19
32 E 57th St
New York, NY   10022-8562   212-759-4212
                                        Fax: 212-888-4531

June Noble Larkin, Owner
June Larkin, Owner

3103   Epilepsy Foundation of Long Island
1500 Hempstead Turnpike
East Meadow, NY   11554
516-739-7733
888-672-7154
Fax: 516-739-1860
efli.org

Thomas Hopkins, President & CEO
Paul Giotis, Chief Operating Officer
Lawrence Boord, Chief Financial Officer
Gladys Brown, Director of Intake Coordination
Provides education, counseling and residential care to Long Island residents with epilepsy and related conditions.

3104   Episcopal Charities
1047 Amsterdam Avenue
New York, NY   10025-1747
212-316-7575
episcopalcharities@dioceseny.org
episcopalcharities-newyork.org

John Talty, President
Lorraine A. LaHuta, Vice President
Evan A. Davis, Secretary
John P Banning, Treasurer
Provides funding and support to a broad range of community-based human service programs throughout the Diocese of New York. These programs, sponsored by Episcopal congregations, serve disadvantaged individuals, youth and families on a non-sectarian basis.

3105   Esther A & Joseph Klingenstein Fund
125 Park Avenue
Suite 1700
New York, NY   10017-5529
212-492-6195
kathleen.pomerantz@klingenstein.com
www.klingfund.org

Charles D. Gilbert, Chairman
Andrew D. Klingenstein, President
Kathleen Pomerantz, Vice President
Supports young investigators engaged in basic or clinical research that may lead to a better understanding of epilepsy

3106   Fay J Lindner Foundation
189 Wheatley Road
Brookville, NY   11545
516-686-4440
www.fayjlindnercenter.org

Terrence Ullrich, President
Dr. Robert Steinberger, Vice President
Thomas F. Moore, Treasurer
Frederick Sterbenz, Secretary

3107   Ford Foundation
320 E 43rd St
New York, NY   10017-4890
212-573-5000
Fax: 212-351-3677
office-of-communications@fordfoundation.org
www.fordfound.org

Darren Walker, President
Kenneth T Monterio, Vice President, Secretary and Ge
Alfred Ironside, Vice President/Communications
Nicholas M. Gabriel, Vice President, Treasurer and Ch
A resource for innovative people and institutions worldwide. Goals are to: strengthen democratic values; reduce poverty and injustice; promote international cooperation; and advance human achievement. While not specific to disabilities, the Ford Foundation operates on several levels that indirectly assist and support those with disabilities through human and civil rights issues, social justice support, economic fairness and opportunity, and access to education involvements.

3108   Fortis Foundation
28 Liberty Street
New York, NY   10005-1401
212-859-7197
Fax: 212-859-7010
Investor.Relations@assurant.com
ir.assurant.com

Elaine D. Rosen, Chair
Howard L. Carver, Director
Melissa Kivett, Senior Vice President, Investor
Suzanne Shepherd, Director, Investor Relations

3109   Foundation Center
79 5th Ave
16th Street
New York, NY   10003-3076
212-620-4230
800-424-9836
Fax: 212-807-3677
communications@foundationcenter.org
foundationcenter.org

Bradford K Smith, President
Lisa Philip, VP, Strategic Philanthropy
Jen Bokoff, Director of GrantCraft
Steven Lawrence, Director of Research
The Foundation Center publishes Foundation Directory Online, with key facts on the US grantmakers and their grants.

3110   Foundation Center Library Services
Foundation Center
79 5th Ave
16th Street
New York, NY   10003-3076
212-620-4230
800-424-9836
Fax: 212-807-3677
communications@foundationcenter.org
foundationcenter.org

Bradford K Smith, President
Lisa Philip, VP, Strategic Philanthropy
Jen Bokoff, Director of GrantCraft
Steven Lawrence, Director of Research
The Center disseminates current information on foundation and corporate giving through our national collections in New York City and Washington D.C., our field offices in San Francisco and our network of over 180 cooperating libraries in all 50 states and abroad.

3111   Foundation for Advancement in Cancer Therapy
P.O.Box 1242
Old Chelsea Station
New York, NY   10113-1242
212-741-2790
info@rethinkingcancer.org
www.rethinkingcancer.org

Ruth Sackman, Founder
A clearinghouse for information regarding alternative cancer therapies, emphasizing nutritional and metabolic approaches.

3112   Gebbie Foundation
215 Cherry St
Jamestown, NY   14701-5207
716-487-1062
Fax: 716-484-6401
info@gebbie.org
www.gebbie.org

Gregory J Edwards, CEO
Daniel Kathman, President
Jonathan Taber, Vice President
Nancy Gleason, Secretary
Giving in Chautauqua County, and secondly, in neighboring areas of western New York. Giving is offered in other areas only when the project is consonant with program objectives that cannot be developed locally.

3113   Gladys Brooks Foundation
1055 Franklin Avenue
Suite 208
Garden City, NY   11530
kathy@gladysbrooksfoundation.org
www.gladysbrooksfoundation.org

Jessica L Rutledge, Director
The purpose of this Foundation is to provide for the intellectual, moral and physical welfare of the people of this country by establishing and supporting nonprofit libraries, educational institutions, hospitals and clinics. The Foundation will make grants only to private, publicly supported, nonprofit, tax-exempt organizations.

3114   Glickenhaus Foundation
546 5th Ave
New York, NY   10036-5000
212-953-7800
info@glickenhaus.com

Seth M. Glickenhaus, Senior Partner and Chief Investm

3115 Guide Dog Foundation for the Blind
371 East Jericho Turnpike
Smithtown, NY 11787-2976
631-930-9000
800-548-4337
Fax: 631-930-9009
info@guidedog.org
www.guidedog.org

James C. Bingham, Chair
Alphonce J. Brown, Vice Chair
Barbara J. Kelly, Secretary
Donald Dea, Treasurer
Providing mobility through the use of trained guide or service dogs to individuals who are blind or with other special needs.

3116 Hearst Foundations
300 W 57th St
Fl 26
New York, NY 10019-3741
212-649-2000
Fax: 212-887-6855
hearst.com

Steven R. Swartz, President and Chief Executive Of
National philanthropic resources for organziations and institutions working in the fields of education, health, culture and social services. Our goal is to ensure that people of all backgrounds have the opportunity to build healthy, productive and inspiring lives.

3117 Henry and Lucy Moses Fund
405 Lexington Ave
New York, NY 10174-1299
212-554-7800
Fax: 212-554-7700
www.mosessinger.com

Irving Sitnick, President
Provides legal services to many prominent industries, individuals and families in the New York City area.

3118 Herman Goldman Foundation
Fl 18
61 Broadway
New York, NY 10006-2708
212-797-9090
Alan Nisselson, President
A private nonoperating foundation.

3119 Kenneth & Evelyn Lipper Foundation
Fl 6
101 Park Ave
New York, NY 10178
212-883-6333
Kenneth Lipper, Director

3120 Long Island Alzheimer's Foundation
5 Channel Drive
Port Washington, NY 11050-2216
516-767-6856
Fax: 516-767-6864
www.liaf.org

Paul Eibeler, Chairman
Fred Jenny, Executive Director
Sean Phillips, Director of Development
Tiffany Ewald, Program Assistant

3121 Louis and Anne Abrons Foundation
First Manhattan Company
399 Park Avenue
New York, NY 10022-7001
212-756-3300
Fax: 212-223-4175
info@firstmanhattan.com
firstmanhattan.com

David Manischewitz, CEO
Sam Colin, Senior Managing Director
Allan Glick, Senior Managing Director
Neal Sterns, Senior Managing Director

3122 Margaret L Wendt Foundation
Ste 277
40 Fountain Plz
Buffalo, NY 14202-2200
716-855-2146
Fax: 716-855-2149

Robert J Kresse, Manager

3123 Merrill Lynch & Company Foundation
250 Vesey St
New York, NY 10080
212-449-1000
800-637-7455
Fax: 212-449-7969
ml.com

Brian T Moynihan, CEO
John Theil, Head
Andy M Sieg, Managing Director
John Hogarty, Chief Operating Officer
Ongoing support for the arts, health, human services, and civic issues. Merrill Lynch's philanthropic priority is a sustained investment in education. Q992

3124 Metzger-Price Fund
Ste 2300
230 Park Ave
New York, NY 10169
212-867-9500
Fax: 212-599-1759

Isaac A Saufer, Secretary/Treasurer

3125 Milbank Foundation for Rehabilitation
116 Village Boulevard
Suite 200
New York, NY 08540
609-951-2283
Fax: 609-951-2281
fdnweb.org/milbank

Jeremiah M. Bogert, Chairman & Secretary
Jeremiah Milbank III, President and Treasurer
Carl Helstrom, Executive Director
Carmel Mazzola, Administrative Assistant
Awarding grants from trust funds based on a competitive selection process or the preferences of the foundation managers and granters. The foundations mission is to integrate people with disabilities into all aspects of american life. Current priorities include, but are not limited to: consumer-focused initiatives that enable people with disablities to lead fulfilling, independent lives; innovative policy research and education on market-based approaches to health care and rehabilitation...

3126 Morgan Stanley Foundation
1585 Broadway
New York, NY 10036-8293
212-761-4000
Fax: 212-761-0086
mediainquiries@morganstanley.com
morganstanley.com

James P. Gorman, Chairman and Chief Executive Off
Thomas Nides, Vice Chairman
Jeff Brodsky, Chief Human Resources Officer
Jim Rosenthal, Chief Operating Officer
Our overachieving mission is threefold: build the potential of individuals and families, encourage and support our employees charitable efforts, and strengthen relationships with our communities.

3127 National Foundation for Facial Reconstruction
333 East 30th St.
Lobby Office
New York, NY 10016-4974
212-263-6656
Fax: 212-263-7534
info@myface.org
myface.org

Barbara H. Zuckerberg, President
John R. Gordon, Chairman
Sondra Neuschotz, Secretary
Jeremiah M. Bogert, Treasurer
A nonprofit organization whose major purposes are to provide facilities for the treatment and assistance of individuals who are unable to afford private reconstructive surgical care, to train and educate professionals in this surgery, to encourage research in the field and to carry on public education.

3128 National Hemophilia Foundation
7 Penn Plaza
Suite 1204
New York, NY   10001-3212   212-328-3700
                                             800-424-2634
                                        Fax: 212-328-3799
                                        handi@hemophilia.org
                                           hemophilia.org

Jorge de la Riva, Chair
Carol Simonetti, Vice Chair
Mark Borreliz, Secretary
Brian Andrew, Treasurer
Dedicated to finding better treatments and cures for bleeding and clotting disorders to preventing the complications of these disorders through education, advocacy and research.

3129 Neisloss Family Foundation
Ste 7
1737 Veterans Hwy
Central Islip, NY   11749-1533   631-234-1600
                                        Fax: 631-234-1066

Stanley Neisloss, President/Owner

3130 New York Community Trust
909 3rd Ave
22nd Floor
New York, NY   10022-4752   212-686-0010
                                        Fax: 212-532-8528
                                           aw@nyct-cfi.org
                                        nycommunitytrust.org

Lorie A Slutsky, President
Carolyn M Weiss, CFO
Mary Z. Greenebaum, Chief Investment Officer
Eileen Casey, Director of Investment Reporting
Our goal is to out charitable money to work, making grants to the city's nonprofit community and building an endowment to tackle future problems.

3131 New York Foundation
10 E 34th St
10th Floor
New York, NY   10016-4327   212-594-8009
                                           info@nyf.org
                                              nyf.org

Marlene Provizer, Chair
Roger Schwed, Vice Chair
Sue A Kaplan, Secretary
Gail Gordon, Treasurer
Grants are given that involve New York City or a particular neighborhood of the city. Emphasize advocacy and community organizing. Address a critical need or disadvantaged population, particularly youth or the elderly. Are strongly identified with a particular community. Require an amount of funding to which a Foundation grant would make a substantial contribution. And can show a clear role for the Foundation's funds.

3132 Northern New York Community Foundation
120 Washington St
Suite 400
Watertown, NY   13601-3376   315-782-7110
                                        Fax: 315-782-0047
                                           info@nnycf.org
                                           www.nnycf.org

Joseph W. Russell, President
Linda S. Merrell, Vice President
Jacquelyn A. Schell, Secretary
Rande S. Richardson, Executive Director
Raises, manages and administers an endowment and collection of funds for the benefit of the community

3133 Parkinson's Disease Foundation
1359 Broadway
Room 1509
New York, NY   10018-7867   212-923-4700
                                             800-457-6676
                                        Fax: 212-923-4778
                                           info@pdf.org
                                           www.pdf.org

Howard D Morgan, Chair
Constance Atwell, Vice Chair
Isobel Konecky, Secretary
Stephen Ackerman, Treasurer
The Parkinson's Disease Foundation is a leading national presence in Parkinson's disease research, education and public advocacy. We are working for the nearly one million people in the US who live with Parkinson's by funding promising scientific research to find the causes of and a cure for Parkinson's while supporting people with Parkinson's, their families and caregivers through educational programs and support services.

3134 Reader's Digest Foundation
Readers Digest Association
Readers Digest Rd
Pleasantville, NY   10570   914-238-1000
                                        Fax: 914-238-4559
                                           letters@rd.com
                                              rd.com

Mary G Berner, CEO
Dedicated to creating opportunities and promoting efforts that encourage individuals to make a positive difference in their communities, and to supporting programs designed to help young people learn, grow and enrich their lives.

3135 Research to Prevent Blindness
645 Madison Ave
Floor 21
New York, NY   10022-1010   212-752-4333
                                             800-621-0026
                                        Fax: 212-688-6231
                                        inforequest@rpbusa.org
                                           www.rpbusa.org

Diane S. Swift, Chair
Brian F. Hofland PhD, President
David H Brenner, Vice President and Secretary
Richard E. Baker, Treasurer and Assistant Secretar
National voluntary health foundation supported by foundations, corporations and voluntary gifts and bequests from individuals. Established to stimulate basic and applied research into the causes, prevention and treatment of blinding eye diseases.

3136 Rita J and Stanley H Kaplan Foundation
Rm 306
866 United Nations Plz
New York, NY   10017-1822   212-688-1047
                                        Fax: 212-688-6907
                                        www.kaplanfoundation.org

Nancy Kaplan Belsky, President
Susan B. Kaplan, Vice President
Scott Kaplan Belsky, Secretary & Treasurer
Rebecca Tobin, Executive Director

3137 Robert Sterling Clark Foundation
135 E 64th St
New York, NY   10065-7045   212-288-8900
                                        Fax: 212-288-1033
                                           rscf@rsclark.org
                                              rsclark.org

James Allen Smith, Chairman
Vincent McGee, President
Clara Miller, Treasurer
Julie Muraco, Secretary
Giving primarily in New York with emphasis on advocacy, research, and public education aimed at informing New York City of state policies.

3138 Skadden Fellowship Foundation
4 Times Sq
New York, NY 10036-6518   212-735-3000
                                 Fax: 212-735-2000
                                 info@skadden.com
                                 www.skadden.com

Alan C Myers, Director
William Schumann, Legal Assistant
The aim of the Foundation is to give Fellows the freedom to pursue public intrest work, thus the Fellows create their own projects at public interest organizations with at least 2 lawyers on staff before they apply.

3139 St George's Society of New York
216 E 45th St
Suite 901
New York, NY 10017-3304   212-682-6110
                                 Fax: 212-682-3465
                                 info@stgeorgessociety.org
                                 stgeorgessociety.org

John Shannon, Almoner
Anna Titley, Director of Operations and Commu
Samantha Hamilton, Director of Development and Memb
Daisy Rowan, Operations Executive
St George's Society provides monthly stipends to the elderly and the handicapped.

3140 Stanley W Metcalf Foundation
Ste 503
120 Genesee St
Auburn, NY 13021-3672   315-252-3634
Walter Lowe, Owner

3141 Stonewall Community Foundation
446 West 33rd Street
New York, NY 10001-1913   212-367-1155
                                 Fax: 212-367-1157
                                 stonewall@stonewallfoundation.org
                                 www.stonewallfoundation.org

Dante Mastri, President
Neill Coleman, Vice President
Chris Davis, Secretary
Tina Salandra, Treasurer
Mission is to promote the well being of lesbian, gay, bisexual, and transgender (LGBT) individuals and strengthen the LGBT community. We do this by increasing resources; targeting those resources strategically to areas of greatest need; and by serving as a catalyst and clearinghouse for ideas and solutions. Through grant-making donor-advised funds, endowment funds and charitable education, Stonewall supports LGBT organizations and helps donors realize their philanthropic goals.

3142 Surdna Foundation
330 Madison Ave
30th Floor
New York, NY 10017-5016   212-557-0010
                                 grants@surdna.org
                                 surdna.org

Jocelyn Downie, Chairperson
Peter B Benedict, Vice Chairperson
Lawrence S.C Griffth, Secretary & Treasurer
Jonathan Goldberg, Director of Grants Management, L
The Foundation makes grants in the areas of environment, community revitalization, effective citizenry, the arts and the nonprofit sector.

3143 The Adaptive Sports Foundation
100 Silverman Way
PO Box 266
Windham, NY 12496   518-734-5070
                                 Fax: 518-734-6740
                                 info@adaptivesportsfoundation.org
                                 www.adaptivesportsfoundation.org

Robert W Stubbs, Chair
Todd Munn, Executive Director
Pam Greene, Program Director
Ginny Scahill, Administrative Director

The Adaptive Sports Foundation is a non-profit organization providing programs for children and adults with physical and cognitive disabilities. Programs center around outdoor physical activities and sports, including skiing and snowboarding, canoeing and cycling.

3144 Tisch Foundation
Fl 19
655 Madison Ave
New York, NY 10065-8043   212-521-2930
                                 Fax: 212-521-2983
Mark J Krinsky, VP

3145 Van Ameringen Foundation
509 Madison Avenue
New York, NY 10022-5501   212-758-6221
                                 Fax: 212-688-2105
                                 info@vanamfound.org
                                 www.vanamfound.org

Kenneth A. Kind, President / Treasurer
Steadman Westergaard, Vice President and Secretary
Eleanor Sypher, Executive Director
Helaine Williams, Office Manager
From its beginning the Foundation has sought to stimulate prevention, education, and direct care in the mental health field with an emphasis on those individuals and populations having an impoverished background and few opportunities, for whom appropriate intervention would produce positive change.

3146 Verizon Foundation
1 Verizon Way
Basking Ridge, NJ 07920-1097   866-247-2687
                                 Fax: 908-630-2660
                                 www.verizon.com

Lowell C McAdam, Chairman & CEO
Roy H Chestnutt, Executive Vice President
James J Gerace, Chief Communications Officer
Craig Silliman, Executive Vice President
Mission is to improve education, literacy, family safety and healthcare by supporting Verizon's commitment to deliver technology that touches life. We focus our philanthropic efforts on 3 areas: Education, Safety and Health. & Volunteerism.

3147 Western New York Foundation
11 Summer St
Third Floor
Buffalo, NY 14209-2256   716-839-4225
                                 Fax: 716-883-1107
                                 bgosch@wnyfoundation.org
                                 www.wnyfoundation.org

Jennifer S. Johnson, Chairman
James A. W. McLeod, President
John N. W. Walsh III, Vice President
Theodore V. Buerger, Treasurer
The Western New York Foundation makes grants in the seven counties of Western New York State: Erie, Niagra, Genesee, Wyoming, Allegany, Cattaraugus and Chautauqua

3148 William T Grant Foundation
570 Lexington Avenue
18th Floor
New York, NY 10022-6837   212-752-0071
                                 Fax: 212-752-1398
                                 info@wtgrantfdn.org
                                 wtgrantfoundation.org

Adam Gamoran, President
Vivian Tseng, Vice President, Program
Deborah McGinn, Vice President, Finance and Admi
Vivian Louie, Program Officer
Purpose is to further the understanding of human behavior through research. The mission focuses on improving the lives of youth ages 8 to 25 in the United States.

North Carolina

3149   Arc of North Carolina
343 East Six Forks Rd.
Suite 320
Raleigh, NC   27609   919-782-4632
                                            800-662-8706
                                       Fax: 919-782-4634
                                          info@arcnc.org
                                            www.arcnc.org

Adonis Brown, President
Robert Rusty Bradstock, Senior Vice President
Rhonda Schandevel, Secretary
Ed McShane, Treasurer
Committed to securing for all people with mental retardation and other developmental disabilities the opportunity to choose and realize their goals of where and how they learn, live, work, and play.

3150   Bob & Kay Timberlake Foundation
1660 E Center Street Ext
Lexington, NC   27292-1309   336-243-7777
                                            800-776-0822
                                       Fax: 336-249-2469
                                        bobtimberlake.com

Daniel Timberlake, President

3151   Duke Endowment
800 East Morehead Street
Charlotte, NC   28202-4012   704-376-0291
                                       Fax: 704-376-9336
                                            info@tde.org
                                        dukeendowment.org

Eugene W. Cochrane Jr., President
Arthur E. Morehead IV, Vice President/General Counsel
Susan L. McConnell, Director of Higher Education
Terri W. Honeycutt, Corporate Secretary
Mission is to serve the people of North Carolina and South Carolina by supporting selected programs of higher education, health care, children's welfare, and spiritual life.

3152   First Union Foundation
301 S College St
Charlotte, NC   28288   704-383-0525
                                       Fax: 704-374-2484

Judy Allison, Director

3153   Foundation for the Carolinas
220 N. Tryon Street
Charlotte, NC   28202   704-973-4500
                                            800-973-7244
                                       Fax: 704-973-4599
                                        mmarsicano@fftc.org
                                            fftc.org

Michael Marsicano, Ph.D., President & CEO
Brian Collier, Executive Vice President
Debra S. Watt, SVP, Information Technology
Laura Smith, Executive Vice President
Giving primarily to organizations serving the citizens of North and South Carolina.

3154   Kate B Reynolds Charitable Trust
128 Reynolda Village
Winston Salem, NC   27106-5123   336-397-5500
                                            800-485-9080
                                       Fax: 336-723-7765
                                                kbr.org

Karen McNeil-Miller,, President
Lori Fuller, Director, Evaluation and Learnin
Joel Beeson, Director, Operations
Nora Ferrell, Director, Communications
Mission is to improve the quality of life and quality of health for the financially needy of North Carolina. Grants resricted to the state of North Carolina only.

3155   Mary Reynolds Babcock Foundation
2920 Reynolda Rd
Winston Salem, NC   27106-3016   336-748-9222
                                       Fax: 336-777-0095
                                           info@mrbf.org
                                               mrbf.org

Jennifer Barksdale, Finance Officer
Toshawia Bruner, Office Assistant
Lavastian Glenn, Network Officer
Justin Maxson, Executive Director
For 1994, this foundation is committed to an extensive educational and planning process to better understand the Southeast and to articulate the role the foundation seeks to play in the region into the twenty-first century.

3156   Triangle Community Foundation
324 Blackwell St
Suite 1220
Durham, NC   27701-3690   919-474-8370
                                       Fax: 919-941-9208
                                      info@trianglecf.org
                                           trianglecf.org

Lacy M. Presnell, Chair
Pat Nathan, Secretary
C. Perry Colwell, Assistant Secretary
James A. Stewart, Treasurer
Triangle Community Foundation connects philanthropic resources with community needs, creates opportunity for enlightned change and encourages philanthropy as a way of life.

North Dakota

3157   Alex Stern Family Foundation
4141 28th South Avenue
Suite 102
Fargo, ND   58104-8403   701-271-0263
                                       Fax: 701-271-0408
                                  alexsternfamilyfoundation.org

Don Scott, Executive Director
Rondi McGovern, Trustee
Dan Carey, Trustee
The Foundation supports the arts, social welfare/human services, education, youth recreation, civic projects and health issues for the benefit of the greater Fargo-Moorhead area.

3158   Arc of North Dakota
2500 DeMers Avenue
Grand Forks, ND   58201-2420   701-772-6191
                                            877-250-2022
                                       Fax: 701-772-2195
                                        thearc@arcuv.com
                                  www.thearcuppervalley.com

Peggy Johnson, President
Joan Karpenko, First Vice President
Ruth Jenny, Secretary
Pam Heyd, Treasurer
Mission is to work in partnership with our constituents, members and affiliated chapters to ensure that children and adults with intellectual and developmental disabilities have the supports, benefits, and services they need, and are accepted, respected and fully included in their communities.

3159   North Dakota Community Foundation
309 N Mandan Street
309 N Mandan Street, Suite 2
P.O.Box 387
Bismarck, ND 58502-0387   701-222-8349
                                        kdvorak@ndcf.net
                                            www.ndcf.net

Kevin J Dvorak, CFP, President & CEO
Amy N. Warnke, CFRE, Development Director East
Kara L. Geiger, Development Director West
Cynthia Kaip, Accountant/Administrator
The mission of the North Dakota Community Foundation is to improve the quality of life for North Dakota's citizens through charitable giving and promothing philanthropy.

Ohio

3160 Akron Community Foundation
345 W Cedar St
Akron, OH   44307-2407
330-376-8522
Fax: 330-376-0202
jpetures@akroncf.org

Mark Alio, Chair
Steven Cox, Vice Chair
Dr. Sandra Selby, Secretary
Paul Belair, Treasurer
Mission is to improve the quality of life in the Greater Akron area by building permanent endowments, and providing philanthropic leadership that enables donors to make lasting investments in the community.

3161 Albert G and Olive H Schlink Foundation
49 Benedict Avenue, Suite C
Norwalk, OH   44857
curtis@hwak.com
www.schlinkfoundation.org

3162 Arc of Ohio
1335 Dublin Rd
Suite 100-A
Columbus, OH   43215-7037
614-487-4720
800-875-2723
Fax: 614-487-4725
info@thearcofohio.org
thearcofohio.org

Gary Tonks, Executive Director
John Hannah, President
Connie Calhoun, Vice President
Josh Ebling, Treasurer
The mission of The Arc of Ohio is to advocacte for human rights, personal dignity and community participation of individuals with mental retardation and other developmental disabilities, through legislative and social action, information and education, local chapter support and family involvement.

3163 Bahmann Foundation
8041 Hosbrook Rd
Suite 210
Cincinnati, OH   45236-2909
513-891-3799
Fax: 513-891-3722
info@bahmann.org
www.bahmann.org

John Gatch, Executive Director
The mission of the Bahmann Foundation is to reduce isolation of low-income older adults through technology.

3164 Cleveland Foundation
1422 Euclid Ave
Suite 1300
Cleveland, OH   44115-2063
216-861-3810
Fax: 216-861-1729
Hello@CleveFdn.org
clevelandfoundation.org

James A. Ratner, Chairman
Paul J. Dolan, Vice Chairman
Ronald B. Richard, President and CEO
Robert E. Eckardt, Executive Vice President
In general, grants are made in (but not restriced to) the areas of arts and culture, community development, economic development, education, environment, health and human services.

3165 Columbus Foundation and Affiliated Organizations
1234 E Broad St
Columbus, OH   43205-1453
614-251-4000
Fax: 614-251-4009
info@columbusfoundation.org
columbusfoundation.org

Doug F. Kridler, President & CEO
Raymond J. Biddiscombe, CPA, Senior Vice President - Finance
Lisa Schweitzer Courtice, P, EVP - Community Research and Gra
Alicia Szempruch, Scholarship Manager

The Columbus Foundation offers a range of charitable fund types that can be used for individuals, families and businesses.

3166 Eleanora CU Alms Trust
Fifth Third Bank
Department 00864
9990 Montgomery Rd
Cincinnati, OH   45263
513-793-2200
Robert W Laclair, President
Giving is limited to Cincinnati, OH.

3167 Eva L And Joseph M Bruening Foundation
Foundation Management Services
1422 Euclid Ave
Suite 966
Cleveland, OH   44115-1952
216-621-2901
Fax: 216-621-8198
www.fmscleveland.com

Janet E. Narten, Founder
Cristin N. Slesh, President
Valerie Schramm, Operations Assistant
Kara L. McCullough, Manager, Grants and Office Opera
Charitable foundation providing grants to noprofit organizations located inCuyahoga county Ohio. No grant are awarded to inviduals.

3168 Fred & Lillian Deeks Memorial Foundation
P.O.Box 1118
Cincinnati, OH   45201-1118
937-339-2329
Fax: 937-339-1861

3169 GAR Foundation
277 East Mill Street
Akron, OH   44308
330-576-2926
Fax: 330-294-5315
info@garfdn.org
www.garfdn.org

Christine Amer Mayer, President
Kirstin S. Toth, Senior Vice President
Candace Campbell Jackson, Consulting Program Officer
Brittany G. Zaehringer, Senior Program Officer
The mission of the Foundation is to strengthen communities in our region through discerning and creative support of worthy organizations.

3170 George Gund Foundation
1845 Guildhall Building
45 Prospect Avenue, West
Cleveland, OH   44115-1008
216-241-3114
Fax: 216-241-6560
info@gundfdn.org
gundfoundation.org

Geoffrey Gund, President & Treasurer
Ann L. Gund, Vice President
David T. Abbott, Executive Director
Catherine Gund, Secretary
The George Gund Foundation was established in 1952 as a private, nonprofit institution with the sole purpose of contributing to human well-being and the progress of society.

3171 Greater Cincinnati Foundation
200 West Fourth St.
Cincinnati, OH   45202-2775
513-241-2880
Fax: 513-852-6886
info@gcfdn.org
www.gcfdn.org

Kathryn e. Merchant, President/CEO
Terri Masur, Executive Assistant
Elizabeth Reiter Benson, APR, Vice President for Communic
Shiloh Turner, Vice President for Community Inv
Offers a wide variety of giving tools to help people achieve their charitable goals and create lasting good work in their communities.

3172   HCR Manor Care Foundation
333 N. Summit St.
P.O.Box 10086
Toledo, OH   43699-0086   419-252-5500
                                       Fax: 419-252-6404
                          foundation@hcr-manorcare.com
                                       hcr-manorcare.com
Paul A Ormond, Chairman, President and CEO
An independent, not-for-profit corporation that provides funding
for organizations and programs that address the needs of the el-
derly and individuals requiring post-acute care services.

3173   HWH Foundation
Canton, OH   330-818-1300
                          contacthwh@hwhfoundation.org
                                       www.hwhfoundation.org
Elizabeth Lacey Hoover, Chairman
Colton Hoover Chase, Vice Chairman
Mark Butterworth, Executive Director
Caiti Pomerance, Esq, Program & Outreach Director
The Herbert W Hoover Foundation funds unique opportunities
that provide solutions to issues related to the Community, Educa-
tion and the Environment.

3174   Harry C Moores Foundation
100 South Third Street
Columbus, OH   43215-4291   614-227-2300
                                       Fax: 614-227-2390
                                       info@bricker.com
                                       bricker.com
Kurtis A Tunnell, Managing Partner
Ahmad Sino, Chief Information Officer
Steve P Odum, Chief Financial Officer
Angela M Gelst, Chief Human Resources Officer

3175   Helen Steiner Rice Foundation
1301 Western Ave.
Cincinnati, OH   45203   513-287-7022
                                       800-877-2665
                          hrice@cincymuseum.org
                                       helensteinerrice.com
Virginia J. Ruehlmann, Creative Consultant
Dorothy C. Lingg, Office Manager
Willis D. Gradison, Jr., Board of Trustee
Gregory Ionna, Board of Trustee
Non-profit corporation whose purpose is to award grants to wor-
thy charitable programs that aid the poor, the needy, and the el-
derly.

3176   Nationwide Foundation
One Nationwide Plaza
Columbus, OH   43215-2220   614-249-7111
                                       800-882-2822
                                       Fax: 614-249-5721
                                       www.nationwide.com
Kirt A. Walker, President and COO Nationwide Fin
Mark A. Pizzi, President and Chief Operating Of
Stephen S. Rasmussen, Chief Executive Officer, Nationw
W. Kim Austen, President and COO, Allied Group,
The Nationwide Foundation is an independent corporation
funded by Nationwide Companies to help positively impact the
quality of life in communities where our associates, agents and
their families live and work.

3177   Nordson Corporate Giving Program
28601 Clemens Rd
Westlake, OH   44145-1148   440-892-1580
                                       Fax: 440-892-9507
                                       kladiner@nordson.com
                                       nordson.com
Michael F. Hilton, President and Chief Executive O
Gregory A. Thaxton, Senior Vice President, Chief Fin
John J. Keane, Senior Vice President, Advanced
Gregory P. Merk, Senior Vice President, Adhesive
Nordson Corporation encourages individual financial support of
nonprofit organizations, colleges, and universities

3178   Parker-Hannifin Foundation
6035 Parkland Blvd
Cleveland, OH   44124-4141   216-896-3000
                                       800-272-7537
                                       Fax: 216-896-4000
                                       parker.com
Donald E. Washkewicz, Chairman, Chief Executive Office
Lee C. Banks, Executive Vice President and Ope
Robert P. Barker, Executive Vice President, Operat
Jon P. Marten, Executive Vice President - Finan
To be a leading worldwide manufacturer of components and sys-
tems for the builders and users of durable goods.

3179   Reinberger Foundation
30000 Chagrin Blvd.
Suite 300
Cleveland, OH   44124-4439   216-292-2790
                                       Fax: 216-292-4466
                          info@reinbergerfoundation.org
                                       www.reinbergerfoundation.org
Karen R. Hooser, President
Sally R. Dyer, Trustee
Richard H. Oman, Trustee
William C. Reinberger, Trustee
Committed to enhancing the quality of life for individuals from
all walks of life. To achieve this goal, proposals in the areas of the
arts, education, healthcare, and social service are favored.

3180   Robert Campeau Family Foundation
7 West Seventh Street
Cincinnati, OH   45202-2424   513-579-7000
                                       Fax: 513-579-7555
                                       federated-fds.com
Terry J Lundgren, Chairman and Chief Executive Officer

3181   Sisler McFawn Foundation
P.O.Box 149
Akron, OH   44309   330-849-8887
                                       Fax: 330-996-6215
Charlotte M Stanley, Grants Manager
Our trust restricts giving to certain programs and types of organi-
zations. You can see recent giving has been by referring to the list
of grants approved and paid during the past year. Call foundation
office to request a guidelines brochure and list.

3182   Stark Community Foundation
400 Market Ave North
Suite 200
Canton, OH   44702-1557   330-454-3426
                                       Fax: 330-454-5855
                                       info@starkcf.org
                                       www.starkcommunityfoundation.org
Mark Samolczyk, President
Patricia Quick, VP/ CFO
Chris Decker, Finance and Systems Officer
Bridgette Neisel, Vice President of Advancement
Stark Community Foundation is dedicated to promoting the bet-
terment of Stark County and enhancing the quality of life of all its
citizens.

3183   Stocker Foundation
201 Burns Road
Elyria, OH   44035   440-366-4884
                                       Fax: 440-366-4656
                          contact@stockerfoundation.org
                                       stockerfoundation.org
Brenda Norton, President
Dawn Dobras, Treasurer
Patricia O'Brien, Executive Director
Melanie R Wilson, Office Manager
The Stocker Foundation seeks creative ideas and projects that are
catalysts for constructive change in the community through arts
and culture, community needs, education, health social services
and women's issues.

3184 **Toledo Community Foundation**
300 Madison Avenue
Suite 1300
Toledo, OH 43604-1583   419-241-5049
Fax: 419-242-5549
toledocf@toledocf.org
www.toledocf.org

David F. Waterman, Chair
Dr. Anthony Armstrong, Vice Chair
Rita N.A. Mansour, Secretary
Scott A Estes, Treasurer
The Toledo Community Foundation is a public, charitable foundation which exists to improve the quality of life in the region.

3185 **William J and Dorothy K O'Neill Foundation**
7575 Northcliff Ave.
Suite 205
Cleveland, OH 44144   216-831-4134
Fax: 216-378-0594
info@oneill-foundation.org
www.oneillfdn.org

Leah S Gary, President & CEO
Symone R McClain, Manager of Grants & Office Opera
Timothy M. McCue, MPH, Senior Program Officer

3186 **Youngstown Foundation**
100 Federal Plaza East, Suite 101
P.O.Box 1162
Youngstown, OH 44503-1162   330-744-0320
Fax: 330-744-0344
Jan@youngstownfoundation.org
www.youngstownfoundation.org

Jan Strasfeld, Executive Director
Crissi Jenkins, Program Coordinator
Rena Colarossi, Admin. Assistant
Funds proposals that provide direct services to children with medically diagnosed disabilities. Grants are awarded to Ohio non-profit agencies that are qualified under the Internal Revenue Service Code 501 (c) (3) for the care of such children in the greater Youngstown Area.

Oklahoma

3187 **Anne and Henry Zarrow Foundation**
401 S Boston Ave
Suite 900
Tulsa, OK 74103-4012   918-295-8004
Fax: 918-295-8049
bmajor@zarrow.com
www.zarrow.com

3188 **Sarkeys Foundation**
530 East Main St
Norman, OK 73071-5823   405-364-3703
Fax: 405-364-8191
angela@sarkeys.org
sarkeys.org

Kim Henry, Executive Director
Lori Sutton, Facilities Manager
Angella Holladay, Director of Grants Management
Susan C. Frantz, Senior Program Officer
Improves the quality of life in Oklahoma. Offers contributions in the areas of social services, arts and cultural programs, educational funding and health care and medical research. Funding only in agencies in the state of Oklahoma.

Oregon

3189 **Arc of Oregon**
2405 Front Street NE
Suite 120
Salem, OR 97301-4342   503-581-2726
877-581-2726
Fax: 503-363-7168
info@arcoregon.org
www.thearcoregon.org

Marcie Ingledue, Executive Director
Tiffany Tombleson, Administrative Assistant
Paula Boga, OSNT Program Director
Cici Gaynor, OSNT Administrative Assistant
Guardianship, Advocacy and Planning Services. Oregon special needs trust; information and referral.

3190 **Chiles Foundation**
1614 Mahan Center Boulevard
Suite 104
Tallahassee, Fl 32308   805-385-7800
Fax: 805-385-7808
kchiles@lawtonchiles.org
chilesfoundation.org

Kitty Chiles, Executive Director
Bud Chiles, President
Dr. Wil J. Blechman, Board Member
Todd Abernethy, Chief Financial Officer
Giving in Oregon, with emphasis on Portland, and the Pacific Northwest.

3191 **Jackson Foundation**
P.O.Box 3168
Portland, OR 97208-3168   503-275-4414
march.voyles@usbank.com
www.thejacksonfoundation.com
Robert H Depew, Vice President & Senior Trust Of
Libby Voyles, Trust Relationship Associate
Purpose is to respond to the requests deemed appropriate to promote the welfare of the public of the city of Portland or the State of Oregon or both.

3192 **Leslie G Ehmann Trust**
P.O.Box 3168
Portland, OR 97208-3168   503-275-5929
800-522-9100
Fax: 503-275-4117
William Dolan, Trustee

Pennsylvania

3193 **Air Products Foundation**
7201 Hamilton Blvd
Allentown, PA 18195-9642   610-481-4911
Fax: 610-481-5900
gigmrktg@airproducts.com
www.airproducts.com

Seifi Ghasemi, Chairman & CEO
M. Scott Crocco, Senior Vice President and Chief
Guillermo Novo, Senior Vice President
Corning F. Painter, Executive Vice President
Giving primarily in areas of company operations throughout the US.

3194   Arc of Pennsylvania
301 Chestnut Street
Suite 403
Harrisburg, PA   17101-2535   717-234-2621
                                           800-692-7258
                                      Fax: 717-234-2622
                                      info@thearcpa.org
                                           thearcpa.org

Maureen Cronin, Executive Director
Pam Klipa, Government Relations Director
Gwen Adams, Operations Director
Ashlinn Masland-Sarani, Policy and Development Director
The Arc's mission is to work to include all children and adults
with cognitive, intellectual, and developmental disabilities in ev-
ery community. We promote active citizenship and inclusion in
every community.

3195   Arcadia Foundation
105 E Logan St
Norristown, PA 19401-3058   202-747-0876
Marilyn L Steinbright, President
Robert Carmona-Borjas, Founder

3196   Brachial Plexus Palsy Foundation
210 Springhaven Cir
Royersford, PA   19468-1178 www.brachialplexuspalsyfoundation.org

3197   Columbia Gas of Pennsylvania Corporate Giving
650 Washington Rd
Pittsburgh, PA 15228-2702   412-572-7104
                                     Fax: 412-572-7140
                          www.columbiagaspamd.com/html/
Rosemary Martinelli, Manager Corporation

3198   Connelly Foundation
100 Front Street,
Suite 1450
West Conshohocken, PA 19428-2873   610-834-3222
                                     Fax: 610-834-0866
                                     info@connellyfdn.org
                                          connellyfdn.org
Josephine C. Mandeville, Chair & President
Emily C Riley, Executive Vice President
Lewis W Bluemle, Senior Vice President
Carol L. Cromie, Executive Assistant
Seeks to foster learning and to improve the quality of life in the
Greater Philadelphia area. The Foundation supports local
non-profit organizations in the fields of education, health and hu-
man services, arts and culture and civic enterprise.

3199   Dolfinger-McMahon Foundation
30 South 17th Street
Philadelphia, PA 19103-4196   215-979-1768
                         www.dolfingermcmahonfoundation.org
Sheldon M. Bonovitz, Trustee
David E. Loder, Trustee
Frank G. Cooper, Counsel
Sharon M. Renz, Executive Secretary

3200   Heinz Endowments
Howard Heinz Endowment
625 Liberty Ave
30 Dominion Tower
Pittsburgh, PA 15222- 3115   412-281-5777
                                     Fax: 412-281-5788
                                     bobbyvagt@heinz.org
                                          heinz.org
Grant Oliphant, President
Edward Kolano, Vice President Finance and Admin
Ann C. Plunkett, Director, Human Resources
Donna Evans Sebastian, Executive Assistant
Mission is to help our region thrive as a whole community-eco-
nomically, ecologically, educationaly, and culturaly while ad-
vancing the state of knowledge and practice in the fields in which
we work.

3201   Henry L Hillman Foundation
310 Grant Street
Suite 2000
Pittsburgh, PA   15219   412-338-3466
                                     foundation@hillmanfo.com
                                     hillmanfamilyfoundations.org
David K Roger, President
Lisa R Johns, Treasurer and Senior Program Off
Lauri K. Fink, Senior Program Officer
D.Tyler Gourley, Program Officer
Established with a broad purpose to improve the quality of life in
Pittsburgh and southwestern Pennsylvania.

3202   Jewish Healthcare Foundation of Pittsburgh
650 Smithfield Street
Suite 2400
Pittsburgh, PA 15222- 3915   412-594-2550
                                     Fax: 412-232-6240
                                          info@jhf.org
                                               jhf.org
Karen Wolk Feinstein, PhD, President and Chief Executive Of
Carla Barricella, Communications Director
Lindsey Kirstatter Hartle, Accounting Manager
Millie Greene, Executive Assistant
The mission of the JHF is to support and foster the provision of
healthcare services, healthcare education, and, when appropriate, medical and scientific research, and to respond to the
health-related needs of elderly, underprivileged, indigent, and
undeserved persons in both the Jewish and general community
throughout Western Pennsylvania. .

3203   Juliet L Hillman Simonds Foundation
310 Grant Street
Suite 2000
Pittsburgh, PA   15219   412-338-3466
                                     Fax: 412-338-3520
                                     foundation@hillmanfo.com
                                     hillmanfamilyfoundations.org
David K. Roger, President
Lisa R. Johns, Treasurer and Senior Program Off
Lauri K. Fink, Senior Program Officer
D.Tyler Gourley, Program Officer

3204   Oberkotter Foundation
1600 Market St
Suite 3600
Philadelphia, PA   19103-7212   215-751-2601
                                     Fax: 215-751-2678
                                     info@oberkotterfoundation.org
                                          oberkotterfoundation.org
George H Nofer, Executive Director
Mildred L. Oberkotter, M.S.W., Trustee
Bruce A. Rosenfield, J.D., Trustee
David A. Pierson, Ph.D., Trustee
The Oberkotter Foundation focuses its efforts on supporting fam-
ilies who have chosen listening and spoken language for their
child and on opportunities for children learning listening and
spoken language to develop their social, emotional, language and
educational skills.

3205   PECO Energy Company Contributions Program
Fl 7toorh
2301 Market St
Philadelphia, PA   19103-1338   215-841-4000
                                          800-494-4000
                                     Fax: 215-841-6830
                                          www.peco.com
Denis P O'Brien, SVP/ CEO
Michael A. Innocenzo, SVP/ COO
Phillip S. Barnett, SVP/ CFO/ Treasurer
Scott A. Bailey, VP/ Controller

3206 PNC Bank Foundation
249 5th Ave
Pittsburgh, PA 15222-2707   412-762-2000
Fax: 412-762-7829
marianna.hallett@pnc.com
www.pncbank.com

Samuel R Patterson, Senior VP
The PNC Foundation's priority is to form partnerships with community-based nonprofit organizations within the markets PNC serves in order to enhance educational opportunities for children, particularly underserved pre-K children though our signature, PNC Grow Uo Great Program, and to promote the growth of targeted communities through economic development initiatives.

3207 Philadelphia Foundation
1234 Market St
Suite 1800
Philadelphia, PA 19107-3704   215-563-6417
Fax: 215-563-6882
philafound.org

R Andrew Swinney, President
Pat Meller, Vice President for Finance & Adm
Andrea Congo, Executive Assistant
Betsy Anderson, Communications Director
The Philadelphia Foundation improves our community by advancing change, leading on issues of importance, forging meaningful relationships and providing knowledge, resources and stewardship.

3208 Pittsburgh Foundation
Five PPG Place
Suite 250
Pittsburgh, PA 15222-5405   412-391-5122
Fax: 412-391-7259
oliphantg@pghfdn.org
pittsburghfoundation.org

Maxwell King, President and CEO
Jonathan Brelsford, Vice President of Investments
Jay Donato, Senior Investment Analyst
Marianne Cola, Special Assistant
The Pittsburgh Foundation works to improve the quality of life in the Pittsburgh region by evaluating and addressing community issues, promoting responsible philanthropy, and connecting donors to the critical needs of the community.

3209 Shenango Valley Foundation
7 West State Street
Suite 301
Sharon, PA 16146-2713   724-981-5882
866-901-7204
Fax: 724-983-9044
comm-foundation.org

Lawrence E. Haynes, Executive Director
Amy Atkinson, Associate Director
Shelly Mason, Chief Financial Officer
Tristan Rice, Development Coordinator
Mission is to promote the betterment of our region and enhancement of the quality of life for all of its citizens.

3210 Staunton Farm Foundation
650 Smithfield Street
Suite 210
Pittsburgh, PA 15222- 3907   412-281-8020
Fax: 844-281-8020
office@stauntonfarm.org
stauntonfarm.org

Joni S. Schwager, Executive Director
Bethany Hemingway, Program Officer
Jason Fate, Office Manager
Robert Musca, Financial Manager
Dedicated to improving the lives of people who live with mental illness.

3211 Stewart Huston Charitable Trust
50 South First Avenue
Coatesville, PA 19320-3418   610-384-2666
Fax: 610-384-3396
admin@stewarthuston.org
stewarthuston.org

Scott G. Huston, Executive Director
Charles L. Huston III, Trustee
Shelton P Sanford, Trustee
Elinor Lashley, Trustee
The purpose of the Trust is to provide funds, technical assistance and collaboration on behalf of non-profit organizations engaged exclusively in religious, charitable or educational work; to extend opportunities to deserving needs persons and, in general, to promote any of the above causes.

3212 Teleflex Foundation
155 S Limerick Rd
Limerick, PA 19468-1603   610-948-5100
Fax: 610-948-5101
teleflex.com

Jeffrey P Black, CEO
The Teleflex Foundation strives to create an impact on the quality of life in Teleflex communities and build supportive relationships among our stakeholders. The Foundation places a priority on progrmas that have the commitmenet and volunteer involvement of Teleflex communities.

3213 USX Foundation
600 Grant St
Pittsburgh, PA 15219-2702   412-433-1121
Fax: 412-433-6847
www.ussteel.com

CD Mallick, General Manager
Patricia Funaro, Program Manager
Giving primarily in areas of company operations located within the United States.

3214 William B Dietrich Foundation
Duane Morrs Llt
30 S 17th St
Philadelphia, PA 19103-4001   215-979-1000
Fax: 215-979-1020
www.duanemorris.com

William B Dietrich, President

3215 William Talbott Hillman Foundation
310 Grant Street
Suite 2000
Pittsburgh, PA 15219   412-338-3466
Fax: 212-792-2677
foundation@hillmanfo.com
hillmanfamilyfoundations.org

David K. Roger, President
Lisa R. Johns, Treasurer and Senior Program Off
Lauri K. Fink, Senior Program Officer
D.Tyler Gourley, Program Officer

3216 William V and Catherine A McKinney Charitable Foundation
20 Stanwix St
Pittsburgh, PA 15222-4802   412-644-8332
Fax: 412-644-6058
verizon.com

William M Schmidt, Senior Vice President

Rhode Island

3217 Arc South County Chapter
2 Barber Avenue
Warwick, RI 02886-3549   401-480-9355
paul@pence.com
www.riroads.com

3218   Arc of Blackstone Valley
500 Prospect St.
Wing B, Suite 203
Pawtucket, RI   02860- 4332   401-727-0150
                                          800-257-6092
                                   Fax: 401-727-1545
                                   contact@bvcriarc.org
                                      www.bvcriarc.org

Kathleen O'Neill, President
Thomas E. Hodge, Vice President
John J. Padien III, Chief Executive Officer
Katherine S. Hunt, Chief Operating Officer
A private nonprofit organization providing residential, developmental, employment and recreational programs and services to more then 400 individuals with intellectual and related disabilities

3219   Arc of Northern Rhode Island
The Homestead Group Administrative Offices
68 Cumberland St
Suite 200
Woonsocket, RI   02895-3323   401-765-3700
                                   Fax: 401-765-1124
                                           arcofnri.org

3220   Champlin Foundations
2000 Chapel View Boulevard
Suite 350
Cranston, RI   02920   401-944-9200
                                   Fax: 401-944-9299
                              www.champlinfoundations.org
Jonathan K. Farnum, Distribution Committee
John Gorham, Distribution Committee
Dione D. Kenyon, Distribution Committee
Lisa P. Koelle, Distribution Committee
Giving in the Rhode Island area. Champlin does not give grants to individuals, only to RI tax-exempt organizations.

3221   CranstonArc
The Keystone Group
PO Box 20130
Cranston, RI   02920-942   401-941-1112
                                   Fax: 401-383-8751
                                   info@accesspointri.org
                                     www.accesspointri.org

Thomas Kane, President & CEO
Kevin McHale, Chief Operating Officer
Maureen Russo, Director of Human Resources
Gary Paulhus, Director of Clinical Services
Mission is to empower persons with differing ablilites to claim and enjoy their right to dignity and respect through their lives.

3222   Down Syndrome Society of Rhode Island
4635 Post Road
Warwick, RI   02818   401-463-5751
                                   Fax: 401-463-5337
                                   TTY:800-745-5555
                              coordinatordssri@verizon.net
                                         www.dssri.org
Claudia M. Lowe, Coordinator
Marilyn Blanche
Jeff DiMillio
Gail Doyle
The Down Syndrome Society of Rhode Island (DSSRI) is dedicated to promoting the rights, dignity and potential of all individuals with Down syndrome through advocacy, education, public awareness, and support.

3223   Frank Olean Center
93 Airport Rd
Westerly, RI   02891-3420   401-596-2091
                                   Fax: 401-596-3945
                                   info@oleancenter.org
                                       oleancenter.org

Joan Gradilone, President
Tony Vellucci, Executive Director
Rick Harley, Vice President
Christine Martone, Secretary

A non-profit organization representing and providing services and supports to persons with developmental disabilities and their families throughout Southern Rhode Island and Southeastern Connecticut.

3224   Horace A Kimball and S Ella Kimball Foundation
23 Broad Street
Westerly, RI   02891-1879   401-348-1238
                                   Fax: 401-364-3565
                                   www.hkimballfoundation.org
Thomas F Black III, President
Norman D. Baker, Jr., Secretary and Treasurer
Edward C. Marth, Foundation Trustees
Makes grants almost exclusively to Rhode Island operatives (charities) or those benefitting Rhode Island residents and causes.

3225   James L. Maher Center
120 Hillside Avenue
Newport, RI   02840   401-846-0340
                                   Fax: 401-849-4267
                                      www.mahercenter.org
Jack Casey, President
William Maraziti, Executive Director
Barbara Burns, President
John S Dugan, Secretary
The mission is to advance independence and opportunity for children and adults with developmental disabilities and their families.

3226   Rhode Island Arc
99 Bald Hill Rd
Cranston, RI   02920-2647   401-463-9191
                                   Fax: 401-463-9244
                                   riarc@compuserve.com
Mary Lou Mc Caffray, Executive Director

3227   Rhode Island Foundation
One Union Station
Providence, RI   02903-1758   401-274-4564
                                   Fax: 401-331-8085
                                   info@rifoundation.org
                                          rifoundation.org
Neil Steinberg, President & CEO
Wendi DeClercq, Executive Assistant
James S. Sanzi, Esq., Vice President of Development
Pamela Tesler Howitt, Senior Development Officer
The Rhode Island Foundation works to build a better Rhode Island as a philanthropic resource, for people, communities, organizations, and programs.

South Carolina

3228   Arc of South Carolina
1202 12th Street
Cayce, SC   29033   803-748-5020
                                   Fax: 803-445-1026
                                   TheArc@ArcSC.org
                                         www.arcsc.org
Margie Williamson, Executive Director
Caroline Kistler, Project Director
Carly Prince, Case Manager
Hilary Bell, Case Manager
The Arc of South Carolina advocates for and alongside people with cognitive, intellectual and developmental disabilities and their families.

3229   Center for Disability Resources
University of South Carolina
8301 Farrow Rd
Columbia, SC   29208-1   803-935-5231
                                   Fax: 803-935-5059
                              David.Rotholz@uscmed.sc.edu
                                        uscm.med.sc.edu

Dr. David A. Rotholz, Director

A University Affiliated Program which develops model programs designed to serve persons with disabilities and to train students in fields related to disabilities.

3230 Colonial Life and Accident Insurance Company Contributions Program
1200 Colonial Life Blvd W
Columbia, SC 29210-7670   803-798-7000
                                    Fax: 803-731-2618

Randy Horn, President and Chief Executive Of
Bill Deeham, Senior Vice President of Sales
Tim Arnold, Senior Vice President of Sales a
John Garrison, Vice President, General Counsel

Tennessee

3231 Arc of Anderson County
728 Emory Valley Road, Suite 42
P.O.Box 4823
Oak Ridge, TN 37831-4823   865-481-0550
                                    arc@arcaid.org
                                www.thearcandersoncounty.com

Sally Browning, President
Dargie Arwood, Executive Director
Ginny Miceli, President
Elizabeth Bonner, Vice President

The Arc of Anderson County provides support and advocacy to people with cognitive, intellectual and developmental disabilities. The Arc provides support, information and training for families and caregivers of adults and children with these disabilities.

3232 Arc of Davidson County
111 N Wilson Blvd
Nashville, TN 37205-2411   615-248-4112
                                    Fax: 615-322-9184
                                    arcdc.org

Kate Deitzer, President
Cynthia Gardner, Vice President
Thom Druffel, Treasurer
Elizabeth Ralph, Secretary

Provides services to adults and children with intellectual and developmental disabilities through a contract with the Tennessee Departmant of Mental Retardation Services Medicaid Waiver Program.

3233 Arc of Hamilton County
4613 Brainerd Rd
Chattanooga, TN 37411-3826   423-624-6887
                                    800-624-6887
                                    Fax: 423-624-3974
                                    arcofhamilton@aol.com
                                    thearchc.org

Shawn Ellis, Executive Director

Provides assistance to individuals and families with mental retardation and related disabilities, in the form of advocacy, information, and support coordination

3234 Arc of Tennessee
151 Athens Way
Suite 100
Nashville, TN 37228-1367   615-248-5878
                                    800-835-7077
                                    Fax: 615-248-5879
                                    info@thearctn.org
                                    thearctn.org

John Lewis, President
John Shouse, Vice President
Donna Lankford, Secretary
Ann Curl, Treasurer

Advocacy, information, referral and support for people with intellectual and developmental disabilities and their families.

3235 Arc of Washington County
110 East Mountcastle Drive
Johnson City, TN 37601-7557   423-928-9362
                                    Fax: 423-928-7431
                                    kim@arcwc.org
                                    www.arcwc.org

Malessa Fleenor, Executive Director
Kim Reid, Human Resources, Quality Assuran
Kim Wheeler, Respite Coordinator
Linda Tilson, Family Support Program Manager

Is a non-profit organization that serves individuals with disabilities and their families. They have an independent support coordination service, as well as, early intervention, family support and respite services.

3236 Arc of Williamson County
129 W Fowlkes St
Suite 151
Franklin, TN 37064-3562   615-790-5815
                                    Fax: 615-790-5891
                                    sbbarc@thearcwc.org
                                    thearcwc.org

Donna Isbell, President
Steve Cassidy, Vice President
Ashley Coulter, Secretary
Jan Lincoln, Treasurer

The Arc is a family-based organization committed to securing for all people with intellectual, developmental, or other disabilities the opportunity to choose and realize their goals of where and how they live, learn, work, and play.

3237 Arc-Diversified
453 Gould Dr
Cookeville, TN 38506   931-432-5981
                                    800-239-9029
                                    Fax: 931-432-5987
                                    www.arcdiversified.com

3238 Benwood Foundation
736 Market St
Suite 1600
Chattanooga, TN 37402-4812   423-267-4311
                                    Fax: 423-267-9049
                                    info@benwood.org
                                    benwood.org

Sarah Morgan, President
Kristy Huntley, Program & Financial Officer
Connie Perrin, Accounting & Grants Manager
Jeff Pfitzer, Program Officer

Benwood Foundation seeks to stimulate creative and innovative efforts to build and strengthen the Chattanooga community.

3239 Community Foundation of Greater Chattanooga
1270 Market St
Chattanooga, TN 37402-2713   423-265-0586
                                    Fax: 423-265-0587
                                    info2@cfgc.org
                                    cfgc.org

Peter T. Cooper, President
Rebecca Underwood, Vice President, Finance & Admini
Marty Robinson, Vice President, Donor Relations
Rebecca Smith, Director of Scholarships

A non-profit organization which receives, holds, invests and distributes assets contributed by individuals and organizations for the benefit of Chattanooga, its citizens and its institutions.

3240 Education and Auditory Research Foundation
PO Box 330867
Nashville, TN 37203-7506   615-627-2724
                                    800-545-4327
                                    Fax: 615-627-2728
                                    info@carfoundation.org
                                    www.carfoundation.org

Michael Glasscock, President

Provides the general public support services promoting the integration of the hearing and balance impaired into mainstream society; to provide practicing ear specialists continuing medical education courses and related programs specifically regarding re-

319

habilitation and hearing preservation; to educate young people and adults about hearing preservation and early detection of hearing loss, enabling them to prevent at an early age hearing and balance disorders.

3241   International Paper Company Foundation
6400 Poplar Ave
Memphis, TN 38197
901-419-9000
800-207-4003
Fax: 901-419-4439
internationalpaper.comm@ipaper.com
internationalpaper.com

Mark S Sutton, Chairman & CEO
David J Bronczek, President & CEO
C. Cato Ealy, Senior Vice President, Corporate
William P. Hoel, Senior Vice President
The Foundation's primary focus is education-specifically environmental education, iliteracy programs for young children and minority career development opportunities for college bound youth.

3242   Montgomery County Arc
1825 K Street
NW, Suite 1200
Washington, DC 20006-2145
202-534-3700
800-433-5255
Fax: 202-534-3731
info@thearc.org
www.thearc.org

Ronald Brown, President
Elise McMillan, Vice President
Peter V Berns, Chief Executive Officer
M.J. Bartelmay, Secretary
Organization works to ensure that the estimated 7.2 million Americans with intellectual and developmental disabilities have the services and supports they need to grow, develop and live in communities across the nation.

Texas

3243   Abell-Hangar Foundation
P.O.Box 430
Midland, TX 79702-0430
432-684-6655
Fax: 432-684-4474
abell-hanger.org

David L Smith, Executive Director
The Foundation makes grants to nonprofit organizations, which are involved in such undertakings for public welfare, including but not limited to, education, health services, human services, arts and cultural activities and community or social benefit.

3244   Albert & Bessie Mae Kronkosky Charitable Foundation
112 East Pecan
Suite 830
San Antonio, TX 78205-1574
210-475-9000
888-309-9001
Fax: 210-354-2204
kronkosky.org

Palmer Moe, Managing Director
Mission is to produce profound good that is tangible and measurable in Bandera, Bexar, Comal, and Kendall counties in Texas by implimenting the Kronkosky's charitable purposes.

3245   American Express Foundation
P.O. Box 981540
El Paso, TX 79998-1540
800-528-4800
TTY:800-221-9950
americanexpress.com

Kenneth I Chenault, Chairman and Chief Executive Off
L. Kevin Cox, Chief Human Resources Officer
Marc D. Gordon, Executive Vice President and Chi
John D. Hayes, Executive Vice President and Chi
Grants are awarded in the three program areas: Community Service, Cultural Heritage, and Economic Independence. Most grants are made for projects operating where the company has a major employee or market presence.

3246   Arc of Texas, The
8001 Centre Park Dr
Suite 100
Austin, TX 78754-5118
512-454-6694
800-252-9729
Fax: 512-454-4956
www.thearcoftexas.org

Charlie Huber, President
John Schneider, Vice President
Amy Mizcles, Executive Director
Terri Schonfeld, Secretary
The Arc of Texas creates opportunities for all people with intellectual and developmental disabilities to actively participate in their communities and make the choices that affect their lives in a positive manner.

3247   BA and Elinor Steinhagen Benevolent Trust
Chase Bank of Texas
700 North St.
Suite D
Beaumont, TX 77701-3928
409-832-6565
Fax: 409-832-7532
www.setxnonprofit.org

Jean Moncla, CTFA, President
Ivy Pate, Treasurer
Chester Jourdan, Executive Director
Kristi Stott, Administrative Assistant

3248   Brown Foundation
P.O.Box 130646
Houston, TX 77219-0646
713-523-6867
Fax: 713-523-2917
bfi@brownfoundation.org
brownfoundation.org

Nancy Pittman, Executive Director
The purpose of the Brown Foundation is to distribute funds for public charitable purposes, principally for support, encouragement and assistance to education, the arts and community service.

3249   CH Foundation
P.O.Box 94038
Lubbock, TX 79493-4038
806-792-0448
Fax: 806-792-7824
ksanford@chfoundation.com
www.chfoundationlubbock.com

Kay Sanford, Executive Director
Heather Hocker, Grants Administrator
Cheryl Sanford, Administrative Assistant
Mission of the CH foundation is to significantly improve human services and cultural and educational opportunities for the residents of the South Plain of Texas.

3250   Cockrell Foundation
1000 Main St
Suite 3250
Houston, TX 77002-6338
713-209-7500
foundation@cockrell.com

Ernest H. Cockrell, President
Nancy Williams, Executive Vice President
Purpose is for giving for higher education at the University of Texas at Austin; support also for cultural programs, social services, youth services and health care. Limitations are giving in Houston, Texas and no grants are awarded to individuals.

3251   Communities Foundation of Texas
5500 Caruth Haven Ln
Dallas, TX 75225-8146
214-750-4222
Fax: 214-750-4210
jsmith@cftexas.org
cftexas.org

Brent E. Chrisopher, President and Chief Executive Of
Elizabeth W. Bull, Senior Vice President and Chief
Jeverley R. Cook, Ph.D., Executive Director, W.W. Caruth,
John Fitzpatrick, Executive Director
Mission is to improve lives, we serve the community by investing wisely and making effective charitable grants.

3252   Community Foundation of North Texas
306 West 7th
Suite 1045
Fort Worth, TX   76102-4906   817-877-0702
                                                   Fax: 817-632-8711
                                                   cfntx.org

Nancy E. Jones, President
Rob Miller, Director of Finance
Vicki Andrews, Director of Operations/Donor Ser
Rose Bradshaw, Executive Vice President
Community Foundation is a tax exempt organization that provides stewardship for many individual charitable funds. With its specialized services, Community Foundation of North Texas gives donors efficient charitable fund administration.

3253   Cullen Foundation
601 Jefferson St
40th Floor
Houston, TX   77002-7900   713-651-8837
                                               Fax: 713-651-2374
                                               cullenfdn.org

Isaac Arnold, Jr, President
Wilhelmina E Robertson, Vice President and Secretary
Meredith T Cullen, Assistant Secretary
Bert L. Campbell, Director
Grants are restricted to Texas-based organizations for programs in Texas, primarily in the Houston area.

3254   Curtis & Doris K Hankamer Foundation
Ste 530
9039 Katy Fwy
Houston, TX   77024-1656   713-461-8140
Gregory A Herbst, Manager

3255   Dallas Foundation
3963 Maple Avenue
Ste. 390
Dallas, TX   75219-4447   214-741-9898
                                                Fax: 214-741-9848
                                         info@dallasfoundation.org
                                               dallasfoundation.org

Mary M Jalonick, President & CEO
Gary W. Garcia, Senior Director of Development
Dawn Townsend, Director of Marketing & Communic
William T. Solomon, Jr., Chief Financial Officer
Serves as a leader, catalyst and resource for philanthropy by providing donors with a flexible means of making gifts to charitable causes that enhance our community.

3256   David D & Nona S Payne Foundation
P.O.Box 174
Pampa, TX   79066-174   806-665-0063
Vanessa G Buzzard, Director
The David & Nona S Payne Foundation was established in August 1980. Mrs Payne established the foundation and did much of her charitable giving in honor of her late husband.

3257   El Paso Natural Gas Foundation
P.O.Box 2511
Houston, TX   77252-2511   713-420-2600
                                                Fax: 713-420-5312
                                           foundation@elpaso.com
                                              www.kindermorgan.com

Douglas Foshee, CEO
Focuses on the areas in locations where we have significant facilities or concentrated employees. Primary area of focus is Civic and Community, Education and Health and Human Services. Secondary area of focus is Arts and Culture and Environment.

3258   Epilepsy Foundation of Southeast Texas
2401 Fountain View Dr
Suite 900
Houston, TX   77057-4821   713-789-6295
                                                888-548-9716
                                                info@eftx.org
                                           www.epilepsy.com/texas

Donna Stahlhut, CEO
Rebecca Moreau, Program Director
Amanda Walker Rockwell, Senior Development Coordinator
Shannon Robbins, Assistant Director
The Epilepsy Foundation of Southeast Texas is a non-profit organization devoted to improving the lives of people with epilepsy in Texas. Services offered by the foundation include public education programs, medical care, therapy and recreation programs.

3259   Epilepsy Foundation: Central and South Texas
10615 Perrin Beitel Rd
Suite 602
San Antonio, TX   78217   210-653-5353
                                                888-606-5353
                                         Fax: 210-653-5355
                                               staff@efcst.org
                                               www.efcst.org

Ariel Robbins, Program Manager
The Epilepsy Foundation of Central & South Texas is a voluntary health organization serving people with epilepsy. Services offered include youth programs, seizure clinics, support groups, referrals and more.

3260   Harris and Eliza Kempner Fund
2201 Market St
12th Floor
Galveston, TX   77553-1529   409-765-6671
                                                Fax: 409-765-9098
                                       information@kemperfund.org
                                               kempnercapital.com

Diana L. Bartula, Vice President, Chief Compliance
V. Delynn Greene, Vice President, Head Trader, Ope
Mission is to further the vision and heritage of the Kemper Family's commitment to philanthropy and sense of responsibility to society.

3261   Hillcrest Foundation
Bank of America
P.O.Box 830241
Dallas, TX   75283   214-209-1965
Daniel Kelly, VP

3262   Hoblitzelle Foundation
5556 Caruth Haven Lane
Suite 200
Dallas, TX   75225-8020   214-373-0462
                                            kstone@hoblitzelle.org
                                             www.hoblitzelle.org

William T Solomon, Chairman
Caren H. Prothro, Vice Chairman
J. McDonald Williams, Treasurer
Karl Hoblitzelle, Founder
Grants made by the directors are usually focused on specific, non-recurring needs of the educational, social service, medical, cultural, and civic organizations in Texas, particularly in the Dallas area.

3263   Houston Endowment
600 Travis St
Suite 6400
Houston, TX   77002-3003   713-238-8100
                                                Fax: 713-238-8101
                                             houstonendowment.org

Ann B Stern, President
Sheryl L Johns, Vice President for Admin
F. Xavier Pena, Vice President for Finance and G
Lisa A. Hall, Vice President for-Programs
A private philanthropic foundation that improves life for people of the greater Houston area through its contributions to charitable organizations and educational institutions.

3264 John G & Marie Stella Kennedy Memorial Foundation
555 N Carancahua
Suite 1700, Tower II
Corpus Christi, TX 78401-0851   361-887-6565
                                  Fax: 361-887-6582

Judge J. A. Garcia, President and Director
Marc A. Cisneros, Chief Executive Officer
Sylvia Whitmore, Chief Operating Officer
Gloria Hicks, Secretary and Director
To advance and nurture activities that contribute to the foundation's core, Catholic values.

3265 John S Dunn Research Foundation
3355 West Alabama
Suite 990
Houston, TX 77098-1722   713-626-0368
                             Fax: 713-626-3866
                             jsdrf@swbell.net
                          johnsdunnfoundation.org

J. Dickson Rogers, President
Dan S. Wilford, Vice President
John R. Wallace, Secretary and Treasurer
John S. Dunn, Trustee

3266 Lola Wright Foundation
515 Congress Avenue
10th Floor
Austin, TX 78701   512-397-2001
                       amber.carden@ustrust.com
                       fdnweb.org/lolawright

Wilford Flowers, President and Director
Paul Hilgers, Vice-President and Director
Ron Oliveira, Secretary and Director
Jay Stewart, Director

3267 Meadows Foundation
3003 Swiss Ave
Dallas, TX 75204-6049   214-826-9431
                              800-826-9431
                         Fax: 214-827-7042
                              www.mfi.org

Linda P Evans, President and CEO
Tom Gale, Vice President and Chief Investm
Paula Herring, Vice President and Treasurer
Laura Bowers, Corporate Secretary
The Meadows Foundation exists to assist people and institutions of Texas improve the quality and circumstances of life for themselves and future generations.

3268 Moody Foundation
2302 Post Office St
Suite 704
Galveston, TX 77550-1994   409-797-1500
                             colleent@moodyf.org
                                  moodyf.org

Frances Moody-Dahlderg, Executive Director
Jamie G. Williams, Human Resources Director
Garrik Addison, Chief Financial Officer
Samantha Seale, Scholarship Administrator
Created for the perpetual benefit of present and future generations.

3269 Pearle Vision Foundation
2534 Royal Ln
Dallas, TX 75229-3884   214-821-7770
                             www.pearlevision.com

Leo Priolo Jr, Owner
Organization dedicated to sight preservation through vision research and education.

3270 San Antonio Area Foundation
303 Pearl Parkway
Suite 114
San Antonio, TX 78215   210-225-2243
                          Fax: 210-225-1980
                              info@saafdn.org
                                  saafdn.org

Marie Smith, Chair
G.P. Singh, Vice Chair
Michelle R. Scarver, Secretary
Luis de la Garza, Treasurer
The San Antonio Area Foundation aspires to significantly enhance the quality of life in our community by providing outstanding service to donors, producting significant asset growth, strengthning community collaboration and managing an exemplary grants program.

3271 Shell Oil Company Foundation
40 Bank Street
London, TX 77252-2463   281-544-7171
                          Fax: 713-241-3329
                        info@shellfoundation.org
                        www.shellfoundation.org

Malcolm Brinded, Chairman
Ben van Beurden, Trustee
William Kalema, Trustee
Hugh Mitchell, Trustee
A not-for-profit foundation funded by donations from Shell Oil Company and other participating Shell companies and subsidiaries.

3272 South Texas Charitable Foundation
P.O.Box 2459
Victoria, TX 77902   512-573-4383
Rayford L Keller, Secretary

3273 Sterling-Turner Foundation
5850 San Felipe Street
Suite 125
Houston, TX 77057-3292   713-237-1117
                             Fax: 713-223-4638
                        jeannie.arnold@stfdn.org
                        www.sterlingturnerfoundation.org

T. R. Reckling, President
Isla C. Reckling, Treasurer
Patricia Stilley, Executive Director
Christiana R McConn, Secretary
Sterling Turner Foundation is a private trust which can assist any Section 501 (c) (3) organization in the state of Texas. The Foundation is not permitted to assist any individuals

3274 TLL Temple Foundation
109 Temple Blvd
Lufkin, TX 75901-7321   936-639-5197
Wayne Corley, Executive Director

3275 William Stamps Farish Fund
Ste 1250
1100 Louisiana St
Houston, TX 77002-5232   713-757-7313
Terry Ward, Manager

Utah

3276 Arc of Utah
18585 Coastal Hwy # 19
Rehoboth Beach, DE 19971   801-364-5060
                              800-371-3060
                         Fax: 801-364-6030
                        gacosta@dunndunn.com
                        www.bewitchedtattoos.com

Kathy Scott, Executive Director
The Arc of Utah advocates for and with cognitive, intellectual and developmental disabilities and their families through awareness, outreach, education, support and public policy.

3277   Marriner S Eccles Foundation
79 S Main St
Salt Lake City, UT 84111-1929   801-532-0934
Shannon K Toronto

3278   Questar Corporation Contributions Program
333 South State Street
P.O. Box 45433
Salt Lake City, UT 84145-0433   801-324-5000
                                                  www.questar.com

Ronald W Jibson, President & CEO
Craig C Wagstaff, Executive vice president
Micheal Dunn, Executive vice president
Brady Rasmussen, Executive Vice President
Focuses on promoting a healthy environment by investing in and
fulfilling its corporate responsibility to support the well-being of
communitites where Questar and its subsidiaries conduct
business.

Vermont

3279   Vermont Community Foundation
3 Court Street
Middlebury, VT 05753   802-388-3355
                                              Fax: 802-388-3398
                                              info@vermontcf.org
                                              www.vermontcf.org

Stuart Comstock-Gay, President
Nina McDonnell, Grants Administrator
Janet McLaughlin, Special Projects Director
Jen Peterson, Vice President for Program and G
Helps build and manage charitable funds created by individuals,
families, groups, organizations, and institutions to improve the
quality of life in Vermont.

Virginia

3280   Arc of Virginia
2147 Staples Mill Road
Richmond, VA 23230   804-649-8481
                                              Fax: 804-649-3585
                                              info@thearcofva.org
                                              www.thearcofva.org

Howard Cullum, President
Shareen Young-Chavez, President-Elect
Marisa Laios, Vice President
Donalda Lovelace, Secretary
The Arc of Virginia advocactes for individuals with mental retar-
dation and developmental disabilities and their families, so they
may all lead productive and fulfilling lives.

3281   Camp Foundation
P.O.Box 813
Franklin, VA 23851   757-562-3439
Bobby B Worrell, CEO

3282   Community Foundation of Richmond & Central Virginia
7501 Boulder View Drive
Suite 110
Richmond, VA 23225- 4047   804-330-7400
                                              Fax: 804-330-5992
                                              info@tcfrichmond.org
                                              tcfrichmond.org

Darcy Oman, President
Bobby Thalhimer, Senior Advisor
Molly Dean Bittner, Vice President
Lisa Pratt O'Mara, Vice President
The Community Foundation provides effective stewardship of
philanthropic assets entrusted to its care by donors who wish to
enhance the quality of community life.

3283   John Randolph Foundation
112 North Main Street
P.O.Box 1606
Hopewell, VA 23860- 1161   804-458-2239
                                              Fax: 804-458-3754
                                      lsharpe@johnrandolphfoundation.org
                                          www.johnrandolphfoundation.org

Lisa H. Sharpe, Executive Director
M. Stephen Cates, Director of Finance and Accounti
Kiffy Werkheiser, Development Program Officer
Tammy E. McCollum, Administrative Associate
The John Randolph Foundation is a community-based Founda-
tion working to improve the health and quality of life for resi-
dents of Hopewell and surrounding areas through Grants and
Scholarships.

3284   Norfolk Foundation
101 W. Main Street,
Suite 4500
Norfolk, VA 23510-2103   757-622-7951
                                              Fax: 757-622-1751
                                      mbrunson@hamptonroadscf.org
                                          www.hamptonroadscf.org

Deborah M DiCroce, Ed.D., President and CEO
Tim McCarthy, Chief Financial Officer
Kay A. Stine, CFRE, Vice President for Development
Lynn Watson Neumann, Director of Gift Planning
The mission of the Norfolk Foundation is to inspire philanthropy
and transform the quality of life in southeastern Virginia.

3285   Robey W Estes Family Foundation
Robey W Estes Jr
3901 West Broad Street
P.O. Box 25612
Richmond, VA 23230-5612   866-378-3748
                                              estes-express.com

Robey W Estes Jr, President and CEO

3286   Virginia Beach Foundation
Suite 4500
101 W. Main Street,
Virginia Beach, VA 23454   757-422-5249
                                              Fax: 757-422-1849
                                      mbrunson@hamptonroadscf.org
                                          www.hamptonroadscf.org

Deborah M DiCroce, President
Tim McCarthy, Chief Financial Officer
Mission is to stimulate the establishment of endowments to serve
the people of Virgina Beach now and in the future. Respond to
changing, emerging, community needs. Provide a vehicle and a
service for donors with varied interests. Serve as a resource, bro-
ker, catalyst and leader in the community.

Washington

3287   Arc of Washington State
2638 State Avenue NE
Olympia, WA 98506-4880   360-357-5596
                                                  888-754-8798
                                              Fax: 360-357-3279
                                              info@arcwa.org
                                              arcwa.org

Cindy O'Neill, Board President
Sue Elliott, Executive Director
Angie Ziska, Secretary
Martha Schulte, Treasurer
Mission is to advocacte for the rights and full participation of all
people with intellectual and developmental disabilities.

323

3288   Ben B Cheney Foundation
3110 Ruston Way
Suite A
Tacoma, WA 98402-5308   253-572-2442
Info@benbcheneyfoundation.org
benbcheneyfoundation.org
Bradbury F. Cheney, President
Piper Cheney, Vice President
Carolyn J. Cheney, Secretary Treasurer
Allan L. Undem, Board Member
The Foundation makes grants in communities where the Cheney
Lumber Company was active. The Foundation's goal is to im-
prove the quality of life in those communities by making grants to
a wide range of activities.

3289   Community Foundation of North Central Washington
9 South Wenatchee Ave
Wenatchee, WA 98801-3332   509-663-7716
Fax: 888-317-8314
info@cfncw.org
www.cfncw.org
Beth Stipe, Executive Director
Kristy Harris, Chief Financial Officer
Lila R. Edlund, Director of Administration
Jennifer Dolge, Director of Donor Services and C
Assists donors by helping identify their specific charitable and
goals and provide grants and scholarships that help groups and
people address critical issues in North Central Washington

3290   Glaser Progress Foundation
1601 Second Avenue
Suite 1080
Seattle, WA 98101-9223   206-728-1050
Fax: 206-728-1123
Martin Collier, Executive Director
Mitchell Fox, Program Officer
Melessa Rogers, Operations Manager
The Glaser Prograss Foundation focuses on four program areas:
measuring progress, animal advocacy, independent media and
global HIV/AIDS.

3291   Greater Tacoma Community Foundation
950 Pacific Avenue
Suite 1100
Tacoma, WA 98402-4423   253-383-5622
Fax: 253-272-8099
info@gtcf.org
www.gtcf.org
Rose Lincoln Hamilton, President and CEO
Shirley Brockmann, CPA, Vice President Finance & Adminis
Elyse Rowe, Chief of Strategy and Community
Gina Anstey, Vice President, Grants
Mission is fostering generosity by connecting people who care
with causes that matter, forever enriching our community.

3292   Inland Northwest Community Foundation
421 West Riverside Avenue
Suite 606
Spokane, WA 99201- 0405   509-624-2606
888-267-5606
Fax: 509-624-2608
admin@inwcf.org
www.inwcf.org
Mark Hurtubise, Ph.D., J.D., President and CEO
Troy Braga, CPA, Controller
P J Watters, Director of Gift Planning
Molly Sanchez, Director of Community Engagement
Serving 20 counties throughout Eastern Washington and North-
ern Idaho, mission is to foster vibrant and sustainable communi-
ties in the Inland Northwest.

3293   Medina Foundation
801 2nd Ave
Suite 1300
Seattle, WA 98104-1517   206-652-8783
Fax: 206-652-8791
info@medinafoundation.org
www.medinafoundation.org
Jennifer Teunon, Executive Director
Jessica Case, Program Officer
Aana Lauckhart, Program Officer
Alexia Cameron, Grants Administrator
A family foundation that works to foster positive change in the
Greater Puget Sound area. The Foundation strives to improve the
human condition by supporting organizations that provide criti-
cal services to those in need.

3294   Norcliffe Foundation
999 3rd Ave
Suite 1006
Seattle, WA 98104-4001   206-682-4820
Fax: 206-682-4821
arline@thenorcliffefoundation.com
www.thenorcliffefoundation.com
Arline Hefferline, Foundation Manager
Nora P. Kenway, President
Geographic area of funding limited to the Puget Sound Region in
and around Seattle, Washington.

3295   Stewardship Foundation
1145 Broadway
Suite 1500
Tacoma, WA 98402-1278   253-620-1340
Fax: 253-572-2721
info@stewardshipfdn.org
www.stewardshipfdn.org
William T. Weyerhaeuser, Chair
Gail T. Weyerhaeuser, Vice Chair and Treasurer
Chi- Dooh, Director
J. Derek McNeil, Director
Christian, evangelical organizations - national or international
impact.

3296   Weyerhaeuser Company Foundation
33663 Weyerhaeuser Way South
Federal Way, WA 98003   253-924-2345
800-525-5440
www.weyerhaeuser.com
Daniel S Fulton, President & CEO
Patricia M Bedient, EVP & CFO
Sandy D McDade, SVP & General Counsel
John A Hooper, SVP, Human Resources
Although the foundation does fund programs for disabled persons from time to time, it is not a specific priority for the foundation. Since it was formed in 1948, the foundation has given more
than $81.1 million to nonprofit organizations and is one of the
oldest funds for corporate philanthropy in the country. Nearly all
of its contributions have been made within the communities
where Weyerhaeuser employees live and work and awards approximately 600 grants annually.

West Virginia

3297   Arc Of West Virginia, The
912 Market Street
Parkersburg, WV 26101-4737   304-422-3151
christina.smith@arcwd.org
www.thearcwv.org

3298 Bernard McDonough Foundation
311 Fourth Street
Parkersburg, WV 26101-5315   304-424-6280
                                      Fax: 304-424-6281
                                www.mcdonoughfoundation.org
Robert W Stephens, Ed.D., President
Mary Riccobene, Vice President
Francis C. McCusker, Treasurer
Katrina Valentine, Corporate Secretary
Directors and officers continue the legacy of the McDonoughs by
providing grants that create a healthier, more educated and cultur-
ally appreciative citizenry.

Wisconsin

3299 Arc of Dunn County
2602 Hils Court
Menomonie, WI 54751-4160   715-235-7373
                                      Fax: 715-233-3565
                                   www.arcofdunncounty.org
Rebecca Cooper, Executive Director
Kathy Lausted, Guardianship Director
Advocating for the rights of citizens with disabilities.

3300 Arc of Eau Claire
4800 Golf Road
Suite 450
Eau Claire, WI 54701-6130   715-833-1735
                                      Fax: 715-833-1215
                                          frcec@frcec.org
                                           www.frcec.org
Brook Steele, President
Melanie Koehler, Vice President
Dr. Jennifer Eddy, Secretary
Dr. Emily Smith-Nguyen, Treasurer
Mission is to provide programs and services that build on family
strengths through prevention, education, support and networking
in collaboration with other resources in the community.

3301 Arc of Fox Cities
211 E. Franklin St.
Suite A
Appleton, WI 54911   920-735-0943
                                      Fax: 920-725-1531
                                    info@arcfoxcities.com
                                         arcfoxcities.com
Laura McCormick, President
Todd Klauer, Vice President
Bryan Mueller, Secretary
Rico Tomasi, Treasurer
Mission statement is to utilize advocacy, respect and concern to
empower all people with disabilities to have the opportunity to
choose and realize their goal of a full life and a secure future.

3302 Arc of Racine County
6214 Washington Ave
Suite C-6
Racine, WI 53404-3350   262-634-6303
                                    info@thearcofracine.org
                                     www.thearcofracine.org
Peggy Foreman, Executive Director
Alison Henry, Program Manager
Ross Gietzel, Program Assistant
The Arc of Racine's mission is to advocate for and provide infor-
mation and services to improve lives.

3303 Arc of Wisconsin Disability Association
2800 Royal Ave
Suite 202
Monona, WI 53713-1518   608-222-8907
                                         877-272-8400
                                      Fax: 608-222-8908
                                           arcw@att.net
John Beisbier, President
Donna Auchue, Vice President
Tina Beauprey, Secretary

The Arc-Wisconsin strives to be a major force in advocating and
promoting self-determined quality of life opportunities for
poeple with developmental and related disabilities and their
families.

3304 Arc-Dane County
6602 Grand Teton Plz
Madison, WI 53719-1091   608-833-1199
                                      Fax: 608-833-1307
                                    arcdanecounty@gmail.com
                                       arcdanecounty.org
Ken Hobbs, President
John Leemkuil, Vice President
Mark Lederer, Secretary
Todd Grundahl, Treasurer
The Arc-Dane County is a non-profit organization whose primary
objective is to support children and adults with developmental
disabilities and their families through advocacy to assure these
individuals are offered the same opportunities and have the rights
due all people. The Arc-Dane County provides numerous services through education, overall support, and legislation that assists those individuals with developmental disabilities be it
within their homes, communities, or at work.

3305 Faye McBeath Foundation
101 W. Pleasant Street
Suite 210
Milwaukee, WI 53212- 3157   414-272-2626
                                      Fax: 414-272-6235
                                      www.fayemcbeath.org
P. Michael Mahoney, Chair
Mary T. Kellner, Vice Chair
Gregory M. Wesley, Secretary
Scott E. Gelzer, Executive Director
A private independent foundation providing grants to tax exempt
nonprofit organizations principally the metropolitan Milwaukee
area.

3306 Helen Bader Foundation
233 North Water Street
4th Floor
Milwaukee, WI 53202- 5761   414-224-6464
                                      Fax: 414-224-1441
                                            info@hbf.org
                                            www.hbf.org
Daniel J. Bader, President/CEO
Lisa G. Hiller, VP, Administration
Maria Lopez Vento, VP, Programs and Partnerships
Robert Tobon, Director, Foundation Relations
Strives to be a philanthropic leader in improving the quality of
life of the diverse communities in which it works. The Founda-
tion makes grants, convenes partners, and shares knowledge to
affect emerging issues in key areas.

3307 Johnson Controls Foundation
5757 N Green Bay Ave
P.O. Box 591
Milwaukee, WI 53201- 4408   414-524-1200
                                         800-333-2222
                                      Fax: 414-524-2077
                                        johnsoncontrols.com
Stephen A Molinaroli, Chairman, President and CEO
Dr. Breda Bolzenius, Vice President, Vice Chairman
Kim Metcalf-Kupres, Vice President and Chief Marketi
R. Bruce McDonald, Executive Vice President and CF
Organized and directed to be operated for charitable purposes
which include the distribution and application of financial sup-
port to soundly managed and operated organizations or causes
which are fundamentally philanthropic.

3308 **Lynde and Harry Bradley Foundation**
1241 N Franklin Pl
Milwaukee, WI 53202-2901   414-291-9915
Fax: 414-291-9991
www.bradleyfdn.org

Dennis J. Kuester, Chairman
David V. Uihlein, Vice Chairman
Michael W. Grebbe, President and CEO
Patrick J. English, Chief Investment Officer
The Foundation's programs support limited, competent government; a dynamic marketplace for economic, intellectual and cultural activity; a vigorus defense at home and abroad, of American ideas and institutions; and scholarly studies and academic achievement.

3309 **Milwaukee Foundation**
101 W Pleasant St
Suite 210
Milwaukee, WI 53212-3963   414-272-5805
Fax: 414-272-6235
info@greatermilwaukeefoundation.org
www.greatermilwaukeefoundation.org
Ellen M Gilligan, President and CEO
Marcus White, Vice President
Kathryn J. Dunn, Vice President
Danae Davis, Executive Director
Guided by three tenets- helping donors create personal legacies of giving that last beyond their lifetimes, investing donor funds for maximum return with minimal risk, and playing a leadership role tackling the communities most challenging needs.

3310 **Northwestern Mutual Life Foundation**
720 E Wisconsin Ave
Milwaukee, WI 53202-4703   414-271-1444
www.northwesternmutual.com
John E Schlifske, Chairman and CEO
Gregory C. Oberland, President
Michael G. Carter, Executive Vice President and CFO
Joann M. Eisenhart, Senior Vice President - Human Re

3311 **Patrick and Anna M Cudahy Fund**
70 E. Lake St.,
Suite 1120
Chicago, Il 60601   312-422-1442
Fax: 312-641-5736
laurenkrieg@cudahyfund.org
cudahyfund.org
Janet S Cudahy MD, President
Lauren Krieg, Executive Director
A general purpose foundation which primarily supports organizations in Wisconsin and the metropolitan Chicago area. Interests are social service, youth, and education with some giving for the arts, and other areas.

3312 **SB Waterman & E Blade Charitable Foundation**
Marshall & Ilsley Trust Company
111 E. Kilbourn Ave.,
Milwaukee, WI 53202-2980   414-287-8700
Fax: 414-765-8200
Thomas C Boettcher, Director
Giving primarily to health associations. Geographical focus is Wisconsin.

Wyoming

3313 **Arc of Natrona County**
314 W. Midwest Ave
P.O. Box 393
Casper, WY 82601   307-577-4913
800-433-5255
Fax: 307-577-4014
info@thearc.org
arcofnatronacounty.org
Beau Covert, President
Dr. Nathan Edwards, Vice President
Kelley Reimer, Treasurer
Colbi Maddox, Secretary
Organization works to ensure that the estimated 7.2 million Americans with intellectual and developmental disabilities have the services and supports they need to grow, develop and live in communities across the nation.

Funding Directories

3314 **Chronicle Guide to Grants**
318 S. Lee Street
Alexandria, DC 20037-1146   202-466-1200
800-287-6072
Fax: 202-452-1033
help@philanthropy.com
heideninc.com
Phil Semas, Manager
Edward J. Heiden, President
A computerized research tool, on floppy disks or a CD-ROM, for immediate use on any IBM compatible personal computer. Offers electronic listings of 10,000 grants from hundreds of foundations, with a subscription that offers 1,000 plus new listings every two months. Each listing offers grant information as well as names, addresses and phone numbers of the grant-making organizations. *$295.00*

3315 **College Student's Guide to Merit and Other No-Need Funding**
Reference Service Press
5000 Windplay Dr
Suite 4
El Dorado Hills, CA 95762-9319   916-939-9620
Fax: 916-939-9626
info@rspfunding.com
www.rspfunding.com
Gail Schlachter, Founder
R. David Weber, Editor
Sandy Hirsh, Editor
Sandy Perez, Funding Finder
More than 1,200 funding opportunities for currently-enrolled or returning college students are described in this directory. *$32.50*
450 pages
ISBN 1-588410-41-2

3316 **Community Health Funding Report**
CD Publications
8204 Fenton St
Silver Spring, MD 20910-4502   301-588-6380
800-666-6380
Fax: 301-588-6385
subscriptions@cdpublications.com
www.cdpublications.com
Michael Gerecht, President
The once twice-monthly report is now web-based to allow for breaking news updates and up the the minute information about funding, including: public and private grant announcements; reports on successful health programs nationwide; interviews with grant officials; plus national news on health policy topics affecting various organizations. *$439.00*
Web-based

3317   Directory of Financial Aids for Women
Reference Service Press
2310 Homestead Rd
Suite C1 #219
Los Altos, CA   94024   650-861-3170
                                          Fax: 650-861-3171
                                          info@rspfunding.com
                                          www.rspfunding.com

Gail Schlachter, Founder
R. David Weber, Editor
Sandy Hirsh, Editor
Sandy Perez, Funding Finder
Funding programs listed support study, research, travel, training,
career development, or innovative effort at any level; descriptions of more than 1,700 funding programs - representing billions
of dollars in financial aid set aside for women; also an annotated
bibliography of 60 key directories that identify even more financial aid opportunities and a set of indexes that let you search the
directory by title, sponsor, researching, tenability, subject, and
deadline. *$45.00*
578 pages Biennial
ISBN 1-588410-00-5

3318   Disability Funding News
8204 Fenton St
Silver Spring, MD   20910-4502   301-588-6380
                                                800-666-6380
                                          Fax: 301-588-6385
                                          www.cdpublications.com

Michael Gerecht, President

3319   FC Search
Foundation Center
79 fifth Avenue
New York, NY   10003-3034   212-620-4230
                                                800-424-9836
                                          Fax: 212-807-3677
                                          order@foundationcenter.org
                                          foundationcenter.org

Bradford K Smith, President
Lisa Philip, Vice President for Strategic Phi
Jen Bokoff, Director of GrantCraft
Lawrence T. McGill, Vice President for Research
Provides access to the Foundation Center's comprehensive data-
base of funders in a convenient CD-ROM format. *$1845.00*

3320   Federal Grants & Contracts Weekly
LRP Publications
360 Hiatt Drive
Palm Beach Gardens, FL   33418-1718   800-341-7874
                                          Fax: 561-622-2423
                                          custserve@lrp.com
                                          www.lrp.com

Kelly Sullivan, Editor
Kenneth F. Kahn, President
The latest funding announcements of federal grants for project
opportunities in research, training and services. Provides profiles
of key programs, tips on seeking grants, updates on legislation
and regulations, budget developments and early alerts to upcoming funding opportunities. *$340.00*
Weekly

3321   Financial Aid for Asian Americans
Reference Service Press
2310 Homestead Rd
Suite C1 #219
Los Altos, CA   94024   650-861-3170
                                          Fax: 650-861-3171
                                          info@rspfunding.com
                                          www.rspfunding.com

Gail Schlachter, Founder
R. David Weber, Editor
Sandy Hirsh, Editor
Sandy Perez, Funding Finder

This is the source to use if you are looking for financial aid for
Asian Americans; nearly 1,000 funding opportunities are described. *$35.00*
336 pages
ISBN 1-588410-02-1

3322   Financial Aid for Hispanic Americans
Reference Service Press
2310 Homestead Rd
Suite C1 #219
Los Altos, CA   94024   650-861-3170
                                          Fax: 650-861-3171
                                          info@rspfunding.com
                                          www.rspfunding.com

Gail Schlachter, Founder
R. David Weber, Editor
Sandy Hirsh, Editor
Sandy Perez, Funding Finder
Nearly 1,300 funding programs open to Americans of Mexican,
Puerto Rican, Central American, or other Latin American heri-
tage are described here. *$37.50*
472 pages
ISBN 1-588410-03-X

3323   Financial Aid for Native Americans
Reference Service Press
2310 Homestead Rd
Suite C1 #219
Los Altos, CA   94024   650-861-3170
                                          Fax: 650-861-3171
                                          info@rspfunding.com
                                          www.rspfunding.com

Gail Schlachter, Founder
R. David Weber, Editor
Sandy Hirsh, Editor
Sandy Perez, Funding Finder
Detailed information is provided on 1,500 funding opportunities
open to American Indians, Native Alaskans, and Native Pacific
Islanders. *$37.50*
562 pages
ISBN 1-588410-04-8

3324   Financial Aid for Research and Creative Activities Abroad
Reference Service Press
2310 Homestead Rd
Suite C1 #219
Los Altos, CA   94024   650-861-3170
                                          Fax: 650-861-3171
                                          info@rspfunding.com
                                          www.rspfunding.com

Gail Schlachter, Founder
R. David Weber, Editor
Sandy Hirsh, Editor
Sandy Perez, Funding Finder
Described here are 1,200 funding programs (scholarships, fel-
lowships, grants, etc.) available to support research, profes-
sional, or creative activities abroad. *$45.00*
378 pages
ISBN 1-588410-82-5

**3325   Financial Aid for Veterans, Military Personnel and their
          Dependents**
Reference Service Press
2310 Homestead Rd
Suite C1 #219
Los Altos, CA   94024   650-861-3170
                                          Fax: 650-861-3171
                                          info@rspfunding.com
                                          www.rspfunding.com

Gail Schlachter, Founder
R. David Weber, Editor
Sandy Hirsh, Editor
Sandy Perez, Funding Finder

According to Reference Book Review, this directory (with its 1,100 entries) is the most comprehensive guide available on the subject. *$40.00*
392 pages
ISBN 1-588410-43-9

3326 Financial Aid for the Disabled and Their Families
Reference Service Press
2310 Homestead Rd
Suite C1 #219
Los Altos, CA   94024   650-861-3170
                                          Fax: 650-861-3171
                                          info@rspfunding.com
                                          www.rspfunding.com
Gail Schlachter, Founder
R. David Weber, Editor
This directory, which Children's Bookwatch calls invaluable describes more than 1,100 financial aid opportunities available to support persons with disabilities and members of their families. Updated every 2 years. *$37.50*
508 pages Every other yr.
ISBN 1-588410-01-3

3327 Foundation & Corporate Grants Alert
LRP Publications
360 Hiatt Drive
Palm Beach Gardens, FL   33418-1718   800-341-7874
                                          Fax: 561-622-2423
                                          custserve@lrp.com
                                          www.lrp.com
Kelly Sullivan, Editor
Kenneth F. Kahn, President
A complete guide to foundation and corporate grant opportunities for nonprofit organizations. Tracks developments and trends in funding and provides notification of changes in foundations' funding priorities. *$245.00*
Monthly
ISSN 1062-46 6

3328 Foundation 1000
Foundation Center
79 fifth Avenue
New York, NY   10003-3076   212-620-4230
                                              800-424-9836
                                          Fax: 212-807-3691
                                          order@foundationcenter.org
                                          www.foundationcenter.org
Bradford K Smith, President
Lisa Philip, Vice President for Strategic Phi
Jen Bokoff, Director of GrantCraft
Lawrence T. McGill, Vice President for Research
Offers comprehensive information on the 1000 largest foundations in the US. *$195.00*

3329 Foundation Directories
Foundation Center
79 fifth Avenue
New York, NY   10003-3034   212-620-4230
                                              800-424-9836
                                          Fax: 212-807-3677
                                          order@foundationcenter.org
                                          foundationcenter.org
Bradford K Smith, President
Lisa Philip, Vice President for Strategic Phi
Jen Bokoff, Director of GrantCraft
Lawrence T. McGill, Vice President for Research
Lists key facts on the top 20,000 US foundations. *$125.00*
ISBN 0-87954 -36-1

3330 Foundation Grants to Individuals
Foundation Center
79 fifth Avenue
New York, NY   10003-3034   212-620-4230
                                              800-424-9836
                                          Fax: 212-807-3677
                                          order@foundationcenter.org
                                          foundationcenter.org
Bradford K Smith, President
Lisa Philip, Vice President for Strategic Phi
Jen Bokoff, Director of GrantCraft
Lawrence T. McGill, Vice President for Research
The only publication that provides extensive coverage of foundation funding prospects for individual grantseekers. *$40.00*
Biennially

3331 From the State Capitals: Public Health
Wakeman/Walworth
P.O.Box 7376
Alexandria, VA   22307-376   703-768-9600
                                          Fax: 703-768-9690
                                          newsletters@statecapitals.com
                                          www.statecapitals.com
Mark Willen, Editor
Digest of state and municipal health care financing and cost containment measures, includes medical legislation, disease control, etc. *$245.00*
6 pages

3332 Grant Guides
Foundation Center
79 fifth Avenue
New York, NY   10003-3034   212-620-4230
                                              800-424-9836
                                          Fax: 212-807-3677
                                          order@foundationcenter.org
                                          foundationcenter.org
Bradford K Smith, President
Lisa Philip, Vice President for Strategic Phi
Jen Bokoff, Director of GrantCraft
Lawrence T. McGill, Vice President for Research
Provides descriptions of actual foundation grants awarded in various subject fields. *$35.00*
ISBN 0-87954 -90-6

3333 Guide to Funding for International and Foreign Programs
79 fifth Avenue
New York, NY   10003-3034   212-620-4230
                                              800-424-9836
                                          Fax: 212-807-3677
                                          order@foundationcenter.org
                                          foundationcenter.org
Bradford K Smith, President
Lisa Philip, Vice President for Strategic Phi
Jen Bokoff, Director of GrantCraft
Lawrence T. McGill, Vice President for Research
Grantmakers featured in this guide provide funding for international relief, disaster assistance, human rights, civil liberties, community development, conferences, and education. *$190.00*

3334 Guide to US Foundations their Trustees, Officers and Donors
Foundation Center
79 fifth Avenue
New York, NY   10003-3034   212-620-4230
                                              800-424-9836
                                          Fax: 212-807-3677
                                          order@foundationcenter.org
                                          foundationcenter.org
Bradford K Smith, President
Lisa Philip, Vice President for Strategic Phi
Jen Bokoff, Director of GrantCraft
Lawrence T. McGill, Vice President for Research
Provides crucial facts on grantmaking. Each entry includes contact information, current assets, annual contributions, officers, donors and more. *$135.00*

3335 High School Senior's Guide to Merit and Other No-Need Funding
Reference Service Press
2310 Homestead Rd
Suite C1 #219
Los Altos, CA 94024
650-861-3170
Fax: 650-861-3171
info@rspfunding.com
www.rspfunding.com
Gail Schlachter, Founder
R. David Weber, Editor
Sandy Hirsh, Editor
Sandy Perez, Funding Finder
Here's your guide to 1,100 funding programs that never look at income level when making awards to college bound high school seniors. *$29.95*
400 pages
ISBN 1-588410-44-X

3336 How to Pay for Your Degree in Business & Related Fields
Reference Service Press
2310 Homestead Rd
Suite C1 #219
Los Altos, CA 94024
650-861-3170
Fax: 650-861-3171
info@rspfunding.com
www.rspfunding.com
Gail Schlachter, Founder
R. David Weber, Editor
Sandy Hirsh, Editor
Sandy Perez, Funding Finder
If you need funding for an undergraduate or graduate degree in business or related fields, this is the directory to use (500+ funding programs described). *$30.00*
290 pages
ISBN 1-588411-45-1

3337 How to Pay for Your Degree in Education& Related Fields
Reference Service Press
2310 Homestead Rd
Suite C1 #219
Los Altos, CA 94024
650-861-3170
Fax: 650-861-3171
info@rspfunding.com
www.rspfunding.com
Gail Schlachter, Founder
R. David Weber, Editor
Sandy Hirsh, Editor
Sandy Perez, Funding Finder
Here's hundreds of funding opportunities available to support undergraduate and graduate students preparing for a career in education, guidance etc. *$30.00*
250 pages
ISBN 1-588411-46-x

3338 National Directory of Corporate Giving
Foundation Center
79 fifth Avenue
New York, NY 10003-3034
212-620-4230
800-424-9836
Fax: 212-807-3677
order@foundationcenter.org
foundationcenter.org
Bradford K Smith, President
Lisa Philip, Vice President for Strategic Phi
Jen Bokoff, Director of GrantCraft
Lawrence T. McGill, Vice President for Research
Offers over 2,000 corporate funders, current giving reviews and profiles of sponsoring companies. *$195.00*

3339 Older Americans Report
Business Publishers
2222 Sedwick Drive
Durham, NC 27713-1995
240-514-0600
800-223-8720
Fax: 800-508-2592
custserv@bpinews.com
www.bpinews.com
Leonard Eiser, Publisher
Follows all programs and funding sources in education, housing, job training, therapy, Social Security Supplemental Security Income, Medicare, Medicaid and more of importance to persons with disabilities. Also covers the latest on the Americans with Disabilities Act. Publishes a newsletter. *$327.00*

3340 Student Guide
US Department of Education
400 Maryland Avenue SW
Washington, DC 20202
202-401-2000
800-872-5327
Fax: 202-401-0689
TTY: 800-437-0833
customerservice@inet.ed.gov
ed.gov
Arne Duncan, Secretary of Education
Jim Shelton, Deputy Secretary
Ted Mitchell, Under Secretary
Describes the major student aid programs the US Department of Education administers and gives detailed information about program procedures.
74 pages

Minnesota

3602 Burnett Foundation
P.O. Box 633
Northfield, MN 55057-6881
817-877-3344
tomburnettfamilyfoundation@msn.com
www.tomburnettfoundation.org
V Neils Agather, Executive Director

Government Agencies

Federal

3341 Administration on Aging
One Massachusetts Ave NW
Washington, DC 20001   202-401-4634
                                    Fax: 202-357-3555
                                    aclinfo@acl.hhs.gov

Kathy Greenlee, Administrator
Sharon Lewis, Principal Deputy Administrator
Aaron Bishop, Commissioner
John Wren, Deputy Administrator
Administers the Older Americans Act of 1965 to assist states and
local communities to develop programs for older persons.

3342 Administration on Children, Youth and Families
370 L Enfant Promenade SW
Washington, DC 20447   202-401-4634
                                         800-422-4453
                                    TTY:800-787-3224
                                        www.acf.hhs.gov

William H. Bentley, Associate Commissioner
Jeannie Chaffin, Director
Naomi Goldstein, Director
Mathew McKearn, Director
Responsible for federal programs that promote the economic and
social well-being of families, children, individuals and
communities.

3343 Administration on Developmental Disabilities
U S Department of Health and Human Services
One Massachusetts Ave NW
Washington, DC 20001   202-401-4634
                                         800-422-4453
                                    TTY:800-787-3224
                                     aclinfo@acl.hhs.gov
                            www.acf.hhs.gov/programs/add
William H. Bentley, Associate Commissioner
Jeannie Chaffin, Director
Eskinder Negash?, Director
Mathew McKearn?, Director
Ensures that individuals with developmental disabilities and
their families participate in the design of and have access to cul-
turally competent services, supports, and other assistance and op-
portunities that promote independence, productivity, and
integration and inclusion into the community.

3344 Americans with Disabilities Act Informationn
US Department of Justice
950 Pennsylvania Avenue NW
Washington, DC 20530   202-282-8000
                                         800-514-0301
                                    Fax: 202-307-1197
                                    TTY: 800-514-0383
                                          www.ada.gov
Gregory B. Friel, Chief
The ADA assures that Americans with disabilities have the same
opportunities as all Americans. To this end, the Justice Department produces publications and conducts programs to increase
compliance of the ADA nationwide.

3345 Civil Rights Division/Disability Rights Section
US Department Of Justice
950 Pennsylvania Avenue NW
Washington, DC 20530   202-282-8000
                                         800-514-0301
                                    Fax: 202-307-1197
                                    TTY: 800-514-0383
                                          www.ada.gov
Gregory B. Friel, Chief
The US Department of Justice answers questions about the Amer-
ican Disabilities Act (ADA) and provides free publications by
mail and fax through its ADA Information Line.

**3346 Committee for Purchase from People Who Are Blind or
Severely Disabled**
1401 S. Clark Street
Suite 715
Arlington, VA 22202-3259   703-603-7740
                                         800-999-5963
                                    Fax: 703-603-0655
                                      info@abilityone.gov
                                       www.abilityone.gov
Tina Ballard, Executive Director & CEO
J Anthony Poleo, Chairperson
Kimberly Zeich, Deputy Executive Director & Chie
Angela Phifer, Chief of Staff
A federal agency that administers the Javits-Wagner-O'Day Pro-
gram, directing federal agencies to purchase products and ser-
vices from nonprofit agencies that employ people who are blind
or have other severe disabilities. Provides a wide range of voca-
tional options to individuals with severe disabilities.

3347 Equal Opportunity Employment Commission
131 M Street NE
Washington, DC 20507-100   202-663-4599
                                         800-669-4000
                                    Fax: 202-419-0739
                                        info@eeoc.gov
                                         www.eeoc.gov
Jenny R Yang, Chair
Constance S Barker, Commissioner
Chai R Feldblum, Commissioner
David Lopez, General Counsel
This agency is responsible for drafting and implementing the reg-
ulations of Title I of the ADA.

3348 Federal Communications Commission
445 12th Street SW
Washington, DC 20554   888-225-5322
                                         888-835-5322
                                    Fax: 866-418-0232
                                       fccinfo@fcc.gov
                                            fcc.gov
Tom Wheeler, Chairman
Mignon Clyburn, Commissioner
Jessica Rosenworcel, Commissioner
Ajit Pai, Commissioner
Enforces ADA telecommunications provisions which require
that companies offering telephone service to the general public
must offer telephone relay services to individuals who use text
telephones or similar devices. Also enforces closed captioning
rules, hearing compatibility and access to equipment and services
for people with disabilities.

3349 Health Care Financing Administration
200 Independence Ave SW
Washington, DC 20201-4   202-690-6726
                                    Fax: 202-690-6262
                            www.federalregister.gov/agencies/
William Roper, Administrator
Thomas Scully, President
Through the Social Security administration, it administers the
Medicare program under Title XVIII of the Social Security Act.
Administers grants to the states for Medicaid under Title XIX of
the Social Security Act for individuals who are medically
indigent.

3350 National Care Planning Council
PO Box 1118
Centerville, UT 84014   801-298-8676
                                         800-989-8137
                                    Fax: 801-295-3776
                                  info@longtermcarelink.net
                                   www.longtermcarelink.net
Thomas E Day, Director
Roxanne Pope, Office Manager
The National Care Planning Council's mission is to help families
with long term care planning for seniors. Some services offered
by them include eldercare articles, books, workshops and seminars, networking and more.

3351 National Coalition of Federal Aviation Employees with Disabilities
Federal Aviation Administration
800 Independence Avenue, SW
Washington, DC   20591   405-954-4709
                                                    866-835-5322
                                               Fax: 405-954-4490
                                               TTY: 405-954-4587

Becky Pritchett, Treasurer
Alan Jones, President of Aeronautical Center
NCFAED is working on: 1) improvement of work conditions for employees; 2) expansion on National Coalition to serve all FAA employees; 3) promote equal opportunity for people with disabilities in the FAA workplace; 4) assist the FAA in its commitment to remove physical and attudinal barriers which inhibit opportunities for people with disabilities; 5) align with internal and external organizations to attract future generations of people with disabilities to the FAA as employees.

3352 National Council on Disability
1331 F Street Northwest
Suite 850
Washington, DC   20004- 1138   202-272-2004
                                               Fax: 202-272-2022
                                               TTY:202-272-2074
                                                    www.ncd.gov

Jeff Rosen, Chairperson
Kartherine D Seelman, Co Vice Chair
Rebecca Cokley, Executive Director
Joan M Durocher, General Counsel
Federal agency led by 15 members appointed by the President of the United States and confirmed by the United States Senate. The overall purpose of the National Council is to promote policies, programs, practices and procedures that guarantee equal opportunities to persons with disabilities.

3353 National Division of the Blind and Visually Impaired
330 C St NW
Washington, DC   20001   202-205-8520
Chester Avery, Director
Develops methods, standards and procedures to assist state agencies in the rehabilitation of blind persons. Administers the Randolph-Sheppard Act, which assures priority for blind persons in the operation of vending facilities on federal property and serves as a program manager for the Helen Keller National Center for Youth who are deaf-blind.

3354 National Institute on Aging
31 Center Dr, MSC 2292
Building 31, Room 5C27
Bethesda, MD 20892   800-222-2225
                                            TTY:800-222-4225
                                            niaic@nia.nih.gov
                                            www.nia.nih.gov
Patrick Shirdon, Director of Management
Michael O'Donnell, Chief Administrative Officer
Luigi Ferrucci, M.D., Ph.D, Scientific Director
The National Institute on Aging (NIA) is the primary Federal agency engaged in researching Alzheimer's disease, providing resources to scientists and educating the public on the results of studies.

3355 National Institutes of Health: National Eye Institute
31 Center Drive MSC 2510
Bethesda, MD   20892-2510   301-496-5248
                                                 800-411-1222
                                            2020@nei.nih.gov
                                               www.nei.nih.gov
Paul A. Sieving, Director
As part of the federal government's National Institutes of Health (NIH), the National Eye Institute finances intramural and extramural research on eye diseases and visual disorders.

3356 Office of Policy
Social Security Administration
1100 West High Rise
6401 Security Blvd
Baltimore, MD 21235   202-293-9138
                                                 800-772-1213
                                            TTY:800-325-0778
                                               www.ssa.gov/policy
Michael J Astrue, Commissioner
Edward Demarco, Assitant Deputy Commissioner
Serge Harrison, Executive Officer
Administers grants to the states for social services under Title XX of the Social Security Act to welfare recipients and others likely to become them.

3357 Office of Special Education Programs: Department of Education
400 Maryland Avenue SW
Washington, DC   20202-7100   202-401-2000
                                                 800-872-5327
                                            Fax: 202-401-0689
                                            TTY: 800-437-0833
                                        customerservice@inet.ed.gov
                        www2.ed.gov/about/offices/list/osers/osep
Arne Duncan, Secretary of Education
Jim Shelton, Deputy Secretary
Ted Mitchell, Under Secretary
The Office of Special Education Programs (OSEP) is dedicated to improving results for infants, toddlers, children and youth with disabilities ages birth through 21 by providing leadership and financial support to assist states and local districts.

3358 President's Committee on People with Intellecutual Disabilities
370 L Enfant Promenade SW
Washington, DC   20447   202-619-0364
                                                 800-422-4453
                                            TTY:800-787-3224
                                                www.acf.hhs.gov
George Sheldon, Acting Assistant Secretary
Laverdia Roach, Acting Executive Director
Formerly the President's Committee on Mental Retardation, a federal advisory committee, estalished by the presidential executive order to adivse the President of the United States and the Secretary of the Department of Health and Human Services on issues concerning citizens with intellectual disabilities, coordinate activities between different federal agencies and assess the impact of their policies upon the lives of citizens with intellectual disabilities and their families.

3359 Rehabilitative Services Administration
400 Maryland Ave SW
Washington, DC   20202-7100   202-401-2000
                                                 800-872-5327
                                            Fax: 202-401-0689
                                            TTY: 800-437-0833
                                        customerservice@inet.ed.gov
                                                   www2.ed.gov
Arne Duncan, Secretary of Education
Jim Shelton, Deputy Secretary
Ted Mitchell, Under Secretary
The Rehabilitation Services Administration (RSA) oversees formula and discretionary grant programs that help individuals with physical or mental disabilities to obtain employment and live more independently through the provision of such supports as counseling, medical and psychological services, job training and other individualized services.

3360 Social Security Administration
5 Park Center Court
Suite 100
Owing Mills, MD   21117   410-965-6114
                                                 800-772-1213
                                            Fax: 410-966-2027
                                                    www.ssa.gov
Bill Vitek, Manager
Administers old age, survivors, and disability insurance programs under Title II of the Social Security Act. Also administers

the federal income maintenance program under Title XVI of the Social Security Act. Maintains network of local/regional offices nationwide.

3361   US Department of Education: Office of Civil Rights
400 Maryland Avenue SW
Washington, DC   20202-1100

800-421-3481
800-877-8339
Fax: 202-453-601
TTY: 800-437-0833
OCR@ed.gov

Catherine E Lhamon, Assistant Secretary
Seth Galanter, Principal Deputy Asst Secretary
Sandra Battle, Deputy Assistant Secretary
James Ferg Cadima, Senior Counsel
Prohibits discrimination on the basis of disability in programs and activities funded by the Department of Education. Investigates complaints and provides technical assistance to individuals and entities with rights and responsibilities under Section 504.

3362   US Department of Labor: Office of Federal Contract Programs
200 Constitution Ave NW
Washington, DC   20210

866-487-2365
TTY: 877-889-5627
webmaster@dol.gov
www.dol.gov/ofccp

Thomas E. Perez, Secretary of Labor
Christopher Lu, Deputy Secretary of Labor
Mathew Colangelo, Chief of Staff
James Moore, Deputy Assistant Secretary
Prohibits discrimination on the basis of disability and requires federal contractors and sub-contractors with contracts of $2,500 or more to take affirmative action to employ and advance individuals with disabilities.

3363   US Department of Transportation
1200 New Jersey Ave SE
Washington, DC   20590

202-366-4000
855-368-4200
TTY: 800-877-8339
www.dot.gov

Anthony Foxx, Secretary of Transportation
Peter Rogoff, Secretary for Police
Kathryn Thomson, General Counsel
Greg Winfree, Assistant Secretary for Research
Enforces ADA provisions that require nondiscrimination in public and private mass transportation systems and services.

3364   US Office of Personnel Management
1900 E St NW
Washington, DC   20415-1000

202-606-1800
Fax: 202-606-0909
TTY: 202-606-2532
Informationquality@opm.gov
opm.gov

Katherine Archuleta, Director
Ann Marie Habershaw, Chief of Staff & Director Extern
Angela Bailey, Chief Operating Officer
Jen Mason, Director, Office of Public Engag
Establishes policies for employment of the handicapped within the federal service. Administers a merit system for the federal employment that includes recruiting, examining, training, and promoting people on the basis of knowledge and skills, regardless of sex, race, religion or other factors.

3365   Alabama Council For Developmental Disabilities
RSA Union Building
RSA Union Building
PO Box 301410
Montgomery, AL   36130- 1410

334-242-3973
800-232-2158
Fax: 334-242-0797
Myra.Jones@mh.alabama.gov
www.acdd.org

Stefan Eisen, Jr., Chair, Parent Advocate
Sophia Whitted, Fiscal Manager
Elmyra Jones-Banks, Executive Director
Shungulla Moorey, Office Manager
Serves as an advocate for Alabama's citizens with developmental disabilities and their families; to empower them with the knowledge and opportunity to make informed choices and exercise control over their own lives; and to create a climate for positive socialchange to enable them to be respected, independent and productive integrated members of society.

3366   Alabama Department of Public Health
The RSA Tower, 201 Monroe Street
PO Box 303017
Montgomery, AL   36130-3017

334-206-5300
800-ALA-1818
www.adph.org

Kathy Vincent, Staff Assistant
Donald E Williamson, Administrator
Provides professional services for the improvement and protection of the public's health through disease prevention and the assurance of public health services to resident and transient populations of the state regardless of social circumstances or the ability to pay.

3367   Alabama Department of Rehabilitation Services
602 S Lawrence St
Montgomery, AL   36104

334-293-7500
800-441-7607
Fax: 334-293-7383
cary.boswell@rehab.alabama.gov
www.rehab.alabama.gov

Cary F Boswell, Commissioner
Jim Carden, Deputy Commissioner
Jim Harris Iii, Assistant Commissioner
Winona Nelson, Cheif Financial Officer
To enable Alabama's children and adults with disabilities to achieve their maximum potential.

3368   Alabama Department of Senior Services
201 Monroe Street
RSA Tower Suite 350
Montgomery, AL 36140

334-242-5743
877-425-2243
Fax: 334-242-5594
Ageline@adss.alabama.gov

Irene Collins, Executive Director
Thomas Ray Edwards, Board Chairman
Dr. Horace Patterson, Vice-Chair
The mission of the Alabama Department of Senior Services is to promote the independence and dignity of those we serve through a comprehensive and coordinated system of quality services

3369   Alabama Disabilities Advocacy Program
University of Alabama
P.O.Box 870395
Tuscaloosa, AL 35487-0395

205-348-4928
800-826-1675
Fax: 205-348-3909
adap@adap.ua.edu

Anita Davidson, Legal Assistant
Janet Owens, Accounting Specialist
James Tucker, Director
Rosemary Beck, Information Systems Administrato
The federally mandate statewide protection and advocacy system serving eligible individuals with disabilities in Alabama. ADAP

has five program components: Protection and Advocacy for persons with developmental disabilities (PADD), Protection and Advocacy for Individuals with Mental Illness (PAIMT), Protection and Advocacy of Individual Rights (PAIR), Protection and Advocacy for Assistive Technology (PAAT) and Protection & Advocacy For Beneficiaries of Social Security (PABSS).

3370 Alabama Division of Rehabilitation and Crippled Children
602 S Lawrence Street
Montgomery, AL 36104   334-293-7500
800-441-7607
Fax: 334-293-7383
www.rehab.state.al.us

Cary F Boswell, Commissioner
Steven Kayes, Board Member
Jimmie Varnado, Board Member

3371 Alabama Governor's Committee on Employment of Persons with Disabilities
602 S Lawrence St
Montgomery, AL 36104   334-293-7500
800-441-7607
Fax: 334-293-7383
www.rehab.alabama.gov

Jimmie Varnado, Board Chairperson
Stacy Mitchell, Board Member
Stephen G Keys, Board Member
Andrea Collett, Board Member
The Alabama Governor's Committee on Employment of People with Disabilities (AGCEPD) is a program of the Alabama Department of Rehabilitation Services (ADRS).

3372 Alabama State Department of Human Resources
Childcare Services Division
50 North Ripley Street
Montgomery, AL 36130   334-242-1310
Fax: 334-353-1115
barry.spear@dhr.alabama.gov
www.dhr.state.al.us

Nancy T. Buckner, Commissioner
Nancy Jinright, Chief of Staff/Ethics Officer
John Hardy, Communications
Conitha King, Finance
Partners with communities to promtoe family stability and provide for the safety and self-sufficiency of vulnerable Alabamians.

3373 Client Assistance Program: Alabama
400 South Union Street
Suite 465
Montgomery, AL 36104   334-263-2749
800-288-3231
Fax: 334-230-9765
rachel.hughes@rehab.alabama.gov
www.sacap.alabama.gov

Rachel Hughes, Director/Advocate

3374 Disability Determination Service: Birmingham
P.O.Box 830300
Birmingham, AL 35283-0300   205-989-2100
800-292-8106
Fax: 205-989-2295
ssa.gov

Tommy Warren, Executive Director
Janet Cox, Owner

3375 Social Security: Mobile Disability Determination Services
PO Box 2371
Mobile, AL 36652-2371   251-433-2820
800-292-6743
Fax: 251-436-0599
www.ssa.gov

Tommy Warren, Executive Director
Jack Miller, Office Manager

3376 Workers Compensation Board Alabama
649 Monroe Street
Montgomery, AL 36131   334-242-2868
800-528-5166
Fax: 334-353-8262
webmaster@labor.alabama.gov
labor.alabama.gov/wc

Charles DeLamar, Director
Al Pelham, Supervisor
Sandy Hallmark, Supervisor
Peggy Barton, Supervisor
The Workers' Compensation Division is responsible for the administration of the Alabama Workers' Compensation Law to ensure proper payment of benefits to employees injured on the job and encourage safety in the work place

Alaska

3377 ATLA
2217 E Tudor Rd
Ste 4
Anchorage, AK 99507-1068   907-563-2599
800-723-2852
Fax: 907-563-0699
atla@atla.biz
www.atla.biz

Kathy Privratsky, Executive Director
Mystie Rail, Commissioner
Margaret Cisco, AT Specialist
Assistive Technology sales and services. ATLA is Alaska's only assistive technology resource center.

3378 Alaska Commission on Aging
150 Third Street #103
PO Box 110693
Juneau, AK 99811-0693   907-465-3250
Fax: 907-465-1398
denise.daniello@alaska.gov
dhss.alaska.gov/acoa

Mary Shields, Chair
Rolf Numme, Vice Chair
Denise Daniello, Executive Director
Sherice Cole, Admin Assistant II
Works to promote and protect the health and well-being of Alaskans.

3379 Alaska Department of Handicapped Children
Ste 314
1231 Gambell St
Anchorage, AK 99501-4664   907-346-1995
Gregory Lee, CEO

3380 Alaska Division of Vocational Rehabilitation:
801 W. 10th Street,
Suite A
Juneau, AK 99801-1878   907-465-2814
800-478-2815
Fax: 907-465-2856
dawn.duval@alaska.gov
labor.alaska.gov

Dianne Blummer, Commissioner
David G Stone, Deputy commissioner
John Cannon, Director
Provides comprehensive services to people with disabilities to assist in achieving an employment outcome.

3381 Client Assistance Program: Alaska
2900 Boniface Pkwy
Ste 100
Anchorage, AK 99504-3195   907-333-2211
800-478-0047
Fax: 907-333-1186
www.icdri.org/legal/AlaskaCAP.htm

Pam Stratton, Executive Director
We provide informatory referral to other programs in Alaska that are funded under the Rehabilitation Act of 1973 as amended; In-

dividual assistance or advocacy, if an individual with disability has applied for or received services from an agency funded under the Rehabilitation Act and has concerns or questions we will work with them to help resolve their concerns with the agency.

3382 Department Of Health & Social Services - Division Of Behaviorial Health
350 Main Street
Suite 214
Juneau, AK 99801-1149　　　　　907-465-3370
　　　　　　　　　　　　　　　　800-465-4828
　　　　　　　　　　　　　　Fax: 907-465-2668
　　　　　　　　　　　　　albert.wall@alaska.gov
　　　　　　　　　　　　　　www.alaska.gov

Albert E. Wall, Director
Stacy Toner, Division Operations Manager
Liz Clement, Program Coordinator
The division plans for and provides appropriate prevention, treatment and support for families impacted by mental disorders or developmental disabilities while maximizing self-determination. Community based services are provided by grantees. Inpatient services are provided in two division operated facilities.

3383 Governor's Committee on Employment and Rehabilitation of People with Disabilities
Division of Vocational Rehabilitation (DVR)
801 W 10th Street
Suite A
Juneau, AK 99801-1878　　　　　907-465-2814
　　　　　　　　　　　　　　　　800-478-2815
　　　　　　　　　　　　　　Fax: 907-465-2815
　　　　　　　　　　　　　dawn.duval@alaska.gov
　　　　　　　　　　　　www.labor.state.ak.us/dvr

Cheryl Walsh, Executive Director
Carries on a continuing program to promote the employment and rehabilitation of citizens with disabilities in the State of Alaska. Advocates for a comprehensive statewide system for access to assistive technology. Obtains and maintains cooperation with public and private groups and individuals in this field.

3384 Governor's Council on Disabilities and Special Education
3601 C Street
Suite 740
Anchorage, AK 99524-0249　　　　907-269-8990
　　　　　　　　　　　　　　　　888-269-8990
　　　　　　　　　　　　　　Fax: 907-269-8995
　　　　　　　　　　　　　　GCDSE@alaska.gov
　　　　　　　　　　　www.hss.state.ak.us/gcdse/

Patrick Reinhart, Executive Director
Rich Sanders, Planner III
Britteny M Howell, M.A., ABD, Research Analyst III
Lanny Mommsen, Health Program Manager
The Governor's Council on Disabilities & Special Education was created to meet Alaska's diverse needs.

3385 Protection & Advocacy System: Alaska
Disability Law Center of Alaska
3330 Arctic Blvd
Ste 103
Anchorage, AK 99503-4580　　　　907-565-1002
　　　　　　　　　　　　　　　　800-478-1234
　　　　　　　　　　　　　　Fax: 907-565-1000
　　　　　　　　　　　　　　akpa@dlcak.org

Deborah Smith, President
James M Shine Sr
Deals with rights of the disabled. Works in conjunction with agencies, law offices and family members.

3386 Protection & Advocacy for Persons with Developmental Disabilities: Alaska
Advocacy Services of Alaska
Ste 101
615 E 82nd Ave
Anchorage, AK 99518-3100　　　　907-222-2652
　　　　　　　　　　　　　　　　866-275-7273
　　　　　　　　　　　　　　Fax: 907-677-8777
　　　　　　　　　　　　　　TTY: 866-232-4525

Greg Schomaker, Manager

3387 Workers Compensation Division
Department of Labor & Workforce Development
PO Box 115512
Juneau, AK 99811-5512　　　　　907-465-2790
　　　　　　　　　　　　　　Fax: 907-465-2797
　　　　　　　　　　　　workerscomp@alaska.gov
　　　　　　　　　　　www.labor.state.ak.us/wc

Clark Bishop, Commissioner
Trena Heikes, Division Director
Michael Monagle, Director
The Division of Workers' Compensation is the agency charged with the administration of the Alaska Workers' Compensation Act (Act). The Act provides for the payment by employers or their insurance carriers of medical, disability and reemployment benefits to injured workers

Arizona

3388 Arizona Department of Economic Security
1717 W Jefferson
Phoenix, AZ 85007　　　　　　　602-542-4791
　　　　　　　　　　　　　　　　www.azdes.gov

Michael Trailor, Director
The Department of Economic Security is a human service agency providing services in six areas: Aging and Community Services, Benefits and Medical Eligibility, Child Support Enforcement, Children and Family Services, Developmental Disabilities and Employment and Rehabilitation Services.

3389 Arizona Department of Health Services
150 North 18th Avenue
Ste 330
Phoenix, AZ 85007-3243　　　　　602-542-1025
　　　　　　　　　　　　　　Fax: 602-542-0883
　　　　　　　　　　　　　　　www.azdhs.gov

Will Humble, Director
Neal Young, Director
Lynne Smith, Chief Exeuctive Officer
Rex Critchfield, Manager
The mission of Children's Rehabilitative Services is to improve the quality of life for children by providing family-centered medical treatment, rehabilitation, and related support services to enrolled individuals who have certain medical, handicapping, or potentially handicapping conditions.

3390 Arizona Division of Aging and Adult Services
1789 West Jefferson Street
Site Code 950A
Phoenix, AZ 85007-3202　　　　　602-542-4446
　　　　　　　　　　　　　　Fax: 602-542-6655
　　　　　　　　　　　　　　　www.azdes.gov

Rex Critchfield, Manager
Neal Young, Director
Lynne Smith, Chief Executive Officer
Will Humble, Director
The Division supports at-risk Arizonans to meet their basic needs and to live safely, with dignity and independence.

3391 Arizona Rehabilitation State Services for the Blind and Visually Impaired
4620 N 16th St, B-106
Ste 100
Phoenix, AZ 85016-5121　　　　　602-266-9579
　　　　　　　　　　　　　　Fax: 602-264-7819
　　　　　　　　　　　　　　　www.azdes.gov

Paul Howell, Vocational Rehab Supervisor
Suzanne Sayre f, Rehab Counselor for Blind
Offers clients a conservation program, eye examinations, treatments, counseling, social work, psychological testing and evaluation, professional training, computer training and more for the visually impaired. The staff includes 56 full time employees.

3392   Developmental Disability Council: Arizona
2828 N Country Club Rd
Ste 100
Tucson, AZ   85716-3202   602-542-4049
                                           800-889-5893
                                      Fax: 602-542-5320
                                           www.cpes.com

David A Berns, Manager
Nebal Chavez, Executive Director
Susan Madison, Manager

The mission of the GovernorOs Council on Developmental Disabilities is to bring together persons with disabilities representing Arizona cultural diversity and their families and other community members, to protect rights, eliminate barriers, and jointly promote equal opportunities

3393   Governor's Council on Developmental Disabilities
1700 West Wasington Street
Suite 420
Phoenix, AZ   85007   520-325-9688
                                           877-665-3176
                                      Fax: 520-325-3561
                                         lclausen@azdes.gov
                                        azgovernor.gov/DDPC/

Larry Clausen, Executive Director
Shelly Adams, Executive Secretary

The purpose of the council is to advocate for and assure that individuals with developmental disabilities and their families participate in the design of and have access to culturally competent services, supports and provides opportunities to become integrated and included in the community.

3394   International Dyslexia Association: Arizona Branch
Meredith Puls AZ-IDA
985 W. Silver Spring Place
Oro Valley, AZ   85755-6548   480-941-0308
                                      arizona.ida@gmail.com
                                        www.dyslexia-az.org

Meredith Puls, President
Rebekah Dyer, Vice President
Melissa A. L. Pallister, Treasurer
Sue Noel, Secretary

Provides free information and referral services for diagnosis and tutoring for parents, educators, physicians, and individuals with dyslexia. Membership includes yearly journal and quarterly newsletter, and Pennsylvania newsletter; discounts to conferences and events.

3395   Protection & Advocacy for Persons with Disabilities: Arizona
Arizona Center for Disability Law
5025 E Washington St
Suite 202
Phoenix, AZ   85034   602-274-6287
                                           800-927-2260
                                      Fax: 602-274-6779
                                      TTY: 602-274-6287
                                     center@azdisabilitylaw.org
                                       www.azdisabilitylaw.org

Anthony DiRienzi, President
Art Gode, Vice President
J. J. Rico, Executive Director
John Chalmers, Treasurer

The Center provides disability-related legal information and advice to individuals who need their services and assistance. In addition to limited legal representation, their goal is to provide efficient, streamlined services to educate people with disabilities and their support on how to enforce their legal rights through self-advocacy. Guides and documents are available online by selecting Self-Advocacy Materials button on the homepage.

3396   Social Security: Phoenix Disability Determination Services
Social Security Admission
4000 North Central Avenue
Suite 1800
Phoenix, AZ   85714   520-638-2000
                                           800-772-1213
                                      TTY:800-325-0778
                                           www.ssa.gov

3397   Social Security: Tucson Disability Determination Services
4710 South Palo Verde Road
Tucson, AZ   85714-2030   520-638-2000
                                           800-772-1213
                                      TTY:800-325-0778
                                           www.ssa.gov

Arkansas

3398   Arkansas Assistive Technology Projects
Increasing Capabilities Access
900 W.7th Street
Little Rock, AR   72201-4538   501-666-8868
                                           800-828-2799
                                      Fax: 501-666-5319
                                         info@ar-ican.org
                                        www.arkansas-ican.org

Eddie Schmeckenbecher, Supervisor
Essie Hardin, Secretary
Bryan Ayres, Advisory Counsel
Billy Altom, Advisory Counsil

A consumer responsive ,statewide program promoting assistive technology devices and sources for persons of all ages with all disabilities. Referral and information services provide information about devices, where to obtain them and their cost.

3399   Arkansas Division of Aging & Adult Services
Department of Human Services
PO Box 1437
Slot-S-530
Little Rock, AR   72203-1437   501-682-2441
                                      Fax: 501-682-8155
                                    aging.services@arkansas.gov
                                      www.state.ar.us/dhs/aging

Craig Cloud, Director
Stephenie Blocker, Assistant Director
Brad Nye, Assistant Director
Brian Bowen, Assistant Director

The division provides services geared for adults and the elderly including supervised living, home delivered meals, adult day care, senior centers, personal care, household chores, and adult protective services.

3400   Arkansas Division of Developmental Disabilities Services
Donaghey Plaza
PO Box 1437
Little Rock, AR   72203-1437   501-682-1001
                                      Fax: 501-682-8820

Charlie Green, Manager

State agency to assist persons with developmental disabilities and their family in obtaining appropriate assistance and services.

3401   Arkansas Division of Services for the Blind
Department Of Health and Human Services
700 Main St
Little Rock, AR   72203-4608   501-682-5463
                                           800-960-9270
                                      Fax: 501-682-0366
                                      TTY: 800-285-1131
                                      humanservices.arkansas.gov/dsb

Terry Sheeler, Chairman
Dickie Walker, Vice Chairman
Sandy Edwards, Secretary
Harold Brewer, Ex-Officio Member

State program which offers services in the areas of health, counseling, social work, self help and education for the visually and multihandicapped. The staff includes 4 full time and 13 part time members including mobility specialists and rehabilitation teachers.

3402   Arkansas Governor's Developmental Disabilities Council
5800 West 10th Street
Suite 805
Little Rock, AR   72204- 1763
501-661-2589
855-627-7580
Fax: 501-661-2399
ddcouncil.org

Regina Wilson, Executive Director
Teresa Sandar, Family Services Coordinator
Lee Russell, Information Oficer
Michelle Boyd, Administrative Assistant
A federally-funded state agency established to bring the perspective of individuals with developmental disabilities and his or her family or natural support system to policy makers and make improvements to the service system.

3403   Baptist Health Rehabilitation Institute
Baptist Heath
9601 Baptist Health Dr.
Little Rock, AR   72205-7299
501-202-1839
888-BAP-TIST
Fax: 501-202-7352
www.baptist-health.com

Ellen Callaway, Director, Rehabilition Therapy
Acute rehab facility serving patients with ortho, spinal cord injury, brain injury, CVA, arthritis, cardiac and generalized weakness; JCAHO and CARF accredited; 17 outpatient therapy centers throughout central Arkansas.

3404   Children's Medical Services
P.O.Box 1437
Little Rock, AR   72203-1437
501-682-8207
800-482-5850
Fax: 501-682-8247
www.cms-kids.com

Nancy Holder, Program Director
Iris Fehr, Nursing Director
Rodney Farley, Parent Activities Coordinator
A collection of programs for eligible children with special needs. Each one of our programs and services are family-centered and designed to help children with a variety of conditions and needs.

3405   President's Committee on People with Disabilities: Arkansas
7th & Main St
Little Rock, AR   72203

3406   Social Security: Arkansas Disability Determination Services
701 Pulaski Street
Little Rock, AR   72201-3990
501-682-3030
800-772-1213
Fax: 501-682-7553
www.socialsecurity.gov

Arthur Boutiette, COO

California

3407   California Department of Aging
1300 National Drive
Suite 200
Sacramento, CA   95834-1992
916-419-7500
Fax: 916-928-2267
TTY:800-735-2929
webmaster@aging.ca.gov
aging.ca.gov

Lora Connoly, Director
Diane Paulsen, Chief Deputy Director
Anna Esparza, Executive Assistant
Chisorom Okwuosa, Chief Counsel
The Department contracts with the network of Area Agencies on Aging, who directly manage a wide array of federal and state-funded services that help older adults find employment; support older and disabled individuals to live as independently as possible in the community; promote healthy aging and commu-

nity involvement; and assist family members in their vital care giving role

3408   California Department of Handicapped Children
714 P Street
Rm 323
Sacramento, CA   95814-6401
916-445-4171
Maridee Gregory
Diana Bonta, Chief Executive Officer

3409   California Department of Rehabilitation
721 Capitol Mall
Sacramento, CA   95814-3510
916-324-1313
800-952-5544
TTY:916-558-5807
externalaffairs@dor.ca.gov
www.rehab.cahwnet.gov

Joe Xavier, Director
David Supkofl, Manager
Assists people with disabilities, particularly those with severe disabilities, in obtaining and retaining meaningful employment and living independently in their communities. The department develops, purchases, provides and advocates for programs and services in vocational rehabilitation, habilitation and independent living with a priority on serving persons with all disabilities, especially those with the most severe disabilities.

3410   California Governor's Committee on Employment of People with Disabilities
Employment Development Department
800 Capitol Mall
PO Box 826880
Sacramento, CA   94280-0001
916-654-8055
800-695-0350
Fax: 916-654-9821
TTY: 916-654-9820
www.edd.ca.gov

Charlie Kaplan, Staff Director
GCEPD works to eliminate the barriers that preclude equal consideration for employment opportunities for people with disabilities. The Governor's Committee is responsible for providing leadership to increase the numbers of people with disabilities in the California workforce.

3411   California Protection & Advocacy: (PAI) A Nonprofit Organization
Protection and Advocacy (PA I)
1831 K Street
Sacramento, CA   95811-4114
916-504-5800
800-776-5746
Fax: 916-504-5802
SERVICES@DISABILITYRIGHTSCA.ORG
www.disabilityrightsca.org

Catherine Blakemore, Executive Director
Andrew Mudryk, Deputy Director
Alan Gildestein, Managing Attorney
Sujatha Branch, Associate Managing Attorney
Advancing the human and legal rights of people with disabilities.

3412   California State Council on Developmental Disabilities
1507 21st Street
Suite 210
Sacramento, CA   95811-5297
916-322-8481
866-802-0514
Fax: 916-443-4957
council@scdd.ca.gov
www.scdd.ca.gov

April Lopez, Chairperson
Jenny Ning Yang, Interim Vice-Chairperson
Tammy Eudy, Office Assistant
Robin Maitino, Executive Assistant
The State Council on Developmental Disabilities (SCDD) is established by state and federal law as an independent state agency to ensure that people with developmental disabilities and their families receive the services and supports they need.

3413 Client Assistance Program: California
CA Health and Human Services Agency Dept of Rehab
721 Capitol Mall
PO Box 944222
Sacramento, CA 95814

916-324-1313
800-952-5544
Fax: 916-558-5391
TTY:916- 558-580
capinfo@dor.ca.gov
www.dor.ca.gov

Tony P Sauer, Director
We have a three-pronged mission to provide services and advocacy that assist people with disabilities to live independently, become employed and have equality in the communities in which they live and work.

3414 International Dyslexia Association: Central California Branch
4594 E Michigan Ave
Fresno, CA 93703-1556

559-251-9385
800-222-3123
Fax: 599-252-1216
www.interdys.org

Joy Moody, President
Provides free information and referral services for diagnosis and tutoring for parents, educators, physicians, and individuals with dyslexia. Membership includes yearly journal and quarterly newsletter, and Pennsylvania newsletter; discounts to conferences and events.

3415 Long Beach Department of Health and Human Services
2525 Grand Avenue
Long Beach, CA 90815-1765

562-570-4000
Fax: 562-570-4049
www.longbeach.gov/health/

Ron Arias, Executive Director
Michael Johnson, Manager
The Long Beach Department of Health and Human Services (Health Department) has been improving the health of the Long Beach community for over a century.

3416 Los Angeles County Department of Health Services
313 N Figueroa Street
Los Angeles, CA 90012-2602

213-240-8101
800-427-8700
Fax: 213-250-4013

Mitchell H Katz, MD, Director
Hal F. Yee, Jr., M.D., Ph.D., Chief Medical Officer
Allan Wecker, Chief Financial Officer
Alexander Li, M.D., Deputy Director
Los Angeles County Department of Health Services is one of the US's largest publicly supported health systems.The system is the main provider of health care for the area's poor and uninsured. It provides general medical and surgical care and is affiliated with the medical school at USC. The system also manages the Emergency Medical Services (EMS) Agency and the Community Health Plan HMO, a low-cost managed care plan for members of Medicaid and other state-funded programs.

3417 Social Security: California Disability Determination Services
3164 Garrity Way
Richmond, CA 94806-1983

800-772-1213
TTY:800-325-0778
www.ssa.gov

Sally Keen, San Francisco Regional PDF Coord

3418 Social Security: Fresno Disability Determination Services
Social Security
1052 C St
Fresno, CA 93706-3245

559-487-5391
800-772-1213
Fax: 510-970-2947
TTY: 800-325-0778
www.ssa.gov

Sally Keen, Regional PDF Coordinator

3419 Social Security: Oakland Disability Determination Services
P.O. Box 24225
Oakland, CA 94623-1225

510-622-3506
800-772-1213
TTY:800-325-0778
www.ssa.gov

3420 Social Security: Sacramento Disability Determination Services
P.O. Box 997121
Suite A
Sacramento, CA 95899-7121

916-515-4400
800-772-1213
Fax: 916-263-5310
TTY: 916-381-9445
ssa.gov

3421 Social Security: San Diego Disability Determination Services
P.O. Box 85326
San Diego, CA 92186-5326

619-278-4300
800-772-1213
Fax: 619-278-4303
TTY: 800-325-0778
www.ssa.gov

Colorado

3422 Colorado Department of Aging & Adult Services
1575 Sherman St
10th Floor
Denver, CO 80203-1702

303-866-5700
Fax: 303-620-2696
cdhs.communications@state.co.us

Reggie Bicha, Executive Director
A department providing services to the elderly.

3423 Colorado Developmental Disabilities Council
1120 Lincoln
Suite 706
Denver, CO 80203

720-941-0176
Fax: 720-941-8490
cddpc.email@state.co.us
coddc.org

Katherine Carol, Chairperson
Irene Aguilar, Colorado Senate
Marcia Tewell, Executive Director
Lionel Llewellyn, Administrative Assistant
The mission is to advocate in collaboration with and on behalf of people with developmental disabilities for the establishment and implementation of public policy which will further their independence, productivity and integration.

3424 Colorado Division of Mental Health
3824 W. Princeton Circle
Denver, CO 80236-3111

303-866-7400
Fax: 303-866-7428
colorado.gov

Patrick K. Fox, Director
Administration of public health program

3425 Colorado Health Care Program for Children with Special Needs
4300 Cherry Creek Drive south
Denver, CO 80246-1530

303-692-2370
800-886-7689
Fax: 303-753-9249
cdphe.psdrequests@state.co.us
www.colorado.gov/cdphe/hcp

Christopher Stanley, Board member
Angie Goodger, HCP Consultant
Kelsey Minor, HCP Consultant
Jennie Munthali, HCP Section Manager
Provides information and state aid to children with disabilities.

3426   Division of Workers' Compensation Dapartment of Labor & Employment
633 17th Street
Suite 201
Denver, CO   80202-3660   303-318-8700
                                                800-388-5515
                                                888-390-7936
                                           Fax: 303-575-8882
                        cdle_workers_compensation@state.co.us
                                            www.colorado.gov/cdle
Ellen Golombek, Executive Director
Infomation regarding Division Rules and procedures for Claimants, Employers, Adjusters, and parties to claim.

3427   Eastern Colorado Services for the Disabled
P. O. Box 1682
617 South 10th Avenue
Sterling, CO 80751-3168   970-522-7121
                                           Fax: 970-522-1173
                                                rhonda@ecsdd.org
                                    www.easterncoloradoservices.org
Rhonda Roth, Executive Director
Traci Schrade, Finance Director
Melissa Dassaro, Case Management Director
Dave Fast, PHR, Human Resources
Case coordination, infant stimulation, family support, residential and vocational programs.

3428   International Dyslexia Association: Rocky Mountain Branch
740 Yale Rd.
Boulder, CO   80305-5010   303-721-9425
                                                855-5ID- RMB
                                           Fax: 303-721-9425
                                              ida_rmb@yahoo.com
                                            www.dyslexia-rmbida.org
Karen Leopold, President
Lynn Kuhn, Secretary
Yona Sammartino, Administrative Director
Julie Bottom, Board of Director
Provides free information and referral services for diagnosis and tutoring for parents, educators, physicians, and individuals with dyslexia. Membership includes yearly journal and quarterly newsletter, and Pennsylvania newsletter; discounts to conferences and events.

3429   Legal Center for People with Disabilities& Older People
455 Sherman St
Ste 130
Denver, CO   80203-4403   303-722-0300
                                                800-288-1376
                                           Fax: 303-722-0720
                                           TTY: 303-722-3619
                                        tlcmail@thelegalcenter.org
                                              thelegalcenter.org
John R. Posthumus, President
Stephen P. Rickles, Vice President
Nancy Tucker, Secretary
John Paul Anderson, Treasurer
Uses the legal system to protect and promote the rights of people with disabilities and older people in Colorado through direct legal representation, advocacy, education and legislative analysis. The Legal Center is Colorado's Protection and Advocacy System. We are also the State Ombudsman for nursing homes and assisted living facilities. Call for a free publications and products list.

Connecticut

3430   Connecticut Board of Education and Servicefor the Blind
184 Windsor Avenue
Windsor, CT   06095-4536   860-602-4000
                                                800-842-4510
                                           Fax: 860-602-4020
                                           TTY: 860-602-4221
                                           brian.sigman@CT.GOV
                                      www.ct.gov/besb/site/default.asp
Amy Porter, Commissioner

Offers rehabilitative services and information for persons with legal blindness and childrenwhonare visually impaired that are residents of Connecticut.

3431   Connecticut Commission on Aging
210 Capitol Avenue
Hartford, CT   06106   860-240-5200
                                           Fax: 860-240-5204
                                                coa@cga.ct.gov
Julia Evans Starr, Executive Director
Deborah Migneault, Senior Policy Analyst
Alyssa Norwood, Project Manager
Christianne Kovel, Communications Specialist
Advocates on beha;f of elderly persons in Connecticut by regularly monitoring their status, assessing the impact of current and propsed initiatives, and conducting activities which promote the interests of these individuals and report to the Governor and the Legislature.

3432   Connecticut Department of Children and Youth Services
505 Hudson Street
Hartford, CT   06106   860-550-6300
                                           Fax: 860-724-2001
                                         Commissioner.dcf@ct.gov
                                                www.ct.gov
Gary Scappini, Manager
Bruce Douglas, Executive Director

3433   Connecticut Developmental Disabilities Council
263 Farmington Avenue
Farmington, CT   6030   860-679-1561
                                                800-653-1134
                                           Fax: 860-679-1571
                                           TTY: 860-679-1502
                                                ctkasa.org
Ed Preneta, Executive Director
Kids As Self Advocates (KASA) is a national grassroots network that helps youth with special needs and their friends become self-advocates, helps other people in the community understand what it's like to live with special health care needs.

3434   Connecticut Office of Protection and Advocacy for Persons with Disabilities
60B Weston Street
Suite B
Hartford, CT   06120-1551   860-297-4300
                                                800-842-7303
                                           Fax: 860-566-8714
                                           TTY: 860-297-4320
                                    OPA-Information@po.state.ct.us
                                            www.ct.gov/opapd
Craig B Henrici, Executive Director
Alexandria Bode, Board Member
Thomas Behrendt, Board Member
John Clausen, Board Member
Provides information, referrals, advocacy assistance & limited legal services to people with disabilities in the state of Connecticut whose civil rights have been violated or who are experiencing the difficulty securing relevant support services. P & A supports the development of community advocacy groups by providing training & technical assistance. P & A is responsible for investigating abuse & neglect of all individuals with intellectual disability ages 18-59.

3435   Social Security: Hartford Area Office
960 Main Street
2nd Floor
Hartford, CT   06103-1228   877-619-2851
                                                800-772-1213
                                           Fax: 860-566-1795
                                           TTY: 860-525-4967
                                                www.ssa.gov
Jan Gilbert, Professional Relations Coord.

Delaware

3436 Delaware Assistive Technology Initiative(DATI)
461 Wyoming Road
Newark, DE 19716-0269
302-831-0354
Fax: 302-831-4690
TTY:800-870-3284
dati@asel.udel.edu
www.dati.org

Beth Mineo, Project Director
Joann McCafferty, Staff Assistant
The Delaware Assistive Technology Initiative (DATI) connects Delawareans who have disabilities with the tools they need in order to learn, work, play and participate in community life safely and independently. DATI services include: Equipment demonstration centers in each county; no-cost, short-term equipment loans that let you try before you buy; Equipment Exchange Program; AT workshops and other training sessions; advocacy for improved AT access policies and funing and several more.

3437 Delaware Client Assistance Program
United Cerebral Palsy Association
254 E Camden Wyoming Ave
Camden, DE 19934-1303
302-698-9336
800-640-9336
Fax: 302-698-9338
icdri.org/legal/DelawareCAP.htm

Melissa Shahan, Executive Director
Provides advocacy services for persons involved with programs covered under the Rehabilitation Act of 1973 as amended, information and referrals on ADA, Title I.

3438 Delaware Department of Health and Social Services
Administration Building D HS S Campus
1901 N Du pont Highway
Main Building
New Castle, DE 19720-1160
302-255-9040
800-464-4357
Fax: 302-255-4429
TTY: 302-744-4556
dhssinfo@state.de.us
www.dhss.delaware.gov

Rita Landgraf, Cabinet Secretary
Henry Smith III, Deputy secretary
Provides most of the human services available through Delaware State Government, including Medicaid, the Children's Health Insurance Program, food stamps, welfare-to-work, vaccines for children, child support enforcement, public health programs, and general services for the aging. Also for individuals with developmental and physical disabilities, visual impairements, mental illness and other vulnerable populations.

3439 Delaware Department of Public Instructing
Townsend Building
401 Federal Street
Dover, DE 19901- 1402
302-735-4000
800-433-5292
Fax: 302-739-4654
deeds@doe.k12.de.us
http://www.doe.k12.de.us

Mark T. Murphy, Secretary of Education
David J. Blowman, Deputy Secretary
Mary Kate McLaughlin, Chief of Staff
Penny Schwinn, Chief Accountability Officer
A publicly funded, state agency that gives information about local facilities and administers supplemental funds for visually handicapped students in local schools. It also maintains special teachers of sight conservation and braille programs for both children and adults.

3440 Delaware Developmental Disability Council
410 Federal Street 2nd Floor
Suite 2
Dover, DE 19901- 3640
302-739-3333
800-464-4357
Fax: 302-739-2015
pat.maichle@state.de.us
www.ddc.delaware.gov

Barbara Monaghan, Council Chair
Patricia L. Maichle, Senior Administrator
Kristin Cosden, Social Service Administrator
Stefanie Lancaster, Administrative Officer
Working to ensure that people with developmental disabilities enjoy the same quality of life as the rest of society.

3441 Delaware Division for the Visually Impaired
1901 North Dupont Highway
New Castle, DE 19720-1160
302-255-9800
Fax: 302-255-4441
dhssinfo@state.de.us
www.dhss.delaware.gov/dvi/

Rita Landgraf, Secretary
Henry Smith, Deputy Secretary
Betsy Deldeo, Office Manager
State agency serving the visually impaired persons from birth, with or without other handicaps. Services offered include vocational rehabilitation, independent living, orientation and mobility, technology assessment, transition from school to work.

3442 Delaware Protection & Advocacy for Persons with Disabilities
Arc of Delaware
144 E Market St
Georgetown, DE 19947-1411
302-856-6019
Fax: 302-856-6133

Becky Allen, Executive Director

3443 Delaware Workers Compensation Board
Industrial Accident Board de dept
4425 North Market Street
Wilmington, DE 19802-1307
302-761-8085
Fax: 302-761-6601
www.delawareworks.com

James Cagle, Manager
The Office of Workers' Compensation administers and enforces state laws, rules and regulations regarding industrial accidents and illnesses.

3444 Social Security: Wilmington Disability Determination
U S Department of Health and Human Services
1528 S 16th Street
Wilmington, NC 28401-3908
866-964-6227
800-772-1213
Fax: 910-254-3444
TTY: 910-815-4695
www.socialsecurity.gov

J Allen Murphy, Founder
Vickie O'Brien, Manager

3445 The Division for the Visually Impaired
Herman M. Holloway, Sr. Campus
1901 N Dupont Hwy
New Castle, DE 19720
302-255-9800
Fax: 302-255-4441
dhssinfo@state.de.us
dhss.delaware.gov

Alan Wingrove, General Manager
Romy Mikhail, Customer Service, Quality & ISO Manager
The Division for the Visually Impaired provides educational, vocational and technical support to people with visual impairments. Some programs offered include education, employment support, guidance for living independently and using assistive devices, business enterprise programs, volunteer opporunities and more.

District of Columbia

3446 District of Columbia Department of Handicapped Children
D C General Hospital
Bldg 10
1900 Massachusetts Ave SE
Washington, DC 20003- 2542   202-541-6337
                                      Fax: 202-675-7694

Jacqueline Mcmorris, Acting Chief
Nayab Ali, MD

3447 District of Columbia Office on Aging
500 K Street NE
Washington, DC 20002-2714   202-724-5622
                                      Fax: 202-724-4979
                                      TTY:202-724-8925
                                      dcoa@dc.gov
                                      dcoa.dc.gov

John M Thompson, Executive Director
Deborah Royster, General Counsel
Tanya Reid, Executive Assistant
Camile Williams, Chief of Staff
Serves the District of Columbia residents 60 years of age and
older. Contact the Information and Assistance Unit for more in-
formation about innovative programs and services offered by the
Office.

3448 Information, Protection & Advocacy for Persons with
Disabilities
IPACHI
220 I Street, N.E.
Suite 130
Washington, DC 20002   202-547-0198
                                Fax: 202-547-2083
                                jbrown@uls-dc.org
                www.acf.hhs.gov/programs/add/states/pas.html
Jane Brown, Executive Director
Ronald Tyson, Information/Referral
Offers services and support for persons with disabilities in the
Washington, DC area.

3449 Information, Protection and Advocacy Center for
Handicapped Individuals
220 I Street, N.E.
Suite 130
Washington, DC 20002-2340   202-547-0198
                                      Fax: 202-547-2083
                                      jbrown@uls-dc.org
                www.acf.hhs.gov/programs/add/states/pas.html
Jane Brown, Executive Director
Serves all persons with disabilities in the DC, Maryland and Vir-
ginia areas offering them legal representation and advocacy, in-
formation and referrals and several publications.

3450 International Dyslexia Association of DC
40 York Rd., 4th Floor
Baltimore, MD 21204-1016   410-296-0232
                                      800-222-3123
                                      Fax: 410-321-5069
                                      info@interdys.org
                                      www.interdys.org

Ruth R Tifford LCSW, President
Provides free information and referral services for diagnosis and
tutoring for parents, educators, physicians, and individuals with
dyslexia. Membership includes yearly journal and quarterly
newsletter, and Pennsylvania newsletter; discounts to
conferences and events.

3451 Wage and Hour Division of the Employment Standards
Administration
US Department of Labor
200 Constitution Ave NW
Washington, DC 20210-1   202-693-5000
                                  866-487-2365
                                  Fax: 202-219-8822
                                  TTY: 877-889-5627
                                  webmaster@dol.gov
                                  www.dol.gov

Hilda Solis, Secretary of Labor
Seth Harris, Deputy Secretary
Elizabeth Kim, Executive Secretariat Director
Betsey Stevenson, Chief Economist
Administers regulations governing the employment of individu-
als with disabilities in sheltered workshops and the disabled
workers industries.

3452 Washington Hearing and Speech Society
2150 N 107th St, Suite 205
Seattle, WA 98133-2633   206-209-5271
                                  Fax: 206-367-8777
                                  office@wslha.org
                                  www.wslha.org

Paul Diez, President
Judith Bernier, Secretary
Julie Leonardo, Treasurer
Lesley Stephens, Clinical SLP
Offers individuals with hearing or speech impairments, in the DC
area, speech, reading classes, audiological services and new aids.

3453 Well Mind Association of Greater Washington
18606 New Hampshire Ave
Ashton, MD 20861-9789   301-774-6617
                                 Fax: 301-946-1402

3454 Workers Compensation Board: District of Columbia
4058 Minnesota Avenue, NE,
Washington, DC 20019-5626   202-724-7000
                                      202-698-4817
                                      Fax: 202-673-6993
                                      does@dc.gov
Deborah A Carroll, Director
The Workers' Compensation Program processes claims and monitors the payment of benefits to injured private-sector employees
in the District of Columbia

Florida

3455 ARC Gateway
3932 North 10th Avenue
Pensacola, FL 32503-2807   850-434-2638
                                     Fax: 850-438-2180
                                     info@arc-gateway.org
                                     www.arc-gateway.org

Peter Mougey, President
Patricia Young, Vice President
Lynn Erickson, Secretary
Donna Fassett, Executive Director
ARC Gateway is a non-profit organization that serves children
who have or are at risk of developmental disabilities as well as
adults with developmental disabilitie

3456 Advocacy Center for Persons with Disabilities
2473 Care Drive
Suite 200
Tallahassee, FL 32308-5020   850-488-9071
                                       800-342-0823
                                       Fax: 850-488-8640
                                       TTY: 800-346-4127
                                       www.disabilityrightsflorida.org

Catherine Piecora, Chair
Maryellen McDonald, Executive Director
Carol Stachurski, Program Operations Manage
Paige Morgan, Executive Assistant

Disability Rights Florida is the designated protection and advocacy system for individuals with disabilities in the State of Florida.

3457 Assistive Technology Educational Network of Florida
1207 S Mellonville Avenue
Sanford, FL 32771-2240   800-558-6580
                                        Fax: 407-320-2379
                            Diane_Penn@scps.k12.fl.us
            www.icdri.org/Assistive%20Technology/aten.htm
Dee Wright, Executive Secretary
Diane Penn, MA, Technology Specialist
Provides state-wide information, awareness and training for students, family members, teachers and other professionals in the area of assisted technology; a quarterly newsletter and a network of specialists (Local Assistive Technology Specialists) trained by ATEN to provide support at the district level.

3458 Bureau Of Exceptional Education And Student Services
325 West Gaines Street Suite 614
Tallahassee, FL 32399   850-245-0475
                                        Fax: 850-245-0953
                            Monica.Verra-Tirado@fldoe.org
                                            www.fldoe.org
Pam Stewart, Education Commissioner
Monica Verra Tirado, Bureau Chief
Chatherine Aponte Gray, Administrative Assistant
Tonya Milton, Program Planner
Provides consultative services for the establishment and operation of school programs for visually impaired students. Provides assistance for in-service teacher training through state or regional workshops or technical assistance to individual programs.

3459 Department of Health & Rehabilitative Services
1317 Winewood Blvd
Building 1
Tallahassee, FL 32399-700   850-487-1111
                                        Fax: 850-922-2993
                                            www.dcf.state.fl.us
David Wilkins, Secretary
Ramin Kouzehkanani, Deputy Secretary
John Bryant, Manager
The Florida Department of Children and Families has adopted an integrated approach to programs and services as we work to help improve the lives of individuals and families.

3460 Division of Workers Compensation
200 East Gaines Street
Tallahassee, FL 32399-0318   850-413-3089
                                            877-693-5236
                                        Fax: 850-413-2950
                    Tanner.Holloman@myfloridacfo.com
                                            www.fldfs.com
Tanner Holloman, Division Director
Andrew Sabolic, Assistant Director
Terry Kester, Chief Information Officer
Robin Delaney, Bureau Chief of Compliance
To actively ensure the self-execution of the workers' compensation system through education and informing all stakeholders of their rights and responsibilities, leveraging data to deliver exceptional value to our customers and stakeholders, and holding parties accountable for meeting their obligations.

3461 Florida Adult Services
1317 Winewood Boulevard
Building 1, Room 202
Tallahassee, FL 32399-700   850-488-2881
                                            800-962-2873
                                            800-273-8255
                                        Fax: 850-922-4193
                                            www.myflfamilies.com
Robert Anderson, State Director
Jan Chaney, Administrative Assistant
Roy Car, Data/Systems
Lindsay Conrad, HCDA and CCDA
The Florida Department of Children and Families has adopted an integrated approach to programs and services as we work to help improve the lives of individuals and families.

3462 Florida Department of Handicapped Children
4030 Esplanade Way
Suite 380
Tallahassee, FL 32399-7016   850-488-4257
                                            866-273-2273
                                        Fax: 850-245-1075
                                apd_info@apd.state.fl.us
                                            www.apd.myflorida.com
Mike Gresham, Executive Director
John Bryant, Manager
The APD works in partnership with local communities and private providers to assist people who have developmental disabilities and their families.

3463 Florida Department of Mental Health and Rehabilitative Services
1317 Winewood Blvd
Building 1
Tallahassee, FL 32399-700   850-487-1111
                                        Fax: 850-922-2993
                                            www.dcf.state.fl.us
David Wilkins, Secretary
Ramin Kouzehkanani, Deputy Secretary

3464 Florida Developmental Disabilities Council
124 Marriott Drive
Suite 203
Tallahassee, FL 32301-2981   850-488-4180
                                            800-580-7801
                                        Fax: 850-922-6702
                                        TTY: 888-488-863
                                            fddc@fddc.org
                                            fddc.org
Sylvia James Miller, Council Chair & Parent Advocate
Tricia Riccardi, Council Vice-Chair
Debra Dowds, Executive Director
Vanda Bowman, Staff Assistant
To advocate and promote meaningful participation in all aspects of life for Floridians with developmental disabilities.

3465 Florida Division of Vocational Rehabilitation
4070 Esplanade Way
Building 1
Tallahassee, FL 32399- 7016   850-245-3399
                                            800-451-4327
                                        Fax: 850-245-3316
                                        TTY: 850-488-2867
                                            rehabworks.org
Bill Palmer, Manager
Linda Parnell, Manager
Aleisa Mckinlay, Director
Don Chester, Counsil Member
State agency serving individuals with physical or mental disabilities that interfere with them keeping or maintaining employment.

3466 Florida's Protection and Advocacy Programs for Persons with Disabilities
2473 Care Drive
Suite 200
Tallahassee, FL 32308   850-488-9071
                                            800-342-0823
                                        Fax: 850-488-8640
                                        TTY: 800-346-4127
                                            www.disabilityrightsflorida.org
Catherine Piecora, Chair
Maryellen McDonald, Executive Director
Carol Stachurski, Program Operations Manager
Paige Morgan, Executive Assistant
The Center is a non-profit organization providing protection and advocacy services in the State of Florida. The Center's mission is to advance the dignity, equality, self-determination and expressed choices of individuals with disabilities.

3467 International Dyslexia Association: Florida Branch
40 York Rd., 4th Floor
Baltimore, MD   21204-3896
　　　　　　　　　　　　　　　410-296-0232
　　　　　　　　　　　　　　　800-222-3123
　　　　　　　　　　　　　　　Fax: 410-321-5069
　　　　　　　　　　　　　　　ear228@aol.com
　　　　　　　　　　　　　　　www.interdys.org
Kristen Penczek, Executive Director
David Holste, Director Of Operations
Stacy Friedman, Manager of Operation
Cyndi Powers, Office Manager
Provides free information and referral services for diagnosis and
tutoring for parents, educators, physicians, and individuals with
dyslexia.   Membership includes yearly journal and quarterly
newsletter, and Pennsylvania newsletter; discounts to
conferences and events.

3468 Social Security Administration
2002 Old Saint Augustine Rd
Suite B12
Tallahassee, FL 32301-4861
　　　　　　　　　　　　　　　850-942-8978
　　　　　　　　　　　　　　　800-772-1213
　　　　　　　　　　　　　　　Fax: 850-942-8980
　　　　　　　　　　　　　　　ssa.gov
Carrie Tucker, Operations Supervisor
Sheila Lee, Management Support Specialist
Administers the Title II and Title XVII disability programs. To be
insured for Title II benefits, applicants must have worked in covered employment for at least five of the last ten years prior to becoming disabled. To be eligible for Title XVII disability benefits,
applicants must meet an income and resource test.

3469 Social Security: Miami Disability Determination
Social Security
11401 W Flagler St
Miami, FL   33174-1023
　　　　　　　　　　　　　　　305-226-0449
　　　　　　　　　　　　　　　800-772-1213
　　　　　　　　　　　　　　　TTY:800-325-0778
　　　　　　　　　　　　　　　www.ssa.gov
Robert L Meekins, Deputy General for Executive Ope

3470 Social Security: Orlando Disability Determination
Social Security
P.O. Box 144040
Orlando, FL   32814-2231
　　　　　　　　　　　　　　　407-648-6673
　　　　　　　　　　　　　　　800-342-2065
　　　　　　　　　　　　　　　TTY:407-245-7057
　　　　　　　　　　　　　　　www.ssa.gov
John C Massolio Jr, Founder
Neil Bush, President

3471 Social Security: Tampa Disability Determination
Social Security Administration
PO Box 340572
Tampa, FL   33694-572
　　　　　　　　　　　　　　　813-878-2906
　　　　　　　　　　　　　　　800-772-1213
　　　　　　　　　　　　　　　www.dbsatampabay.org
John Balcomb, President
Carol Yaros, 1st Vice President
Cheryl McGhan , 2nd Vice President
Neil Bush, Treasurer
The Depression and Bipolar Support Alliance Tampa Bay , is a
nonprofit and all volunteer organization for individuals, family
and friends of those who have been diagnosed with bipolar disor-
der, depression and other affective disorders.

Georgia

3472 ADA Technical Assistance Program
Southeast Disability & Business Technical Assist.
1419 Mayson Street NE
Atlanta, GA   30324
　　　　　　　　　　　　　　　404-541-9001
　　　　　　　　　　　　　　　800-949-4232
　　　　　　　　　　　　　　　Fax: 404-541-9002
　　　　　　　　　　　　　　　ADAsoutheast@law.syr.edu
　　　　　　　　　　　　　　　www.sedbtac.org
Pamela Williamson, Project Director
Cheri Hofmann, Information Specialist
Cyndi Smith, Office Assistant
Marsha Schwanke, Web Manager
One of ten regional centers funded by NIDRR, to provide infor-
mation and technical assistance to assist in voluntary compliance
with the Americans with Disabilities Act, and accessible educa-
tion-based information technology.

3473 Division of Birth Defects and Developmental Disabilities
1600 Clifton Road
Atlanta, GA   30333-4027
　　　　　　　　　　　　　　　404-498-3800
　　　　　　　　　　　　　　　800-232-4636
　　　　　　　　　　　　　　　TTY:888-232-6348
　　　　　　　　　　　　　　　cdcinfo@cdc.gov
　　　　　　　　　　　　　　　www.cdc.gov
Coleen A Boyle, Director
The mission of CDC's National Center on Birth Defects and Developmental Disabilities (NCBDDD) is to promote the health of
babies, children and adults and to enhance the potential for full,
productive living.

3474 Georgia Advocacy Office
150 East Ponce De Leon Avenue
Suite 430
Decatur, GA 30030-2547
　　　　　　　　　　　　　　　404-885-1234
　　　　　　　　　　　　　　　800-537-2329
　　　　　　　　　　　　　　　Fax: 404-378-0031
　　　　　　　　　　　　　　　info@thegao.org
　　　　　　　　　　　　　　　thegao.org
Ruby Moore, Executive Director
Crystal Rasa, Program Manager
Mona Givens, Director of Investigation
Olwyn Mayer, Chief Operating Officer
Protection and advocacy services for Georgians with disabilities.

3475 Georgia Client Assistance Program
Division of Rehabilitation Services
2 Peachtree Street NW
Suite 29-250
Atlanta, GA   30303- 3141
　　　　　　　　　　　　　　　404-656-4507
　　　　　　　　　　　　　　　800-822-9727
　　　　　　　　　　　　　　　Fax: 404-651-6880
　　　　　　　　　　　　　　　connect.georgia.gov
　　　　　　　　　　　　　　　dhs.georgia.gov/
Mark Trail, Manager
Robertiena Fletcher, Chair
Franklin G Auman, Vice Chair
Monica Walters, Secretary
Helps eligible persons with complaints, appeals and understanding available benefits under the 1992 Rehabilitation Act Amendments and Title I of the Americans with Disabilities Act. CAP
investigates complaints, mediates conflict, represents complain-
ants in appeals, provides legal services if warranted, advocates
for due process, identifies and recommends solutions to system
problems, advises of benefits available under the 1992 Rehab Act
Amendments and Americans with Disabilities Act.

3476 **Georgia Council On Developmental Disabilities**
2 Peachtree St N.W.
26th Floor, Suite 246
Atlanta, GA 30303-3141   404-657-2126
                                             888-275-4233
                                        Fax: 404-657-2132
                                        TTY:404-657-2133
                                    eric.jacobson@gcdd.ga.gov
                                             www.gcdd.org

Eric E. Jacobson, Executive Director
Caitlin Childs, Organizing Director
Dottie Adams, Family/Individual Support Dir.
Valerie Meadows Suber, Public Information Director
The Georgia Council on Developmental Disabilities collaborates with Georgia's citizens, public and private advocacy organizations and policymakers to positively influence public policies that enhance the quality of life for people with disabilities and their families. GCDD provides this through education and advocacy activities, program implementation, funding and public policy analysis and research.
Quartlery

3477 **Georgia Department of Aging**
2 Peachtree Street NW
33rd Floor
Atlanta, GA 30303-3142   404-657-5258
                                             866-552-4464
                                        Fax: 404-657-5285
                                         dhs.georgia.gov/

Stephen Dolinger, President
Andrea Fuller-Ruffin, Administrator
The Division of Aging Services (DAS) works to continuously improve the effectiveness and efficiency of services.

3478 **Georgia Department of Handicapped Children**
2600 Skyland Dr NE
Atlanta, GA 30319-3640   404-679-1625
                                        Fax: 404-679-1630

Ron Jackson, Manager
Frank Koues, Auditor

3479 **Georgia Division of Mental Health, Developmental Disabilities & Addictive Diseases**
Two Peachtree Drive NW
24th Floor
Atlanta, GA 30303-3142   404-657-2252
                                             800-715-4225
                                        Fax: 404-657-2310
                                     mhddad.dhr.georgia.gov

Kimberly Ryan, Board Member
David Glass, Board member
Ellice P. Martin, Board Member
Kimberly Carroll-Hawkins, Board Member
MHDDAD provides treatment and support services to people with mental illnesses and addictive diseases, and support to people with mental retardation and related developmental disabilities. MHDDAD serves people of all ages with the most severe and likely to be long-term conditions.

3480 **Georgia State Board of Workers' Compensation**
270 Peachtree St NW
Atlanta, GA 30303-1299   404-656-3875
                                             800-533-0682
                                        Fax: 404-657-1767
                                         sbwc.georgia.gov

Frank McKay, Chairman
Elizabeth Gobeil, Director
Delece A. Brooks, Executive Director
Martine Schweitzer, Administrative Assistant
To provide superior access to the Georgia Workers' Compensation program for injured workers and employers in a manner that is sensitive, responsive, and effective and to insure efficient processing and swift, fair resolution of claims, while encouraging workplace safety and return to work.

3481 **International Dyslexia Association: Georgia Branch**
1951 Greystone Rd.
Atlanta, GA 30318   404-256-1232
                                            info@idaga.org
                                            www.idaga.org

Jennifer Kopp, President
jennings Miller, Vice-President
Robert Moore, Treasurer
Susie McDaniel, Corresponding Secretary
Provides free information and referral services for diagnosis and tutoring for parents, educators, physicians, and individuals with dyslexia. Membership includes yearly journal and quarterly newsletter, and Pennsylvania newsletter; discounts to conferences and events.

3482 **Social Security: Atlanta Disability Determination**
401 W Peachtree St NW
Suite 2860 Flr 28
Atlanta, GA 30308-3538   800-772-1213
                                        TTY:800-325-0778
                                        www.socialsecurity.gov

3483 **Social Security: Decatur Disability Determination**
2853 Candler Rd
Suite 8
Decatur, GA 30034-1421   800-772-1213
                                        TTY:800-325-0778
                                                  ssa.gov

Hawaii

3484 **Assistive Technology Resource Centers of Hawaii**
200 North Vineyard Boulevard
Suite 430
Honolulu, HI 96817-5362   808-532-7110
                                             800-645-3007
                                        Fax: 808-532-7120
                                        TTY: 808-532-7113
                                        atrc-info@atrc.org
                                             www.atrc.org

Barbara Fischlowitz-Leong, Executive Director
Jodi Asato, Deputy Director
Edna Kaahaaina, Office Manager
Joseph Go, Assistive Technology Trainer
Provides information and referral to anyone interested in assistive technology devices and services. Operates equipment loan. Bank Provides training to consumer and professional groups including self-advocacy skills for consumers and family members. Works to ensure that schools, vocational rehabilitation agencies and health insurers provide assessments, funding and training in the use of assistive technology devices and services for their clients. Low-interest loan programs available.

3485 **Diabetes Network of East Hawaii**
1221 Kilauea Ave
Suite 70
Hilo, HI 96720-4264   808-935-1673
                                        Fax: 808-935-6760

Steve Fukunada, Manager

3486 **Disability and Communication Access Board**
1010 Richards St
Suite 118
Honolulu, HI 96813   808-586-8121
                                        Fax: 808-586-8129
                                        dcab@doh.hawaii.gov
                                        hawaii.gov/health/dcab

Francine Wai, Executive Director
Bill-Wayne Nakamatsu, Parking Program Specialist
Provides ADA coordination for state & county government; reviews state & county construction documents to appropriate federal & state accessibility guidelines; credentials American sign language interpreters; coordinates parking for persons with disabilities; coordinates information & referral for consumers, parents and others seeking disability related information.

3487 **Hawaii Assistive Technology Training and**
200 North Vineyard Boulevard
Suite 430
Honolulu, HI 96817-5362   808-532-7110
                                        800-645-3007
                                   Fax: 808-532-7120
                                        atrc-info@atrc.org
                                        www.atrc.org

Barbara Fischlowitz-Leong, Executive Director

3488 **Hawaii Department for Children With Special Needs**
Department of Health
741 Sunset Avenue
Honolulu, HI 96816-2343   808-733-9070
                                   Fax: 808-733-9068
                                        patricia.heu@doh.hawaii.gov
                                        health.hawaii.gov

Patricia Heu, Manager
Karen Mak, Manager
Children with Special Health Needs Branch(CSHNB) is working
to assure that all children and youth with special health care needs
(CSHCN) will reach optimal health, growth, and development,
by improving access to a coordinated system of family-centered
health care services and improving outcomes, through systems
development, assessment, assurance, education, collaborative
partnerships, and family support,

3489 **Hawaii Department of Health, Adult Mental Health Division**
P.O.Box 3378
Honolulu, HI 96801-3378   808-586-4686
                                   Fax: 808-586-4745

3490 **Hawaii Department of Human Services**
Hawaii Department of Human Serv
P.O. Box 339
Honolulu, HI 96813   808-586-4892
                                   Fax: 808-586-4890
                                        dhs@dhs.hawaii.gov
                                        humanservices.hawaii.gov

Rachael Wong, Director
Pankaj Bhanot, Deputy Director
Lisa Nakao, Admin Assis. & Legislative Coor.
Scott Nakasone, Acting Administrator
To provide timely, efficient and effective programs, services and
benefits for the purpose of achieving the outcome of empowering
Hawaii's most vulnerable people; and to expand their capacity for
self-sufficiency, self-determination, independence, healthy
choices, quality of life, and personal dignity.

3491 **Hawaii Disability Compensation Division Department of Labor and Industrial Relations**
830 Punchbowl Street
Room 209
Honolulu, HI 96813-5095   808-586-9200
                                   Fax: 808-586-9219
                                        dlir.director@hawaii.gov
                                        hawaii.gov/labor

Walter Kawamura, Administrator
Clyde Imada, Workers Comp Chief
The Disability Compensation Division (DCD) administers the
Workers' Compensation (WC) law, the Temporary Disability Insurance (TDI) law, and the Prepaid Health Care (PHC) law. All
employers with one or more employees, whether working
full-time or part-time, are directly affected.

3492 **Hawaii Disability Rights Center**
1132 Bishop Street
Suite 2102
Honolulu, HI 96813-3701   808-949-2922
                                        800-882-1057
                                   Fax: 808-949-2928
                                        info@hawaiidisabilityrights.org
                                        hawaiidisabilityrights.org

John Dellera, Executive Director
Ann Collins, Director Of Operations
IT IS THE POLICY OF HDRCto advocate for as many people
with disabilities in the State of Hawaii, on as wide a range of disability rights issues, as our resources allow; and to resolve rights
violations with the lowest feasible level of intervention; but, if
necessary, to also provide full legal representation to protect the
rights of people with disabilities, consistent with authorizing
statutes and Center priorities.

3493 **Hawaii Executive Office on Aging**
250 South Hotel Street
Suite 406
Honolulu, HI 96813-2831   808-586-0100
                                        800-468-4644
                                   Fax: 808-586-0185
                                        hawaii.gov/health/eoa

Noemi Pendleton, Manager
Virginia Pressler, Director
Keith Y. Yamamoto, Deputy Director
Danette Wong Tomiyasu, Deputy Director
State unit on aging responsible for policy formulation, program
development, planning, information dissemination, advocacy
and other activities, for persons age 60 and over.

3494 **Hawaii State Council on Developmental Disabilities**
919 Ala Moana Blvd
Suite113
Honolulu, HI 96814-4920   808-586-8100
                                   Fax: 808-586-7543
                                        council@hiddc.org
                                        www.hiddc.org

Waynette K Y Cabral, Executive Administrator
Joe Shacter, Planner
Debbie Miyasaka Gushiken, Community & Legislative Liaison
Susan Kawano, Secretary
The mission of the council is to support people with developmental disabilities to control their own destiny and determine the
quality of life they desire. The Council: engages in analysis and
policy development; provides training in legislative advocacy
and leadership development for individuals with disabilities and
their families; demonstrates new approaches to services and supports; informs policymakers about developmental disability
issues; and fosters interagency collaboration.

3495 **International Dyslexia Association: Hawaii Branch**
913 Alewa Dr.
Honolulu, HI 96817-1610   808-538-7007
                                        hida@dyslexia-hawaii.org
                                        dyslexia-hawaii.org

Charles Bering, President
Deborah Knight, Vice President
Laurie Moore, Treasurer
Margaret Higa, Executive Director
Provides free information and referral services for diagnosis and
tutoring for parents, educators, physicians, and individuals with
dyslexia. Membership includes yearly journal and quarterly
newsletter. Call for conference dates.

3496 **Social Security: Honolulu Disability Determination**
Social Security
300 Ala Moana Blvd
Honolulu, HI 96850-1   808-541-3600
                                        800-772-1213
                                        TTY:800-825-0778
                                        hivrsbd@kestrok.com
                                        www.ssa.gov

Neil Shim, Administrator

3497 **State Planning Council on Developmental Disabilities**
919 Ala Moana Blvd
Room 101
Honolulu, HI 96814-4920   808-586-8121
                                   Fax: 808-586-8129
                                        TTY:808-586-8121
                                        dcab@doh.hawaii.gov
                                        hawaii.gov/health/dcab

Michael Okamoto, Chairperson
Peter Fritz, Vice Chairperson
Francine Wai, Executive Director
Debbra Jackson, Planning and ADA Cooordinator
Consists of 25 Hawaii residents appointed by the governor. The
council addresses the needs of the people with developmental

disabilities: specifically, develops a state plan that sets the priorities for persons with developmental disabilities.

Idaho

3498 Idaho Commission on Aging
341 W Washington
Boise, ID 83702-1   208-334-3833
                                           800-926-2588
                                     Fax: 208-334-3033
                                   ICOA@aging.idaho.gov
                                       www.idahoaging.com

Sam Haws, Administrator
Cathy Hart, State Ombudsman
Jeff Weller, Deputy Administrator
Raul Enriquez, Program Specialist
There number one priority is to provide the best possible service through this single point of entry website where people of all incomes and ages can obtain information on a full range of long-term care support programs and services.

3499 Idaho Council on Developmental Disabilities
Health and Wellfare
700 W. State Street
Suite 119
Boise, ID 83702-5868   208-334-2178
                                           800-544-2433
                                     Fax: 208-334-3417
                                      info@icdd.idaho.gov
                                          icdd.idaho.gov

Jim Baugh, Council Member
Christine Pisani, Executive Director
Tracy Warren, Program Specialist/Planner
Deborah Daniels, Management Assistant
The mission of the Idaho Council on Developmental Disabilities is to promote the capacity of people with developmental disabilities and their families to determine, access, and direct the services and/or support they need to live the lives they choose, and to build the communities ability to support their choices.

3500 Idaho Department of Handicapped Children
Statehouse
Boise, ID 83720-1   208-334-8000
Thomas Bruck, Chief
Sandy Frazier, Manager

3501 Idaho Disability Determinations Service
PO Box 21
Boise, ID 83707-0021   208-327-7333
                                           800-626-2681
                                     Fax: 208-327-7331
                                    TTY: 800-377-3529
                                          labor.idaho.gov

Roger B Madsen, Director
Rogelio Valdez, Executive Director
Under contract with the Social Security Administration, makes determinations of medical eligibility for disability benefits.

3502 Idaho Industrial Commission
P.O. Box 83720
Boise, ID 83720-0041   208-334-6000
                                           800-950-2110
                                     Fax: 208-334-2321
                                  mholbrook@iic.idaho.gov
                                       www.iic.idaho.gov

Mindy Montgomery, Manager
Beth Kilian, Commission Secretary
Free rehabilitation services to workers' who have suffered on the job injuries in Idaho. Field offices throughout the state.

3503 Idaho Mental Health Center
1720 Westgate Dr
Boise, ID 83704-7164   208-334-0808
                                           800-926-2588
                                     Fax: 208-334-0828

Richard Armstrong, Director
Darrell Kerby, Chairperson
Tom Stroschein, Vice Chair
Stephen Weeg, Board Member
The State of Idaho provides state funded and operated community based mental health care services through Regional Behavioral Health Centers (RBHC) located in each of the seven geographical regions of the state. Each RBHC provides mental health services through a system of care that is both community-based and consumer-guided.

Illinois

**3504 Attorney General's Office: Disability Rights Bureau &
Health Care Bureau**
100 W Randolph Street
Chicago, IL 60601-3218   312-814-3000
                                           877-305-5145
                                     Fax: 312-793-0802
                                    TTY: 800-964-3013
                                  illinoisattorneygeneral.gov

Lisa Madigan, Manager
Raymond Throlkeld, Chief Health Care Bureau
Information on Illinois' Comprehensive Health Insurance Plan and architectural accessibility. Enforcement of Illinois' access law and standards and other disability rights laws. Information on initiatives such as: Opening the Courthouse Doors to People with Disabilities; the abuse, neglect or financial exploitation of people with disabilities and voter accessibility. Other information and referrals.

3505 Client Assistance Program (CAP)
Illinois State Board of Education
100 South Grand Ave. E.
Springfield, IL 62794   217-524-0695
                                           800-641-3929
                                           888-460-5111
                                     Fax: 217-524-1184
                                   dhs.cap@illinois.gov
                                      www.dhs.state.il.us

James T. Dimas, Secretary
Francisco Alvarado, Manager
Quinetta L. Wade, Rehabilitation Services
The Client Assistance Program (CAP) helps people with disabilities receive quality Vocational Rehabilitation services by advocating for their interests and helping them identify resources, understand procedures, resolve problems, and protect their rights in the rehabilitation process, and employment.

3506 Equip for Equality
20 North Michigan Avenue
Suite 300
Chicago, IL 60602- 4861   312-341-0022
                                           800-537-2632
                                     Fax: 312-541-7544
                                    TTY: 800-610-2779
                              contactus@equipforequality.org
                                      equipforequality.org

Zena Naiditch, President/CEO
Barry C Taylor, Vice President
Lia Burkey, Administrative Assistant
Thomas Fischer, Special Assistant to President
Equip for equality is an independent, private, not-for-profit organization designated by the Governor in 1985 to implement the federally mandated Protection and Advocacy (P&A) System in Illinois. The mission of Equip for Equality is to advance the human and civil rights of children and adults with disabilities in Illinois.

3507 Equip for Equality - Carbondale Office
300 East Main St
Suite 18
Carbondale, IL 62901

618-457-7930
800-758-0559
Fax: 618-457-7985
TTY: 800-610-2779
contactus@equipforequality.org
equipforequality.org

Zena Naiditch, President/CEO
Barry C Taylor, Vice President
Lia Burkey, Administrative Assistant
Thomas Fischer, Special Assistant to President
Equip for equality is an independent, private, not-for-profit organization designated by the Governor in 1985 to implement the federally mandated Protection and Advocacy (P&A) System in Illinois. The mission of Equip for Equality is to advance the human and civil rights of children and adults with disabilities in Illinois.

3508 Equip for Equality - Moline Office
1515 Fifth Ave
Suite 420
Moline, IL 61265

309-786-6868
800-758-6869
Fax: 309-797-8710
TTY: 800-610-2779
contactus@equipforequality.org
equipforequality.org

Zena Naiditch, President/CEO
Barry C Taylor, Vice President
Lia Burkey, Administrative Assistant
Thomas Fischer, Special Assistant to President
Equip for equality is an independent, private, not-for-profit organization designated by the Governor in 1985 to implement the federally mandated Protection and Advocacy (P&A) System in Illinois. The mission of Equip for Equality is to advance the human and civil rights of children and adults with disabilities in Illinois.

3509 Equip for Equality - Springfield Office
1 West Old State Capitol Plaza
Suite 816
Springfield, IL 62701

217-544-0464
800-758-0464
Fax: 217-523-0720
TTY: 800-610-2779
contactus@equipforequality.org
equipforequality.org

Zena Naiditch, President/CEO
Barry C Taylor, Vice President
Lia Burkey, Administrative Assistant
Thomas Fischer, Special Assistant to President
Equip for equality is an independent, private, not-for-profit organization designated by the Governor in 1985 to implement the federally mandated Protection and Advocacy (P&A) System in Illinois. The mission of Equip for Equality is to advance the human and civil rights of children and adults with disabilities in Illinois.

3510 Illinois Assistive Technology Project
1 West Old State Capitol Plaza
Suite 100
Springfield, IL 62701-1200

217-522-7985
800-852-5110
Fax: 217-522-8067
TTY: 217-522-9966
iatp@iltech.org
iltech.org

Wilhelmina Gunther, Executive Director
Shelly Lowe, Finance/Personnel Manager
Yvonne Miller, Administrative Assistant
Barbara Howell, Administration
Directed by and for people with disabilities and their family members. As a federally mandated program, IATP strives to break down barriers and change policies that make getting and using technology difficult. IATP offers solutions to help people find what is available in products and services that will best meet their needs, where to find it, and how to get it.

3511 Illinois Council on Developmental Disability
State of Illinois Center
100 W Randolph St
16-100
Chicago, IL 60601-3218

312-814-2121
800-843-6154
Fax: 312-814-7441
www2.illinois.gov

Sheila T. Romano, Executive Director
Dennis Sienko, Manager
The Illinois Council on Developmental Disabilities (ICDD) is dedicated to leading change in Illinois so that all people with developmental disabilities are able to exercise their rights to freedom and equal opportunity.

3512 Illinois Department of Mental Health and Developmental Disabilities
Suite 3b
314 E Madison
Springfield, IL 62701

217-782-6680
Fax: 217-524-3834

Karen Perrin, Manager
Lori Stone, Director

3513 Illinois Department of Rehabilitation
100 South Grand Avenue East
Springfield, IL 62762-1304

217-782-6680
800-843-6154
Fax: 217-524-3834
TTY: 800-447-6404
DHS.WEBBITS@ILLINOIS.GOV
www.dhs.state.il.us/page.aspx?item=29736

Robert Kilbury, Director
Timothy Martin, Manager
DHS's Division of Rehabilitation Services is the state's lead agency serving individuals with disabilities. DRS works in partnership with people with disabilities and their families to assist them in making informed choices to achieve full community participation through employment, education, and independent living opportunities.

3514 Illinois Department on Aging
One Natural Resources Way
Suite 100
Springfield, IL 62702-1271

217-785-2870
800-252-8966
Fax: 217-785-4477
TTY: 888-206-1327
www2.illinois.gov

John K. Holton, Director
Jennifer Reif, Deputy Director
Matthew Ryan, Chief of Staff
Bradley A. Rightnowar, General Counsil
The MISSION of the Illinois Department on Aging is to serve and advocate for older Illinoisans and their caregivers by administering quality and culturally appropriate programs that promote partnerships and encourage independence, dignity, and quality of life.

3515 International Dyslexia Association: Illinois Branch
751 Roosevelt Rd.
Suite 116
Glen Ellyn, IL 60137

630-469-6900
Fax: 630-469-6810
info@readibida.org
www.readibida.org

Jo Ann Paldo, President
Foley Burckardt, Vice President
Joan Budovec, Treasurer
Sherry Grobe, Secretary
Provides free information and referral services for diagnosis and tutoring for parents, educators, physicians, and individuals with dyslexia in Illinois. Membership includes yearly journal and quarterly newsletter.

3516 **Social Security: Springfield Disability Determination**
3112 CONSTITUTION DR
Springfield, IL 62704-1323   877-279-9504
                                           800-772-1213
                                        TTY:800-325-0778
                                                 ssa.gov

3517 **Workers Compensation Board Illinois**
100 W Randolph St
Ste 8-200
Chicago, IL 60601-3227   312-814-6611
                                           866-352-3033
                                       Fax: 312-814-6523
                            infoquestions.wcc@illinois.gov
                                          www2.illinois.gov

Joann Fratianni, Chairman
The Illinois Workers' Compensation Commission resolves disputes between employees and employers regarding work-related injuries and illnesses.

Indiana

3518 **Indiana Client Assistance Program**
4701 N. Keystone Avenue
Suite 222
Indianapolis, IN 46204-1191   317-722-5555
                                           800-622-4845
                                       Fax: 317-722-5564
                                       TTY: 317-722-5555
                         www.icdri.org/legal/IndianaCAP.htm

Michael Burks, Chairman
Wen Lu, Secretary and Treasurer

3519 **Indiana Developmental Disability Council**
402 West Washington Street
Room E145
Indianapolis, IN 46204-2801   317-232-7770
                                       Fax: 317-233-3712
                                        GPCPD@gpcpd.org
                                              www.in.gov

Katrina Gossett, Chair
Dawn Adams JD, Agency representative
Suellen Jackson-Boner, Executive Director
Christine Dahlberg, Deputy Director
The Indiana Governor's Council is an independent state agency that facilitates change. Our mission is to promote public policy which leads to the independence, productivity and inclusion of people with disabilities in all aspects of society

3520 **Indiana Protection & Advocacy Services Commission**
4701 N. Keystone Avenue
Suite 222
Indianapolis, IN 46205-1561   317-722-5555
                                           800-622-4845
                                       Fax: 317-722-5564
                            ExecutiveDirector@ipas.in.gov
                                          www.in.gov/ipas

Dawn Adams, Executive Director
Milo Gray, Client & Legal Services Director
Gary Richter, Support Services Director
Karen Pedevilla, Education/Training Director
An independent state agency established to protect and promote the rights of individuals with disabilities through empowerment and advocacy.

3521 **Indiana State Commission for the Handicapped**
P.O.Box 1964
Indianapolis, IN 46206   317-233-1292

3522 **International Dyslexia Association: Indiana Branch**
Fisher, IN 46038   317-926-1450
                                          www.ida-indiana.org

Kim Haughee, President
Sara Silvey, Vice President
Ginger Lentz, Secretary
Woody Sears, Treasurer

The Indiana Branch was formed to help the members of the learning disabilities community in Indiana. Promotes understanding and facilitate treatment of the Specific Language Disability (Dyslexia) in children and adults, promotes teacher training and educational intervention strategies for dyslexic students and to foster effective teaching, supports research in the field and early identification of dyslexia, serves as a clearinghouse for information and to actively disseminate knowledge.

Iowa

3523 **Governor's Developmental Disability Council**
617 East Second Street
Des Moines, IA 50309-1831   515-281-9082
                                           800-452-1936
                                       Fax: 515-281-9087
                             fmorris@dhs.state.ia.us
                                      http://idaction.com/

Becky Harker, Executive Director
Rik Shannon, Public Policy Manager
Janet Shoeman, Program Planner/Contract Manager
Fran Morris, Council Secretary
The Council identifies, develops and promotes public policy and support practices through capacity building, advocacy, and systems change activities. The purpose is to ensure that people with developmental disabilities and their families are included in planning, decision making, and development of policy related to services and supports that affect their quality of life and full participation in communities of their choice.

3524 **International Dyslexia Association: Iowa Branch**
P.O. Box 11188
Cedar Rapids, IA 52410-1188   765-507-9432
                                         info@iowaida.org
                                       ia.dyslexiaida.org

Denise Little, President
Tricia Krsek, Vice President
Genevieve Monthie, Secretary
Wayne Wunschel, Treasurer
The purpose of the Iowa Branch of IDA is to increase awareness of dyslexia and promote services that address the importance of diagnosis and remediation for those not meeting their reading potential. Providese services and assistance in a way that promotes unity, support, and cooperation among those who work with these individuals so that all communities in Iowa benefit from the skills and talents of its citizens.

3525 **Iowa Child Health Specialty Clinics**
100 Hawkins Drive
Room 247 CDD
Iowa City, IA 52242-1016   319-356-1117
                                           866-219-9119
                                       Fax: 319-356-3715
                              kathy-colbert@uiowa.edu
                                           www.chsciowa.org

Jeffrey Lobas, Director
Brian Wilkes, Director Of Operations
Child Health Specialty Clinics has a mission to improve the health, development, and well-being of Iowa's children and youth with special health care needs in partnership with families, service providers, and communities.

3526 **Iowa Commission of Persons with Disabilities**
Department of Human Rights
Lucas State Office Bldg, 2nd Floor
Des Moines, IA 50319- 2006   515-242-6171
                                           888-219-0471
                                       Fax: 515-242-6119
                                       TTY: 888-219-0471
                                          www.state.ia.us/dhr/pd

Jill Fulitano-Avery, Administrator
To equalize opportunities for full participation in employment and other areas of the state's economic, educational, social and political life for Iowans with disabilities.

3527 Iowa Compass
Center for Disabilities & Development
100 Hawkins Dr
Suite S295
Iowa City, IA 52242-1011   800-779-2001
                                        TTY:877-686-0032
                                    iowa-compass@uiowa.edu
                                       www.iowacompass.org
Michael Lightbody, Project Director
Carolyn Petitgout, CRS, Admin Services Coordinator & Database Editor
Iowa Compass offers free information and program referrals to thousands of unique local, state and national organizations serving people with complex health related conditions and disabilities.
BiMonthly

3528 Iowa Department for the Blind
State Of Iowa
524 4th Street
Des Moines, IA 50309-2364   515-281-1333
                                             800-362-2587
                                         Fax: 515-281-1263
                                        TTY: 515-281-1355
                                  information@blind.state.ia.us
                                          www.IDBonline.org
Richard Sorey, Director
Jodi Aldini, Library Support Staff
Julie Aufdenkamp, Transition Specialist, Transitio
Jessica Badding, Vocational Rehabilitation Counse
Mission is to be the means for persons who are blind to obtain univeral access and full participation as citizens in whatever roles they may choose.

3529 Iowa Department of Human Services
1305 E Walnut St
Des Moines, IA 50319-114   515-242-6510
                                             800-972-2017
                                         Fax: 515-281-4597
                                    mfinkel@dhs.state.ia.us
                                        www.dhs.state.ia.us
Terry E Branstad, Governor
Charles M Palmer, Director
Sally Titus, Deputy Director
Richard Shults, Division Administrator
Help individuals and families to achieve stable and healthy lives.

3530 Iowa Department on Aging
510 E 12th Street
Suite 2
Des Moines, IA 50319-9025   515-725-3333
                                             800-532-3213
                                         Fax: 866-236-1430
                                        www.aging.iowa.gov
Donna K. Harvey, Director
Danika Welch, Executive Secretary
Joel Wulf, Administrator
Jeanne Yordi, State Long Term Care Ombudsman

3531 Iowa Protection & Advocacy for the Disabled
400 East Court Avenue
Suite 300
Des Moines, IA 50309   515-278-2502
                                             800-779-2502
                                         Fax: 515-278-0539
                                           info@DRIowa.org
                                       disabilityrightsiowa.org
Christine Glosser, President
Todd Lantz, Vice President
Jane Hudson, Executive Director
Cyndy Miller, Senior Staff Attorney
Disability Rights IOWA aims to defend and promote the human and legal rights of Iowans who have disabilities and mental illness.

3532 Social Security: Des Moines Disability Determination
Social Security Administration
Riverpoint Office Complex
455 SW 5TH ST STE F
Des Moines, IA 50309-2115   515-284-4260
                                             800-772-1213
                                         Fax: 515-284-4394
                                        TTY: 800-325-0778
                                                  ssa.gov
Leroy Brown, Manager

3533 Workers Compensation Board Iowa
1000 East Grand Avenue
Des Moines, IA 50319-0209   515-281-5387
                                         Fax: 515-281-6501
                                     IWD.DWC@iwd.iowa.gov
                                      www.iowaworkforce.org
Joseph S Cortese II, Commissioner
Janna E. Martin, Commissioner
Sandy Breckenridge, Administrative Secretary
Jolene Doll, Support Staff
The Workers' Compensation Act is a part of the Iowa Code designed to provide certain benefits to employees who receive injury (85), occupational disease (85A) or occupational hearing loss (85B) arising out of and during the course of their employment.

Kansas

3534 Beach Center on Families and Disability
University of Kansas
1200 Sunnyside Ave
Room 3136
Lawrence, KS 66045-7600   785-864-7600
                                             866-783-3378
                                         Fax: 785-864-7605
                                        beachcenter@ku.edu
                                         www.beachcenter.org
Michael Wehmeyer, Co-Director
Ann Turnbull, Co-Founder
Shonda Anderson, Project Coordinator
Peter Griggs, Evaluation Coordinator
A federally funded center that conducts research and training in the factors that contribute to the successful functioning of families with members who have disabilities.

3535 International Dyslexia Association: Kansas/Missouri Branch
16628 Bond St.
Overland Park, KS 66221   816-945-2665
                                      ksmoida@gmail.com
                                     ksmo.dyslexiaida.org
Cathy Denesia, President
Holly Aranda, Vice President
Nora Wolf, Treasurer
Richard Bradford, Regional Representative
Provides free information and referral services for diagnosis and tutoring for parents, educators, physicians, and individuals with dyslexia in Illinois. Membership includes yearly journal and quarterly newsletter.

3536 Kansas Advocacy and Protective Services
214 SW 6th Ave.,
Ste 100
Topeka, KS 66603-3726   785-273-9661
                                             877-776-1541
                                         Fax: 785-273-9414
                                        TTY: 877-335-3725
                                        www.drckansas.org/
Rocky Nichols, Executive Director
Debbie White, Deputy Director
Lane Williams, Deputy Director
Catherine Johnson, Disability Rights Attorney
Protection and advocacy for persons with disabilities.

3537 Kansas Client Assistance Program
635 SW Harrison
Suite 100
Topeka, KS 66603 785-273-9661
877-776-1541
Fax: 785-273-9414
TTY: 877-335-3725
rocky@drckansas.org
www.icdri.org/legal/KansasCAP.htm

3538 Kansas Commission on Disability Concerns
900 SW Jackson
Suite 100
Topeka, KS 66612-1246 785-296-1722
800-295-5232
Fax: 785-296-1795
KCDCoffice@ks.gov
kcdcinfo.ks.gov
Martha Gabehart, Executive Director
Kerrie Bacon, Employment Liaison
The Kansas Commission on Disability Concerns provides disability-related supports and information to the people of Kansas. The commission offers legislative advocacy, education and resource networking to ensure full and equal citizenship for all Kansans with disabilities.

3539 Kansas Department on Aging
503 S Kansas Ave
New England Building
Topeka, KS 66603- 3404 785-296-4986
800-432-3535
Fax: 785-296-0256
TTY: 785-291-3167
wwwmail@kdads.ks.gov
www.kdads.ks.gov
Kathy Greenlee, Manager
Barbara Conant, Public Information Officer
Kari Bruffett, Secretary
Services and information for Kansas seniors, over age 60.

3540 Kansas Developmental Disability Council
Disability Rights Center of Kansas
915 SW Harrison
DSOB Rm 141
Topeka, KS 66612-3726 785-296-2608
877-431-4604
Fax: 785-296-2861
TTY: 877-335-3725
sgieber@kcdd.org
www.kcdd.org/
Steve Gieber, Executive Director
Craig Knutson, Public Policy Coordinator
Charline Cobbs, Senior Administrative Assistant
The purpose of the Kansas Council on Developmental Disabilities (KCDD) is to support people of all ages with developmental disabilities so they have the opportunity to make choices regarding both their participation in society, and their quality of life.

Kentucky

3541 Kentucky Council on Developmental Disability
1151 So. Fourth Street
Louisville, KY 40203 502-584-1239
800-372-2973
Fax: 502-584-1261
info@councilondd.org
councilondd.org
Richard Bush, President
Dave Fowler, Treasurer
Missy Kinnaird, Secretary
Donovan Fornwalt, Chief Executive Officer
Implementation of Developmental Disabilities Planning Council responsible under P.L. 101-496.

3542 Kentucky Department for Mental Health and Mental Retardation Services
275 E. Main St.,
1E-B
Frankfort, KY 40621 502-564-4527
Fax: 502-564-5478
chfs.ky.gov
Deborah Anderson, Commissioner
Chris Harbeck, Executive Secretary
Marnie Mountjoy, Staff Assistant
Kristi Gentry, Executive Staff Advisor
The Department for Mental Health and Mental Retardation Services contracts with fourteen regional community mental health and mental broads to provide an array of community based mental health services; operates three psychiatric hospitals and contracts with two additional hospitals; operates or contracts for 10 ICFs/MR; also operates two nursing facilities.

3543 Kentucky Department for Mental Health:
275 E. Main St.,
1E-B
Frankfort, KY 40621 502-564-4527
Fax: 502-564-5478
chfs.ky.gov
Deborah Anderson, Commissioner
Chris Harbeck, Executive Secretary
Marnie Mountjoy, Staff Assistant
Kristi Gentry, Executive Staff Advisor
The Department for Mental Health and Mental Retardation Services contracts with fourteen regional community mental health and mental broads to provide an array of community based mental health services; operates three psychiatric hospitals and contracts with two additional hospitals; operates or contracts for 10 ICFs/MR; also operates two nursing facilities.

3544 Kentucky Office for the Blind
275 E Main St
Frankfort, KY 40621 502-564-4754
800-321-6668
Fax: 502-564-2951
TTY: 502-564-2929
amy.mefford@ky.gov
blind.ky.gov
Cora McNabb, Executive Director
Deanna Doll, Vocational Rehabilitation Counselor
Tonisha Everhart, Vocational Rehabilitation Counselor
Provides career services and assistance to adults with severe visual handicaps who want to become productive in the home or work force. The office also runs a Client Assistance Program established to provide advice, assistance and information available from rehabilitation programs to persons with handicaps.

3545 Kentucky Office of Aging Services
Cabinet for Health Services
275 East Main Street
Suite 1E-B
Frankfort, KY 40621 502-564-6930
Fax: 502-564-4595
TTY:888-642-1137
David.Boswell@ky.gov
www.kcdd.ky.gov
Deborah Anderson, Commissioner
Chris Harbeck, Executive Secretary
Marnie Mountjoy, Staff Assistant
Kristi Gentry, Executive Staff Advisor
The Kentucky Office of Aging Services is the state agency directly responsible for programs and services for people with disabilities. Efforts are made to fully integrate the service response information that considers broad farmiliar implications.

3546 Kentucky Protection & Advocacy
100 Fair Oaks Ln 3rd Fl
Frankfort, KY 40601-1108 502-564-2967
800-372-2988
Fax: 502-564-0848
kypa.net
Marsha Hockensmith, Executive Director

Protection and advocacy, Kentucky's federally-mandated protection and advocacy system, protects & promotes the disability rights of individuals through free legally-based advocacy, technical assistance, and education.

3547 Social Security: Frankfort Disability Determination
Social Security
140 Flynn Avenue
Frankfort, KY   40601   866-964-1724
                                               800-772-1213
                                          Fax: 502-226-4519
                                          TTY: 502-226-4519
                                               www.ssa.gov
Stephen Jones, Director
Burton Sisk, Manager

3548 Social Security: Louisville Disability Determination
Social Security
601 W Broadway
Room 101
Louisville, KY   40202-2227   866-716-9671
                                               800-772-1213
                                           TTY:502-582-5238
                                                   ssa.gov

Louisiana

3549 Advocacy Center
8325 Oak Street
New Orleans, LA   70118   504-237-2337
                                               800-960-7705
                                          Fax: 504-522-5507
                                          TTY: 855-861-3577
                               advocacycenter@advocacyla.org
                                               advocacyla.org
Lois Simpson, Executive Director
Susan Gibbens, Volunteer
Laurie Peller, Attorney
John Felt, Chief Information Officer
The Advocacy Center is Louisiana's protection and advocacy system. AC provides free legal services to people with disabilities in designated priority areas. In addition, AC also provides legal assistance to people residing in nursing homes in Louisiana and people over 60 in Orleans, Plaquemines and St. Tammany parishes. AC ombudsmen advocate for the rights of group home and nursing home residents. Benefits specialists help people who receive public benefits to return to work or go to work.

3550 Louisiana Assistive Technology Access Network
3042 Old Forge Dr.
P O Box 14115
Baton Rouge, LA   70898   225-925-9500
                                               800-270-6185
                                          Fax: 225-925-9560
                                           cporciau@latan.org
                                               www.latan.org/
Jim Parks, President & CEO
Sandee Winchell, Executive Director
An information and training resource on Assistive Technology for the State of Louisiana. LATAN operates three regional centers to provide better access for consumers.

3551 Louisiana Center for Dyslexia and Related Learning Disorders
PO Box 2050
Thibodaux, LA   70310-1   985-448-4214
                                          Fax: 985-448-4423
                                  karen.chauvin@nicholls.edu
                                               www.nicholls.edu
Karen Chauvin, Director
Jason Talbot, Assessment & Research Coor
Ashley D Munson, Senior Program Coordinator
Sue Benoit, Administrative Coordinator 3
Provides free information and referral services for diagnosis and tutoring for parents, educators, physicians and individuals with dyslexia. The voice of our membership is heard in 48 countries.

Membership includes yearly journal and quarterly newsletter. Call for conference dates.

3552 Louisiana Department of Aging
Office of Elderly Affairs
PO Box 629
Baton Rouge, LA   70821-0629   225-342-9500
                                          Fax: 225-342-5568
                                         robin.wagner@la.gov
                                          new.dhh.louisiana.gov/
Tara LeBlanc, Assistant Secretary
Robin Wagner, Deputy Assistant Secretary
Kirsten Clebart, Director
Annie Olivier, Director-Program Operation
Serves as a focal point for Louisiana's senior citizens and administers a broad range of home and community based services through a network of 37 Area Agencies on Aging. Serve as the focal point for the development, implementation, and administration of the public policy for the state of Louisiana, and address the needs of the state's elderly citizens.

3553 Louisiana Department of Health - Mental Health Services
PO Box 629
Baton Rouge, LA   70821-0629   225-342-9500
                                               888-342-6207
                                          Fax: 225-342-5568
                                             ldhinfo@la.gov
                                          new.dhh.louisiana.gov
Rebekah Gee, Ph.D, Secretary
Michelle Alletto, Deputy Secretary
Jimmy Guidry, Ph.D, State Health Officer
Andrew Tuozzolo, Chief of Staff
The Office of Behavioral Health's mental health services provide a variety of treatments for people who have different types of mental illnesses. Also offered are treatment clinics and family support services.

3554 Louisiana Developmental Disability Council
PO Box 3455
626 Main Street, Suite A
Baton Rouge, LA 70821-3455   225-342-6804
                                               800-450-8108
                                          Fax: 225-342-1970
                                         shawn.fleming@la.gov
                                               www.laddc.org
Sandra Sam Beech, Chairperson
Brenda Cosse, Vice Chairperson
Sandee Winchell, Executive Director
Shawn Fleming, Deputy Director
The Council's mission is to lead and promote advocacy, capacity building, and systemic change toimprove the quality of life for individualswith developmental disabilities and their families.

3555 Louisiana Learning Resources System
2525 Wyandotte St
Baton Rouge, LA   70805-6464   225-355-6197
                                          Fax: 225-357-3508
Bobbie Robertson, Administrator
Provides consultation on educational seOrvices for local schools, offers psychological testing and evaluation, maintains resource rooms in district schools and more for the blind and handicapped throughout the state.

3556 Social Security: Baton Rouge Disability Determination
Department of Social Services
5455 Bankers Ave
Baton Rouge, LA   70808   866-613-3070
                                               800-772-1213
                                          Fax: 225-219-9399
                                          TTY: 225-382-2090
                                   adren.wilson@dss.state.la.us
                                               www.ssa.gov
Shirley Williams, Director
Ann Williamson, Manager

3557 Workers Compensation Board Louisiana
1001 North 23rd Street
Post Office Box 94094
Baton Rouge, LA 70804-9094   225-342-3111
                                           800-259-5154
                                      Fax: 225-342-7960
                                       owd@lwc.la.gov
                                       www.laworks.net

Curt Eysink, Executive Director
Carey Foy, Deputy Executive Director
Renee Ellender Roberie, Chief Financial Officer
Bryan Moore, Director
The Louisiana Workforce Commission's vision is to make Louisiana the best place in the country to get a job or grow a business, and our goal is to be the country's best workforce agency.

Maine

3558 Maine Assistive Technology Projects
University of Maine at Augusta
Georgia Institute of Technology
490 Tenth Street
Atlanta, GA 30332-0156   404-894-4960
                                      Fax: 404-894-9320
                                       catea@coa.gatech.edu
                                       assistivetech.net

3559 Maine Bureau of Elder and Adult Services
11 State House Station
41 Anthony Avenue
Augusta, ME 04333   207-287-9200
                                           800-262-2232
                                      Fax: 207-287-9229
                                       www.maine.gov

Ricker Hamilton, Director
AnnMarie Stevens, Administrative Assistant
Lois Emerson, Office Specialist I
Maureen Hill, Office Associate II
Adult Protective Services (APS), is responsible for providing or arranging for services to protect incapacitated and/or dependent adults in danger.

3560 Maine Department of Health and Human Services
221 State Street
Augusta, ME 04333-0040   207-287-3707
                                      Fax: 207-287-3005
                                       brenda.harvey@maine.gov
                                       www.maine.gov/dhhs

Mary C. Mayhew, Commissioner
Sam Adolphsen, Chief Operating Officer
Ricker Hamilton, Deputy Commissioner of Programs
Alec Porteous, Deputy Commissioner of Finance
Provision of an array of services to people with nental illness, substance abuse issues, children with special needs and people with developmental disabilities.

3561 Maine Developmental Disabilities Council
225 Western Avenue
Suite 4
Augusta, ME 04330   207-287-4213
                                           800-244-3990
                                      Fax: 207-287-8001
                                       nancy.e.cronin@maine.gov
                                       www.maineddc.org

Nancy Cronin, Executive Director
Rachel Dyer, Associate Director
Erin Howes, Office Manager
The MDDC is a partnership of people with disabilities, their families, and agencies which identifies barriers to community inclusion, self-determination, and independence, and acts to effect positive change.

3562 Maine Division for the Blind and Visually Impaired
21 Enterprise Dr
Suite 2
Augusta, ME 04333-0073   207-624-5120
                                           800-760-1573
                                      Fax: 207-624-5133
                                       TTY: 800-633-0770
                                       mdol@maine.gov
                                       www.maine.gov/rehab/dbvi

Harold Lewis, Director
Sandra Cavanaugh, Executive Director
Works to bring about full access to employment, independence and community integration for people with disabilities in Maine.

3563 Maine Office of Elder Services
State of Maine
11 State House Station
41 Anthony Avenue
Augusta, ME 04333   207-287-9200
                                           800-262-2232
                                      Fax: 207-287-9229
                                       TTY: 800-606-0215
                                       mdol@maine.gov
                                       www.maine.gov/dhhs/oads/aging

James Martin, Director
Gary Wolcott, Associate Director
Romaine Turyn, Aging Service Manager
Elizabeth Gattine, Long Term Care Service Manager
The Office of Elder Services (OES), an Office within the Maine Department of Health and Human Services, promotes programs and services for older adults, their families and for people with disabilities.

3564 Maine Workers' Compensation Board
27 State House Station
Augusta, ME 04333   207-287-3751
                                           888-801-9087
                                      Fax: 207-287-7198
                                       TTY:877-832-5525
                                       www.maine.gov/wcb

Paul H Sighinolfi, Executive Director
Lindsay Lizzotte, Secretary Specialist
Gary Koocher, Management Representative
Ron Green, Labor Representative
The general mission of the Maine Workers' Compensation Board is to serve the employees and employers of the State fairly and expeditiously by ensuring compliance with the workers' compensation laws, ensuring the prompt delivery of benefits legally due, promoting the prevention of disputes, utilizing dispute resolution to reduce litigation and facilitating labor-management cooperation.

3565 Social Security: Maine Disability Determination
330 Civic Center Dr
Suite 4
Augusta, ME 04330-6325   866-882-5422
                                           800-772-1213
                                       TTY:207-623-4190
                                       ssa.gov

Louis Tepin, Manager
This office makes the medical determination about whether a consumer is disabled and, therefore, medically eligible for Social Security benefits. Legally, an individual is considered disabled if he or she is unable to do any substantial gainful work activity because of a medical condition (or conditions), that has lasted, or can be expected to last for at least 12 months, or that is expected to result in death.

Maryland

3566 Health Resources & Services Administration: State Bureau of Health
Federal Government
5600 Fishers Lane
Rockville, MD   20857

301-443-2216
888-275-4772
ask@hrsa.gov
www.hrsa.gov

Diana Espinosa, Deputy Administrator
Jim Macrae, Acting Administrator
Deborah Parham Hopson, Senior Advisor
Sarah Linde, Chief Public Health Officer
Through appropriated funds, supports education programs, credentialing analysis, and development of human resources needed to staff the U.S. health care system.

3567 International Dyslexia Association: Maryland Branch
International Dyslexia Association
P.O. Box 233
Brookland, MD   21022-0233

800-509-4980
info@idamd.org
md.dyslexiaida.org

Annette Fallon, President
Karen Fallon, Vice President
Timothy Yearick, Secretary
Jonathan Grimmel, Treasurer
Nonprofit organization providing free information and referral services for diagnosis and tutoring for parents, educators, physicians, and individuals with dyslexia. Membership includes yearly journal and quarterly newsletter. Call for conference dates.

3568 Maryland Client Assistance Program Division of Rehabilitation Services
2301 Argonne Drive
Baltimore, MD   21218-1628

410-554-9442
888-554-0334
Fax: 410-554-9362
TTY: 443-798-2840
dors@maryland.gov
dors.maryland.gov

Suzanne R. Page, DORS Director
Helps individuals with disabilities understand the rehabilitation process and receives appropriate and quality services from the Division of Rehabilitation Services and other programs and facilities providing services under the Rehabilitation Act of 1973.

3569 Maryland Department of Aging
State Office Building
301 West Preston Street
Suite 1007
Baltimore, MD   21201- 2393

410-767-1100
800-243-3425
Fax: 410-333-7943
www.mdoa.state.md.us/

Stuart Rosenthal, Chair
Sharonlee J. Vogel, Vice-Chair
Rona E. Kramer, Secretary
Sandie Callis, Commissiom Member
The Department of Aging protects the rights and quality of life of older persons in Maryland. To meet the needs of senior citizens, the Department administers programs throughout the State, primarily through local area agencies on aging.

3570 Maryland Department of Handicapped Children
201 W Preston St
Unit 50
Baltimore, MD   21201-2301

410-335-6470
www.msa.md.gov

Judson Force, Director
Children's Medical Services is a joint federal/state/local program which assists in obtaining specialized medical, surgical and related habilitative/rehabilitative evaluation and treatment services for children with special health care needs and their families. To be eligible for the program's services, an individual must be a resident of Maryland, younger than 22 years, have or be suspected of having an eligible medical condition and meet both medical and financial criteria.

3571 Maryland Developmental Disabilities Council
217 E Redwood Street
Suite 1300
Baltimore, MD   21202-3313

410-767-3670
800-305-6441
Fax: 410-333-3686
BrianC@md-council.org
www.md-council.org

Brian Cox, Executive Director
Catherine Lyle, Deputy Director
Rachel London, Director, Children & Family Poli
Kelley Malone, Director of Communications
A public policy organization comprised of people with disabilities and family members who are joined by state officials, service providers and other designated partners. The Council is an independent, self-governing organization that represents the interests of people with developmental disabilities and their families.

3572 Maryland Division of Mental Health
201 W. Preston Street
Baltimore, MD   21201

410-767-6500
877-463-3464
dhmh.healthmd@maryland.gov

Norma Pinette, Executive Director
Van T. Mitchell, Secretary
Our Public Health Services Division oversees vital public services to Maryland residents including infectious disease and environmental health concerns, family health services and emergency preparedness and response activities.

3573 National Maternal and Child Health Bureau
Rm 1805
5600 Fishers Ln
Rockville, MD   20852-1750

301-443-2216
888-275-4772
hrsa.gov

Michael C. Lu, Associate Administrator
Laura Kavanagh, Deputy Associate Administrator
Natasha Coulouris, Senior Advisor
Angela Hooten, Executive Officer
Offers information, books and pamphlets to professionals, parents and children facing health issues or disabilities.

3574 Social Security: Baltimore Disability Determination
711 West 40th Street
Ste 415 Rotunda Mall
Baltimore, MD 21211-2120

800-772-1213
TTY:800-325-0778
ssa.gov

3575 Workers Compensation Board Maryland
10 East Baltimore Street
Baltimore, MD   21202-1641

410-864-5100
800-492-0479
Fax: 410-333-8122
info@wcc.state.md.us
www.wcc.state.md.us

R. Karl Aumann, Chairperson
Mary K. Ahearn, Chief Executive Officer
David E. Jones, Chief Financial Officer
Joyce McNemar, Chief Information Officer

Massachusetts

3576 Center for Public Representation
22 Green Street
Northampton, MA 01060-3708
413-586-6024
Fax: 413-586-5711
info@cpr-ma.org
centerforpublicrep.org

Bob Agoglia, President
Nickie Chandler, Clerk/Treasurer
Bob Riedel, Director
Neal Rosen, Esq., Director
The Center seeks to improve the quality of lives of people with mental illness and other disabilities through the systemic enforcement of their legal rights while promoting improvements in services for citizens with disabilities

3577 Massachusetts Assistive Technology Partnership
Children s Hospital Boston
1295 Boylston St
Suite 310
Boston, MA 02215-3407
617-355-7820
800-848-8867
Fax: 617-355-6345

Marylyn Howe, Project Director
Pat Hill, Training Coordinator
A statewide program promoting assistive technology devices and services for persons with all disabilities.

3578 Massachusetts Client Assistance Program
Massachusetts Office on Disability
1 Ashburton Pl
Suite 1305
Boston, MA 02108-1518
617-727-7440
800-322-2020
james.aprea@state.ma.us
www.mass.gov/anf/employment-equal-access-disa
Barbara Lybarger, Assistant Director
Myra Berloff, Director
Michael Dumont, Assistant Director
Jeffrey Dougan, Assistant Director
Provides advocacy and information services.

3579 Massachusetts Department of Mental Health
25 Staniford St.
Boston, MA 02114-2503
617-626-8000
TTY:617-727-9842
dmhinfo@massmail.state.ma.us
www.mass.gov/dmh
Joan Mikula, Commissioner
The Massachusetts Department of Mental Health, as the State Mental Health Authority, assures and provides access to services and supports to meet the mental health needs of individuals of all ages, enabling them to live, work and participate in their communities. The Department establishes standards to ensure effective and culturally competent care to promote recovery. The Department sets policy, promotes self-determination, protects human rights and supports mental health training and research.

3580 Massachusetts Developmental Disabilities Council
100 Hancock Street
Second Floor, Suite 201
Quincy, MA 02169-4398
617-770-7676
Fax: 617-770-1987
TTY:617-770-9499
adelia.deltrecco@state.ma.us
www.state.ma.us/mddc/
Daniel Shannon, Executive Director
Faith Behum, Disability Policy Specialist
Kristin Britton, Director of Public Policy
Adelia DelTrecco, Member Services Coordinator
Group of citizens which analyzes needs of people with severe, lifelong disabilities and works to improve public policy. MDDC produces several publications and has committees and a grants program to study and advocate for changes in the service system.

3581 Social Security: Boston Disability Determination
110 Chauncy Street
Boston, MA 02111
617-727-7600
800-772-1213
TTY:800-882-2040
www.socialsecurity.gov
Michael F. Bertrand, Commissioner

3582 Workers Compensation Board Massachusetts
Rm 211
1 Ashburton Pl
Boston, MA 02108-1518
617-626-7122
Fax: 617-727-1090
www.state.ma.us/dia
Russell Gilfus, Manager
The Massachusetts Workers' Compensation system is in place to make sure that workers are protected by insurance if they are injured on the job or contract a work-related illness. Under this system, employers are required by Massachusetts General Laws c. 152, 25A to provide workers' compensation (WC) insurance coverage to all their employees.

Michigan

3583 Department of Blind Rehabilitation
Western Michigan University
1903 W Michigan Ave
Kalamazoo, MI 49008-5218
269-387-3455
Fax: 269-387-3567
g.dennis@wmich.edu
www.wmich.edu/visionstudies
James Leja, Chair
Charles Adams, Faculty Specialist I
Gayla Dennis, Office Coordinator
Jeannyne Depoian, Office Associate
The Department of Blindness and Low Vision Studies at Western Michigan University is recognized internationally as the oldest, largest and best program of its kind. It originated in 1961 with a graduate degree in Orientation and Mobility, responding to the need for professionals to rehabilitate the many military personnel blinded during World War Two and the Korean War.

3584 Michigan Association for Deaf and Hard of Hearing
5236 Dumond Court
Suite C
Lansing, MI 48917-6001
517-487-0066
800-968-7327
Fax: 517-487-0202
TTY: 517-487-2586
info@madhh.org
www.madhh.org
Nancy Asher, Executive Director
Pat Walton, Office Manager
MADHH is a statewide collaboration agency dedicated to improving the lives of people who are deaf and hard of hearing through leadership in education, advocacy & services. Interpreter IC print-out, assistive devices available.

3585 Michigan Association for Deaf, and Hard of Hearing
5236 Dumond Court
Suite C
Lansing, MI 48917-6001
517-487-0066
800-968-7327
Fax: 517-487-2586
info@madhh.org
www.madhh.org
Nancy Asher, Executive Director
Pat Walton, Office Manager
MADHH is a statewide collaboration agency dedicated to improving the lives of people who are deaf and hard of hearing through leadership in education, advocacy and services.

3586 Michigan Client Assistance Program
4095 Legacy Pkwy
Ste 500
Lansing, MI   48911-4264   517-487-1755
                                                      800-288-5923
                                               Fax: 517-487-0827
                                               TTY: 800-288-5923
                                               molson@mpas.org
                                               www.mpas.org

Kate Pew Wolters, President
Thomas Landry, 1st Vice President
John McCulloch, 2nd Vice President
Elmer L. Cerano, Executive Director
The Client Assistance Program (CAP) assists people who are seeking or receiving services from Michigan Rehabilitation Services, Consumer Choice Programs, Michigan Commission for the Blind, Centers for Independent Living, and Supported Employment and Transition Programs. The CAP program is part of Michigan Protection and Advocacy Service, Inc.

3587 Michigan Coalition for Staff Development and School Improvement
12236 6 1/2 Mile Road
MCES
Battle Creek, MI   49014-1062   269-967-2086
                                                      800-444-2014
                                               Fax: 517-371-1170
                                               michigances.org

3588 Michigan Commission for the Blind - Gaylord
Ste 102
209 W 1st St
Gaylord, MI   49735-1386   989-732-2448
                                                      800-292-4200
                                               Fax: 989-731-3587
                                               www.michigan.gov

Judy Terwilliger, Manager
The mission of the Michigan Commission for the Blind (MCB) is to provide opportunity to individuals who are blind or visually impaired to achieve employability and/or function independently in society. The MCB vision is that someday it will be said that Michigan is a great place for blind people to live, learn, work, raise a family, and enjoy life

3589 Michigan Commission for the Blind
Michigan Dept Of Energy, Labor & Economic Growth
PO Box 30652
Lansing, MI   48909-8152   517-373-2062
                                                      800-292-4200
                                               Fax: 517-335-5140
                                               TTY: 517-373-4025
                                               turneys@michigan.gov
                                               www.michigan.gov/mcb

Patrick Cannon, State Director
The Michigan Commision for the blind is a state government agency that provides state and federally funded training and other services to individuals who are legally blind (blind and visually impaired). Services are provided to people of all ages throughout the state of Michigan toward the goal of employment and/or independence.

3590 Michigan Commission for the Blind Training Center
PO Box 30652
Lansing, MI   48909   517-373-2062
                                                      800-292-4200
                                               Fax: 517-335-5140
                                               TTY: 517-373-4025
                                               mossc@michigan.gov
                                               www.michigan.gov/mcb

Cheryl L Heibeck, Director
Bruce Schultz, Assistant Director
Residential facility that provides instruction to legally blind adults in braille, computer operation and assistive technology, handwriting, cane travel, cooking, personal management, industrial arts and also crafts. During training students will develop career plans which may include work experience, internships, volunteer opprtunities and even part-time paid employment.

3591 Michigan Commission for the Blind: Escanaba
305 Ludington St
State Office Bldg., 1st Floor
Escanaba, MI   49829-4029   906-786-8602
                                                      800-323-2535
                                               Fax: 906-786-4638
                                               michigan.gov/mcb

Bernie Kramer, Manager
The mission of the Michigan Commission for the Blind (MCB) is to provide opportunity to individuals who are blind or visually impaired to achieve employability and/or function independently in society. The MCB vision is that someday it will be said that Michigan is a great place for blind people to live, learn, work, raise a family, and enjoy life

3592 Michigan Commission for the Blind: Flint
125 E Union St
Seventh Floor
Flint, MI   48502-2041   810-760-2030
                                                      800-292-4200
                                               Fax: 810-760-2032

Debbie Wilson, Manager
Vocational and Independent living skills training for individuals who are legally blind.

3593 Michigan Commission for the Blind: Grand Rapids
250 Ottawa Avenue
Grand Rapids, MI   49503-4029   906-786-8602
                                                      800-323-2535
                                               Fax: 906-786-4638
                                               michigan.gov/mcb

Bernie Kramer, Manager
The mission of the Michigan Commission for the Blind (MCB) is to provide opportunity to individuals who are blind or visually impaired to achieve employability and/or function independently in society. The MCB vision is that someday it will be said that Michigan is a great place for blind people to live, learn, work, raise a family, and enjoy life

3594 Michigan Council of the Blind and Visually Impaired (MCBVI)
Neal Freeling
350 Ottawa Ave NW
Grand Rapids, MI   49503-2316   616-356-0180
                                                      800-292-4200
                                               Fax: 616-356-0199
                                               michigan.gov/mcb

Bernie Kramer, Manager
MCBVI is a diverse group of very friendly people from around the state working together to improve the lives of all citizens who are blind or visually impaired.

3595 Michigan Department of Handicapped Children
3423 N Martin Luther King Jr Blvd
Lansing, MI   48906-2934   517-484-9312
                                               Fax: 517-484-9836

Alan Curtiss, President
Bobbie Butler, Manager

3596 Michigan Developmental Disabilies Council
201 Townsend Street
Suite 120
Lansing, MI   48910-1646   517-335-3158
                                               Fax: 517-335-2751
                                               TTY:517-335-3171
                                               mdch-dd-council@michigan.gov
                                               www.michigan.gov/ddcouncil

Nick Lyon, Director
Nancy Grijalva, Assistant
Tim Becker, Chief Deputy Director
Trish Ray, Assistant
The Michigan DD Council is a group of citizens from across the state. Its membership is made up of: people with developmental disabilities; people from families who have, among their members, people with developmental disabilities; and professionals from state and local agencies charged with assisting people with developmental disabilities.

3597 Michigan Office of Services to the Aging
P.O.Box 30676
Lansing, MI 48909-8176   517-373-8230
                                           Fax: 517-373-4092
                                       OSAInfo@michigan.gov
                                       www.michigan.gov/osa

Wendi Middleton, Division Director
Kari Sederburg, Director
Carol Dye, Senior Executive Assistant
Annette Gamez, Executive Assistant
State unit on aging; allocates and monitors state and federal funds for the Older American Act services: nutrition, community services, administers home and community based waiver, develops programs through Area Agencies on Aging, advocates on behalf of seniors with legislature, governor, state departments, federal government, responsible for state planning of aging services, develops formula for distribution of state and federal funds.

3598 Michigan Protection & Advocacy Service
4095 Legacy Pkwy
Ste 500
Lansing, MI 48911-4264   517-487-1755
                                                 800-288-5923
                                           Fax: 517-487-0827
                                          molson@mpas.org
                                             www.mpas.org

Kate Pew Wolters, President
Thomas Landry, 1st Vice President
John McCulloch, 2nd Vice President
Elmer L. Cerano, Executive Director
People with disabilities have to deal with a wide variety of issues. TThey try to answer any questions you may have relating to disability. They have experience in the following areas: discrimination in education, employment, housing, and public places; abuse and neglect; Social Security benefits; Medicaid, Medicare and other insurance; housing; Vocational Rehabilitation; HIV/AIDS issues; and many other disability-related topics

3599 Michigan Rehabilitation Services
300 N. Washington Sq.
Lansing, MI 48913   517-335-4590
                                                 888-784-7328
                                           Fax: 517-373-0059
                                           TTY: 517-373-4035
                                       zimmermanng@michigan.org
                                             www.michigan.org

George Zimmermann, Vice President
Michelle Begnoche, Communications Specialist
Bonnie Fink, Travel Consultant Coordinator
David Lorenz, Public and Industry Relations Ma
A state and federally funded program that helps persons with disabilities prepare for and fund a job that matches their interests and abilities. Assistance is also available to workers with disabilities who are having difficulty keeping a job. A person is eligible for MRS services if he or she has a disability, is unemployed and needs vocational rehabilitation services to prepare for and find a job or independent living services.

3600 Social Security Administration
1100 West High Rise
6401 Security Blvd.
Baltimore, MD 21235-3878   517-393-3876
                                                 800-772-1213
                                           Fax: 517-393-4686
                                           TTY: 800-325-0778
                                       jennifer.bower@ssa.gov
                                                   ssa.gov

Tiffany L. Flick, Executive Secretary
Michael J. Astrue, Commissioner
Carolyn W. Colvin, Deputy Commissioner
We deliver services through a nationwide network of over 1,400 offices that include regional offices, field offices, card centers, teleservice centers, processing centers, hearing offices, the Appeals Council, and our State and territorial partners, the Disability Determination Services. We also have a presence in U.S. embassies around the globe. For the public, we are the face of the government. The rich diversity of our employees mirrors the public we serve.

3601 State of Michigan Workers' Compensation Agency
PO Box 30016
Lansing, MI 48909-7516   888-396-5041
                                           Fax: 517-322-1808
                                          wcinfo@michigan.gov
                                       www.michigan.gov/wca/

Mark C. Long, Director
Jack A. Nolish, Deputy Director
Julie Lenneman, Administrative Assistant
Ted Day, Division Manager
Michigan's injured workers and their employers are governed by the Workers' Disability Compensation Act. This Act was first adopted in 1912 and provides compensation to workers who suffer an injury on the job and protects employers' liability. The mission of the Workers' Compensation Agency is to efficiently administer the Act and provide prompt, courteous and impartial service to all customers.

Minnesota

3603 International Dyslexia Association: Upper Midwest Branch
International Dyslexia Association
5021 Vernon Ave. S
Suite 159
Minneapolis, MN 55436-2102   612-486-4242
                                       info.umw@dyslexiaida.org
                                           umw.dyslexiaida.org

Tom Strewler, President
Donna Burns, Member at Large
Jennifer Bennett, Secretary
Brian Pittenger, Treasurer
The Upper Midwest Branch of the International Dyslexia Association serves the residents of Minnesota, North Dakota, South Dakota, and Winnipeg, Canada. They offer local educational conferences about dyslexia and related subjects, Orton-Gillingham training for teachers, tutors, and parents, quarterly speaker series, member discounts on conferences, information line, and tutor referral.

3604 Minnesota Assistive Technology Project
STAR
358 Centennial Office Building
658 Cedar Street
Saint Paul, MN 55155-1402   651-201-2640
                                                 888-234-1267
                                                 800-627-3529
                                           Fax: 651-282-6671
                                       star.program@state.mn.us

Chuck Rassbach, Program Director
Kim Moccia, Program Coordinator
Jennie Delisi, Resource Specialist
Joan Gillum, Contracts Coordinator
A statewide program promoting assistive technology devices and services for persons of all ages with all disabilities.

3605 Minnesota Board on Aging
P.O. Box 64976
Saint Paul, MN 55164-0976   651-431-2500
                                                 800-882-6262
                                                 800-333-2433
                                           Fax: 651-431-7453
                                          TTY:800-627-3529
                                             www.mnaging.org

Don Samuelson, Chair
Jean Wood, Executive Director
Leonard Axelrod, Board Member
Tracy Keibler, Board Member
A state unit on aging for the state of Minnesota. Funds 14 area agencies on aging throughout the state that provide services at the local level. The mission is to keep older people in the homes or places of residence for as long as possible.

3606 Minnesota Children with Special Needs, Minnesota Department of Health
P.O.Box 64882
Saint Paul, MN 55164-0882
651-201-3650
800-728-5420
Fax: 651-201-3655
TTY: 651-201-5797
health.cyshn@state.mn.us
www.health.state.mn.us/mcshn

Dr. Edward Ehlinger, Commissioner
Daniel L. Pollock, Deputy Commissioner
Jeanne F. Ayers, Assistant Commissioner
Barb Dalbec, Director
Minnesota Children with Special Health Needs (MCSHN) provides leadership through partnerships with families and other key stakeholders to improve the access and quality of all systems impacting children and youth with special health care needs and their families.

3607 Minnesota Department of Labor & Industry Workers Compensation Division
443 Lafayette Rd N
Saint Paul, MN 55155-4301
651-284-5005
800-342-5354
TTY:651-297-4198
dli.communications@state.mn.us
doli.state.mn.us

Ken Petersom, Commissioner
Jessica Looman, Deputy Commissioner
James Honerman, Communications
Wendy Legge, General Counsil
To reduce the impact of work related injuries for employees and employers. Advice is given and questions answered on the toll-free number.

3608 Minnesota Disability Law Center
430 1st Avenue North
Suite 300
Minneapolis, MN 55401- 1780
612-334-5970
800-292-4150
Fax: 612-334-5755
TTY: 612-332-4668
website@mylegalaid.org
mylegalaid.org/about/our-work/disability-law
Mary L. Knoblauch, Chair
Cathy Haukedahl, Executive Director
Andrea Kaufman, Director of Development
Lisa Cohen, Deputy Director of Operations
Provides free, civil, legal assistance to Minnesotans with disabilities on issues related to their disability.

3609 Minnesota Governor's Council on Developmental Disabilities
370 Centennial Office Building
658 Cedar St
Saint Paul, MN 55155
651-296-4018
877-348-0505
Fax: 651-297-7200
TTY: 800-627-3529
admin.dd@state.mn.us
mn.gov/mnddc
John Hoffman, Chair
Colleen Wieck, PhD, Executive Director
Andrei Hahn, Planner
The mission of the Minnesota Governor's Council on Developmental Disabilities is to provide information, education, and training that will lead to increased independence, productivity, integration and inclusion for people with developmental disabilities and their families.

3610 Minnesota Mental Health Division
Human Services Building
PO Box 64981
Saint Paul, MN 55164-0981
651-431-2225
800-366-5411
Fax: 651-431-7418
TTY: 800-627-3529
dhs.info@state.mn.us
www.dhs.state.mn.us

Lucinda Jesson, Commissioner
Anne M. Barry, Deputy Commissioner
Jennifer DeCubellis, Assistant Commissioner
Loren Colman, Assistant Commissioner
Oversees the provision of services to people with mental illness in the state of Minnesota. Services are provided on the local level through a network of 87 county social service departments.

3611 Minnesota Protection & Advocacy for Persons with Disabilities
Minnesota Disability Law Center
2324 University Avenue West
Suite 101B
Saint Paul, MN 55114-1742
651-228-9105
800-292-4150
Fax: 651-222-0745
statesupport@mnlegalservices.org
Mary Kaczorek, Supervising Attorney
Ann Conroy, Office Manager
Elsa Marshall, Education for Justice Coordinato
Emily Good, Legal Project Manager
Provide public legal information on legal issues impacting the rights of low-income Minnesotans

3612 Minnesota State Council on Disability(MSCOD)
121 E 7th Place
Suite 107
Saint Paul, MN 55101-2114
651-361-7800
800-945-8913
Fax: 651-296-5935
council.disability@state.mn.us
www.disability.state.mn.us

Joan Willshire, Executive Director
Linda Gremillion, Business Operations Manager
Margot Imdieke Cross, Accessibility Specialist
David Fenley, Legislative Coordinator
The MSCOD collaborates, advocates, advises and provide technical information to expand opportunities, increase the quality of life and empower all persons with disabilities. This mission is accomplished by: providing information, referral and technical assistance to thousands of individuals every year via email, letter or telephone; through trainings on a variety of disability related topics; through publications and its web site; and through its advocacy and advisory work.

3613 Minnesota State Services for the Blind
2200 University Avenue West
Suite 240
Saint Paul, MN 55114-1840
651-539-2300
800-652-9000
Fax: 651-649-5927
TTY: 651-642-0506
star.program@state.mn.us
http://mn.gov/deed/job-seekers/blind-visual-i
Richard Strong, Executive Director
Kenneth Trebelhorn, Council Member
Jan Bailey, Chair
Steve Jacobson, Council Member
State agency serving blind and visually impaired persons with rehabilitation, information access, assistive technology, training and job placement services. Extensive older blind program.

3614 Social Security: St. Paul Disability Determination
5210 Perry Robinson
Lansing, MI   48911-3878
877-512-5944
800-772-1213
Fax: 517-393-4686
TTY: 800-325-0778
jennifer.bower@ssa.gov
www.ssa.gov

Karena L. Kilgore, Executive Secretary
Carolyn W. Colvin, Commissioner
Carolyn W. Colvin, Deputy Commissioner
James A. Kissko, Chief of Staff

We deliver services through a nationwide network of over 1,400 offices that include regional offices, field offices, card centers, teleservice centers, processing centers, hearing offices, the Appeals Council, and our State and territorial partners, the Disability Determination Services. We also have a presence in U.S. embassies around the globe. For the public, we are the face of the government. The rich diversity of our employees mirrors the public we serve.

Mississippi

3615 International Dyslexia Association: Louisiana Branch
1217 N. 32nd Ave.
Hattiesburg, MS   39401
601-467-1662
carla.carlos4dys@gmail.com
la.dyslexiaida.org

Carla Carlos, President
Lisa Best, Treasurer
Gale Pick, Secretary
Georgann Mire, Vice President of Education

Provides free information and referral services for diagnosis and tutoring for parents, educators, physicians, and individuals with dyslexia in Illinois. Membership includes yearly journal and quarterly newsletter.

3616 Mississippi Assistive Technology Division
1281 Highway 51
PO Box 1698
Jackson, MS   39215-1698
601-853-5160
800-443-1000
Fax: 601-853-5158
www.mdrs.ms.gov

Jean Massey, Superintendent of Education
Carey Wright, Superintendent of Education
Jack Virden, Chairman
Diana Mikula, Executive Director

A statewide program promoting assistive technology devices and services for persons of all ages with all disabilities.

3617 Mississippi Bureau of Mental Retardation
1101 Robert E. Lee Bulding
239 North Lamar Street
Jackson, MS   39201
601-359-1288
877-210-8513
Fax: 601-359-6295
TTY: 601-359-6230
ed.legrand@dmh.state.ms.us
www.dmh.state.ms.us

Sampat Shivangi, M.D., Chair
George Harrison, Vice Chair
Edwin C. Legrand, Executive Director
Kris Jones, Bureau Director of Quality Manag

Since its inception in 1974, the Mississippi Department of Mental Health has endeavored to provide services of the highest quality through a statewide service delivery system. As one of the major state agencies in Mississippi, the Department of Mental Health provides a network of services to persons who experience problems with mental illness, alcohol and/or drug abuse/dependence, or who have intellectual and developmental disabilities. Services are provided through an array of facilities and ag

3618 Mississippi Client Assistance Program
Mississippi Department of Rehabilitation Services
500-G East Woodrow Wilson Drive
P.O. Box 4958
Jackson, MS 39296
601-982-7051
Fax: 601-982-1951
www.msdisabilities.com

Dr. Ken Cleveland, President
Presley Posey, Executive Director
Dr. Michael Ogburn, Executive Director
David Cleland, Executive Director

Advocacy program for clients/client applicants for state of MS vocational services.

3619 Mississippi Department of Mental Health
1101 Robert E Lee Bldg
239 North Lamar Street
Jackson, MS 39201
601-359-1288
877-240-8513
Fax: 601-359-6295
TTY: 601-359-6230
ed.legrand@dmh.state.ms.us

Sampat Shivengi, M.D., Chair
George N. Harrison, Vice Chair
Edwin C. Legrand, Executive Director
Kris Jones, Bureau Director of Quality Manag

Administers Mississippi's public programs of serving persons with mental illness, mental retardation, alcohol and substance abuse problems, and alzheimer's disease and related dementia.

3620 Mississippi Division of Aging and Adult Services
Mississippi Department Of Human Services
750 North State Street
Jackson, MS   39202-3033
601-355-5536
800-345-6347
877-882-4916
Fax: 601-359-3664
webspinner@mdhs.state.ms.us
www.mdhs.state.ms.us/

Donald R. Taylor, Executive Director
Julia M. Todd, Director
Judy Collins, Director
Mary Scott, Director

Protects the rights of older citizens while expanding their opportunities and access to quality services.

3621 Mississippi State Department of Health
Children s Medical Program
570 East Woodrow Wilson Drive
Post Office Box 1700
Jackson, MS   39216-1700
601-576-7400
866-458-4948
Fax: 601-364-7447
web@HealthyMS.com
www.msdh.state.ms.us

Larry Clark, Director
Vickey Berryman, Director, Bureau of Licensure
Jim Craig, Director, Office of Health Pro
Tim Darnell, Director, MSDH Field Services

Financial assistance to families of children with physical handicaps. Rehabilitative in nature and has as its goal the correction or reduction of physical handicaps. Eligibility determined by diagnosis and provided to children from birth to age twenty-one. Financial eligibility is determined by factors of family income, family size, estimated cost of treatment and family liabilities. Categories include, but are not limited to: orthopedic, congenital heart defects, cerebral palsy, etc.

3622   Mississippi: Workers Compensation Commission
1428 Lakeland Dr
P.O. Box 5300, 39296-5300
Jackson, MS 39216-4718   601-987-4200
                                           866-473-6922
                                      Fax: 601-987-4220
                                      www.mwcc.state.ms.us

Liles Williams, Chairman
John Junkin, Commissioner
Debra Gibbs, Commissioner
Cindy Polk Wilson, Administrative Judge
Our goal is to provide the public with useful information regarding Workers' Compensation in the state of Mississippi.

Missouri

3623   Institute for Human Development
University of Missouri-Kansas City
215 W. Pershing Road
6th floor
Kansas City, MO 64108- 2639   816-235-1770
                                         800-444-0821
                                    Fax: 888-503-3107
                                    TTY: 800-452-1185
                                    beckmanncc@umkc.edu
                                    www.ihd.umkc.edu

Carl F. Calkins, Ph.D., Director
Kay Conklin, Training Director
Cindy Beckmann, Assistant to the Director
Kathy Fuger, Director, Early Childhood and Yo
A statewide program promoting person-centered planning and services for persons of all ages with all disabilities.

3624   Missouri Division Of Developmental Disabilities
Missouri Department Of Mental Health
1706 E. Elm St.
P.O.Box 687
Jefferson City, MO   65102   573-751-4122
                                        800-364-9687
                                   Fax: 573-751-8224
                                   ddmail@dmh.mo.gov
                                   www.dmh.mo.gov

Jay Nixon, Governor
Keith Schafer, Ed.D., Director
Bob Bax, Deputy Director
Rikki J. Wright, J.D., General Counsel
The Missouri Department of Mental Health was first established as a cabinet-level state agency by the Omnibus State Government Reorganization Act, effective July 1, 1974. State law provides three principal missions for the department: (1) the prevention of mental disorders, developmental disabilities, substance abuse, and compulsive gambling; (2) the treatment, habilitation, and rehabilitation of Missourians who have those conditions; and (3) the improvement of public understanding and attitudes

3625   Missouri Protection & Advocacy Services
925 S Country Club Dr
Jefferson City, MO   65109-4510   573-893-3333
                                        866-777-7199
                                   Fax: 573-893-4231
                                   TTY: 800-735-2966
                                   mopasjc@embarqmail.com
                                   moadvocacy.org

Joe Wrinkle, Chair
Barbara H. French, Vice Chair
Shawn De Loyola, Executive Director
Susan Pritchard-Green, Secretary/Treasurer
MO P&A potects the rights of individuals with disabilities by providing advocacy and legal services for disability related issues. As Missouri's Protection and Advocacy system, Mo P&A investigates allegations of abuse, neglect, death, and violations of rights against individuals with disabilities. Those who contact Mo P&A can receive information, referrals, advocacy services or legal counsel provided through one of nine federally-funded programs.

3626   Missouri Rehabilitation Services for the Blind
615 Howerton Court
PO Box 2320
Jefferson City, MO 65102-2320   573-751-3221
                                        800-592-6004
                                   Fax: 573-751-3091
                                   askrsb@dss.mo.gov
                                   www.dss.mo.gov/fsd/rsb/

Mark Laird, Executive Director
Ronald J. Levy, Director
Brian Kinkade, Deputy Director
Jennifer Tidball, Division Director
Offers services for the totally blind, legally blind, visually impaired, including counseling, educational, recreational, rehabilitation, computer training and professional training services.

3627   Social Security: Jefferson City Disability Determination
129 SCOTT STATION ROAD
Jefferson City, MO   65101-4421   877-405-9803
                                        800-772-1213
                                   Fax: 517-393-4686
                                   TTY: 800-325-0778
                                   jennifer.bower@ssa.gov
                                   www.ssa.gov

Karena L. Kilgore, Executive Secretary
Carolyn W. Colvin, Commissioner
Carolyn W. Colvin, Deputy Commissioner
James A. Kissko, Chief of Staff
We deliver services through a nationwide network of over 1,400 offices that include regional offices, field offices, card centers, teleservice centers, processing centers, hearing offices, the Appeals Council, and our State and territorial partners, the Disability Determination Services. We also have a presence in U.S. embassies around the globe. For the public, we are the face of the government. The rich diversity of our employees mirrors the public we serve.

3628   Workers Compensation Board Missouri
Department of Labor and Industrial Realtions
421 East Dunkin Street
P.O. Box 58
Jefferson City, MO 65102-0058   573-751-4231
                                        800-775-2667
                                        800-320-2519
                                   Fax: 573-751-4945
                                   workerscomp@labor.mo.gov
                                   labor.mo.gov/DWC/

Butch Albert, Chairman
James Avery, Commissioner
Curtis E. Chick, Commissioner
Ryan McKenna, Department Director
The Missouri Division of Workers' Compensation administers the programs providing services to all stake holders including workers who have been injured on the job or been exposed to occupational disease arising out of and in the course of employment. The Division makes sure that an injured worker receives benefits that he/she is entitled to under the Missouri Workers' Compensation law. The Division's Administrative Law Judges have the authority to approve settlements or issue awards after a hear

Montana

3629   Addictive & Mental Disorders Division
555 Fuller Ave
PO Box 202905
Helena, MT 59620-2905   406-444-3964
                                   Fax: 406-444-4435
                                   lothompson@mt.gov
                                   http://www.dphhs.mt.gov/amdd/

Lou Thompson, Administrator
Joan Cassidy, Chemical Dependency Bureau Chief
E. Lee Simes, Medical Director
Deb Matteucci, Behavioral Health Program Facili
The mission of the Addictive and Mental Disorders Division (AMDD) of the Montana Department of Public Health and Hu-

man Services is to implement and improve an appropriate state-wide system of prevention, treatment, care, and rehabilitation for Montanans with mental disorders or addictions to drugs or alcohol.

3630 Disability Rights Montana
1022 Chestnut Street
Helena, MT 59601-890
406-449-2344
800-245-4743
Fax: 406-449-2418
TTY: 406-449-2344
advocate@disabilityrightsmt.org
www.disabilityrightsmt.org/janda3/
Bernadette Franks-Ongoy, Executive Director
Kelli Kaufman, Director of Finance & Administra
Steve Heaverlo, Director of Programs/Advocacy Sp
Laurie t Danforth, Paralegal/Executive Suppor
Protects and advocates the human and legal rights of Montanans with mental and physical disabilities while advancing dignity, equality, and self-determination. Designated federal P&A, with AT, CAP, PADD, PAIMI and PAIR programs. Advocacy and legal services for abuse, neglect, rights violations, access, discrimination in employment, accommodations and housing, and assistance with vocational rehabilitation/visual services.

3631 MonTECH
700 SW Higgins Ave.
Suite 250
Missoula, MT 59803
406-243-5751
877-243-5511
Fax: 406-243-4730
montech@ruralinstitute.umt.edu
montech.ruralinstitute.umt.edu/
Kathleen Laurin, Program Director
Chris Clasby, Program Coordinator
Leslie Mullette
Specialzing in Assistive Technology and oversee a variety of AT related grants and contracts. The overall goal is to develop a comprehensive, statewide system of assistive technology related assistance. Striving to ensure that all people in Montana with disabilities have equitable access to assistive technology devices and services in order to enhance their independence, productivity and quality of life.

3632 Montana Blind & Low Vision Services
111 N Last Chance Gulch, Suite 4C
PO Box 4210
Helena, MT 59604-4210
406-444-2590
877-296-1197
Fax: 406-444-3632
lothompson@mt.gov
dphhs.mt.gov
Lou Thompson, Administrator
Joan Cassidy, Chemical Dependency Bureau Chief
E. Lee Simes, Medical Director
Deb Matteucci, Behavioral Health Program Facili
Mission: promoting work and independence for Montanans with disabilities.

3633 Montana Council on Developmental Disabilities
2714 Billings Ave
Helena, MT 59601-9767
406-443-4332
866-443-4332
Fax: 406-443-4192
www.mtcdd.org
Deborah Swingley, CEO/Executive Director
Dee Burrell, Contract Manager
The Council is made up of Montanans both with and without developmental disabilities, who believe in improving the lives of Montana's citizens who have a disability. We concentrate on issues related to self-determination, education, employment, transportation, housing, recreation, health care, community inclusion and the overall quality of life of people with developmental disabilities. As a Council we are committed to both question, and action as we work to discover and promote creative ways t

3634 Montana Department of Aging
Room 210
111 Sanders
Helena, MT 59604
406-444-7734
Fax: 406-444-3465
www.agingcare.com
Keith Messmer, Manager
Jeff Sturm, President

3635 Montana Department of Handicapped Children
111 North Sanders Street
Helena, MT 59620
406-444-7734
Fax: 406-444-3465
dphhs.mt.gov
Keith Messmer, Manager

3636 Montana Protection & Advocacy for Persons with Disabilities
1022 Chestnut Street
Helena, MT 59601-820
406-449-2344
800-245-4743
Fax: 406-449-2418
TTY: 406-449-2344
advocate@disabilityrightsmt.org
www.disabilityrightsmt.org/janda3/
Susie McIntyre, President
Will Warberg, Sales and Marketing Manager
Bernadette Franks-Ongoy, Executive Director
Kelli Kaufman, Director of Finance & Administra
Disability Rights Montana is the federally-mandated civil rights protection and advocacy system for Montana. We have the legal authority to represent almost any person with a disability.

3637 Montana State Fund
P.O.Box 4759
Helena, MT 59604-4759
406-495-5000
800-332-6102
Fax: 406-495-5020
TTY: 406-495-5030
www.montanastatefund.com
Elizabeth Best, Chairman
Montana State Fund is committed to the health and economic prosperity of Montana through superior service, leadership and caring individuals, working in an environment of teamwork, creativity and trust.

3638 Social Security: Helena Disability Determination
10 W 15th St
Ste 1600
Helena, MT 59626-9704
406-441-1270
800-772-1213
TTY:406-441-1278
www.socialsecurity.gov
Karena L. Kilgore, Executive Secretary
Carolyn W. Colvin, Commissioner
Carolyn W. Colvin, Deputy Commissioner
James A. Kissko, Chief of Staff
Social Security offers online information and services to third parties who do business with them.

Nebraska

3639 Nebraska Advocacy Services
134 S 13th St
Suite 600
Lincoln, NE 68508-1930
402-474-3183
800-422-6691
Fax: 402-474-3274
info@disabilityrightsnebraska.org
www.disabilityrightsnebraska.org
Jill Flagel, Chairperson
Mary Angus, Vice-Chairperson
Timothy F. Shaw, Chief Executive Officer
Eric Evans, Chief Operating Officer
Offers protection and advocacy services to people with developmental disabilities or mental illness. Direct assistance provided if

issue within broad case priorities. Sliding scale fee. Information and referral at no cost.

3640 Nebraska Client Assistance Program
301 Centennial Mall South
P. O. Box 94987
Lincoln, NE 68509-4987

402-471-3656
800-742-7594
Fax: 402-471-3656
victoria.rasmussen@nebraska.gov
www.cap.state.ne.us/

3641 Nebraska Commission for the Blind & Visually Impaired
4600 Valley Rd
Suite 100
Lincoln, NE 68510-4844

402-471-2891
877-809-2419
Fax: 402-471-3009
kathy.stephens@nebraska.gov
ncbvi.state.ne.us

Pearl Van zandt, Executive Director
Carlos Servan, Deputy Director
Bob Deaton, Deputy Director
Barbara Loos, Chairman
Offers services for the totally blind, legally blind, visually impaired, mentally retarded blind and more with health, counseling, educational, recreational, rehabilitation, computer training and professional training services.

3642 Nebraska Department of Health & Human Services of Medically Handicapped Children's Prgm
301 Centennial Mall S
5TH Floor
Lincoln, NE 68508-2529

402-471-3121
800-383-4278
Fax: 402-471-3577
mary.gordon@nebraska.gov
dhhs.ne.gov

Kerry Winterer, Chief Executive Officer
Amy Borer, Admininstrative Assistant,Divisi
Dan Howell, CEO,Beatrice State Developmental
Maternal and child health, Title V, children with special health care needs; community based, statewide programs to facilitate diagnoses and care of children with disabilities and chronic medical conditions.

3643 Nebraska Department of Health and Human Services, Division of Aging Services
P.O.Box 95026
301 Centennial Mall South
Lincoln, NE 68509-5026

402-471-2115
800-942-7830
Fax: 402-471-3577
mary.gordon@nebraska.gov
dhhs.ne.gov

Kerry Winterer, Chief Executive Officer
Amy Borer, Admininstrative Assistant,Divisi
Dan Howell, CEO,Beatrice State Developmental
The Council focuses on persons who experience a severe disability that occurs before the individual attains the age of 22, which includes persons with physical disabilities, mental/behavioral health conditions and persons that are served by the current state developmental disabilities system.

3644 Nebraska Department of Mental Health
4545 South 86th Street
Lincoln, NE 68526-2529

402-483-6990
888-210-8064
Fax: 402-483-7045
www.nmhc-clinics.com

Jill Zlomke McPherson, Executive Director
Thomas I. McPherson, Technical Coordinator
Lee Zlomke, Clinical Director
Lisa Logsden, Staff Psychologist
Nebraska Mental Health Centers is a family mental health clinic for people from all walks of life. Among the many services we provide are psychological evaluations, individual and group counseling, substance abuse care, neuropsychological services,

domestic violence group intervention and help for victims of domestic violence, treatment for eating disorders, an ADHD clinic, Women's Counseling and much more.

3645 Nebraska Planning Council on Developmental Disabilities
Department of Health and Human Services
P.O.Box 95026
Lincoln, NE 68509-5026

402-471-2115
Fax: 402-471-3577
TTY:402-471-9570
dhhs.ne.gov/developmental_disabilities/Pages/

Mary Gordon, Executive Director
Kerry Winterer, Chief Executive Officer
Amy Borer, Admininstrative Assistant,Divisi
Dan Howell, CEO,Beatrice State Developmental
The Council focuses on persons who experience a severe disability that occurs before the individual attains the age of 22, which includes persons with physical disabilities, mental/behavioral health conditions and persons that are served by the current state developmental disabilities system.

3646 Nebraska Workers' Compensation Court
State of Nebraska
P.O.Box 98908
Lincoln, NE 68509-8908

402-471-6468
800-599-5155
Fax: 402-471-8231
www.wcc.ne.gov/

Glenn W. Morton, Administrator
Susan K. Davis, Public Information Manager
Jacqueline J Boesen, General Counsel
Randall Cecrle, Information Technology Manager
It is the web site of the Nebraska Workers' Compensation Court. The court maintains this web site to enhance public access and provide general information regarding workers' compensation in Nebraska.

3647 Social Security: Lincoln Disability Determination
Department of Education
P.O.Box 94987
Lincoln, NE 68509-4987

402-471-2295
800-772-1213
TTY:402-471-3659
www.socialsecurity.gov

Karena L. Kilgore, Executive Secretary
Carolyn W. Colvin, Commissioner
Carolyn W. Colvin, Deputy Commissioner
James A. Kissko, Chief of Staff
Social Security offers online information and services to third parties who do business with them.

Nevada

3648 Aging and Disability Services Division
3416 Goni Rd
Suite D 132
Carson City, NV 89706-8008

775-687-4210
800-992-0900
Fax: 775-687-0574
adsd@adsd.nv.gov
adsd.nv.gov

Jane Gruner, Administrator
Tina Gerber-Winn, Deputy Administrator
Michele Ferral, Deputy Administrator
Jill Berntson, Deputy Administrator
Provides services for seniors in Nevada including community based care. advocacy and volunteer programs. Call write or e-mail for more information.

3649 Nevada Assistive Technology Project
Ste 32
3656 Research Way
Carson City, NV 89706-7932

775-687-4452
888-337-3839
Fax: 775-687-3292

Todd Butterworth, Manager

Serves all ages and all disabilities through partnerships with community organizations. The NATP provides training, advocacy, funding, information and referral services, a newsletter and weekly television show.

3650   Nevada Bureau of Vocational Rehabilitation
500 East Third Street
Carson City, NV   89713
775-684-0400
Fax: 775-684-4184
TTY:775-684-0360
detr.state.nv.us

Maureen Cole, Administrator
Melaine Mason, Deputy Administrator, Operations
Janice John, Deputy Administrator, Programs
Mechelle Merrill, Rehabilitation Chief II
Bureau of Vocational Rehabilitation is a state and federally funded program designed to help people with disabilities become employed and to help those already employed perform more successfully through training, counseling and other support methods.

3651   Nevada Community Enrichment Program (NCEP)
2550 University Avenue
Suite 330N
Saint Paul, MN   55114
651-645-7271
, 800-466-7722
Fax: 651-645-0541
TTY: 800-627-352
info@accessiblespace.org

Mark E. Hamel, Esq., Chair
Kay Knutson, Vice Chair
John W. Adams, MBA, Secretary
Mary Lindgren, Board Member
Comprehensive neurological rehabilitation and life skills training.

3652   Nevada Developmental Disability Council
896 W. Nye Ln.
Suite 202
Carson City, NV   89703
775-687-8619
Fax: 775-684-8626
smanning@dhhs.nv.gov
www.nevadaddcouncil.org

Jodi Thornley, Chairman
Santa Perez, Vice Chairman
Sherry Manning, Executive Director
Kari.Horn, Project Manager
The mission of the Nevada Developmental Disabilities Council is to provide resources at the community level which promote equal opportunity and life choices for people with disabilities through which they may positively contribute to Nevada society.

3653   Nevada Disability Advocacy and Law Center -Sparks/Reno Office
2820 West Charleston
Boulevard #11
Las Vegas, NV   89102
702-257-8150
888-349-3843
Fax: 702-257-8170
lasvegas@ndalc.org
www.ndalc.org

Reggie Bennettr, Secretary/Treasurer
Jana Spoor, President
John Miller, Vice President
Bob Bennett, Chairman
Nevada's protection and advocacy system for the human legal and service rights of individuals with disabilities. NDALC has offices in Reno/Sparks and Las Vegas, with services provided statewide.

3654   Nevada Division for Aging: Las Vegas
175 Berkeley Street
Boston, MA   02116
888-398-8924
libertymutual.com

Michael J. Babcockrs, Director
Marian L. Heard, Director
Martn P. Slark, Director

Develops, coordinates and delivers a comprehensive support service system in order for Nevada' senior citizens to lead independent, meaningful and dignified lives.

3655   Nevada Division of Mental Health and Developmental Services
5865 Lakeshore Road
Buford, GA   30518
770-945-4441
Fax: 678-482-1965

Keith Mixon, CEO/President
Offers treatment, prevention, education, habitation and rehabilitation for mental disorders. Works with advocacy groups, families, agencies and the community.

3656   Social Security: Carson City Disability Determination
1170 Harvard Way
Reno, NV   89502-2107
775-784-5221
800-772-1213
Fax: 775-784-5501
TTY: 800-325-0778
www.socialsecurity.gov

Karena L. Kilgore, Executive Secretary
Carolyn W. Colvin, Commissioner
Carolyn W. Colvin, Deputy Commissioner
James A. Kissko, Chief of Staff
Social Security offers online information and services to third parties who do business with them.

3657   State of Nevada Client Assistance Program
1631 W. Craig Rd.
Suite # 9-162
North Las Vegas, NV 89032-3767
702-635-4020
800-633-9879
800-633-9879
Fax: 702-642-7020
TTY:800-633-9879

3658   Workers Compensation Board Nevada
1301 North Green Valley Parkway
Suite 200
Henderson, NV 89074
702-486-9000
Fax: 775-687-6305
dirweb.state.nv.us

New Hampshire

3659   New Hampshire Workers Compensation Board
46 Donovan St
Concord, NH   03301-2624
603-225-2841
800-698-2364
Fax: 603-226-6903
www.nhprimex.org

Ty Gagne, CEO
Jonathan Kipp, Operations Manager
Julie Converse, Director of Finance
Carl Weber, Director of Member Services
Primex3 stands ready to provide our school, municipal, and county government members with the most comprehensive coverages and services available to New Hampshire local government.

3660   New Hampshire Assistive Technology Partnership Project
Department of Education
10 West Edge Drive
Suite 101
Durham, NH   03824
603-862-4320
Fax: 603-862-0555
atinnh.org

Jan Nisbet, Director
Mary Schuh, Associate Director
Eve Fralick, Associate Director
The goal of the New Hampshire Assistive Technology Partnership Project is to increase access to assistive technology through the creation and support of consumer driven systems for the provision of state-of-the-art assistive technology products and services for citizens with disabilities in the state of New Hampshire.

361

3661 New Hampshire Bureau of Developmental Services
Department of Health and Human Services
129 Pleasant St
Concord, NH   03301-3852   603-271-5034
                                   Fax: 603-271-5166
                                   www.dhhs.nh.gov

Matthew Ertas, Director
Peggy Sue Greenwood, Administrative Assistant
Developmental Services promotes opportunities for normal life experiences for persons with developmental disabilities and aquired brain disorders in all areas of community life: employment, housing, recreation, social relationships and community association. Services and supports are organized throught a central state office and ten private nonprofit community area agencies. Family support is provided to families of children with chronic health conditions or are developmentally disabled.

3662 New Hampshire Client Assistance Program
121 South Fruit Street
Suite 101
Concord, NH   03301-8518   603-271-2773
                                        800-852-3405
                                   Fax: 603-271-2837
                                   Disability@nh.gov
                   www.state.nh.us/disability/caphomepage.html
Bill Hagy, Ombudsman
John Richards, Executive Director
Jillian Shedd, Accessibility Coordinator
Gayle Baird, Accountant
The Commission's goal is to remove the barriers, architectural, attitudinal or programmatic, that bar persons with disabilities from participating in the mainstream of society.

3663 New Hampshire Commission for Human Rights
64 South Street
Concord, NH   03301-8501   603-225-3431
                                        800-735-2964
                                   Fax: 603-224-3766
                                   webmaster@nh.gov
                                   www.nh.gov

Peggy Mc Allister, Executive Director
Enforces New Hampshire law against discrimination in housing, employment or public accomodations. Disability discrimination is prohibited under New Hampshire law. Takes formal charges and investigates them.

3664 New Hampshire Department of Mental Health
129 Pleasant Street
Concord, NH   03301-3852   603-226-0111
                                   Fax: 603-271-5058
                                   www.dhhs.nh.gov

Donald Shumway, Director
Paul Garmon
Tim Rourke, Religious Leader

3665 New Hampshire Developmental Disabilities Council
2 1/2 Beacon Street
21 Fruit Street
Concord, NH   03301- 4447   603-271-3236
                                        800-852-3345
                                        800-852-3236
                                   Fax: 603-271-1156
                                   TTY:800-735-2964
                                   nhddc.org

Kristen McGraw, Chairman
Katherine Epstein, Vice-Chair
Carol Stamatakis, Executive Director
David Ouellette, Project Director
Offers information, referral and support services to disabled persons. A federally funded state agency.

3666 New Hampshire Division of Elderly and Adult Services
Bureau of Elderly & Adult Services
129 Pleasant St
Concord, NH   03301-3852   603-271-4680
                                        800-351-1888
                                   Fax: 603-271-4643
                                   pio@dhhs.state.nh.us
                                   www.dhhs.state.nh.us

Nicholas A. Toumpas, Comissioner
Mary Maggioncaida, Administrator
Marilee Nihan, Deputy Commissioner
Sheri Rockburn, Chief Financial Officer
The Bureau of Elderly and Adult Services provides a variety of social and long-term supports to adults age 60 and older and to adults between the ages of 18 and 60 who have a chronic illness or disability. These services range from home care, meals on wheels, care management, transportation assistance and assisted living to nursing home care.

3667 New Hampshire Governor's Commission on Disability
121 South Fruit Street
Suite 101
Concord, NH   03301-8518   603-271-2773
                                        800-852-3405
                                   Fax: 603-271-2837
                                   Disability@nh.gov
                                   www.nh.gov/disability

Paul Van Blarigan, Chairman
Charles J. Saia, Executive Director
Michael Coe, Accessibility Coordinator
Carol Conforti-Adams, Information and Referral Special
The Commission's goal is to remove the barriers, architectural, attitudinal or programmatic, that bar persons with disabilities from participating in the mainstream of socie

3668 New Hampshire Protection & Advocacy for Persons with Disabilities
Disabilities Rights Center, Inc
64 North Main Street
Suite 2, 3rd Floor
Concord, NH 03301-4913   603-228-0432
                                        800-834-1721
                                   Fax: 603-225-2077
                                   TTY: 800-834-1721
                                   advocacy@drcnh.org
                                   drcnh.org

Paul Levy, President
Joanne Malloy, Vice President
Richard Cohen, Executive Director
Aaron Ginsberg, Staff Attorney
Legal services for individuals with disabilities; I & R.

3669 Social Security: Concord Disability Determination
Ste 100
70 Commercial St
Concord, NH   03301-5005   603-224-1939
                                        800-772-1213
                                   TTY:800-325-0778
                                   www.ssa.gov

Karena L. Kilgore, Executive Secretary
Carolyn W. Colvin, Commissioner
Carolyn W. Colvin, Deputy Commissioner
James A. Kissko, Chief of Staff
Social Security offers online information and services to third parties who do business with them.

3670 Workers Compensation Board New Hampshire
PO Box 2076
95 Pleasant Street
Concord, NH   03301   603-271-3176
                                        800-272-4353
                                   Fax: 603-271-2668
                                   workerscomp@labor.state.nh.us
                                   www.nh.gov/labor

Kathryn J. Barger, Director, Workers' Compensation
George N. Copadis, Commissioner of Labor
David M. Wihby, Deputy Commissioner

The Department of Labor monitors Employers, Workers Compensation, and Insurance Carriers to insure that they are in compliance with NH Labor laws. These laws range from minimum wage, overtime, safety issues and workers compensation.

New Jersey

3671 Division of Developmental Disabilities
210 South Broad Street
3rd Floor
Trenton, NJ 08608   609-292-9742
                                          800-922-7233
                                     Fax: 609-777-0187
                                     TTY: 609-633-7106
                                     advocate@drnj.org
                                     www.njpanda.org

James W Smith Jr, Executive Director
New Jersey's designated protection and advocacy system for poeple with disabilities and provides legal, nonlegal individual and systems advocacy.

3672 International Dyslexia Association: New Jersey Branch
P.O. Box 32
Long Valley, NJ 07853   908-876-1179
                                     Fax: 908-876-3621
                                     njida@msn.com
                                     nj.dyslexiaida.org

Patricia Barden, President
Provides free information and referral services for diagnosis and tutoring for parents, educators, physicians, and individuals with dyslexia in Illinois. Membership includes yearly journal and quarterly newsletter.

3673 New Jersey Commission for the Blind and Visually Impaired
153 Halsey St, Fl 6
PO Box 47017
Newark, NJ 7101-4701   973-648-3333
                                          877-685-8878
                                     Fax: 973-693-5046
                                     Vito.DeSantis@dhs.state.nj.us
                                     www.state.nj.us/humanservices/cbvi

Daniel B. Frye, J.D., Executive Director
Bernice Davis, Executive Assistant
Edward Szajdecki, Manager
John Walsh, Chief of Program Administration
The mission of the New Jersey Commission for the Blind and Visually Impaired is to promote and provide services in the areas of education, employment, independence and eye health through informed choice and partnership with persons who are blind or visually impaired, their families and the community. Serves Bergen, Essex, Hudson, Morris, Passaic, Sussex and Warren Counties.

3674 New Jersey Department of Aging
210 South Broad Street
3rd Floor
Trenton, NJ 08608   609-292-9742
                                          800-922-7233
                                     Fax: 609-777-0187
                                     TTY: 609-633-7106
                                     advocate@drnj.org
                                     www.drnj.org

Walter Anthony Woodberry, Chairman
Andrew McGeady, Vice Chairman
Linda K. Soley, Treasurer
Leah Ziskin, Secretary

3675 New Jersey Department of Health/Special Child Health Services
New Jersey Department of Health and Senior Service
P.O.Box 360
Trenton, NJ 08625-0360   609-777-7778
                                     Fax: 609-292-3580
                                     plisciotto@doh.state.nj.us
                                     www.nj.gov/health/fhs/sch/

Jennifer Velez, ESQ, Commissioner
Provides services for New Jersey children that will prevent or reduce the effects of a developmental delay, chronic illness or behavioral disorder.

3676 New Jersey Division of Mental Health Services
Department Human Services
222 South Warren Street
P.O. Box 700
Trenton, NJ 8625- 700   609-292-3717
                                          800-382-6717
                                     Fax: 609-341-3333
                                     www.state.nj.us/humanservices

Jennifer Velez, ESQ, Commissioner
Lynn A. Kovich, Assistant Commissioner
Oversees the public mental health system for the state of New Jersey. Operates six regional and specialty psychiatric hospitals, and contracts with over 125 not-for-profit agencies to provide a comprehensive system of community mental health services throughout all counties in the state.

3677 New Jersey Governor's Liaison to the Office of Disability Employment Policy
1 John Fitch Plaza
P. O.Box 110
Trenton, NJ 08625-110   609-659-9045
                                     Fax: 609-633-9271
                                     Constituent.Relations@dol.state.nj.us
                                     lwd.state.nj.us/labor

Harold J. Wriths, Commissioner
Frederick J. Zavaglia, Chief of Staff
Aaron R. Fichtner, Ph.D., Deputy Commissioner
Brian T. Murray, Director of Communications & Mar
The Division of Vocational Rehabilitation Services provides vocational rehabilitation services to prepare and place in employment eligilbe individuals with disabilities who, because of their disabling conditions, would otherwise be unable to secure and/or mantain employment

3678 New Jersey Protection & Advocacy for Persons with Disabilities
210 South Broad Street
3rd Floor
Trenton, NJ 08608   609-292-9742
                                          800-922-7233
                                     Fax: 609-777-0187
                                     TTY: 609-633-7106
                                     advocate@drnj.org
                                     www.drnj.org

Walter Anthony Woodberry, Chairman
Andrew McGeady, Vice Chairman
Linda K. Soley, Treasurer
Leah Ziskin, Secretary

3679 Regional ADA Technical Assistance Center
United Cerebral Palsy Associations of New Jersey
201 Dolgen Hall
Ithaca, NY 14853   607-255-6686
                                          800-949-4232
                                     Fax: 607-255-2763
                                     northeastada@cornell.edu
                                     www.northeastada.org

LaWanda H. Cook, Ph.D., Extension Associate/Training Spe
Hannah Rudstam, Ph.D., Director of Training
Erin Sember-Chase, Project Coordinator and Technic
Luz Semeah, Technical Assistance

3680 Social Security Administration
1100 West High Rise
6401 Security Blvd.
Baltimore, MD 21235

800-772-1213
TTY:800-325-0778
www.ssa.gov

Karena L. Kilgore, Executive Secretary
Carolyn W. Colvin, Commissioner
Carolyn W. Colvin, Deputy Commissioner
James A. Kissko, Chief of Staff

Social Security disability is a social insurance program that workers and employers pay for with their Social Security taxes. Eligibility is based on your work history, and the amount of your benefit is based on your earnings. Social Security also has a disability program for people with limited income and resources- the Supplemental Security Income (SSI) program. For more information on these federal programs, please call our nationwide toll-free number.

New Mexico

3681 New Mexico Aging and Long-Term Services Department
2550 Cerrillos Rd
P.O. Box 27118
Santa Fe, NM 87505-3260

505-476-4799
866-451-2901
Fax: 505-476-4836
www.nmaging.state.nm.us

Miles Copeland, Deputy Secretary
Retta Ward, Secretary
Jason Sanchez, Administrative Services Division
Greg Rockstroh, IT Manager

Information and services for seniors, people with disabilities and their families.

3682 New Mexico Client Assistance Program
1720 Louisiana Blvd NE
Site 204
Albuquerque, NM 87110- 7070

505-256-3100
800-432-4682
Fax: 505-256-3184
info@drnm.org
www.drnm.org

Katie Toledo, Chairperson
Cyndy Costanza, Vice Chairperson
Jeanne A. Hamrick, President
Larry Rodriguez, Vice President

The mission of Disability Rights New Mexico (DRNM) is to protect, promote and expand the legal and civil rights of persons with disabilities. DRNM is an independent, private nonprofit agency operating federally mandated and other advocacy programs in pursuit of this mission.

3683 New Mexico Commission for the Blind
2905 Rodeo Park Dr E
Bldg 4, Suite 100
Santa Fe, NM 87505-6342

505-476-4479
888-513-7968
Fax: 505-476-4475
greg.trapp@state.nm.us
www.cfb.state.nm.us/

Arthur A. Schreiber, Chairman
Jim Babb, Commissioner
Dallas Allen, Commissioner
Greg Trapp, Executive Director

Offers services for the totally blind, legally blind, visually impaired, mentally retarded blind and more with health, counseling, educational, recreational, rehabilitation, computer training and professional training services.

3684 New Mexico Department of Health: Children's Medical Services
1190 S Saint Francis Dr
Santa Fe, NM 87505-4173

505-841-6100
800-797-3260
Fax: 505-827-2530

Gloria Bonner, Program Manager
Susan Baum, Medical Director
Freida Adams, Nurse Coordinator
Kim Love, Operations Manager

Title V MCH Program for children with special health care needs from birth to age 21 years. Services provided include: diagnosis, medical intervention, clinics and service coordination.

3685 New Mexico Governor's Committee on Concerns of the Handicapped
491 Old Santa Fe Trl
Santa Fe, NM 87501-2753

505-476-0412
877-696-1470
Fax: 505-827-6328
gcd@state.nm.us
www.gcd.state.nm.us/

Susan Gray, Chair
Curtiss Wilson, Vice Chair
Jim Parker, Director
Karen Courtney-Peterson, Chief Financial Officer

3686 New Mexico Protection & Advocacy for Persons with Disabilities
1720 Louisiana Blvd NE
Site 204
Albuquerque, NM 87110- 7070

505-256-3100
800-432-4682
Fax: 505-256-3184
info@drnm.org
www.drnm.org

Katie Toledo, Chairperson
Cyndy Costanza, Vice Chairperson
Jeanne A. Hamrick, President
Larry Rodriguez, Vice President

The mission of Disability Rights New Mexico (DRNM) is to protect, promote and expand the legal and civil rights of persons with disabilities. DRNM is an independent, private nonprofit agency operating federally mandated and other advocacy programs in pursuit of this mission.

3687 New Mexico Technology Assistance Program
435 Saint Michaels Dr
Ste D
Santa Fe, NM 87505-7679

505-827-8535
800-866-2253
Fax: 505-954-8608
TTY: 800-659-4915

Julie Martinez, Program Director

Examines and works to eliminate barriers to obtaining assistive technology in New Mexico. Has established a statewide program for coordinating assistive technology services; is designed to assist people with disabilities to locate, secure, and maintain assistive technology.

3688 New Mexico Workers Compensation Administration
2410 Centre Avenue SE
P.O.Box 27198
Albuquerque, NM 87125-7198

505-841-6000
800-255-7965
Fax: 505-841-6009
www.workerscomp.state.nm.us/

Ned S. Fuller, Director
Robert E. Doucette, Executive Deputy Director
Darin A. Childers, General Counsel
Thomas E. Dow, Executive Deputy Director

Regulates workers' compensation in New Mexico.

3689 Social Security: Santa Fe Disability Determination
6401 Security Blvd.
Baltimore, MD 21235
800-772-1213
TTY:800-325-0778
www.socialsecurity.gov

Karena L. Kilgore, Executive Secretary
Carolyn W. Colvin, Commissioner
Carolyn W. Colvin, Deputy Commissioner
James A. Kissko, Chief of Staff

3690 Southwest Branch of the International Dyslexia Association
International Dyslexia Association
3915 Carlisle Blvd. NE
Albuquerque, NM 87107
505-255-8234
800-222-3123
Fax: 505-262-8547
swida@southwestida.org
southwestida.com

Carolee Dean, President
Claudia Gutierrez, Vice President
Michelle Wick, Recording Secretary
Erin Brown, Corresponding Secretary
Provides free information and referral services for diagnosis and tutoring for parents, educators, physicians, and individuals with dyslexia. The voice of our membership is heard in 48 countries. Membership includes yearly journal and quarterly newsletter. Call for conference dates.

3691 Workers Compensation Board New Mexico
2410 Centre Avenue SE
P.O.Box 27198
Albuquerque, NM 87125-7198
505-841-6000
800-255-7965
Fax: 505-841-6009
www.workerscomp.state.nm.us/

Ned S. Fuller, Director
Robert E. Doucette, Executive Deputy Director
Darin A. Childers, General Counsel
Thomas E. Dow, Executive Deputy Director
Regulates workers' compensation in New Mexico.

New York

3692 Albany County Department for Aging and Albany Social Services
112 State Street
Room 900
Albany, NY 12207-2304
518-447-7000
Fax: 518-447-7188
aging@albanycounty.com
albanycounty.com

George Brown, Commissioner
Judy L. Coyne, Commissioner
Kathleen M. Dalton, Ph.D., Commissioner
The Point of Entry access line provides information and assistance and comprehensive referrals, and or assessments for the elderly, adults and children with disabilities, their family, or service providers.

3693 Jawonio
260 N Little Tor Road
New City, NY 10956-2627
845-708-2000
Fax: 845-634-7731
TTY:845-639-3521
www.jawonio.org

Jill A. Warner, Executive Director & CEO
Matthew Shelly, Chief Program Officer
Diana Hess, Chief Communications Officer
Joseph Bloss, Chief Financial Officer
A dedicated community resource providing services to more than 500 children and adults annually. Provide early intervention, day care and pre-school special ed to our children. Job training, day habilitation, recreation, medical and service coordination for adults.

3694 Jawonio Vocational Center
260 N Little Tor Rd
New City, NY 10956-2627
845-708-2000
Fax: 845-634-7731
TTY:845-639-3521
jawonio.org

Jill A. Warner, Executive Director & CEO
Matthew Shelly, Chief Program Officer
Diana Hess, Chief Communications Officer
Joseph Bloss, Chief Financial Officer
A dedicated community resource providing services to more than 500 children and adults annually. Provide early intervention, day care and pre-school special ed to our children. Job training, day habilitation, recreation, medical and service coordination for adults.

3695 NYS Commission on Quality of Care & Advocacy for Persons with Disabilities
401 State St
Schenectady, NY 12305-2300
518-388-2892
Fax: 518-388-2890
marcelc@cqc.state.ny.us

Andrew M. Cuomo, Governor
Roger Bearden, Chair
Bruce Blower, Member
Patricia Okoniewski, Member

3696 NYSARC
393 Delaware Ave
Delmar, NY 12054-3094
518-439-8311
800-724-2094
Fax: 518-439-1893
info@nysarc.org
nysarc.org

Laura J. Kennedy, President
Patricia Campanella, Senior Vice President
Joseph M. Bognanno, Vice President
Lori Martindale, Treasurer

3697 National Alliance on Mental Illness of New York State
99 Pine Street
Suite 302
Albany, NY 12207-1336
518-462-2000
800-950-3228
Fax: 518-462-3811
info@naminys.org
www.naminys.org

Sherry Grenz, President
Wend Burch, Executive Director
Sharon Clairmont, Finance & Business Office Dir.
Matthew Shapiro, Development/Events Coordinator

3698 New State Office of Mental Health Agency
Office of Mental Health
44 Holland Ave
Albany, NY 12229
518-474-4403
800-597-8481
Fax: 518-474-2149
www.omh.ny.gov

Mike Hogan, Commissioner
Promoting the mental health of all New Yorkers with a particular focus on providing hope and recovery for adults with serious mental illness and children with serious emotional disturbances.

3699 New York Client Assistance Program
855 Central Avenue
Suite 110
Albany, NY 12206
518-459-6422
Fax: 518-459-7847
TTY:518-459-6422
www.nls.org

3700   New York Department of Handicapped Children
Department of Heath Education
Corning Tower
Empire State Plaza
Albany, NY   12237   518-456-0665
                                        866-881-2809
                                        Fax: 518-456-1126
                                        www.health.ny.gov

Andrew M. Cuomo, Governor
Dr James B. Crucetti, MD, MPH, Commissioner
Howard Zucker, Acting Commissioner

3701   New York State Commission for the Blind
52 Washington St
Rensselaer, NY   12144-2796   518-473-7793
                                        866-871-3000
                                        Fax: 518-486-7550
                                        www.ocfs.state.ny.us

Madeline Raciti, Manager
Offers services for the totally blind, legally blind, visually impaired, mentally retarded blind and more with health, counseling, educational, recreational, rehabilitation, computer training and professional training services.

3702   New York State Commission on Quality of Care
401 State St
Schenectady, NY   12305-2300   518-388-2892
                                        Fax: 518-388-2890
                                        marcelc@cqc.state.ny.us
                                        www.cqc.state.ny.us

Andrew M. Cuomo, Governor
Roger Bearden, Chair
Bruce Blower, Member
Patricia Okoniewski, Member

3703   New York State Congress of Parents and Teachers
1 Wembley Ct
Albany, NY   12205-6258   518-452-8808
                                        877-569-7782
                                        Fax: 518-452-8105
                                        pta.office@nyspta.org
                                        nyspta.org

Bonnie Russell, President
Gracemarie Rozea, First Vice President
Judy Van Harren, Secretary
Penny Hollister, Vice President
Parent Teacher Association and PTA are registered service marks of the National Congress of Parents and Teachers (National PTA). Only those groups chartered by the New York State PTA are entitled to use the name PTA. Any other use constitutes trademark infringement.

3704   New York State Office of Advocates for Persons with Disabilities
Ste 1001
1 Empire State Plz
Albany, NY   12223-1100   518-449-7860
                                        800-522-4369
                                        Fax: 518-473-6005
                                        www.oapwd.org

Gary O'Brien, Chair Commissioner
Provides information and referral services; administers NYS Tech Art Project; promotes implementation of disability-related laws.

3705   New York State Office of Mental Health
44 Holland Ave
Albany, NY   12229-1   518-474-4403
                                        800-597-8481
                                        Fax: 518-474-2149
                                        www.omh.state.ny.gov in

Michael Hogan, Ph.D.
Promoting the mental health of all New Yorkers with a particular focus on providing hope and recovery for adults with serious mental illness and children with serious emotional disturbances.

3706   New York State TRAID Project
New York State Commisionon Qualityof Careand Advoc
Ste 1001
1 Empire State Plz
Albany, NY   12223-1100   518-449-7860
                                        800-522-4369
                                        Fax: 518-473-6005

Cliff Sigfride, Manager

3707   Parent to Parent of New York State
500 Balltown Rd
Schenectady, NY   12304-2247   518-381-4350
                                        800-305-8817
                                        Fax: 518-393-9607
                                        mjuda@ptopnys.org
                                        parenttoparentnys.org

Louise Nitto, President
Jim Costello, Vice President
Elizabeth Smithmeyer, Secretary
Michele Juda, Executive Director
Parent to Parent of NYS, which began in 1994, is a statewide not for profit organization established to support and connect families of individuals with special needs. The 13 offices, located throughout NYS, are staffed by Regional Coordinators, who are parents or close relatives of individuals with special needs.

3708   Protection and Advocacy Agency of NY
401 State St
Schenectady, NY   12305-2303   518-388-2892
                                        Fax: 518-388-2890

Andrew M. Cuomo, Governor
Roger Bearden, Chair
Bruce Blower, Member
Patricia Okoniewski, Member

3709   Regional Early Childhood Director Center
89 Washington Ave.
Room 580 EBA
Albany, NY   12234   518-474-2925
                                        800-222-5627
                                        accesadm@mail.nysed.gov
                                        www.acces.nysed.gov

3710   Schools And Services For Children With Autism Spectrum Disorders.
116 E 16th St
5th Floor
New York, NY   10003-2164   212-677-4650
                                        Fax: 212-254-4070
                                        info@resourcesnyc.org
                                        www.resourcesnyc.org

Ellen Miller-Wachtel, Chairman
Shon E. Glusky, President
Owen P. J. King, Treasurer
Rachel Howard, Executive Director
This publication fun resource for children provides extreme coverage of services for children with autism, asbergez syndrome, and/or PDD.

3711   Singeria/Metropolitan Parent Center
2082 Lexington Ave.
4th Floor
New York, NY   10035   212-643-2840
                                        866-867-9665
                                        Fax: 212-496-5608
                                        intake@sinergiany.org
                                        sinergiany.org

Len Torres, President
Johnny C. Rivera, Vice President
Paola Jordan, Treasurer
Donald Lash, Executive Director

3712 **Social Security: Albany Disability Determination**
1 Clinton Ave
Albany, NY 12207   518-431-4051
                                         800-772-1213
                                         TTY:518-431-4050
                                         www.ssa.gov

Karena L. Kilgore, Executive Secretary
Carolyn W. Colvin, Commissioner
Carolyn W. Colvin, Deputy Commissioner
James A. Kissko, Chief of Staff

3713 **State Agency for the Blind and Visually Impaired**
52 Washington St
Rensselaer, NY 12144-2834   518-473-7793
                                         866-871-3000
                                         Fax: 518-486-7550
                                         info@ocfs.state.ny.us
                                         www.ocfs.state.ny.us

3714 **State Education Agency Rural Representative**
89 Washington Avenue
Albany, NY 12234   518-474-3852
                                         Fax: 518-473-2860
                                         RegentsOffice@mail.nysed.gov
                                         www.nysed.gov
Merryl H. Tisch, Chancellor
Anthony S. Bottar, Vice Chancellor

3715 **State Mental Health Representative for Children and Youth**
44 Holland Ave
Albany, NY 12229   518-473-6328
                                         www.rcybc.ca
David Woodlock, Deputy Commissioner

3716 **State Mental Retardation Program**
44 Holland Ave
Albany, NY 12229   518-474-6601
                                         Fax: 518-473-1271
Diana Ritter, Manager

3717 **United We Stand of New York**
98 Moore St
Brooklyn, NY 11206-3326   718-302-4313
                                         Fax: 718-302-4315
                                         uwsofny@aol.com
Lourdes Rivera-Putz, Executive Director
Lourdes Figueroa, Intake/Receptionist
Carmen Soltero, Outreach/Trainer
Martha Vizcarrondo, Family Support Associate
Assists families with improving the quality of life for all individuals with disabilities.

3718 **University Afiliated Program/Rose F Kennedy Center**
1971
1300 Morris Park Avenue
Bronx, NY 10461   718-430-2000
                                         information@einstein.yu.edu
                                         www.einstein.yu.edu
Maris D. Rosenberg, Interim Director
Christine M. Baric, Assistant Director
John J. Foxe, Director
Robert W. Marion, Director

3719 **University of Rochester Medical Center**
601 Elmwood Ave
Rochester, NY 14642   585-275-8762
                                         Fax: 585-275-3366
                                         phil_davidson@urmc.rochester.edu
                                         www.rochester.edu
Brad Berk, MD, PhD, CEO

3720 **VESID**
New York State Education Department
89 Washington Ave.
Room 580 EBA
Albany, NY 12234   800-222-5627
                                         Fax: 518-474-8802
                                         accesadm@mail.nysed.gov
                                         www.acces.nysed.gov/vr/
Dr Rebecca Cort, Deputy Commissioner
Vocational and educational services for individuals with disabilities.

3721 **VSA Arts of New York City**
2700 F Street, NW
Washington, DC 20566   202-467-4600
                                         800-444-1324
                                         Fax: 717-225-6305
                                         bbvsanyc@msn.com
David M. Rubenstein, Chairman
Deborah F. Rutter, President
Christoph Eschenbach, Music Director
Roger L. Stevens, Founding Chairman
Provides art, educational and creative expression experiences to thousands of children, youth, and adults with disabilities who reside in the five boroughs of New York City. It provides opportunities for people with disabilities to demonstrate their accomplishments in the arts and foster increased understanding and acceptance.

3722 **Westchester Institute for Human Development**
Cedarwood Hall
Valhalla, NY 10595   914-493-8150
                                         info@WIHD.org
                                         www.wihd.org
William H. Bave, Chairman
Pamela Thornton, Vice Chairman
Ansley Bacon PhD, President/CEO
David M.C. Stern, Treasurer
WIHD advances policies and practices that foster the healthy development and ensure the safety of all children, strengthen families and communities, and promote health and well-being among people of all ages with disabilities and special health care needs.

3723 **Workers Compensation Board New York**
PO Box 5205
328 State Street
Schenectady, NY 12305-2318   518-462-8880
                                         877-632-4996
                                         Fax: 518-473-1415
                                         general_information@wcb.ny.gov
                                         www.wcb.ny.gov
Andrew M. Cuomo, Governor
Robert E. Beloten, Chairman
Richard A. Bell, Commissioner

North Carolina

3724 **Developmental Disability Services Section**
Building 325n
Albemarle
Raleigh, NC 27699   919-420-7901
                                         Fax: 919-420-7917
                                         www.dhhs.state.nc.us/mhddsas/
Diana Simmons, Human Resources Manager
Ureh N. Lekwauwa, Chief, Clinical Policy
Courtney Cantrell, Acting Director
Jim Jarrard, Deputy Director
Makes policies and monitors public services and supports to people with mental illness, developmental disabilities and substance abuse throughout North Carolina.

3725 **International Dyslexia Association: North Carolina Branch**
NC   nc.dyslexiaida.org
Kris Cox, President

Provides free information and referral services for diagnosis and tutoring for parents, educators, physicians, and individuals with dyslexia in Illinois. Membership includes yearly journal and quarterly newsletter.

3726 North Carolina Workers Compensation Board
4340 Mail Service Center
Raleigh, NC 27699-4340　　　　　919-807-2501
　　　　　　　　　　　　　　　　800-688-8349
　　　　　　　　　　　　　　Fax: 919-508-8210
　　　　　　　　　　　　　　infospec@ic.nc.gov
　　　　　　　　　　　　　　www.ic.nc.gov

Julian Bunn, Owner

3727 North Carolina Assistive Technology Project
1110 Navaho Dr
Suite 101
Raleigh, NC 27609-7322　　　　　919-872-2298
　　　　　　　　　　　　　　Fax: 919-850-2792
　　　　　　　　　　　　　　ncatp.org

Ricki Cook, Project Director
Annette Lauber, Funding Specialist
Jacquelyne Gordon, Consumer Resource Specialist
Tony Hiatt, Executive Director
The North Carolina Assistive Technology Project exists to create a statewide, consumer-responsive system of assistive technology services for all North Carolinians with disabilities. The project's activities impact children and adults with disabilities across all aspects of their lives.

3728 North Carolina Children & Youth Branch
North Carolina Publc of Health
1928 Mail Service Ctr
Raleigh, NC 27699-1900　　　　　919-839-6262
　　　　　　　　　　　　　　Fax: 919-733-8034
　　　　　　　　　　　　　　cathy.kluttz@nemail.net

Lawrence J Wheeler, Manager
Cathy Kluttz, Unit Manager Special Service
Dianne Tyson, Help Line Manager
Ran Coble, Executive Director

3729 North Carolina Client Assistance Program
2806 Mail Service Ctr
Raleigh, NC 27699-2806　　　　　919-855-3600
　　　　　　　　　　　　　　800-215-7227
　　　　　　　　　　　　　　Fax: 919-715-2456
　　　　　　　　　　　　　　nccap@dhhs.nc.gov
　　　　　　　　　　　　　　cap.state.nc.us

John Marens, Director
Diane Rawdarowicz, Client Advocate
Sharon Wisner, Client Advocate
Tami Andrews, Processing Assistant
A federally funded program designed to assist individuals with disabilities in understanding and using rehabilitation services. CAP serves as an integral part of the rehabilitation system by advising and informing individuals of all services and benefits available to them through programs authorized under both the Rehabilitation Act and Title 1 of the Americans with Disabilities Act.

3730 North Carolina Developmental Disabilities
3125 Poplarwood Court
Suite 200
Raleigh, NC 27604-7368　　　　　919-850-2901
　　　　　　　　　　　　　　800-357-6916
　　　　　　　　　　　　　　Fax: 919-850-2915
　　　　　　　　　　　　　　Info@nccdd.org
　　　　　　　　　　　　　　www.nc-ddc.org

Caroline Valand, Executive Director
A planning council established to assure that individuals with developmental disabilities and their families participate in the planning of and have access to culturally competent services, supports, and other assistance and opportunities that promote independence, productivity, and integration and inclusion into the community; and to promote, through systemic change, capacity building and advocacy activities, a consumer and family-centered comprehensive system.

3731 North Carolina Division of Aging
2101 Mail Service Ctr
Raleigh, NC 27699-2001　　　　　919-855-4800
　　　　　　　　　　　　　　Fax: 919-733-0443
　　　　　　　　　　　　　　ncdhhs.gov

Dennis Streets, Manager
Jim Slate, Director
Laketha Miller, Controller
Emery Edwards Milliken, General Counsel

3732 North Carolina Industrial Commission
4340 Mail Service Center
Raleigh, NC 27699-4340　　　　　919-807-2501
　　　　　　　　　　　　　　800-688-8349
　　　　　　　　　　　　　　Fax: 919-508-8210
　　　　　　　　　　　　　　infospec@ic.nc.gov
　　　　　　　　　　　　　　www.ic.nc.gov

J Howard Bunn Jr, Chairman
Peg Dorer, Executive Director

3733 Social Security Administration
4701 Old Wake Forest Rd
Raleigh, NC 27609-4919　　　　　877-803-6311
　　　　　　　　　　　　　　800-772-1213
　　　　　　　　　　　　　　800-325-0778
　　　　　　　　　　　　　　Fax: 919-790-2860
　　　　　　　　　　　　　　TTY:919-790-2773
　　　　　　　　　　　　　　www.socialsecurity.gov

Karena L. Kilgore, Executive Secretary
Carolyn W. Colvin, Commissioner
Carolyn W. Colvin, Deputy Commissioner
James A. Kissko, Chief of Staff
Provides information on how to obtain social security through a disability.

North Dakota

3734 Division of Mental Health and Substance Abuse
600 East Boulevard Avenue
Dept 325
Bismarck, ND 58505- 0250　　　　701-328-2310
　　　　　　　　　　　　　　800-472-2622
　　　　　　　　　　　　　　Fax: 701-328-2359
　　　　　　　　　　　　　　dhseo@nd.gov
　　　　　　　　　　　　　　www.nd.gov/humanservices

Dennis Goetz, Executive Director
Kerry Wicks, Executive Director
Andrew J. McLean, Medical Director
Alex Schweitzer, Superintendent
The Department of Human Services' Mental Health and Substance Abuse Services Division provides leadership for the planning, development, and oversight of a system of care for children, adults, and families with severe emotional disorders, mental illness, and/or substance abuse issues.

3735 North Dakota Workers Compensation Board
50 E Front Ave
Bismarck, ND 58504　　　　　　701-328-3800
　　　　　　　　　　　　　　800-777-5033
　　　　　　　　　　　　　　Fax: 701-329-9911
　　　　　　　　　　　　　　TTY: 701-328-3786

Brent Edison, Director

3736 North Dakota Client Assistance Program
400 East Broadway
Suite 409
Bismarck, ND 58501-4071　　　　701-328-2950
　　　　　　　　　　　　　　800-472-2670
　　　　　　　　　　　　　　Fax: 701-328-3934
　　　　　　　　　　　　　　panda@nd.gov
　　　　　　　　　　　　　　www.ndpanda.org/cap

Dennis Lyon, CEO
Janelle Olson, Advocate
Paula Rustad, Office Assistant
Angie Dubovoy, Advocate

CAP assists clients and client applicants of North Dakota Vocational Rehabilitation services, Tribal Vocational Rehabilitation, or Independent Living services.

3737 North Dakota Department of Human Resources
1237 W Divide Ave
Suite 6
Bismarck, ND 58501-1208

701-328-5300
800-451-8693
Fax: 701-328-5320
dhsaging@nd.gov
www.nd.gov

Shane Goettle, Manager

3738 North Dakota Department of Human Services
600 E Boulevard Ave
Dept 325
Bismarck, ND 58505-0250

701-328-2310
800-472-2622
Fax: 701-328-2359
dhseo@nd.gov
www.nd.gov/dhs

Carol K Olson, Executive Director
Dennis Goetz, Executive Director
Kerry Wicks, Executive Director
Andrew J. McLean, Medical Director
Provides services that help vulnerable North Dakotans of all ages to maintain or enhance their quality of life, which may be threatened by lack of financial resources, emotional crises, disabling conditions, or an inability to protect themselves.

3739 Protection & Advocacy Project
1984
400 East Broadway
Suite 409
Bismarck, ND 58501-4071

701-328-2950
800-472-2670
Fax: 701-328-3934
panda@nd.gov
ndpanda.org

Teresa Larsen, Executive Director
Janelle Olson, Advocate
Paula Rustad, Office Assistant
Angie Dubovoy, Advocate
The Protection and Advocacy is a state agency whose purpose is to advocate for and protect the rights of people with disabilities. The Protection and Advocacy Project has programs to serve people with developmental disabilities, mental illnesses and other types of disabilities. The projects programs and services are free to eligible individuals.

3740 Social Security: Bismarck Disability Determination
1680 E Capitol Ave
Bismarck, ND 58501-5603

701-250-4200
800-772-1213
TTY:701-250-4620
ssa.gov

Karena L. Kilgore, Executive Secretary
Carolyn W. Colvin, Commissioner
Carolyn W. Colvin, Deputy Commissioner
James A. Kissko, Chief of Staff

3741 Workers Compensation Board North Dakota
1600 East Century Avenue
Suite 1
Bismarck, ND 58503-649

701-328-3800
800-777-5033
Fax: 701-328-3820
www.workforcesafety.com

Sandy Blunt, CEO

3742 Epilepsy Council of Greater Cincinnati
Ste 550
895 Central Ave
Cincinnati, OH 45202-5700

513-721-2905
877-804-2241
Fax: 513-721-0799
ecgc@fuse.net

Kathy Stewart, Executive Director

3743 International Dyslexia Association: Central Ohio Branch
P.O. Box 1601
Westerville, OH 43086

614-899-5711
info@cobida.org
coh.dyslexiaida.org

Mike McGovern, President
Blythe Wood, Vice President
Chris Lowe, Secretary
Diana McGovern, Treasurer
Provides free information and referral services for diagnosis and tutoring for parents, educators, physicians, and individuals with dyslexia. Membership includes yearly journal and quarterly newsletter.

3744 Ohio Bureau for Children with Medical Handicaps
Ohio Department of Health
246 N. High St
P.O. Box 1603
Columbus, OH 43215-1603

614-466-3543
800-755-4769
Fax: 614-728-3616
bcmh@odh.ohio.gov
www.odh.ohio.gov

John R. Kasich, Governor
James Bryant Md, Bureau Chief
Alvin Jackson, MD, Director
Lance D. Himes, Interim Director
Provides funding for the diagnosis, treatment and coordination of services for eligible Ohio children, under age 21, with medical handicaps; conducts quality assurance activities to establish standards of care and determine unmet needs of children with handicaps and their families; collaborates with public health nurses to increase access to care; and assists families to access and use third party resources. Conducts a separate program for adults with cystic fibrosis.

3745 Ohio Bureau of Worker's Compensation
30 W Spring St
Columbus, OH 43215-2256

800-335-0996
Fax: 877-321-9481
TTY:614-292-4833
ombudsperson@bwc.state.oh.us
www.bwc.ohio.gov

Stephen Buehrer, Administrator/CEO
Dale Hamilton, Chief Operating Officer (COO)
Kevin Abrams, Chief of Employers Services
Toni Brokaw, Chief of Human Resources
To provide a quality, customer-focused workers' compensation insurance system for Ohio's employers and employees.

3746 Ohio Client Assistance Program
50 W. Broad St.
Suite 1400
Columbus, OH 43215-5923

614-466-7264
800-282-9181
Fax: 614-752-4197
TTY: 614-728-2553
www.olrs.ohio.gov

Donald Bishop, Executive Director

3747 Ohio Department of Aging
1982
50 W Broad St
Fl 9
Columbus, OH   43215-3363   614-466-5500
                                         866-243-5678
                                         888-243-5678
                                         Fax: 614-466-5741
                                         TTY:614-466-6191
                                         www.aging.ohio.gov

Bonnie Kantor-Burman, Director
John Ratliff, Public Information Officer
The department serves and represents about 2 million Ohioans
age 60 & older. They advocate for the needs of all older citizens
with emphasis on improving the quality of life, helping senior citizens live active, healthy, & independent lives, & promoting positive attitudes toward aging & older people. Committed to helping
the frail elderly who choose to remain at home by providing home
& community based services, their goal is to promote the level of
choice, independence & self-care.

3748 Ohio Department of Mental Health
30 E Broad St
8th Floor
Columbus, OH   43215-3414   614-466-4775
                                         877-275-6364
                                         Fax: 614-752-8410
                                         uhricks@mh.state.oh.us

Michael Hogan, Director
Christine Vincenty, Manager

3749 Ohio Developmental Disabilities Council
899 E Broad St, Ste 203
Columbus, OH   43205   614-466-5205
                                         800-766-7426
                                         Fax: 614-466-0298
                                         www.ddc.ohio.gov

Carolyn Knight, Executive Director
Mark Seifarth, Chair
Robert Shuemak, Vice Chair
Kimberly Stults, Secretary
The Ohio Developmental Disabilities Council is one of 55 councils found in all states and territories which provides funding for
systems change grant projects. The DD Council is a planning and
advocacy agency that seeks to improve the lives of Ohioans with
disabilities.

3750 Ohio Developmental Disability Council (ODDC)
899 E Broad St, Ste 203
Columbus, OH   43205   614-466-5205
                                         800-766-7426
                                         Fax: 614-466-0298
                                         www.ddc.ohio.gov

Carolyn Knight, Executive Director
Mark Seifarth, Chair
Robert Shuemak, Vice Chair
Kimberly Stults, Secretary

3751 Ohio Governor's Council on People with Disabilities
400 E Campus View Blvd
Columbus, OH   43235-4685   614-438-1200
                                         800-282-4536
                                         RSC.Webmaster@rsc.state.oh.us
                                         gcpd.ohio.gov

Jacqueline Romer-Sensky, Chairman
Jack Licate, Vice Chairman
Kevin Miller, Executive Director
Bill Bishilany, Assistant Executive Director
The Governor's Council on People with Disabilities exists to:
Advise the Governor and General Assembly on statewide disability issues, promote the value of diversity, dignity and the quality
of life for people with disabilities, be a catalyst to create systemic
change promoting awareness of disability-related issues that will
ultimately benefit all citizens of Ohio, Educate and advocate for:
partnerships at the local, state and national level, promotion of
equality, access and independence.

3752 Ohio Rehabilitation Services Commission
400 E Campus View Blvd
Columbus, OH   43235-4604   614-438-1200
                                         800-282-4536
                                         ohio.gov

Kevin Miller, Executive Director
RSC is Ohio's state agency that provides vocational rehabilitation (VR) services to help people with disabilities become employed and independent. We also offer a variety of services to
Ohio businesses, resulting in quality jobs for individuals who
have disabilities.

**3753 Ohio Women, Infants, & Children Program - Ohio
Department of Health**
246 N High St
Columbus, OH   43215-2406   614-644-8006
                                         Fax: 614-564-2470

Michele Frizzell, Chief, Bureau of Nutrition Svcs.

3754 Social Security: Columbus Disability Determination
90 E Washington Bridge Rd
Suite 140
Worthington, OH 43085   614-888-5339
                                         800-772-1213
                                         TTY:614-288-0226
                                         www.socialsecurity.gov

Karena L. Kilgore, Executive Secretary
Carolyn W. Colvin, Commissioner
Carolyn W. Colvin, Deputy Commissioner
James A. Kissko, Chief of Staff

Oklahoma

3755 Oklahoma Workers Compensation Board
Department of Labor
3017 N. Stiles, Suite 100
Oklahoma City, OK   73105   405-521-6100
                                         888-269-5353
                                         Fax: 405-521-6018
                                         labor.info@labor.ok.gov
                                         www.ok.gov/odol

Jim Marshall, Chief of Staff
Mark Costello, Commissioner of Labor
Lizzette McNeill, Communications Director
Stacy Bonner, Deputy Commissioner

**3756 Oklahoma Client Assistance Program/Office of Disability
Concerns**
2401 NW 23rd Street
Suite 90
Oklahoma City, OK   73107- 2431   405-521-3756
                                         800-522-8224
                                         Fax: 405-522-6695
                                         www.ok.gov

Todd Lamb, Governor
Gary Jones, Auditor and Inspector
E. Scott Pruitt, Attorney General
Ken Miller, Treasurer
CAP informs and advises applicants and consumers about the vo-
cational rehabilitation process and services available under the
Federal Rehabilitation Act, including services provided by DVR
and DVS. CAP staff can help you communicate concerns to the
DVR/DVS and assist you with administrative, mediation, fair
hearing, legal and other solutions

**3757 Oklahoma Department of Human Services Aging Services
Division**
25 Sigourney Street, 10th Floor
Hartford, CT   06106   405-521-3646
                                         866-218-6621
                                         800-522-7233
                                         Fax: 860-424-5301

Margaret Ger Murkette, MSW, Director
Ed Lake, Director

3758   Oklahoma Department of Labor
3017 N. Stiles
Suite 100
Oklahoma City, OK   73105-5206   405-521-6100
                                              888-269-5353
                                        Fax: 405-521-6018
                                        www.labor.ok.gov

Mark Castello, Commissioner
Jim Marshall, Chief of Staff
Stacy Bonner, Deputy Commissioner
Don Schooler, General Counsel

**3759   Oklahoma Department of Mental Health & Substance
Abuse Services**
1200 NE 13th Street
P.O.Box 53277
Oklahoma City, OK 73152-3277   405-522-3908
                                              800-522-9054
                                        Fax: 405-522-3650
                                        TTY: 405-522-3851
                                        www.odmhsas.org

J. Andy Sullivan, Chairperson
Gail Henderson, Vice-Chair
Terri White, Commissioner
Durand Crosby, Chief Operating Officer
State agency providing mental helath , substance abuse and do-
mestic violence services.

3760   Oklahoma Department of Rehabilitation Services
3535 NW 58th St.
Suite 500
Oklahoma City, OK   73112-4824   405-951-3400
                                              800-845-8476
                                        Fax: 405-951-3529
                                        info@okdrs.gov
                                        www.okdrs.gov
Noel Tyler, Director
The Oklahoma Department of Rehabilitation Services (DRS)
provides assistance to Oklahomans with disabilities through vocational rehabilitation, employment, independent living, residential and outreach programs, and the determination of medical
eligibility for disability benefits.

3761   Workers Compensation Board Oklahoma
1915 N Stiles Ave
Oklahoma City, OK   73105-4918   405-522-8600
                                              800-522-8210

Leroy E Young, D.O., Chairman
Joyce Sanders, Supervisor
Michael J. Harkey, Vice Presiding Judge
Katrina Stephenson, Assistant Court Clerk

Oregon

3762   International Dyslexia Association: Oregon Branch
International Dyslexia Association
P.P. Box 2609
Portland, OR   97208-2609   503-228-4455
                                        info@orbida.org
                                        or.dyslexiaida.org

Jane Cooper, President
Danielle Thompson, Vice President
Anne Mauboussin, Treasurer
Christy Coss, Secretary
Provides free information and referral services for diagnosis and
tutoring for parents, educators, physicians, and individuals with
dyslexia. Membership includes yearly journal and quarterly
newsletter.

3763   Office of Vocational Rehabilitation Services (OVRS)
500 Summer St NE
Salem, OR   97301-1063   503-945-5944
                                        Fax: 503-378-2897
                                        TTY:503-945-6214
                                        www.oregon.gov/dhs

Erinn Kelley-Siel, Director
Gene Evans, Communication Director
Eric Moore, Chief Financial Officer
Jim Scherzinger, Chief Operating Officer
The mission of OVRS to assist Oregonians with disabilities to
achieve and maintain employment and independence.

3764   Oregon Advocacy Center
620 SW 5th Ave
5th Floor
Portland, OR   97204-1428   503-243-2081
                                              800-452-6094
                                        Fax: 503-243-1738
                                        TTY: 800-556-5351
                                        welcome@oradvocacy.org
                                        oradvocacy.org

Robert Joondeph, Executive Director
Barbara Herget, Operations Director
The protection and advocacy system for Oregon.

3765   Oregon Client Assistance Program
620 SW 5th Ave
5th Floor
Portland, OR   97204-1420   503-243-2081
                                        Fax: 503-243-1738
                                        TTY:800-556-5351
                                        oradvocacy.org

Robert Joondeph, Executive Director

3766   Oregon Department of Mental Health
500 Summer St NE
Salem, OR   97301-1063   503-945-5944
                                        Fax: 503-378-2897
                                        TTY:503-945-6214
                                        www.oregon.gov/DHS

Erinn Kelley-Siel, Director
Gene Evans, Communication Director
Eric Moore, Chief Financial Officer
Jim Scherzinger, Chief Operating Officer
Sets out the purpose and guides the activities of our large, com-
plex organization. Vision is for better outcomes for clients and
communities through collaboration, integration and shared
responsibility.

3767   Oregon Technology Access for Life
2225 Lancaster Drive NE
Salem, OR   97305-1396   503-361-1201
                                              800-677-7512
                                        Fax: 503-370-4530
                                        TTY: 503-361-1201
                                        www.accesstechnologiesinc.org

Laurie Brooks, President
A statewide program promoting assistive technology devices and
services for persons of all ages with all disabilities.

3768   Social Security: Salem Disability Determination
90 E Washington Bridge Rd
Suite 140
Worthington, OH 43085-3772   614-888-5339
                                              800-722-1213
                                        TTY:614-288-0226
                                        www.socialsecurity.gov

Karena L. Kilgore, Executive Secretary
Carolyn W. Colvin, Commissioner
Carolyn W. Colvin, Deputy Commissioner
James A. Kissko, Chief of Staff

3769 Vocational Rehabilitation Agency: Oregon Commission for the Blind
535 SE 12th Ave.
Portland, OR 97214-2408
971-673-1588
888-202-5463
Fax: 503-234-7468
ocb.mail@state.or.us
www.oregon.gov/blind

Dacia Johnson, Executive Director
A resource for visually impaired Oregonians, as well as their families, friends, and employers. Nationally recognized programs and staff that make a difference in people's lives every day.

3770 Washington County Disability, Aging and Veteran Services
Ste 208
180 E Main St
Hillsboro, OR 97123-4054
503-640-3489
Fax: 503-693-6124
www.co.washington.or.us/aging

Jeff Hill, Director
Janet Long, Support Staff
Provides services to individuals through the Older Americans Act, state in home care services and represent, veterans in benefit claims process with Federal VA.

Pennsylvania

3771 Disability Rights of Pennsylvania (DRP)
Harrisburg Office
301 Chestnut St
Suite 300
Harrisburg, PA 17101
717-839-5235
800-692-7443
Fax: 717-236-0192
TTY: 877-375-7139
ldo@disabilityrightspa.org
www.disabilityrightspa.org

Jeneice Davis, Chairman
Peri Jude Radecic, CEO
Kelly Darr, Legal Director
Judy Banks, Programs Director
The Disability Rights of Pennsylvania is a statewide, non-profit corporation dedicated to advancing and protecting the civil rights of adults and children with disabilities by ensuring access to community services, a full and inclusive education and the freedom to live free of discrimination, abuse and neglect.

3772 International Dyslexia Association: Pennsylvania Branch
1062 E. Lancaster Ave.
Suite 15A
Rosemont, PA 19010
610-527-1548
855-220-8885
www.pbida.org

Lisa Goldstein, President
Tracy Bowes, Office Manager
Provides free information and referral services for diagnosis and tutoring for parents, educators, physicians, and individuals with dyslexia. Membership includes yearly journal and quarterly newsletter, and Pennsylvania newsletter.

3773 Mental Health Association in Pennsylvania
1414 N Cameron St
1st Floor
Harrisburg, PA 17103-1049
717-346-0549
855-220-8885
Fax: 717-236-0192
mfo@mhapa.org
www.mhapa.org

Julia Walker, Esq., President
Michael Brody, President & CEO
Marge Dailey, Director of Human Resources
Anthony Schweitzer, Treasurer
The Mental Health Association in Pennysylvania is a non-profit providing services to those struggling with mental health issues. Services include advocacy, education and public policy.

3774 Pennsylvania Workers Compensation Board
651 Boas Street
Room 1700
Harrisburg, PA 17121-2510
717-787-5279
Fax: 717-772-0342
dli.state.pa.us

Joseph Brimmeier, CEO

3775 Pennsylvania Bureau of Blindness & Visual Services
Department of Pennsylvania
1521 N 6th St
Harrisburg, PA 17102
717-787-3201
800-622-2842
Fax: 717-787-3210
www.dli.state.pa.us

David Denotaris, Director
Jennifer Cave, Clerk Typist 3
Offers services for the totally blind, legally blind, visually impaired, mentally retarded blind and more with health, counseling, educational, recreational, rehabilitation, computer training and professional training services.

3776 Pennsylvania Client Assistance Program
1515 Market Street
Suite 1300
Philadelphia, PA 19102- 1819
215-557-7112
888-745-2357
Fax: 215-557-7602
www.equalemployment.org

Stephen S. Pennington, Executive Director
Jamie C Ray, Assistant Director
Margaret Passio-McKenna, Senior Advocate
Lee Lippi, Advocate
The Pennsylvania Client Assistance Program is dedicated to ensuring that the rehabilitation system in Pennsylvania is open and responsive to your needs. CAP help is provided to you at no charge, regardless of income. CAP helps people who are seeking services from the Office of Vocational Rehabilitation, Blindness and Visual Services, Centers for Independent Living and other programs funded under federal law.

3777 Pennsylvania Department of Aging
555 Walnut St
5th Floor
Harrisburg, PA 17101-1919
717-783-1550
Fax: 717-783-6842
aging@pa.gov
www.aging.state.pa.us

Nora Eisenhower, Manager

3778 Pennsylvania Department of Children with Disabilities
P.O. Box 2675
Harrisburg, PA 17105-2675
717-787-2600
Fax: 717-772-0323
www.pachildren.state.pa.US

Tom Corbett, Governor
Shelly Yanoff, Commission Chair

3779 Pennsylvania Developmental Disabilities Council
605 South Drive
Room 561
Harrisburg, PA 17120
717-789-6057
877-685-4452
TTY:717-705-0819
www.paddc.org

Amy High, Vice Chairperson
Graham Mulholland, Executive Director
Sandra Amador Dusek, Deputy Director

3780 Public Interest Law Center of Philadelphia
United Way Building, 2nd Floor
1709 Benjamin Franklin Parkway
Philadelphia, PA   19103-5153   215-627-7100
                                        Fax: 215-627-3183
                                        general@pilcop.org
                                        pilcop.org

Eric J. Rothschild, Chair
Brian T. Feeney, Vice Chair
Jennifer R. Clarke, Executive Director
Latrice Brooks, Director of Administration
A non-profit, public interest law firm with a Disabilities Project
specializing in class action suits brought by individuals and orga-
nizations.

3781 Social Security: Harrisburg Disability Determination
Suite 160
90 E Washington Bridge Rd
Worthington, OH 17101-1925   614-888-5339
                                        800-722-1213
                                        TTY:614-288-0226
                                        ssa.gov

Karena L. Kilgore, Executive Secretary
Carolyn W. Colvin, Commissioner
Carolyn W. Colvin, Deputy Commissioner
James A. Kissko, Chief of Staff

3782 Workers Compensation Board Pennsylvania
651 Boas Street
Room 1700
Harrisburg, PA   17121-2510   717-787-5279
                                        Fax: 717-772-0342
                                        www.dli.state.pa.us

Tom Corbett, Governor
Julia K. Hearthway, Secretary
Joseph Brimmeier, CEO

Rhode Island

3783 Department of Mental Health, Retardation and Hospitals of Rhode Island
Goverment of Rhode Isalnd
14 Harrington Rd
Cranston, RI   02920-3080   401-462-2339
                                        Fax: 401-462-3204
                                        Craig.Stenning@bhddh.ri.gov
                                        www.bhddh.ri.gov/

Craig S. Stenning, Director
Ellen Nelson, Manager
Kathleen Spangler, Manager
State department responsible for creating and administering systems of care for individuals with disabilities, specifically focused
on mental health and mental illness; developmental disabilities,
substance abuse and long term hospital care.

3784 Rhode Island Department Health
3 Capitol Hl
Providence, RI   02908-5097   401-222-3855
                                        Fax: 401-222-6548

Mary Salerno, Manager
Patricia Nolan, Executive Director
Pamela Corcoran, Disability Health Program

3785 Rhode Island Department of Elderly Affairs
74 West Road
Hazard Bldg, 2nd Floor
Cranston, RI   02920- 3001   401-462-3000
                                        Fax: 401-462-0740
                                        www.dea.state.ri.us

Corrine Russo, Manager

3786 Rhode Island Department of Mental Health
Cottage 405 Court B
Cranston, RI   02920   401-462-2003
                                        Fax: 401-462-2008
                                        www.butler.org

George W. Shuster, Chairman
Dennis D. Keefe, President & CEO
Reed Cosper, Manager

3787 Rhode Island Developmental Disabilities Council
400 Bald Hill Rd
Suite 515
Warwick, RI   02886-1692   401-737-1238
                                        Fax: 401-737-3395
                                        TTY:401-737-1238
                                        riddc@riddc.org
                                        www.riddc.org

Charles Zawacki, Chairperson, Individual & Family
John Susa, Chairperson, Executive Committee
Anne Frank, Chairperson, Individual & Family
Mary Okero, Executive Director
The Rhode Island Developmental Disabilities Council works to
make Rhode Island a better place for people with developmental
disabilities to live, work, go to school, and be part of their
community.

3788 Rhode Island Disability Law Center
275 Westminster St
Suite 401
Providence, RI   02903-3434   401-831-3150
                                        800-733-5332
                                        Fax: 401-274-5568
                                        TTY: 401-831-5335
                                        info@ridlc.org
                                        www.ridlc.org

Raymond A Marcaccio, Esq., Chair
Raymond L Bandusky, Executive Director
Darby Castigliego, Director of Finance & Administration
Minerva Doti, Intake Advocate
The Rhode Island Disability Law Center (RIDLC) provides free
legal assistance to persons with disabilities. Services include individual representation to protect rights or to secure benefits and
services, self-help information, educational programs and administrative and legislative advocacy.

3789 Rhode Island Governor's Commission on Disabilities
John O Pastore Center
Warwick City Hall
3275 Post Road
Warwick, RI   02920-3049   401-738-2000
                                        Fax: 401-462-0106
                                        www.warwickri.gov

Bob Cooper, Executive Secretary
The Commision is responsible for: coordinating compliance by
state agencies with federal and state disablity right laws; approv-
ing or modifying state and local goverment agency's open meeting accessibility for persons with disabilities transition plans;
assisting local boards of canvassers to ensure accessible polling
places locations; aproving or rejecting requests to waive the state
building code's standards for accessibility at facilities to be
leased by state agencies...

3790 Rhode Island Parent Information Network
1210 Pontiac Avenue
Cranston, RI   02920   401-270-0101
                                        800-464-3399
                                        Fax: 401-270-7049
                                        info@ripin.org
                                        ripin.org

Kathleen DiChiara, Chairman
Ammala Douangsavanh, Vice Chairman
Stephen Brunero, Executive Director
Matthew Cox, Associate Exeutive Director
A nonprofit organization established by parents and concerned
professionals providing culturally appropriate information,
training and support for families and professionals designed to
improve educational and life outcomes for all children. Serving
the State of Rhode Island.

3791 Rhode Island Services for the Blind and Visually Impaired
40 Fountain St
Providence, RI   02903-1830
401-421-7005
800-752-8088
Fax: 401-421-9259
TTY: 401-421-7016
www.ors.ri.gov

Kathleen Grygiel, Administrator
Ronald Racine, Associate Director
Laurie DiOrio, Acting Associate Director
JoAnn Nannig, Assistant Administrator of VR
Offers services for the totally blind, legally blind, visually impaired, mentally retarded blind and more with health, counseling, educational, recreational, rehabilitation, computer training and professional training services.

3792 Services for the Blind and Visually Impaired
40 Fountain St
Providence, RI   02903-1830
401-421-7005
Fax: 401-222-1328
TTY:401-421-7016
www.ors.ri.gov

Kathleen Grygiel, Administrator
Ronald Racine, Associate Director
Laurie DiOrio, Acting Associate Director
JoAnn Nannig, Assistant Administrator of VR
Offers services for the blind and visually impaired.

3793 Social Security: Providence Disability Determination
Social Security
40 Fountain Street
6th Floor
Providence, RI   02903-3246
401-222-3182
800-772-1213
Fax: 401-222-3868
TTY: 401-273-6648
Deborah.A.Cannon@ssa.gov
www.ssa.gov

Karena L. Kilgore, Executive Secretary
Carolyn W. Colvin, Commissioner
Carolyn W. Colvin, Deputy Commissioner
James A. Kissko, Chief of Staff
We deliver services through a nationwide network of over 1,400 offices that include regional offices, field offices, card centers, teleservice centers, processing centers, hearing offices, the Appeals Council, and our State and territorial partners, the Disability Determination Services. We also have a presence in U.S. embassies around the globe. For the public, we are the face of the government. The rich diversity of our employees mirrors the public we serve.

3794 Workers Compensation Board Rhode Island
1 Dorrance Plz
Providence, RI 02903-3973
401-458-5000
Fax: 401-222-3121

George E Healy Jr, Manager
George Healy Jr, Manager

South Carolina

3795 Protection & Advocacy for People with Disabilities
Ste 208
3710 Landmark Dr
Columbia, SC   29204-4034
803-782-0639
866-275-7273
Fax: 803-790-1946
TTY: 866-232-4525
info@pandasc.org
protectionandadvocacy-sc.org

Gloria Prevost, Executive Director
Anne Trice, Director of Administration
J. Ashley Twombley, Chair
Sherry Williams, Vice-Chair
An independent, nonprofit organization responsible for safe guarding rights of South Carolinians with disabilities and other handicapped individuals without regard to age, income, severity of disability, sex, race, or religion.

3796 Social Security: West Columbia Disability Determination
P.O. Box 60
Columbia, SC   29171-0060
803-896-6400
800-772-1213
Fax: 803-822-4318
TTY: 800-325-0078
Kenneth.Norris@ssa.gov
www.socialsecurity.gov

Karena L. Kilgore, Executive Secretary
Carolyn W. Colvin, Commissioner
Carolyn W. Colvin, Deputy Commissioner
James A. Kissko, Chief of Staff
We deliver services through a nationwide network of over 1,400 offices that include regional offices, field offices, card centers, teleservice centers, processing centers, hearing offices, the Appeals Council, and our State and territorial partners, the Disability Determination Services. We also have a presence in U.S. embassies around the globe. For the public, we are the face of the government. The rich diversity of our employees mirrors the public we serve.

3797 South Carolina Assistive Technology Project
Midlands Center
8301 Farrow Road
Columbia, SC   29203
803-935-5263
800-915-4522
Fax: 803-935-5342
TTY: 803-935-5263
jjendron@usit.net
www.sc.edu/scatp/

Carol Page, Ph.D, CCC-SLP, A, Program Director
Janet Jendron, Program Coordinator
Mary Alice Bechtler, Program Coordinator
Lydia Durham, Administrative Assistant
A statewide program promoting assistive technology devices and services for persons of all ages with all disabilities. Recently a statewide AT resource, demonstrations and equipment loan center and lab annual expo and training and workshops on a variety of disabilities and technology topics.

3798 South Carolina Client Assistance Program
Governor's Office oe Executive Policy & Programs
1205 Pendleton St
Columbia, SC   29201-3756
803-734-0285
800-868-0040
Fax: 803-734-0546
TTY: 803-734-1147
cap@oepp.sc.gov

Denise Riley Pensmith, MSW, Executive Director
Cindy Popenhagen, Administrative Assistant
The Client Assistance Program (CAP) helps citizens of the State by acting as advocates regarding services provided by the Vocational Rehabilitation Department (VR), Commission for the Blind, and all Independent Living programs and projects funded under the Rehabilitation Act of 1973. As advocates, CAP staff can investigate, negotiate, mediate, and pursue administrative, and other remedies to ensure that clients' rights are protected.

3799 South Carolina Commission for the Blind
1430 Confederate Avenue
P. O. Box 2467
Columbia, SC 29202-79
803-898-8731
800-922-2222
888-335-5951
Fax: 803-898-8800
publicinfo@sccb.sc.gov
www.sccb.state.sc.us

James Kirby, Commissioner
Peter Smith, Board Member
Dr. Julianne Kleckley, Board Member
Dr. Julia Barnes, Board Member
Offers services for the totally blind, legally blind, visually impaired, mentally retarded blind and more with health, counseling, educational, recreational, rehabilitation, computer training and professional training services.

3800 South Carolina Department of Children with Disabilities
2600 Bull St
Columbia, SC 29201-1708   803-434-4260
Miroslav Cuturic, Director
Peter Getz, Administrator

3801 South Carolina Department of Mental Healthand Mental Retardation
Administration Building
2414 Bull Streets
Columbia, SC 29202-485   803-898-8581
                                  800-273-8255
                          Fax: 864-297-5130
                          webmaster@scdmh.org
                          www.state.sc.us/dmh

John H. Magill, State Director
Mark Binkley, Deputy Director
David Schaefer, Director
Eleanor Odom, Director
The S.C. Department of Mental Health gives priority to adults, children, and their families affected by serious mental illnesses and significant emotional disorders. We are committed to eliminating stigma and promoting the philosophy of recovery, to achieving our goals in collaboration with all stakeholders, and to assuring the highest quality of culturally competent services possible.

3802 South Carolina Developmental Disabilities Council
Office of the Governor
1205 Pendleton St
Suite 461
Columbia, SC 29201-3756   803-734-0465
                          Fax: 803-734-1409
                          TTY:803-734-1147
                          jvancleave@oepp.sc.gov
                          www.scddc.state.sc.us

Valarie Bishop, Executive Director
Cheryl English, Program Information Coordinator
Kimberly Johnson Fontanez, Grants Administrator
Esther Williams, Administrative Support Specialis
The mission of the South Carolina Developmental Disabilities Council is to provide leadership in advocating, funding and implementing initiatives which recognize the inherent dignity of each individual, and promote independence, productivity, respect and inclusion for all persons with disabilities and their families.

3803 Workers Compensation Board: South Carolina
PO Box 1715
Columbia, SC 29202-1715   803-737-5700
                          Fax: 803-737-5768
                          www.state.sc.us/wcc

Gary Cannon, Executive Director
Kim Balleutine, Admin. Assistant

South Dakota

3804 Children's Special Health Services Program
600 E Capitol Ave
Pierre, SD 57501-2536   605-773-3361
                                  800-738-2301
                          Fax: 605-773-5683
                          DOH.info@state.sd.us
                          www.doh.sd.gov
Dianne Weyer, Manager
Barb Hemmelman, Program Manager
Health KiCC is a program, funded through federal and state monies, that provides financial assistance for medical appointments, procedures, treatments, medications and travel reimbursement for children with certain chronic health conditions.

3805 Division of Labor and Management
South Dakota Department of Labor
700 Governors Dr
Pierre, SD 57501-2291   605-773-3101
                          Fax: 605-773-6184
                          jamesmarsh@state.sd.us
                          dlr.sd.gov

Sara Minton, Executive Director
Pamela S Roberts, Secretary
Marcia Hultman, Deputy Secretary of Labor and D
Lyle Harter, Director of Administrative Servi
Our mission is to promote economic opportunity and financial security for individuals and businesses through quality, responsive and expert services; fair and equitable employment solutions; and safe and sound business practices.

3806 Health KiCC
South Dakota Department of Health
600 E Capitol Ave
Pierre, SD 57501-2536   605-773-3361
                                  800-738-2301
                          Fax: 605-773-5683
                          DOH.info@state.sd.us
                          www.doh.sd.gov
Dianne Weyer, Manager
Health KiCC is a program, funded through federal and state monies, that provides financial assistance for medical appointments, procedures, treatments, medications and travel reimbursement for children with certain chronic health conditions.

3807 South Dakota Advocacy Services
221 S Central Ave
Ste. 38
Pierre, SD 57501-2479   605-224-8294
                                  800-658-4782
                          Fax: 605-224-5125
                          sdas@sdadvocacy.com
                          sdadvocacy.com

Sandy Stocklin Hook, Partners Coordinator
Designated protection and advocacy progam for South Dakota providing legal, administrative, mediation and other services to elgible persons with disabilities in the state.

3808 South Dakota Department of Aging
700 Governors Dr
Pierre, SD 57501-2291   605-773-3656
                                  866-854-5465
                          Fax: 605-773-4085

Marilyn Kinsman, Division Director
Lynne Valenti, Deputy Secretary
Amy Iversen-Pollreisz, Deputy Secretary
Kristin Kellar, Communications Director
The Division of Adult Services and Aging (ASA) provides home and community service options to individuals 60 years of age and older and 18 years of age and older with physical disabilities, regardless of income.

3809 South Dakota Department of Human Services Division of Community Behavioral Health
South Dakota of Human Services
700 Governors Drive
Hillsview Properties Plaza
Pierre, SD 57501-5007   605-773-3165
                                  800-265-9684
                          Fax: 605-773-7076
                          infoMH@state.sd.us
                          http://dss.sd.gov/behavioralhealthservices
Shawna Fullerton, Division Director
South Dakota's state mental health authority.

3810 South Dakota Developmental Disability Council
Hillsview Plaza 3800 E Highway 34
c/o 500 East Capital Avenue
Pierre, SD 57501   605-773-5990
                                              800-265-9684
                                         Fax: 605-773-5483
                                         TTY: 605-773-6412
                                       infodhs@state.sd.us
                                           www.state.sd.us

Dan Lusk, Director
Laurie R. Gill, Secretary
Carol Ruen, Assistant Director
Lindsay Dummer, Program Specialist II
To assist individuals with developmental disabilities to control
their own destiny and to achieve the quality of life they desire.

3811 South Dakota Division of Rehabilitation
700 Governors Dr
Pierre, SD 57501-2291   605-773-3101
                                         Fax: 605-773-6184
                                     jamesmarsh@state.sd.us
                                           www.sdjobs.org

Sara Minton, Executive Director
Pamela S Roberts, Secretary
Marcia Hultman, Deputy Secretary of Labor and D
Lyle Harter, Director of Administrative Servi
Offers diagnosis, evaluation and physical restoration services,
counseling, social work, educational and professional training,
employment and rehabilitation services for the disabled.

3812 Workers Compensation Board: South Dakota
700 Governors Dr
Pierre, SD 57501-2291   605-773-3101
                                         Fax: 605-773-6184
                                           www.sdjobs.org

Sara Minton, Executive Director
Marcia Hultman, Secretary
Lyle Harter, Director of Administrative Servi
Bret Afdahi, Director of the Division of Bank
Our mission is to promote economic opportunity and financial se-
curity for individuals and businesses through quality, responsive
and expert services; fair and equitable employment solutions;
and safe and sound business practices.

Tennessee

3813 Disability Determination Services
400 Deaderick St
Nashville, TN 37243-1403   800-342-1117
                               DHS.CustomerService@tn.gov
                                         www.tennessee.gov

Thea Smith, Human Resources Program Specialist
Wendy Davis, Finance & Administration
Cherrell Campbell-Street, Assistant Commissioner
The Disability Determination Services is a branch of the Division
of Rehabilitation Services in the Department of Human Services.
Its main responsibility is to process Social Security and Supple-
mental Security Income disability claims.

3814 International Dyslexia Association: Tennessee Branch
Knoxville, TN   865-207-4918
                                      msamwood@bellsouth.net
                                           www.tnida.org

Emily Dempster, President
Erin Alexander, Senior Vice President
Nikki Davis, Secretary
Sharon Dytrt, Treasurer
The Tennessee Branch of the International Dyslexia Association
(TN-IDA) was formed to increase awareness about Dyslexia in
the state of Tennessee. TN-IDA supports efforts to provide information regarding appropriate language arts instruction to those
involved with language-based learning differences and to encourage the identity of these individuals at-risk for such
disorders as soon as possible.

3815 Tennessee Assistive Technology Projects
Citizens Plaza State Office Buildin
511 Union St.
Nashville, TN 37219-1403   615-313-5183
                                              800-732-5059
                                        TTY:615-313-5695
                                           TN.TTAP@tn.gov
                                               www.tn.gov

Bill Haslam, Governor
Raquel Hatter, Commissioner
Beth White, Manager
Julie Oden, Manager
A statewide program promoting assistive technology devices and
services for persons of all ages with all disabilities.

3816 Tennessee Client Assistance Program
Tennessee Protection and Advocacy
P.O.Box 121257
Nashville, TN 37212-1257   615-298-1080
                                              800-342-1660
                                         Fax: 615-298-2046
                                           www.tpainc.org

Shirley Shea, Executive Director
Doris Lopez, Assistant Executive Director

3817 Tennessee Commission on Aging and Disability
502 Deaderick Street
9th Floor
Nashville, TN 37243-860   615-741-2056
                                         Fax: 615-741-3309
                                         cindy.warf@tn.gov
                                      www.tn.gov/comaging

Richard M. Honn, Executive Director
Ryan Ellis, Aging Info. & Data Director
Kathy Zamata, Aging Program Director
Richard Presler, Fiscal Director

3818 Tennessee Council on Developmental Disabilities
500 James Robertson Pkwy
1st Floor
Nashville, TN 37243   615-532-6615
                                         Fax: 615-532-6964
                                            tnddc@tn.gov
                                             tn.gov/cdd

Wanda Willis, Executive Director
Lynette Porter, Deputy Director
Alicia Cone, Director of Grant Program
Lauren Pearcy, Director of Public Policy
The council is a state agency that leads initiatives to improve disability policies by educating policymakers and the public about
best practices in disability services, facilitating collaboration
across organizations, and producing educational publications on
the subject.

3819 Tennessee Department of Children with Disabilities
511 Union St.
Nashville, TN 37219-9004   615-741-9701
                                              800-861-1935
                                         Fax: 615-253-5216
                                          dcs.email@tn.gov
                                               www.tn.gov

Ruth S Letson, Manager
Haticile Buchanan, Manager
Mary Beth Franklyn, CS Program Director
Kristi Faulkner, Special Counsel to the Commissio
Tennessee's children thrive in safe, healthy and stable families.
Families thrive in healthy, safe and strong communities. Tennes-
see's citizens benefit from the best child welfare and juvenile jus-
tice agency in the country.

3820 **Tennessee Department of Mental Health**
500 Deaderick Street
Nashville, TN 37243-3400 615-532-6597
800-560-5767
Fax: 615-532-6514
www.state.tn.us/mental
Doug Varney, Commissioner
Grant Lawrence, Director Office of Communication
Bob Grunow, Deputy Commissioner
Howard Burley, Asst Commissioner Clinical Ldrsp
TDMH is the state's mental health and substance abuse authority.
Its mission is to plan for and promote the availability of a comprehensive array of quality prevention, early intervention, treatment, habilitation, and rehabilitation services and supports based on the needs and choices of individuals and families served. Responsible for policy, and oversight, and for advocacy of the consumer within the state.

3821 **Tennessee Division of Rehabilitation**
400 Deaderick St
Nashville, TN 37243-1403 615-313-4700
800-270-1349
TTY:615-313-5695
http://www.tn.gov
Patsy Matthews, Commissioner
Randall Beasley, Manager
Raquel Hatter, Commissioner
Bill Haslam, Givernor
Offers rehabilitation, medical and therapeutic information and referrals to the disabled.

3822 **Workers Compensation Division Tennessee**
Dept of Labor & Workforce Development
220 French Landing Drive
1st Floor
Nashville, TN 37243- 1002 615-741-6642
800-332-2667
Fax: 615-532-1468
wc.info@tn.gov
www.tn.gov/labor-wfd/wcomp.html
Karla Davis, Commissioner
Alisa Malone, Deputy Commissioner
Stephanie Mitchell, General Counsel
Ron Jones, Administrator of Fiscal Services
We administer the workers' compensation system and promote a better understanding of the program's benefits by informing employees and employers of their rights and responsibilities. Workers' Compestation administers a mediation program for disputed claims, encourage workplace safety, participate in a public awareness campaign concerning fraud, and oversee an information awareness program for educating the public on laws and regulations which define workers' compensation requirements. We ensure

Texas

3823 **Disability Policy Consortium**
2222 West Braker Lane
Austin, TX 78758-1024 512-454-4816
800-252-9108
Fax: 512-323-0902
dpctexas@advocacyinc.org
www.disabilityrightstx.org
Mary Faithful, Executive Director
Roberta Rosenberg-Roque, Manager
An independent group of statewide advocacy organizations that strives to achieve the development and full implementation of public policy that promotes and supports the rights, inclusion, integration and independence of Texans with disabilities.

3824 **Division of Special Education**
1701 Congress Ave.
Austin, TX 78701-1402 512-463-9414
Fax: 512-463-9838
teainfo@tea.state.tx.us
www.tea.state.tx.us
Cory Green, Federal & State Education Policy
Donna Bahorich, Chair
Ruban Cortez Jr., Secretary
The Texas Education Agency is the state agency that oversees primary and secondary public education. It is headed by the commissioner of education. The mission of TEA is to provide leadership, guidance and resources to help schools meet the educational needs of all students

3825 **Easter Seal of Greater Dallas, TX**
233 South Wacker Drive
Suite 2400
Chicago, IL 60606-4743 972-394-8900
800-580-4718
800-221-6827
Fax: 972-394-6266
wjohnson@dallas.easterseals.com
easterseals.com
Richard W. Davidson, Chairman
Sandra L. Bouwman, 1st Vice Chairman
Joseph G. Kern, 2nd Vice Chairman
Bennett Leventhal, M.D., President
Easter Seals has a longstanding history in our community of providing a wealth of unique programs and services for individual with a wide variety of disabilities, including Autism Spectrum Disorder, Alzheimer's disease, Down syndrome, Cerebral Palsy, Mental and Developmental Delays, and a wealth of other disabilities. We provide programs and services, education, outreach, and advocacy so that people living with disabilities can live, learn, work and play in our communities.

3826 **Easter Seals Greater NW Texas**
1424 Hemphill Street
Fort Worth, TX 76104-8130 817-332-717
888-617-7171
Fax: 817-332-7601
wjohnson@dallas.easterseals.com
www.easterseals.com/northtexas
Donna Dempsey, President and Chief Executive Of
Nancy Robinson, Executive Vice President & Chief
Nancy Swartz, Vice President of Development an
Lenee Bassham, Vice President Community Living
Easter Seals has a longstanding history in our community of providing a wealth of unique programs and services for individual with a wide variety of disabilities, including Autism Spectrum Disorder, Alzheimer's disease, Down syndrome, Cerebral Palsy, Mental and Developmental Delays, and a wealth of other disabilities. We provide programs and services, education, outreach, and advocacy so that people living with disabilities can live, learn, work and play in our communities.

3827 **El Valle Community Parent Resource Center**
Ste J
530 S Texas Blvd
Weslaco, TX 78596-6262 956-969-0215
800-680-0255
Fax: 956-968-7102
Robert Garza, Owner

3828 **Grassroots Consortium**
Greenroots Consortium
6202 Belmark St
Houston, TX 77087-6324 713-643-9576
Fax: 713-643-6291
Speckids@aol.com
Agnes A Johnson, Director

3829 International Dyslexia Association: Austin Branch
Austin, TX   512-452-7658
aus.dyslexiaida.org

Mary Bach, President
Karen Monteith, Vice President
Herman H. Klare, Treasurer
Kristie Beavers, Executive Director
Provides free information and referral services for diagnosis and
tutoring for parents, educators, physicians, and individuals with
dyslexia in Illinois. Membership includes yearly journal and
quarterly newsletter.

3830 NAMI Texas
FOUNTAIN Park Plaza III
P.O. Box 300817
Austin, TX 78703-5700   512-693-2000
800-633-3760
Fax: 512-693-8000
namitexas.org

Andrea Hazlitt, President
Ed Dickey, Vice President
Chris Scroggin, Executive Director
Kelly Jeschke, Membership Coordinator
NAMI Texas has a variety of programs directed to mental health
consumers, family members, friends, professionals, other stake
holders and the community at large to address the mental health
needs of Texans. NAMI Texas works to inform the public about
mental illness by distributing information about mental illness
through every means of communication. Interviews are produced
on television, stories are featured in newspapers, brochures are
distributed, referrals are provided and more.

3831 Parent Connection
1020 Riverwood Ct
Conroe, TX   77304-2811   936-756-8321
800-839-8876
parentCNCT@aol.com
http://www.parentingaspergerscommunity.com/pu
Dave Angel, Founder
Includes parenting help and Aspergers advice, including
parenting tips, tricks and techniques to help your child with
Aspergers. Our worldwide membership base is helping parents to
understand their child with Aspergers better and make their home
& family life a better place to be.

3832 Parents Supporting Parents Network
8001 Centre Park Drive
Suite 100
Austin, TX   78754   512-454-6694
800-252-9729
Fax: 512-454-4956
secretary@thearcoftexas.org
www.thearcoftexas.org

Charlie Huber, President
John Schneider, Vice-President
Nancy Lepley, Treasurer
Terri Schonfeld, Secretary
Since our founding in 1950 by a group of parents of children with
intellectual and developmental disabilities, The Arc at the local,
state and national level has been instrumental in the creation of
virtually every program, service, right, and benefit that is now
available to more than half a million Texans with intellectual and
developmental disabilities. Today, The Arc continues to advocate
for including people with intellectual and developmental
disabilities in all aspects of society.

3833 Partners Resource Network
Ste B
1090 Longfellow Dr
Beaumont, TX   77706-4819   409-898-4684
800-866-4726
Fax: 409-898-4869
partnersresource@sbcglobal.net
partnerstx.org

Janice Meyer, Executive Director
Statewide network of three parent training and information centers.

3834 Social Security: Austin Disability Determination
P.O. Box 149198
Austin, TX   78714-9198   512-437-8311
800-772-1213
800-252-9627
Fax: 512-437-8595
TTY:512-916-5958
dan.tippit@ssa.gov
www.ssa.gov

Karena L. Kilgore, Executive Secretary
Carolyn W: Colvin, Commissioner
Carolyn W. Colvin, Deputy Commissioner
James A. Kissko, Chief of Staff
We deliver services through a nationwide network of over 1,400
offices that include regional offices, field offices, card centers,
teleservice centers, processing centers, hearing offices, the Appeals Council, and our State and territorial partners, the Disability Determination Services. We also have a presence in U.S.
embassies around the globe. The rich diversity of our employees
mirrors the public we serve.

3835 Statewide Information at Texas School for the Deaf
1102 S Congress Ave
Austin, TX   78704-1728   512-462-5353
Fax: 512-462-5353
webmaster@tsd.state.tx.us
www.tsd.state.tx.us

Sonia Karimi Bridges, Video Communication Specialist
Avonne Brooker-Rutowski, Program Specialist
David Coco, Program Specialist
Lisa Crawford, Parent Liason
Welcome to Texas School for the Deaf, a place where students
who are deaf or hard of hearing including those with additional
disabilities, have the opportunity to learn, grow and belong in a
culture that optimizes individual potential and provides accessible language and communication across the curriculum. Our educational philosophy is grounded in the belief that all children who
are deaf and hard of hearing deserve a quality language and com-
munication-driven program that provides education tog

3836 Texas Advocates Supporting Kids with Disabilities
P.O.Box 162685
Austin, TX   78716-2685   512-310-2102
Fax: 512-310-2102
ASKTASK@aol.com
www.main.org/task/

3837 Texas Commission for the Blind
P.O. Box 149198
Austin, TX   78714-9198   512-459-8575
800-252-5204
Fax: 512-424-4730
DARS.Inquiries@dars.state.tx.us
www.dars.state.tx.us

Canzata Crowder, Manager
Offers services for the totally blind, legally blind, and visually
impaired, with counseling, educational, recreational, rehabilitation, computer training and professional training services.

3838 Texas Commission for the Deaf and Hard of Hearing
D AR S
P.O. Box 149198
Austin, TX   78714-9198   512-407-3250
800-628-5115
Fax: 512-424-4730
TTY: 512-407-3251
DARS.Inquiries@dars.state.tx.us
www.dars.state.tx.us

Veronda L. Durden, Commissioner
Glenn Neal, Deputy Commissioner
David Myers, Executive Director
Daniel Bravo, Chief Operating Officer

3839 Texas Council for Developmental Disabilities
6201 E Oltorf St
Suite 600
Austin, TX   78741-7509   512-437-5432
                                                800-262-0334
                                          Fax: 512-437-5434
                                          TTY: 512-437-5431
                                          tcdd@tcdd.texas.gov
                                          txddc.state.tx.us

Mary Durheim, Chairman
Andrew D. Crim, Vice Chairman
Roger Webb, Executive Director
Koren Vogel, Executive Assistant
The Texas Council for Developmental Disabilities is a 27-member board dedicated to ensuring that all Texans with developmental disabilities, about 411,479 individuals, have the opportunity to be independent, productive and valued members of their communities. The mission of the Texas Council for Developmental Disabilities is to create change so that all people with disabilities are fully included in their communities and exercise control over their own lives.

3840 Texas Department of Human Services
701 W 51st St
P.O. Box 149030
Austin, TX   78751-2312   512-438-3011
                                                888-834-7406
                                          Fax: 512-472-0603
                                          TTY: 888-425-6889
                                          mail@dads.state.tx.us
                                          www.dads.state.tx.us

Jon Weizenbaum, Commissioner
Kristi Jordan, Associate Commissioner
Chris Adams, Deputy Commissioner
Elisa J. Garza, Assistant Commissioner for Acces

3841 Texas Department of Mental Health & Mental Retardation
P.O.Box 12668
Austin, TX   78711-2668   512-472-4138
                                          Fax: 512-472-0603

Bill West, Manager
Randy Fritz, Chief Operating Officer

3842 Texas Department on Aging
701 W 51st St
P.O. Box 149030
Austin, TX   78751-2312   512-438-3011
                                                800-252-9240
                                          mail@tdoa.state.tx.us
                                          www.dads.state.tx.us

Jon Weizenbaum, Commissioner
Kristi Jordan, Associate Commissioner
Chris Adams, Deputy Commissioner
Elisa J. Garza, Assistant Commissioner for Acces

3843 Texas Federation of Families for Children's Mental Health
Ste 505
7701 N Lamar Blvd
Austin, TX   78752-1000   512-407-8844
                                                866-893-3264
                                          Fax: 512-407-8266
                                          www.txffcmh.org
Patti Derr, Executive Director
Pat Calley, Chairperson
S Barron, Operations Director

3844 Texas Governor's Committee on People with Disabilities
1100 San Jacinto Blvd
P.O. Box 12428
Austin, TX   78701- 1935   512-463-2000
                                          Fax: 513-463-5745
                                          www.governor.state.tx.us/disabilities
Angela English, LPC, LMFT, Executive Director
Erin Lawler, JD, MS, Accessibility and Disability Rig
Nancy Van Loan, Executive Assistant
Jo Virgil, MS, Community Outreach and Informati
The Governor's Committee on People with Disabilities is within the office of the Governor. The committee's mission is to further opportunities for persons with disabilities to enjoy full and equal access to lives of independence, productivity, and self-determination. The committee is composed of 12 members appointed by the governor and of nonvoting ex officio members.

3845 Texas Protection & Advocacy Services for Disabled Persons
Advocacy
2222 West Braker Lane
Austin, TX   78758-1024   512-454-4816
                                                800-252-9108
                                                800-315-3876
                                          Fax: 512-323-0902
                                          dpctexas@advocacyinc.org
                                          www.disabilityrightstx.org
Mary Faithful, Executive Director
Roberta Rosenberg-Roque, Manager
A federally funded, independent, nonprofit agency that advocates for the legal, human and service rights of persons with disabilities. Publishes 'Special Edition' newsletter, at a small fee and 'It's a Good Idea!' a parent manual for $10, plus many other handouts free of charge.

3846 Texas Respite Resource Network
P.O. Box 149030
710 West 51st Street
Austin, TX   78714- 9030   512-438-5555
                                          Fax: 512-438-4374
                                          archrespite.org

Jill Kagan, Program Director
Liz Newhouse, Assistant Director
Mike Mathers, Executive Director
Maggie Edgar, Senior Consultant
A state clearinghouse and technical assistance network for respite in Texas. TRRN identifies, initiates and improves respite options for families caring for individuals with disabilities on the local, state and national levels. TRRN provides training/technical assistance to programs/groups wanting to establish respite services.

3847 Texas Technology Access Project
Center for Disabilities Studies
10100 Burnet Rd
Austin, TX   78758-4445   512-232-0740
                                                800-828-7839
                                          Fax: 512-232-0761
                                          TTY: 512-232-0762
                                          rogerlevy@austin.utexas.edu
                                          techaccess.edb.utexas.edu
Roger Levy, Program Director
Darlene West, Assistive Technology Coordinator
Steve Thomas, Operations and External Relation
Darlene West, Assistive Technology Specialist
Their mission is to increase access for people with disabilities to assistive technology that provides them more control over their immediate environments and an enhanced ability to function independently.

3848 Texas UAP for Developmental Disabilities
University of Texas
1 University Station
Austin, TX   78712   512-471-3434
                                                800-828-7839
                                          www.utexas.edu

Gregory L. Fences, President
Judith H. Langlois, Executive Vice President and Pr
Gregory J. Vincent, Vice President
Patricia C. Ohlendorf, Vice President
Welcome to The University of Texas at Austin. Founded in 1883, UT is one of the largest and most respected universities in the nation. Ours is a diverse learning community, with students from every state and more than 100 countries. We're a university with world talent and Texas traditions. Discover more about us online and come visit our beautiful campus in person.

3849 Texas Workers Compensation Commission
333 Guadalupe
P.O. Box 149104
Austin, TX 78701-1645
512-676-6000
800-578-4677
800-252-3439
Fax: 512-804-4401
TTY:512-322-4238
WebStaff@tdi.state.tx.us
www.tdi.texas.gov

Robert Shipe, Executive Director
Rod Bordelon, Commissioner
Workers' compensation is a state-regulated insurance program that pays medical bills and replaces some lost wages for employees who are injured at work or who have work-related diseases or illnesses.

3850 United Cerebral Palsy of Texas
National Cerebral Palsy of American
Ste 145
1016 La Posada Dr
Austin, TX 78752-3828
512-472-8696
800-798-1492
Fax: 512-472-8026
info@ucptexas.org
ucptexas.org

Jean Langendorf, Executive Director
Offers a unique array of programs and services designed for one specific purpose: to ensure that people with cerebral palsy and similar disabilities have the opportunity to participate fully and equally in every aspect of our society.

Utah

3851 Access Utah Network
Ste 100
155 S 300 W
Salt Lake City, UT 84101-1288
801-533-4636
800-333-8824
Fax: 801-533-3968
accessut.org

Mark L. Smith, Information Specialist
Access Utah Network is Utah's prime source for information and referral for individuals with disabilities and their caregivers since 1990. Our operators can provide you with the information you need to find accessible housing, assistive technology and financial and social supports needed to live independently with a disability. Call us or explore our web site today to see how Access Utah Network can help you become more independent.

3852 Social Security: Salt Lake City Disability Determination
Social Security
P.O. Box 144032
Salt Lake City, UT 84111-4032
801-321-6500
800-772-1213
800-221-3493
Fax: 801-321-6599
TTY:801-524-5047
Dave.Carlson@ssa.gov
www.ssa.gov

Karena L. Kilgore, Executive Secretary
Carolyn W. Colvin, Commissioner
Carolyn W. Colvin, Deputy Commissioner
James A. Kissko, Chief of Staff
We deliver services through a nationwide network of over 1,400 offices that include regional offices, field offices, card centers, teleservice centers, processing centers, hearing offices, the Appeals Council, and our State and territorial partners, the Disability Determination Services. We also have a presence in U.S. embassies around the globe. The rich diversity of our employees mirrors the public we serve.

3853 Utah Assistive Technology Projects
Utah State University
6855 Old Main Hl
Logan, UT 84322-6855
435-797-3824
800-524-5152
TTY:435-797-2355
www.uatpat.org

Sachin Pavithran, Program Director
Alma Burgess, UATP Data Collection Coordinator
Clay Christensen, Lab Coordinator
Marilyn ' Hammond, Executive Director
A statewide program promoting assistive technology devices and services for persons of all ages with all disabilities.

3854 Utah Client Assistance Program
205 N 400 W
Salt Lake City, UT 84103-1125
801-363-1347
800-662-9080
Fax: 801-363-1437
www.disabilitylawcenter.org

Bryce Fifield Ph.D, President
Jared Fields, Vice President
Barbara M. Campbell, Treasurer
Kevin Murphy, Board Member
Since 1979, the Disability Law Center (DLC) has helped thousands of Utahns with disabilities and their families. The DLC has broad statutory powers to safeguard the human and civil rights of persons with disabilities. We provide self-advocacy assistance, legal services, disability rights education, and public policy advocacy on behalf of the more than 400,000 Utah residents with disabilities. Our services are available statewide and without regard for ability to pay.

3855 Utah Department of Aging
195 North 1950 West
Salt Lake City, UT 84116
801-538-3910
877-424-4640
Fax: 801-538-4395
debooth@utah.gov

Nels Holmgren, Director
Michael S. Styles, Assistant Director
Michelle Benson, Director
Sarah Brenna, Director
We administer a wide variety of home and community-based services for Utah residents who are 60 or older. Programs and services are primarily delivered by a network of 12 Area Agencies on Aging which reach all geographic areas of the state. Our goal is to provide services that allow people to remain independent.

3856 Utah Department of Human Services: Division of Services for People with Disabilities
Utah Department of Human Services
195 North 1950 West
Salt Lake City, UT 84116
801-538-3910
877-424-4640
Fax: 801-538-4395
debooth@utah.gov
www.hsdspd.utah.gov

Paul T. Smith, Division Director
Clay Hiatt, Fiscal Management
Information and referral services for people with disabilities, including DD/MR, brain injury and physical disabilities throughout the state of Utah.

3857 Utah Division Of Substance Abuse & Mental Health
Utah Department of Human Services
195 No. 1950 West
Salt Lake City, UT 84116-1550
801-538-4171
Fax: 801-538-4016
WWW.DHS.UTAH.GOV

Lana Stohl, Executive Director

3858 Utah Division of Services for the Disabled
195 North 1950 West
Salt Lake City, UT 84116
801-538-3910
877-424-4640
Fax: 801-538-4395
dirdhs@utah.gov

Paul T. Smith, Division Director
Clay Hiatt, Fiscal Management
Offers services for the totally blind, legally blind, visually impaired, mentally retarded blind and more with health, counseling, educational, recreational, rehabilitation, computer training and professional training services.

3859 Utah Governor's Council for People with Disabilities
155 S 300 W
Suite 100
Salt Lake City, UT 84101-1288
801-533-4636
Fax: 801-533-3968
www.gcpd.org/

Mark Smith, Manager
Angela Allen, Administrative Secretary

3860 Utah Labor Commission
160 E 300 S
3rd Floor
Salt Lake City, UT 84114-6600
801-530-6800
800-222-1238
Fax: 801-530-6390
laborcom@utah.gov
laborcommission.utah.gov

Jaceson R Maughan, Commissioner
Alison Adams-Perlac, Director
Britton Beims, Employment Discrimination Investigation
Michael Barrett, MSHR, Outreach & Education Coordinator
The Utah Labor Commission is a regulatory agency that works to ensure safety in the workplace. The commission also offers services related to workplace injuries, wage issues, descrimination and industrial accidents.

3861 Utah Protection & Advocacy Services for Persons with Disabilities
Disability Law Center
205 N 400 W
Salt Lake City, UT 84103-1125
801-363-1347
800-662-9080
Fax: 801-363-1437
www.disabilitylawcenter.org

Bryce Fifield Ph.D, President
Jared Fields, Vice President
Barbara M. Campbell, Treasurer
Kevin Murphy, Board Member
Since 1979, the Disability Law Center (DLC) has helped thousands of Utahns with disabilities and their families. The DLC has broad statutory powers to safeguard the human and civil rights of persons with disabilities. We provide self-advocacy assistance, legal services, disability rights education, and public policy advocacy on behalf of the more than 400,000 Utah residents with disabilities. Our services are available statewide and without regard for ability to pay.

Vermont

3862 Disability Law Project
57 N Main St
Rutland, VT 05701-3246
800-889-2047
Fax: 802-775-0022
nbreiden@vtlegalaid.org
vtlegalaid.org

Nanci Smith, President
Jessica Porter, Vice President/Secretary
John Holme, Treasurer
Eric Avildsen, Executive Director
Legal services (protection and advocacy) for people with disabilities on legal issues arising from disability. Statewide. Adults and children. Employment, education, discrimination, housing, public benefits, health care.

3863 Disability Rights Vermont
141 Main Street
Suite 7
Montpelier, VT 05602-2916
802-229-1355
800-834-7890
Fax: 802-229-1359
TTY: 800-889-2047
info@disabilityrightsvt.org
www.disabilityrightsvt.org

Sarah Wendell-Launderville, President
David Gallagher, Vice president
Crocker Paquin, Treasurer
Michael Sabourin, Secretary
Advocacy and legal services for people with mental illness on legal issues arising, out of disabilities. Children and adults.

3864 Social Security: Vermont Disability Determination Services
Ste 6
93 Pilgrim Park Rd
Waterbury, VT 05676-1729
802-241-2463
800-734-2463
800-772-1213
Fax: 802-241-2492
www.ssa.gov

Karena L. Kilgore, Executive Secretary
Carolyn W. Colvin, Commissioner
Carolyn W. Colvin, Deputy Commissioner
James A. Kissko, Chief of Staff
We deliver services through a nationwide network of over 1,400 offices that include regional offices, field offices, card centers, teleservice centers, processing centers, hearing offices, the Appeals Council, and our State and territorial partners, the Disability Determination Services. We also have a presence in U.S. embassies around the globe. The rich diversity of our employees mirrors the public we serve.

3865 Vermont Assistive Technology Projects
103 S Main St
Weeks Building
Waterbury, VT 05671-2305
800-750-6355
800-750-6355
Fax: 802-871-3048
TTY: 802-241-1464
atp.vermont.gov

Amber Fulcher, Program Director
Sharon Alderman, Assistive Technology Reuse Coord
Emma Cobb, Assistive Technology Services Co
Dan Gilman, ATP, Assistive Technology Access Spec
Increase awareness and change policies to insure assistive technology (AT) is available to all Vermonters with disabilities. Our Commitment is to enable Vermonters with disabilities to have greater independence, productivity, and confidence. To provide them with a clear and direct avenue toward integration and inclusion within the work force and community.

3866 Vermont Client Assistance Program
57 N Main St
Rutland, VT 05701-3246
802-775-0021
800-769-7459
www.vocrehabvermont.org/html/clientassistance

Patrick Flood, Commissioner
The Client Assistance Program (CAP) is an independent advocacy program to help if you are applying for or receiving services from one of the following sources: Division of Vocational Rehabilitation (VR); Vermont Center for Independent Living (VCIL); Division for the Blind and Visually Impaired (DBVI); Vermont Association of Business, Industry & Rehabilitation (VABIR); Vermont Association for the Blind and Visually Impaired (VABVI); Supported Employment Programs; Transition Programs.

3867 Vermont Department of Aging
103 S Main St
Weeks Building
Waterbury, VT 05671-1601   802-241-2401
Fax: 802-871-3281
TTY:802-241-3557
AHS-DAIL-DeptWebMaster@state.vt.us
dail.vermont.gov
Susan Wehry, Commissioner
Marybeth McCaffrey, Director
Linda Henzel, Executive Staff Assistant
Adele Edelman, Assistant Division Director

3868 Vermont Department of Developmental and
103 S Main St
Weeks Building
Waterbury, VT 05671-1601   802-241-2401
Fax: 802-871-3281
TTY:802-241-3557
dail.vermont.gov
Jonathan Wood, Manager

3869 Vermont Department of Disabilities, Aging and Independent Living
Aging and Disabilities
103 S Main St
Waterbury, VT 05671-1601   802-241-2401
Fax: 802-241-2325
dail.vermont.gov
Susan Wehry, Commissioner
Camille George, Deputy Commissioner

3870 Vermont Department of Health: Children with Special Health Needs
Vermont Department Of Health
108 Cherry Street
Burlington, VT 05402-70   802-863-7200
800-464-4343
Fax: 802-865-7754
healthvermont.gov
Harry Chen, M.D., Commissioner
Barbara Cimaglio, Deputy Commissioner for Alcohol
Tracy Dolan, Deputy Commissioner for Public H
Dixie Henry, Esq., Senior Policy and Legal Advisor
Multidisciplinary clinics and family support for children with chronic conditions, birth to age 21 years.

3871 Vermont Developmental Disabilities Council
103 S Main St
Waterbury, VT 05671-9800   082-241-2220
vtddc@upgate1.ahs.state.vt.us
www.ahs.state.vt.us/vtddc
Cynthia D LaWare, Secretary
The mission of VTDDC is to facilitate connections and to promote supports that bring people with developmental disabilities into the heart of Vermont Communities.

3872 Vermont Division for the Blind & Visually Impaired
Agency of Human Svcs Dept Disabilities, Aging & IL
103 S Main St
Weeks Building
Waterbury, VT 5671-2304   802-871-3038
800-405-5005
888-405-5005
Fax: 802-871-3048
www.dbvi.vermont.gov
Fred Jones, Director
Scott Langley, Counselor
Heather Allen, Administrative Assistant
Paul Putnam, Rehabilitation Associate
Offers services for the totally blind, legally blind, visually impaired, mentally retarded blind and more with health, counseling, educational, recreational, rehabilitation, computer training and professional training services.

3873 Vermont Division of Disability & Aging Services
103 S Main St
Weeks Building
Waterbury, VT 05671-1601   802-241-2401
Fax: 802-871-3281
TTY:802-241-3557
www.dail.vermont.gov
Susan Wehry, Commissioner
Marybeth McCaffrey, Director
Linda Henzel, Executive Staff Assistant
Adele Edelman, Assistant Division Director
Provides services to adults and children with developmental disabilities all to the aging.

3874 Workers Compensation Board Vermont
Department of Labor
5 Green Mountain Drive
PO Box 488
Montpelier, VT 05601- 0488   802-828-4000
Fax: 802-828-4022
labor.vermont.gov
Deborah Bruce, Human Resource Administrator
Allen Evans, Executive Director Workforce Dev
Annie Noonan, Commissioner
Erika Wolf?ng, Principal Assistant
Welcome to the Vermont Department of Labor's website. VDOL's primary focus is to provide services that assist businesses, workers, and job seekers.

Virginia

3875 Aging & Disability Services

3876 Aging and Disability Services
2100 Washington Blvd
4th Floor
Arlington, VA 22204   703-228-1700
TTY:703-228-1788
arlaaa@arlingtonva.us
aging-disability.arlingtonva.us
Anita Friedman, Director, Department of Human Services
The Aging and Disability Services Division offers care coordination, home care, and supportive services to the aging residents of Arlington. Services are provided to adults over 60, adults with developmental disabilities and their caregivers.

3877 International Dyslexia Association: Virginia Branch
3126 West Cary St.
Suite 102
Richmond, VA 23221   866-893-0583
va.dyslexiaida.org
Lisa Snidery, President
Lisa Harrah, Vice President
Robin Hegner, Secretary
Mark Whitehurst, Treasurer
Provides free information and referral services for diagnosis and tutoring for parents, educators, physicians, and individuals with dyslexia in Illinois. Membership includes yearly journal and quarterly newsletter.

3878 Virginia Department for the Blind and Vision Impaired
397 Azalea Ave
Richmond, VA 23227-3623   804-371-3140
800-622-2155
Fax: 804-371-3157
Kimberley.Jennings@dbvi.virginia.gov
www.vdbvi.org
Robert S. Dendy, Chair
Raymond E. Hopkins, Commissioner
Dr. Rick L. Mitchell, Deputy Commissioner
James R. Meehan, Deputy Commissioner
Offers services for the totally blind, legally blind, visually impaired, mentally retarded blind and more with health, counseling, educational, recreational, rehabilitation, computer training and professional training services.

3879 Virginia Department of Mental Health
P.O.Box 1797
Richmond, VA 23218-1797 804-786-3921
Fax: 804-371-6638
TTY:804-371-8977
jim.stewart@dbhds.virginia.gov
www.dbhds.virginia.gov

Debra Ferguson, Commissioner
John Pezzoli, Deputy Commissioner
Daniel Herr, Assistant Commissioner of Behavi
Connie Cochran, Assistant Commissioner of Develo
Available to citizens statewide, Virginia's public mental health, intellectual disability and substance abuse services system is comprised of 16 state facilities and 40 locally-run community services boards (CSBs) The CSBs and facilities serve children and adults who have or who are at risk of mental illness, serious emotional disturbance, intellectual disabilities, or substance abuse disorders.

3880 Virginia Developmental Disability Council
103 S Main St
Waterbury, VT 05671-9800 082-241-2220
Cynthia D LaWare, Secretary
The mission of VTDDC is to facilitate connections and to promote supports that bring people with developmental disabilities into the heart of Vermont Communities.

3881 Virginia Office Protection and Advocacy for People with Disabilities
1512 Willow Lawn
Suite 100
Richmond, VA 23230-3034 804-225-2042
800-552-3962
Fax: 804-662-7057
info@dLCV.org
disabilitylawva.org

Coleen Miller, Executive Director
LaToya Blizzard, Deputy Director
Mickie Chapman, IT Specialist
Melissa Charnes-Gibson, Staff Attorney
Through zealous and effective advocacy and legal representation to: protect and advance legal, human, and civil rights of persons with disabilities; combat and prevent abuse, neglect, and discrimination; and promote independence, choice, and self-determination by persons with disabilities.

3882 Virginia Office for Protection & Advocacy
5005 Mitchelldale
Suite #100
Houston, TX 77092-3034 713-574-5287
866-964-2867
Fax: 281-476-7800
info@dLCV.org
vopa.state.va.us

V Coleen Miller, Executive Director
Rusty Hill, Administrative Assistant
LaToya Blizzard, Deputy Director for Fiscal and O
Mickie Chapman, Information Technology Specialis
An independent state agency that helps ensure that the rights of persons with disabiltiies in the Commonwealth are protected. The mission of DRVD is to provide zealous and effective advocacy and legal representation to protect and advance legal, human and civil rights of persons with disabilities, combat and prevent abuse, neglect and discrimination, and promote independence, choice and self-determination by persons with disabilities.

3883 Virginia Office for Protection and Advocacy
5005 Mitchelldale
Suite #100
Houston, TX 77092-3034 713-574-5287
866-964-2867
Fax: 281-476-7800
info@dLCV.org

V Coleen Miller, Executive Director
Rusty Hill, Administrative Assistant
LaToya Blizzard, Deputy Director for Fiscal and O
Mickie Chapman, Information Technology Specialis

An independent state agency that helps ensure that the rights of persons with disabiltiies in the Commonwealth are protected. The mission of DRVD is to provide zealous and effective advocacy and legal representation to protect and advance legal, human and civil rights of persons with disabilities, combat and prevent abuse, neglect and discrimination, and promote independence, choice and self-determination by persons with disabilities.

3884 Virginia's Developmental Disabilities Planning Council
Stae Agency
1100 Bank Street
7th Floor
Richmond, VA 23219-3426 804-786-0016
800-846-4464
Fax: 804-662-7662
TTY: 800-811-7893
info@vbpd.virginia.gov
www.vaboard.org

Korinda Rusinyak, Chairman
Charles Meacham, Vice Chairman
Dennis Manning, Secretary
Heidi L. Lawyer, Executive Director
To create a Commonwealth that advances opportunities for independence, personal decision-making and full participation in community life for individuals with developmental disabilities.

Washington

3885 DSHS/Aging & Adult Disability Services Administration
P.O.Box 45130
Olympia, WA 98504-5130 360-902-7797
800-737-0617
Fax: 360-902-7848
TTY: 800-737-7931

Dan Murphy, Director
Bea Rector, Project Director
Tamarra Paradee, Executive Secretary
Bill Moss, Director
The Aging and Disability Services Administration assists children and adults with developmental delays or disabilities, cognitive impairment, chronic illness and related functional disabilities to gain access to needed services and supports by managing a system of long-term care and supportive services that are high quality, cost effective, and responsive to individual needs and preferences.

3886 Disability Rights: Washington
315 5th Avenue South
Suite 850
Seattle, WA 98104-2691 206-324-1521
800-562-2702
Fax: 206-957-0729
TTY: 206-957-0728
info@dr-wa.org
www.disabilityrightswa.org

Mark Stroh, Executive Director
David Carison, Director of Legal Advocacy
Emily Cooper, Staff Attorney
Charlotte Cunningham, Staff Attorney
WPAS is a private, non-profit right protection agency for persons with disabilities residin in Washington state. Our advocacy services include information referral, technical assistance, training, publications and systemic advocacy.

3887 International Dyslexia Association: Washington State Branch
P.O. Box 27435
Seattle, WA 98165 info@wabida.org
wabida.org

Kristie English, President
Jessica Ruger, Vice President
Beverly Wolf, Treasurer
Bonnie Meyer, Secretary
Provides free information and referral services for diagnosis and tutoring for parents, educators, physicians, and individuals with

dyslexia in Arkansas, Idaho, Montana and Washington state. Membership includes yearly journal and quarterly newsletter.

3888   Social Security: Olympia Disability Determination
Social Security
P.O. Box 9303-MS-45550
Olympia, WA 98507
                    360-664-7356
                    800-772-1213
                    800-562-6074
                    Fax: 360-586-0851
                    TTY:800-325-0778
                    Jennifer.Elsen@ssa.gov
                    www.ssa.gov

Karena L. Kilgore, Executive Secretary
Carolyn W. Colvin, Commissioner
Carolyn W. Colvin, Deputy Commissioner
James A. Kissko, Chief of Staff
We deliver services through a nationwide network of over 1,400 offices that include regional offices, field offices, card centers, teleservice centers, processing centers, hearing offices, the Appeals Council, and our State and territorial partners, the Disability Determination Services. We also have a presence in U.S. embassies around the globe. The rich diversity of our employees mirrors the public we serve.

3889   WA Department of Services for the Blind
4565 7th Avenue SE
PO Box 40933
Lacey, WA 98503
                    360-725-3830
                    800-552-7103
                    Fax: 360-407-0679
                    info@dsb.wa.gov
                    www.dsb.wa.gov

Sue Ammeter, council chair
Nancy Kim
Veronica Baca, Council Member
Michael Cunningham, Council Member
Vocational rehabilitation for the blind.

3890   Washington Client Assistance Program
2531 Rainier Ave S
Seattle, WA 98144-5328
                    206-721-5999
                    800-544-2121
                    888-721-6072
                    Fax: 206-721-4537
                    TTY:206-721-6072
                    www.washingtoncap.org

Jerry Johnson, Executive Director
Bob Huven, rehabilitation coordinator
Advocacy and information assistance for persons of disability seeking services through vocational rehabilitation or other program under the 1973 Rehabilitation Act as commented. We provide counseling.

3891   Washington Developmental Disability
2600 Martin Way E
Suite F
Olympia, WA 98506-4974
                    360-586-3560
                    800-634-4473
                    Fax: 360-586-2424
                    Ed.Holen@ddc.wa.gov
                    www.ddc.wa.gov

Diana Zottman, Chairman
Ed Holen, Executive Director
Brain Dahl, Support Coordinator
Aziz Aladin, Budget & Fiscal Director
Developmental Disabilities Council members are appointed by the Governor to plan comprehensive services for the State of Washington's citizens with developmental disabilities.

3892   Washington Governor's Committee on Disability Issues & Employment
605 Woodland Square Loop SE
Lacey, WA 98503
                    360-438-3168
                    Fax: 928-447-6579
                    gcdetz@gmail.com
                    www.gcde.org

Martin Haule, Director
Toby Olson, Manager

3893   Washington Office of Superintendent of Public Instruction
600 Washington St. S.E.
P. O. Box 47200
Olympia, WA 98504-7200
                    360-725-6000
                    TTY:360-644-3631
                    www.k12.wa.us

Randy Dorn, State Superintendent
Gil Mendoza, Deputy Superintendent
JoLynn Berge, Assistant Superintendent
Ken Kanikeberg, Chief of Staff
The Office of Superintendent of Public Instruction (OSPI) is the primary agency charged with overseeing K-12 education in Washington state. OSPI works with the state's 296 school districts to administer basic education programs and implement education reform on behalf of more than one million public school students.

3894   Washington State Developmental Disabilities Council
2600 Martin Way E
Suite F
Olympia, WA 98506-4974
                    360-586-3560
                    800-634-4473
                    Fax: 360-586-2424
                    Ed.Holen@ddc.wa.gov
                    www.ddc.wa.gov

Diana Zottman, Chairman
Ed Holen, Executive Director
Brain Dahl, Support Coordinator
Aziz Aladin, Budget & Fiscal Director
Developmental Disabilities Council members are appointed by the Governor to plan comprehensive services for the State of Washington's citizens with developmental disabilities.

3895   Workers Compensation Board Washington
State of Washington
7273 Linderson Way SW
Tumwater, WA 98501-5414
                    360-902-5800
                    800-547-8367
                    Fax: 360-902-5798
                    TTY: 360-902-5797
                    www.lni.wa.gov

Judy Schurke, Director
Lisa Rodriguez, Executive Assistant
Vickie Kennedy, Special Assistant
Tamara Jones, Dir of Government Relations
&I is a diverse state agency dedicated to the safety, health and security of Washington's 3.2 million workers. We help employers meet safety and health standards and we inspect workplaces when alerted to hazards. As administrators of the state's workers' compensation system, we are similar to a large insurance company, providing medical and limited wage-replacement coverage to workers who suffer job-related injuries and illness. Our rules and enforcement programs also help ensure workers are pai

West Virginia

3896 Bureau of Employment Programs Division of Workers' Compensation
State of West Virginia
407 Virginia Street East
Charleston, WV 25301-2531
304-357-0101
800-628-4265
Fax: 304-357-0788
helpdesk@kanawha.us
kanawha.us

Patricia Starkey, Manager
Vern Cormick, Manager
Michael ' Campbell, Director of IT
Larry McDonnell, Chief Webmaster
Kanawha County today is an exciting technology center that is earning recognition in information technology, medical research, chemical synthesis research, and telecommunications.

3897 Disability Determination Section
Ste 500
500 Quarrier St
Charleston, WV 25301-2913
304-343-5055
800-772-1213
800-344-5033
Fax: 304-353-4212
Kenneth.Lim@ssa.gov
www.ssa.gov

Karena L. Kilgore, Executive Secretary
Carolyn W. Colvin, Commissioner
Carolyn W. Colvin, Deputy Commissioner
James A. Kissko, Chief of Staff
We deliver services through a nationwide network of over 1,400 offices that include regional offices, field offices, card centers, teleservice centers, processing centers, hearing offices, the Appeals Council, and our State and territorial partners, the Disability Determination Services. We also have a presence in U.S. embassies around the globe. The rich diversity of our employees mirrors the public we serve.

3898 Social Security: Charleston Disability Determination
Social Security
500 Quarrier Street
Suite 500
Charleston, WV 25301-2913
304-343-5055
800-772-1213
800-344-5033
Fax: 304-353-4212
www.ssa.gov

Karena L. Kilgore, Executive Secretary
Carolyn W. Colvin, Commissioner
Carolyn W. Colvin, Deputy Commissioner
James A. Kissko, Chief of Staff
We deliver services through a nationwide network of over 1,400 offices that include regional offices, field offices, card centers, teleservice centers, processing centers, hearing offices, the Appeals Council, and our State and territorial partners, the Disability Determination Services. We also have a presence in U.S. embassies around the globe. The rich diversity of our employees mirrors the public we serve.

3899 West Virginia Advocates
1207 Quarrier St
Suite 400
Charleston, WV 25301-1826
304-346-0847
800-950-5250
Fax: 304-346-0867
kellie.l.aikman@wv.gov
wvadvocates.org

Terry Dilcher, President
John Galloway, Treasurer
Don Neurman, Secretary
Clarice Hausch, Executive Director
West Virginia Advocates, Inc. (WVA) is the federally mandated protection and advocacy system for people with disabilities in West Virginia. WVA is a private, nonprofit agency. Our services are confidential and free of charge.

3900 West Virginia Client Assistance Program
West Virginia Advocates
1900 Kanawha Blvd E
Room 9
Charleston, WV 25305-1
304-558-3780
Fax: 304-558-4092

Clarice Hausch, Executive Director

3901 West Virginia Department of Aging
1900 Kanawha Blvd. East
Charleston, WV 25305
304-558-3317
877-987-3646
Fax: 304-558-5609
www.wvseniorservices.gov

Robert E. Roswall, Commissioner
Nel Kimble
The information we offer is tailored to those who are seeking to locate programs and services for themselves or their loved ones and also for professionals who may be looking for up-to-date information relating to the field of aging.

3902 West Virginia Department of Children with Disabilities
Children with Special Health Care Needs
One Davis Square
Suite 100 East
Charleston, WV 25301- 1757
304-558-0684
Fax: 304-558-1130
DHHRSecretary@wv.gov
www.dhhr.wv.gov

Douglas M. Robinson, Deputy Commissioner
Virginia Mahan, Executive Secretary
Karen Villanueva-Matkovich, General Counsel
Melissa Rosen, CFO
The Bureau for Public Health directs public health activities at all levels within the state to fulfill the core functions of public health: the assessment of community health status and available resources; policy development resulting in proposals to support and encourage better health; and assurance that needed services are available, accessible, and of acceptable quality.

3903 West Virginia Department of Health
One Davis Square
Suite 100 East
Charleston, WV 25301
304-558-0684
Fax: 304-558-1130
DHHRSecretary@wv.gov
www.dhhr.wv.gov

Douglas M. Robinson, Deputy Commissioner
Virginia Mahan, Executive Secretary
Karen Villanueva-Matkovich, General Counsel
Melissa Rosen, CFO
The Bureau for Public Health directs public health activities at all levels within the state to fulfill the core functions of public health: the assessment of community health status and available resources; policy development resulting in proposals to support and encourage better health; and assurance that needed services are available, accessible, and of acceptable quality.

3904 West Virginia Developmental Disabilities Council
110 Stockton St
Charleston, WV 25387
304-558-0416
Fax: 304-558-0941
TTY:304-558-2376
dhhrwvddc@wv.gov
www.ddc.wv.gov

Diana Zottman, Chairman
Ed Holen, Executive Director
Brain Dahl, Support Coordinator
Laurie Bahr, Budget & Fiscal Director
Working to assure that West Virginians with developmental disabilities receive the services, supports, and other forms of assistance they need to exercise self-determination and achieve independence, productivity, integration, and inclusion in the community.
6-8 pages Quarterly Newsl

3905 West Virginia Division of Rehabilitation Services
107 Capitol Street
Charleston, WV 25301-2609
304-356-2060
800-642-8207
www.wvdrs.org

Donna L. Ashworth, Acting Director
Kay Goodwin, Cabinet Secretary
DRS' mission is to enable and empower individuals with disabilities to work and to live independently.

Wisconsin

3906 Disability Rights Wisconsin: Milwaukee Office
Ste 3230
6737 W Washington St
Milwaukee, WI 53214-5651
414-773-4646
800-708-3034
Fax: 414-773-4647
TTY: 888-758-6049
info@drwi.org
disabilityrightswi.org

Ted Skemp, President
Beth Moss, Vice President
Susan Gramling, Secretary
Dan Idzikowski, Executive Director
The protection and advocacy agency for people with disabilities in Wisconsin. DRW provides guidance, advice, investigation, negotiation and in some cases legal representation to people with disabilities and their families. Local and state level systems advocacy and training are also provided.

3907 International Dyslexia Association: Wisconsin Branch
1616 Graham Ave.
Eau Claire, WI 54701
608-355-0911
wi.dyslexiaida.org

Tammy Tillotson, President
Kimberly Chan, Treasurer
Pattie Huse, Secretary
Ann Malone, Director
Provides free information and referral services for diagnosis and tutoring for parents, educators, physicians, and individuals with dyslexia in Illinois. Membership includes yearly journal and quarterly newsletter.

3908 Social Security: Madison Field Office
6011 Odana Rd
Madison, WI 53719-1101
866-770-2262
800-772-1213
Fax: 608-270-1021
TTY: 800-325-0778
wi.fo.madison@ssa.gov
www.ssa.gov

3909 West Virginia Department of Health
One Davis Square
Suite 100 East
Charleston, WV 25301
304-558-0684
800-441-4576
Fax: 304-558-1130
DHHRSecretary@wv.gov
www.dhhr.wv.gov

Rocco S. Fucillo, Cabinet Secretary
Susan Shelton Perry, Deputy Secretary for Legal Servi
Ellen Cannon, Privacy Officer
Virginia Mahan, Executive Secretary
The Department of Health and Family Services operates the federal Title V Maternal and Child Health Block Grant Program for Children with Special Health Care Needs. The program provides program monitoring, consultation and technical assistance to five regional CSHCN centers throughout Wisconsin; a Birth Defects Monitoring and Surveillance Program and a Universal Newborn Hearing Screening Program.

3910 Wisconsin Board for People with Developmental Disabilities (WBPDD)
201 W Washington Ave
Suite 111
Madison, WI 53703-2796
608-266-7826
888-332-1677
Fax: 608-267-3906
TTY:608-266-6660
wcdd.org

Jennifer Ondrejka, Manager
Joshua Ryf, Office Manager
Statewide systems advocacy group for people with developmental disabilities in Wisconsin.

3911 Wisconsin Bureau of Aging
State Office of Wisconsin
1 West Wilson Street
Madison, WI 53703
608-266-1865
Fax: 608-267-3203
TTY:888-701-1251
DHSwebmaster@wisconsin.gov

Donna Mc Dowell, Executive Director
Gail Schwersenska, Section Chief
Dennis G. Smith, Secretary
Keeps and updates information and printed materials on senior housing directories, nursing home listings, and home care agencies.

3912 Wisconsin Coalition for Advocacy: Madison Office
16 N Carroll St
Suite 400
Madison, WI 53703-2762
608-267-0214
800-928-8778
Fax: 608-267-0368

Kim Hogan, Intake Specialist
Mr Lynn Breedlove, Executive Director
The protection and advocacy agency for people with disabilities in Wisconsin. WCA provides guidance, advice, investigation, negotiation and in some cases legal representation to people with disabilities and their families. Local and state level systems advocacy and training are also provided.

3913 Wisconsin Governor's Committee for People with Disabilities
1 West Wilson Street
Madison, WI 53703
608-266-1865
877-865-3432
Fax: 608-266-3386
TTY: 888-701-1251
DHSwebmaster@wisconsin.gov

Donna Mc Dowell, Executive Director
Gail Schwersenska, Section Chief
Dennis G. Smith, Secretary
To advise the Governor and state agencies on problems faced by people with disabilities; to review legislation affecting people with disabilities; to promote effective operation of publicly-administered or supported programs serving people with disabilities; to promote the collection, dissemination and incorporation of adequate information about persons with disabilities for purposes of public planning at all levels of government.

3914 Workers Compensation Board Wisconsin
Room C100, 201 E. Washington Avenue
P. O. Box 7901
Madison, WI 53707-7901
608-266-1340
Fax: 608-267-0394
dwd.wisconsin.gov/wc

Reggie Newson, Secretary
Jonathan Barry, Deputy Secretary
John Metcalf, Division Administrator
Brain Krueger, Deputy Administrator
The Worker's Compensation Division administers programs designed to ensure that injured workers receive required benefits from insurers or self-insured employers; encourage rehabilitation and reemployment for injured workers; and promote the reduction of work-related injuries, illnesses, and deaths.

Wyoming

3915 Social Security: Cheyenne Disability Determination
Social Security
821 W Pershing Blvd
Cheyenne, WY 82002-1
307-777-7341
800-438-5788
Fax: 307-637-0247
Jeff.Graham@ssa.gov
ssa.gov

Karena L. Kilgore, Executive Secretary
Carolyn W. Colvin, Commissioner
Carolyn W. Colvin, Deputy Commissioner
James A. Kissko, Chief of Staff
We deliver services through a nationwide network of over 1,400 offices that include regional offices, field offices, card centers, teleservice centers, processing centers, hearing offices, the Appeals Council, and our State and territorial partners, the Disability Determination Services. We also have a presence in U.S. embassies around the globe. The rich diversity of our employees mirrors the public we serve.

3916 WY Department of Health: Mental Health and Substance Abuse Service Division
401 Hathaway Building
Cheyenne, WY 82002-1
307-777-7656
800-535-4006
Fax: 307-777-7439
TTY: 307-777-5581
www.health.wyo.gov

Thomas O. Forslund, Director
Lee Clabots, Deputy Director
Bob Peck, Chief Financial Officer
Heather Babbitt, Senior Administartor
State office responsible for purchase of service and program development policy.

3917 Workers Compensation Board Wyoming
350 South Washington Street
PO Box 1068
Afton, WY 83110-3004
307-886-9260
Fax: 307-886-9269

3918 Wyoming Client Assistance Program
Protection and Advocacy System
2nd Fl
320 W 25th St
Cheyenne, WY 82001-3069
307-632-2682
877-854-5041
Fax: 307-638-0815
wypanda@vcn.com
ap.org

Jeanne Thobro, Manager
Jeanne A Thobro, Executive Director

3919 Wyoming Department of Aging
State Department of Wyoming
401 Hathaway Building
Cheyenne, WY 82002-1
307-777-7656
800-442-2766
Fax: 307-777-7439
wyaging@wyo.gov
health.wyo.gov

Thomas O. Forslund, Director
Lee Clabots, Deputy Director
Bob Peck, Chief Financial Officer
Heather Babbitt, Senior Administartor
The Wyoming Department of Health's Aging Division is committed to providing care, ensuring safety and and promoting independent choices for Wyoming's older adults

3920 Wyoming Developmental Disability Council
122 W 25th St
1st. Fl. West, Herschler Building,
Cheyenne, WY 82002
307-777-7230
800-438-5791
Fax: 307-777-5690
wgcdd@wyo.gov

Shannon Buller, Executive Director
Von Maul, Administrative Assistant
Sam Janney, Public Information Officer
Calob Taylor, Grants & Policy Analyst
Our purpose is to assure that individuals with developmental disabilities and their families participate in and have access to needed community services, individualized supports and other forms of assistance that promote independence, productivity, integration and inclusion in all facets of community life.

3921 Wyoming Protection & Advocacy for Persons with Disabilities
7344 Stockman Street
Cheyenne, WY 82009
307-632-3496
Fax: 307-638-0815
wypanda@wypanda.com
wypanda.com

Tori Rosenthal, President
Jeanne A Thobro, Executive Director
Wyoming Protection & Advocacy System, Inc. (P&A), established in 1977, is the official non-profit corporation authorized to implement certain mandates of several federal laws. Enacted by Congress, these laws provide various protection and advocacy services.

Independent Living Centers

Alabama

3922 Birdie Thornton Center
2350 Hine Street
Athens, AL 35611 256-232-0366
Fax: 256-230-9398

Kristy Allen King, Program Director
Heather Mereidth, Program Professional, QMRP
Rabieb Clem, Senior Aid
Kay Green, Training Specialist
The Birdie Thornton Center is devoted to providing care, education, and training to adults with developmental delays and disabilities.

3923 Independent Living Center of Mobile
5301 Moffett Rd
Suite 110
Mobile, AL 36618-2926 251-460-0301
Fax: 251-341-1267
TTY:251-460-2872
Michaeld@ilcmobile.org
ilcmobile.org

Michael Davis, Executive Director
Darmita Flood, Administrative Assistant
Barbara Hattier, ILS/Transportation Coordinator
James Flora, ILS/Outreach Specialist
Helping people with disabilities become independent.

3924 Independent Living Resources Of Greater Birmingham: Alabaster
120 Plaza Cir, Suite C
P. O. Box 2048
Alabaster, AL 35007-7034 205-685-0570
Fax: 205-251-0605
TTY:205-685-0570
gwen.brown@drradvocates.org
www.ilrgb.org

Kathy Lovell, President
Phil Klebine, Vice President
Susan Parker, Secretary
Milton Moats, Treasurer
The mission of this Independent Living Center is to empower people with disabilities to fully participate in the community.

3925 Independent Living Resources of Greater Birmingham: Jasper
300 Birmingham Ave
PO Box 434
Jasper, AL 35502-3811 205-387-0159
Fax: 205-387-0162
TTY:205-387-0159
www.ilrgb.org

Kathy Lovell, President
Phil Klebine, Vice President
Susan Parker, Secretary
Milton Moats, Treasurer
The purpose of this Independent Living Center is to empower people with disabilities to fully participate in the community.

3926 Independent Living Resources of Greater Birmingham
1418 6th Avenue North
Birmingham, AL 35203-1317 205-251-2223
Fax: 205-251-0605
TTY:205-251-2223
www.ilrgb.org

Kathy Lovell, President
Phil Klebine, Vice President
Susan Parker, Secretary
Milton Moats, Treasurer
The mission of this Independent Living Center is to empower people with disabilities to fully participate in the community.

3927 Montgomery Center for Independent Living
600 S Court St
Montgomery, AL 36104-4106 334-240-2520
Fax: 334-240-6869
TTY:334-240-2520
mcil@bellsouth.net
www.cilmontgomery.org

Scott Renner, Executive Director
Barbara F. Crozier, President
Kenneth Marshall, Vice President
Vickie P. FitzGerald, Secretary
Encourgaes people with disabilities to support one another in reaching their own independent living goals.

Alaska

3928 Access Alaska: ADA Partners Project
1217 East 10th Ave
Suite 105
Anchorage, AK 99501-2044 907-248-4777
800-770-4488
888-462-1444
Fax: 907-263-1942
TTY:907-248-8799
info@accessalaska.org
accessalaska.org

Lorali Simon, President
Mike O'Neill, Vice President
Jim Duffield, Treasurer
Eric Spangler, Member
Assisting Alaskans with disabilities to live independently in the community of their choice.

3929 Access Alaska: Fairbanks
526 Gaffney Rd
Suite 100
Fairbanks, AK 99701-4914 907-479-7940
800-770-7940
Fax: 907-474-4052
TTY: 907-474-8619
info@accessalaska.org
accessalaska.org

Lorali Simon, President
Mike O'Neill, Vice President
Jim Duffield, Treasurer
Eric Spangler, Member
A local non profit agency using its resources to actively promote a society where persons with disabilities can live and work independently in the community of their choice.

3930 Access Alaska: Mat-Su
1075 Check St,
Suite 109
Wasilla, AK 99654-6937 907-357-2588
800-770-0228
Fax: 907-357-5585
info@accessalaska.org
accessalaska.org

Lorali Simon, President
Mike O'Neill, Vice President
Jim Duffield, Treasurer
Eric Spangler, Member
Provides independent living services to persons with significant disabilities. Mission is to encourage and promote the total integration of persons with disabilities into the community of their choice. Services include independent living skills training, information and referral, advocacy, peer support, and at home modifications.

3931 Alaska SILC
Ste 206
1217 East 10th Ave
Anchorage, AK   99501-1760   907-248-4777
                                      800-770-4488
                                      888-294-7452
                                  Fax: 907-263-1942
                                  info@accessalaska.org
                                     www.alaskasilc.org

Jim Beck, Executive Director
Lorali Simon, President
Mike O'Neill, Vice President
Jim Duffield, Treasurer
The Alaska Statewide Independent Living is committed to promoting a philosophy of consumer control, peer support, self help, self determination, equal access, and individual and systems advocacy, in order to maximize leadership, empowerment, independence, productivity, and to support full inclusion and integration of individuals with disabilities into the mainstream of American society.

3932 Arctic Access
P.O.Box 930
Kotzebue, AK   99752-930   907-412-0695
                                     877-442-2393
                                  TTY:907-442-2393
                             arcticaccesskotz@gci.net

Roger Wright Jr, Executive Director
Russell Williams, Jr,, Elder & Disability Resource Coor
Audrey Aanes
The Arctic Access Independent Living Center provides services and opportunities for elders and others with disabilities so they may remain in their village and be as active as possible with their families and commuties in the North West Arctic and Bering Straits Regions of Alaska.

3933 Hope Community Resources
540 W Intl Airport Rd
Anchorage, AK   99518-1105   907-561-5335
                                     800-478-0078
                                  Fax: 907-564-7429
                                   info@hopealaska.org
                                       hopealaska.org

Robert Owens, President
John Dittrich, Vice President
Eugene 'Gene' Bates, Treasurer
Stephen P. Lesko, Executive Director
Provider of services to individuals who experience a disability.

3934 Kenai Peninsula Independent Living Center
265 E. Pioneer Suite 201
P.O.Box 2474
Homer, AK   99603- 2474   907-235-7911
                                     800-770-7911
                                  Fax: 907-235-6236
                                  info@peninsulailc.org
                                       peninsulailc.org

Candy Norman, President
Mike Harmer, Vice President
Offers peer counseling, disability education and awareness, attendant care registry and information on accessible housing.

3935 Kenai Peninsula Independent Living Center: Seward
201 Third Avenue, Suite 101Bs
P. O. Box 3523
Seward, AK 99664-3523   907-224-8711
                                  Fax: 907-224-7793
                                  info@peninsulailc.org
                                     www.peninsulailc.org

Candy Norman, President
Mike Harmer, Vice President
Offers peer counseling, disability, education and awareness, attendant care registry and information on accessible housing.

3936 Keni Peninsula Independent Living Center: Central Peninsula
47255 Princeton Avenue
Suite 8
Soldotna, AK   99669   907-262-6333
                                  Fax: 907-260-4495
                                     www.peninsulailc.org

Candy Norman, President
Mike Harmer, Vice President
Offers peer counseling, disability education and awareness, attendant care registry and information on accessible housing.

3937 Southeast Alaska Independent Living
3225 Hospital Drive
Suite 300
Juneau, AK   99801-7863   907-586-4920
                                     800-478-7245
                                  Fax: 907-586-4980
                                  TTY: 907-523-5285
                                     info@sailinc.org
                                         sailinc.org

Robert Purvis, President
Jeff Irwin, Vice President
Suzanne Williams, Secretary
Mary Gregg, Treasurer
To empower consumers with disabilities by providing services and information to support them in making choices that will positively affect their independence and productivity in society.

3938 Southeast Alaska Independent Living: Ketchikan
602 Dock St
Suite 107
Ketchikan, AK   99901-6574   907-225-4735
                                     888-452-7245
                                  Fax: 907-247-4735
                                  ketchikan@sailinc.org
                                      www.sailinc.org

Robert Purvis, President
Jeff Irwin, Vice President
Suzanne Williams, Secretary
Mary Gregg, Treasurer
To empower consumers with disabilities by providing services and information to support them in making choices that will positively affect their independence and productivity in society.

3939 Southeast Alaska Independent Living: Sitka
514 Lake St
Suite C
Sitka, AK   99835-7405   907-747-6859
                                     888-500-7245
                                  Fax: 907-747-6783
                                    sitka@sailinc.org
                                      www.sailinc.org

Robert Purvis, President
Jeff Irwin, Vice President
Suzanne Williams, Secretary
Mary Gregg, Treasurer
To empower consumers with disabilities by providing services and information to support them in making choices that will positively affect their independence and productivity in society.

Arizona

3940 ASSIST! to Independence
P.O.Box 4133
Tuba City, AZ   86045-4133   928-283-6261
                                     888-848-1449
                                  Fax: 928-283-6284
                                  TTY: 928-283-6672
                                  assist01@frontiernet.net
                                www.assisttoindependence.org

Michael Blatchford, Executive Director
Priscilla Lane, IL Services Coordinator/Dep Dir
A community based, American Indian owned and operated non-profit agency that was established by and for people with dis-

abilities and chronic health conditions to help fill some of the gaps in service delivery.

3941   Arizona Bridge to Independent Living
5025 E Washington St
Suite 200
Phoenix, AZ   85034-7439
602-256-2245
800-280-2245
Fax: 602-254-6407
boardofdirectors@abil.org
www.abil.org

Mary Slaughter, Chairman
Brad Wemhaner, Vice Chairman
Michael Somsan, Secretary
Jim Winterton, Treasurer
ABIL offers and promotes programs designed to empower people with disabilities to take personal responsibility so they may achieve or continue independent lifestyles within the community.

3942   Arizona Bridge to Independent Living: Phoenix
1229 E.Washington St.
Suite D405
Phoenix, AZ   85034
602-296-0551
800-280-2245
Fax: 602-256-0184
TTY: 602-296-0591
boardofdirectors@abil.org
www.abil.org

Mary Slaughter, Chairman
Brad Wemhaner, Vice Chairman
Michael Somsan, Secretary
Jim Winterton, Treasurer
ABIL offers and promotes programs designed to empower people with disabilities to take personal responsibility so they may achieve or continue independent lifestyles within the community.

3943   Arizona Bridge to Independent Living: Mesa
2150 S Country Club Dr
Suite 10
Mesa, AZ   85210-6879
480-655-9750
800-280-2245
Fax: 480-655-9751
TTY: 480-655-9750
boardofdirectors@abil.org
www.abil.org

Mary Slaughter, Chairman
Brad Wemhaner, Vice Chairman
Michael Somsan, Secretary
Jim Winterton, Treasurer
ABIL offers and promotes programs designed to empower people with disabilities to take personal responsibility so they may achieve or continue independent lifestyles within the community.

3944   Community Outreach Program for the Deaf
268 W Adams St
Tucson, AZ   85705-6534
520-792-1906
Fax: 520-770-8554
TTY:520-792-1906
request@copdaz.org
copdaz.org

Anne Levy, Executive Director
A non-profit organization, which has been serving the needs of people in Southern Arizona who are deaf or hard of hearing.

3945   DIRECT Center for Independence
1023 N Tyndall Ave
Tucson, AZ   85719-4446
520-624-6452
800-342-1853
Fax: 520-792-1438
TTY: 520-624-6452
direct@directilc.org
www.directilc.org

Ron Trozzi, President
Marrill Eisenberg, Vice President
Steve Fristoe, Treasurer
Loretta Alvarez, Secretary
A non-consumer directed, community-based advocacy organization, that promotes independent living and offers a variety of pro-

grams for all people with disabilities which encourage them to achieve their full potential and to participate in the community.

3946   New Horizons Independent Living Center: Prescott Valley
8085 E Manley Dr
Prescott Valley, AZ   86314-6154
928-772-1266
800-406-2377
Fax: 928-772-3808
TTY: 928-772-1266
ltoone@newhorizonsilc.org
www.newhorizonsilc.org

Deborah Henderson, Office Manager
Liz Toone, Executive Director
Nick Perry, President
Jim Stobbs, Vice President
To provide services and advocacy which empower and enable people with disabilities to self-determine the goals and activities of their lives.

3947   Services Maximizing Independent Living and Empowerment (SMILE)
1931 South Arizona Ave
Suite 4
Yuma, AZ   85364-5721
928-329-6681
855-209-8363
Fax: 928-329-6715
TTY: 928-782-7458
info@smile-az.org
www.smile-az.org

Laura Duval, Executive Director
Brenda Howard, Finance Manager/ Admin Assistant
Shawnnita Miranda, Advocate/ Home modification Mana
Brandon Howard, Outreach Coordinator, Technology
SMILE continually advocates for the Independent Living Philosophy, both individually and system wide. The Board and staff constantly strives to improve the system by writing letters, training staff, providing services, and creating public awareness as to the services and opportunities open to people who have disabilities.

3948   Sterling Ranch: Residence for Special Women
Sterling Ranch
P.O.Box 36
Skull Valley, AZ   86338-36
928-442-3289
Fax: 928-442-9272
www.sterlingranch.info

Russell Dryer, Executive Director
Trent Nichel, Manager
A nonprofit residence for women with developmental disabilities which has been in operation since 1947. As a small facility (19 residents) the orientation is personal and family-like. Offers activities that range from gardening, quilting, academics, sign-language, crafts and a myriad of field trips and excursions. Private rooms and spacious living on 4 1/2 acres.

Arkansas

3949   Arkansas Independent Living Council
11324 Arcade Drive
Suite 7
Little Rock, AR   72212
501-372-0607
800-772-0607
Fax: 501-372-0598
arkansasilc@att.net
www.ar-silc.org

Sha Stephens, Executive Director
Cheryl , Director
Brenda Stinebuck, Chair
Liz Adams, Vice Chair
A non-profit organization promoting independent living for people with disabilities.

3950 Delta Resource Center for Independent Living
11324 Arcade Drive
Little Rock, AR 72212-6249
501-372-0607
800-772-0607
Fax: 501-372-0598
drcilar@yahoo.com
www.ar-silc.org

Sha Stephens, Executive Director
Katy Morris, Director
Cheryl , Director
Brenda Stinebuck, Chair
Provides services, support, and advocacy which enables people with severe disabilities to live as independently as possible within their family and community.

3951 Mainstream
300 S Rodney Parham Rd
Suite 5
Little Rock, AR 72205- 4774
501-280-0012
800-371-9026
Fax: 501-280-9267
TTY: 501-280-9262
mainstreamilrc.com

Rita Byers, Executive Director
Vincent McKinney
Vincent Acklin
Debbie Gillespie
A non residential, consumer driven independent living resource center for persons with disabilities. Mainstream operates with conviction that people with disabilities have the right and responsibility to make choices, to control their lives and to participate fully and equally in the community.

3952 Our Way: The Cottage Apt Homes
9175 Greenback Lane
Orangevale, CA 95662-6616
501-225-5030
888-879-9584
Fax: 501-225-5190
rentthecottages.com

Katrina Williams, Manager
Crystal Brown, Assistant Manager
Advocacy and information services. One bedroom apartments for mobility impaired and elderly 62 years or older persons.
Based on income

3953 Sources for Community IL Services
1918 N Birch Ave
Fayetteville, AR 72703-2408
479-442-5600
888-284-7521
Fax: 479-442-5192
TTY: 479-251-1378
jmather@arsources.org
www.arsources.org

Brent Williams, PhD, President
Elise Burt, Treasurer
Burke Fanari, Secretary
Jim Mather, Executive Director
Provides services, support, and advocacy for individuals with disabilities, their families and the community.

3954 Spa Area Independent Living Services
621 Albert Pike
Hot Springs, AR 71913
501-624-7710
800-255-7549
Fax: 501-624-7003

Dejan S. Vojnovic, President
Joseph E. Anderson, Vice President - Real Estate
Bryan S. Cox, Vice President - Technology
Brenda Stinebuck, Executive Director
Provides services and advocacy by and for persons with all types of disabilities. The goal is to assist individuals with disabilities to achieve thier maximum potential within their families and communities.

California

3955 Access Center of San Diego
8885 Rio San Diego Dr
Suite 131
San Diego, CA 92108-1625
619-293-3500
800-300-4326
Fax: 619-293-3508
TTY: 619-293-7757
info@a2isd.org
www.a2isd.org

Louis Frick, Executive Director
Derek Parker, Chair
Jacquelyn E. Nash, Vice Chair
Nick Bradley, Treasurer
Access to Independence is an independent living center (ILC), a nonresidential, cross-disability, non-profit corporations that provide services to people with disabilities to help maximize their independence and fully integrate into their communities. Access to Independence is one of 391 ILCs across the country and one of 29 serving Californians. Like all ILCs, Access to Independence offers required federal and state programs and services to people of all disability types and ages at no charge.

3956 Access to Independence
8885 Rio San Diego Drive
Suite 131
San Diego, CA 92108- 1625
619-293-3500
800-300-4326
Fax: 619-293-3508
TTY: 619-293-7757
info@a2isd.org
www.a2isd.org

Louis Frick, Executive Director
Derek Parker, Chair
Jacquelyn E. Nash, Vice Chair
Nick Bradley, Treasurer
A community resource for people with disabilities to lead independent lives.

3957 Access to Independence of Imperial Valley
101 Hacienda Drive
Suite 13
Calexico, CA 92231-2875
760-768-2044
866-976-3515
Fax: 760-768-4977
TTY: 619-293-7757
info@a2isd.org
www.a2sid.org

Louis Frick, Executive Director
Derek Parker, Chair
Jacquelyn E. Nash, Vice Chair
Nick Bradley, Treasurer
A community resource for people with disabilities to lead independent lives.

3958 Access to Independence of North County
209 E Broadway
Vista, CA 92084-6005
760-643-0447
Fax: 760-435-9206
info@a2isd.org

Louis Frick, Executive Director
Derek Parker, Chair
Jacquelyn E. Nash, Vice Chair
Nick Bradley, Treasurer
A community resource for people with disabilities to lead independent lives.

3959 Beaumont Senior Center: Community Access Center
1310 Oak Valley Parkway
Beaumont, CA 92223-2218
951-769-8524
Fax: 951-769-8519
TTY:909-769-2794
ilser5@ilcac.org
www.ci.beaumont.ca.us

Laurie Hoirup, Director

A non profit organization; one of 29 similar programs throughout the state of California CAC is a community resource, advocate, and educator for Riverside County residents with disabilities.

3960 California Foundation For Independent Living Centers
1234 H Street
Suite 100
Sacramento, CA 95814-1912
916-325-1690
Fax: 916-325-1699
TTY:916-325-1695
cfilc@cfilc.org
www.cfilc.org

Robert Hand, Chairperson
Ana Acton, Vice Chairperson
Tink Miller, Executive Director
Kim Cantrell, Program Director
Community Rehabilitation Services, Inc. (CRS) is a private, non-profit agency established in 1974 to assist persons with disabilities within the East/North East areas of Los Angeles County to enhance their options for living independently. Any person who is 18 yrs of age or more with physical, sensory, mental/emotional or developmental disabilities can work with us to become more self-sufficient. Our intake procedures provide an orientation to the staff, facilities and services at CRS.

3961 California Foundation for Independent Living Centers
1235 H Street
Suite 100
Sacramento, CA 95814-1913
916-325-1690
Fax: 916-325-1699
TTY:916-325-1695
cfilc@cfilc.org
www.cfilc.org

Robert Hand, Chairperson
Ana Acton, Vice Chairperson
Tink Miller, Executive Director
Kim Cantrell, Program Director
CFILC's mission is to support independent living centers in their local communities through advocating for systems change and promoting access and integration for people with disabilities.

3962 California State Independent Living Council (SILC)
1235 H Street
Suite 100
Sacramento, CA 95814-4010
916-325-1690
866-866-7452
Fax: 916-325-1699
TTY: 866-745-2889
www.calsilc.org

Susan M. Madison, Chairman
Eli Gelardin, Vice Chairman
Liz Pazdral, Executive Director
Caroline Kuhn, Staff Services Analyst
To maximize options for independence for persons with disabilities

3963 Center for Independence of the Disabled
Suite 103
2001 Winward Way
San Mateo, CA 94404-3062
650-645-1780
Fax: 650-645-1785
TTY:650-522-9313
http://www.cidsanmateo.org

Brad Friedman, Co-President
Laura Whitsitt Hillyard, Co-President
Thomas J. Devine, Vice President
John Horgan, Secretary
Increase the social, educational, and economic participation of persons with disabilities in San Mateo County, and to encourage, support, and provide options for self determination, equal access and freedom of choice.

3964 Center for Independence of the Disabled- Daly City
Ste 256
355 Gellert Blvd
Daly City, CA 94015-2675
650-991-5124
Fax: 650-757-2075
TTY:650-991-5182
dalycity5@aol.com
www.cidbelmont.org

Kent Mickelson, Director
The Daly City Branch office fulfills its mission by serving disabled consumers in Brisbane, Colma, Daly City, El Granada, Half Moon Bay, Montara, Moss Beach, Pacifica, Pescadero, Princeton and South San Francisco. Our mission is to increase the social, educational, economic, social and political participants of persons with disabilities in San Mateo county, California.

3965 Center for Independent Living
Suite 103
2001 Winward Way
San Mateo, CA 94404
650-645-1780
Fax: 650-645-1785
TTY:510-522-9313
bburgess@cilberkeley.org
www.cidsanmateo.org

Beatrice Burgess, Interim Executive Director
Jody Yarborough, President
Michael Levinson, Vice President
The Center for Independent Living, Inc (CIL) is a national leader in helping people with disabilities live independently and become productive members of society. Advocates for greater accessibility in communities, designing techniques in independent living and providing direct services to people with disabilities.
1972

3966 Center for Independent Living: East Oakland
Suite 100
3075 Adeline Street
Berkeley, CA 94703-2403
510-841-4776
Fax: 510-841-6168
info@cilberkeley.org
www.cilberkeley.org

Melissa Male, Chair
Bea Worthen, Vice-Chair
Paul Hippolitus, Secretary
A national leader in helping people with disabilities live independently and become productive, fully participating members of society.

3967 Center for Independent Living: Oakland
Suite 100
3075 Adeline Street
Berkeley, CA 94703-1285
510-841-4776
Fax: 510-841-6168
TTY:510-444-1837
info@cilberkeley.org
cilberkeley.org

Melissa Male, Chair
Bea Worthen, Vice-Chair
Paul Hippolitus, Secretary
Ted Dienstfrey, Finance Committee
A national leader in supporting disabled people in their efforts to lead independent lives.

3968 Center for Independent Living: Tri-County
2822 Harris Street
Eureka, CA 95503
707-445-8404
877-576-5000
Fax: 707-445-9751
TTY: 707-445-8405
aa@tilinet.org
www.tilinet.org

Gail Pascoe, President
Linda Arnold, Vice President
Kevin O'Brien, Treasurer
Chris Jones, Executive Director

3969   Center for Independent Living:Fresno
3475 Wesy Shaw Ave
Suite 101
Fresno, CA   93711   559-276-6777
                                              Fax: 559-276-6778
                                              TTY:559-276-6779
                                              www.cil-fresno.org

Bob Hand, Manager

3970   Center for Independent Living; Oakland
1904 Franklin Street
Suite 320
Oakland, CA   94612-2324   510-763-9990
                                              Fax: 510-763-4910
                                              TTY:510-536-2271
                                              info@cilberkeley.org
                                              cilberkeley.org

Melissa Male, Chair
Bea Worthen, Vice-Chair
Hank Stratford, Treasurer
Paul Hippolitus, Secretary
Independent living center to maximise the options for independence for persons with disabilities.

3971   Center of Independent Living: Visalia
121 E Main
Suite 101
Visalia, CA   93291-6262   559-622-9276
                                              Fax: 559-622-9638
Fran Phillips, Executive Directorram Manager
Renee Ezelle, Manager

3972   Central Coast Center for IL: San Benito
1234 H Street
Suite 100
Sacramento, CA   95814-1914   916-325-1690
                                              Fax: 916-325-1699
                                              TTY:916-325-1695
                                              cfile@cfilc.org
                                              www.cfilc.org

Ana Acton, Chairperson
Larry Grable, Vice Chairperson
Nayana Shah, Treasurer
Jessie Lorenz, Secretary
To advocate for barrier-free access and equal opportunity for people with disabilities to participate in the community life by increasing the capacity of Independent Living Centers to achieve their missions.

3973   Central Coast Center for Independent Living
318 Cayuga St.
Suite 208
Salinas, CA   93901-2600   831-757-2968
                                              Fax: 831-757-5549
                                              TTY:831-757-3949
                                              cccil@cccil.org
                                              cccil.org

Jennifer L. Williams, President
Elsa Quezada, Executive Director
Brenda Cardoza, Information and Referral Special
Gabriel Garcia, Independent Living Specialist
CCCIL promotes the independence of people with disabilities by supporting their equal and full participation in community life. CCCIL provides advocacy, education and support to all people with disabilities, their families and the community.

3974   Central Coast Center: Independent Living - Santa Cruz Office
1350 - 41st Avenue
Suite 101
Capitola, CA   95010-3930   831-462-8720
                                              Fax: 831-462-8727
                                              TTY:831-462-8729
                                              cccil@cccil.org
                                              www.cccil.org

Jennifer L. Williams, President
Elsa Quezada, Executive Director
Brenda Cardoza, Information and Referral Special
Gabriel Garcia, Independent Living Specialist
CCCIL promotes the independence of people with disabilities by supporting their equal and full participation in community life. CCCIL provides advocacy, education and support to all people with disabilities, their families and the community.

3975   Central Coast for Independent Living
1111 San Felipe Rd
Suite 107
Hollister, CA   95023-2814   831-636-5196
                                              Fax: 831-637-0478
                                              TTY:831-637-6235
                                              cccil@cccil.org
                                              www.cccil.org

Jennifer L. Williams, President
Elsa Quezada, Executive Director
Brenda Cardoza, Information and Referral Special
Gabriel Garcia, Independent Living Specialist
CCCIL promotes the independence of people with disabilities by supporting their equal and full particpation in community life. CCCIL provides advocacy, education and support to all people with disabilities, their families and the community.

3976   Central Coast for Independent Living: Watsonville
18 W. Beach St.
Suite Y
Watsonville, CA   95076-4371   831-724-2997
                                              Fax: 831-724-2915
                                              TTY:831-786-0915
                                              www.cccil.org

Jennifer L. Williams, President
Elsa Quezada, Executive Director
Brenda Cardoza, Information and Referral Special
Gabriel Garcia, Independent Living Specialist
An advocacy and information center organized by and for people with disabilities that strives to make our communities more accessible and to empower people with disabilities with information and skills to live fulfilling lives in our communities.

3977   Communities Actively Living Independent and Free
634 S Spring St
2nd Floor
Los Angeles, CA   90014-3921   213-627-0477
                                              Fax: 213-627-0535
                                              TTY:213-623-9502
                                              info@calif-ilc.org
                                              califilc.webs.com

Lillibeth Navarro, Founder & Executive Director
Alex San Martin, Temporary Chair
Fernando Roldan, Board Secretary
Ben Rockwell, Temporary Board Treasurer
Envisions a culturally diverse independent living center designed to empower the Disability Community.

3978   Community Access Center
6848 Magnolia Ave
Suite 150
Riverside, CA   92506-2858   951-274-0358
                                              Fax: 951-274-0833
                                              TTY:951-274-0834
                                              execdir@ilcac.org
                                              www.ilcac.org

Mark Dyer, President
Janet Newcomer, Vice President
Perry Halteman, Secretary
Chuck Reutter, Treasurer

A non-profit organization; one of 29 similar programs throughout the state of California. CAC is a community resource, advocate, and educator for Riverside County residents with disabilities.

3979 Community Access Center: Indio Branch
83233 Indio Blvd
Indio, CA 92201-4748   760-347-4888
                                                Fax: 760-347-0722
                                                TTY:760-347-6802
                                                pmgr3@ilcac.org
                                                www.ilcac.org

Mark Dyer, President
Janet Newcomer, Vice President
Perry Halteman, Secretary
Chuck Reutter, Treasurer
To empower persons with disabilities to control their own lives, create an accessible community and advocate to achieve complete social, economic, and political integration. We implement this vision by providing information, supportive services and independent living skills training.

3980 Community Access Center: Perris
371 Wilkerson Ave
Perris, CA 92570-2241   951-443-1158
                                                Fax: 951-443-2608
                                                TTY:951-443-1158
                                                www.ilcac.org

Mark Dyer, President
Janet Newcomer, Vice President
Perry Halteman, Secretary
Chuck Reutter, Treasurer
Community Access Center empowers persons with disabilities to control their own lives, create an accessible community and advocate to achieve complete social, economic, and political integration. CAC also implements this vision by providing information, suportive services and independent living skills training.

3981 Community Rehabilitation Services
844 E. Mission Road
Suite A & B
San Gabriel, CA 91776- 2759   323-266-0453
                                                Fax: 626-614-1590
                                                TTY:323-266-3016

Frances Garcia, Executive Director
CRS is an independent living center that provides free services to persons with disabilities in the areas of advocacy, housing and independent living skills; assistive technology, employment, personal assistant services, peer counseling and information and referral.

3982 Community Resources for Independence: Mendocino/Lake Branch
Ste B
415 Talmage Rd
Ukiah, CA 95482-7486   707-463-8875
                                                Fax: 707-463-8878
                                                TTY:707-463-4498
                                                www.cri-dove.org

Tanner Silva, Manager
A non-profit corporation established by a group of disabled and non-disabled individuals to advance the rights of persons with disabilities to equal justice, access, opportunity and participation in the communities.

3983 Community Resources for Independence: Napa
Ste 208
1040 Main St
Napa, CA 94559-2605   707-258-0270
                                                Fax: 707-258-0275
                                                TTY:707-257-0274
                                                cri-dove.org

Tyler Stanley, Manager
Matthew Shultz, Independent Living Advocate
A non-profit corporation established by a group of disabled and non-disabled individuals to advance the rights of persons with disabilities to equal justice, access, opportunity and participation in the communities.

3984 Community Resources for Independent Living: Hayward
3311 Pacific Ave
Livermore, CA 94550-5013   925-371-1531
                                                Fax: 925-373-5034
                                                TTY:925-371-1533
                                                info@cril-online.org
                                                crilhayward.org

Sheri Burns, Executive Director
Michael Galvan, PhD., Program Director
April Monroe, Finance Director
Esperanza Diaz-Alvarez, IL Coor - Travel Trainer & PAS
CRIL offers independent living services at no charge to persons with disabilities living in southern and eastern Alameda county. CRIL is also a resource for disability awareness education and training, advocacy and technical advice.

3985 Community Resources for Independent Living
39155 Liberty St
Suite A100
Fremont, CA 94538-1503   510-794-5735
                                                info@cril-online.org
                                                crilhayward.org

Sheri Burns, Executive Director
Michael Galvan, PhD., Program Director
April Monroe, Finance Director
Esperanza Diaz-Alvarez, PAS Coordinator/Benefits Advocat
Community Resources for Independent Living is a peer-based disability organization that advocates and provides resources for people with disabilities to improve lives and make communities fully accessible.

3986 DRAIL (Disability Resource Agency for Independent Living)
501 W Weber Ave
Ste 200-A
Stockton, CA 95203-6239   209-477-8143
                                                Fax: 209-477-7730
                                                TTY:209-465-5643
                                                barry@drail.org
                                                www.drail.org

Terry Gray, President
Michael Kim Cornelius, Treasurer
Adeline Bagwell, Secretary
Barry Smith, Executive Director
A non-profit corporation that is community based, consumer controlled, consumer choice, cross disability center for independent living.

3987 Dayle McIntosh Center: Laguna Niguel
24031 El Toro Road
Suite 300
Laguna Hills, CA 92653-3632   949-460-7784
                                                800-422-7444
                                                Fax: 949-334-2302
                                                TTY: 800-735-2929
                                                www.daylemc.org

Libby Partain, President
Cindy McLeroy, Vice President
Eva Casas-Sarmiento, Secretary
Michael Ryan, Treasurer
DMC advances empowerment and inclusion of all persons with disabilities. DMC is the largest Independent Living Center in California, and was named in memory of a young woman with a severe physical disability who worked to found the center.

3988 Disability Resource Agency for Independent Living: Modesto
920-12th Street
Modesto, CA 95354-543   209-521-7260
                                                Fax: 209-521-4763
                                                TTY:209-576-2409
                                                larry@drail.org
                                                www.drail.org

Terry Gray, President
Michael Kim Cornelius, Treasurer
Adeline Bagwell, Secretary
Barry Smith, Executive Director

A non-profit corporation that is community based, consumer controlled, consumer choice, cross disability center for independent living.

3989   Disability Services & Legal Center
521 Mendocino Ave.
Santa Rosa, CA 95401-1649   707-528-2745
                                          Fax: 707-528-9477
                                          TTY:707-528-2151
                          www.disabilityserviceandlegal.org

Adam Brown, Chairman
Shirley Johnson-Foell, Board President
Jack Geary, Board Member
Ben Karpilow, Board Secretary
A non-profit corporation established by a group of disabled and non-disabled individuals to advance the rights of persons with disabilities to equal justice, access, opportunity and participation in the communities.

3990   Disabled Resources Center
2750 E Spring St
Suite 100
Long Beach, CA 90806-2263   562-427-1000
                                          Fax: 562-427-2027
                                          TTY:562-427-1366
                                          info@drcinc.org
                                          drcinc.org

C. Timothy Lashlee, President
Dora Hogan, Vice President
Finola Campbell, Treasurer
Dolores Nason, Executive Director
To empower people with disabilities to live independently in the community, to make their own decisions about their lives and to advocate on their own behalf.

3991   FREED Center for Independent Living
2059 Nevada City Hwy
Suite 102
Grass Valley, CA 95945- 3227   530-477-3333
                                          800-655-7732
                                          Fax: 530-477-8184
                                          TTY: 530-477-8194
                                          contact-04@freed.org
                                          freed.org

Ana Acton, Executive Director
To eliminate barriers to full equality for people with disabilities through programs which promote independent living.

3992   FREED Center for Independent Living: Marysville
508 J St
Marysville, CA 95901-5636   530-742-4476
                                          TTY:530-742-4474
                                          freed.org
Claudia Hallis, Manager
To eliminate barriers to full equality for people with disabilities through programs which promote independent living.

3993   First Step Independent Living
1174 Nevada St
Redlands, CA 92374-2893   800-362-0312

3994   Independent Living Center of Kern County
5251 Office Park Dr
Suite 200
Bakersfield, CA 93309   661-325-1063
                                          877-688-2079
                                          800-529-9541
                                          Fax: 661-325-6702
                                          TTY:661-325-6702
                                          info@ilcofkerncounty.org
                                          www.ilcofkerncounty.org

Jimmie Soto, Executive Director
Tammy Hartsch, Finance Manager
Harvey Clowers, Special Projects and AT Coordina
Olivia Kent, Systems Change Advocate
A consumer-based consumer-directed non-profit agency assisting persons with disabilities to live independently in their com-munity. The ILCKC presently offers a wide range of services to a growing population of persons with disabilities.

3995   Independent Living Center of Lancaster
606 East Avenue K4
Lancaster, CA 93535-2844   661-942-9726
                                          Fax: 661-945-5690
                                          TTY:661-723-2509
                                          www.ilcsc.org

Taura Jacob, Manager
Marcy Hernandez
Niyanta Dave
ILCSC is a non-profit, consumer based, non-residential agency providing a wide range of services to a growing population of people with disabilities. ILCSC is dedicated to empowering persons with disabilities to exercise indpendence-pofessionally, personally and creatively-while striving to educate the community on their needs.

3996   Independent Living Resource Center
7425 El Camino Real
Suite R
Atascadero, CA 93422-4656   805-464-3203
                                          Fax: 805-462-1166
                                          TTY:805-462-1162
                                          info@ilrc-trico.org
                                          www.ilrc-trico.org

Kit McMillion, President
Larry Laborde, Vice President
Dani Anderson, Executive Director
Jennifer Griffin, Business Manager
To assist and encourage individuals to achieve their optimal level of self-sufficiency while eliminating the architectural, communication and attitudinal barriers which prevent them from full participation in the community.

3997   Independent Living Resource Center: Santa Barbara
423 W Victoria St
Santa Barbara, CA 93101-3619   805-284-9051
                                          Fax: 805-963-1350
                                          TTY:805-963-0595
                                          info@ilrc-trico.org
                                          www.ilrc-trico.org

Kit McMillion, President
Larry Laborde, Vice President
Dani Anderson, Executive Director
Jennifer Griffin, Business Manager
To assist and encourage individuals to achieve their optimal level of self-sufficiency while eliminating the architectural, communication and attitudinal barriers which prevent them from full participation in the community.

3998   Independent Living Resource Center: San Francisco
825 Howard Street
San Francisco, CA 94103-4128   415-543-6222
                                          Fax: 415-543-6318
                                          TTY:415-543-6698
                                          info@ilrcsf.org
                                          ilrcsf.org

Juma Byrd, President
Kolya Kirienko, Vice President
Ben MacMullan, Treasurer
Will Simpson, Secretary
To ensure that people with disabilities are full social and economic partners, both within their families and in a fully accessible community.

3999 Independent Living Resource Center: Santa Maria Office
327 East Plaza Dr
Suite 3A
Santa Maria, CA 93454-6930   805-354-5948
                                               Fax: 805-349-2416
                                               TTY:805-925-0015
                                               info@ilrc-trico.org
                                               www.ilrc-trico.org

Kit McMillion, President
Larry Laborde, Vice President
Dani Anderson, Executive Director
Jennifer Griffin, Business Manager
To assist and encourage individuals to achieve their optimal level of self-sufficiency while eliminating the architectural, communication and attitudinal barriers which prevent them from full participation in the community.

4000 Independent Living Resource Center: Ventura
1802 Eastman Ave
Suite 112
Ventura, CA 93003-5759   805-256-1036
                                               Fax: 805-650-9278
                                               TTY:805-650-5993
                                               info@ilrc-trico.org
                                               www.ilrc-trico.org

Kit McMillion, President
Larry Laborde, Vice President
Dani Anderson, Executive Director
Jennifer Griffin, Business Manager
An organization of, by and for persons with disabilities who reside or work in the service area. Purpose is to assist and encourage individuals to achieve their optimal level of self-sufficiency while eliminating the architectural, communication and attitudinal barriers which prevent them from full participation in the community.

4001 Independent Living Resource of Contra Coast
1850 Gateway Blvd
Suite 120
Concord, CA 94520-3293   925-363-7293
                                               Fax: 925-363-7296
                                               www.ilrscc.org

Sarah BirdwelL, Board President
Kathy Mitsopoulos, Board Vice President
Teri Ruggiero, Board Secretary
Susan Rotchy, Executive Director
Offers workshops, services are accessible to individuals with cognitive disabilities, physical disabilities, deaf and hard of hearing, emotional disabilities, visual impairments, learing disabilities and seniors.

4002 Independent Living Resource of Fairfield
470 Chadbourn Rd
Ste. B
Fairfield, CA 94534   707-435-8174
                                               Fax: 707-435-8177
                                               www.ilrscc.org

Sarah BirdwelL, Board President
Kathy Mitsopoulos, Board Vice President
Teri Ruggiero, Board Secretary
Susan Rotchy, Executive Director
To empower people with disabilities to: control their own lives, provide advocacy and support for individuals with disabilities to live independently, create an accessible community free of physical and attitudinal barriers.

4003 Independent Living Resource: Antioch
3727 Sunset Lane
#103
Antioch, CA 94509-1761   925-754-0539
                                               TTY:925-755-0934
                                               www.ilrscc.org

Sarah BirdwelL, Board President
Kathy Mitsopoulos, Board Vice President
Teri Ruggiero, Board Secretary
Susan Rotchy, Executive Director
Non-profit organizations run and controlled by persons with disabilities. They are non-residential, community-based centers where people with disabilities can receive assistance with a variety of daily living issues and learn the skills they need to take controll of their lives from people who have had similar experiences living with a disability.

4004 Independent Living Resource: Concord
1850 Gateway Blvd
Suite 120
Concord, CA 94520-3293   925-363-7293
                                               Fax: 925-363-7296
                                               gilc@ilrccc.org
                                               www.ilrscc.org

Sarah BirdwelL, Board President
Kathy Mitsopoulos, Board Vice President
Teri Ruggiero, Board Secretary
Susan Rotchy, Executive Director
To empower people with disabilities to: control their own lives, provide advocacy and support for individuals with disabilities to live independently, create an accessible community free of physical and attitudinized barriers.

4005 Independent Living Resources (ILR)
Bldg 2a
101 Broadway
Richmond, CA 94804-1945   510-233-7400
                                               info@ilrccc.org

Marvin Dyson, Manager
Provides services to meet the diverse needs of people who have a variety of disabilities in all age groups.

4006 Independent Living Service Northern California: Redding Office
169 Hartnell Ave
Suite 128
Redding, CA 96002-1849   530-242-8550
                                               800-464-8527
                                               Fax: 530-241-1454
                                               TTY: 530-242-8550
                                               info@ilsnc.org
                                               actionctr.org

Lauri Evans, President
Frank Smith, Vice President
Evan Levang, Executive Director
Tracy Barker, Program Manager
Independent Living Services of Northern California is a private non profit organization that provides support services to help empower community members with disabilities.

4007 Independent Living Services of Northern California
Jennifer Roberts Building
1161 East Ave
Chico, CA 95926-1018   530-893-8527
                                               800-464-8527
                                               Fax: 530-893-8574
                                               TTY: 530-893-8527
                                               actionctr.org

Lauri Evans, President
Frank Smith, Vice President
Evan Levang, Executive Director
Tracy Barker, Program Manager
Independent Living Services of Northern California is a private, non profit organization that provides support services to help empower community members with disabilities.

4008 Marin Center for Independent Living
710 4th St
San Rafael, CA 94901-3213   415-459-6245
                                               Fax: 415-459-7047
                                               TTY:415-459-7027
                                               marincil.org

Chris Schultz, President
Joe Brnnett, Vice President
Eli Gelardin, Executive Director
Susan Malardino, Deputy Director
A non-profit organization that provides advocacy and services for seniors and persons with disabilities.

4009 Mother Lode Independent Living Center(DRAIL: Disability Resource Agency for Independent
Living)
67 Linoberg St
Suite A.
Sonora, CA 95370-4646 209-532-0963
Fax: 209-532-1591
TTY:209-288-3309
barry@drail.org
www.drail.org

Terry Gray, President
Michael Kim Cornelius, Treasurer
Adeline Bagwell, Secretary
Barry Smith, Executive Director
DRAIL is a non-profit, community based, consumer controlled, cross disability center for independent living.

4010 Placer Independent Resource Services
11768 Atwood Rd
Suite 29
Auburn, CA 95603 530-885-6100
800-833-3453
Fax: 530-885-3032
TTY: 530-885-0326
lbrewer@pirs.org
pirs.org

Eldon Luce, President
Michael Cummings, Vice President
Dan Roye, Director
Peter Beckh, Treasurer
A non profit independent living center whose mission is to advocate, empower, educate and provide services for people with disabilities that would enable them to live more independently.

4011 Resources for Independent Living
420 i St, Level B.
Suite 3
Sacramento, CA 95814-2319 916-446-3074
Fax: 916-446-2443
leonc@ril-sacramento.org
www.ril-sacramento.org

Ramona Garcia, Board Chairperson
Francisco Godoy, Vice Chairperson
Joanne Bodine, Treasurer
Frances Gracechild, Executive Director
Promoting the socio-economic independence of persons with disabilities by providing peer-supported, consumer-directed independent living services and advocacy.

4012 Rolling Start
570 W 4th St
Suite 107
San Bernardino, CA 92401-1438 909-884-2129
Fax: 909-386-7446
TTY:909-884-7396
www.rollingstart.org

John Anaya, Chairperson
Kathi Pryor, Treasurer
Francis Bates, Executive Director
Tony Chavez, Deputy Director
Empowers and educates people with disabilities to achieve the independent life of their choice.

4013 Rolling Start: Victorville
17330 Bear Valley Road
Suite A102
Victorville, CA 92395 760-843-7959
Fax: 760-843-7977
TTY:760-951-8175
www.rollingstart.org

John Anaya, Chairperson
Kathi Pryor, Treasurer
Francis Bates, Executive Director
Tony Chavez, Deputy Director
Empowers and educates people with disabilities to achieve the independent life of their choice.

4014 Services Center For Independent Living
107 S Spring Street
Claremont, CA 91711-549 909-621-6722
800-491-6722
Fax: 909-445-0727
TTY: 949-445-0726
www.scil-ilc.org

Larry Grable, Executive Director
Janice Ornelas, Independent Living Specialist
Angela Nwokike, System Change Advocate
Albert Gonzales, Benefits Specialist
Dedicated to expanding access, information and resources to help increase independence and enhance the quality of life for the East San Gabriel Valley residents with disabilities.

4015 Silicon Valley Independent Living Center
2202 N. First St.
San Jose, CA 95131-1115 408-894-9041
Fax: 408-894-9050
TTY:408-894-9012
info@svilc.org
svilc.org

Patricia Kokes, President
Richard A. Wentz, Vice President
Gabe Lopez, Treasurer
Nayana Shah, Executive Director
A private, consumer-driven, nonprofit corporation that offers quality services to individuals with disabilities in Silicon Valley.

4016 Silicon Valley Independent Living Center: South County Branch
7881 Church Street
Suite C
Gilroy, CA 95020-7346 408-843-9100
Fax: 408-842-4791
TTY:408-842-2591
info@svilc.org
svilc.org

Patricia Kokes, President
Richard A. Wentz, Vice President
Gabe Lopez, Treasurer
Nayana Shah, Executive Director
A private, consumer-driven, non-profit corporation that offers quality services to individuals with disabilities in Silicon Valley.

4017 Southern California Rehabilitation Services
7830 Quill Dr
Suite D
Downey, CA 90242-3440 562-862-6531
Fax: 562-923-5274
TTY:562-869-0931
scrs-ilc.org

Lisa Hayes, President
Michael Strong, Vice President
Carol Trees, Secretary/Treasurer
Chad Williams, Board Member
Empowers persons with disabilities to achieve their personalized goals through community education and individualized services that provide the knowledge, skills, and confidence building to maximize their quality of life.

4018 Through the Looking Glass
3075 Adeline St.
Ste. 120
Berkeley, CA 94703 510-848-1112
800-644-2666
Fax: 510-848-4445
TTY: 510-848-1005
tlg@lookingglass.org
www.lookingglass.org

Maureen Block, J.D., Board President
Thomas Spalding, Board Treasurer
Alice Nemon, D.S.W., Board Secretary
Karen Fessel, Ph.D., Executive Director
To create, demonstrate and encourage non-pathological and empowering reesources and model early intervention services for families with disability issues in parent or child which integrate

expertise derived from personal disability experience and disability culture.

4019   Tri-County Independent Living Center
2822 Harris Street
Eureka, CA   95503

707-445-8404
877-576-5000
Fax: 707-445-9751
TTY: 707-445-8405
aa@tilinet.org
www.tilinet.org

Gail Pascoe, President
Linda Arnold, Vice President
Kevin O'Brien, Treasurer
Chris Jones, Executive Director
Promotes the philosophy of independent living, to connect individuals to services, and to create and accessible community, so that people with disabilities can have control over their lives and full access to the communities in which they live.

4020   Westside Center for Independent Living
12901 Venice Blvd
Los Angeles, CA   90066-3509

310-390-3611
888-851-9245
Fax: 310-390-4906
TTY: 310-398-9204
development@wcil.org
www.wcil.org

David Geffen, President
Chris Knauf, 1st Vice President
Brenda Green, Secretary
Aliza Barzilay, Executive Director
The Westside Center for Independent Living (WCIL) helps people living with disabilities maintain self-sufficient and productive lives through non-residential peer support services and training programs. Independent Living promotes self-determination, community living, full participation in community life and access to the same opportunities and resources available to people without disabilities.

Colorado

4021   Atlantis Community
201 S Cherokee St
Denver, CO   80223-1836

303-733-9324
Fax: 303-733-6211
TTY: 303-733-0047
info@atlantiscommunity.org

David Hays, Manager
Provide direct services, and to empower people with disabilities integrating, with full and equal rights, into all parts of society including employment, affordable, accessible, housing, transportation, recreation, communication, education, and public places while exercising and exerting choice and self determination.

4022   Center for Independence
740 Gunnison Ave
Grand Junction, CO   81501-3222

708-588-0833
Fax: 708-588-0406
center-for-independence.org

Linda Taylor, Executive Director
The Center for Independence works to promote community solutions and to empower individuals with disabilities to live independently.

4023   Center for People with Disabilities
615 Main St
Longmont, CO   80501-4983

303-772-3250
Fax: 303-772-5125
TTY: 303-772-3250
info@cpwd.org
www.cpwd-ilc.org

Dale Gaar, Board President
Deborah.A Conley, Board Vice President
Nancy Phares-Zook, Board Secretary
Tony Adams, Board Treasurer

Provides resources, information, and advocacy to assist people with disabilities in overcoming barriers to independent living.

4024   Center for People with Disabilities: Pueblo
1304 Berkley Ave
Pueblo, CO   81004-3002

719-546-1271
800-659-3656
Fax: 719-546-1374
ivaleneamidei@yahoo.com
www.ilcpueblo.org

Larry Williams, Executive Director
One of the 10 centers for independent living in Colorado founded under Title VII of the Rehabilitation Act of 1973 as amended in 1978. All new centers under this Independent Living (CIL) Title of the Act received initial and ongoing grants through this new Federal Program created by the Act.

4025   Center for People with Disabilities: Boulder
1675 Range St
Boulder, CO   80301-2722

303-442-8662
888-929-5519
Fax: 303-442-0502
info@cpwd.org
www.cpwd-ilc.org

Dale Gaar, Board President
Deborah.A Conley, Board Vice President
Nancy Phares-Zook, Board Secretary
Tony Adams, Board Treasurer
Providing resources, information and advocacy to people with disabilities. Assist people with disabilities in transitioning from nursing homes to independent living in the community. Also provide personal assistance services.

4026   Colorado Springs Independence Center
729 South Tejon Street
Colorado Springs, CO   80903

719-471-8181
Fax: 719-471-7829
TTY: 719-471-2076
www.theindependencecenter.org

Billy A. , Chair Elect
Billy B. , Secretary
Dean C. , Treasurer
To empower persons with disabilities to maximize their independence within the community and to remove barriers which impact their quality of life, while encouraging them to live independently in their community.

4027   Connections for Independent Living
1331 8th Avenue
Greeley, CO   80631-4027

970-352-8682
800-887-5828
Fax: 970-353-8058
TTY: 970-352-8682
pattid4z@yahoo.com
www.connectionsforindependentliving.org

Beth Danielson, Executive Director
Michael Stevens, Director of Services
Alicia Garza, Director
Dianna Shmidl, Community Transition Specialist
Certified IL Center, I and R advocacy, peer support, skills training, sign language interpretations, reader services, housing. Cross-disability, all ages.

4028   Denver CIL
Ste 100
777 Grant St
Denver, CO   80203-3501

303-837-1020
Fax: 303-837-0859
www.denverhousing.org

Greg Beran, Owner
Ismael Guerrero, Executive Director
Joshua Crawley, Agency Counsel
Nichole Ford, Chief Financial Officer
Provides resources, information, and advocacy to assist people with disabilities in overcoming barriers to independent living.

4029 Disability Center for Independent Living
4821 East 38th Avenue
Denver, CO 80207-1232   303-320-1345
                                Fax: 303-320-1345
                                TTY:303-322-2330
                                avillasenor.dcil@gmil.com
                                www.accil.net

Larry Williams, Executive Director
John Wooster, Consultant
Anthony Gonzales, Housing Coordinator
Jenna Emery, OBI Specialist
Independent living center providing quality services for people with disabilities.

4030 Disabled Resource Services
1017 Robertson Street
Unit B
Fort Collins, CO 80524-3915   970-482-2700
                                Fax: 970-449-6972
                                TTY:970-407-7060
                                drs@frii.com
                                disabledresourceservices.org

George Tremblay, Chairman
John Weins, Vice Chairman
Nancy Jackson, Executive Director
Marj Grell, Office Manager
To empower individuals with disabilities to achieve their maximum level of independence and to gain personal dignity within society. Disabled Resource Services, as a private non-profit state certified center for independent living, is dedicated to working with individuals with all types of disabilities in Larimer County to promote their independence and equality through services which support advocacy, awareness and access to their community.

4031 Disbled Resource Services
640 E Eisenhower Blvd
Loveland, CO 80537-3954   970-667-0816
                                Fax: 970-593-6582
                                drs@frii.com
                                disabledresourceservices.org

George Tremblay, Chairman
John Weins, Vice Chairman
Nancy Jackson, Executive Director
Marj Grell, Office Manager
To empower individuals with disabilities to achieve their maximum level of independence and to gain personal dignity within society.

4032 Greeley Center for Independence
2780 28th Ave
Greeley, CO 80634-7803   970-339-2444
                                800-748-1012
                                Fax: 970-339-0033
                                gciinc@gciinc.org
                                www.gciinc.org

Chari Armagost, Chief Financial Officer
Sarita Reddy, PH. D, Executive Director
Rob Rabe, Director of Outpatient Service
Dee Seekamp, Director of Nursing
Provides places of growth, transition and encouragement, where people with temporary and permanent disabilities can reach toward their maximum potential of personal independence and wellness.

4033 Independent Life Center
P.O.Box 612
Craig, CO 81626-612   970-826-0833
                                888-526-0833
                                Fax: 970-826-0832
                                TTY: 970-826-0833
                                www.accil.net

Larry Williams, Executive Director
John Wooster, Consultant
Anthony Gonzales, Housing Coordinator
Jenna Emery, OBI Specialist
Provides resources, information, and advocacy to assist people with disabilities in overcoming barriers to independent living.

4034 Pueblo Goodwill Industries
15810 Indianola Drive
Rockville, MD 20855   240-333-5590
                                800-GOO-WILL
                                contactus@goodwill.org
                                www.goodwill.org

Debi Diaz, CEO
Lauren Lawson-Zilai, Director of Public Relations
Charlene Sarmiento, Senior Specialist, Public Relati
PGoodwill works to enhance the dignity and quality of life of individuals and families by strengthening communities, eliminating barriers to opportunity, and helping people in need reach their full potential through learning and the power of work.

4035 Southwest Center for Independence
3473 Main Avenue
#23
Durango, CO 81301-5474   970-259-1672
                                866-962-2158
                                Fax: 970-259-0947
                                TTY: 970-259-1672
                                swindependence.org/

Martha Mason, Executive Director
Mariellen Walz, Chair
Patricia Ziegler, Assistant Director
Jason Armstrong, Treasurer
Empowering individuals with disabilities and their families to achieve their maximum level of independence in work, play and other areas of life.

4036 Southwest Center for Independence: Cortez
2409 East Empire Street
PO Box 640
Cortez, CO 81321-9164   970-570-8001
                                866-962-2158
                                Fax: 970-565-7169
                                director@swilc.org
                                swindependence.org/

Mariellen Walz, Chair
Johnny Bulson, Vice Chair
Jason Armstrong, Treasurer
Martha Mason, Executive Director
Empowers individiuals with disabilities and their families to achieve their maximum level of independence in work, play and other areas of life.

Connecticut

4037 Center for Disability Rights
764-B Campbell Ave
764 Campbell Ave
W Haven, CT 06516- 3786   203-934-7077
                                Fax: 203-934-7078
                                TTY:203-934-7079
                                info@cdr-ct.org
                                cdr-ct.org

Marc Gallucci, Executive Director
Chris Zurcher, Consumer Relations
Dana Canevari, I&R Specialist
Susan St. John, Administrative Assistant
Resources, information, and advocacy to assist people with disabilities in overcoming barriers to independent living.

4038 Center for Independent Living SC
26 Palmers Hill Rd
Stamford, CT 06902-2113   203-353-8550
                                Fax: 203-353-1423
                                TTY:203-353-8550

Dana Canevari, Director
Provides resources, information, and advocacy to assist people with disabilities in overcoming barriers to independent living.

4039 Chapel Haven
1040 Whalley Ave
New Haven, CT 06515-1740   203-397-1714
                                    Fax: 203-937-2466
                              admissions@chapelhaven.org
                                    chapelhaven.org

Michael Storz, President
The only combined state-accredited special education facility and independent living facility for adults with cognitive disabilities.

4040 Connecticut State Independent Living Council
151 New Park Ave
Hartford, CT 06106   860-523-0126
                                    Fax: 860-523-5603
                                    info@ctsilc.org
                                    ctsilc.org

Katherine Pellerin, President
Keith Mullinar, Vice President
Alexia Bouckoms, Treasurer
Daria Smith, Executive Director
The mission of the council is to promote equal access, opportunities, and social inclusion for people with disabilities in all spheres of society.

4041 Disabilities Network of Eastern Connecticut
19 Ohio Avenue
Suite 2
Norwich, CT 06360-2111   860-823-1898
                                    Fax: 860-886-2316
                                    CFerry@dnec.org
                                    dnec.org

Katherine Pellerin, President
Robert Davidson, Vice President
Jane O'Friel, Secretary/Treasurer
Cathy Ferry, Executive Director
Dedicated to supporting and advancing the rights of individuals with disabilities. The goal is to creat a completely inclusive society where people live together in communities regardless of their abilities.

4042 Disability Resource Center of Fairfield County
80 Ferry Blvd
Suite 205
Stratford, CT 06615-6079   203-378-6977
                                    Fax: 203-375-2748
                                    TTY:203-378-3248
                                    www.accessinct.org
Ethel M R, President
Thomas D, Vice-President
Anthony Lacava, Executive Director
Glenn Calaffin, Program Director
A crosss-disability resource and advocacy organization for people with disabilities that has provided unique, consumer-directed services both for individuals and for the communities of Fairfield County.

4043 Independence Northwest Center for Independent Living
1183 New Haven Rd
Suite 200
Naugatuck, CT 06770-5033   203-729-3299
                                    Fax: 203-729-2839
                                    TTY:203-729-1281
                              info@independencenorthwest.org
                              www.independencenorthwest.org
Maureen Mayo, President
Tom Ford, Vice President
Charles Marino, Treasurer
Jaff Laliberte, Secretary
Provides services in such areas as peer counseling, advocacy, independent living skills training and information and referral.

4044 New Horizons Village
37 Bliss Rd
Unionville, CT 06085   860-673-8893
                                    Fax: 860-675-4369
                       Michael.Shaw@NewHorizonsVillage.com
                                 newhorizonsvillage.com
Carolyn Fields, Administrator
A 68 unit apartment complex designed for people who have severe physical disabilities.

Delaware

4045 Freedom Center for Independent Living
400 N Broad St
Middletown, DE 19709-1089   302-376-4399
                                    866-687-3245
                                    Fax: 302-376-4395
                                    TTY: 302-376-4397
                                    info@fcilde.org
                                    fcilde.org
Hersernest Cole, Executive Director
Lillian Evans, Independent Living Specialist
Protects the Civil Rights and promote the empowerment of persons with disabilities and their families through our independent living philosophy.

4046 Independent Living
Apt 210
1800 N Broom St
Wilmington, DE 19802-3854   302-429-6693
                                    Fax: 302-429-8031
                                    TTY:302-429-8034
Susan Cycyk, Executive Director
Providing skilled support and caring guidance to adults with disabilities. Our case management services include: daily living skills training, medical coordination, transportation assistance, financial management, housing assistance, and vocational/educational planning.

4047 Independent Resource Georgetown
Ste 37
410 S Bedford St
Georgetown, DE 19947-1850   302-854-9330
                                    Fax: 302-854-9408
                                    TTY:302-854-9340
Larry Henderson, Director
Pat Boyd, Manager
Provides independent living services to persons who experience a significant disability. Offers skills training, individually and in small groups, peer support/peer counseling and information and referral services. Strives to remove the architectural and attitudnal barriers through individual and systems advocacy.

4048 Independent Resources: Dover
154 South Governor's Avenue
Dover, DE 19904-7311   302-735-4599
                                    Fax: 302-735-5623
                                    TTY:302-735-5629
                          lhenderson@independentresources.org
                                    www.iri-de.org
Tes DelTufo, Office Director
Carolyn Miller, IL Specialist
Debbie Justice, IL Specialist
Barty Rochester, Peer Support Coordinator
Private, non-profit, consumer-controlled, community based organization providing services and advocacy by and for persons with all types of disabilities. Their goal is to assist individuals with disabilities to achieve their maximum potential within their families and communities.

4049 Independent Resources: Wilmington
6 Denny Rd
Suite 101
Wilmington, DE 19809-3444   302-765-0191
                                              Fax: 302-765-0195
                                              TTY:302-765-0194
                                                www.iri-de.org

Larry D Henderson, Executive Director
Phyllis Farrare, Director of Operations
Private, non-profit, consumer-controlled, community based organization providing services and advocacy by and for persons with all types of disabilities. Their goal is to assist individuals with disabilities to achieve their maximum potential within their families and communities.

4050 Mosaic Of De
4980 S. 118TH ST
Omaha, NE 68137   302-456-5995
                                                    877-366-7242
                                              Fax: 402-896-1511
                                              info@mosaicinfo.org
                                                mosaicinfo.org

Terry Olson, Executive Director
Linda Timmons, President and CEO
Raul Saldivar, Chief Operating Officer
Cindy Schroeder, Chief Financial Officer
Provides services to adults with developmental disabilities who reside in homes and apartments. Services are designed to provide them with opportunities for choices and participation in the life of their communities. Supports are geared to assist each individual in becoming more independent in activities of daily living, vocational skills, community mobility and transportation, and recreation and leisure activities.

District of Columbia

4051 District of Columbia Center for Independent Living
1400 Florida Ave NE
Washington, DC 20002-5032   202-388-0033
                                              Fax: 202-398-3018
                                                info@dccil.org
                                                  dccil.org
Rev. Patric Hailes Fears, President
Dr. John Thompson, Vice President
Carl Bartels, Treasurer
Angela Washington, Secretary
Mission is to maximize the leadership, empowerment, independence, and productivity of individuals with disabilities, and to integrate these individuals into the mainstream of American society.

4052 National Council on Independent Living
2013 H St. NW
6th Flr
Washington, DC 20006-3007   202-207-0334
                                                    844-778-7961
                                              Fax: 202-207-0341
                                                 ncil@ncil.org
                                                  www.ncil.org

Kelly Buckland, Executive Director
Lou Ann Kibbee, President
Sarah Launderville, Vice President
Derrel Christenson, Treasurer
NCIL advances independent living and the rights of people with disabilities through consumer-driven advocacy.

Florida

4053 Ability 1st
1300 E. Green Street
Pasadena, CA 91106   626-396-1010
                                                    877-768-4600
                                              Fax: 626-396-1021
                                              info@abilityfirst.org
                                                abilityfirst.org

Steve Brockmeyer, Chairman
John Kelly, Vice Chairman
Lori.E Gangemi, President
Kevin Schaffels, CFO
To empower persons with disabilities to live independently and participate actively in their community.

4054 Adult Day Training
Goodwill Industries - Suncoast
10596 Gandy Blvd N
St Petersburg, FL 33702-1422   727-523-1512
                                                    888-279-1988
                                              Fax: 727-563-9300
                                              TTY:727-579-1068
                                   gw.marketing@goodwill-suncoast.com
                                          www.goodwill-suncoast.org
Oscar J. Horton, Chairman
Martin W. Gladysz, Vice Chairman
Heather Ceresoli, Vice Chairman
Deborah.A Passerini, President
An innovative program which uses job skills to teach self-help, daily living, communication, mobility, travel, decision-making, behavioral and social skills. This focus provides concrete, transferable experiences to help prepare individuals for greater community inclusion by achieving the highest possible degree of independence in their daily life, increasing their confidence and supporting their successful transitions to less structured, self-sufficient environments.

4055 CIL of Central Florida
720 N Denning Dr
Winter Park, FL 32789-3020   407-623-1070
                                              Fax: 407-623-1390
                                              info@cilorlando.org
                                                cilorlando.org

Jason Vennings, Development Director
Kim Byerly, Chair
Cheryl Stone, Secretary
Don Pirozzoli, M.S., Programs Director
A private, non-profit organization dedicated to helping people with disabilities achieve their self-determined goals for independent living.

4056 Caring and Sharing Center for Independent Living
12552 Belcher Rd S
Largo, FL 33773-3014   727-539-7550
                                                    866-539-7550
                                              Fax: 727-539-7588
                                              cascil@cascil.org
                                  www.disabilityachievementcenter.org

Barbara Dandro, Treasurer
Mary Bucca, Secretary
Patricia Bell, Director
Dennis Shelt, Director
Empowering people with disabilities.

4057 Caring and Sharing Center: Pasco County
12552 Belcher Rd S
Largo, FL 33773-3014   727-539-7550
                                                    866-539-7550
                                              Fax: 727-539-7588
                                  www.disabilityachievementcenter.org

Barbara Dandro, Treasurer
Mary Bucca, Secretary
Patricia Bell, Director
Dennis Shelt, Director
Empowering people with disabilities.

4058   Center for Independent Living in Central Florida
720 N Denning Dr
Winter Park, FL 32789-3095   407-623-1070
                                          Fax: 407-623-1390
                                          info@cilorlando.org
                                          cilorlando.org

Jason Vennings, Development Director
Kim Byerly, Chair
Cheryl Stone, Secretary
Don Pirozzoli, M.S., Programs Director
In partnership with the community, promotes personal right snad
responsiblities among people with all disabilities.

4059   Center for Independent Living of Broward
4800 N State Road 7
Suite 102
Lauderdale Lakes, FL 33319-5811   954-722-6400
                                              888-722-6400
                                          Fax: 954-735-1958
                                          cilb@cilbroward.org
                                          www.cilbroward.org

Craig Lilienthal, President
Christopher Sharp, VP
Shea Smith, Treasurer
Laurie Menekou, Secretary
Offers assistance to people with disabilities in fulfilling the goals
of independence and self-sufficiency.

4060   Center for Independent Living of Florida Keys
103400 Overseas Hwy
Suite 243
Key Largo, FL 33037-2849   305-453-3491
                                              877-335-0187
                                          Fax: 305-453-3488
                                          TTY: 305-453-3491
                                          cilkeys@cilkeys.org
                                          www.cilofthekeys.org

Brenda K Pierce, Executive Director
Offers assistance to persons with disabilities in acquiring independent living and self-advocacy skills in order to obtain and
maintain independence and self-sufficiency.

4061   Center for Independent Living of N Florida
1823 Buford Ct
Tallahassee, FL 32308-4465   850-575-9621
                                          Fax: 850-575-5740
                                          TTY:850-575-5245
                                          cilnf@nettally.com
                                          www.ability1st.info

Judith Barrett, Executive Director
Offers assistance to persons with disabilities in acquiring independent living and self-advocacy skills in order to obtain and
maintain independence and self-sufficiency

4062   Center for Independent Living of NW Florida
3600 N Pace Blvd
Pensacola, FL 32505-4240   850-595-5566
                                              877-245-2457
                                          Fax: 850-595-5560
                                          cil-drc@cil-drc.org
                                          cil-drc.org

James Hicks, President
Kathleen Wilks, Secretary
John Bouchard, Treasurer
Frank Cherry, Executive Director
Provides services such as information and referral, peer counsel-
ing, housing, advocacy, training, independent living skills train-
ing, free wheelchairs, loan locker, assistive technology.

4063   Center for Independent Living of North Central Florida
3445 NE 24th Street
Ocala, FL 34470-9214   352-368-3788
                                              877-232-8261
                                          Fax: 352-629-0098
                                          www.cilncf.org

Joe Dyke, President
Robert Miller, Vice President
David Christie, Treasurer
Jim Gorske, Secretary
Empowers people with disabilities to exert their individual rights
to live as independently as possible, make personal life choices
and achieve full community inclusion.

4064   Center for Independent Living of North Central Florida
222 SW 36th Ter
Gainesville, FL 32607-2863   352-378-7474
                                              800-265-5724
                                          Fax: 352-378-5582
                                          TTY: 352-372-3443
                                          www.cilncf.org

Joe Dyke, President
Robert Miller, Vice President
David Christie, Treasurer
Jim Gorske, Secretary
Empowering people with disabilities to exert their individual
rights to live as independently as possible, make personal life
choices and achieve full community inclusion.

4065   Center for Independent Living of S Florida
6660 Biscayne Blvd
Miami, FL 33138-6285   305-751-8025
                                          Fax: 305-751-8944
                                          TTY:305-751-8891
                                          info@soflacil.org
                                          soflacil.org

Alvin W. Roberts, President
Gregg Goldfarb, Vice President
Timothy Werner, Ph.D, Secretary
Jay Weiss, M.B.A., Treasurer
A community based non for profit, independent living center
serving people of all ages with any type of disability. Services:
Basic education, GED preperation, American sign language advocacy, peer support, information and referral, independent living skills training, housing assistance, transportation assistance,
home modiifications, transition from nursing facility to the community assisatnace filing ADA complaints, accessibility surveys,
diability awareness traing.

4066   Center for Independent Living of SW Florida
2321 Bruner Ln
Fort Myers, FL 33912-1904   239-277-1447
                                              800-435-7352
                                          Fax: 239-277-1647

Ronald J Muschong, Interim Executive Director
Helping people with disabilities achieve independence and
self-determination in their lives.

4067   Coalition for Independent Living Options: Okeechobee
1680 SW Bayshore Boulevard
Suite 231
Port St. Lucie, FL 34984   772-878-3500
                                          Fax: 772-878-3344
                                          www.cilo.org

Scott Shoemaker, President
Sharon D'Eusanio, Vice President
Joseph Fields Jr., Esquire, Secretary
Genevieve Cousminer,Esq, Executive Director
Private non-profit promoting independences for people with disabilities in Palm Beach, Martin, St. Lucie & Okeechobee Counties. Services include advocacy, independent living skills &
training, peer support, after school & summer programs for teens,
crime victim support services, and veterans transition services.

4068 Coalition for Independent Living Options: Fort Pierce
6800 Forest HIll Boulevard
West Palm Beach, FL 33413
561-966-4288
Fax: 561-966-0441
www.cilo.org

Scott Shoemaker, President
Sharon D'Eusanio, Vice President
Joseph Fields Jr., Esquire, Secretary
Genevieve Cousminer,Esq, Executive Director
Private non-profit promoting independences for people with disabilities in Palm Beach, Martin, St. Lucie & Okeechobee Counties. Services include advocacy, independent living skills & training, peer support, after school & summer programs for teens, crime victim support services, and verterans transition services.

4069 Coalition for Independent Living Options
6800 Forest HIll Boulevard
West Palm Beach, FL 33413-3310
561-966-4288
Fax: 561-966-0441
www.cilo.org

Scott Shoemaker, President
Sharon D'Eusanio, Vice President
Joseph Fields Jr., Esquire, Secretary
Genevieve Cousminer,Esq, Executive Director
Private non-profit promoting independences for people with disabilities in Palm Beach, Martin, St. Lucie & Okeechobee Counties. Services include advocacy, independent living skills & training, peer support, after school & summer programs for teens, crime victim support services, and verterans transition services.

4070 Coalition for Independent Living Options: Stuart
1680 SW Bayshore Boulevard
Suite 231
Port St. Lucie, FL 34984
772-878-3500
Fax: 772-878-3344
www.cilo.org

Scott Shoemaker, President
Sharon D'Eusanio, Vice President
Joseph Fields Jr., Esquire, Secretary
Genevieve Cousminer,Esq, Executive Director
Private non-profit promoting independences for people with disabilities in Palm Beach, Martin, St. Lucie & Okeechobee Counties. Services include advocacy, independent living skills & training, peer support, after school & summer programs for teens, crime victim support services, and verterans transition services.

4071 Disability Resource Center
300 W. 5th St.
Panama City, FL 32401-4704
850-769-6890
Fax: 850-769-6891
outreach@drcpc.org
www.drcpc.org

Robert Cox, Executive Director
Becky Cadwell, Independent Living Specialist
They are commiteed to collaborating with other disability/consumer-focused organizations in their community

4072 Lakeland Adult Day Training
3033 Drane Field Rd
Suite 5
Lakeland, FL 33811-3305
863-701-1351
TTY:863-701-1356
gw.marketing@goodwill-suncoast.com
www.goodwill-suncoast.org

Oscar J. Horton, Chairman
Martin W. Gladysz, Vice Chairman
Heather Ceresoli, Vice Chairman
Deborah.A Passerini, President
An innovative program which uses job skills to teach self-help, daily living, communication, mobility, travel, decision-making, behavioral and social skills. This focus provides concrete, transferable experiences to help prepare individuals for greater community inclusion by achieving the highest possible degree of independence in their daily life, increasing their confidence and supporting their successful transitions to less structured, self-sufficient environments.

4073 Lighthouse Central Florida
215 E New Hampshire St
Orlando, FL 32804-6403
407-898-2483
Fax: 407-895-5255
lvaneepoel@lcf-fl.org
www.lighthousecentralflorida.com

Alex B. Hull, Chair
David Stahl, Vice Chair
Paul Prewitt, Secretary
Nancy L. Urbach, Treasurer
Promote the independence and success of people living with vision impairment.

4074 Miami-Dade County Disability Services and Independent Living (DSAIL)
701 NW 1st Court
Miami, FL 33136-1647
786-469-4600
Fax: 305-547-7355
www.miamidade.gov

Michael Moxam, Manager
Lucia Davis-Raiford, Director
Offers information and referral services serving all types of disabilities with the goal of assisting the disabled acquiring independence and control over their lives. Teaches independent living skills, job readiness and placement, home health care, sensitivity training, training in ASL and Braille, counsel people with disabilities or wide range of problems.

4075 Ocala Adult Day Training
2920 W Silver Springs Blvd
Ocala, FL 34475-5654
352-629-0456
TTY:352-629-0874
gw.marketing@goodwill-suncoast.com
www.goodwill-suncoast.org

Oscar J. Horton, Chairman
Martin W. Gladysz, Vice Chairman
Heather Ceresoli, Vice Chairman
Deborah.A Passerini, President
An innovative program which uses job skills to teach self-help, daily living, communication, mobility, travel, decision-making, behavioral and social skills. This focus provides concrete, transferable experiences to help prepare individuals for greater community inclusion by achieving the highest possible degree of independence in their daily life, increasing their confidence and supporting their successful transitions to less structured, self-sufficient environments.

4076 Pinellas Park Adult Day Training
7601 Park Blvd
Pinellas Park, FL 33781-3704
727-541-6205
TTY:727-544-5835
gw.marketing@goodwill-suncoast.com
www.goodwill-suncoast.org

Oscar J. Horton, Chairman
Martin W. Gladysz, Vice Chairman
Heather Ceresoli, Vice Chairman
Deborah.A Passerini, President
An innovative program which uses job skills to teach self-help, daily living, communication, mobility, travel, decision-making, behavioral and social skills. This focus provides concrete, transferable experiences to help prepare individuals for greater community inclusion by achieving the highest possible degree of independence in their daily life, increasing their confidence and supporting their successful transitions to less structured, self-sufficient environments.

4077 SCCIL at Titusville
571-W Haverty Court
Rockledge, FL 32955
321-633-6011
Fax: 321-633-6472
TTY:706-724-6324
jilldunham9@gmail.com
www.virtualcil.net

Jill Dunham-Schuller, Executive Director
Directory of Independent Living Centers throughout the United States.

4078 **Self Reliance**
8901 N Armenia Ave
Tampa, FL 33604-1041 813-375-3965
Fax: 813-375-3970
TTY:813-375-3972
bruehl@self-reliance.org
www.self-reliance.org
Finn Kavanagh, Executive Director
Michele Pineda, Director of Finance & Operations
Gary Martoccio, Programs Director
Kim Albritton, Chairperson
A cross disability agency providing services to both children and adults with disabilities to identify and overcome barriers to independence in their lives. Self Reliance also promotes independence through empowering persons with disabilities and improving the communities in which they live.

4079 **Space Coast Center for Independent Living**
571 Haverty Court, Suite W.
Rockledge, FL 32955 321-633-6011
Fax: 321-633-6472
spacecoastcil.org
Michael Lavoie, President
Howard Fetes, VP
Jason Miller, Treasurer/Secretary
Provides overall services for individuals with al types of disabilities. Offers peer support, advocacy, skills training, accessibility surveys, support groups, transportation, specialized equipment and sign language interpreter referral services and home modifications.

4080 **Suncoast Center for Independent Living, Inc.**
3281 17th Street
Sarasota, FL 34235 941-351-9545
Fax: 941-316-9320
Info@scil4u.org
www.scil4u.org
Kevin Sanderson, Chair
Michael Fluker, Executive Director
Vicke Mack, Treasurer
Scott Biehler, Secretary
Helping people with disabilities live independently.

4081 **disAbility Solutions for Independent Living**
119 S Palmetto Ave
Suite 180
Daytona Beach, FL 32114- 4369 386-255-1812
866-310-1039
Fax: 386-255-1814
TTY: 386-252-6222
info@dsil.org
www.dsil.org
Julie M Shaw, Executive Director
To maximize the leadership, empowerment, independence and productivity of individuals with disabilities, to promote and attain integration and full inclusion of individuals with disabilities in all aspects of our society; accomplished through consumer control, peer support, education, self-determination, equal access and individual and systems advocacy

Georgia

4082 **Arms Wide Open**
5036 Snapfinger Woods Drive
Ste 205
Decatur, GA 30035- 1677 678-404-7696
Fax: 770-498-2778
kenmorris@armswideopen.org
www.armswideopen.org
Ken Morris, Director
Arms Wide Open operates a durable medical equipment loan program and a life care program. The mission of Arms Wide Open is to provide support services to the aged, disabled and chronically ill for the purpose of helping them to avoid institutional placement.

4083 **Bain, Inc. Center For Independent Living**
316 W Shotwell St.
Bainbridge, GA 39819-3906 229-246-0150
888-830-1530
Fax: 229-246-1715
TTY: 888-830-1530
bain@surfsouth.com
www.baincil.org
Virginia Harris, Executive Director
Malissa Thompson, Program Manager
Tomonia Becon, Nursing Home Transition Coordina
Dameca Fillingame, President
A non-residential Center for Independent Living serving eleven counties throughout Southwest. BAIN is a non-profit, community based resource and advocacy center run by and for individuals with disabilities.

4084 **Disability Connections**
170 College St
Macon, GA 31201-1656 478-741-1425
800-743-2117
Fax: 478-755-1571
disabilityconnections.com
Jerilyn Leverett, Executive Director
A private non-profit organization that looks to enable all people with disabilities to attain and have access to all opportunities in life.

4085 **Division of Rehabilitation Services**
Georgia Department of Labor
410 Mall Blvd
Suite B
Savannah, GA 31406-4869 912-356-2226
Fax: 912-356-2875
TTY:912-356-2940
dol.state.ga.us
Mark Bultler, Commissioner
Jody Lane, Manager
George Foley, Manager
Vocational rehabilitation services.

4086 **Living Independence for Everyone (LIFE)**
5105 Paulsen Street
Suite 143-B
Savannah, GA 31405 912-920-2414
800-948-4824
Fax: 912-920-0007
www.lifecil.com
Mark Schreiber, President
Stuart Klugler, Vice President
John Paul Berlon, Secretary
Cheryl Brackin, Board Member
The Southeast's Regional disability resource center that offers a wide range of resources, education, and advocacy to the community to help level the playing field for people with disabilities to create a world in which everyone can fully participate.

4087 **Multiple Choices Center for Independent Living**
145 Barrington Dr.
Athens, GA 30605-3133 706-850-4025
www.multiplechoices.us
Doug Hatch, President
Donald Veater, VP
Elllen Des Jardines, Secretary
William Holley, Executive Director
To break down all barriers to inclusion by enhancing the equality of life and empowering people with disabilities through advocacy, education and training.

4088 **North District Independent Living Program**
Ste 209
311 Green St NW
Gainesville, GA 30501-3364 770-535-5930
Sharon McCurry, Coordinator
Cindy Hanna, Executive Director
Information and referral, advocacy, peer counseling, service coordination and ADA consultation.

4089 Southwest District Independent Living Program
P.O.Box 1606
Albany, GA   31702-1606   229-430-4170
                                      Fax: 229-430-4466
Bill Layton, Director
Diane Davis, Executive Director
Offers peer counseling, disability education and awareness, attendant care registry, and information on accessible home for the disabled.

4090 Statewide Independent Living Council of Georgia
315 West Ponce de Leon Avenue
Suite 600
Decatur, GA 30030-2617   770-270-6860
                                           888-288-9780
                                      Fax: 770-270-5957
                                      shellys5@hotmail.com
                                           silcga.org
Steve Oldaker, President
Angela Denise Davis, Vice President
Mark Schreiber, Treasurer
Scott Osborne, Secretary
Founded to ensure that people with disabilities have opportunities to live as independently as possible.

4091 Walton Options for Independent Living
948 Walton Way
Augusta, GA   30901-519   706-724-6262
                                           877-821-8400
                                      Fax: 706-724-6729
                                      TTY: 706-724-6262
                                      tjohnston@waltonoptions.org
                                      www.waltonoptions.org
Tiffany Cilford, Executive Director
Ann Campbell-Kelly, Special Projects Coordinator
Alyson Schwartz, Special Projects Coordinator
Sam Creech, Director-Information Technology
Services include individual and systems advocacy, peer support, skills training (including basic computer and return to work skills), information and referral services and transition from institutions back to the community.

4092 disABILITY LINK: Rome
1901 Montreal Road
Suite 102
Tucker, GA   30084   404-687-8890
                                      Fax: 404-687-8298
                                      disabilitylink.org
Kim Gibson, Executive Director
Travis Evans, Health, Wellness and Resource Sp
Larry Brown, Finance Director
Hillary Elliott, Independent Living Services Prog
Committed to promoting the rights of all people with disabilities.

Hawaii

4093 Center For Independent Living- Kauai
State Office Building 3060 Eiwa Str
Lihue, HI   96766-6529   808-274-3484
                                      Fax: 808-245-3485
                                      kauaiddc@pixi.com
                                      hiddc.org/kauai.htm
Humberto Blanco, Administrator
Teri Yamashiro, IL Specialist
Offers peer counseling, disability education, attendant care registry, outreach services and advocacy.

4094 Hawaii Center For Independent Living
1055 Kinoole Street
Suite 105le St
Hilo, HI   96720-3872   808-935-3777
                                           800-420-6928
                                      TTY: 808-935-7888
                                      info@pacificil.org
                                      www.cil-hawaii.org
Gordon Fuller, Executive Director

Provides an array of support services for people with all types of disabilities of any age.

4095 Hawaii Center for Independent Living-Maui
220 Imi Kala Street
Suite 103
Wailuku, HI   96793-1209   808-242-4966
                                           866-303-4245
                                           800-420-6928
                                      Fax: 808-244-6978
                                      TTY: 808-242-4968
                                      www.cil-hawaii.org
Clytie Nishihara, Manager
T Lay , Administrative Assistant
Offers disability education and awareness, advocacy and counseling.

4096 Hawaii Centers for Independent Living
200 N. Vineyard Blvd Bldg. A501
Honolulu, HI   96817-3950   808-522-5400
                                           800-420-6928
                                      Fax: 808-522-5427
                                      www.cil-hawaii.org
Cheryl Mizusaawa, Executive Director
M.J. (Kimo) Keawe, COO & Executive Director
Our staff and Board of directors are excellent advocates with the disabled community. We will connect you with resources to make your own choices for housing, employment, and personal care and to find assistive devices and technology to improve quality of life. On both the islands of Oahu and Hawaii, we have an independent living specialist who is fluent in American sign language and is well known in the deaf community.

4097 Kauai Center for Independent Living
4340 Nawiliwili Rd.
Lihue, HI   96766-6529   808-246-4800
                                           800-420-6928
                                      Fax: 808-245-7218
                                      www.cil-hawaii.org
Laurao Tobosa, Program Coordinator
Provides a variety of support services for people with all types of disabilities.

Idaho

4098 American Falls Office: Living Independently for Everyone (LIFE)
250 S. Skyline
Idaho Falls, ID   83402-4508   208-529-8610
                                      Fax: 208-529-6804
                                      diane@idlife.org
                                      www.idlife.org
Dean Nilson, Executive Director
Tina Noreen, Programs Coordinator
Mickey Palmer, Fiscal Intermediary Manager
Enables people with disabilities to manage their own lives, make their own choices, and give information and knowledge to assist in living with dignity and bravado.

4099 Dawn Enterprises
280 Cedar Street P.O.Box 388
Blackfoot, ID   83221-388   208-785-5890
                                      Fax: 208-785-3095
                                      dawnent.org
Donna Butler, Executive Director
Teresa Oakes, Assistant Director/Fiscal Coordi
To assist individuals of Southeastern Idaho with mental, physical or social disabilities in achieving independence through employment training, skill training, social development, or living enhancements up to each individual's maximum capability.

4100 Disability Action Center NW
505 N Main St
Moscow, ID 83843-2615
208-883-0523
800-475-0070
Fax: 208-883-0524
www.dacnw.org

Larry Topp, President
Jean Coil, Vice President
Mark Leeper, CEO
Karl Johanson, Treasurer
A non-profit community partnership working to promote the independence and equality of all individuals with disabilities in all aspects of society. *$45.00*

4101 Disability Action Center NW: Coeur D'Alene
7560 N Government Way
Suite 1
Coeur D Alene, ID 83815- 4069
208-664-9896
800-854-9500
Fax: 208-666-1362
www.dacnw.org

Larry Topp, President
Jean Coil, Vice President
Mark Leeper, CEO
Karl Johanson, Treasurer
A non-profit community partnership working to promote the independence and equality of all individuals with disabilities in all aspects of society.

4102 Disability Action Center NW: Lewiston
330 5th Street
Suite A1
Lewiston, ID 83501-2086
208-746-9033
800-746-9033
Fax: 208-746-1004
www.dacnw.org

Larry Topp, President
Jean Coil, Vice President
Mark Leeper, CEO
Karl Johanson, Treasurer
A non-profit community partnership working to promote the independence and equality of all individuals with disabilities in all aspects of society.

4103 Idaho Falls Office: Living Independently for Everyone (LIFE)
250 S. Skyline
Idaho Falls, ID 83402-3702
208-529-8610
800-631-2747
Fax: 208-232-2753
diane@idlife.org
www.idlife.org

Dean Nielson, Executive Director
Tina Noreen, Programs Coordinator
Mickey Palmer, Fiscal Intermediary Manager
Enables people with disabilities to manage their own lives, make their own choices, and give information and knowledge to assist in living with dignity and bravado.

4104 LIFE: Fort Hall
1333 Moursund
Houston, TX 77019
713-520-0232
Fax: 713-520-5785
TTY:713-520-0232
www.ilru.org

Lex Frieden, Director
Linda CoVan, Grant Coordinator
Diego Demaya, Legal Specialist
Marisa Demaya, Training & Information Coor.
Enables people with disabilities to manage their own lives, make thier own choices, and give information and knowledge to assist in living with dignity and bravado.

4105 Living Independence Network Corporation
1878 W Overland Rd
Boise, ID 83705-3142
208-336-3335
Fax: 208-384-5037
info@lincidaho.org
lincidaho.org

Roger Howard, Executive Director
A non-profit organization empowering people with disabilities to achieve their desired level of independence.

4106 Living Independence Network Corporation: Twin Falls
1182 Eastland Dr North
Suite C
Twin Falls, ID 83301-8972
208-733-1712
Fax: 208-733-7711
info@lincidaho.org
www.lincidaho.org

Melva Heinrich, Executive Director
A non-profit organization empowering people with disabilities to achieve their desired level of independence.

4107 Living Independence Network Corporation: Caldwell
1609 Kimball Ave
Ste. 201
Caldwell, ID 83605-6965
208-454-5511
Fax: 208-454-5515
TTY:208-454-5511
info@lincidaho.org
www.lincidaho.org

Heidi Caldwell, Executive Director
A non-profit organization empowering people with disabilities to achieve their desired level of independence.

4108 Living Independent for Everyone (LIFE): Pocatello Office
640 Pershing Ave
PO Box 4185
Pocatello, ID 83201-3702
208-232-2747
800-631-2747
Fax: 208-232-2753
TTY: 208-232-2747
tracy@idlife.org
www.idlife.org

Dean Nielson, Executive Director
Mickey Palmer, Fiscal Intermediary Manager
Tina Noreen, Programs Coordinator
Enables people with disabilities to manage thier own lives, make their own choices, and give information and knowledge to assist in living with dignity and bravado.

4109 Living Independently for Everyone (LIFE): Blackfoot Office
Living Independently for Everyone (LIFE): Pocate
570 W. Pacific
P.O.Box 86
Blackfoot, ID 83221-86
208-785-9648
Fax: 208-785-2398
lori@idlife.org
www.idlife.org

Dean Nielson, Executive Director
Tina Noreen, Programs Coordinator
Mickey Palmer, Fiscal Intermediary Manager
Enable people with disabilities to manage their own lives, make their own choices, and give information and knowledge to assist in living with dignity and bravado.

4110 Living Independently for Everyone: Burley
2311 Park Ave
Suite 7
Burley, ID 83318-2170
208-678-7705
Fax: 208-678-7771
hotwheels@idlife.org
www.idlife.org

Dean Nielson, Executive Director
Mickey Palmer, Fiscal Intermediary Manager
Tina Noreen, Programs Coordinator
Enables people with disabilities to manage their own lives, make their own choices, and give information and knowledge to assist in living with dignity and bravado.

4111 Southwestern Idaho Housing Authority
1108 W Finch Dr
Nampa, ID 83651-1732   208-467-7461
                               Fax: 208-463-1772

David W Patten, Manager
Offers housing for rent and section/8

Illinois

4112 Access Living of Metropolitan Chicago
115 W Chicago Ave
Chicago, IL 60654-3209   312-640-2100
                                 800-613-8549
                            Fax: 312-640-2101
                            TTY: 312-640-2102
                        info@accessliving.org
                              accessliving.org

Marca Bristo, CEO
Bhuttu Mathews, Disability Resources Coordinator
Gary Arnold, Public Relations Coordinator
Daisy Feidt, Executive Vice President
Established in 1980, access living is a change agent commited to fostering an incusive society that enables Chicagoans with disabilities to live fully engaged and self-directed lives. Nationally recognized as a leading force in the disability community. Access Living challenges stereotypes, protects civil rights, and champions social reform.

4113 Center on Deafness
3444 Dundee Rd
Northbrook, IL 60062-2258   847-559-0110
                               Fax: 847-559-8199
                               TTY:847-559-9493
                          www.centerondeafness.org

Bonnie Simon, Executive Director
Donna Gomez, Residential Services/ Adult Plac
Brandi Buie, School Intake
David Wood, Coordinator
COD is dedicated to providing quality services for persons who are deaf or hard of hearing and their families, through educational, vocational, and residential services in a therapuetic, community-based environment

4114 Community Residential Alternative
Coleman Tri- County Services
22 Veterans Drive, ST. A
P.O. Box 869
Harrisburg, IL 62946-2017   618-252-0275
                               Fax: 618-252-2389
                               TTY:618-269-4211
                          cts.62946@frontier.com
                          colemantricounty.tripod.com

Samantha Austin, Executive Director
Six bed group home that provides a residential alternative for the developmentally disabled adult. This program is designed to promote independence in daily living skills, economic self-sufficiency, and integration into the community.

4115 Division of Rehabilitation Services
Department of Human Services
100 South Grand Avenue East
Springfield, IL 62762-2625   217-782-2093
                                 800-843-6154
                            Fax: 217-524-2471
                        DHS.WebBits@illinois.gov
                              www.dhs.state.il.us

Carol Adams, President
Provides medical, therapeutic and counseling services for the disabled, as well as employment services.

4116 DuPage Center for Independent Living
3130 Finley Rd.
Ste. 500
Downers Grove, IL 60515-5877   630-469-2300
                                   Fax: 630-469-2606
                                   TTY:630-469-2300
                                      www.dupagecil.org

Charles Stack, Board President
Bette Lawrence Water, Vice President
John Lausas, Treasurer
Jeff Gullang, Secretary
A non residential, community based, not for profit agency wich provides advocacy and services to persons with disabilities in DuPage County.

4117 Fite Center for Independent Living
1230 Larkin Ave
Elgin, IL 60123-6200   847-695-5818
                           Fax: 847-695-5892
                              info@fitecil.org
                               www.fitecil.org

Linda Bradford-Foster, Chairman, Board Treasurer
Gracia Bittner, Board Secretary
Provides services to people with disabilities in Kane, Kendall and McHenry counties. Our non-residential agency provides independent living skills training, advocacy, systemic + individual peer counseling, information and referral and housing services. Also provides technical assistance to businesses and agencies to work with people with disabilities. Locations in Elgin and Aurora. Please call for further details.

4118 Illinois Department of Rehab Services
Department of Human Services
100 South Grand Avenue East
Springfield, IL 62762-1   217-782-2093
                              800-843-6154
                         Fax: 217-524-2471
                     DHS.WebBits@illinois.gov
                           www.dhs.state.il.us

Carol Adams, President
Karen Perrin, Manager
The state's lead agency serving individuals with disabilities. DRS works in partnership with people with disabilities and their families to assist them in making informed choices to achieve full community participation through employment, education, and independent living opportunities.

4119 Illinois Valley Center for Independent Living
18 Gunia Dr
La Salle, IL 61301-9780   815-224-3126
                              800-822-3246
                         Fax: 815-224-3576
                             ivcil@ivcil.com
                                  ivcil.com

John Hurst, President
Gary Rydleski, Vice President
Sue Faber, Secretary
Danielle Furar, Treasurer
A nonprofit service and advocacy organization that assists persons with disabilities in opening doors to their independence.

4120 Illinois and Iowa Center for Independent Living
501 11th St.
PO Box 6156
Rock Island, IL 61231-6156   309-793-0090
                                 877-541-2505
                                 855-744-8918
                            Fax: 309-793-5198
                                  www.iicil.com

Liz Sherwin, Executive Director
Alfonso Ayew-Ew, Blind Independent Living Skill S
Eddie Williams, CommunityReintegration Advocate
Hershel Jackson, Deaf & Hard of Hearing Advocate
To create and maintain independence options for people with disabilities by advocating for civil rights, providing services, and promoting full participation of disabled individuals in all aspects of the community.

4121 Impact Center for Independent Living
2735 E Broadway
Alton, IL 62002-1859
618-462-1411
888-616-4261
Fax: 618-474-5309
staff@impactcil.org
impactcil.org

Susy Woods, President
Judy O'Malley, Vice President
Bishop Samuel White, Treasurer
Cathy Contarino, Executive Director
Promotes pride and respect for people with disabilities by sharing the tools that are necessary to take control of one's own life.

4122 Jacksonville Area CIL: Havana
220 W Main St
Havana, IL 62644-1138
309-543-6680
877-759-2187
Fax: 309-543-6711
info@jacil.org
www.jacil.org

Phil Foxworth, President
Mark Arnold, Vice President
Ruth Lanier, Secretary
Joe Vieira, Treasurer
Committed to enabling persons with disabilities to gain effective control and director of their own lives in the home, in the workplace and in the community.

4123 Jacksonville Area Center for Independent Living
15 Permac Road
Jacksonville, IL 62650-2071
217-245-8371
Fax: 217-245-1872
TTY:217-245-8371
info@jacil.org
www.jacil.org

Phil Foxworth, President
Mark Arnold, Vice President
Ruth Lanier, Secretary
Joe Vieira, Treasurer
Committed to enabling persons with disabilities to gain effective control and direction of their own lives in the home, in the workplace and in the community.

4124 LIFE Center for Independent Living
Ste 1
2201 Eastland Dr
Bloomington, IL 61704-7923
309-663-5433
888-543-3245
Fax: 309-663-7024
TTY:309-663-5433
gail@lifecil.org
lifecil.org

Gail Kear, Executive Director
Jill Doran, Associate Director
Brianne Anderson, Office Manager
Rickielee Benecke, Disability Rights Advocate
A community-based, not-for-profit, non-residential organization that promotes disability rights, equal access, and full community participation for persons with disabilities.

4125 LINC-Monroe Randolph Center
Ste 4
1514 S Main St
Red Bud, IL 62278-1382
618-282-3700
Fax: 618-282-2740
TTY:618-282-3700

Violete Nast, Manager

4126 Lake County Center for Independent Living
377 N Seymour Ave
Mundelein, IL 60060-2322
847-949-4440
Fax: 847-949-4445
TTY:847-949-0641
lindsey@lccil.org
www.lccil.org

Kelli Brooks, Executive Director
Andy Balint, Director of Finance
Lety Cruz, Bilingual Program Assistant
Jenny Farley, Youth Leadership Advocate
Lake County Center for Independent Living is a disability rights organization governed and staffed by a majority of people with disabilities. LCCIL offers services and advocacy that promote a fully accessible society, which expects participation by persons with disabilities.

4127 Life Center for Independent Living: Pontiac
318 West Madison Street
Pontiac, IL 61764-1785
815-844-1132
Fax: 815-844-1148
lifecil@lifecil.org
lifecil.org

Gail Kear, Executive Director
Jill Doran, Associate Director
Brianne Anderson, Office Manager
Rickielee Benecke, Disability Rights Advocate
A community-based, not-for-profit, non-residential organization that promotes disability rights, equal access, and full community participation for persons with disabilities.

4128 Living Independently Now Center (LINC)
120 E a St
Belleville, IL 62220-1401
618-235-9988
Fax: 618-233-3729
TTY:618-235-9988
info@lincinc.org
www.lincinc.org

Linda Conley, President
Ron Tialdo, Vice-President
Lynn Jarman, Executive Director
Robert Rahlfs, Treasurer
Empowers persons with disabilities to live independently and to promote accessibility and inclusion in all areas.

4129 Living Independently Now Center: Sparta
Western Egyptian Building
207 West 4th Street
Waterloo, IL 62298
618-317-4028
info@lincinc.org
www.lincinc.org

Linda Conley, President
Ron Tialdo, Vice-President
Lynn Jarman, Executive Director
Robert Rahlfs, Treasurer
Empowers persons with disabilities to live independently and to promote accessibility and inclusion in all areas.

4130 Living Independently Now Center: Waterloo
Western Egyptian Building
207 West 4th Street
Waterloo, IL 62298-1336
618-317-4028
info@lincinc.org
www.lincinc.org

Linda Conley, President
Ron Tialdo, Vice-President
Lynn Jarman, Executive Director
Robert Rahlfs, Treasurer
Empowers persons with disabilities to live independently and to promote accessibility and inclusion in all areas.

4131 Mosaic: Pontiac
4980 S. 118th St.
Omaha, NE 68137 877-366-7242
Fax: 402-896-1511
www.mosaicinfo.org

Max Miller, Chairperson
James Zils, Vice Chairperson
Lisa Negstad, 2nd Vice Chairperson
Kathy Patrick, Secretary
A faith-based organization serving people with developmental disabilities.

4132 Opportunities for Access: A Center for Independent Living
4206 Williamson Pl
Suite 3
Mount Vernon, IL 62864-6705 618-244-9212
Fax: 618-244-9310
TTY:618-244-9575
spud@ofacil.org
ofacil.org

Michael Egbert, Executive Director
Serves, trains and provides information to persons with disabilities, family members and significant others and service providers. Services include: advocacy, information and referral, peer support, skills training, volunteer programs and other related services. Services are free. A cross disability community based, nonresidential, nonprofit organization serving Clay, Clinton, Edwards, Effingham, Fayette, Hamilton, Jasper, Jefferson, Marion, Wabash, Washington, Wayne and White Counties.

4133 Options Center for Independent Living: Bourbonnais
22 Heritage Dr
Suite 107
Bourbonnais, IL 60914-2510 815-936-0100
Fax: 815-936-0117
TTY:815-936-0132
optionscil@optionscil.com
www.optionscil.org

Mark Mantarian, President
Ronald D. Smith, Vice President
Dina Raymond, Co-Secretary
Daniel Brough, Treasurer
A non-residential, not-for-profit, community-based organization that promotes independent living for people with disabilities.

4134 Options Center for Independent Living: Watseka
103 Laird Ln
Suite 103
Watseka, IL 60970 815-432-1332
Fax: 815-432-1360
TTY:815-432-1361
www.optionscil.com

Mark Mountain, President
Ronald D. Smith, Vice President
Dina Raymond, Co-Secretary
Daniel Brough, Treasurer
A non-residential, not-for-profit, community-based organization that promotes independent living for people with disabilities.

4135 PACE Center for Independent Living
1317 E Florida Ave
Urbana, IL 61801-6007 217-344-5433
Fax: 217-344-2414
TTY:217-344-5024
info@pacecil.org
pacecil.org

Evelyn Brown, President
Fred Neubert, Vice President
Nancy McClellan-Hickey, Executive Director
Arland Stratton, Treasurer
Promotes the full participation of people with disabilities in the rights and responsibilities of society. Provides services, which assist people with disabilities in achieving or maintaining independence.

4136 Progress Center for Independent Living
7521 Madison St
Forest Park, IL 60130-1407 708-209-1500
Fax: 708-209-1735
TTY:708-209-1826
info@progresscil.org
www.progresscil.org

Anne Gunter, Independent Living Advocate
Kim Liddell, Independent Living Advocate
Horacio Esparza, Executive Director
Art Johnson, Home Services Team Coordinator
A community-based, non-profit, non-residential, service and advocacy organization operated for people with disabilities, by people with disabilities.

4137 Progress Center for Independent Living: Blue Island
12940 Western Ave
Blue Island, IL 60406-3766 708-388-5011
Fax: 708-388-5016
TTY:708-389-8250
info@progresscil.org
www.progresscil.org

Horacio Esparza, Executive Director
Anne Gunter, Independent Living Advocate
Kim Liddell, Independent Living Advocate
Art Johnson, Home Services Team Coordinator
A community-based, non-profit, non residential, service and advocacy organization operated for people with disabilities, by people with disabilities.

4138 Regional Access & Mobilization Project
202 Market St
Rockford, IL 61107-3954 815-968-7467
Fax: 815-968-7612
TTY:815-968-2401
rampcil.org

Shari Snyder, President
Tina Kaatz, Vice President
Craig Fetty, Secretary
Sharon Wyland, Treasurer
To promote an accessible society that allows and expects full participation by people with disabilities.

4139 Regional Access & Mobilization Project: Belvidere
530 S State St
Suite 103
Belvidere, IL 61008-3711 815-544-8404
Fax: 815-544-1896
TTY:815-544-8404
rampcil.org

Shari Snyder, President
Tina Kaatz, Vice President
Craig Fetty, Secretary
Sharon Wyland, Treasurer
Promote an accessible society that allows and expects full participation by people with disabilities.

4140 Regional Access & Mobilization Project: De Kalb
115 N First Street
Dekalb, IL 60115-3055 815-756-3202
Fax: 815-756-3556
TTY:815-756-4263
rampcil.org

Shari Snyder, President
Tina Kaatz, Vice President
Craig Fetty, Secretary
Sharon Wyland, Treasurer
Promotes an accessible society that allows and expects full partiipation by persons with disabilities.

4141 Regional Access & Mobilization Project: Freeport
2155 W Galena Ave
Freeport, IL 61032-3013
815-233-1128
Fax: 815-233-0743
TTY:815-233-1128
rampcil.org

Shari Snyder, President
Tina Kaatz, Vice President
Craig Fetty, Secretary
Sharon Wyland, Treasurer
Promotes an accessible society that allows and expects full
partiipation by persons with disabilities.

4142 Soyland Access to Independent Living(SAIL)
2449 E Federal Dr
Decatur, IL 62526-2160
217-876-8888
800-358-8080
Fax: 217-876-7245
TTY: 217-876-8888
jwooters@decatursail.com
www.decatursail.com

Jeri J Wooters, Executive Director
Betty Watkins, Rural Outreach Coordinator
A community-based, non-residential Center for Independent Living whose purpose is to promote and practice independent living
for all people with disabilities.

4143 Soyland Access to Independent Living: Charleston
757 Windsor Rd
Charleston, IL 61920-7474
217-345-7245
Fax: 217-345-7226
TTY:217-345-7245
triplec@consolidated.net
www.decatursail.com

Betty Watkins, Rural Outreach Coordinator
Jeri J Wooters, Executive Director
A community-based, non-residential Center for Independent Living whose purpose is to promote and practice independent living
for all people iwth disabilities.

4144 Soyland Access to Independent Living: Shelbyville
1810 W.S. 3rd ST P.O.Box 650
Shelbyville, IL 62565-650
217-774-4322
Fax: 217-774-4368
TTY:217-774-4322
sailsel@consolidated.net
www.decatursail.com

Jeri J Wooters, Executive Director
Betty Watkins, Rural Outreach Coordinator
A community-based, non-residential Center for Independent Living whose purpose is to promote and practice independent living
for all people with disabilities.

4145 Soyland Access to Independent Living: Sullivan
1102 W Jackson St
Sullivan, IL 61951-1067
217-728-3186
Fax: 217-728-2299
TTY:217-728-3186
sulsail@wireless111.com
www.decatursail.com

Betty Watkins, Rural Outreach Coordinator
Jeri J Wooters, Executive Director
A community-based, non-residential Center for Independent Living whose purpose is to promote and practice independent living
for all people with disabilities.

4146 Springfield Center for Independent Living
330 South Grand Ave W
Springfield, IL 62704-3716
217-523-4032
800-447-4221
Fax: 217-523-0427
TTY: 217-523-4032
scil@scil.org
scil.org

Pete Roberts, Executive Director
Susan Coopers, Program Director
Denise Groesch, Reintegration Coordinator
Kathryn Cline, Business Manager

To increase opportunities for equality, integration and independence for all persons with disabilities through advocacy, services,
and public education.

4147 Stone-Hayes Center for Independent Living
39 N Prairie St
Galesburg, IL 61401-4613
309-344-1306
888-347-4245
Fax: 309-344-1305
TTY: 309-344-1306

Vanya Peterson, Executive Director
Michael Bohnenkamp, Associate Director
John Hunigan, Office Manager
Lynn Voeller, Independent Living Associate
The purpose of INCIL is to facilitate the collaboration of all Cen-
ters for Independent Living in Illinois for promoting, through the
Independent Living Movement, equal opportunities and civil
rights for all persons with disabilities.

4148 West Central Illinois Center for Independent Living
639 York St.
Suite 204
Quincy, IL 62301-1065
217-223-0400
Fax: 217-223-0479
TTY:217-223-0475
info@wcicil.org
www.wcicil.org

Glenda Hackemack, Executive Director
Dale Winner, Information & Referral Coordinat
Dustin Gorde Director of Community, Jenny
Kelly Transition Co-Ordinato
A not-for-profit advocacy center funded by state and federal
grants to provide services to people with disabilities.

**4149 West Central Illinois Center for Independent Living:
Macomb**
440 N Lafayette St
Macomb, IL 61455-1512
309-833-5766
Fax: 309-833-4690
TTY:217-223-0475
info@wcicil.org
www.wcicil.org

Glenda Hackemack, Executive Director
Dale Winner, Information & Referral Coordinat
Dustin Gorde Director of Community, Jenny
Kelly Transition Co-Ordinato
A not-for-profit advocacy center funded by state and federal
grants to provide services to people with disabilities.

4150 Will Grundy Center for Independent Living
2415 W Jefferson St
Suite A
Joliet, IL 60435-6464
815-729-0162
Fax: 815-729-3697
TTY:815-729-2085
will-grundycil.org

Elaine Sommer, President
Chris Boyk, Vice President
Dianne Mundle, Treasurer
Rhonda Price, Secretary
A cross-disability, community based organization that strives for
equalityand empowerment of persons with disabilities in the Will
and Grundy County areas.

Indiana

4151 Assistive Technology Training and Information Center (ATTIC)
1721 Washington Ave
Vincennes, IN 47591-4823
812-886-0575
877-96A-8842
Fax: 812-886-1128
inbox@atticindiana.org
www.atticindiana.org

Patricia Stewart, Executive Director
Rebecca Anderson, Assistant Director
Mark Schmitt, Fiscal Controller
Jackie Evans, Independent Living Coordinator
ATTIC provides support, information and education for individuals with disabilities and for families of children with special needs, and the professionals who assist these families. All disabilities, all ages.

4152 DAMAR Services
6067 Decatur Blvd.
Indianapolis, IN 46241
317-856-5201
Fax: 317-856-2333
info@damar.org
damar.org

Gail Shiel, Chairman
Rick Torbeck, Vice Chairman
Jim Dalton, Psy.D., HSPP, President and CEO
Richard L. Harcourt, Vice President & CFO
Builds better futures for children and adults facing life's greatest developmental and behavioral challenges.

4153 Everybody Counts Center for Independent Living
3616 Elm St
Room 3
East Chicago, IN 46410-7097
219-229-5055
888-769-3636
Fax: 219-769-5326
TTY:219-756-3323
info@everybodycounts.org
everybodycounts.org

Teresa Torres, Executive Director
Emma Lewis Sullivan, On Loan Consultant
Mark Torres, Systems Manager
Jodi Hawn, Administrative Assistant
A nonprofit corporation dedicated to the achievement of maximum independence and enhanced quality of life for persons with disabilities.

4154 Four Rivers Resource Services
Hwy. 59 South
P.O. Box 249
Linton, IN 47441-249
812-847-2231
Fax: 812-847-8836
fourrivers@frrs.org
frrs.org

Stephen Sacksteder, Executive Director
Robin Duncan, Chief Financial Officer
Dean Dorrell, Information Systems Director
Jessica Davis, Development Coordinator
FRRS is established to enable individuals with disabilities and other challenges to attain self independence and natural interdependence, inclusion in normal life experiences and opportunities, and general life enrichment, by working in partnership with them, their families and the communities in and around Greene, Sullivan, Daviess, and Martin Counties.

4155 Future Choices Independent Living Center
309 N High St
Muncie, IN 47305-1618
765-741-8332
866-741-3444
Fax: 765-741-8333
futurechoices.org

Beth Y. Quarles, President
Provides unlimited options for minorities, youth, and Hoosiers with disabilities.

4156 Independent Living Center of Eastern Indiana (ILCEIN)
1818 W Main St
Richmond, IN 47374-3822
765-939-9226
877-939-9226
Fax: 765-935-2215
www.ilcein.org

Jim McCormick, Executive Director
Dean Turner, Administrative Director
Ann Barnhart, Compliance Manager
Michelle Satterfield, Service Coordinator
Serving Fayette, Franklin, Henry, Decatur, Rush, Union and Wayne Counties.

4157 Indianapolis Resource Center for Independent Living
5302 East Washington Street
Indianapolis, IN 46219
317-926-1660
866-794-7245
Fax: 317-926-1687
info@abilityindiana.org
www.abilityindiana.org

Judy Townsend, President
Dave Trulock, Vice President
Jacqueline Troy, Treasurer
Don Lane, Secretary
Provides services, support and information to people with disabilities to help insure equal access to all aspects of community life.

4158 League for the Blind and Disabled
5821 S Anthony Blvd
Fort Wayne, IN 46816-3701
260-441-0551
800-889-3443
Fax: 260-441-7760
TTY: 800-889-3443
the-league@the-league.org
the-league.org

David A. Nelson, CEO/President
Catherine Collins, Chair
Anne Palmer, Administrative Assistant
Kevin Showalter, Youth Services Coordinator
To provide and promote opportunities that empower people with disabilities to achieve their potential.

4159 Martin Luther Homes of Indiana
Mosaic
26 N Brown Ave
Terre Haute, IN 47803-1523
812-235-3399
Fax: 812-235-1590

4160 Ruben Center for Independent Living
5302 East Washington Street
Indianapolis, IN 46219-3227
317-926-1660
Fax: 317-926-1687
TTY:219-397-6496
info@abilityindiana.org
www.abilityindiana.org

Judy Townsend, President
Dave Trulock, Vice President
Jacqueline Troy, Treasurer
Don Lane, Secretary
An independent living center providing support, information and education.

4161 SILC, Indiana Council on Independent Living (ICOIL)
P.O.Box 7083
Indianapolis, IN 46207-7083
317-232-1303
800-545-7763
Fax: 317-232-6478
nancy.young@fssa.in.gov
www.icoil.org

Nancy Young, Program Director
Richard Simers, SILC Chairperson

4162 Southern Indiana Center for Independent Living
1494 W. Main Street
PO Box 308
Mitchell, IN   47446-1943   812-277-9626
                                                   800-845-6914
                                              Fax: 812-277-9628
                                                  sicilindiana.org

Al Tolbert, Executive Director
Darlene Webster, Independent Living Center Direct
SICIL is a consumer controlled, community based, cross-disability, non-residential and not for profit organization that promotes and practices the philosophy of independent living: consumer control, peer support, self-help, self-determination, equal access, and individual and community advocacy. SICIL also promotes accesible and affordable housing, recreation and transportation.

4163 Wabash Independent Living Center & Learning Center (WILL)
1 Dreiser Square
Terre Haute, IN   47807   812-298-9455
                                                   877-915-9455
                                              Fax: 812-299-9061
                                              TTY: 877-915-9455
                                              info@thewillcenter.org
                                              www.thewillcenter.org

Don Rogers, Chairman
Jody Pomfret, Vice Chairman
Kevin Burke, Treasurer
Peter Ciancone, Secretary-Executive Director
To empower people with disabilities to ensure that they have full and complete access to community resources to promote their independence

Iowa

4164 Black Hawk Center for Independent Living
2800 Falls Ave.
P.O. Box 2275
Waterloo, IA   50701-2275   319-291-7755
                                                   888-291-7754
                                              Fax: 319-291-7781
                                              TTY:800-735-2942
                                              blackhawkcenter.org

4165 Central Iowa Center for Independent Living
655 Walnut St
Suite 131
Des Moines, IA   50309-3930   515-243-1742
                                                   888-503-2287
                                              Fax: 515-243-5385

Bob Jeppesen, Executive Director
Frank Strong, Associate Director
Crystal Toman, Office Coordinator
Dee Howard, Independent Living Specialist
CICIL is a community based, non-profit, non-residential program serving persons with disabilities. CICIL assists all persons, regardless of disability in making choices about their own lives and in experiencing success in achieving independence.

4166 Evert Conner Rights & Resources CIL
730 S Dubuque St
Iowa City, IA   52240-4202   319-338-3870
                                                   800-982-0272
                                              Fax: 319-354-1799

Scott Gill, Executive Director
Provides community services like disability awareness training and classroom presentations. Individual services include independent living skills training and peer counseling. All services are custom designed to support the independence of people with disabilities in their own community.

4167 Hope Haven
1800 19th St
PO Box 70
Rock Valley, IA   51247-1098   712-476-2737
                                              Fax: 712-476-3110
                                                  hopehaven.org

Dr. Kent Eric Eknes, President
Ron Boote, Vice President
David Vanningen, Executive Director
Calvin Helmus, Chief Operating Officer
Unleashes the potential in people through work and life skills so that they may enjoy a productive life in their community.

4168 League of Human Dignity, Center for Independent Living
1520 Avenue M
Council Bluffs, IA   51501-1185   712-323-6863
                                              Fax: 712-323-6811
                                     Cinfo@leagueofhumandignity.com
                                     www.leagueofhumandignity.com

Carrie England, Director
League of Human Dignity actively promotes the full integration of individuals with disabilities into society. To this end, the League will advocate their needs and rights, and provide quality services to involve these persons in becoming and remaining independent citizens.

4169 Martin Luther Homes of Iowa
P.O. Box 2316
Princeton, NJ   08543-2316   877-843-7953
                                              Fax: 563-568-3992
                                                    www.rwjf.org

Mary Lynn ReVoir, Project Director
Fred Naumann III, Communications
Richard Wicks, Executive Director

4170 South Central Iowa Center for Independent Living
117 1st Ave W
Oskaloosa, IA   52577-3243   641-672-1867
                                                   800-651-7911
                                              Fax: 641-672-1867
                                              brookie43@gmail.com
                                     www.iowasilc.org/cilinfo.html

Deb Philpot, Executive Director
Provides services, support, information and referral to people with disabilities to help insure equal access to all aspects of community life.

4171 Three Rivers Center for Independent Living
900 Rebecca Avenue
Pittsburgh, PA   15221-2938   412-371-7700
                                                   800-633-4588
                                              Fax: 412-371-9430
                                              TTY: 412-371-6230
                                                  lgray@trcil.org

Stanley A. Holbrook, President & Executive Director
Lisa Wilson, HR Program Manager
Rachel Rogan, Director of Waiver Services
Charles Keenan, TRCIL Real Properties Board
Providing a wide array of services to assist individuals and families in achieving positive life goals.

Kansas

4172 Advocates for Better Living For Everyone(A.B.L.E.)
Ste C
521 Commercial St
Atchison, KS   66002   913-367-1830
                                                   888-845-2879
                                              Fax: 913-367-1830

Ken Gifford, President & CEO
A not for profit agency providing services within the State of Kansas. ABLE looks to assist people with disabilities as well as any other member of the community to live an integrated, quality life with dignity, respect, and independence.

4173   Center for Independent Living SW Kansas: Liberal
1023 N Kansas Ave
Suite 2
Liberal, KS   67901-2655   620-624-5500
                                            800-327-4048
                                            Fax: 620-624-6576
                                            TTY: 620-624-5500
                                            www.cilswks.org

Victor Otero, Manager
Crystal Tharp, Independent Living Advocate
Dedicated to helping people achieve full participation in society.

4174   Center for Independent Living Southwest Kansas
P.O.Box 2090
Garden City, KS   67846-2090   620-276-1900
                                            800-736-9443
                                            Fax: 620-271-0200
                                            www.cilswks.org

Troy Horton, Executive Director
Dedicated to helping people achieve full participation in society.

4175   Center for Independent Living Southwest Kansas: Dodge City
2601 Central Ave
Dodge City, KS   67801-6200   620-227-6660
                                            800-326-1366
                                            Fax: 620-227-8185
                                            TTY: 620-227-6660

Mary Jane Sandoval, Independent Living Advocate
Dedicated to helping people achieve full participation in society

4176   Coalition for Independence
4911 State Ave
Kansas City, KS   66102-1749   913-321-5140
                                            866-201-3829
                                            Fax: 913-321-5182
                                            TTY: 913-321-5216
                                            cfi-kc.org

Clarence Smith, Executive Director
Laarni Sison, Executive Assistant
Claire Marr, Lead Independent Living Speciali
Shauna Garrett, Lead Accountant
Facilitates positive and responsible independence for all people with disabilities by acting as an advocate for individuals with disabilities, providing services, and promoting accessibility and acceptance.

4177   Cowley County Developmental Services
P.O.Box 618
Arkansas City, KS   67005-618   620-442-5270
                                            866-442-5270
                                            Fax: 620-442-5623

Bill Brooks, Executive Director
Provides services for persons with developmental disabilities in Cowley County..

4178   Independence
2001 Haskell Ave
Lawrence, KS   66046-3249   785-841-0333
                                            888-824-7277
                                            Fax: 785-841-1094
                                            comment@independenceinc.org
                                            independenceinc.org

Karen McGrath, President
Bruce Passman, Vice President
Sandra London, Lieb
Athena Johnson, Secretary
Provides advocacy, services, and education for people with disabilities and our communities.

4179   Independent Connection
1710 W. Schilling Road
P.O.Box 1160
Salina, KS   67402- 1160   785-827-9383
                                            800-526-9731
                                            Fax: 785-823-2015
                                            TTY: 785-827-9383
                                            www.occk.com

Shelia Nelson-Stout, President/CEO
Deanna L. Lamer, Senior Director,Human Resources
Tasha Suppes, Human Resources Coordinator
Dedicated to helping people with physical or mental disabilities remove barriers to employment, independent living, and full participation in their communities.

4180   Independent Connection: Abilene
Suite 221
300 N. Cedar St.
Abilene, KS   67410   785-263-2208
                                            Fax: 785-263-3795
                                            TTY:785-263-2208
                                            www.occk.com

Shelia Nelson-Stout, President/CEO
Deanna L. Lamer, Senior Director,Human Resources
Tasha Suppes, Human Resources Coordinator
Dedicated to helping people with physical or mental disabilities remove barriers to employment, independent living, and full participation in their communities.

4181   Independent Connection: Beloit
501 W 7th St
Beloit, KS   67420-2107   785-738-5423
                                            Fax: 785-738-3320
                                            TTY:785-738-5423
                                            www.occk.com

Shelia Nelson-Stout, President/CEO
Deanna L. Lamer, Senior Director,Human Resources
Tasha Suppes, Human Resources Coordinator
Dedicated to helping people with physical or mental disabilities remove barriers to employment, independent living, and full participation in their communities.

4182   Independent Connection: Concordia
1502 Lincoln St
Concordia, KS   66901-4830   785-243-1977
                                            Fax: 785-243-4524
                                            TTY:785-243-1977
                                            www.occk.com

Shelia Nelson-Stout, President/CEO
Dedicated to helping people with physical or mental disabilities remove barriers to employment, independent living, and full participation in their communities.

4183   Independent Living Resource Center
3033 W 2nd St N
Wichita, KS   67203-5357   316-942-6300
                                            800-479-6861
                                            Fax: 316-942-2078
                                            ilrcks.org

Jean Shuler, President
Angie Schmidt, Vice Chairman
Derrick Prichard, Secretary/Treasurer
James Thayer, Board Member
Empower people with disabilities to lead independent lives by providing advocacy, education and direct services. Serve people with all types of disabilities; permanent or temporary, physical disabilities, mental disabilities, and developmental disabilities.

4184   Kansas Services for the Blind & Visually Impaired
2601 SW East Circle Dr N
Topeka, KS   66606-2445   785-296-3738
                                            800-547-5789
                                            Fax: 785-291-3138
                                            rehab@srskansas.org
                                            srskansas.org

Dennis Ford, Manager
Michael Donnelly, Director

Helps persons who are blind or visually to improve their quality of life. KSBVI provides people with an array of services and experiences aimed at overcoming not only the physical difficulties brought on by the loss of vision, but also the fear of change associated with vision loss. KSBVI can also help with job search and retention activities; life skills training; access to medical services; and technical assistance..

4185 LINK: Colby
505 N Franklin Ave
Suite G
Colby, KS 67701-2342
785-462-7600
800-736-9418
TTY:785-462-7600
brianatwell@linkinc.org
www.linkinc.org

Brian Atwell, Executive Director
Promotes and supports the civil rights of people with disabilities and empowers them to achieve a life of independence and equality..

4186 Living Independently in Northwest Kansas: Hays
2401 E 13th St
Hays, KS 67601-2663
785-625-6942
800-596-5926
Fax: 785-625-2334
TTY: 785-625-6942
brianatwell@linkinc.org
www.linkinc.org

Brian Atwell, Executive Director
Promotes and supports the civil rights of people with disabilities and empowers them to achieve a life of independence and equality.

4187 Prairie IL Resource Center
103 W 2nd St
Pratt, KS 67124-2644
620-672-9600
Fax: 620-672-9601
info@pilr.org
www.pilr.org

Dave Mullins, President
Stephanie Guthrie, Vice President
Chris Owens, Executive Director
Roger Frischenmeyer, Independent Living Specialist
To achieve the full inclusion and acceptance of people with disabilities through education and advocacy

4188 Prairie Independent Living Resource Center
17th S Main St
Hutchinson, KS 67501
620-663-3989
888-715-6818
Fax: 620-663-4711
TTY:620-663-9920
info@pilr.org
www.pilr.org

Dave Mullins, President
Stephanie Guthrie, Vice President
Chris Owens, Executive Director
Roger Frischenmeyer, Independent Living Specialist
To achieve the full conclusion and acceptance of people with disabilities through education and advocacy

4189 Resource Center for Independent Living
104 S. Washington Ave.
Iola, KS 66749-8805
620-365-8144
877-944-8144
Fax: 620-365-7726
rcilinc.org

Chad Wilkins, Executive Director
Committed to working with individuals, families, and communities to promote independent living and individual choice to persons with disabilities.

4190 Resource Center for Independent Living, Inc. (RCIL)
409 Columbia St.
Utica, NY 13503-210
315-797-4642
800-580-7245
Fax: 315-797-4747
TTY: 315-797-5837
rcilinc.org

Chad Wilkins, Executive Director
Committed to working with individuals, families, and communities to promote independent living and individual choice to persons with disabilities. As a center for independent living in Kansas, we provide advocacy, peer counseling, information and referral, independent living skills training and deinstitutionalization. In addition to these services, we also provide HOBS payroll services and a variety of programs benefiting individuals with disabilities.

4191 Resource Center for Independent Living: Emporia
215 West Sixth Avenue
Suite 202
Emporia, KS 66801-2886
620-342-1648
888-261-4024
Fax: 620-342-1821
info@rcilinc.org
rcilinc.org

Deone Wilson, Executive Director
Beth Combes, Information & Outreach Coordinat
Amy Richardson, Targeted Case Manager
Trevor Larson, Office Assistant
Committed to working with individuals, families, and communities to promote independent living and individual choice to persons with disabilities.

4192 Resource Center for Independent Living: Arkansas City
P.O. Box 257
1137 Laing
Osage City, KS 66523
785-528-3105
800-580-7245
Fax: 785-528-3665
TTY: 785-528-3106
info@rcilinc.org
rcilinc.org

Deone Wilson, Executive Director
Tania Harrington, Director of Quality Assurance
Adam Burnett, Director of Core Services
Mike Pitts, Finance Committee Chairperson
Committed to working with individuals, families, and communities to promote independent living and individual choice to persons with disabilities.

4193 Resource Center for Independent Living: Burlington
P.O. Box 257
1137 Laing
Osage City, KS 66523
785-528-3105
800-580-7245
Fax: 785-528-3665
TTY: 785-528-3106
info@rcilinc.org
rcilinc.org

Deone Wilson, Executive Director
Tania Harrington, Director of Quality Assurance
Adam Burnett, Director of Core Services
Mike Pitts, Finance Committee Chairperson
Committed to working with individuals, families, and communities to promote independent living and individual choice to persons with disabilities.

4194 Resource Center for Independent Living: Coffeyville
P.O. Box 257
1137 Laing
Osage City, KS 66523

785-528-3105
800-580-7245
Fax: 785-528-3665
TTY: 785-528-3106
info@rcilinc.org
rcilinc.org

Deone Wilson, Executive Director
Tania Harrington, Director of Quality Assurance
Adam Burnett, Director of Core Services
Mike Pitts, Finance Committee Chairperson
Committed to working with individuals, families, and communities to promote independent living and individual choice to persons with disabilities.

4195 Resource Center for Independent Living: El Dorado
615 1/2 N Main St
El Dorado, KS 67042-2027

316-322-7853
800-960-7853
Fax: 316-322-7888
info@rcilinc.org
rcilinc.org

Macy Gaines, Independent Living Specialist
Doris Hammons, Targeted Case Manager
Shirley Mullin, Targeted Case Manager
Barbara Ehret, Office Assistant
Committed to working with individuals, families, and communities to promote independent living and individual choice to persons with disabilities.

4196 Resource Center for Independent Living: Ft Scott
P.O. Box 257
1137 Laing
Osage City, KS 66523

785-528-3105
800-580-7245
Fax: 785-528-3665
TTY: 785-528-3106
info@rcilinc.org
rcilinc.org

Deone Wilson, Executive Director
Tania Harrington, Director of Quality Assurance
Adam Burnett, Director of Core Services
Mike Pitts, Finance Committee Chairperson
Committed to working with individuals, families, and communities to promote independent living and individual choice to persons with disabilities.

4197 Resource Center for Independent Living: Ottawa
233 W 23rd Street
Ottawa, KS 66067-3533

785-242-1805
800-995-1805
Fax: 785-242-1448
rcilinc.org

Chad Wilkins, Executive Director
Committed to working with individuals, families, and communities to promote independent living and individual choice to persons with disabilities.

4198 Resource Center for Independent Living: Overland Park
Ste 100
10200 W 75th St
Shawnee Mission, KS 66204-2242

913-362-6618
877-439-2847
Fax: 913-677-2742
rcilinc.org

Chad Wilkins, Executive Director
RCIL is committed to working with individuals, families, and communities to promote independent living and individual choice to persons with disabilities.

4199 Resource Center for Independent Living: Topeka
1507 S.W. 21stStreet
Suite 203
Topeka, KS 66604-2356

785-267-1717
877-719-1717
Fax: 785-267-1711
info@rcilinc.org
rcilinc.org

Rosie Cooper, Director of Independent Living S
Stuart Jones, Assistive Technology Specialist
Mikel McCary, Assistive Technology Specialist
Mandy Smith, Finance Committee Chairperson
Committed to working with individuals, families, and communities to promote independent living and individual choice to persons with disabilities.

4200 Southeast Kansas Independent Living (SKIL)
1801 Main
P.O. Box 957
Parsons, KS 67357-957

620-421-5502
800-688-5616
Fax: 620-421-3705
TTY: 620-421-0983
skil@skilonline.com
www.skilonline.com

Nancy Varner, Chairman
Janet Spillman, Vice Chairman
Shari Coatney, CEO/President
Olivia Lyons, Secretary/Treasurer
To empower, integrate and maximize independence for all persons with disabilities.

4201 Southeast Kansas Independent Living: Independence
107 East Main
P.O.Box 944
Independence, KS 67301-944

620-331-1006
866-927-1006
Fax: 620-331-1257
TTY: 620-331-1006
skilindy@skilonline.com
www.skilonline.com

Nancy Varner, Chairman
Janet Spillman, Vice Chairman
Shari Coatney, CEO/President
Olivia Lyons, Secretary/Treasurer
To empower, integrate and maximize independence for all persons with disabilities.

4202 Southeast Kansas Independent Living: Chanute
2 W. Main
P.O.Box 645
Chanute, KS 66720-645

620-431-0757
866-927-0757
Fax: 620-431-7274
TTY: 620-431-0757
skilchanute@skilonline.com
www.skilonline.com

Nancy Varner, Chairman
Janet Spillman, Vice Chairman
Shari Coatney, CEO/President
Olivia Lyons, Secretary/Treasurer
To empower, integrate and maximize independence for all persons with disabilities.

4203 Southeast Kansas Independent Living: Columbus
123 N. Kansas
P.O. Box 478
Columbus, KS 66725-1801

620-429-3600
866-927-3600
Fax: 620-429-1027
skilcolumbus@skilonline.com
www.skilonline.com

Nancy Varner, Chairman
Janet Spillman, Vice Chairman
Shari Coatney, CEO/President
Olivia Lyons, Secretary/Treasurer
To empower, integrate and maximize independence for all persons with disabilities.

4204 **Southeast Kansas Independent Living: Fredonia**
623 Monroe
P.O.Box 448
Fredonia, KS 66736-448 620-378-4881
866-927-4881
Fax: 620-378-4851
TTY: 620-378-4881
skilfredonia@skilonline.com
www.skilonline.com

Nancy Varner, Chairman
Janet Spillman, Vice Chairman
Shari Coatney, CEO/President
Olivia Lyons, Secretary/Treasurer
To empower, integrate and maximize independence for all persons with disabilities.

4205 **Southeast Kansas Independent Living: Hays**
510 W. 29thStreet, Suite A
PO Box 366
Hays, KS 67601-366 785-628-8019
800-316-8019
Fax: 785-628-3116
TTY: 785-628-3128
skilhays@skilonline.com
www.skilonline.com

Nancy Varner, Chairman
Janet Spillman, Vice Chairman
Shari Coatney, CEO/President
Olivia Lyons, Secretary/Treasurer
To empower, integrate and maximize independence for all persons with disabilities.

4206 **Southeast Kansas Independent Living: Pittsburg**
1403 N. Broadway
P.O.Box 1706
Pittsburg, KS 66762-1706 620-231-6780
866-927-6780
Fax: 620-232-9915
TTY: 620-231-6780
skilpittsburg@skilonline.com
www.skilonline.com

Nancy Varner, Chairman
Janet Spillman, Vice Chairman
Shari Coatney, CEO/President
Olivia Lyons, Secretary/Treasurer
To empower, integrate and maximize independence for all persons with disabilities.

4207 **Southeast Kansas Independent Living: Sedan**
113 West Main
P.O.Box 340
Sedan, KS 67361-340 620-725-3990
866-906-3990
Fax: 620-725-3942
TTY: 620-725-3990
skilsedan@skilonline.com
www.skilonline.com

Nancy Varner, Chairman
Janet Spillman, Vice Chairman
Shari Coatney, CEO/President
Olivia Lyons, Secretary/Treasurer
To empower, integrate and maximize independence for all persons with disabilities.

4208 **Southeast Kansas Independent Living: Yates Center**
119 W. Butler
P.O.Box 129
Yates Center, KS 66783-129 620-625-2818
866-927-2818
Fax: 620-625-2585
www.skilonline.com

Nancy Varner, Chairman
Janet Spillman, Vice Chairman
Shari Coatney, CEO/President
Olivia Lyons, Secretary/Treasurer
To empower, integrate and maximize independence for all persons with disabilities.

4209 **Three Rivers Independent Living Center**
504 Miller Drive
P.O.Box 408
Wamego, KS 66547-0408 785-456-9915
800-555-3994
Fax: 785-456-9923
TTY: 785-456-9915
reception@threeriversinc.org
www.threeriversinc.org

Audrey Schremmer-Philips, Executive Director
Keyna Steinbrock, IL Specialist
Erica Christie, Director of Supports & Services
Rebel Eichelberger, Senior Accountant
A nonprofit organization promoting the self reliance of individuals with disabilities through education, advocacy, training and support.

4210 **Three Rivers Independent Living Center: Clay**
719 5th Street
P.O.Box 33
Clay Center, KS 67432-0033 785-632-6117
Fax: 785-632-6117
TTY:785-632-6117
reception@threeriversinc.org
www.threeriversinc.org

Audrey Schremmer-Philips, Executive Director
Keyna Steinbrock, IL Specialist
Erica Christie, Director of Supports & Services
Rebel Eichelberger, Senior Accountant
A non-profit organization promoting the self reliance of individuals with disabilities through, education, advocacy, training and support.

4211 **Three Rivers Independent Living Center: Manhattan**
401 Houston St.
Manhattan, KS 66502 785-776-9294
800-432-2703
Fax: 785-776-9479
reception@threeriversinc.org
www.threeriversinc.org

Audrey Schremmer-Philips, Executive Director
Keyna Steinbrock, IL Specialist
Erica Christie, Director of Supports & Services
Rebel Eichelberger, Senior Accountant
A non profit organization promoting the self reliance of individuals with disabilities through education, advocacy, training and support.

4212 **Three Rivers Independent Living Center: Seneca**
416 Main St
Seneca, KS 66538-1926 785-336-0222
Fax: 785-336-0288
reception@threeriversinc.org
www.threeriversinc.org

Audrey Schremmer-Philips, Executive Director
Keyna Steinbrock, IL Specialist
Erica Christie, Director of Supports & Services
Rebel Eichelberger, Senior Accountant
A non profit organization promoting the self reliance of individuals with disabilities through education, advocacy, training and support.

4213 **Three Rivers Independent Living Center: Topeka**
P.O.Box 4152
Topeka, KS 66604-4152 785-273-0249
Fax: 785-273-0249
reception@threeriversinc.org
www.threeriversinc.org

Audrey Schremmer-Philips, Executive Director
Keyna Steinbrock, IL Specialist
Erica Christie, Director of Supports & Services
Rebel Eichelberger, Senior Accountant
A non profit organization promoting the self reliance of individuals with disabilities through education, advocacy, training and support.

4214 Topeka Independent Living Resource Center
501 SW Jackson St
Suite 100
Topeka, KS   66603-3300   785-233-4572
                                            Fax: 785-233-1561
                                            TTY:785-233-4572
                                            tilrcweb@tilrc.org
                                                 tilrc.org

Mike Oxford, Executive Director
Evan Korynta, Operations Manager
Angie Harter, Independent Living Advocacy Staf
Carol Doss, Independent Living Advocacy Staf
A civil and human rights organization that advocates for justice, equality and essential services for a fully integrated and accessible society for all people with disabilities.

4215 Whole Person: Nortonville
7301 Mission Road
Suite 135
Prairie Village, KS   66208- 3006   913-262-1294
                                                 877-767-8896
                                            Fax: 913-262-2392
                                            info@thewholeperson.org
                                            www.thewholeperson.org

Rick O'Neal, President
Jim Atwater, Vice President
MIchelle Ford, Secretary
Timothy L. Urban, Treasurer
Assists people with disabilities to live independently and encourages change within the community to expand opportunities for independent living.

4216 Whole Person: Nortonville, The
7301 Mission Road
Suite 135
Prairie Village, KS   66208- 3006   913-262-1294
                                                 877-767-8896
                                            Fax: 913-262-2392
                                            info@thewholeperson.org
                                            www.thewholeperson.org

Rick O'Neal, President
Jim Atwater, Vice President
MIchelle Ford, Secretary
Timothy L. Urban, Treasurer
Assists people with disabilities to live independently and encourages change within the community to expand opportunities for independent living.

4217 Whole Person: Prairie Village
7301 Mission Rd
Prairie Village, KS   66208-3006   913-262-1294
                                            Fax: 913-262-2392
                                            info@thewholeperson.org
                                            www.thewholeperson.org

Rick O'Neal, President
Jim Atwater, Vice President
MIchelle Ford, Secretary
Timothy L. Urban, Treasurer
Assists people with disabilities to live independently and encourages change within the community to expand opportunities for independent living.

4218 Whole Person: Prairie Village, The
7301 Mission Road
Suite 135
Prairie Village, KS   66208- 3006   913-262-1294
                                                 877-767-8896
                                            Fax: 913-262-2392
                                            info@thewholeperson.org
                                            www.thewholeperson.org

Rick O'Neal, President
Jim Atwater, Vice President
MIchelle Ford, Secretary
Timothy L. Urban, Treasurer
Assists people with disabilities to live independently and encourages change within the community to expand opportunities for independent living.

4219 Whole Person: Tonganoxie
7301 Mission Road
Suite 135
Prairie Village, KS   66208- 3006   913-262-1294
                                                 877-767-8896
                                            Fax: 913-262-2392
                                            info@thewholeperson.org
                                            www.thewholeperson.org

Rick O'Neal, President
Jim Atwater, Vice President
MIchelle Ford, Secretary
Timothy L. Urban, Treasurer
Assists people with disabilities to live independently and encourages change within the community to expand opportunities for independent living.

Kentucky

4220 Center for Accessible Living
501 S. 2nd Street
Ste 200
Louisville, KY   40202-2121   502-589-6620
                                                 888-813-8497
                                            Fax: 502-589-3980
                                            TTY:502-589-6690
                                            info@calky.org
                                            www.calky.org

Jan Day, CEO
Michael Markiewicz, Chief Financial Officer
Jeanne M. Gallimore, Branch Director
Susan Tharpe, Coordinator of Services
To assist the individuals with disabilities who seek to live independently.

4221 Center for Accessible Living: Murray
1051 N 16th St
Suite C
Murray, KY   42071-8511   270-753-7676
                                                 888-261-6194
                                            Fax: 270-753-7729
                                            TTY:270-767-0549
                                            www.calky.org

Jeanne M. Gallimore, Branch Director
Susan Tharpe, Coordinator of Services
Jan Day, CEO
Michael Markiewicz, Chief Financial Officer
To assist the individuals with disabilities who seek to live independently.

4222 Center for Independent Living: Kentucky Department for the Blind
Independent Living Office
Rear
409 N Miles St
Elizabethtown, KY   42701-1834   270-766-5126
Buel E Stalls Jr, Office Manager and IL Specialist
Nancy Bachuss, Manager
Offers peer counseling, attendant care registry and other services to the community as they relate to the blind community. The Murray office is an independent living regional office which covers 20 far western counties of Kentucky..

4223 Disability Coalition of Northern Kentucky
Ste 219
525 W 5th St
Covington, KY   41011-1293   859-431-7668
                                            Fax: 859-431-7688
                                            TTY:800-648-6057

Kitt Heeg, Executive Director
Empowering people with disabilities through education, networking, and positive attitudes..

4224 Disability Resource Initiative
624 Eastwood St
Bowling Green, KY 42103-1602   270-796-5992
                                        877-437-5045
                                    Fax: 270-796-6630
                                        www.dri-ky.org

Marilyn Mitchell, Executive Director
Tracy Cole, Independent Living Specialist
Steve Burchett, IT Specialist
Jenny McCallister, Administrative Assistant
One of the most important premises in Independent Living is that people with disabilities are the most knowledgable about their own needs. Because of this all of their services are designed to be consumer-driven. Within each service, Center Staff work with both participant and provider to achieve and maintain an Independent Lifestyle.

4225 Independence Place
1093 S. Broadway
Suite 1218
Lexington, KY 40504-1787   859-266-2807
                                     877-266-2807
                                Fax: 859-335-0627
                                 TTY: 800-648-6056
                        info@independenceplaceky.org
                        www.independenceplaceky.org

Michael Fein, Chairman
Carla Webster, Vice Chairwoman
Pamela Roark-Glisson, Executive Director
Orissa Mason, Consumer Services Coordinator
To assist people with disabilities to achieve their full potential for community inclusion through improving access, choice and equal opportunity.

4226 Pathfinders for Independent Living
105 E Mound St
Harlan, KY 40831-2355   606-573-5777
                                    877-340-PATH
                                Fax: 606-573-5739
                                 TTY: 606-573-5777

Sandra Goodwyn, Executive Director
Andrew Saylor, Director of IT (Internal) and Fi
Stacy Marple, Director of IT (External)
Ron Walker, Public Affairs Specialist
They publish a newsletter called LifeLine 4-5 times a year. Most articles are written by Sandra Goodwyn. Editor is Andrew Saylor. Serves people with disabilities to maintain as much independence as they desire

4227 SILC Department of Vocational Rehabilitation
209 Saint Clair St
Frankfort, KY 40601-1817   502-564-4440
                                     800-372-7172
                                Fax: 502-564-6745
                        sarahf.richardson@ky.gov
                                www.ovr.ky.gov

Sarah Richardson, SILC Liaison
We recognize and respect the contributions of all individuals as a necessary and vital part of a productive society..

Louisiana

4228 New Horizons: Central Louisiana
Ste 18
2406 Ferrand St
Monroe, LA 71201-3236   318-323-4374
                                     800-428-5505
                                Fax: 318-323-5445
                                    nhilc@nhilc.org
                                    www.nhilc.org

Alan Loosley, President
Sharon Geddes, Vice-President
Clint Snell, Vice-President for Finance
Mary Russell, Secretary

A private, non-profit, non-residential, consumer-controlled, community-based organization that enables people with disabilities to live independently.

4229 New Horizons: Northeast Louisiana
3717 Government Street
Suite 7
Alexandria, LA 71301-4037   318-484-3596
                                     888-361-3596
                                Fax: 318-484-3640
                                    nhilc@nhilc.org
                                    www.nhilc.org

Alan Loosley, President
Sharon Geddes, Vice-President
Clint Snell, Vice-President for Finance
Mary Russell, Secretary
A private, non-profit, non-residential, consumer controlled, community based organization that enables people with disabilities to live independently.

4230 New Horizons: Northwest Louisiana
1111A Hawn Avenue
Shreveport, LA 71106-6144   318-671-8131
                                     877-219-7327
                                Fax: 318-688-7823
                                    nhilc@nhilc.org
                                    www.nhilc.org

Alan Loosley, President
Sharon Geddes, Vice-President
Clint Snell, Vice-President for Finance
Mary Russell, Secretary
A private, non-profit, non-residential, consumer-controlled, community based organization that enables people with disabilities to live independently.

4231 Resources for Independent Living: Baton Rouge
New Orleans Resources for Independent Living
3233 South Sherwood Forest Blvd.
Suite 101A
Baton Rouge, LA 70816   225-753-4772
                                     877-505-2260
                                Fax: 225-753-4831
                                    contact@noril.org
                                    www.noril.org

Yavonka G. Archaga, Executive Director
Alisha S. Hammond, Assistant Director
Rosie Calvin, Program Manager
Deonne T. Bailey, Core Service Manager
RIL provides quality services to individuals with disabilities to assist with living independent. RIL also offers services to inculde information and referral, advocacy, peer support and independent living skills training.

4232 Resources for Independent Living: Metairie
2001 21st Street Kenner
Kenner, LA 70062   504-522-1955
                                     877-505-2260
                                Fax: 504-522-1954
                                    www.noril.org

Yavonka G. Archaga, Executive Director
Alisha S. Hammond, Assistant Director
Rosie Calvin, Program Manager
Deonne T. Bailey, Core Service Manager
RIL provides quality services to individuals with disabilities to assist with living independently. RIL also offers an array of services to include information and referral, advocacy, peer support and independent living skills training.

4233 Southwest Louisiana Independence Center: Lake Charles
2016 Oak Park Boulevard
Lake Charles, LA 70601-5391   337-477-7198
                                     888-403-1062
                                Fax: 337-477-7198
                                 TTY: 337-477-7198
                                    www.slic-la.org

4234 Southwest Louisians Independence Center: Lafayette
850 Kaliste Saloom Rd
Suite 118
Lafayette, LA 70508-4230   337-269-0027
                                                   888-516-5009
                                             Fax: 337-233-7660
                                                   www.slic-la.org

4235 Volunteers of America of Greater New Orleans
4152 Canal St.
New Orleans, LA 70119   504-482-2130
                                             Fax: 504-482-1922
                                                   voagno.org
Robert C. Rhoden, Chair
Wayne M. Baquet, Chair Elect
James M. Le Blanc, President/CEO
Geoffrey C. Artigues, Treasurer
Volunteers of America Greater New Orleans offers many services
that aim to improve the lives of children, youth, and families.

4236 W Troy Cole Independent Living Specialist
Ste H
1900 Lamy Ln
Monroe, LA 71201-9200   318-323-4374
Katherine Carnell, Manager

Maine

4237 Alpha One: Bangar
3300 Ponce de Leon Blvd.
Coral Gables, FL 33134   305-567-9888
                                                   877-228-7321
                                             Fax: 305-567-1317
                                             info@alpha-1foundation.org
                                                   www.alpha1.org
John W. Walsh, President & CEO, Co-founder
Marcia F. Ritchie, Vice President/ COO
Marsha A. Carnes, Director of Program Evaluation
Robert Campbell, Communications Manager
Committed to being a leading enterprise providing the community with information, services and products that create opportunities for people with disabilities to live independently. Provides
many services including adaptive and mobility equipment selection, peer support, advocacy, information and referral services,
adapted drive evaluation and training, and consumer directed
personal assistance.

4238 Alpha One: South Portland
127 Main St
South Portland, ME 04106-2647   207-767-2189
                                                   800-640-7200
                                             Fax: 207-799-8346
                                             TTY: 207-767-5387
                                                   www.alphaonenow.com
Dennis Stubbs, Chairman
Bob McPhee, Vice-Chairman
Darlene Stewart, Independent Living Specialist
Ketra S Crosson, Aroostook County Coordinator
Committed to being a leading enterprise providing the community with information, services and products that create opportunities for people with disabilities to live independently. Offers
adaptive equipment loan program, independent living skills instruction, adapted driver evaluation and training, information
and referral services, peer support, advocacy, access design
consultation, and more.

4239 Motivational Services
71 Hospital Street
P.O.Box 229
Augusta, ME 04332-0229   207-626-3465
                                             Fax: 207-626-3469
                                             TTY:207-621-2542
                                                   www.mocomaine.com
Connie Dunn, President
Grace Leonard, Vice President/Secretary
Faith Madore, Treasurer
Richard Weiss, Executive Director
Improving the lives of people with disabilities through housing,
employment and community support.

4240 Shalom House
106 Gilman St
Portland, ME 04102-3034   207-874-1080
                                             Fax: 207-874-1077
                                             TTY:207-842-6888
                                             generalmail@shalomhouseinc.org
                                                   shalomhouseinc.org
Megan Lewis, Human Resources Manager
Mary Haynes-Rodgers, Executive Director
Kristine Lausier, Quality Assurance Administrator
Jane Collette, Accounting Manager
Offers hope for adults living with severe mental illness by provid-
ing a choice of quality housing and support services that help peo-
ple lead stable and fulfilling lives in the community.

Maryland

4241 Broadmead
13801 York Rd
Cockeysville, MD 21030-1899   410-527-1900
                                                   877-STA-HOME
                                                   www.broadmead.org
Ann H. Heaton, Chair
John E. Howl, Chief Executive Officer
Patricia Gordon, Chief Financial Officer/Treasure
Douglas Bareis, Director of Support Services
To provide continuing care services to a diverse group of seniors
in a warm, congenial community founded and operated in the
spirit of the Religious Society of Friends.

4242 Eastern Shore Center for Independent Living
309 Sunburst Highway
Suite 13
Cambridge, MD 21613-2050   410-221-7701
                                                   800-705-7944
                                             Fax: 410-221-7714
                                             TTY: 410-221-4150
                                                   www.autismspeaks.org
Liz Feld, President
Alec M. Elbert, Chief Strategy & Dev Officer
Jamitha Fields, VP, Community Affairs
Lisa Goring, EVP, Programs and Services
ESCIL provides services to people with all disabilities regardless
of age, religion, gender, ethnicity, race or national origin. In addition to the core services of information and referral, skills training, peer support and advocacy, ESCIL also offers assistance with
accessibility modifications, Americans with Disabilities Act education and training, housing referrals and counseling, transportation referral and information, Brailling capabilities, Personal
Attendent Services referral, and more.

4243 Freedom Center
14 W. Patrick Street
Suite 10
Frederick, MD 21701   301-846-7811
                                             Fax: 301-846-9070
                                             advocate@thefreedomcenter-md.org
                                                   thefreedomcenter-md.org
Jamey George, Executive Director
Russell Holt, President
Patrick Mcmurtray, Vice-President
Craig Shafer, Treasurer

A walk in center for independent living, provides services and supports to empower individuals with disabilities to lead self-directed, independent, and productive lives in a barrier-free community.

4244 Housing Unlimited
Ste G1
1398 Lamberton Dr
Silver Spring, MD 20902-3435 301-592-9314
Fax: 301-592-9318
information@housingunlimited.org
www.housingunlimited.org
Nancy Cohen, President Emerita
Russell Phillips, President
Robyn S. Raysor, Vice President
Johnnie Mae Armstrong, Treasurer
To address the housing crisis for adults with psychiatric disabilities who reside in Montgomery County, Maryland.

4245 Independence Now
Ste 101
12301 Old Columbia Pike
Silver Spring, MD 20904-1656 301-277-2839
Fax: 301-625-9777
info@innow.org
innow.org
Sarah Sorensen, Executive Director
Trish Foley, Director of Community Services
Todd Thorpe, Director of Operations
Robert Watson, President
A nonprofit organization created by people with disabilities and provides services that promote independence and the inclusion of people with disabilities in their communities.

4246 Independence Now: The Center for Independent Living
12301 Old Columbia Pike
Suite 101
Silver Spring, MD 20904 301-277-2839
Fax: 301-625-9777
info@innow.org
innow.org
Robert Watson, President
Sarah Sorensen, Executive Director
Todd Thorpe, Operations & IT Manager
Denise Sosbe, Employment Services Coordinator
A nonprofit organization created by people with disabilities to provide services that promote independence and the inclusion of people with disabilities within their communities. Some of their services include employment support, nursing home outreach, assistive technology and a youth leadership forum.

4247 Making Choices for Independent Living
Ste 202
1118 Light St
Baltimore, MD 21230-4152 410-234-8195
888-560-2221
andreab@mcil-md.org
www.mcil-md.org
Jimmie Joku Cooper, Owner
Provides services to help empower people with disabilities to lead self-directed, independent and productive lives in the community and protect their civil rights.OUTOF ORDER.

4248 Resources for Independence
30 N. Mechanic Street
Unit B
Cumberland, MD 21502-2705 301-784-1774
800-371-1986
Fax: 301-784-1776
www.rficil.org
Lori Magruder, Executive Director
John Michaels, Assistant Director
Robert Cannon, Benefits Counselor
Sherry Williams, Finance Director
Private, non-profit, consumer-controlled, community-based organization providing services and advocacy by and for persons with all type of disabilities. Their goal is to create opportunities for independence, and to assist individuals with disabilities to

achieve their maximum level of independent functioning within their families and communities.

4249 Southern Maryland Center for LIFE
P.O.Box 657
Charlotte Hall, MD 20622-657 301-884-4498
Fax: 301-884-6099
www.somd.com
Marie Robinson, Executive Director
Carrie Lanthier, Administrative Assistant
A non-profit community based organization which provides services to disabled people who live or work in the tri-county area. Our mission is to empower people with disabilities to lead self-directed, independent, and productive lives in their community.

Massachusetts

4250 Adlib
215 North St
Pittsfield, MA 01201-4644 413-442-7047
800-232-7047
Fax: 413-443-4338
adlib@adlibcil.org
adlibcil.org
Linda Febles, President
Michael Hinkley, Vice President
Allison Bedard, Treasurer
Shannon Miller, Secretary/Clerk
Offers information and referral services, independent living skills training, peer counseling, individual and group advocacy services available to all people with disabilities. Access consultation provided to businesses, agencies and institutions in accordance to the Americans with Disabilities Act.

4251 Arc of Cape Cod
P.O.Box 428
171 Main Street
Hyannis, MA 02601-428 508-790-3667
Fax: 508-775-5233
info@arcofcapecod.org
www.arcofcapecod.org

4252 Boston Center for Independent Living
5th Floor
60 Temple Place
Boston, MA 02111-1324 617-338-6665
Fax: 617-338-6661
TTY:617-338-6662
info@bostoncil.org
www.bostoncil.org
Sergio Goncalves, Chairman
Linda Landry, Vice Chairman
Stacey Zelbow, Treasurer
Bill Henning, Executive Director
A frontline civil rights organization led by people with disabilities that advocates to eliminate discrimination, isolation and segregation by providing advocacy, information and referral, peer support, skills training, and PCA services in order to enhance the independence of people with disabilities.

4253 Cape Organization for Rights of the Disabled (CORD)
106 Bassett Lane
Hyannis, MA 2601 508-775-8300
800-541-0282
Fax: 508-775-7022
TTY: 800-541-0282
cordinfo@cilcapecod.org
www.cilcapecod.org
Coreen Brinkerhoff, Executive Director
The Cape Organization for the Rights of the Disabled (CORD) has been aggresively working since 1984 to advance the independence, productivity, and integration of people with disabilities into mainstream society. CORD is the Center for Independent Living (CIL) and is a member of the Aging and Disability Resources Consortium (ADRC) servinf Cape Cod and the Islands.

4254   Center for Living & Working: Fitchburg
76 Summer Street
Suite 110
Fitchburg, MA   01420-5785   978-345-1568
                                        TTY:978-345-1568
                                    centerlwA@centerlw.org
                                           www.centerlw.org

Cindy Purcell, Board President
Mary Ann Donovan, Treasurer
Ed Roth, Secretary
Jim O'Day, Advisor to CLW Board of Director
The Center for Living and Working is a non-profit Independent Living Center which takes its direction from persons with disabilities. The Center advocates to empower persons with disabilities to take active roles in their lives and in their community in which they live. Also provides comprehensive and innovative programs and services in order to maximize individual independence and opportunities.

4255   Center for Living & Working: Framingham
484 Main St
Suite 345
Worcester, MA   01608-1824   508-798-0350
                                        Fax: 508-797-4015
                                        TTY:508-755-1003
                                    opsearch@centerlw.org
                                           www.centerlw.org

Cindy Purcell, Board President
Mary Ann Donovan, Treasurer
Ed Roth, Secretary
Jim O'Day, Advisor to CLW Board of Director
The Center for Living and Working is a non-profit Independent Living Center which takes its direction from persons with disabilities. The Center advocates to empower persons with disabilities to take active roles in their lives and in their community in which they live. Also provides comprehensive and innovative programs and services in order to maximize individual independence and opportunities.

4256   Center for Living & Working: Worcester
484 Main St
Suite 345
Worcester, MA   01608-1824   508-798-0350
                                        Fax: 508-797-4015
                                        TTY:508-755-1003
                                    opsearch@centerlw.org
                                           www.centerlw.org

Cindy Purcell, Board President
Mary Ann Donovan, Treasurer
Ed Roth, Clerk/Secretary
Jim O'Day, Advisor to CLW Board of Director
The Center for Living and Working is a non-profit Independent Living Center which takes its direction from persons with disabilities. The Center advocates to empower persons with disabilities to take active roles in their lives and in their community in which they live. Also provides comprehensive and innovative programs and services in order to maximize individual independence and opportunities.

4257   Developmental Evaluation and Adjustment Facilities
215 Brighton Ave
Allston, MA   02134-2013   617-254-4041
                                           800-886-5195
                                        Fax: 617-254-7091
                                    info@deafinconline.org
                                        deafinconline.org

Sharon L. Applegate, Executive Director
Kelly Kim, President
John Sullivan, Treasurer
Kendra Timko-Hochkeppel, Vice President
Encourages and empowers deaf, hard of hearing, deafblind and late-deafened individuals to lead independent and productive lives.

4258   Independence Associates
100 Laurel Street
1st Suite 122
East Bridgewater, MA 02301-4012   508-583-2166
                                           800-649-5568
                                        Fax: 508-583-2165
                                           info@iacil.org
                                               iacil.org

Mark Lewis, President
James Clark, Treasurer
Anita Ashdon, Secretary
Steven Higgins, Executive Director
Provides comprehensive services which will enhance the range of acceptable options available to the consumer and improve the quality of life of persons with disabilities; to work on behalf of the objective of the disablility rights and independent living movement.

4259   Independent Living Center of Stavros: Greenfield
55 Federal St
Greenfield, MA   01301-2546   413-774-3001
                                           www.stavros.org

Glenn Hartmann, President
Nancy Bazanchuk, Vice President
Donna M. Bliznak, Treasurer
Greta Biagi, Clerk
Promoting independence and access in the communities for persons with disabilities and deaf people.

4260   Independent Living Center of Stavros: Springfield
210 Old Farm Road
Amherst, MA   01002-2704   413-256-0473
                                           800-804-1899
                                        Fax: 413-256-0190
                                           www.stavros.org

Glenn Hartmann, President
Nancy Bazanchuk, Vice President
Donna M. Bliznak, Treasurer
James Kruidenier, Executive Director
Promoting independence and access in the communities for persons with disabilities and deaf people.

4261   Independent Living Center of the North Shore & Cape Ann
27 Congress St
Suite 107
Salem, MA   01970-5577   978-741-0077
                                           888-751-0077
                                        Fax: 978-741-1133
                                    information@ilcnsca.org
                                           ilcnsca.org

Mary Margaret Moore, Executive Director
Marion A Dawicki, President
Patricia Cox, Vice President
Joe Karaman, Treasurer
A service and advocacy center run by and for people with disabilities that supports the struggle of people who have all types of disabilities to live independently and participate fully in community life.

4262   MetroWest Center for Independent Living
280 Irving Street
Framingham, MA   01702-7306   508-875-7853
                                        Fax: 508-875-8359
                                        TTY:508-875-7853
                                           info@mwcil.org
                                               mwcil.org

Youcef J. Bellil, President
Michael Kennedy, Vice President
Edward J. Carr, Treasurer
Penny Kelley, Secretary
To help individuals with disabilities become productive and contributing members of the community and to eliminate barriers within the community that impede this process.

4263   Multi-Cultural Independent Living Center of Boston
329 Centre Street
Jamaica Plain, MA   02130-1232   617-942-8060
                                         Fax: 617-942-8630
                                         TTY:617-288-2707
                                         info@milcb.org
                                         milcb.org

Derrick Dominique, Executive Director
Ana Ortiz, Director of Services
Eleanor Slaughter, Senior IL Advocate
Louise Beach, Community Outreach Coordinator
Seeks to create opportunities for people with disabilities and
their families in unserved/under-served populations and cultures
who reside in Boston's inner city.

4264   Northeast Independent Living Program
20 Ballard Rd
Lawrence, MA   01843-1018   978-687-4288
                                         Fax: 978-689-4488
                                         TTY:978-687-4288
                                         help@nilp.org
                                         nilp.org

June Cowen, Executive Director
Nanette Goodwin, Assistant Director
Lisa DiGiuseppe, Director of Finance
Jim Lyons, Director, Community Development
A consumer controlled Independent Living Center providing Ad-
vocacy and Services to people with all disabilities in the greater
Merrimack Valley who wish to live as independently as possible
in the comunity.

4265   Renaissance Clubhouse
176 Walker St
2nd Floor
Lowell, MA   01854-3126   978-454-7944
                                         Fax: 978-937-7867
                                         renclub1@gmail.com
                                         www.renclublowell.org

Elaine Walker, Executive Director
Pammy Sadoie, Assistant Director
Offers daily structure, assistance wtih jobs, retirement, and hous-
ing.

4266   Southeast Center for Independent Living
66 Troy Street
Suite 3
Fall River, MA   02720-3023   508-679-9210
                                         Fax: 508-677-2377
                                         TTY:508-679-9210
                                         scil@secil.org
                                         secil.org

Lisa M Pitta, Executive Director
Damase Cote, President
Paul Remy, Vice President
Debbie Pacheco, Treasurer / Secretary
The Philosophy of Independent Living, maintains that individuals with disabilities have the right to choose services and make
decisions for themselves. This belief is the foundation and guiding principle of all of SCIL's policies and operations. SCIL provides training, information and support to help consumers
achieve individual goals, experience personal growth and
participate fully in community life.

4267   Student Independent Living Experience Massachusetts
Hospital School
560 Harrison Avenue
Suite 600
Boston, MA   02118-2447   617-338-6409
                                         800-843-5879
                                         TTY:800-328-3202
                                         www.mass.gov

4268   Ann Arbor Center for Independent Living
3941 Research Park Drive
Ann Arbor, MI   48108-6852   734-971-0277
                                         Fax: 734-971-0826
                                         www.annarborcil.org

Carolyn Grawi, Executive Director
Chris Baty, Theater Coordinator
Bryan Wilkinson, Director of Operations and Sales
Shirley Coombs, Chief Financial Officer
AACIL assists people with disabilities and their families in living
full and productive lives. AACIL assures the equality of opportu-
nity, full participation, independent living and economic
self-sufficiency of people with disabilities in the community.

4269   Arc Michigan
1325 S Washington Ave
Lansing, MI   48910-1652   517-487-5426
                                         800-292-7851
                                         Fax: 517-487-0303
                                         dhoyle@arcmi.org
                                         arcmi.org

Donald Teegarden, President
Laurel Robb, Vice President
Dohn Hoyle, Executive Director
Sherri Boyd, Associate Director
Exists to empower local chapters of The ARC to assure that citi-
zens with developmental disabilities are valued and that they and
their families can participate fully in and contribute to the life of
their community.

4270   Arc/Muskegon
601 Terrace Street
Suite 101
Muskegon, MI   49440-2197   231-777-2006
                                         Fax: 231-777-3507
                                         info@arcmuskegon.org
                                         www.arcmuskegon.org

Tim Michalski, President
Brenda McCarthy Wiener, Vice President
Margaret O'Toole, Executive Director
Janis Milliron, Administrative Assistant
Offers information and referral, advocacy services and peer
counseling.

4271   Bad Axe: Blue Water Center for Independent Living
614 N Port Crescent Street
P.O. Box 29
Bad Axe, MI 48413-1207   989-269-5421
                                         810-987-9337
                                         Fax: 989-269-5422
                                         info@bwcil.org
                                         www.bwcil.org

Karen Massaro-Mundt, President
Chuck Wanninger, Treasurer
Jim Whalen, Executive Director
Bill Farris, Administrative Assistant
A non-profit, consumer-based organization that advocates,
informs and supports persons with disabilities in the community.

4272   Bay Area Coalition for Independent Living
Ste 17
701 S Elmwood Ave
Traverse City, MI   49684-3185   231-929-4865
                                         Fax: 231-929-4896
                                         steve@bacil.org

Steve Wade, Director

4273   Capital Area Center for Independent Living
2812 N. Martin Luther King Jr. Blvd
Lansing, MI   48906
517-999-2760
877-652-3777
Fax: 517-999-2767
TTY: 800-649-3777
www.cacil.org

Mark Pierce, Executive Director
Jeffrey Gass, Financial Manager
Justine Bond, Independent Living Specialist
Jean Harris, Program Coordinator
CACIL provide training, mentoring, and referrals to help people with disabilities and their families live productive lives.

4274   Caro: Blue Water Center for Independent Living
1184 Cleaver Rd
Caro, MI   48723-1143
989-673-3678
810-987-9337
Fax: 989-673-3656
info@bwcil.org
www.bwcil.org

Karen Massaro-Mundt, President
Chuck Wanninger, Treasurer
Jim Whalen, Executive Director
Bill Farris, Administrative Assistant
A non-profit, consumer-based organization that advocates, informs and supports persons with disabilities in the community.

4275   Center for Independent Living of Mid-Michigan
3941 Research Park Drive
Ann Arbor, MI   48108-6832
734-971-0277
Fax: 734-971-0826
www.annarborcil.org
Carolyn Grawi, Executive Director
Chris Baty, Theater Coordinator
Bryan Wilkinson, Director of Operations and Sales
Shirley Coombs, Chief Financial Officer
Comprised of over 51 percent of people with disabilities, and advocates for the rights of people with disabilities in the Mid-Michigan area. Call for information on disability issues or for assistance in obtaining services, within your community..

4276   Community Connections of Southwest Michigan
5671 N. Skeel Ave.
Suite 8
Oscoda, MI   48750
989-569-6001
800-578-4245
Fax: 269-925-7141
Kathy Ellis, Director
An advocacy organization that teaches and empowers people with disabilities to make choices about living life to the fullest, controlling and directing their own lives and asserting their rights and responsibilites within their Berrien County communities..

4277   Cristo Rey Handicappers Program
1717 N High St
Lansing, MI   48906-4529
517-372-4700
Fax: 517-372-8499
info@cristo-rey.org
www.cristo-rey.org
Marlene M Berens, Manager
To care for the spiritual and social needs of individuals and families by offering services that encourage self-sufficiency and recognize the dignity of the human person..

4278   Detroit Center for Independent Living
1042 Griswold
Suite 2
Port Huron, MI   48060
810-987-9337
810-987-9337
Fax: 810-987-9548
info@bwcil.org
www.bwcil.org

Karen Massaro-Mundt, President
Chuck Wanninger, Treasurer
Jim Whalen, Executive Director
Bill Farris, Administrative Assistant

BWCIL is a consumer-based organization designed to serve persons with disabilities who have physical, psychiatric, sendory, cognitive, and multiple disabilities through the provision of advocacy, information and referral, service provision, and the promotion of needed services so to maximize the individual's optimal level of independence.

4279   Disability Advocates of Kent County
3600 Camelot Drive SE
Grand Rapids, MI   49546-8103
616-949-1100
Fax: 616-949-7865
contact@dakc.us
disabilityadvocates.us

David Bulkowski, JD, Executive Director
Denise Borges, Employment Specialist
Jackson Botsford, Accessibility Specialist
Katie Foreman, Independent Living Specialist
Exists to advocate, assist, educate and inform on independent living options for persons with disabilities and to create a barrier-free society for all.

4280   Disability Connection
27 E. Clay Avenue
Muskegon, MI   49442
231-722-0088
866-322-4501
Fax: 231-722-0066
dcilmi.org

John Wahlberg, President
Michael Hamm, Vice President
Tamera Collier, Executive Director
Tom Munn, Associate Director
To advocate, educate, empower, and provide resources for persons with disabilities and promote accessible communities.

4281   Disability Network Southwest Michigan
517 E Crosstown Pkwy
Kalamazoo, MI   49001-2867
269-345-1516
Fax: 269-345-0229
info@dnswm.org
www.dnswm.org

Cameron J. Lambe, Chair
Cheri Stoltzner, Vice Chair
Joel W Cooper, President
Kevin Klute, Treasurer
To educate and empower people with disabilities to create change intheir own lives, and to advocate for social change to create inclusive communities. As a center for independent living, they are part of the disability rights movement.

4282   Disability Network of Mid-Michigan
1705 S. Saginaw Road
Midland, MI   48640-6825
989-835-4041
800-782-4160
Fax: 989-835-8121
dnmm.org

Tom Provoast, President
Dr. Barbara Gibson, Vice President
David Emmel, Executive Director
Steven Locke, Associate Director
To promote and encourage independence for all people with disabilities.

4283   Disability Network of Oakland & Macomb
16645 15 Mile Rd
Clinton Township, MI   48035-2206
586-268-4160
800-284-2457
Fax: 586-285-9942
info@dnom.org
dnom.org

Andrew Maurer, Chairperson
Randy Charon, Vice Chairperson
Kellie Boyd, Executive Director
Kelly Winn, Director of Operations
Commited to advancing personal choice, independence, and positive social change for persons with disabilities through advocacy, education and outreach.

4284 Disability Network/Lakeshore
426 Century Lane
Holland, MI 49423-2200   616-396-5326
                                            800-656-5245
                                       Fax: 616-396-3220
                                       TTY: 616-396-5326
                                       info@dnlakeshore.org
                                       dnlakeshore.org

Michelle Chaney, President
Amber Marcy, Vice President
Brian Dykhuis, Treasurer
Todd Whiteman, Executive Director
A cross-disability, community-based organization providing advocacy, education, and information and referral to persons with disabilities in Ottawa and Allegan counties.

4285 Grand Traverse Area Community Living Management Corporation
935 Barlow St
Traverse City, MI 49686-4250   231-932-9030
                                       www.gtaclmc.org

Mary Jean Brick, Administrative Director
We are a training home for individuals with developmental disabilities over the age of 18

4286 Great Lakes/Macomb Rehabilitation Group
Apt 104
4 E Alexandrine St
Detroit, MI 48201-2032   313-832-3371
                                       Fax: 313-832-3850

Jeannie Meece-Brooks, Contact
Independent living center. .

4287 JARC
30301 Northwestern Hwy
Suite 100
Farmington Hills, MI 48334-3277   248-538-6611
                                            877-767-7781
                                       Fax: 248-538-6615
                                       jarc@jarc.org
                                       jarc.org

Ronald Applebaum, President
Richard A. Loewenstein, Chief Executive Officer
Randy P. Baxter, Chief Financial Officer
Rena Friedberg, CFRE, Chief Development Officer
A nonprofit, nonsecretarian agency dedicated to enabling people with disabilities to live full, dignified lives in the community, and to providing support and advocacy for their families.

4288 Lapeer: Blue Water Center for Independent Living
392 West Nepessing Street
Lapeer, MI 48446-2192   810-664-9098
                                            810-987-9337
                                       Fax: 810-664-0937
                                       info@bwcil.org
                                       www.bwcil.org

Karen Massaro-Mundt, President
Chuck Wanninger, Treasurer
Jim Whalen, Executive Director
Bill Farris, Administrative Assistant
A non-profit, consumer-based organization that advocates, informs and supports persons with disabilities in the community.

4289 Livingston Center for Independent Living
3075 E Grand River Ave
Suite 108
Howell, MI 48843-6585   517-545-1741
                                       Fax: 517-548-1751
                                       www.virtualcil.net

Dan Durci, Director
Independent living skills training and empowerment training for persons with disabilities..

4290 Michigan Commission for the Blind: Independent Living Rehabilitation Program
235 S. Grand Ave.
P.O. Box 30037
Lansing, MI 48909-1254   989-758-1765
                                            800-292-4200
                                       Fax: 989-758-1405
                                       www.michigan.gov

Debbie Wilson, Manager
Patrick Cannon, Agency Director
Rehabilitation teaching, independent living skills for persons over 55 with severe vision loss.

4291 Michigan Commission for the Blind: Detroit
Ste 4-450
3038 W Grand Blvd
Detroit, MI 48202-6012   313-456-1646
                                       Fax: 313-456-1645
                                       mcnealg@michigan.gov

Gwen McNeal, Supervisor
Shawnese Laury-Johnson, Assistant East Region Manager
Promotes the inclusion of people with legal blindness into our communities on a full and equal basis through empowerment, education, participation, and choice..

4292 Monroe Center for Independent Living
1285 N Telegraph Rd
Monroe, MI 48162-3368   734-242-5919
                                       mrawlings@aacil.org
                                       monroecil.tripod.com

Linda Maier, Manager
To act as a catalyst for personal and social change through the empowerment of people with disabilities; and, to replace the perception of disability as tragic with a disability culture promoting pride, power and personal style.

4293 Port Huron: Blue Water Center for Independent Living
1042 Griswold St
Suite 2
Port Huron, MI 48060-5431   810-987-9337
                                            810-987-9337
                                       Fax: 810-987-9548
                                       info@bwcil.org
                                       bwcil.org

Karen Massaro-Mundt, President
Chuck Wanninger, Treasurer
Jim Whalen, Executive Director
Bill Farris, Administrative Assistant
A non-profit, consumer-based organization that advocates, informs and supports persons with disabilities in the community.

4294 Sandusky: Blue Water Center for Independent Living
103 East Sanilac Road
Suite 3
Sandusky, MI 48471-1615   810-648-2555
                                            810-987-9337
                                       Fax: 810-648-2583
                                       info@bwcil.org
                                       www.bwcil.org

Karen Massaro-Mundt, President
Chuck Wanninger, Treasurer
Jim Whalen, Executive Director
Bill Farris, Administrative Assistant
A non-profit, consumer-based organization that advocates, informs and supports persons with disabilities in the community.

4295 Southeastern Michigan Commission for the Blind
4450 Grandy St
Detroit, MI 48207   313-456-0334
                                            877-932-6424
                                       Fax: 313-456-1645
                                       www.michigan.gov

Patrick Cannon, Executive Director
Pat Bragg, Manager
Vocational rehabilitation agency. Personal adjustment vocational assessment and training, job placement and follow-up services. .

4296 Superior Alliance for Independent Living(SAIL)
1200 Wright Street
Suite A
Marquette, MI   49855

906-228-5744
800-379-7245
Fax: 906-228-5573
TTY: 906-228-5744
www.upsail.com

Elgie Dow, President
Aaron Andres, Vice President
Amy Maes, Executive Director
Judy Vivian, Finance Director
Promotes the inclusion of people with disabilities into our communities on a full and equal basis through empowerment, education, participation and choice.

4297 disAbility Connections
409 Linden Ave
Jackson, MI   49203-4065

517-782-6054
Fax: 517-782-3118
www.disabilityconnect.org

Michael Jackson, President
James Gorse, Vice President
Lesia Pikaart, Executive Director
Joann Lucas, Associate Director
Supporting Jackson County residents in their efforts to lead independent, fulfilling, productive lives.

Minnesota

4298 Accessible Space, Inc.
2550 University Avenue West
Suite 330N
Saint Paul, MN 55114-1085

651-645-7271
800-466-7722
Fax: 651-645-0541
TTY: 800-627-3529
info@accessiblespace.org
www.accessiblespace.org

Mark E. Hamel, Esq., Chairman
Kay Knutson, Vice Chairman
Steve Schugel, Treasurer
John W. Adams, Secretary
Accessible, rent-subsidized apartments for very low-income adults with qualifying physical disabilities as well as seniors. Accessible Space, Inc., sponsors, develops and manages housing & ASI apartments are rent based on income and are located across the country.

4299 Accessnorth CIL of Northeastern MN: Aitkin
1309 East 40th Street
Hibbing, MN   55746-1821

218-262-6675
800-390-3681
Fax: 218-262-6677
TTY: 218-262-6675
info@accessnorth.net
www.accessnorth.net

Mary Ribich, Chair
David Hohl, Vice-Chair
Donald Brunette, Executive Director
Cathy Baudeck, Program Manager
Assists individuals to live independently, pursue meaningful goals, and have equal opportunities and choices.

4300 Accessnorth CIL of Northeastern MN: Duluth
118 East Superior Street
Duluth, MN   55802-2155

218-625-1400
888-625-1401
Fax: 218-625-1401
info@accessnorth.net
www.accessnorth.net

Mary Ribich, Chair
David Hohl, Vice-Chair
Donald Brunette, Executive Director
Cathy Baudeck, Program Manager
Assisting individuals with disabilities to live independently, puruse meaningful goals, and have equal opportunities and choices.

4301 Center for Independent Living of NE Minnesota
1309 East 40th Street
Hibbing, MN   55746-1821

218-262-6675
800-390-3681
Fax: 218-262-6677
TTY: 218-262-6675
info@accessnorth.net
accessnorth.net

Mary Ribich, Chair
David Hohl, Vice-Chair
Donald Brunette, Executive Director
Cathy Baudeck, Program Manager
Assisting individuals with disabilities to live independently, pursue meaningful goals, and have an equal opportunities and choices

4302 Courage Center
800 E. 28th St.
Minneapolis, MN   55407-4298

612-863-4200
866-880-3550
Fax: 763-520-0577
TTY: 763-520-0245
couragekenny@allina.com
www.allinahealth.org

Jan Malcolm, CEO
Alice Johnson, Chief Financial Officer
Stephen Bariteau, Chief Development Officer
Pamela J. Lindemoen, Executive Vice President of Oper
A nonprofit rehabilitation and resource center that advances the lives of children and adults experiencing barriers to health and independence. Specialize in treating brain injury, spinal cord injury, stroke, chronic pain, autism and disabilities experienced since birth.

4303 Freedom Resource Center for Independent Living: Fergus Falls
125 W Lincoln Avenue
Suite 7
Fergus Falls, MN   56537-2152

218-998-1799
800-450-0459
Fax: 218-998-1798
freedom@freedomrc.org
www.freedomrc.org

Nate Aalgaard, Executive Director
Angie Bosch, Office Coordinator
Mark Mark Bourdon Bourdon, Program Director
Andrea Nelson, Independent Living Advocate
Freedom Resource Center assists people in working towards goals they establish for themselves.

4304 Metropolitan Center for Independent Living
Ste 16
1600 University Ave W
Saint Paul, MN   55104-3825

651-646-8342
Fax: 651-603-2006
TTY:651-603-2001
homeramps@gmail.com

4305 Minnesota Association of Centers for Independent Living
215 North Benton Drive
Sauk Rapids, MN   56379

320-529-9000
888-529-0743
Fax: 320-529-0747
ilicil@independentlifestyles.org
independentlifestyles.org

Cara Ruff, Executive Director
Jay Keller, Board Chairman
Pamela Kotzenmacher, Treasurer
Autumn Gould, Attorney
A non-profit organization whose purpose is to advocate for the independent living needs of people with disabilities who are citizens of the State of Minnesota

4306 OPTIONS
Ste B
123 S Main St
Crookston, MN 56716-1970   218-281-5722
                                    Fax: 218-281-5722
                                    TTY:218-281-5722
                                    options3@rrv.net

Gordie Haug, Manager
Provides people with disabilities advocacy, information, skills training and peer mentoring relationships to help them achieve their personal goals of how and where they live their lives.

4307 Options Interstate Resource Center for Independent Living
2200 2nd Street SW
Rochester, MN 55902-1887   507-285-1815
                                    800-726-3692
                                    Fax: 218-773-7119
                                    TTY: 218-773-6100
                                    options@myoptions.info
                                    www.macil.org

Vicki Dalle Molle, President
Randy Sorensen, Executive Director
Located in Minnesota, but also serves North Dakota..

4308 Perry River Home Care
330 High Way Pen S
Saint Cloud, MN 56304   320-255-1882
                                    Fax: 320-255-5137

Berna Florentine, CEO
Ken Figge, President
Courtney Salzi, Administrator
Offers skilled nursing services RN, LPN, TV Therapy, Pediatrics, Rehabilitation Services, PT, OT, ST, Paraprofessional staff, Home Health Aides, Homemakers, Personal Care Attendents, Companions, Live-ins, Sleep overs, Respite care, Extended hours.

4309 SMILES
820 Winnebago Ave
Suite 1
Fairmont, MN 56031-3619   507-345-7139
                                    888-676-6498
                                    Fax: 507-235-3488
                                    www.smilescil.org

Brain Koch, President
Doug Robinson, Vice President
Alan Augustin, Executive Director
Helen Mitchell, Administrative Assistant
A nonprofit organization committed to providing a wide array of services that assist individuals with disabilities that live independently, pursue meaningful goals, and enjoy the same opportunities and choices as all persons.

4310 SMILES: Mankato
709 S. Front Street
Suite 7
Mankato, MN 56001-3887   507-345-7139
                                    888-676-6498
                                    Fax: 507-345-8429
                                    smiles@smilescil.org
                                    smilescil.org

Brain Koch, President
Doug Robinson, Vice President
Alan Augustin, Executive Director
Helen Mitchell, Administrative Assistant
A nonprofit organization committed to providing a wide array of services that assist individuals with disabilities that live independently, pursue meaningful goals, and enjoy the same oportunities and choices as all persons.

4311 Southeastern Minnesota Center for Independent Living: Red Wing
2200 2nd Street SW
Rochester, MN 55902   507-285-1815
                                   888-460-1815
                                   Fax: 507-288-8070
                                   semcil@semcil.org
                                   www.semcil.org

Brian Koch, President
Doug Robinson, Vice President
Alan Augustin, Executive Director
Helen Mitchell, Administrative Assistant
Non profit organization that assists people with disabilities to become independent and productive community members.

4312 Southeastern Minnesota Center for Independent Living: Rochester
2200 Second Street SW
Rochester, MN 55902-3980   507-285-1815
                                   888-460-1815
                                   Fax: 507-288-8070
                                   semcil@semcil.org
                                   www.semcil.org

Brain Koch, President
Doug Robinson, Vice President
Alan Augustin, Executive Director
Helen Mitchell, Administrative Assistant
A non profit organization that assists people with disabilities to become independent and productive community members.

4313 Southwestern Center for Independent Living
2864 S Nettleton Ave
Suite 700
Springfield, MO 65807   417-886-1188
                                   800-676-7245
                                   Fax: 417-886-3619
                                   TTY: 417-886-1188
                                   scil@swcil.org
                                   www.swcil.org

Randy Custer, Board President
Emilio Vela, CEO
Shannon Porter, Deputy Director
Lacee Thompson, Director of Operations
SWCIL is a private, non-profit community-based organization providing independent living services to assist people with disabilities in obtaining and maintaining the greatest control over their lives. Services are available in southwestern Minnesota to persons of all ages, with any disability. Services include community access, education & outreach, mental health counseling, youth services, transition services and more.

4314 Vinland Center Lake Independence
3675 Ihduhapi Road
Loretto, MN 55357-308   763-479-3555
                                   866-956-7612
                                   Fax: 763-479-2605
                                   vinland@vinlandcenter.org
                                   www.vinlandcenter.org

Gerald Seck, President
Mary Roehl, Executive Director
Colleen Larson, Operations Manager
Debbie Larson, Accounting Manager
A Minnesota based rehabilitation center which offers services in three distinct service areas: vocational rehabilitation; inclusive community programs; and for people with cognitive disabilities, specially adapted chemical dependency treatment.

Mississippi

4315 Alpha Home Royal Maid Association for the Blind
PO Drawer 30
Hazlehurst, MS 39083-30   601-894-1771
                                   Fax: 601-894-2993

Howard Becker, Director
Offers attendant care registry, information on accessible housing and referrals.

4316 Gulf Coast Independent Living Center
18 JM Tatum Industrial Drive
Hattiesburg, MS 39401-8341   601-544-4860
                                          Fax: 601-582-2544

Albert Holifield, Executive Director
Independent living center.

4317 Jackson Independent Living Center
1981 Hollywood Dr
Jackson, TN 38305-2131   731-668-2211
                                               800-848-0298
                                          Fax: 731-668-0406
                                          TTY: 601-351-1585
                                  information@jcil.tn.org
                                  www.j-cil.com/contact-us.html

Denea Smith, Director
Timothy Jackson
Provides services to consumers with severe disabilities.

4318 LIFE of Mississippi
1304 Vine St
Jackson, MS 39202-3429   601-969-4009
                                               800-748-9398
                                          Fax: 601-969-1662
                                          TTY: 800-748-9398
                                          www.lifeofms.com

Augusta Smith, Executive Director
Margie Moore, Project Coordinator
Densie Smith, Assistant
Christine Woodell, ADA Consultant
To empower people wit significant disabilities to be as independent and as fully involved in their communities as they can and want to be.

4319 LIFE of Mississippi: Biloxi
2030 Pass Road
Suite C
Biloxi, MS 39531   228-388-2401
                                          Fax: 228-338-2413
                                          www.lifeofms.com

Augusta Smith, Executive Director
Ruby Jackson, I.L. Specialist
Kim Allison, IL Specialist/ B2I
Christine Woodell, ADA Coordinator
To empower people with significant disabilities to be as independent and as fully involved in their communities as they can and want to be.

4320 LIFE of Mississippi: Greenwood
502a W Park Ave
Greenwood, MS 38930-2906   662-453-9940
                                          Fax: 662-453-9934
                                          www.lifeofms.com

Augusta Smith, Executive Director
Pam Wraggs, I.L. Specialist
Ruth Elliott, IL Specialist Assistant
Christine Woodell, ADA Consultant
To empower people with significant disabilities to be as independent and as fully involved in their communities as they can and want to be.

4321 LIFE of Mississippi: Hattiesburg
710 Katie Ave
Hattiesburg, MS 39401-4377   601-583-2108
                                          www.lifeofms.com

Augusta Smith, Executive Director
Margie Moore, Project Coordinator
Densie Smith, Assistant
Christine Woodell, ADA Consultant
To empower people with significant disabilities to be as independent and as fully involved in their communities as they can and want to be.

4322 LIFE of Mississippi: McComb
915-A S. Locust Street
McComb, MS 39648-4817   601-684-3079
                                          www.lifeofms.com

Augusta Smith, Executive Director
Margie Moore, Project Coordinator
Densie Smith, Assistant
Christine Woodell, ADA Consultant
To empower people with significant disabilities to be as independent and as fully involved in their communities as they can and want to be.

4323 LIFE of Mississippi: Meridian
Ste 103a
2440 N Hills St
Meridian, MS 39305-2653   601-485-7999
                                          www.lifeofms.com

Augusta Smith, Executive Director
Margie Moore, Project Coordinator
Densie Smith, Assistant
Christine Woodell, ADA Consultant
To empower people with significant disabilities to be as independent and as fully involved in their communities as they can and want to be.

4324 LIFE of Mississippi: Oxford
Ste 5
404 Galleria Dr
Oxford, MS 38655-4383   662-234-7010
                                          www.lifeofms.com

Augusta Smith, Executive Director
Margie Moore, Project Coordinator
Densie Smith, Assistant
Christine Woodell, ADA Consultant
To empower people with significant disabilities to be as independent and as fully involved in their communities as they can and want to be.

4325 LIFE of Mississippi: Tupelo
1051 Cliff Gookin Blvd
Tupelo, MS 38801-6739   662-844-6633
                                          Fax: 662-844-6803
                                          www.lifeofms.com

Emily Word, Regional Coordinator
Ronnie Jernigan, I.L. Specialist/HOT
Wayne Lauderdale, I.L. Specialist
Tara Christian, I.L. Specialist Assistant
To empower people with significant disabilities to be as independent and as fully involved in their communities as they can and want to be.

Missouri

4326 Access II Independent Living Center
101 Industrial Parkway
Gallatin, MO 64640-1280   660-663-2423
                                               888-663-2423
                                          Fax: 660-663-2517
                                          access@accessii.org
                                          www.accessii.org

Heather Swymeler, Executive Director
Brandy Gannan, Program Manager
Amber Wells, Financial Director
Dawn Ernat, In-Home Director
The mission of Access II is to remove architectural and attitudinal barriers that limit the independence of persons with disabilities, promote a positive change in attitudes about disability and persons with disabilities, and encourage greater independence for persons with disabilities within our communities. As a Center for Independent Living, Access II is comitted to the provision of a full range of independent living services.

4327 Bootheel Area Independent Living Services
PO Box 326
Kennett, MO 63857-326

573-888-0002
888-449-0949
Fax: 573-888-0708
TTY: 573-888-0002
tshaw@bails.org
www.bails.org

Tim Shaw, Executive Director
BAILS goal is to foster an open, barrier free society flor all people regardless of their disability. BAILS service area is predominantly rural and includes the Southeast Missouri counties of: Dunklin, New Madrid, Pemiscot and Stoddard.

4328 Coalition for Independence: Missouri Branch Office
6724 Troost Ave
Ste. 408
Kansas City, MO   66131

816-822-7432
Fax: 816-363-3469
TTY: 913-321-5126

Clarenece Smith, Executive Director
Coalition For Independence (CFI) is to facilitate positive and responsible independence for all people with disabilities by acting as an advocate for individuals with disabilities, providing services, and promoting accessibility and acceptance.

4329 Delta Center for Independent Living
PO Box 550
Suite #107
St. Peters, MO   63376-5608

636-926-8761
866-727-3245
Fax: 636-447-0341
info@dcil.org
www.dcil.org

Jennifer Mueller-Sparrow, President
Don Whalen, Vice President
Otis Pitts, Secretary
Bob Zeffert, Treasurer
A non profit corporation which assists people with significant disabilities who want to live more independently.

4330 Disability Resource Association
130 Brandon Wallace Way
Festus, MO   63028-1726

636-931-7696
Fax: 636-931-4863
TTY: 636-937-9016
dra@disabilityresourceassociation.org
www.disabilityresourceassociation. org
Craig Henning, Executive Director
Nancy Pope, Assistant Director
Suzan Weller, Director/Resource Developer
Independent Living Cener.

4331 Independent Living Center of Southeast Missouri
511 Cedar St
Poplar Bluff, MO   63901-7301

573-686-2333
888-890-2333
Fax: 573-686-0733
TTY: 573-776-1178
info@ilcsemo.org
www.ilcsemo.org
Bruce Lynch, Executive Director
Debbie Hardin, Independent Living Director
To make Southeast Missouri barrier free for all persons with disabilities, enabling them to live more independently, extending their rights to control and direct their own lives and empowering them to live more producitve lives.

4332 Life Skills Foundation
10176 Corporate Square Drive
Suite #150
Saint Louis, MO 63132-2935

314-432-6200
Fax: 314-432-8894
TTY: 314-802-5299
intake@lifeskills-stl.org
www.eastersealsmidwest.org

Christopher Wittanauer, Chair
Sean Donlin, Vice Chair
Wendy Sullivan, President
Marian Nunn, Secretary
Assists people with disabilities live and work with dignity in the community.

4333 Midland Empire Resources for Independent Living (MERIL)
4420 South 40th St
Saint Joseph, MO   64503-2157

816-279-8558
800-637-4548
Fax: 816-279-1550
TTY: 816-279-4943
www.meril.org

Dr. Robert Bush, Chair
Jaren Pippitt, Vice Chair
Wayne Crawford, Secretary
J. Robert Brown, Treasurer
Designed to promote independent living and to enhance the quality of life for persons with disabilities by empowering them to control and direct their lives.

4334 Northeast Independent Living Services
909 Broadway
Suite 350
Hannibal, MO   63401

573-221-8282
877-713-7900
Fax: 573-221-9445
www.neilscenter.org

Rose McNally, President
Dawn Davis, Vice President
Brooke Kendrick, Executive Director
Tara Fortner, Finance Director
To empower persons with disabilities to live as full and productive members of society.

4335 On My Own
428 E Highland Ave
Nevada, MO   64772-2609

417-667-7007
800-362-8852
Fax: 417-667-6262
www.omoinc.org

Jennifer Gundy, Executive Director
A non profit independent living center.

4336 Ozark Independent Living
109 Aid Ave
West Plains, MO   65775-3529

417-257-0038
888-440-7500
Fax: 417-257-2380
TTY: 888-440-7500
info@ozarkcil.com
ozarkcil.com

Michael Conner, Vice Chair
Scott Schneider, Secretary/Treasurer
Cindy Moore, Executive Director
Jane Kramer, Special Education Teacher
OIL?was created to provide independent living services to persons with disabilities who reside in the following counties in Missouri: Oregon Ozark, Shannon, Wright, Howell, Texas, and Douglas. OIL is non-profit, on-residential supported by grants, donations, and volunteers

4337   Paraquad
5240 Oakland Ave
Saint Louis, MO   63110-1436   314-289-4200
                                       Fax: 314-289-4201
                                       TTY:314-289-4252
                                       contactus@paraquad.org
                                       www.paraquad.org

Robert Funk, Executive Director
Paraquad works to empower people with disabilities to increase
their independence through choice and opportunity.

4338   Places for People
4130 Lindell Blvd
Saint Louis, MO   63108-2914   314-535-5600
                                       Fax: 314-535-6037
                                       contact@placesforpeople.org
                                       www.placesforpeople.org

Kevin Kissling, President
Robin Kolker Adkins, Vice President
Joe Yancey, Executive Director
Dennis Wells, Secretary
Places for People provides individualized, high quality and effective services to adults with serious and persistent mental disorders to assist them in living, working and socializing
responsibility to serve those individuals who rely on public
funding.

4339   RAIL
3024 Dupont Circle
Jefferson City, MO   65109   573-526-7039
                                            877-222-8963
                                            888-667-2117
                                       Fax: 573-751-1441
                                       mo.silc@vr.dese.mo.gov
                                       www.mosilc.org

Chris Camene, Chairperson
Jessica Hatfield, Vice-Chairperson
Barnnie Cooper, Secretary/Treasurer
Teresa Myers, Executive Director
RAIL is an Independent Living Center, one of twenty-two in the
State of Missouri, RAIL's Mission is to assist persons with dis-
abilities to live as independently as they choose within the com-
munities of their choice. RAIL offers four core services which
are: Advocacy, Peer Support, Information & Referral, and Inde-
pendent Living Skills Training. RAIL is a Consumer Services
Directed Program vendor

4340   SEMO Alliance for Disability Independence
1913 Rusmar St
Cape Girardeau, MO   63701-7623   573-651-6464
                                            800-898-7234
                                       Fax: 573-651-6565
                                       TTY: 573-651-6464
                                       www.sadi.org

Timothy D. Woodard, President
Michelle Spooler, Vice-President
Leemon Priest, Secretary
Janet Wilson, Treasurer
A community based, non-profit, nonresidential center for inde-
pendent living that is committed to providing services to persons
with disabilities to enable them to remain in their own home and
community, not an institution.

4341   Services for Independent Living
1401 Hathman Place
Columbia, MO   65201-5552   573-874-1646
                                            800-766-1968
                                       Fax: 573-874-3564
                                       TTY: 573-874-4121
                                       sil@silcolumbia.org
                                       www.silcolumbia.org

Dan Dunham, President
Bonnie Gregg, Vice President
Amy Henderson, Treasurer
Barbara Hammer, Secretary
A non-residential, community-based center for independent living. Provides individualized and group services to persons with
severe disabilities in the Mid-Missouri area; works to help people
with disabilities achieve their highest potential in independent
living and community life.

4342   Southwest Center for Independent Living (S CIL)
2864 S Nettleton Ave
Springfield, MO   65807-5970   417-886-3619
                                            800-676-7245
                                       Fax: 417-886-3619
                                       TTY: 417-886-1188
                                       scil@swcil.org
                                       www.swcil.org

Amy C. Lewis, President
Mark Grantham, Vice President
Gary Maddox, Chief Executive Officer
Lacee Thompson, Administrative Assistant
Provides services, advocacy, and resources for people with any
disability in Christian, Dallas, Greene, Lawrence, Polk, Stone,
Taney and Webster Counties of Southwest Missouri.

4343   Tri-County Center for Independent Living
1420 HWY 72 East
Rolla, MO   65401   573-368-5933
                                       Fax: 573-368-5991
                                       TTY:573-368-5933
                                       www.tricountycenter.com

Victoria Evans, Executive Director
Mission is to eliminate physical and attitudinal barriers through
the power of advocacy, enlightenment, and reformation.

4344   West Central Independent Living Solutions
610 N Ridgeview Dr
Suite B
Warrensburg, MO   64093-9323   660-422-7883
                                            800-236-5175
                                       Fax: 660-422-7895
                                       TTY: 660-422-7894
                                       info@w-ils.org
                                       www.w-ils.org

David De Frain, President
James Piatt, Vice President
Kathy Kay, Executive Director
Julie Steele, Director of Operations
Works to empower people with disabilities to become more inde-
pendent by providing independent living skills training, peer
support, information and referral and advocacy. West Central In-
dependent Living Solutions now has satellite offices in Sedalia,
MO and Lexington.

4345   Whole Person, The
3710 Main Street
Kansas City, MO   64111-7501   816-225-0301
                                            800-878-3037
                                       Fax: 816-931-0529
                                       TTY: 816-561-0304
                                       info@thewholeperson.org
                                       www.thewholeperson.org

Rick O'Neal, President
Jim Atwater, Vice President
Julie Dejean, CEO
Mike Wiley, COO
The Whole Person, assists people with disabilities to live inde-
pendently and encourages change within the community to ex-
pand opportunities for independent living.

4346   Whole Person: Kansas City
3710 Main Street
Kansas City, MO   64111-7501   816-561-0304
                                            800-878-3037
                                       Fax: 816-931-0529
                                       TTY: 816-627-2202
                                       info@thewholeperson.org
                                       www.thewholeperson.org

Rick O'Neal, President
Jim Atwater, Vice President
Julie Dejean, CEO
Mike Wiley, COO

Assists people with disabilities to live independently and encourages change within the community to expand opportunities for independent living.

Montana

4347 Living Independently for Today and Tomorrow
1201 Grand Avenue
Suite 1
Billings, MT 59102-2033 406-259-5181
800-669-6319
Fax: 406-259-5259
TTY: 406-245-1225
www.liftt.org

Bobbie Becker, Executive Director
Martha Carstensen, Program Director
LIFTT's Independent living program works with people with disabilities so they can live independently and have access to the community. LIFTT staff, most of whom have disabilities, serve as mentors to people as they work to achieve the goals they have set for themselves.

4348 Montana Independent Living Project, Inc.
825 Great Northern Blvd
Suite 105
Helena, MT 59601-4715 406-442-5755
800-735-6457
Fax: 406-442-1612
TTY: 406-442-5755
bmaffit@milp.us
www.milp.us

Bob Maffit, Executive Director
Les Clark, Independent Living Specialist
Charlene White, Financial Manager
Marie Largent, Office Manager
A not-for-profit agency that provides services that promote independence for people with disabilities.

4349 North Central Independent Living Services
1120 25th Ave
Black Eagle, MT 59414-1037 406-452-9834
800-823-6245
Fax: 406-453-3940
ncils.osborn@sofast.net

Tom Osborn, Executive Director
North Central Independent Living Services is located in Great Falls and provides services from Glacier County across the Hi-Line to the North Dakota border. A satellite office is set up in Glasgow.

4350 Summit Independent Living Center: Kalipsell
1203 Highway 2 W.
Suite #35
Kalispell, MT 59901-6020 406-257-0048
800-995-0029
Fax: 406-257-0634
TTY: 406-257-0048
webmaster@bils.org
www.summitilc.org

Steve Hackler, President
Larry Riley, Vice President
Jenny Montgomery, Secretary
Flo Kiewel, Manager
To promote community awareness, equal access, and the independence of people with disabilities through advocacy, education, and the advancement of civil rights.

4351 Summit Independent Living Center: Hamilton
316 North 3rd St
Suite #113
Hamilton, MT 59840-2479 406-363-5242
800-398-9013
Fax: 406-375-9035
webmaster@bils.org
www.summitilc.org

Steve Hackler, President
Larry Riley, Vice President
Jenny Montgomery, Secretary
Joanne Berwolf, Manager
To promote community awareness, equal access, and the independence of people with disabilities through advocacy, education, and the advancement of civil rights.

4352 Summit Independent Living Center: Missoula
700 SW Higgins Ave
Suite #101
Missoula, MT 59803-1489 406-728-1630
800-398-9002
Fax: 406-829-3309
missoula@summitilc.org
www.summitilc.org

Steve Hackler, President
Larry Riley, Vice President
Jenny Montgomery, Secretary
Mike Mayer, Executive Director
To promote community awareness, equal access, and the independence of people with disabilities through advocacy, education, and the advancement of civil rights.

4353 Summit Independent Living Center: Ronan
124 Main St.
Ronan, MT 59864-2718 406-215-1604
866-230-6936
Fax: 406-552-1028
ronan@summitilc.org
www.summitilc.org

Steve Hackler, President
Larry Riley, Vice President
Jenny Montgomery, Secretary
Gary Stevens, Manager
To promote community awareness, equal access, and the independence of people with disabilities through advocacy, education, and the advancement of civil rights.

Nebraska

4354 Center for Independent Living of Central Nebraska
3335 West Capital Street
Grand Island, NE 68803-1730 308-382-9255
877-400-1004
Fax: 308-384-7832
TTY: 308-382-9255
jthomas@cilne.org
www.cilne.org

Joni Thomas, Executive Director
Irene Britt, Western Program Manager
Lesia Gracia, Independent Living Specialist
Mike Niece, Driving Program Coordinator
Offers independent living skills training, peer sharing, information and referral, housing counseling and referral, accessibility and barrier removal consultation including ADA training and technical assistance, driver education and training, assistive technology services including demonstration and equipment loan, and a free lending library of adapted toys and ability switches for children with severe disabilities. Serves all diabilities and all ages.

4355 League of Human Dignity: Lincoln
1701 P St
Lincoln, NE 68508-1799 402-441-7871
888-508-4758
Fax: 402-441-7650
TTY:402-441-7871
info@leagueofhumandignity.com
www.leagueofhumandignity.com
Mike Schafer, CEO
The mission of the League of Human Dignity is to actively promote the full integration of individuals with disabilities into society. To this end, we will advocate their needs and rights, and provide quality services to involve these persons in becoming and remaining independent citizens.

4356 League of Human Dignity: Norfolk
400 Elm Ave
Norfolk, NE 68701-4033 402-371-4475
800-843-5785
Fax: 402-371-4625
TTY: 402-371-4475
ninfo@leagueofhumandignity.com
leagueofhumandignity.com
Mike Shafer, CEO
Jean M. Kloppenborg, Norfolk CIL Director
The mission of the League of Human Dignity is to actively promote the full integration of individuals with disabilities into society. To this end, we will advocate their needs and rights, and provide quality services to involve these persons in becoming and remaining independent citizens.

4357 League of Human Dignity: Omaha
5513 Center St
Omaha, NE 68106-3001 402-595-1256
800-843-5784
Fax: 402-595-1410
oinfo@leagueofhumandignity.com
www.leagueofhumandignity.com
Mike Schafer, CEO
Bob Gomez, Executive Director
The mission of the League of Human Dignity is to actively promote the full integration of individuals with disabilities into society. To this end, we will advocate their needs and rights, and provide quality services to involve these persons in becoming and remaining independent citizens.

4358 Mosaic of Axtell Bethpage Village
1044 23rd Rd.
PO Box 67
Axtell, NE 68924 308-743-2401
Fax: 308-743-2659
www.mosaicinfo.org/axtell
Max Miller, Chairperson
James Zils, Vice Chairperson
Linda Timmons, President/ CEO
Raul Saldivar, COO
Provides services that respect the human dignity and rights of each person. An interdisciplinary team of family, staffmembers and professional consultatns support individuals served in developing personal goals and programs, helping them to fully participate in Axtell's community life. Mosaic at Axtell offers residential and community services.

4359 Mosaic of Beatrice
722 S. 12th St.
PO Box 607
Beatrice, NE 68310-607 402-223-4066
Fax: 402-223-4951
jerry.campbell@mosaicinfo.org
www.mosaicinfo.org/beatrice
Max Miller, Chairperson
James Zils, Vice Chairperson
Linda Timmons, President/ CEO
Raul Saldivar, COO
Provides individualized services, living options, work choices, spiritual nurture and advocacy to people with disabilities in more than 250 communities across 14 states and Great Britain through the work of 4,800 employees.

4360 Mosaic: York
220 W South 21st St
York, NE 68467-9316 402-362-2180
Fax: 402-362-2961
www.mosaicinfo.org
Max Miller, Chairperson
James Zils, Vice Chairperson
Linda Timmons, President/ CEO
Raul Saldivar, COO
Providing a wide array of services to assist individuals and families in achieving positive life goals. Services to persons with disabilities and other special needs include community living options, training and employment options, spiritual growth and development options, training and counseling support.

Nevada

4361 Carson City Center for Independent Living
900 Mallory Way
Carson City, NV 89701 775-841-2580
Sandra Coyle, Owner
Helps consumers continue to live independently in the community through a variety of individual and community services.

4362 Northern Nevada Center for Independent Living: Fallon
1919 Grimes St
Suite B
Fallon, NV 89406-3100 775-423-4900
800-885-3712
Fax: 775-423-1399
TTY: 775-423-4900
nncilf@cccomm.net
www.nncil.org
Lisa Bonie, Executive Director
Hilda Velasco, Operations Manager
Joni Inglis, Independent Living Advocate
Deb Maijala, Rural Services Coordinator
Independent Living Center.

4363 Rural Center for Independent Living
1895 E Long St
Carson City, NV 89706-3214 775-841-2580
Fax: 775-841-2580
ruralcil@yahoo.com
Dee Dee Foremaster, Executive Director
Advocacy, Benefit Assistance, social security assistance, peer support, housing information and home-less day drop-in center for individuals with disabilities.

4364 Southern Nevada Center for Independent Living: North Las Vegas
3100 E Lake Mead Blvd
North Las Vegas, NV 89030-7380 702-649-3822
800-398-0760
Fax: 702-649-5022
TTY: 702-649-3822
sncilnv@aol.com
www.sncil.org
Connie Kratky, President
Elliot Yug, Vice - President
Pamela Rake, Secretary
William Sheehan, Treasurer
SNCIL is committed to removing barriers preventing indpendent living by providing services designed to empower people with disabilities.

4365 Southern Nevada Center for Independent Living: Las Vegas
2950 S. Rainbow Blvd.
Suite 220
Las Vegas, NV   89146-5611
702-889-4216
800-870-7003
Fax: 702-889-4574
TTY: 702-889-4216
sncil2@aol.com
www.sncil.org

Connie Kratky, President
Elliot Yug, Vice - President
Pamela Rake, Secretary
William Sheehan, Treasurer
SNCIL is committed to removing barriers preventing Independent Living by providing services designed to empower people with disabilities.

New Hampshire

4366 Granite State Independent Living Foundation
21 Chenell Drive
Concord, NH   3301-4079
603-228-9680
800-826-3700
Fax: 603-444-3128
TTY: 603-228-9680
info@gsil.org
www.gsil.org

Ken Traum, Chair
Lorna D. Greer, Vice Chair
Clyde E. Terry, CEO
Deborah Krider, COO
GSIL is a statewide non-profit that recognizes the fact that all of us will need some type of support in the course of the lives. GSIL offers tools and resources so that individuals can participate as fully as the choose in their lives, families and communities. Contact the Independent Living Foundation for referrals to living situations.

New Jersey

4367 Alliance Center for Independance
Alliance for Disabled in Action
629 Amboy Ave, First Floor
Edison, NJ   08837-3579
732-738-4388
Fax: 732-738-4416
TTY: 732-738-9644
adacil@adacil.org
www.adacil.org

Colleen Roche, Chair
Bernard Zuckerman, Treasurer
Carole Tonks, Executive Director
Luke Koppisch, Deputy Director
Alliance for Disabled in Action is a private, not-for-profit center for independent living serving people in Middlesex, Somerset and Union Counties of New Jersey. ADA's mission is to support and promote choice, self-direction and independent living in the lives of people with disabilities, with the right of individuals to inclusion in the community as the primary goal.

4368 Camden City Independent Living Center
2600 Mount Ephraim Ave
Camden, NJ   8104-3236
856-966-0800
Fax: 856-966-0832
TTY: 856-966-0830
vedasmithccilc@aol.com
www.camdencityilc.org

Bruce Smith, Chairperson
John Quann, Vice Chairperson
Tanya Brown, Treasurer
Veda Smith, Executive Director
Provides services designed to empower people with disabilities. To provide services to individuals with significant disabilities. Services include information referral, advocacy, peer support, and independent living skills training. CCILC services individuals in Camden City

4369 Center for Independent Living: Long Branch
279 Broadway
Suite #201
Long Branch, NJ   7740-6940
732-571-4884
Fax: 732-571-4003
TTY: 732-571-4878
www.moceanscil.org

Jennifer Sterner, Vice Chair
Maureen Poling, Secretary
Stan Soden, Director IL Services
Susan Pniewski, IL Transition Specialist
Offers peer support, disability education and personal assistant services. Serving Monmouth and Ocean Counties with information and referrals, advocacy, peer support and independent living instructions.

4370 Center for Independent Living: South Jersey
1150 Delsea Drive
Suite #1
Westville, NJ   8093-2251
856-853-6490
800-413-3791
Fax: 856-853-1466
TTY: 856-853-7602

Hazel Lee-Briggs, Executive Director
Danuta Debicki, Program Manager
Terryama Davis, Independent Living Specialist
Dedicated to providing people with disabilities in Gloucester and Camden counties the opportunity to actively participate in society, to provide freedom of choice, to work, to own a home, raise a family and in general, to participate to the fullest extent in day-to-day activities. The center provides information and referrals, advocacy, peer support, and independent living skills training.

4371 DAWN Center for Independent Living
66 Ford Road
Suite 121
Denville, NJ   7834-1235
973-625-1940
888-383-3296
Fax: 973-625-1942
TTY: 973-625-1932
info@dawncil.org
www.dawncil.org

Elizabeth Lehmann, President
Gabrielle Waldman, Vice President
Carmela Slivinski, Executive Director
Caroleen Marano, Independent Living Program
DAWN is the Center for Independent Living serving Morris, Sussex and Warren counties. DAWN empowers people with disabilities to strive for equality and to take control of their own lives by providing the tools that encourage independence and self-advocacy, promoting public awareness of the needs, desires and rights to individuals living with disabilities, and offering community activities that create new experiences and opportunities.

4372 Dial: Disabled Information Awareness & Living
2 Prospect Village Plaza
Floor 1
Clifton, NJ   7013-1918
973-470-8090
866-277-1733
Fax: 973-470-8171
TTY: 973-470-2521
info@dial-cil.org
www.dial-cil.org

Cynthia DeSouza, President
Anthony Gianduso, Vice President
John Petix, Executive Director
Tim Burns, Secretary
Promotes the full inclusion of all people living with disabilities into society and encourage the consumers and the community at large to seek involvement in this self-governing organization to the fullest extent.

4373   Disability Rights New Jersey
New Jersey Protection and Advocacy
210 S. Broad Street
Floor 3
Trenton, NJ   08608-2407   609-292-9742
                                             800-922-7233
                                        Fax: 609-777-0187
                                        TTY: 609-633-7106
                                        advocate@drnj.org
                                             www.drnj.org

Walter Anthony Woodberry, Chair
Andrew McGeady, Vice Chair
Linda K. Soley, Treasurer
Leah Ziskin, Secretary
Assistive Technology Advocacy Center provides assistance to
persons with disabilities in helping them to obtain assistive tech-
nology devices and/or services.

4374   Family Resource Associates
35 Haddon Ave
Shrewsbury, NJ   7702-4007   732-747-5310
                                        Fax: 732-747-1896
                                        info@frainc.org
                                             www.frainc.org

Allan Proske, President
Bill Sheeser, Vice President
John Feeney, Treasurer
Judy Fuller, Secretary
FRA is dedicated to helping children, adolescents and people of
all ages with disabilities to reach their fullest potential. FRA also
connects individuals to independence through modern therapies
and advanced technology. FRA provides direct services to those
in the greater Nonmouth/Ocean County area.

4375   Heightened Independence and Progress: Hackensack
131 Main St
Suite #120
Hackensack, NJ   7601-7182   201-996-9100
                                        Fax: 201-996-9422
                                        TTY:201-966-9424
                                        ber@hipcil.org
                                             www.hipcil.org

Eileen Goff, President/CEO
Trish Carney, Finance and Development Director
Empowers people with disabilities to achieve independent living
through outreach, advocacy and education.

4376   Heightened Independence and Progress: Jersey City
35 Journal Square
Suite #703
Jersey City, NJ   7306-4105   201-533-4407
                                        Fax: 201-533-4421
                                        TTY:201-533-4409
                                        hud@hipcil.org
                                             www.hipcil.org

Jean Csaposs, Board Chair
Lottie Esteban, First Vice Chair
Eileen Goff, President/CEO
Trish Carney, Finance and Development Director
Empowering People with Disabilities to Achieve Independent
Living through Outreach, Advocacy, and Education.

4377   Progressive Center for Independent Living
3525Quakerbridge Rd.
Suite 904
Hamilton, NJ   8619-3710   609-581-4500
                                             877-917-4500
                                        Fax: 609-581-4555
                                        TTY: 609-581-4550
                                        info@pcil.org
                                             www.pcil.org

Norman Smith, President
John Witman, Vice President
Scott Elliott, Executive Director
Jerry Carbone, Training Coordinator
Advocates for the rights of people with disabilities to achieve and
maintain independent lifestyles. The Center has programs to as-

sist with employment, transition from school to adult life, and
emergency preparedness.

4378   Progressive Center for Independent Living: Flemington
4 Walter E Foran Blvd
Suite 410
Flemington, NJ   8822-4669   908-782-1055
                                             877-376-9174
                                        Fax: 908-782-6025
                                        TTY: 908-782-1081
                                        info@pcil.org
                                             pcil.org

Norman Smith, President
John Witman, Vice President
Scott Elliott, Executive Director
Jerry Carbone, Training Coordinator
Advocates for the rights of people with disabilities to achieve and
maintain independent lifestyles.

4379   Project Freedom
223 Hutchinson Rd
Robbinsville, NJ   8691-3457   609-448-2998
                                        Fax: 609-448-7293
                                   ProjectFreedom1@aol.com
                                        www.projectfreedom.org

Tim Doherty, Executive Director
Norman A. Smith, Assoc Ex Director
Elizabeth Maxwell, Office Manager
Paul Campanella, Property Manager
Dedicated to developing, supporting, and advocating opportuni-
ties for independent living persons with disabilities.

4380   Project Freedom: Hamilton
715 Kuser Rd
Hamilton, NJ   8619-3924   609-588-9919
                                        Fax: 609-588-8831
                                   cfunk@projectfreedom.org
                                        www.projectfreedom.org

Cecilia Funk, Social Service Coordinator
Judy Wilkinson, Office Manager
Paul Campanella, Property Manager
Dedicated to developing, supporting, and advocating opportuni-
ties for independent living persons with disabilities.

4381   Project Freedom: Lawrence
1 Freedom Blvd
Lawrence, NJ   8648-4531   609-278-0075
                                        Fax: 609-278-1250
                                   jelsowiny@projectfreedom.org
                                        www.projectfreedom.org

Jacklene Elsowiny, Social Serv Coordinator
Tim Doherty, Executive Director
Stephen Schaefer, CFO
Tracee Battis, Director of Housing Development
Dedicated to developing, supporting, and advocating opportuni-
ties for independent living persons with disabilities.

4382   Total Living Center
6712 Washington Ave
Egg Harbor Township, NJ   8234-1999   609-645-9547
                                        Fax: 609-813-2318
                                        TTY:609-645-9593
                                             www.tlcenter.org

Jo Hudson, President
Cliff Anderson, Vice President
Cathy Shaner, Secretary
Julia Bonelli, Executive Director
Total Living Center is a non-profit organization whose mission is
to empower individuals with significant disabilities to maximize
their potential for independence and productivity, to live as fully
as possible within the community, taking responsibility for themselves, and sharing this commitment with others.

New Mexico

4383 Ability Center
715 E. Idaho Ave
Building 3E
Las Cruces, NM 88001-4702   575-526-5016
800-376-4372
Fax: 575-526-1202
TTY: 505-526-5016
freedom@theabilitycenter.org
www.theabilitycenter.org

Vincent Montano, Executive Director
Cesar Rodriguez, Vice-President
C. Neil Gibbs, Treasurer
The Ability Center is a private, nonresidential, nonprofit, New Mexico corporation. As a center for independent living (CIL) TACIL provides a variety of services to promote independence, self-reliance, and community integration. Our professional staff and active board of directors are dedicated to helping our consumers maintain their personal freedom at home, in the community, and throughout the state.

4384 CASA Inc.
116 West Baltimore Street
Hagerstown, MD 21740   301-739-4990
Fax: 301-790-0064
casa4@myactv.net
www.casaabq.com

Sherry Donovan, President
Linda Davis, Vice-President
Melinda Marsden, Treasurer
Laura Allis, Secretary
Offers peer counseling and information and referral services.

4385 CHOICES Center for Independent Living
200 E 4th St.
Suite #200
Roswell, NM 88201-6237   575-627-6727
800-387-4572
Fax: 575-627-6754
TTY: 505-627-6727

Julia Calvert, Executive Director
Offers many core services including independent living skills training, peer support, information and referral, advocacy and transition.

4386 New Mexico Technology Assistance Program
625 Silver Ave. SW
Ste. 100 B
Albuquerque, NM 87102   505-841-4464
877-696-1470
Fax: 505-841-4467
TTY: 800-659-4915
Tracy.Agiovlasitis@state.nm.us
www.tap.gcd.state.nm.us

Julie Martinez, Program Director
Tracy Agiovlasitis, Supervisor
Samuel Castillo, Coordinator
Jesse Armijo, Specialist
Examines and works to eliminate barriers to obtaining assistive technology in New Mexico. Has established a statewide program for coordinating assistive technology services; is designed to assist people with disabilities to locate, secure, and maintain assistive technology.

4387 New Vistas
1205 Parkway Dr.
Suite A
Santa Fe, NM 87501-2483   505-471-1001
Fax: 505-471-4427
info@newvistas.org
www.newvistas.org

Victor Ortega, President
Libby Gonzales, Vice-President
Gay Romero, Secretary/Treasurer

Partners with and supports people with disabilities and families of children with special needs to enrich their quality of life in New Mexico.

4388 San Juan Center for Independence
1204 San Juan Blvd
Farmington, NM 87401   505-566-5827
877-484-4500
Fax: 505-566-5842
TTY: 505-566-5827
sjci@sjci.org
www.sjci.org

Patricia Ziegler, Executive Director
Tim Carver, CFO
SJCI is a New Mexico private non residential, nonprofit corporation that serves people with disabilities. The purpose of SJCI is to provide a variety of community based, consumer driven service to people with disablties to promote independence, self-residence and intergration into the community.

New York

4389 AIM Independent Living Center: Corning
271 E 1st St
Corning, NY 14830-2924   607-962-8225
Fax: 607-937-5125
TTY: 607-962-8225
troche@aimcil.com
www.aimcil.com

Rene Snyder, Executive Director
Sabrina Mineo-O'Connell, President
George Spisack, Vice President
Barbara Squires, Treasurer
AIM is a non-profit organization dedicated to people with disabilities, their families, friends, the businesses that serve them and those with an interest in disabilities. The mission of AIM is to support the individuals ability to make independent, self-directing choices through education, advocacy, information and referral.

4390 AIM Independent Living Center: Elmira
650 Baldwin St.
Elmira, NY 14901-2216   607-733-3718
Fax: 607-733-0180
TTY: 607-733-7764
troche@aimcil.com
www.aimcil.com

Rene Snyder, Executive Director
Sabrina Mineo-O'Connell, President
George Spisack, Vice President
Barbara Squires, Treasurer
AIM's goal is to enable the consumer to live an independent and comfortable lifestyle in the security of their home environment so they may feel dignity and pride in their achievements while controling their own care.

4391 ARISE
635 James St
Syracuse, NY 13203-2661   315-472-3171
Fax: 315-472-9252
TTY: 315-479-6363
info@ariseinc.org
www.ariseinc.org

Tania Anderson, President
Sue Judge, Vice President
Michael Cook, Treasurer
Tom McKeown, Executive Director
Founded in 1979, ARISE's mission is to work with people of all abilities to create a fair and just community in which everyone can fully participate. As a center for independent living, ARISE is a non-profit organization run by and for individuals with disabilities. ARISE serves over 3,000 children and adults with disabilities each year through our programs and services in several broad areas including advocacy, employment, independent living/integrated recreation programs, and much more.

4392   ARISE: Oneida
131 Main St
Suite #107
Oneida, NY   13421-1644   315-363-4672
                                        Fax: 315-363-4675
                                        TTY:315-363-2364
                                        info@ariseinc.org
                                        www.ariseinc.org

Tania Anderson, President
Sue Judge, Vice President
Michael Cook, Treasurer
Tom McKeown, Executive Director
A consumer controlled, non-profit Independent Living Center
that promotes the full inclusion of people with disabilities in the
community.

4393   ARISE: Oswego
9 Fourth Avenue
Oswego, NY   13126-1803   315-342-4088
                                        Fax: 315-342-4107
                                        TTY:315-342-8696
                                        info@ariseinc.org
                                        www.ariseinc.org

Tania Anderson, President
Sue Judge, Vice President
Michael Cook, Treasurer
Tom McKeown, Executive Director
A consumer controlled, non-profit Independent Living Center
that promotes the full inclusion of people with disabilities in the
community.

4394   ARISE: Pulaski
2 Broad St
Pulaski, NY   13142-4446   315-298-5726
                                        Fax: 315-298-5729
                                        info@ariseinc.org
                                        www.ariseinc.org

Tania Anderson, President
Sue Judge, Vice President
Michael Cook, Treasurer
Tom McKeown, Executive Director
A consumer controlled, non-profit Independent Living Center
that promotes the full inclusion of people with disabilities in the
community.

4395   Access to Independence of Cortland County, Inc.
26 N Main St
Cortland, NY   13045-2198   607-753-7363
                                        Fax: 607-756-4884
                                        info@aticortland.org
                                        www.aticortland.org

Judy Bentley, Chair
Peter Morse-Ackley, Vice Chair
Chad W. Underwood, CEO
Mary E. Ewing, Program Manager
Access to Independence is Cortland County's foremost disability
resource. It empowers people to lead independent lives in their
community and strives to open doors to full participation and
access for all.

4396   Action Toward Independence: Middletown
130 Dolson Avenue
Suite 35
Middletown, NY   10940-6563   845-343-4284
                                        Fax: 845-342-5269
                                        actiontowardindependence.org

Stephen McLaughlin, Executive Director
Joann Hargabus, Services Director, Orange Cnty.
Gilles Malkine, Services Director, Sullivan Cnty
Cheryl Babcock, Fiscal Manager
Independent living center that serves Orange & Sullivan counties. Provides programs and services to individuals who have disabilities and to their families. These services include peer
counseling, individual & systems advocacy, independent living,
skills training, information and referral, benefits advisement,
recreation and a drop in center. We are designed to enable people
with disabilities to achieve independence, inclusion and
participation in their communities.

4397   Action Toward Independence: Monticello
309 E Broadway
Suite A
Monticello, NY   12701-8810   845-794-4228
                                        Fax: 845-794-4475
                                        TTY:845-794-4228
                                        www.atitoday.org

Steve McLaughlin, Executive Director
Joann Hargabus, Director of Services
A not-for-profit, non residential, peer run, referral and advocacy
agency for persons with disaiblities in Orange and Sullivan counties. Our services are aimed at promoting accessibility, community integration, and equal opportunity in all aspects of society
for persons with all types of disabilities.

4398   BRiDGES
873 Route 45
Suite 108
New City, NY   10956   845-624-1366
                                        Fax: 845-624-1369
                                        info@bridgesrc.org
                                        www.bridgesrc.org

Patricia Ranieri, President
David Jacobsen, Ph.D, Psy.D, Executive Director
Michael Coleman, Director of Finance & Controller
Nanci Goldman, Director of Human Resources
BRiDGES is a community-based non-profit organization that
serves people with disabilities. Services provided by them in-
clude personal assistance self-employers, independent living ser-
vices, volunteer opportunities, advocacy and more.

4399   Bronx Independent Living Services
4419 Thrid Avenue
Suite 2C
Bronx, NY   10457   718-515-2800
                                        Fax: 718-515-2844
                                        TTY:718-515-2803
                                        webmaster@bils.org
                                        www.bils.org

Barbara Linn, President
Anita Richichi, Vice President
Sheldon Mann, Treasurer
Brett L. Eisenberg, Executive Director
BILS is a not-for-profit community agency serving people with
all kinds of disabilities. The mission is to empower people with
disabilities toward living independent lives. BILS assists individuals by providing advocacy, peer counseling, housing information, and independent living training/counseling.

4400   Brooklyn Center for Independence of the Disabled
27 Smith Street
Suite #200
Brooklyn, NY   11201   718-998-3000
                                        Fax: 718-998-3743
                                        TTY:718-998-7406
                                        advocate@bcid.org
                                        www.bcid.org

Joan Peters, Executive Director
Sandrina Kingston, Program Director
Princess Davis, Office Manager
Stanley Stephen, Office Assistant
Operated by a majority of people with disabilities, BCID is dedi-
cated to guaranteeing the civil rights of people with disabilities.
BCID exists to improve the quality of life of brooklyn residents
with disabilities thgouh programs that empower them to gain
greater control of their lives and achieve full and equal
integration into society.

4401 Capital District Center for Independence
845 Central Ave
South 3
Albany, NY   12206-1342   518-459-6422
                                      Fax: 518-459-7847
                                      TTY:518-459-6422
                                      info@cdciweb.com
                                      www.cdciweb.com

Laurel Kelley, Executive Director
Dawn Werner, Deputy Director
Judy Zuchero, Program Director
G. W. Barr, Advocate
One of 37 Independent Living Centers in New York State, the Center is a non-residential, community based organization, which primarily serves Albany and Schenetady Counties. The Center's mission is to assist people with disabilities to acquire self-advocacy skills and by teaching through example, consumers achieve greater control over the direction of their lives.

4402 Catskill Center for Independence
6104 State Highway 23
Oneonta, NY   13820   607-432-8000
                                      Fax: 607-432-6907
                                      TTY:607-432-8000
                                      ccfi@ccfi.us
                                      www.ccfi.us

Chris Zachmeyer, Executive Director
Christine Worden, Assistant Director
One of 37 community-based independent living centers located throughout the state of New York. As an advocacy agency, we provide a vareity of services to people with disabilities, their friends and family members. In addition, we provide advocacy, training, and technical assistance to our community members, organizations, businesses and state and local governments in a variety of disability related areas. Serves Otsego, Delaware and Schoharie counties.

4403 Center for Community Alternatives
115 E Jefferson St
Suite #300
Syracuse, NY   13202-2018   315-422-5638
                                      Fax: 315-471-4924
                                      cca@communityalternatives.org
                                      www.communityalternatives.org

Kwame Johnson, President
Susan R. Horn, Esq., Vice-President
Carole A. Eady, Secretary
Marsha Weissman, Executive Director
Promotes reintegrative justice and a reduced reliance on incarceration through advocacy, services and public policy development in pursuit of civil and human rights.

4404 Center for Independence of the Disabled of New York
80-02 Kkew Garden Rd.
Suite 107
Kew Gardens, NY   11415   646-442-1520
                                      Fax: 347-561-4883
                                      TTY:718-886-0427
                                      info@cidny.org
                                      www.cidny.org

Martin Eichel, President
Anne M. Davis, Vice President
John O'Neill, Vice President
Susan Dooha, Executive Director
To ensure full integration, independence and equal opportunity for all people with disabilities by removing barriers to the social, economic, cultural and civic life of the community.

4405 Center for Independence of the Disabled of New York
841 Broadway
Suite #301
New York, NY   10003-4708   212-674-2300
                                      Fax: 212-254-5953
                                      TTY:212-674-5619
                                      info@cidny.org
                                      www.cidny.org

Martin Eichel, President
Anne M. Davis, Vice President
John O'Neill, Vice President
Susan Dooha, Executive Director
To ensure full integration, independence and equal opportunity for all people with disabilities by removing barriers to the social, economic, cultural and civic life of the community.

4406 DD Center/St Lukes: Roosevelt Hospital Center
St Lukes Roosevelt
1000 10th Ave
New York, NY   10019-1192   212-473-2045
                                      Fax: 212-473-0501

Charles Raimondo, VP
Farooq Chaudry, MD
Independent living center that advocates for people with disabilities by assisting with the application process of housing, benefits, etc.

4407 Finger Lakes Independence Center
215 5th St
Ithaca, NY   14850-3403   607-272-2433
                                      Fax: 607-272-0902
                                      TTY:607-272-2433
                                      flic@clarityconnect.com
                                      www.fliconline.org

Lenore Schwager, Executive Director
FLIC assists all people with disabilities, their families and friends to promote independence and make informed decisions in pursuit of their goals. The servides provided are free of charge, and services are primarily served to residents of Tompkins, Schyler counties.

4408 Harlem Independent Living Center
289 St. Nicholas Avenue
Suite #21
New York, NY   10027- 4805   212-222-7122
                                      800-673-2371
                                      Fax: 212-222-7199
                                      harlemilc@aol.com
                                      www.hilc.org

Christina Curry, Executive Director
Edward Randolph, Resource Specialist
Dr. Herbert Thornhill, Emeritus
Vanessa J. Young, Chair
A non-profit agency that advocates for people with disabilities by assisting with the application process of housing, benefits, etc. Our services are free of charge.
Monthly

4409 Independent Living
5 Washington Terrace
Newburgh, NY   12550   845-565-1162
                                      Fax: 845-565-0567
                                      TTY:845-565-0337
                                      info@myindependentliving.org
                                      www.myindependentliving.org

Doug J Hovey, President & CEO
Shannon Zawiski, Chief Operating Officer
Emily Robisch, Chief Financial Officer
Julie Stainton, Community Relations & Marketing Manager
A non-profit agency run by people with disabilities for others with disabilities. The agency offers programs and services to enhance quality of life, including benefits advising, personal assistance services, advocacy, employment and mental health services, recovery center, supportive housing and more.

4410 Long Island Center for Independent Living
3601 Hempstead Tpke
Suites 208 & 500
Levittown, NY 11756-1331   516-796-0144
Fax: 516-520-1247
TTY:516-796-0135
licil@aol.com
www.licil.net

Joan Lynch, Executive Director
LICIL is committed to the empowerment of consumers with disabilities. LICIL staff functions as ambassadors to the belief that individuals with disabilities have a responsibility to take an active role in their own lives and self determined view of their futures.

4411 Massena Independent Living Center
156 Center St.
Massena, NY 13662-1495   315-764-9442
877-397-9613
Fax: 315-764-9464
mindepli@twcny.rr.com
www.milcinc.org

Jeff Reifensnyder, Executive Director
Provides a variety of non-residential direct services as well as educating the public through community awareness campaigns. Also seeks to address the current appropriate unmet needs of persons experiencing a disability.

4412 NYS Independent Living Council
111 Washington Ave
Suite #101
Albany, NY 12210-2280   518-427-1060
877-397-4126
Fax: 518-427-1139
bradw@nysilc.org
www.nysilc.org

Brad Williams, Executive Director
Patty Black, Administrative Assistant
Provides support and technical assistance to 37 independent living centers-community-based organizations directed by and for people with disabilities.

4413 Nassau County Office for the Physically Challenged
60 Charles Lindberg Blvd
Uniondale, NY 11553-4812   516-227-7399
www.nassaucountyny.gov

Edward P. Mangano, County Executive
This agency serves as the ADA compliance coordinating office for all Nassau County governmental facilities, programs and services. It also serves in an advisory capacity to local, regional and national policy-making organizations, planning committees and legislative bodies and conducts advocacy as well as direct programs and services to enhance inclusion by people with disabilities to employment, consumerism and transportation.

4414 North Country Center for Independent Living
80 Sharron Avenue
Plattsburgh, NY 12901-3827   518-563-9058
Fax: 518-563-0292
TTY:518-563-9058
andrew@ncci-online.com
www.ncci-online.com

Ted Graser, President
Kathy Latinville, Vice President
Robert Poulin, Executive Director
Deb Piper, Program Director
To empower people with disabilities to live more independent and productive lives, and to promote beneficial policies and community understanding of disability issues.

4415 Northern Regional Center for Independent Living: Watertown
210 Court St
Suite #107
Watertown, NY 13601-4546   315-785-8703
800-585-8703
Fax: 315-785-8612
TTY: 315-785-8704
nrcil@nrcil.net
www.nrcil.net

Ronald Griffin, Chair
Michael Simmons, Vice Chair
Melanie Adkins, Secretary
Aileen Martin, Executive Director
A disability rights and resource center that promotes community efforts to end discrimination, segregation, and prejudice against people with disabilities.

4416 Northern Regional Center for Independent Living: Lowville
7632 N State St
Lowville, NY 13367-1318   315-376-8696
Fax: 315-376-3404
TTY:315-376-8696
karenb@nrcil.net
www.nrcil.net

Ronald Griffin, Chair
Michael Simmons, Vice Chair
Melanie Adkins, Secretary
Aileen Martin, Executive Director
A disability rights and resource center that promotes community efforts to end discrimination, segregation, and prejudice against people with disabilities.

4417 Options for Independence: Auburn
75 Genesee St
Auburn, NY 13021-3667   315-255-3447
Fax: 315-255-0836
gguy@optionsforindependence.org
www.ariseinc.org

Tania Anderson, President
Sue Judge, Vice President
Michael Cook, Treasurer
Tom McKeown, Executive Director
Options for Independence is an Independent Living Center which assists people with disabilities to gain opportunities, make their own decisions, pursue activities and become part of comunity life. Options provides a variety of services to all people with disabilities, their families, friends, and service providers in Cayuga and Seneca Counties.

4418 Putnam Independent Living Services
1961 Route 6
2nd Floor
Carmel, NY 10512-2324   845-228-7457
Fax: 845-228-7460
TTY:866-933-5390
info@wilc.org
www.putnamils.org

Joe Bravo, Executive Director
Mildred Caballero-Ho, Deputy Executive Director
Margaret Valenzuela, Program Director, IL Services
Jessica Baumann, Program Director, Educational Ad
A non-profit, community-based advocacy and resource center that serves people with all types of disabilities.

4419 Regional Center for Independent Living
497 State St
Rochester, NY 14608-1642   585-442-6470
Fax: 585-271-8558
TTY:585-442-6470
bdarling@rcil.org
www.rcil.org

Shelly Perrin, Chairperson
Bobbi Wallach, Vice Chairperson
Bruce E Darling, Executive Director
Jennifer Smouse, Director of Finance
To empower people with disabilities to self-advocate, to live independently and to enhance the quality of community life.

4420 Resource Center for Accessible Living
727 Ulster Ave
Kingston, NY 12401-1709
845-331-0541
Fax: 845-331-2076
TTY:845-331-4527
office@rcal.org
www.rcal.org

Paul Scarpati, President
Paula Kindos-Carberry, Co-Vice President
Bernadette Mueller, Co-Vice President
Susan Hoger, RCAL Executive Director
RCAL is a non-profit, community based service and advocacy run by and for people with any type of disability. RCAL is dedicated to assisting and empowering individuals, of all ages, to live independently and participate in all aspects of community life.

4421 Resource Center for Independent Living
347 W Main St
Amsterdam, NY 12010-2225
518-842-3561
Fax: 518-842-0905
TTY:518-842-3593

Shelly Perrin, Chairperson
Bobbi Wallach, Vice Chairperson
Bruce E Darling, Executive Director
Jennifer Smouse, Director of Finance
Peer counseling, advocacy, independent living skills training, information and referral services, self-advocacy training, ADA consultation, home and community based services, community education, benefits advisement and more. All programs and services are available in English and Spanish.

4422 Southern Adirondack Independent Living
418 Geyser Rd
Country Club Plaza
Ballston Spa, NY 12020-6002
518-584-8202
Fax: 518-584-1195
sail@sail-center.org
www.sail-center.org

Karen Thayer, Executive Director
Anna Livingston, Assistant Director
Barbara Potvin, Executive Assistant
Michele Nicholson, Administrative Assistant
To assist individuals with disabilities to become independent empowered self-advocates.

4423 Southern Adirondack Independent Living Center
71 Glenwood Ave
Queensbury, NY 12804-1728
518-792-3537
Fax: 518-792-0979
TTY:518-792-0505
www.sail-center.org

Karen Thayer, Executive Director
Anna Livingston, Assistant Director
Shirley Dumont, Director of Advocacy
Barbara Potvin, Executive Assistant
To assist individuals with disabilities to become independent empowered self-advocates.

4424 Southern Tier Independence Center
135 E Frederick St
Binghamton, NY 13904-1224
607-724-2111
Fax: 607-772-3600
TTY:607-724-2111
stic@stic-cil.org
www.stic-cil.org

Maria Dibble, Executive Director
Frank Pennisi, Accessibility Services
STIC provides assistance and services to all people with disabilities of all ages to increase their independence in all aspects of integrated community life. STIC also serves their families and friends, and businesses, agencies, and governments to enable them to better meet the needs of people with disabilities, and finally STIC educates and influences the community in pursuit of full inclusion of people with disabilities.

4425 Southwestern Independent Living Center
843 N Main St
Jamestown, NY 14701-3546
716-661-3010
Fax: 716-661-3011
TTY:716-661-3012
info@ilc-jamestown-ny.org

Marie T Carrubba, Executive Director
Linda Rumbaugh, Independent Living Specialist
Christine Ahlstrom, Independent Living Specialist
Helen Kern, Independent Living Specialist
A non-residential, private, nonprofit agency established to provide services throughout Chautauqua County that will assist individuals with disabilities in reaching maximum independence and an enriched quality of life.

4426 Staten Island Center for Independent Living, Inc.
470 Castleton Ave
Staten Island, NY 10301
718-720-9016
Fax: 718-720-9664
TTY:718-720-9870
ldesantis@siciliving.org
www.siciliving.org

Lorraine DeSantis, Executive Director
Claudia J. Stanton, Office Manager
Michelle Sabatino, Independent Living Specialist
John Mastellone, Community Consultant / Benefits
Mission is to provide all individuals with disabilities the information, life skills training, and facilitative assistance which contributes to independence, individuality, and integration in the community and provides the skills and knowledge necessary to function in the least restrictive, personally fulfilling, most self reliant and productive manner.

4427 Suffolk Independent Living Organization(SILO)
2111 Lakeland Ave.
Suite A
Ronkonkoma, NY 11779
631-880-7929
Fax: 631-946-6377
TTY:631-946-6585
www.siloinc.org/?

Edward Ahern, Manager
Glenn Campbell, Co-Executive Director
A not-for-profit organization that helps the disabled become more independent and more involved in the community by providing them with information on referrals on Housing, Education, Employment and Benefits.

4428 Taconic Resources for Independence
82 Washington St
Suite #214
Poughkeepsie, NY 12601-2305
845-452-3913
866-948-1094
Fax: 845-485-3196
tri@taconicresources.org
www.taconicresources.org

Cynthia L. Fiore, Executive Director
Patrick Muller, Program Director
Diane Barkstrom, Program Director/Staff Interpret
Jeanine Byrnes, Coordinator of Deaf & Hard of He
A center for independent living, benefits advisement information, and referral, advocacy, independent living skills, peer counseling, parent advocacy, sign language interpreters.

4429 Westchester Disabled on the Move
984 N. Broadway
Suite LL-10
Yonkers, NY 10701-1320
914-968-4717
Fax: 914-968-6137
info@wdom.org
www.wdom.org

Gail Cartenuto Cohn, President
Mattie Trupia, Vice President
Sandra Dolman, Secretary
Chandra Sookdeo, Assistant Recording Secretary
WDOM empowers people with disabilities to control their own lives; advocates for civil rights and a barrier free society; encourages people with disabilities to participate in the political process; educates government, business, other entities, and a society

as a whole to understand, accept, and accommodate people with disabilities; creates an environment that inspires self-respect

4430 Westchester Independent Living Center
200 Hamilton Avenue
2nd Floor
White Plains, NY 10601- 1809
914-682-3926
Fax: 914-682-8518
TTY:866-933-5390
Contact@wilc.org
www.wilc.org

Joseph Bravo, Executive Director
A not-for-profit, community-based advocacy and resource center that serves people with all types of disabilities.

North Carolina

4431 Disability Awareness Network
609 Country Club Dr.
Suite C
Greenville, NC 27834-6210
252-353-5522
Fax: 252-353-5160
DAWNpittco@aol.com

Jackie Hansley, Owner
Information and referral for diabled persons; peer counseling for diabled persons; advocacy on ADA issues; independent living skills and training.

4432 Disability Rights & Resources
5801 Executive Center Dr.
Suite #101
Charlotte, NC 28212-8870
704-537-0550
800-755-5749
Fax: 704-566-0507
TTY: 704-537-0550
mailto@disability-rights.org
www.disability-rights.org

Maura Chavez, President
Marta Fales, Vice President
Holly Howell, Secretary
Rick Griffiths, Treasurer
To guard the civil rights of people wtih disabilities by empowering ourselves and others to live as we choose.

4433 Joy: A Shabazz Center for Independent Living
235 N Greene St
Greensboro, NC 27401-2410
336-272-0501
Fax: 336-272-0575
TTY:336-272-0501

Aaron Shabazz, Executive Director
James Wells, President
Stephen Simpson, Vice-President
B. J. Gerald Covington, Secretary/Treasurer
A non-profit, consumer oriented, Center for Independent Living (CIL) providing advocacy, peer counseling and peer support, independent living skills, training, information and referrals, with other related services for persons with disabilites.

4434 Live Independently Networking Center
P.O.Box 1135
Newton, NC 28658-1135
828-464-0331
Fax: 828-464-7375
TTY:828-464-2838
www.linconline.org

Donavon Kirby, Deputy Director
Private, nonprofit, federally funded center for independent living located in Western North Carolina.

4435 Live Independently Networking Center: Hickory
2830 16th St NE
Apt. 17
Hickory, NC 28601-8606
828-464-0331
Fax: 828-464-7375

4436 Pathways for the Future Center for Independent Living
525 Mineral Springs Dr
Sylva, NC 28779-9077
828-631-1167
Fax: 828-631-1169
TTY:828-631-1167
bdavis@pathwayscil.org
www.pathwayscil.org

Barbara Davis, Executive Director
Dedicated to increasing independence, changing attitudes, promoting equal access and building a peer support network in western North Carolina through the use of community education, independent living services and advocacy.

4437 Western Alliance Center for Independent Living
30b London Rd
Asheville, NC 28803-2706
828-274-0444
Fax: 828-274-4461
westernalliance.org

Katy Hollingsworth, Manager
Jerry Brewton, Independent Living Specialist
.

4438 Western Alliance for Independent Living
108 New Leicester Highway
Asheville, NC 28806
828-298-1977
Fax: 828-298-0875
khollingsworth@disabilitypartners.org
www.disabilitypartners.org

Kathy Hollingsworth, Associate Director
Rosemary Weaver, Independent Living Specialist
Mechelle Holt, Volunteer/Program Coordinator
Eva Reynolds, Emploment Network Coordinator

North Dakota

4439 Dakota Center for Independent Living: Dickinson
26-1st street East
Suite 103
Dickinson, ND 58601-5103
701- 48- 436
800-489-5013
Fax: 701- 48- 436
TTY: 800489501363
dcil@ndsupernet.com
www.dakotacil.org

Robin Were, President
Claudia Ziegler, Vice president
Carol Mihulka, Secretary/Treasurer
Royce Schultze, Executive Director
Believes in self-determination for people with disabilities and creates the environment in which it is achieved.

4440 Dakota Center for Independent Living: Bismarck
3111 E Broadway Ave
Bismarck, ND 58501-5085
701-222-3636
800-489-5013
Fax: 701-222-0511
TTY: 701-222-3636
maryr@dakotacil.org
www.dakotacil.org

Robin Were, President
Cladia Ziegler, Vice president
Carol Mihulka, Secretary/Treasurer
Royce Schultze, Executive Director
Believes in self-determination for people with disabilities and creates the environment in which it is achieved.

4441 Fraser
2902 University Drive South
Fargo, ND 58103-6053
701-232-3301
Fax: 701-237-5775
fraser@fraserltd.org
fraserltd.org

Sandra Leyland, Executive Director
Mark Brodshaug, President
Michael Kirk, Vice President
David A. Laske, Treasurer

Private non-profit, federally funded center for independent living

4442   Freedom Resource Center for Independent Living: Fargo
2701 9th Ave S
Suite H
Fargo, ND   58103-8712

701-478-0459
800-450-0459
Fax: 701-478-0510
TTY: 701-478-0459
freedom@freedomrc.org
www.freedomrc.org

Nate Aalgaard, Executive Director
Angie Bosch, Office Coordinator
Mark Mark Bourdon Bourdon, Program Director
Andrea Nelson, Independent Living Advocate
To work toward equality and inclusion for people with disabilities through programs of empowerment, community education, and systems change.

4443   Resource Center for Independent Living: Minot
300 3rd Ave SW
Suite F
Minot, ND   58701-4346

701-839-4724
800-377-5114
Fax: 701-838-1677
TTY: 701-839-4724
independencecil@independencecil.org
www.independencecil.org/?

Susan Ogurek, Chair
Scott Burlingame, Executive Director
Dee Tischer, Senior Independent Living Specia
Jamie Hardt, Youth Transition Specialist
A resource center for independent living. Mission is to advocate for the freedom of choice for individuals with disabilities to live independently through the removal of all barriers.

Ohio

4444   Ability Center of Greater Toledo
5605 Monroe St
Sylvania, OH   43560-2702

419-885-5733
866-885-5733
Fax: 419-882-4813
TTY: 419-885-5733
www.abilitycenter.org

Tim Harrington, Executive Director
Lisa Justice, Executive Assistant
Dale Abell, Director of Programme Developmen
Debbie Keller, Tomorrow Planning Specialist
To assist people with disabilities to live, work and socialize within a fully accessible community.

4445   Ability Center of Greater Toledo: Defiance
5605 Monroe St
Sylvania, OH   43560-2702

419-885-5733
866-885-5733
Fax: 419-882-4813
TTY: 419-885-5733
www.abilitycenter.org

Tim Harrington, Executive Director
Lisa Justice, Executive Assistant
Dale Abell, Director of Programme Developmen
Debbie Keller, Tomorrow Planning Specialist
To assist people with disabilities to live, work and socialize within a fully accessible community.

4446   Ability Center of Greater Toledo: Port Clinton
1848 East Perry Street
Suite #110
Port Clinton, OH   43452-1802

419-734-0330
877-734-0330
Fax: 419-732-6864
TTY: 419-734-0330
www.abilitycenter.org

Tim Harrington, Executive Director
Lisa Justice, Executive Assistant
Dale Abell, Director of Programme Developmen
Debbie Keller, Tomorrow Planning Specialist
To assist people with disabilities to live, work and socialize within a fully accessible community.

4447   Access Center for Independent Living
901 S Ludlow St
Dayton, OH   45402-2614

937-341-5202
Fax: 937-341-5217
TTY:937-341-5218
info@acils.com
www.acils.com/?

Darrell Price, IL Team Co-Leader
Tonya Banther, IL Team Co-Leader
Melody Burba, Information & Referral Specialis
John Dixon, Information & Referral Specialis
Offers peer counseling, disability education and other services to the community.

4448   Center for Independent Living Options
2031 Auburn Avenue
Cincinnati, OH   45219-2436

513-241-2600
Fax: 513-241-1707
TTY:513-241-7170
cilo.net

Lin Laing, Executive Director
Justin Bifro, President
Brian Frazier, Vice-President
Ed Klene, Treasurer
The oldest center for independent living in Ohio serving individuals with disabilities in the Greater Cincinnati/Northern Kentucky region.

4449   Fairfield Center for Disabilities and Cerebral Palsy
681 E 6th Ave
Lancaster, OH   43130-2602

740-653-5501
Fax: 740-653-6046
fcdcp@sbcglobal.net
www.fcdcp.org

David Macioci, President
David Welsh, Vice-President
Mary Snider, Treasurer
Edwin R. Payne, Secretary
Adult Day Program and Transportation. The mission of the Fairfield Center for disabilities and Cerebral Palsy, Inc, is to create a better future for people with a disability by increasing and enhancing their lifestyle opportunities.

4450   Linking Employment, Abilities and Potential
2545 Lorain Ave.
Cleveland, OH   44113-3102

216-696-2716
Fax: 216-687-1453
www.leapinfo.org

Charles Heindrichs, President
Brian Roof, Vice President
Vincent Shemo, Treasurer
Betsey Kamm, Secretary
Consumer-directed to ensure a society of equal opportunity for all persons, regardless of disability.

4451 **Mid-Ohio Board for an Independent Living Environment (MOBILE)**
690 S High St
Columbus, OH 43206-1016

614-443-5936
Fax: 614-443-5954
TTY:614-443-5957
info@mobileonline.org
www.mobileonline.org

Darry Moore, President
Thomas Shapaka, Vice-President
Mark Morton, Treasurer
Warren King, Secretary

A non-profit Center for Independent Living directed by persons with disabilities. MOBILE was founded on principles that affirm the right of persons with disabilities to live their lives with a full measure of liberty and human dignity.

4452 **Ohio Statewide Independent Living Council**
670 Morrison Road
Suite 200
Gahanna, OH 43230-5324

614-892-0390
800-566-7788
Fax: 614-861-0392
www.ohiosilc.org

Kay Grier, Executive Director
Eugene Iacovetta, Special Projects Coordinator
Mary Butler, Systems Change Coordinator
Janae Miller, Office Manager

Committed to promoting a philosophy of consumer control, peer support, self-help, self-determination, equal acess, and individual and systems advocacy, in order to maximize leadership, empowerment, independence, productivity and to support full inclusion and integration of individuals with disabilities into the mainstream of American society.

4453 **Rehabilitation Service of North Central Ohio**
270 Sterkel Blvd
Mansfield, OH 44907-1508

419-756-1133
800-589-1133
Fax: 419-756-6544
info@therehabcenter.org
www.therehabcenter.org

Veronica L. Groff, President/CEO
Susan Baker, Chairman
Dan Wiegand, Vice-Chairman
Scott Donnenwirth, Secretary

Private nonprofit organization providing coordinated, team-oriented comprehensive outpatient rehabilitation services to children and adults of all ages. Serves 8 counties in N/C Ohio. Four umbrella areas of service include medical rehabilitation services, vocational rehabilitation services, behavioral health service and drug and alcohol addiction services. Medical rehabilitation services include physical therapy, occupational therapy, speech therapy and audiology.

4454 **Samuel W Bell Home for Sightless**
3775 Muddy Creek Rd
Cincinnati, OH 45238-2055

513-241-0720
Fax: 513-241-1481
swbellhome@fuse.net
www.samuelbell.org

Timothy Lighthal, President
Kevin Kappa, Vice-President
Miles L.Hoff, Treasurer
James Witte, Secretary

Offers a residential, independent living environment for blind and legally blind adults.

4455 **Services for Independent Living**
25100 Euclid Ave
Suite #105
Cleveland, OH 44117-2663

216-731-1529
Fax: 216-731-3083
TTY:216-731-1529
www.sil-oh.org

Lynn Hildebrand, Executive Director

Offers support ADA, consultation and education, advocacy, transitional education services, independent living skills training, information and referrals.

4456 **Society for Equal Access: Independent Living Center**
1458 5th St NW
New Philadelphia, OH 44663-1224

330-343-9292
888-213-4452
Fax: 330-602-7425
TTY:330-602-2557
www.seailc.org

Scott Huston, President
Edna Fillinger, Vice-President
Victoria Eichel, Secretary
Twyla Mccartney, Treasurer

The Society works with individuals to become more independent. Our agency assists with peer support, advocacy, information and referral, independent living skills and transportation. Our goal is to move those with challenges in the direction ofn independence.

Oklahoma

4457 **Ability Resources**
823 S Detroit Ave
Suite #110
Tulsa, OK 74120-4223

918-592-1235
800-722-0886
Fax: 918-592-5651
webadmin@ability-resources.org
www.ability-resources.org

Carla Lawson, Executive Director

To assist people with disabilities in attaining and maintaining their personal independence.

4458 **Green County Independent Living Resource Center**
4100 S.E. Adams Rd
Suite C-106
Bartlesville, OK 74006- 8409

918-335-1314
800-559-0567
Fax: 918-333-1814
TTY: 918-335-1314

Vicki Haws, Executive Director

Independent living skills training, information and referrals, advocacy, a loan library of adaptive equipment and books. Services available to all individuals with disabilities and their family members who reside in Northeastern Oklahoma.

4459 **Oklahomans for Independent Living**
601 East Carl Albert Parkway
McAlester, OK 74501-5410

918-426-6220
800-568-6821
Fax: 918-426-3245
TTY: 918-426-6263
info@oilok.org
www.oilok.org

Pam Pulchny, Executive Director/ADAspecialist
Terry Yates, Administrative Assistant/Bookke
Leanna Amos, Service Management Specialist
Stephen Strickland, Living Choice Coordinator

OIL encourages individuals of all ages, with all types of disabilities to increase: personal dependence; empowerment and self determiation; and ful integration and participation in their work, community, school and home activities.

4460 **Progressive Independence**
121 N Porter Avenue
Norman, OK 73071-5834

405-321-3203
800-801-3203
Fax: 405-321-7601
TTY: 405-321-2942
www.progind.org

Scott Spray, Chairperson
Teresa Tisdell, Vice Chair
Mark Newman, Treasurer
Mary Dulan, Secretary

Preovides four cores services of Information & Referral, Individaul& Systems Advocacy, Peer Counseling, and Skills Training; in addition, offers accessible computer lab, short term DME loans, ande benefits counseling for SSI/SSDI.

Oregon

4461   Abilitree
2680 NE Twin Knolls Dr.
Suite 3
Bend, OR   97701
                                                541-388-8103
                                                Fax: 541-389-2337
                                                TTY:541-388-8103
                                                www.abilitree.org

Tim Johnson, Executive Director
Greg Sublett, Director of Operations
April O'Meara, Marketing Director
Jen Michelson, Access Manager
CORIL empowers people with disabilities to maximize their independence, productivity and inclusio in community life. CORIL envisions a society where all people have the opportunity to develop their full capabilities with independence, productivity and more meaningful involvment in local community events and activities.

4462   Eastern Oregon Center for Independent Living
1021 SW 5th Ave
Ontario, OR   97914-3301
                                                541-889-3119
                                                866-248-8369
                                                Fax: 541-889-4647
                                                eocil@eocil.org
                                                www.eocil.org
Kirt Toombs, Executive Director
EOCIL is a nonprofit community based resource and advocacy center that promotes independent living and equal access for all persons with disabilities. EOCIL serves consumers in the counties of: Baker, Gilliam, Grant, harney, Malheur, Morrow, Umatilla, Union, Wallowa and Wheeler.

4463   HASL Independent Abilities Center
305 NE 'E' Street
Grants Pass, OR   97526
                                                541-479-4275
                                                800-758-4275
                                                Fax: 541-479-7261
                                                TTY: 541-479-3588
                                                haslstaff@yahoo.com
                                                www.haslonline.org
Randy Samuelson, Executive Director
To promote public awareness of the special needs and legal rights of individuals with cross-disabilities; to facilitate their integration into society and provide support through advocacy, peer counseling, skills training and information and referral to encourage independence.

4464   Independent Living Resources
1839 NE Couch Street
Portland, OR   97232-5308
                                                503-232-7411
                                                Fax: 503-232-7480
                                                TTY:503-232-8404
                                                info@ilr.org
                                                www.ilr.org/?
Barry Fox-Quamme, Executive Director
May Altman, LCSW, Associate Director
Barbara Norris, Office Manager, Executive Assist
Amy Camp, Independent Living Specialist, R
ILR looks to promote the philosophy of Independent Living by creating opportunities, encouraging choices, advancing equal access, and furthering the level of independence for all people with disabilities

4465   Laurel Hill Center
2145 Centennial Plaza
Eugene, OR   97401-2474
                                                541-485-6340
                                                Fax: 541-984-3124
                                                TTY:541-684-6822
                                                info@laurel.org
                                                www.laurel.org
Tom Fauria, President
DAVE Burtner, Vice-President
EDUARDO Sifuentez, Secretary
Lt. Jennifer Bills, Special operations
Provides natoinall-recognized, recovery-focused rehabilitation services in Lane County, Oregon, for people with severe and persistent mental illnesses

4466   Progressive Options
611 S.W. Hurbert Street
Suite A
Newport, OR   97365-9678
                                                541-265-4674
                                                Fax: 541-574-4313
                                                TTY:541-574-1927
                                                progop541@yahoo.com
                                                www.progressive-options.org
Rhonda Walker, Executive Director
Progressive Options seeks to provide free services and support to people with disabilities of all kinds to help them achieve and maintain maximum independence and self-sufficiency in Lincoln County and surrounding areas in Oregon.

4467   SPOKES Unlimited
1006 Main St
Klamath Falls, OR   97601-6029
                                                541-883-7547
                                                Fax: 541-885-2469
                                                TTY:541-883-7547
                                                www.spokesunlimited.org
Wendy Howard, Executive Director
Mission is to enhance the ability of people with disabilities to live more independently.

4468   Umpqua Valley Disabilities Network
736 SE Jackson Street
Roseburg, OR   97470-110
                                                541-672-6336
                                                Fax: 541-672-8606
                                                TTY:541-440-2882
                                                uvdn@uvdn.org
                                                www.uvdn.org
David Fricke, Executive Director
Heather Vialpando, Executive Assistant
UVDN's mission is to promote independent living and community inclusion for people with disabilities.

Pennsylvania

4469   Abilities in Motion
210 N 5th St
Reading, PA   19601-3304
                                                610-376-0010
                                                888-376-0120
                                                Fax: 610-376-0021
                                                TTY: 610-228-2301
                                                www.abilitiesinmotion.org
Terry Graul, Board President
David Lerch, Vice-President
Bonnie Milke, Treasurer
Ralph Trainer, Executive Director
Dedicated to advancing the rights of persons with disabilities in orer to promote a full life in the community through the prevention and elimination of physical, psychological, social and attitudinal barriers which serve to deny them the rights and privileges common to the general public.

4470   Anthracite Region Center for Independent Living
Pennsylvania Council on Independent Living
8 West Broad St
Suite 228
Hazleton, PA   18201-6418   570-455-9800
                                              800-777-9906
                                         Fax: 570-455-1731
                                          TTY: 570-455-9800
                                  dcorcoran@anthracitecil.org
Irene Mordosky, President
Margo Madden, Vice-President
Rand Martin, Treasurer
Tracy Clark, Secretary
Enables individuals with disabilities to attain their highest possible level of independence.

4471   Brian's House
757 Springdale Dr.
Exton, PA   19341-8531   610-399-1175
                                       ekihara@brianshouse.org
                                              brianshouse.org
Diana L. Ramsay, MPP, OTR, FAOT, Resident and Chief Executive Off
Peter M. Shubiak, MA, Executive Vice President and Chi
Lori Plunkettt, Executive Director
A non-profit organization that provides residential, vocational and recreational/respite programs for children and adults with intellectual and developmental disabilities.

4472   Community Resources for Independence
3410 W 12th St
Erie, PA   16505-3649   814-838-7222
                                              800-530-5541
                                         Fax: 814-838-8491
                                          TTY: 814-838-8115
                                              www.crinet.org
Timothy Finegan, Executive Director
William Essigmann, Administrative Program Manager
Carl Berry, Human Resources Director
Marty Pushchak, Controller
A community based, nonprofit, nonresidential organization that offers services and assistance to enable people with disabilities to expand their options, pursue their goals, and achieve and maintain self-sufficient and producitve lives in the community.

4473   Community Resources for Independence, Inc., Bradford
3410 West 12th Street
Erie, PA   16505   814-838-7222
                                              800-530-5541
                                         Fax: 814-838-8491
                                          TTY: 814-838-8115
                                                 crinet.org
Timothy J. Finegan, Executive Director
William Essigmann, Administrative Program Manager
Carl Berry, Human Resources Director
Marty Pushchak, Controller
Community Resources for Independence, Inc is committed to preserve, enhance and enrich the quality of life for all people with disabilities.

4474   Community Resources for Independence: Lewistown
33 East Hale Street
Suite L
Lewistown, PA   17044-2160   717-248-8011
                                              800-309-0989
                                         Fax: 717-248-8029
                                              www.crinet.org
Timothy Finegan, Executive Director
William Essigmann, Administrative Program Manager
Carl Berry, Human Resources Director
Marty Pushchak, Controller
A community based, nonprofit, nonresidential organization that offers services and assistance to enable people with disabilities to expand their options, pursue their goals, and achieve and maintain self-sufficient and producitve lives in the community.

4475   Community Resources for Independence: Altoona
1331 Twelth Ave
Suite #103
Altoona, PA   16601   814-994-2645
                                              866-944-2645
                                         Fax: 814-944-2683
                                              www.crinet.org
Timothy Finegan, Executive Director
William Essigmann, Administrative Program Manager
Carl Berry, Human Resources Director
Marty Pushchak, Controller
A community based, nonprofit, nonresidential organization that offers services and assistance to enable people with disabilities to expand their options, pursue their goals, and achieve and maintain self-sufficient and producitve lives in the community.

4476   Community Resources for Independence: Clarion
1200 Eastwood Drive
Suite #1
Clarion, PA   16214-8824   814-297-7141
                                              800-372-0140
                                         Fax: 814-297-7161
                                              www.crinet.org
Timothy J. Finegan, Executive Director
William Essigmann, Administrative Program Manager
Carl Berry, Human Resources Director
Marty Pushchak, Controller
A community based, nonprofit, nonresidential organization that offers services and assistance to enable people with disabilities to expand their options, pursue their goals, and achieve and maintain self-sufficient and producitve lives in the community.

4477   Community Resources for Independence: Clearfield
209 E Locust St
Clearfield, PA   16830-2422   814-765-6405
                                              866-619-6405
                                         Fax: 814-765-1269
                                              www.crinet.org
Timothy Finegan, Executive Director
William Essigmann, Administrative Program Manager
Carl Berry, Human Resources Director
Marty Pushchak, Controller
A community based, nonprofit, nonresidential organization that offers services and assistance to enable people with disabilities to expand their options, pursue their goals, and achieve and maintain self-sufficient and producitve lives in the community.

4478   Community Resources for Independence: Hermitage
3875 East State St
Suite B
Hermitage, PA   16148-3415   724-347-4121
                                         Fax: 724-347-5966
                                              www.crinet.org
Timothy J. Finegan, Executive Director
William Essigmann, Administrative Program Manager
Carl Berry, Human Resources Director
Marty Pushchak, Controller
A community based, nonprofit, nonresidential organization that offers services and assistance to enable people with disabilities to expand their options, pursue their goals, and achieve and maintain self-sufficient and producitve lives in the community.

4479   Community Resources for Independence: Lewisburg
11 Reitz Blvd
Suite #105
Lewisburg, PA   17837-1493   570-524-4314
                                              800-332-4135
                                         Fax: 570-524-9236
                                              www.crinet.org
Timothy J. Finegan, Executive Director
William Essigmann, Administrative Program Manager
Carl Berry, Human Resources Director
Marty Pushchak, Controller
A community based, nonprofit, nonresidential organization that offers services and assistance to enable people with disabilities to expand their options, pursue their goals, and achieve and maintain self-sufficient and producitve lives in the community.

4480 Community Resources for Independence: Oil City
250 Elm St
Oil City, PA 16301-1413   814-677-4655
866-209-3882
Fax: 814-677-4915
www.crinet.org

Tim Finegan, Executive Director
William Essigmann, Administrative Program Manager
Carl Berry, Human Resources Director
Marty Pushchak, Controller
A community based, nonprofit, nonresidential organization that offers services and assistance to enable people with disabilities to expand their options, pursue their goals, and achieve and maintain self-sufficient and producitve lives in the community.

4481 Community Resources for Independence: Warren
1003 Pennsylvania Ave W
Warren, PA 16365-1837   814-726-3404
866-579-3404
Fax: 814-726-3428
www.crinet.org

Timothy Finegan, Executive Director
William Essigmann, Administrative Program Manager
Carl Berry, Human Resources Director
Marty Pushchak, Controller
A community based, nonprofit, nonresidential organization that offers services and assistance to enable people with disabilities to expand their options, pursue their goals, and achieve and maintain self-sufficient and producitve lives in the community.

4482 Community Resources for Independence: Wellsboro
38 Plaza Ln
Wellsboro, PA 16901-1766   570-724-5852
866-401-7911
Fax: 570-724-3945
www.crinet.org

Timothy Finegan, Executive Director
William Essigmann, Administrative Program Manager
Carl Berry, Human Resources Director
Marty Pushchak, Controller
A community based, nonprofit, nonresidential organization that offers services and assistance to enable people with disabilities to expand their options, pursue their goals, and achieve and maintain self-sufficient and producitve lives in the community.

4483 Freedom Valley Disability Center
3607 Chapel Road
Suite B
Newtown Square, PA 19073-3602   610-353-6640
800-427-4754
Fax: 610-353-6753
TTY: 610-353-8900

Ann Cope, Executive Director
Assists persons with disabilities in the achievement of independent living goals. Also promotes individual and community options to maximize independence for persons with disabilities. Serves people with disabilities in Chester, Delaware, and Montgomery Counties.

4484 Institute on Disabilities At Temple Univ.
Temple University
1755 N. 13th St
Student Center, Rm. 4115
Philadelphia, PA 19122-6099   215-204-1356
Fax: 215-204-6336
iod@temple.edu
www.disabilities.temple.edu

James Earl Davis, Phd, Interim Executive Director
Celia Feinstein, Co-Executive- Director
Amy Goldman, Co-Executive- Director
Ann Marie White, Deputy- Director
Leads by example, creating connections and promoting networks within and among communitites so that people with disabilities are recognized as integral to the fabric of community life.

4485 Lehigh Valley Center for Independent Living
713 North 13th Street
Allentown, PA 18102-9121   610-770-9781
800-495-8245
Fax: 610-770-9801
TTY: 610-770-9789
info@lvcil.org
www.lvcil.org

Scott Berman, President
Michelle Mitchell, Vice President
Amy Beck, Executive Director
Cara Steidel, Fiscal Coordinator
Serves persons in Lehigh and Northampton Counties with any type of disability and/or his/her family.

4486 Liberty Resources
714 Market St
Suite #100
Philadelphia, PA 19106-2337   215-634-2000
888-634-2155
Fax: 215-634-6628
TTY: 215-634-6630
lrinc@libertyresources.org
www.libertyresources.org

Edwin Bomba, Chairman
Mary Ellen Caffrey, Chairman
Estelle B. Richman, Vice-Chairman
Thomas H. Earle, CEO
A non-profit, consumer driven organization that advocates and promotes Independent Living for persons with disabilities.

4487 Life and Independence for Today
503 E Arch St
Saint Marys, PA 15857-1779   814-781-3050
800-341-5438
Fax: 814-781-1917
TTY: 814-781-3050
lift@liftcil.org
www.liftcil.org

Stephen DePrater, President
Linda McKinstry, Vice-President
Larry Caggeso, Treasurer
Hope Weichman, Deputy Director
Offers services to enable people with disabilities to achieve new goals and broaden their horizons. It enables them to achieve and maintain self-sufficient and productive lives.

4488 Northeastern Pennsylvania Center for Independent Living
1142 Sanderson Ave
Suite #1
Scranton, PA 18509   570-344-7211
800-344-7211
Fax: 570-344-7218
TTY: 570-344-5275
nepacilinfo@nepacil.org
www.nepacil.org

Robert Treptow, President
Michael Sporer, Secretary
Chris Armone, Esq, Treasurer
Established to assist in removing barriers and expanding independent living options available to people with disabilities.

4489 South Central Pennsylvania Center for Independence Living
1019 Logan Blvd
Altoona, PA 16602-2434   814-949-1905
800-237-9009
Fax: 814-949-1909
TTY: 814-949-1912
cilscpa@cilscpa.org
www.cilscpa.org

Susan Estep, Executive Director
The missio of the Center for Independent Living of South Central PA is to empower people with disabilities to lead independent lives in their commnuitites. The Center covers Bedford, Blair, cambria, Fulton, Huntingdon, Indiana and Somerset counties.

4490   Three Rivers Center for Independent Living: New Castle
900 Rebecca Ave
Pittsburgh, PA   15221-9383   412-371-7700
                                           800-633-4588
                                           Fax: 412-371-9430
                                           TTY: 412-371-6230
                                           lgray@trcil.org
                                           www.trcil.myfastsite.net/
Kourtney T. Diaz, Chairperson
Shanicka Kennedy, Esq, Vice-Chairperson
Stanley A Holbrook, President
Rachel Rogan, Chief Executive Officer
To empower people with disabilities to enjoy self-directed, per-
sonally meaningful lives by providing outstanding consumer
controlled services and by advocating for effective community
college.

4491   Three Rivers Center for Independent Livi ng: Washington
900 Rebecca Ave
Pittsburgh, PA   15221-4425   412-371-7700
                                           800-633-4588
                                           Fax: 412-371-9430
                                           TTY: 412-371-6230
                                           lgray@trcil.org
                                           www.trcil.myfastsite.net/
Stanley A Holbrook, President
Kourtney T. Diaz, Chairperson
Shanicka Kennedy, Esq, Vice-Chairperson
Roxanne Huss, Director of Waiver Services
To empower people with disabilities to enjoy self-directed, per-
sonally meaningful lives by providing outstanding consumer
controlled services and by advocating for effective community
college.

4492   Three Rivers Center for Independent Living
900 Rebecca Ave
Pittsburgh, PA   15221-2938   412-371-7700
                                           800-633-4588
                                           Fax: 412-371-9430
                                           TTY: 412-371-6230
                                           lgray@trcil.org
                                           www.trcil.myfastsite.net/
Stanley A Holbrook, President
Kourtney T. Diaz, Chairperson
Shanicka Kennedy, Esq, Vice-Chairperson
Roxanne Huss, Director of Waiver Services
To empower people with disabilities to enjoy self-directed, per-
sonally meaningful lives by providing outstanding consumer
controlled services and by advocating for effective community
college.

4493   Tri-County Patriots for Independent Living
69 East Beau St
Washington, PA   15301-4711   724-223-5115
                                          877-889-0965
                                          Fax: 724-223-5119
                                          TTY: 724-228-4028
                                          www.tripil.com
Kathleen Kleinmann, Chief Executive Officer
Maxine Berton, Administrative Assistant
Jeffry D. Woods, Chief Information Officer
Jan Crockett, Chief Financial Officer
Brings together individuals who share common problems in
equal access, education, housing, employment, attendant care,
transportation, and access to technology.

4494   Voices for Independence
1107 Payne Ave
Erie, PA   16503-1741   814-874-0064
                                          866-407-0064
                                          Fax: 814-874-3497
                                          TTY: 814-874-0064
                                          web@vficil.org
                                          www.vficil.org
Shona Eakin, Executive Director
Edna Anabui, Executive Administrative Assista
Doug McClintock, Director of Finances
Colleen Porath, Accountant

To empower people with disabilities and promote independent
living.

Rhode Island

4495   Arc of Blackstone
500 Prospect St.
Wing B, Suite 203
Pawtucket, RI   2860- 4396   401-727-0150
                                          800-257-6092
                                          Fax: 401-727-1545
                                          contact@bvcriarc.org
                                          www.bvcriarc.org
Kathleen O'Neill, President
Thomas E. Hodge, Vice-President
Joseph F. McEnness, Treasurer
A. Melanie Cherry, Secretary
Committed to supporting people with developmental disabilities
secure the opportunity to choose and realize their goals of where
and how they live, learn, work and play

4496   Franklin Court Assisted Living
180 Franklin St
Bristol, RI   2809-3352   401-253-3679
                                          Fax: 401-253-5855
                                          www.ebcdc.org
Michelle Belmore Cabana, Chief Financial Officer
Brenda Marshall, Administrator
Lynn A. Marshall, Property Manager
Jennifer Morra, Administrative Assistant
Offers local seniors an affordable assisted living option with
first-rate services and gracious accommodations.

4497   IN-SIGHT Independent Living
43 Jefferson Blvd
Warwick, RI   2888-1078   401-941-3322
                                          Fax: 401-941-3356
                                          cbutler@in-sight.org
                                          www.in-sight.org
Jean Saylor, Chairman
Robert Tyler, Vice-Chairman
James Hahn, Treasurer
Karl Sherry, Secretary
Creating opportunities and choices for people who are blind and
visually impaired

4498   Ocean State Center for Independent Living
1944 Warwick Avenue
Warwick, RI   2889-2448   401-738-1013
                                          866-857-1161
                                          Fax: 401-738-1083
                                          TTY: 401-738-1015
                                          info@oscil.org
                                          www.oscil.org
Lorna Ricci, Executive Director
OSCIL is a consumer controlled, community based, nonprofit organization established to provide a range of independent living
services to enhance, through self direction, the quality of life of
Rhode Islander with significant disability and to promote integration into the community.

4499   Office of Rehabilitation Services
40 Fountain St
Suite #4B
Providence, RI   2903-1898   401-421-7005
                                          Fax: 401-421-7016
                                          www.ors.ri.gov
Ronald Racine, Associate Director
Kathleen Brown, Acting Administrator ORD
Ron Racine, Deputy Administrator Blind
John Microulis, Deputy Administrator Disability
Their goal is to help individuals with physical and mental disabil-
ities prepare for and obtain appropriate employment.

4500 PARI Independent Living Center
500 Prospect St
Pawtucket, RI 2860-6259

401-725-1966
Fax: 401-725-2104
TTY:401-725-1966
info@pari-ilc.org
www.pari-ilc.org

Leo Canuel, Executive Director
Sue Bilodau, Program Director
Offers information and referral services, personal care attendant services, home modifications, advocacy services and peer counseling, independent living skills training, and recycled equipment.

South Carolina

4501 Columbia Disability Action Center
136 Stonemark Lane
Suite #100
Columbia, SC 29210

800-681-6805
Fax: 803-779-5114
TTY:803-779-0949
www.able-sc.org/

David Dawson, President
Rochelle Gadson, Vice President
Joe Butler, Treasurer
Angela Jacildone, Secretary
A non-profit consumer governed Center for Independent Living. Programs and services support persons with disabilities in taking full advantage of community resources, enhancing personal opportunities, and determining the direction of their lives.

4502 Disability Action Center
330B Pelham Rd
Suite 100 A
Greenville, SC 29615-3116

864-235-1421
800-681-7715
Fax: 864-235-2056
TTY: 864-235-8798
amayne@dacsc.org
www.able-sc.org/

David Dawson, President
Rochelle Gadson, Vice President
Joe Butler, Treasurer
Angela Jacildone, Secretary
Empowering people with disabilities to reach their highest level of independence.

4503 Graham Street Community Resources
306 Graham St
Florence, SC 29501-4735

843-665-6674
Fax: 843-665-6674
Faye Thompson, Manager
Promotes independent living and empowers people with disabilities to reach their highest level of independence.

4504 South Carolina Independent Living Council
136 Stonemark Lane
Suite #100
Columbia, SC 29210-7318

803-217-3209
800-994-4322
Fax: 803-731-1439
TTY: 803-217-3209
scilc@scilconline.org
www.scsilc.com

Mike Le Fever, President
Committed to equal opportunity, equal access, self determination, independence, and choice for all people with disabilities and pursues these goals by the means available.

4505 Walton Options for Independent Living: North Augusta
325 Georgia Ave
North Augusta, SC 29841-3848

803-279-9611
Fax: 803-279-9135
tjohnston@waltonoptions.org
www.waltonoptions.org
Cynthia Anzek, Executive Director
Empowers persons of all ages with all types of disabilities to reach their highest level of independence, community inclusion and employment.

South Dakota

4506 Adjustment Training Center
607 N 4th St
Aberdeen, SD 57401-2733

605-229-0263
Fax: 605-225-3455
www.aspiresd.org

Jennifer Gray, Executive Director
Arlette Keller, Director of Service Coordination
Angela Huffman, Director of Nursing
Paul Schumacher, Director of Vocational Services
Offers peer counseling, attendant care registry and referrals.

4507 Black Hills Workshop & Training Center
Black Hills Workshop
3650 Range Road
PO Box 2104
Rapid City, SD 57709-2104

605-343-4550
Fax: 605-343-0879
TTY:800-877-1113
drosby@bhws.com
www.blackhillsworks.org

Brad Saathoff, Chief Executive Officer
Janet Niehaus, VP of Finance
Michelle Aman, VP of Residential Services
Helen Usera, VP of Development
Offers job placement, housing options, case coordination, supported employment and supported living for all disability groups, as well as specialized services for brian injury victims.

4508 Communication Service for the Deaf: Rapid City
200 W Cesar Chavez St
Suite 650
Austin, TX 78701-694

844-222-0002
800-642-6410
Fax: 605-394-6609
TTY: 866-273-3323
csd@csd.org
www.c-s-d.org

Dr. Benjamin Soukup, Founder, Chairman & CEO
Christopher Soukup, President
Brad Hermes, Chief Financial Officer
Christina Kokenge, Vice President, Human Resources
A private, nonprofit organization dedicated to providing broad-based services, ensuring public accessibility and increasing public awareness of issues affecting deaf and hard of hearing inividuals.

4509 Native American Advocacy Program for Persons with Disabilities
P.O.Box 527
Winner, SD 57580-527

605-842-3977
800-303-3975
Fax: 605-842-3983
TTY: 605-842-3977

Marla Bull Bear, Executive Director
Charles Bull Bear, Specialist
Betty Farr, Il Specialist
Megan L. Garcia, Prevention Specialist
The mission is to encourage a healthy organization that assists Native Americans with disabilities, by providing prevention, education and training, advocacy, support, independent living skills and referrals.

4510   Prairie Freedom Center for Independent Living: Sioux Falls
4107 S Carnegie Cr
Suite #9
Sioux Falls, SD 57106-3100   605-362-3550
                                      Fax: 605-367-5639
                                      i-l-c@ilcchoices.org
                                      www.ilcchoices.org

Steve Tripp, President
Cheri Raymond, Vice President
Matt Cain, Executive Director
Laura Staebner, Treasurer
Established to provide basic skills so many of us take for granted:
to take care of our own needs and to make our own decisions to be
independent.

4511   Prairie Freedom Center for Independent Li ving: Madison
4107 S Carnegie Cr
411 SE 10th St
Sioux Falls, SD 57106-3570   605-362-3550
                                      Fax: 605-256-5071
                                      i-l-c@ilcchoices.org
                                      www.ilcchoices.org

Steve Tripp, President
Cheri Raymond, Vice President
Matt Cain, Executive Director
Laura Staebner, Treasurer
Established to provide basic skills so many of us take for granted:
to take care of our own needs and to make our own decisions to be
independent.

4512   Prairie Freedom Center for Independent Living: Yankton
4107 S Carnegie Cr
Suite #107
Sioux Falls, SD 57106-2800   605-362-3550
                                      Fax: 605-668-3060
                                      TTY:605-668-3060
                                      i-l-c@ilcchoices.org
                                      www.ilcchoices.org

Steve Tripp, President
Cheri Raymond, Vice President
Matt Cain, Executive Director
Laura Staebner, Treasurer
Established to provide basic skills so many of us take for granted:
to take care of our own needs and to make our own decisions to be
independent.

4513   South Dakota Assistive Technology Project: DakotaLink
1161 Deadwood Ave N
Suite #5
Rapid City, SD 57702-382   605-394-6742
                                      800-645-0673
                                      Fax: 605-394-6744
                                      TTY: 605-394-6742
                                      atinfo@dakotalink.net

Pat Czerny, Manager
Patrick Czerny, Technical Services Coordinator
David Scherer, Program Coordinator
DakotaLink, the South Dakota Assistive Technology Program,
provides resources and supports to individuals of all ages to ensure greater access to and acquisition of assistive technology devices and services.

4514   Western Resources for dis-ABLED Independence
405 East Omaha St
Suite D
Rapid City, SD 57701-2974   605-718-1930
                                      888-434-4943
                                      Fax: 605-718-1933
                                      TTY: 605-718-1930
                                      chad@wril.org
                                      www.wril.org

Jeff Wangen, President
Dennis Coull, Vice-President
Linda Lockner, Secretary
Mike Pendo, Treasurer
WRDI advocates for the rights of equal inclusion of people with
disabilities in all aspects of community life. WRDI also strives to
identify and promote access to existing resources and to advocate

for the development of new resources, which may enable people
with disabilities to live more independently.

Tennessee

4515   Center for Independent Living of Middle Tennessee
955 Woodland St
Nashville, TN   37206-3753   615-292-5803
                                      866-992-4568
                                      Fax: 615-383-1176
                                      TTY: 615-292-7790

Tom Hopton, Executive Director
Tria Bridgeman, Benefits Analyst-Jackson
Dylan Brown, Benefits Analyst-Nashville
Pattrick Gallaher, Employment Assistant-Nashville

CILMT provides persons with disabilities opportunities to be self
advocates and make their own decisions regarding living arrangements, means of transportation, employment, social and
recreational activities, as well as other aspects of everyday life.
Serves Davidson, Cheatham, Wilson, Robertson, Rutherford,
Sumner and Williamson Counties.

4516   DisAbility Resource Center: Knoxville
900 E Hill Ave
Suite 205
Knoxville, TN   37915-2567   865-637-3666
                                      Fax: 865-637-5616
                                      TTY:865-637-6976
                                      drc@drctn.org
                                      www.drctn.org

Lillian Burch, Executive Director
Nicole Craig, Programme Director
Katherine Moore, Independent Living Specialist
Basil Farris, Employment Coach
DRCTN mission is to empower people with disabilities to fully
integrate and participate in the community. DRC is a community-based non-residential program of services designed to assist
people with disabilities to gain independence and to assist the
community in eliminating barriers of independence.

4517   Jackson Center for Independent Living
1981 Hollywood Drive
Jackson, TN   38305-4388   731-668-2211
                                      Fax: 731-668-0406
                                      TTY:731-664-3970
                                      www.j-cil.com

Glen Barr, Executive Director
JCIL works with people with significant disabilities and the Deaf
Community in achieving their Independent Living Goals while
assisting the community in eliminating barriers to Independent
Living.

4518   Memphis Center for Independent Living
1633 Madison Ave
Memphis, TN   38104-2506   901-726-6404
                                      800-848-0298
                                      Fax: 901-726-6521
                                      TTY: 901-726-6404
                                      info@mcil.org
                                      www.mcil.org

Kevin Lofton, Chairman
Marvin Glenn Bailey, Vice-Chairman
Charles M. Weirich, Jr., Board Counsel
MCIL is a community based non-profit organization whose pri-
mary mission is to facilitate the full integration of persons with
disabilities into all aspects of community life.

4519   Tennessee Technology Access Program (TTAP)
400 Deaderick St
14th Fl
Nashville, TN   37243-1403   615-313-5183
                                               800-732-5059
                                          Fax: 615-532-4685
                                          TTY: 615-313-5695
                                         tn.ttap@state.tn.us
                        www.state.tn.us/humanserv/rehab/ttap.html
Kevin Wright, Director
TTAP's mission is to maintain a statewide program of technology-rated assistance that is timely, comprehensive and consumer driven to ensure that all Tennesseans with disabilities have the information, services and deices that they need to make choices about where and how they spend their time as independently as possible. .

4520   Tri-State Resource and Advocacy Corporation
6925 Shallowford Rd
#300
Chattanooga, TN   37421   423-892-4774
                                               800-868-8724
                                          Fax: 423-892-9866
                                          TTY: 423-892-4774
                                         4trac@bellsouth.net
                                              www.1trac.org
Mark Woofall, Executive Director
Pam Jackson, Independent Living Facilitator
TRAC is dedicated to improving opportunities for individuals wuth disabilities.

Texas

4521   ABLE Center for Independent Living
1931 E 37th
St # 1
Odessa, TX   79762-6906   432-580-3439
                                         info@ablecenterpb.org
                                          www.ablecenterpb.org
Marilyn Hancock, Executive Director
Kathleen Story MA, Independent Living Specialist
Britni Veretto, HR Manager
To promote independent living for people with disabilities.

4522   Austin Resource Center for Independent Living
825 E. Rundberg Ln
Suite E6
Austin, TX   78753-4813   512-832-6349
                                               800-414-6327
                                          Fax: 512-832-1869
                                            arcil@arcil.com
                                              www.arcil.com
Ross Davis, Chair
Linda Loach, Vice-Chair
Sylvia Davis, Secretary/Treasurer
Vonnye Gardner, Member
Serving people with disabilities, their families and communities throughout Travis and surrounding counties.

4523   Austin Resource Center: Round Rock
525 Round Rock West
Suite A120
Round Rock, TX   78681-5020   512-828-4624
                                          Fax: 512-828-4625
                                            sally@arcil.com
                                              www.arcil.com
Ross Davis, Chair
Linda Loach, Vice-Chair
Sylvia Davis, Secretary/Treasurer
Vonnye Gardner, Member
Serving peole with disabilities, their families and communities throughout Travis and surrounding counties.

4524   Austin Resource Center: San Marcos
618 South Guadalupe St
Suite #103
San Marcos, TX   78666- 6977   512-396-5790
                                               800-572-2973
                                          Fax: 512-396-5794
                                         sanmarcos@arcil.com
                                              www.arcil.com
Ross Davis, Chair
Linda Loach, Vice-Chair
Sylvia Davis, Secretary/Treasurer
Vonnye Gardner, Member
Serving people with disabilities, their families and communities throughout Travis and surounding counties.

4525   Brazoria County Center For Independent Living
1104D East Mullberry Street
Suite D
Angleton, TX   77515- 3952   979-849-7060
                                               888-872-7957
                                          Fax: 979-849-8465
                                          TTY: 979-849-7060
                                           bccil@neosoft.com
                                              www.hcil.cc
Chamane Barrow, Manager
To promote the full inclusion, equal opportunity and participation of persons with disabilities in every aspect of community life. We believe that people with disabilities have the right to make choices affecting their lives, a right to take risks, a right to fail, and a right to succeed.

4526   Centre, The
3550 West Dallas Rd
Houston, TX   77019   713-525-8400
                                          Fax: 713-525-8444
                                          thecenterhouston.org
Bill Coorsh, President
Richard Rosenberg, Vice-President
Lisa F. Schott, Secretary
Glen Shepherd, Treasurer
Provides services for more than 600 children and adults with mental retardation and other developmental disabilities. The Center also offers a wide array of programs including education, vocational training and job placement services, three different residential options representing both urban and rural living environments, special programs designed to meet the needs of older adults, and a variety of therapeutic support services.

4527   Crockett Resource Center for Independent Living
1020 Loop 304 East
Crockett, TX   75835-1806   936-544-2811
                                          Fax: 936-544-7315
                                          TTY:936-544-2811
                                         crcil@windstream.net
                                    www.crockettresourcecenter.org
Sara Minton, Executive Director
Mary Killough, Chief Financial Officer
Cathy Newsome, Information/Outreach Coordinator
Debbie Oliver, Information and Outreach Coor.
Provides independent living services to cross-disability groups to increase their personal self-determination and minimize dependence on others. Maintain comprehensive information on availability of resources and provides referrals to such resources. Provides instruction to assist people with disabilities to gain skills that would empower them to live independently. Peer counseling, advocacy - both individual and community by assisting to obtain support services to make changes in society.

4528   Houston Center for Independent Living (HCIL)
6201 Bonhomme Rd.
Suite 150-South
Houston, TX   77036   713-974-4621
                                          Fax: 713-974-6927
                                           hcil@neosoft.com
                                              www.hcil.cc
Sandra Bookman, Executive Director
Advocacy organization created by and for people with disabilities (PWD) to empower and protect their rights. Services include

but not limited to: peer to peer support, individual and systems advocacy, independent living skills training, information and referral, disability cultural awareness, ASL and Braille classes, ADA technical assistance, Relocation/Transition to Community Services, computer technology training, SSA Work Incentives Technical Assistance, equipment loan program.

4529 Independent Life Styles
215 North Benton Drive
Sauk Rapids, MN   56379-1874
320-529-9000
888-529-0743
Fax: 320-529-0747
ilicil@independentlifestyles.org
www.independentlifestyles.org
Karen Ahles, Chair
Jay Keller, Educator
Cara Ruff, Executive Director
Chad Hansen, Community Member
Offers peer counseling, advocacy and other services to the community.

4530 Independent Living Research Utilization Project
Institute For Rehabilitation & Research
1333 Moursund
Houston, TX   77030
713-520-0232
Fax: 713-520-5785
TTY:713-520-0232
ilru@ilru.org
www.ilru.org
Lex Frieden, Director
Linda CoVan, Grant Coordinator
Maria Del Bosque, Project Associate
Diego Demaya, Legal Specialist
ILRU is a national center for information, training, research and technical assistance in independent living. Its goal is to expand the body of knowledge in independent living and to improve utilization of results of research programs and demonstration projects in this field. ILRU is a program of The Institute for Rehabilitation and Research, a nationally recognized medical rehabilitation facility for persons with disabilities. TTY phone number: (713) 520-5136.

4531 LIFE/ Run Centers for Independent Living
8240 Boston Avenue
Lubbock, TX   79423-2342
806-795-5433
Fax: 806-795-5607
TTY:806-795-5433
wilmacrain@yahoo.com
www.liferun.org
Michelle Crain, Executive Director
Committed to providing individuals with disabilities the information and skills necessary to become independent and to achieve full inclusion in every aspect of their life.

4532 Office for Students with Disabilities, University of Texas at Arlington
701 South Nedderman Drive
Arlington, TX   76019-1
817-272-3364
800-735-2989
Fax: 817-272-1447
TTY: 800-735-2989
helpdesk@uta.edu
www.uta.edu/disability
Penny Acrey, Director
Demarice Ferguson, MS, CRC, Associate Director
Scott Holmes, Assistant Director for Testing
Gilda Williams, BSW, Office Manager
Offers disability counseling and academic accomodation to UT Arlington community.

4533 Palestine Resource Center for Independent Living
421 Avenue a St
Palestine, TX   75801-2903
903-729-7505
888-326-5166
Fax: 903-729-7540
TTY:903-729-7505
prcil@embarqmail.com
www.palestineresourcecenter.org/?
Sara Minton, Executive Director
Mary Killough, Chief Financial Officer
Cathy Newsome, Information/Outreach Coordinator
Debbie Oliver, Information and Outreach Coor.
Provides independent living services to cross-disability groups to increase their personal self-determination and minimize dependence on others. Maintain comprehensive information on availability of resources and provides referrals to such resources. Provides instruction to assist people with disabilities to gain skills that would empower them to live independently. Peer counseling, advocacy - both individual and community by assisting to obtain support services to make changes in society.

4534 Panhandle Action Center for Independent Living Skills
417 W. 10th Avenue
Amarillo, TX   79101-4316
806-374-1400
Fax: 806-374-4550
TTY:806-374-2774
info@panhandleilc.org
www.panhandleilc.org
Joe Rogers, Executive Director
Alma Benavides, Employment Director
Chris White, Development Director
Cynthia Hammett, Consumer Coordinator & Youth Tra
PILC is a non profit organization dedicated to the advancement of full participation in all aspects of life. PILC services are developed, directed, delivered, and governed primarily by individuals with disabilities.

4535 REACH of Dallas Resource Center on Independent Living
8625 King George Drive
Suite 210
Dallas, TX   75235-2286
214-630-4796
Fax: 214-630-6390
TTY:214-630-5995
reachdallas@reachcils.org
www.reachcils.org
Charlotte A. Stewart, Executive Director
Kevan Johnson, Employment Consultant
Janie Peachee, Information & Referral Specialis
Kiowanda Jasso, Information & Referral Specialis
Information and referral, peer support/peer counseling, independent living skills training and advocacy assistance.

4536 REACH of Denton Resource Center on Independent Living
405 S. Elm St
Suite 202
Denton, TX   76201-6068
940-383-1062
Fax: 940-383-2742
reachden@reachcils.org
www.reachcils.org
Charlotte A. Stewart, Executive Director
Missy Dickenson, Assistant Director
Murphy Hardinger, IL Skills Training & ADA Special
Becky Teal, Office Manager
To provide for people with disabilities so that they are enabled to lead self-directed lives and to educate the general public about disability-related topics in order to promote a barrier free community.

4537 **REACH of Fort Worth Resource Center on Independent Living**
1000 Macon Street
Suite 200
Fort Worth, TX 76102-4527 817-870-9082
Fax: 817-877-1622
TTY:817-870-9086
reachftw@reachcils.org
www.reachcils.org

Charlotte A. Stewart, Executive Director
Missy Dickenson, Assistant Director
Murphy Hardinger, IL Skills Training & ADA Special
Becky Teal, Office Manager
To provide services for people with disabilities so that they are enabled to lead self-directed lives and to educate the general public about disability-related topics in order to promote a barrier free community.

4538 **RISE-Resource: Information, Support and Empowerment**
755 11th Street
Suite 101
Beaumont, TX 77701-3723 409-832-2599
Fax: 409-838-4499
TTY:409-832-2599
www.risecil.org

Jim Brocato, Executive Director
Amanda Powe, Relocation Services Specialist
Cheryl Bass, Program Director
Gracie Jackson, Independent Living Specialist
A non-profit center for independent living.

4539 **SAILS**
1028 S Alamo St
San Antonio, TX 78210-1170 210-281-1878
800-474-0295
Fax: 210-281-1759
TTY: 210-281-1878
kbrietzke@sailstx.org
www.sailstx.org

Patricia Byrd, Chair
Dennis Wolf, Vice Chair
Jerry D. King, Treasurer
Donna McBee, Member
SAILS advocates for the rights and empowerment of people with disabilities in San Antonio; as well as surrounding areas. Services are provided to people with disabilities in the following counties: Atacosa, Bandera, Bexar, Calhoun, Comal, DeWitt, Dimmit, Edwards, Frio, Gillespie, Goliad, Gonzalez, Guadalupe, Jackson, Karnes, La Salle, Kendall, Kerr, Kinney, Lavaca, Maverick, Medina, Real, Uvalde, Val Verde, Victoria, Wilson and Zavala.

4540 **Texas Department of Assistive and Rehabilitative Services**
4800 N. Lamar Blvd
Austin, TX 78756 512-472-4138
800-628-5115
Fax: 512-472-0603
TTY: 866-581-9328
dars.inquiries@dars.state.tx.us
www.dars.state.tx.us

Bill West, Manager
Daniel Bravo, Chief Operating Officer
Rebecca Trevino, Chief Financial Officer
Glenn Neal, Deputy Commissioner
Provides technical assistance and other support services to the state's Independent Living Council, Independent Living Centers and Independent Living Counseling programs.

4541 **VOLAR Center for Independent Living**
1220 Golden Key Circle
El Paso, TX 79925-5825 915-591-0800
800-591-0800
Fax: 915-591-3506
TTY: 915-591-0800
volar@volarcil.org
www.volarcil.org

Luis Chew, Executive Director
Danny Monroe, Chief Financial Officer
Nena Garcia, Records Manager/ Bookkeeper
Thelma Hernandez, Office Manager
VOLAR is committed to providing independent living ervices and information and referral, and to developing community options for persons with cross disabilities to empower them to live the kind of lives they choose. VOLAR is an organization of and for people with disabilities, advocating human and civil rights, community options and empowering people to live the lives they choose. Newsletter available.

4542 **Valley Association for Independent Living (VAIL)**
3012 N McColl Road
McAllen, TX 78501 956-668-8245
866-400-8245
Fax: 956-878-1601
info@vailrgv.org
vailrgv.org

Woodie Johnston, Executive Director
Offers information and referral, peer couseling, MS supprt group, independent living skills training, and advocacy, work incentives planning and assistance, transitioning people with disabilities from the nursing home into the community.

4543 **Valley Association for Independent Living: Harlingen**
1824 W. Jefferson Ave
Suite B
Harlingen, TX 78550-5247 956-428-1126
866-400-8245
Fax: 956-428-4339
www.valleyassociation.org

Soledad Myers, Manager
Provides information and referral, peer counseling, support groups, independent living skills training, community rehab program and advocacy

Utah

4544 **Active Re-Entry**
10 S Fairgrounds Rd
Price, UT 84501 435-637-4950
Fax: 435-637-4952
TTY:435-637-4950
active@arecil.org
www.arecil.org

Nancy Bentley, Executive Director
Active Re-Entry is a community based program which assists individuals with disabilities to acheive or maintain self-sufficient and productive live in their own communities. Active Re-Entry is committed to promoting the rights, dignity, and quality of life for all persons with disabilities.

4545 **Active Re-Entry: Vernal**
10 S Fairgrounds Rd
Price, UT 84501-9727 435-637-4950
Fax: 435-789-6090
TTY:435-789-4021
active@arecil.org
www.arecil.org

Heather Moore, President
Active Re-Entry is a community based program which assists individuals with disabilities to achieve or maintain self-sufficient and productive lives in their own communities. We are committed to promoting the rights, dignity, and quality of life for all persons with disabilities.

4546 Central Utah Independent Living Center
3445 S Main St
Salt Lake City, UT   84115-2824   801-466-5565
                                                  877-421-4500
                                          Fax: 801-466-2363
                                          TTY: 801-373-5044
                                          uilc@uilc.org
                                          www.uilc.org

Debra Mair, Executive Director
Kim Meichle, Assistant Director
Patty Trent, Fiscal Manager
Shauna Brock, Independent Living Specialist
Empowers people with disabilities to reach their full potential in community settings through peer support, advocacy, and education.

4547 OPTIONS for Independence
Northern Utah Center for Independent Living
106 East 1120 N
Logan, UT   84341-2215   435-753-5353
                                          Fax: 435-753-5390
                                          TTY:435-753-5353
                                          www.optionsind.org

Cheryl Atwood, Executive Director
OPTIONS for Independence, the Northern Utah Center for Independent Living serves people of all ages with all types of disabilities. OPTIONS is a nonresidential Center that provides services to individuals with disabilities to facilitate their full participation in the community and raise the understanding of disability issues and access to the community. The Independent Living philosophy is strictly adhered to: consumer control and choice being the focus.

4548 OPTIONS for Independence: Brigham Satellite
106 East 1120 N
Logan, UT   84341-3379   435-753-5353
                                          Fax: 435-753-5390
                                          TTY:435-723-2171
                                          dcrockett@qwestoffice.net
                                          www.optionsind.org

Cheryl Atwood, Executive Director
Deanna Crockett, Manager
OPTIONS is a nonresidential Independent Living Center where people with disabilities can learn skills to gain more control and independence over their lives. OPTIONS raises the vision and capability of the community at large to the point where people of all abilities will have equal access.

4549 Red Rock Center for Independence
515 W 300 N
Suite A
Saint George, UT   84770-4578   435-673-7501
                                          800-649-2340
                                          Fax: 435-673-8808
                                          rrci@rrci.org
                                          www.rrci.org

Barbara Lefler, Executive Director
Jerry Salkowe, President
Celeste Sorensen, Secretary
Joseph Gordon, Treasurer
Red Rock Center for Independence assists people with disabilities to live and participate independently.

4550 Tri-County Independent Living Center
P.O.Box 428
Ogden, UT   84402-428   801-612-3215
                                          866-734-5678
                                          Fax: 801-612-3732
                                          TTY: 801-612-3215
                                          www.uilc.org

Richard Fox, Chairperson
Kim Price, Vice-Chairperson
Greg Killpack, Secretary/Treasurer
Debra Mair, Executive Director
The mission of the Tri-County ILC is to enhance independence for all people with disabilities. Serves Davis, Weber and Morgan Counties.

4551 Utah Assistive Technology Program (UTAP) Utah State University
6855 Old Main Hill
Logan, UT   84322-6855   435-797-3811
                                          800-524-5152
                                          Fax: 435-797-2355
                                          www.uatpat.org

Sachin Pavithran, UATP Program Director
Marilyn Hammond, Utah Assistive Technology Founda
Lois Summers, UATP Staff Assistant/UATF Busine
Alma Burgess, Data Collection Coordinator
Provides expertise, resources, and a structure to enhance and expand AT services provided by private and public agencies in Utah. Occcurs through monitoring, coordination, information dissemination, empowering individuals, the identification and removal of barriers, and expanding state resources.

4552 Utah Independent Living Center
3445 S Main St
Salt Lake City, UT   84115-4453   801-466-5565
                                          800-355-2195
                                          Fax: 801-466-2363
                                          TTY: 801-466-5565
                                          uilc@uilc.org
                                          www.uilc.org

Debra Mair, Executive Director
Kim Meichle, Assistant Director
Julie Beckstead, Program Coordinator
Patty Trent, Fiscal Manager
Offers information and referral services. To assist persons with disabilities achieve independence by providing services and activities which enhance independent living skillspromote the public's understanding, accomodation, and acceptance of their rights, needs and abilities.

4553 Utah Independent Living Center: Minersville
P.O.Box 168
Minersville, UT   84752-168   435-691-7724
                                          rrci@rrci.org
                                          www.rrci.org

Barbara Lefler, Executive Director
Jerry Salkowe, President
Celeste Sorensen, Secretary
Joseph Gordon, Treasurer
To enhance independence for all people with disaibilities.

4554 Utah Independent Living Center: Tooele
42 S Main St
Tooele, UT   84074-2132   435-843-7353
                                          Fax: 435-843-7359
                                          TTY:435-843-7353
                                          www.uilc.org

Debra Mair, Executive Director
Kim Meichle, Assistant Director
Julie Beckstead, Program Coordinator
Patty Trent, Fiscal Manager
Mission is to assist persons with disabilities achieve greater independence by providing services and activities which enhance independent living skills and promote the public's understanding, accomodation, and acceptance of their rights, needs and abilities.

Vermont

4555 Vermont Assistive Technology Program
Department of Aging and Independent Living
100 State Street
Montpelier, VT   05602-2305   802-871-3353
                                          800-750-6355
                                          Fax: 802-871-3048
                                          TTY: 802-241-1464
                                          www.atp.vermont.gov/tryout-centers

Julie Tucker, Program Director
David Punia ATP, Information/Education Specialist
Encompasses a state coordinating council for assistive technology issues, regional centers for demonstration, trial and technical

support with computer and augmentative communication equipment and regional seating and positioning centers.

4556   Vermont Center for Independent Living: Bennington
601 Main St
Bennington, VT   5201-2875

802-447-0574
800-639-1522
info@vcil.org
www.vcil.org

Colleen Arcodia, Peer Advocate Counselor
Michelle Grubb, Finance & Operations Officer
Sarah Launderville, Executive Director
Sue Booth, Business Office Coordinator
Believes that individuals with disabilities have the right to live with dignity and with appropriate support in their own homes, fully participate in their communities, and to control and make decisions about their lives.

4557   Vermont Center for Independent Living: Chittenden
11 East State Street
Montpelier, VT   05602

802-229-0501
800-639-1522
Fax: 802-229-0503
TTY: 802-229-0501
info@vcil.org
www.vcil.org

Colleen Arcodia, Peer Advocate Counselor
Nathan Besio, Peer Advocate Counselor
Chanda Beun, Receptionist/Admin Specialist
Sue Booth, Business Office Coordinator
Believes that individuals with disabilities have the right to live with dignity and with appropriate support in their own homes, fully participate in their communities, and to control and make decisions about their lives.

4558   Vermont Center for Independent Living: Montpelier
11 E State St
Montpelier, VT   05602-3008

802-229-0501
800-639-1522
Fax: 802-229-0503
info@vcil.org
vcil.org

Colleen Arcodia, Peer Advocate Counselor
Denise Bailey, Direct Services Coordinator
Dhiresha Blose, Development Officer
Sue Booth, Business Office Coordinator
Believes that individuals with disabilities have the right to live with dignity and with appropriate support in their own homes, fully participate in their communities, and to control and make decisions about their lives.

Virginia

4559   Access Independence
324 Hope Dr
Winchester, VA   22601-6800

540-662-4452
Fax: 540-662-4474
TTY: 540-662-5556
askai@accessindependence.org
www.accessindependence.org

Donald Price, Executive Director
Brenda Ernst, Independent Living Specialist
Joan Davis, Manager Operations/Rep Payee
Michaela Zaraszczak, Executive Administrative Assis.
Offers support services to persons with disabilities to assist in maintaining or increasing their independence and self-determination. Includes housing assistance, independent living skills training, information, referral services, assistance and representative payee and advocacy.

4560   Appalachian Independence Center
230 Charwood Dr
Abingdon, VA   24210-2566

276-628-2979
Fax: 276-628-4931
TTY: 276-676-0920
aicadmin@ntelos.net
aicadvocates.org

Greg Morrell, Executive Director
Donna Buckland, Development Director
Scarlett Cox, Operations Director
Mission is to advocate for and with people with disabilities to promote full participation in society

4561   Blue Ridge Independent Living Center
Ste B
1502 Williamson Rd NE
Roanoke, VA   24012-5100

540-342-1231
Fax: 540-342-9505
TTY: 540-342-1231
brilc@brilc.org
brilc.org

Karen Michalski-Karn, Executive Director
Dana Jackson, Program Services Director
Lottie Diomedi, Independent Living Coordinator
Sallee Ebbett, Finance Manager
BRILC assists people with disabilities to live independently. The Center also serves the community at large by helping to create and environment that is accessible to all. BRILC offers a variety of services ranging from referrals to community resources, support services, and direct services. These include peer counseling, support groups, training and seminars, advocacy, education, support services, awareness, aid in obtaining specialized equipment, and much more.

4562   Blue Ridge Independent Living Center: Christianburg
210 Pepper Street S
Christiansburg, VA   24073-3571

540-381-8829
Fax: 540-381-8833
TTY: 540-381-9149
brilc@brilc.org
brilc.org

Karen Michalski-Karney, Executive Director
Dana Jackson, Program Services Director
Lottie Diomedi, Independent Living Coordinator
Sallee Ebbett, Finance Manager
Assists people with disabilities to live independently. The center also serves the community at large by helping to create an environment that is accessible to all.

4563   Blue Ridge Independent Living Center: Low Moor
P.O.Box 7
Low Moor, VA   24457-7

540-862-0252
Fax: 540-862-0252
TTY: 540-862-0252
brilc.org

Karen Michalski-Karney, Executive Director
Dana Jackson, Program Services Director
Lottie Diomedi, Independent Living Coordinator
Sallee Ebbett, Finance Manager
Assists to help people with disabilities to live independently. The center also serves the community at large by helping to create an environment that is accessible to all.

4564   Clinch Independent Living Services
1139C Plaza Drive
Grundy, VA   24614-6780

276-935-6088
800-597-2322
Fax: 276-935-6342
TTY: 276-935-6088
cils@clinchindependent.org

Betty Bevins, Executive Director
Nonprofit organization providing information and referral, peer counseling, advocacy and independent living skills training to persons with disabilities.

4565 Disability Resource Center
409 Progress St
Fredericksburg, VA 22401-3337
540-373-2559
800-648-6324
Fax: 540-373-8126
TTY: 540-373-5890
drc@cildrc.org

Debe Fults, Executive Director
Eric Barnes, Equipment Connection Assistant
Grace Marshall, Community Integration Coor.
Janet Lutkewitte, Accounting/IT
Mission is to assist people with disabilities, those who support them, and the community, through information, education and resources, to achieve the highest potential and benefit of independent living.

4566 ENDependence Center of Northern Virginia
2300 Claredon Blvd.
Suite 3305
Arlington, VA 22201-3367
703-525-3268
866-849-3852
Fax: 703-525-3585
TTY: 703-525-3553
info@ecnv.org
www.ecnv.org

Cynthia Evans, Director of Community Services
Layo Oyewole, Director of Medicaid Programs
Doris Ray, Director of Advocacy and Outreac
Brewster Thackeray, Executive Director
ECNV is a community-based resource and advocacy enter which is managed by and for people with disabilities. ENCV promotes independent living philosophy and equal access for all persons with disabilities and, like the nearly 400 centers for independent living across the country, ECNV grew from local disability rights and self-help movements.

4567 Equal Access Center for Independence
4031 University Drive
Suite #301
Fairfax, VA 22030-3409
703-934-2020
TTY: 703-277-7730

David Sharp, Executive Director
Provides information and referral, peer counseling, advocacy and independent living skills training to persons with disabilities.

4568 Independence Empowerment Center
8409 Dorsey Circle
Suite 101
Manassas, VA 20110-4414
703-257-5400
Fax: 703-257-5043
TTY: 703-257-5400
info@ieccil.org
www.ieccil.org

Mary D Lopez, Executive Director
Roberta McEachern, Program Director
Sheree Thomas, Grants Coordinator
Alan Smiley, Service Facilitator
A non-profit Center for Independent Living. One of over 500 centers in the United States with roots in civil rights models of the 1960's.

4569 Independence Resource Center
815 Cherry Ave
Charlottesville, VA 22903-3448
434-971-9629
Fax: 434-971-8242
TTY: 434-971-9629
tvandever@ntelos.net
www.charlottesvilleirc.org

Tom Vandever, Executive Director
Brenda Gianniny, Administrator
Carolyn Berry, Participant Services Coordinator
Nate Brown, Senior Peer Advocate
Information and referral services.

4570 Independent Living Center Network: Department of the Visually Handicapped
Ste 300
1809 Staples Mill Rd
Richmond, VA 23230-3515
Fax: 804-355-9297
Robert W Partin, Director
Robert Kastenbaum, Partner
Information and referral services.

4571 Junction Center for Independent Living
P.O.Box 1210
Norton, VA 24273-913
276-679-5988
Fax: 276-679-6569
TTY: 276-679-5988
jcil1@junctioncenter.org
junctioncenter.org

Dennis Horton, Executive Director
Cindy Mefford, Assistant to the Executive Direc
Joe Brady, Deaf and Hard of Hearing Coordin
Brenda Cowden, Housing Specialist
To assist those who have significant disabilities so that they migh live independently in the least restrictive and most integrated environment possible.

4572 Junction Center for Independent Living: Duffield
P.O.Box 408
Duffield, VA 24244-408
276-431-1195
Fax: 276-431-1196
TTY: 276-431-1195
jcil1@junctioncenter.org
junctioncenter.org

Dennis Horton, Executive Director
Cindy Mefford, Assistant to the Executive Direc
Joe Brady, Deaf and Hard of Hearing Coordin
Brenda Cowden, Housing Specialist
To assist those who have significant disabilities so that they might live independently in the least restrictive and most integrated environment possbile.

4573 Lynchburg Area Center for Independent Living
500 Alleghany Ave
Suite #520
Lynchburg, VA 24501-2610
434-528-4971
Fax: 434-528-4976
TTY: 434-528-4972
www.lacil.org

Phil Theisen, Executive Director
LACIL is a private non-profit, non-residential consumer driven organization that promotes the efforts of persons with disabilities to live independently in the community and supports the efforts of the community to be open and accessible to all citizens.

4574 Peidmont Independent Living Center
Piedmont Living Center
601 S. Belvidere Street
Richmond, VA 23220
804-782-1986
800-828-1140
Fax: 877-VHD- 123
www.vhda.com

Kit Hale, Chairman
Timothy M. Chapman, Vice Chairman
Susan Dewey, Executive Director
Tammy Neale, Chief Learning Officer
Empowering indiviuals with disabilities to become self-sufficient and independent within their communities.

4575 Peninsula Center for Independent Living
2021-A Cunningham Drive
Suite #2
Hampton, VA 23666-3320
757-827-0275
Fax: 757-827-0655
TTY: 757-827-8800
iepcil@hvacil.org
www.hvacil.org

Ralph Shelman, Executive Director
IEPCIL is a private non-profit non-residential Agency established to provide services to people with disabilities. The Centers

Philosophy is that people with a disability should play a major role in deciding their future. The center provides services to people with disabilities in the cities of Hampton, Newport News, Poquoson, Williamsburg, and counties of James City, York, and Gloucester.

4576   Piedmont Independent Living Center
1045 Main Street
Suite #2
Danville, VA   24541-1800   434-797-2530
                                                    Fax: 434-797-2568
                                                    TTY:434-797-2530

Clarence Dickerson, Executive Director
Jeanette King, ILS Coordinator/BPAD
Lori Penn, Office Manager
Empowering indiviuals with disabilities to become self-sufficient and independent within their communities.

4577   Resources for Independent Living
4009 Fitzhugh Ave
Richmond, VA   23230-3953   804-353-6503
                                                    Fax: 804-358-5606
                                                    TTY:804-353-6583
                                                    info@ril-va.org
                                                    www.ril-va.org

Gerald O'Neill, Executive Director
Marcia Guardino, Program Manager
Kelly Hickok, Community Services Manager
Tom Allen, Chair
Assisting persons who are severly disabled to live independently in the community and to encourage necessary change within the community so independent living is a possibility.

4578   Valley Associates for Independent Living (VAIL)
Shenandoah Valley Workforce Investment Board
3210 Peoples Drive
Suite 220
Harrisonburg, VA   22801-869   540-433-6513
                                                         888-242-8245
                                                    Fax: 540-433-6313
                                                    vail@govail.org
                                                    www.govail.org

Marcia Du Bois, Executive Director
Bob Satterwhite, Executive Director
VAIL is a not-for-profit, private Center for Independent Living providing advocacy, information and referral, independent living skills training, supported employment, and peer counseling to individuals with disabilities in our planning district.

4579   Valley Associates for Independent Living: Lexington
205-B South Liberty St
Harrisonburg, VA   22801-3638   540-433-6513
                                                         888-242-8245
                                                    Fax: 540-433-6313
                                                    TTY:540-438-9265
                                                    vail@govail.org
                                                    www.govail.org

Marcia Du Bois, Executive Director
Promoting self-direction among people with disabilities and removing barriers to independence in the community.

4580   Woodrow Wilson Rehabilitation Center Training Program
243 Woodrow Wilson Avenue
Fishersville, VA   22939-1500   540-332-7000
                                                         800-345-9972
                                                    Fax: 540-332-7132
                                                    TTY: 800-811-7893
                                                    WWRCInfo@wwrc.virginia.gov
                                                    www.wwrc.net

Rick Sizemore, Executive Director
Information & referral services. Six week Virginia residential programs and evaluation services.

Washington

4581   Alliance for People with Disabilities: Seattle
1120 E. Terrace St
Suite 100
Seattle, WA   98122   206-545-7055
                                                         866-545-7055
                                                    Fax: 206-545-7059
                                                    TTY: 206-632-3456
                                                    info@disabilitypride.org
                                                    www.disabilitypride.org

Kimberly Heymann, Executive Director
Elizabeth Kennedy, Executive Assistant
Bhelle Ollero, IL Specialist
Hope Drumond, Program Manager
The Alliance promotes equality and choice for people with disabilities. They provide advocacy, peer support, idependent living skills training, information and referral, transition assistance for youth, civil rights legal aid, assistive technology, training and nursing home transition back into the community.

4582   Alliance of People with Disabilities: Redmond
East King County Office
1150 140th Ave NE
Suite 101
Bellevue, WA   98005-3537   425-558-0993
                                                         800-216-3335
                                                    Fax: 425-558-4773
                                                    TTY: 425-861-4773
                                                    info@disabilitypride.org
                                                    www.disabilitypride.org

Kimberly Heymann, Executive Director
Elizabeth Kennedy, Executive Assistant
Bhelle Ollero, IL Specialist
Hope Drumond, Program Manager
Services include: information and referral, independent living skills training, peer groups, disAbility law project (DLP), access reviews, health insurance advising, and systems advocacy.

4583   Community Services for the Blind and Partially Sighted
Store: Sight Connection
9709 Third Ave NE
Suite #100
Seattle, WA   98115-2027   206-525-5556
                                                         800-458-4888
                                                    Fax: 206-525-0422
                                                    info@sightconnection.org
                                                    www.sightconnection.org

Mary Lewis, Secretary
Shannon Grady Martsolf, President/CEO
Miles Otoupal, Chair
Jonathan Avedovech, Vice Chair
Over 300 practical products for living with vision loss selected by certified vision rehabilitation specialists from Community Services for the Blind and Partially Sighted. Easy-to-use online store features large print, large photos, secure transactions, and links to other vision-related resources.

4584   disAbility Resource Connection: Everett
607 SE Everett Mall Way
Suite 6C
Everett, WA   98208-3210   425-347-5768
                                                         800-315-3583
                                                    Fax: 425-710-0767
                                                    TTY: 425-347-5768
                                                    www.drconline.net

Charley Lane, Executive Director
disAbility Resource Connection is all about living your life as you choose. The staff is committed to assisting every individual to connect to resources, connect to skills, connect to life.

4585 Kitsap Community Resources
845 8th St
Bremerton, WA 98337-1517 360-478-2301
Fax: 360-415-2706
info@kcr.org
www.kcr.org

Larry Eyer, Executive Director
Irmgard Davis, Fiscal Officer
Rudy Taylor, Board President
Kurt Wiest, Board Vice President
Kitsap Community Resources is a local, non-profit organization dedicated to helping people in need. KCR creates hope and opportunity for low-income Kitsap County Residents by providing resources that promote self-sufficiency.

4586 Spokane Center for Independent Living
8817 E. Mission Ave.
Suite 106
Spokane Valley, WA 99212 509-326-6355
Fax: 509-327-2420
info@scilwa.org
www.scilwa.org

William Kane, Executive Director
To improve the self-determination and self-reliance of people with disabilities through systems and individual advocacy, education and independent living services.

4587 Tacoma Area Coalition of Individuals with Disabilities
6315 S 19th St
Tacoma, WA 98466-6217 253-565-9000
877-538-2243
Fax: 253-565-5578
TTY: 253-565-3486
www.tacid.org

Ken Gibson, Executive Director
Steve Pierce, CFO
Jo Ann Maxwell, Deputy Executive Director - Phil
Marsha Doman-Masters, Executive Assistant - Administra
Promotes the independence of individuals with disabilities.

West Virginia

4588 Appalachian Center for Independent Living
4710 Chimney Drive
Suite # C
Charleston, WV 25302-4841 304-965-0376
800-642-3003
Fax: 304-965-0377
TTY: 800-642-3003
acil@yahoo.com
www.mtstcil.org

Ann Weeks, President and CEO
Adam Elmer, Chief Financial Officer
Georgetta Stevens, VP, Corporate Operations
Debbie Conley, Board Chair
A resource center for persons with disabilities and their communities. Serves Kanawha, Clay, Boone and Putnam counties.

4589 Appalachian Center for Independent Living: Spencer
811 Madison Avenue
Suite #106
Spencer, WV 25276-1900 304-927-4080
Fax: 304-927-4330
TTY:800-642-3003
susanacil@yahoo.com
www.mtstcil.org

Ann Weeks, President and CEO
Adam Elmer, Chief Financial Officer
Georgetta Stevens, VP, Corporate Operations
Debbie Conley, Board Chair
A resource center for persons with disabilities and their communities. Serves Jackson, Roane, and Calhoun counties.

4590 Mountain State Center for Independent Living
329 Prince St
Beckley, WV 25801-4515 304-255-0122
Fax: 304-255-0157
TTY:304-255-0122
aoweeks@mtstcil.org
www.mtstcil.org

Ann Weeks, President and CEO
Adam Elmer, Chief Financial Officer
Georgetta Stevens, VP, Corporate Operations
Debbie Conley, Board Chair
This office provides individual and systems advocacy, independent living skills development, information and referral, peer support, personal assistance services, housing referral and training, transportation. Serves Raleigh counties.

4591 Mountain State Center for Independent Living
821 Fourth Avenue
Huntington, WV 25701-1406 304-525-3324
866-687-8245
Fax: 304-525-3360
TTY: 304-525-3324
aoweeks@mtstcil.org
www.mtstcil.org

Ann Weeks, President and CEO
Adam Elmer, Chief Financial Officer
Georgetta Stevens, VP, Corporate Operations
Debbie Conley, Board Chair
Services provided are: individual and systems advocacy, independent living skills development, information and referral, peer support, personal assistance services, supported employment, community integration program, housing referral and training, transportation. Serves Cabell and Wayne counties.

4592 Northern West Virginia Center for Independent Living
601-603 East Brockway
Suite A & B
Morgantown, WV 26501 304-296-6091
800-834-6408
Fax: 304-292-5217
TTY: 304-296-6091
nwvcil@nwvcil.org
www.mtstcil.org

Ann Weeks, President and CEO
Adam Elmer, Chief Financial Officer
Georgetta Stevens, VP, Corporate Operations
Debbie Conley, Board Chair
NWVCIL is committed to the philosophy that all persons have equal access and unconditional value, that all individuals shall be respected for their uniqueness and shall have the right to live within the community of their choice, having equal access to participate in and contribute to that community.

Wisconsin

4593 Center for Independent Living of Western Wisconsin
2920 Schneider Avenue East
Menomonie, WI 54751-2331 715-233-1070
800-228-3287
Fax: 715-233-1083
TTY: 800-228-3287
www.cilww.com

Tim Sheehan, Executive Director
Kay Sommerfeld, Assistant Director
Tammy Grage, Fiscal & HR Manager
Noelle Johnson, Resource Counselor Camp Quest
Advocates for the full participation in society of all persons with disabilities. Our goal is empowering individuals to exercise choices to maintain or increase their indpendence. Our strategy is providing consumer-driven services at no cost to persons with disiabilities in Western Wisconsin

4594 Independence First
540 South 1st Street
Milwaukee, WI 53204-1516   414-291-7520
                            Fax: 414-291-7525
                            TTY:414-297-7520
                            lschulz@independencefirst.org
                            www.independencefirst.org
Lee Schulz, President and CEO
John Schmid, Chair
Judy Murphy, Vice Chair
Judi Wisla, Secretary
A non-profit agency directed by, and for the benefit of, persons with disabilities, primarily serving the four county metropolitan Milwaukee area.

4595 Independence First: West Bend
735 S Main St
West Bend, WI 53095-3965   262-306-6717
                            lschulz@independencefirst.org
                            www.independencefirst.org
Lee Schulz, President and CEO
John Schmid, Chair
Judy Murphy, Vice Chair
Judi Wisla, Secretary
A non-profit agency directed by, and for the benefit of, persons with disabilities, primarily serving the four county Metropolitan Milwaukee area.

4596 Inspiration Ministries
N2270 State Road 67
Walworth, WI 53184-948   262-275-6131
                          Fax: 262-275-3355
                          IMinfo@InspirationMinistries.org
                          inspirationministries.org
Robin Knoll, President
Richard Hall, Executive Vice President
Craig Pape, VP Ministry Services
Michael Scholl, VP Development
Formerly known as Christian League for the Handicapped, Inspiration Ministries is a vibrant community of adults with disabilities engaged in living, working, leisure and faith activities designed to provide a complete living experience. The campus consists of a modern residential facility offering a range of living accomodations; a work center and resale shop; and Inspiration Center, a retreat/camping center designed to be 100% wheelchair accessible.

4597 Mid-State Independent Living Consultants: Wausau
3262 Church Street
Suite #1
Stevens Point, WI 54481-5321   715-344-4210
                                800-382-8484
                                Fax: 715-344-4414
                                TTY: 800-382-8484
                                milc@milc-inc.org
                                www.milc-inc.org
Tom Vandehey, President
Becky Paulson, Independent Living Consultant
Working for persons with disabilities towards empowerment to make informed choices.

4598 Mid-state Independent Living Consultants: Stevens Point
3262 Church Street
Suite #1
Stevens Point, WI 54481-5321   715-344-4210
                                800-382-8484
                                Fax: 715-344-4414
                                TTY: 800-382-8484
                                milc@milc-inc.org
                                www.milc-inc.org
Jenny Fasula, Executive Director
Karalyn Peterson, Resource Director
Committed to enhancing personal and community relationships, providing opportunities for growth, and helping people with varying abilities achieve their personal goals.

4599 North Country Independent Living
69 N 28th St.
Suite 28
Superior, WI 54880-5138   715-392-9118
                           800-924-1220
                           Fax: 715-392-4636
                           john@northcountryil.com
                           northcountryil.com
John Nousaine, Executive Director
Gloria Hakkila-Johnson, Assistant Director
Jim Glaeser, Accountant
Russ Stover, Office Assistant
Empowers people with disabilities.

4600 North Country Independent Living: Ashland
422 3rd St. W.
Suite #114
Ashland, WI 54806-1553   715-682-5676
                          800-499-5676
                          Fax: 715-682-3144
                          TTY: 715-682-5676
                          northcountryil.com
John Nousaine, Director
Empowers people with disabilities.

4601 Options for Independent Living
555 Country Club Road
Green Bay, WI 54307-1967   920-490-0500
                            888-465-1515
                            Fax: 920-490-0700
                            TTY:920-490-0600
                            info@optionsil.com
                            www.optionsil.com
Thomas Diedrick, Executive Director
Kathryn C. Barry, Assistant Director
Sandra L. Popp, Independent Living Coordinator
Vicky Lasch, Independent Living Coordinator
A non-profit organization committed to empowering people with disabilities to lead independent and productive lives in their community through advocacy, the provision of information, education, technology and related services.

4602 Options for Independent Living: Fox Valley
820 West College Ave
Suite #5
Appleton, WI 54914   920-997-9999
                      888-465-1515
                      Fax: 920-997-9381
                      TTY:920-490-0600
                      www.optionsil.com
Thomas Diedrick, Executive Director
Kathryn C. Barry, Assistant Director
Sandra L. Popp, Independent Living Coordinator
Vicky Lasch, Independent Living Coordinator
A non-profit organization committed to empowering people with disabilities to lead independent and productive lives in their community through advocacy, the provision of information, education, technology and related services.

4603 Society's Assets: Elkhorn
615 E Geneva St
Elkhorn, WI 53121-2301   262-723-8181
                          800-261-8181
                          Fax: 262-723-8184
                          TTY: 866-840-9763
                          info@societysassets.org
                          www.societysassets.org
Bruce Nelson, Director
Jill Vigueres, Manager
To ensure the rights of all persons with disabilities to live and function as independently as possible in the community of their choice, through supporting individual's efforts to achieve control over their lives and become integrated into community life.

4604 **Society's Assets: Kenosha**
5455 Sheridan Road
Suite 101
Kenosha, WI 53140-4103   262-657-3999
                                            800-317-3999
                                      Fax: 262-657-1672
                                       TTY: 866-840-9762
                                 info@societysassets.org
                                 www.societysassets.org

Sue Liu, Manager
Bruce Nelsen, Executive Director
To ensure the rights of all persons with disabilities to live and function as independently as possible in the community of their choice, through supporting individuals efforts to achieve controll over their lives and become integrated into community life. Offers home care and independent living services.

4605 **Society's Assets: Racine**
5200 Washinton Ave
Suite #225
Racine, WI 53406-4238   262-637-9128
                                            800-378-9128
                                      Fax: 262-637-8646
                                       TTY: 886-840-9761
                                 info@societysassets.org
                                 www.societysassets.org

Deb Pitsch, Administrator
Karen Olufs, Director Independent Living
Jean Rumachik, Director Home Care Services
Society's Assets assists people with disabilities to live as independently as possible. A non-profit human services agency, Society's Assets provides information and referral, independent living skills training, peer support, advocacy, and supportive home care. Home health care is provided by SAI Home Health Care. The agency serves 5 counties in southeastern Wisconsin and also provides information about interpreters, employment, benefits, home modifications, assistive equipment and accessibility.
Fees vary

Wyoming

4606 **RENEW: Gillette**
35 Fairgrounds Road
Newcastle, WY 82701   307-746-4733
                                            888-253-4653
                                      Fax: 307-746-9701
                                      www.renew-wyo.com

Donna Bombeck, Chairwoman
Carolyn Holso, Vice Chairwoman
Renee Nack, Secretary
Bryan Bergstreser, Treasurer
Empowering persons with disabilities to enrich their lives.

4607 **RENEW: Rehabilitation Enterprises of North Eastern Wyoming**
1969 S Sheridan Ave
Sheridan, WY 82801-6108   307-672-7481
                                            888-309-2020
                                      Fax: 307-674-5117
                                       pr@renew-wyo.com
                                      www.renew-wyo.com

Donna Bombeck, Chairwoman
Carolyn Holso, Vice Chairwoman
Renee Nack, Secretary
Bryan Bergstreser, Treasurer
Multi-disciplinary organization dedicated to the highest possible economic and social independence for persons with disabilities. Extensive referral service, specialized employment placement, occupational therapy, psychological services, evaluation services, and coordination of external services as needed to meet client plans and objectives.

4608 **Rehabilitation Enterprises of North Eastern Wyoming: Newcastle**
35 Fairgrounds Rd
Newcastle, WY 82701-2625   307-746-4733
                                            888-693-9245
                                      Fax: 307-746-9701
                                       pr@renew-wyo.com
                                      www.renew-wyo.com

Donna Bombeck, Chairwoman
Carolyn Holso, Vice Chairwoman
Renee Nack, Secretary
Bryan Bergstreser, Treasurer
Empowering persons with disabilities to enrich their lives.

4609 **Wyoming Services for Independent Living**
1156 South 2nd
Lander, WY 82520-3905   307-332-4889
                                            800-266-3061
                                      Fax: 307-332-2491
                                       TTY: 307-332-7582
                                            www.wysil.org

Susan Hoesel, Business Manager
Donna Langelier, Program Manager
Marcia Henthorn, Program Manager
Valentina Knutson, Independent Living Specialist
Committed to enhancing personal and community relationships, providing opportunities for growth, and helping people with varying abilities achieve thier personal goals.

Law

Associations & Referral Agencies

4610 ADA In Details: Interpreting the 2010 Americans with Disabilities Act Stands
Wiley Publishing
111 River St
Hoboken, NJ 07030-5774   201-748-6000
                                 Fax: 201-748-6088
                                 info@wiley.com
                                 www.wiley.com

Matthe S. Kissner, Chief Executive Officer
Christopher Caridi, Senior Vice President
Helps readers understand the facilities requirements of the Americans with Disabilities Act Accessibility Guidelines. Presents the technical requirements for accessible elements and spaces in new construction, alterations and additions. *$40.00*
304 pages Paperback 1917
ISBN 9-781119-27-7

4611 AIDS Legal Council of Chicago
17 North State Street
Suite 900
Chicago, IL 60602   312-427-8990
                            Fax: 312-427-8419
                            aidslegal.com

Tom Yates, Executive Director
Mike Sullivan, President
Jena Levin, Vice President
Andrew Skiba, CRSP, Treasurer
The AIDS Legal Council of Chicago provides legal assistance for people with HIV/AIDS related issues.

4612 AIDSLAW of Louisiana
2601 Tulane Avenue
Suite 630
New Orleans, LA 70119   225-302-5968
                                info@aidslaw.org
                                www.aidslaw.org

Don Paul Landry, Executive Director
Stacy Morris, Deputy Executive Director
Joshua Holmes, Full-time Staff Attorney
Louise Bienvenu, Supervising Attorney
The mission of AIDSLaw is to provide excellent, specialized legal services for people living with HIV/AIDS in Louisiana, to improve their quality of life and access to health care, related to their HIV/AIDS status.
1989

4613 Center for Disability and Elder Law, Inc.
205 W. Randolph
Suite 1610
Chicago, IL 60606   312-376-1880
                            Fax: 312-376-1885
                            info@cdelaw.org
                            www.cdelaw.org

Mark Hellner, Executive Director
Caroline Manley, Supervising Attorney
Thomas Wendt, Chief Legal Officer
A not-for-profit legal services organization which provids legal services to low income persons residing in Chicago and Cook County, Il., who are either elderly and/or persons with disabilities. CDEL provides legal services by matching qualified candidates with volunteer attorneys who represent them, pro-bono, in a wide range of civil legal matters; and through special initiatives including the Senior Center Initiative (SCI) and the Senior Tax Opportunity program.

4614 Chicago Lawyers' Committee for Civil Rights Under Law
100 N LaSalle Street
Suite 600
Chicago, IL 60602-2400   312-630-9744
                                 Fax: 312-630-1127
                                 info@clccrul.org
                                 www.clccrul.org

Bonnie Allen, Executive Director
Donna J. Vobornik, President
Lauren Loew, Treasurer
Timma Axel, Communications Manager
Promotes and protects civil rights of low-income, minority and disadvantaged people in the social, economic, and political systems of the nation.

4615 DNA People's Legal Services
PO Box 306
Window Rock, AZ 86515   928-871-4151
                                Fax: 928-871-5036
                                www.dnalegalservices.org

Kathy Gallagher, Development Director
Tom Parker, Development Assistant
A nonprofit legal aid organization working to protect civil rights, promote tribal sovereignty and alleviate civil legal problems for people who live in poverty in the Southwestern United States.
1967

4616 Disability Law Colorado
455 Sherman St.
Suite 130
Denver, CO 80203   303-722-3619
                           800-288-1376
                           Fax: 303-722-0720
                           tlcmail@thelegalcenter.org
                           disabilitylawco.org

Stephen P. Rickles, Esq., President
Mary Anne Harvey, Executive Director
Alison Butler Daniels, Esq., Director of Legal Services
Protects and promotes the rights of people with disabilities and older people in Colorado through direct legal representation, advocacy, education and legislative analysis.

4617 Disability Rights Advocates
2001 Center St
4th Floor
Berkeley, CA 94704-1204   510-665-8644
                                  Fax: 510-665-8511
                                  frontdesk@dralegal.org
                                  dralegal.org

Laurel Ackerson, Paralegal
Julia Calagiovanni, Development & Communications Assistant
Jodi Grigas, Human Resources & Office Manager
Maria Pryputniewicz, Accounting Manager
Disability Rights Advocates is a non-profit legal center representing people with disabilities, advocating for them when their civil rights have been violated. Their clients include those with mobility, sensory, cognitive, and psychiatric disabilities.

4618 Disability Rights Education and Defense Fund
3075 Adeline Street
Suite 210
Berkeley, CA 94703   510-644-2555
                             Fax: 510-841-8645
                             info@dredf.org
                             dredf.org

Susan Henderson, Executive Director
Arlene B. Mayerson, Directing Attorney
Claudia Center, President/Chair
Ann C. Freeman, Secretary/Treasurer
Nonprofit organization dedicated to advancing the civil rights of individuals with disabilities through legislation, litigation, informal and formal advocacy and education and training of lawyers, advocates and clients with respect to disability issues. DREDF also provides training, advocacy, technical assistance and referrals for parents of disabled children.

4619   Disability Rights Texas
2222 West Braker Lane
Austin, TX   78758-1024   512-454-4816
                                            866-362-2851
                                        Fax: 512-323-0902
                                    www.disabilityrightstx.org
Mary Faithfull, Executive Director
A federally designated legal protection and advocacy agency
(P&A) for people with disabilities in Texas. Helps people with
disabilities understand and exercise their rights under the law, en-
suring their full and equal participation in society.

4620   Equal Employment Advisory Council
1501 M Street NW
Suite 400
Washington, DC   20005   202-629-5650
                                        Fax: 202-629-5651
                                            info@eeac.org
                                            www.eeac.org
Joseph S. Lakis, President
Rae T. Vann, Vice President and General Counsel
Valerie Vickers, Chair
Dana Baughns, Vice Chair
Nonprofit employer association providing guidance to its mem-
ber companies on understanding and complying with their EEO
and affirmative action obligations.
1976

4621   Guardianship Services Associates
41A South Blvd
Oak Park, IL   60302-2777   708-386-5398
                                        Fax: 708-386-5970
                                    GSAoakpark@sbcglobal.net
Robert R. Wohlgemuth, Executive Director
Information and counseling on guardianship and its alternatives.
Can provide direct assistance in obtaining guardianship for dis-
abled adults in Cook County. Also provides information and di-
rect assistance on durable powers of attorney.

4622   Independence Economic Development
201 N Forest Avenue
Suite 120
Independence, MO   64050- 2753   816-252-5777
                                        Fax: 816-254-1641
                                        tlesnak@inedc.biz
                                            www.iced.org
Tom Lesnak, President
Jodi Krantz, Vice President
Lee Langerock, Executive Director
Jason Snodgrass, Chairman
A non-profit, public/private partnership established for the pur-
pose of supporting and enhancing the economic growth of inde-
pendence.

4623   Independent Living Research Utilization
1333 Moursund
Houston, TX   77030-7031   713-520-0232
                                        Fax: 713-520-5785
                                        TTY:713-520-0232
                                            ilru@ilru.org
                                            ilru.org
Lex Frieden, Director
George Powers, Legal Specialist
Edward Elms, Research Associate
Darell Jones, Program Director
The ILRU is a national center for information, training, research,
and technical assistance in independent living. Its goal is to ex-
pand the body of knowledge in independent living and to improve
utilization of results of research programs and demonstration
projects in this field.

4624   Judge David L Bazelon Center for Mental Health Law
1101 15th Street NW
Suite 1212
Washington, DC   20005   202-467-5730
                                        Fax: 202-223-0409
                                        TTY:202-467-4232
                                    communications@bazelon.org
                                            www.bazelon.org
Ira Burnim, Director
Mark Murphy, Managing Attorney
Nikki Heidepriem, Chair
David Apatoff, Treasurer
A nonprofit organization devoted to improving the lives of peo-
ple with mental illnesses through changes in policy and law.

4625   Legal Action Center
810 1st Street
Suite 200
Washington, DC   20002-4980   202-544-5478
                                        Fax: 202-544-5712
                                    nationalpolicy@lac.org
                                            www.lac.org
Brad S. Karp, Chairman
Mary Beth Forshaw, Vice Chair
Sally Friedman, Legal Director
The only non-profit law and policy organization in the United
States whose sole mission is to fight discrimination against peo-
ple with histories of addiction, HIV/AIDS, or criminal records,
and to advocate for sound public policies in these areas.

4626   Legislative Handbook for Parents
NAPVI
250 W 64th St
New York, NY   10023   800-284-4422
                                    napvi@lighthouseguild.org
                                            www.napvi.org
Alan R. Morse, President/CEO
Mark G. Ackermann, Executive Vice President
James M. Dubin, Chairman
Joseph A. Ripp, Vice Chairman
A publication for parents who make direct contact with public of-
ficials on behalf of their children. Sample letters,
do's-and-dont's, and a glossary of legislative terms are some of
the topics that are contained in this manual. *$5.50*
24 pages Paperback

4627   National Health Law Program (NHeLP)
3701 Wilshire Blvd
Suite 750
Los Angeles, CA   90010   310-204-6010
                                        Fax: 213-368-0774
                                        www.healthlaw.org
Amy Chen, Senior Attorney
Abigail Coursolle, Senior Attorney
Elizabeth G. Taylor, Executive Director
Jane Perkins, Legal Director
A national public interest law firm that seeks to improve health
care for America's working and unemployed poor, minorities, the
elderly and people with disabilities. NHeLP serves legal services
programs, community-based organizations, the private bar, providers and individuals who work to preserve a health care safety
net for the millions of uninsured or underinsured low-income
people.
1970

4628   National Right to Work Legal Defense Foundation
8001 Braddock Rd.
Springfield, VA   22160   703-321-8510
                                            800-336-3600
                                        Fax: 703-321-9319
                                            nrtw.org
Raymond LaJeunesse, Legal Director
Byron S. Andrus, Staff Attorney
Matthew B. Gilliam, Staff Attorney
Amanda K. Freeman, Staff Attorney
The National Right to Work Legal Defense Foundation is a non-
profit, charitable organization. Its mission is to eliminate coer-

cive union power and compulsory unionism abuses through strategic litigation, public information, and education programs. *1968*

4629 REACH/Resource Centers on Independent Living
8625 King George
Suite 210
Dallas, TX 75235-2286
214-630-4796
Fax: 214-630-5995
TTY:214-630-6390
www.reachcils.org
Julia Charlker, President
Joyce Tepley, Vice President
Patt Bourland, Secretary
Gordon Meredith, Treasurer
Providing services for people with disabilities so that they are empowered to lead self-directed lives and educating the general public on disability-related topics in order to promote a barrier-free community.

4630 Summaries of Legal Precedents & Law Review
Through the Looking Glass
3075 Adeline St
Suite 120
Berkeley, CA 94703
510-848-1112
800-644-2666
Fax: 510-848-4445
TLG@lookingglass.org
www.lookingglass.org
Megan Kirshbaum, Executive Director
Summarizes legal precedents and law review articles relevant to marital custody and child protection situations of parents with diverse disabilities. *$25.00*
24 pages

4631 TASH Connections
TASH
1875 Eye St. NW
Suite 582
Washington, DC 20006
202-429-2080
Fax: 202-540-9019
info@tash.org
www.tash.org
Julia M. White, Editor
Ruite-Marie Beckwith, Executive Director
Dawn Brown, Development Director
Raquel Rosa, Special Projects Manager
Connections is the online magazine written exclusively for, and by, TASH members. Each issue contains provocative articles on breakthroughs in the disability field, and challenges readers to rethink some of the toughest issues affecting people with disabilities, their families and advocates.
Quarterly

Resources for the Disabled

4632 ABDA/ABMPP Annual Conference
American Board of Disability Analysts
4525 Harding Road
2nd Floor
Nashville, TN 37205
615-327-2984
Fax: 615-327-9235
americanbd@aol.com
www.americandisability.org
Alexander E. Horowitz, Executive Officer Emeritus
Kenneth N. Anchor, Administrative Officer/Editor
Gabriel Sella, Education Coordinator
Lela Boggs, Business Manager
February workshop. Workshop leader: Dr. William Tsushima.

4633 Americans with Disabilities Act Manual
US Department of Justice
950 Pennsylvania Ave NW
Washington, DC 20530-9
202-307-0663
800-514-0301
Fax: 202-307-1197
TTY: 800-514-0383
www.ada.gov
Rebecca B. Bond, Chief
Zita Johnson Betts, Deputy Chief
Sally Conway, Deputy Chief
James Bostrom, Deputy Chief
An in-depth analysis of the legal and practical implications of the ADA using non-technical language. *$20.00*

4634 Americans with Disabilities Act: Selected Resources for Deaf
Gallaudet University Bookstore
800 Florida Avenue NE
Washington, DC 20002-3695
202-651-5000
800-621-2736
Fax: 202-651-5508
clerc.center@gallaudet.edu
www.gallaudet.edu
Priscilla O'Donnell, Bookstore Manager
Iva Williams, Bookstore Secretary
Elaine Vance, Human Resources Director
Marteal Pitts, Circulation Coordinator
This resource identifies programs and publications specific to the ADA and deafness and also lists ADA materials and programs for people with any disability.

4635 Approaching Equality
T J Publishers
Ste 108
2544 Tarpley Rd
Carrollton, TX 75006-2288
972-416-0800
800-999-1168
Fax: 301-585-5930
TJPubinc@aol.com
Frank Bowe, Author
Public education laws guarantee special education for all deaf children, but may find the special education system confusing, or are unsure of their rights under current laws. For anyone with an interest in education, advocacy and the deaf community, this book reviews dramatic developments in education of deaf children, youth and adults since COED's 1988 report, Toward Equality.. *$12.95*
112 pages
ISBN 0-93266 -39-6

4636 Assessment of the Feasibility of Contracting with a Nominee Agency
Mississippi State University
PO Drawer 6189
Mississippi State, MS 39762
662-325-2001
Fax: 662-325-8989
rrtc@colled.msstate.edu
www.blind.msstate.edu
Michelle Capella McDonnall, Interim Director
Stephanie Hall, Business Manager
Douglas Bedsaul, Research and Training Coordinator
Jacqui Bybee, Research Associate II
Only five State Licensing Agencies currently utilize nominee agreements. This study compared the Pennsylvania BE program with four states that utilize nominee agencies and four states that do not. *$20.00*
152 pages Paperback

4637 **Bluebook: Explanation of the Contents of the ADA**
Disability Rights Education and Defense Fn
3075 Adeline Street
Suite 210
Berkeley, CA   94703   510-644-2555
                                                        800-348-4232
                                                  Fax: 510-841-8645
                                                  TTY: 510-841-8645
                                                     info@dredf.org
                                                         dredf.org

Claudia Center, President and Chair
Ann Cupolo Freeman, Secretary and Treasurer
Susan Henderson, Executive Director
Arlene B. Mayerson, Directing Attorney
Written in narrative form for both professionals and lay people,
DREDF's bluebook offers detailed, thorough analysis of all of
the law's provisions, encompassing ADA legislative history, the
statute and regulations. Available in alternative formats. *$100.00*
214 pages

4638 **Can America Afford to Grow Old?**
Brookings Institution
1775 Massachusetts Ave NW
Washington, DC   20036-2103   202-797-6000
                                                  Fax: 202-797-6004
                                                bibooks@brookings.edu
                                                www.brookings.edu

William Antholis, Managing Director
Steven Bennett, Vice President and Chief Operating Officer
Kimberly Churches, Vice President for Development
Kemal Dervis, Vice President and Director, Global Economy and
Development
Social security laws and regulations. *$8.95*
144 pages Paperback
ISBN 0-815700-43-1

4639 **Childcare and the ADA**
Eastern Washington University
Rm 223
705 W 1st Ave
Spokane, WA   99201-3909   509-623-4200
                                                  Fax: 509-623-4230
                                              susan.vanmeter@mail.ewu.edu
Nancy Ashworth, Director Child Development
Allen Barrom, Manager
Provides information on how childcare providers must comply
with the ADA. Eight videotapes plus an instructional manual
with examples of situations and problems.. *$85.00*
Set

4640 **Common ADA Errors and Omissions in New Construction**
and Alterations
US Department of Justice
950 Pennsylvania Ave NW
Washington, DC   20530   202-307-0663
                                                        800-574-0301
                                                  Fax: 202-307-1197
                                                         www.ada.gov
Rebecca B. Bond, Chief
Zita Johnson Betts, Deputy Chiefs
James Bostrom, Deputy Chiefs
Sally Conway, Deputy Chiefs
Lists a sampling of common accessibility errors or omissions that
have been identified through the Department of Justice's ongoing
enforcement efforts.
13 pages

4641 **Commonly Asked Questions About Child Care Centers and**
the Americans with Disabilities Act
US Department of Justice
950 Pennsylvania Ave NW
Washington, DC   20530   202-307-0663
                                                        800-574-0301
                                                  Fax: 202-307-1197
                                                         www.ada.gov
Rebecca B. Bond, Chief
Zita Johnson Betts, Deputy Chiefs
James Bostrom, Deputy Chiefs
Sally Conway, Deputy Chiefs
Explains how the requirements of the ADA apply to Child Care
Centers. Also describes some of the Department of justice's on-
going enforncement efforts in the child care area and it provides
a resource list on sources of information on the ADA.
13 pages

4642 **Commonly Asked Questions About Title III of the ADA**
US Department of Justice
950 Pennsylvania Ave NW
Washington, DC   20530-9   202-307-0663
                                                        800-574-0301
                                                  Fax: 202-307-1197
                                                  TTY: 800-514-0383
                                                         www.ada.gov
Rebecca B. Bond, Chief
Zita Johnson Betts, Deputy Chief
Sally Conway, Deputy Chief
James Bostrom, Deputy Chief
A 6-page publication providing information for state and local
governments about ADA requirements for ensuring that people
with disabilities receive the same services and benefits as
provided to others.
on-line

4643 **Commonly Asked Questions About the ADA and Law**
Enforcement
US Department of Justice
950 Pennsylvania Ave NW
Washington, DC   20530-9   202-307-0663
                                                        800-574-0301
                                                  Fax: 202-307-1197
                                                  TTY: 800-514-0383
                                                         www.ada.gov
Rebecca B. Bond, Chief
Zita Johnson Betts, Deputy Chief
Sally Conway, Deputy Chief
James Bostrom, Deputy Chief
A publication explaining ADA requirements for ensuring that
people with disabilities receive the same law enforcement ser-
vices and protections as provided to others.
13 pages on-line

4644 **Complying with the Americans with Disabilis Act**
Greenwood Publishing Group
130 Cremona Drive
Santa Barbara, CA   93117   805-968-1911
                                                        800-368-6868
                                                  Fax: 866-270-3856
                                            CustomerService@abc-clio.com
                                                  www.greenwood.com
Don Fresh, Author
Peter W Thomas, Co-Author
John Gosden, Library Resource Consultants
Lina Gosden, Library Resource Consultants
A guidebook for management and people with disabilities. This
unique guidebook presents a comprehensive analysis of the new
Americans with Disabilities Act (ADA), the most significant fed-
eral civil rights law in almost 30 years, and its impact on over four
million American businesses, state and local governments, non-
profit associations, 87 percent of American's private sector jobs,
and 22.7 million working-age people with disabilities. *$117.95*
280 pages Hardcover
ISBN 0-899307-14-0

4645 **Court-Related Needs of the Elderly and Persons with Disabilities**
Mental Health Commission
2700 Martin Luther King Jr Ave SE
Washington, DC 20032-2601 202-282-0027
Fax: 202-373-7982
276 pages

4646 **Criminal Law Handbook on Psychiatric & Psychological Evidence & Testimony**
New York City Bar
42 West 44th Street
New York, NY 10036-6604 212-382-6600
Fax: 212-768-8116
phynes@nycbar.org
www.nycbar.org

Bret Parker, Executive Director
Debra Raskin, President
Alan Rothstein, General Counsel
Maria Cilenti, Director Legislative Affairs
The Criminal Law Handbook provides lawyers, judges and forensic experts with comprehensive, in-depth treatment of admissibility (and limitations on admissibility) of psychiatric and psychological evidence and testimony pertaining to key criminal mental health law standards. *$47.00*

4647 **Department of Justice ADA Mediation Program**
US Department of Justice
950 Pennsylvania Ave NW
Washington, DC 20530 202-307-0663
800-574-0301
Fax: 202-307-1197
TTY: 800-514-0383
www.ada.gov

Rebecca B. Bond, Chief
Zita Johnson Betts, Deputy Chiefs
James Bostrom, Deputy Chiefs
Sally Conway, Deputy Chiefs
Provides an overview of the Department's Mediation Program and examples of successfully mediated cases.
6 pages

4648 **Dimensions of State Mental Health Policy**
Greenwood Publishing Group
130 Cremona Drive
Santa Barbara, CA 93117 805-968-1911
800-368-6868
Fax: 866-270-3856
CustomerService@abc-clio.com
www.greenwood.com

Christopher Hudson, Author
Arthur J Cox, Co-Author
John Gosden, Library Resource Consultants
Lina Gosden, Library Resource Consultants
Introduces students to the emerging field of state mental health policy, its history, current policies, organizational models and required programming knowledge. *$86.95*
320 pages Hardcover
ISBN 0-275932-52-7

4649 **Disability Compliance for Higher Education**
LRP Publications
360 Hiatt Dr
Palm Beach Gardens, FL 33418 561-622-6520
800-341-7874
Fax: 561-622-0757
lrpitvp@lrp.com
www.lrp.com

Kenneth Kahn, CEO
Gives guidance on the most difficult issues faced, such as supporting students with psychological disabilities, ensuring accessibility, understanding OCR rulings, and more. *$57.29*
300 pages

4650 **Disability Discrimination Law, Evidence and Testimony**
ABA Commission on Mental & Physical Disability Law
1050 Connecticut Ave. N.W.
Suite 400
Washington, DC 20036 202-662-1000
800-285-2221
Fax: 202-442-3439
cmpdl@americanbar.org
www.americanbar.org

John W Parry JD, Author
Explains and analyzes key aspects of disability discriminiation law from several different perspectives to guide you through the myriad federal and state statutes, court cases, and regulations. *$105.00*
694 pages Paperback
ISBN 1-604420-12-8

4651 **Disability Law in the United States**
William Hein & Company
2350 North Forest Rd.
Getzville, NY 14068-1296 716-882-2600
800-828-7571
Fax: 716-883-8100
mail@wshein.com
www.wshein.com

Dr Bernard D Reams Jr, Author
Peter J McGovern, Co-Author
Jon S Schultz, Co-Author
Offers thousands of pages of information on the laws and legislation affecting the disabled in the United States. Its purpose is to provide a clear and comprehensive mandate to end discrimination against individuals with disabilities and to bring disabled persons into the economic and social midstream of American Life. *$675.00*
5750 pages
ISBN 0-899417-97-3

4652 **Disability Rights Now**
Disability Rights Education and Defense Fund
3075 Adeline Street
Suite 210
Berkeley, CA 94703 510-644-2555
800-348-4232
Fax: 510-841-8645
TTY: 510-841-8645
info@dredf.org
dredf.org

Claudia Center, President and Chair
Ann Cupolo Freeman, Secretary and Treasurer
Susan Henderson, Executive Director
Arlene B. Mayerson, Directing Attorney
Free quarterly publication describing the activities of the Disability Rights Education and Defense Fund, available in alternative formats.
Quarterly

4653 **Disability Under the Fair Employment & Housing Act: What You Should Know About the Law**
California Department of Fair Employment & Housing
2218 Kausen Drive
Suite 100
Elk Grove, CA 95758 916-478-7251
800-884-1684
Fax: 916-227-2870
contact.center@dfeh.ca.gov
www.dfeh.ca.gov

Phyllis W Cheng, Director
Intended to highlight and summarize workplace disability laws enforced by the California Department of Fair Employment and Housing. It will familiarize people with the content of these laws, including recent changes and amendments to state statutes and attendent accommodation responsibilities.

4654 Discrimination is Against the Law
California Department of Fair Employment & Housing
2218 Kausen Drive
Suite 100
Elk Grove, CA 95758 916-478-7251
800-884-1684
Fax: 916-227-2870
contact.center@dfeh.ca.gov
www.dfeh.ca.gov
Phyllis Cheng, Director
Enforces California state laws that prohibit harassment and discrimination in employment, housing, and public accomodations and that provide for pregnancy leave and family and personal leave.

4655 Education of the Handicapped: Laws, Legislative Histories and Administrative Document
William S Hein & Co Inc
2350 North Forest Rd.
Getzville, NY 14068-1296 716-882-2600
800-828-7571
Fax: 716-883-8100
mail@wshein.com
www.wshein.com
Bernard D Reams Jr, Editor
Focuses upon Elementary and Secondary Education Act of 1965 and its amendment, Education For All Handicapped Children Act of 1975 and its amendments and acts providing services for the blind, deaf, mentally retarded, etc. *$2950.00*
55 volumes
ISBN 0-899411-57-6

4656 ElderLawAnswers.com
150 Chestnut Street
4th Floor, Box 15
Providence, RI 02903 617-267-9700
866-267-0947
support@elderlawanswers.com
www.elderlawanswers.com
Harry S Margolis, Founder/President
Mark Miller, Director of Product and Business Development
Ken Coughlin, Managing Editor
Supports seniors, their families and their attorneys in achieving their goals by providing

4657 Employment Discrimination Based on Disability
California Department of Fair Employment & Housing
2218 Kausen Drive
Suite 100
Elk Grove, CA 95758 916-478-7251
800-884-1684
Fax: 916-227-2870
contact.center@dfeh.ca.gov
www.dfeh.ca.gov
Phyllis W Cheng, Director
Prohibits employment discrimination and harassment based on a person's disability or perceived disability. Also requires employers to reasonably accommodate individuals with mental or physical disabilities unless the employer can show that to do so would cause an undue hardship.

4658 Employment Standards Administration Department of Labor (ESA)
200 Constitution Ave NW
Washington, DC 20210-1 800-321-6742
TTY:877-889-5627
osha.gov
David Michaels, Assistant Secretary
Jordan Barab, Deputy Assistant Secretary
Richard Fairfax, Deputy Assistant Secretary
Deborah Berkowitz, Chief of Staff
Monitors compliance with sub-minimum wage requirements for handicapped workers in sheltered workshops, competitive industry and hospitals and institutions under Section 14 of the Fair Labor Standards Act of 1938.

4659 Enforcing the ADA: A Status Report from the Department of Justice
US Department of Justice
950 Pennsylvania Ave NW
Washington, DC 20530 202-307-0663
800-514-0301
Fax: 203-307-1197
www.ada.gov
Rebecca B. Bond, Chief
Zita Johnson Betts, Deputy Chiefs
James Bostrom, Deputy Chiefs
Sally Conway, Deputy Chiefs
A brief report issued by the Justice Department each quarter providing timely information about ADA cases and settlements, building codes that meet ADA accessibility standards, and ADA technical assistance activities.

4660 Federal Laws of the Mentally Handicapped: Laws, Legislative Histories and Admin. Documents
William Hein & Company
2350 North Forest Rd.
Getzville, NY 14068-1296 716-882-2600
800-828-7571
Fax: 716-883-8100
mail@wshein.com
www.wshein.com
Bernard D Reams Jr, Editor
Chronological compilation of all relevant federal laws dealing with the mentally handicapped along with supporting documentation necessary to create a complete legislative history. *$3500.00*
42 Volume/Set
ISBN 0-899411-06-1

4661 Formed Families: Adoption of Children with Handicaps
Haworth Press
711 Third Avenue
New York, NY 10017 212-216-7800
800-354-1420
Fax: 212-244-1563
subscriptions@tandf.co.uk
www.haworthpress.com
William Cohen, Owner
Provides broad coverage of the issues relating to the adoption of children with handicaps. Concerned professionals can find here all the answers about clinical programs, legal issues, estimates of frequency, and important factors related to positive and negative outcomes of these adoptions. *$74.95*
242 pages Hardcover
ISBN 0-866569-14-6

4662 Free Appropriate Public Education: The Law and Children with Disabilities
Love Publishing Company
9101 E Kenyon Avenue
Suite 2200
Denver, CO 80237 303-221-7333
Fax: 303-221-7444
lpc@lovepublishing.com
www.lovepublishing.com
H Rutherford Turnbull III, Author
Matthew J Stowe, Co-Author
Nancy E Huerta, Co-Author
Includes the 2004 IDEA reauthorization and the proposed regulations. This up-to-the-minute resource brings you the most recent developments in legislation, case law techniques, due process, parent participation and much, much more. *$78.00*
448 pages Hardcover
ISBN 0-891083-25-2

4663 Health Care Quality Improvement Act of 1986
William Hein & Company
2350 North Forest Rd.
Getzville, NY 14068-1296   716-882-2600
                                      800-828-7571
                                  Fax: 716-883-8100
                                      mail@wshein.com
                                      www.wshein.com
Bernard D Reams Jr, Editor
In order to encourage more stringent peer review by doctors and
hospitals, and to protect reporting physicians and institutions
from retaliatory lawsuits, Congress enacted The Health Care
Quality Improvement Act. The Act was also intended to address
the increasing incidence of medical malpractice and to prevent
the ease with which incompetent practitioners moved from state
to state. Hardcover. *$125.00*
721 pages
ISBN 0-899416-93-4

4664 Housing and Transportation of the Handicapped
William Hein & Company
2350 North Forest Rd.
Getzville, NY 14068-1296   716-882-2600
                                      800-828-7571
                                  Fax: 716-883-8100
                                      mail@wshein.com
                                      www.wshein.com
Bernard D Reams Jr, Editor
National laws, recognizing the problems encountered by the
handicapped in the areas of Housing and Transportation and providing assistance in an effort to surmount those problems, span
more than half a century. *$1552.50*
30000 pages 250 documents
ISBN 0-899412-47-5

**4665 Human Resource Management and the Americans with
Disabilities Act**
Greenwood Publishing Group
130 Cremona Drive
Santa Barbara, CA 93117   805-968-1911
                                       800-368-6868
                                   Fax: 866-270-3856
                              CustomerService@abc-clio.com
                                     www.greenwood.com
John G Veres, Author
Ronald R Sims, Co-Author
John Gosden, Library Resource Consultants
Lina Gosden, Library Resource Consultants
Concrete advice for human resource professionals on how to cope
with the vague, often obscure provisions of the Americans with
Disabilities Act. *$107.95*
232 pages Hardcover
ISBN 0-899308-57-9

4666 International Handbook on Mental Health Policy
Greenwood Publishing Group
130 Cremona Drive
Santa Barbara, CA 93117   805-968-1911
                                       800-368-6868
                                   Fax: 866-270-3856
                              CustomerService@abc-clio.com
                                     www.greenwood.com
John Gosden, Library Resource Consultants
Lina Gosden, Library Resource Consultants
Steve Pearson, Library Resource Consultants
Lou Pingitore, Library Resource Consultants
The first major reference book for academics and practitioners
that provides a systematic survey and analysis of mental health
policies in twenty representative countries. *$179.95*
512 pages Hardcover
ISBN 0-313275-67-8

4667 Knowing Your Rights
A AR P Fulfillment
601 E St NW
Washington, DC 20049-1   202-434-3525
                                       800-687-2277
                                  Fax: 202-434-3443
                                  TTY: 877-434-7598
                                      member@aarp.org
                                      www.aarp.org
William D. Novelli, CEO
Lynn Smith, Director of Human Resources
Describes how changes in Medicare's reimbursement policies are
designed to reduce health care costs and suggests steps that
Medicare beneficiaries, their families and friends can take to assure that they continue to receive quality care under the Prospective Payment System.
19 pages

4668 Law Center Newsletter
Public Interest Law Center of Philadelphia
1709 Benjamin Franklin Parkway
United Way Building
Philadelphia, PA 19103   215-627-7100
                                   Fax: 215-627-3183
                                      www.pilcop.org
Eric J Rothschild, Chair
Brian T Feeney, Vice Chair
Jennifer R. Clarke, Executive Director
Ellen S Friedell, Treasurer
Information on mental health, foster care and public education.
Provides all updates concerning the law in these areas.

4669 Legal Center for People with Disabilities& Older People
455 Sherman St
Suite 130
Denver, CO 80203   303-722-0300
                                       800-288-1376
                                   Fax: 303-722-0720
                                  TTY: 303-722-3619
Mary Anne Harvey, Executive Director
John R. Posthumus, President
Stephen P. Rickles, Vice President
John Paul Anderson, Treasurer
Uses the legal system to protect and promote the rights of people
with disabilities and older people in Colorado through direct le-
gal representation, advocacy, education and legislative analysis.
The Legal Center is Colorado's Protection and Advocacy System.
We are also the State Ombudsman for nursing homes and assisted
living facilities. Call for a free publications and products list.

**4670 Legal Right: The Guide for Deaf and Hard of Hearing
People**
National Association of the Deaf
8630 Fenton Street
Suite 820
Silver Spring, MD 20910- 3819   301-587-1789
                                   Fax: 301-587-1791
                                  TTY:301-587-1789
                                      www.nad.org
Christopher Wagner, Board Chair
Howard A. Rosenblum, Chief Executive Officer
Marc P. Charmatz, Staff Attorney
Lizzie Sorkin, Director of Communications
This revised fifth edition is in easy-to-understand language, of-
fering the latest state and federal statues and administrative pro-
cedures that prohibit discrimination against the deaf, hard of
hearing and other physically challenged people. *$32.50*
264 pages Paperback
ISBN 1-563680-00-9

4671 Legal Rights of Persons with Disabilities
LRP Publications
360 Hiatt Dr
Palm Beach Gardens, FL 33418-7106   561-622-6520
                                           800-341-7874
                                      Fax: 561-622-0757
                                           lrpitvp@lrp.com
                                           www.lrp.com
Kenneth Kahn, CEO
Shows what is required, permitted and guaranteed by federal disability laws-including the ADA, Section 504 of the Rehabilitation Act and the IDEA. Explores the boundaries of accceptable behavior under disability laws and provides guidelines to help clients fulfill their legal obligations. *$365.00*
2722 pages

4672 Legislative Network for Nurses
Business Publishers
2222 Sedwick Drive
Durham, NC 27713   800-223-8720
                     Fax: 800-508-2592
                          custserv@bpinews.com
                          www.bpinews.com
8 pages Newsl./BiMonthly

4673 Loving Justice
Exceptional Parent Library
P.O.Box 1807
Englewood Cliffs, NJ 7632-1207   201-947-6000
                                        800-535-1910
                                   Fax: 201-947-9376
                                        eplibrary@aol.com
                                        www.eplibrary.com

4674 Making News: How to Get News Coverage of Disability Rights Issues
Advocado Press
PO Box 406781
Louisville, KY 40204   888-739-1920
                         Fax: 502-899-9562
                              www.advocadopress.org
Tari Susan Hartman, Author
Mary Johnson, Co-Author
This book gives examples and tips on how to fight back and get on the front pages, lead the newscasts and influence public debate. *$10.95*
165 pages Paperback
ISBN 0-962706-43-4

4675 Medicare and Medicaid Patient and Program Protection Act of 1987
William Hein & Company
2350 North Forest Rd.
Getzville, NY 14068-1296   716-882-2600
                                  800-828-7571
                             Fax: 716-883-8100
                                  mail@wshein.com
                                  www.wshein.com
Bernard D Reams Jr, Editor
Enables the HHS to protect patients and federal health care programs from censured practitioners. The Act broadens the authority of HHS to exclude practitioners from Medicare and Medicaid programs; strengthens the monetary penalities HHS may impose on violators; provides for criminal penalties in certain cases; and requires states to inform HHS regarding sanctions against health care providers. *$195.00*
3 Volumes
ISBN 0-899416-95-0

4676 Mental & Physical Disability Law Reporter
American Bar Association
1050 Connecticut Ave. N.W.
Suite 400
Washington, DC 20036-1019   202-662-1570
                                   800-285-2221
                              Fax: 202-442-3439
                                   cmpdl@abanet.org
                                   www.abanet.org
Robert M Carlson, Chair
James R Silkenat, President
Jack L Rives, Executive Director
G. Nicholas Casey, Treasurer
Contains over 2,000 summanes per year of federal and state court decisions and legislation that affect persons with mental and physical disabilities. Includes bylined articles by experts in the field regarding disability law developments and trends. *$384.00*
350+ pages BiMonthly

4677 Mental Disabilities and the Americans with Disabilities Act
Greenwood Publishing Group
130 Cremona Drive
Santa Barbara, CA 93117   805-968-1911
                                 800-368-6868
                            Fax: 866-270-3856
                                 CustomerService@abc-clio.com
                                 www.greenwood.com
John Gosden, Library Resource Consultants
Lina Gosden, Library Resource Consultants
Steve Pearson, Library Resource Consultants
Lou Pingitore, Library Resource Consultants
A clear, practical compliance guide, written by a psychologist, to help organizations conform to provisions on mental disabilities in the Americans with Disabilities Act. Hardcover. *$91.95*
216 pages Hardcover
ISBN 0-899308-26-5

4678 Mental Disability Law, Evidence and Testimony
ABA Commission on Mental & Physical Disability Law
1050 Connecticut Ave. N.W.
Suite 400
Washington, DC 20036-1019   202-662-1000
                                   800-285-2221
                                   www.abanet.org
Robert M Carlson, Chair
James R Silkenat, President
Jack L Rives, Executive Director
G. Nicholas Casey, Treasurer
Provides a comprehensive analysis of federal and state statues and case law with a disability discrimination focus. *$95.00*
491 pages Paperback
ISBN 1-590318-32-3

4679 Mental Health Law Reporter
Business Publishers
2222 Sedwick Drive
Durham, NC 27713   240-514-0600
                          800-223-8720
                     Fax: 800-508-2592
                          custserv@bpinews.com
                          www.bpinews.com
Leonard A Eiserer, Publisher
Jeremy Bond, Editor MHLR
Bob Grupe, Editor MHLR
Adam Goldstein, President
MHLR brings you the most timely, focused and thorough information on the legal issues that concern mental health practitioners in mental health litigation. Topics include: malpractice litigation, patient-therapist confidentiality, sexual victimization of patients, the insanity defense, social security administrative case law and much more.. *$286.00*
8 pages Monthly

4680 Mental and Physical Disability Law Reporter
American Bar Association
1050 Connecticut Ave. N.W.
Suite 400
Washington, DC 20036-1019   202-662-1000
                                  800-285-2221
                          service@americanbar.org
                             www.americanbar.org
Wm T Robinson III, President
The only periodical that comprehensively covers civil and criminal mental disability law and disability discrimination law. *$324.00*
150+ pages Bimonthly

4681 Mentally Disabled and the Law
William S Hein & Company
2350 North Forest Rd.
Getzville, NY 14068-1296   716-882-2600
                                  800-828-7571
                            Fax: 716-883-8100
                               mail@wshein.com
                                 www.wshein.com

Samuel Brakel, Author
John Parry, Co-Author
Barbara A Weiner, Co-Author
Chapters retained from 1961 and 1971 editions have been substantially rewritten. Two subjects-sterilization and sexual psychopathy-have been integrated into chapters on family law. Three new chapters on treatment rights, provider-patient relationship and rights of mentally disabled persons in the community. Sixteen new tables supplement the existing revised 41. *$92.00*
845 pages
ISBN 0-910059-05-5

4682 Myths and Facts
US Department of Justice
950 Pennsylvania Ave NW
Washington, DC 20530-9   202-307-0663
                                  800-514-0301
                            Fax: 202-307-1197
                            TTY: 800-514-0383
                                 www.ada.gov

Rebecca B. Bond, Chief
Zita Johnson Betts, Deputy Chief
Sally Conway, Deputy Chief
James Bostrom, Deputy Chief
A 3-page publication dispelling some common misconceptions about the ADA's requirements and implementation.

4683 NAD Broadcaster
National Association of the Deaf
8630 Fenton Street
Suite 820
Silver Spring, MD   20910- 3819   301-587-1789
                            Fax: 301-587-1791
                            TTY:301-587-1789
                               nad.info@nad.org
                                  www.nad.org

Christopher Wagner, Board Chair
Howard A. Rosenblum, Chief Executive Officer
Marc P. Charmatz, Staff Attorney
Lizzie Sorkin, Director of Communications
National newspaper published 11 times a year by the nation's largest organization safeguarding the accessbility and civil rights of 28 million deaf and hard of hearing Americans in education, employment, health care, and telecommunications. Membership: individual $30 per year. *$7.00*

4684 No Longer Disabled: the Federal Courts & the Politics of Social Security Disability
Greenwood Publishing Group
130 Cremona Drive
Santa Barbara, CA 93117   805-968-1911
                                  800-368-6868
                            Fax: 866-270-3856
                        CustomerService@abc-clio.com
                              www.greenwood.com

John Gosden, Library Resource Consultants
Lina Gosden, Library Resource Consultants
Steve Pearson, Library Resource Consultants
Lou Pingitore, Library Resource Consultants
This book is a case study of judicial policy making. It focuses on the role of adjudication in the making and refining of federal policy. *$107.95*
208 pages Hardcover
ISBN 0-313254-24-9

4685 Nolo's Guide to Social Security Disability Getting and Keeping Your Benefits
NOLO
950 Parker St
Berkeley, CA 94710-2524   800-955-4775
                            Fax: 800-645-0895
                                  www.nolo.com

David Morton, Author
This guide demystifies the program and tells you everything you need to know about qualifying and applying for benefits, maintaining your benefits, and appealing the denial of a claim. *$25.49*
512 pages paperback
ISBN 1-413311-04-4

4686 Opening the Courthouse Door: An ADA Access Guide for State Courts
American Bar Association
1050 Connecticut Ave. N.W.
Suite 400
Washington, DC 20036-1019   202-662-1000
                                  800-285-2221
                          service@americanbar.org
                             www.americanbar.org
Wm T Robinson III, President
Practical step-by-step guide walks the reader through the courthouse and court process, presenting a menu of straightforawrd access ideas to enhance communications in court, make the facility more accessbile, and nodify rules and procedures. *$12.00*
78 pages

4687 PAL News
Parent Professional Advocacy League
45 Bromfield Street
10th Floor
Boston, MA 02108-4106   866-815-8122
                            Fax: 617-542-7832
                                 info@ppal.net
                                 www.ppal.net

Earl N. Stuck, Chair
Lisa Lambert, Executive Director
Deborah A. Fauntleroy, Associate Director
Anne Metzger, Treasurer
Parent/Professional Advocacy Leage (PPAL) is an organization that promotes a strong voice for families of children and adolescents with mental health needs. PAL advocates for supports, treatment and policies that enable families to live in their communities in an environment of stability and respect.
Quarterly

4688 Power of Attorney for Health Care
Center for Public Representation
P.O.Box 260049
Madison, WI 53726-49   608-251-4008
                                  800-369-0388
                            Fax: 606-251-1263

132 pages
ISBN 0-93262 -38-0

4689 Title II & III Regulation Amendment Regarding Detectable Warnings
U S Department of Justice
950 Pennsylvania Ave NW
Washington, DC 20530-9
202-307-0663
800-514-0301
Fax: 202-307-1197
TTY: 800-514-0383
www.ada.gov

Rebecca B. Bond, Chief
Zita Johnson Betts, Deputy Chief
Sally Conway, Deputy Chief
James Bostrom, Deputy Chief
This document suspends the requirements for detectable warnings at curb ramps, hazardous vehicular areas, and reflecting pools.

4690 Title II Complaint Form
US Department of Justice
950 Pennsylvania Ave NW
Washington, DC 20530
202-307-0663
800-514-0301
Fax: 202-307-1197
www.ada.gov

Rebecca B. Bond, Chief
Zita Johnson Betts, Deputy Chiefs
James Bostrom, Deputy Chiefs
Sally Conway, Deputy Chiefs
Standard form for filing a complaint under title II of the ADA or section 504 of the Rehabilitation Act of 1973, which prohibit discrimination on the basis of disability by State and local governments and by recipients of federal financial assistance.

4691 Title II Highlights
US Department of Justice
950 Pennsylvania Ave NW
Washington, DC 20530
202-307-0663
800-514-0383
Fax: 202-307-1197
www.ada.gov

Rebecca B. Bond, Chief
Zita Johnson Betts, Deputy Chiefs
James Bostrom, Deputy Chiefs
Sally Conway, Deputy Chiefs
Outline of the key requirements of the ADA for State and local governments. Provides detailed information in bullet format for quick reference.
8 pages

4692 Title III Technical Assistance Manual and Supplement
U S Department of Justice
950 Pennsylvania Ave NW
Washington, DC 20530
202-307-0663
800-574-0301
Fax: 202-307-1197
www.ada.gov

Rebecca B. Bond, Chief
Zita Johnson Betts, Deputy Chiefs
James Bostrom, Deputy Chiefs
Sally Conway, Deputy Chiefs
Explains in lay terms what businesses and non-profit agencies must do to ensure access to their goods, services, and facilities.
83 pages

4693 Toward Independence
National Council on Disability
81 E. Main Street
Xenia, OH 45385
937-376-3996
Fax: 937-376-2046
info@ti-inc.org
www.ti-inc.org

Mary Rose Zink, Chair
Paul Osterfeld, Vice Chair
Mark Schlater, Executive Director
Bob Groskopf, Treasurer
A 1986 report to the U.S. Congress on the federal laws and programs serving people with disabilities, and recommendations for legislation.

4694 UCP Washington Wire
United Cerebral Palsy
1825 K Street NW
Suite 600
Washington, DC 20006-1601
202-776-0406
800-872-5827
Fax: 202-776-0414
info@ucp.org
www.ucp.org

Stephen Bennett, President/CEO
Publication that provides a comprehensive source of information on federal legislation, agency regulations, court decisions and other issues of interest to the disability community.
weekly

4695 US Department of Health and Human Services Office for Civil Rights
200 Independence Ave SW
Room 509F, HHH Building
Washington, DC 20201
202-619-0403
800-368-1019
TTY:800-537-7697
ocrmail@hhs.gov
www.hhs.gov

Georgina Verdugo, Director
The Department's civil rights and health privacy law enforcement agency, OCR investigates complaints, enforces rights, and promulgates regulations, develops policy and provides technical assistance and public education to ensure understanding of and compliance with non-discrimination and health information privacy laws.

4696 US Department of Labor
200 Constitution Ave NW
Washington, DC 20210
866-487-2365
www.dol.gov

Hilda L Solis, Secretary of Labor
Seth D Harris, Deputy Secretary
To foster, promote, and develop the welfare of the wage earners, job seekers, and retirees of the United States; improve working conditions, advance opportunities for profitable employment; and assure work-related benefits and rights.

4697 US Department of Labor Office of Federal Contract Compliance Programs
200 Constitution Ave NW
Washington, DC 20210
312-596-7010
866-487-2365
Fax: 312-596-7044
OFCCP-MW-PreAward@dol.gov
www.dol.gov

Melissa L Speer, Interim Regional Director
To enforce, for the benefit of job seekers and wage earners, the contractual promise of affirmative action and equal employment opportunity required of those who do business with the Federal government.

4698 University Legal Services AT Program
Ste 130
220 i St NE
Washington, DC 20002-4364
202-547-4747
877-221-4638
Fax: 202-547-2083
TTY: 202-547-2657
atpdc@uls-dc.org
dcpanda.org

Jane Brown, Executive Director
Designed to empower individuals with disabilities; to promote consumer involvement and advocacy, and provide information, referral and training as they relate to accessing assistive technology services and devices; and to identify and improve access to funding resources..

4699 **William S Hein & Company**
2350 North Forest Rd.
Getzville, NY 14068-1296

716-882-2600
800-828-7571
Fax: 716-883-8100
mail@wshein.com
www.wshein.com

Kevin Marmion, President
Offers a catalog of periodicals, publications and reprints, microforms and government publications on medical, handicapped and health law.

Libraries & Research Centers

Alabama

4700 Alabama Institute for Deaf and Blind Library and Resource Center
205 E South Street
P.O. Box 698
Talladega, AL 35160   256-761-3206
                                 Fax: 256-761-3352
                                            aidb.org

Dr. John Mascia, President
Teresa Lacy, Director, Library & Resource Center
Book collection includes discs, cassettes, braille and large print. Also closed-circuit TV and magnifiers. Offers braille production and binding.

4701 Alabama Radio Reading Service Network(ARRS)
Public Radio WBHM 90.3 FM
650 11th St S
Birmingham, AL 35233-1   205-934-2606
                                         800-444-9246
                                 Fax: 205-934-5075
                                            wbhm.org

Audrey Atkins, Marketing Manager
Scott E Hanley, General Manager
Theresa Kidd, Office Manager
Michael Krall, Program Director
Services and readings are broadcast over a subcarrier service of public radio WBHM. This is a statewide service devoted to Alabama's blind and handicapped community.

4702 Alabama Regional Library for the Blind and Physically Handicapped
Alabama Public Library Service
6030 Monticello Dr
Montgomery, AL 36130-1   334-213-3906
                                         800-392-5671
                                 Fax: 334-213-3993
                                 revans@apls.state.al.us
                                 webmini.apls.state.al.us
Mike Coleman, Blind & Physically Handicapped Division
Tim Emmons, Blind & Physically Handicapped Division
Nancy Pack, Director
Kelyn Ralya, Assistant Director
Recreational reading in special format for persons unable to use standard print. Reference materials offered include materials on blindness and other handicaps, films, local subjects and authors.

4703 Dothan Houston County Library System
Formerly Houston-Love Memorial Library
445 N Oates St
Dothan, AL 36303   334-793-9767
                                    dhcls@dhcls.org
                                       www.dhcls.org
Jason DeLuc, Library Director
Charlotte Mitchell, Main Library Manager
Offers magnifiers, summer reading programs and more for the blind and physically handicapped. Scanner, software, jaws for Windows.

4704 Huntsville Subregional Library for the Blind & Physically Handicapped
Huntsville-Madison County Public Library
915 Monroe St SW
Huntsville, AL 35804-0000   256-532-5980
                                 Fax: 256-532-5994
                                 bphdept@hmcpl.org
                                       www.hmcpl.org
Laurel Best, Executive Director
Talking books for people who are blind or disabled offering reference materials on the blind and other disabilities, large-print photocopier, thermaform duplicator and more.

4705 Public Library Of Anniston-Calhoun County
108 E 10th St
Anniston, AL 36201   256-237-8501
                                 library@publiclibrary.cc
                                       publiclibrary.cc

4706 Technology Assistance for Special Consumers
UCP Huntsville
1856 Keats Drive
Huntsville, AL 35810   256-859-8300
                                 Fax: 256-859-4332
                                 tasc@ucphuntsville.org
                                       ucphuntsville.org
Cheryl Smith, Chief Executive Officer
Provide individuals with disabilities, their families and/or advocates, and associated professionals access to assistive technology devices and services to increase independence at home, school, and work.

Alaska

4707 Alaska State Library Talking Book Center
State of Alaska
344 W 3rd Ave
Ste 125
Anchorage, AK 99501-2338   907-465-1304
                                         888-820-4525
                                 Fax: 907-269-6580
                                 tbc@alaska.gov
                                 talkingbooks.alaska.gov
Patience Frederiksen, Director, Division of Libraries, Archives & Museums
Freya Anderson, Requisitions Librarian
Ginny Jacobs, Library Assistant
The Alaska State Library Talking Book Center is a cooperative effort between the Library of Congress National Library Service for the Blind and Physically Handicapped and the Alaska State Library to provide print handicapped Alaskans with talking book and Braille service. The Talking Book Center has 55,000 audiobooks that can be checked out to eligible Alaskans whose visual or physical handicap prevents them from reading standard print materials.

Arizona

4708 Arizona Braille and Talking Book Library
Arizona State Library
1030 N 32nd St
Phoenix, AZ 85008-5108   602-255-5578
                                         800-255-5578
                                 Fax: 602-286-0444
                                       www.azlibrary.gov
Linda Montgomery, Director
Audio and braille books and magazines, summer reading program, volunteer-produced audio books, audo described, films and more.

4709 Books for the Blind of Arizona
Unit A107
6120 E 5th St
Tucson, AZ 85711-2536   602-792-9153
                                 Fax: 520-886-9839
Betty Evans, Chairperson
Offers large print photocopier, textbooks, recreational, career, vocational, braille books, talking books, cassettes, large print books and more for the visually impaired K-12, college students and adults..

4710 Children's Center for Neurodevelopmental Studies
5430 W Glenn Dr
Glendale, AZ 85301-2628
623-915-0345
Fax: 623-937-5425
admin@ccnsaz.org
www.thechildrenscenteraz.org

Kent Rideout, Executive Director
Dawna Sterner, Preschool & Education Informatio
Catherine Orsak, Therapy Information
Alicia Bolan, Teaching Staff
The Center is a non-profit school and therapy center for children with autism and other developmental delays specializing in the use of sensory integration.

4711 Flagstaff City-Coconino County Public Library
300 W Aspen Ave
Flagstaff, AZ 86001-5304
928-779-7670
TTY:928-214-2417
www.flagstaffpubliclibrary.org

4712 Fountain Hills Lioness Braille Service
P.O.Box 18332
Fountain Hills, AZ 85269-8332
480-837-3961
Jean Hauck, Chairperson
Braille and large print books on the subjects of recreation, career and vocations, religion, novels and cookbooks for the visually impaired..

4713 Prescott Public Library
215 E Goodwin St
Prescott, AZ 86303-3911
928-777-1500
Fax: 928-771-5829
prescottlibrary.info

Roger Saft, Director
Martha Baden, Public Services Manager
Teresa Vonk, Support Services Manager
Lisa Zierke, Technical Services
Large print, braille and audio books; magnifiers; text to voice scanner; talking book machine application; toy library for children with special needs; special needs product catalogs; home book delivery; descriptive videos; 43 point PC monitor..

4714 Special Needs Center/Phoenix Public Library
1221 N Central Ave
Phoenix, AZ 85004-1867
602-262-4636
TTY:602-254-8205
www.phoenixpubliclibrary.org

4715 World Research Foundation
P.O. Box 20828
Sedona, AZ 86341-8804
928-284-3300
Fax: 928-284-3530
info@wrf.org
wrf.org

Steven A Ross, President
LaVerne Boeckmann, Co-Founder
Large research library of alternative medicine; offers a computer search and printout of specific health issues for a nominal fee.

Arkansas

4716 Arkansas Regional Library for the Blind and Physically Handicapped
900 West Capitol Avenue
Suite 100
Little Rock, AR 72201-3108
501-682-2053
www.library.arkansas.gov

J D Hall, Manager of BPH Services
Dwain Gordon, Deputy Director
Danny Koonce, Public Information Specialist
Ruth Hyatt, Manager of Extension Services
Public library books in recorded or braille format. Popular fiction and nonfiction books for all ages, books and players are on free loan, sent to patrons by mail and may be returned postage free. Anyone who cannot see well enough to read regular print with glasses on or who has a disability that makes it difficult to hold a book or turn the pages is eligible.

4717 Arkansas School for the Blind
P.O.Box 668
Little Rock, AR 72203-668
501-296-1810
800-362-4451
Fax: 501-296-1831
www.arkansasschoolfortheblind.org

Khayyam Eddings, Chairperson
Jennifer Benedetti, Elementary Principal
Teresa Doan, Special Education Supervisor
William Harrison, Technology Director
Students at the ASB receive a quality education from specially trained instructors of the Visually Impaired in all academic areas. ASB features a comprehensive Music and Art program, as well as extensive extra-curricular activities. ASB is a proud member of the Arkansas Activities Association and The North Central Association of Schools for the Blind.

4718 Educational Services for the Visually Impaired
2402 Wildwood Avenue
Suite 112
Sherwood, AR 72120-5085
501-835-5448
Fax: 501-835-6840
Angyln.Young@arkansas.gov
www.esvi.org

Angyln Young, State Coordinator
Cindy Lester, Data Management Specialist
Cynthia Kelly, ESVI Office Manager
Offers textbooks, braille books and more to the visually impaired grades K-12 in the Arizona area.

4719 Library for the Blind and Physically Handicapped SW Region of Arkansas
P.O.Box 668
2057 North Jackson St
Magnolia, AR 71754-668
870-234-1991
Fax: 870-234-5077
library@cocolib.org
www2.youseemore.com/Columbia

Rhonda Rolen, Director
Dana Thornton, Assistant Director
Becky Verschage, Processing Clerk
Lisa Lewis, Bookkeeping
A free library service that serves adults and children who meet the eligiblity requirements, offers free loan of cassette machine and recorded books, which meet the reading preferences of a highly diverse clientele.

4720 Northwest Ozarks Regional Library for the Blind and Handicapped
Fayetteville, AR 72701
479-575-2000
www.uark.edu

California

4721 Braille Institute Library
741 N Vermont Ave
Los Angeles, CA 90029-3594
323-663-1111
800-808-2555
Fax: 323-663-0867
la@brailleinstitute.org
brailleinstitute.org

Leslie E. Stocker, President
Sally H. Jameson, Vice President of Programs and S
Peter A. Mindnich, Executive Vice President
Reza Rahman, Vice President of Finance/Chief
Braille Institute provides an environment of hope and encouragement for people who are blind and visually impaired through integrated educational, social and recreational programs and services.

4722 Braille Institute Santa Barbara Center
2031 De La Vina St
Santa Barbara, CA 93105-3895   805-682-6222
                                        800-272-4553
                                    Fax: 805-687-6141
                                    sb@brailleinstitute.org
                                    brailleinstitute.org

Leslie E. Stocker, President
Sally H. Jameson, Vice President of Programs and S
Peter A. Mindnich, Executive Vice President
Reza Rahman, Vice President of Finance/Chief
Offers programs, services and information for persons with visual impairments.

4723 Braille Institute Sight Center
741 N Vermont Ave
Los Angeles, CA 90029-3594   323-663-1111
                                      800-808-2555
                                  Fax: 323-663-0867
                                  la@brailleinstitute.org
                                  brailleinstitute.org

Sally H. Jameson, Vice President of Programs and S
Leslie E Stocker, President
Peter A. Mindnich, Executive Vice President
Reza Rahman, Vice President of Finance/Chief
Offers help, programs, services and information to the blind and visually impaired children and adults.

4724 Braille and Talking Book Library: California
P.O. Box 942837
Sacramento, CA 94237-0001   916-654-0640
                                      800-952-5666
                          www.library.ca.gov/services/btbl.html

Stacey A. Aldrich, State Librarian
Debbie Newton, Bureau Chief, Administrative Ser
Phyllis Smith, Manager, Human Resources and Bus
Sharleen Finn, Budget Officer, Fiscal Services
Free service for eligible Northern California residents.

4725 California State Library Braille and Talking Book Library
PO Box 942837
Sacramento, CA 94237-0001   916-654-0640
                                      800-952-5666
                                  btbl@library.ca.gov
                                  www.btbl.ca.gov

4726 Clearinghouse for Specialized Media and Translations
1430 N St
Ste 3207
Sacramento, CA 95814-5901   916-319-0800
                                  Fax: 916-323-9732
                                  www.cde.ca.gov/re/pn/sm

Jonn Paris-Salb, Manager
Provides materials in accessible formats; aural media, braille, large print, digital talking books and electronic media access technology.

4727 Dental Amalgam Syndrome (DAMS) Newsletter
725-9 Tramway Ln NE
Albuquerque, NM 87122-1672   505-291-8239
                                  Fax: 505-294-3339

4728 Fresno County Free Library Blind and Handicapped Services
2420 Mariposa Street
Fresno, CA 93721-3640   559-600-7323
                                  800-742-1011
                          wendy.eisenberg@fresnolibrary.org
                          www.fresnolibrary.org/tblb

Wendy Eisenberg, Manager
Laurel Prysiazny, County Librarian
Magnifiers, home visits, volunteer-produced cassette books, discs and cassettes.

4729 Glaucoma Research Foundation
251 Post St
Ste 600
San Francisco, CA 94108-5017   415-986-3162
                                        800-826-6693
                                    Fax: 415-986-3763
                                    question@glaucoma.org
                                    glaucoma.org

Tom Brunner, President and CEO
Nancy Graydon, Executive Director of Development
Andrew L. Jackson, Director of Communications
Catalina San Agustin, Director of Operations
Clinical and laboratory studies of glaucoma. We work to prevent vision loss from glaucoma by investing in innovative research, education and support with the ultimate goal of finding a cure..

4730 Herrick Health Sciences Library
Alta Bates Medical Center
2001 Dwight Way
Berkeley, CA 94704-2608   510-869-6777
                                  Fax: 510-204-4091
                                  www.altabatessummit.org

Laurie Bagley, Librarian
Carol Hirsch-Butler, Administrator
Carolyn Kemp, Regional Manager of Public Relations
Information on rehabilitation, psychiatry and psychoanalysis.

4731 Kuzell Institute for Arthritis and Infectious Diseases
Medical Research Institute Of San Francisco
2200 Webster St.
San Francisco, CA 94115-1821   415-561-1734
Edward Byrd, Owner
One of seven units comprising the Medical Research Institute of San Francisco that offers basic and applied research in arthritis and related diseases.

4732 New Beginnings: The Blind Children's Center
4120 Marathon St
Los Angeles, CA 90029-3584   323-664-2153
                                      800-222-3566
                                  Fax: 323-665-3828
                                  blindchildrenscenter.org

Lena French, Executive Director
Kimberlee Jones, Director of Development
Ross Vergara, Director of Finance
Manuel Ayala, Director of Facilities
The purpose of the Center is to turn initial fears into hope. Helps children and their families become independent by creating a climate of safety and trust. Children learn to develop self confidence and to master a wide range of skills. Services include an infant stimulation program, educational preschool, interdisciplinary assessment services, family services, correspondence program, toll free national hotline and a publication and research service.

4733 Research & Training Center on Mental Health for Hard of Hearing Persons
California School of Professional Psychology
Ste 140
6215 Ferris Sq
San Diego, CA 92121-3279   619-282-4443
                                    800-HEA-R619
                                  Fax: 800-642-0266

Raymond J Trybus, Director
Thomas J Goulder, Associate Director
Funded by the National Institute on Disability and Rehabilitation Research, this training center aims to address issues of psychological relevance to persons who are hard of hearing or late deafened (as distinct from prelingually, culturally deaf persons). Also serves as information clearinghouse on this topic.

4734 Rosalind Russell Medical Research Center for Arthritis
Suite 600
350 Parnassus Ave
San Francisco, CA 94117   415-476-1141
                                        Fax: 415-476-3526
                                    rrac@medicine.ucsf.edu
                            www.rosalindrussellcenter.ucsf.edu
Ephraim P Engleman, MD, Center Director
David Wofsy, MD, Associate Director
Paula R. Gambs, Chair
Christine Abele, Volunteer
Arthritis research and its probable causes.

4735 San Francisco Public Library for the Blindand Print Handicapped
100 Larkin St
San Francisco, CA 94102-4705   415-557-4400
                                        Fax: 415-557-4252
                                    TTY:415-557-4433
                                    webmail@sfpl.org
                                        www.sfpl.org
Toni Cordova, Chief of Communications, Program
Toni Bernardi, Special Projects Manager
Laura Lent, Chief of Collections & Technical
Edward Melton, Chief of Branches
Foreign-language books on cassette, children's books on cassettes and more.

4736 San Jose State University Library
150 E San Fernando St
San Jose, CA 95112-3580   408-808-2000
                                        Fax: 408-924-1118
                                        www.sjlibrary.org
Don W Kassing, President
Jane Light, Library/Executive Director
Jeff Barber, Security Officer
Luann Budd, Administrative Officer
Information on physical disabilities, accessibility and learning disabilities.

Colorado

4737 AMC Cancer Research Center
3401 Quebec Street
Suite 3200
Denver, CO 80207   303-233-6501
                                        800-321-1557
                                    Fax: 303-239-3400
                                    contactus@amc.org
                                        amc.org
Gary Kortz, Chairman
Steven D. Toltz, Treasurer
Cheryl Kisling, Secretary
Karen Padgett, President and CEO
Provides trained counselors who provide understanding and support for cancer patients; information and referral services; and screening programs.

4738 Boulder Public Library
1001 Arapahoe Ave
Boulder, CO 80302-6015   303-441-3100
                                        www.boulderlibrary.org
Melinda Mattling, Manager
Priscilla Hudson, Manager
Offers braille books, cassettes, talking books, large print photocopier, large print books and more for the visually impaired.

4739 Colorado Talking Book Library
180 Sheridan Blvd
Denver, CO 80226-8101   303-727-9277
                                        800-685-2136
                                    Fax: 303-727-9281
                                    ctbl.info@cde.state.co.us
                            www.cde.state.co.us/ctbl/index.htm
Debbie Macleod, Executive Director

Provides free library service to Coloradans of all ages who are unable to read standard print due to visual, physical or learning disabilities whether permanent or temporary. Provides audio, braille and large-print books and magazines.

4740 National Jewish Medical & Research Center
1400 Jackson St
Denver, CO 80206-2762   303-388-4461
                                        877-225-5654
                                    www.nationaljewish.org
Michael Salem, MD, President and CEO
Richard A. Schierburg, Chair
Robin Chotin, Vice Chair
Robin Chotin, Secretary
The only medical center in the country whose research and patient care resources are dedicated to respiratory and immunologic diseases.

Connecticut

4741 Connecticut Braille Association
107 Vanderbilt Ave
West Hartford, CT 6110-1514   860-953-4445
                                        Fax: 860-378-0205
Nick Martino, Owner
Offers textbooks, cassettes, large print books, braille books and more.

4742 Connecticut Library for the Blind and Physically Handicapped
231 Capitol Avenue
Hartford, CT 06106-1569   860-757-6500
                                        860-866-4478
                                    Fax: 860-721-2056
                                    ctaylor@cslib.org
                                        www.cslib.org
Kendall Wiggin, State Librarian
Ursula Hunt, Administrative Assistant
Shelley Delisle, IT Manager
Jane Beaudoin, Administrative Assistant
Network library of the National Library Service for the Blind and Physically Handicapped, Library of Congress. Lends books and magazines in Braille or recorded formats along with the necessary playback equipment, free, for any Connecticut adult or child who is unable to read regular print due to a visual or physical disability. All materials are mailed to and from library patrons by postage-free mail

4743 Connecticut State Library
Connecticut State Government
231 Capitol Ave
Hartford, CT 06106-1569   860-757-6500
                                        866-866-4478
                                    Fax: 860-721-2056
                                    isref@cslib.org
                                        www.cslib.org
Kendall Wiggin, State Librarian
Ursula Hunt, Administrative Assistant
Shelley Delisle, IT Manager
Jane Beaudoin, Administrative Assistant
Discs, cassettes, braille, reference materials on blindness and other handicaps, closed-circuit TV and large-print photocopier.

4744 Connecticut Tech Act Project: Connecticut Department of Social Services
Bureau of Rehabilitations Services
25 Sigourney St
11th Floor
Hartford, CT 06106-5041   860-424-4881
                                        800-537-2549
                                    Fax: 860-424-4850
                                    TTY: 860-424-4839
                                    arlene.lugo@ct.gov
                                        www.cttechact.com
Arlene Lugo, Program Director

Single point of entry, advocacy, information and referral, peer counseling, and access to objective expert advice and consultation for people with disabilities.

4745   Prevent Blindness Connecticut
101 Whitney Avenue
New Haven, CT   06510   203-722-4653
                                                800-850-2020
                                       Fax: 203-722-4691
                             info@preventblindnesstristate.org
Kathryn Garre-Ayars, President and CEO
Tahesha Bryan, Administrative Assistant
Naomi Hayner, Connecticut Program Manager
Maria Giarratana, Grants Manager
The mission of Prevent Blindness Connecticut is to save sight and prevent blindness through eye screenings, education, safety activities and research.

4746   Yale University: Vision Research Center
310 Cedar St, LH 108
PO Box 208023
New Haven, CT   06520- 8023   203-785-2759
                                                800-395-7949
                                       Fax: 203-785-7303
                             pamela.berkheiser@yale.edu
                             medicine.yale.edu/pathology
George Shafranov, Chairman
Pam Burkheiser, Manager
Robert J. Alpern, Dean
Vision including studies on growth and development.

Delaware

4747   Delaware Assistive Technology Initiative (DATI)
Alfred I. duPont Hospital for Children
461 Wyoming Road
Newark, DE   19716-0269   302-831-0354
                                                800-870-3284
                                       Fax: 302-831-4690
                                       TTY: 302-651-6794
                             dati@asel.udel.edu
                             www.dati.org
Beth Mineo Mollica, Director
Sonja Rathel, Project Coordinator
The Delaware Assistive Technology Initiative (DATI) connects Delawareans who have disabilities with the tools they need in order to learn, work, play and participate in community life safely and independently. DATI services include: Equipment demonstration centers in eah county; no-cost, short-term equipment loans that let you try before you buy; Equipment Exchange Program; AT workshops and other training sessions; advocacy for improved AT access policies and funding and several more.

4748   Delaware Library for the Blind and Physically Handicapped
Government
121 Duke of York Street
Dover, DE   19901-7430   302-739-4748
                                                800-282-8676
                                       Fax: 302-739-6787
                                       debph@lib.de.us
                                       libraries.delaware.gov
Dr. Annie E. Norman, Director
Sonja Brown, Administrative Specialist
Beth-Ann Ryan, Deputy Director
Diann Colose, Administrative Librarian
Books on cassette and playback equipment are provided to patrons who are unable to read regular printed books.

4749   Elwyn Delaware
111 Elwyn Road
Elwyn, PA   19063-3499   610-891-2000
                                       Fax: 302-654-5815
                                       info@elwyn.org
                                       www.elwyn.org
Vicki Haschak, Contact
Kendra Johnson, Contact

Provides work training, job placement and supported employment, and elder care services.

District of Columbia

4750   District of Columbia Public Library: Services for the Deaf Community
District of Columbia Public Library
901 G St NW, Room 215
Washington, DC   20001-4531   202-727-0321
                                       Fax: 202-727-0321
                                       TTY:202-559-5368
                             library_deaf_dc@yahoo.com
                             dclibrary.org
Venetia Demson, Chief Adaptive Services
Janice Roseu, Library for the Deaf Community
Offers reference services through videophone, signers for library programs, sign language classes, information about deafness, print and non-print materials for persons who have hearing disabilities. Book talks on deaf culture and American Sign Language story hours for kids, and Saturday sessions on employment-related skills are offered. Videophones for public use are available at the MLK Library.

4751   District of Columbia Regional Library for the Blind and Physically Handicapped
901 G St NW
Washington, DC   20001-4531   202-727-0321
                                       Fax: 202-727-1129
                                       TTY:202-727-2145
                             lbphb_2000@yahoo.com
                             www.dclibrary.org
Richard Reyes-Gavilan, Executive Director
Jonathan Butler, Director of Business Services
Barbara Kirven, Director of Human Resources
Joi Mecks, Director of Communications
Regional library/RPH is network library in the Library of Congress, National Library Services for the Blind and Physically Handicapped.

4752   Georgetown University Center for Child and Human Development
P.O.Box 571485
Washington, DC   20057-1485   202-687-5000
                                       Fax: 202-687-8899
                                       TTY:202-687-5000
                             gucdc@georgetown.edu
                             gucchd.georgetown.edu
Phyllis R Magrab, Phd, Director
John J DeGioia, President
Established over four decades ago to improve the quality of life for all children and youth, especially those with, or at risk for, special needs and their families. Located in the nation's capital, this center both directly serves vulnerable children and their families, as well as influences local, state, national and international programs and policy.

4753   National Institute on Disability and Rehabilitation Research
U S Department of Education
400 Maryland Ave SW
Washington, DC   20202-1   202-401-2000
                                                800-872-5327
                                       Fax: 202-401-0689
                                       TTY: 800-437-0833
                             customerservice@inet.ed.gov
                             ed.gov
Arne Duncan, Secretary of Education
Jim Shelton, Deputy Secretary
Ted Mitchell, Secretary
A national leader in sponsoring research. Mission is to generate, disseminate and promote new knowledge to improve the options available to disabled persons.

Florida

4754   Brevard County Talking Books Library
Brevard County Libraries
2725 Judge Fran Jamieson Way
Viera, FL 32940   321-633-2000
                                     Fax: 321-633-1964
                                     TTY:321-633-1838
                                     kbriley@brev.org
                           www.brevardcounty.us/PublicLibraries
Camille Johnson, Manager
Catherine J Schweinsburg, Library Services Director
Subregional library for the blind and physically handicapped,
assistive reading devices collection, reference materials on
blindness and other handicaps, descriptive videos, CCTV, phonic
ear, reading edge and LOUD-R assistive listening devices
available.

4755   Broward County Talking Book Library
100 S Andrews Ave
Fort Lauderdale, FL 33301-1830   954-357-7444
                                     Fax: 954-357-5548
                                     www.broward.org
Robert E. Cannon, Director
Carolyn Kayne, Manager
Reference materials on blindness and other handicaps, films,
closed-circuit TV, discs, cassettes and a book discussion group is
offered.

4756   Dade County Talking Book Library
Miami Dade Public Library System
101 West Flagler Street
Miami, FL 33130   305-375-2665
                                          800-451-9544
                                     Fax: 305-757-8401
                                     talkingbooks@mdpls.org
                                     www.mdpls.org
Raymond Sanpiago, Executive Director
Lainey Brooks, Development Officer
Sylvia Mora Oria, Assistant Director
Ian D. Rosenior, Operations Administrator
A free Outreach Service of the Miami-Dade Public Library Sys-
tem. A network library, or subregional, of the National Library
Service for the Blind and Physically Handicapped, Library of
Congress, and of the Florida Bureau of Braille and Talking Books
Library Service.

4757   Florida Division of Blind Services
Regional Library
325 West Gaines Street
Turlington Building, Suite 1114
Tallahassee, FL 32399-0400   850-245-0300
                                          800-342-1828
                                     Fax: 850-245-0363
                                     dbs.myflorida.com
Mike Gunde, Manager
Susan Roberts, Bureau Chief
Robert Doyle, Director
Edward Hudson, Bureau Chief
Discs, cassettes, closed-circuit TV, large-print photocopier,
films, children's books on cassettes and more.

**4758   Florida Instructional Materials Center for the Visually
Impaired (FIMC-VI)**
4210 W Bay Villa Ave
Tampa, FL 33611-1206   813-837-7826
                                          800-282-9193
                                     Fax: 813-837-7979
                                     FloridaBrailleChallenge@gmail.com
                                     www.fimcvi.org
Mary Stoltz, Database Manager
Jeffrey Fitterman, Technology Specialist
Teresa Gutierrez, Administrative Secretary
Kay Ratzlaff, Coordinator
Operates a clearinghouse depository and production center for
braille, large print and digital texts. Provides assistance in assess-
ment of materials and specialized apparatus, organizes and trains

volunteers for material production for the visually impaired, and
provides professional development for teachers of the visually
impaired. Provides electronic texts to NIMAS-eligible students
in Florida.

**4759   Hillsborough County Talking Book Library
Tampa-Hillsborough County Public Library**
900 N Ashley Dr
Tampa, FL 33602-3704   813-273-3652
                                     Fax: 813-273-3707
                                     TTY:813-273-3610
                                     www.hcplc.org
Joe Stines, Director of Libraries
Marcee Challener, Assitant Director
David Wullschleger, Chief of Operations
Linda Gillon, Manager of Staff & Administrativ
Serves as the reference hub and resource center for all citzens of
Hillsborough County and as the flagship library of the
Tampa-Hillsborough County Public Library System.

4760   Jacksonville Public Library: Talking Books/Special Needs
303 N Laura St
Jacksonville, FL 32202-3505   904-630-2665
                                     Fax: 904-630-0604
                                     www.jpl.coj.net/lib/talkingbooks.html
Barbara Gubbin, Executive Director
Offers cassettes and digital books, reference materials on blindness and ADA issues, newsline, descriptive videos, and some
assistive devices.

4761   Lee County Library System: Talking Books Library
2001 N. Tamiami Trail N.E.
North Fort Myers, FL 33903-4855   239-533-4320
                                          800-854-8195
                                     Fax: 239-485-1146
                                     TTY: 239-995-2665
                                     talkingbooks@leegov.com
                                     www.lee-county.com/library
Cynthia N Cobb, Director
Terri Crawford, Deputy Director
Debbie Parrott, Manager
Karen McLeish-Delgado, Librarian
Provides free books and magazines to Lee County residents of all
ages who have any disability that prevents them from reading
printed material. Books are played on special players provided
free by the National Library Service. Circulates low tech
assistive aids and devices for temporary loan to Lee County Library card holders. Directs people to assistive technology and
disability related resources.

**4762   Louis de la Parte Florida Mental Health Institute Research
Library**
University of South Florida
4202 E. Fowler Ave. LIB122
Tampa, FL 33620   813-974-2729
                                     Fax: 813-974-7242
                                     lib.usf.edu/fmhi
William A. Garrison, Dean
Florence Jandreau, CAP, Senior Assistant to the Dean
Claudia Dold, Assistant University Librarian
Tomaro Taylor, Associate University Librarian / Certified Archivist
Information offered on mental illness, autism and pervasive de-
velopment disabilities mental health research and archives
management.

4763   Orange County Library System: Audio-Visual Department
101 E Central Blvd
Orlando, FL 32801-2429   407-835-7323
                                     Fax: 407-835-7649
                                     TTY:407-835-7641
                                     comments@ocls.info
                                     www.ocls.info
Ted Maines, President
Lisa Franchina, Vice President
Bob Tessier, Comptroller
Craig Wilkins, Public Service Administrator
Serves the residents of the Orange County Library District, with
headquarters in downtown Orlando.

4764   Pearlman Biomedical Research Institute
Mt Sinai Medical Center
1600 NW 10th Ave
Miami Beach, FL   33140   305-674-2121
                                       Fax: 305-674-2198
                        william-abraham@msmc.com

William Abraham, Director
A 32,000 square feet facility located on the main campus of
Mount Sinai. The institute consists of laboratory space, research
and administrative offices. The studies conducted within the facility are primarily pre-clinical research.

**4765   Pinellas Talking Book Library for the Blind and Physically
Handicapped**
1330 Cleveland St
Clearwater, FL   33755-5103   727-441-8408
                                       Fax: 727-441-8398
                                       TTY:727-441-3168
                                       contactus@pplc.us
                                       www.pplc.us

William Horne, Chair
Cheryl Morales, Executive Director
David Saari, Facilities Manager
Rosa Rodriguez, Deaf Literacy Coordinator at Saf
The Pinellas Public Library Cooperative serves Pinellas County
residents in member cities and the unincorporated county. The
Cooperative Office provides cooridination of activities and fund-
ing as well as marketing services for the the member counties.
The Talking Book Library servces Pinellas, Manatee, and
Sarasota counties.

4766   Talking Book Service: Mantatee County Central Library
1112 Manatee Avenue West
Bradenton, FL   34206-1000   941-748-4501
                                       Fax: 941-751-7098
                                       www.mymanatee.org

Patricia Schubert, Manager
Offers children's books on disc and cassette and more reference
materials for the blind and physically handicapped.

**4767   Talking Books Library for the Blind and Physically
Handicapped**
Palm Beach County Library
3650 Summit Blvd
West Palm Beach, FL   33406-4114   561-233-2600
                                       888-780-4962
                                       Fax: 561-233-2627
                                       webmaster@pbclibrary.org
                                       www.pbclibrary.org

John Callahan, Executive Director
Bill Rautenberg, Chair
Harriet Helfman, Vice Chair
John Callahan III, Library Director
Established in 1967, today the County Library system serves
Palm Beach County through the Main Library, 2 Regional Librar-
ies, 11 Branch Libraries, a Bookmobile and a library annex. It
continues to expand through our involvement with library net-
works, the Internet, and the World Wide Web.

4768   Talking Books/Homebound Services
Brevard County Library System
2725 Judge Fran Jamieson Way
Viera, FL   32940   321-633-2000
                                       Fax: 321-633-1838
                                       kbriley@brev.org
                        www.brevardcounty.us/PublicLibraries

Kay Briley, Librarian
Camille Johnson, Executive Director
Offers reference materials on blindness and other handicaps.
Subregional library for the blind and physically handicapped,
assistive reading devices collection, reference materials on
blindness and other handicaps; CCTV, phonic ear, reading edge
and LOUD-R assistive listening devices available.

4769   University of Miami: Bascom Palmer Eye Institute
Department Of Ophthalmalogy
900 NW 17th St
Miami, FL   33136-1119   305-243-2020
                                       888-845-0002
                                       Fax: 305-326-7000
                                       www.bascompalmer.org

Michael Gittelman, CEO
Teresa Spaulding, Manager
Eduardo C. Alfonso, M.D., Professor and Chairman
Jennifer Cohen, Executive Director
Clinical and basic research into blindness and visual impair-
ments.

**4770   University of Miami: Mailman Center for Child
Development**
1601 NW 12th Ave
Miami, FL   33136-1005   305-243-6395
                                       Fax: 305-326-7594
                                       pedsinformation@med.miami.edu
                                       pediatrics.med.miami.edu

William Donelan, Vice President for Medical Admin
William W. O'Neill, M.D., Executive Dean, Chief Medical Of
Pascal J. Goldschmidt, M.D., SVP, Dean, CEO
Steven Falcone, M.D., Executive Dean
Focuses on birth defects and children's illnesses.

4771   West Florida Regional Library
200 W Gregory St
Pensacola, FL   32502-4822   850-436-5060
                                       Fax: 850-436-5039
                                       TTY:850-436-5063
                                       hhudson@ci.pensacola.fl.us

Eugene Fischer, Executive Director
Helen Hudson, Outreach Librarian
Offers children's print/braille books.

Georgia

**4772   Athens Talking Book Center-Athens-Clarke County
Regional Library**
2025 Baxter St
Athens, GA   30606-6331   706-613-3655
                                       800-531-2063
                                       Fax: 706-613-3660

Stacey Chandler, Manager
Discs, cassettes, large print books, reference materials on blindness, descriptive videos, films, closed-circuit TV, magnifiers,
braille writer, summer reading programs, cassette books and
magazines and more.

4773   Augusta Talking Book Center
823 Telfair Street
Augusta, GA   30901-2232   706-821-2600
                                       Fax: 706-724-6762
                                       TTY:706-722-1639
                                       www.ecgrl.org

Lillie Hamilton, Board Of Trustee
Audrey Bell, Manager
Loran Gray, Board Of Trustee
Brenda Morton, Board Of Trustee
Discs, cassettes, braille writer, films, large print books, summer
reading program, magnifiers and reference materials on blind-
ness and other handicaps.

**4774   Bainbridge Subregional Library for the Blind & Physically
Handicapped**
S W Georgia Regional Library
301 S Monroe St
Bainbridge, GA   39819-4029   229-248-2665
                                       800-795-2680
                                       Fax: 229-248-2670
                                       lbph@swgrl.org
                                       www.swgrl.org

Susans Wittle, Manager
Kathy Hutchins, Supervisor

The library houses a large collection of recorded materials as well as reference materials. For recorded and Braille materials that are provided by the National Library Service (NLS) but not currently in stock at the Bainbridge Library, the Regional Library in Atlanta can be contacted to Interlibrary Loan the requested materials.

4775   Columbus Subregional Library For The Blind And Physically Handicapped
1120 Bradley Dr
Columbus, GA   31906-2813

706-649-0780
800-652-0782
Fax: 706-649-1914
TTY: 706-649-0974

Dorothy Bowen, Librarian
Braille writer, magnifiers, closed-circuit TV, large-print photocopier, cassette books and magazines, children's books on cassette, home visits and other reference materials on blindness and other handicaps.

4776   Emory Autism Resource Center
Emory University
1551 Shoup Ct
Decatur, GA   30033

404-727-8350
Fax: 404-727-3969
tohannon@emory.edu
www.emory.edu/HOUSING/CLAIRMONT/autism.html

James W. Wagner, President
Larry Hagan, IT Manager
Paul B. Pruett, MD, Director of Residency Education
Terri Trotter, Coordinator of Residency Educati
Offers on-line bulletin boards which are relevant to autism.

4777   Emory University Laboratory for Ophthalmic Research
1365b Clifton Rd NE
Atlanta, GA   30322-1013

404-778-4530
Fax: 404-778-4002
pbennet@emory.edu
www.eyecenter.emory.edu

James W. Wagner, President
Larry Hagan, IT Manager
Paul B. Pruett, MD, Director of Residency Education
Terri Trotter, Coordinator of Residency Educati
Various studies into the aspects of blindness.

4778   Georgia Library for the Blind and Physically Handicapped
Georgia Public Library
1800 Century Place
Suite 150
Atlanta, GA   30345-4304

404-235-7200
800-248-6701
Fax: 404-756-4618
dscott@georgialibraries.org
georgialibraries.org

Stella Cone, Director
Deborah Scott, Business Manager
Dr. Lamar Veatch, Librarian
Julie Walker, State Librarian
Discs, cassettes, braille, films, closed-circuit TV, braille writer, large-print photocopier, cassette books and magazines.

4779   Hall County Library: East Hall Branch and Special Needs Library
127 Main St NW
Gainesville, GA   30501-3614

770-532-3311
Fax: 770-532-4305
TTY:770-531-2520
info@hallcountylibrary.org
www.hallcountylibrary.org

Adrian Mixson, Manager
Summer reading programs, braille writer, magnifiers, scanners and readers, audio described videos, closed captioned videos, closed-circuit TV, large-print photocopier, cassette books and magazines, large print books, children's books on cassette, home visits and other reference materials on blindness and other handicaps.

4780   Macon Library for the Blind and Physically Handicapped
Washington Memorial Library
1180 Washington Ave
Macon, GA   31201-1762

478-744-0800
Fax: 478-742-3161
jonest@bibblib.org
www.co.bibb.ga.us/library

Thomas Jones, Director
Leila Brittain, Finance Officer
Hannah Warren, Office Manager
Viveca Jackson, Librarian, West Bibb Branch
Summer reading programs, braille writer, magnifiers, closed-circuit TV, large-print photocopier, cassette books and magazines, children's books on cassette, home visits and other reference materials on blindness and other handicaps.

4781   National Center on Birth Defects and Developmental Disabilities
Centers for Disease Control and Prevention
1600 Clifton Rd NE
MS E-87
Atlanta, GA   30333

404-639-3311
800-232-4636
Fax: 404-498-3070
TTY: 888-232-6348
cdcinfo@cdc.gov
www.cdc.gov/ncbddd/

Coleen A. Boyle, PhD, MSHyg, Director
Stephanie Dulin, MBA, Deputy Director
Vicki Kipreos, PMP, Management Officer
Lisa Richardson, MD, Director, Division of Blood Diso
Promotes child development, prevents birth defects and developmental disabilities.

4782   North Georgia Talking Book Center
LaFayette-Walker Public Library
305 S Duke St
La Fayette, GA   30728-2936

706-638-8312
888-506-0509
888-506-0509
Fax: 706-638-4028
www.chrl.org

Tim York, Manager
June DeLong, Library Assistant
Martha McKeehan, Library Assistant
Kaylee Smith, Library Assistant
We offer books on cassette for the visual and physically disabled induvidual, books in braille, magazines on cassette, zoom text screen magnifier, computer voice program, large-print photocopier, summer reading program, home visits na dother reference materials on blindness and other disabilities.

4783   Oconee Regional Library
801 Bellevue Ave
Dublin, GA   31021-4847

478-272-5710
Fax: 478-275-5381
georgialibraries.org

Stella Cone, Director
Deborah Scott, Business Manager
Dr. Lamar Veatch, Librarian
Leard Daughety, Director
Summer reading programs, braille writer, magnifiers, closed-circuit TV, large-print photocopier, cassette books and magazines, children's books on cassette, home visits and other reference materials on blindness and other handicaps.

4784   Rome Subregional Library for the Blind and Physically Handicapped
205 Riverside Pkwy
Rome, GA   30161-2922

706-236-4611
888-263-0769
Fax: 706-236-4631
TTY: 706-236-4618

Diana Mills, Librarian
Delana Hickman, Manager
The regional library system serves Floyd and Polk counties. System headquarters are located in Rome, Georgia, within the Rome/Floyd County Library Branch.

4785 South Georgia Regional Library-Valdosta Talking Book Center
300 Woodrow Wilson Dr
Valdosta, GA 31602-2532
229-333-0086
Fax: 229-333-0364
commissioner@lowndescounty.com
sgrl.org

Chuck Gibson, Manager
Summer reading programs, Braille writer, magnifiers, closed-circuit TV, large print photocopier, cassette books and magazines, children's books on cassette, home visits and other reference materials on blindness and other handicaps.

4786 Talking Book Center Brunswick-Glynn County Regional Library
208 Gloucester St
Brunswick, GA 31520-7007
912-267-1212
Fax: 912-267-9597
www.trrl.org

Betty Ransom, Librarian
Joe Shinnick, Executive Director
The Three Rivers Regional Library system is named for 3 rivers that flow through all 7 counties of the library system. The Three Rivers Regional Library system serves patrons in Brantley, Camden, Charlton, Glynn, Long, McIntosh, and Wayne counties in southeast Georgia.

Hawaii

4787 Assistive Technology Resource Centers of Hawaii (ATRC)
200 North Vineyard Boulevard
Suite 430
Honolulu, HI 96817-5362
808-532-7110
800-645-3007
Fax: 808-532-7120
TTY: 808-532-7110
atrc-info@atrc.org
www.atrc.org

Barbara Fischlowitz-Leong, Executive Director
Jeff Ah Sam, Technical Assisstant
Jodi Asato, Deputy Director
Edna Kaahaaina, Office Manager
Provides information and training on assistive technology devices, services, and funding resources. Conducts presentations and demonstrations in the community to increase AT awareness and promote self-advocacy among people with disabilities.

4788 Hawaii State Library for the Blind and Physically Handicapped
874 Dillingham Blvd
Honolulu, HI 96817-4505
808-845-9221
800-559-4096
Fax: 808-733-8449
honcclib@hawaii.edu
www2.honolulu.hawaii.edu/library

Fusako Miyashiro, Manager
Supported by the Hawaii State Public Library System and the National Library Service for the Blind and Physically Handicapped, Library of Congress. Staff with knowledge of sign language; Special interest periodicals; Books on deafness and sign language; captioned media; Special Services: Radio Reading Service, Talking Books Reader's Club, educational and cultural programs, machine lending agency. Braille, cassette and large type. Regional and National service, quarterly newsletter.

Idaho

4789 Idaho Assistive Technology Project
University of Idaho
121 West Sweet Ave
Moscow, ID 83843-2268
208-885-3557
800-432-8324
Fax: 208-885-6145
idahoat@uidaho.edu
www.idahoat.org

Janice Carson, Project Director
Irene Lunsford, Loan Program Manager
Julie Magelky, Loan Program Coordinator
Dan Dyer, Training Coordinator
A federally funded program managed by the Center on Disbailities and Human Development at the University of Idaho. The goal of the IATP is to increase the availability of assistive technology devices and services for Idahoans with disabilities. The IATP offers free trainings and technical assistance, a low-interest loan program, assistive technology assessments for children and agriculture workers, and free informational materials.

4790 Idaho Commission for Libraries: Talking Book Service
325 W State St
Boise, ID 83702-6055
208-334-2150
800-458-3271
Fax: 208-334-4016
talkingbooks@libraries.idaho.gov
www.libraries.idaho.gov/tbs

Ann Joslin, Manager
Irene Lunsford, Library Consultant
David Harrell, IT & Telecommunications Resources Manager
Erica Compton, Project Coordinator
Offers audio and braille books and magazines, equipment, and accessories. All materials are mailed free to users' homes. Service is available free to all Idaho residents with a disability which limits their ability to use print materials.

Illinois

4791 Chicago Public Library Talking Book Center
400 S State St
Chicago, IL 60605-1216
312-747-4300
800-757-4654
Fax: 312-747-4962
dtaylor@chipublib.org
www.chipublib.org

Linda Johnson Rice, President
Christopher Valenti, Vice President
Cristina Benitez, Secretary
Joselyn Bell, Director, Finance
Summer reading programs, braille writer, closed-circuit TV, large print photocopier, cassette books and magazines, children's books on cassette, home visits and other reference materials on blindness and other handicaps. Three assistive technology centers designed and equipped for the blind and visually impaired, funded by the National Library Service for the Blind and Handicapped, a division of the Library of Congress. All services FREE!

4792 Department of Ophthalmology and Visual Science
1855 W Taylor St
Chicago, IL 60612-7242
312-996-7000
800-625-2013
Fax: 312-996-7770
TTY: 312-413-0123
www.uic.edu

Paula Allen-Meares, Chancellor
Lon S. Kaufman, Vice Chancellor for Academic Aff
Mitra Dutta, Vice Chancellor for Research
Barbara Henley, Vice Chancellor for Student Affa
Offers help, support, information and research for persons with vision problems, including Retinitis Pigmentosa.

4793 Guild for the Blind
65 E. Wacker Place
Suite 1010
Chicago, IL 60601-7463   312-236-8569
                                      Fax: 312-236-8128
                              info@guildfortheblind.org
                                    www.second-sense.org

Brett Christenson, President
Laura Rounce, Vice President
Michael P. Wagner, Treasurer
Toria Emas, Secretary
provides worship on vision rehabilitation, training on computers and other adaptive technology, career counseling, and professional development workshops and offers assistive devices for sale.

4794 Horizons for the Blind
125 Erick St.
A103
Crystal Lake, IL 60014   815-444-8800
                                          800-318-2000
                                      Fax: 815-444-8830
                                 mail@horizons-blind.org
                                   www.horizons-blind.org

Camille Caffarelli, Executive Director
Jeff T. Thorsen, First Vice President & Treasurer
Keith Myers, Second Vice President
Maryann Bartkowski, Secretary
Horizons for the Blind is a nonprofit organization working to improve the quality of life for people who are blind or visually impaired by increasing access to consumer products, services, culture, arts, education, and recreation.

4795 Illinois Early Childhood Intervention Clearinghouse
51 Gerty Drive
Champaign, IL 61820-7469   217-333-1386
                                          877-275-3227
                                      Fax: 217-244-7732
                                 Illinois-eic@illinois.edu
                                 www.eiclearinghouse.org

Charlton Brandt, Manager
Patricia Traylor, Project Associate
Free lending library of materials related to early childhood and disability. Books, audiovisuals and articles available. Computerized database with more than 31,000 items available to Illinois residents.

4796 Illinois Machine Sub-Lending Agency
607 S Greenbriar Rd
Carterville, IL 62918-1602   618-985-8375
                                          800-455-2665
                                      Fax: 618-985-4211
                                  imsastaff@imsa.lib.il.us

Loretta Broomfield, Director
The Illinois Machine Sublending Agency (IMSA) is a division of the Illinois Network of Talking Book and Braille Libraries. The primary responsibility of IMSA is to maintain Talking Book equipment and accessories and to issue Talking Book equipment and accessories to Illinois residents who are registered for the service. IMSA is also the support center for patrons in need of assistance with the Braille and Audio Reading Download (BARD) service.

4797 Illinois Regional Library for the Blind and Physically Handicapped
1055 W Roosevelt Rd
Chicago, IL 60608-1559   312-746-9210
                                          800-331-2351
                                      Fax: 312-746-9192

Shawn Thomas, Reference Librarian
Barbara Perkins, Acting Director
Summer reading programs, braille writer, magnifiers, closed-circuit TV, large-print photocopier, cassette books and magazines, descriptive videos, children's books on cassette, home visits and other reference materials on blindness and other handicaps.

4798 Mid-Illinois Talking Book Center
600 High Point Ln
East Peoria, IL 61611-9396   309-694-9200
                                          800-426-0709

Rose Chenoweth, Director
Michelle Moran, Assistant
Rebecca Rollings, Assistant
Jane Furrh, Assistant
Providing a free library service to anyone unable to read regular print because of a visual or physical disability. There are books and magazines on tape and playback equipment; and also in Braille. Books and magazines are mailed free to and from library patrons, wherever they reside.

4799 National Eye Research Foundation (NERF)
Ste 207a
910 Skokie Blvd
Northbrook, IL 60062-4033   847-564-4652
                                          800-621-2258
                                      Fax: 847-564-0807
                                        info@nerf.org
                                         www.nerf.org

Joel Tenner, Manager
Dedicated to improving eye care for the public and meeting the professional nees of eye care practitioners; sponsors eye research projects on contact lens applications and eye care problems. Special study sections in such fields as orthokertology, primary eyecare, pediatrics, and through continuing education programs. Provides eye care information for the public and professionals. Educational materials including pamphlets. Program activities include education and referrals.

4800 National Lekotek Center
2001 N. Clybourn
Chicago, IL 60614   773-528-5766
                                          800-366-7529
                                      Fax: 773-537-2992
                                    lekotek@lekotek.org
                                       www.lekotek.org

Elaine D. Cottey, Chair
Joanna Horsnail, Chair Elect
Eric Gastevich, Treasurer
Carol Neiger, Secretary
Toy library and play-centered programs for children with special needs and their families with branches in 17 states. Sliding fee scale. Lekotek also has a Toy Resource Helpline that provides individualized assistances in the selection of toys and play materials and general resources for families with children with disabilities.

4801 Northwestern University Multipurpose Arthritis & Musculoskeletal Center
420 East Superior Street
Chicago, IL 60611-4296   312-503-8194
                                      Fax: 312-503-1204
                              www.feinberg.northwestern.edu
Cynthia Barnard, MBA, Director, Quality Strategies
John Vozenilek, MD, Assistant Professor
Eric G. Neilson, MD, Vice President for Medical Affairs
Sherri L. LaVela, PhD, MPH, MBA, Assistant Professor
Conducts biomedical, educational and health services research into musculoskeletal diseases.

4802 Skokie Accessible Library Services
Skokie Public Library
5215 Oakton St
Skokie, IL 60077-3680   847-673-7774
                                      Fax: 847-673-7797
                                  TTY:847-673-8926
                                    www.skokie.lib.il.us

Carolyn A. Anthony, Director
John J. Graham, President
Diana Hunter, Vice President/President Emerita
Karen Parrilli, Secretary
Library services for people with disabilities, including electronic aids, materials in special formats, programs and special services.

4803 University of Illinois at Chicago: Lions of Illinois Eye Research Institute
University of Illinois at Chicago
1855 West Taylor Street, m/c 648
Room 3.138
Chicago, IL 60612   312-996-6591
Fax: 312-996-7770
eyeweb@uic.edu
www.uic.edu

Rolanda Geddis, Manager
Paula Alen Meares, Chancellor
Jerry Bauman, Vice President for Health Affairs
James Schmidt, Director of Athletics
Visual impairments and blindness research, including glaucoma studies.

4804 Voices of Vision Talking Book Center at DuPage Library System
125 Tower Drive
Burr Ridge, IL 60527-2771   630-734-5055
800-426-0709
Fax: 630-208-0399
info@illinoistalkingbooks.org
www.illinoistalkingbooks.org

Karen L. Odean, Director
Provides library service to persons who are unable to use standard printed material because of visual or physical disabilities. Part of the Illinois network of Talking Book Libraries. The service is free to those who are eligable. Provides books and magazines on audio-cassettes. Special playback equipment needed to use the books is also loaned. Braille books and magazines are also available. The collection includes popular books, classics and children's literature.

Indiana

4805 Allen County Public Library
900 Library Plaza
Fort Wayne, IN 46802-3699   260-421-1200
Fax: 260-421-1386
TTY:260-421-1302
Genealogy@ACPL.Info
www.acpl.lib.in.us

Jeffrey R. Krull, Director
Martin E. Seifert, President
Alan McMahan, Vice President
Paul G. Moss, Secretary
Summer reading programs, braille writer, magnifiers, closed-circuit TV, large-print photocopier, cassette books and magazines, children's books on cassette, home visits and other reference materials on blindness and other handicaps.

4806 Bartholomew County Public Library
536 5th St
Columbus, IN 47201-6225   812-379-1255
Fax: 812-379-1275
library@barth.lib.in.us
barth.lib.in.us

Beth Poor, Executive Director
Summer reading programs, braille writer, magnifiers, closed-circuit TV, large-print photocopier, cassette books and magazines, children's books on cassette, home visits and other reference materials on blindness and other handicaps.

4807 Elkhart Public Library for the Blind and Physiclly Handicapped
300 S 2nd St
Elkhart, IN 46516-3109   574-522-2223
800-622-4970
Fax: 574-522-2174
webmaster@myepl.org
www.myepl.org/epl

Connie Jo Ozinga, Executive Director
Barbara G. Anderson, President
Janice E. Dean, Vice-President
Krystal Anderson, Secretary

Summer reading programs, braille writer, magnifiers, closed-circuit TV, large-print photocopier, cassette books and magazines, children's books on cassette, home visits and other reference materials on blindness and other handicaps.

4808 Indiana Resource Center for Autism
2853 E 10th St
Bloomington, IN 47408-2696   812-855-6508
800-825-4733
Fax: 812-855-9630
TTY: 812-855-9396
iidc@indiana.edu
www.iidc.indiana.edu/irca

Dr Cathy Pratt Ph.D., BCBA, Director
Donna Beasley, Administrative Program Secretary
Pamela Anderson, Outreach/Resource Specialist
Marci Wheeler, M.S.W., Social Work Specialist
The Indiana Resource Center for Autism staff conduct outreach training and consultations, engage in research and develop and disseminate information focused on building the capicity of local communities, organizations, agencies and families to support children and adults across the autism spectrum in typical work, school, home and community settings. Please check our website for a complete list of publications.

4809 Indiana University: Multipurpose Arthritis Center
School Of Medicine, Rheumatology Division
509 E. 3rd Street
Bloomington, IN 47401-3654   812-855-0516
Fax: 812-855-9943
research.iu.edu

Dr. Kenneth Brandt MD, Director
Carmichael Center, Vice President for Research
Steven A Martin, Associate Vice President for Research
Marisa Pratt, Executve Financial & Operations Officer
The mission of the center is to pursue major biomedical research interests relevant to the rheumatic diseases. Current areas of emphasis include; articular cartilage biology, pathogenesis of articular cartilage breakdown in osteoarthritis, causes of pain and disability in QA, the pathogenesis and treatment of various forms of amyloidosis, the pathogenesis of dermatomyositis, and immunologic and biochemical markers of cartilage breakdown and repair.

4810 Lake County Public Library Talking Books Service
1919 W 81st Ave
Merrillville, IN 46410-5488   219-769-3541
Fax: 219-769-0690
www.lcplin.org

Larry Acheff, Manager
Large-print books, descriptive videos, braille writer, magnifiers, closed-circuit TV, large-print photocopier, cassette books and magazines, children's books on cassette, and other reference materials on blindness and other handicaps.

4811 Special Services Division: Indiana State Library
140 N Senate Ave
Indianapolis, IN 46204-2207   317-232-3675
800-622-4970
Fax: 317-253-3209
TTY: 317-232-7763
delivery@statelib.lib.in.us
www.in.gov/isloutage

Roberta Brooker, Manager
Barbara Maxwell, State Librarian
C Ewick, Manager
Circulates a collection of braille, recorded, and large print books and magazines and the special equipment needed to play the recorded materials to anyone in Indiana who cannot read regular print due to a visual or physical disability.

4812 St. Joseph Hospital Rehabilitation Center
700 Broadway
Fort Wayne, IN 46802-1402   260-425-3000
Fax: 260-425-3741
www.stjoehospital.com

Kirk Ray, CEO
Bob Hailes, Vice President

Information offered on rehabilitation.

4813 Talking Books Service Evansville Vanderburgh County Public Library
200 SE Martin Luther King Jr Blvd
Evansville, IN 47713- 1802
812-428-8200
866-645-2536
Fax: 812-428-8397
tbs@evpl.org
www.evpl.org

Marcia Learned Au, COO
Connie Davis, Vice President
Marcia Au, Executive Director
Barbara Shanks, Talking Book Manager
The Talking Book Service of the Evansville Vanderburgh Public Library is part of a nationwide network of cooperating libraries headed by the National Library Service & a division of the Library of Congress. This free program provides library services and materials in alternative formats to person who are unable to use standard print material due to a visual or physical handicap.

Iowa

4814 Iowa Department for the Blind Library
State Of Iowa
524 4th Street
Des Moines, IA 50309-2364
515-281-1333
800-362-2587
Fax: 515-281-1263
TTY: 515-281-1355
contact@blind.state.ia.us
www.IDBonline.org

Richard Sorey, Director
Mike Hoenig, Chair
Steve Hagemoser, Commision Board Member
Peggy Elliott, Commision Board Member
Summer reading programs, large print, disc, Braille and cassette books and magazines, descriptive videos and reference materials on blindness and other handicaps.

4815 Iowa Registry for Congenital and Inherited Disorders
University of Iowa
Department of Epidemiology, Univers
100 BVC, Room W260
Iowa City, IA 52242-5000
319-335-4107
866-274-4237
Fax: 319-335-4030
ircid@uiowa.edu
www.public-health.uiowa.edu/ircid/

Paul Romitti, Ph.D, Director
Kim Keppler-Noreuil, M.D, Clinical Director for Birth Defects
Katherine. Mathews, M.D, Clinical Director for Neuromuscular Disorders
James Torner, Ph.D., Chair
The mission of the Iowa Registry for Congenital and Inherited Disorders is; maintain statewide surveillance for collecting information on selected congenital and inherited disorders in Iowa, monitor annual trends in occurrence and mortality of these disorders, provide data for research studies and educational activities for the prevention and treatment of these disorders.

4816 Library Commission for the Blind
State Of Iowa
524 4th Street
Des Moines, IA 50309-2364
515-281-1333
800-362-2587
Fax: 515-281-1263
TTY: 515-281-1355
contact@blind.state.ia.us

Karen A Keninger, Director
Aldini Jodi, Library Support Staff
Barber Kim, Independent Living Supervisor
Bauer Marcia, Rehabilitation Teacher
Summer reading programs, Braille writer, magnifiers, closed-circuit TV, large print photocopier, cassette books and magazines,

children's books on cassette and other reference materials on blindness and other handicaps.

Kansas

4817 Center for the Improvement of Human Functioning
3100 N Hillside St
Wichita, KS 67219-3904
316-682-3100
Fax: 316-682-5054
information@riordanclinic.org
www.riordanclinic.org

Hugh D Riordan, President
Ron Hunninghake MD, Chief Medical Officer
Brian Riordan, Chief Executive Officer
Danae , Certified Medical Assistant
Medical, research, and educational facility specializing in the treatment of chronic illness.

4818 Central Kansas Library Systems Headquarters (CSLS)
1409 Williams St
Great Bend, KS 67530-4020
620-792-4865
800-362-2642
Fax: 620-793-7270
cbobbitt@ckls.org
www.ckls.org

Harry Williams, Administrator
Vickie Herl, Adminstrative Manager
Marquita Boehnke, Department Head
Connie Bobbitt, Assistant
Summer reading programs, braille writer, magnifiers, closed-circuit TV, large-print photocopier, cassette books and magazines, children's books on cassette, home visits and other reference materials on blindness and other handicaps. Assistive technology available. Serving 17 counties in Central Kansas.

4819 Manhattan Public Library
629 Poyntz Ave
Manhattan, KS 66502-6131
785-776-4741
800-432-2796
Fax: 785-776-1545
refstaff@mhklibrary.org
manhattan.lib.ks.us

Linda Knupp, Director
John Pecoraro, Assistant Director
Brice Hobrock, President
Thomas Giller, Vice President
Summer reading programs, Braille writer, magnifiers, closed-circuit TV, large-print photocopier, cassette books and magazines, children's books on cassette, home visits and other reference materials on blindness and other disabilities.

4820 Northwest Kansas Library System Talking Books
2 Washington Square
Norton, KS 67654-1615
785-877-5148
800-432-2858
Fax: 785-877-5697
www.nwkls.org

George Seamon, Director
Alice Evans, Business Manager & Acquisitions
David Fischer, Technology Consultant
Marry Boller, Children's and Talking Book Consultant
Offers books on disc and cassette. Library of Congress talking book and program for qualified individuals. Also offers descriptive videos to eligible persons.

4821 South Central Kansas Library System
321 North Main Street
South Hutchinson, KS 67505-1145
620-663-3211
800-234-0529
Fax: 620-663-9797
sckls.info

Paul Hawkins, Director
Sharon Barnes, Technology Consultant
Larry Papenfuss, Director of Information Technology
Jill Stern, Continuing Education Specialist

Serving public, school, academic and special libraries in 12 counties since 1968, the South Central Kansas Library System (SCKLS) is the "go to" resource for innovative services, quality member awareness and assistance.

4822   State Library of Kansas
Esu Memorial Union
300 SW 10th Ave.
Room 312-N
Topeka, KS 66612-1593

620-341-6280
800-362-0699
KTB@ks.gov
kslib.info/talking-books

Cindy Roupe, State Librarian
Michael Lang, Director
Kansas Talking Books provides personalized library support and materials in a specialized format to eligible Kansas residents to ensure that all may read. Features: Audiobooks, magazines and audio equipment mailed directly to your house and returned postage free; special equipment lent to you at no charge; downloadable books from the Braille and Audio Reading Download (BARD) website or by using the new BARD app.

4823   Topeka & Shawnee County Public Library Talking Books Service
1515 SW 10th Ave
Topeka, KS 66604-1374

785-580-4400
800-432-2925
Fax: 785-580-4496
TTY: 785-580-4544
www.tscpl.org

Stephanie Hall, Manager
Gina Millsap, Chief Executive Officer
Robert Banks, Chief Operating Officer
Sheryl Weller, Chief Financial Officer
Talking books is a free service that provides cassette and digital books and equipment to people who are unable to read or use standard print materials because of a visual or physical impairment. There are no fees. To apply for Talking Books you must fill out and submit an application, have it certified by the appropriate authority and return it to the library. You can find an application on our website or have one mailed out to you by contacting our office.

4824   Wichita Public Library/Talking Book Service
Wichita Public Library
223 S Main St
Wichita, KS 67202-3795

316-261-8500
Fax: 316-262-4540
TTY: 316-262-3972
admin@wichita.lib.ks.us
www.wichita.lib.ks.us

Cynthia Berner-Harris, Executive Director
Eric J. Larson, Member of the Board
Furnish recorded reading material (books and magazines) for visually and physically challenged citizens.

4825   Wichita Public Library/Talking Book Service
223 S Main St
Wichita, KS 67202-3795

316-261-8500
Fax: 316-262-4540
TTY: 316-262-3972
admin@wichita.lib.ks.us

Cynthia Berner-Harris, Executive Director
Eric J. Larson, Member of the Board
Furnish recorded reading material (books and magazines) for visually and physically challenged citizens.

Kentucky

4826   EnTech: Enabling Technologies of Kentuckiana
Spaulding University
851 South 3rd Street
Louisville, KY 40203-2115

502-585-9911
800-896-8941
Fax: 502-585-7103
admissions@spalding.edu
www.spalding.edu

Laura Strickland, Manager
Mary Kaye Steinmietz, Outreach Coordinator
Tori Murden McClure, President
Assistive technology resource and demonstration center, serving persons of all ages and disabilities in Kentucky and Southern Indiana. Services include: assistive technology information, demonstration, evaluation, training, technical support and short-term loan of equipment.

4827   Kentucky Talking Book Library - Kentucky Dept. for Libraries and Archives
300 Coffee Tree Road
PO Box 537
Frankfort, KY 40602-0537

502-564-8300
800-372-2968
Fax: 502-564-5773
ktbl.mail@ky.gov
www.kdla.ky.gov

Barbara Penegor, Regional Librarian
Lauren Abner, Field Services
Katherine K. Adelberg, E-Rate Coordinator
Jackie Arnold, Local Records Regional Administrator
Provides library service to those who are physically unable to read print. Audio and braille books and magazines are available via mail or download.

4828   Louisville Free Public Library
301 York Street
Louisville, KY 40203-2257

502-574-1611
Fax: 502-574-1666
lfpl.org

Craig Buthod, Manager
Summer reading programs, braille writer, magnifiers, closed-circuit TV, large-print photocopier, cassette books and magazines, children's books on cassette, home visits and other reference materials on blindness and other handicaps.

Louisiana

4829   Central Louisiana State Hospital Medical and Professional Library
P.O.Box 5031
Pineville, LA 71361-5031

318-484-6200
Fax: 318-484-6501
www.doa.la.gov

Patrick Kelly, CEO
Carol Gee, Manager
Information offered on psychiatry, psychology and mental health.

4830   Louisiana State Library
701 North 4th St
Baton Rouge, LA 70802-5345

225-342-4913
800-543-4702
Fax: 225-219-4804
admin@state.lib.la.us
www.state.lib.la.us

Rebecca Hamilton, Assistant Secretary, State Libra
Diane Brown, Deputy State Librarian
Beverly Dugas, Business Manager
Meg Placke, Associate State Librarian
Summer reading programs, braille writer, magnifiers, closed-circuit TV, large-print photocopier, cassette books and magazines, children's books on cassette. Descriptive videoss and other reference materials on blindness and other handicaps.

4831 Louisiana State University Genetics Section of Pediatrics
533 Bolivar St
New Orleans, LA 70112-1349   504-568-6151
                                    Fax: 504-568-8500
                                    postmaster@lsuhsc.edu
                                    www.medschool.lsuhsc.edu

Steve Nelson, MD, Dean
Janis Letourneau, MD, Associate Dean for Faculty & Ins
Cathi Fontenot, MD, Associate Dean for Alumni Affair
Charles Hilton, MD, Associate Dean for Academic Affa
Our goal is to continue building a strong department in which all of the faculty are successful in attracting funding, and committed to establishing productive programs that bring credit to the Department and to the Health Sciences Center as a whole.

4832 State Library of Louisiana: Services for the Blind and Physically Handicapped
701 North 4th St
Baton Rouge, LA 70802-5345   225-342-4913
                                    800-543-4702
                                    Fax: 225-219-4804
                                    www.state.lib.la.us

Rebecca Hamilton, Assistant Secretary, State Libra
Diane Brown, Deputy State Librarian
Beverly Dugas, Business Manager
Meg Placke, Associate State Librarian
Summer reading programs, braille publications, cassette books and magazines, children's books on cassette and other reference materials on blindness and other handicaps. Louisiana Hotlines - quarterly newsletter. Affiliated with National Library Service for the Blind and Physically Handicapped, Washington, DC. Louisiana Voices recording program uses volunteers to record books for the blind.

Maine

4833 Bangor Public Library
145 Harlow St
Bangor, ME 04401-4900   207-947-8336
                                Fax: 207-945-6694
                                bpill@bpl.lib.me.us
                                www.bpl.lib.me.us

Barbara Mc Dade, Executive Director
Norman Minsky, President
Franklin E. Bragg II, MD, Vice President
Lee Chick, Treasurer
Summer reading programs, braille writer, magnifiers, closed-circuit TV, large-print photocopier, cassette books and magazines, children's books on cassette, home visits and other reference materials on blindness and other handicaps.

4834 Cary Library
107 Main Street
Houlton, ME 04730-2196   207-532-1302
                                 Fax: 207-532-4350
                                 www.cary.lib.me.us

Iva Sussman, Chair
Forrest Barnes, Treasurer
Gary Hagan, Secretary
Linda Faucher, Library Director
Summer reading programs, braille writer, magnifiers, closed-circuit TV, large-print photocopier, cassette books and magazines, children's books on cassette, home visits and other reference materials on blindness and other handicaps.

4835 Lewiston Public Library
200 Lisbon St
Lewiston, ME 04240-7234   207-513-3004
                                  Fax: 207-784-3011
                                  TTY:207-200-1511
                                  LPLReference@LewistonMaine.gov
                                  lplonline.org

Rick Speer, Library Director
Marcela Peres, Adult Services Librarian
David Moorhead, Children's Librarian
Beth Martel, Circulation Services Supervisor

Summer reading programs, braille writer, magnifiers, closed-circuit T.V., large-print photocopier, cassette books and magazines, children's books on cassette, home visits and other reference materials on blindness and other handicaps.

4836 Maine State Library
Maine State
64 State House Sta
Augusta, ME 04333-64   207-287-5650
                               800-762-7106
                               Fax: 207-287-5624
                               TTY: 888-577-6690
                               benitad@ursus3.ursus.maine.edu
                               maine.gov

Chris Boynton, Manager
J Gary Nichols, State Librarian
Melora Norman, Manager
Summer reading programs, cassette books and magazines, children's books on cassette, home visits and other reference materials on blindness and other handicaps.
Newsl./BiAnnual

4837 New England Regional Genetics Group
P.O.Box 920288
Needham, MA 02492-4   781-444-0126
                              Fax: 781-444-0127
                              mfgnergg@verizon.net
                              www.nergg.org

Marinell Newtown, President
Jennifer Walsh, Secretary
Merrill Henderson, Treasurer
Mary Frances Garber, MS, CGC, Executive Director
New Englands primary network for collaborative exchange of genetic health information and education.

4838 Portland Public Library
5 Monument Sq
Portland, ME 04101-4072   207-871-1700
                                  Fax: 207-871-1703
                                  reference@portland.lib.me.us
                                  portlandlibrary.com

Stephen J. Podgajny, Executive Director
Clare E. Hannan, Head of Finance and Operations
Linda Albert, Head of Human Resources
Linda Putnam, Head of Reference and Informatio
Summer reading programs, magnifiers, closed-circuit T.V., large-print photocopier, cassette books and magazines, children's books on cassette, home visits and other reference materials on blindness and other handicaps.

4839 Waterville Public Library
73 Elm Street
Waterville, ME 04901-6078   207-872-5433
                                    Fax: 207-873-4779
                                    wplhelpdesk@waterville.lib.me.us
                                    www.watervillelibrary.org

Sarah Sugden, Executive Director
Marnie Terhune, President
William Grant, Treasurer
Cindy Jacobs, Secretary
Summer reading programs, braille writer, magnifiers, closed-circuit T.V., large-print photocopier, cassette books and magazines, children's books on cassette, home visits and other reference materials on blindness and other handicaps.

Maryland

4840 Johns Hopkins University Dana Center for Preventive Ophthalmology
Wilmer Ophthalmology Institute
600 N Wolfe St
Wilmer Suite 122
Baltimore, MD 21287-9019 410-955-2777
Fax: 410-955-2542
boland@jhu.edu

Harry Quigley, Director
Emily W. . Gower, Ph.D, Director
Joanne . Katz, Sc.D, Director/Professor and Associate Chair
Oliver D. Schein, M.D., MPH, MBA, Director
Established in 1979, the Dana Center for Preventive Ophthalmology is dedicated to improving knowlege of risk factors for ocular disease and public health approaches to the prevention of these diseases and their ensuing visual impairment and blindness worldwide.

4841 Johns Hopkins University: Asthma and Allergy Center
5501 Hopkins Bayview Cir
Baltimore, MD 21224-6821 410-550-0545
Fax: 410-550-1733
jhuallergy@jhmi.edu
hopkins-arthritis.org

Lawrence Lichtenstein, Director
Studies of allergic diseases and individuals with allergic disease, pulmonary diseases and diseases involving inflammation and immunological processes.

4842 Maryland State Library for the Blind and Physically Handicapped
Maryland State Department of Education
415 Park Avenue
Baltimore, MD 21201-3603 410-230-2424
800-964-9209
Fax: 410-333-2095
TTY: 800-934-2541
referenc@lbph.lib.md.us

Jill Lewis, Manager
Diana Jarvis, Administrative Specialist
LaTarsha Wilson, Secretary
Provide comprehensive library services to the eligible blind and physically handicapped residents of the State of Maryland. The vision is to provide innovative and quality services to meet the needs and expectations of the patrons of Maryland.

4843 Montgomery County Department of Public Libraries/Special Needs Library
6400 Democracy Blvd
Bethesda, MD 20817-1638 240-777-0922
TTY:301-897-2203
montgomerycountymd.gov

Susan F Cohen, Assistant Head Librarian
James Montgomery, Owner
Joseph Eagan, Branch Manager
Serves the library information and reading needs of people with disabilities, family members, students and service providers. Some of its services include books, periodicals, and videos on disability issues, adaptive technology, community information; the National Library for the Blind and Physically Handicapped Talking Book program; large print books; and computer room with adaptive technology.

4844 National Epilepsy Library (NEL)
Epilepsy Foundation
8301 Professional Pl
Landover, MD 20785-7223 866-330-2718
800-332-1000
Fax: 877-687-4878
ContactUs@efa.org
www.epilepsyfoundation.org

Marl A Finucane, Executive Vice President
Patty Dukes, Vice President Operations/Human
Mimi Browne, Director, HRSA programs
Chad Hartman, Director of Major Gifts

Contains information about epilepsy and seizure disorders and serves physicians and other health professionals. Provides in-house bibliographic database (ESDI), searches and documents delivery and interlibrary loans. Maintains the Albert and Ellen Grass Archives.

4845 National Federation of the Blind Jernigan Institute
200 E. Wells St.
at Jernigan Place
Baltimore, MD 21230 410-659-9314
Fax: 410-685-5653
nfb@nfb.org
nfb.org/jernigan-institute

Anil Lewis, Executive Director, NFB Jernigan Institute
Patricia Maurer, Director of Reference, Jacobus tenBroek Library
Cutting-edge research and training is conducted through the NFB Jernigan Institute to address the real problems of blindness, such as model education and rehabilitation methods to empower the blind or improved instruction in Braille.

4846 National Institute on Aging
31 Center Dr, MSC 2292
Building 31, Room 5C27
Bethesda, MD 20892 800-222-2225
TTY:800-222-4225
niaic@nia.nih.gov
www.nia.nih.gov

Luigi Ferrucci, M.D., Ph.D, Scientific Director
Patrick Shirdon, Director of Management
Michael O'Donnell, Chief Administrative Officer
The National Institute on Aging (NIA) is the primary Federal agency engaged in researching Alzheimer's disease.

4847 National Rehabilitation Information Center(NARIC)
8400 Corporate Drive
Suite 500
Landover, MD 20785-2245 301-459-5984
800-346-2742
Fax: 301-459-4263
TTY: 301-459-5984
naricinfo@heitechservices.com
www.naric.com

Heidi W Gerding, CEO
Mark X. Odum, Project Director
Jessica H. Chaiken, Media and Information Services Manager
Birgitta Chaiken, Research Associate
NARIC is a federally-funded library and information center that focuses on disability and rehabilitation information.

4848 Red Notebook
Friends of Libraries for Deaf Action
2930 Craiglawn Rd
Silver Spring, MD 20904-1816 301-572-5168
Fax: 301-572-5168
TTY:301-572-5168
folda86@aol.com
www.folda.net

Alice L Hagemeyer, MLS, Founder/President
Merrie A. Davidson, Associate
Ricardo Lopez, MS, Associate
Joan Naturale, M.Ed, MLIS, Associate
A binder containing fact sheets, library reprints, announcements and other printed informational materials that are related to both deaf and library issues. It is designed to help build communication among individuals and groups within the deaf community. The focus is on assisting libraries in providing cost-effective and efficient library and information services to these consumers in a unbiased fashion.

4849 Social Security Library
U S Social Security Administration
6401 Security Blvd
Baltimore, MD 21235-6401 800-772-1213
TTY:800-325-0778
www.socialsecurity.gov

Bill Vitek, Manager
Jo B Barnhart, Chief Executive Officer
Information on social security and disability insurance.

4850 Warren Grant Magnuson Clinical Center
National Institue Health
9000 Rockville Pike
Bethesda, MD   20892-1   301-496-2563
                                     800-411-1222
                                 Fax: 301-480-2984
                                 TTY: 866-411-1010
                                 prpl@mail.cc.nih.gov
                                 www.cc.nih.gov

John I Gallin, MD, Clinical Center Director
Clare Hastings, PhD, RN, FAA, Chief Nurse Officer
Maureen E. Gormley, MPH, MA, RN, Chief Operating Officer
Maria D. Joyce, MBA, CPA, Chief Financial Officer
Established in 1953 as the research hospital of the National Institutes of Health. Designed so that patient care facilities are close to research laboratories so new findings of basic and clinical scientists can be quickly applied to the treatment of patients. Upon referral by physicians, patients are admitted to NIH clinical studies.

Massachusetts

4851 Boston University Arthritis Center
Boston University
715 Albany St
Boston, MA   02118-2526   617-638-4640
                                 Fax: 617-638-5226
                                 www.bumc.bu.edu

Karen Antman, Dean & Provost, Medical School
Meg Aranow, Director
Barbara A. Cole, Associate VP for Research Admin
Christopher Dorney, Director
The Arthritis Center focuses its educational, research and patient care efforts on the diagnosis and treatment of rheumatic diseases. These include the many forms of arthritis; the auto-immune diseases such as Scleroderma, Systemic Lupus, Erythematosus, Rheumatoid Arthritis; localized pain syndromes such as tendonitis, bursitis, and carpal tunnel syndrome; and metabolic bone disorders such as osteoporosis.

4852 Boston University Center for Human Genetics
840 Memorial Drive
Suite 101
Cambridge, MA   02139   617-638-7083
                                 Fax: 617-638-7092
                                 amilunsk@bu.edu
                                 www.chginc.org

Aubrey Milunsky, Co-Director
Jeff Milunsky, M.D., F.A.C., Director of Clinical Genetics
Research and molecular diagnosis.

4853 Boston University Robert Dawson Evans Memorial Dept. of Clinical Research
75 East Newton St
Boston, MA   02118-2657   617-247-5019
                                 Fax: 617-638-8728

Norman G Levinsky, Director
Jack Ansel, MD
Integral unit of the University Hospital specializing in arthritis and connective tissue studies.

4854 Braille and Talking Book Library, Perkins School for the Blind
175 North Beacon Street
Watertown, MA 02472-2751   617-972-3434
                                     800-852-3133
                                 Fax: 617-926-2027
                                 Info@Perkins.org
                                 www.perkins.org

Frederic M. Clifford, Chairman
Philip L. Ladd, Vice Chairman
Dave Power, CEO & President
Michael Schnitman, Secretary
The Braille and Talking Book Library loans braille and recorded reading materials and the playback equipment necessary to use

them. You are eligible for services if you are unable to read print due to a disability.

4855 Brigham and Women's Hospital: Asthma and Allergic Disease Research Center
75 Francis St
Boston, MA   02115-6110   617-732-5500
                                     855-278-8010
                                 Fax: 617-730-2858
                                 arc@partners.org

Matthew H Liang, Director
Elizabeth G Nabel, President
Arthur Mombourquette, Vice President of Support Servic
Joel T. Katz, M.D., Director
Integral unit of the hospital focusing research attention on asthma and allergy related disorders.

4856 Brigham and Women's Hospital: Robert B Brigham Multipurpose Arthritis Center
Brigham and Women s Hospital
75 Francis St
Boston, MA   02115-6110   617-732-5500
                                     855-278-8010
                                 Fax: 617-432-0979
                                 www.brighamandwomens.org

Matthew H Liang, Director
Elizabeth G Nabel, President
Arthur Mombourquette, Vice President of Support Servic
Joel T. Katz, M.D., Director
Research studies into arthritis and rheumatic diseases.

4857 Caption Center
Media Access Group at WGBH
One Guest St.
Boston, MA   02135   617-300-3600
                                 Fax: 617-300-1020
                                 access@wgbh.org
                                 www.wgbh.org/caption

Pat McDonald, Director
The Caption Center was the world's first captioning agency providing access to television for viewers who are visually impaired and/or hard of hearing. The Center develops new solutions and uses closed captioning and descriptive video to promote access to technology .

4858 Center for Interdisciplinary Research on Immunologic Diseases
Childrens Hospital Medical Center
300 Longwood Avenue
Boston, MA   02115-5724   617-355-6000
                                     800-355-7944
                                 Fax: 617-355-0443
                                 TTY: 617-730-0152
                                 webteam@tch.harvard.edu
                                 www.childrenshospital.org

Sandra L. Fenwick, President and Chief Executive Officer
Kevin Churchwell, MD, Executive Vice President
Dick Argys, Senior Vice President and Chief Administrative Officer
Jean Mixer, Vice President, Strategy
Organizational research unit of the Children's Hospital that focuses on the causes, prevention and treatments of asthma, infections and allergies.

4859 Harvard University Howe Laboratory of Ophthalmology
Massachusetts Eye & Ear Infirmary
243 Charles Street
Boston, MA   02114-3002   617-523-7900
                                 Fax: 617-573-4380
                                 TTY:617-573-5498
                                 richard.godfrey@schepens.harvard.edu
                                 www.masseyeandear.org/

Wycliffe Grousbeck, Chairman
John Fernandez, President and CEO
Jonathan Uhrig, Treasurer
Lily H. Bentas, Secretary
Development ophthalmology and eye research.

4860 Laboure College Library
303 Adams Street
Dorchester Center, MA 02124-5698   617-296-8300
                                             Fax: 617-296-7947
                                             admissions@laboure.edu
                                             laboure.edu
Andrew Callo, Manager
Maureen A. Smith, President
Offers information on physical disabilities, independent living, peer counseling and advocacy.

4861 Massachusetts Rehabilitation Commission
600 Washington Street
Boston, MA 02111   617-204-3603
                                             800-245-6543
                                             Fax: 617-727-1354
                                             TTY: 800-245-6543
                                             www.mass.gov/mrc
Elmer C Bartels, Commissioner
Deval L. Patrick, Governor
Timothy P. Murray, Lieutenant Governor
John Polanowicz, Secretary
Vacational Rehabilitation and Independent Living for people with disabilities.

4862 Schepens Eye Research Institute
20 Staniford Street
Boston, MA 02114-2508   617-912-0100
                                              Fax: 617-912-0118
                                              geninfo@vision.eri.harvard.edu
John Fernandez, President and CEO
Debra Rogers, Vice President for Ophthalmology
Alan A Ryan, Director Research Finance
Frances Ng, M.B.A., Director of Human Resources
Prominent center for research on eye, vision, and blinding diseases; dedicated to research that improves the understanding, management, and prevention of eye diseases and visual deficiencies; fosters collaboration among its faculty members; trains young scientists and clinicians from around the world; promotes communication with scientists in allied fields; leader in the worldwide dispersion of basic scientific knowledge of vision.

4863 Talking Book Library at Worcester Public Library
3 Salem Sq
Worcester, MA 01608-2015   508-799-1730
                                              800-762-0085
                                              Fax: 508-799-1676
                                              talkbook@cwmars.org
                                              www.worcpublib.org
James Izatt, Dept Head
Braille embosser, magnifiers, closed-circuit TV, adapted computers, cassette books and magazines, children's books on cassette, reference materials on blindness and other disabilities.

Michigan

4864 Artificial Language Laboratory
Michigan State University
220 Trowbridge Rd
East Lansing, MI 48824-1042   517-353-5940
                                              Fax: 517-353-4766
                                              finaid@msu.edu
                                              www.msu.edu
Dr. John B Eulenberg, Phd, Director
Stephen R. Blosser, BSME, Technical Director
Shawn A. Miller, Laboratory Manager
Rebecca Ann Baird, Editor, Communication Outlook
Multidisciplinary research center in the Audiology & Speech Science department, Michigan State University. Its basic research program includes speech analysis and synthesis. Applied research is carried out on computer-based systems for persons who are blind and for persons with cerebral palsy and head injury. The laboratory develops physical, cognitive and linguistic assessment technology.

4865 Burger School for the Autistic
31735 Maplewood St.
Garden City, MI 48135-1993   734-793-1830
                                              Fax: 734-762-8533
                                              garden-city.lib.mi.us
James B Lenze, Library Director
Dan Lodge, Adult Librarian
Lindsay Fricke, Youth Librarian
Marti Boyn Tamaroglio, Library Aide
Burger school for students with autism is the largest public school in the United States that specializes in the education of students with autism.

4866 Chi Medical Library
Ingham Regional Medical Center
401 West Greenlawn
Lansing, MI 48910-2819   517-975-6000
                                              irmc.org
Judy Barnes, Manager
Consumer health and patient education collection in books, videotapes, pamphlets. Open to the public.

4867 Glaucoma Laser Trial
Sinai Hospital of Detroit: Dept. of Opthalmology
31 Center Drive
Bethesda, MI 20892-2510   301-496-5248
                                              kcl@nei.nih.gov
                                              www.nei.nih.gov
Paul A. Sieving, M.D., Ph.D., Director
The purpose of the trial is to compare the safety and long-term efficacy of argon laser treatment of the trabecular meshwork with standard medical treatment for primary open-angle glaucoma.

4868 Grand Traverse Area Library for the Blind and Physically Handicapped
610 Woodmere Ave
Traverse City, MI 49686-3103   231-932-8500
                                              877-931-8558
                                              Fax: 231-932-8578
                                              webmaster@tadl.tcnet.org
                                              www.tadl.org
Metta Lansdale, Library Director
Thomas Kachadurian, President
Jason Gillman, Vice President
Jerry Beasley, Secretary
The LBPH was established as a sub-regional library in 1972 and currently provides services for 783 registered individuals in 16 counties, 171 of these registrants are Grand Traverse County residents. Anyone unable to read regular printed materials because of visual or physical limitations may be eligible.

4869 Kent District Library for the Blind and Physically Handicapped
814 West River Center Dr. NE
Comstock Park, MI 49321-3420   616-784-2007
                                              877-243-2466
                                              Fax: 616-336-3256
                                              WyomingYouthStaff@kdl.org
                                              www.kdl.org
Charles R Myers, Chair
Vickie Hoekstra, Vice Chair
Carol Simpson, Secretary
Lance Werner, Director
Summer reading programs, braille writer, magnifiers, large-print photocopier, cassette books and magazines, children's books on cassette, and other reference materials on blindness and other handicaps.

4870 Macomb Library for the Blind & Physically Handicapped
40900 Romeo Plank
Clinton Township, MI 48038-1132   586-226-5020
800-203-5274
Fax: 586-286-0634
mlbph@cmpl.org
www.cmpl.org

Larry Neal, Library Director
Fred L. Gibson, Jr., President
Peter M. Ruggirello,, Vice Chairman
Barbara S. Brown, Treasurer
Braille writer, closed-circuit T.V., large-print books, cassette books and magazines, children's books on cassette, other reference materials on blindness and other handicaps, descriptive videos and bifokal kits. Assistive technology including JAWS, Zoomtext, OpenBook, and Duxbury.

4871 Michigan Braille and Talking Book Library
P.O. Box 30007
702 W. Kalamazoo St
Lansing, MI 48909-7507   517-373-5614
800-992-9012
Fax: 517-373-5865
btbl@michigan.gov
www.michigan.gov/btbl

Sue Chinault, Manager
Provides library service to people with visual or physical disabilities that are unable to utilize standard print materials. Digital book cartridges (audio books) and/or braille books are sent directly to the patron's home, completely free of charge. This program is available to all Michigan residents.

4872 Michigan Library for the Blind and Physically Handicapped
Genesee District Library
G-4195 Pasadena Rd.
Flint, MI 48504   810-732-1120
866-732-1120
fun@thegdl.org
www.thegdl.org/services/talking-book-center

William Delaney, Chair
David Conklin, Director
Amy Goldyn, Finance Manager
Jerilyn Klich, Human Resources Manager
Offers Genesee County residents with visual or physical impairments a service allowing them to borrow talking books application through the Talking Book Center.

4873 Michigan's Assistive Technology Resource
Physically Impaired Association of Michigan
1023 S Us Highway 27
Saint Johns, MI 48879-2423   989-224-0333
800-274-7426
Fax: 989-224-0330
matr@edzone.net
www.cenmi.org

Jeff Diedrich, Manager
Maryann Jones, Coordinator
Barbara Warren, Information Specialist
Provides information services, support materials, technical assistance, and training to local and intermediate school districts in michigan to increase their capacity to address the needs of students with disabilities for assistive technology.

4874 Mideastern Michigan Library Co-op
503 S Saginaw St
Suite 711
Flint, MI 48502   810-232-7119
800-641-6639
Fax: 810-232-6639
dhooks@mmlc.info
www.mmlc.info

Denise Hooks, Director
Irene Bancroft, Administrative Specialist
Provides resources and supports for member libraries in the areas of funding, advocacy, educational opportunities for librarians and networking with other libraries. Its members include Library for the Blind and Physically Handicapped, and Braille and Talking Book Library.

4875 Muskegon Area District Library for the Blind and Physically Handicapped
4845 Airline Rd
Unit 5
Muskegon, MI 49444-4503   231-737-6248
877-569-4801
Fax: 231-737-6307
TTY: 231-722-4103
mclsm@llcoop.org
madl.org

Stephen Dix, Director
Richard Schneider, Assistant Director
Brenda Hall, Business Manager
Michele Wittkopp, Youth Services Coordinator
Braille typewriter, magnifiers, closed-circuit TV, large-print photocopier, cassette books and magazines, children's books on cassette, home visits and other reference materials on blindness and other handicaps, The Reading Edge, and large print books.

4876 Northland Library Cooperative
Library Cooperative/ Library for the blind
220 W. Clinton St.
Charlevoix, MI 49720   231-855-2206
webmaster@nlc.lib.mi.us
www.nlc.lib.mi.us

Jennifer Dean, Director
Christine Johnston, Executive Director
Roger Mendel, Director
Summer reading programs, Braille writer, magnifiers, closed-circuit TV, large-print photocopier, cassette books and magazines, children's books on cassette and other reference materials on blindness and other handicaps.

4877 Oakland County Library for the Visually & Physically Impaired
1200 N Telegraph Rd
Pontiac, MI 48341-1032   248-858-5050
800-774-4542
Fax: 248-858-1153
TTY: 248-452-2247
www.oakgov.com/lvpi

Dave Conklin, Manager
The Oakland County Library for the Visually and Physically Impaired was established in 1974 to provide access to free library service for County residents who are unable to read standard printed material because of a visual impairment or physical limitation.

4878 St. Clair County Library Special Technologies Alternative Resources (S.T.A.R.)
210 McMorran Blvd
Port Huron, MI 48060-4014   810-982-3600
800-272-8570
Fax: 810-982-3600
TTY: 810-455-0200
www.sccl.lib.mi.us/LBPH.aspx

Arnold H. Larson, Chairperson
Arlene M. Marcetti, Trustee
Kathleen J. Wheelihan, Trustee
Laurie Crisenbery, Trustee
Offers library services to the blind, deaf and blind, visually disabled, phsyically disabled, and reading disabled.

4879 University of Michigan: Orthopaedic Research Laboratories
1500 E. Medical Center Drive
Ann Arbor, MI 48109   734-936-6641
800-211-8181
Fax: 734-647-0003
www.med.umich.edu

Steve Goldstein, Lab Director
Paul Castillo, C.P.A., Chief Financial Officer
Michael ME Johns, M.D., Interim Executive Vice President for Medical Affairs
Quinta Vreede, Chief Administrative Officer,
Develops and studies the causes and treatments for arthritis including new devices and assistive aids.

4880 **Upper Peninsula Library for the Blind**
1615 Presque Isle Ave
Marquette, MI 49855-2811   906-228-7697
                                  800-562-8985
                             Fax: 906-228-5627
                             TTY: 906-228-7697
                     webmaster@uproc.lib.mi.us
                            www.uplibraries.org

Suzanne Dees, Executive Director
Summer reading programs, braille writer, magnifiers, closed-circuit T.V., large-print photocopier, cassette books and magazines, children's books on cassette, home visits and other reference materials on blindness and other handicaps.

4881 **Washtenaw County Library for the Blind & Physically Handicapped**
P.O.Box 8645
Ann Arbor, MI 48107-8645   734-222-6860
                             Fax: 734-222-6803
                                    ewashtenaw.org

Mary Udoji, Manager
Michigan Subregional Library, Library of Congress National Library Service network. General library service for persons unable to use standard print materials for various physical reasons. Lends audio books and listening equipment, large type books, descriptive videos. Provides reference information and programs. Kurzweil scanner with components which convert standard print to Braille, large type or audio and closed circuit TV magnifier on site.

4882 **Wayne County Regional Library for the Blind**
30555 Michigan Ave
Westland, MI 48186-5310   734-727-7300
                                  888-968-2737
                             Fax: 734-727-7333
                             TTY: 734-727-7330

Vanessa Morris, Regional Librarian
Sue Steiger, Librarian
Rebecca Farmer, Student Intern
Mariya Webb, Student Intern
Summer reading programs, braille writer, magnifiers, closed-circuit T.V., large-print photocopier, cassette books and magazines, children's books on cassette, and other reference materials on blindness and other handicaps.

4883 **Wayne State University: CS Mott Center for Human Genetics and Development**
42. W. Warren Avenue
Detroit, MI 48202-1405   313-577-1485
                             Fax: 313-577-8554
                            rsokol@med.wayne.edu
                             www.media.wayne.edu

Robert Sokol, Director
Matthew Lockwood, Director of Communications
Tom Reynolds, Associate Director of Public Relations
Mike Brinich, Associate Director of Communicaitons
Human growth and development disorders.

Minnesota

4884 **Century College**
3300 Century Ave North
White Bear Lake, MN 55110-1252   651-779-3300
                                  800-228-1978
                             Fax: 651-779-3417
                             TTY: 651-773-1715
                                    century.edu

Dr. Ron Anderson, President
Steven Ritt, Vice President
Harold M. Johnson, Treasurer
Ralph Olsen, Jr., Secretary
Programs of study - Orthotic Practitioner, Orthotic Technician, Prosethetic Practitioner, Prosthetic Technician. In addition, Century College offers more than 50 other programs in liberal arts, career and occupational programs.

4885 **Communication Center/Minnesota State Services for the Blind**
Services for the Blind
332 Minnesota Street
Suite 200
Saint Paul, MN 55101-1351   651-642-0500
                                  800-652-9000
                             Fax: 651-649-5927
                     DEED.CustomerService@state.mn.us
                            www.mnssb.org

Katie Clark Sieben, Commissioner
Brian Allie, Chief Information Officer
Kim Babine, Director Government Affairs
Richard Strong, Executive Director
Special library service for the blind and physically handicapped providing tape and Braille transcription of textbooks and vocational materials; Minnesota Radio Talking Book providing current newspaper, magazines and best selling books; Dial-in-News, a touch tone phone accessed newspaper service; Library of Congress cassette and phonograph talking book equipment; repair services for special audio reading equipment, with most services free to Minnesota Residents.

4886 **Duluth Public Library**
520 W Superior St
Duluth, MN 55802-1578   218-730-4200
                             Fax: 218-723-3822
                            www.duluth.lib.mn.us

Carla Powers, Library Manager
Renee Zurn, Digital & Outreach Manager
Davis Ouse, Public Services Manager
Dave Lull, Technical Services Manager
Main library computer lab contains one Sorenson Relay and accessibility computer with zoom text JAWS software.

4887 **Minnesota Library for the Blind and Physically Handicapped**
Department of Education
1500 Highway 36 West
Roseville, MN 55113   651-582-8200
                                  800-722-0550
                             Fax: 507-333-4832
                     charlene.briner@state.mn.us
                            education.state.mn.us

Catherine A. Durivage, Manager
Rene Perrance, Librarian
Charlene Briner, Chief of Staff
Dr. Brenda Cassellius, Commissioner
Provides books and magazines in Braille, large print, records, and cassettes to qualified residents of Minnesota who have a visual or physical impairment, including reading disabilities due to an organic cause certified by a medical doctor, that prevents residents from reading standard print or physically handling a book. Equipment for in-house use include magnifiers, braillers, listening equipment, and CCTV. Reference collection for in-house use only on visual impairment topics.

4888 **Special U**
University of Minnesota
P.O.Box 721-Umhc
Minneapolis, MN 55455   612-625-3846
                                  800-276-8642
                             Fax: 612-624-0997
                            kdwb-var@umn.edu

Mississippi

4889 Blind and Physically Handicapped Library Services
Mississippi Library Commission
3881 Eastwood Dr
Jackson, MS 39211-6473
601-432-4492
877-594-5733
Fax: 601-432-4478
mlcref@mlc.lib.ms.us
www.mlc.lib.ms.us

Shellie Zeigler, BPHLS Director
Christy Williams, Director of Administrative Services Bureau
Gloria Washington, Public Relations Director
Jennifer Walker, Director of Development Services Bureau
BPHLS serves as the MS Regional Library for the Library of Congress, NLS for the Blind and Physically Handicapped. Book collections include audio cassette, CDs, digital books, Braille, large print, children's 18-20 point large print, and standard print reference collection. Descriptive videos, magazines in Braille or on cassette are available, as well as equipment: adaptive workstation, Braille embosser, closed-circuit TV, magnifier, speech input/output, and more. Check for eligibility.

4890 Mississippi Library Commission
3881 Eastwood Dr
Jackson, MS 39211-6473
601-432-4111
800-647-7542
Fax: 601-354-4181
TTY: 601-354-6411
mslib@mlc.lib.ms.us
www.mlc.lib.ms.us/index.html

Susan Cassagne, Executive Director
Katherine Buntin, Senior Library Consultant
Tracy Carr, Library Services Bureau Director
David Collins, Grant Program Director
Summer reading programs, braille writer, magnifiers, closed-circuit T.V., large-print photocopier, cassette books and magazines, children's books on cassette, home visits and other reference materials on blindness and other handicaps.

4891 Mississippi Library Commission\Talking Book and Braille Services
3881 Eastwood Dr
Jackson, MS 39211-6473
601-432-4111
800-446-0892
Fax: 601-354-4181
mslib@mlc.lib.ms.us
www.mlc.lib.ms.us/index.html

Susan Cassagne, Executive Director
Katherine Buntin, Senior Library Consultant
Tracy Carr, Library Services Bureau Director
David Collins, Grant Program Director
Library service for the print handicapped braille, cassette and disc materials (books & periodicals) for children and adults. Large print RG production (copier & printer), braille embosser and other handicaps.

Missouri

4892 Assemblies of God Center for the Blind
1445 N Boonville Ave
Springfield, MO 65802-1894
417-862-2781
855-642-2011
Fax: 417-863-6614
blind@ag.org
www.blind.ag.org

Paul Weingartner, Director
Caryl Weingartner, Office Administrator
Sarah Sykes, Certified Braille Transcriber
Sharron Stevens, Librarian
Offers braille and electronic text lending library, Sunday School materials for all ages, braille and audio periodicals, resource assistance, and resources for blind children and children of blind parents. Children's braille books with tactile graphics are also

avaiable for purchase or loan, as well as books in digital media for adaptive reading services.

4893 Church of the Nazarene
Nazarene Publishing House
P.O. Box 843116
Kansas City, MO 64184-3116
816-333-7000
800-877-0700
Fax: 800-849-9827
it@nazarene.org
www.nazarene.org

Dr.Eugenio R Duarte, Board of General Superintendents
Dr.Jerry D. Porter, Board of General Superintendents
Dr. David A Busic, Board of General Superintendents
Dr. David W. Graves, Board of General Superintendents
Offers braille and large print books. Also offers a lending library and cassettes for the blind.

4894 Judevine Center for Autism
1333 W Lockwood Avenue
Saint Louis, MO 63132-3252
314-432-6200
800-780-6545
Fax: 888-507-4453
judevine@judevine.org
www.judevine.org

Becky Blackwell, President
Evaluations and assessments, parent and professional training programs, consultations, workshops, seminars, family support, clinical therapies, adult programs and support, residential services.

4895 Lutheran Blind Mission
7550 Watson Rd
Saint Louis, MO 63119-4409
314-918-0415
888-215-2455
Fax: 314-963-0738
blind.mission@blindmission.org

Sherry Lambing, Manager
Dave Andrus, Executive Director
Nancy Crawford, Manager
Offers Christian books in braille and large print books and cassettes for the blind and visually impaired, on loan, as well as Christian periodicals in braille, large print and cassette tape.

4896 University of Missouri: Columbia Arthritis Center
University of Missouri
1 Hospital Dr
Columbia, MO 65212-1
573-882-4141
Fax: 573-884-3996
webeditor@missouri.edu
www.muhealth.org

James Ross, Chief Executive Officer
Mitch Wasden, Chief Operating Officer
Anita Larsen, Chief Nurse Executive
Jeri Doty, Chief Planning Officer
Research into arthritis and rheumatic diseases. One of the most comprehensive health-care networks in Missouri, our 5 hospitals and numerous clinics, all staffed by University Physicians, offer the finest primary, secondary, and tertiary health-care services. We also provide education for future health-care providers and participate in important research.

4897 Wolfner Talking Book & Braille Library
Secretary State Office
600 West Main Street
PO Box 387
Jefferson City, MO 65101-387
573-751-4936
800-392-2614
Fax: 573-526-2985
TTY: 800-347-1379
wolfner@sos.mo.gov
www.sos.mo.gov/wolfner/

Richard J Smith, Division Director
Paul Mathews, Reader Advisor, A-CO
Brandon Kempf, Reader Advisor, CP-G & Wi-Z
Virginia Ryan, Reader Advisor, H-L
Wolfner Library provides reading material for Missouri State residents unable to read standard print due to a visual or physical dis-

ability. Book formats are recorded books on digital cartridge and cassette, braille and some childrens books in large print. Wolfner Library also lends out descriptive videos, playback equipment for the cartridges and cassettes are also on loan.

Montana

4898 MonTECH, Montana's Statewide Assistive Technology Program
700 SW Higgins Ave
Suite 250
Missoula, MT 59803
406-243-5751
877-243-5511
montech@ruralinstitute.umt.edu
montech.ruralinstitute.umt.edu

Kathy Laurin PhD, Project Director
Chris Clasby MSW MATP, Project Coordinator
James Poelstra MA, Info Technology Specialist
Specializing in Assistive Technology and oversee a variety of AT related grants and contracts. The overall goal is to develop a comprehensive, statewide system of assistive technology related assistance. Striving to ensure that all people in Montana with disabilities have equitable access to assistive technology devices and services in order to enhance their independence, productivity, and quality of life.

4899 Montana State Library-Talking Book Library
1515 East 6th Ave
P.O. Box 201800
Helena, MT 59620-1800
406-444-2064
800-332-5087
Fax: 406-444-0266
TTY: 406-444-4799
mtbl@mt.gov
msl.mt.gov/talking_book_library
Christie Briggs, Regional Librarian/Supervisor
Erin Harris, Director Recording and Volunteer Programs
Carolyn Meier, Library Clerk/Circulation
Martin Landry, Readers' Advisor
The Library offers FREE alternative audio and Braille reading materials for Montana citizens who cannot read standard print materials because of a visual, physical or reading handicap. Over 50,000 titles on 4-track cassette, WebBraille, Web0pac, WebBlud, summer reading programs, braille writer, magnifiers, closed-circuit T.V., large-print photocopier, cassette books and magazines, children's books on cassette, home visits and other reference materials on blindness and other handicaps.

Nebraska

4900 Nebraska Assistive Technology Partnership Nebraska Department of Education
Ste C
5143 S 48th St
Lincoln, NE 68516-2261
402-471-0734
888-806-6287
888-806-6287
Fax: 402-471-6052
TTY:402-471-0734
nlc.nebraska.gov/tbbs/
Steve Miller, Manager
Lilly Blase, Program Coordinator
Provides statewide assistive technology and home modification services for Nebraskans of all ages and disabilities.

4901 Nebraska Library Commission: Talking Book and Braille Service
Talking Book and Braille Service
Ste 120
1200 N St
Lincoln, NE 68508-2020
402-471-4016
800-307-2665
Fax: 402-471-6244
TTY: 402-471-4083
talkingbook@nlc.state.ne.us
nlc.nebraska.gov
David Oertli, Executive Director
Kay Goehring, Reader Services Coordinator
Bill Ainsley, Audio Production Studio Manager
Scott Scholz, Circulation & Audio Prod. Coor.
Summer reading programs, braille writer, magnifiers, closed-circuit T.V., large-print photocopier, audio books and magazines, children's audio books, and in braille and reference materials on blindness and other disabilities.

Nevada

4902 Las Vegas-Clark County Library District
7060 W. Windmill Lane
Las Vegas, NV 89113
702-734-7323
Fax: 702-507-6187
www.lvccld.org
Keiba Crear, Chair
Michael Saunders, Vice Chair
Randy Ence, Secretary
Ydoleena Yturralde, Treasurer
Summer reading programs, braille writer, magnifiers, closed-circuit T.V., large-print photocopier, cassette books and magazines, children's books on cassette, home visits and other reference materials on blindness and other handicaps.

4903 Nevada State Library and Archives
100 North Stewart Street
Carson City, NV 89701-4285
775-684-3313
800-922-2880
Fax: 775-684-3330

Michael Fischer, Director
Ann Brinkmeyer, Head of Government Publications
Kathy Edwards, Government Publications Libraria
Sherry Glick, Library Assistant
Summer reading programs, braille writer, magnifiers, closed-circuit T.V., large-print photocopier, cassette books and magazines, children's books on cassette, home visits and other reference materials on blindness and other handicaps.

New Hampshire

4904 New Hampshire State Library: Talking Book Services
117 Pleasant St
Concord, NH 03301-3852
603-271-3429
800-491-4200
Fax: 603-271-8370
TTY: 800-735-2964
michael.york@dcr.nh.gov
www.nh.gov/nhsl/talking_books
Michael York, State Librarian
Janet Eklund, Administrator of Library Operations
Donna Gilbreth, Supervisor
Marilyn Stevenson, Supervisor
Regional Library for National Library Service for the Blind & Physically Handicapped offers digital and cassette books, magazines on cassette, children's books on digital and on cassette, descriptive videos, playaways, and downloadable digital audio books, and Braille services.

New Jersey

4905   Autism New Jersey
500 Horizon Dr.
Suite 530
Robbinsville, NJ   08691   609-588-8200
800-4AU-TISM
Fax: 609-588-8858
information@autismnj.org
www.autismnj.org

Suzanne Buchanan, Executive Director
Ellen Schisler, Associate Executive Director
Elena Graziosi, Manager of Information Services
Autism New Jersey is the largest statewide network of parents
and professionals dedicated to improving lives of individuals
with autism spectrum disorders. Self-advocates, families, the
professionals who work with them, government officials, the media, and concerned state residents all turn to Autism New Jersey
for information, compassionate support, and training.

**4906   Children's Specialized Hospital Medical Library - Parent
Resource Center**
150 New Providence Rd
Mountainside, NJ   07092-2590   908-518-5806
888-244-5373
Fax: 908-233-4176
jbrooks@childrens-specialized.org
www.childrens-specialized.org

Amy B Mansue, President and CEO
Robin A. Walton, Chairwoman
Victoria Wicks, Treasurer
Sueanne D. Korn, Secretary
Contains some 3,000 books, and journals specializing in nursing,
pediatrics, child neurology, and rehabilitation. Also provides a
Parent Resource Center, a special collection of books, videos and
pamphlets designed to meet the information needs of parents and
families, as well as the local community.

4907   Christopher & Dana Reeve Foundation
636 Morris Turnpike
Suite 3A
Short Hills, NJ   07078   973-379-2690
800-225-0292
Fax: 973-912-9433
infospecialist@christopherreeve.org
www.christopherreeve.org

John M Hughes, Chairman
John E McConnell, Vice Chairman
Peter Wilderotter, President & CEO
Maggie Goldberg, Vice President, Policy & Programs
A national clearinghouse for information, referral and educa-
tional materials on paralysis. The foundation also offers a free
book titled 'Paralysis Resource Guide' in English or Spanish, as
well as a free library.

4908   Eye Institute of New Jersey
New Jersey Medical School
Suite 6100
PO Box 1709
Newark, NJ   07101-1709   973-972-2065
Fax: 973-972-2068

Jacinta Ogbonna, Administrative director
Department A
Tatiana Forofonova, Program Coordinator
Ophthamology, including research into cornea, retina and
neuro-ophthamalogy.

4909   Mycoclonus Research Foundation
Apt 17d
200 Old Palisade Rd
Fort Lee, NJ   7024-7060   201-585-0770
Fax: 201-585-0770
http://www.pspinformation.com/index.html

Mark Seiden, VP
Supports clinical and basic research into the cause and treatment
of myoclonus; four international workshops facilitated the sharing of information by physicians, scientists, and investigators active in the field, resulted in three publications; supports promising research projects, clinical neurological fellows, with special
emphasis on posthypoxic myoclonus and encourages all who are
interested in futhering the understanding, treatment, and cure of
myoclonus.

4910   New Jersey Library for the Blind and Handicapped
2300 Stuyvesant Ave
Trenton, NJ   8618-3226   609-530-4000
800-792-8322
Fax: 609-406-7181
TTY: 609-530-4000
tbbc@njstatelib.org
njlbh.org

Adam Szczepaniak, Director
Maria Baratta, Assistant Director
Information Technology
Summer reading programs, braille writer, magnifiers, closed-circuit T.V., large-print, cassette, braille books and magazines, children's books on cassette, and other reference materials on
blindness and other handicaps. Provides reading material on audio, cassette, large print and braille to eligible NJ residents.

New Mexico

**4911   New Mexico State Library for the Blind and Physically
Handicapped**
1209 Camino Carlos Rey
Santa Fe, NM   87507-4400   505-476-9700
1 -0 -6 5
Fax: 505-476-9776
TTY: 800-659-4915
lbph@state.nm.us
www.nmstatelibrary.org

David L. Caffey, Chairperson
Norice Lee, Vice Chairperson
Eugene Gant, Public Education Department Appointee
Dean Smith, Professional Member
Summer reading programs, braille writer, magnifiers, closed-cir-
cuit T.V., large-print photocopier, cassette books and magazines,
children's books on cassette, home visits and other reference ma-
terials on blindness and other handicaps.

New York

4912   Andrew Heiskell Braille and Talking Book Library
New York Public Library
40 W 20th St
New York, NY   10011-4211   212-206-5400
Fax: 212-206-5418
TTY:212-206-5458
ahlbph@nypl.org
www.nypl.org/locations/heiskell

Tony Marx, President and CEO
Mary Lee Kennedy, Chief Library Officer
Anne L. Coriston, Vice President for Public Service
Jeff Roth, Vice President for Finance and Strategy
The library provides talking books and talking book players to the
five boroughs of New York City, and braille books to New York
City and Long Island. These items may be circulated in person or
through the mail without charge to the borrower. Deposit collections may be arranged with agencies that provide service to people with visual impairments. The library also circulates large
print books and materials in other formats.

4913   Center on Human Policy: School of Education
Syracuse University
302 Huntington Hall
Syracuse, NY   13244   315-443-3851
800-894-0826
Fax: 315-443-4338
thechp@syr.edu
thechp.syr.edu

Alan Foley, Director

The Center on Human Policy is an organization that works to ensure the rights of people with disabilities. This is accomplished through research, teaching, and advocacy in policy.

4914   DREAMMS for Kids
190 Whispering Oaks Dr
Longs, SC   29568-6973   607-539-3027
                                       Fax: 607-539-9930
                                       janet@dreamms.org
                                       www.dreamms.org
Janet Hosmer, Executive Director
DREAMMS is committed to increasing the use of computers, high quality instructional technology, and assistive technologies for students with special needs in schools, homes and the workplace.

4915   Ehrman Medical Library
New York University Medical Center
577 First Avenue
Room 117
New York, NY   10016-6402   212-263-5394
                                       Fax: 212-263-6534
                                       HSL_admin@nyumc.org
                                       hsl.med.nyu.edu
N. Rambo, Chair/Director
D. Peters, Executive Assistant
N. Romanosky, Department

Administrator
J. Williams, Associate Director

Our mission of the Fredrick L. Ehrman Library is to enhance learning, research and patient care and New York University Medical Center by effectively managing knowledge-based resources, providing client-centered information services and education, and extending access through new initiatives in information technology.

4916   Finger Lakes Developmental Disabilities Service Office
44 Holland Avenue
Albany, NY   12229-0001   518-474-3625
                                       866-946-9733
                                       Fax: 585-461-8764
              www.opwdd.ny.gov/opwdd_contacts/local_
Mike Feeney, Director
Carolyn Bassett, Manager
Andrew M Cuomo, Governor
Information on mental retardation and developmental disabilities.

4917   Helen Keller International
Fl 12
352 Park Ave S
New York, NY   10010-1723   212-532-0544
                                       877-535-5374
                                       Fax: 212-532-6014
                                       info@hki.org
                                       hki.org
Henry C. Barkhorn III, Chairman
Desmond G. FitzGerald, Vice Chairman
Mary Crawford, Secretary
Nonprofit international organization whose mission is to combat the causes and consequences of blindness and malnutrition.

4918   Helen Keller National Center for Deaf - Blind Youths And Adults
141 Middle Neck Rd
Sands Point, NY   11050-1218   516-944-8900
                                       Fax: 516-944-7302
                                       TTY:516-944-8637
                                       hkncinfo@hknc.org
                                       www.hknc.org
Joseph McNulty, Executive Director

HKNC is the only national vocational and rehabilitation program providing services exclusively to youth and adults who are deaf-blind.

4919   Institute for Basic Research in Developmental Disabilities
1050 Forest Hill Rd
Staten Island, NY   10314-6399   718-494-0600
                                       Fax: 718-698-3803
                                       ibr@opwdd.ny.gov
                                       opwdd.ny.gov
Khalid Iqbal, Department Chairman
Joseph J Maturi, Acting Director
Wojciech Kaczmarski, Research Scientist
Maureen Marlow, Editor, Grants Manager, Communications
The Institute for Basic Research in Developmental Disabilities offers services to New Yorkers with developmental disabilities. Services include research, clinical studies, education, publications, employment supports and more.

4920   Institute for Visual Sciences
221 E 71st St
New York, NY   10021-4139   212-517-0400
                                       Fax: 212-472-0295
                                       www.mmm.edu/
Judson R. Shaver, Ph.D., President
Paul Ciraulo, Executive Vice President for Administration and Finance
Carol L Jackson, Vice President for Student Affairs and Dean of Students
David Podell, Vice President for Academic Affairs & Dean of the Faculty
Ophthalmology with emphasis on the development of care for the eye.

4921   JGB Cassette Library International
15 W 65th St
New York, NY   10023-6601   212-769-6200
                                       800-284-4422
                                       Fax: 212-769-6266
                                       info@guildhealth.org
                                       www.guildhealth.org
Jerry Bechhofer, President
Summer reading programs, braille writer, magnifiers, closed-circuit T.V., large-print photocopier, cassette books and magazines, children's books on cassette, home visits and other reference materials on blindness and other handicaps.

4922   Nassau Library System
900 Jerusalem Ave
Uniondale, NY   11553-3097   516-292-8920
                                       Fax: 516-565-0950
                                       outreach@nassaulibrary.org
                                       nassaulibrary.org
Ken Ulric, President
Barbara Behrens, Vice President
Kathy Seyfried, Treasurer
Joe Carroll, Secretary
Information about public library services in Nassau County, including services for people with disabilities and the Senior Connections volunteer project (information and referral for seniors and their families).

4923   National Braille Association
95 Allens Creek Road
95 Allens creek road
Suite 202
Rochester, NY   14618   585-427-8260
                                       Fax: 585-427-0263
                                       nbaoffice@nationalbraille.org
                                       www.nationalbraille.org
David Shaffer, Executive Director
Jan Carroll, President
Cindi Laurent, Vice President
Heidi Lehmann, Secretary
Only national organization dedicated to the professional development of individuals who prepare and produce braille materials.

4924 New York State Talking Book & Braille Library
New York State Library and Education
Cultural Education Center
222 Madison Avenue
Albany, NY 12230-1   518-474-5930
                                          800-342-3688
                                     Fax: 518-474-5786
                                     tbbl@mail.nysed.gov
Loretta Ebert, Research library director
Lends audio and braille books and specialized playback equipment to eligible borrowers with print disabilities. Service is completely free. Serves 55 counties of upstate NY (Westchester and above). Also provides service to schools, nursing homes, and other facilities.

4925 Postgraduate Center for Mental Health
124 E 28th St
New York, NY 10016-8402   212-576-4150
                                     Fax: 212-696-1679
                          www.dvguide.com/newyork/postgrad.html
Marge Slobetz, Assistant Director
Marie Serrano, Manager
Evaluations and psychotherapy by social workers psychologists for children, adolescents, families and couples. Neuropsychological testing and remedation for learning disabilities.

4926 Rehabilitation Research Library
Human Resources Center
Albertson, NY 11507   516-741-2010
                                     Fax: 516-746-3298
Amnon Tishler, Research Librarian
Susan Feifer, Manager
Information on rehabilitation and occupational rehabilitation.

4927 State University of New York Health Sciences Center
450 Clarkson Avenue
Brooklyn, NY 11203-2098   718-270-1000
                                     Fax: 718-778-5397
                                     www.downstate.edu
Meg O'Sullivan, Assistant Vice President
Jennifer Hayes, Staff Assistant
Child psychiatry research programs.

4928 Suffolk Cooperative Library System: Long Island Talking Book Library
Long Island Talking Book Library System
2 Penn Plaza
Suite 1102
New York, NY 10121   212-502-7600
                                          888-545-8331
                                     Fax: 631-286-1647
                                     TTY: 631-286-4546
                                     communications@afb.net
                                          www.afb.org
Carl R Augusto, President & CEO
Kelly Bleach, Chief Administrative Officer
Rick Bozeman, Chief Financial Officer
Robin Vogel, Vice President Resource Development
Offers a variety of support services to its 55 member libraries and other patrons including, an extensive talking book program, assistive technology and other services for people with disabilities.

4929 United Spinal Association
75-20 Astoria Blvd
Suite 100
East Elmhurst, NY 11370- 1177   718-803-3782
                                          800-404-2898
                                     Fax: 718-803-0414
                                     info@unitedspinal.org
                                     www.unitedspinal.org
Lex Frieden, Chairman of the Board
Denise A. Mc Quade, Vice Chairman of the Board
Michael B. Kinne, Secretary
Paul J. Tobin, President

United Spinal Association's mission is to improve the quality of life of all people living with spinal cord injuries and disorders (SCI/D).

4930 Wallace Memorial Library
Rochester Institute Of Technology
90 Lomb Memorial Dr
Rochester, NY 14623-5603   585-475-2551
                                     Fax: 585-475-7220
                                     TTY:585-475-2760
                                     twc@rit.edu
                                     wallacecenter.rit.edu
Lynn Wild, Associate Provost for Faculty Development
Shirley Bower, Director RIT Libraries
Julia Lisuzzo, Director of TWC Administration
Steven Wunrow, Director of RIT Production Services
Information on physical disabilities and deafness.

4931 Xavier Society for the Blind
Two Penn Plaza,
Suite 1102
New York, NY 10121-4595   212-473-7800
                                          800-637-9193
                                     Fax: 212-473-7801
                          info@xaviersocietyfortheblind.org
                          www.xaviersocietyfortheblind.org
Fr. John Sheehan, SJ, Chairman of the Board / CEO
Fr. Claudio Burgaleta, SJ, Vice-President
Mr. Victor Gainor, Secretary
Ms.Margaret O'Brien, Operations Manager
Provides spiritual and inspirational reading material to visually impaired persons in suitable format: braille, large print and cassette, throughout U.S. and Canada. Services are provided both by way of regular periodical publications sent through the mail and non-returnable; and by means of a lending library where books are returned. All services are provided free.

North Carolina

4932 Genova Diagnostics
63 Zillicoa St
Asheville, NC 28801-1038   828-253-0621
                                          800-522-4762
                                     Fax: 828-252-9303
                                          gdx.net
Ted Hull, President and Chief Executive Officer
Darrly Landis, Vice President and Chief Medical Officer
Ceco Ivanov, Chief Information Officer
Jennifer Gillen, Director of Marketing
Laboratory serves over 8000 primary/specialty physicians and healthcare providers, offering over 125 specialized diagnostic assessments. These innovative tests cover a wide range of physiological areas, including digestive, immune, nutritional, endocrine, and metabolic function. To date, the lab has performed over 2 million individual diagnostic tests.

4933 North Carolina Library for the Blind and Physically Handicapped
109 East Jones Street
Raleigh, NC 27635-1   919-807-7450
                                          888-388-2460
                                     Fax: 919-733-6910
                                     TTY: 919-733-1462
                                     nclbph@ncdcr.gov
                                     statelibrary.dcr.state.nc.us
Francine Martin, Manager
Carl Ginger Rush, Secretary
James Benton, President
Dennis Thurman, Vice president
Free loan of large print, braille, and cassette tape books and magazines and specialized playback equipment to registered eligible North Carolinians. Call for an application form. Collection contains general fiction and nonfiction titles. Registered borrowers may subscribe to receive descriptive videos for a one time fee.

4934 Pediatric Rheumatology Clinic
Duke Medical Center
P.O.Box 3212
Durham, NC   27708-3212   919-684-8111
Fax: 919-684-6616
rabin001@mc.duke.edu
www.duke.edu

Rebecca H. Buckley, Medical Director
Michael Duke, Owner
Clinical and laboratory pediatric rheumatoid studies.

4935 University of North Carolina at Chapel Hill: Neuroscience Research Building
115 Mason Farm Road
Chapel Hill, NC   27599-7250   919-843-8536
Fax: 919-966-9605
www.med.unc.edu/ophth/

Ricky D. Bass, MBA, MHA, Associate Chair for Administration
Sandy Scarlett, Development Director
Cassandra J. Barnhart, MPH, Manager of Research Administration
An interdepartmental research center on the campus of the UNC-Chapel Hill School of Medicine. Mission is to promote neuroscience research with specific emphasis on developmental, cellular, and disease-related processes.

North Dakota

4936 North Dakota State Library Talking Book Services
604 E Boulevard Ave
Bismarck, ND   58505-0800   701-328-4622
800-472-2104
Fax: 701-328-2040
TTY: 800-892-8622
ndsl.lib.state.nd.us

Doris Ott, Manager
Hullen E. Bivins, State Lbirarian
Susan Hammer-Schneider, Head Disability Serves
The Talking Books Program provides patrons with free access to cassette books and magazines. The Talking Books Program is administered by the National Library Service for the Blind and Physically Handicapped.

Ohio

4937 Case Western Reserve University
10900 Euclid Ave
Cleveland, OH   44106-4901   216-368-2000
president@case.edu
www.case.edu

Barbara R. Snyder, President
Stanton L. Gerson, MD
W.A. Bud Baeslack, Provost and Executive Vice President
Steven M. Altschuler, M, Chief Executive Officer
Programs which encompass the arts and sciences, engineering, health sciences, law, management, and social work.

4938 Case Western Reserve University Northeast Ohio Multipurpose Arthritis Center
11100 Euclid Ave
Cleveland, OH   44106-1716   216-844-3969
888-844-8447
www.uhhs.com

Fred Rothstein, Executive Director
Basic and clinical research into the causes, diagnosis and treatment of arthritis.

4939 Cincinnati Children's Hospital Medical Center
University Of Cincinnati Uap
3333 Burnet Ave
Cincinnati, OH   45229-3026   513-636-4200
800-344-2462
Fax: 513-636-2837
TTY: 513-636-4900
www.cincinnatichildrens.org

James Anderson, CEO
James M Anderson, Chief Executive Officer
David Schonfeld, Executive Director
Richard G Azizkhan, Member of the Board
Dedicated to providing the highest level of pediatric care. As Greater Cincinnati's only pediatric hospital, Cincinnati Children's is committed to bringing the very best medical care to children in our community.

4940 Cleveland FES Center
11000 Cedar Ave
Suite 230
Cleveland, OH   44106-3056   216-231-3257
Fax: 216-231-3258
TTY:216-231-3257
fescenter.case.edu

Robert Kirsch, Executive Director
Peckham P Hunter, Director
Research and development center on functional electrical stimulation. Houses the FES Information Center, a resource center with a library. Publications, newsletters and videotapes for persons with disabilities and others interested in electrical stimulation are offered.

4941 Cleveland Public Library
325 Superior Ave E
Cleveland, OH   44114-1271   216-623-2800
Fax: 216-623-2800
cpl.org

Felton Thomas, Executive Director
Thomas D. Corrigan, President
Maritza Rodriguez, Vice President
Alan Seifullah, Secretary
Summer reading programs, braille writer, magnifiers, closed-circuit T.V., large-print photocopier, cassette books and magazines, children's books on cassette, and other reference materials on blindness and other handicaps.

4942 Ohio Regional Library for the Blind and Physically Handicapped
National Library Office
800 Vine St
Cincinnati, OH   45202-2009   513-369-6900
800-582-0335
Fax: 513-369-3111
TTY: 516-665-3384
www.cincinnatilibrary.org

Kimber L. Fender, Director
Ross A Wright, President
Paul G Sittenfeld, Vice President
Elizabeth H LaMachhia, Secretary
Summer reading programs, braille writer, magnifiers, closed-circuit T.V., large-print photocopier, cassette books and magazines, children's books on cassette, and other reference materials on blindness and other handicaps.

4943 State Library of Ohio: Talking Book Program
National Library Service in Washington
Ste 100
274 E 1st Ave
Columbus, OH   43201-3692   614-644-7061
800-686-1531
Fax: 614-466-3584
library.ohio.gov

Jo Budler, Manager
Jim Buchman, Dir Patron & Catalog Services
Peter Bates, Deputy Director
A machine-lending agency for the visually impaired. Provides free recorded books, and magazines to approximately 26,000 eli-

493

gible blind, visually impaired, physically handicapped, and reading disabled Ohio residents.

Oklahoma

4944 Oklahoma Library for the Blind & Physically Handicapped
300 NE 18th St
Oklahoma City, OK 73105-3296

405-521-3514
800-523-0288
Fax: 405-521-4582
TTY: 405-521-4672
library@drs.state.ok.us
www.library.state.ok.us

Paul Adams, Library Director
Vicky Golightly, Public Information Officer
Braille writer, magnifiers, closed-circuit T.V., large-print photocopier, cassette books and magazines, children's books on cassette, home visits and other reference materials on blindness and other handicaps.

4945 Oklahoma Medical Research Foundation
825 NE 13th St
Oklahoma City, OK 73104-5097

405-271-6673
800-522-0211
Fax: 405-271-7510
contact@omrf.org
www.omrf.org

Dr. Stephen Prescott, President
Mike D. 'Chip' Morgan, Executive VP and COO
Adam Cohen, Senior VP and General Counsel
Lisa Day, VP of Business and Government Affairs
Focuses on arthritis and muscoloskeletal disease research.

4946 Tulsa City-County Library System: Outreach Services
Tulsa City: County Library System
400 Civic Centre
Tulsa, OK 74103-3857

918-549-7323
os@tulsalibrary.org
www.tulsalibrary.org

Tracy Warren, Director
Tulsa City-County Library's Outreach Services Department provides library services to individuals that are unable to regularly visit a library, including monthly bookmobile visits and deliveries to residents of senior sites, along with mailing materials to homebound individuals/caretakers residing in their own homes.

Oregon

4947 Oregon Health Sciences University, Elks' Children's Eye Clinic
Casey Eye Institute
3181 S.W. Sam Jackson Park Rd.
Portland, OR 97239-3098

503-494-3000
888-222-8311
Fax: 503-494-4286
www.ohsucasey.com

Earl A Palmer, Director
Eleen Reyster, Clinic Manager
James Rosenbaum, Manager
The elks children's eye clinic is the major charitable project of the Oregon State Elks association. The clinic would not be possible without the organization's dedication and commitment to providing eye care for babies and children.

4948 Oregon Talking Book & Braille Services
250 Winter St NE
Salem, OR 97301-3950

503-378-5389
800-452-0292
Fax: 503-585-8059
TTY: 503-378-4334
tbabs.info@state.or.us
www.oregon.gov/OSL/TBABS/Pages/index.aspx

Mary Kay Dahlgreen, Interim State Librarian
Robin Speer, Fund Development Officer
Susan Westin, Program Manager
Joel Henderson, Admin Program Coordinator
We serve the blind and physically disabled. Cassette books and magazines, Braille books-magazines, for children and adults. Descriptive videos. Audiocassette machines are provided free of charge. Call us for an application.

4949 Talking Book & Braille Services Oregon State Library
250 Winter St NE
Salem, OR 97301-3950

503-378-5389
800-452-0292
Fax: 503-585-8059
TTY: 503-378-4334
tbabs.info@state.or.us
www.oregon.gov/OSL/TBABS/Pages/index.aspx

Mary Kay Dahlgreen, Interim State Librarian
Robin Speer, Fund Development Officer
Susan Westin, Program Manager
Joel Henderson, Admin Program Coordinator
Braille writer, magnifiers, large-print photocopier, cassette books and magazines, children's books on cassette and braille books.

Pennsylvania

4950 Associated Services for the Blind and Visually Impaired
919 Walnut St.
Philadelphia, PA 19107

215-627-0600
Fax: 215-922-0692
asbinfo@asb.org
www.asb.org

Patricia C. Johnson, President & Chief Executive Officer
Kate Slattery Parghi, Director, Development
Associated Services for the Blind and Visually Impaired (ASB), is a private, nonprofit organization working to provide services, education, training, and resources to promote self-esteem, independence, and self determination in people who are blind or visually impaired. In addition, ASB advocates for the rights of blind and visually impaired persons through community actions and public education.

4951 Carnegie Library of Pittsburgh Library for the Blind & Physically Handicapped
4400 Forbes Ave
Pittsburgh, PA 15213-4007

412-622-3114
800-242-0586
Fax: 412-687-2442
info@carnegielibrary.org
carnegielibrary.org

Cathy Chaparro, Manager
Sue Murdock, Manager
Jane Dayton, Assistant Director
Jacqueline Flanagan, Executive Director
Loans recorded books/magazines and playback equipment, large print books and described videos to western PA residents unable to use standard printed materials due to a visual, physical, or physically-based reading disability.

4952 Free Library of Philadelphia: Library for the Blind and Physically Handicapped
1901 Vine Street
Philadelphia, PA 19103   215-686-5322
reardons@freelibrary.org
www.library.phila.gov
Tobey Gordon Dichter, Chair
Richard A. Greenawalt, First Vice Chair
Miriam Spector, Vice Chair
Siobhan A. Reardon, President and Director
Summer reading programs for children and teens. Closed-circuit T.V. for enlarging print for low vision; computers with screen readers and large print; cassette books and magazines; braille books and magazines; and descriptive videos for the blind and visually impaired. Unique and acclaimed adult education program for all disabilities. State of the art book recording facilities.

4953 Pennsylvania College of Optometry Eye Institute
8360 Old York Rd
Elkins Park, PA 19027-1598   215-780-1400
Fax: 215-780-1336

4954 Reading Rehabilitation Hospital
Box 250
Rr 1
Reading, PA 19607   610-796-6297
Fax: 610-796-6353
rehab.fsnhospitals.com/USA/PA/Pottstow
Richard Kruczek, CEO
Doug Mehrkam, Owner
Information on physical disabilities, stroke, head injuries, aging and spinal cord injuries.

Rhode Island

4955 Office Of Library & Information Services for the Blind and Physically Handicapped
1 Capitol Hill
4th Floor
Providence, RI 02908-5803   401-574-9300
Fax: 401-574-9320
olis.webmaster@olis.ri.gov
www.olis.ri.gov
Howard Boksenbaum, Chief Library Officer
Chaichin Chen, Library Program Specialist: LORI
Debbie Cullerton, Information Services Technician:
Jeremy Cutler, Information Services Technician
Offers information and services for the visually impaired including reference materials, braille printers, braille writers, large-print books and more.

4956 Talking Books Plus
Library for the Blind & Physically Handicapped
1 Capitol Hill
4th Floor
Providence, RI 02908-5803   401-574-9300
Fax: 401-574-9320
olis.webmaster@olis.ri.gov
www.olis.ri.gov
Howard Boksenbaum, Chief Library Officer
Chaichin Chen, Library Program Specialist: LORI
Debbie Cullerton, Information Services Technician:
Jeremy Cutler, Information Services Technician
Offers talking book services for the blind and physically handicapped. Collection includes reference materials, braille printer, braille writer, large-print books, adaptive computer workstations and referrals to appropriate agencies/programs for other services.

South Carolina

4957 Medical University of South Carolina Arthritis Clinical/Research Center
171 Ashley Avenue
Charleston, SC 29425-100   843-792-1414
800-424-MUSC
Fax: 843-792-7121
academicdepartments.musc.edu/musc/
Jennie Ariail, Director
Tom Gasque Smith, Associate Director
Dr. David Cole, President
Mark S Sothmann, Ph.D., Vice President for Academic Affairs and Provost
Offers patient care services and basic and clinical research on various types of arthritis and connective tissue diseases.

4958 South Carolina State Library
1500 Senate Street
P.O.Box 11469
Columbia, SC 29211-1469   803-734-8026
Fax: 803-734-4757
reference@statelibrary.sc.gov
statelibrary.sc.gov
Debbie Anderson,, Administrative Coordinator
Flora A. DuBose, Administrative Specialist
Leesa Benggio, Acting Director
Paula James, Director of Finance and Administration
Summer reading programs, braille writer, magnifiers, closed-circuit T.V., large-print photocopier, cassette books and magazines, children's books on cassette, home visits and other reference materials on blindness and other handicaps.

South Dakota

4959 South Dakota State Library
800 Governors Dr
Pierre, SD 57501-2294   605-773-3131
800-423-6665
Fax: 605-773-6962
TTY: 605-773-4950
library@state.sd.us
library.sd.gov
Dr. Lesta V. Turchen, President
Monte Loos, Vice President
Sarah Easter, Secretary
Daria Bossman, State Librarian
Summer reading programs, braille writer, magnifiers, closed-circuit T.V., large-print photocopier, cassette books and magazines, children's books on cassette, home visits and other reference materials on blindness and other handicaps.

Tennessee

4960 Tennessee Library for the Blind and Physically Handicapped
Tennessee State Library Archives
403 7th Ave N
Nashville, TN 37243-1409   615-741-3915
800-342-3308
Fax: 615-532-8856
tlbph.tsla@tn.gov
www.tennessee.gov/tsla/lbph/
Ruth Hemphill, Director
Ed Byrne, Assistant Director
Blake Fontenay, Communications Director
Provides free public library service to residents of Tennessee who are unable to read standard print due to a physical disability. Cooperating library with national network of libraries serving people with print disabilities, operating under the auspices

Texas

4961 Baylor College of Medicine Birth Defects Center
One Baylor Plaza
Houston, TX 77030-2348   713-798-4951
                                      Fax: 832-825-3141
                                      www.bcm.edu/obgyn/tcfs
Frank Greenberg, Director
Dr. Paul Klotman, President
One of the few centers in the world that performs fetal surgery.
Provides integrated, multidisciplinary care for mothers, carrying
babies with genetic or anatomic birth defects requiring therapy
before or immediately after birth. This collaboration enable.

4962 Baylor College of Medicine: Cullen Eye Institute
Baylor College of Medicine
One Baylor Plaza
Houston, TX 77030-2743   713-798-4951
                                           888-562-3937
                                      Fax: 713-798-1521
                          http://www.bcm.edu/eye/index.cfm?pmid=0
Dan B. Jones, Professor and Chair
Al Vaughan, Manager
Michael Cassidy, Plant Manager
Dr. Paul Klotman, President
Research activities focus on restoring vision and preventing
blindness through a better understanding of the disease.

4963 Brown-Heatly Library
4800 N Lamar Blvd
P O Box 149198
Austin, TX 78756-2316   800-252-5204
                                           800-628-5115
                                 DARS.Inquiries@dars.state.tx.us
                                      www.dars.state.tx.us
Veronda L. Durden, Commissioner
Glenn Neal, Deputy Commissioner
Daniel Bravo, Chief Operating Officer
Rebecca Trevino, Chief Financial Officer
Houses a collection of books, audio and video tapes and periodi-
cals focusing on rehabilitation, disabilities, employment skills
and practices and management for the Texas Rehabilitation Com-
mission. Houses materials on developmental and other
disabilities.

4964 Center for Research on Women with Disabilities
Baylor College of Medicine
One Baylor Plaza
Houston, TX 77030-3411   713-798-5782
                                           800-443-7693
                                      Fax: 713-798-4688
                                      crowd@bcm.tmc.edu
                                      www.bcm.edu/crowd
Kathy Fire, Administrator
Margaret A. Nosek, Executive Director
Martha Mendez, Secretary
Susan Robin Whelen, Investigator
Research organization dedicated to conducting research and pro-
moting, developeing, and disseminating information to expand
the life choices of women with disabilities. Conducts research
and training activities on issues related to the health,
independence

4965 Christian Education for the Blind
Suite 702
4200 S Freeway Dr
Fort Worth, TX 76115   817-920-0044
                                      Fax: 817-920-0777
                                      bceb@evl.net
Rodger Dyer, Executive Director
Offers braille and large print books and cassettes for the visually
impaired.

4966 Houston Public Library: Access Center
500 McKinney St
Houston, TX 77002-5000   832-393-1313
                                      Fax: 832-393-1474
                                      TTY:832-393-1539
                                      website@hpl.lib.tx.us
                                      houstonlibrary.org
Rhea Brown Lawson, Director
Roosevelt Weeks, Deputy Director
Greg Simpson, Assistant Director
Offers full library services to the visually and hearing impaired in
Houston, TX at no charge. Houses unique and critical services for
its users including online access to the Internet in a private and
secure area.

4967 Talking Book Program/Texas State Library
Talking Book Program
1201 Brazos St.
PO Box 12927
Austin, TX 78711-2927   512-463-5458
                                           800-252-9605
                                      Fax: 512-936-0685
                                      tbp.services@tsl.state.tx.us
                                      www.texastalkingbooks.org
Ava M Smith, Director
Providing free library service to Texans of all ages who are unable
to read standard print material due to visual, physical, or reading
disabilities-whether permanent or temporary. The program offers
more than 80,000 titles in fiction and nonfiction, plus 80 national
magazines for adults and children.

**4968 University of Texas Southwestern Medical Center/Allergy &
Immunology**
5323 Harry Hines Blvd
Dallas, TX 75390-7208   214-648-3111
                                      www.utsouthwestern.edu
Diane Jeffries, Director
Priscilla Alderman, Executive Assistant
Daniel K Podolsky, President
Mission is to improve the health care in our community, Texas,
our nation, and the world through innovation and education. To
educate the next generation of leaders in patient care, biomedical
science and disease prevention. To conduct high-impact, intern

4969 University of Texas at Austin Library
101 E 21st St
Austin, TX 78712-900   512-495-4350
                                      Fax: 512-495-4347
                                      webform@lib.utexas.edu
                                      www.lib.utexas.edu
Douglas Dempster, Manager
Sheldon Ekland-Olson, Chief Executive Officer
Dr. Fred Heath, Vice Provost and Director
Provides access to information for all users, including those with
disabilities, in accordance with the overall mission of the General
Libraries of the University of Texas at Austin.

Utah

**4970 Utah State Library Division: Program for the Blind and
Disabled**
250 North 1950 West
Suite A
Salt Lake City, UT 84116- 7901   801-715-6789
                                           800-662-5540
                                      Fax: 801-715-6767
                                      TTY: 801-715-6721
                                      blind@utah.gov
                                      www.blindlibrary.utah.gov
Donna Morris, Director
Lisa Nelson, Program Manager
Michael Sweeney, Readers Advisor Librarian
Scott Brooks, Multistate Manager
The Program for the Blind and Disabled provides the kinds of ma-
terials found in public libraries in formats accessible to the blind
and disabled. Books and magazines are available in braille, in

large print, on audio cassettes, and on audio digital books. Services are provided by the Utah State Library Division in cooperation with the Library of Congress, National Library Service for the Blind and Physically Handicapped. Services are provided free of charge to eligible readers.

Vermont

4971   National Center for PTSD
VA Medical Center (116D)
215 N Main St
White River Junction, VT   05009
802-296-5132
802-296-6300
Fax: 802-296-5135
ncptsd@va.gov
www.ptsd.va.gov

Paula P Schnurr, PhD, Executive Director
Cybele Merrick, MA, MS, Associate Director for Education
Nancy Bernardy, PhD, Associate Director of Clinical Networking
Lauren Sippel, PhD, Associate Director for Research
The National Center for PTSD works to improve care for America's Veterans and others who suffer from trauma or PTSD. The center engages in researchand provides education and training for diagnosis and treatment of the disorder.

4972   Vermont Department of Libraries - Special Services Unit
578 Paine Tpke N
Berlin, VT   05602
802-828-3273
800-479-1711
Fax: 802-828-3109
www.libraries.vermont.gov/ssu

Teresa Faust, Special Services Librarian
Sara Blow, Library Assistant
Jennifer Hart, Librarian
Aidan Sammis, Library Assistant
Regional network library pf the National Library Service for the Blind & Physically Handicapped. The SSU makes available reading material in large print and NLS talking book formats, including these special collections: children's print braille books, audio described videos and DVDs.

4973   Vermont Department of Libraries -Special Services Unit
578 Paine Tpke N
Berlin, VT   05602-9139
802-828-3273
800-479-1711
Fax: 802-828-3109
www.libraries.vermont.gov/ssu

Teresa Faust, Special Services Librarian
Sara Blow, Library Assistant
Jennifer Hart, Librarian
Aidan Sammis, Library Assistant

Virginia

4974   Access Services
Fairfax County Public Library
12000 Government Center Pkwy
Suite 123
Fairfax, VA 22035-1
703-324-7329
Fax: 703-222-3193
TTY:703-324-8365
access@fairfaxcounty.gov
fairfaxcounty.gov

Janice Kuch, Branch Manager
Beena Pandey, Volunteer Coordinator
Ken Plummer, Outreach Manager
Offers talking books, TDD access, assistive devices such as decoders for three-week loans, support groups for people who are visually impaired, adapted computer work station with braille printer and assistive listening devices.

4975   Alexandria Library Talking Book Service
5005 Duke St
Alexandria, VA   22304-2903
703-746-1702
Fax: 703-519-5917
TTY:703-519-5911
www.alexandria.lib.va.us

Rose T. Dawson, Director
Renee DiPilato, Deputy Director
Linda Wesson, Communications Officer
Kym Robertson, Talking Book Service
Summer reading programs, braille writer, magnifiers, closed-circuit T.V., large-print photocopier, cassette books and magazines, children's books on cassette, home visits and other reference materials on blindness and other handicaps.

4976   Arlington County Department of Libraries
Arlington County Library
1015 N Quincy St
Arlington, VA   22201-4603
703-228-5990
Fax: 703-228-7720
TTY:703-228-6320
libraries@arlingtonva.us
arlingtonva.us

Diane Kresh, Director
Margaret Brown, Chief
Anne Gable, Administrative Services/Technology Division Chief
Peter Golkin, Public Information Officer
Summer reading programs, braille writer, magnifiers, closed-circuit T.V., large-print photocopier, cassette books and magazines, children's books on cassette, home visits and other reference materials on blindness and other handicaps.

4977   Braille Circulating Library for the Blind
2700 Stuart Ave
Richmond, VA   23220-3305
804-359-3743
Fax: 804-359-4777
bclministries.org

Rev. Brian J Barton, Sr., Executive Director
Offers library materials for the blind and visually impaired on a free-loan basis. Serves the entire USA and 41 foreign countries with cassette tapes, reel to reel tapes, braille books, large print books along with talking book records.

4978   Central Rappahannock Regional Library
1201 Caroline St
Fredericksburg, VA   22401-3701
540-372-1144
Fax: 540-899-9867
TTY:540-371-9165
webmaster@crrl.org
www.librarypoint.org

Donna Cote, Executive Director
Alison Heartwell, Librarian
Offers reference materials on blindness and other disabilities.

4979   Council for Exceptional Children
2900 Crystal Dr.
Suite 1000
Arlington, VA   22202-3557
888-232-7733
TTY:866-915-5000
service@cec.sped.org
www.cec.sped.org

Alexander T. Graham, Executive Director
Sharon Rodriguez, Senior Executive Assistant
Craig Evans, Director of Operations
The largest international professional organization dedicated to improving the educational success of individuals with disabilities and/or gifts and talents. Advocates for appropriate governmental policies, sets professional standards, provides professional development, advocates for individuals with exceptionalities, and helps professionals obtain conditions and resources necessary for effective professional practice.

4980 James Branch Cabell Library
Virginia Commonwealth University
901 Park Avenue
PO Box 842033
Richmond, VA 23284-2033

804-828-1110
866-828-2665
866-828-2665
Fax: 804-828-0151
library@vcu.edu
www.library.vcu.edu

John Birch, Media Specialist II
Wesley Chenault, Head
Yuki Hibben, Assistant Head
Ray Bonis, Coordinator
Provides individualized orientations and assistance with library
research and equipment.

4981 Newport News Public Library System
2400 Washington Ave
3rd Floor
Newport News, VA 23607- 4301

757-926-8000
Fax: 757-926-1365
icieszyn@ci.newport-news.va.us
newportnewsva.com

Thomas P. Herbert, P.E., Chair
Wendy C. Drucker, Vice Chair
Sam Workman, Assistant Director of Development
Matt Johnson, Business Retention Coordinator
Summer reading programs, braille writer, magnifiers, closed-cir-
cuit T.V., large-print photocopier, cassette books and magazines,
children's books on cassette, home visits and other reference ma-
terials on blindness and other handicaps.

**4982 Northern Virginia Resource Center for Deafand Hard of
Hearing Persons**
3951 Pender Dr
Suite 130
Fairfax, VA 22030-6035

703-352-9056
Fax: 703-352-9058
TTY:703-352-9056
info@nvrc.org
nvrc.org

William Boyd, Chair
Jim Faughnan, Vice Chair
Steve Williams, Treasurer
Donna Grossman, Secretary
Empowering deaf and hard of hearing individuals and their fami-
lies through education, advocacy and community involvement.

4983 Roanoke City Public Library System
706 S Jefferson St
Roanoke, VA 24016-5191

540-853-2473
Fax: 540-853-1781
main.library@roanokeva.gov
www.roanokegov.com/library

Michael L. Ramsey, President
Barbara Lemon, Vice President
Summer reading programs, braille writer, magnifiers, closed-circuit T.V., large-print photocopier, cassette books and magazines,
children's books on cassette, home visits and other reference materials on blindness and other handicaps.

4984 Staunton Public Library Talking Book Center
1 Churchville Ave
Staunton, VA 24401-3229

540-885-6215
800-995-6215
Fax: 540-332-3906
www.talkingbookcenter.org

Lisa Eye, Reader Advisor
Lynn Harris, President
Daniel Swift, Treasurer
Betsy Little, Secretary
Offers free library service by circulating recorded books, maga-
zines, and playback equipment to individuals unable to use stan-
dard print materials because of visual or physical impairment.

**4985 University of Virginia Health System General Clinical
Research Group**
P.O.Box 800787
Charlottesville, VA 22908-0787

434-924-2394
Fax: 434-924-9960
gcrc.med.virginia.edu

Pamela Sprouse, Administrator
Eugene J. Barrett, Program Director
Mary Lee Vance, Associate Director
Provides investigators with the specialized resources necessary
to conduct advanced clinical research. The facility includes ten
inpatient beds, skilled research nurses, a core assay laboratory, a
metabolic kitchen, outpatient facilities, computing and st

4986 Virginia Autism Resource Center
4100 Price Club Blvd
PO Box 842020
Richmond, Virginia, VA 23284-2020

804-674-8888
877-667-7771
877- -
Fax: 804-276-3970
www.varc.org

Carol Schall, Ph.D., Director
Florence McLeod, Administrative Assistant
Dawn Hendricks, Ph.D., Faculty/instructor
VARC promotes and facilitates best practices for those diagnosed
within the autism spectrum. Information, resources, and education and training help parents, educators, service providers and
medical professionals provide effective support from early
childhood through adulthood.

4987 Virginia Beach Public Library Special Services Library
936 Independence Blvd
Virginia Beach, VA 23455-6006

757-385-2680
Fax: 757-464-6741
spaddock@vbgov.com
www.vbgov.com/dept/library

Marcy Sims, Library Director
David Palmer, Public Services Manager
Susan Paddock, Library Manager
A public library for people with visual and physical disabilities,
braille writer, magnifiers, closed-circuit T.V., large-print photocopier, cassette books and magazines, children's books on cassette, and other reference materials on blindness and other d

4988 Virginia Chapter of the Arthtitis Foundation
2201 W. Broad St
Suite 100
Richmond, VA 23220-3937

800-365-3811
800-456-4687
Fax: 804-359-4900
cmogel@arthritis.org
www.arthritis.org/virginia

Gail Norman, Interim President/CEO
Terri Harris, Chief Financial Officer
Nick Turvas, Senior VP of Health/Wellness
Cecil Wallace, Senior VP Policy and Communication
Provides free information, services and counseling to the public.
Services include assistance in locating and accessing govern-
ment and other health care programs for persons with arthritis, re-
ferral to doctors specializing in the treatment of arthritis,

**4989 Virginia State Library for the Visually and Physically
Handicapped**
395 Azalea Ave
Richmond, VA 23227-3623

804-266-2477
800-552-7015
Fax: 804-266-2478
barbara.mccarthy@dbvi.virginia.gov
virginiavoice.org

Paula I. Otto, President
Susan C. Rucker, Secretary/Treasurer
Nicholas B Morgan, Executive Director
Rebecca Emmett, Office Manager
Summer reading programs, braille writer, magnifiers, closed-cir-
cuit T.V., large-print photocopier, cassette books and magazines,
children's books on cassette, home visits and other reference ma-
terials on blindness and other handicaps.

Washington

4990 Meridian Valley Clinical Laboratory
801 SW 16th St
Suite 126
Renton, WA 98057-2632
425-271-8689
855-405-8378
Fax: 425-271-8674
meridian@meridianvalleylab.com
www.meridianvalleylab.com

Dr. Jonathan Wright, Medical Director
A clinical test facility dedicated to providing the most accurate and informative data for patient diagnosis and therapeutic monitoring. With our current research and up-to-date information and various aspects of clinical nutritional medicine, our methodo

4991 Ophthalmic Research Laboratory Eye Institute/First Hill Campus
747 Broadway
Seattle, WA 98122-4307
206-386-6000
800-833-8879
TTY:206-386-2022
www.swedish.org

Bryan Mueller, CEO
Dan Harris, CFO
Heidi Aylsworth, Chief Strategy Officer
Naren Balasubramaniam, Chief Human Resources Officer
Color vision physiology, vision disorders and blindness research.

4992 Washington Talking Book and Braille Library
2021 9th Ave
Seattle, WA 98121-2783
206-615-0400
800-542-0866
Fax: 206-615-0437
TTY: 206-615-0418
wtbbl@sos.wa.gov
wtbbl.org

Danielle Miller, Director and Regional Librarian
Amy Ravenholt, Assistant Program Manager
Mandy Gonnsen, Youth Services Librarian
David Gonnsen, Volunteer and Outreach Services
Summer reading programs, braille writer, magnifiers, closed-circuit T.V., large-print photocopier, cassette books and magazines, children's books, and other reference materials on blindness and other handicaps, online catalog, reference station with assis

West Virginia

4993 Cabell County Public Library/Talking Book Department/Subregional Library for the Blind
455 9th St
Huntington, WV 25701-1417
304-528-5700
Fax: 304-528-5739
cabell.lib.wv.us

Judy K. Rule, Director
Angela Straight, Assistant Director
Mary Lou Pratt, Adult Services Coordinator
Breana Brown, Youth Service Manager
Summer reading programs, Braille writer, magnifiers, closed-circuit TV, cassette books and magazines, children's books on cassette reference materials on blindness and other handicaps, enlargers and Arkenstone Reader.

4994 Division of Rehabilitation Services: Staff Library
107 Capitol St
Charleston, WV 25301-2609
304-356-2060
800-642-8207
Fax: 304-766-4913
wvdrs.org

Carol Johnson, Manager
Specialized library with information on disabilities and the rehabilitation there of special collections: deaf and hard of hearing, visually impaired/blind, wellness center, literacy and career. The library has assistive devices such as CCTV, scanner and

4995 Kanawha County Public Library
123 Capitol St
Charleston, WV 25301-2686
304-343-4646
Fax: 304-348-6530
kanawha.lib.wv.us

Cheryl Morgan, President
Jennifer Pauer, First Vice President
Elizabeth O. Lord, Second Vice President
Michael Albert, Board Member
Summer reading programs, large print PC option, magnifiers, large type books, cassette books, and magazines, children's books on cassette, home visits and other reference materials on blindness and other handicaps

4996 Ohio County Public Library Services for the Blind and Physically Handicapped
52 16th St
Wheeling, WV 26003-3671
304-232-0244
Fax: 304-232-6848
wheeling.weirton.lib.wv.us

Jimmie McCamic, Chairman
Michael Baker, Secretary-Treasurer
Greg Marquart, Trustee
Anthony Werner, Trustee
The Ohio Public Library exists to provide books and related materials that will assist the residents of the community in the pursuit of knowledge, information, education, research, and recreation in order to promote an enlightned citizenry and to enrich t

4997 Talking Book Department, Parkersburg and Wood County Public Library
3100 Emerson Ave
Parkersburg, WV 26104-2414
304-420-4587
Fax: 304-420-4589

Lindsay Place, Talking Books Dept. Coordinator
Brian Raitz, Director
Free program loaning recorded books and magazines, braille books and magazines to people who are unable to read or use standard print due to a visual or physical impairment.

4998 West Virginia Autism Training Center
Marshall University College Of Educational & Human
Old Main 316
1 John Marshall Drive
Huntington, WV 25755-1
304-696-2332
800-344-5115
Fax: 304-696-2846
www.marshall.edu/atc/

Amanda Plumley, Executive Office Manager
Ginny Painter, Communications Director
Joe Ciccarello, Associate Executive Director
J. T. Schneider, Grants Officer
Provides education, training, and treatment programs for W Virginians who have autism, pervasive developmental disorders or Asperger's disease and have formally been registered with the center.

4999 West Virginia Library Commission
1900 Kanawha Blvd E
Charleston, WV 25305-9
304-558-2041
800-642-9021
Fax: 304-558-2044
www.librarycommission.wv.gov

Karen Goff, Secretary
Deborah McNeal, Personnel Officer
Steve Tyler, Supervisor
Denise Seabolt, Library Administrative Services Director
Summer reading programs, braille writer, magnifiers, closed-circuit T.V., large-print photocopier, cassette books and magazines, children's books on cassette, home visits and other reference materials on blindness and other handicaps.

5000 West Virginia School for the Blind Library
301 E Main St
Romney, WV 26757-1828   304-822-4840
                                          Fax: 304-822-3370
                                   cjohn@access.mountain.net
                                          wvde.state.wv.us

Patsy Shank, Administrator
Cynthia Johnson, Librarian
Summer reading programs, braille writer, magnifiers, closed-circuit T.V., large-print photocopier, cassette books and magazines, children's books on cassette, home visits and other reference materials on blindness and other handicaps.

Wisconsin

5001 Brown County Library
Central Library Downtown
515 Pine Street
Green Bay, WI 54301-3743   920-448-4400
                                          Fax: 920-448-4376
                                          TTY:920-448-4400
                                     bc_library@co.brown.wi.us
                                      www.co.brown.wi.us/library

Terry Watermelon, President
Kathy Pletcher, Vice President
Carla Buboltz, Secretary
John Hickey, Financial Secretary
Summer reading programs, braille writer, magnifiers, closed-circuit TV, large-print photocopier, cassette books and magazines, children's books on cassette, home visits and other reference materials on blindness and other handicaps.

5002 Eye Institute of the Medical College of Wisconsin and Froedtert Clinic
925 N 87th St
Milwaukee, WI 53226-4812   414-456-2020
                                          Fax: 414-456-6300
                                          eyecare@mcw.edu
                                          doctor.mcw.edu

Jane D Kivlin, Director
Richard Schultz, MD, Director
A national leader as a full-service academic opthalmology program. Dedicated to the highest quality patient care, education, and vision research, the faculty and staff strive to provide state-of-the-art clinical and surgical patient care in a compassionat

5003 Trace Research and Development Center
2107 Ecb
Madison, WI 53706   608-262-6966
                                          Fax: 608-262-8848
                                          info@trace.wisc.edu
                                          trace.wisc.edu

Kate Vanderheiden, Program Manager
Research focused on how standard information and communication technology products may be designed so that more people with disabilities can use them.

5004 Wisconsin Regional Library for the Blind& Physically Handicapped
813 W Wells St
Milwaukee, WI 53233-1436   414-286-3045
                                          800-242-8822
                                          Fax: 414-286-3102
                                          TTY: 414-286-3548
                                          lbph@mpl.org

Marsha J Valance, Manager
Meredith Wittmann, Regional Librarian
Circulates recorded materials, playback equipment and braille materials to print-handicapped Wisconsin residents.

Wyoming

5005 Wyoming Services for the Visually Impaired
Wyoming Department of Education
2300 Capitol Ave
Cheyenne, WY 82002-0050   307-777-7690
                                          Fax: 307-777-6234
                                          jackie.miller@wyo.gov
                          edu.wyoming.gov/in-the-classroom/special-prog
Ron Micheli, Chairman
Scotty Ratliff, Vice-Chair
Pete Ratliff, Treasurer
Cindy Hill, Superintendent
Services for the Visually Impaired assists people of all ages who have low vision or are blind. The goal is to provide information, education, and support to individuals with low vision in order that they may lead enjoyable and productive lives with maxim

5006 Wyoming's New Options in Technology(WYNOT) - University of Wyoming
1000 E University Ave
Laramie, WY 82071-2000   307-766-2761
                                          888-989-9463
                                          Fax: 307-766-2763
                                          TTY: 800-908-7011
                                          wind.uw@uwyo.edu
                                          wind.uwyo.edu/wynot
William MacLean Jr., Ph.D., Executive Director
Designed to develop and implement a consumer oriented statewide system of technology-related assistance for people with disabilities of all ages.

Media, Print

Children & Young Adults

5007 Assistive Technology for Infants and Toddlers with Disabilities Handbook
Idaho Assistive Technology Project
University of Idaho
1187 Alturas Dr.
Moscow, ID 83843- 2268
800-432-8324
Fax: 208-885-6102
idahoat@uidaho.edu
www.idahoat.org

LaRae Rhoads, Author
Ron Seiler, Author
This handbook is designed as a guide for parents and families in Idaho who have infants and toddlers with developmental delays or disabilities.

5008 Assistive Technology for School-Age Children with Disabilities - Handbook
Idaho Assistive Technology Project
University of Idaho
1187 Alturas Dr.
Moscow, ID 83843- 2268
208-885-3557
800-432-8324
Fax: 208-885-6102
idahoat@uidaho.edu
www.idahoat.org

LaRae Rhoads, Author
Ron Seiler, Author
Michelle Doty, Author
A handbook designed to provide guidance and information for parentswho have school-aged children with disabilities, focusing on resources for assistive technologies available for their children.

5009 Children's Understanding of Disability
Routledge (Taylor & Francis Group)
711 Third Ave.
New York, NY 10017
212-216-7800
800-634-7064
Fax: 202-564-7854
enquiries@taylorandfrancis.com
www.routledge.com

Ann Lewis, Author
Children's Understanding of Disability is a valuable addition to the debate surrounding the integration of children with special needs into ordinary schools. Taking the viewpoint of the children themselves, it explores how pupils with severe learning difficulties and their non-disabled classmates interact.Ann Lewis examines what happens when non-disabled children and pupils with severe learning difficulties work together regularly over the course of a year.
Hardcover

5010 Complete IEP Guide: How to Advocate for Your Special Ed Child (8th Edition)
NOLO (Internet Brands)
909 N. Sepulveda Blvd
11th Fl.
El Segundo, CA 90245
310-280-4000
www.nolo.com

Lawrence Siegel, Attorney/Author
This all-in-one guide will help you understand special education law, identify your child's needs, prepare for meetings, develop the IEP and resolve disputes.
384 pages

5011 Don't Call Me Special: A First Look at Disability
Barron's Educational Series
250 Wireless Blvd
Hauppauge, NY 11788
800-645-3476
Fax: 631-494-3723
barrons@barronseduc.com
www.barronseduc.com

Pat Thomas, Author
This picture book explores questions and concerns about physical disabilities in a simple and reassuring way. Youger children can find out about individual disabilities, special equipment that is available to help the disabled, and how people of all ages can deal with disabilities and live happy and full lives.
Paperback

5012 Everything Parent's Guide to Special Education
Adams Media
4868 Innovation Dr
Bldg 2
Fort Collins, CO 80525
855-278-0402
www.adamsmediastore.com

Amanda Morin, Author
This handbook offers parents assistance, advice, and aid on navigating special education for their child, with information on assessment, evaluation, specific needs for specific disabilities, current law, and dealing with parent-school conflict. It includes worksheets, forms, and sample documents to help parents be effective advocates for their child's learning.

5013 It isn't Fair!: Siblings of Children with Disabilities
Praeger - ABC-CLIO
130 Cremona Dr
Santa Barbara, CA 93117
805-968-1911
800-368-6868
Fax: 866-270-3856
CustomerService@abc-clio.com
www.abc-clio.com/praeger

Stanley D. Klein, Editor
Maxwell J. Schleifer, Editor
This book presents a wide range of perspectives on the relationship of siblings to children with disabilities. These perspectives are written in the first person by parents, young adult siblings, younger siblings, and professionals.
200 pages

5014 Life Beyond the Classroom: Transition Strategies for Young People with Disabilities
Brookes Publishing
P.O.Box 10624
Baltimore, MD 21285-0624
410-337-9580
800-638-3775
Fax: 410-337-8539
custserv@brookespublishing.com
www.brookespublishing.com

Paul Wehman, Author
This textbook is an essential guide to planning, designing, and implementing successful transition programs for students with disabilities.
616 pages

5015 Mayor of the West Side
Fanlight Productions
32 Court St
21st Fl.
Brooklyn, NY 11201
718-488-8900
800-876-1710
Fax: 718-488-8642
info@fanlight.com
www.fanlight.com

Judd Ehrlich, Director
What happens when love gets in the way of letting go? As a teenager with multiple disabilities prepares for his Bar Mitzvah, his family and community consider what Mark's life will be like when they are no longer able to protect him.

5016 New Horizons Independent Living Center
8085 E Manley Dr
Prescott Valley, AZ   86314-6154
928-772-1266
800-406-2377
Fax: 928-772-3808
TTY: 928-772-1266
www.nhilc.org

Gale Dean, Executive Director
Alan Loosley, President
Sharon Geddes, Vice President
Mary Russell, Secretary
The mission of New Horizons Independent Living Center is to provide programs and services in Northern Arizona which encourage and empower people with disabilities to self-determine the goals and activities of their lives.

5017 Rolling Along with Goldilocks and the Three Bears
Woodbine House
6510 Bells Mill Rd
Bethesda, MD   20817
800-843-7323
info@woodbinehouse.com
www.woodbinehouse.com

Cindy Meyers, Author
Carol Morgan, Illustrator
The familiar fairytale with a special needs twist. Ages 3-7.
28 pages

5018 Shriner's Hospitals for Children Newsletter
3101 SW Sam Jackson Park Rd
Portland, OR   97201
503-241-5090
Fax: 503-221-3498
mthoreson@shrinenet.org
www.shrinershospitalforchildren.org

5019 Sibling Forum: A FRA Newsletter
Family Resource Associates
35 Haddon Ave
Shrewsbury, NJ   07702-4007
732-747-5310
Fax: 732-747-1896
info@frainc.org
www.frainc.org

Quarterly

5020 Sibshops: Workshops for Siblings of Children with Special Needs
Sibling Supporting Project
322-6512 23rd Ave NW
Seattle, WA   98117
206-297-6368
info@siblingsupport.org
www.siblingsupport.org

Don Meyer, Author
Patricia Vadasy, Author
Sibshops is a program that brings together 8-to 13-year-old brothers and sisters of children with special needs. The siblings receive support and information in a recreational setting, so they have fun while they learn.
264 pages

5021 Special Education Report
LRP Publications
360 Hiatt Dr
Dept. 150F
Palm Beach Gardens, FL   33418
800-341-7874
Fax: 561-622-2423
custserv@lrp.com
www.lrp.com

Monthly Newsletter

5022 Special Format Books for Children and Youth Ages 3-19
New York State Talking Book and Braille Library
Cultural Education Center
222 Madison Ave
Albany, NY 12230-0001
518-474-5935
800-342-3688
Fax: 518-474-7041
tbbl@nysed.gov
www.nysl.nysed.gov/tbbl/index.html

5023 The Sibling Slam Book: What It's Really Like To Have a Brother or Sister with Special Needs
Sibling Support Project
6512 23rd Ave NW
Ste 322
Seattle, WA   98117
206-297-6368
info@siblingsupport.org
www.siblingsupport.org

Don Meyer, Author
A brutally honest, non-PC look at the lives, experiences, and opinions of siblings without disabilities who have siblings with disabilities. Formatted like the slam books passed around in many junior high and high schools, this one poses a series of 50 personal questions, with responses drawn from the author's interviews with over 80 teens from across the United States. It reflects experiences that range from positive to negative.

5024 The Sibling Survival Guide
Sibling Support Project
6512 23rd Ave. NW
Ste 322
Seattle, WA   98117
206-297-6368
info@siblingsupport.org
www.siblingsupport.org

Don Meyer, Author
Emily Holl, Author
Edited by experts in the field of disabilities and sibling relationships, The Sibling Survival Guide focuses on the topmost concerns identified in a survey of hundreds of siblings.

5025 Views from Our Shoes
Sibling Support Project
6512 23rd Ave NW
Ste 322
Seattle, WA   98117
206-297-6368
www.siblingsupport.org

Don Meyer, Author
Siblings share what it is like to have a brother or sister with a disability. Age 9 and up.
106 pages Paperback

5026 What About Me? Growing Up with a Developmentally Disabled Sibling
Da Capo Press/ Perseus Books Group
Order Department
210 American Dr
Jackson, TN   38301
800-343-4499
Fax: 800-351-5073
www.perseusbooksgroup.com

Bryna Siegel, Author
Stuart Silverstein, Author
A compassionate and accessible guide on living with and caring for a developmentally disabled sibling.
316 pages Paperback

5027 What It's Like to be Me
Friendship Press
P.O.Box 37844
Cincinnati, OH   45222-844
513-948-8733
Fax: 513-761-3722

Community

5028 'Cultural Life,' Disability, Inclusion, and Citizenship: Moving Beyond Leisure in Isolation
Routledge (Taylor & Francis Group)
711 Third Ave
New York, NY   10017
212-216-7800
800-634-7064
Fax: 202-564-7854
enquiries@taylorandfrancis.com
www.routledge.com

Simon Darcy, Editor
Jerome Singleton, Editor

This book concentrates on disability citizenship in leisure.
90 pages Hardback

5029   Active Citizenship and Disability: Implementing the Personalization of Support
Cambridge University Press
Shaftesbury Rd
Cambridge, UK   CB2-8BS   information@cambridge.org
www.cambridge.org

Andrew Power, Author
Janet E. Lord, Author
Allison S. DeFranco, Author
This book provides an international comparative study of the implementation of disability rights law and policy focused on the emerging principles of self-determination and personalisation. The case studies examine how different jurisdictions have reformed disability law and policy and reconfigured how support is administered and funded to ensure maximum choice and independence is accorded to people with disabilities.
518 pages Paperback; Hardcover

5030   California Community Care News
Community Residential Care Association of CA
1924 Alhambra Blvd
P.O. Box 163270
Sacramento, CA 95816-9270   916-455-0723
Fax: 916-455-7201
www.crcac.com

Charles W Skoien Jr, Director/Lobbyist
Denise Johnson, Consultant
Forum for the exchange of ideas, information and opinions among clients, families and service providers. Information regarding services and assisted living programs for the elderly, mentally ill and disabled.
Monthly

5031   Community Disability Services: An Evidence-Based Approach to Practice
Purdue University Press
Stewart Center 190
504 W State St
West Lafayette, IN 47907-2058   265-494-2038
pupress@purdue.edu
www.thepress.purdue.edu

Ian Dempsey, Editor
Karen Nankervis, Editor
Articles by an array of international experts provide as an excellent resource for professionals and students involved in the area of disability studies. The book is divided into three parts: (1) disability and modern society; (2) working with people who are challenged; and (3) working within a disability-services environment. This approach mirrors the contemporary debate within a practice framework reflecting how individuals, organizations, and communities deal with the problem and solutions.
304 pages Paperback

5032   Comprehensive Care Coordination for Chronically Ill Adults
Wiley-Blackwell
111 River St
Hoboken, NJ 07030-5774   201-748-6000
877-762-2974
Fax: 201-748-6088
info@wiley.com
www.wiley.com

Cheryl Schraeder, Editor
Paul S. Shelton, Editor
A combination of theory and case studies, this book presents the growing demographic of chronically ill adults in the U.S., offering models for change and improvement in quality of care; recommendations on relevant and current literature; and descriptions of successful care outcomes.
440 pages Paperback

5033   Hallmarks and Features of High-Quality Community-Based Services
Independent Living Research Utilization (ILRU)
1333 Moursund
Houston, TX   77030   713-520-0232
Fax: 713-520-5785
ilru@ilru.org
ilru.org

5034   Human Exceptionality: School, Community,and Family (12th Edition)
Cengage Learning
20 Channel Center St
Boston, MA   02210   617-289-7700
Fax: 617-289-7844
www.cengage.com/us

Michael L. Hardman, Author
M. Winston Egan, Author
Clifford J. Drew, Author
An evidence-based testament to the critical role of cross-professional collaboration in enhancing the lives of exceptional individuals and their families. This text's unique lifespan approach combines powerful research, evidence-based practices, and inspiring stories, engendering passion and empathy and enhancing the lives of individuals with exceptionalities.
544 pages Hardcover

5035   Inclusive Leisure Services (3rd Edition)
Venture Publishing Inc.
1999 Cato Ave
State College, PA   16801   814-234-4561
Fax: 814-234-1651
www.venturepublish.com
John Dattilo, Author
This text will educate future and current leisure services professionals about attitude development and actions that promote positive attitudes about people who have experienced discrimination and segregation. It provides strategies that will facilitate meaningful leisure participation by all participants, while respecting their rights.
560 pages Hardcover

5036   Independent Living for Persons with Disabilities and Elderly People
IOS Press
6751 Tepper Dr
Clifton, VA   20124   703-830-6300
Fax: 703-830-2300
sales@iospress.com
www.iospress.nl
Mounir Mokhtari, Editor
Discusses the need for assistive technology in making homes more accessible for the elderly and people with disabilities. Goes on to suggest the application of these technologies in other areas of the community, such as hospitals and schools, which allow those with disabilities and the elderly to live their lives with some independence and autonomy.
216 pages Softcover

5037   Independent Living for Physically Disabled People
People With Disabilities Press (iUniverse)
1663 Liberty Dr
Bloomington, IN   47403   812-330-2909
800-288-4677
Fax: 812-355-4085
media@iuniverse.com
www.iuniverse.com
Nancy M. Crewe, Author
Irving Kenneth Zola, Author
This book describes the philosophy of independent living, from legislative strides to community centres, as well as future trends.
436 pages

5038   Pathways To Inclusion (2nd Edition)
Captus Press
1600 Steeles Ave W
Concord, ON, Canada   L4K-4M2   416-736-5537
                                    Fax: 416-736-5793
                                    info@captus.com
                                    www.captus.com

John Lord, Author
Peggy Hutchison, Author
Pathways to Inclusion 2nd edition addresses the organizational
strategies that have been used in the past and highlights areas for
change. Human service organizations are examined, pinpointing
common characteristics that have led to improved quality of life
for people with disabilities and other vulnerable citizens.
328 pages Paperback

Employment

**5039   A Supported Employment Workbook: Individual Profiling
and Job Matching**
Jessica Kingsley Publishers
73 Collier St
London, UK   N19BE   hello@jkp.com
                                www.jkp.com

Steve Leach, Author
Created with the goal of helping job developers, this guide offers
practical tools and strategies to help job development professionals assist their clients. The workbook includes vocational forms,
job analysis forms, and support review charts, and offers aid to
professionals in assisting disabled persons to find and secure
stable jobs in their communities.
224 pages Paperback

5040   Career Success for Disabled High-Flyers
Jessica Kingsley Publishers
73 Collier St
London, UK   N19BE   hello@jkp.com
                                www.jkp.com

Sonali Shah, Author
Drawing on case studies of 31 disabled adults, this book suggests
that individual traits and patterns of behaviour are key factors in
career success, and shows that it is often society rather than impairment that hinders professional progression. It will provide
role models and valuable insights for young career-minded
disabled people.
208 pages Paperback

5041   Job Success for Persons with Developmental Disabilities
Jessica Kingsley Publishers
73 Collier St
London, UK   N19BE   hello@jkp.com
                                www.jkp.com

David B. Wiegan, Author
This book provides a comprehensive approach to developing a
successful jobs program for persons with developmental disabilities, drawn from the author's extensive experience and real
success.
160 pages Paperback

**5042   Making News: How to Get News Coverage of Disability
Rights Issues**
The Advocado Press

                                contact145@advocadopress.org
                                www.advocadopress.org

165 pages

5043   Making Self-Employment Work for People with Disabilities
Brookes Publishing
P.O.Box 10624
Baltimore, MD   21285-0624   410-337-9580
                                    800-638-3775
                                    Fax: 410-337-8539
                                    custserv@brookespublishing.com
                                    www.brookespublishing.com

Cary Griffin, Author
David Hammis, Author
Beth Keeton, Author
Molly Sullivan, Author
Practical support for individuals with significant disabilities in
starting and maintaining a small business. Covers building a
business plan; pinpointing interests, strengths, and goals; and
finding helpful information and support
288 pages

**5044   Road Ahead: Transition to Adult Life for Persons with
Disabilities (3rd Edition)**
IOS Press
6751 Tepper Dr
Clifton, VA   20124   703-830-6300
                                    Fax: 703-830-2300
                                    sales@iospress.com
                                    www.iospress.nl

Keith Storey, Editor
Dawn Hunter, Editor
Explores transition planning, assessment, instructional strategies, career development and support, social life, quality of life,
supported living, and post-secondary education for people with
disabilities.
318 pages

**5045   The Job Developer's Handbook: Practical Tactics for
Customized Employment**
Brookes Publishing
P.O. Box 10624
Baltimore, MD   21285-0624   410-337-9580
                                    800-638-3775
                                    Fax: 410-337-8539
                                    custserv@brookespublishing.com
                                    www.brookespublishing.com

Cary Griffin, Author
David Hammis, Author
Tammara Geary, Author
Michael Callahan, Author
One of the most practical employment books available, this for-
ward-thinking guide walks employment specialists step by step
through customized job development for people with disabilities,
revealing the best ways to build a satisfying, meaningful job
around a person's preferences, skills, and goals.
264 pages

General Disabilities

5046   A Guide to Disability Rights Laws
U.S. Department of Justice
950 Pennsylvania Ave NW
Washington, DC   20530-0001   202-514-2000
                                    www.ada.gov

Available in Large Print & Braille

5047   A Practical Guide to Art Therapy Groups
Routledge (Taylor & Francis Group)
711 Third Ave
New York, NY   10017   212-216-7800
                                    800-634-7064
                                    Fax: 202-564-7854
                                    enquiries@taylorandfrancis.com
                                    www.routledge.com

Diane Fausek, Author
Unique approaches, materials, and device will inspire you to tap
into your own well of creativity to design your own treatment
plans. It lays out the ingredients and the skills to get the results
you want. Includes strategies that have been used for people with

Alzheimer's, geri-psychiatric conditions and developmental disabilities.
124 pages Hardcover; Paperback

5048 A World Awaits You
Mobility International USA
132 E. Broadway
Ste 343
Eugene, OR 97401   541-343-1284
                           Fax: 541-343-6812
                           info@miusa.org
                           www.miusa.org

Yearly

5049 ADA Guide for Small Businesses
U.S. Department of Justice, Civil Rights Division
950 Pennsylvania Ave NW
Washington, DC 20530-0001   202-514-4609
                                 Fax: 202-307-1197
                                 TTY:202-514-0716
                                 www.ada.gov

5050 ADA Information Services
U.S. Department of Justice, Civil Rights Division
950 Pennsylvania Ave NW
Washington, DC 20530-0001   202-514-4609
                                 800-514-0301
                                 Fax: 202-307-1197
                                 TTY: 800-514-0383
                                 www.ada.gov

5051 ADA Pipeline
DRTAC: Southeast ADA Center
1419 Mayson Street NE
Atlanta, GA 30324   404-385-0636
                                 800-949-4232
                                 Fax: 404-385-0641
                                 www.sedbtac.org

Cyndi Smith, B.S., Office Assistant
Mary Morder, Information Technology Support
Sally Z. Weiss, B.A., Director
Rebecca Williams, B.A., M.S., Information Specialist / Technical Assistance
16 pages Quarterly

5052 ADA Questions and Answers
U.S. Department of Justice, Civil Rights Division
950 Pennsylvania Ave NW
Washington, DC 20530-0001   202-514-4609
                                 800-514-0301
                                 Fax: 202-307-1197
                                 TTY: 800-514-0383
                                 www.ada.gov

5053 ADA Tax Incentive Packet for Business
US Department of Justice
950 Pennsylvania Ave NW
Washington, DC 20530-9   202-586-5000
                                 800-574-0301
                                 Fax: 202-307-1197
                                 TTY: 800-514-0383
                                 www.ada.gov

James Bostrom, Deputy Chiefs
Zita Johnson Betts, Deputy Chiefs
Sally Conway, Deputy Chiefs
Jana Erickson, Deputy Chiefs
A 13-page packet of information to help businesses understand and take advantage of the tax credit and deduction available for complying with the ADA.

5054 ADA and City Governments: Common Problems
US Department of Justice
950 Pennsylvania Ave NW
Washington, DC 20530-9   202-586-5000
                                 800-574-0301
                                 Fax: 202-307-1197
                                 TTY: 800-514-0383
                                 www.ada.gov

James Bostrom, Deputy Chiefs
Zita Johnson Betts, Deputy Chiefs
Sally Conway, Deputy Chiefs
Jana Erickson, Deputy Chiefs
A 9-page document that contains a sampling of common problems shared by city governments of all sizes, provides examples of common deficiencies and explains how these problems affect persons with disabilities.

5055 ADA-TA: A Technical Assistance Update from the Department of Justice
US Department of Justice
950 Pennsylvania Ave NW
Washington, DC 20530-9   202-586-5000
                                 800-574-0301
                                 Fax: 202-307-1197
                                 TTY: 800-514-0383
                                 www.ada.gov

James Bostrom, Deputy Chiefs
Zita Johnson Betts, Deputy Chiefs
Sally Conway, Deputy Chiefs
Jana Erickson, Deputy Chiefs
A serial publication that answers Common Questions about ADA requirements and provides Design Details illustrating particular design requirements. The first edition addresses Readily Achievable Barrier Removal and Van Accessible Packing Spaces.

5056 AEPS Family Report: For Children Ages Birth to Three
Brookes Publishing
P.O.Box 10624
Baltimore, MD 21285-0624   410-337-9580
                                 800-638-3775
                                 Fax: 410-337-8539
                                 custserv@brookespublishing.com
                                 www.brookespublishing.com

Diane Bricker, Author
Betty Capt, Author
JoAnn Johnson, Author
Kristine Slentz, Author
This is a 64-item questionnaire that asks parents to rank their child's abilities on specific skills. In packages of 10.
28 pages Saddle-stiched

5057 ARC's Government Report
Arc of the District of Columbia
817 Varnum St NE
Washington, DC 20017-2144   202-636-2950
                                 Fax: 202-636-2996
                                 www.arcdc.net

Mary Lou Meccariello, Executive Director
Ed Cabatic, Director of Finance
Randy Shingler, Chief Operating Officer
Denize Stanton-Williams, Director of Supports & Services
Reports on government activities related to individuals with disabilities with a focus on persons with mental retardation. *$ 50.00*

5058 ARCA Newsletter
ARCA - Dakota County Technical College
1300 145th St E
Rosemount, MN 55068-2932   651-423-8301
                                 877-937-3282
                                 Fax: 651-423-7028
                                 dctc.edu

Ron Thomas, President
Offers information on support groups, conventions, books, manuscripts and programs for the rehabilitation professional and the disabled.
Monthly

5059   Accent on Living Magazine
Cheever Publishing
P.O.Box 700
Bloomington, IL 61702-700   309-378-2961
                                          800-787-8444
                                     Fax: 309-378-4420
Julie Cheever, Marketing Manager
A magazine published for forty four years, serves physically disabled people, with general interest, travel, and home modification features. *$12.00*
112 pages Quarterly

5060   Access Design Services: CILs as Experts
Independent Living Research Utilization ILRU
1333 Moursund
Houston, TX 77030   713-520-0232
                                     Fax: 713-520-5785
                                          ilru@ilru.org
                                          ilru.org
Lex Frieden, Director, ILRU
Richard Petty, Consultant
Rose Shepard, Office Manager
Featuring the Access Design Services of Alpha One in Maine, this month's Readings is another of the winners of the recent competition for innovative CIL programs.
10 pages

5061   Access To Independence Inc.
Access to Independence
3810 Milwaukee Street
Madison, WI 53714   608-242-8484
                                          800-362-9877
                                     Fax: 608-242-0383
                                     TTY: 608-242-8485
                                     info@accesstoind.org
                                     www.accesstoind.org
Dee Truhn, Executive Director
Jason Belaungy, Assistant Director
Geri , Finances/HR
Janie , Administrative Assistant
Independent Living Center serving people of any age and all types of disabilities in south-central Wisconsin. Empower people with disabilities, through advocacy, education, and support.
24 pages Semi-Annual

5062   Access for 911 and Telephone Emergency Services
US Department of Justice
950 Pennsylvania Ave NW
Washington, DC 20530-9   202-586-5000
                                          800-574-0301
                                     Fax: 202-307-1197
                                     TTY: 800-514-0383
                                          www.ada.gov
James Bostrom, Deputy Chiefs
Zita Johnson Betts, Deputy Chiefs
Sally Conway, Deputy Chiefs
Jana Erickson, Deputy Chiefs
A 10-page publication explaining the requirements for direct, equal access to 911 for persons who use teletypewritters (TTYs).

5063   Achieving Diversity and Independence
Independent Living Research Utilization ILRU
1333 Moursund
Houston, TX 77030   713-520-0232
                                     Fax: 713-520-5785
                                          ilru@ilru.org
                                          ilru.org
Lex Frieden, Director, ILRU
Richard Petty, Consultant
Rose Shepard, Office Manager
10 pages

5064   Activity-Based Intervention: 2nd Edition
Brookes Publishing
P.O.Box 10624
Baltimore, MD 21285-0624   410-337-9580
                                          800-638-3775
                                     Fax: 410-337-8539
                                     custserv@brookespublishing.com
                                          readplaylearn.com
Paul H. Brooks, Chairman
Jeffrey D. Brookes, President
Melissa A. Behm, Executive Vice President
This 14 minute video illustrates how activity-based intervention can be used to turn everyday events and natural interactions into opportunities to promote learning in young children who are considered at risk for developmental delays or who have mild to significant disabilities. *$39.00*
ISBN 1-55766 -86-3

5065   Ad Lib Drop-In Center: Consumer Management, Ownership and Empowerment
Independent Living Research Utilization ILRU
1333 Moursund
Houston, TX 77030   713-520-0232
                                     Fax: 713-520-5785
                                          ilru@ilru.org
                                          ilru.org
Lex Frieden, Director, ILRU
Richard Petty, Consultant
Rose Shepard, Office Manager
Joe describes how Ad Lib ensured consumer control in their Drop-In Center: the DIC came about because of consumer input, and consumers are involved in planning the program; members can choose to become volunteers or paid staff members. All of the staff at the DIC are consumers; and active consumer advisory board helps develop policies and programs and provides input to the Ad Lib board.
10 pages

5066   Adobe News
Santa Barbara Foundation
15 E Carrillo St
Santa Barbara, CA 93101-2706   805-963-1873
                                          805-966-2345
                                     Fax: 805-966-2345
Ron Gallo, CEO
8 pages Bi-Annually

5067   Advocate
Arc Massachusetts
217 South St
Waltham, MA 02453-2710   781-891-6270
                                     Fax: 781-891-6271
                                     arcmass@arcmass.org
                                          www.arcmass.org
Leo V. Sarkissian, Executive Director
Judy Zacek, Associate Editor
Beth Rutledge, Production Coordinator/Ad
Brenda Asis, Director of Development
Advocate is The Arc of Massachusetts' quarterly newsletter. This is one of the ways in which we inform and educate people about current topics in the field of developmental disabilities. *$20.00*
8-12 pages Quarterly

5068   American Herb Association Newsletter
P.O.Box 353
Nevada City, CA 95959-353   530-265-9552
                                     Fax: 530-274-3140
                                          www.ahaherb.com

5069   Americans with Disabilities Act Checklist for New Lodging Facilities
US Department of Justice
950 Pennsylvania Ave NW
Washington, DC   20530-9   202-586-5000
                                            800-574-0301
                                       Fax: 202-307-1197
                                       TTY: 800-514-0383
                                            www.ada.gov

James Bostrom, Deputy Chiefs
Zita Johnson Betts, Deputy Chiefs
Sally Conway, Deputy Chiefs
Jana Erickson, Deputy Chiefs
This 34-page checklist is a self-help survey that owners, franchisors, and managers of lodging facilities can use to identify ADA mistakes at their facilities.

5070   Americans with Disabilities Act Handbook
Aspen Publishers
76 9th Ave
7th Floor
New York, NY   10011-4962   212-790-2000
                                       Fax: 212-771-0885
                          customerservice@aspenpublishers.com
                                    www.aspenpublishers.com

Henry H Perritt Jr Esq, Author
Bob Lemmond, President and CEO
Gustavo Dobles, Vice President & Chief Content Officer
Susan Pikitch, Vice President & CFO
The Americans With Disabilities Act (ADA) Handbook provides comprehensive coverage of the ADA's employment, commercial facilities, and public accommodations provisions as well as coverage of the transportation, communication, and federal, local, and state government requirements. *$599.00*
1671 pages 2X per year
ISBN 0-735531-48-X

5071   An Interdisciplinary Journal for the Social Study of Health, Illness and Medicine
Sage Publications
2455 Teller Rd
Thousand Oaks, CA   91320-2218   805-499-0721
                                            800-818-7243
                                       Fax: 805-499-0871
                                       hea.sagepub.com

Alan Radley, Editor
Blaise Simqu, Chief Executive Officer
Quarterly

5072   Annual Report Sarkeys Foundation
530 E Main St
Norman, OK   73071-5823   405-364-3703
                                       Fax: 405-364-8191
                                       susan@sarkeys.org
                                            sarkeys.org

Kim Henry, Executive Director
Lorri Sutton, Executive Assistant
Susan C. Frantz, Senior Program Officer
Linda English Weeks, Senior Program Officer
Yearly

5073   Applied Kinesiology: Muscle Response in Diagnosis, Therapy and Preventive Medicine
Inner Traditions
P.O.Box 388
Rochester, VT   05767-388   802-767-3174
                                            800-246-8648
                                       Fax: 802-767-3726
                                  orders@innertraditions.com
                                    www.InnerTraditions.com

Jessica Arsenault, Sales Associate
Rob Meadows, VP Sales & Marketing
$12.95
144 pages
ISBN 0-892813-28-8

5074   Arc Connection Newsletter
Arc of Tennessee
151 Athens Way
Suite 100
Nashville, TN   37228-1367   615-248-5878
                                            800-835-7077
                                       Fax: 615-248-5879
                                       pcooper@thearctn.org
                                            thearctn.org

Carrie Hobbs Guiden, Executive Director
Peggy Cooper, Membership, Chapter and Communications Manager
Nicole Davidson, Business Manager
Lori Israel, Office Manager
The Arc of Tennessee is a nonprofit organization that offers advocacy, information, referral and support to people with intellectual or developmental disabilities and their families. This is their publication. It is free to members. *$10.00*
12 pages Quarterly

5075   Aromatherapy Book: Applications and Inhalations
2526 Martin Luther King Jr. Way
Berkeley, CA   94704   510-549-4270
                                       Fax: 510-549-4276
                                   info@northatlanticbooks.com
                                    www.northatlanticbooks.com

Minda Armstrong, Print Production Manager
Richard Grossinger, Founding Publisher
Janet Levin, Director of Sales & Distribution
Alla Spector, Director of Finance & Office Operations
A book of practical and researched information about aromatherapy. *$18.95*
400 pages
ISBN 1-556430-73-6

5076   Aromatherapy for Common Ailments
Simon & Schuster
100 Front St
Delran, NJ   8075-1181   856-461-6500
                                            800-323-7445
                                       Fax: 856-824-2402
                                       www.simonsays.com

David Schaeffer, VP
Explains aromatherapy with emphasis on medicinal uses.
96 pages
ISBN 0-671731-34-3

5077   As I Am
Fanlight Productions
32 Court Street
21st Floor
Brooklyn, NY   11201   718-488-8900
                                            800-876-1710
                                       Fax: 718-488-8642
                                       info@fanlight.com
                                            www.fanlight.com

Ben Achtenberg, Owner
Anthony Sweeney, Marketing Director
Three young people with developmental disabilities speak for themselves about their lives, the problems they face and their hopes and expectations for the future. *$99.00*
ISBN 1-572950-58-7

5078   Attitudes Toward Persons with Disabilities
Springer Publishing Company
11 West 42nd Street
15th Floor
New York, NY   10036   212-431-4370
                                            877-687-7476
                                       Fax: 212-941-7842
                                   marketing@springerpub.com
                                       www.springerpub.com

James C. Costello, Vice President, Journal Publishing
Diana Osborne, Production Manager
Megan Larkin, Managing Editor, Journals
Theodore C. Nardin, Chief Executive Officer and Publisher

This volume examines what is known of people's complex and multifaceted attitudes toward persons with disabilities. Divided into five areas of concern: theory, origin of attitudes, attitude measurement, attitudes of specific groups and attitude change. *$38.95*

352 pages Hardcover
ISBN 0-82616-90-1

5079   Authoritative Guide to Self- Help Resourcein Mental Health
Guilford Press
72 Spring St
New York, NY   10012-4019   212-431-9800
                                                       800-365-7006
                                                    Fax: 212-966-6708
                                                    info@guilford.com
                                                    www.guilford.com

Linda F Campbell PhD, Author
Thomas P Smith PsyD, Author
Robert Sommer PhD, Author
Bob Matloff, President
Reviews and rates 600+ self-help books, autobiographies, and popular films, and evaluates hundreds of Internet sites. Addresses 28 of the most prevalent clinical disorders and life challenges- from ADHD, Alzheimer's, and anxiety disorders, to marital problems, mood disorders and weight management. Also in cloth at $45.00 (ISBN# 1-57230-506-1) *$25.00*

377 pages Paperback
ISBN 1-572305-80-0

5080   AwareNews
Services for Independent Living
26250 Euclid Ave
Suite 801
Euclid, OH   44132   216-731-1529
                                                    Fax: 216-731-3083
                                                       sil@stratos.net
                                                       www.sil-oh.org

Molly Foos, Executive Director
Katherine Foley, Director of Advocacy
Lisa Marn, Assistant Director
Laura A. Gold, Director
12 pages Quarterly

5081   Bach Flower Therapy: Theory and Practice
Inner Traditions
1 Park St
Rochester, VT   05767   802-767-3174
                                                    Fax: 802-767-3726
                                       customerservice@InnerTraditions.com
                                                    www.innertraditions.com

Ehud Sperling, Owner
Contemporary study of Bach's techniques, intended for practitioners and lay readers alike. Includes lists of symptoms to facilitate diagnosis, ans aims to provide an understanding of psychosomatic elements in relation to physical complaints.
ISBN 0-892812-39-7

5082   Barrier Free Travel: A Nuts and Bolts Guide for Wheelers and Slow Walkers (3rd Edition)
Demos Health Publishing
11 W 42nd St
15th Fl
New York, NY   10036   212-683-0072
                                                     barrierfreetravel.net

Candy Harrington, Author
Billed as the definitive guide to accessible travel, this indispensable resource contains detailed information about the logistics of planning accessible travel by plane, train, bus and ship. *$19.95*

200 pages Paperback
ISBN 1-932603-83-2

5083   Beliefs, Values, and Principles of Self Advocacy
Brookline Books
34 University Rd
Brookline, MA   02445-4533   800-666-2665
                                                    Fax: 617-734-3952
                                                    brbooks@yahoo.com
                                                    www.brooklinebooks.com

48 pages Paperback
ISBN 0-57129-22-2

5084   Beliefs: Pathways to Health and Well Being
Metamorphous Press
P.O.Box 10616
Portland, OR   97296-616   503-228-4972
                                                    Fax: 503-223-9117

David Balding, Publisher
Explores behavioral technologies and belief change strategies that can alter beliefs that support unhealthy habbits such as smoking, overeating, and drug use. Also covers the changing of thinking processes that create phobias and unreasonable fears, retraining the immune system to eliminate allergies and to deal optinally with cancer, AIDS, and other diseases. Includes strategies to transform unhealthy beliefs into lifelong constructs of wellness.

5085   Bench Marks
Govennor's Council on Developmental Disabilities
1717 W Jefferson St
Phoenix, AZ   85007-3202   602-542-4049
                                                       800-889-5893
                                                    Fax: 602-542-5320

Micheal Ward, Executive Director
Susan Madison, Manager
Quarterly

5086   Bodie, Dolina, Smith & Hobbs, P.C.
21 W Susquehanna Ave
Suite 110
Towson, MD   21204-5218   410-823-1250
                                                       877-739-1013
                                                    Fax: 443-901-0802
                                                    chobbs@bodie-law.com
                                                    www.bodie-law.com

Chester Hobbs, Esquire
Thomas G. Bodie, Lawyer
Wallace Dann, Lawyer
Thomas J. Dolina, Lawyer
Law firm; provides estates, trusts and guardianship administration, estate planning, elder law, tax issues, bankruptcy, foreclosures, and real estate issues. *$25.00*
Quarterly

5087   Body Reflexology: Healing at Your Fingertips
Parker Publishing Company
Ste 2605
1501 Broadway
New York, NY   10036-5600   212-869-6350
Hy Dubin, President
Features step-by-step instructions of how to send healing flows of energy through the body to relieve back pain, headaches, arthritis, and other afflictions. Illustrated.
343 pages Hardcover
ISBN 0-132997-36-3

5088   Body Silent: The Different World of the Disabled
WW Norton & Company
324 State St
Santa Barbara, CA   93101-2362   800-333-6867
                                                    Fax: 805-962-5087
                                                    www.specialneeds.com/store/

256 pages
ISBN 0-393320-42-1

5089 Body of Knowledge/Hellerwork
406 Berry St
Mount Shasta, CA 96067-2548 530-926-2500
theheller@aol.com
www.josephheller.com

Joseph Heller, Owner
Information, referral directory, training and certification.

5090 Bridge Newsletter
Arizona Bridge to Independent Living
1229 E Washington St
Phoenix, AZ 85034-1101 602-256-2245
800-280-2245
Fax: 602-254-6407
abil.org

Phil Pangrazio, President & CEO
Regina Mitzel, V. P. & Chief Administrative Officer
Amina Kruck, V.P. of Advocacy
Ann Pasco, V.P. of Operations
12 pages Monthly

5091 Bridging the Gap: A National Directory of Services for Women & Girls with Disabilities
Educational Equity Concepts
71 Fifth Avenue
New York, NY 10016-5506 212-725-1803
Fax: 212-725-0947
TTY: 212-725-1803
www.edequity.org

Ellen Rubin, Coordinator Disability Programs
Merle Froschl, Editor
Contains a resource section of publications and videos geared specifically to women and girls with disabilities. Available in print, on cassette, and also in braille. *$24.95*
ISBN 0-931629-16-0

5092 Bulletin of the Association on the Handicapped
Assoc. on Handicapped Student Service Program
P.O.Box 21192
Columbus, OH 43221-0192 614-365-5216
Fax: 614-365-6718

5093 CDR Reports
Council for Disability Rights
Ste 1540
20 N Wacker Dr
Chicago, IL 60606-2903 312-201-4800
Fax: 312-444-1977
www.disabilityrights.org

Jo Holzer, Executive Director/Editor
Bruce Moore, Employment Specialist
 $15.00
8 pages Monthly

5094 California Financial Power of Attorney
NOLO
950 Parker St
Berkeley, CA 94710-2524 510-549-1976
800-955-4775
Fax: 510-548-5902
www.nolo.com

Maira Dizgalvis, Trade Customer Service Manager
Susan McConnell, Director Sales
Natasha Kaluza, Sales Assistant
David Rothenberg, CEO
A plain-English book packed with forms and instructions to give a trusted person the legal authority to handle your financial affairs.
Paperback

5095 Caring for America's Heroes
Oklahoma City VA Medical Center
921 NE 13th St
Oklahoma City, OK 73104-5007 405-270-0501
Fax: 405-270-1560
www.oklahoma.va.gov

Steven Gentlin, Director
Kathleen Fogarty, Associate Director
D Robert McCaffree MD, Chief of Staff
Tom Duchene, Plant Manager

5096 Center for Health Research: Eastern Washington University
Showalter 209a
Cheney, WA 99004 509-359-2279
800-221-9369
Fax: 509-359-2778
sharon.wilson@mail.ewu.edu

5097 Center for Libraries and Educational Improvement
400 Maryland Ave SW
Washington, DC 20202-1 202-260-2226
800-872-5327
Fax: 202-401-0689
TTY: 800-437-0833
www.ed.gov

5098 Centering Corporation Grief Resources
7230 Maple Street
Omaha, NE 68134 402-553-1200
866-218-0101
Fax: 402-533-0507
j1200@aol.com
www.centering.org

Joy Johnson, Founder
Dr. Marvin Johnson, Founder
Janet Roberts, Executive Director
Kelsey Novacek, Director of Marketing
A full catalog of all our available bereavement resources. We are a small, non-profit organization providing help to families in crisis situations.
32 pages BiAnnually

5099 Centers for Disease Control and Prevention
US Department of Health and Human Services
1600 Clifton Rd NE
Atlanta, GA 30329-4018 404-639-3311
800-232-4636
Fax: 404-498-1177
inquiry@cdc.gov
www.cdc.gov

Robert Delaney, Plant Manager
Publishes an annually updated list of infectious and communicable diseases transmitted through the handling of food in accordance with Section 103 of Title I.

5100 Child With Special Needs: Encouraging Intellectual and Emotional Growth
Addison-Wesley Publishing Company
Ste 300
75 Arlington St
Boston, MA 02116-3988 617-848-7500
800-238-9682
Fax: 617-944-7273
www.awprofessional.com

Bill Barke, CEO
Covering all kinds of disabilities — including cerebral palsy, autism, retardation, ADD, and language problems — this guide offers parents specific ways of helping all special needs chidren reach their full intellectual and emotional potential. *$32.00*
496 pages
ISBN 0-201407-26-4

5101 Chinese Herbal Medicine
Shambhala Publications
300 Massachusetts Avenue
Boston, MA 02115   617-424-0030
                          Fax: 617-236-1563
                          editors@shambhala.com
                          shambhala.com

Richard Reoch, President
Gives an in-depth look into herbal medicine.
176 pages
ISBN 0-877733-98-8

5102 Christian Approach to Overcoming Disability: A Doctor's Story
Haworth Press
10 Alice St
Binghamton, NY 13904-1503   607-722-5857
                               800-429-6784
                               Fax: 607-722-6362
                               orders@haworthpress.com
                               www.haworthpress.com

William Cohen, Owner
$29.95
128 pages
ISBN 0-789022-57-5

5103 Closing the Gap
526 Main Street
P.O.Box 68
Henderson, MN 56044-68   507-248-3294
                               Fax: 507-248-3810
                               info@closingthegap.com
                               www.closingthegap.com

Dolores Hagen, Founder
Delores Hagen, Founder
Connie Kneip, Vice President
Megan Turek, Managing Editor
Explores use of microcomputers as personal and educational tools for persons with disabilities.
36+ pages BiMonthly

5104 Conference of the Association on Higher Education & Disability
AHEAD
107 Commerce Center Dr.
Suite 204
Huntersville, NC 28078   704-947-7779
                               Fax: 704-948-7779
                               information@ahead.org
                               www.ahead.org

Jamie Axelrod, President
Gaeir Dietrich, Treasurer
Stephan Smith, Executive Director
Katy Washington, Secretary
An annual conference focused on aiding and meeting the needs of persons with disabilities attending higher education institutions.

5105 Constellations
Minnesota STAR Program
Ste 309
50 Sherburne Ave
Saint Paul, MN 55155-1402   651-296-2771
                               800-657-3862
                               Fax: 651-282-6671
                               star.program@state.mn.us

Chuck Rassbach, Executive Director
Free quarterly publication from the Minnesota STAR Program.
8 pages Quarterly

5106 Consumer Buyer's Guide for Independent Living
American Occupational Therapy Association (AOTA)
4720 Montgomery Ln
Bethesda, MD 20814-5320   301-652-2682
                               800-SAY-AOTA
                               Fax: 301-652-7711
                               TTY: 800-377-8555
                               www.aota.org

Florence Clark, President
A buyer's directory of products and publications for the general public listing suppliers' names, addresses and telephone numbers. This directory lists AOTA publications on numerous topics (back pain, Alzheimers, Carpal Tunnel Syndrome, etc.) and suppliers of equipment to assist in activities of daily living for individuals with disabilities.
60 pages Annual

5107 Coping+Plus: Dimensions of Disability
Greenwood Publishing Group
130 Cremona Drive
Santa Barbara, CA 93117   805-968-1911
                               800-368-6868
                               Fax: 866-270-3856
                               CustomerService@abc-clio.com
                               www.abc-clio.com

Matt Laddin, Vice President of Marketing
Mike Saltzman, Director-Eastern Territories & National Accounts
James Lingle, International Sales & Marketing
Everyone can learn new or more effective coping skills and strategies to deal with times of loss, crisis and disability. $55-$59.95
280 pages Hardcover
ISBN 0-275945-44-8

5108 Council News
Northern Nevada Center for Independent Living
999 Pyramid Way
Sparks, NV 89431-4471   775-353-3599
                               Fax: 775-353-3588
                               www.nncil.org

Lisa Bonie, Executive Director
Hilda Velasco, Operations Manager
Joni Inglis, Independent Living Advocate
Patti Rodriguez, Life Skills Coordinator
NNCIL was founded in 1982 by a small group of people with disabilities, who believe that each person, regardless of the severity of his or her disability, has the potential to grow, develop and share fully the joys and responsibilities of our society.
12 pages Quarterly

5109 Counseling in Terminal Care & Bereavement
Brookes Publishing
P.O.Box 10624
Baltimore, MD 21285-0624   410-337-9580
                               800-638-3775
                               Fax: 410-337-8539
                               custserv@brookespublishing.com
                               readplaylearn.com

Paul H. Brooks, Chairman
Jeffrey D. Brookes, President
Melissa A. Behm, Executive Vice President
Provides practical suggestions for addressing the needs of patients and family members who are anticipating or currently dealing with grief and bereavement, such as hospice care, hospitals, or at home care. $34.00
210 pages Paperback
ISBN 1-85433-78-7

5110 Creating Wholeness: Self-Healing Workbook Using Dynamic Relaxation, Images and Thoughts
Plenum Publishing Corporation
233 Spring St
7th Floor
New York, NY 10013-1522   212-620-8000
                                           800-644-4831
                                           Fax: 212-460-1575
                                           ainy@aveda.com
                                           www.aveda.edu

232 pages
ISBN 0-306441-72-1

5111 DRS Connection
Disabled Resource Services
Ste 101
424 Pine St
Fort Collins, CO 80524-2421   970-482-2700
                                          Fax: 970-407-7072

Nancy Jackson, Executive Director
4 pages Quaterly

5112 Demand Response Transportation Through a Rural ILC
Independent Living Research Utilization ILRU
1333 Moursund
Houston, TX 77030   713-520-0232
                                          Fax: 713-520-5785
                                          ilru@ilru.org
                                          ilru.org

Lex Frieden, Director, ILRU
Richard Petty, Consultant
Rose Shepard, Office Manager
Oklahomans for Independent Living's transportation program was selected as exemplary becuase they marketed it by emphasizing people with disabilities as economic constituency.
10 pages

5113 Developing Organized Coalitions and Strategic Plans
Independent Living Research Utilization ILRU
1333 Moursund
Houston, TX 77030   713-520-0232
                                          Fax: 713-520-5785
                                          ilru@ilru.org
                                          ilru.org

Lex Frieden, Director, ILRU
Richard Petty, Consultant
Rose Shepard, Office Manager
10 pages

5114 Dictionary of Congenital Malformations& Disorders
Informa Healthcare
Fl 16
52 Vanderbilt Ave
New York, NY 10017-3846   212-520-2777
                                          Fax: 212-661-5052
                                          orders@crcpress.com
                                          www.tandfonline.com

193 pages
ISBN 0-850705-77-1

5115 Dictionary of Developmental Disabilities Terminology
Brookes Publishing
P.O.Box 10624
Baltimore, MD 21285-0624   410-337-9580
                                          800-638-3775
                                          Fax: 410-337-8539
                                          custserv@brookespublishing.com
                                          www.brookespublishing.com

Paul H. Brooks, Chairman
Jeffrey D. Brookes, President
Melissa A. Behm, Executive Vice President
George S. Stamathis, Vice President & Publisher
With more than 3,000 easy-to-understand entries, this dictionary provides thorough explanations of terms associated with developmental disabilities and disorders. *$55.95*
368 pages Hardcover
ISBN 1-557662-45-2

5116 Directory of Members
American Network of Community Options & Resources
1101 King St
Suite 380
Alexandria, VA 22314-2962   703-535-7850
                                          Fax: 703-535-7860
                                          ancor@ancor.org
                                          ancor.org

Dave Toeniskoetter, President
Chris Sparks, Vice President
Julie Manworren, Secretary/Treasurer
Wendy Swager, Past president
The Directory lists over 600 agencies that provide residential services and supports in 48 states and the District of Columbia. The listings include the name of the Executive Directors, the name, address, and phone number of the agency, describe the types of services that are provided and how many individuals receive services from that agency. *$25.00*
189 pages

5117 Disability Awareness Guide
Central Iowa Center for Independent Living
655 Walnut St
Suite 131
Des Moines, IA 50309-3930   515-243-1742
                                          Fax: 515-243-5385

Bob Jeppesen, Executive Director
Frank Strong, Assistant Director Programs
Bob Jepson, Manager
The Disability Awareness Guide contains information about our center; who we are and what we do. It also contains the telephone numbers of local and national agencies and resources available for people with disabilities.

5118 Disability Rights Movement
Children's Press
Sherman Tpke
Danbury, CT 6813   800-621-1115
                                          Fax: 800-374-4329

Elena Rockman, Marketing Manager
Author Deborah Kent illuminates both the history of the National Disability Rights Movement and the inspiring personal stories of individuals with various disabilities. *$18.00*
32 pages Hardcover
ISBN 0-53106-32-3

5119 Disabled People's International Fifth World Assembly as Reported by Two US Participants
Independent Living Research Utilization ILRU
1333 Moursund
Houston, TX 77030   713-520-0232
                                          Fax: 713-520-5785
                                          ilru@ilru.org
                                          ilru.org

Lex Frieden, Director, ILRU
Richard Petty, Consultant
Rose Shepard, Office Manager
This report describes the international conference on independent living held in Mexico City in December 1998 as experienced by staff members from two U.S. centers. Kaye Beneke interviewed Luis Chew and Marco Antonio Coronado for this edition of Readings in Independent Living.
10 pages

5120 Disabled We Stand
Brookline Books
34 University Rd
Brookline, MA 02445-4533   800-666-2665
                                          Fax: 617-734-3952
                                          brbooks@yahoo.com
                                          www.brooklinebooks.com

Paperback
ISBN 0-25331 -80-0

5121 Disabled, the Media, and the Information Age
Greenwood Publishing Group
130 Cremona Drive
Santa Barbara, CA   93117   805-968-1911
                                                    800-368-6868
                                              Fax: 866-270-3856
                                      CustomerService@abc-clio.com
                                              www.abc-clio.com
Matt Laddin, Vice President of Marketing
Mike Saltzman, Director-Eastern Territories & National Accounts
James Lingle, International Sales & Marketing
A short and easy-to-read overview of how disabled Americans
have been portrayed by the media and how images and the role of
the handicapped are changing. *$55.00*
264 pages Hardcover
ISBN 0-313284-72-5

5122 Discovery Newsletter
North Dakota State Library Talking Book Services
Dept 250
604 E Boulevard Ave
Bismarck, ND   58505-605   701-328-2000
                                                    800-843-9948
                                              Fax: 701-328-2040
                                          sbschneider@nd.gov
                          ndsl.lib.state.nd.us/DisabilityServices.html
Doris Ott, Manager
The North Dakota State Library Disability Services produces the
Doscovery Newsletter containing information on services,
books, catalogs and of interest to the patron.
6 pages Bi-Annually

5123 EP Resource Guide
Exceptional Parent Library
P.O.Box 1807
Englewood Cliffs, NJ   7632-1207   201-947-6000
                                                    800-535-1910
                                              Fax: 201-947-9376
                                          eplibrary@aol.com
                                              www.eplibrary.com

5124 ESCIL Update Newsletter
Eastern Shore Center for Independent Living
9 Sunburst Ctr
Cambridge, MD   21613-2057   410-221-7701
                                                    800-705-7944
                                              Fax: 410-221-7714
Shirley Tarbox, Executive Director
Jean Reed, Administrative Assistant
Lisa Morgan, Director IL Services
6 pages Quarterly

**5125 Easy Things to Make Things Simple: Do It Yourself
Modifications for Disabled Persons**
Brookline Books
34 University Rd
Brookline, MA   02445-4533   800-666-2665
                                              Fax: 617-734-3952
                                          brbooks@yahoo.com
                                              www.brooklinebooks.com
160 pages Paperback
ISBN 1-571290-24-9

**5126 Enabling Romance: A Guide to Love, Sex & Relationships
for the Disabled**
Ken Kroll, Author
Erica Levy Klein, Author
An uncensored, illustrated guide to intimacy and sexual expres-
sion for persons with physical disabilities.

5127 Encyclopedia of Disability
Sage Publications
2455 Teller Rd
Thousand Oaks, CA   91320-2218   805-499-0721
                                          info@sagepub.com
                                              www.sagepub.com
Gary L Albrecht, Editor
Blaise Simqu, Chief Executive Officer
A five volume set that covers disabilities A-Z *$850.00*
2500 pages
ISBN 0-761925-65-1

**5128 EveryBody's Different: Understanding and Changing Our
Reactions to Disabilities**
Brookes Publishing
P.O.Box 10624
Baltimore, MD   21285-0624   410-337-9580
                                                    800-638-3775
                                              Fax: 410-337-8539
                                      custserv@brookespublishing.com
                                              readplaylearn.com
Paul H. Brooks, Chairman
Jeffrey D. Brookes, President
Melissa A. Behm, Executive Vice President
This book discusses the emotions, questions, fears, and stereo-
types that people without disabilities sometimes experience
when they interact with people who do have disabilities. The au-
thor teaches readers to become more at ease with the concept of
disability and to communicate more effectively with each other.
Features activities and exercises that encourage self-examina-
tion, helping people to create more enriching personal relationships and work toward a fully inclusive society.
Paperback
ISBN 1-55766 -59-9

5129 Everybody's Guide to Homeopathic Medicines
Jeremy P Tarcher
375 Hudson St
New York, NY   10014-3658   212-366-2000
                                          academic@penguin.com
                                              www.us.penguingroup.com
John Makinson, Chairman and CEO
Coram Williams, CFO
Covers alternative treatments in homeopathic medicines.
375 pages
ISBN 0-874778-43-3

**5130 Everyday Social Interaction: A Program for People with
Disabilities**
Brookes Publishing
P.O.Box 10624
Baltimore, MD   21285-0624   410-337-9580
                                                    800-638-3775
                                              Fax: 410-337-8539
                                      custserv@brookespublishing.com
                                              readplaylearn.com
Paul H. Brooks, Chairman
Jeffrey D. Brookes, President
Melissa A. Behm, Executive Vice President
This source guides teachers and human services professionals in
helping people with disabilities acquire social interaction skills
and develop satisfying relationships. Included is a checklist and
task analyses that shows how complex skills can be broken down
into major components for easy performance monitoring accompanied by tips on social courtesies, rewards, praise, and criticism.
$41.95
342 pages Paperback
ISBN 1-55766 -58-4

5131 Family Challenges: Parenting with a Disability
Aquarius Health Care Videos
P.O.Box 1159
Sherborn, MA   01770-7159   508-650-1616
                                             888-440-2963
                                        Fax: 508-650-4216
                                       aqvideos@tiac.net
                               www.aquariusproductions.com
Lesile Kussmann, Owner
When a parent has a disability, everyone in the family is affected. For children, these experiences may profoundly influence their lives and views of the world. In this sensitive film, you will hear about different roles that all the family members take on at varying times. *$195.00*

5132 Force A Miracle
Writer's Showcase Press
244 pages
ISBN 0-595226-88-4

5133 Forum
Coalition for the Education of Disabled Children
165 W Center St
Marion, OH   43302-3742   740-382-7362
                                             800-374-2806
                                        Fax: 740-382-3428
Tracie Wilson, Manager
Leeann Derugen, Manager
Forum is a newsletter reporting on legislative and other developments affecting persons with disabilities.
Quarterly

5134 Foundation Fundamentals for Nonprofit Organizations
Foundation Center
Department Ze
79 5th Ave
New York, NY   10003-3034   212-620-4230
                                             800-424-9836
                                        Fax: 212-807-3677
                              order@foundationcenter.org
                                     www.fdncenter.org
Bradford K. Smith, President
Lisa Philip, Vice President for Strategic Philanthropy
Lawrence T. McGill, Vice President for Research
Lisa Brooks, Director of Knowledge Management Systems
This video is designed to give fundraisers a general overview of the foundation funding process and to introduce them to the many resources available through our libraries and cooperating collections. The video gives clear, step-by-step instructions on how to build a fundraising program. *$24.00*
Video

5135 Four-Ingredient Cookbook
Laurel Designs
Apt A
1805 Mar West St
Belvedere Tiburon, CA   94920-1962   *Fax:* 415-435-1451
Janet Sawyer, Owner
Lynn Montoya, Owner
Simple, easy to follow recipes, each containing four ingredients. Particularly suited to persons with limited physical ability. Includes 400 recipes, appetizers to desserts. *$9.00*

5136 Frequently Asked Questions About Multiple Chemical Sensitivity
Independent Living Research Utilization ILRU
1333 Moursund
Houston, TX   77030   713-520-0232
                                        Fax: 713-520-5785
                                           ilru@ilru.org
                                              ilru.org
Lex Frieden, Director, ILRU
Richard Petty, Consultant
Rose Shepard, Office Manager
This FAQ covers important information about multiple chemical sensitivity and environmental illness. The FAQ describes the conditions, recommends strategies for improving access, and lists resources for CILs and other organizations. As the fact sheet states, centers must set an example in assuring that all people can enter their offices.
10 pages

5137 Genetic Disorders Sourcebook
Omnigraphics
155 W. Congress
Suite 200
Detroit, MI   48226-3900   313-961-1340
                                             800-234-1340
                                        Fax: 800-875-1340
                                contact@omnigraphics.com
                                     www.omnigraphics.com
Paul Rogers, Publicity Associate
Georgiann Fratoni, Customer Service Manager
Provides information on hereditary diseases and disorders. *$7800.00*
650 pages
ISBN 0-789892-41-1

5138 Genetic Nutritioneering
McGraw-Hill Company
2460 Kerper Blvd
Dubuque, IA   52001-2224   563-588-1451
                                             800-338-3987
                                        Fax: 614-755-5654
                                www.mhhe.com/hper/physed
Kurt Strand, VP
Describes how to modify the expression of genetic traits, potentially preventing heart disease, cancer, arthritis, and hormone-related problems. Features how to slow biological aging and reduce the risk of age-related diseases. *$16.95*
288 pages
ISBN 0-879839-21-X

5139 Going to School with Facilitated Communication
Syracuse University, School of Education
230 Huntington Hall
Syracuse, NY   13244-1   315-443-4752
                                        Fax: 315-443-2258
                                          jhrusso@syr.edu
                                          www.soe.syr.edu
Shirley Adamczyk, Administrative Assistant
Rachael Gazdick, Executive Director
Isabelle M. Glod, Administrative Assistant
Angela Flanagan, Development Assistant
A video in which students with autism and/or severe disabilities illustrate the use of facilitated communication focusing on basic principles fostering facilitated communication.
Video

5140 Grief: What it is and What You Can Do
Centering Corporation
7230 Maple Street
Omaha, NE   68134   402-553-1200
                                             866-218-0101
                                        Fax: 402-533-0507
                                          j1200@aol.com
                                          www.centering.org
Joy Johnson, Founder
Dr. Marvin Johnson, Founder
Janet Roberts, Executive Director
Kelsey Novacek, Director of Marketing
General grief information for all grief issues. *$3.50*
32 pages Paperback

5141 Guidelines on Disability
US Department of Housing & Urban Development
451 7th St SW
Washington, DC   20410-1   202-708-1112
                                       TTY:202-708-1455
                              portal.hud.gov/hudportal/HUD
Shaun Donovan, Secretary
Helen R. Kanovsky, Acting Deputy Secretary
Jennifer Ho, Senior Advisor to the Secretary
Mike Anderson, Chief Human Capital Officer

Contains information on housing and accessibility for persons with disabilities.

5142 Handbook of Services for the Handicapped
Greenwood Publishing Group
130 Cremona Drive
Santa Barbara, CA 93117
805-968-1911
800-368-6868
Fax: 866-270-3856
CustomerService@abc-clio.com
www.abc-clio.com
Matt Laddin, Vice President of Marketing
Mike Saltzman, Director-Eastern Territories & National Accounts
James Lingle, International Sales & Marketing
A handy reference book offering information and services for disabled individuals. $59.95-$65.00.
291 pages Hardcover
ISBN 0-313213-85-2

5143 Healing Herbs
Rodale Press
33 E Minor St
Emmaus, PA 18098-1
610-967-5171
Fax: 610-967-8963
www.rodale.com
Maria Rodale, Chairman/Chief Executive Officer
Scott D. Schulman, President
Heather Rodale, Board Member/Vice President/ Leadership Development
Thomas A. Pogash, EVP/Chief Financial Officer
Covers everything from growing the herbs to home remedies.

5144 Helen Keller National Center for Deaf- Blind Youths And Adults
141 Middle Neck Rd
Sands Point, NY 11050-1218
516-944-8900
Fax: 516-944-7302
hkncinfo@hknc.org
www.hknc.org
Joseph McNulty, Executive Director
HKNC is the only national vacational and rehabilitation program providing services exclusively to youth and adults who are deaf-blind.

5145 Hospice Alternative
Harper Collins Publishers/Basic Books
10 E 53rd St
New York, NY 10022-5244
212-207-7000
800-242-7737
Fax: 212-207-7203
Jane Friedman, CEO
An account of the hospice experience. An innovative and humane way of caring for the terminally ill. *$8.95*
256 pages
ISBN 0-46503 -61-0

5146 How to File a Title III Complaint
US Department of Justice
950 Pennsylvania Ave NW
Washington, DC 20530-9
202-307-0663
800-574-0301
Fax: 202-307-1197
TTY: 800-514-0383
www.ada.gov
Rebecca B. Bond, Chief
Zita Johnson Betts, Deputy Chiefs
Sally Conway, Deputy Chiefs
James Bostrom, Deputy Chiefs
This publication details the procedure for filing a complaint under Title III of the ADA.

5147 How to Live Longer with a Disability
Accent Books & Products
PO Box 700
Bloomington, IL 61702-700
309-378-2961
800-787-8444
Fax: 309-378-4420
acmtlvng@aol.com
Raymond C Cheever, Publisher
Betty Garee, Editor
Eleven chapters to help you enjoy every aspect of your life, and live easier and happier. Includes sexuality and disability, getting more from the medical community and benefit programs. Co-authored by Robert Mauro, sociologist and Elle Becker, counselor and psychologist, both disabled. *$11.50*
266 pages Paperback
ISBN 0-19570 -38-8

5148 Ideas for Kids on the Go
Accent Books & Products
PO Box 700
Bloomington, IL 61702-700
309-378-2961
800-787-8444
Fax: 309-378-4420
acmtlvng@aol.com
Raymond C Cheever, Publisher
Betty Garee, Editor
This guide shows kids with physical disabilities how to go for it! Lists products and where to get them, and includes tips from others for having fun and getting ahead. Ages 1-18. *$6.95*
69 pages Paperback
ISBN 0-91570 -17-5

5149 If I Only Knew What to Say or Do
AARP Fulfillment
601 E St NW
Washington, DC 20049-1
202-434-2277
800-424-3410
Fax: 202-434-3443
TTY: 877-434-7598
member@aarp.org
www.aarp.org
Carol Raphael, Chair
Ronald E. Daly, Sr., Board Vice Chair
Jeannine English, President
A. Barry Rand, Chief Executive Officer
Provides a concise discussion of how to help a friend in crisis. Learn what to say and what not to say.

5150 If it Weren't for the Honor: I'd Rather Have Walked
Accent Books & Products
PO Box 700
Bloomington, IL 61702-700
309-378-2961
800-787-8444
Fax: 309-378-4420
acmtlvng@aol.com
Raymond C Cheever, Publisher
Betty Garee, Editor
Revealing, often humorous, highly interesting and important reading. This book offers an account told by the author who was on the scene and actually saw and participated in many events that paved the way for progress for all those with disabilities. *$14.50*
262 pages Paperback
ISBN 0-91570 -41-8

5151 Imagery in Healing Shamanism and Modern Medicine
Shambhala Publications
300 Massachusetts Avenue
Horticultural Hall
Boston, MA 02115
617-424-0030
888-424-2329
Fax: 617-236-1563
editors@shambhala.com
www.shambhala.com
Richard Reoch, President

Patients use self imagery to fight sickness and pain throughout their lives. *$15.95*
272 pages
ISBN 1-570629-34-x

5152   Independence
Easter Seals
1219 Dunn Ave
Daytona Beach, FL   32114-2405   386-255-4568
                                          877-255-4568
                                       Fax: 386-258-7677
                        www.easterseals-volusiaflagler.org

Jeff Blass, Chairman
Austin Brownlee, Chair-Elect
Becky Rutland, Vice Chair
Lynn Sinnott, President/ CEO
4-6 pages Quarterly

5153   Independent Living Centers and Managed Care: Results of an ILRU Study on Involvement
Independent Living Research Utilization ILRU
1333 Moursund
TIRR Memorial Hermann Research Cent
Houston, TX   77030-7031   713-520-0232
                                       Fax: 713-520-5785
                                          ilru@ilru.org
                                          www.ilru.org

Lex Frieden, Director, ILRU
Richard Petty, Program Director
Vinh Nguyen, Program Director
Roxy Funchess, Administrative Secretary
This month's Readings presents findings from an ILRU study of roles centers are taking vis-a-vis managed care. Initiated in spring 1998, we asked Drew Batavia to take the lead in conducting this study for us. We were interested in collecting data on frequency with which centers are contacted by consumers with managed care problems. This is a study that will need to be repeated periodically as our experiences with managed care evolves. Meanwhile, here are the initial findings.
10 pages

5154   Independent Living Challenges the Blues
Independent Living Research Utilization ILRU
1333 Moursund
TIRR Memorial Hermann Research Cent
Houston, TX   77030-7031   713-520-0232
                                       Fax: 713-520-5785
                                          ilru@ilru.org
                                          www.ilru.org

Lex Frieden, Director, ILRU
Richard Petty, Program Director
Vinh Nguyen, Program Director
Roxy Funchess, Administrative Secretary
Patricia's article highlights the Georgia SILC's health care advocacy efforts: the Georgia legislature passed a bill enabling Georgia Bleu to convert to for-profit status without a distribution of assets to similar nonprofit corporations; the Georgia SILC joined other health care advocates in filing a class action law suit to challenge the legality of the conversion; the Georgia SILC continues advocacy efforts to involve people with disabilities in developing and monitoring health care policy.
10 pages

5155   Independent Living Office
Department of Housing & Urban Development (HUD)
451 7th St SW
Washington, DC   20410-1   202-863-2800
                                          www.portal.hud.gov
Ted Tozer, President
Rafael Diaz, Chief Information Officer/Chief Information Officer
Mike Anderson, Chief Human Capital Officer
Shaun Donovan, Secretary
This office within HUD is charged with encouraging the construction of housing that is accessible to handicapped persons. The Office of Independent Living encourages modifications of apartments and other dwellings so that handicapped persons can enter without assistance.

5156   Independent Newsletter
Easter Seals Nebraska
12565 West Center Road
Suite 100
Omaha, NE   68144-8144   402-345-2200
                                          800-650-9880
                                       Fax: 402-345-2500
                                          www.easterseals.com/ne/
James C. Summerfelt, President/Chief Executive Officer
Angela Howell, Vice President
Lily Sughroue, Director of Camp
Terrific fun for campers and a much needed respite for families and care givers from the daily challenges of caring for special needs indviduals
4 pages Quarterly

5157   Information Services for People with Developmental Disabilities
Greenwood Publishing Group
130 Cremona Drive
Santa Barbara, CA   93117   805-968-1911
                                          800-368-6868
                                       Fax: 866-270-3856
                           CustomerService@abc-clio.com
                                          www.abc-clio.com

Matt Laddin, Vice President of Marketing
Mike Saltzman, Director - Eastern Territories
James Lingle, International Sales & Marketing
Overviews the information needs of people with developmental disabilities and tells librarians how to meet them. $65.oo-$75.00.
368 pages Hardcover
ISBN 0-313287-80-5

5158   Innovative Programs: An Example of How CILs Can Put Their Work in Context
Culture
1333 Moursund
TIRR Memorial Hermann Research Cent
Houston, TX   77030-7031   713-520-0232
                                       Fax: 713-520-5785
                                          ilru@ilru.org
                                          www.ilru.org

Lex Frieden, Director, ILRU
Richard Petty, Program Director
Vinh Nguyen, Program Director
Roxy Funchess, Administrative Secretary
Another winner in the innovative CIL competition- Steve Brown describes the Talking Books Program of Southeast Alaska Independent Living, discussing their efforts to record the oral history and life experiences of people with disabilities in the larger context of disability culture.
10 pages

5159   Insurance Solutions: Plan Well, Live Better
Demos Medical Publishing
11 West 42nd Street
15th Floor
New York, NY   10036   212-683-0072
                                          800-532-8663
                                       Fax: 212-683-0118
                          support@demosmedical.com
                                          www.demosmedpub.com
Paul Choi, Vice-President of Finance and Operations
Matt Conmy, Sr. Director of Sales
Thomas Hastings, Marketing Manager
Beth Kaufman Barry, Publisher
Learn how to look at various insurance options from a new perspective — including life, disability, health, and long-term care. Concrete information for dealing with potential problems in your coverage, to secure your financial future. *$24.95*
192 pages 2002
ISBN 1-888799-55-2

5160 International Directory of Libraries for the Disabled
KG Saur/Division of RR Bowker
121 Chanlon Rd
New Providence, NJ 7974-1541   908-286-1090
                                             800-521-8110
Michael Cairns, CEO
An essential resource for improving the quality and quantity of
materials available to the print-handicapped audience. Featuring
talking books, braille books, large print books as well as production centers for these materials. *$46.00*
257 pages
ISBN 3-59821 -81-1

5161 Issues in Independent Living
Independent Living Research Utilization
1333 Moursund
TIRR Memorial Hermann Research Cent
Houston, TX 77030-7031   713-520-0232
                                         Fax: 713-520-5785
                                             ilru@ilru.org
                                             www.ilru.org
Laurie Redd, Executive Director
Lex Frieden, Manager
Vinh Nguyen, Program Director
Roxy Funchess, Administrative Secretary
This booklet is a report of the National Study Group on the Impli-
cations of Health Care Reform for Americans with Disabilities
and Chronic Health Conditions.
30 pages

5162 JAMA: The Journal of the American Medical Association
American Medical Association
PO Box 10946
Chicago, IL 60654-4820   312-670-7827
                                             800-262-2350
                                         Fax: 312-464-5909
                                  subscriptions@jamanetwork.com
                                         jama.jamanetwork.com
Howard Bauchner, MD, Editor-in-Chief
Articles cover all aspects of medical research and clinical medi-
cine. *$66.00*

5163 JCIL Advocate Times
Jackson Center for Independent Living
409 Linden Ave
Jackson, MI 49203-4065   517-782-6054
                                         Fax: 517-782-3118
Lesia Pikaart, Executive Director
JoAnn Lucas, Associate Director
Quarterly

5164 Jason & Nordic Publishers, Inc.
PO Box 441
Hollidaysburg, PA 16648-441   814-696-2929
                                         Fax: 814-696-4250
Norma Mc Phee, Owner/CEO
Norma Phee
Turtle Books for children with disabilities present heroes who
look like them, have problems like theirs, have similar doubts and
feelings in non-threatening, fun stories. They are motivational,
bridge the gap and promote understanding among peers and siblings. 22 children's books (grades preK-3) plus Sensitivity and
Awareness Guide containing lesson plans, activities, background
information keyed to the series. Disabilities include: Down syndrome, cerebral palsy, blindness, deafness and more.

5165 Journal of Social Work in Disabilty & Rehabilitation
Haworth Press
10 Alice St
Binghamton, NY 13904-1503   607-722-5857
                                             800-429-6784
                                         Fax: 607-722-6362
                                      orders@haworthpress.com
                                         www.haworthpress.com
William Cohen, Owner
John T Oardeck PhD, Editor
S Harrington-Miller, Advertising

Presents and explores issues related to disabilities and social policy, practice, research, and theory. Reflecting the broad scope of
social work in disabilty practice, this interdisciplinary journal
examines vital issues aspects of the field — from innovative practice methods, legal issues, and literature reviews to program descriptions and cuttinf-edge practice research.
Quarterly

5166 Just Like Everyone Else
World Institute on Disability
3075 Adeline Street
Suite 155
Oakland, CA 94703-1520   510-225-6400
                                         Fax: 510-225-0477
                                         TTY:510-225-0478
                                             wid@wid.org
                                             www.wid.org
Paul W. Schroeder, Chair
Linda M. Dardarian, Vice Chair
Mary Brooner, Treasurer
Cassandra Malry, Secretary
The oversize-format publication, intended for general audiences,
provides perspective, inspiration and information about the Inde-
pendent Living Movement and the Americans with Disabilities
Act. *$5.00*
16 pages

**5167 Keep the Promise: Managed Care and People with
Disabilities**
American Network of Community Options & Resource
1101 King St
Ste 380
Alexandria, VA 22314-2962   703-535-7850
                                         Fax: 703-535-7860
                                             ancor@ancor.org
                                             www.ancor.org
Dave Toeniskoetter, President
Chris Sparks, Vice President
Julie Manworren, Secretary/Treasurer
Renee L. Pietrangelo, PhD, Chief Executive Officer
This publication presents a detailed review of the process and the
lessons learned. Details a way for all stake holders to work to-
gether for a state or local system.
119 pages $18 - $22

5168 Keeping Our Families Together
Through the Looking Glass
3075 Adeline St.
Ste. 120
Berkeley, CA 94703-2212   510-848-1112
                                             800-644-2666
                                         Fax: 510-848-4445
                                         TTY: 510-848-1005
                                       tlg@lookingglass.org
                                       www.lookingglass.org
Maureen Block, J.D., Board President
Thomas Spalding, Board Treasurer
Alice Nemon, D.S.W.,, Board Secretary
Report of the National Task Force on parents with disabilities and
their families. Available in braille, large print or cassette. *$2.00*
12 pages

5169 Learn About the ADA in Your Local Library
US Department of Justice
950 Pennsylvania Ave NW
Washington, DC 20530-9   202-307-0663
                                             800-574-0301
                                         Fax: 202-307-1197
                                         TTY: 800-514-0383
                                             www.ada.gov
Rebecca B. Bond, Chief
Zita Johnson Betts, Deputy Chiefs
Sally Conway, Deputy Chiefs
A 10-page annotated list of 95 ADA publications and one video-
tape that are available in 15,000 public libraries throughout the
country.

5170   LifeLines
Disabled & Alone/Life Services for the Handicapped
1440 Broadway
23rd Floor
New York, NY   10018-2326   212-532-6740
                                             800-995-0066
                                        Fax: 212-532-3588
                                      info@disabledandalone.org
                                      www.disabledandalone.org

Leslie D. Park, Chairman
Rex L. Davidson, Vice President
William G. Shannon, J.D., Treasurer
Lee Alan Ackerman, B.A., Executive Director
Newsletter providing current and valuable information about
lifetime care and planning for persons with disabilities and their
families and the organizations serving them. Free upon request.
4-10 pages BiAnnual

**5171   Lifelong Leisure Skills and Lifestyles for Persons with
         Developmental Disabilities**
Brookes Publishing
PO Box 10624
Baltimore, MD   21285-0624   410-337-9580
                                             800-638-3775
                                        Fax: 410-337-8539
                                   custserv@brookespublishing.com
                                        www.readplaylearn.com

Paul H. Brooks, Chairman
Jeffrey D. Brookes, President
Melissa A. Behm, Executive Vice President
This instructional manual offers ideas and detailed examples that
describe how to guide individuals of all ages through popular activities using adaptations that foster skill acquisition and inclusion. Some of the concepts explored are home-school-community
collaboration, choice making and the dignity of risk, and leisure
skill acquisition for the life span. *$35.00*
352 pages Paperback
ISBN 1-55766 -47-2

5172   Livin'
Lehigh Valley Center for Independent Living
435 Allentown Dr
Allentown, PA   18109-9121   610-770-9781
                                        Fax: 610-770-9801
                                             info@lvcil.org
                                             www.lvcil.org

Amy Beck, Executive Director
Cara Steidel, Director of Finance
Greg Bott, Director of Development
Jessica DeMaio, Administrative Services Coordinator
4 pages Quarterly

5173   Living in a State of Stuck
Brookline Books
8 Trumbull Rd
Suite B-001
Northampton, MA   01060   413-584-0184
                                             800-666-2665
                                        Fax: 413-584-6184
                                         brbooks@yahoo.com
                                        www.brooklinebooks.com

3rd ed., paper
ISBN 1-571290-27-3

5174   Living in the Community
Independent Living Research Utilization ILRU
1333 Moursund
TIRR Memorial Hermann Research Cent
Houston, TX   77030-7031   713-520-0232
                                        Fax: 713-520-5785
                                             ilru@ilru.org
                                             www.ilru.org

Lex Frieden, Director, ILRU
Richard Petty, Program Director
Vinh Nguyen, Program Director
Roxy Funchess, Administrative Secretary

James, Lori, and Jamey describe the elements of their successful
program to move people out of nursing homes and into the community: providing funding for deposits, first month's rent and
other neccessities, including assistive technology; providing
training and the other core services before and after consumers
leave the nursing home; developing relationships with housing
and other service providers.
10 pages

5175   Loud, Proud and Passionate
Mobility International USA
132 E. Broadway, Suite 343
PO Box 10767
Eugene, OR   97401   541-343-1284
                                        Fax: 541-343-6812
                                             info@miusa.org
                                             www.miusa.org

Susan Sygall, CEO
Cerise Roth-Vinson, COO
Cindy Lewis, Director of Programs
Stephanie Gray, Program Managers
A resource book for international development and women's or-
ganization about including women with disabilities in projects in
the community. Informs women sith disabilities about the efforts
and successes of their peers worldwide. *$30.00*

5176   Love: Where to Find It, How to Keep It
Accent Books & Products
PO Box 700
Bloomington, IL   61702-700   309-378-2961
                                             800-787-8444
                                        Fax: 309-378-4420
                                          acmtlvng@aol.com

Raymond C Cheever, Publisher
Betty Garee, Editor
Offers ideas such as how to meet other single people, avoid the
wrong type; communications skills and much more for the disabled person wanting to date. *$6.95*
104 pages Paperback
ISBN 0-91570 -31-0

5177   MOOSE: A Very Special Person
Brookline Books
8 Trumbull Rd
Suite B-001
Northampton, MA   01060   413-584-0184
                                             800-666-2665
                                        Fax: 413-584-6184
                                         brbooks@yahoo.com
                                        www.brooklinebooks.com

Paperback
ISBN 0-91479 -73-5

5178   Mainstream Magazine
2973 Beech St
San Diego, CA   92102-1529   619-232-2727
                                        Fax: 619-234-3155
                                        www.mainstream-mag.com

Cyndi Jones, Executive Director
The authoritative, national voice of people with disabilities, publishes in-depth reports on employment, education, new products
and technology, legislation and disability rights advocacy, recreation and travel, disability arts and culture, plus personality profiles and challenging commentary. *$24.00*
Monthly

5179   Making Changes: Family Voices on Living Disabilities
Brookline Books
8 Trumbull Rd
Suite B-001
Northampton, MA   01060   413-584-0184
                                             800-666-2665
                                        Fax: 413-584-6184
                                         brbooks@yahoo.com
                                        www.brooklinebooks.com

216 pages Paperback
ISBN 0-91479 -93-

5180 Making Informed Medical Decisions: Where to Look and How to Use What You Find
Patient-Centered Guides
1005 Gravenstein Highway North
Sebastopol, CA 95472-3836 707-827-7019
800-889-8969
Fax: 707-824-8268
orders@oreilly.com
www.patientcenters.com

Tim O'Reilly, CEO
Making Informed Medical Decisions acts like a friendly reference librarian, explaining: tips for researching for someone else; medical journal articles; statistics and risk; standard treatment options; clinical trial; making an ally of your doctor; and determining your own best course. Authors Oster, Thomas, and Joseff-a patient advocate, medical librarian, and medical doctor-also share examples and stories. *$17.95*
280 pages Paperback
ISBN 1-565924-59-2

5181 Making Wise Decisions for Long-Term Care
AARP Fulfillment
601 E St NW
Washington, DC 20049-1 202-434-2277
800-424-3410
Fax: 202-434-3443
TTY: 877-434-7598
member@aarp.org
www.aarp.org

Carol Raphael, Chair
Ronald E. Daly, Sr., Board Vice Chair
Jeannine English, President
A. Barry Rand, Chief Executive Officer
Here's a comprehensive consumer education effort in the area of long-term care.
28 pages

5182 Making a Difference
Georgia Council On Developmental Disabilities
2 Peachtree St N.W.
Suite 26-246
Atlanta, GA 30303-3141 404-657-2126
888-275-4233
Fax: 404-657-2132
TTY: 404-657-2133
eejacobson@dhr.state.ga.us
www.gcdd.org

Eric E Jacobson, Executive Director
Pat Nobbie, Deputy Director
Dottie Adams, Family/Individual Support Dir.
Valerie Meadows Suber, Public Information Director
The Georgia Council on Developmental Disabilities collaborates with Georgia's citizens, public and private advocacy organizations and policymakers to positively influence public policies that enhance the quality of life for people with disabilities and their families. GCDD provides this through education and advocacy activities, program implementation, funding and public policy analysis and research.

5183 Making a Difference: A Wise Approach
Easter Seals
233 South Wacker Drive
Suite 2400
Chicago, IL 60606-4703 312-726-0653
800-221-6827
Fax: 312-726-1494
www.easterseals.com

Richard W. Davidson, Chairman
Sandra L. Bouwman, 1st Vice Chairman
Joseph G. Kern, 2nd Vice Chairman
Ralph F. Boyd, Jr., Treasurer
The town of Wise, Virginia, and its leading citizen, Virgil Craft, personify what Making a Difference is all about when a community supports implementing the provisions of the Americans with Disabilities Act. Craft, a person with a disability, has spent his life giving back to the community. The community, in turn, has supported Craft's efforts to improve the environment, education,

healthcare and access for disabled persons. A must buy for companies of all sizes, clubs and organizations. *$50.00*

5184 Managing Your Activities
Arthritis Foundation
PO Box 78423
Atlanta, GA 30357-0669 404-237-8771
800-933-7023
Fax: 404-872-0457
help@arthritis.org
www.arthritis.org

John H Klippel, CEO/ President

5185 Managing Your Health Care
Arthritis Foundation
PO Box 78423
Atlanta, GA 30357-0669 404-237-8771
800-933-7023
Fax: 404-872-0457
help@arthritis.org
www.arthritis.org

John H Klippel, CEO/ President

5186 Medical Aspects of Disability: A Handbook For The Rehabilitation Professional
Springer Publishing Company
11 West 42nd Street
15th Floor
New York, NY 10036 212-431-4370
877-687-7476
Fax: 212-941-7842
cs@springerpub.com
www.springerpub.com

Ursula Springer, President
Theodore C. Nardin, CEO/Publisher
Jason Roth, VP/Marketing Director
James C. Costello, Vice President, Journal Publishing
$62.92
744 pages
ISBN 0-826179-71-1

5187 Meeting the Needs of Employees with Disabilities
Resources for Rehabilitation
22 Bonad Road
Ste 19a
Winchester, MA 01890-4330 781-368-9080
Fax: 781-368-9096
orders@rfr.org
www.rfr.org

Susan Greenblatt, Editor
Provides information to help people with disabilities retain or obtain employment. Information on government programs and laws, supported employment, training programs, environmental adaptations and the transition from school to work are included. Chapters on mobility impairment, vision impairment and hearing and speech impairments. *$ 47.95*
167 pages Biennial
ISBN 0-92971 -13-5

5188 NCD Bulletin
National Council on Disability
1331 F Street Northwest
Suite 850
Washington, DC 20004- 1138 202-272-2004
Fax: 202-272-2022
ncd@ncd.gov
www.ncd.gov

Jeff Rosen, Chairperson
Kamilah Oni Martin-Proctor, Co-Vice Chair
Lynnae Ruttledge, Co-Vice Chair
Rebecca Cokley, Executive Director
Reports on the latest issues and news affecting people with disabilities.
2 pages Monthly

5189 NCDE Survival Strategies for Oversease Living for People with Disabilities
National Clearinghouse on Disability and Exchange
132 E. Broadway, Suite 343
PO Box 10767
Eugene, OR 97401 541-343-1284
Fax: 541-343-6812
info@miusa.org
www.miusa.org

Susan Sygall, CEO
Cerise Roth-Vinson, COO
Cindy Lewis, Director of Programs
Stephanie Gray, Program Managers
This book will provide individuals with disabilities information, resources and guidance on pursuing international exchange opportunities. It addresses disability-related aspects of the international exchange process such as choosing a program, applying, preparing for the trip, adjusting to a new country and returning home.

5190 NOD E-Newsletter
National Organization on Disability
77 Water St.
Suite 204
New York, NY 10005 646-505-1191
Fax: 646-505-1184
www.nod.org

Carol Glazer, President
Lindsay Beltzer, Chief of Staff
Amber Cecil, Communications Manager
Howard Green, Deputy Director
Monthly E-Newsletter from the National Organization on Disability. The subscription to this newsletter is free.
3 pages Monthly

5191 National Hookup
ISC
16 Liberty St
Larkspur, CA 94939-1520 415-924-3549
Fax: 415-927-9556

Russ Bohlke, Manager
Newsletter published by ISC, a national organization of people with physical disabilities. *$6.00*
12-16 pages Quarterly

5192 New Horizons in Sexuality
Accent Books & Products
PO Box 700
Bloomington, IL 61702-700 309-378-2961
800-787-8444
Fax: 309-378-4420
acmtlvng@aol.com

Raymond C Cheever, Publisher
Betty Garee, Editor
This manual helps both males and females progress toward a satisfying post-injury relationship. *$7.95*
50 pages Paperback
ISBN 0-91570 -42-6

5193 New Voices: Self Advocacy By People with Disabilities
Brookline Books
8 Trumbull Rd
Suite B-001
Northampton, MA 01060 413-584-0184
800-666-2665
Fax: 413-584-6184
brbooks@yahoo.com
www.brooklinebooks.com

274 pages Paperback
ISBN 1-57129 -04-4

5194 North Star Community Services
3420 University Ave
Waterloo, IA 50701-2050 319-236-0901
888-879-1365
Fax: 319-236-3701
jmuller@northstarcs.org
www.northstarcs.org

Mark Witmer, Executive Director
Matt Hinders, Director of Operations & Safety
Bridget Hartmann, Director of Human Resources
Terri Davis, Director of Financial Services
North Star Community Services is a rehabilitative services organization with home office in Waterloo, IA and several branch offices in Northeast, Northern and Central Iowa. North Star helps indiviuals with disabilities live and work in their communities. Services include: adult day services, supported community living services, employment services, and case management/service coordination.

5195 Nothing is Impossible: Reflections on a New Life
Ballantine Books
1745 Broadway
10th Floor
New York, NY 10019 212-782-9000
rhkidspublicity@randomhouse.com
www.atrandom.com

Edward Warren, Owner
Reeve offers a uniquely powerful message of hope on topics ranging from the controversial stem cell debate to the mind-body connection he credits with his recent physical improvements. *$6.99*
224 pages
ISBN 0-345470-73-7

5196 Nutritional Desk Reference
Keats Publishing
P.O.Box 876
New Canaan, CT 06840 203-966-8721
800-323-4900

5197 Nutritional Influences on Illness:
Third Line Press
4751 Viviana Dr
Tarzana, CA 91356-5038 818-996-0076
third-line.com

Melvyn R Werbach, Owner
A comprehensive summary of the world's knowledge concerning the relationship between dietary and nutrtional factors and illness. This book does not try to promote any particular school of thought. Instead of the author telling readers his opinion as to what research says, he makes it easy for them to see data for themselves and then form their own opinions.
504 pages
ISBN 0-879835-31-1

5198 Oregon Perspectives
Oregon Council on Developmental Disabilities
540 24th Pl NE
Salem, OR 97301-4517 503-945-9941
800-292-4154
Fax: 503-945-9947
ocdd@ocdd.org
www.ocdd.org

Laura Bronson, Office Manager
Beth Kessler, Planning & Communications Coordi
A quarterly publication from the Oregon Council on Developmental Disabilities.

5199 Organ Transplants: Making the Most of Your Gift of Life
Patient-Centered Guides
1005 Gravenstein Highway North
Sebastopol, CA 95472-3836 707-827-7000
800-998-9938
Fax: 707-824-8268
orders@oreilly.com

Linda Lamb, Series Editor
Shawnde Paull, Marketing
Tim O'Reilly, CEO

Over 64,000 people in the US are awaiting an organ transplant. Although transplant surgeries are now fairly routine and can give their recipients the gift of new life, the road to getting a transplant can be long and harrowing. Living with immunosuppressive drugs and strong emotional responses can also be more challenging than families imagine. Medical journalist Robert Finn answers the concerns of these families, with the latest facts about transplantation - as well as the stories behind them. *$19.95*
326 pages Paperback
ISBN 1-565926-34-X

5200 PEAK Parent Center
611 N Weber St
Suite 200
Colorado Springs, CO 80903-1072   719-531-9400
                                          800-284-0251
                                     Fax: 719-531-9452
                                     info@peakparent.org
                                     www.peakparent.org

Barbara Buswell, Executive Director
PEAK Parent Center is a federally-designated Parent Training and Information Center (PTI). As a PTI, PEAK supports and empowers parents, providing them with information and strategies to use when advocating for their children with disabilities. PEAK works one-on-one with families and educators helping them realize new possibilities for children with disabilities by expanding knowledge of special education and offering new strategies for success.

5201 Parallels in Time
MN Governor's Council on Development Disabilities
658 Cedar St
Saint Paul, MN 55155-1603   651-296-4018
                                          877-348-0505
                                     Fax: 651-297-7200
                                     admin.dd@state.mn.us
                                     www.mncdd.org

Colleen Wieck PhD, Executive Director
Parallels in Time traces present attitudes and the treatment of people with disabilities, and supplements the first weekend session of Partners in Policymaking. This CD-ROM includes the History of the Parent Movement and the History of the Independent Living Movement, as well as personal stories of self advocates, leaders in the self advocacy movement.

5202 Part of the Team
Easter Seals
Ste 1800
230 W Monroe St
Chicago, IL 60606-4851   312-726-6800
                                     Fax: 312-726-1494

Janet D Jamieson, Communications Manager
James Williams Jr, Chief Executive Officer
Designed for employers of all sizes, rehabilitation organizations and all others concerned with the employment of people with disabilities. It addresses managers' concerns and questions about supervising persons with disabilities and can be used as a discussion/team-building tool for employees with and without disabilities. The video recognizes people with disabilities as strong contenders for almost any job. *$15.00*

5203 Partnering with Public Health: Funding& Advocacy Opportunities for CILs and SILCs
Independent Living Research Utilization ILRU
1333 Moursund
Houston, TX 77030-7031   713-520-0232
                                     Fax: 713-520-5785
                                     ilru@ilru.org
                                     ilru.org

Lex Frieden, Director, ILRU
Richard Petty, Program Director
Roxy Funchess, Administrative Secretary
George Powers, Legal Specialist
Laura Rauscher discusses how CILs and SCILs can use funding from the Centers for Disease Control and partnerships with public health agencies to provide innovative programs promoting the health of people with disabilities.
10 pages

5204 Peer Counseling: Roles, Functions, Boundaries
Independent Living Research Utilization ILRU
1333 Moursund
Houston, TX 77030-7031   713-520-0232
                                     Fax: 713-520-5785
                                     ilru@ilru.org
                                     ilru.org

Lex Frieden, Director, ILRU
Richard Petty, Program Director
Roxy Funchess, Administrative Secretary
George Powers, Legal Specialist
In this article, the following points were discussed: describing peer support as counseling suggests safeguards and expectations which cannot be provided by nonprofessionals; the purpose of peer counseling is to promote the independent living philosophy and encourage consumers to embrace it; peer counseling cannot and is not intended to help individuals deal with intense emotional stress, whether it is related to their disability or to something else.
10 pages

5205 Peer Mentor Volunteers: Empowering People for Change
Independent Living Research Utilization ILRU
1333 Moursund
Houston, TX 77030-7031   713-520-0232
                                     Fax: 713-520-5785
                                     ilru@ilru.org
                                     ilru.org

Lex Frieden, Director, ILRU
Richard Petty, Program Director
Roxy Funchess, Administrative Secretary
George Powers, Legal Specialist
Arizona Bridge to Independent Living (ABIL) in Phoenix, featured in this issue, is another winner in the innovative CIL program competition.
10 pages

5206 People and Families
New Jersey Council on Developmental Disabilities
20 West State Street, 6th Floor
P.O.Box 700
Trenton, NJ 08625-0700   609-292-3745
                                          800-792-8858
                                     Fax: 609-292-7114
                                     TTY: 609-777-3238
                                     njcdd@njcdd.org
                                     www.njcdd.org

Elaine Buchsbaum, Chairman
Christopher Miller, Vice Chair
Alison M. Lozano, Ph.D, Executive Director
Shirla Rufo Simpson, M.A., DRCC, Deputy Director
A free magazine for people with disabilities, their families and the public about disability topics such as personal assistance, deinstitutionalization, health care and community living. Published by the New Jersey council on Developmental Disabilities, a federally funded advocacy and policy advisory body. The council has 25 members - 15 consumer/product volunteers and 10 professionals.
48 pages Quarterly

5207 People with Disabilities & Abuse: Implications for Center for Independent Living
Independent Living Research Utilization ILRU
1333 Moursund
P.O.Box 700
Houston, TX 77030-7031   713-520-0232
                                     Fax: 713-520-5785
                                     ilru@ilru.org
                                     ilru.org

Lex Frieden, Director, ILRU
Richard Petty, Program Director
Roxy Funchess, Administrative Secretary
George Powers, Legal Specialist
10 pages

5208 People with Disabilities Who Challenge the System
Brookes Publishing
P.O.Box 10624
Baltimore, MD 21285-0624   410-337-9580
                                          800-638-3775
                                    Fax: 410-337-8539
                   custserv@brookespublishing.com
                                readplaylearn.com

Paul H. Brooks, Chairman
Jeffrey D. Brookes, President
Melissa A. Behm, Executive Vice President
Jeffrey D. Brookes, President
Helpful forms, tables, and case studies plus an emphasis on self-determination point the way to the development of supports so that people who are deaf-blind, have severe to profound physical and cognitive disabilities, or have serious behavior problems can be fully included in the classroom, workplace, and community. *$34.00*
464 pages Paperback
ISBN 1-55766 -29-0

5209 People's Voice
Independence CIL
300 3rd Ave SW
Suite F
Minot, ND 58701-4346   701-839-4724
                                          800-377-5114
                                    Fax: 701-838-1677
                   independencecil@independencecil.org
                                 independencecil.org

Susan Ogurek, Chair
Heather Wittliff, Vice Chair
Scott Burlingame, Executive Director
Emily Rodacker, Secretary/Treasurer
8 pages Quarterly

5210 Personal Perspectives on Personal Assistance Services
World Institute on Disability
3075 Adeline Street
Suite 155
Berkeley, CA 94703   510-225-6400
                                    Fax: 510-225-0477
                                    TTY:510-225-0478
                                        wid@wid.org
                                        www.wid.org

Anita Shafer Aaron, Executive Director
Thomas Foley, Deputy Director
Bruce Curtis, International Program Director
Marsha Saxton, Director of Research and Training.
This collection of personal essays explores a wide range of perspectives on Personal Assistance Services. Family issues and PAS concerns for people with various different disabilities, of different ages and as members of minority groups are addressed. *$5.00*
80 pages Paperback

5211 Perspectives
National Assoc of State Directors of DD Services
113 Oronoco St
Alexandria, VA 22314-2015   703-683-4202
                                    Fax: 703-684-1395
                                    dberland@nasddds.org

Nancy Thaler, Executive Director
Nancy Thaler, Executive Director
Provides a concise summary of national policy developments and initiatives affecting persons with devlopmental disabilities and the programs that serve them. From bills pending before Congress, to the growth in Medicaid-funded services, to changes in federal-state Medicaid policies and the shift of responsibility from Washington to the states, keeps readers in tune with the latest national issues shaping publically funded disability services. *$95.00*
Monthly

5212 Place to Live
Accent Books & Products
P.O.Box 700
Bloomington, IL 61702-700   309-378-2961
                                          800-787-8444
                                    Fax: 309-378-4420
                                     acmtlvng@aol.com

Raymond C Cheever, Publisher
Betty Garee, Editor
Raymond C Cheever, Publisher
Many disabled people have found that group housing or accessible apartments are the best alternative to living in a nursing home. These articles tell about some of the alternatives people have found so they can live independently. Just one idea might be the answer for better living for you. *$4.95*
64 pages Paperback
ISBN 0-91570 -30-2

5213 Psychological & Social Impact of Disability
Springer Publishing Company
11 West 42nd Street
15th Floor
New York, NY 10036   212-431-4370
                                          877-687-7476
                                    Fax: 212-941-7842
                                   cs@springerpub.com
                                  www.springerpub.com

James C. Costello, Vice President, Journal Publishing
Diana Osborne, Production Manager
Megan Larkin, Managing Editor, Journals
$49.95
488 pages
ISBN 0-826122-13-2

5214 Psychology and Health
Springer Publishing Company
11 West 42nd Street
15th Floor
New York, NY 10036   212-431-4370
                                          877-687-7476
                                    Fax: 212-941-7842
                                   cs@springerpub.com
                                  www.springerpub.com

James C. Costello, Vice President, Journal Publishing
Diana Osborne, Production Manager
Megan Larkin, Managing Editor, Journals
Content of this book spans a wide range of clinical conditions, including somatization disorders, chronic pain, migraine, anxiety and cancer. *$29.95*
256 pages

5215 Psychology of Disability
Springer Publishing Company
11 West 42nd Street,
15th Floor
New York, NY 10036-3915   212-431-4370
                                          877-687-7476
                                    Fax: 212-941-7842
                                   cs@springerpub.com
                                  www.springerpub.com

James C. Costello, Vice President, Journal Publishing
Diana Osborne, Production Manager
Megan Larkin, Managing Editor, Journals
Theodore C Nardin, Chief Executive Officer
Reactions to the disabled. *$27.95*
288 pages
ISBN 0-82613 -40-1

5216   Quality of Life for Persons with Disabilities
Brookline Books
8 Trumbull Road
Suite B-001
Northampton, MA   01060   413-584-0184
                                           800-666-2665
                                      Fax: 413-584-6184
                                      brbooks@yahoo.com
                                      www.brooklinebooks.com
James C. Costello, Vice President, Journal Publishing
Quality of life generally refers to a person's subjective experience of his or her life and focuses attention on how the individual with a disabling condition experiences the world. This book presents a comprehensive and international view of this concept as applied to a broad range of settings in which persons with disabilities live, work and play. *$35.00*
Paperback
ISBN 0-91479 -92-1

5217   REACHing Out Newsletter
REACH of Dallas Resource on Independent Living
8625 King George Drive
Suite 210
Dallas, TX   75235-2286   214-630-4796
                                      Fax: 214-630-6390
                                      TTY:214-630-5995
                                      reachdallas@reachcils.org
                                           reachcils.org
Charlotte A. Stewart, Executive Director
Kiowanda Jasso, Information & Referral Specialist
Kevan Johnson, Employment Consultant
Janie Peachee, Administrative Assistant
Quarterly newsletter from REACH of Dallas Resource Center on Independent Living.
16 pages Quarterly

5218   RTC Connection
Research and Training Center
University of Wisconsin Stou
Menomonie, WI   54751   715-232-2236
                                      Fax: 715-232-2251
                                      menz@uwstout.edu
Julie Larson, Program Assistant
Bi-annual reports on disability and rehabilitation research and policy topics.
Newsletter

5219   Rehabilitation Gazette
Gazette International Networking Institute
4207 Lindell Blvd
Suite 110
Saint Louis, MO   63108-2930   314-534-0475
                                      Fax: 314-534-5070
                                      info@post-polio.org
                                      www.post-polio.org
Joan L Headley, Executive Director
William G. Stothers, President/Chairperson
Saul J. Morse, Vice President
Marny K. Eulberg, Secretary
International journal of independent living for people with disabilities. *$12.00*
8 pages Bi-Annually

5220   Relaxation: A Comprehensive Manual for Adults and Children with Special Needs
Research Press
2612 N. Mattis Ave.
P.O.Box 7886
Champaign, IL   61822- 9177   217-352-3273
                                           800-519-2707
                                      Fax: 217-352-1221
                                      orders@researchpress.com
                                      www.researchpress.com

Paperback
ISBN 0-878221-86-8

5221   Resources for People with Disabilities and Chronic Conditions
Resources for Rehabilitation
Ste 19a
33 Bedford St
Lexington, MA   02420-4330   781-890-6371
                                      Fax: 781-861-7517
Susan Greenblatt
A comprehensive resource directory that helps people with disabilities and chronic conditions achieve their maximum level of independence. Chapters on spinal cord injuries, low back pain, diabetes, hearing and speech impairments, epilepsy, multiple sclerosis. Describes organizations, products and publications. *$49.95*
215 pages Biennial
ISBN 0-92971 -12-7

5222   Role Portrayal and Stereotyping on Television
Greenwood Publishing Group
130 Cremona Drive
P O Box 1911
Santa Barbara,, CA 93117-4208   203-226-3571
                                           800-368-6868
                                           805-968-1911
                                      Fax: 866-270-3856
                                      customerservice@abc-clio.com
                                      www.abc-clio.com

214 pages $55 - $59.95
ISBN 0-313248-55-9

5223   Screening in Chronic Disease
Oxford University Press
2001 Evans Rd
Cary, NC   27513-2009   800-445-9714
                                           877-773-4325
                                      Fax: 919-677-1303
                                      custserv.us@oup.com
                                      global.oup.com
Thomas Carty, Senior Vice President
Early detection, or screening, is a common strategy for controlling chronic disease, but little information has been available to help determine which screening procedures are worthwhile, until this textbook. *$42.50*
256 pages

5224   Sexual Adjustment
Accent Books & Products
P.O.Box 700
Bloomington, IL   61702-700   309-378-2961
                                           800-787-8444
                                      Fax: 309-378-4420
                                      acmtlvng@aol.com
Raymond C Cheever, Publisher
Betty Garee, Editor
Essential information concerning sexual adjustment for the paraplegic male. *$4.95*
73 pages Paperback
ISBN 0-19570 -00-0

5225   Sexuality and Disabilities: A Guide for Human Service Practitioners
Haworth Press
2&4 Park Square
Abingdon, FL   33487-1503   561-994-0555
                                      Fax: 561-241-7856
                                      orders@taylorandfrancis.com
                                      taylorandfrancisgroup.com

159 pages Hardcover
ISBN 1-560243-75-9

5226 Sickened: The Memoir of a Muchausen by Proxy Childhood
Bantam Books
1745 Broadway
10th Floor
New York, NY 10019-4039   212-782-9000
Fax: 212-572-6066
crownpublicity@randomhouse.com
www.randomhouse.com
256 pages Hardcover
ISBN 0-553803-07-7

5227 Socialization Games for Persons with Disabilities
Charles C. Thomas
2600 S First St
Springfield, IL 62704-4730   217-789-8980
800-258-8980
Fax: 217-789-9130
books@ccthomas.com
www.ccthomas.com
Michael P. Thomas, President
This text will assist those who want to teach severely multiple disabled students by providing information on: general principles of intervention and classroom organization; managing the behavior of students; physically managing students and using adaptive equipment; teaching eating skills; teaching toileting, dressing, and hygiene skills; teaching cognition, communication, and socialization skills; teaching independent living skills; and teaching infants and preschool students. *$38.95*
176 pages Paperback
ISBN 0-398067-46-5

5228 Sometimes You Just Want to Feel Like a Human Being
Brookes Publishing
P.O.Box 10624
Baltimore, MD 21285-0624   410-337-9580
800-638-3775
Fax: 410-337-8539
custserv@brookespublishing.com
readplaylearn.com
Paul Brooks, Owner
Case studies of empowering psychotherapy with people with disabilities. This text reveals how counseling can be beneficial to individuals with disabilities of all kinds, including autism, mental retardation, sensory impairment, cerebral palsy, or HIV infection. *$ 26.95*
272 pages Paperback
ISBN 1-55766-96-0

5229 South Carolina Assistive Technology Program
8301 Farrow Road
University Center for Excellence
Columbia, SC 29203-2920   803-935-5263
800-915-4522
Fax: 803-935-5342
carol.page@uscmed.sc.edu
www.sc.edu/scatp/
Carol Page, Ph.D, Program Director
Mary r Alice Bechtle, Program Coordinator
Janet Jendron, Program Coordinator
Lydia Durham, Administrative Assistant
The South Carolina Assistive Technology Program (SCATP) is a federally funded program concerned with getting technology into the hands of people with disabilities so that they might live, work, learn and be a more independent part of the community.We provide an equipment loan and demonstration program, an on-line equipment exchange program, training, technical assistance, publications, an interactive CDROM (SC Curriculum Access through AT), an information listserv and work with various state com
7-8 pages Bi-annually

5230 Space Coast CIL News
Space Coast Center for Independent Living
571 Haverty Court,
Suite W
Rockledge, FL 32955-2566   321-633-6011
Fax: 321-633-6472
TTY:321-784-9008
agrau@bellsouth.net
www.sccil.net
Michael Lavoie, President
Howard Fetes, Vice-President
Non-profit organization that provides services which enable people with disabilities to live as independently as possible.
12 pages Quarterly

5231 Special Needs Trust Handbook
Aspen Publishers
7th Fl
76 9th Ave
New York, NY 10011-4962   301-644-3599
800-638-8437
customerservice@aspenpublishers.com
www.aspenpublishers.com
Bob Lemmond, President and CEO
Gustavo Dobles, Vice President and Chief Content Officer
Susan Pikitch, Vice President and Chief Financial Officer
Alan Scott, Vice President & Chief Marketing Office
The Special Needs Trusts Handbook is the single-volume, comprehensive resource that provides information on how to handle the complex requirements of drafting and administering trusts for clients who are mentally or physically disabled, or who wish to provide for others with disabilities. *$245.00*
900 pages
ISBN 0-735572-88-7

5232 Special Siblings: Growing Up With Someone with A Disability
Brookes Publishing
P.O.Box 10624
Baltimore, MD 21285-0624   410-337-9580
800-638-3775
Fax: 410-337-8539
custserv@brookespublishing.com
readplaylearn.com
Paul Brooks, Owner
The author reveals what she experienced as the sister of a man with cerebral palsy and mental retardation — and shares what others have learned about being and having a special sibling. Weaving a lifetime of memories and reflections with relevant research and interviews with more than 100 other siblings and experts, McHugh explores a spectrum of feelings — from anger and guilt to love and pride — and helps readers understand the issues siblings may encounter. *$21.95*
256 pages Paperback
ISBN 1-557666-07-5

5233 TERI
251 Airport Rd
Oceanside, CA 92058-1321   760-721-1706
teriinc.org
Cheryl Kilmer, CEO & Founder
William E. Mara, Chief Operating Officer
Krysti DeZonia, Ed.D, Director of Education & Research
Joe Michalowski, Chief Financial Officer
A private, nonprofit corporation which has been developing and operating programs for individuals with developmental disabilities since 1980. Offers staff training videos, staff training tools and technique manuals.

5234 That All May Worship: An Interfaith Welcome to People with Disabilities
American Association of People with Disabilities
2013 H St NW
5th Fl
Washington, DC 20006-1207
202-521-4316
800-840-8844
communications@aapd.com
www.aapd.com/publications

5235 The Ultimate Guide to Sex and Disability
Read How You Want Large Print Books
800-797-9277
support@readhowyouwant.com
www.readhowyouwant.com

Miriam Kaufman, Author
For everyone, men and women of all ages and sexual identities, The Ultimate Guide to Sex and Disability covers the span of disabilities - from chronic fatigue and back pain to spinal cord injury, multiple sclerosis, cystic fibrosis, cerebral palsy, and many others.

5236 To Live with Grace and Dignity
World Institute on Disability
3075 Adeline Street
Suite 155
Berkeley, CA 94703-1520
510-225-6400
Fax: 510-225-0477
TTY:510-225-0478
wid@wid.org
www.wid.org

Anita Shafer Aaron, Executive Director
Thomas Foley, Deputy Director
Bruce Curtis, International Program Director
Marsha Saxton, Director of Research and Training.
This unique book combines photographs and essays to allow the reader to enter some of the real day to day relationships that develop between individuals with disabilities and their personal assistants. Looking at and listening to what these relationships are all about is what motivated and inspired this book, says author Lydia Gans. The individuals included in this book represent a wide range of ages, disabilities and cultural backgrounds. *$26.00*
72 pages Paperback

5237 Touch/Ability Connects People with Disabilities & Alternative Health Care Pract.
Independent Living Research Utilization ILRU
1333 Moursund
Houston, TX 77030-7031
713-520-0232
Fax: 713-520-5785
ilru@ilru.org
ilru.org

Lex Frieden, Director, ILRU
Richard Petty, Program Director
Roxy Funchess, Administrative Secretary
George Powers, Legal Specialist
The people at DIRECT center for Independence and Touch/Ability in Tuscon, Arizona, have collaborated to develop a wellness program that makes alternative health care choices available to people with disabilities. The Touch/Ability Wellness program was selected as one of last year's winners in the Innovative CILs competition because of this outcome of increased options open to people with disabilities.
10 pages

5238 US Role in International Disability Activities: A History
World Institute on Disability
3075 Adeline Street
Suite 155
Berkeley, CA 94703-1520
510-225-6400
Fax: 510-225-0477
TTY:510-225-0478
wid@wid.org
www.wid.org

Anita Shafer Aaron, Executive Director
Thomas Foley, Deputy Director
Bruce Curtis, International Program Director
Marsha Saxton, Director of Research and Training.
This study was undertaken to present an initial introduction to US involvement in the field of international rehabilitation and disability. *$12.00*
169 pages Paperback

5239 Understanding and Accommodating Physical Disabilities: Desk Reference
Greenwood Publishing Group
130 Cremona Drive
P O Box 1911
Santa Barbara,, CA 93117-4208
203-226-3571
800-368-6868
805-968-1911
Fax: 866-270-3856
customerservice@abc-clio.com
www.abc-clio.com

200 pages $52.95 - $55
ISBN 0-899308-14-7

5240 Vestibular Disorders Association
Vestibular Disorders Association
5018 NE 15th Ave
PO Box 13305
Portland, OR 97211-305
503-229-7705
800-837-8428
Fax: 503-229-8064
info@vestibular.org
www.vestibular.org

Cynthia Ryan MBA, Executive Director
Tony Staser, Development Director
Kerrie Denner, Outreach Coordinator
Karen Ilari, Administrative Support Coordinator
The mission of the Vestibular Disorders Association is to serve people with vestibular disorders by providing access to information, offering a support network, and elevating awareness of the challenges associated with these disorders. *$15.00*
ISBN 0-963261-15-0

5241 Visions & Values
Idaho Council on Developmental Disabilities
650 W. State St., Room 100
P. O. Box 83720
Boise, ID 83720-5840
208-332-1824
800-544-2433
Fax: 208-334-2307
www.state.id.us/icdd

C. L. Butch Otter, Governor
A quarterly publication from the Idaho Council on Developmental Disabilities.

5242 Weiner's Herbal
Quantum Books
355 Middlesex Avenue
Wilmington, MA 01887-1406
978-988-2470
Fax: 617-577-7282
www.quantumbooks.com

William Szabo, Owner
A-Z index covering all aspects of herbs.
Paperback
ISBN 0-812825-86-1

5243 **When the Brain Goes Wrong**
Fanlight Productions
32 Court Street,
21st Floor
Brooklyn, NY 11201-1731   718-488-8900
                                 800-876-1710
                            Fax: 718-488-8642
                            info@fanlight.com
                            www.fanlight.com

Ben Achtenberg, Owner
Nicole Johnson, Publicity Coordinator
Anthony Sweeney, Marketing Director
An extraordinary and provocative series of seven short films
which profile individuals with a range of brian dysfunctions. The
seven brief segments focus on schizophrenia, manic depression,
epilepsy, head injury, headaches and addiction. In addition to the
personal stories, the segments include interviews with physicians
who speak briefly about what is known about the disorders and
treatment. #131 *$245.00*
ISBN 1-572951-31-1

5244 **Women with Physical Disabilities: Achieving & Maintaining
Health & Well-Being**
Spina Bifida Association of America
1600 Wilson Blvd.
Suite 800
Arlington, VA 22209-4226   202-944-3285
                                 800-621-3141
                            Fax: 202-944-3295
                            sbaa@sbaa.org
                            www.spinabifidaassociation.org
Ana Ximenes, Chair
Sara Struwe, President & CEO
Cindy Brownstein, CEO
George Sturm, Treasurer
Introduces the critical concept of womens health in the context of
physical disabilities. *$42.00*

5245 **Work in the Context of Disability Culture**
Independent Living Research Utilization ILRU
1333 Moursund
Houston, TX 77030-7031   713-520-0232
                            Fax: 713-520-5785
                            ilru@ilru.org
                            ilru.org
Lex Frieden, Director, ILRU
Richard Petty, Program Director
Roxy Funchess, Administrative Secretary
George Powers, Legal Specialist
Another winner in the innovative CIL competition-Steve Brown
describes the Talking Books Program of Southeast Alaska Inde-
pendent Living, discussing their efforts to record the oral history
and life experiences of people with disabilities in the larger context of the disability culture.
10 pages

Parenting: General

5246 **AEPS Family Report: Birth to Three Years**
Brookes Publishing
P.O. Box 10624
Baltimore, MD 21285-0624   410-337-9580
                                 800-638-3775
                            Fax: 410-337-8539
                            custserv@brookespublishing.com
                            www.brookespublishing.com

Diane Bricker, Author
Betty Capt, Author
JoAnn Johnson, Author
Misti Waddell, Author
This Family Report was developed for use in conjunction with the
AEPSr for children birth to 3 years to obtain information from
parents and other caregivers about their children's skills and abil-
ities across major areas of development. Available in packages of
10.
28 pages Saddle-stiched

5247 **AEPS Family Report: For Children Ages Three to Six**
Brookes Publishing
P.O.Box 10624
Baltimore, MD 21285-0624   410-337-9580
                                 800-638-3775
                            Fax: 410-337-8539
                            custserv@brookespublishing.com
                            www.brookespublishing.com
Diane Bricker, Author
Betty Capt, Author
JoAnn Johnson, Author
Elizabeth Straka, Author
This is a 64-item questionnaire that asks parents to rank their
child's abilities on specific skills. In packages of 10 paperback.
28 pages Saddle-stiched

5248 **Adapted Physical Activity**
Human Kinetics
1607 N Market St
P.O.Box 5076
Champaign, IL 61820-5076   800-747-4457
                            Fax: 217-351-1549
                            info@hkusa.com
                            www.humankinetics.com

5249 **Assistive Technology for Parents with Disabilities Handbook**
Idaho Assistive Technology Project
University of Idaho
1187 Alturas Dr.
Moscow, ID 83843- 2268   208-885-3557
                                 800-432-8324
                            Fax: 208-885-6102
                            idahoat@uidaho.edu
                            www.idahoat.org

5250 **Babyface: A Story of Heart and Bones**
Penguin Books USA
375 Hudson St
New York, NY 10014   212-366-2000
                  consumerservices@penguinrandomhouse.com
                            www.penguin.com
Jeanne McDermott, Author
A must read for families that seek insight into coping with a
chronic condition. Many useful resources provided.
288 pages Paperback

5251 **Backyards and Butterflies: Ways to Include Children with
Disabilities in Outdoor Activities**
Brookline Books
8 Trumbull Rd
Ste B-001
Northampton, MA 01060   413-584-0184
                                 800-666-2665
                            Fax: 413-584-6184
                            brbooks@yahoo.com
                            www.brooklinebks.com
Doreen Greenstein, Author
Suzanne Bloom, Author
An illustrated book with dozens of imaginative ways parents can
include children with physical disabilities in outdoor activities.
Offers clear concise, how-to directions for constructing home-
made toys, utensils, and other items that can be enjoyed outside
safely and comfortably.
72 pages Paperback

5252 **Beyond Tears: Living After Losing a Child**
St. Martin's Griffin (Macmillan Publishers)
75 Varick St
New York, NY 10013   212-226-7521
                            press.inquiries@macmillan.com
                            us.macmillan.com/smp
Ellen Mitchell, Author
Meant to comfort and give direction to bereaved parents, Beyond
Tears is written by nine mothers who have each lost a child. This
revised edition includes a new chapter written from the perspec-
tive of surviving siblings. The death of a child is that unimagin-
able loss no parent ever expects to face. In this book, nine mothers

share their individual stories of how to survive in the darkest hour.

5253 Broken Dolls: Gathering the Pieces: Caringfor Chronically Ill Children
St. Paul Press
Jennifer Travis Cox, Author
Told from the point of view of the author, this book tracks the challenges faced by parents and caregivers of chronically ill children - both in terms of medical care and emotional impact. It offers advice based on the author's own experiences caring for her child, as well as insights from other families who have gone through the same experience.
164 pages Paperback

5254 Building the Healing Partnership: Parents, Professionals and Children
Brookline Books
8 Trumbull Road
Suite B-001
Northampton, MA 01060
413-584-0184
800-666-2665
Fax: 413-584-6184
brbooks@yahoo.com
www.brooklinebooks.com
Paperback
ISBN 0-91479-63-8

5255 Children with Disabilities
Brookes Publishing
P.O.Box 10624
Baltimore, MD 21285-0624
410-337-9580
800-638-3775
Fax: 410-337-8539
custserv@brookespublishing.com
www.brookespublishing.com
Mark L Batshaw MD, Editor
Paul Brooks, Owner
Lauren Rohe, Regional Sales Consultant
Cary Gold, Educational Sales Representative
Extensive coverage of genetics, heredity, pre- and postnatal development, specific disabilities, family roles, and intervention. Features chapters on substance abuse, HIV and AIDS, Down syndrome, fragile X syndrome, behavior management, transitions to adulthood, and health care in the 21st century. Also reveals the causes of many conditions that can lead to developmental disabilities. *$69.95*
912 pages Hardcover
ISBN 1-557665-81-8

5256 Conditional Love: Parents' Attitudes Toward Handicapped Children
Greenwood Publishing Group
130 Cremona Drive
P O Box 1911
Santa Barbara,, CA 93117-4208
203-226-3571
800-368-6868
805-968-1911
Fax: 866-270-3856
customerservice@abc-clio.com
www.abc-clio.com
312 pages
ISBN 0-89789-24-7

5257 Coordinacion De Servicios Centrado En La Familia
Brookline Books
8 Trumbull Road
Suite B-001
Northampton, MA 01060
413-584-0184
800-666-2665
Fax: 413-584-6184
brbooks@yahoo.com
www.brooklinebooks.com
34 pages Paperback
ISBN 0-91479-90-5

5258 Developing Personal Safety Skills in Children with Disabilities
Brookes Publishing
P.O.Box 10624
Baltimore, MD 21285-0624
410-337-9580
800-638-3775
Fax: 410-337-8539
custserv@brookespublishing.com
readplaylearn.com
Paul Brooks, Owner
A guide for teachers, parents, and caregivers, this volume explores the issue of personal safety for children with disabilities and offers strategies for empowering and protecting them at home and in school. Recognizing that children with disabilities are vulnerable to abuse, this work explores why children with disabilities need personal safety skills, offers, curriculum ideas and exercises, and advocates the development of self-esteem and assertiveness so that children can protect themselves. *$34.00*
220 pages Paperback
ISBN 1-557661-84-7

5259 Developmental Disabilities in Infancy and Childhood
Brookes Publishing
P.O.Box 10624
Baltimore, MD 21285-0624
410-767-6100
800-638-3775
Fax: 410-767-5850
custserv@brookespublishing.com
readplaylearn.com
Paul Brooks, Owner
This two volume set explores advances in assessment and treatment, retains a clinical focus, and incorporates recent developments in research and theory. Can be purchased individually or as a set (Vol. 1: Neurodevelopmental Diagnosis and Treatment Vol. 2: The Spectrum of Developmental Disabilities). *$210.00*
Hardcover
ISBN 1-55766O-CA-P

5260 Dictionary of Developmental Disabilities Terminology
Brookes Publishing
P.O.Box 10624
Baltimore, MD 21285-0624
410-337-9580
800-638-3775
Fax: 410-337-8539
custserv@brookespublishing.com
readplaylearn.com
Paul Brooks, Owner
Answers thousands of questions for medical or human services professionals, parents or advocates of children with disabilities, or students preparing for their careers. Provides thorough explanations of the most common terms associated with disabilities. *$55.95*
368 pages Hardcover
ISBN 1-557662-45-2

5261 Encyclopedia of Genetic Disorders & Birth Defects
Facts on File
132 W 31st St
17th Floor
New York, NY 10001-3406
800-322-8755
Fax: 800-678-3633
custserv@factsonfile.com
www.infobasepublishing.com/
Mark Donnell, President
Layperson-accessible entries on genetic terminology and genetically-influenced conditions. *$71.50*
474 pages
ISBN 0-816038-09-0

5262 Exceptional Parent Magazine
Psy-Ed Corporation
416 Main Street
Johnstown, PA   15901-2032   814-361-3860
                                          877-372-7368
                                    Fax: 814-361-3861
                                    www.eparent.com

Vanessa B Ira, Contributing Writer / Editor
Joseph M. Valenzano, Jr., President, CEO & Publisher
Rick Rader, MD, Editor-in-Chief
Lois Keegan, Human Resources Manager
Magazine that provides information, support, ideas, encouragement, and outreach for parents and families of children with disabilities and the professionals who work with them. *$39.95*
85 pages Monthly

5263 Face of Inclusion
Special Needs Project
Ste H
324 State St
Santa Barbara, CA   93101-2364   805-962-8087
                                          800-333-6867
                                    Fax: 805-962-5087
                                    eplibrary@aol.com
                                    www.eplibrary.com

Hod Gray, Owner
A unique and moving parents' perspective of inclusion for administrators, teachers, and parents of children with disabilities. *$99.00*

5264 Families Magazine
New Jersey Developmental Disabilities Council
20 West State Street, 6th Floor
P.O.Box 700
Trenton, NJ 08625-0700   609-292-3745
                                          800-792-8858
                                    Fax: 609-292-7114
                                    TTY: 609-777-3238
                                    njcdd@njcdd.org
                                    www.njddc.org

Elaine Buchsbaum, Chairman
Christopher Miller, Vice Chair
Alison M. Lozano, Ph.D, Executive Director
Shirla Rufo Simpson, M.A., DRCC, Deputy Director
Quarterly magazine for people with disabilities, their families and the public, features family profiles, news, columns and the New Jersey Family support councils newsletter.
Quarterly

5265 Families, Illness & Disability
Through the Looking Glass
3075 Adeline St
Ste. 120
Berkeley, CA   94703-2212   510-848-1112
                                          800-644-2666
                                    Fax: 510-848-4445
                                    TTY: 510-848-1005
                                    tlg@lookingglass.org
                                    www.lookingglass.org

Maureen Block, J.D., Co-Founder
Karen Fessel, Ph.D., Executive Director
$35.00
320 pages

5266 Family Interventions Throughout Disability
Springer Publishing Company
11 West 42nd Street,
15th Floor
New York, NY   10036-3915   212-431-4370
                                          877-687-7476
                                    Fax: 212-941-7842
                                    cs@springerpub.com
                                    www.springerpub.com

Theodore C Nardin, Chief Executive Officer
James C. Costello, Vice President, Journal Publishing
Diana Osborne, Production Manager
Megan Larkin, Managing Editor, Journals

Family attitudes throughout chronic illness and disability.
$31.95
320 pages
ISBN 0-82615 -80-4

5267 Family-Centered Service Coordination: A Manual for Parents
Brookline Books
8 Trumbull Road
Suite B-001
Northampton, MA   01060   413-584-0184
                                          800-666-2665
                                    Fax: 413-584-6184
                                    brbooks@yahoo.com
                                    www.brooklinebooks.com

34 pages Paperback
ISBN 0-91479 -90-5

5268 Handbook About Care in the Home
AARP Fulfillment
601 E St NW
Washington, DC   20049-1   202-434-2277
                                          888-687-2277
                                    TTY:877-434-7598
                                    member@aarp.org
                                    www.aarp.org

24 pages

5269 LifeLines
Disabled & Alone/Life Services for the Handicapped
1440 Broadway,
23rd Floor
New York, NY   10006-2734   212-532-6740
                                          800-995-0066
                                    Fax: 212-532-6740
                                    info@disabledandalone.org
                                    www.disabledandalone.org

Leslie D. Park, Chairman
Rex L Davidson, Vice President
Disabled and Alone is a national, nonprofit organization whose sole purpose is to assure the well being of disabled individuals, particularly those whose families have died and have engaged Disabled and Alone to provide advocacy and oversight for the lifetime of their disabled children. This newsletter provides information about 'future planning' for a person with a disability.
8-16 pages Bi-annual

5270 Living with a Brother or Sister with Special Needs: A Book for Sibs
Sibling Support Project
6512 23rd Ave NW
Ste 322
Seattle, WA   98117   206-297-6368
                                    info@siblingsupport.org
                                    www.siblingsupport.org

Don Meyer, Author
Patricia Vadasy, Author
Living with a Brother or Sister with Special Needs focuses on the intensity of emotions that brothers and sisters experience when they have a sibling with special needs, and the hard questions they ask. It talks about the good and not-so-good parts of having a brother or sister who has special needs, and offers suggestions for how to make life easier for everyone in the family.
144 pages Paperback

5271 Loving & Letting Go
Centering Corporation
7230 Maple Street
Omaha, NE   68134-5064   402-553-1200
                                          866-218-0101
                                    Fax: 402-533-0507
                                    j1200@aol.com
                                    www.centering.org

Joy Johnson, Founder
Dr. Marvin Johnson, co-Founder

For parents who decide to turn away from aggressive medical intervention for their critically ill newborn. *$5.95*
48 pages Paperback

5272 Mobility Training for People with Disabilities
Charles C. Thomas
2600 S First St
Springfield, IL 62704-4730
217-789-8980
800-258-8980
Fax: 217-789-9130
books@ccthomas.com
www.ccthomas.com

Michael P. Thomas, President

5273 Mother to Be
Through the Looking Glass
3075 Adeline St
Ste. 120
Berkeley, CA 94703-2212
510-848-1112
800-644-2666
Fax: 510-848-4445
TTY: 510-848-1005
tlg@lookingglass.org
www.lookingglass.org

Maureen Block, J.D., Co-Founder
Karen Fessel, Ph.D., Executive Director
Guide to pregnancy and birth for women with disabilities. *$34.00*
410 pages

5274 New Language of Toys: Teaching Communication Skills to Children with Special Needs
Spina Bifida Association of America
1600 Wilson Blvd.
Suite 800
Arlington, VA 22209-4226
202-944-3285
800-621-3141
Fax: 202-944-3295
sbaa@sbaa.org
www.spinabifidaassociation.org

Ana Ximenes, Chair
Sara Struwe, President & CEO
Cindy Brownstein, CEO
George Sturm, Treasurer
A guide for parents and teachers and a reader-friendly resource guide that provides a wealth of information on how play activities affect a child's language development and where to get the toys and materials to use in these activities. *$19.00*

5275 NewsLine
Federation for Children with Special Needs
45 Bromfield Street
10th Floor
Boston, MA 02108
866-815-8122
Fax: 617-542-7832
info@ppal.net
www.ppal.net

Lisa Lambert, Executive Director
Deborah A. Fauntleroy, MSW, Associate Director
Offers information for parents and families on resources, medical updates, activities, fund-raising events and association news for their disabled children.
Quarterly

5276 On the Road to Autonomy: Promoting Self- Competence in Children & Youth with Disabilities
Brookes Publishing
P.O.Box 10624
Baltimore, MD 21285-0624
410-337-9580
800-638-3775
Fax: 410-337-8539
custserv@brookespublishing.com
readplaylearn.com

Paul Brooks, Owner
This book provides detailed conceptual, practical, and personal information regarding the promotion of self-esteem, self-deter-

mination, and coping skills among children and youth with and without disabilities. *$48.00*
432 pages Paperback
ISBN 1-55766 -35-5

5277 Pain Erasure
M Evans and Company
216 E 49th St
New York, NY 10017-1546
212-979-0880
Fax: 212-486-4544

Mary Evans, Owner
This book explains Bonnie Prudden's method for pain relief using myotherapy, a method hailed by doctors and patients.
ISBN 0-345331-02-8

5278 Parent Centers and Independent Living Centers: Collectively We're Stronger
Independent Living Research Utilization ILRU
1333 Moursund
Houston, TX 77030-7031
713-520-0232
Fax: 713-520-5785
ilru@ilru.org
ilru.org

Lex Frieden, Director, ILRU
Richard Petty, Program Director
Roxy Funchess, Administrative Secretary
George Powers, Legal Specialist
This article describes several examples of effective working relationships of PTIs and CILs. The examples highlight how parent and consumer organizations have identified complimentary strengths and formed partnerships to better support children with disabilities and their families. These partnerships can also be a very important way of involving youth in the disability movement so they may become leaders of tomorrow.
10 pages

5279 Parent-Child Interaction and Developmental Disabilities
Greenwood Publishing Group
130 Cremona Drive
P O Box 1911
Santa Barbara,, CA 93117
800-368-6868
805-968-1911
Fax: 866-270-3856
customerservice@abc-clio.com
www.abc-clio.com

395 pages Hardcover
ISBN 0-275928-35-7

5280 Parenting
Accent Books & Products
P.O.Box 700
Bloomington, IL 61702-700
309-378-2961
800-787-8444
Fax: 309-378-4420
acmtlvng@aol.com

Raymond C Cheever, Publisher
Betty Garee, Editor
Experienced parents (who are disabled) discuss: raising children from infant to teens, balancing career and motherhood, discipline methods and more when both parents are disabled. *$7.95*
83 pages
ISBN 0-91570 -26-4

5281 Parenting with a Disability
Through the Looking Glass
3075 Adeline St
Ste. 120
Berkeley, CA 94703-2212
510-848-1112
800-644-2666
Fax: 510-848-4445
TTY: 510-848-1005
tlg@lookingglass.org
www.lookingglass.org

Maureen Block, J.D., Board President
Rusty Hendlin, M.A., LMFT, Director of Medi-Cal Services
Thomas Spalding, Board Treasurer
Alice Nemon, D.S.W., Board Secretary

International newsletter. Available in braille, large print or cassette.
3 per year

5282 Perspectives on a Parent Movement
Brookline Books
8 Trumbull Rd
Suite B-001
Northampton, MA 1060-4533

413-584-0184
800-666-2665
Fax: 413-584-6184
brbooks@yahoo.com
www.brooklinebooks.com

Paperback
ISBN 0-91479 -74-3

5283 Sexuality and the Developmentally Handicapped
Edwin Mellen Press
P.O.Box 450
Lewiston, NY 14092-450

716-754-2266
Fax: 716-754-4056
jrupnow@mellenpress.com
mellenpress.com

Herbert Richardson, Owner
Presents the knowledge, attitudes, and skills pertinent to responding to the sexual problems of developmentally handicapped persons, their families and communities. Details fully documented cases, issues concerning the law, and resource materials available. *$89.95*
245 pages Hardcover
ISBN 0-88946 -32-5

5284 Shattered Dreams-Lonely Choices: Birth Parents of Babies with Disabilities
Greenwood Publishing Group
130 Cremona Drive
Santa Barbara, CA 93117-4208

203-226-3571
800-368-6868
805-968-1911
Fax: 866-270-3856
customerservice@abc-clio.com
www.abc-clio.com

208 pages Hardcover
ISBN 0-897892-86-0

5285 Since Owen, A Parent-to-Parent Guide for Care of the Disabled Child
Special Needs Project
Ste H
324 State St
Santa Barbara, CA 93101-2364

818-718-9900
800-333-6867
Fax: 818-349-2027
editor@specialneeds.com
www.specialneeds.com

Hod Gray, Owner
Against the background of his experience as the parent of a severely disabled young man, Callahan writes conscientiously to other parents. *$16.95*
486 pages

5286 Sleep Better! A Guide to Improving Sleep for Children with Special Needs
Brookes Publishing
P.O.Box 10624
Baltimore, MD 21285-624

410-337-9580
800-638-3775
Fax: 410-337-8539
custserv@brookespublishing.com
readplaylearn.com

Paul Brooks, Owner
This book offers step-by-step, how to instructions for helping children with disabilities get the rest they need. For problems ranging from bedtime tantrums to night waking, parents and caregivers will find a variety of widely tested and easy-to-implement

techniques that have already helped hundreds of children with special needs. *$21.95*
288 pages Paperback
ISBN 1-55766 -15-7

5287 Something's Wrong with My Child!
Charles C. Thomas
2600 S First St
Springfield, IL 62704-4730

217-789-8980
800-258-8980
Fax: 217-789-9130
books@ccthomas.com
www.ccthomas.com

Michael P. Thomas, President
This text provides professionals and parents with the opportunity to gain insights into a family that has benefited positively and constructively from the presence of a member with a disability. The author presents a compilation of easy-to-read material that's based on real-life experiences. *$39.95*
234 pages Paperback 1998
ISBN 0-398068-99-8

5288 Sometimes I Get All Scribbly
Exceptional Parent Library
P.O.Box 1807
Englewood Cliffs, NJ 7632-1207

201-947-6000
800-535-1910
Fax: 201-947-9376
eplibrary@aol.com
www.eplibrary.com

5289 Son-Rise: The Miracle Continues
2080 South Undermountain Road
Sheffield, MA 01257-9643

413-229-2100
877-766-7473
Fax: 413-229-3202
sonrise@option.org
www.son-rise.org

Barry Neil Kaufman, Co-Founder/ Co-Originator/Senior Teacher/Trainer
Samahria Lyte Kaufman, Co-Founder/ Co-Originator/Senior Teacher/Trainer
Bryn Hogan, ATCA Senior Staff
William Hogan, ATCA Senior Staff
Documents Raun Kaufman's astonishing development from a lifeless, autistic, retarded child into a highly verbal, lovable youngster with no traces of his former condition. Details Raun's extraordinary progress from the age of four into young adulthood, also shares moving accounts of five families that successfully used the Son-Rise Program to reach their own special children.
372 pages
ISBN 0-915811-53-7

5290 Special Kids Need Special Parents: A Resource for Parents of Children With Special Needs
Berkley Publishing Group
375 Hudson Street
New York, NY 10014-3657

212-366-2372
Fax: 212-366-2933
ecommerce@us.penguingroup.com
www.us.penguingroup.com

319 pages Paperback
ISBN 0-425176-62-2

5291 Special Parent, Special Child
Exceptional Parent Library
P.O.Box 1807
Englewood Cliffs, NJ 7632-1207

201-947-6000
800-535-1910
Fax: 201-947-9376
eplibrary@aol.com
www.eplibrary.com

Hardcover

5292 Strategies for Working with Families of Young Children with Disabilities
Brookes Publishing
P.O.Box 10624
Baltimore, MD 21285-624   410-337-9580
                                  800-638-3775
                                  Fax: 410-337-8539
                                  custserv@brookespublishing.com
                                  readplaylearn.com
Paul Brooks, Owner
This text offers useful techniques for collaborating with and supporting families whose youngest members either have a disability or are at risk for developing a disability. The authors address specific issues such as cultural diversity, transitions to new programs, and disagreements between families and professionals. *$33.00*
272 pages Paperback
ISBN 1-55766-57-6

5293 That's My Child
Exceptional Parent Library
P.O.Box 1807
Englewood Cliffs, NJ 7632-1207   201-947-6000
                                     800-535-1910
                                     Fax: 201-947-9376
                                     eplibrary@aol.com
                                     www.eplibrary.com

5294 The Complete Guide to Creating a Special Needs Life Plan
Jessica Kingsley Publishers
73 Collier St
London, UK N19BE   hello@jkp.com
                               www.jkp.com
Hal Wright, Author
The purpose of special needs planning is to create the best possible life for an adult with a disability. This book provides comprehensive guidance on creating a life plan to transition a special needs child to independence or to ensure they are well cared for in the future.
360 pages

5295 They Don't Come with Manuals
Fanlight Productions
32 Court Street, 21st Floor
Brooklyn, NY 11201-1731   718-488-8900
                                  800-876-1710
                                  Fax: 718-488-8642
                                  orders@fanlight.com
                                  www.fanlight.com
Ben Achtenberg, Owner
Anthony Sweeney, Marketing Director
Nicole Johnson, Publicity Coordinator
The parents and adoptive parents in this video speak candidly of their day to day experiences caring for children with physical and mental disabilities. *$145.00*

5296 They're Just Kids
Aquarius Health Care Videos
30 Forest Road
P.O. Box 249
Millis, MA 02054-7159   508-376-1244
                                Fax: 508-376-1245
                                aqvideos@tiac.net
                                www.aquariusproductions.com
Lesile Kussmann, President
Joyce Farmer, Assistant Director
The importance and value of inclusion, excellent for anyone working with kids with disabilities. The documentary explores the advantages of the inclusion of disabled children in the classroom, cub scouts and other extracurricular activities. *$99.00*
Video

5297 To a Different Drumbeat
Alliance for Parental Involvement in Education
P.O.Box 59
East Chatham, NY 12060-59   518-392-6900
                                    Fax: 518-392-6900

5298 Uncommon Fathers
Woodbine House
6510 Bells Mill Rd
Bethesda, MD 20817-1636   301-897-3570
                                  800-843-7323
                                  info@woodbinehouse.com
                                  woodbinehouse.com
Irv Shapell, Owner
Nineteen fathers talk about the life-altering experience of having a child with special needs and offer a welcome, seldom-heard perspective on raising kids with disabilities, including autism, cerebral palsy, and Down syndrome. Uncommon Fathers is the first book for fathers by fathers, but it is also helpful to partners, family, friends, and service providers. *$14.95*
206 pages Paperback
ISBN 0-933149-68-9

5299 We Can Speak for Ourselves: Self Advocacy by Mentally Handicapped People
Brookline Books
8 Trumbull Rd
Suite B-001
Northampton, MA 1060-4533   413-584-0184
                                    800-666-2665
                                    Fax: 413-584-6184
                                    brbooks@yahoo.com
                                    www.brooklinebooks.com
246 pages Paperback
ISBN 0-25336-65-9

5300 You May Be Able to Adopt
Through the Looking Glass
3075 Adeline St
Ste. 120
Berkeley, CA 94703-2212   510-848-1112
                                  800-644-2666
                                  Fax: 510-848-4445
                                  TTY: 510-848-1005
                                  tlg@lookingglass.org
                                  www.lookingglass.org
Maureen Block, J.D., Board President
Rusty Hendlin, M.A., LMFT, Director of Medi-Cal Services
Thomas Spalding, Board Treasurer
Alice Nemon, D.S.W., Board Secretary
A guide to the adoption process for prospective mothers with disabilities and their partners. Available in braille, large print or cassette. *$10.00*
112 pages

5301 You Will Dream New Dreams
Kensington Publishing
119 West 40th Street
New York, NY 10018   800-221-2647
                             www.kensingtonbooks.com
Steven Zacharius, Chairman, President & CEO
A parent's support group in print. The shared narratives come from those with newly diagnosed children, adult disabled children, and everything in between. *$13.00*
278 pages Paperback
ISBN 1-575665-60-3

5302 Your Child Has a Disability: A Complete Sourcebook of Daily and Medical Care
Brookes Publishing
P.O.Box 10624
Baltimore, MD 21285-624   410-337-9580
                                  800-638-3775
                                  Fax: 410-337-8539
                                  custserv@brookespublishing.com
                                  readplaylearn.com
Paul Brooks, Owner
Offers expert advice on a wide range of issues-from finding the right doctor and investigating the medical aspects of a child's condition to learning care techniques and fulfilling education requirements. *$24.95*
368 pages Paperback
ISBN 1-557663-74-2

Parenting: Specific Disabilities

5303 **Cancer Clinical Trials: A Commonsense Guide to Experimental Cancer Therapies and Trials**
DiaMedica Inc.
2 Carlson Pkwy N
Ste 165
Minneapolis, MN 55447
763-270-0603
Fax: 763-710-4456
info@diamedica.com
www.diamedica.com

Tomasz M. Beer, Author
Larry W. Axmaker, Author
Cancer Clinical Trials is a comprehensive, no-nonsense, and readable guide for anyone who is considering therapeutic options in addition to standard cancer therapy. The book seeks to share knowledge about cancer clinical trials with people living with cancer, their families and loved ones. It will help readers decide if a clinical trial is a good option for them, to choose an appropriate trial, and to navigate through the clinical trial process.
192 pages

5304 **Different Dream Parenting: A Practical Guide to Raising a Child with Special Needs**
Discovery House Publishers
3000 Kraft Ave SE
P.O. Box 3566
Grand Rapids, MI 49512
800-653-8333
support@dhp.org
dhp.org

Jolene Philo, Author
In Different Dream Parenting, author Jolene Philo offers guidance and encouragement through biblical insights and her own personal experiences. Find spiritual wisdom, practical resources, and tools that can help you become an extraordinary advocate for your child. Discover how you can move beyond the challenges and experience the joy of being your childs biggest and best supporter.
336 pages

5305 **Essential First Steps for Parents of Children with Autism**
Woodbine House
6510 Bells Mill Rd
Bethesda, MD 20817
301-897-3570
800-843-7323
info@woodbinehouse.com
www.woodbinehouse.com

Lara Delmolino, Author
Sandra L. Harris, Author
When autism is diagnosed or suspected in young children, overwhelmed parents wonder where to turn and how to begin helping their child. Drs. Delmolino and Harris, experienced clinicians and ABA therapists, eliminate the confusion and guesswork by outlining the pivotal steps parents can take now to optimize learning and functioning for children ages 5 and younger.
154 pages Paperback

5306 **Final Report: Challenges and Strategies of Disabled Parents: Findings from a Survey (1997)**
Through the Looking Glass
3075 Adeline St
Ste. 120
Berkeley, CA 94703-2212
510-848-1112
800-644-2666
Fax: 510-848-4445
TTY: 510-848-1005
tlg@lookingglass.org
www.lookingglass.org

Linda Toms Barker, Author
Vida Maralani, Author
This milestone TLG-directed report presents findings from the first national survey of parents with disabilities. The report includes a description of parents with disabilities, barriers to parenting among adults with disabilities, transportation issues, personal assistance, adaptive parenting equipment, housing, as well as recommendations for legal and service system changes.

5307 **Pervasive Developmental Disorders: Findinga Diagnosis and Getting Help**
Patient-Centered Guides/O'Reilly Media
1005 Gravenstein Hwy N
Sebastopol, CA 95472
707-827-7019
800-889-8969
Fax: 707-824-8268
orders@oreilly.com
shop.oreilly.com

Mitzi Waltz, Author
This unique book encompassess both the practical aspects as well as ther personal stories and emotional facets of living with PDD-NOS, the most common pervasive developmental disorder. Parents of an undiagnosed child may suspect many things, from autism to servere allergies. Pervasive Developmental Disorders is for parents (or newly diagnosed adults) who struggle with this neurological condition that profoundly impacts the life of child and family.
580 pages Paperback 1999

5308 **Teaching Children with Down Syndrome about Their Bodies, Boundaries, and Sexuality**
Woodbine House
6510 Bell Mills Rd
Bethesda, MD 20817
800-843-7323
info@woodbinehouse.com
www.woodbinehouse.com

Terri Couwenhoven, Author
Drawing on her unique background as both a sexual educator and mother of a child with Down syndrome, the author blends factual information and practical ideas for teaching children with Down syndrome about their bodies, puberty, and sexuality. This book gives parents the confidence to speak comfortably about these sometimes difficult subjects.
332 pages Paperback

5309 **Thinking Differently: An Inspiring Guidefor Parents of Children with Learning Disabilities**
William Morrow Paperbacks (HarperCollins)
195 Broadway
New York, NY 10007
212-207-7000
orders@harpercollins.com
www.harpercollins.com

David Flink, Author
An innovative, comprehensive guide—the first of its kind—to help parents understand and accept learning disabilities in their children, offering tips and strategies for successfully advocating on their behalf and helping them become their own best advocates.

5310 **Your Child in the Hospital: A Practical Guide for Parents (3rd Edition)**
Childhood Cancer Guides/O'Reilly Media
1005 Gravenstein Hwy N
Sebastopol, CA 95472
707-827-7019
800-889-8969
Fax: 707-824-8268
orders@oreilly.com
shop.oreilly.com

Nancy Keene, Author
This book offers advice from dozens of veteran parents on how to cope with a child's hospitalization, relieving anxious parents so they can help dispel their child's fears and concerns. Parents will find easy-to-read tips on preparing their child, handling procedures without trauma, and preventing insurance snafus. The second edition features a journal to help open communication and give the child a measure of control over the experience.
176 pages Paperback

Parenting: School

5311   Allergy & Asthma Today
Allergy & Asthma Network
8229 Boone Blvd
Ste 260
Vienna, VA 22182   800-878-4403
                                      Fax: 703-288-5271
                       canderson@allergyasthmanetwork.org
                              www.allergyasthmanetwork.org
Tonya Winders, President
Charmayne Anderson, Director, Advocacy
Gary Fitzgerald, Managing Editor
Laurie Ross, Associate Editor
Practical, medical,information for school patients, physicians,
caregivers and families.

**5312   Carolina Curriculum for Infants and Toddlers with Special
         Needs (3rd Edition)**
Brookes Publishing
P.O.Box 10624
Baltimore, MD 21285-0624   410-337-9580
                                           800-638-3775
                                      Fax: 410-337-8539
                          custserv@brookespublishing.com
                                 www.brookespublishing.com
Nancy M. Johnson-Martin, Author
Susan M. Attermeier, Author
Bonnie J. Hacker, Author
This book includes detailed assessment and intervention se-
quences, daily routine integration strategies, sensorimotor adaptations, and a sample 24-page Assessment Log that shows readers
how to chart a child's individual progress.
504 pages Spiral-bound

**5313   Choosing Outcomes and Accommodations for Children
         (COACH) (2nd Edition)**
Brookes Publishing
P.O.Box 10624
Baltimore, MD 21285-0624   410-337-9580
                                           800-638-3775
                                      Fax: 410-337-8539
                          custserv@brookespublishing.com
                                 www.brookespublishing.com
Michael F. Giangreco, Author
Chigee J. Cloninger, Author
Virginia Salce Iverson, Author
A guide to educational planning for students with disabilities,
second edition. Focuses on life outcomes such as social relationships and participation in typical home, school, and community
activities.
232 pages Spiral bound

**5314   Complete IEP Guide: How to Advocate for Your Special Ed
         Child (8th Edition)**
NOLO (Internet Brands)
909 N. Sepulveda Blvd
11th Fl.
El Segundo, CA 90245   310-280-4000
                                            www.nolo.com
Lawrence Siegel, Author/Attorney
This all-in-one guide will help you understand special education
law, identify your child's needs, prepare for meetings, develop
the IEP and resolve disputes.
384 pages

5315   Exceptional Student in the Regular Classroom (6th Edition)
Pearson
330 Hudson St
New York, NY 10013   212-641-2400
                                          www.pearsoned.com
Bill R. Gearheart, Author
Mel W. Weishan, Author
Carol J. Gearheart, Author

Offers good, solid information through a practical understandable presentation unencumbered by specialized jargon. Covers
topics associated with special learners.
517 pages

**5316   Study Power Workbook: Exercises in Study - Skills to
         Improve Your Learning and Your Grades**
Brookline Books
8 Trumbull Rd
Ste B-001
Northampton, MA 1060-4533   413-584-0184
                                           800-666-2665
                                      Fax: 413-584-6184
                                      brbooks@yahoo.com
                                    www.brooklinebks.com
Sara Beth Huntley, Author
William Luckie, Author
Wood Smethurst, Author
The techniques in the easy-to-use, self-teaching manual have
yielded remarkable success for students from elementary to medi-
cal school, at all levels of intelligence and achievement. Key
skills covered include: listening, note taking, concentration,
summarizing, reading comprehension, memorization, test taking, preparing papers and reports, time management, and more.
These abilities are vital to success throughout every stage of
learning; the benefits will last a lifetime.

Parenting: Spiritual

**5317   A Good and Perfect Gift: Faith, Expectations, and a Little
         Girl Named Penny**
Bethany House Publishers (Baker Publishing Group)
6030 E Fulton Rd
Ada, MI 49301   616-676-9185
                                           800-877-2665
                                      Fax: 616-676-9573
                               bakerpublishinggroup.com
Amy Julia Becker, Author
When her first baby, Penny, is given a frightening diagnosis, Amy
Julia's world comes crashing down. Could she continue to trust
God's goodness through what felt like personal tragedy? But
challenging surprises often lead to unforeseen joy, and disap-
pointments can turn into blessings. This wise and beautiful book
is more than a courageous story of raising a child against the
odds—it is a journey through the unexpected ups and downs of
life and the discoveries that come along the way.
240 pages

5318   Before and After Zachariah
Chicago Review Press
814 N Franklin St
Chicago, IL 60610   312-337-0747
                                           800-888-4741
                                      Fax: 312-337-5110
                               www.chicagoreviewpress.com
Fern Kupfer, Author
This intimate chronicle of one family's life with a severely brain
damaged child is recently back in print.
247 pages 1982

**5319   Bethy and the Mouse: A Father Remembers His Children
         with Disabilities**
Brookline Books
8 Trumbull Rd
Ste B-001
Northampton, MA 1060-4533   413-584-0184
                                           800-666-2665
                                      Fax: 413-584-6184
                                      brbooks@yahoo.com
                                    www.brooklinebks.com
Donald C. Bakely, Author
A moving collection of poetry, photographs, and prose following
a father's experiences with two disabled children—one with
Down Syndrome and one with an underdeveloped brain.
184 pages Paperback 1999

5320 Disabled God: Toward a Liberatory Theology of Disability
Abingdon Press
2222 Rosa L. Parks Blvd
Nashville, TN 37288
615-749-6615
800-251-3320
orders@abingdonpress.com
www.abingdonpress.com
Nancy L. Eisland, Author
Draws on themes of the disability rights movement to identify people with disabilities as members of a socially disadvantaged minority group rather than as individuals who need to adjust. Highlights the history of people with disabilities in the church and society.
139 pages Paperback 1994

5321 Farewell, My Forever Child
CreateSpace, an Amazon Company
4900 Lacross Rd
North Charleston, SC 29406
843-760-8000
www.createspace.com
Kalila Smith, Author
Based on her own experiences following the loss of her 29-year-old daughter, Kalila Smith discusses the complex grief felt by parents who have lost a developmentally disabled child, and offers strategies to help families achieve peace and deal with the loss.
134 pages

5322 In Time and with Love: Caring for the Special Needs Infant and Toddler
William Morrow Paperbacks (HarperCollins)
195 Broadway
New York, NY 10007
212-207-7000
orders@harpercollins.com
www.harpercollins.com
Marilyn Segal, Author
Roni Leiderman, Author
Wendy S. Masi, Author
For families and caregivers of preteen and handicapped children in their first three years - more than one hundred tips for adjusting and coping. Part of the Your Child At Play series.
240 pages

5323 Journal of Disability & Religion
Routledge (Taylor & Francis Group)
711 Third Ave
New York, NY 10017
212-216-7800
800-354-1420
Fax: 202-564-7854
orders@taylorandfrancis.com
www.tandfonline.com
Quarterly

5324 Spiritually Able: A Parents Guide to Teaching Faith To Children with Special Needs
Loyola Press
3441 N Ashland Ave
Chicago, IL 60657
800-621-1008
Fax: 773-281-0555
customerservice@loyolapress.com
www.loyolapress.com
David Rizzo, Author
Both memoir and manual, Spiritually Able: A Parent's Guide to Teaching the Faith to Children with Special Needs is a life-preserver to parents who are seeking ways to grow and nourish a deeper relationship to God and their faith for their child with special needs. Full of tips, advice, and personal accounts, Spiritually Able helps bridge the gap and invites all into the welcoming embrace of the Church.
140 pages

5325 The Spiritual Art of Raising Children with Disabilities
Judson Press
P.O. Box 851
Valley Forge, PA 19482
800-458-3766
www.judsonpress.com
Kathleen Deyer Bolduc, Author

In The Spiritual Art of Raising Children with Disabilities, Bolduc uses the metaphor of the mosaic to life as parents of children with disabilities. Readers are walked through the process using the spiritual disciplines to help you recognize God's presence in your life and regain the balance we all need. this book offers readers the unique perspective of a parent raising a child with disabilities and dealing with it through faith and spiritual direction.
192 pages Paperback

5326 Worst Loss: How Families Heal from the Death of a Child
Holt Paperbacks (Macmillan Publishers)
75 Varick St
New York, NY 10013
212-226-7521
press.inquiries@macmillan.com
us.macmillan.com/henryholt
Barbara D. Rosof, Author
Combines anecdotal case histories and the latest research to help bereaved parents cope with the loss of a child, offering practical and comforting advice on how to overcome the disabling symptoms of grief.
304 pages 1995

Professional

5327 American Journal of Physical Medicine & Rehabilitation
Lippincott, Williams & Wilkins
2001 Market St
Ste 5
Philadelphia, PA 19103-1551
215-521-8300
800-638-3030
Fax: 215-521-8902
orders@lww.com
www.lww.com
Walter R. Frontera, MD, PHD, Editor-in-Chief
Journal of the Association of Academic Psychiatrists. Articles covering research and clinical studies and applications of new equipment, procedures and therapeutic advances.
Monthly

5328 American Journal of Psychiatry
American Psychiatric Association
1000 Wilson Blvd
Ste 1825
Arlington, VA 22209-3924
703-907-7322
800-368-5777
Fax: 703-907-1091
ajp@psych.org
ajp.psychiatryonline.org
Robert Freedman, Editor
Peer-reviewed articles focus on developments in biological psychiatry as well as on treatment innovations and forensic, ethical, economic, and social topics.
Monthly

5329 American Journal of Public Health
American Public Health Association
800 I St NW
Washington, DC 20001
202-777-2471
888-320-2742
Fax: 202-777-2534
TTY: 202-777-2500
www.apha.org
Alfredo Morabia, Editor-in-Chief
Association journal containing professional articles and sections such as Notes from the Field and Association News.
Monthly

5330 Art Therapy
American Art Therapy Association
4875 Eisenhower Ave
Ste 240
Alexandria, VA   22304-3302
703-548-5860
888-290-0878
Fax: 703-783-8468
info@arttherapy.org
www.arttherapy.org

Quarterly

5331 CAREERS & the disABLED Magazine
Equal Opportunity Publications
445 Broad Hollow Rd
Ste 425
Melville, NY   11747-3615
631-421-9421
Fax: 631-421-1352
info@eop.com
www.eop.com

Barbara Capella Loehr, Editor
A career magazine for professional career seekers who have disabilities. Profiles disabled people who have achieved successful careers. Features a career section in Braille, career guide.

**5332 Clinician's Practical Guide to
Attention-Deficit/Hyperactivity Disorder**
Brookes Publishing
P.O.Box 10624
Baltimore, MD   21285-0624
410-337-9580
800-638-3775
Fax: 410-337-8539
custserv@brookespublishing.com
www.brookespublishing.com

Marianne Mercugliano, Author
Quick reference volume with comprehensive data on psychoeducational and neuropsychological assessment, related symptoms, drug and counseling therapies and critical issues.
368 pages

**5333 Counseling Parents of Children with Chronic Illness or
Disability**
Wiley
111 River St
Hoboken, NJ   07030-5774
201-748-6000
877-762-2974
Fax: 201-748-6088
info@wiley.com
www.wiley.com

Hilton Davis, Author
This book aims to help medical staff and carers relate to parents in ways that facilitate their adaptation to their child's illness. The key to this is in effective communication.
148 pages Paperback

**5334 Creating Options for Family Recovery: A Provider's Guide
to Promoting Parental Mental Health**
Employment Options Inc.
82 Brigham St
Marlboro, MA   01752-3137
508-485-5051
Fax: 508-485-8807
options@employmentoptions.org
www.employmentoptions.com

Joanne Nicholson, Author
Toni Wolf, Author
Chip Wilder, Author
Kathleen Biebel, Author
This book seeks to advise professionals and providers on strategies to use when working with families who are dealing with mental illness, assisting them with the promotion of a healthy recovery. The resources in this guide are drawn from over 20 years of research and practice, and the lived experiences of parents, children and family members.
120 pages Paperback

5335 Cystic Fibrosis: Medical Care
Lippincott, Williams & Wilkins
16522 Hunters Green Pkwy
Hagerstown, MD   21740
301-223-2300
800-638-3030
Fax: 301-223-2400
orders@lww.com
www.lww.com

David M. Orenstein, Author
Beryl J. Rosenstein, Author
Robert C. Stern, Author
A guide to the medical community to the principles and practices of cystic fibrosis care. After chapters on the molecular and cellular bases of CF and its diagnosis, they cover the major organ systems affected by CF and deal with surgery for CF patients, transplantation (lung and liver), hospitalization, and terminal care. Also included are chapters on special populations, exercise, and laboratory testing.
365 pages

5336 Disability & Rehabilitation Journal
Taylor & Francis Online
6000 Broken Sound Pkwy NW
Ste 300
Boca Raton, FL   33487
212-216-7800
800-634-7064
Fax: 212-564-7854
enquiries@taylorandfrancis.com
www.taylorandfrancis.com

Dave Muller, Editor-in-Chief
Peer-reviewed journal offering the latest news, research, and insights on disability and rehabilitation medicine.
Bi-weekly

**5337 Disability Analysis Handbook: Tools for Independent
Practice**
American Board of Disability Analysts
4525 Harding Rd
2nd Fl
Nashville, TN   37205
americanbd@aol.com
www.americandisability.org

Kenneth N. Anchor, Editor
Handbook providing information on physical and mental disabilities, including: diabetes, substance abuse, aging, nonverbal learning, chronic pain, etc.
396 pages

**5338 Enhancing Everyday Communication for Children with
Disabilities**
Brookes Publishing
P.O.Box 10624
Baltimore, MD   21285-0624
410-337-9580
800-638-3775
Fax: 410-337-8539
custserv@brookespublishing.com
www.brookespublishing.com

Jeff Sigafoos, Author & Editor
Michael Arthur-Kelly, Author
Nancy Butterfield, Author
Practical and concise, this introductory guide is filled with real-world tips and strategies for anyone working to improve the communication of children with moderate, severe, and multiple disabilities. Emphasizing the link between behavior and communication, three respected researchers transform up-to-date research and proven best practices into instructional procedures and interventions ready for use at home or in school.
176 pages Paperback

5339 Ethical Issues In Home Health Care (2nd Edition)
Charles C. Thomas
2600 S First St
Springfield, IL 62704-4730   217-789-8980
                                                     800-258-8980
                                            Fax: 217-789-9130
                                            books@ccthomas.com
                                            www.ccthomas.com
Sheri Smith, Author
Rosalind Ekman Ladd, Author
Lynn Pasquerella, Author
This book will help to answer some of the growing number of ethical questions and more complex issues that home health care nurses face. The cases presented in each chapter of the book are fictionalized situations based on interviews conducted with home health care nurses in both hospital-sponsored and private agencies, in hospices, and in urban and rural settings. Each chapter of the book is devoted to one of the main areas of concern for home health care nurses.
258 pages

5340 Journal of Public Health
Oxford Journals, Oxford University Press
2001 Evans Rd
Cary, NC 27513   919-677-0977
                                                     800-852-7323
                                            Fax: 919-677-1714
                                            www.oxfordjournals.org
Eugene Milne, Editor
Ted Schrecker, Editor
Scholarly articles on issues that relate to public health and the healthcare system.

5341 National Rehabilitation Association Annual Report
National Rehabilitation Association (NRA)
633 S Washington St
P.O. Box 150235
Alexandria, VA 22315-4109   703-836-0850
                                                     888-258-4295
                                            Fax: 703-836-0848
                                            TTY: 703-836-0849
                                            info@nationalrehab.org
                                            www.nationalrehab.org
Fredric Schroeder, Executive Director
Sandra Mulliner, Administrative Assistant
Association newsletter containing news, programs and information of interest to the Association and its members.
Annual

5342 PM&R Journal
American Academy of Physical Medicine & Rehab
9700 W Bryn Mawr Ave
Ste 200
Rosemont, IL 60018-5701   847-737-6000
                                                     877-227-6799
                                            Fax: 847-737-6001
                                            TTY: 800-437-0833
                                            info@aapmr.org
                                            www.pmrjournal.org
Stuart M. Weinstein, Editor-in-Chief
Cathy Mendelsohn, Managing Editor
Covers medical, social and employment aspects of vocational rehabilitation. The content of PM&R includes articles that are contemporary and important to both research and clinical practice. The various sections of the journal include original research such as clinical trials, outcomes studies, and clinically relevant translational science; reviews (narrative and analytical); case presentations; point/counterpoint debates; ethical/legal topics; practice management updates; and statistical themes.
Monthly

5343 Provider Magazine
American Health Care Association
1201 L St NW
Washington, DC 20005-4024   202-842-4444
                                                     888-656-6669
                                            Fax: 202-842-3860
                                            sales@ahca.org
Joanne Erickson, Editor-in-Chief
Amy Mendoza, Managing Editor
Magazine for long-term healthcare professionals.
Monthly

5344 Public Health Reports
Association of Schools & Programs of Public Health
1900 M St NW
Ste 710
Washington, DC 20036   202-296-1099
                                            Fax: 202-296-1252
                                            support@publichealthreports.org
                                            www.publichealthreports.org
Frederic E. Shaw, Editorn-in-Chief
Sasha M. Ruiz, Acting Managing Editor
PHR is a peer-reviewed journal published on a bi-monthly basis. Each issue offers recurring guest columns such as Local Acts, Global Health Matters, ASPPH From the Schools and Programs of Public Health, Law and the Public's Health, Public Health Chronicles, NCHS Dataline, and the Surgeon General's Perspectives.
Bi-monthly

5345 Sociopolitical Aspects of Disabilities(2nd Edition)
Charles C. Thomas
2600 S First St
Springfield, IL 62704-4730   217-789-8980
                                                     800-258-8980
                                            Fax: 217-789-9130
                                            books@ccthomas.com
                                            www.ccthomas.com
Willie V. Bryan, Author
Provides understanding of the social and political histories of people with disabilities in the United States. This understanding is pivotal in working with persons with disabilities, to provide background and perspective on current policies and attitudes.
284 pages

5346 Starting and Sustaining Genetic Support Groups
Johns Hopkins University Press
2715 N Charles St
Baltimore, MD 21218-4363   410-516-6900
                                            Fax: 410-516-6968
                                            webmaster@jhupress.jhu.edu
                                            www.press.jhu.edu
Joan O. Weiss, Author
Jayne S. Mackta, Author
Guide to the establishment and maintenance of genetic support groups for individuals with genetic disorders and their families. For therapists and group leaders. Discusses practical matters including finding a leader, fund-raising, organizing peer support training programs.
152 pages

5347 The Essential Brain Injury Guide (5th Edition)
Brain Injury Association of America
1608 Spring Hill Rd
Ste 110
Vienna, VA 22182   703-761-0750
                                            Fax: 703-761-0755
                                            customerservice2@biausa.org
                                            shop.biausa.org

5348 What Psychotherapists Should Know about Disabilty
Guilford Press
370 Seventh Ave
Ste 1200
New York, NY 10001-1020   800-365-7006
                                 Fax: 212-966-6708
                                 info@guilford.com
                                 www.guilford.com
Rhoda Olkin, Author
This comprehensive volume provides the knowledge and skills that mental health professionals need for more effective, informed work with clients with disabilities. Topics addressed include etiquette with clients with disabilities; special concerns in assessment, evaluation, and diagnosis. Filled with clinical examples and observations, the volume also discusses strategies for enhancing teaching, training, and research.
368 pages

5349 Women with Visible & Invisible Disabilitiees: Multiple Intersections, Issues, Therapies
Routledge (Taylor & Francis Group)
711 Third Ave
New York, NY 10017   212-216-7800
                                 800-634-7064
                                 Fax: 202-564-7854
                                 enquiries@taylorandfrancis.com
                                 www.routledge.com
Martha E. Banks, Editor
Ellyn Kaschak, Editor
Addresses the issues faced by women with disabilities, examines the social construction of disability, and makes suggestions for the development and modification of culturally relevant therapy to meet the needs of disabled women.
414 pages Hardcover; Paperback

Specific Disabilities

5350 inMotion Magazine
Amputee Coalition
9303 Center St
Ste 100
Manassas, VA 20110   865-524-8772
                                 888-267-5669
                                 www.amputee-coalition.org
Bi-monthly

Vocations

5351 Ability Magazine
P.O. Box 10878
Costa Mesa, CA 92627   www.abilitymagazine.com
Bi-monthly

5352 Chemists with Disabilities Committee - American Chemical Society
American Chemical Society
1155 16th St NW
Washington, DC 20036   202-872-4600
                                 800-227-5558
                                 Fax: 202-872-4574
                                 cwd@acs.org
                                 www.acs.org
John Johnston, Ph.D, MBA, Chair
James Schiller, Chair Elect
Paula Christopher, Staff Liaison
Promotes the full involvement of individuals with physical and learning disabilities in educational and career opportunities in the chemical and allied sciences. CWD members help individuals with disabilities to connect with employers and educators of persons with disabilities.

5353 Demystifying Job Development: Field-Based Approaches to Job Development for the Disabled
Training Resource Network
266 Roaring Dr.
St. Augustine, FL 32084   *Fax:* 904-823-3554
                                 www.trn-store.com
David Hoff, Author
Cecilia Gandolfo, Author
Marty Gold, Author
Melanie Jordan, Author
A guide to successful placement of individuals with severe disabilities in quality jobs in the community.
105 pages

5354 Hiring Idahoans with Disabilities
Idaho Assistive Technology Project
University of Idaho
1187 Alturas Dr.
Moscow, ID 83843- 8331   208-885-3557
                                 800-432-8324
                                 Fax: 208-885-6102
                                 idahoat@uidaho.edu
Jane Frederickson, Author
Kristen Hagen, Author
The purpose of this handbook is to inform employers in Idaho business and industry about the promise of hiring Idahoans with disabilities.

5355 Life Beyond the Classroom: Transition Strategies for Young People with Disabilities
Brookes Publishing
P.O.Box 10624
Baltimore, MD 21285-0624   410-337-9580
                                 800-638-3775
                                 Fax: 410-337-8539
                                 custserv@brokespublishing.com
                                 www.brokespublishing.com
Paul Wehman, Author
Specialists in a variety of disciplines use creative and practical techniques to ensure careful transition planning, to build young people's confidence and competence in work skills, and to foster support from businesses and community organizations for training and employment programs.
616 pages

5356 More Than a Job: Securing Satisfying Careers for People with Disabilities
Brookes Publishing
P.O. Box 10624
Baltimore, MD 21285-0624   800-638-3775
                                 Fax: 410-337-8539
                                 custserv@brookespublishing.com
                                 www.brookespublishing.com
Paul Wehman, Editor
John Kregel, Editor
This book transforms job placement into career counseling for people with physical and developmental disabilities. It presents step-by-step guidelines for helping people with disabilities to identify their own interests.
384 pages 1998

5357 OT Practice Magazine
American Occupational Therapy Association
4720 Montgomery Ln
Bethesda, MD 20814-3449   301-652-6611
                                 800-729-2682
                                 Fax: 301-652-7711
                                 TTY: 800-377-8555
                                 otpractice@aota.org
                                 www.aota.org/publications-news.aspx

5358 **Occupational Therapy and Vocational Rehabilitation**
Wiley
111 River St
Hoboken, NJ 07030-5774

201-748-6000
877-762-2974
Fax: 201-748-6088
info@wiley.com
www.wiley.com

Joanne Ross
This book introduces the occupational therapist to the practice of vocational rehabilitation. As rehabilitation specialists, Occupational Therapists work in a range of diverse settings with clients who have a variety of physical, emotional and psychological conditions. This book highlights the contribution, which can be made by occupational therapists in assisting disabled, ill or injured workers to access, remain in and return to work.
280 pages Paperback

5359 **Work and Disability: Contexts, Issues & Strategies for Enhancing Employment Outcomes**
PRO-ED Inc.
8700 Shoal Creek Blvd
Austin, TX   78757-6897

512-451-3246
800-897-3202
Fax: 800-397-7633
general@proedinc.com
www.proedinc.com

Edna Mora Szymanski, Editor
Randall M. Parker, Editor
492 pages

Media, Electronic

Audio/Visual

5360 **A Place for Me**
Educational Productions
9000 SW Gemini Dr
Beaverton, OR 97008-7151
503-644-7000
800-950-4949
Fax: 503-350-7000
custserve@edpro.com
www.teachingstrategies.com
Diane Trister Dodge, Founder/President/Lead Author
Arnitra Duckett, VP, Sales & Strategic Marketing
In this video, parents discuss the issues they face in planning for their child's future. This program is designed to stimulate discussion of these issues and help increase awareness of the options available in your local community.

5361 **Able to Laugh**
Fanlight Productions
32 Court St.
21st Floor
Brooklyn, NY 11201-4421
718-488-8900
800-876-1710
Fax: 718-488-8642
info@fanlight.com
www.fanlight.com
Jonathan Miller, President
Patricio Guzman, Director
Meredith Miller, Sales Manager
Anthony Sweeney, Acquisitions
An exploration of the world of disability as interpreted by six professional comedians who happen to be disabled. It is also about the awkward ways disabled and able-bodied people relate to one another. *$199.00*
ISBN 1-572951-05-2

5362 **Acting Blind**
Fanlight Productions
32 Court St.
21st Floor
Brooklyn, NY 11201-4421
718-488-8900
800-876-1710
Fax: 718-488-8642
info@fanlight.com
www.fanlight.com
Jonathan Miller, President
Patricio Guzman, Director
Meredith Miller, Sales Manager
Anthony Sweeney, Acquisitions
Takes audiences behind the scenes as a company of non-professional actors rehearse a play about life without sight. The performers have no problem imagining themselves in these roles: they are blind themselves. *$229.00*

5363 **Adaptive Baby Care**
Through the Looking Glass
3075 Adeline St
Suite 120
Berkeley, CA 94703-2577
510-848-1112
800-644-2666
Fax: 510-848-4445
TTY: 510-848-1005
tlg@lookingglass.org
www.lookingglass.org
Megan Kirshbaum, Executive Director
Paul Preston, Assoc. Dir
This publication is presented as a catalyst for problem-solving regarding the development of adaptive baby care equipment. This newest publication is designed for parents, family members and professionals. It includes: guidelines for problem-solving baby care barriers; photographs and descriptions of prototypes and resources for adaptive baby care equipment; adaptive baby care techniques; adaptive baby care equipment checklist; commercial

product safety commission guidelines; and local and natio
$250.00

5364 **Adaptive Baby Care Equipment Video and Book Through the Looking Glass**
Through the Looking Glass
3075 Adeline St
Suite 120
Berkeley, CA 94703-2577
510-848-1112
800-644-2666
Fax: 510-848-4445
TTY: 510-848-1005
tlg@lookingglass.org
www.lookingglass.org
Stephanie Miyashiro, Board President
Thomas Spalding, Board Treasurer
Alice Nemon, D.S.W., Board Secretary
Christina Jopes, Board Members
Includes Adaptive Baby care Equipment: Guide Lines; Prototypes and Resources, plus a twelve minute video. Available in braille, large print or cassette. *$79.00*

5365 **All About Attention Deficit Disorders, Revised**
Parent Magic
800 Roosevelt Rd
B-309
Glen Ellyn, IL 60137-5839
630-208-0031
800-442-4453
Fax: 630-208-7366
ordercenter@parentmagic.com
www.parentmagic.com
Nancy Roe, Administrator/Exec Admin
Thomas Phelan, Owner/President/CEO
A psychologist and expert on ADD outlines the symptoms, diagnosis and treatment of this neurological disorder. Video ($49.95 - 2 parts) and audio cassette ($24.95). Also in DVD format (1 disk-$39.93).

5366 **Autism**
Aquarius Health Care Media
30 Forest Rd
PO Box 249
Millis, MA 2054-1511
508-376-1244
Fax: 508-376-1245
www.nmm.net
Lesile Kussmann, Owner/President/Producer
Kathy Newkirk, Director
Jane Hutchinson, Assoc. Director
This video takes you into the lives of autistic people and their families to understand more about autism. What defines autism and how can we help those living with the disability? Children, teens, and adults are also profiled and we begin to see the varying levels of development and new technology to help these people communicate. Preview Available. *$149.00*
Video

5367 **Basic Course in American Sign Language(B100) Harris Communications, Inc.**
Harris Communications
15155 Technology Dr
Eden Prairie, MN 55344-2273
952-906-1180
800-825-6758
Fax: 952-906-1099
TTY: 800-825-9187
info@harriscomm.com
www.harriscomm.com
Robert Harris, Owner/President
Kevin Horsky, Business Director
Randall Moore, Manager
This series of four one-hour tapes is designed to illustrate the various exercises and dialogues in the text. *$39.95*
Video

5368   Beginning ASL Video Course
Harris Communications
15155 Technology Dr
Eden Prairie, MN   55344-2273   952-906-1180
                                                 800-825-6758
                                          Fax: 952-906-1099
                                          TTY: 800-825-9187
                                          info@harriscomm.com
                                          www.harriscomm.com

Robert Harris, Owner/President
Kevin Horsky, Business Director
Randall Moore, Manager
You'll watch a family teach you to learn American Sign Language during funny and touching family situations. A total of 15 tapes in the course. *$599.40*
Video

5369   Blindness
Landmark Media
3450 Slade Run Dr
Falls Church, VA   22042-3940   703-241-2030
                                                 800-342-4336
                                          Fax: 703-536-9540
                                          info@landmarkmedia.com
                                          www.landmarkmedia.com

Michael Hartogs, President/Owner
Joan Hartogs, Owner/Vice President
Peter Hartogs, Vice President
Richard Hartogs, Vice President
Landmark Media is an independent family-owned company currently celebrating our 28th anniversary. We have been fortunate to be able to offer the finest quality educational DVDs available. *$250.00*
Video

5370   Boy Inside, The
Fanlight Productions
32 Court St.
21st Floor
Brooklyn, NY   11201-4421   718-488-8900
                                                 800-876-1710
                                          Fax: 718-488-8642
                                          info@fanlight.com
                                          www.fanlight.com

Jonathan Miller, President
Patricio Guzman, Director
Meredith Miller, Sales Manager
Anthony Sweeney, Acquisitions
Filmmaker Marianne Kaplan tells the personal and often distressing story of her son Adam, a 12-year-old with Asperger Syndrome, during a tumultuous year in the life of their family.

5371   Braille Documents
Metrolina Association for the Blind
704 Louise Ave
Charlotte, NC   28204-2128   704-887-5118
                                                 800-926-5466
                                          Fax: 704-372-3872
                                          bschmiel@mabnc.org
                                          www.mabnc.org

Robert Scheffel, President
Richard Hartness, Vice President, Product Design & Development
Barbara Schmiel, Vice President, Accessible Braille Services
Chris Wilkins, Vice President, Information Technology
This production shop creates Braille and large-print documents. We work with our clients to find the most cost effective solutions for their needs. Unlike other modified statement service providers, we accept your existing style of statement or allow you to design your own statement.Documents may be received in electronic data files as encrypted data sent over public networks, data sent to a file transfer protocol drop box, or data sent over a dedicated data line. ABS also accepts paper hardcopi

5372   Bringing Out the Best
PO Box 9177
Dept. 11W
Champaign, IL   61826-9177   217-352-3273
                                                 800-519-2707
                                          Fax: 217-352-1221
                                          orders@researchpress.com
                                          www.researchpress.com

David Parkinson, Chairman
Russell Pence, President
Gail Salyards, Dir. Of Marketing/President

5373   Business as Usual
Fanlight Productions
32 Court St.
21st Floor
Brooklyn, NY   11201-4421   718-488-8900
                                                 800-876-1710
                                          Fax: 718-488-8642
                                          info@fanlight.com
                                          www.fanlight.com

Jonathan Miller, President
Patricio Guzman, Director
Meredith Miller, Sales Manager
Anthony Sweeney, Acquisitions
An enlightening documentary, brings a unique international perspective to this struggle. This film examines five innovative programs which create opportunities for people with mental and physical disabilities to own and operate their own businesses. *$145.00*

5374   Buying Time: The Media Role in Health Care
Fanlight Productions
32 Court St.
21st Floor
Brooklyn, NY   11201-4421   718-488-8900
                                                 800-876-1710
                                          Fax: 718-488-8642
                                          info@fanlight.com
                                          www.fanlight.com

Jonathan Miller, President
Patricio Guzman, Director
Meredith Miller, Sales Manager
Anthony Sweeney, Acquisitions
This video program is a thoughtful and disturbing examination in the role of the media in determining the allocation of health care resources. This program is a powerful tool on ethics, policy, journalism, sociology, medicine and nursing as well as for professional workshops, and continuing education programs. *$99.00*

5375   Caring for Persons with Developmental Disabilities
PO Box 9177
Dept. 11W
Champaign, IL   61826-9177   217-352-3273
                                                 800-519-2707
                                          Fax: 217-352-1221
                                          www.researchpress.com

David Parkinson, Chairman
Russell Pence, President
Gail Salyards, Dir. Of Marketing/President

5376   Clockworks
Learning Corporation of America
6493 Kaiser Dr
Fremont, CA   94555-3610   510-490-7311
Oonchia Chia, Owner
Scotty, who has Down Syndrome, is fascinated by clocks. This film follows him on his adventures of employment in the clock shop.
Film

5377 Close Encounters of the Disabling Kind
Mainstream
6930 Carroll Ave
Suite 204
Takoma Park, MD 20912-4468   301-891-8777
Fax: 301-891-8778
info@mainstreaminc.org

Lillie Harrison, Information Programs Clerk
Fritz Rumpel, Editor
A training video that provides a hiring manager with information on how to learn the basics of disability etiquette and, by the end of the video, seems much better prepared and willing to interview qualified individuals with disabilities. Includes trainer and trainee guides. *$99.95*
Video

5378 Deaf Children Signers
Harris Communications
15155 Technology Dr
Eden Prairie, MN 55344-2273   952-906-1180
800-825-6758
Fax: 952-906-1099
TTY: 800-825-9187
info@harriscomm.com
www.harriscomm.com

Robert Harris, Owner
Kevin Horsky, Business Director
Randall Moore, Manager
Graduate to voicing for Deaf children ages 5-11. Adding new meaning to the phrase, Out of the mouths (hands?) of babes..., this unique tape lets eleven young children demonstrate their abilities by signing about what is important to them. *$39.95*
Video

5379 Deaf Culture Series
Harris Communicatin
15155 Technology Dr
Eden Prairie, MN 55344-2273   952-906-1180
800-825-6758
Fax: 952-906-1099
TTY: 800-825-9187
info@harriscomm.com
www.harriscomm.com

Robert Harris, Owner
Kevin Horsky, Business Director
Randall Moore, Manager
Each video in this five-part series features a topic dealing with the unique culture of deaf people. It is an excellent resource for deaf studies programs, Interpreter Preparation programs and Sign Language programs. *$49.95*
Video

5380 Deaf Mosaic
Harris Communications
15155 Technology Dr
Eden Prairie, MN 55344-2273   952-906-1180
800-825-6758
Fax: 952-906-1099
TTY: 800-825-9187
info@harriscomm.com
www.harriscomm.com

Robert Harris, Owner
Kevin Horsky, Business Director
Randall Moore, Manager
Deaf Mosaic: Deaf President Now documents the most extraordinary week in deaf history, including interviews with student leaders; exclusive footage of the demonstrations; and an interview with Gallaudet president, Dr. I. King Jordan. *$29.95*
Video

5381 Do You Hear That?
Alexander Graham Bell Association
3417 Volta Pl. NW
Washington, DC 20007   202-337-5220
Fax: 202-337-8314
info@agbell.org
www.agbell.org

Ted A. Meyer, Chair
Catharine McNally, Chair-Elect
Susan Lenihan, Secretary
Emilio Alonso Mendoza, Chief Executive Officer
This video shows auditory-verbal therapy sessions of a therapist working individually with 11 children who range in age from 7 months to 7 years old and have hearing aids or cochlear implants.
Video

5382 Doing Things Together
Britannica Film Company
345 4th St
San Francisco, CA 94107-1206   415-928-8466
Fax: 415-928-5027

Dave Bekowich, Owner
Steve went with his parents to an amusement park. He met another boy named Martin who at first was shocked by Steve's prosthetic hand.
Film

5383 Emerging Leaders
Mobility International USA
132 E. Broadway
Suite 343
Eugene, OR 97401-2767   541-343-1284
Fax: 541-343-6812
info@miusa.org
www.miusa.org

Susan Sygall, CEO/Founder
Susan Dunn, Exec. Asst./Project Specialist
Cindy Lewis, Director of Programs
Estelle Coreris-Moore, Financial Manager
Pioneering short-term international disability leadership programs in the U.S. and abroad with 2,000 youth, young adults and professionals from over 100 countries. *$49.00*
Video

5384 Face First
Fanlight Productions
32 Court St.
21st Floor
Brooklyn, NY 11201-4421   718-488-8900
800-876-1710
Fax: 718-488-8642
info@fanlight.com
www.fanlight.com

Jonathan Miller, President
Patricio Guzman, Director
Meredith Miller, Sales Manager
Anthony Sweeney, Acquisitions
In this documentary, the stories told reflect the reality faced by all those who are seen as different. Despite their difficult experiences, the survival of the profiled individuals affords comic relief &, by adulthood, they possess unusual strengths that shape their careers in pediatrics, disability care, public speaking, and journalism. *$ 195.00*

5385 Family-Guided Activity-Based Intervention for Toddlers & Infants
Brookes Publishing
PO Box 10624
Baltimore, MD 21285-0624   410-337-9580
800-638-3775
Fax: 410-337-8539
custserv@brookespublishing.com
www.readplaylearn.com

Paul Brooks, Owner
This 20-minute video was created to assist early childhood professionals to incorporate therapeutic intervention into daily living. It includes a discussion and demonstration of how

intervention professionals actively may involve caregivers in the planning and implementation of activities aimed at encouraging development of a child's target skills *$37.00*

20 Minutes

ISBN 1-55766-19-3

5386   Filmakers Library
124 E 40th St
Suite 901
New York, NY   10016-1798   212-808-4980
                                          Fax: 212-808-4983
                                          info@filmakers.com
                                          www.filmakers.com

Sue Oscar, Co-President
Linda Gottesman, Co-President
Andrea Traubner, Dir., Broadcast Sales

Filmakers Library has been a leading source of outstanding films for the education, library, and non-theatrical markets. Now, as an imprint of award-winning online publisher Alexander Street Press, Filmakers Library is able to offer online streaming access to most of our titles, ensuring that our films receive the greatest possible exposure and accessibility through the most flexible delivery platforms. We market and promote our films throughout the world by direct mail, print advertising, exhib

5387   Filmakers Library: An Imprint Of Alexander Street Press
124 E 40th St
Suite 901
New York, NY   10016-1798   212-808-4980
                                          Fax: 212-808-4983
                                          info@filmakers.com
                                          www.filmakers.com

Sue Oscar, Co-President
Linda Gottesman, Co-President
Andrea Traubner, Dir., Broadcast Sales

Filmakers Library has been a leading source of outstanding films for the education, library, and non-theatrical markets. Now, as an imprint of award-winning online publisher Alexander Street Press, Filmakers Library is able to offer online streaming access to most of our titles, ensuring that our films receive the greatest possible exposure and accessibility through the most flexible delivery platforms. We market and promote our films throughout the world by direct mail, print advertising, exhib

$100 - $300

5388   Films & Videos on Aging and Sensory Change
Lighthouse International
111 E 59th St
New York, NY   10022-1202   212-821-9200
                                              800-829-0500
                                          Fax: 212-821-9706
                                          info@lighthouse.org

Joanna Mellor, VP Information Services
Tara Cortes, President

An annotated list of over 80 films and videos dealing with age-related sensory change, divided into sections on vision impairment, hearing impairment, and multiple sensory impairments. *$5.00*

5389   Heart to Heart - Blind Childrens Center, Inc
Blind Children's Center
4120 Marathon St
Los Angeles, CA   90029-3584   323-664-2153
                                              800-222-3567
                                          Fax: 323-665-3828
                                    info@blindchildrenscenter.org
                                    www.blindchildrenscenter.org

Lena French, Executive Director
Fernanda Armenta-Schmitt, PhD, Director of Education & Family Services/Assistant Executive
Muriel Scharf, Director of Development
Ross Vergara, Director of Finance

Parents of blind and partially sighted children talk about their feelings. *$35.00*

Video

5390   Helping Hands
Fanlight Productions
32 Court St.
21st Floor
Brooklyn, NY   11201-4421   718-488-8900
                                              800-876-1710
                                          Fax: 718-488-8642
                                          info@fanlight.com
                                          www.fanlight.com

Jonathan Miller, President
Patricio Guzman, Director
Meredith Miller, Sales Manager
Anthony Sweeney, Acquisitions

The ADA mandates equal access and opportunity for the 43 million people with disabilities in the United States. These individuals may have limited speech, sight or mobility; a developmental disability; or a medical condition which limits some life activities. Many, however, are ready, willing and very able to join the workforce. This video demonstrates that many modifications or adaptations can be made simply by using ingenuity or common sense — such as keeping the aisles clear, etc. *$145.00*

37 Minutes

5391   Home is in the Heart: Accommodating Peoplewith Disabilities in the Homestay Experience
Mobility International USA
132 E. Broadway
Suite 343
Eugene, OR   97401-2767   541-343-1284
                                          Fax: 541-343-6812
                                          info@miusa.org
                                          www.miusa.org

Susan Sygall, CEO/Founder
Susan Dunn, Exec. Asst./Project Specialist
Cindy Lewis, Director of Programs
Estelle Coreris-Moore, Financial Manager

Provides information and ideas for exchange organizations. Discusses how to recruit homestay families, meet accessibility needs and accommodate international participants with disabilities. *$49.00*

Video

5392   How Difficult Can This Be ? (Fat City) - Rick Lavoie
CACLD
PO Box 210
Barnstable, MA   02630-210   508-362-1052
                                    scheduling@ricklavoie.com
                                    www.ricklavoie.com

Rick Lavoie, Film Maker

This unique program allows viewers to experience the same frustration, anxiety and tension that children with learning disabilities face in their daily lives. Teachers, social workers, psychologists, parents and friends who have participated in Richard Lavoie's workshop reflect upon their experience and the way it changed their approach to L.D. children. 1989.

5393   How We Play
Fanlight Productions
32 Court St.
21st Floor
Brooklyn, NY   11201-4421   718-488-8900
                                              800-876-1710
                                          Fax: 718-488-8642
                                          info@fanlight.com
                                          www.fanlight.com

Jonathan Miller, President
Patricio Guzman, Director
Meredith Miller, Sales Manager
Anthony Sweeney, Acquisitions

Though most of the people in this new, short documentary are in wheelchairs, and one is blind, they are anything but handicapped. Playing tennis, snorkeling, whitewater canoeing, practicing karate - they are living proof that a disability can be a challenge, not an obstacle. *$99.00*

5394   I'm Not Disabled
Landmark Media
3450 Slade Run Dr
Falls Church, VA   22042-3940   703-241-2030
                                                 800-342-4336
                                            Fax: 703-536-9540
                                          info@landmarkmedia.com
                                          www.landmarkmedia.com
Michael Hartogs, President
Joan Hartogs, Vice President
Peter Hartogs, Vice President
Richard Hartogs, Vice President
Young people talk about their disabilities and the importance of
sports in their lives. The afflictions range from blindness and
missing limbs to paralysis. Through physical education and ther-
apy they enjoy freedom of movement and participate in sports
such as tennis, basketball, kayaking, skiing, and swimming.
$195.00
Video

5395   Imagery Procedures for People with Special Needs
Research Press
PO Box 9177
Dept. 11W
Champaign, IL   61826-9177   217-352-3273
                                                 800-519-2707
                                            Fax: 217-352-1221
                                          rp@researchpress.com
                                          www.researchpress.com
David Parkinson, Chairman
Russell Pence, President
Gail Salyards, Dir. Of Marketing/President
This video was developed at the Groden Center and illustrates imagery based procedures including the use of positive reinforcement, covert modeling, and a self-control triad to assists
individuals to self-regulate their behaviors in stressful situations
or under conditions that may evoke extreme fear. Recommended
for professionals and family members interested in teaching
self-control strategies that individuals with autism spectrum disorders can use in community settings. $195.00
32 Minutes

5396   Include Us
Exceptional Parent Library
PO Box 1807
Englewood Cliffs, NJ   7632-1207   201-947-6000
                                                 800-535-1910
                                            Fax: 201-947-9376
                                          eplibrary@aol.com
                                          www.eplibrary.com

5397   Intensive Early Intervention and Beyond
PO Box 9177
Dept. 11W
Champaign, IL   61826-9177   217-352-3273
                                                 800-519-2707
                                            Fax: 217-352-1221
                                          www.researchpress.com
David Parkinson, Chairman
Russell Pence, President
Gail Salyards, Dir. Of Marketing/President

5398   Invisible Children
Learning Corporation of America
6493 Kaiser Dr
Fremont, CA   94555-3610   510-490-7311
Oonchia Chia, Owner
Renaldo was blind, Mandy was deaf, and Mark had Cerebral
Palsy and used a wheelchair. These child-size puppet characters
interacted with non-handicapped puppets.
Film

5399   Look Who's Laughing
Aquarius Health Care Videos
30 Forest Rd
PO Box 249
Millis, MA   2054-1511   508-376-1244
                                            Fax: 508-376-1245
                                          aqvideos@tiac.net
                                          www.aquariusproductions.com
Lesile Kussmann, Owner/President/Producer
Kathy Newkirk, Director
Jane Hutchinson, Assoc. Director
This video is packed with laugh-out-loud comedic moments, but
is also full of intelligent and inspiring messages. Look Who's
Laughing introduces viewers to some of today's funniest comedians - who just happen to be physically disabled. We hear them talk
openly and honestly about their limitations as well as their abilities and talents. Helpful for those who work with the disabled and
motivational to both the disabled and able-bodied. Preview option available. $95.00
Video

5400   My Body is Not Who I Am
Aquarius Health Care Videos
30 Forest Rd
PO Box 249
Millis, MA   2054-1511   508-376-1244
                                            Fax: 508-376-1245
                                          aqvideos@tiac.net
                                          www.aquariusproductions.com
Lesile Kussmann, Owner/President/Producer
Kathy Newkirk, Director
Jane Hutchinson, Assoc. Director
This thought-provoking video introduces viewers to people who
openly discuss the struggles and triumphs they have experienced
living in a body that is physically disabled. They talk honestly
about the social stigma of their disability and the problems they
face in terms of mobility, health care and family relationships, as
well as the challenges of emotional and sexual intimacy. Preview
option available. $195.00
Video

5401   My Country
Aquarius Health Care Videos
30 Forest Rd
PO Box 249
Millis, MA   2054-1511   508-376-1244
                                            Fax: 508-376-1245
                                          aqvideos@tiac.net
                                          www.aquariusproductions.com
Lesile Kussmann, Owner/President/Producer
Kathy Newkirk, Director
Jane Hutchinson, Assoc. Director
By telling the stories of three people with disabilities and their
struggle for equal rights under the law, this film draws a powerful
parallel between the efforts of disability rights activists and the
civil rights struggle of the 1960s. Great for disability awareness
programs, and for discussions of disability rights issues. Should
be part of every college curriculum on disabilities. Awarded Best
of Show Superfest 98. Preview option available. $195.00
Video

5402   No Barriers
Aquarius Health Care Videos
30 Forest Rd
PO Box 249
Millis, MA   2054-1511   508-376-1244
                                            Fax: 508-376-1245
                                          aqvideos@tiac.net
                                          www.aquariusproductions.com
Lesile Kussmann, Owner/President/Producer
Kathy Newkirk, Director
Jane Hutchinson, Assoc. Director
Everyone faces the world with different abilities and disabilities.
But everyone has at least one goal in common...to break through
their own barriers says Mark Wellman. Mark, a paraplegic, knows
this well. No Barriers takes us into Mark's world where he defies
the odds for most able bodied individuals by climbing Yosemite's
Half Dome and El Capitan. This video is more than inspiring and

fun to watch...it helps one make that paradigm shift from can't do to can do! Preview option available *$90.00*
Video

5403   On The Spectrum
Fanlight Productions
32 Court St.
21st Floor
Brooklyn, NY   11201-4421   718-488-8900
                                                                      800-876-1710
                                                              Fax: 718-488-8642
                                                              info@fanlight.com
                                                              www.fanlight.com

Jonathan Miller, President
Patricio Guzman, Director
Meredith Miller, Sales Manager
Anthony Sweeney, Acquisitions
Adults living with Asperger syndrome describe the ways AS has affected their lives, their work and their relationships. They discuss learning to cope with the disorder and the comfort and reinforcement of participating with others 'like them' in an Asperger's support group. 53 min. *$199.00*

5404   Open for Business
Disability Rights Education and Defense Fund
3075 Adeline Street
Suite 210
Berkeley, CA   94703-2219   510-644-2555
                                                                      800-841-8645
                                                              Fax: 510-841-8645
                                                              info@dredf.org
                                                              www.dredf.org

Sue Henderson, Executive Director
Jenny . Kern, Esq, President/Chair
Claudia Center, Esq, Treasurer
Vikki Davis, Secretary
Documentary video captures the drama and emotions of the historic civil rights demonstration of people with disabilities in 1977, resulting in the signing of the 504 Regulations, the first Federal Civil Rights Law protecting people with disabilities. Includes contemporary news footage and news interviews with participants and demonstration leaders. *$179.00*

5405   Open to the Public
Aquarius Health Care Videos
30 Forest Rd
PO Box 249
Millis, MA   2054-1511   508-376-1244
                                                              Fax: 508-376-1245
                                                              aqvideos@tiac.net
                                                      www.aquariusproductions.com

Lesile Kussmann, Owner/President/Producer
Kathy Newkirk, Director
Jane Hutchinson, Assoc. Director
Provides an overview of the Americans with Disabilities Act as it applies to state and local governments. The ADA doesn't provide recommendations for solving common problems, but this film could provide enough information for governments to solve some common problems without turning to high-priced consultants. Preview option available. *$125.00*
Video

5406   Our Own Road
Aquarius Health Care Videos
30 Forest Rd
PO Box 249
Millis, MA   2054-1511   508-376-1244
                                                              Fax: 508-376-1245
                                                              aqvideos@tiac.net
                                                      www.aquariusproductions.com
Lesile Kussmann, Owner/President/Producer
Kathy Newkirk, Director
Jane Hutchinson, Assoc. Director
This video shows the disabled helping other people who are disabled and portrays the sense of pride they get from helping others. This multicultural program features many different healing techniques, and teaches the importance of helping those who are disabled become independent and productive. *$99.00*

5407   Outsider: The Life and Art of Judith Scott
Fanlight Productions
32 Court St.
21st Floor
Brooklyn, NY   11201-4421   718-488-8900
                                                                      800-876-1710
                                                              Fax: 718-488-8642
                                                              info@fanlight.com
                                                              www.fanlight.com

Jonathan Miller, President
Patricio Guzman, Director
Meredith Miller, Sales Manager
Anthony Sweeney, Acquisitions
Judith Scoot has Down Syndrome, is deaf, and does not speak. Yet after 35 years of institutionalization, with the help of a sister who never gave up on her, she emerged to create a series of sculptures that have fascinated and mystified art experts and collectors around the world. 26 minutes. *$199.00*

5408   Passion for Justice
Fanlight Productions
32 Court St.
21st Floor
Brooklyn, NY   11201-4421   718-488-8900
                                                                      800-876-1710
                                                              Fax: 718-488-8642
                                                              info@fanlight.com
                                                              www.fanlight.com

Jonathan Miller, President
Patricio Guzman, Director
Meredith Miller, Sales Manager
Anthony Sweeney, Acquisitions
An unusually penetrating examination of the question of inclusion, this is an engaging portrait of Bob Perske, the author of Unequal Justice, and a crusader for the legal rights of people with developmental disabilities. A Passion for Justice asks challenging questions about society's responsibility to this population, and about ways to protect everyone's rights to equality and justice. *$99.00*
29 Minutes

5409   Phoenix Dance
Fanlight Productions
32 Court St.
21st Floor
Brooklyn, NY   11201-4421   718-488-8900
                                                                      800-876-1710
                                                              Fax: 718-488-8642
                                                              info@fanlight.com
                                                              www.fanlight.com

Jonathan Miller, President
Patricio Guzman, Director
Meredith Miller, Sales Manager
Anthony Sweeney, Acquisitions
A heroic journey of transformation and healing, Phoenix Dance challenges our expectations of what it means to be disabled. In March, 2001, renowned dancer Homer Avila discovered that the pain in his hip was cancer. A month later, his right leg and most of his hip were amputated. *$199.00*

5410   Pool Exercise Program - Arthritis Water Exercise / Arthritis Foundation
Arthritis Foundation Distribution Center
PO Box 932915
Atlanta, GA   31193-2915   440-872-7100
                                                                      800-283-7800
                                                              Fax: 404-872-0457
                                                              aforders@arthritis.org
                                                              www.arthritis.org

John Klippel, President/CEO
This video features water exercises that will help you increase and maintain joint flexibility, strengthen and tone muscles, and increase endurance. All exercises are performed in water at chest level. No swimming skills are necessary. *$19.50*

5411 Potty Learning for Children who Experience Delay
Exceptional Parent Library
PO Box 1807
Englewood Cliffs, NJ   7632-1207   201-947-6000
                                         800-535-1910
                                    Fax: 201-947-9376
                                    eplibrary@aol.com
                                    www.eplibrary.com

5412 Pushin' Forward
Fanlight Productions
32 Court St.
21st Floor
Brooklyn, NY   11201-4421   718-488-8900
                                         800-876-1710
                                    Fax: 718-488-8642
                                    info@fanlight.com
                                    www.fanlight.com

Jonathan Miller, President
Patricio Guzman, Director
Meredith Miller, Sales Manager
Anthony Sweeney, Acquisitions
Growing up poor and Latino, James Lilly was a gang member and
drug dealer until, at fifteen, he was shot in the back and paralyzed.
Today, he shares his story with inner city kids, and tells them
about one thing that helped him move on; wheelchair racing. In
Pushin' Forward he takes on the world's longest wheelchair race,
from Fairbanks to Anchorage, Alaska, in six days! 39 minutes.
$229.00

5413 Recognizing Children with Special Needs
Films Media Group
132 W. 31st St
16th Fl.
New York, NY   10001   800-322-8755
                                    Fax: 800-678-3633
                                    custserv@films.com
                                    www.films.com

DVD/Video

5414 Relaxation Techniques for People with Special Needs
Research Press
PO Box 9177
Dept. 11W
Champaign, IL   61826-9177   217-352-3273
                                         800-519-2707
                                    Fax: 217-352-1221
                                    rp@researchpress.com
                                    www.researchpress.com

David Parkinson, Chairman
Russell Pence, President
Gail Salyards, Dir. Of Marketing/President
The developers discuss and demonstrate how to use special relaxation procedures with children and adolescents who have developmental disabilities. They emphasize the need for students to
learn relaxation as a means of coping with stress and developing
self-control. During the scenes of Dr June Groden conducting relaxation training, viewers will see how to correctly use the training procedures, how to use reinforcement during training and
how to use guided imagery. 23 minutes. Includes book. *$195.00*
Video

5415 Right at Home
Aquarius Health Care Videos
30 Forest Rd
PO Box 249
Millis, MA   2054   508-376-1244
                                    Fax: 508-376-1245
                                    aqvideos@tiac.net
                                    www.aquariusproductions.com

Lesile Kussmann, Owner/President/Producer
Kathy Newkirk, Director
Jane Hutchinson, Assoc. Director
Shows simple solutions for complying with the Fair Hoiusing Act
amendments. Emphasizes low-cost, practical solutions, and
working with people with disabilities to find the best applicable
solution. Ideal for people with disabilities and their families, as

well as housing providers, university courses, and disability
awareness organizations. Preview option is available. *$99.00*
Video

5416 Seat-A-Robics
PO Box 630064
Little Neck, NY   11363-64   718-631-4007
Daria Alinovi, President
Offers a variety of safe, affordable and medically approved video
exercise programs that are listed in our video chapter. In addition
the company offers two resources. The first Healthy Eating &
Facts For Kids is geared specifically to health professionals and
educators that work with disabled children ($39.95). The second
is a recreational resource guide that stimulates children to be creative and get involved. It keeps them actively engaged while
having fun and getting fit ($29.95).

5417 Shining Bright: Head Start Inclusion
Brookes Publishing
PO Box 10624
Baltimore, MD   21285-624   410-337-9580
                                         800-638-3775
                                    Fax: 410-337-8539
                                    custserv@brookespublishing.com
                                    www.readplaylearn.com

Paul Brooks, Owner
This documentary depicts the collaborative efforts of a Head
Start and a local education agency to include children with severe
disabilities in a Head Start program. This video addresses issues
such as support for children with severe health impairments, benefits of participating in Head Start, ability of teachers with a general education background to serve children with severe
disabilities, and staff relations. Includes a 28-page sad-
dle-stitched booklet. *$45.00*
23 Minutes
ISBN 1-55766 -95-9

5418 Small Differences
Aquarius Health Care Videos
30 Forest Rd
PO Box 249
Millis, MA   2054-1511   508-376-1244
                                    Fax: 508-376-1245
                                    aqvideos@tiac.net
                                    www.aquariusproductions.com

Lesile Kussmann, Owner/President/Producer
Kathy Newkirk, Director
Jane Hutchinson, Assoc. Director
What happens when you give children with and without disabili-
ties a camera and ask them to produce a video about disabilities?
The result is an uplifting, award-winning disability video that
both children and adults can relate to. The kids interviewed adults
and children with physical and sensory disabilities. A top-quality
production that increases understanding and awareness. Winner,
Columbus International Film & Video Festival. Winner, National
Education Media Network. Preview option availabe *$110.00*
Video

5419 Someday's Child
Educational Productions
9000 SW Gemini Dr
Beaverton, OR   97008-7151   503-644-7000
                                         800-950-4949
                                    Fax: 503-350-7000
                                    custserv@edpro.com
                                    www.edpro.com

Diane Trister Dodge, Founder/President/Lead Author
Arnitra Duckett, VP, Sales & Strategic Marketing
This video focuses on three families' search for help and informa-
tion for their children with disabilities.

5420 Sound & Fury
Aquarius Health Care Videos
30 Forest Rd
PO Box 249
Millis, MA 2054-1511   508-376-1244
                                Fax: 508-376-1245
                          aqvideos@tiac.net
                      www.aquariusproductions.com
Lesile Kussmann, Owner/President/Producer
Kathy Newkirk, Director
Jane Hutchinson, Assoc. Director
This film takes viewers inside the seldom seen world of the deaf
to witness a painful family struggle over a controversial medical
technology called the cochlear implant. Some of the family mem-
bers celebrate the implant as a long overdue cure for deafness
while others fear it will destroy their language and way of life.
This documentary explores this seemingly irreconcilable conflict
as it illuminates the ongoing struggle for identity among deaf
people today. *$195.00*
Video

5421 Special Children/Special Solutions
Option Indigo Press
2080 S Undermountain Rd
Sheffield, MA 1257-9643   413-229-8727
                                   800-714-2779
                                Fax: 413-229-8727
                          indigo@option.org
                      www.optionindigo.com
Barry Kaufmans, Owner/Founder/Author
Samahria Kaufmans, Owner/Founder
This four-tape audio series presents concrete, down-to-earth,
no-nonsense alternatives which are full of love and acceptance
for the special child while being wholly supportive of parents,
professionals and helpers who want to reach out. The accepting
(nonjudgmental) attitude presented is the basis of all Samahria's
work and is the foundation for the nurturing teaching process that
has encouraged and helped parents, children and others to accomplish more than most would have believed. *$55.00*
Audio

5422 Technology for the Disabled
Landmark Media
3450 Slade Run Dr
Falls Church, VA 22042-3940   703-241-2030
                                   800-342-4336
                                Fax: 703-536-9540
                          info@landmarkmedia.com
                          landmarkmedia.com
Michael Hartogs, President
Joan Hartogs, Vice President
Peter Hartogs, Vice President
Richard Hartogs, Vice President
Physically disabled people cope with the frustrations of a body
they cannot control. The computer age has made many disabled
more self-reliant; armless feed themselves, the blind read news-
papers and the voiceless speak through marvelous technological
breakthroughs. *$195.00*
Video

5423 Three R's for Special Education: Rights, Resources, Results
Brookes Publishing
PO Box 10624
Baltimore
MD, 21 0624-624   410-337-9580
                                   800-638-3775
                                Fax: 410-337-8539
                          custserv@brookespublishing.com
Paul Brooks, Owner
This is a guide for parents, and a tool for educators. Through this
video parents learn how to work through the steps of the special
education system and work toward securing the best education
and services for their children. Reviews the laws to protect children with disabilities in easy to understand language. Also provides a list of national organizations that can offer resources,
information and advice to parents. *$49.95*
50 Minutes
ISBN 0-96461-80-7

5424 Tools for Students
Aquarius Health Care Videos
30 Forest Rd
PO Box 249
Millis, MA 2054-1511   508-376-1244
                                Fax: 508-376-1245
                          aqvideos@tiac.net
                      www.aquariusproductions.com
Lesile Kussmann, Owner/President/Producer
Kathy Newkirk, Director
Jane Hutchinson, Assoc. Director
Provides a series of 26 fun occupational therapy sensory processing activities. Designed as an in-home, in-workshop, and in-class
exercise leader with students. Activities include: Strenghten the
muscles necessary for normal activities, provide the muscles necessary to enhance alertness and concentration, increase the ability to use good posture, help social skills and fitting in and
increase coordination; concludes with emphasis on team collaboration between the student, teacher, and parents. *$99.00*
Video

5425 Video Guide to Disability Awareness
Aquarius Health Care Videos
30 Forest Rd
PO Box 249
Millis, MA 2054-1511   508-376-1244
                                Fax: 508-376-1245
                          aqvideos@tiac.net
                      www.aquariusproductions.com
Lesile Kussmann, Owner/President/Producer
Kathy Newkirk, Director
Jane Hutchinson, Assoc. Director
President Clinton opens and concludes this informative video
about disability awareness. A series of candid interviews with
people who have a wide range of disabilities provide personal in-
sights into the issues surrounding visual, hearing, physical and
mental disabilities. Video comes with written reference guide and
is also available with open or closed captioning. Preview option
available. *$195.00*
Video

5426 Video Intensive Parenting
Systems Unlimited/LIFE Skills
1556 S 1st Ave
Iowa City, IA 52240-6007   319-356-5412
Geoffrey Lauer, Program Director
Bill Gorman, President
Ginny Kirschling, Public Information Specialist
Parents who have children with special needs share their reac-
tions to their child's diagnosis and how they have learned to cope
with their feelings. *$69.95*

5427 Vital Signs: Crip Culture Talks Back
Fanlight Productions
32 Court St.
21st Floor
Brooklyn, NY 11201-4421   718-488-8900
                                   800-876-1710
                                Fax: 718-488-8642
                          info@fanlight.com
                          www.fanlight.com
Jonathan Miller, President
Patricio Guzman, Director
Meredith Miller, Sales Manager
Anthony Sweeney, Acquisitions
This edgy, raw video documentary explores the politics of dis-
ability through the performances, debates and late-night conver-
sations of artists at a recent national conference of disabilities
and the art's. Vital Signs conveys the intensity, variety and vital-
ity of disability culture today. *$225.00*
Video

5428 What About Me?
Educational Productions
9000 SW Gemini Dr
Beaverton, OR   97008-7151   503-644-7000
                                                    800-950-4949
                                              Fax: 503-350-7000
                                           custserve@cdpro.com
                                        www.teachingstrategies.com
Diane Trister Dodge, Founder/President/Lead Author
Arnitra Duckett, VP, Sales & Strategic Marketing
This video focuses on two siblings of children with disabilities.
The siblings (Brian and Julie) share their perspectives, their wor-
ries, concerns and victories about living with a sibling with a
disability.

5429 When Billy Broke His Head...and Other
Fanlight Productions
32 Court St.
21st Floor
Brooklyn, NY   11201-4421   718-488-8900
                                                    800-876-1710
                                              Fax: 718-488-8642
                                             info@fanlight.com
                                               www.fanlight.com

Jonathan Miller, President
Patricio Guzman, Director
Meredith Miller, Sales Manager
Anthony Sweeney, Acquisitions
When Billy Golfus, an award-winning journalist, became brain
damaged as the result of a motor scooter accident, he joined the
ranks of the 43 million Americans with disabilities, this country's
largest and most invisible minority. He helped create this video,
which blends humor with politics and individual experience with
a chorus of voices, to explain what it is really like to live with a
disability in America. #136 *$195.00*
ISBN 1-57295-36-2

5430 When I Grow Up
Britannica Film Company
345 4th St
San Francisco, CA   94107-1206   415-928-8466
                                              Fax: 415-928-5027

Dave Bekowich, Owner
At a costume party each child was to come as what they wanted to
be when they grew up. Some of the children had handicaps, and
they talked about why their handicaps would not prevent them
from fulfilling their desires.
Film

5431 When Parents Can't Fix It
Fanlight Productions
32 Court St.
21st Floor
Brooklyn, NY   11201-4421   718-488-8900
                                                    800-876-1710
                                              Fax: 718-488-8642
                                             info@fanlight.com
                                               www.fanlight.com

Jonathan Miller, President
Patricio Guzman, Director
Meredith Miller, Sales Manager
Anthony Sweeney, Acquisitions
This documentary looks at the lives of five families who are raising children with disabilities - the problems they face, how they
have learned to cope, and the rewards and stresses of adapting to
their child's condition. It explores the medical complexities and
financial pressures families encounter, the emotional and physical toll on parents and siblings, and the dangers of child abuse in
this population. It offers a very realistic look at different family
strengths and coping styles.
58 Min. DVD/VHS
ISBN 1-572958-76-6

5432 White Cane and Wheels
Fanlight Productions
32 Court St.
21st Floor
Brooklyn, NY   11201-4421   718-488-8900
                                                    800-876-1710
                                              Fax: 718-488-8642
                                             info@fanlight.com
                                               www.fanlight.com

Jonathan Miller, President
Patricio Guzman, Director
Meredith Miller, Sales Manager
Anthony Sweeney, Acquisitions
Carmen and Steve once dreamed of lives on stage and screen, but
their plans were cut short by her blindness and his muscular dystrophy. This program is a funny and touching exploration of a relationship filled with frustration, but held together with patience,
stubborness, forgiveness, and love. 26 minutes. *$169.00*

5433 Why My Child
976 Lake Baldwin Lane
Suite 104
Orlando, FL   32814   407-895-0802
                                                   800-313-ABDC
                                             staff@birthdefects.org
                                               www.birthdefects.org

---

Web Sites

5434 ADA Questions and Answers
U.S. Department of Justice, Civil Rights Division
950 Pennsylvania Ave NW
Washington, DC   20530-0001   202-514-4609
                                              Fax: 202-307-1197
                                             TTY:202-514-0716
                                                      www.ada.gov

5435 Ability Jobs
Ability Magazine
P.O. Box 10878
Costa Mesa, CA   92627   www.abilityjobs.com

**5436 AbleApparel - Affordable Adaptive Clothing and
Accessories**
2121 Hillside Ave
New Hyde Park, NY   11040-2712   516-873-6552
                                              Fax: 516-248-7308
                                             sales@abledata.com
                                              www.ableapparel.com

Mary Ann Tenaglia, Partner
Marie Harmon, Partner
Donna Lo Monica, Partner/Designer
AbleApparel is always designing and creating new products that
will make Matty's life and others with disabilities a little easier.
Most of the people spoken to regardless of age want to be able to
wear clothes that are functional, affordable and, above all,
fashionable.

5437 AbleData
103 W Broad St
Suite 400
Falls Church, VA   22046   301-608-8998
                                                    800-227-0216
                                              Fax: 301-608-8958
                                             TTY: 301-608-8912
                                         abledata@neweditions.net
                                                www.abledata.com

Katherine Belknap, Director
David Johnson, Publications Director
AbleData provides objective information on assistive technology
and rehabilitation equipment available from domestic and international sources to consumers, organizations, professionals, and
caregivers within the United States. AbleData serves the nation's
disability, rehabilitation and senior communities.

5438 Access Unlimited
570 Hance Rd
Binghamton, NY   13903-5700
607-669-4822
800-849-2143
Fax: 607-669-4595
www.accessunlimited.com

Thomas Egan, President/Owner
Tom 'TC' Cole, National Sales Manager
Adaptive transportation and mobility equipment for people with disabilities. ccess Unlimited products empower people with disabilities to regain control of their mobility.

5439 Ai Squared
130 Taconic Business Park
Manchester Center, VT   05255-9752
802-362-3612
800-859-0270
Fax: 802-362-1670
sales@aisquared.com
www.aisquared.com

David Wu, CEO
Jost Eckhardt, VP of Engineering
Doug Hacker, VP of Business Development
Scott Moore, VP of Marketing
Ai Squared has been a leader in the assistive technology field for over 20 years. Our flagship product, ZoomText, is the world's best magnification and reading software for the vision impaired. We pride ourselves on delivering the highest quality software products and superior technical support.

5440 Alternatives in Education for the Hearing Impaired (AEHI)
9300 Capitol Drive
Wheeling, IL   60090-7207
847-850-5490
Fax: 847-850-5493
info@agbms.org
www.agbms.org

Sandra L. Mosetick, Board President Emeritus
Bridget Chevez, Board President
Daniel Konopacki, Treasurer
Debra Trude-Suter, Ph.D., CEO/Executive Director
AEHI is a program of the Alexander Graham Bell Montessori School in Mt. Prospect, IL, that fosters literacy and empowers people with hearing impairments to achieve their full potential through unique educational options. AEHI provides Cued Speech workshops, individualized parental training and support, educational consulting, professional development opportunities, and access to a wide variety of information on Cued Speech and its benefits.

5441 American Academy of Audiology
11480 Commerce Park Drive
Suite 220
Reston, VA   20190- 4748
800-222-2336
Fax: 703-476-5157
infoaud@audiology.org
www.audiology.org

Cheryl Kreider Carey, Executive Director
Edward Sullivan, Deputy Executive Director
Deborah Carlson, PhD, President
Shilpi Banerjee, PhD, Board Member
The American Academy of Audiology is the world's largest professional organization of, by, and for audiologists. The active membership of more than 11,000 is dedicated to providing quality hearing care services through professional development, education, research, and increased public awareness of hearing and balance disorders.

5442 American Association of People with Disabilities
2013 H Street, NW
5th Floor
Washington, DC   20006-1675
202-457-0046
800-840-8844
Fax: 866-536-4461
www.aapd.com

Mark Perriello, President/CEO
Henry Claypool, Executive Vice President
Ginny Thornburgh, Director of Interfaith Initiative
TaKeisha Walker, Director of Workplace & Leadership Initiatives
The American Association of People with Disabilities is the nation's largest disability rights organization. We promote equal opportunity, economic power, independent living, and political participation for people with disabilities. Our members, including people with disabilities and our family, friends, and supporters, represent a powerful force for change.

5443 American Botanical Council
6200 Manor Rd
PO Box 144345
Austin, TX   78723-4345
512-926-4900
800-373-7105
Fax: 512-926-2345
abc@herbalgram.org
www.abc.herbalgram.org

Mark Blumenthal, Founder/Executive Director
Gayle Engels, Special Projects Director
Matthew Magruder, Art Director
Denise Meikel, Development Director
Provide education using science-based and traditional information to promote responsible use of herbal medicine - serving the public, researchers, educators, healthcare professionals, industry and media.

5444 American College of Rheumatology, Researchand Education Foundation
2200 Lake Boulevard NE
Atlanta, GA   30319-5310
404-633-3777
Fax: 404-633-1870
acr@rheumatology.org
www.rheumatology.org

Audrey B. Uknis, MD, President
David I. Daikh, MD, PhD, Foundation President
Jan K. Richardson, PT, PhD, O, ARHP President
E. William St.Clair, MD, Treasurer
The American College of Rheumatology's mission is advancing rheumatology.The organization represents over 8,500 rheumatologists and rheumatology health professionals around the world. The ACR offers its members the support they need to ensure that they are able to continue their innovative work by providing programs of education, research, advocacy , and practice support.

5445 American Liver Foundation
39 Broadway
Suite 2700
New York, NY   10006-3054
212-668-1000
Fax: 212-483-8179
www.liverfoundation.org

Ryan Reczek, National Director, Field Development
Rolf Taylor, National Director, Corporate Relations
Pritha Kuchaculla, National Director, Programs
David Ticker, Chief Financial Officer
Is the only national voluntary health organization dedicated to preventing, treating, and curing hepatitis and other liver and gall bladder diseases through research and education.

5446 American Mobility: Personal Mobility Solutions
60 Island St
Lawrence, MA   1840-1835
978-794-3030
www.americanmobility.com

David Lacroix, President
Source of Pride Scooters, Jazzy Power Chairs, personal mobility vehicles, and lift and recline chairs.

5447   American Speech-Language and Hearing Association
2200 Research Blvd
Rockville, MD   20850-3289
301-296-5700
800-638-8255
Fax: 301-296-8580
TTY: 301-296-5650
actioncenter@asha.org
www.asha.org

Wayne A. Foster, PhD, CCC-SLP/A, Chair, Audiology Advisory Council
Patricia A. Prelock, PhD, CCC-SLP, President
Carolyn W. Higdon, EdD, CCC-SLP, Vice President for Finance
Howard Goldstein, PhD, CCC-SL, Vice President for Science and Research
Exhibits by companies specializing in alternative and augmentative communications products, publishers, software and hardware compinies, and hearing aid testing equipment manufacturers.

5448   Americans with Disabilities Act: ADA Home Page
800-514-0301
TTY:800-514-0383
webmaster@usdoj.gov
www.ada.gov

5449   Appliance 411
www.appliance411.com

5450   Arc of the United States
1825 K Street, NW
Suite 1200
Washington, DC   20006-5689
202-534-3700
800-433-5255
Fax: 202-534-3731
info@thearc.org
www.thearc.org

Gary Bass, Director
Carol Wheeler, Director
Nancy Webster, President
Ronald Brown, Vice President
We are the largest national community-based organization advocating for and serving people with intellectual and developmental disabilities and their families. We encompass all ages and all spectrums from autism, Down syndrome, Fragile X and various other developmental disabilities.

5451   Association for the Cure of Cancer of the Prostate (CaP CURE)-Prostate Cancer Foundation
1250 Fourth St
Suite 360
Santa Monica, CA   90401-1444
310-570-4700
800-757-2873
Fax: 310-570-4701
info@pcf.org
www.pcf.org

Mike Milken, Founder/Chairman
Jonathon Simons, MD, President/CEO
Ralph Finerman, Chief Financial Officer/Treasurer/Secretary
Howard R. Soule, PhD, Executive Vice President /Chief Science Officer
CURE is a nonprofit public charity that is dedicated to supporting prostate cancer research and hastening the conversion of research into cures or controls.

5452   Asthma and Allergy Foundation of America
8201 Corporate Drive
Suite 1000
Landover, MD   20785-2266
800-727-8462
info@aafa.org
www.aafa.org

Lynn Hanessian, Chair
Michele Abu Carrick, LICSW, Co-Chair, Governance
Judi McAuliffe, RN, Co-Chair, Programs & Services
Calvin Enderson, Chair/Finance/Treasurer

AAFA is dedicated to improving the quality of life for people with asthma and allergic diseases through education, advocacy and research.

5453   Auditory-Verbal International
Alexander Graham Bell Association
3417 Volta Pl. NW
Washington, DC   20007
202-204-4700
Fax: 202-337-8314
academy@agbell.org
www.agbell.org

Ted A. Meyer, Chair
Catharine McNally, Chair-Elect
Susan Lenihan, Secretary
Emilion Alonso Mendoza, Chief Exectuive Officer
Focus on education, guidance, advocacy, family support and the rigorous application of techniques to promote optimal acquision of spoken language.

5454   BDRC Newsletter
Birth Defect Research for Children
976 Lake Baldwin Ln
Ste. 104
Orlando, FL   32814
407-895-0802
Fax: 407-895-0824
staff@birthdefects.org
www.birthdefects.org

Betty Mekdeci, Executive Director
A monthly electronic newsletter offering the latest news, research, and updates on birth defects.
Monthly

5455   Cancer Immunotherapy and Gene Therapy
www.skcc.org

5456   Cancer Research Institute
29 Broadway
4th Floor
New York, NY   10006
212-688-7515
800-992-2623
Fax: 212-832-9376
info@cancerresearch.org
www.cancerresearch.org

Jill O'Donnell-Tormey, CEO & Director of Scientific Affair
Lynne Harmer, Director of Grants Administration and Special Events
Alfred R. Massidas, Chief Financial Officer and Director of Human Resources
Alexandra S. Mulvey, Associate Director of Communications
Nonprofit organization dedicated to cancer immunotherapy.

5457   Center on the Social & Emotional Foundations for Early Learning (CSEFEL)
Vanderbilt University 110 Magnolia
Box 328 GPC
Nashville, TN   37203
615-322-8150
Fax: 615-343-1570
ml.hemmeter@vanderbilt.edu
csefel.vanderbilt.edu

Mary-Louise Hemmeter, Principal Investigator
Rob Corso, Project Coordinator
Tweety Yates, Project Coordinator
Glen Dunlap, Key Center Personnel
The center will: focus on promoting the social and emotional developmental of children as a means of preventing challenging behaviors; collaborate with existing T/TA providers for the purpose of ensuring the implementation and sustainability of practices at the local level; provide ongoing identification of training needs and preferred delivery formats of local programs and T/TA providers; disseminate evidence-based practices.

5458 Damon Runyon Cancer Research Foundation
Walter Winchell Foundation
One Exchange Plaza, 55 Broadway
Suite 302
New York, NY 10006-3720 212-455-0500
877-722-6237
info@damonrunyon.org
www.damonrunyon.org
Lorraine Egan, President/Chief Executive Officer
Elizabeth Portland, Director of Development
Marialice C. Pagnotta, Director of the Damon Runyon Broadway Tickets Service
Kimberly Kubert, Director of Special Events
The Damon Runyon Cancer Research Foundation funds early career cancer researchers who have the energy, drive and creativity to become leading innovators in their fields. We identify the best young scientists in the nation and support them through four award programs: our Fellowship, Pediatric Cancer Fellowship, Clinical Investigator and Innovation Awards.

5459 DisAbility Information and Resources

jlubin@eskimo.com
www.makoa.org
Jim Lubin, Creator/Owner
Offers dozens of links to sites with information, services and products for the disabled.

5460 Disability Rights Activist

www.disrights.org

5461 DisabilityAdvisor.com
37 North Orange Ave.
Suite 500
Orlando, FL 32801 321-332-7800
888-393-1010
Fax: 888-985-6060
joeram@disabilityadvisor.com
www.disabilityadvisor.com
Joseph E. Ram, Publisher
Kay Derochie, Editor
Jackie Booth, Ph.D., Editor
Lisa Nuss, Writer
DisabilityAdvisor.com provides free information on federal and state disability benefits programs and other resources for readers and their families. This includes disabled children and students, military veterans, injured workers and disabled seniors. Readers are encouraged to submit their questions and comments online. The website also offers information on managing finances, education, parenting, relationships and other issues of interest to the disabled and their friends and families.

5462 DisabilityResources.org
Four Glatter Lane
Dept. IN
Centereach, NY 11720-1032 631-585-0290
Fax: 631-585-0290
Julie Klauber, Co-founder/Managing Editor
Avery Klauber, Co-Founder/Executive Director
Sally Rosenthal, Contributing Editor
Ruth Porfert, Editorial Assistant
Disability Resources, inc. is a nonprofit 501(c)(3) organization established to promote and improve awareness, availability and accessibility of information that can help people with disabilities live, learn, love, work and play independently.

5463 Discover Technology
Houston, TX 713-885-1519
dtinc8888@hotmail.com
www.discovertechnology.com
Amantha Cole, Founder
The primary mission of Discover Technology, Inc. is to create and administer computer labs for persons with disabilities, to encourage communication between persons with and without disabilities and to educate the general population about the disabled population.

5464 Dynamic Living
125 Old Iron Ore Road
Bloomfield, CT 06002-1315 860-683-4442
888-940-0605
Fax: 860-243-1910
info@dynamic-living.com
www.dynamic-living.com
Andrea Tannenbaum, Owner
Kitchen products, bathroom helpers, and unique daily living products that provide a convienient, comfortable, and safe environment for people with disabilities.

5465 ElderLawAnswers.com
150 Chesnut St
4th Floor, Box #15
Providence, RI 02903 866-267-0947
support@elderlawanswers.com
www.elderlawanswers.com
Harry S. Margolis, Founder/President
Ken Coughlin, Editor
Mark Miller, Director of Product and Business Development
Wendy Miki Glaus, Attorney
Provides information about legal issues facing senior citizens and a searchable directory of attorneys.

5466 Exploring Autism: A Look at the Genetics of Autism
Box 3445 DUMC
Durham, NC 27710 *Fax:* 919-684-0952
Chantelle Wolpert, Project Director
Dedicated to helping families who are living with the challenges of autism stay informed about the exciting breakthroughs involving the genetics of autism. Report and explain new genetic research findings. Explain genetic principles as they relate to autism, provide the latest research news, and seek your imput.

5467 FHI 360
1825 Connecticut Ave., NW
Suite 800
Washington, DC 20009-5721 202-884-8000
Fax: 202-884-8400
CareerCenterSupport@fhi360.org
www.fhi360.org
Willard Cates Jr, MD, MPH, President Emeritus
Albert J. Siemens, PhD, Chief Executive Officer
Patrick C. Fine, MS, Chief Operating Officer
Robert S. Murphy, MBA, Chief Financial Officer
FHI 360 is a nonprofit human development organization dedicated to improving lives in lasting ways by advancing integrated, locally driven solutions.

5468 Foundation Fighting Blindness
7168 Columbia Gateway Dr.
Suite 100
Columbia, MD 21046 410-423-0600
800-683-5555
TTY:410363713951
info@FightBlindness.org
www.blindness.org
William T. Schmidt, Chief Executive Officer
Valerie Navy-Daniels, Chief Development Officer
Stephen M. Rose, PhD, Chief Research Officer
The Foundation Fighting Blindness (FFB) works to promote research in order to prevent, treat and restore vision. FFB is currently the world's leading private funder of retinal disease research, funding over 100 research grants and 150 researchers.

5469 Freedom Scientific
11830 31st Court North
St. Petersburg, FL 33716-1805 727-803-8000
800-444-4443
Fax: 727-803-8001
info@freedomscientific.com
www.freedomscientific.com
Lee Hamilton, President/CEO/Chairman
Mike Self, Sales Representative
Joseph McDaniel, Sales Representative
Bobby Lakey, Sales Representative

Assistive technology for blind and visually impaired computer users.

5470   Gallaudet University Press
800 Florida Ave, NE
Washington, DC 20002-3695

202-651-5488
Fax: 202-651-5489
gupress@gallaudet.edu
www.gupress.gallaudet.edu

5471   Glaucoma Research Foundation
251 Post Street
Suite 600
San Francisco, CA 94108-5017

415-986-3162
800-826-6693
question@glaucoma.org
www.glaucoma.org

Andrew Iwach, MD, Board Chair/Executive Director
Thomas r M. Brunne, President/CEO
H. Allen Bouch, Vice Chair
Fred H. Brinkmann, Treasurer
Our mission is to prevent vision loss from glaucoma by investing in innovative research, education, and support with the ultimate goal of finding a cure.

5472   HealthyWomen
P.O. Box 430
Red Bank, NJ 07701

732-530-3425
877-986-9472
Fax: 732-865-7225
info@healthywomen.org
www.healthywomen.org

Oxana K Pickeral, Ph.D, MBA, Chair
Beth Battaglino, CEO
Phyllis E Greenberger, MSW, Senior Vice President, Science & Health Policy
Amy Takis, Director of Communications & Development
Website providing information for women with disabilities, health professionals, researchers, and caretakers.

5473   Herb Research Foundation
5589 Arapahoe Ave
Suite 205
Boulder, CO 80303-8115

303-449-2265
www.herbs.org

Rob McCaleb, President
John Lowe, Director of Research
Research and public education on the health benefits of medicinal plants. Dedicated to world health through the informed use of herbs.

5474   Hypokalemic Periodic Paralysis Resource Page
155 West 68th St
Suite 1732
New York, NY 10023-5830

407-339-9499
lfeld@cfl.rr.com
www.periodicparalysis.org

Jacob Levitt, President/Medical Director
Linda Feld, Vice President
Provides understandable information on HKPP, dynamia linkage to several additional sources of helpful information on the Internet, and offers several online networking opportunities.

5475   INCLUDEnyc
Formerly Resources for Children with Special Needs
116 E. 16th St.
5th Fl.
New York, NY 10003

212-677-4650
Fax: 202-254-4070
info@includenyc.org
www.includenyc.org

Barbara Glassman, Executive Director
Todd Dorman, Senior Director of Communications and Outreach
Mariko Sakita, Director of Parent & Family Services
Lori Podvesker, Senior Manager of Disability and Education Policy
Provides free services and resources for youth and families with disabilities in all five state boroughs. Organizational services include: Parenting & Advocacy; School and Community Activities; Parent counseling and Training for students with Autism; Medicaid Waiver services; Transition and Adult Services; and Social skills and building relationships.

5476   Innovation Management Group
179 Niblick Road
Suite 454
Paso Robles, CA 93446-4845

818-701-1579
800-889-0987
Fax: 818-936-0200
sales@imgpresents.com
www.imgpresents.com

5477   Interstitial Cystitis Association
1760 Old Meadow Road
Suite 500
McLean, VA 22102-2651

703-442-2070
800-435-7422
Fax: 703-506-3266
icamail@ichelp.org
www.ichelp.org

Barbara Gordon, Co-Chair/Executive Director
Eric Zarnikow, MBA, Co-Chair
Marilynn Schreibstein, CFO
F. Neal Thompson, Treasurer
The Interstitial Cystitis Association (ICA) advocates for interstitial cystitis (IC) research dedicated to discovery of a cure and better treatments, raises awareness, and serves as a central hub for the healthcare providers, researchers and millions of patients who suffer with constant urinary urgency and frequency and extreme bladder pain called IC. (IC is also referred to as painful bladder syndrome, bladder pain syndrome, and chronic pelvic pain.)

5478   LD OnLine - WETA Public Television
2775 S. Quincy Street
Arlington, VA 22206-2269

703-998-2060
Fax: 703-998-2060
ldonline@weta.org
www.ldonline.org

Noel Gunther, Executive Director
Christian Lindstrom, Director
Tina Chovanec, Director
Shalini Anand, Senior Mangager
LD OnLine seeks to help children and adults reach their full potential by providing accurate and up-to-date information and advice about learning disabilities and ADHD. The site features hundreds of helpful articles, multimedia, monthly columns by noted experts, first person essays, children's writing and artwork, a comprehensive resource guide, very active forums, and a Yellow Pages referral directory of professionals, schools, and products.

5479   Lyme Disease Foundation
PO Box 332
Tolland, CT 6084-332

860-870-0070
Fax: 860-870-0080
info@lyme.org
www.lyme.org

Karen Forschuer, Chairman
Thomas Forschuer, Executive Director
Provides critical information about tick-borne disease prevention, improves healthcare and funds research for solutions. 500,000 children, adults, and professionals assisted 25 countries.

5480   Mainstream Living
333 SW 9th St
Des Moines, IA 50309

515-243-8115
Fax: 515-243-5017
www.mainstreamliving.org

5481   Mainstream Online Magazine of the Able-Disabled

www.mainstream-mag.com

Cyndi Jones, Publisher
William G. Stothers, Editor

The leading news, advocacy and lifestyle magazine for people with disabilities.

5482 Microsoft Accessibility Technology for Everyone
One Microsoft Way
Redmond, WA 98052-6399
425-882-8080
800-642-7676
Fax: 425-936-7329
TTY: 800-892-5234
www.microsoft.com/enable

William Gates III, Chairman
Steven Ballmer, CEO/Director
Information about accessibility features and options included in Microsoft products.

5483 MossRehab ResourceNet
1200 West Tabor Road
Philadelphia, PA 19141-3099
215-456-9900
800-225-5567
www.mossresourcenet.org

John Whyte, Owner
Ruth Lefton, COO
Anthony Allonardo, Director of Technology
MossRehab, a modern, 147-bed facility, offers comprehensive care to people with a broad range of conditions—including stroke, brain injury, orthopaedic and musculoskeletal disabilities, spinal cord dysfunction, pulmonary disorders, amputations, and other forms of disability.

5484 Multiple Sclerosis National Research Institute
11350 SW Village Parkway
Port St. Lucie, FL 34987-2352
858-597-3872
866-676-7400
Fax: 858-597-3804
info@ms-research.org
www.ms-research.org

Robin Offord, Chairman
Richard Houghten, President/CEO
Donald B. Cooper, C.F.O
Karen Douthitt, VP & Corporate Secretary
Multiple Sclerosis National Research Institute is a division of Torrey Pines Institute for Molecular Studies, a not-for-profit basic research center dedicated to the discovery and development of innovative research methods that lead to treatments for major medical conditions, including multiple sclerosis, AIDS, Alzheimer's disease, pain, heart disease, many types of cancer, and more.

5485 National Alliance of the Disabled(NAOTD)
www.naotd.wheelboat.com

Walton Dutcher, Executive Director/Operations
Fred Temple, Director
Spike Spikberg, Director
Donna Eustice, Director
The National Alliance OF The DisAbled is an online informational and advocacy organization dedicated to working towards gaining equal rights for the disAbled in all areas of life.

5486 National Association for Visually Handicapped Lighthouse International
111 E 59th St
New York, NY 10022-1202
212-821-9497
800-829-0500
Fax: 212-821-9707
TTY: 212-821-9713
www.lighthouse.org/navh

Karen Campbell, Director of Social Services
Mark Ackermann, President/CEO
Jonathan Wainwright, VP & Secretary
Since 1905, Lighthouse International has led the charge in the fight against vision loss through prevention, treatment and empowerment.

5487 National Brain Tumor Foundation - National Brain Tumor Society
55 Chapel Street
Suite 200
Newton, MA 02458-2599
617-924-9997
800-770-8287
Fax: 617-928-9998
info@braintumor.org
www.braintumor.org

Jeffrey Kolodin, Chair
Michael Nathanson, Vice Chair
N. Paul TonThat, Executive Director
Michele Rhee, Director of Program Initiatives
An organization serving people whose lives are affected by brain tumors. The organization is dedicated to promoting a cure for brain tumors, improving the quality of life and giving hope to the brain tumor community by funding meaningful research and providing patient resources, timely information and education.

5488 National Business & Disability Council
201 I.U. Willets Road
Albertson, NY 11507-1516
516-465-1516
lfrancis@viscardicenter.org
www.business-disability.com
Michael C. Pascucci, Executive Leadership Team Chairman
Laura Francis, Executive Director
John D. Kemp, President
The NBDC is the leading resource for employers seeking to integrate people with disabilities into the workplace and companies seeking to reach them in the consumer marketplace.

5489 National Organization on Disability
77 Water St.
Suite 204
New York, NY 10005
646-505-1191
Fax: 646-505-1184
info@nod.org
www.nod.org

Carol Glazer, President
Lindsay Beltzer, Chief of Staff
Amber Cecil, Communications Manager
Howard Green, Deputy Director
The National Organization on Disability promotes the full and equal participation of men, women and children with disabilities in all aspects of American life.

5490 National Rehabilitation Information Center
8400 Corporate Drive
Suite 500
Landover, MD 20785-2266
301-459-5900
800-346-2742
Fax: 301-459-4263
TTY: 301-459-5984
www.naric.com

Mark X. Odum, Director
Jessica H. Chaiken, Media and Information Services Manager
Natalie J. Collier, Library and Acquisitions Manager
Tamara J. Pyle, Library and Information Services Coordinator
Serves both professionals and the general public intersted in disability and rehabilitation.

5491 NeuroControl Corporation
8333 Rockside Rd
Valley View, OH 44125-6134
216-912-0101
800-378-6955
Fax: 216-912-0129
www.neurocontrol.com

5492 Newsletter of PA's AT Lending Library
Temple University Institute on Disabilities
1755 N 13th Street
Student Center, Room 411S
Philadelphia, PA 19122-6024   215-204-1356
                                      800-204-PIAT
                                  Fax: 215-204-6336
                                  TTY: 215-204-1805
                                  iod@temple.edu
                        www.disabilities.temple.edu/atlend
Celia Feinstein, Co-Executive Director of the Institute on Disabilities
Amy Goldman, Co-Executive Director of the Institute on Disabilities
Ann Marie, Deputy Director
Kristin Ahrens, PA Consumer & Family Training Project Assistant Director
Newsletter from the Assistive Technology Lending Library in
Pennsylvania. It is produced quarterly, is free of charge, and is
available online only.
4-8 pages Quarterly

5493 Office of Juvenile Justice and Delinquency Prevention
810 Seventh St NW
Washington, DC 20531-3718   202-307-5911
                                      800-851-3420
                                  Fax: 301-519-5600
                                  www.ojjdp.gov
Kathi Grasso, Director, Concentration of Federal Efforts Program
Robert Listenbee, Jr., Administrator
Melodee Hanes, Principal Deputy Administrator
Nancy Ayers, Deputy Administrator for Operations
The Office of Juvenile Justice and Delinquency Prevention
(OJJDP) provides national leadership, coordination, and resources to prevent and respond to juvenile delinquency and victimization. OJJDP supports states and communities in their
efforts to develop and implement effective and coordinated prevention and intervention programs and to improve the juvenile
justice system so that it protects public safety, holds offenders accountable, and provides treatment and rehabilitative services
tailored

5494 Osteogenesis Imperfecta Foundation
804 W. Diamond Ave.
Suite 210
Gaithersburg, MD 20878- 1414   301-947-0083
                                      800-981-2663
                                  Fax: 301-947-0456
                                  bonelink@oif.org
                                  www.oif.org
Mary Beth Huber, Director of Program Services
Tom Costanzo, Director of Finance & Administration
*Erika r Ruebensaal Carte, Director of Communications & Develop-
ment*
Tracy Smith Hart, Chief Executive Officer
Strives to improve the quality of life for indivduals with this brit-
tle bone disorder through research, education, awareness, and
mutual support.

5495 Quantum Technologies
25242 Arctic Ocean Drive
Lake Forest, CA 92630-6217   949-930-3400
                                  Fax: 949-399-4600
                                  www.qtww.com
Dale Rasmussen, Chairman
Alan Niedzwieck, President/Director
W. Brian Olson, Chief Executive Officer
Bradley J. Timon, Chief Financial Officer
Provides access to information and tools for independence to
serve the visually impaired and those with a learning disability.

5496 Regional Resource Centers Program
1 Quality Street
Suite 721
Lexington, KY 40507   859-257-4921
                                  Fax: 859-257-4353
                                  TTY:859-257-2903
                                  mike.abell@uky.edu
                                  www.rrcprogram.org
Shauna Crane, RRCP Coordinator
Perry Williams, OSEP, Team Member
Mike Abell, Team Member
Betty Beale, Team Member
The Regional Resource Centers Program provides service to all
states as well as the Pacific jurisdictions, the Virgin Islands, and
Puerto Rico. The six regional program centers are funded by the
federal Office of Special Education Programs (OSEP) to assist
state education agencies in the systemic improvement of educa-
tion programs, practices, and policies that affect children and
youth with disabilities.

5497 Research!America
1101 King Street
Suite 520
Alexandria, VA 22314-2960   703-739-2577
                                      800-366-2873
                                  Fax: 703-739-2372
                                  info@researchamerica.org
                                  www.researchamerica.org
Hon. John Edward Porter, Chair
Hon. Michael Castle, Vice Chair
Mary Woolley, President/CEO
Barbara Love, Executive Assitant to the President
Builds active public support for more government and private-in-
dustry research to find treatments and cures for both physical and
mental disorders.

5498 Social Security Online
5 Park Centre Court
Suite 100
Owings Mills, MD 21117-1   800-772-1213
                                  TTY:800-325-0778
                                  www.ssa.gov
Carolyn W. Colvin, Commissioner
James A. Kissko, Chief of Staff
Katherine A. Thornton, Deputy Chief of Staff
*Karena L. Kilgore, Executive Secretary,Office of Executive
Operations*
Official website of the Social Security Administration.

5499 Special Clothes for Children
PO Box 333
E. Harwich, MA 02645-333   508-430-2410
                                  Fax: 508-430-2410
                                  TTY:508-430-2410
                                  lou@lnrmusic.com
                                  www.special-clothes.com
A catalog of adaptive clothing for children with disabilities -
helping boys and girls with special needs meet the world with
pride and confidence since 1987.

5500 V Foundation for Cancer Research
106 Towerview Court
Cary, NC 27513-3595   919-380-9505
                                      800-454-6698
                                  info@jimmyv.org
                                  www.jimmyv.org
Sherrie Mazur, Director of Marketing & Communication
Danielle Smith, Director of Corporate and Market Development
*Mark Steudel, Associate Director of Development for Prospect Re-
search*
Nick Valvano, President Emeritus
Named after basketball coach and broadcaster, Jim Valvano. The
V Foundation funds critical stage research conducted by young
researchers at NCI approved cancer research facilities.

5501 **ValueOptions**
240 Corporate Blvd.
Norfolk, VA 23502-4900   757-459-5100
                                Fax: 501-707-0940
                                TTY:877-334-0077
                                www.valueoptions.com

Heyward R. Donigan, President/CEO
Scott Tabakin, Chief Financial Officer
Kyle A. Raffaniello, Executive Vice President and Chief Strategy Officer
Paul Rosenberg, Executive Vice President and General Counsel
Serves over 22 million people in behavioral healthcare through publicaly funded, federal, and commercial contracts.

5502 **Wardrobe Wagon: The Special Needs Clothing Store**
258B Route 46 E
Fairfield, NJ 7004-2324   973-244-2414
                                 800-992-2737
                                 wardrobew@aol.com
                                 www.wardrobewagon.com

E Oppenberg, President
Bonnie Oppenberg
Jerome Oppenberg, Owner
Wearing apparel for individuals with special clothing needs.

5503 **We Magazine**
130 William St
New York, NY 10038   646-769-2722
                                 Fax: 212-375-6266
                                 TTY:212-375-6235
                                 sales@wemedia.com

5504 **We Media**
1801 Reston Parkway
Suite 300
Reston, VA 20190-4303   703-880-2659
                                 help@wemedia.com
                                 www.wemedia.com

Andrew Nachison, Founder
Dale Peskin, Founder
Online network for people with disabilities.

5505 **WebABLE**

                    www.hisoftware.com/press/webable.html

5506 **WheelchairNet**
6425 Penn Ave
Suite 401 BAKSQ, Department of Reha
Philadelphia, PA 15206   412-624-6279
                                 ruffing@pitt.edu
                                 www.wheelchairnet.org

Joseph Ruffing, Communications Specialist
A virtual community of people who care about wheelchairs.

5507 **World Association of Persons with Disabilities**
2441 N Sterling Ave
302W
Oklahoma, OK 73127-2009   405-672-4440
                                 www.wapd.org

Byron R. Kerford, Founder/Leader
Thomas J. Mecke, Executive Director
Sierra Hebron, Director of Human Resources
Ashley Wardle, Director of Internet Marketing
Dedicated to improving the quality of life for those with disabilities.

Toys & Games

General

5508 Age Appropriate Puzzles
7756 Winding Way
Fair Oaks, CA 95628-5735   916-961-3507
                                   Fax: 916-961-0765

Cheryl Meyers, President
These unique puzzles teach numerous concepts: picture, name, color and shape recognition. Each of the two themes (holidays, and clothing) comes with self-adhesive stickers that name each picture in English, Hmong, Russian, Spanish and Vietnamese. A notch at each puzzle piece makes grasping and lifting the pieces easy to use., They are designed for children from 18 months and up. Special needs children, preschool through high school would also benefit. *$9.95*

5509 All-Turn-It Spinner
AbleNet, Inc.
2625 Patton Road
Roseville, MN 55113-1308   651-294-2200
                                   800-322-0956
                                   Fax: 651-294-2222
                        customerservice@ablenetinc.com
                                   www.ablenetinc.com

Jennifer Thalhuber, President/CEO
Cheryl Volkman, Co-founder
Bill Sproull, Chairman of the Board
William Mills, Board of Directors
The All-Turn-It Spinner is a random spinner that comes with a dice overlay allowing user's to participate in any commercially-available game that require dice. Activate the spinner with its built-in switch or connect an external switch. Overlays are interchangeable with AbleNet designed spinner games or create your own overlay. A great inclusion tool!. *$89.00*

5510 Anthony Brothers Manufacturing
Convert-O-Bike
9 Capper Drive
Dailey Industrial Park,
Pacific, MO 63069-5196   636-257-0533
                                   800-346-6313
                                   Fax: 636-257-5473
                                   www.angelesstore.com

Tim Lynch, Director of Sales
David Curry, General Manager
Michelle Vondera, Customer Service Manager
Sally Perrin, National Account Manager
Manufacture wheeled toys and goods for disabled children.

5511 Automatic Card Shuffler
Maxi Aids
42 Executive Blvd
Farmingdale, NY 11735-4710   631-752-0521
                                   800-522-6294
                                   Fax: 631-752-0689
                                   TTY: 631-752-0738
                                   sales@maxiaids.com
                                   www.maxiaids.com

5512 Backgammon Set: Deluxe
Maxi Aids
42 Executive Blvd
Farmingdale, NY 11735-4710   631-752-0521
                                   800-522-6294
                                   Fax: 631-752-0689
                                   TTY: 631-752-0738
                                   sales@maxiaids.com
                                   www.maxiaids.com

5513 Board Games: Snakes and Ladders
Maxi Aids
42 Executive Blvd
Farmingdale, NY 11735-4710   631-752-0521
                                   800-522-6294
                                   Fax: 631-752-0689
                                   TTY: 631-752-0738
                                   sales@maxiaids.com
                                   www.maxiaids.com

5514 Board Games: Solitaire
Maxi Aids
42 Executive Blvd
Farmingdale, NY 11735-4710   631-752-0521
                                   800-522-6294
                                   Fax: 631-752-0689
                                   TTY: 631-752-0738
                                   sales@maxiaids.com
                                   www.maxiaids.com

5515 Braille Playing Cards: Plastic
Maxi Aids
42 Executive Blvd
Farmingdale, NY 11735-4710   631-752-0521
                                   800-522-6294
                                   Fax: 631-752-0689
                                   TTY: 631-752-0738
                                   sales@maxiaids.com
                                   www.maxiaids.com

5516 Braille: Bingo Cards, Boards and Call Numbers
Maxi Aids
42 Executive Blvd
Farmingdale, NY 11735-4710   631-752-0521
                                   800-522-6294
                                   Fax: 631-752-0689
                                   TTY: 631-752-0738
                                   sales@maxiaids.com
                                   www.maxiaids.com

5517 Braille: Rook Cards
Maxi Aids
42 Executive Blvd
Farmingdale, NY 11735-4710   631-752-0521
                                   800-522-6294
                                   Fax: 631-752-0689
                                   TTY: 631-752-0738
                                   sales@maxiaids.com
                                   www.maxiaids.com

5518 Card Holder Deluxe
Maxi Aids
42 Executive Blvd
Farmingdale, NY 11735-4710   631-752-0521
                                   800-522-6294
                                   Fax: 631-752-0689
                                   TTY: 631-752-0738
                                   sales@maxiaids.com
                                   www.maxiaids.com

5519 Cards: Musical
Sense-Sations
919 Walnut St
Philadelphia, PA 19107-5237   215-627-0600
                                   Fax: 215-922-0692
                                   asbinfo@asb.org
                                   www.asb.org

Richard Forsythe, Director
Patricia Johnson, CEO
Robert Bivenour, IT Manager
Brian Rusk, Public Relations Officer
These cards, for all occasions, play music when they are opened, for the visually impaired and blind persons. *$2.50*

5520 **Cards: UNO**
Maxi Aids
42 Executive Blvd
Farmingdale, NY 11735-4710   631-752-0521
                                            800-522-6294
                                       Fax: 631-752-0689
                                        TTY: 631-752-0738
                                      sales@maxiaids.com
                                          www.maxiaids.com

5521 **Checker Set: Deluxe**
Maxi Aids
42 Executive Blvd
Farmingdale, NY 11735-4710   631-752-0521
                                            800-522-6294
                                       Fax: 631-752-0689
                                        TTY: 631-752-0738
                                      sales@maxiaids.com
                                          www.maxiaids.com

5522 **Chess Set: Deluxe**
Maxi Aids
42 Executive Blvd
Farmingdale, NY 11735-4710   631-752-0521
                                            800-522-6294
                                       Fax: 631-752-0689
                                        TTY: 631-752-0738
                                      sales@maxiaids.com
                                          www.maxiaids.com

5523 **Dice: Jumbo Size**
New Vision Store
919 Walnut St
Philadelphia, PA 19107-5237   215-629-2990
                                                www.asb.org

Richard Forsythe, Director
Patricia Johnson, CEO
Robert Bivenour, IT Manager
Brian Rusk, Public Relations Officer
The large white and black dice are over-sized and have grooved
dots to indicate the numbers, for easy reading for the visually
handicapped. *$4.95*

5524 **Early Learning 1**
MarbleSoft
12301 Central Ave NE
Suite 205
Blaine, MN 55434-4902   763-755-1402
                                            888-755-1402
                                       Fax: 763-862-2920
                                      sales@marblesoft.com
                                         www.marblesoft.com

Vicki Larson, Manager
Early learning 2.1 includes four activities that teach prereading
skills. Single and dual-switch scanning are built in and special
prompts allow blind students to use all levels of difficulty. Includes Matching Colors, Learning Shapes, Counting Numbers
and Letter Match. Runs on Windows 98 or later and MAC OS 9 or
OSX (classic not required). *$70.00*

5525 **Enabling Devices**
50 Broadway
Hawthorne, NY 10532-2837   914-747-3070
                                            800-832-8697
                                       Fax: 914-747-3480
                                   info@enablingdevices.com
                                     www.enablingdevices.com

Steven Kanor, Owner
Karen O'Connor, Vice President Operations
Elizabeth Bell, Marketing Manager
Enabling Devices is a company dedicated to developing affordable learning and assistive devices to help people of all ages with
disabling conditions. Founded by Steven E. Kanor, Ph.D. and
orginally known as Toys for Special Children, the company has
been creating innovative communicators, adapted toys and
switches for the physically challenged for more than 35 years.

5526 **Hands-Free Controller**
Nintendo
PO Box 957
Redmond, WA 98073-957   800-255-3700
                                          www.nintendo.com

Yoshio Tsuboike, Editor-in-Chief
Nintendo controller for the physically disabled.

5527 **Let's Count Braille and Tactile Numbers Poster**
Maxi Aids
42 Executive Blvd
Farmingdale, NY 11735-4710   631-752-0521
                                            800-522-6294
                                       Fax: 631-752-0689
                                        TTY: 631-752-0738
                                      sales@maxiaids.com
                                          www.maxiaids.com

5528 **National Lekotek Center**
2001 N. Clybourn Av.
1st Floor
Chicago, IL 60614-3716   773-528-5766
                                            800-366-PLAY
                                       Fax: 773-537-2992
                                        TTY: 773-973-2180
                                      lekotek@lekotek.org
                                            www.lekotek.org

Elaine D. Cottey, Chair
Joanna Horsnail, Chair
Eric Gastevich, Treasurer
Carol Neiger, Secretary
Maximizes the development of children with special needs
through play. Supports families through nationwide family play
centers, toy lending libraries and computer play programs. Pub-
lishes six-page newsletter three times per year.

5529 **New Language of Toys: Teaching Communication Skills to
Children with Special Needs**
Spina Bifida Association of America
4590 MacArthur Blvd,NW,
Suite 250
Washington, DC 20007- 4226   202-944-3285
                                            800-621-314
                                       Fax: 202-944-3295
                                           sbaa@sbaa.org
                                www.spinabifidaassociation.org

Lisa Raman, Director-National Resource Center
Mary Nethercutt, National Walk Director
Christopher Vance, Director of Development
Cindy Brownstein, President /CEO
A guide for parents and teachers and a reader-friendly resource
guide that provides a wealth of information on how play activities
affect a child's language development and where to get the toys
and materials to use in these activities. *$19.00*

5530 **Puzzle Games: Cooking, Eating, Community and Grooming**
PCI
PO Box 34270
San Antonio, TX 78265-4270   210-670-3866
                                            800-594-4263
                                       Fax: 218-210-3771

Janie Haugen, Program Director
Jeff McLane, President/CEO
Rebecca Phillips, Executive Director
Each game has 63 pieces which are 2 inches in size. The completed full color puzzle is 19 inch x 15 inch. Step 1 - Work the puzzle. Step 2 - Match picture or word cards to the correct space on
the puzzle. These puzzles teach basic life skills. *$19.95*

5531   Single Switch Games
MarbleSoft
12301 Central Ave NE
Suite 205
Blaine, MN   55434-4902

763-755-1402
888-755-1402
888-755-1402
Fax: 763-862-2920
sales@marblesoft.com
www.marblesoft.com

Vicki Larson, Manager
Mark Larson
Theres alot of educational software for single switch users, but how about something that's just fun? We've taken some games similar to the ones you enjoyed as a kid and made them work just right for single switch users. Includes Single Switch Maze, A Frog's Life, Switching Lanes, Switch Invaders, Slingshot Gallery and Scurry. Runs on Windows 98 or later and MAC OS9 or OSX (classic not required) *$60.00*

5532   Single Switch Latch and Timer
AbleNet
2625 Patton Road
Roseville, MN   55113-1308

651-294-2200
800-322-0956
Fax: 651- 29- 225
customerservice@ablenetinc.com
www.ablenetinc.com

Bill Sproull, Chairman of the Board
William Mills, Board of Directors, Chair
Jennifer Thalhuber, President/CEO
Paul Sugden, Vice President of Finance, IT & CFO, Trustee
A Single Switch Latch and Timer allows a user to activate a battery-operated toy or appliance in the latch, timed seconds and timed minutes modes of control. Choose for one user and one device at a time. *$63.00*

5533   Socialization Games for Persons with Disabilities
Charles C. Thomas
2600 S First St
Springfield, IL   62704-4730

217-789-8980
800-258-8980
Fax: 217-789-9130
books@ccthomas.com
www.ccthomas.com

Michael P. Thomas, President
Nevalyn Nevil, Author
Marna Beatty, Author
David Moxley, Author
This text will assist those who want to teach severely multiple disabled students by providing information on: general principles of intervention and classroom organization; managing the behavior of students; physically managing students and using adaptive equipment; teaching eating skills; teaching toileting, dressing, and hygiene skills; teaching cognition, communication, and socialization skills; teaching independent living skills; and teaching infants and preschool students. *$38.95*

176 pages Paperback
ISBN 0-398067-46-5

5534   Take a Chance
Speech Bin
1965 25th Ave
Vero Beach, FL   32960-3062

772-770-0007
800-477-3324
Fax: 772-770-0006
info@speechbin.com

Jan J Binney, Senior Editor
Card game for practice of commonly misarticulated speech sounds. *$18.75*

16 pages Book & Cards
ISBN 0-93785 -46-7

5535   Tic Tac Toe
Maxi Aids
42 Executive Blvd
Farmingdale, NY   11735-4710

631-752-0521
800-522-6294
Fax: 631-752-0689
TTY: 631-752-0738
sales@maxiaids.com
www.maxiaids.com

5536   Turnabout Game
Maxi Aids
42 Executive Blvd
Farmingdale, NY   11735-4710

631-752-0521
800-522-6294
Fax: 631-752-0689
TTY: 631-752-0738
sales@maxiaids.com
www.maxiaids.com

Travel & Transportation

Newsletters & Books

5537 **A Guide for the Wheelchair Traveler**
Access for Disabled Americans
3240 Burnt Mill Drive
Orinda, CA 94563-2317 925-254-1499
Fax: 925-254-6167
psmither@aol.com

Neal Smither, President
Patricia Smither, Editor/Secretary
All you need to know when traveling in a wheelchair. *$30.00*
165 pages Paperback
ISBN 1-928616-00-3

5538 **A World Awaits You**
Mobility International USA
132 E. Broadway
Suite 343
Eugene, OR 97401-2767 541-343-1284
Fax: 541-343-6812
info@miusa.org
www.miusa.org

Susan Sygall, CEO/Founder
Susan Dunn, Exec. Asst./Project Specialist
Cindy Lewis, Director of Programs
Estelle Coreris-Moore, Financial Manager
A journal of success stories and tips of people with disabilities
participating in international exchange programs.
40 pages Yearly

5539 **Access Travel: Airports**
Consumer Information Center
Department 575a
Pueblo, CO 81009-1 719-948-3334
catalog.pueblo@gsa.gov

Michael Clark, Public Affairs
Alfred Pino, Manager
Tips and suggestions for easier travel for persons with disabilities
and the elderly. Lists designs, facilities, and services at 553 airport terminals worldwide.

5540 **Architectural Barriers Action League**
PO Box 57088
Tucson, AZ 85732-7088 520-628-8118
Martin Floerchinger, Owner
Offers guides to accessible hotels and motels across the country.

5541 **Directory of Travel Agencies for the Disabled**
Twin Peaks Press
PO Box 129
Vancouver, WA 98666-129 206-694-2462
800-637-2256

David Lynch, Director
Directory lists more than 360 travel agents specializing in arrangements for people with disabilities. Handbook provides information about accessibility. *$19.95*
40 pages Paperback
ISBN 0-93326-04-8

5542 **Elderly Guide to Budget Travel/Europe**
Pilot Books
PO Box 2102
Greenport, NY 11944-893 631-477-1094
Fax: 631-661-4379

5543 **Ideas for Easy Travel**
Accent Books & Products
PO Box 700
Bloomington, IL 61702-700 309-378-2961
800-787-8444
Fax: 309-378-4420

Raymond C Cheever, Publisher
Betty Garee, Editor
Ideal for helping the new traveler get started having fun. Points
out favorite accessible high-spots as reported by two travel experts (one is disabled), and offers basic ideas to help wherever
you go. *$3.25*
55 pages Paperback
ISBN 0-91570-36-1

5544 **Sports n' Spokes Magazine**
Paralyzed Veterans of America
801 18th St NW
Washington, DC 20006-3517 202-872-1300
800-424-8200
888-888-2201
Fax: 202-785-4432
TTY:800-795-4327
info@pva.org
www.pva.org

Homer S. Townsend, Jr., Executive Director
Larry Dodson, National Secretary
Bill Lawson, National President
Al Kovach, Jr, Natonal Senior Vice President
Publication of the PVA, a congressionally chartered veterans service organization, with unique expertise on a wide variety of issues involving the special needs of our members— veterans of
the armed forces who have experienced spinal cord injury or
dysfunction.

5545 **Survival Strategies for Going Abroad, A Guide for People
with Disabilites**
132 E. Broadway
Suite 343
Eugene, OR 97401-2767 541-343-1284
Fax: 541-343-6812
info@miusa.org
www.miusa.org

Susan Sygall, Executive Director
Melissa Mitchell, Public Relations
$16.95
225 pages

5546 **Travel Information Service/Moss Rehab Hospital**
Moss Rehabilitation Hospital
1200 W Tabor Rd
Philadelphia, PA 19141-3099 215-456-9900
800-225-5667
www.mossresourcenet.org

John Whyte, Owner
Ruth Lefton, COO
Anthony Allonardo, Director of Technology
Alberto Esquenazi, Plant Manager
Offers information and resources, to telephone callers only, for
persons with special traveling/accessibility needs.

5547 **United States Department of the Interior National Park
Service**
Superintendent of Documents
1849 C St NW
Washington, DC 20240-1 202-208-3100
Fax: 202-619-7302
feedback@ios.doi.gov
www.doi.gov

Mainella, Director
Gale Norton, Chief Executive Officer
Offers an informational packet containing books, guides and
tours for the disabled and elderly.

5548 Wheelin Around
Wheelers Handicapped Accessible Van Rentals
6614 W Sweetwater Ave
Glendale, AZ   85304-1040   602-776-8830
                                         800-456-1371
                                   Fax: 623-412-9920
                              info@wheelersvanrentals.com
                              www.wheelersvanrentals.com

Tammy Smith, President
Ron Smith, Corporate Treasurer
Wheelers has been breaking travel barriers through innovative service and products since 1989. Our mission is to have Wheelers rental affiliates available in every city in the United States, Canada and all around the globe. Wheelers' objective is to connect you to the best possible solution for your transportation challenges and continue to find new and innovative ways in making the world a more accessible place.

5549 Where to Stay USA
Council On International Educational Exchange
633 3rd Ave
New York, NY   10017-6706   212-822-2600
                                         888-COU-NCIL
                                   Fax: 212-822-2649

Priscilla Tovey, Information Services
A guide to low-cost lodging throughout the United States including information on whether the establishment is accessible. *$15.95*
250 pages
ISBN 0-67179-49-5

Associations & Programs

5550 Access America
Northern Cartographic
4050 Williston Rd
South Burlington, VT   5403-6062   802-860-2886
                                   Fax: 802-865-4912

Cynthia Belliveau, President
Offers information on 36 national parks, providing detailed information on accessibility.

5551 Access Yosemite National Park
Special Needs Project
324 State Street
Santa Barbara, CA   93101-2364   805-962-8087
                                         800-333-6867
                              books@specialneeds.com
                              www.specialneeds.com

Hod Gray, Owner
Represents unprecedented combinations of intensive information survey data with high quality cartography. *$7.95*
31 pages

5552 American Hotel and Lodging Foundation
1201 New York Ave NW
Suite 600
Washington, DC   20005-3931   202-289-3100
                                   Fax: 202-289-3199
                              membership@ahla.com
                              www.ahla.com

Barbara DiRocco, Director, Conventions & Events
Katherine Lugar, President/CEO
Pam Inman, IOM, CAE, CMHS, Executive Vice President/COO
Joori Jeon, CPA, CAE, Executive Vice President/CFO, President of AH&LEF
Will disseminate information, develop and conduct a series of seminars for the hotel and motel industry at state-level association conferences, and develop and distribute an ADA Compliance handbook for use by the lodging industry.

5553 Amtrak
50 Massachusetts Ave NE
Washington, DC   20002-4214   202-000-1111
                                         800-872-7245
                                   Fax: 202-906-4564
                                   TTY: 800-523-6590
                                         www.amtrak.com

Joseph H. Boardman, President/CEO
Eleanor D. Acheson, Vice President, General Counsel and Corporate Secretary
Stephen J. Gardner, Vice President, NEC Infrastructure and Investment Developmen
DJ Stadtler, Vice President, Operations
Amtrak is committed to making travel for passengers with disabilities more accessible. Anyone interested should contact Amtrak's Special Services Desk at 1-800-USA-RAIL at least 24 hours in advance to arrange for special assistance. The type of equipment and accessibility vary from train to train and station to station.

5554 Easter Seals Project ACTION
1425 K St NW
Suite 200
Washington, DC   20005-3508   202-347-3066
                                         800-659-6428
                                   Fax: 202-737-7914
                                   TTY: 202-347-7385
                        project_action@easterseals.com
                              www.projectaction.org

Judy Shanley,Ph. D, Director
Donna Smith, Director of Training
C. Marie Maus, Assistant Director
Mary Leary, Vice President
A national technical assistance program designed to improve access to transportation services for people with disabilities and assist transit providers in implementing the Americans with Disabilities Act. Publishes quarterly newsletter.

5555 General Motors Mobility Program for Persons with Disabilities
GM Mobility Program
PO Box 5053
Troy, MI   48007   800-323-9935
                                   TTY:800-833-9935
                              www.gmmobility.com

Frederick A Henderson, CEO
GM Mobility Program provides up to $1000 reimbursement toward mobility adaptations for drivers or passengers and/or vehicle alerting devices for drivers who are deaf or hard of hearing. Provided on eligible new Chevrolet, Pontiac, Oldsmobile, Buick, Cadillac, and GMC vehicles. Complete GMC financing available. GM Mobility also offers free resource information, including list of area adaptive equipment installers, plus free resource video.

5556 Kenny Foundation
21700 Northwestern Hwy
Suite 730
Southfield, MI   48075- 4930   810-552-0202
                                         800-237-3422
                                   comnet@uwcs.org

Susan Burstein, Executive Director
Provides education, advocacy & direct services to people with mobility impairments throughout Michigan. Services include Equipment Connection, a database, available online, that connects buyers & sellers of used adaptive equipment; Attitudes is a disability awareness program for 1st & 2nd graders; Information & Referral services; and Accessbility, a program that uses volunteer labor and donated materials to buid ramps for people who can't afford them.

5557 MedEscort International
PO Box 8766
Allentown, PA   18105-8766   610-791-3111
                                         800-255-7182
                                   Fax: 610-791-9189
                                   www.medescort.com

Craig Poliner, President

MedEscort International was founded over a decade ago with these basic principles and philosophies as its foundation. MedEscort has served the health care community, throughout the world, and has strived to perfect the techniques of moving patients from one place to another. Our medical staff includes registered nurses, respiratory therapists, paramedics, and physicians. MedEscort has developed comprehensive, individual aeromedical services to meet each patient's needs with a personal touch.

5558   Nantahala Outdoor Center
13077 Highway 19 W
Bryson City, NC   28713-9165
828-488-2176
888-905-7238
Fax: 828-488-2498
TTY:800-877-8339
rafting@noc.com
www.noc.com

Sutton Bacon, CEO
Nantahala Outdoor Center, the leader in outdoor recreation and education for more than 30 years, strongly encourages and supports participants with disabilities. We offer whitewater rafting adventures on six rivers in the Southeast for all skill and thrill levels for groups, also kayak and canoe adaptive instruction. NOC will tailor a whitewater program to your skill and ability level, modify the gear, and pace instruction for you. We also offer a Ropes Challenge Course and team building program

5559   Paralysis Society of America
Paralyzed Veterans of America
801 18th St NW
Washington, DC   20006-3517
202-872-1300
800-424-8200
Fax: 202-785-4432
TTY: 800-795-4327
info@pva.org
www.pva.org

Homer S. Townsend, Jr., Executive Director
Larry Dodson, National Secretary
Bill Lawson, National President
Al Kovach, Jr, Natonal Senior Vice President
A national organization whose members are people with spinal cord injury or disease, their family members and caregivers, health-care professionals, and others with an interest in the disciplines of spinal cord medicine and paralsis. One year membership includes NewsWheels, a quarterly newsletter.

5560   Shilo Inns & Resorts
11707 NE Airport Way
Portland, OR   97220-5995
503-252-7500
800-222-2244
Fax: 503-254-0794
franchiseinfo@shiloinns.com
www.shiloinns.com

Mark S. Hemstreet, Founder/Owner
Ivan Mc Affee, VP
Shilo Inns offers affordable excellence with special assist rooms at many of our locations throughout the western United States. These rooms include larger sized bathrooms equipped with assistance railings and wheelchair access. Special assist dogs are welcome free of charge ar most Shilo Inns. Call 1-800-222-2244 for details or make reservations or check out www.shiloinns.com

5561   Travelers Aid International
1612 K St. NW
Suite 206
Washington, DC   20006-2849
202-546-0599
Fax: 202-546-9112
info@travelersaid.org
www.travelersaid.org

Joan Lowden, Chair
Brian Rogers, Vice Chair
Edward Powers, Vice Chair
Jessica M. Rooney, Treasurer
Provides crisis intervention and casework services, limited financial assistance, protective travel assistance and information and referrals for travelers, transients and newcomers.

5562   US Airways/America West Airlines
4000 E Sky Harbor Blvd
Phoenix, AZ   85034-3802
480-693-0800
800-327-7810
Fax: 480-693-3702
TTY: 800-245-2966
www.usairways.org

Douglas Parker, CEO
This airline trains employees to make sure that passengers with disabilities enjoy convenient, safe and comfortable travel.

5563   US Servas
1125 16th Street
Suite 201
Arcata, CA   95521-5585
707-825-1714
Fax: 707-825-1762
info@usservas.org
www.usservas.org

Judy Sears, Administrator
International network that links travelers with hosts in 130+ countries with the hope of building world peace through understanding and friendship.
Quarterly

5564   Westin Hotels and Resorts
270 West 43rd Street
New York, NY   10036
212-201-2700
Fax: 212-201-2701
info@westinny.com

Sue A Brush, Senior VP
Westin Hotels & Resortsr indulge our guests in elements of well-being. Our refreshing ambience, innovative programs and thoughtful amenities help provide a stay that leaves you feeling better than when you arrived.

5565   Wheelers Handicapped Accessible Van Rentals
6614 W Sweetwater Ave
Glendale, AZ   85304-1040
602-418-5076
800-456-1371
Fax: 623-412-9920
info@wheelersvanrentals.com
www.wheelersvanrentals.com

Tammy Smith, President
Rental wheelchairs and scooter accessible vans. Technically advanced engineering features bring a world of independence to the user. Locations throughout the U.S. call 800-456-1371 to make reservations at any of our locations nationwide.

5566   Wilderness Inquiry
808 14th Ave SE
Minneapolis, MN   55414-1516
612-676-9400
800-728-0179
Fax: 612-676-9401
TTY: 612-676-9475
info@wildernessinquiry.org
www.wildernessinquiry.org

Greg Lais, Executive Director
Lee Friedman, Business and Outreach Director
Megan O'Hara, Youth Outdoor Employment Director
Beth Dooley, Communications Director
Allows people of all ages and abilities to share the adventure of wilderness travel. This nonprofit organization was formed in 1978 and conducts tours to some of the most beautiful and remote parts of the world.

Tours

5567   Able Trek Tours
P.O. Box 384
Reedsburg, WI   53959
608-524-3021
800-205-6713
Fax: 608-524-8302
info@abletrektours.com
abletrektours.com

5568 AccessToThePlanet
Accessible Journeys
35 W Sellers Ave
Ridley Park, PA 19078-2113

610-521-0339
800-846-4537
Fax: 610-521-6959
sales@disabilitytravel.com
www.accessiblejourneys.com

Howard Mc Coy, Owner
Kathy Pagliei, Director
Howard J. McCoy, President/CEO
Contains new product announcements, organizing land groups
and world travel news.
Monthly

5569 Accessible Journeys
35 West Sellers Ave
Ridley Park, PA 19078-2113

610-521-0339
800-846-4537
Fax: 610-521-6959
sales@accessiblejourneys.com
www.accessiblejourneys.com

Howard Mc Coy, Owner
Kathy Pagliei, Director
Howard J. McCoy, President/CEO
Accessible Journeys is a vacation planner and tour operator ex-
clusively for wheelchair travelers, their families and friends.

**5570 American The Beautiful; National Parks & Federal
Recreation Lands**
National Parks Service
1849 C St NW
Washington, DC 20240-1

202-208-6843
888-275-8747
Fax: 202-219-0910
webteam@ios.doi.gov
www.nps.gov

Mary A Bomar, CEO
A free lifetime passport to federally operated parks, monuments,
historic sites, recreation areas and wildlife refuges for persons
who are blind or permanently disabled.

5571 Anglo California Travel Service
4250 Williams Rd
San Jose, CA 95129-3344

408-257-2257
Fax: 408-257-2664

Audrey Cooper, President
Plans for one and two week accessible tours.

5572 Cunard Line
24305 Town Center Drive
Suite 200
Valencia, CA 91355- 2079

305-463-3000
800-528-6273
Fax: 305-463-3010
www.cunard.com

Pamela C Conover, CEO
Cunard Line, one of the world's most recognized brand names
with a classic British heritage, operated by Cunard Line Limited,
has provided the ultimate in deluxe ocean travel experience for
the past 158 years. The fleet consists of famed liner Queen Elizabeth 2 and the Caronia, a classic ship formerly identified as
Vistafjord. The Cunard Line brand, the epitome of British essence, focuses on recalling the golden age of sea travel for those
who missed the first.

5573 Dell Rapids Sportsmens Club
PO Box 126
Dell Rapids, SD 57022-126

605-428-3522
Fax: 605-428-5502
billybuckww@sio.midco.net
www.sdshootingsports.org

Wayne Coffaa, President
Pat Weinacht, Vice President
Bill Weber, Secretary/Treasurer
Robin Anderson, Board Member

Offers leage shooting for trap, as well as shooting on individual
basis for archery, trap and pistol.

5574 Diabetic Cruise Desk
Hartford Holidays
500 Old Country Rd
Suite 110
Garden City, NY 11530-536

516-746-6670
800-828-4813
Fax: 516-746-6690
info@hartfordholidays.com
www.hartfordholidays.com

Scott M. Kertes, President
Les Kertes, Chief Executive Officer
Stacey Ganca, Chief Financial Officer
*Sally Kertes, Business Development Manager / Senior Travel
Counselor*
Offers a seven-day cruise to Alaska for people with diabetes. In-
cludes seminars on diabetes, self management, planning, special
guidance for exercise classes and individual dietary advice.

5575 Dialysis at Sea Cruises
2504 Merchant Ave
Odessa, FL 33556-3468

813-775-4040
800-544-7604
001-813-775
Fax: 727-372-7396
info@dialysisatsea.com
www.dialysisatsea.com

Steve Debroux, Owner
Been in the business of providing travel opportunities for persons
on hemodialysis and CAPD since 1977. Handle all aspects of
their travel and medical requirements. Not Sold Through Travel
Agents! Make all reservations and coordinates the total set-up
and operation of an onboard ship mobile dialysis clinic. Cruises
run from seven days to three weeks and have departures from cities around the world on a variety of cruise lines.

5576 Directions Unlimited Acccessible Tours
Empress Travel
720 N. Bedford Rd
Bedford Hills, NY 10507-1508

914-241-1700
800-533-5343
Fax: 914-241-0243

Lois Bonanni, Director
Charles Digiacomo, Manager
Arrange vacations throughout the world for all disabilities including accessible cruises, African safari, rafting and scuba diving, European and Caribbean vacations.

5577 Dvorak Expeditions
17921 Us Highway 285
Nathrop, CO 81236-9701

719-539-6851
800-824-3795
Fax: 719-539-3378
info@dvorakexpeditions.com
www.dvorakexpeditions.com

Bill Dvorak, Owner
Jaci Dvorak, Co-Owner
This organization does river trips for people who are deaf, visually impaired, physically or mentally disabled. Rafting trips with
groups and families and whitewater instruction.

5578 Environmental Traveling Companions
Fort Mason Center, 2 Marina Blvd.
Bldg. C
San Francisco, CA 94123

415-474-7662
Fax: 415-474-3919
info@etctrips.org
www.etctrips.org

Diane Poslosky, Executive Director
Maureen O'Hagan, Associate Director
Jessica Heyman, Development Manager
Davido Crow, River Program Manager
Aids travelers regardless of physical or financial limitations to
experience the beauty and challenge of the wilderness.

5579 **Flying Wheels Travel**
143 W. Bridge St.
PO Box 382
Owatonna, MN 55060-382   507-451-5005
                                 877-451-5006
                            Fax: 507-451-1685
                      barbaraj@flyingwheelstravel.com
                         www.flyingwheelstravel.com

Barbara Jacobson, Owner
Timothy Holtz
Arranges worldwide custom independent travel and cruises for
the physically challenged.

5580 **Guide Service of Washington**
734 15th St NW
Suite 701
Washington, DC 20005-1023   202-628-2842
                               Fax: 202-638-2812
                          sales@dctourguides.com
                           www.dctourguides.com

Neil Amrine, President
A guide service offering tours of Washington DC and vicinity.

5581 **Guided Tour for Persons 17 & Over with Developmental
and Physical Challenges**
7900 Old York Rd
Suite 111-B
Elkins Park, PA 19027-2310   215-782-1370
                                     800-783-5841
                                Fax: 215-635-2637
                             gtour400@aol.com
                              www.guidedtour.com

Irv Segal, DCSW, LSW, Owner/Director
Jon Fash, Administration
Lynsey Trohoske, Office/Program Co-ordinator
The Guided Tour is a very special program that offers opportuni-
ties for personal growth, recreation and socialization through
travel.

5582 **Hostelling North America**
Hostelling International
8401 Colesville Road
Suite 600
Silver Spring, MD 20910- 6339   301-495-1240
                                   Fax: 240-650-2094
                           netanya.trimboli@hiusa.org
                                  www.hiusa.org

Russ Hedge, CEO
Demetria Trent, Manager
Netanya Trimboli, Communications & PR Manager
Hostels are very inexpensive accommodations for travelers of all
ages. They provide dorm-style sleeping rooms with separate
quarters for males and females, fully equipped self-service kitchens, dining areas and common rooms for relaxing and socializing.
HI-AYH has hostels in major cities, in national and state parks,
near beaches and in the mountains. Send for a copy of Hostelling
North America, a directory of hostels in U.S. and Canada, which
lists hostels that are handicap accessible. *$ 3.00*
400 pages Yearly

5583 **New Courier Travel**
532 Duane St
Glen Ellyn, IL 60137-4695   630-469-0511
                                    888-777-4453
                               Fax: 630-469-7390

Fred Mueller, Owner
Offers specialized assistance for independent travel or tours for
persons with disabilities including cruises and travel in the USA
and abroad. Fee charged for out-of-state clients, long-distance
calls and clients who have free air.

5584 **New Directions For People With Disabilities, Inc.**
5276 Hollister Avenue
Suite 207
Santa Barbara, CA 93111-3068   805-967-2841
                                      888-967-2841
                                 Fax: 805-964-7344
                          hello@newdirectionstravel.org
                             www.newdirectionstravel.org

Dee Duncan, Executive Director
Jeanne Mohle, Director of Operations
Danna Mead, Program Director
Colette Piacentini, Business Manager
A non-profit organization providing high quality local, national,
and international travel vacations and holiday programs for peo-
ple with mild to moderate developmental disabilities.

5585 **Norwegian Cruise Line**
7665 Corporate Center Drive
Miami, FL 33126-1201   866-234-0292
                               800-327-7030
                          Fax: 305-436-4117
                               www.ncl.com

Tan Sri Lim Kok Thay, Director
David Chua Ming Huat, Director
Marc J. Rowan, Director
Steve Martinez, Director
Has accessible cabins but urges mobility impaired passengers to
travel in the same cabin with a person who is not mobility im-
paired. Cruise fares vary.

5586 **ROW Adventures**
202 Sherman Ave
PO Box 579
Coeur D Alene, ID 83816   208-765-0841
                                  800-451-6034
                             Fax: 208-667-6506
                          info@rowadventures.com
                           www.rowadventures.com

*Brad Moss, Adventure Administration - Director - Marketing &
Sales*
Betsy Bowen, Adventure Administration - Founder
*Morag Prosser, Adventure Administration - International Sales
Manager*
Candy Bening, Adventure Administration - Domestic Sales Manager
Offers one to six day rafting trips to physically disadvantaged
people. Designs custom itineraries, or trips with a special focus
for small groups. For those with special dietary needs, they pre-
pare special meals. So come ride the rapids and enjoy life. They
also offer canoe trips aboard 34' voyager canoes along the trail of
Lewis and Clark on Montana's upper Missouri River. Free
brochure upon request.

5587 **Sundial Special Vacations**
750 Marine Dr.
Suite 100
Astoria, OR 97103   503-325-4536
                            800-547-9198
                       Fax: 503-325-4536
                    thomas@sundial-travel.com
                        www.sundialtour.com

Terry Conner, VP
Provides special vacations for developmentally disabled persons. Provides quality vacations for persons with developmental
disabilities. Ratio is 1 for 7 or 1 for 5 depending on tour. Only two
people to a room. Exciting destinations. 3 to 4 star properties.
Great fun.

5588 **Trips Inc.**
P.O. Box 10885
Eugene, OR 97440   541-686-1013
                           800-686-1013
                      Fax: 541-465-9355
                        trips@tripsinc.com
                          www.tripsinc.com

Jim Peterson, President & Founder
Leslie Peterson, Executive Director
Trips Inc. Special Adventures provides travel outings to adults of
various abilities in a safe, respectful and fun atmosphere. Our

trips are designed for people with developmental disabilities and special needs who require staff assistance for a safe and enjoyable vacation.

5589 Ventures Travel
3600 Holly Lane N.
Suite 95
Plymouth, MN 55447-1619
952-852-0107
866-692-7400
Fax: 952-852-0123
vt@venturestravel.org
www.venturestravel.org

Nikki Adegun, Director
Lisa Moore, Director
Maggie Venell

A limited liability company is a service of Friendship Ventures-a nonprofit organization that has been enriching the lives of people with mental retardation and related developmental disabilities since 1985. Contact us to learn about our other programs, employment information, volunteer openings or donor opportunities.

5590 Wheelchair Getaways
PO Box 1098
Mukilteo, WA 98275-1098
425-353-8213
800-536-5518
Fax: 425-355-6159
info@wheelchairgetaways.com
www.wheelchairgetaways.com

Edward Van Artsdalen, Director

Wheelchair Getaways, the largest wheelchair/scooter accessible van rental company in the US, has 50 franchise locations serving major cities and airports throughout the continental US and Hawaii. Rentals by the day, week, month or longer. Delivery/pickup available.

5591 Wilderness Inquiry
808 14th Ave SE
Minneapolis, MN 55414
612-676-9400
Fax: 612-676-9401
info@wildernessinquiry.org
www.wildernessinquiry.org

Greg Lais, Executive Director
Jenny Lavine, Associate Director
Nell Holden, Programs Director
Jonathan Houlihan, Business Operations Director

Wilderness Inquiry is a non-profit adventure travel organization on a mission to connect everyone to great places through activities such as sea kayaking, canoeing, rafting, hiking, safaris and dogsledding. Adventures provide high-quality experiences featuring carefully crafted itineraries, excellent food, top-notch gear and, highly-skilled trail guides who aim to provide the very best experience possible.

Vehicle Rentals

5592 ABC Union, ACE, ANLV, Vegas Western Cab
5010 S Valley View Blvd
Las Vegas, NV 89118-1705
702-798-3498
Fax: 702-736-8813
www.lvcabs.com

Phyllis Frias, President
Charles Frias, President

Taxi service in Las Vegas that uses vans with wheelchair lifts at regular taxi rates.

5593 Accessible Vans Of America

866-224-1750
www.accessiblevans.com

5594 Avis Rent A Car
379 Parsippany Road
Parsippany, NJ 07054-5111
973-428-3900
TTY:800-331-2323
access@avis.com

F Robert Salerno, President

Avis Access is a program of Avis Rent A Car that provides a full range of complementary products and services to drivers and passengers with physical disabilities. Renters can simply call the designated Avis Access Reservation line (888-TRY-HARDER) at 24 hours in advance. Products or services include transfer boards, hand controls, swivel seats, and more.

5595 Consulting & Engineering for the Handicapped (CEH)
4457 63rd Cir
Pinellas Park, FL 33781-5981
727-522-0364
866-244-1150
Fax: 727-522-9024
www.liftsandramps.com

Al Crisp, Owner
Brenda Crisp, Owner

New vans, used vans, specializing in quad conversions, all types of handicap equipment. Celebrating 33 years in business. Hand controls, lifts & ramps, porch lifts, hand-crank bikes.

5596 Mobile Care
6201 Riverdale Rd
Suite 101
Riverdale, MD 20737-2174
301-277-7371
Fax: 301-699-1865
jaklimo@aol.com

Maurice Naccache, Manager

Specializing in non-emergency wheelchair service for the elderly and physically challenged.

5597 National Car Rental System
600 Terminal Drive
Suite 202
Fort Lauderdale, FL 33315- 3618
954-359-3020
877-222-9058
888-826-6890
Fax: 954-359-8313
www.nationalcar.com

William Decker, Manager

Accommodates special requests subject to availability. Offers hand controls, bench seats, extra mirrors and vans with lifts at many major locations.

5598 Northwest Limousine Service
9950 Lawrence Ave
Suite 314
Schiller Park, IL 60176-1216
847-698-0000
800-376-5466
chiohare@aol.com
www.oharelimousine.com

Sam Malas, Manager

Offers wheelchair accessible mini vans, sedans, stretch and super stretch limousines for hourly or daily rental.

5599 Over the Rainbow Disabled Travel Services& Wheelers Accessible Van Rentals
186 Mehani Cir
Kihei, HI 96753-8072
808-879-5521
800-303-3750
Fax: 808-871-7533

David McKown, VP

Offers the disabled traveler Hawaii airport arrangements and ticketing accessible accommodations, hotels and condos including roll-in showers, Wheelers' Accessible Van Rentals on Maui and Honolulu or cars with hand controls, personal care attendants, medical or recreational equipment rentals and activities such as: helicopter rides, luau's, whalewatching, boating and more. Airfare varies from departure points and time of the year.

5600 Public Technology
US Department of Transportation
1301 Pennsylvania Ave NW
Washington, DC 20004
202-626-2400
Fax: 202-626-2498

J Rutter, CEO

One of a series of reports concerned with improving transportation for elderly and disabled persons.
28 pages

5601 Rehabiliation Engineering Center for Personal Licensed Transportation
University Of Virginia School Of Engineering
PO Box 400246
Charlottesville, VA 22904-4246   434-924-3072
Tom Connors, VP
Mitch Rosen, Director

5602 Wheelchair Getaways Wheelchair/Scooter Accessible Van Rentals
4443 Dixie Highway
PO Box 1098
Mukilteo, WA 98275-2864   425-353-8213
                                          800-536-5518
                                     Fax: 425-355-6159
                          info@wheelchairgetaways.com
                          www.wheelchairgetaways.com

Jennifer Richardson, Owner
Dale Richardson, Owner
Rebecca Heim, Manager
Moon Ko, Owner
Rents wheelchair/scooter accessible vans by the day, week, month or longer and offers delivery to major airports and other convenient locations in more than 200 cities in 42 states and Puerto Rico. Also offers full size and mini vans with automatic lifts and ramps. Some vans are equipped with hand controls, six-way power seats and remote controls for powered door operation and lifts.

5603 Wheelers - Marauatha Baptist Church
9120 N 95th Avenue
Peoria, AZ 85345-2501   623-937-7866
                                          800-456-1371
                                     Fax: 623-934-3971

Greg Iehl, Religious Leader, Pastor
Gene Noel, Assn't Pastor
Offers delivery to airports in 29 states and Washington, D.C. In about 40 cities, Wheelers works directly with Avis Rent-a-Car. Wheelers offers a variety of van configurations with capacity for up to three wheelchairs, automatic ramps or lifts and nylon tie-downs, hand controls or other modifications.

5604 Wheelers Handicapped Accessible Van Rentals
6614 W Sweetwater Ave
Glendale, AZ 85304-1040   602-418-5076
                                          800-456-1371
                                     Fax: 623-412-9920
                          info@wheelersvanrentals.com
                          www.wheelersvanrentals.com

Tammy Smith, President
Ron Smith, Corporate Treasurer
Wheelers has been breaking travel barriers through innovative service and products since 1989. Our mission is to have Wheelers rental affiliates available in every city in the United States, Canada and all around the globe. Wheelers' objective is to connect you to the best possible solution for your transportation challenges and continue to find new and innovative ways in making the world a more accessible place.

Veteran Services

National Administrations

5605 **Department of Medicine and Surgery Veterans Administration**
810 Vermont Ave NW
Washington, DC 20420   202-273-8504
                              800-827-1000
                              www.va.gov

David J. Shulkin, Secretary
Vivieca Wright, Chief of Staff
Provides hospital and outpatient treatment as well as nursing home care for eligible veterans in Veterans Administration facilities. Services elsewhere provided on a contract basis in the United States and its territories. Provides non-vocational inpatient residential rehabilitation services to eligible legally blinded veterans of the armed forces of the United States.

5606 **Department of Veterans Affairs Regional Office - Vocational Rehab Division**
810 Vermont Ave NW
Washington, DC 20420   202-273-8504
                              800-827-1000
                              www.va.gov

David J. Shulkin, Secretary
Vivieca Wright, Chief of Staff
Vocational rehabilitation is a program of services administered by the Department of Veterans Affairs for service members and veterans with service-connected physical or mental disabilities. If persons are compensibly disabled and are found in need of rehabilitation services because they have an employment handicap, this program can prepare them for a suitable job; get and keep that job; assist persons to become fully productive and independent.

5607 **Department of Veterans Benefits**
810 Vermont Ave NW
Washington, DC 20420   202-461-6913
                              800-827-1000
                              www.va.gov

David J. Shulkin, Secretary
Vivieca Wright, Chief of Staff
Furnishes compensation and pensions for disability and death to veterans and their dependents. Provides vocational rehabilitation services, including counseling, training, assistance and more towards employment, to blinded veterans disabled as a result of service in the armed forces during World War II, Korea and the Vietnam era; also provides rehabilitation services to certain peace-time veterans.

5608 **Disabled American Veterans Headquarters**
3725 Alexandria Pike
Cold Spring, KY 41076   877-426-2838
                              feedback@davmail.org
                              www.dav.org

David W Riley, Chairman
Barry Jesinoski, Executive Director
James Killen, Associate National Communications Director
Randy Reese, Director of Human Resources
Serves America's disabled veterans and their families. Direct services include legislative advocacy; professional counseling about compensation, pension, educational and job training programs and VA health care; and assistance in applying for those entitlements.

5609 **Federal Benefits for Veterans and Dependents**
810 Vermont Ave NW
Washington, DC 20420   202-273-6763
                              800-827-1000
                              www.benefits.va.gov

David J. Shulkin, Secretary
Viveca Wright, Chief of Staff
Offers information on benefits for veterans and their families.
93 pages
ISBN 0-16048 -58-

5610 **US Department of Veterans Affairs National Headquarters**
810 Vermont Ave NW
Washington, DC 20420   202-273-5400
                              800-827-1000
                              www.va.gov

David J. Shulkin, Secretary
Vivieca Wright, Chief of Staff
A federal agency that provides healthcare services to military veterans at VA medical centers and outpatient clinics located throughout the country; several non-healthcare benefits including disability compensation, vocational rehabilitation, education assistance, home loans, and life insurance; and provides burial and memorial benefits to veterans and family members at 135 national cemeteries.
80 pages

5611 **Veteran's Voices Writing Project**
406 W 34th St
Suite 103
Kansas City, MO 64111-3043   816-701-6844
                              veteransvoices@sbcglobal.net
                              www.veteransvoices.com

Deann Mitchell, President
Sheryl Liddle, Vice President
Marianne Watson, Treasurer
Margaret Clark, Editor in Chief
Individuals and organizations united to encourage veterans to write for pleasure and rehabilitation. The organization also maintains speakers' bureau and audio tape versions for the blind. Also offered are numerous monetary awards, articles, book reviews, cartoons and drawings, light verse, poetry and short stories.
$15.00
64 pages Magazine
ISSN 0504-07 9

Alabama

5612 **Alabama VA Benefits Regional Office - Montgomery**
U.S. Department of Veteran Affairs
345 Perry Hill Rd
Montgomery, AL 36109   800-827-1000
                              Fax: 334-213-3565
                              montgomery.query@vba.va.gov
                              www.va.gov

Cory A. Hawthorne, Director
Erica P. Worthington, Assistant Director
Jamie Bozeman, Vocational Rehabilitation & Employment Officer
Lolita McClung-Shepherd, Veterans Service Center Manager
The Veterans Benefits Administration (VBA) provides a variety of benefits and services to Servicemembers, Veterans, and their families.

5613 **Alabama VA Medical Center - Birmingham**
Veterans Health Administration U.S. Dept. of VA
700 S. 19th St
Birmingham, AL 35233   205-933-8101
                              www.birmingham.va.gov

Thomas Smith, Director
Veterans medical clinic offering disabled veterans medical treatments.

5614 **Central Alabama Veterans Healthcare System**
Veterans Health Administration, U.S. Dept. of VA
215 Perry Hill Rd
Montgomery, AL 36109-3798   334-272-4670
                              800-214-8387
                              www.centralalabama.va.gov

Paul Bockelman, Interim Director
Thomas Huettemann, Associate Director for Resources
Linda Townsend-Green, Acting Associate Director, Operations
Vic Malabonga, Chief of Staff
CAVHCS exists to provide excellent services to veterans across the continuum of healthcare. We take pride in providing delivery of timely quality care by staff who demonstrate outstanding customer service, the advancement of health care through research, and the education of tomorrow's health care providers.

5615 Tuscaloosa VA Medical Center
Veterans Health Administration, U S Dept. of V A
3701 Loop Rd E
Tuscaloosa, AL   35404-5015   205-554-2000
                                           888-269-3045
                                      Fax: 205-554-2845
                                      www.tuscaloosa.va.gov

John F. Merkle, Medical Center Director
David L. Carden, Associate Director, Nursing & Patient Care Services
Carlos Berry, Chief of Staff
To serve America's Heroes by improving their health and well-being through Veteran and Family Centered Care.

Alaska

5616 Alaska VA Healthcare System - Anchorage
1201 North Muldoon Road
Ste 115
Anchorage, AK   99504-5914   907-257-4700
                                          888-353-7574
                                     Fax: 907-561-7183
                                     www.alaska.va.gov

Linda L. Boyle, Interim Director
Shawn Bransky, Associate Director
Veterans medical clinic offering disabled veterans medical treatments.

5617 DAV Department of Alaska
2925 Debarr Rd
Room 3101
Anchorage, AK   99508-2983   907-257-4803
                                     Fax: 907-258-9828
                                     www.davmembersportal.org

Pamela F. Beale, Alaska Commander
Robert W. Bingham, Membership Chairman

5618 Veteran Benefits Administration - Anchorage Regional Office
U.S. Department of Veteran Affairs
1201 Muldoon Rd
Anchorage, AK   99504   907-257-4803
                                          800-827-1000
                                     anchorage.query@vba.va.gov
                                     www.benefits.va.gov/anchorage
Robert A. McDonald, Secretary of Veterans
Robert D. Snyder, Chief of Staff
The Anchorage Regional Office is remotely managed by the Salt Lake City Regional Office. The VBA operation includes a one-stop Veterans Service Center made up of the merged Adjudication and Veterans Service Divisions. There is also a one person Loan Guaranty Division and a Vocational Rehabilitation and Employment Division.

Arizona

5619 Carl T Hayden VA Medical Center
Veterans Health Administration, U S Dept. of V A
650 E Indian School Rd
Phoenix, AZ   85012-1839   602-277-5551
                                          800-554-7174
                                     Fax: 602-222-6472
                                     g.vhacss@forum.va.gov
                                     www.phoenix.va.gov
D Gregg Gordon, President
Marva Greene, Vice President
John Fears, CEO
Linda Herrly MSW, LCSW, Caregiver Support Coordinator

5620 Northern Arizona VA Health Care System
Veterans Health Administration, US Dept. of VA
500 Hwy 89N
Prescott, AZ   86313-5001   928-445-4860
                                          800-949-1005
                                     Fax: 928-768-6076
                                     g.vhacss@forum.va.gov
                                     www.prescott.va.gov
Deborah Thompson, Manager

5621 Southern Arizona VA Healthcare System
Veterans Health Administration, U S Dept. of V A
3601 S 6th Ave
Tucson, AZ   85723   520-792-1450
                                          800-470-8262
                                     Fax: 520-629-1818
                                     g.vhacss@forum.va.gov
                                     www.tucson.va.gov
Jonathan H. Gardner, MPA, FACHE, Director
Jennifer S Gutowski, MHA, FACHE, Associate Director
Katie A. Landwehr, MBA, Assistant Director
Fabia Kwiecinski, MD, FACP, Chief of Staff
The Southern Arizona VA Health Care System (SAVAHCS) located in Tucson AZ serves over 170,000 Veterans located in eight counties in Southern Arizona and one county in Western New Mexico.

Arkansas

5622 Eugene J Towbin Healthcare Center
Veterans Health Administration, U S Dept. of V A
2200 Fort Roots Dr
North Little Rock, AR   72114-1706   501-257-1000
                                          800-827-1000
                                     Fax: 501-257-1779
                                     g.vhacss@forum.va.gov
                                     www.littlerock.va.gov
Michael R. Winn, Director
Toby T. Mathew, MHA/MBA, Deputy Director
Cyril O. Ekeh, MHA, Associate Director
Julie A. Brandt, MSN, RN, CNA-B, Associate Director for Patient Care Service/Nurse Executive
CAVHS is reaching out to veterans through its community-based outpatient clinics in Mountain Home, El Dorado, Hot Springs, Mena, Pine Bluff, Searcy, Conway, Russellville, its Home Health Care Service Center in Hot Springs, and a VA Drop-In Day Treatment Center for homeless veterans in downtown Little Rock.

5623 Fayetteville VA Medical Center
Veterans Health Administration, US Dept. of VA
1100 N College Ave
Fayetteville, AR   72703-1944   479-443-4301
                                          800-691-8387
                                     g.vhacss@forum.va.gov
                                     www.fayettevillear.va.gov
W. Todd Grams, Chief Financial Officer
Glenn D. Haggstrom, Principal Executive Director
Stephen W. Warren, Principal Deputy Assistant Secretary
Honor America's Veterans by providing exceptional health care that improves their health and well-being.

5624 John L McClellan Memorial Hospital
Veterans Health Administration, US Dept. of VA
4300 W 7th St
Little Rock, AR   72205-5446   501-257-1000
                                          800-827-1000
                                     g.vhacss@forum.va.gov
                                     www.littlerock.va.gov
Michael R. Winn, Director
Toby T. Mathew, MHA/MBA, Deputy Director
Cyril O. Ekeh, MHA, Associate Director
Julie A. Brandt, MSN, RN, CNA-B, Associate Director for Patient Care Service/Nurse Executive
CAVHS is reaching out to veterans through its community-based outpatient clinics in Mountain Home, El Dorado, Hot Springs, Mena, Pine Bluff, Searcy, Conway, Russellville, its Home Health

Care Service Center in Hot Springs, and a VA Drop-In Day Treatment Center for homeless veterans in downtown Little Rock. Throughout its rich 90 year history, CAVHS has been widely recognized for excellence in education, research, and emergency preparedness, and -first and foremost -for a tradition of quality an

5625   North Little Rock Regional Office
Veterans Benefits Administration, U S Dept. of V A
2200 Fort Roots Drive
Building 65
N Little Rock, AR 72114-1756   501-370-3820
                                                800-827-1000
                                            Fax: 501-370-3829
                                    littlerock.query@vba.va.gov
                                                    www.va.gov

Eric K. Shinseki, Secretary
Stephen W. Warren, Principal Deputy Assistant Secretary
W. Todd Grams, Chief Financial Officer
Glenn D. Haggstrom, Principal Executive Director
The Little Rock VA Regional Office offers services to veterans in the State of Arkansas and the city of Texarkana in Bowie County, Texas. Based on 2004 information provided by the Office of Policy, Planning, and Preparedness, the veteran population of Arkansas is 268,000 and the city of Texarkana, Texas, has a veteran population of 3,545. With a staff of approximately 124 employees, the Regional Office determines entitlement to disability compensation and pension, survivors' benefits, vocational

California

5626   Jerry L Pettis Memorial VA Medical Center
Veterans Health Administration, U S Dept. of V A
11201 Benton St
Loma Linda, CA 92357-1000   909-825-7084
                                                800-741-8387
                                    g.vhacss@forum.va.gov
                                        www.lomalinda.va.gov
Barbara Fallen, RD, MPA, FACHE, Acting Director
Prachi V. Asher, FACHE, Assistant Director
Dwight C. Evans, M.D., Chief of Staff
Shane M. Elliott, MBA, AD for Administration
Since 1977, VA Loma Linda Healthcare System has been improving the health of the men and women who have so proudly served our nation. We consider it our privilege to serve your health care needs in any way we can.

5627   Long Beach VA Medical Center
Veterans Health Administration, U S Dept. of V A
5901 E 7th St
Long Beach, CA 90822-5201   562-826-8000
                                                800-827-1000
                                                888-769-8387
                                    g.vhacss@forum.va.gov
                                        www.longbeach.va.gov
Isabel Duff, Medical Center Director
John M. Tryboski, MSN, Associate Director
Anthony DeFrancesco, FACHE, Associate Director
Sherrie Schuldheis, Ph.D., RN, Assistant Director, Systems Redesign

5628   Los Angeles Regional Office
Veterans Benefits Administration, U S Dept. of V A
11000 Wilshire Blvd
Los Angeles, CA 90024-3602   800-827-1000
                                    losangeles.query@vba.va.gov
                                                    www.va.gov
Eric K. Shinseki, Secretary
Stephen W. Warren, Principal Deputy Assistant Secretary
W. Todd Grams, Chief Financial Officer
Glenn D. Haggstrom, Principal Executive Director
The Los Angeles Regional Office (RO) provides benefits and services to approximately 706,000 veterans residing in the Southern California counties of Los Angeles, San Bernardino, Riverside, Ventura, Santa Barbara, San Luis Obispo, and Kern. VA benefits expenditures for veterans residing within the jurisdiction of the

RO exceed $800 million annually. All Loan Guaranty activities for the six counties are under jurisdiction of the Phoenix Regional Office.

5629   Martinez Outpatient Clinic
Veterans Health Administration, U S Dept. of V A
150 Muir Rd
Martinez, CA 94553-4668   925-372-2000
                                                800-382-8387
                                    g.vhacss@forum.va.gov
                                                    www.va.gov
John H Simms, Director
Brian E. Schuman, Chief of Police
The Martinez Outpatient Clinic offers a full range of medical, surgical, mental health, and diagnostic outpatient services, including nuclear medicine, ultrasound, CT and MRI. The Center for Rehabilitation and Extended Care is located adjacent to the outpatient clinic.

5630   Oakland VA Regional Office
Veterans Benefits Administration U S Dept. of V A
1301 Clay Street
12th Floor
Oakland, CA 94612-5217   800-827-1000
                                    oakland.query@vba.va.gov
                                    www.benefits.va.gov/oakland
Geri Spearman, Director
The jurisdiction includes all Northern California, except for Modoc, Lassen, Alpine and Mono counties, which are assigned to the Reno Regional Office. All Loan Guaranty activities are under the jurisdiction of the Phoenix Regional Office. Seven service organizations are collocated on the eleventh floor of the Federal Office building occupied by the regional office.

5631   Rehabilitation Research and Development Center
Department of Veteran s Affairs
810 Vermont Avenue, NW
Washington, DC 94304-1207   202-443-0575
                                            Fax: 202-495-6153
                                    tiffany.asqueri@va.gov
                                    www.rehab.research.va.gov
Patricia A. Dorn, Ph.D., Acting Director, Rehab R&D Service
Ricardo Gonzalez, Administrative Officer
Gloria Winford, Staff Assistant
Sarah Armstrong, Budget Technician
The VA Center of Excellence on Mobility in Palo Alto, CA is dedicated to developing innovative clinical treatments and assistive devices for veterans with physical disabilities to increase their independence and improve their quality of life. The clinical emphasis of the center is to improve mobility, either ambulation or manipulation, in individuals with neurologic impairments or orthopaedic impairments. We do not publish any printed books, journals or periodicals.

5632   Sacramento Medical Center
Veterans Health Administration U S Department of V
10535 Hospital Way
Mather, CA 95655-4200   916-843-7000
                                                800-382-8387
                                    g.vhacss@forum.va.gov
                                    www.northerncalifornia.va.gov
David G. Mastalski, Interim Director
Donna Iatarola, RN, MSN, Associate Director
William T. Cahill, MD, Chief of Staff
It is an integrated health care delivery system, offering a comprehensive array of medical, surgical, rehabilitative, mental health and extended care to veterans in Northern California. The health system is comprised of a medical center in Sacramento; a rehabilitation and extended care facility in Martinez, and seven outpatient clinics.

5633 San Diego VA Regional Office
Veterans Benefits Administration, U S Dept. of V A
8810 Rio San Diego Dr
San Diego, CA   92108-1698   858-552-8585
                                          800-827-1000
                                     Fax: 858-552-7436
                             oakland.query@vba.va.gov
                             www.benefits.va.gov/sandiego
Janet M Peyton, Administrative Officer
The San Diego VA Regional Office provides benefit services for
over 600,000 Veterans and their dependents in the Southern California Counties of Imperial, Orange, Riverside and San Diego.
Since the Regional Office shares occupancy of the building with
a VA Outpatient Clinic and the Employment Development Department of the State of California, it truly offers a one stop
Service Center.

5634 VA Central California Health Care System
Veterans Health Administration, U S Dept. of V A
2615 E Clinton Ave
Fresno, CA   93703-2223   559-225-6100
                                          888-826-2838
                                     Fax: 559-268-6911
                             g.vhacss@forum.va.gov
                             www.fresno.va.gov
Joanne Krumberger, Director
Susan Shyshka, Associate Director
Patricia Richardson Ed.D, RN, N, Nursing Executive
Wessel Meyer MB ChB, FCP (SA), Chief of Staff
VA Central California Health Care System (VACCHCS) has been
improving the health of the men and women who have so proudly
served our nation. We consider it our privilege to serve your
health care needs in any way we can.

5635 VA Greater Los Angeles Healthcare System
Veterans Health Administration U S Deptartment of
11301 Wilshire Blvd
Los Angeles, CA   90073-1003   310-478-3711
                                          800-827-1000
                                     Fax: 310-268-4848
                             g.vhacss@forum.va.gov
                             www.losangeles.va.gov
Donna M. Beiter, RN, MSN, Director
Christopher Sandles, Assistant Director
*Marlene Brewster, RN, MSN, Acting Associate Director, Nursing
and Patient Care Services*
*Carrie J Dekorte, Associate Director for Administration /
Operations*
The VA Greater Los Angeles Healthcare System is the largest,
most complex healthcare system within the Department of Veterans Affairs.GLA consists of three ambulatory care centers, a tertiary care facility and 10 community based outpatient clinics.
GLA serves veterans residing throughout five counties: Los Angeles, Ventura, Kern, Santa Barbara, and San Luis Obispo. There
are 1.4 million veterans in the GLA service area. GLA is affiliated
with both UCLA School of Medicine and USC School of Medici

5636 VA Northern California Healthcare System
Veterans Health Administration, U S Dept. of V A
150 Muir Rd
Martinez, CA   94553-4668   925-372-2000
                                          800-382-8387
                             g.vhacss@forum.va.gov
                             www.northerncalifornia.va.gov
David G. Mastalski, Interim Director
Donna Iatarola, RN, MSN, Associate Director
William T. Cahill, MD, Chief of Staff
VA Northern California Health Care System (VANCHCS) is an
integrated health care delivery system, offering a comprehensive
array of medical, surgical, rehabilitative, mental health and extended care to veterans in Northern California. The health system
is comprised of a medical center in Sacramento; a rehabilitation
and extended care facility in Martinez, and seven outpatient
clinics.

5637 VA San Diego Healthcare System
Veterans Health Administration, U S Dept. of V A
3350 La Jolla Village Dr
San Diego, CA   92161   858-552-8585
                                          800-331-8387
                             g.vhacss@forum.va.gov
                             www.sandiego.va.gov
Jeffrey T. Gering, FACHE, Director
Cynthia Abair, MHA, Associate Director
Robert M. Smith, MD, Chief of Staff/Medical Director
*Sandra Solem, PhD, RN, Associate Director, Patient Care Ser-
vices/Nurse Executive*
We provide medical, surgical, mental health, geriatric, spinal
cord injury, and advanced rehabilitation services. VASDHS has
296 authorized beds, including skilled nursing beds and operates
several regional referral programs including cardiovascular sur-
gery and spinal cord injury. The facility also supports three Vet
Centers at the following locations: Chula Vista, San Diego, and
San Marcos.

Colorado

5638 Boulder Vet Center
4999 Pearl East Circle
Suite 106
Boulder, CO   80301   303-440-7306
                                          877-927-8387
                                     Fax: 303-449-3907
                             www.va.gov
Gail N Bennett, Office Manager
Michael J Pantaleo, Team Leader
Annette Matlock, Counselor
Collette M Archibald, Counselor
Offers trauma and readjustment from military and civilian life
counseling and assistance with disability claims, military bene-
fits and employment are provided.

5639 Colorado/Wyoming VA Medical Center
Veterans Benefits Administration U S Dept. of V A
155 Van Gordon St
Suite 395
Lakewood, CO   80225   303-914-2680
                                          800-827-1000
                             denver.query@vba.va.gov
                             www.denver.va.gov
Forest Farley Jr, Medical Center Director
Thomas E Bowen, Chief of Staff

5640 Denver VA Medical Center
Veterans Health Administration, U S Dept. of V A
1055 Clermont St
Suite 6A138
Denver, CO   80220-3808   303-393-2869
                                          888-336-8262
                             judi.guy@va.gov
                             www.denver.va.gov
Lynnette Roth, Executive Director
Peggy Kearns MS, RD, FACHE, Associate Director
*Judith Burke RN, MS, NEA-BC, Associate Director, Patient Care
Services*
Rebecca Keough MPA, VHA-CM, Assistant Director
Construction of our 1.1m sq foot, $800m replacement facility is
well under way! Concrete is being poured, steel is being put in,
and we're working hard to open in 2015.

5641 Grand Junction VA Medical Center
Veterans Health Administration
2121 North Ave
Grand Junction, CO   81501-6428   970-242-0731
                                          866-206-6415
                                     Fax: 970-244-1300
                                     g.vhacss@forum.va.gov
                                     www.grandjunction.va.gov

Patricia A. Hitt, MS, Acting Director
Michael Murphy, Manager
Randal France, M.D., Chief Psychiatry Service/ Int. Chf. of Staff
Angela T Brothers, AD/ Patient Care Svcs
The VAMC operates 53 beds comprised of 23 acute care and 30 Transitional Care Unit beds. The VAMC provides primary and secondary care including acute medical, surgical, and psychiatric inpatient services, as well as a full range of outpatient services.

Connecticut

5642 Hartford Regional Office
Veterans Benefits Administration U S Department of
555 Willard Ave
Building 2E
Newington, CT   6111-2631   860-666-6951
                                          800-827-1000
                                     hartford.query@vba.va.gov

Jeanette A Chirico Post, Network Director
The Hartford Regional Office now provides one-stop service to veterans and their families seeking assistance in compensation, pension, and vocational rehabilitation and employment in an accessible campus environment.

5643 Hartford Vet Center
25 Elm St
Suite A
Rocky Hill, CT   06067-2305   860-563-8800
                                          877-927-8387
                                     Fax: 860-563-8805
                                     donna.hryb@med.va.gov
                                     www.va.gov

Donna Hryb LCSW, Team Leader
Pedro Ortiz, Counselor
Amy Otzel, Counselor
Laura Hall, Military Sexual Trauma Counselor
A U.S. Department of Veterans Affairs counseling center offering counseling to Vietnam era and combat veterans. Sexual trauma/harassment counseling, medical screening and benefit referral is available to all veterans.

5644 VA Connecticut Healthcare System: Newington Division
Veterans Health Administration U S Department. of
555 Willard Ave
Newington, CT   6111-2631   860-666-6951
                                          800-827-1000
                                     Fax: 860-667-6764
                                     g.vhacss@forum.va.gov
                                     www.connecticut.va.gov

Janice M. Boss, MS, Director
Margaret Veazey, RN, MSN, Associate Director for Patient Care Services
John Callahan, Associate Director
Al Montoya, Assistant Director
The mission of VA Connecticut Healthcare Systems is to fulfill a nation's commitment to its veterans by providing quality healthcare, promoting health through prevention and maintaining excellence in teaching and research. Provides primary, secondary and tertiary care in medicine, geriatrics, neurology, psychiatry and surgery with an operating capacity of 211 hospital beds.

5645 VA Connecticut Healthcare System: West Haven
Veterans Health Administration, U S Dept. of V A
950 Campbell Ave
West Haven, CT   06516-2770   203-932-5711
                                          800-827-1000
                                     Fax: 203-937-3868
                                     g.vhacss@forum.va.gov
                                     www.connecticut.va.gov

Janice M. Boss, MS, Director
Margaret Veazey, RN, MSN, Associate Director for Patient Care Services
John Callahan, Associate Director
Al Montoya, Assistant Director
The mission of VA Connecticut Healthcare Systems is to fulfill a nation's commitment to its veterans by providing quality healthcare, promoting health through prevention and maintaining excellence in teaching and research. Provides primary, secondary and tertiary care in medicine, geriatrics, neurology, psychiatry and surgery with an operating capacity of 211 hospital beds.

Delaware

5646 Delaware VA Regional Office
Veterans Benefits Administration U S Dept. of V A
1601 Kirkwood Hwy
Wilmington, DE   19805-4917   302-994-2511
                                          800-461-8262
                                     Fax: 302-633-5516
                                     wilmington.query@vba.va.gov
                                     www.wilmington.va.gov

Daniel D. Hendee, FACHE, MHA, Director
Mary Alice Johnson, MS, RN, Associate Director for Patient Care Services
William E. England, Associate Director for Finance and Operations
Enrique Guttin, MD, MMM, CPE,, Chief of Staff
We offer comprehensive services ranging from preventive screenings to long-term care. Wilmington VAMC proudly serves Veterans in multiple locations for convenient access to the services we provide.

5647 Wilmington VA Medical Center
Veterans Health Administration, US Dept. of VA
1601 Kirkwood Hwy
Wilmington, DE   19805-4917   302-994-2511
                                          800-461-8262
                                     Fax: 302-633-5516
                                     g.vhacss@forum.va.gov
                                     www.wilmington.va.gov

Daniel D. Hendee, FACHE, MHA, Director
Mary Alice Johnson, MS, RN, Associate Director for Patient Care Services
William E. England, Associate Director for Finance and Operations
Enrique Guttin, MD, MMM, CPE,, Chief of Staff
We offer comprehensive services ranging from preventive screenings to long-term care. Wilmington VAMC proudly serves Veterans in multiple locations for convenient access to the services we provide.

5648 Wilmington Vet Center
2710 Centerville Road
Suite 103
Wilmington, DE   19808- 4917   302-994-1660
                                          877-927-8387
                                     Fax: 302-994-8361
                                     www.va.gov

Joan Spencer, Team Leader
Patricia Elwood, Office Manager
Valerie Feeley, Counselor
Barbara F Blevins, Counselor
Veterans counseling program offering individual counseling services, advocacy services and group counseling. The focus is the counseling of all veterans coping with the aftermath of war, sexual abuse/harassment in the military and all veterans of the Vietnam era. The center also has an active outreach program to seek veterans needing services. Hours of operation are between 8:00

AM - 4:30 PM, Monday - Friday and other times by appointment only. Services are free.

District of Columbia

5649   Disabled American Veterans
Legislative HQ
807 Maine Ave SW
Washington, DC   20024
202-554-3501
Fax: 202-554-3581
feedback@davmail.org
www.dav.org

David W Riley, Chairman
Delphine Metcalf-Foster, National Commander
J. Marc Burgess, National Adjutant
Garry J Augustine, Executive Director
Serves America's disabled veterans and their families. Direct services include legislative advocacy; professional counseling about compensation, pension, educational and job training programs and VA health care; and assistance in applying for those entitlements.

5650   PVA Sports and Recreation Program
Paralyzed Veterans of America
801 18th St NW
Washington, DC   20006-3517
202-872-1300
800-424-8200
888-888-2201
Fax: 202-785-4432
TTY:800-795-4327
info@pva.org
www.pva.org

Randy Pleva, President
Homer S. Townsend, Jr., Executive Director
Larry Dodson, National Secretary
Bill Lawson, National President
Today, the work continues to create an America where all veterans and people with disabilities, and their families, have everything they need to live full and productive lives.

5651   VA Medical Center, Washington DC
50 Irving St NW
Washington, DC   20422-1
202-745-8000
800-827-1000
877-328-2621
g.vhacss@forum.va.gov
www.washingtondc.va.gov

Brian A. Hawkins, MHA, Medical Center Director
Bryan C. Matthews, MBA, Associate Medical Center Director
Natalie Merckens, Assistant Medical Center Director
Ross D. Fletcher, MD, Chief of Staff
Acute general and specialized services in medicine, surgery, neurology, and psychiatry.

5652   Washington DC VA Medical Center
Veterans Health Administration, U S Dept. of V A
50 Irving St NW
Washington, DC   20422-1
202-745-8000
800-827-1000
877-328-2621
Fax: 202-754-8530
g.vhacss@forum.va.gov
www.washingtondc.va.gov

Brian A. Hawkins, MHA, Medical Center Director
Bryan C. Matthews, MBA, Associate Medical Center Director
Natalie Merckens, Assistant Medical Center Director
Ross D. Fletcher, MD, Chief of Staff
Acute general and specialized services in medicine, surgery, neurology, and psychiatry.

Florida

5653   Bay Pines VA Medical Center
Veterans Health Administration, U S Dept. of V A
10000 Bay Pines Blvd
PO Box 5005
Bay Pines, FL   33744
727-398-6661
800-827-1000
888-820-0230
g.vhacss@forum.va.gov
www.baypines.va.gov

Suzanne M. Klinker, Medical Center Director
Kristine Brown, MPH, Associate Director
Teresa Kumar, RN, MSN, CPHQ,, Associate Director for Patient / Nursing Services
Keith Neeley, FACHE, Assistant Director
Since 1933, Bay Pines VA Healthcare System has been improving the health of the men and women who have so proudly served our nation. We consider it our privilege to serve your health care needs in any way we can. Our services are available to Veterans living in a ten county catchment area in west central Florida.

5654   Gainesville Division, North Florida/South Georgia Veterans Healthcare System
Veterans Health Administration, U S Dept. of V A
1601 SW Archer Rd
Gainesville, FL   32608-1611
352-376-1611
800-324-8387
Fax: 352-379-7445
g.vhacss@forum.va.gov
www.northflorida.va.gov/northflorida

Thomas Wisnieski, MPA, FACHE, Director
Nancy Reissener, Deputy Director
Maureen Wilkes, Associate Director
LeAnne Whitlow, RN, MSHSA, MB, Associate Director, Nursing Service
In addition to our medical centers in Gainesville and Lake City, we offer services in three satellite outpatient clinics and several community-based outpatient clinics across North Florida and South Georgia.

5655   James A Haley VA Medical Center
Veterans Health Administration, U S Dept. of V A
13000 Bruce B Downs Blvd
Suite T72
Tampa, FL   33612-4745
813-972-2000
800-827-1000
888-811-0107
g.vhacss@forum.va.gov
www.tampa.va.gov

Kathleen R. Fogarty, Director
Roy L. Hawkins Jr., Deputy Director
David J. VanMeter, Associate Director
Suzanne Tate, Assistant Director
Comprehensive health care is provided through primary care, tertiary care, and long-term care in areas of medicine, surgery, psychiatry, physical medicine and rehabilitation, spinal cord injury, neurology, oncology, dentistry, geriatrics, and extended care.

5656   Miami VA Medical Center
Veterans Health Administration, U S Dept. of V A
1201 NW 16th St
Suite B822
Miami, FL   33125-1693
305-575-7000
800-827-1000
888-276-1785
Fax: 305-575-3266
g.vhacss@forum.va.gov
www.miami.va.gov

Paul M. Russo, Director
Mark E. Morgan, Associate Director
Marcia Lysaght, Associate Director, Patient Care Services
P. Gwendolyn Findley, Ph.D., Assistant Director
The Miami VA is an accredited comprehensive medical provider, providing general medical, surgical, inpatient and outpatient mental health services, the Miami VA Healthcare System includes an AIDS/HIV center, a prosthetic treatment center, spinal

cord injury rehabilitative center, and Geriatric Research, Education, and Clinical Center (GRECC).

5657   St. Petersburg Regional Office
Veterans Benefits Administration, U S Dept. of V A
9500 Bay Pines Blvd
St Petersburg, FL   33708   727-319-7492
                                                             800-827-1000
                                                    stpete.query@vba.va.gov
                                                                www.va.gov

Warren McPherson, Executive Director

5658   West Palm Beach VA Medical Center
Veterans Health Administration, U S Dept. of V A
7305 N Military Trl
West Palm Beach, FL   33410-7417   561-422-8262
                                                             800-972-8262
                                                        Fax: 561-882-6707
                                                   g.vhacss@forum.va.gov
                                                  www.westpalmbeach.va.gov
Charleen R. Szabo, FACHE, Medical Center Director
Cristy McKillop, FACHE, MHA, Medical Center Associate Director
Gloria A. Bays, MSN, ARNP, NE-BC, Associate Director for Patient Care Services
Deepak Mandi, MD, Chief of Staff
The medical center is a general medical, psychiatric and surgical facility. It is a teaching hospital, providing a full range of patient care services, with state-of-the-art technology as well as education and limited research. Comprehensive healthcare is provided through primary care and long-term care in the areas of dentistry, extended care, medicine, neurology, oncology, pharmacy, physical medicine, psychiatry, rehabilitation and surgery. The West Palm Beach VA Medical Center operates a Blin

Georgia

5659   Atlanta Regional Office
Veterans Benefits Administration, U S Dept. of V A
1700 Clairmont Road
Decatur, GA   30033-1210   404-463-3100
                                                             800-827-1000
                                                        Fax: 404-929-5819
                                                   atlanta.query@vba.va.gov
                                                                www.va.gov

Chick Krautler, Executive Director
The Atlanta VA Regional Office is responsible for delivering non-medical VA benefits and services to Georgia Veterans and their dependent family members. This is accomplished through the administration of comprehensive and diverse benefit programs established by Congress. Our goal is to deliver these benefits and services in a timely, accurate, and compassionate manner.

5660   Atlanta VA Medical Center
Veterans Health Administration, U S Dept. of V A
1670 Clairmont Rd
Decatur, GA   30033-4004   404-321-6111
                                                             800-827-1000
                                                        Fax: 404-728-7734
                                                   g.vhacss@forum.va.gov
                                                          www.atlanta.va.gov

Leslie B. Wiggins, Director
Tom Grace, MBA/MHA, Associate Director
Sheila Meuse, PhD, Assistant Director
Sandy Leake, MSN, RN, Associate Director for Nursing/Patient Services
The Atlanta VA Medical Center (VAMC), located on 26 acres in Decatur, is one of eight medical centers in the VA Southeast Network. It is a teaching hospital, providing a full range of patient care services complete with state-of-the-art technology, education, and research.

5661   Augusta VA Medical Center
Veterans Health Administration, U S Dept. of V A
950 15th Street Downtown/1 Freedom
Augusta, GA   30904-6258   706-733-0188
                                                             800-827-1000
                                                        Fax: 706-731-7227
                                                   g.vhacss@forum.va.gov
Robert U. Hamilton, MHA, FACHE, Medical Center Director
Richard Rose, Associate Director
Michelle Cox-Henley, MS, RN, Associate Director for Nursing/Patient Services
Luke M. (Mik Stapleton, MD, Chief of Staff
The Charlie Norwood VA Medical Center is a two-division Medical Center that provides tertiary care inmedicine, surgery, neurology, psychiatry, rehabilitation medicine, and spinal cord injury. The Downtown Division is authorized 155 beds (58 medicine, 37 surgery, and 60 spinal cord injury). The Uptown Division, located approximately three miles away, is authorized 315 beds (68 psychiatry, 15 blind rehabilitation and 40 medical rehabilitation. In addition, a 132-bed Restorative/Nursing Home C

5662   Carl Vinson VA Medical Center
Veterans Health Administration, U S Dept. of V A
1826 Veterans Blvd
Dublin, GA   31021-3699   478-272-1210
                                                        Fax: 478-277-2717
                                                   dana.doles@med.va.gov
                                                          www.dublin.va.gov

John S. Goldman, Director
Gerald M. DeWorth, Associate Director
Sue Preston, RN, Associate Director for Patient and Nursing Services
Nomie Finn, M.D, Chief of Staff
Since 1948, Carl Vinson VA Medical Center has been improving the health of the men and women who have so proudly served our nation. We consider it our privilege to serve your health care needs in any way we can. Services are available to veterans living in the Middle Georgia area.

5663   Southeastern Paralyzed Veterans of America(PVA)
4010 Deans Bridge Rd
U.S. Highway 1
Hephzibah, GA 30815-5616   706-796-6301
                                                             800-292-9335
                                                        Fax: 706-796-0363
                                                   homercpva@gmail.com
                                                  www.southeasternpva.org
Dr. Chuck Turek, National Director
Linda Hutchinson, Advocacy & Legislative Director for North and South Carolina
Homer Cole, Chapter President
Larry Dodson, Chapter Vice President
Works to maximize the quality of life for its members and all people with SCI/D as a leading adovocate for healthcare, SCI/D research and education, veteran's benefits, and rights, accessibility and the removal of architectural barriers, sports programs, and disability rights.

Hawaii

5664   Hilo Vet Center
70 Lanihuli St
Suite 102
Hilo, HI   96720-2067   808-969-3833
                                                             877-927-8387
                                                        Fax: 808-969-2025
                                                                www.va.gov

Felipe Sales, Team Leader
Samuelito Labasan, Office Manager
Peter Ehlich, Counselor
Nancy G Waller, Counselor
Veterans medical clinic offering disabled veterans medical treatments, readjustment and PTSD counseling to combat veterans

5665 Honolulu VBA Regional Office
Veterans Benefits Administration, U S Dept. of V A
459 Patterson Road, E-Wing
Honolulu, HI   96819-1522   808-566-1412
                                           800-827-1000
                                           Fax: 808-433-0478
                                           honolulu.query@vba.va.gov
                                           www.vba.va.gov/ro/honolulu

Claude M Kicklighter, Chief of Staff
Alan Furuno, Manager
Alvin Kalawe, Elderly Program Coordinator
Karin Frazier, Women Veteran's Program Coordinator
The Honolulu Regional Office is responsible for administering
VA's benefit programs under the leadership and direction of the
Under Secretary for Benefits for the Veterans Benefits Adminis-
tration. Formerly part of the Honolulu VA Medical & Regional
Office Center (VAMROC), the Honolulu Regional Office (RO)
was renamed as a stand alone RO on June 2, 2003. The office is
co-located with the Spark M. Matsunaga Pacific Islands Health
Care System medical center, on the grounds of the Tripler Army
Medic

5666 Pacific Islands Health Care System
Veterans Health Administration, US Dept. of VA
459 Patterson Rd
Honolulu, HI   96819-1522   808-433-0600
                                           800-214-1306
                                           Fax: 808-433-0390
                                           g.vhacss@forum.va.gov
                                           www.hawaii.va.gov

William F. Dubbs, M.D., Acting Director
Brandon K. Yamamoto, Acting Associate Director
Jane Wellman, APRN, Associate Director of Patient Care Services
David M. Bernstein, M.D, Acting Chief of Staff
The VA Pacific Islands Health Care System (VAPIHCS) Honolulu provides a broad range of medical care services, serving an
estimated 127,600 veterans throughout Hawaii and the Pacific Islands. The VAPIHCS provides outpatient medical and mental
health care through a main Ambulatory Care Clinic on Oahu (Honolulu) and through five Community Based Outpatient Clinics
(CBOCs) on the neighboring islands including: Hawaii (Hilo and
Kona), Maui, Kauai, and Guam. Traveling clinicians also
provide episodi

Idaho

5667 Boise Regional Office
Veterans Benefits Administration, U S Dept. of V A
444 W. Fort Street
Boise, ID   83702-4531   800-827-1000
                                           boise.query@vba.va.gov
                                           www.va.gov

Jim Vance, Director
Pat Teague, Service Officer
Tom Ressler, Manager
The Boise Regional Office administers monetary benefits to
17,283 veterans in Idaho, Utah, and Oregon. The Regional Office
issued monthly disability and death benefit payments of over $15
million in January 2007. VBA's annual compensation and pension benefits for veterans residing within the RO's jurisdiction
now exceed $185 million

5668 Boise VA Medical Center
Veterans Health Administration, U S Dept. of V A
500 W Fort St
Boise, ID   83702-4531   208-422-1000
                                           800-827-1000
                                           Fax: 208-422-1326
                                           g.vhacss@forum.va.gov
                                           www.boise.va.gov

Jennifer T Shalz, Chief of Staff
We truly hope to improve your health and well-being and will
make your visit or stay as pleasant as possible. We are committed
to veterans and the nation and strive to continually enhance the
care we provide. We also train future healthcare professionals,
conduct research and support our nation in times of emergency.

In all of these activities, our employees will respect and support
your rights as a patient.

Illinois

5669 Edward Hines Jr Hospital
Veterans Health Administration, U S Dept. of V A
5000 South 5th Avenue
Hines, IL   60141   708-202-8387
                                           800-827-1000
                                           Fax: 708-202-2684
                                           g.vhacss@forum.va.gov
                                           www.hines.va.gov

Joan Ricard, FACHE, Hospital Director
Dr. Daniel Zomchek, Associate Director
Carol A. Gouty, RN, MSN, PhD, Associate Director of Patient Care
Karandeep Sraon, Assistant Director
Specialized clinical programs include Blind Rehabilitation, Spinal Cord Injury, Neurosurgery, Radiation Therapy and Cardiovascular Surgery. The hospital also serves as the VISN 12
southern tier hub for pathology, radiology, radiation therapy, human resource management and fiscal services. Hines VAH currently operates 471 beds and six community based outpatient
clinics in Elgin, Kankakee, Oak Lawn, Aurora, LaSalle, and
Joliet.

5670 Marion VA Medical Center
Veterans Health Administration U S Department of V
2401 W Main St
Marion, IL   62959-1188   618-997-5311
                                           800-827-1000
                                           kimberly.travelstead@va.gov
                                           www.marion.va.gov

Paul Bockelman, Medical Center Director
Frank Kehus, Associate Director
The VA Medical Center in Marion, Illinois, is a general medical
and surgical facility that operates 55 acute care beds and a 60 bed
Community Living Center. Ten Outpatient Clinics that provide
primary care and behavioral medicine services are located in Har-
risburg; Carbondale; Effingham; and Mt. Vernon, IL; Paducah;
Hanson; Owensboro; and Mayfield, Kentucky; Vincennes and
Evansville, IN.

5671 North Chicago VA Medical Center
Veterans Health Administration, U S Dept. of V A
3001 North Green Bay Rd
North Chicago, IL   60064-3048   847-688-1900
                                           800-393-0865
                                           g.vhacss@forum.va.gov
                                           www.lovell.fhcc.va.gov

Patrick L. Sullivan, Director
Captain Jos, A. Acosta, MC, US, Commanding Officer/Deputy Di-
rector
Captain Jami Kersten, Associate Director
Dr. Sarah Fouse, Associate Director of Patient Services/Nurse
Executive
The arrangement incorporates facilities, services and resources
from the North Chicago VA Medical Center (VAMC) and the Na-
val Health Clinic Great Lakes (NHCGL). A combined mission of
the health care center means active duty military, their family
members, military retirees and veterans are all cared for at the
facility.

5672 VA Illiana Health Care System
Veterans Health Administration, U S Dept. of V A
1900 E Main St
Danville, IL   61832-5198   217-554-3000
                                           800-320-8387
                                           Fax: 217-554-4552
                                           g.vhacss@forum.va.gov
                                           www.danville.va.gov

Emma Metcalf, MSN, RN,, Director
Diana Carranza, Associate Director
Alesia Coe, MSN, RN,, Associate Director for Patient Care Services
Nirmala Rozario, M.D., Ph.D, Chief of Staff

Since 1898, our buildings, facilities, patients, and missions have changed, but remaining constant is VA Illiana Health Care System's endeavor in improving the health of the men and women who have so proudly served our nation. Being the 8th oldest VA facility, we consider it our privilege to serve your health care needs in any way we can.

Indiana

5673 Indianapolis Regional Office
Veterans Benefits Administration U S Department of
575 N Pennsylvania St
Indianapolis, IN   46204-1563
317-226-7860
800-827-1000
TTY:800-829-4833
indianapolis.query@vba.va.gov
www.benefits.va.gov/indianapolis

5674 Richard L Roudebush VA Medical Center
Veterans Health Administration, U S Dept. of V A
1481 W 10th St
Indianapolis, IN   46202-2803
317-554-0000
800-827-1000
Fax: 317-554-0127
g.vhacss@forum.va.gov
www.indianapolis.va.gov

Thomas Mattice, Director
Jeff Nechanicky, Associate Director
Kimberly Radant, Associate Director for Patient Care Services
Cathy Lee, Assistant Director
Since 1932, Richard L. Roudebush VA Medical Center has been improving the health of the men and women who have so proudly served our nation. We consider it our privilege to serve your health care needs in any way we can. Services are available to more than 196,000 veterans living in a 45-county area of Indiana and Illinois.

5675 VA North Indiana Health Care System: Fort Wayne Campus
Veterans Health Administration, U S Dept. of V A
2121 Lake Ave
Fort Wayne, IN   46805-5100
260-426-5431
800-360-8387
g.vhacss@forum.va.gov
www.northernindiana.va.gov

Denise M. Deitzen, Medical Center Director
Audrey L. Frison, MHA, RN, Associate Director
Helen Rhodes MPA, RN, Associate Director for Operations
Ajay Dhawan MD FACHE, Chief of Staff
The Fort Wayne Campus offers primary and secondary medical and surgical services. Primary care clinics are available at both medical center campuses and at Community Based Outpatient Clinics (CBOCs) located in South Bend, Goshen, Peru and Muncie Indiana. Recently completed renovations and construction, and continuous maintenance, ensure an attractive, state-of-the-art healthcare environment.

5676 VA Northern Indiana Health Care System: Marion Campus
Veterans Health Administration, U S Dept. of V A
1700 E 38th St
Marion, IN   46953-4568
765-674-3321
800-360-8387
g.vhacss@forum.va.gov
www.northernindiana.va.gov

Denise M. Deitzen, Medical Center Director
Audrey L. Frison, MHA, RN, Associate Director
Helen Rhodes MPA, RN, Associate Director for Operations
Ajay Dhawan MD FACHE, Chief of Staff
The Marion Campus offers a full range of mental health, nursing home care, and extended care services. Primary care clinics are available at both medical center campuses and at Community Based Outpatient Clinics (CBOCs) located in South Bend, Goshen, Peru and Muncie Indiana.

Iowa

5677 Des Moines VA Medical Center
Veterans Health Administration, U S Dept. of V A
3600 30th St
Des Moines, IA   50310-5753
515-699-5999
800-294-8387
Fax: 515-699-5862
g.vhacss@forum.va.gov
www.centraliowa.va.gov

Donald Cooper, Director
Susan Martin, Associate Director for Resources and Operations
Tammy Neff, RN, MBA, MSN, M, Acting Associate Director for Patient Services/Nurse Executi
Fredrick Bahls, MD, Chief of Staff
The VA Central Iowa Health Care System (VACIHCS) operates a Veterans Health Administration (VHA) medical facility in Des Moines, with Community Based Outpatient Clinics (CBOCs) in Mason City, Fort Dodge, Knoxville, Marshalltown and Carroll. The medical center provides acute and specialized medical and surgical services, residential outpatient treatment programs in substance abuse and post-traumatic stress and a full range of mental health and long-term care services, as well as sub-acute and r

5678 Des Moines VA Regional Office
Veterans Benefits Administration, U S Dept. of V A
210 Walnut Street
Des Moines, IA   50309-2115
515-323-7580
800-827-1000
Fax: 515-323-7580
leander@vba.va.gov
www.va.gov

Rich Anderson, Service Director
The Des Moines VA Regional Office provides Compensation, Pension and Vocational Rehabilitation and Counseling services for all military veterans in the State of Iowa. The Des Moines VA Regional Office currently provides approximately $260 million in benefits to the approximately 270,000 veterans in Iowa.

5679 Iowa City VA Medical Center
Veterans Health Administration, U S Dept. of V A
601 Highway 6 West
Iowa City, IA   52240-2202
319-338-0581
800-637-0128
866-687-7382
Fax: 319-339-7171
g.vhacss@forum.va.gov
www.iowacity.va.gov

Barry Sharp, Director
Timothy McMurry, Associate Director for Operations
Dawn Oxley, RN, Associate Director Patient Care Services/Nurse Executive
Stanley Parker, MD, Acting Chief of Staff
Tertiary care facility, affiliated teaching hospital, and research center seving an aging veteran populatiaon in eastern Iowa and western Illinois. Satellite clinics are located in Bettendord, Dubuque, and Waterloo, Iowa and in Quincy and Galesburg, Illinois.

5680 Knoxville VA Medical Center
Veterans Health Administration, U S Dept. of V A
1515 W Pleasant St
Knoxville, IA   50138-3399
641-842-3101
800-816-8878
Fax: 641-828-5124
g.vhacss@forum.va.gov
www.centraliowa.va.gov

Claudia M Kicklighter

5681 **VA Central Iowa Health Care System**
3600 30th St
Des Moines, IA   50310-5753   515-699-5999
                                                800-294-8387
                                          Fax: 515-699-5862
                                          www.centraliowa.va.gov

Donald Cooper, Director
Susan Martin, Associate Director for Resources and Operations
Tammy Neff, RN, MBA, MSN, M, Acting Associate Director for Patient Services/Nurse Executi
Fredrick Bahls, MD, Chief of Staff
The VA Central Iowa Health Care System (VACIHCS) operates a Veterans Health Administration (VHA) medical facility in Des Moines, with Community Based Outpatient Clinics (CBOCs) in Mason City, Fort Dodge, Knoxville, Marshalltown and Carroll. The medical center provides acute and specialized medical and surgical services, residential outpatient treatment programs in substance abuse and post-traumatic stress and a full range of mental health and long-term care services, as well as sub-acute and r

Kansas

5682 **Colmery-O'Neil VA Medical Center**
Veterans Health Administration, U S Dept. of V A
2200 SW Gage Blvd
Topeka, KS   66622   785-350-3111
                                                800-574-8387
                                          g.vhacss@forum.va.gov
                                          www.topeka.va.gov
A. Rudy Klopfer, FACHE, Director
John Moon, Associate Director
Nelson L. Dean, RN, BSN, MA, Associate Director for Patient Care Services
Christine M Kleckner, MBA, RD, Assistant Director
Since 1946, the staff of the Colmery-O'Neil VA Medical Center has been serving veterans. Today, we proudly serve our nation's veterans with excellent health care as part of the VA Eastern Kansas Health Care System (VAEKHCS). We consider it our privilege to serve your health care needs in any way we can.

5683 **Dwight D Eisenhower VA Medical Center**
Veterans Health Administration, U S Dept. of V A
4101 4th Street Trafficway
Leavenworth, KS   66048-5014   913-682-2000
                                                800-952-8387
                                          g.vhacss@forum.va.gov
                                          www.leavenworth.va.gov
A. Rudy Klopfer, FACHE, Director
John Moon, Associate Director
Nelson L. Dean, RN, BSN, MA, Associate Director for Patient Care Services
Christine M Kleckner, MBA, RD, Assistant Director
Since 1886, the staff of the Dwight D. Eisenhower VA Medical Center has been serving veterans. Today, we proudly serve our nation's veterans with excellent health care as part of the VA Eastern Kansas Health Care System (VAEKHCS). We consider it our privilege to serve your health care needs in any way we can.

5684 **Kansas VA Regional Office**
Veterans Benefits Administration, U S Dept. of V A
5500 E Kellogg Dr
Wichita, KS   67218-1607   800-827-1000
                                          wichita.query@vba.va.gov
                                          www.benefits.va.gov/wichita
Edgar L Tucker, Medical Center Director

5685 **Robert J Dole VA Medical Center**
Veterans Health Administration, U S Dept. of V A
5500 E Kellogg Dr
Wichita, KS   67218-1607   316-685-2221
                                                800-827-1000
                                                888-827-6881
                                          Fax: 316-651-3666
                                          g.vhacss@forum.va.gov
                                          www.wichita.va.gov
Kevin Inkley, MA, Director
Vicki Bondie, MBA, Associate Director
Carol A. Kaster, MA, RN, Associate Director of Patient Care/Nurse Executive
M. Ganga Hematillake, MD, Chief of Staff
For over 70 years, the Dole VA Medical and Regional office center has been honored to serve Kansas area veterans. The center provides a full range of primary and specialty acute and extended care services to veterans in 59 counties of Kansas. Special emphasis programs include substance abuse, post traumatic stress disorder (PTSD), women's health, spinal cord injury, visual impairment, prosthetic and sensory aids, and homeless services.

Kentucky

5686 **Lexington VA Medical Center**
Veterans Health Administration, U S Dept. of V A
1101 Veterans Dr
Lexington, KY   40502-2235   859-281-4900
                                                800-352-4000
                                          g.vhacss@forum.va.gov
                                          www.lexington.va.gov
Martin J. Traxler, Acting Medical Center Director
Patricia Breeden, MD, Acting Chief of Staff
Laura Faulkner, Acting Associate Medical Center Director
Agnes Therady, RN, NEA-BC, F, Acting Associate Director Patient Care Services
The Lexington Veterans Affairs Medical Center is a fully accredited, two-division, tertiary care medical center with an operating bed complement of 199 hospital beds. Acute medical, neurological, surgical and psychiatric inpatient services are provided at the Cooper Division, located adjacent to the University of Kentucky Medical Center. Other available services include: emergency care, medical-surgical units, acute psychiatry, ICU, progressive care unit, (includes Cardiac Cath Lab) ambulatory s

5687 **Louisville VA Medical Center**
Veterans Health Administration, U S Dept. of V A
800 Zorn Ave
Louisville, KY   40206-1433   502-287-4000
                                                800-376-8387
                                          g.vhacss@forum.va.gov
                                          www.louisville.va.gov
Wayne L. Pfeffer, MHSA, FACHE, Medical Center Director
Douglas V Paxton, Sr, Associate Director / Operations
Pamala Thompson, RN, MSA, MSN, Associate Director for Patient Care Services
Marylee Rothschild, M.D., Chief of Staff
Since 1952, Robley Rex VAMC has been improving the health of the men and women who have so proudly served our nation. We consider it our privilege to serve your health care needs in any way we can. Services are available to more than 166,000 veterans living in a 35-county area of the Kentuckiana area.

5688 **Louisville VA Regional Office**
Veterans Benefits Administration, U S Dept. of V A
800 Zorn Avenue
Louisville, KY   40206-1433   502-287-4000
                                                800-376-8387
                                          louisville.query@vba.va.gov
                                          www.louisville.va.gov
Wayne L. Pfeffer, MHSA, FACHE, Medical Center Director
Douglas V Paxton, Sr, Associate Director / Operations
Pamala Thompson, RN, MSA, MSN, Associate Director for Patient Care Services
Marylee Rothschild, M.D., Chief of Staff

Since 1952, Robley Rex VAMC has been improving the health of the men and women who have so proudly served our nation. We consider it our privilege to serve your health care needs in any way we can. Services are available to more than 166,000 veterans living in a 35-county area of the Kentuckiana area.

Louisiana

5689   Alexandria VA Medical Center
Department of Veterans Affairs
2495 Shreveport Highway
Pineville, LA   71360-9004   318-466-4000
                                                    800-375-8387
                                              Fax: 318-483-5029
                                        richard.wright2@va.gov
                                           www.alexandria.va.gov
Martin J. Traxler, Medical Center Director
Yolanda Sanders-Jackson, Associate Director
Jose N Rivera, MD, Acting Chief of Staff
Amy Lesniewski, RN MS, Nurse Executive
The VAMC Alexandria is categorized as a primary and secondary care facility. It is a teaching hospital, providing a full range of primary care services with state-of-the-art technology and education. Comprehensive acute and extended health care is provided on a primary and secondary basis in areas of medicine, surgery, psychiatry, physical medicine and rehabilitation, neurology, oncology, dentistry, geriatrics, and extended care. The Medical Center serves a potential veteran population of over 1

5690   New Orleans VA Medical Center
Veterans Health Administration, U S Dept. of V A
1601 Perdido St
New Orleans, LA   70112-1262   504-412-3700
                                                     800-935-8387
                                              Fax: 504-589-5210
                                        Stacie.Rivera@med.va.gov
                                           www.neworleans.va.gov
John D Church Jr, Medical Director/President
Fernando Rivera, Association Medical Center Direc
Sam Lucero, Special Assistant to Director
Stacie M Rivera, Public Affairs Officer
A teaching hospital, providing a full range of patient care services, with state-of-the-art technology as well as education and research. Comprehensive health care is provided through primary care, tetiary care, and long-term care in areas of medicine, surgery, psychiatry, physical medicine and rehabilitation, neurology, oncology, dentistry, geriatrics, and extended care.

5691   Shreveport VA Medical Center
Veterans Health Administration, U S Dept. of V A
510 E Stoner Ave
Shreveport, LA   71101-4295   318-221-8411
                                                     800-827-1000
                                           www.shreveport.va.gov
Shirley M. Bealer, Medical Center Director
Todd M. Moore, Assistant Medical Center Director
Erik J. Glover, Associate Medical Center Director
Ruth Davis, DNS, Associate Director for Patient Care Services

Maine

5692   Maine VA Regional Office
Veterans Benefits Administration, U S Dept. of V A
1 VA Center
Augusta, ME   4330-6719   207-623-8411
                                                     877-421-8263
                                        togus.query@vba.va.gov
                                                     www.va.gov
Dale Demers, Director
Scott Karczewski, Manager

5693   Togus VA Medical Center
Veterans Health Administration, U S Dept. of V A
1 VA Center
Augusta, ME   04330-6795   207-623-8411
                                                     877-421-8263
                                              Fax: 207-623-5792
                                        g.vhacss@forum.va.gov
Scott Karczewski, Regional Office Director
Denise Benson, Veterans Sevice Center Manager
Gregg Morin, Assistant Veterans Service Center Manager
Tracy Sinclair, Support Services Chief

Maryland

5694   Baltimore Regional Office
Veterans Benefits Administration, U S Dept. of V A
31 Hopkins Plz
Baltimore, MD   21201-2825   800-827-1000
                                        baltimore.query@vba.va.gov
                                                     www.va.gov
Jerry L Calhoun
The Baltimore Regional Office serves 484,013 veterans living in the State of Maryland, 2% of the national veteran population. The Regional Office's jurisdiction includes all counties in the State of Maryland. The Baltimore Regional Office has an assigned staffing of 218. We provide services at the VA Medical Center in Baltimore and Transition Assistance throughout the State. We actively participate in a homeless veterans outreach program based at the Maryland Center for the Veterans Educatio

5695   Baltimore VA Medical Center
Veterans Health Administration, U S Dept. of V A
10 N Greene St
Baltimore, MD   21201-1524   410-605-7000
                                                     800-463-6295
                                              Fax: 410-605-7901
                                        g.vhacss@forum.va.gov
                                           www.maryland.va.gov
Dennis H. Smith, Director
Nancy Quailey-Giannopoulis, Associate Director for Operations
Frederick P. Soetje, Associate Director for Finance
David O. Barrett, Acting Chief of Staff
The Baltimore Medical Center is nationally recognized for its outstanding patient safety and state-of-the-art technology, the VA Maryland Health Care System is proud of its reputation as a leader in veterans' health care, research and education.

5696   Fort Howard VA Medical Center
Veterans Health Administration, U S Dept. of V A
9600 N Point Rd
Fort Howard, MD   21052-3050   410-477-1800
                                                     800-351-8387
                                              Fax: 410-477-7177
                                           www.mdva.state.md.us
Thomas Hutchins, Secretary

5697   Maryland Veterans Centers
10 N Greene St
Baltimore, MD   21201-1524   410-605-7000
                                                     800-463-6295
                                              Fax: 410-605-7901
                                           www.maryland.va.gov
J Y Jacks, Manager
Dennis H Smith, Executive Director
Veterans medical clinic offering disabled veterans medical treatments.

5698 Perry Point VA Medical Center
Veterans Health Administration, U S Dept. of V A
Circle Drive
Perry Point, MD 21902   410-642-2411
                                      800-949-1003
                                 Fax: 410-642-1165
                              g.vhacss@forum.va.gov
                               www.maryland.va.gov

Dennis H. Smith, Director
Nancy Quailey-Giannopoulis, Associate Director for Operations
Frederick P. Soetje, Associate Director for Finance
David O. Barrett, Acting Chief of Staff
It is nationally recognized for its outstanding patient safety and
state-of-the-art technology, the VA Maryland Health Care System
is proud of its reputation as a leader in veterans' health care, re-
search and education.

5699 VA Maryland Health Care System
10 N Greene St
Baltimore, MD 21201-1524   410-605-7000
                                      800-463-6295
                                 Fax: 410-605-7900
                               www.maryland.va.gov

Dennis H. Smith, Director
Nancy Quailey-Giannopoulis, Associate Director for Operations
Frederick P. Soetje, Associate Director for Finance
David O. Barrett, Acting Chief of Staff
A dynamic and exciting health care organization that is dedicated
to providing quality, compassionate and accessible care and service to Maryland's veterans. As a part of one of the largest health
care systems in the United States, the VAMHCS has a reputation
as a leader in veterans' health care, reserch and education. Provides comprehensive service to veterans including medical, surgical, rehabilitative, nurological and mental health care on both
an inpatient and outpatient basis.

Massachusetts

5700 Boston VA Regional Office
Veterans Benefits Administration, U S Dept. of V A
15 New Sudbury Street
JFK Bldg
Boston, MA 2203-9928   617-232-9500
                                      800-827-1000
                              boston.query@vba.va.gov
                                www.boston.va.gov

Liza Catucci, Administrative Officer
Michael Lawson, President

5701 Edith Nourse Rogers Memorial Veterans Hospital
Veterans Health Administration U S Deptartment of
200 Springs Rd Bldg #23
Bedford, MA 1730-1114   781-687-2000
                                      800-827-1000
                                 Fax: 781-687-3536
                              g.vhacss@forum.va.gov
                               www.bedford.va.gov

Michael Mayo-Smith, Manager

5702 Northampton VA Medical Center
Veterans Health Administration, U S Dept. of V A
421 N Main St
Leeds, MA 1062   413-584-4040
                                      800-827-1000
                              g.vhacss@forum.va.gov

Richard Woloss, Manager

5703 VA Boston Healthcare System: Brockton Division
Veterans Health Administration, U S Dept. of V A
940 Belmont St
Brockton, MA 02301-5596   508-583-4500
                                      800-865-3384
                                 Fax: 617-323-7700
                              g.vhacss@forum.va.gov
                                www.boston.va.gov

Vincent Ng, Acting Director
Susan A. MacKenzie, PhD, Associate Director
Cecilia McVey, BSN, MHA, CAN, Associate Director Nursing & Pa-
tient Care Services
VA Boston Healthcare System's consolidated facility consists of
the Jamaica Plain campus, located in the heart of Boston's Longwood Medical Community; the West Roxbury campus, located on
the Dedham line; and the Brockton campus, located 20 miles
south of Boston in the City of Brockton.

5704 VA Boston Healthcare System: Jamaica Plain Campus
Veterans Health Administration, U S Dept. of V A
150 S Huntington Ave
Boston, MA 2130-4817   617-232-9500
                                      800-865-3384
                                 Fax: 617-278-4549
                              g.vhacss@forum.va.gov
                                www.boston.va.gov

Vincent Ng, Acting Director
Susan A. MacKenzie, PhD, Associate Director
Cecilia McVey, BSN, MHA, CAN, Associate Director Nursing & Pa-
tient Care Services
VA Boston Healthcare System's consolidated facility consists of
the Jamaica Plain campus, located in the heart of Boston's Longwood Medical Community; the West Roxbury campus, located on
the Dedham line; and the Brockton campus, located 20 miles
south of Boston in the City of Brockton.

5705 VA Boston Healthcare System: West Roxbury Division
Veterans Health Administration, U S Dept. of V A
1400 VFW Pkwy
West Roxbury, MA 2132-4927   617-323-7700
                                      800-865-3384
                              g.vhacss@forum.va.gov
                                www.boston.va.gov

Susan A Mac Kenzie, Associate Director
VA Boston Healthcare System's consolidated facility consists of
the Jamaica Plain campus, located in the heart of Boston's Longwood Medical Community; the West Roxbury campus, located on
the Dedham line; and the Brockton campus, located 20 miles
south of Boston in the City of Brockton.

Michigan

5706 Aleda E Lutz VA Medical Center
Veterans Health Administration, U S Dept. of V A
1500 Weiss St
Saginaw, MI 48602-5251   989-497-2500
                                      800-827-1000
                                 Fax: 989-791-2428
                              g.vhacss@forum.va.gov
                                www.saginaw.va.gov

Jeff Nechanicky, Acting Medical Center Director
Stephanie Young, Associate Director
Penny Holland, R.N., MSN, Associate Director for Patient Care
Svcs
Robert W. Dorr, D.O., JD, CHCQM,, Chief of Staff
Since 1950, the Aleda E. Lutz VA Medical Center has been improving the health of the men and women who have so proudly
served our nation. We consider it our privilege to serve your
health care needs in any way we can. Services are available to
more than 31,000 veterans living in the Central and Northern 35
counties of Michigan's Lower Peninsula.

5707 Battle Creek VA Medical Center
Veterans Health Administration, U S Dept. of V A
5500 Armstrong Rd
Battle Creek, MI   49037-7314   269-966-5600
                                              888-214-1247
                                              888-214-1247
                                         Fax: 269-966-5483
                                         g.vhacss@forum.va.gov
                                         www.battlecreek.va.gov

Mary Beth Skupien, Director
Edward Dornoff, Associate Director
Kay Bower, Associate Director for Patient Care Services
Dr. Shah, Acting Chief of Staff
Since 1924, the Battle Creek, Michigan VA Medical Center has been improving the health of the men and women who have so proudly served our nation. The Battle Creek VA Medical Center consists of 104 medical and psychiatric beds, 32 residential rehabilitation beds, and 103 nursing home care unit beds. In addition, specialized services offered include a Palliative Care Unit, a Substance Abuse Clinic, a Post Traumatic Stress Disorder Program and a Domicilliary.

5708 Iron Mountain VA Medical Center
Veterans Health Administration, U S Dept. of V A
325 East H Street
Iron Mountain, MI   49801-4760   906-774-3300
                                              800-827-1000
                                         Fax: 906-779-3114
                                         g.vhacss@forum.va.gov
                                         www.ironmountain.va.gov

James W. Rice, Medical Center Director
William Caron, FACHE, Associate Medical Center Director
Andrea Collins, RN, MSN, Associate Director for Nursing and Patient Care Service
Grace L. Stringfellow, M.D., Chief of Staff
OGJVAMC is a primary and secondary level care facility with 17 acute care beds, 13 in the medical/surgical ward and 4 in the intensive care unit (ICU). The main facility provides limited emergency and acute inpatient care, and collaborates with larger VA Medical Centers in Milwaukee and Madison, WI, to provide higher-level emergency and specialty care services. OGJVAMC also provides rehabilitation and extended care, including palliative and hospice care, in its 40-bed Community Living Center.

5709 John D Dingell VA Medical Center
Veterans Health Administration, U S Dept. of V A
4646 John R St
Detroit, MI   48201-1916   313-576-1000
                                              800-827-1000
                                         Fax: 313-576-1112
                                         g.vhacss@forum.va.gov
                                         www.detroit.va.gov

Pamela J. Reeves, M.D., Director
Annette Walker, M.S.H.A., B.S., Associate Director
Ann M. Herm, R.N., B.S.N., M., Associate Director, Patient Care Services
Scott A. Gruber, M.D., Ph.D.,, Chief of Staff
Our mission is to provide timely, compassionate and high quality care to those we serve by encouraging teamwork, education, research, innovation, and continuous improvement.

5710 Michigan VA Regional Office
Veterans Benefits Administration, U S Dept. of V A
477 Michigan Ave
Patrick V McNamara Federal Building
Detroit, MI   48226-1217   800-827-1000
                                         detroit.query@vba.va.gov
                                         www.benefits.va.gov/detroit

David Leonard, Director
Dennis W Paradowski, Assistant Director
The Regional Office Staff are dedicated to providing responsive and timely service to the veterans of Michigan and their families. Their duties include processing and making decisions on claims for disability compensation, and assisting with applications for a wide range of VA benefits.

5711 VA Ann Arbor Healthcare System
Veterans Health Administration, U S Dept. of V A
2215 Fuller Rd
Ann Arbor, MI   48105-2303   734-769-7100
                                              800-361-8387
                                         Fax: 734-761-7870
                                         g.vhacss@forum.va.gov
                                         www.annarbor.va.gov

Robert P. McDivitt, FACHE, Director
Randall E. Ritter, Associate Director
Stacey Breedveld, R.N., Associate Director Patient Care
Ginny Creasman, Assistant Director
Since 1953, the VA Ann Arbor Healthcare System (VAAAHS) has provided state-of-the-art healthcare services to the men and women who have so proudly served our nation. We consider it our privilege to serve your healthcare needs in any way we can.

5712 Vet Center Readjustment Counseling Service
1940 Eastern Ave SE
Grand Rapids, MI   49507-2771   616-285-5795
                                              800-905-4675
                                         Fax: 616-285-5898
                                         www.va.gov

William Busby, Executive Director
Branden K Lyon, Counselor
Lynn Hall, Clinical Coordinator
Providing a broad range of counseling outreach and referral services to eligible veterans in order to help make readjustments to cilvilian life.

Minnesota

5713 Minneapolis VA Medical Center
Veterans Health Administration, U S Dept. of V A
1 Veterans Dr
Minneapolis, MN   55417-2399   612-725-2000
                                              866-414-5058
                                         Fax: 612-725-2049
                                         g.vhacss@forum.va.gov
                                         www.minneapolis.va.gov

Judy Johnson-Mekota, Director
Erik J. Stalhandske, Associate Director
Kent Crossley, Chief of Staff
Helen Pearlman, Nurse Executive
Minneapolis VA Health Care System (VAHCS) is a teaching hospital providing a full range of patient care services with state-of-the-art technology, as well as education and research. Comprehensive health care is provided through primary care, tertiary care and long-term care in areas of medicine, surgery, psychiatry, physical medicine and rehabilitation, neurology, oncology, dentistry, geriatrics and extended care.

5714 St. Cloud VA Medical Center
Veterans Health Administration, U S Dept. of V A
4801 Veterans Dr
Saint Cloud, MN   56303-2015   320-252-1670
                                              800-247-1739
                                         Fax: 320-255-6472
                                         g.vhacss@forum.va.gov
                                         www.stcloud.va.gov

Barry I. Bahl, Director
Cheryl Thieschafer, Associate Director
Meri Hauge, BSN, MSN Nurse, Executive/Associate Director for Patient Care Services
Susan Markstrom, MD, Chief of Staff
Specialty care services include audiology, cardiology, dentistry, hematology, oncology, optometry, orthopedics, podiatry, pulmonology, urology and rheumatology. A new Ambulatory Surgery (same-day) Center opened in the fall of 2011 and will provide access to additional outpatient surgical procedures. The medical center offers extensive mental health programming, including acute psychiatric care, Residential Rehabilitation Treatment programs and an outpatient mental health clinic. The programs u

5715 St. Paul Regional Office
Veterans Benefits Administration, U S Dept. of V A
1 Federal Dr
Fort Snelling, MN 55111-4080   800-827-1000
stpaul.query@vba.va.gov
www.benefits.va.gov/stpaul

Vincent Crawford, Director

5716 Vet Center
405 E Superior St
Ste 160
Duluth, MN 55802-2240   218-722-8654
877-927-8387
Fax: 218-723-8212
www.vetcenter.va.gov

Cynthia Macaulay MEd, Counselor
Rob Evanson, Counselor
Debbie Burt, Office Manager
Counseling, social services and benefits assistance for combat
veterans and those sexually traumatized in the military.

Mississippi

5717 Biloxi/Gulfport VA Medical Center
Veterans Health Administration, U S Dept. of V A
400 Veterans Ave
Biloxi, MS 39531-2410   228-523-5000
800-296-8872
Fax: 228-563-2898
g.vhacss@forum.va.gov
www.biloxi.va.gov

Anthony L. Dawson, Director
Nancy Weaver, Associate Director
Kenneth Shimon, Chief of Staff
Margaret G Givens, Assciate Director

5718 Jackson Regional Office
Veterans Benefits Administration, U S Dept. of V A
1600 E Woodrow Wilson Ave
Jackson, MS 39216-5100   601-364-7000
800-827-1000
Fax: 601-364-7007
jackson.query@vba.va.gov
www.benefits.va.gov/jackson

Neil Anthony Mcphie, Chairman
Barbara Sapin, Vice Chairman

Missouri

5719 Harry S Truman Memorial Veterans' Hospital
Veterans Health Administration, U S Dept. of V A
800 Hospital Dr
Columbia, MO 65201-5275   573-814-6000
800-827-1000
Fax: 573-814-6551
g.vhacss@forum.va.gov
www.columbiamo.va.gov

Sallie Houser-Hanfelder, Director
Robert Ritter, Associate Director
Lana Zerrer, Chief of Staff

5720 John J Pershing VA Medical Center
Veterans Health Administration, U S Dept. of V A
1500 N Westwood Blvd
Poplar Bluff, MO 63901-3318   573-686-4151
888-557-8262
Fax: 573-778-4156
g.vhacss@forum.va.gov
www.poplarbluff.va.gov

Merk Hedstrom, Medical Center Director
Linda Haga, Research Contact

5721 Kansas City VA Medical Center
Veterans Health Administration, U S Dept. of V A
4801 E Linwood Blvd
Kansas City, MO 64128-2226   816-861-4700
800-827-1000
g.vhacss@forum.va.gov
www.kansascity.va.gov

Kenneth Grasing, Research/Development
Ram Sharma, Administrative Officer
Kent Hill, Executive Director
The Kansas City VA Medical Center is a modern, well-equipped
teriary care inpatient and outpatient center. As the third largest
teaching hospital in the metropolitan area, it maintains educa-
tional affiliations with the University of Kansas School of
Medicine.

5722 St. Louis Regional Office
Veterans Benefits Administration, U S Dept. of V A
400 S 18th St
Saint Louis, MO 63103-2265   800-827-1000
stlouis.query@vba.va.gov
www.stlouis.va.gov

5723 St. Louis VA Medical Center
Veterans Health Administration, U S Dept. of V A
915 N Grand Blvd
Saint Louis, MO 63106-1621   314-652-4100
800-228-5459
Fax: 314-289-7009
g.vhacss@forum.va.gov
www.stlouis.va.gov

Dolores Minor, Administrative Officer

Montana

5724 Montana VA Regional Office
3633 Veterans Drive
Fort Harrison, MT 59636-188   406-442-7310
800-827-1000
www.va.gov

5725 V A Montana Healthcare System
U S Dept. of V A
3687 Veterans Drive
PO Box 1500
Fort Harrison, MT 59636-1500   406-442-6410
877-468-8387
Fax: 406-447-7916
ftharrison.query@vba.va.gov
www.montana.va.gov

Christine Gregory, Director
Vicki Thennis, Interim Associate Director
Trena Bonde, Chief of Staff
Norlynn Nelson, Associate Director for Patient Care
This is a complete, medically reliable dictionary of congenital
malformations and disorders. As the authors explain, 'Down syn-
drome is the only common congenital disorder, the other defects
and disorders are rare or very rare, some having been reported
fewer than 20 times worlwide.' This dictionary covers them all.
Examples: Aagenaes syndrome, Acrocallosal syndrome, and
Acrodysostosis

5726 VA Montana Healthcare System
Veterans Health Administration, U S Dept. of V A
1892 William St
Fort Harrison, MT 59636   406-447-7945
800-827-1000
Fax: 406-447-7965
g.vhacss@forum.va.gov
www.montana.va.gov

Joseph Underkofel, Executive Director
Gregory Johnson, MD

5727 Vet Center
Readjusment Counciling Service Western Mountain Re
2795 Enterprise Ave.
Suite 1
Billings, MT 59102-3238   406-657-6071
                                                 Fax: 406-657-6603
                                                      www.va.gov

Bob Phillips, Manager
Luanne Anderson, Office Manager
Barry Osgard MS, Counselor
Readjustment counseling service for counseling veterans who
are having difficulty adjusting from military service especially
those diagnosed with PTSD.

Nebraska

5728 Grand Island VA Medical System
Veterans Health Administration, U S Dept. of V A
2201 N Broadwell Ave
Grand Island, NE 68803-2153   308-382-3660
                                                     866-580-1810
                                              g.vhacss@forum.va.gov

John Hilbert, Executive Director
Daniel L Parker, Deputy Director

5729 Lincoln Regional Office
Veterans Benefits Administration, U S Dept. of V A
3800 Village Dr.
Lincoln, NE 68501-4103   402-471-4444
                                                     800-827-1000
                                                 Fax: 402-479-5124
                                              lincoln.query@vba.va.gov
                                               www.veteranprograms.com

Bill Gibson, CEO
Daniel Parker, Deputy Director

5730 Lincoln VA Medical Center
Veterans Health Administration, U S Dept. of V A
600 S 70th St
Lincoln, NE 68510-2451   402-489-3802
                                                     800-827-1000
                                                 Fax: 402-486-7860
                                              g.vhacss@forum.va.gov
Ryon L Adams, Research/Development Coordinator

5731 VA Nebraska-Western Iowa Health Care System
Veterans Health Administration, U S Dept. of V A
4101 Woolworth Ave
Omaha, NE 68105-1850   402-449-0610
                                                     800-451-5796
                                                 Fax: 402-449-0684
                                               www.nebraska.va.gov

Marci Mylan, Director
Rowen Zetterman, Chief of Staff

Nevada

5732 Las Vegas Veterans Center
1919 S. Jones, Suite A
Las Vegas, NV 89146-905   702-251-7873
                                                 Fax: 702-388-6664
                                                www.lasvegas.va.gov

Daryl Harding, Resident Counselor LCSW
Matt Watson, Team Leader MSW
Veterans clinical counseling center for veterans and their dependent individual and group counseling, marital and family counseling, alcohol and drug assessment referral or treatment.
Community education and consultation, employment
counseling.

5733 Reno Regional Office
Veterans Benefits Administration U S Deptartment o
1000 Locust St
Reno, NV 89502-2597   775-328-1486
                                                     800-827-1000
                                                 Fax: 775-328-1447
                                              reno.query@vba.va.gov
                                                   www.reno.va.gov

Joseph E Dardillo, Administrative Officer

5734 VA Sierra Nevada Healthcare System
Veterans Health Administration, U S Dept. of V A
957 Kirman Ave
Reno, NV 89502-2597   775-786-7200
                                                     888-838-6256
                                                 Fax: 775-328-1816
                                                   www.reno.va.gov

Kurt W. Schlegelmich, Director
Michael C. Tadych, Associate Director
Rachel Crossley, Associate Director
Steve E. Brilliant, Chief of Staff

5735 VA Southern Nevada Healthcare System
Veterans Health Administration, U S Dept. of V A
6900 North Pecos Rd
Las Vegas, NV 89086   702-791-9000
                                                     800-827-1000
                                                 Fax: 707-636-3027
                                              g.vhacss@forum.va.gov
                                                www.lasvegas.va.gov

Isabel M. Duff, Acting Director
Ramu Komanduri, Chief of Staff
Sandra L. Solem, Acting Nurse Executive
John L. Stelsel, Assistant Director

New Hampshire

5736 Manchester Regional Office
Veterans Benefits Administration, U S Dept. of V A
275 Chestnut St
Manchester, NH 3101-2411   800-827-1000
                                           manchester.query@vba.va.gov
                                                      www.va.gov
Jerry Beale, Director

5737 Manchester VA Medical Center
Veterans Health Administration, U S Dept. of V A
718 Smyth Rd
Manchester, NH 03104-7007   603-624-4366
                                                     800-892-8384
                                              g.vhacss@forum.va.gov
                                               www.manchester.va.gov

Susan MacKenzie, Acting Med Center Director
Tammy A. Krueger, Associate Director
Andrew J. Breuder, Chief of Staff
Carol Williams, Associate Director for Patients

5738 New Hampshire Veterans Centers
103 Liberty St
Manchester, NH 3104-3118   603-668-7060
                                                     800-562-3127
                                                 Fax: 603-666-7404
                                                      www.va.gov

Caryl Ahern, Manager
Paulette Landry, Office Manager
Veterans clinic offering combat veterans outpatient counseling

New Jersey

5739 Disabled American Veterans: Ocean County
P.O.Box 1806
Toms River, NJ 8754-1806   732-929-0907
Mary Bencivenga, Contact

5740 East Orange Campus of the VA New Jersey Healthcare System
385 Tremont Ave
East Orange, NJ   07018-1023   973-676-1000
                                        Fax: 973-676-4226
                                        www.newjersey.va.gov

Kenneth Mizrach, Director
Glen Giaquinto, Associate Director
John A. Griffith, Associate Director
Patrick J. Troy, Nurse Executive

5741 Lyons Campus of the VA New Jersey Healthcare System
Veterans Health Administration, U S Dept. of V A
151 Knollcroft Rd
Lyons, NJ   7939-5001   908-647-0180
                                        800-827-1000
                                        Fax: 908-647-3452
                                        g.vhacss@forum.va.gov
                                        www.newjersey.va.gov

James J Farsetta, Director
Donna Henderson, Coordinator

5742 Newark Regional Office
Veterans Benefits Administration, U S Dept. of V A
20 Washington Pl
Newark, NJ   07102-3174   973-645-1441
                                        800-827-1000
                                        newark.query@vba.va.gov
                                        www.newjersey.va.gov

Stephen G Abel, Deputy Commissioner for Veterans

New Mexico

5743 New Mexico State Veterans' Home
992 South Broadway
Truth or Consequences, NM   87901-927   575-894-4200
                                        800-964-3976
                                        Fax: 575-894-4270

Lori S Montgomery, Administrator
Carol B Wilson, Admission Coordinator
Veterans medical clinic offering disabled veterans medical treatments.

5744 New Mexico VA Healthcare System
Veterans Health Administration, US Dept. of VA
1501 San Pedro Dr SE
Albuquerque, NM   87108-5154   505-265-1711
                                        800-465-8262
                                        Fax: 505-256-2855
                                        g.vhacss@forum.va.gov
                                        www.albuquerque.va.gov

George Marnell, Executive Director
Pamela Crowell, Acting Associate Director
Peter Woodbridge, Chief of Staff
Jennifer DeWinne, Acting Assistant Director

New York

5745 Albany VA Medical Center: Samuel S Stratton
Veterans Health Administration, U S Dept. of V A
113 Holland Ave
Albany, NY   12208-3410   518-626-5000
                                        800-233-4810
                                        888-838-7890
                                        Fax: 518-626-5500
                                        g.vhacss@forum.va.gov
                                        www.albany.va.gov

Donald W Stuart, Associate Director (Interim)
Linda W Weiss, Director
Laurdes Irzarry, Chief of Staff
Deborah Spath, Associate Director for Patient/N

5746 Albany Vet Center
Ste 2
17 Computer Dr W
Albany, NY   12205-1618   518-458-7998
                                        Fax: 518-458-8613

Lloyd Mc Omber, Owner
Melodie Krahula, Team Leader
Provides readjustment counseling for combat veterans and also provides benefits and job counseling for all veterans.

5747 Bath VA Medical Center
Veterans Health Administration U S Deptartment of
76 Veterans Avenue
Bath, NY   14810   607-664-4000
                                        877-845-3247
                                        888-823-9659
                                        Fax: 607-664-4000
                                        g.vhacss@forum.va.gov
                                        www.bath.va.gov

Michael Swartz, Medical Center Director
David B. Krueger, Associate Director
Felipe Diaz, Chief of Staff
Shirley A. Pikula, Associate Director for Patient Services

5748 Bronx VA Medical Center
Veterans Health Administration, U S Dept. of V A
130 W Kingsbridge Rd
Bronx, NY   10468-9938   718-584-9000
                                        800-877-6976
                                        Fax: 718-733-1223
                                        g.vhacss@forum.va.gov
                                        www.bronx.va.gov

Eric Langhoff, Director
Vincent F Immiti, Associate Director
Kathleen M. Capitulo, Chief of Staff
Kathleen M Capitulo, Associate Director for Patient C

5749 Brooklyn Campus of the VA NY Harbor Healthcare System
Veterans Health Administration, U S Dept. of V A
800 Poly Place
Brooklyn, NY   11209-7104   718-836-6600
                                        800-827-1000
                                        g.vhacss@forum.va.gov
                                        www.nyharbor.va.gov

Martina A Parauda, Director
Veronica J Foy, Associate Director, Facilities &
Michael S Simberkoff, Executive Chief of Staff
Elizabeth H Weinshel, Deputy Chief of Staff

5750 Buffalo Regional Office - Department of Veterans Affairs
Veterans Benefits Administration
130 South Elmwood Avenue
Buffalo, NY   14202-2465   716-852-3028
                                        800-827-1000
                                        www.va.gov

5751 Canandiagua VA Medical Center
Veterans Health Administration, U S Dept. of V A
400 Fort Hill Ave
Canandaigua, NY   14424-1159   585-394-2000
                                        800-204-9917
                                        g.vhacss@forum.va.gov
                                        www.canandaigua.va.gov

Craig S Howard, Medical Center Director
Margaret Owens, Associate Director
Dr. Robert B Babcock, Chief of Staff
Patricia Hryzak Lind, Associate Director for Patient/N

5752 Castle Point Campus of the VA Hudson Valley Healthcare System
Veterans Health Administration, U S Dept. of V A
Route 9D
Castle Point, NY   12511   845-831-2000
                                          800-827-1000
                                    Fax: 845-838-5193
                                g.vhacss@forum.va.gov
                                www.hudsonvalley.va.gov
Gerald F Culliton, Director
John M. Gary, Associate Director
Patricia A. Burke, Associate Director
Joanne J. Malina, Chief of Staff

5753 New York City Campus of the VA NY Harbor Healthcare System
Veterans Health Administration, U S Dept. of V A
423 E 23rd St
New York, NY   10010-5011   212-686-7500
                                          800-827-1000
                                    Fax: 718-567-4082
                                g.vhacss@forum.va.gov
                                www.nyharbor.va.gov
Camille R Varacchi, Administrative Officer

5754 New York Regional Office
Veterans Benefits Administration, U S Dept. of V A
245 W Houston St
New York, NY   10014-4805   212-714-0699
                                          800-827-1000
                                    Fax: 212-807-4042
                                newyork.query@vba.va.gov
                                www.va.gov
Ronna Brown, President

5755 Northport VA Medical Center
Veterans Health Administration, U S Dept. of V A
79 Middleville Rd
Northport, NY   11768-2296   631-261-4400
                                          800-827-1000
                                    Fax: 631-266-6710
                                g.vhacss@forum.va.gov
                                www.northport.va.gov
Philip C Moschitta, Medical Center Director
Rosie A Chatman, Associate Director for Patient &
Maria Favale, Associate Director
Edward Mack, Chief of Staff

5756 Syracuse VA Medical Center
Veterans Health Administration, U S Dept. of V A
800 Irving Ave
Syracuse, NY   13210-2716   315-425-4400
                                          800-792-4334
                                          888-838-7890
                                g.vhacss@forum.va.gov
                                www.syracuse.va.gov
James Cody, VA Medical Center Director
Judy Hayman, Associate Medical Center Director
William H Marx, Chief of Staff
Nancy Schmid, Associate Director for Patient/N

5757 Torah Alliance of Families of Kids with Disabilities
T AF KI D
1433 Coney Island Ave
Brooklyn, NY   11230-4119   718-252-2236
                                    Fax: 718-252-2216
Juby Shapiro, Manager
Serves over 1k families whose children have a variety of disabilities and special needs. Many of these families are large families in
the low socioeconomic level. Offers monthly meetings, guest lectures, parent matching, information of new developments in software, technology and techniques, sibling support groups, pen pal
lists, audio and video library, alternative medicine and nutrition
information and education on legal awareness and rights of
disabled citizens.

5758 VA Hudson Valley Health Care System
Veterans Health Administration, U S Department of
2094 Albany Post Road
Montrose, NY   10548-1454   914-737-4400
                                    Fax: 845-788-4244
                                www.hudsonvalley.va.gov
James J Farsette, Network Director
Michael Sabo, Executive Director

5759 VA Western NY Healthcare System, Batavia
Veterans Health Administration, U S Dept. of V A
222 Richmond Ave
Batavia, NY   14020-1227   585-297-1000
                                          800-827-1000
                                    Fax: 585-786-1258
                                g.vhacss@forum.va.gov
                                www.va.gov
William F Feeley, Medical Center Director
Miguel Rainstein, Chief of Staff
Jason C Petti, Associate Medical Center Directo
Royce Calhoun, Assistant Director

5760 VA Western NY Healthcare System, Buffalo
Veterans Health Administration, U S Dept. of V A
3495 Bailey Ave
Buffalo, NY   14215-1129   716-834-9200
                                          800-532-8387
                                www.buffalo.va.gov
Brian Stiller, Medical Center Director
Jason C. Petti, Chief of Staff
Royce Calhoun, Associate Medical Center Directo
Miguel Rainstein, Chief of Staff

North Carolina

5761 Asheville VA Medical Center
Veterans Health Administration, U S Dept. of V A
1100 Tunnel Rd
Asheville, NC   28805-2043   828-298-7911
                                          800-932-6408
                                    Fax: 828-299-2502
                                g.vhacss@forum.va.gov
                                www.asheville.va.gov
Cynthia Beyfogle, Executive Director
David A. Pattillo, Assistant Medical Director
James Wells, Chief of Staff
Dennis J. Mehring, Public Affairs Officer

5762 Charlotte Vet Center
2114 Ben Craig Drive
Charlotte, NC   28262-2350   704-549-8025
                                    Fax: 704-549-8261
                                www.va.gov
Loretta Deaton, Team Leader
Cynthia Algra, Office Manager
Billy Moore, Counselor
Melissa L Saunders, Counsilor
Preadjustment Counseling for Combat Veterans with Post Trau-
matic Stress Disorder (PTSD).

5763 Durham VA Medical Center
Veterans Health Administration, U S Dept. of V A
508 Fulton St
Durham, NC   27705-3875   919-286-0411
                                          800-827-1000
                                          888-878-6890
                                    Fax: 919-286-5944
                                leola.jenkins@med.va.gov
                                www.durham.va.gov
Deanne M Seekins, Director
Rudy A Klopfer, Associate Director
John D Shelburne, Chief of Staff
Kathryn Ward-Presson, Associate Director for Nursing P
Since 1953, Durham Veterans Affairs Medical Cetner has been
improving the health of the men and women who have so proudly
served our nation. We consider it our privilege to serve your

health care needs in any way we can. Services are available to more than 200,000 veterans living in a 26-county area of central and eastern North Carolina.

5764   Fayetteville VA Medical Center
Veterans Health Administration, U S Dept. of V A
2300 Ramsey St
Fayetteville, NC   28301-3856   910-488-2120
                                                800-771-6106
                                                Fax: 910-822-7926
                                                g.vhacss@forum.va.gov
                                                www.va.gov

Elizabeth Goolsby, Director
James Galkowski, Associate Director, Operations
Jesse Howard III, Acting Chief of Staff
Joyce Alexander-Hines, Associate Director, Patient Care
Since 1940, the Fayetteville VA Medical Center (VAMC) has improved the health of the men and women who have so proudly served our nation. We consider it our privilege to serve your health care needs in any way we can. Medical, mental health, women's health care and specialty services are available to more than 157,000 veterans living in a 21-county area of North Carolina and South Carolina.

5765   WG Hefner VA Medical Center - Salisbury
Vet Health Administration U S Department of VA
1601 Brenner Ave
Salisbury, NC   28144-2515   704-638-9000
                                                800-469-8252
                                                Fax: 704-638-3395
                                                g.vhacss@forum.va.gov
                                                www.salisbury.va.gov

Kaye Green, Director
Linette Barker, Associate Medical Center Directo
Subbarao Pemmaraju, Chief of Staff (Interim)
Michele Hilll, Associate Director for Patient C
Since 1953, Hefner VAMC has been improving the health of the men and women who have so proudly served our nation. We consider it our privilege to serve your health care needs in any way we can. Primary and secondary inpatient health care are available to more than 287,000 veterans living in a 24-county area of the Central Piedmont Region of North Carolina. This includes the Charlotte area with over 100,000 veterans, and the Winston-Salem area with 65,000 veterans.

5766   Winston-Salem Regional Office
Veterans Benefits Administration, U S Dept. of V A
251 N Main St
Winston-Salem, NC   27155-2   336-768-5560
                                                800-827-1000
                                                Fax: 336-768-7295
                                                TTY: 800-829-4833
                                                winsalem.query@vba.va.gov
                                                www.va.gov

Glenn Cobb, Executive VP

North Dakota

5767   Fargo VA Medical Center
Veterans Health Administration, U S Dept. of V A
2101 North Elm
Fargo, ND   58102-2417   701-232-3241
                                                800-410-9723
                                                Fax: 701-239-7166
                                                g.vhacss@forum.va.gov
                                                www.va.gov

Michael J Murphy, Healthcare Center Director
Dale DeKrey, Associate Director for Operation
J Brian Hancock, Chief of Staff
Julie Bruhn, Associate Director for Patient C

5768   North Dakota VA Regional Office - Fargo Regional Office
Veterans Benefits Administration, U S Dept. of V A
2101 Elm St N
Fargo, ND   58102-2417   701-451-4690
                                                800-410-9723
                                                Fax: 701-451-4690
                                                fargo.query@vba.va.gov
                                                www.fargo.va.gov
Thomas Santoro, Director Research Department

Ohio

5769   Chillicothe VA Medical Center
Veterans Health Administration, U S Dept. of V A
17273 State Route 104
Chillicothe, OH   45601-9718   740-773-1141
                                                 800-358-8262
                                                 888-838-6446
                                                 Fax: 740-772-7023
                                                 g.vhacss@forum.va.gov
                                                 www.chillicothe.va.gov

Wendy J. Hepker, Medical Center Director
Keith Sullivan, Associate Medical Center Directo
Deborah M Meesig, Chief of Staff
Ruth Yerardi, Associate Director for Patient C
The Chillicothe VA Medical Center provides acute and chronic mental health services, primary and secondary medical services, a wide range of nursing home care services, specialty medical services as well as specialized women Veterans health clinics. The facility is an active ambulatory care setting and serves as a chronic mental health referral center for VA Medical Center in southern Ohio and parts of West Virginia and Kentucky

5770   Cincinnati VA Medical Center
Veterans Health Administration, U S Dept. of V A
3200 Vine St
Cincinnati, OH   45220-2213   513-861-3100
                                                 800-827-1000
                                                 888-267-7873
                                                 Fax: 513-475-6500
                                                 g.vhacss@forum.va.gov
                                                 www.cincinnati.va.gov

Linda Smith, Director
David Ninneman, Associate Director
Robert Falcone, Chief of Staff
Katheryn Cook, Nurse Executive

5771   Cleveland Regional Office
Veterans Benefits Administration, U S Dept. of V A
1240 E 9th St
Cleveland, OH   44199-2068   800-827-1000
                                                 Fax: 216-522-8262
                                                 cleveland.query@vba.va.gov
                                                 www.va.gov

P Hunter Peckham, Director
Robert Ruff, Assistant Director
William Bunkley, Minority Veterans Program Coordi

5772   Dayton VA Medical Center
Veterans Health Administration U S Department of V
4100 W 3rd St
Dayton, OH   45428-9000   937-268-6511
                                                 800-368-8262
                                                 888-838-6446
                                                 Fax: 937-262-2170
                                                 g.vhacss@forum.va.gov
                                                 www.dayton.va.gov

Glenn Costie, Acting Director
Mark Murdock, Associate Director
James T. Hardy, Chief of Staff
Anna Jones, Associate Director, Patient Care
The Dayton VAMC is a state of the art teaching facility that has been serving Veterans for 146 years, having accepted its first patient in 1867. The Dayton VA Medical Center provides a full range of health care through medical, surgical, mental health (inpatient and outpatient), home and community health programs,

geriatric (nursing home), physical medicine and therapy services, neurology, oncology, dentistry, and hospice.

5773   Louis Stokes VA Medical Center - Wade Park Campus
Veterans Health Administration, U S Dept. of V A
10701 East Blvd
Cleveland, OH   44106-1702   216-791-3800
                                         877-838-8262
                                         888-838-6446
                                   Fax: 440-838-6017
                                   g.vhacss@forum.va.gov
                                   www.cleveland.va.gov

Susan M Fuehrer, Medical Center Director
Darwin Goodspeed, Associate Medical Center Director
Murray D. Altose, Chief of Staff
Inette Sarduy, Associate Director Patient

Oklahoma

5774   Jack C. Montgomery VA Medical Center
Veterans Benefits Administration, U S Dept. of V A
1011 Honor Heights Dr
Muskogee, OK   74401-1318   918-577-3000
                                         800-827-1000
                                   muskogee.query@vba.va.gov
                                   www.muskogee.va.gov
Alef Nancy Graham, Manager

5775   Jack C. Montomery VA Medical Center
1011 Honor Heights Dr
Muskogee, OK   74401-1318   918-577-3000
                                         800-827-1000
                                   muskogee.query@vba.va.gov
                                   www.muskogee.va.gov
James R. Floyd, Medical Director
Inez Reitz, Acting Associate Director
Thomas D. Schneider, Chief of Staff
Bonnie R Pierce, Associate Director for Patient C

5776   Oklahoma City VA Medical Center
Veterans Health Administration, U S Dept. of V A
921 NE 13th St
Oklahoma City, OK   73104-5007   405-456-1000
                                         800-827-1000
                                   Fax: 405-270-1560
                                   www.oklahoma.va.gov
Jimmy A. Murphy, Director
Debra A. Colombe, Associate Director
Mark Huycke, Chief of Staff
Donna DeLise, Associate Director for Patient C

5777   Oklahoma Veterans Centers Vet Center
3033 N Walnut Ave
Ste W101
Oklahoma City, OK   73105-2833   405-270-5184
                                   Fax: 405-270-5125
Peter Sharp, Manager
Steve Kenzie, Owner
PTSP counseling for all combat Veterans and victims of sexual trauma/sexual harassment.

Oregon

5778   Oregon Health Sciences University
3181 SW Sam Jackson Park Rd
Portland, OR   97239-3098   503-494-8311
                                   ohsu.edu
Joe Robertson, President
James Morgan, Executive Director
Offers services for the totally blind, legally blind, visually impaired, mentally retarded blind and more with health, counseling, educational, recreational, rehabilitation, computer training and professional training services.

5779   Portland Regional Office
Veterans Benefits Administration, U S Dept. of V A
100 SW Main St, Floor 2
Portland, OR   97204-2802   503-373-2388
                                         800-827-1000
                                   portland.query@vba.va.gov
                                   www.va.gov

5780   Portland VA Medical Center
Veterans Health Administration, U S Dept. of V A
3710 SW U.S. Veterans Hospital Rd.
Portland, OR   97239-2964   503-220-8262
                                         800-949-1004
                                   Fax: 503-273-5319
                                   g.vhacss@forum.va.gov
                                   www.portland.va.gov
John E Patrick, Director
David Stockwell, Deputy Director of Administratio
Tom Anderson, Chief of Staff
Kathleen M Chapman, Deputy Director for Patient Care
The Portland VA Medical Center (PVAMC) is a 303-bed consolidated facility with two main divisions. The medical center serves as the quaternary referral center for Oregon, Southern Washington, and parts of Idaho for the U.S. Department of Veterans Affairs. The Portland VAMC is located atop Marquam Hill on 28.5 acres overlooking the city of Portland. In addition to comprehensive medical and mental health services, the Portland VAMC supports ongoing research and medical education, including nati

5781   Roseburg VA Medical Center
Veterans Health Administration, U S Dept. of V A
913 NW Garden Valley Blvd
Roseburg, OR   97471-6523   541-440-1000
                                         800-549-8387
                                   Fax: 541-440-1225
                                   g.vhacss@forum.va.gov
                                   www.roseburg.va.gov
Jim Willis, Director
Mark Traines, MD

5782   Southern Oregon Rehabilitation Center & Clinics
Veterans Health Administration, U S Dept. of V A
8495 Crater Lake Hwy
White City, OR   97503   541-826-2111
                                         800-809-8725
                                   Fax: 541-830-3500
                                   g.vhacss@forum.va.gov
                                   www.southernoregon.va.gov
George Andries, Executive Director

Pennsylvania

5783   Butler VA Medical Center
Veterans Health Administration, U S Dept. of V A
325 New Castle Rd
Butler, PA   16001-2418   724-282-7171
                                         800-362-8262
                                   Fax: 724-282-7640
                                   g.vhacss@forum.va.gov
                                   www.butler.va.gov
John Gennaro, Director
Rebecca Hubscher, Associate Director
Sharon Parson, Nurse Executive
Timothy Burke, Chief of Staff
VA Butler Healthcare is located in the heart of Butler County, on the bus line, and convenient to community support services for Western Pennsylvania and Eastern Ohio-area Veterans. We have been attending to Veterans' total care since 1947 and are the health care choice for over 18,000 Veterans - providing comprehensive Veteran care including primary, specialty, and mental health care - as well as health maintenance plans, management of chronic conditions and preventative medicine needs.

5784   Coatesville VA Medical Center
Veterans Health Administration, U S Dept. of V A
1400 Blackhorse Hill Rd
Coatesville, PA   19320-2040   610-384-7711
                                                      800-290-6172
                                                      888-558-3812
                                             g.vhacss@forum.va.gov
                                                www.coatesville.va.gov

Gary Devansky, Director
Sheila Chelleppa, Chief of Staff
Nancy Schmid, Associate Director Patient Care
Jonathan Eckman, Associate Director

5785   Erie VA Medical Center
Veterans Health Administration, U S Dept. of V A
135 E 38th Street Blvd
Erie, PA   16504-1559   814-868-8661
                                                      800-274-8387
                                                      888-860-2124
                                                 Fax: 814-860-2425
                                             g.vhacss@forum.va.gov
                                                    www.erie.va.gov

Michael Adelman, Medical Center Director
Melissa Sundin, Associate Medical Center Directo
Dr. Anthony Behm, Chief of Staff
Dorene Sommers, Associate Director for Patient C

5786   James E Van Zandt VA Medical Center
Veterans Health Administration, U S Dept. of V A
2907 Pleasant Valley Blvd
Altoona, PA   16602-4377   814-943-8164
                                                      800-827-1000
                                                 Fax: 814-940-7898
                                             g.vhacss@forum.va.gov
                                                         www.va.gov

Cecil B Hengeveld, Director
Gerald Williams, Executive Director

5787   Lebanon VA Medical Center
Veterans Health Administration, U S Dept. of V A
1700 S Lincoln Ave
Lebanon, PA   17042-7597   717-272-6621
                                                      800-409-8771
                                                 Fax: 717-228-5907
                                             g.vhacss@forum.va.gov
                                                 www.lebanon.va.gov

Robert (Bob) Callahan Jr., Director
Robin C. Aube-Warren, Associate Director
Kanan Chatterjee, Chief of Staff
Margaret G Wilson, Associate Director for Patient C

5788   Pennsylvania Veterans Centers
Veterans Health Administration, U S Department of
135 E 38th St
Erie, PA   16504   814-868-8661
                                                      800-274-8387
                                                 Fax: 717-861-8589
                                                    www.erie.va.gov

Michael Aldeman, medical Center Director
Melissa Sundin, Associate Director
Anthony Behm, Chief of Staff
Veterans medical clinic offering disabled veterans medical treatments.

5789   Philadelphia Regional Office and Insurance Center
Veterans Benefits Administration, U S Dept. of V A
5000 Wissahickon Ave
Philadelphia, PA   19144-4867   215-336-3003
                                                      800-827-1000
                                                 Fax: 215-336-5542
                                            phillyro.query@vba.va.gov
                                                         www.va.gov

Sonny Dicrecchio, Executive Director

5790   Philadelphia VA Medical Center
Veterans Health Administration, U S Dept. of V A
3900 Woodland Avenue
Philadelphia, PA   19104   215-823-5800
                                                      800-949-1001
                                             g.vhacss@forum.va.gov
                                               www.philadelphia.va.gov

Joseph M Dalpiaz, Director
Ralph Schapira, Chief of Staff
Margaret O'Shea Caplan, Associate Director for Finance
Patricia O'Kane, Acting Associate Director for Cl

5791   Pittsburgh Regional Office
Veterans Benefits Administration U S Deparment of
1000 Liberty Avenue
Pittsburgh, PA   15222   412-688-6100
                                                      800-827-1000
                                                 Fax: 412-688-6121
                                            pittsburgh.query@vba.va.gov
                                                www.pittsburgh.va.gov

Micahel E Moreland

5792   VA Pittsburgh Healthcare System, University Drive Division
Veterans Health Administration, U S Dept. of V A
University Dr
Pittsburgh, PA   15240-2400   412-688-6000
                                                      866-482-7488
                                                 Fax: 412-688-6901
                                             g.vhacss@forum.va.gov
                                                www.pittsburgh.va.gov

Timothy Mar Carlos, CEO

5793   VA Pittsburgh Healthcare System, Highland Drive Division
Veterans Health Administration, U S Dept. of V A
7180 Highland Dr
Pittsburgh, PA   15206-1206   412-688-6000
                                                      800-827-1000
                                                 Fax: 412-365-4213
                                             g.vhacss@forum.va.gov
                                                www.pittsburgh.va.gov

Kristin Best, Deputy Adjutant General
Roger Sutton, MD

5794   Wilkes-Barre VA Medical Center
Veterans Health Administration, U S Dept. of V A
1111 E End Blvd
Wilkes Barre, PA   18711-30   570-824-3521
                                                      877-928-2621
                                                 Fax: 570-821-7278
                                             g.vhacss@forum.va.gov
                                               www.wilkes-barre.va.gov

William H Mills, Director (Interim)
Douglas V Paxton Sr., Associate Director
Mirza Z Ali, Chief of Staff
Linda Stout, Associate Director for Nursing S

Rhode Island

5795   Providence Regional Office
Veterans Benefits Administration, U S Dept. of V A
380 Westminster St
Providence, RI   2903-3246   401-462-0324
                                                      800-827-1000
                                                 Fax: 401-254-2320
                                            providence.query@vba.va.gov
                                                         www.va.gov

Daniel Evangelista, Acting Associate Director

5796 Providence VA Medical Center
Veterans Health Administration, U S Dept. of V A
830 Chalkstone Ave
Providence, RI 02908-4799   401-273-7100
     866-363-4486
     Fax: 401-457-3360
     g.vhacss@forum.va.gov
     www.providence.va.gov

Vincent W Ng, Medical Center Director
William J Burney, Medical Center Associate Directo
Gregory M Gillette, Medical Center Chief of Staff
Deborah A Clickner, Medical Center Associate Directo
To fulfill President Lincoln's promise To care for him who shall have borne the battle, and for his widow, and his orphan by serving and honoring the men and women who are America's veterans.

South Carolina

5797 Columbia Regional Office
Veterans Benefits Administration, U S Dept. of V A
6437 Garners Ferry Rd
Columbia, SC 29209-2401   803-401-1094
     800-827-1000
     columbia.query@vba.va.gov
     www.va.gov

Jimmie Ruff, Executive Director

5798 Ralph H Johnson VA Medical Center
Veterans Health Administration, U S Dept. of V A
109 Bee St
Charleston, SC 29401-5703   843-577-5011
     800-827-1000
     888-878-6884
     Fax: 843-876-5384
     g.vhacss@forum.va.gov
     www.charleston.va.gov

Carolyn L Adams, Director
Scott Isaacks, Associate Director
Florence N Hutchinson, Chief of Staff
Mary C Fraggos, Associate Director for Patient/N

5799 William Jennings Bryan Dorn VA Medical Center
Veterans Health Administration U S Department of V
6439 Garners Ferry Rd
Columbia, SC 29209-1638   803-776-4000
     800-293-8262
     Fax: 803-695-6739
     Carolyn.Adams@va.gov
     www.columbiasc.va.gov

Carolyn L Adams, Director
Barbara Temeck, Chief of Staff
David L. Omura, Chief of Staff
Ruth Mustard, Director for Patient Care/Nursin

South Dakota

5800 Royal C Johnson Veterans Memorial Medical Center
Veterans Health Administration, U S Dept. of VA
2501 W. 22nd St
Sioux Falls, SD 57105-5046   605-336-3230
     800-316-8387
     Fax: 605-333-6878
     g.vhacss@forum.va.gov
     www.siouxfalls.va.gov

Patrick J Kelly, Director
Sara Ackert, Associate Director
Victor Waters, Chief of Staff
Barbara Teal, Associate Director, Patient Care

5801 Sioux Falls Regional Office
Veterans Benefits Administration, U S Dept. of V A
2501 W. 22nd St
Sioux Falls, SD 57105-5046   605-336-3230
     800-827-1000
     Fax: 605-333-5316
     siouxfalls.query@vba.va.gov
     www.siouxfalls.va.gov

Tennessee

5802 Alvin C York VA Medical Center
Veterans Health Administration, U S Dept. of V A
3400 Lebanon Pike
Murfreesboro, TN 37129-1237   615-867-6000
     800-876-7093
     Fax: 615-867-5768
     g.vhacss@forum.va.gov
     www.tennesseevalley.va.gov

Juan Morales, Medical System Director
Janice Cobb, Associate Director, Nursing Serv
Emma Metcalf, Chief Operating Officer

5803 Memphis VA Medical Center
Veterans Health Administration, U S Dept. of V A
1030 Jefferson Ave
Memphis, TN 38104-2127   901-523-8990
     800-636-8262
     g.vhacss@forum.va.gov
     www.memphis.va.gov

Jay Robinson III, Associate Medical Center Directo
Douglas D Southall, Assistant Medical Center Directo
Margarethe Hagemann, Chief of Staff
Marilyn Kerkhoff, Interim Associate Medical Center

5804 Mountain Home VA Medical Center - James H Quillen VA Medical Center
Veterans Health Administration, US Dept. of VA
Corner of Lamont & Veterans Way
Mountain Home, TN 37684   423-926-1171
     877-573-3529
     g.vhacss@forum.va.gov
     www.mountainhome.va.gov

Charlene S Ehret, Medical Center Director
Jimmy H McGlawn, Associate Director
David R Reagan, Chief of Staff
Linda M McConnell, Associate Director, Patient/Nurs

5805 Nasheville Regional Office
Veterans Benefits Administration, U S Dept. of V A
110 9th Ave S
Nashville, TN 37203-3817   800-827-1000
     nashville.query@vba.va.gov
     www.va.gov

Michael R Walsh, Administrative Officer
Donald H Rubin, Research/Development Coordinator

5806 Nashville VA Medical Center
Veterans Health Administration, US Dept. of VA
1310 24th Ave S
Nashville, TN 37212-2637   615-327-4751
     800-228-4973
     Fax: 615-321-6350
     g.vhacss@forum.va.gov
     www.tennesseevalley.va.gov

Juan Morales, Medical System Director
Michael A Doukas, Chief of Staff
Gary D Trende, Associate Director, Nursing Serv
Gary D Trende, Chief Operating Officer

Texas

5807 Amarillo VA Healthcare System
Veterans Health Administration, U S Dept. of V A
6010 Amarillo Blvd West
Amarillo, TX   79106-1991
806-355-9703
800-687-8262
Fax: 806-354-7869
g.vhacss@forum.va.gov
www.amarillo.va.gov

David Welch, Director
Lance Robinson, Associate Director
Grace Stringfelow, Chief of Staff
Louise Anderson, Executive/Chief, Nursing Service

5808 Amarillo Vet Center
Department of Veterans Affairs
3414 Olsen Blvd
Suite E
Amarillo, TX   79109-3072
806-351-1104
Fax: 806-351-1104
www.va.gov

Pedro Garcia Jr., Team Leader
Simon Camarillo, Counsilor
William C Santer, Family Therapist
Cathy L Williams, Office Manager
Provides individual, group and family counseling to veterans who served in combat theaters of World War II and Korea, veterans of the Vietnam Era, and veterans of conflicts zones in Lebanon, Grenada, Panama, the Persian Guld and Somalia.

5809 El Paso VA Healthcare Center
Veterans Health Administration, U S Dept. of V A
5001 N Piedras
El Paso, TX   79930-4210
915-564-6100
800-672-3782
Fax: 915-564-7920
g.vhacss@forum.va.gov
www.elpaso.va.gov

John A. Mendoza, Director
Elizabeth Lowery, Associate Director
Homer LeMar, Interim Chief of Staff
Timothy McMurry, Associate Director, Patient Care

5810 Houston Regional Office
Veterans Benefits Administration, U S Dept. of V A
6900 Almeda Rd
Houston, TX   77030-4200
713-791-1414
800-827-1000
houston.query@vba.va.gov
www.va.gov

Cecil Aultman, Executive Director
Edgar Tucker, Chief Executive Officer

5811 Michael E. Debakey VA Medical Center
Veterans Health Administration, U S Dept. of V A
2002 Holcombe Blvd
Houston, TX   77030-4211
713-791-1414
800-553-2278
g.vhacss@forum.va.gov
www.houston.va.gov

Adam C Walmus, Director
J Kalavar, Chief of Staff
Francisco Vazquez, Associate Director
Thelma Grey-Becknell, Associate Director for Patient C

5812 South Texas Veterans Healthcare System
Veterans Health Administration, U S Dept. of V A
7400 Merton Minter
San Antonio, TX   78229-4404
210-617-5300
877-469-5300
888-686-6350
g.vhacss@forum.va.gov
www.southtexas.va.gov

Marie L. Wedon, Director
Wade Vlosich, Associate Director
Joe A. Perez, Assistant Director
Julianne Flynne, Chief of Staff

5813 VA North Texas Health Veterans Affairs Care System: Dallas VA Medical Center
Veterans Health Administration, U S Dept. of V A
4500 S Lancaster Rd
Dallas, TX   75216-7167
214-742-8387
800-849-3597
Fax: 214-857-1171
www.northtexas.va.gov/index.asp

Jeffrey Milligan, Director
Peter Dancy, Associate Director
Clark R. Gregg, Chief of Staff
Alan Bernstein, Assistant Director
Health care system which serves veterans with medical care and rehabilitation services including spinal cord injury center. For VA benefit inquiries contact 1-800-827-1000. This system has locations in Bonham, Dallas, and Fort Worth.

5814 Waco Regional Office
Veterans Benefits Administration, U S Dept. of V A
4800 Memorial Dr
Waco, TX   76711-1
254-752-6581
800-423-1111
TTY:800-829-4833
waco.query@vba.va.gov
www.centraltexas.va.gov

William F. Harper, Chief of Staff
Russell E. Lloyd, Associate Director of Resources
Karen Spada, Associate Director for Patients
Andrew Garcia, Assistant Director for Operations
Mission is to honor America's Veterans by providing exceptional health care that improves their health and well being.

5815 West Texas VA Healthcare System
Veterans Health Administration, U S Dept. of V A
300 Veterans Blvd
Big Spring, TX   79720-5566
432-263-7361
800-472-1365
Fax: 915-264-4834
g.vhacss@forum.va.gov
www.bigspring.va.gov

Andrew M. Welch, Interim Director
Kenneth Allensworth, Associate Director
Raul Zambrano, Chief of Staff
Charles V. Silveri, Associate Director
The West Texas VA Health Care System (WTVAHCS) proudly serves Veterans in 33 counties across 53,000 square miles of rural geography in West Texas and Eastern New Mexico. The George H. O'Brien, Jr. VA Medical Center is located in Big Spring, Texas and the six Community Based Outpatient Clinics (CBOC's) that comprise the remainder of the health care system are located in Abilene, TX, Stamford, TX, San Angelo, TX, Odessa, TX, Fort Stockton, TX, and Hobbs, NM.

Utah

5816 Utah Division of Veterans Affairs
Utah Division of Veterans Affairs
550 Foothill Blvd
Ste 202
Salt Lake City, UT 84113-1106   801-582-1565
                                         800-894-9497
                                    Fax: 801-326-2369
                                    www.saltlakecity.va.gov

David J Peifer, Director
Todd Andrews, Assistant to the Director
Karen H. Gribbin, Manager
Our mission is to serve the veteran who served us. The VA Salt
Lake City Health Care System is committed to providing our pa-
tients with the highest Quality of Care in an environment that is
safe. We do this by focusing on Continuous Process Improvement
and by supporting a Culture of Safety

5817 VA Salt Lake City Healthcare System
Veterans Health Administration, U S Dept. of V A
500 Foothill Drive
Salt Lake City, UT 84148-1   801-582-1565
                                       800-613-4012
                                  Fax: 801-584-1289
                                  www.saltlakecity.va.gov

Steven W Young, Director
Warren E Hill, Associate Director
Karen H. Gribbin, Chief of Staff
Shella Stovall, Associate Director, Patient Care
Our mission is to serve the veteran who served us. The VA Salt
Lake City Health Care System is committed to providing our pa-
tients with the highest Quality of Care in an environment that is
safe. We do this by focusing on Continuous Process Improvement
and by supporting a Culture of Safety

Vermont

5818 Vermont VA Regional Office Center
Veterans Benefits Administration U S Department V
215 N Main St
White River Junction, VT 05009-1   802-295-9363
                                        866-687-8387
                                   Fax: 802-290-6354
                                   whiteriver.query@vba.va.gov
                                   www.whiteriver.va.gov

Deborah Amdur, Executive Director
Danielle S. Ocker, Associate Director
Melanie Thompson, Acting Chief of Staff
Laura F. Miraldi, Associate Director for Nursing
The White River Junction VA Medical Center (WRJ VAMC) is re-
sponsible for the delivery of health care services to eligible Veter-
ans in Vermont and the 4 contiguous counties of New Hampshire.
These services are delivered at the Medical Center's main campus
located in White River Junction, Vermont, and at its seven Outpa-
tient Clinics (Bennington, Brattleboro, Colchester, Newport, and
Rutland, Vermont; Keene and Littleton, New Hampshire). The
White River Junction VA is closely affiliated with the Ge

5819 Vermont Veterans Centers
359 Dorset St
South Burlington, VT 05403-6210   802-862-1806
                                        877-927-8387
                                   Fax: 802-865-3319
                                   www.va.gov

Fred Forehand, Team Leader
William Newkirk, Counsilor
George Troutman, Counsilor
Tamara R Thompson, Family Therapist
Veterans medical clinic offering disabled veterans medical treat-
ments.

Virginia

5820 Hampton VA Medical Center
Veterans Health Administration, U S Dept. of V A
100 Emancipation Dr
Hampton, VA 23667-1   757-722-9961
                                        800-827-1000
                                   Fax: 757-728-3135
                                   mike.eisenberg@med.va.gov
                                   www.hampton.va.gov

Deanne M Seekins, Medical Center Director
Benita K Stoddard, Associate Director for Operation
G. Arul, Chief of Staff
Shedale Tindall, Associate Director for Patient C

5821 Hunter Holmes McGuire VA Medical Center
Veterans Health Administration, U S Dept. of V A
1201 Broad Rock Blvd
Richmond, VA 23249-1   804-675-5000
                                        800-784-8381
                                   Fax: 804-675-5236
                                   g.vhacss@forum.va.gov
                                   www.richmond.va.gov

Charles E Sepich, Director
David P Budinger, Associate Director
Julie Beales, Interim Chief of Staff
Rita A Duval, Associate Director for Patient C

5822 Roanoke Regional Office
Veterans Benefits Administration, U S Dept. of V A
116 North Jefferson St
Roanoke, VA 24016-1906   540-362-1999
                                        800-827-1000
                                   Fax: 540-563-4838
                                   www.va.gov

Roger Bohm, Executive
Bert Boyd, COO/Executive Director

5823 Salem VA Medical Center
Veterans Health Administration, U S Dept. of V A
1970 Roanoke Blvd
Salem, VA 24153-6478   540-982-2463
                                        800-827-1000
                                        888-982-2463
                                   Fax: 540-983-1096
                                   g.vhacss@forum.va.gov
                                   www.salem.va.gov

Miguel H LaPuz, Director
Carol S Bogedain, Associate Director
Maureen McCarthy, Chief of Staff
Pearl Washington, Nurse Executive

5824 Virginia Department of Veterans Services
270 Franklin Rd SW
Roanoke, VA 24011-2204   540-857-7102
                                   Fax: 540-857-6437

Colbert Boyd, Manager

Washington

5825 Jonathan M Wainwright Memorial VA Medical Center
Veterans Health Administration, U S Dept. of V A
77 Wainwright Dr
Walla Walla, WA 99362-3975   509-525-5200
                                        888-687-8863
                                   Fax: 509-946-3062
                                   www.va.gov

Michael W Parnicky, R and D Coordinator

5826 Seattle Regional Office
Veterans Benefits Administration U S Department of
915 2nd Ave
Seattle, WA   98174-1060   206-762-1010
                                             800-827-1000
                                    seattle.query@vba.va.gov
                                             www.va.gov

Va Ad Harabanim, Executive Director
Timothy Williams, Chief Executive Officer

5827 Spokane VA Medical Center
Veterans Health Administration, U S Dept. of V A
4815 N Assembly St
Spokane, WA   99205-6185   509-434-7000
                                             800-325-7940
                                    Fax: 509-434-7119
                                    g.vhacss@forum.va.gov
                                    www.spokane.va.gov

Alan Prentiss, Chief of Staff
Dirk Minatre, Coordinator
Joseph Manley, Executive Director

5828 VA Puget Sound Health Care System
Veterans Health Administration, U S Dept. of V A
1660 S Columbian Way
Seattle, WA   98108-1532   206-762-1010
                                             800-329-8387
                                    g.vhacss@forum.va.gov
                                    www.pugetsound.va.gov

Michael Fisher, Director
Michael Tadych, Deputy Director
Walt Dannenberg, Assistant Director
William Campbell, Chief of Staff

West Virginia

5829 Huntington Regional Office
Veterans Benefits Administration, U S Dept. of V A
640 4th Ave
Huntington, WV   25701-1340   304-525-5131
                                             800-827-1000
                                    Fax: 304-399-9344
                                    huntington.query@vba.va.gov
                                             www.va.gov

Mark Bugher, President

5830 Huntington VA Medical Center
Veterans Health Administration, U S Dept. of V A
1540 Spring Valley Dr
Huntington, WV   25704-9300   304-429-6741
                                             800-827-8244
                                    Fax: 304-429-6713
                                    www.huntington.va.gov

Edward H Seiler, Director
Suzanne Jene, Associate Director
Jeffery B Breaux, Chief of Staff
Catherine J Locher, Associate Director for Nursing S

5831 Louis A Johnson VA Medical Center
Veterans Health Administration, U S Dept. of V A
1 Medical Center Drive
Clarksburg, WV   26301-4155   304-623-3461
                                             800-733-0512
                                    Fax: 304-626-7048
                                    g.vhacss@forum.va.gov
                                    www.clarksburg.va.gov

William E Cox, Director
Jeffrey A Beiler II, Associate Director
Glenn R Snider, Chief of Staff
Theresa J White, Nurse Executive

5832 Martinsburg VA Medical Center
Veterans Health Administration, U S Dept. of V A
510 Butler Avenue
Martinsburg, WV   25405-9990   304-263-0811
                                             800-817-3807
                                    Fax: 304-262-7433
                                    g.vhacss@forum.va.gov
                                    www.martinsburg.va.gov

Ann R Brown, Director
Timothy J Cooke, Associate Medical Center Directo
Jonathan E Fierer, Chief of Staff
Susan George, Nursing Programs and Education

5833 US Department Veterans Affairs Beckley Vet Center
200 Veterans Ave
Beckley, WV   25801-4301   304-255-2121
                                             877-902-5142
                                    Fax: 304-254-8711
                                    www.beckley.va.gov

Karin L. McGraw, Director
Vet Center services includes individual and group readjustment counseling, referral for benefits assistance, liason with community agencies, marital and family counseling, substance abuse counseling, job counseling and referral, sexual trauma counseling, and community education.

Wisconsin

5834 Clement J Zablocki VA Medical Center
Veterans Health Administration U S Department of V
5000 W National Ave
Milwaukee, WI   53295-1   414-384-2000
                                             888-827-1000
                                             888-469-6614
                                    Fax: 414-382-5319
                                    www.milwaukee.va.gov

Robert H Beller, Director
Michael D Erdmann, Chief of Staff
Judith A Murphy, Associate Director for Patient/N
In an effort to improve access to veterans in Milwaukee County, the VAMC has deployed a mobile clinic that provides primary care four days a week to veterans. The Medical Center also assists the Vet Center located in the City of Milwaukee. In addition, this Medical Center participates in a four-way partnership with the WDVA, the Center for Veterans Issues, Ltd., and the Social Development Commission, to operate Vets Place Central, a 72-bed transitional housing program.

5835 Tomah VA Medical Center
Veterans Health Administration, U S Dept. of V A
500 E Veterans St
Tomah, WI   54660-3105   608-372-3971
                                             800-872-8662
                                    Fax: 608-372-1224
                                    g.vhacss@forum.va.gov
                                    www.tomah.va.gov

Mario V. DeSanctis, Medical Center Director
David Huffman, Associate Director
David J. Houlihan, Chief of Staff
Judith E. Broad, Associate Director
VAMCTomah has been improving the health of the men and women who have so proudly served our nation. We consider it our privelege to serve your health care needs in any way we can. Services are available to veterans living in a Western/Central area of Wisconsin.

5836   William S Middleton Memorial VA Hospital Center
Veterans Health Administration, U S Dept. of V A
2500 Overlook Ter
Madison, WI 53705-2254

608-256-1901
888-478-8321
888-256-1901
Fax: 608-280-7244
g.vhacss@forum.va.gov
www.madison.va.gov

Judy McKee, Director
John Rohrer, Associate Director
Alan J. Bridges, Chief of Staff
Rebecca Kordahl, Associate Director

5837   Wisconsin VA Regional Office
Veterans Benefits Administration, U S Dept. of V A
5000 W National Ave
Milwaukee, WI 53295-1

414-384-2000
800-827-1000
Fax: 414-382-5374
milwaukee.query@vba.va.gov
www.milwaukee.va.gov

Philip L Cook, Executive Director
Neil S Mandel, Research/Development Coordinator
Glen Grippen, CEO

In an effort to improve access to veterans in Milwaukee County, the VAMC has deployed a mobile clinic that provides primary care four days a week to veterans. The Medical Center also assists the Vet Center located in the City of Milwaukee. In addition, this Medical Center participates in a four-way partnership with the WDVA, the Center for Veterans Issues, Ltd., and the Social Development Commission, to operate Vets Place Central, a 72-bed transitional housing program.

Wyoming

5838   Casper Vet Center
1030 N. Poplar Suite B
Casper, WY 82601-2665

307-261-5355
Fax: 307-261-5439
www.vetcenter.va.gov

James Whipps, Office Manager
Vet Center offering re-adjustment counseling for combat veterans.

5839   Cheyenne VA Medical Center
Veterans Health Administration, U S Dept. of V A
2360 E Pershing Blvd
Cheyenne, WY 82001-5356

307-778-7370
877-927-8387
888-483-9127
Fax: 307-638-8923
g.vhacss@forum.va.gov
www.va.gov

Cynthia McCormack, Medical Center Director
Elizabeth Lowery, Associate Director
Jerry Zang, Chief of Staff
Polly Baird, Associate Director

5840   Sheridan VA Medical Center
Veterans Health Administration, U S Dept. of V A
1898 Fort Rd
Sheridan, WY 82801-8320

307-672-3473
800-827-1000
866-822-6714
Fax: 307-672-1639
www.sheridan.va.gov/index.asp

Debra L Hirschman, Director
Michele Beach, Director
Wendell Robison, Chief of Staff
Jane Votaw, Nurse Executive

5841   Wyoming/Colorado VA Regional Office
Veterans Benefits Administration, U S Dept. of V A
155 Van Gordon St
Lakewood, CO 80228-1709

303-894-7474
800-827-1000
Fax: 303-894-7442
denver.query@vba.va.gov
www.va.gov

E William Belz, Director

Vocational & Employment

Alabama

5842   ADRS Lakeshore
Alabama Department Of Rehabilitation Services
3830 Ridgeway Dr
Birmingham, AL 35259-9127   205-870-5999
                                                800-441-7609
                                           Fax: 205-879-2685
                                           www.rehab.alabama.gov

Stephen G. Kayes, District 1, Mobile
Jimmy Varnado, District 2, Montgomery
Eddie C. Williams, District 5, Huntsville
Roger McCullough, District 6, Birmingham
Rehabilitation offering employment services to severely disabled persons. Programs include Adaptive Driving Training, Assistive Technology; Employability Development, and Vocational Evaluation.

5843   Alabama Goodwill Industries
2350 Green Springs Highway S
Birmingham, AL 35205-6834   205-323-6331
                                           Fax: 205-324-9059
                                       caroline.goodwill@yahoo.com
                                          www.alabamagoodwill.org

Don Smith, President & CEO
Paul Beasley, Chairman
Herbert L. Boring, Vice Chairman
Roger Cartwright, Treasurer
The mission of Goodwill is to provide rehabilitation services, training, employment, and opportunities for personal growth to the disabled/disadvantaged.

5844   Arc of Jefferson County
6001 Crestwood Blvd
Birmingham, AL 35212   205-323-6383
                                           Fax: 205-323-0085
                                             www.arcofjeff.org

Chris B. Stewart, President & CEO
Scarlet Thompson, Vice President, Development
Clarissa McKinney, Director, Day Programs - Jefferson County
Mary Frances Colley, Assistant Director, Development
The ARC has four primary components. The HOPE Program provides early intervention therapy services to developmentally delayed infants and toddlers up to the age of three years. The ARC also provides services to adults ages 21 and over with intellectual disabilities. Adult services provides education, pre-vocational screening, and socialization skills training. Employment services provides vocational training, a sheltered workshop, off-site job skills training, job coach services and more.

5845   Coffee County Training Center
801 Aviation Blvd
P.O.Box 311343
Enterprise, AL 36330   334-393-1732
                                           Fax: 334-347-0252

Vickie Florence, Manager
Clients 21 years and up receive training in Independent Living Skills, Self-Care, Language Skills, Learning, Self-Direction and Economic Self-Sufficiency. Transportation is also provided to clients of the center.

5846   Easter Seals: Achievement Center
Easter Seals of Alabama
510 W Thomason Circle
Opelika, AL 36801-5499   334-745-3501
                                                866-239-2237
                                           Fax: 334-749-5808
                                          www.achievement-center.org

Furrel Bailey, Executive Director
Rick Dudley, Vocational Instructor
Star Wray, Director Of Industrial & Vocational Services
George Dunn, Employment Specialist

Provides vocational development and extended employment programs for physically, mentally, and developmentally disabled individuals and to non-disabled persons who are culturally, socially, or economically disadvantaged.

5847   Easter Seals: Opportunity Center
6300 McClellan Blvd
Anniston, AL 36206   256-820-9960
                                           Fax: 256-820-9592
                                        www.opportunity-center.com

Steven D. Miles, Administrator
Marty Gwin, Assistant Administrator Director of Rehabilitation
Lisa Fincher, Employment Specialist
Debra Wood, Vocational Instructor
A nationally accredited non-profit organization providing vocational evaluation/assessment, paid work training, and employment services for people with disabilities in Calhoun, Cleburne, Clay, Talladega, Coosa and Randolph counties.

5848   Montgomery Career Center: Alabama Employment Services Division
Alabama Department of Labor
649 Monroe St
Montgomery, AL 36131   334-286-1746
                                           Fax: 334-288-7286
                                      montgomery@alcc.alabama.gov
                                          joblink.alabama.gov

5849   Vocational Rehabilitation Service - Opelika
Alabama Department of Rehabilitation Services
520 W Thomason Circle
Opelika, AL 36801   334-749-1259
                                                800-671-6835
                                           Fax: 334-749-8753
                                           TTY: 800-499-1816
                                           www.rehab.state.al.us

5850   Vocational Rehabilitation Service - Dothan
Alabama Department of Rehabilitation Services
795 Ross Clark Circle NE
Ste 2
Dothan, AL 36303   334-699-8600
                                                800-275-0132
                                           Fax: 334-792-1783
                                           www.rehab.state.al.us

5851   Vocational Rehabilitation Service - Homewood
Alabama Department Of Rehabilitation Services
236 Goodwin Crest Dr
Birmingham, AL 35209   205-290-4400
                                                800-671-6837
                                           Fax: 205-290-0486
                                           www.rehab.state.al.us

Roger McCullough, Manager
Availiable through any of the 21 VRS offices statewide, services can include educational services, vocational assesment, evaluation and counseling, job training, assistive technology, orientation and mobility training, and job placement.

5852   Vocational Rehabilitation Service - Huntsville
3000 Johnson Rd SW
Huntsville, AL 35805-5847   256-650-1700
                                                800-671-6840
                                           Fax: 256-650-1795
                                           www.rehab.state.al.us

Eddie C. Williams, Manager
Available through any of the 21 VRS offices statewide, services can include educational services, vocational assesment, evaluation and counseling, job training, assistive technology, orientation and mobility training, and job placement.

5853 Vocational Rehabilitation Service - Jackson
1401 Forest Ave
P.O.Box 1005
Jackson, AL 36545
251-246-5708
800-671-6836
Fax: 251-246-5224
www.rehab.state.al.us

5854 Vocational Rehabilitation Service - Jasper
Alabama Department of Rehabilitation Services
4505 Hwy 78 E
Ste 300
Jasper, AL 35501
205-221-7840
800-671-6841
Fax: 205-221-1062
www.rehab.state.al.us

5855 Vocational Rehabilitation Service - Mobile
Alabama Department of Rehabilitation Services
2419 Gordon Smith Dr
Mobile, AL 36617
251-479-8611
800-671-6842
Fax: 251-478-2197
www.rehab.state.al.us

Stephen G. Kayes, Manger
Available through any of the 21 VRS offices statewide, services can include educational services, vocational assesment, evaluation and counseling, job training, assistive technology, orientation and mobility training, and job placement.

5856 Vocational Rehabilitation Service - Muscle Shoals
Alabama Department of Rehabilitation Services
1450 E Avalon Ave
Muscle Shoals, AL 35661
256-381-1110
800-275-0166
Fax: 256-389-3149
www.rehab.state.al.us

5857 Vocational Rehabilitation Service - Selma
Alabama Department of Rehabilitation Services
722 Alabama Ave
Selma, AL 36701
334-877-2927
888-761-5995
Fax: 334-877-3796
www.rehab.state.al.us

5858 Vocational Rehabilitation Service - Talladega
Alabama Department of Rehabilitation Services
31 Arnold St
Talladega, AL 35160
256-362-1300
800-441-7592
Fax: 256-362-6387
www.rehab.state.al.us

5859 Vocational Rehabilitation Service - Troy
Alabama Department of Rehabilitation Services
1109 Troy Plaza St
Troy, AL 36081
334-566-2491
800-441-7608
Fax: 334-566-9415
www.rehab.state.al.us

5860 Vocational Rehabilitation Service - Tuscaloosa
Alabama Department of Rehabilitation Services
1305 James I Harrison Jr Parkway E
Tuscaloosa, AL 35405
205-554-1300
800-331-5562
Fax: 205-554-1369
www.rehab.state.al.us

William Strickland, Manager
Available through any of the 21 VRS offices statewide, services can include educational services, vocational assessment, evaluation and counseling, job training, assistive technology, orientation and mobility training, and job placement.

5861 Vocational Rehabilitation Service- Gadsden
Alabama Department of Rehabilitation Services
1100 George Wallace Dr
Gadsden, AL 35903-6501
256-547-6974
800-671-6839
Fax: 256-543-1784
www.rehab.state.al.us

5862 Vocational Rehabilitation Service: Scottsboro
Alabama Department of Rehabilitation Services
203 S Market St
P.O. Box 296
Scottsboro, AL 35768-0296
256-574-5813
800-418-8823
Fax: 256-574-6033
www.rehab.alabama.gov

5863 Vocational Rehabilitation Services - Andalusia
Alabama Department of Rehabilitation Services
1082 Village Square Dr
Ste 1
Andalusia, AL 36420
334-222-4114
800-671-6833
Fax: 334-427-1216
www.rehab.state.al.us

5864 Vocational Rehabilitation Services - Anniston
Alabama Department of Rehabilitation Services
1910 Coleman Rd
Anniston, AL 36207
256-240-8800
800-671-6834
Fax: 256-240-6580
www.rehab.state.al.us

5865 Vocational and Rehabilitation Service - Decatur
Alabama Department of Rehabilitation Services
621 Cherry St NE
Decatur, AL 35602
256-353-2754
800-671-6838
Fax: 256-351-2476
www.rehab.state.al.us

5866 Vocational and Rehabilitation Services - Montgomery
Alabama Department of Rehabilitation Services
602 S Lawrence St
Montgomery, AL 36104
334-293-7500
800-441-7578
Fax: 334-293-7372

Jimmy Varnado, Manager
Available through any of the 21 VRS offices statewide, services can include educational services, vocational assessment, evaluation and counseling, job training, assistive technology, orientation and mobility training and job placement.

5867 Wiregrass Rehabilitation Center, Inc.
795 Ross Clark Circle
Dothan, AL 36303
334-792-0022
800-395-7044
Fax: 334-712-7632
www.wrcjobs.com

Ben Slingluff, Chairman
Jeff Coleman, Vice-Chairman
Cynthia Green, Director, Development
Trains individuals to become employable and assists them in finding jobs withing their communities. Also assists individuals who have difficulty maintaining employment, those who are on forms of public assistance such as welfare and those who are employable and underemployed.

5868 Workshops, Inc.
4244 3rd Ave S
Birmingham, AL   35222-2008   205-592-9683
                                               888-805-9683
                                          Fax: 205-592-9687
                                          TTY:205-592-8006
                                     email@workshopsinc.org
                                       www.workshopsinc.org

Susan Crow, Executive Director
Dana Chang, Director, Programs
Kathy Dunn, Director, Operations
Mary Hendley, Director, Development & Marketing
Provides vocational training, sheltered employment and other support services to people with disabilities in central Alabama.

Alaska

5869 Alaska Division of Vocational Rehabilitation
Department of Labor & Workforce Development
1111 W. 8th St
Ste 210
Juneau, AK   99801-1894   907-465-2814
                                               800-478-2815
                                          Fax: 907-465-2856
                                          TTY: 800-478-2815
                                    dol.dvr.info@alaska.gov
                                   www.labor.state.ak.us/dvr

John Cannon, Director
Assist individuals with disabilities to obtain and maintain employment.

5870 Alaska Fair Employment Practice Agency
Alaska State Commission for Human Rights
800 A St
Ste 204
Anchorage, AK   99501-3669   907-276-7474
                                               800-478-4692
                                          Fax: 907-278-8588
                                          TTY: 907-276-3177
                                   www.humanrights.alaska.gov

5871 Alaska Job Center Network
Alaska Department of Labor & Workforce Development
P.O. Box 115509
Juneau, AK   99811-5509   907-465-2712
                                          Fax: 907-465-4537
                                          www.jobs.alaska.gov

Arizona

5872 Downtown Neighborhood Learning Center
1001 W Jefferson St
Phoenix, AZ   85007-2913   602-254-6524
                                               800-869-8521
                                          Fax: 602-256-2524
                                            dnlc@swlink.net
                                            www.swlink.net

Scott Ritchey, Manager
Mattie Johnson, Receptionist
Peg Osinski, El Mirage Learning Lab
Adult education agency providing basic skills, GED, ESOL, life skills, computer skills, resume assistance and career testing.

5873 Fair Employment Practice Agency: Arizona
Arizona Civil Rights Division
1275 W Washington St
Phoenix, AZ   85007-2926   602-542-5025
                                               800-352-8431
                                          Fax: 602-542-4085
                                              www.azag.gov

Virginia Gonzales, Director
Bruna Pedrini, Manager

Provides legal advice to most state agencies. The office also investigates and prosecutes consumer fraud, white collar crime, organized crime, public corruption, and civil rights.

5874 JOBS Administration Job Opportunities & Basic Skills
1717 W Jefferson St
Phoenix, AZ   85007-3202   602-542-9596
                                          Fax: 602-542-5171

Gretchen Evans, Program Administrator
Assist applicants and recipients of temporary assistance to needy families to obtain job training and employment that will lead to economic independence.

5875 TETRA Services
Beacon Group SW Inc
2222 N 24th Street
Phoenix, AZ   85008   602-685-9703
                                          Fax: 602-244-2435
                                        info@tetraservices.org

5876 Vocational and Rehabilitation Agency Rehabilitation Services Administrations
Division of Employment & Rehabilitation Services
1789 W Jefferson St
Phoenix, AZ   85007-3202   602-604-8835
                                               800-563-1221
                                               800-563-1221
                                          Fax: 602-604-8901
                                          TTY:602-542-6049
                                           tazrsa@azdes.gov
                                             azdes.gov/rsa

Michelle Nitschke, Manager
Katharine Levandowsky, Administrator
Moises Gallegos, Manager
This program serves individuals with disabilities seeking jobs and job training.

5877 Yavapai Regional Medical Center-West
1003 Willow Creek Rd
Prescott, AZ   86301-1668   928-445-2700
                                               877-843-9762
                                          Fax: 928-445-0994
                                                   yrmc.org

Tim Barnett, CEO
Widely recognized for the quality and success of the physical, occupational, and speech therapy programs it offers. Provides a wide range of programs and services that enable our patients to reach their maximum level of function and independence- and enjoy the highest possible quality of life.

Arkansas

5878 Arkansas Employment Service Agency and Job Training Program
Arkansas Employment Security Department
Capitol Mall
Ste 2
Little Rock, AR   72201-2981   501-682-2033
                                          Fax: 501-682-2273
                                         www.arkansas.gov/esd

Artee Williams, Manager
Wide range of services including employment services, unemployment insurance, and labor market information.

5879 Easter Seal Work Center
3920 Woodland Heights Rd
Little Rock, AR   72212-2406   501-227-3600
                                          Fax: 501-227-7180
                                      mail@ar.easterseals.com
                                      www.ar.easterseals.com

Lauren Zilk, Administrator
Mission is to provide exceptional services to ensure that all people with disabilities or special needs have equal opportunities to live,learn work and play in their communities.

5880 VCT/A Job Retention Skill Training Program
Arkasas Rehab Services
P.O.Box 1358
Hot Springs, AR 71902-1358   501-624-4411
    Fax: 501-624-0019
Barbara Lewis, Administrator
Mae Robinson, Assistant Administrator
A training program designed for use in rehabilitation and educational settings. Using a social skill training strategy, VCT helps participants learn how to solve on-the-job problems and cope with common supervisory demands.

5881 Vocational and Rehabilitation Agency Division of Services for the Blind
700 Main St
Little Rock, AR 72201-4608   501-686-9433
    800-960-9270
    Fax: 501-686-9418
    TTY: 501-682-0093
    www.state.ar.us
Lyndel Lybarger, Field Adminstrator
James Hudson, Executive Director

5882 Vocational and Rehabilitation Agency for Persons Who Are Visually Impaired
Arkansas Department of Human Services
P.O.Box 3237
Little Rock, AR 72203-3237   501-686-9433
    800-960-9270
    Fax: 501-686-9418
    TTY: 501-324-9271
James C Hudson, Executive Director
Furnishes a wide variety of services to help people with disabilities return to work.

California

5883 ABLE Industries
8127 Avenue 304
Visalia, CA 93291   559-651-8150
    888-813-2253
    Fax: 559-651-0357
    www.ableindustries.org
Wende-Leigh Ayers, Executive Director
Committed to improving the lives of people with disabilities by creating opportunities to maximize their independence.

5884 ARC-Adult Vocational Program
1500 Howard St
San Francisco, CA 94103-2525   415-255-7200
    Fax: 415-255-9488
    www.thearcsanfrancisco.org
Timothy Hornbecker, Executive Director
Job placement programs, remunerative work services and work adjustment training programs.

5885 AbilityFirst
1300 E Green Street
Pasadena, CA 91106   626-396-1010
    877-768-4600
    Fax: 626-396-1021
    info@abilityfirst.org
    www.abilityfirst.org
Lori E Gangemi, President
Steve S. Schultz, CFO
Keri Castaneda, Chief Program Officer
Syed Kazmi, Controller
Provides programs and services to help children and adults with physical and developmental disabilities reach their full potential throughout their lives. Offers a broad range of employment, recreational and socialization programs and operate 12 accessible residential housing complexes.

5886 Achievement House & NCI Affiliates
496 Linne Road
Paso Robles, CA 93446   805-238-6630
    Fax: 805-239-9073
    conact@nciaffiliates.org
    www.achievementhouse.org

5887 Bakersfield ARC
2240 S Union Ave
Bakersfield, CA 93307-4158   661-834-2272
    800-834-3160
    Fax: 661-834-1694
    lplank@barc-inc.org
    www.barc-inc.org
Jim Baldwin, President/CEO
William Froning, Senior VP/CFO
Dave Kyle, Senior VP/Chief Compliance Officer
Mike Grover, Senior VP/Chief Programmes Officer
A non-profit organization that has been providing essential job training, employment and support services for the developmentally disabled and their families.
1949

5888 California Department of Fair Employment& Housing
2218 Kauden Drive
Suite 100
Elk Grove, CA 95758   916-478-7251
    800-884-1684
    contact.center@dfeh.ca.gov
    www.dfeh.ca.gov
Phyllis W Cheng, Director
Annmarie Billotti Esq, Chief Deputy Director
To protect Californians from employment, housing and public accomodation discrimination, and hate violence.

5889 Career Connection Transition Program
Whittier Union High School District
9401 Painter Ave
Whittier, CA 90605-2729   562-698-8121
    Fax: 562-693-4414
    Richard.Rosenberg@wuhsd.k12.ca.us
    www.wuhsd.k12.ca.us
Richard L Rosenberg PhD, Vocational Coordinator
Bonnie Bolton, Transition Department Head
Job placement programs, remunerative work services and work adjustment training programs. Transition services.

5890 Career Development Program (CDP)
260 W Grand Ave
Escondido, CA 92025-2604   760-738-0277
    Fax: 760-741-9452
Richard Brady MD
Wendy Hope, Supported Employment
Jill Hennessy, Independent Living
Work hardening and disciplinary programs.

5891 Colton-Redlands-Yucaipa Regional Occupational Programs
1214 Indiana Ct
PO Box 8640
Redlands, CA 92374-2896   909-793-3115
    Fax: 909-793-6901
    www.cryrop.org
Stephanie Houston, Superintendent
Sandra Moritensen, Manager Student Services
Provides quality hands-on training programs in over 40 high demand career fields to assist high school students and adults in acquiring marketable job skills. Works in cooperation with local high schools, adult education colleges, and employers providing a collaborative team of academic and ROP occupational teachers who integrate academic and vocational competencies to provide sequenced paths within career majors. Support services, career guidance and services are provided to disabled people.

5892 Community Outpatient Rehabilitation Center
2823 Fresno Street
Fresno, CA 93721   559-459-6000
                                      Fax: 559-459-1004
                          complaint@jointcommission.org
                               www.communitymedical.org

Tim A. Joslin, Chief Executive Officer
Thomas Utecht, M.D., Senior Vice President
Craig S. Castro, Senior Vice President
Vicki Anderson, Vice President, Managed Care

Physical, occupational and speech therapy, neuropsychology services available for orthopedic and neurological diagnosis. Lymphedema program.

5893 Desert Haven Enterprises
43437 Copeland Circle
PO Box 2110
Lancaster, CA 93535   661-948-8402
                                      Fax: 661-948-1080
                                       www.deserthaven.org

Jenni Moran, Executive Director
Kathleen Miller, Program Services Director
Lisa Enos, Director Contract Services
Kathy Burcina, Job Developer

A private, nonprofit organization dedicated to developing, enhancing, and promotingthe capabilities of persons with mental retardation and other developmental disabilities.

5894 ESS Work Center
858 Stanton Rd
Burlingame, CA 94010-1404   650-697-2642
                                      Fax: 650-697-2405

Ed Mentzer, Owner
Work adjustment and remunerative work programs.

5895 Employment Service: California
Employment Development Department
800 Capitol Mall
P.O. Box 826880
Sacramento, CA 95814- 0001   916-653-0707
                                             www.edd.ca.gov

5896 Feather River Industries
1811 Kusel Rd
Oroville, CA 95966-9528   530-534-1112
                                      Fax: 530-534-3137
                             www.featherriverindustries.com

Randy Guild, Rehabilitation Counselor
Ed Turner, Production Coordinator
Judy Smith, President
Steve Wattenberg, Vice President

Vocational training for persons with developmental disabilities provided through wood products fabrication and assembly tasks. Instructor to trainer rating ranging from 1 to 12, 1 to 8, 1 to 6, and 1 to 4 depending on individual needs and complexity of tasks.

5897 Fit to Work
Ste 401
3581 Palmer Dr
Cameron Park, CA 95682-8238   530-676-7485
                                      Fax: 530-676-9114
                                          www.trueyellow.com

Helen Cheng
Provides remunerative work.

5898 Fresno City College: Disabled Students Programs and Services
Fresno City College
1101 E University Ave
Fresno, CA 93741   559-442-4600
                                      Fax: 559-499-6051
                          campusnews@fresnocitycollege.edu
                               www.fresnocitycollege.edu

Ryan Blodgett, Department Chair
Heather Beltran, Department Secretary
Sam Alvarado, Counselor
Chris Aldaco-Glass, Learning Disabilities Specialist

The Disabled Students Programs & Services (DSPS) at Fresno City College provides services for students with physical, learning and/or psychological disabilities to successfully pursue their individual educational, vocational and personal goals. Some programs offered include basic computer training, adaptive software training, independent living and consumer skills training, note-taking assistance, special classes and more.

5899 Heartland Opportunity Center
323 N E Street
Madera, CA 93638   559-674-8828
                                      Fax: 559-674-8857
                         kanderson@heartlandopportunity.com
                              www.heartlandopportunity.com

Kristy Anderson, CEO
Maria Alvarado, CFO

Provides employment, job placement, vocational and life skills training to adults with mental, physical and/or emotional disabilities in order to help them reach their personal and vocational goals.

5900 Hollister Workshop
Hope Rehabilitation Services
185 Berry Street
Suite 4000
San Francisco, CA 94107-2536   415-243-4200
                                           888-567-7442
                                           415-764-1622
                                      Fax: 831-637-8726
                                  salesteam@loopnet.com
                                          www.loopnet.com

Fred Saint, President
Wayne Warthen, CTO & SVP, Information Technology
Curtis Kroeker, President, LoopNet Marketplace Verticals
Leah McMurtry, Vice President, Member Services

Work adjustment and remunerative work programs.

5901 Job Training Program Liaison: California
Employment Development Department
800 Capitol Mall
Sacramento, CA 95814-4807   916-654-8210
                                           800-300-5616
                                      Fax: 916-657-5294
                                             edd.ca.gov

Patrick Henning, Manager
Provides information on filing an Unemployment Insurance or Disability Insurance claim, on-line job and resume bank which boasts thousands of job openings.

5902 King's Rehabilitation Center
494 E Hanford-Armona Road
Hanford, CA 93232   559-583-5051
                                      Fax: 559-582-1182
                                        www.kingsrehab.com

Robert Knudseon, President
Steve Mendoza, Executive Director
Pat Vestal, VP
Renee Castro, Treasurer

To enhance the lives of adults with disabilities by providing day program services, vocational training and employment opportunities to assist such persons to attain their full potential.

5903 Morongo Basin Work Activity Center
74325 Joe Davis Dr
Twentynine Palms, CA 92277   760-366-8474
                                           www.guidestar.org

Sheree Fraser
Job placement programs, remunerative work services and work adjustment training programs.

5904 Mother Lode Rehabilitation Enterprises
399 Placerville Dr
Placerville, CA 95667
530-622-4848
Fax: 530-622-0204
www.morerehab.org

Susan Peters, Chair
Henry Jeter, VP Finance
Christa K. Campbell, Secretary
A private, non-profit organization dedicated to supporting persons with disabilities. MORE was established by a group of parents, educators, rehabilitation professionals and concerned citizens and first began serving adults with disabilities in 1973.

5905 Napa Valley PSI Inc.
P.O.Box 600
Napa, CA 94559-600
707-255-0177
Fax: 707-255-0802
admin@napavaleypsi.org
http://www.napavalleypsi.org

Kimberly Alexander-Yarbor, President
Carol Gonsalves , Vice President
Eleanor Cullum, Secretary
Worthy Brooks, Directors
Work adjustment, work training and educational services for developmentally disabled adults. Emphasis is on manufacture of quality wood products, primarily wooden office furniture.

5906 Oakland Work Activity Area
6315 San Leandro St
Oakland, CA 94621-3727
510-639-9350
oaklandlocal.com

Greg Whalley
Dennis Scharssenberg, Manager
Susan Mernit, Editor/Publisher
Abraham Hyatt, Editor
Job placement programs, remunerative work services and work adjustment training programs.

5907 Opportunities for the Handicapped
P.O.Box 322
New York, NY 10040-0322
419-855-2742
www.giveindia.org

Kathy Dodd
Pradeep Jayaraman, President
Harendra Guturu, Secretary
Uttara Diwan, Treasurer
Work adjustment and remunerative work programs.

5908 Orange County ARC
225 W Carl Karcher Way
Anaheim, CA 92801
714-744-5301
Fax: 714-744-5312
jhearn2001@yahoo.com
ocarc.net

Joyce Hearn, CEO
Richard Farmer, VP Finance
Michael Galliano, VP Operations
Patrick Faraday, VP Sales
To provide quality care, training and services to our intellectually/developmentally disabled clients.

5909 PRIDE Industries
10030 Foothills Boulevard
Roseville, CA 95747-7102
916-788-2100
800-550-6005
Fax: 800-888-0447
info@prideindustries.com
http://www.prideindustries.com

Michael Ziegler, CEO
Tim Yamauchi, Executive Vice President and Chi
John Vaughan, Senior Vice President, Manufactu
Pete Berghuis, Senior Vice President, Integrate
Vocational rehabilitation and employment services creating jobs for people with disabilites; services include career counseling, vocational assessment, work adjustment, work services, job seeking skills, job development, job placement, on-the-job sup-

port (coaching), mentoring, independent living skills, transition services and case management.

5910 Parents and Friends, Inc
350 Cypress St
PO Box 656
Fort Bragg, CA 95437
707-964-4940
Fax: 707-964-8536
rmoon@parentsandfriends.org
www.parentsandfriends.org

Rick Moon, Executive Director
Serves people with developmental disabilities.

5911 PathPoint
315 W Haley Street
Ste 102
Santa Barbara, CA 93101
805-966-3310
info@pathpoint.org
www.pathpoint.org

Barbara Stevenson, Chair
Christopher Jones, Vice Chair/Treasurer
Mary E. Tiffany, Secretary
Jeffery Dodds, Director
To provide comprehensive training and support serviceds that empower people with disabilities of disadvantages to live and work as valued members of the community.

5912 People Services, Inc
4195 Lakeshore Blvd
Lakeport, CA 95453
707-263-3810
Fax: 707-263-0552
idumont@nctac.com
www.peopleservices.org

Ilene Dumont, Executive Director
To serve as the local community agency, providing the delivery of quality services for people with disabilities.

5913 Pomona Valley Workshop (PVW)
PVW
4650 Brooks St
Montclair, CA 91763
909-624-3555
Fax: 909-624-5675
ines@pvwonline.org
www.pvwonline.org

Mitch Gariador, Executive Director
Kitty Dubois, Director of Human Resources
Terri Perkins, Director of Work Services
Lucy Yamas-Cortez, Program Director
The Pomona Valley Workshop seeks to assist adults with disabilities to reach their full potential through services such as vocational training, employment preparation and placement services.

5914 Porterville Sheltered Workshop
194 West Poplar Avenue
Porterville, CA 93257-3449
559-784-1399
Fax: 559-781-5651
http://www.portervilleshelteredworkshop.com/

Steve Tree, Executive Director
Work adjustment and remunerative work programs. Mission is to assist disabled individuals achieve a more independent and productive life.

5915 Project Independence
3505 Cadillac Ave
Suite O-103
Costa Mesa, CA 92626
714-549-3464
877-444-0144
Fax: 714-549-3559
info@proindependence.org
www.proindependence.org

Debra Marsteller, Executive Director
Promote civil rights for people with developmental disabilities through services which expand independence and choice.

5916 Sacramento Vocational Services
6950 21st Ave
Sacramento, CA 95820

916-381-1300
Fax: 916-381-9026
info@inallianceinc.com
inallianceinc.com

5917 San Francisco Vocational Services
Ste 600
490 Golf Club Road
Pleasant Hill, CA 94523-1553

925-682-6343
Fax: 925-682-6375
rsnc-centers.org

Gina Chenoweth, Executive Director
Jeffrey Faircloth, Manager Case Management
Rita Hays, Chair/President
William Wilson, Vice Chair

Comprehensive vocational rehabilitation center offering vocational evaluation, rehabilitative counseling, business office training, work experience, and job placement.

5918 Shasta County Opportunity Center
1265 Redwood Blvd
Redding, CA 96003-1965

530-225-5781
Fax: 530-225-5751
oppcenter_info@co.shasta.ca.us
www.co.shasta.ca.us

Del Lockwood, Manager
Leonard Moty, 2012 Chairman
David A. Kehoe, Board of Supervisor
Glenn Hawes, Board of Supervisor

An employment training program for people with disabilities in Shasta County. These individuals perform paid work in a number of different work environments and at the same time learn the skills necessary to obtain competetive employment in the local community.

5919 Social Vocational Services
Ste A104
350 Crenshaw Blvd
Torrance, CA 90503-1725

310-783-0633
Fax: 310-783-0636
nto@svsinc.org

Sabrina Silva, Manager
Dan Strohm, Manager

The leading provider of services for people with developmental disabilities in the state of California

5920 South Bay Vocational Center
1526 W 240th St
Harbor City, CA 90710

310-784-2032
Fax: 310-539-6342
www.sbvc1.com

Corey Sylve, President/CEO
Clare Grey, Vice President/COO
Santiago Lindo, Operations Specialist
Celia Bennett, CFO

A not-for-profit organization that has been providing excellent vocational programs and services for individuals with disabilities.

5921 Tri-County Independent Living Center
2822 Harris Street
Eureka, CA 95503

707-445-8404
877-576-5000
Fax: 707-445-9751
aa@tilinet.org
http://www.tilinet.org

Chris Jones, Executive Director
Allan Daniel, Information & Referral / Indepen
Mary Bullwinkel, Outreach & Resource Development
Cindy Calderon, Systems Change Advocate

To provide programs, services and information for people with disabilities living in Humboldt, Del Norte and Trinity Counties in northern California in an effort to allow choices for individuals to optimize their independence.

5922 Unyeway
Suite E
2330 Main Street
Ramona, CA 92065-2595

760-789-5960
Fax: 760-789-8156
http://www.unyeway.com

Kim Metli, Executive Director
Lisa Oertling, President
Dr. Richard Ferguson, Vice President/Audit Committee C
Pearl Aiello, Director

Job placement programs, remunerative work services and work adjustment training programs.

5923 V-Bar Enterprises
720 Gordon Cir
Suisun City, CA 94585

707-864-1334
government-contractors.findthebest.com

Lu Brunet

Job placement programs, remunerative work services and work adjustment training programs.

5924 Valley Light Industries
5360 Irwindale Avenue
Irwindale, CA 91706

626-332-6200
valleylightind.org

5925 Visalia Workshop
2031 S. Mooney Blvd.
Visalia, CA 93277-6711

559-622-9650
Fax: 866-575-6627
www.buildabear.com

Hortensia Venegas

Work hardening and disciplinary programs.

5926 Westside Opportunity Workshop
9503 Jefferson Blvd
Culver City, CA 90232-2917

310-836-4262
Fax: 310-825-0676
ayokota@mednet.ucla.edu
http://www.semel.ucla.edu

Peter Whybrow, Director
Fawzy Fawzy, Associate Director
Mark Wheeler, Media Relations
Alan Han, Director of Development

Job placement programs, remunerative work services and work adjustment training programs.

5927 Work Training Center
2255 Fair Street
Chico, CA 95928

530-343-7994
Fax: 530-343-4619
carlo@ewtc.org
www.wtcinc.org

Carl Ochsner, Executive Director
Brett Barker, Vocational Services Director
Deb Royat, Rehabilitation Services Director

A nonprofit organization providing services to people with disabilities.

Colorado

5928 Blue Peaks Developmental Services
703 Fourth Street
Alamosa, CO 81101-2638

719-589-5135
Fax: 719-589-0680
http://www.bluepeaks.org

John Kreiner, Director
Randall P. Johnson, Human Resources/Staff Developmen
Brooke Hayden, Residential Director
George Garcia, Operations Director

Provides remunerative work.

5929 Cheyenne Village
6275 Lehman Drive
Colorado Springs, CO 80918
719-592-0200
Fax: 719-548-9947
TTY:719-592-0224
info@cheyennevillage.org
www.cheyennevillage.org

Ann M Turner, Executive Director
B. Jeanne Solze, Business Director
Serves adults with developmental disabilities such as Autism,
Down syndrome, Cerebral Palsy, and Mental Retardation in El
Paso, Teller and Park Counties.

5930 Colorado Civil Rights Divsion
1560 Broadway
Ste 110
Denver, CO 80202
303-894-7855
800-866-7675
Fax: 303-894-7885
www.dora.state.co.us

Barbara J. Kelly, Executive Director
Fred J. Joseph, Banking Division
Steven Chavez, Civil Rights Division
Chris Mykelbust, Division of Financial Services
Embraces the Department's mission of consumer protection and
works to protect individuals from discrimination in employment,
housing and at places of public accommodation through enforce-
ment and outreach consistent with the Colorado Civil Rights
Laws.

5931 Colorado Employment Service
Department of Labor and Employment
Suite 400
1800 Grant Street
Denver, CO 80203-3528
303-860-4200
855-216-7740
Fax: 303-860-4299
employeeservices@cu.edu
www.cu.edu/employee-services

Clara Capano, Manager
Job placement programs, remunerative work services and work
adjustment training programs.

5932 Developmental Training Services
4600 North Fairfax Drive
Suite 402
Arlington, VA 22203
703-465-9388
Fax: 703-465-9344
www.onlinedts.com

Roger Jensen, CEO
Linda Davis, Administrator
Indira Kaur Ahluwalia,, Founder and President
Viresh Desai, Vice President
Residential and employment programs for adults with develop-
mental disabilities.

5933 Dynamic Dimensions
701 Cypress Street
Sulphur, LA 70663
337-527-7034
Fax: 719-346-6010
https://www.wcch.com

Cheryl Reese, Executive Director
Vocational, evaluation and assessment, training and placement
for most disabilities. Group homes and day programs for the developmentally disabled.

5934 Gray Street Workcenter
11177 West 8th Avenue
Lakewood, CO 80215-2821
303-233-3363
Fax: 303-467-2793
http://services.ddrcco.com

Tammy Drumright, Manager
C. David Pemberton, II, President
Neal Berlin, Vice President
Joanne Elliott, M.A., Secretary
Residental and employment programs for adults with develop-
mental disabilities.

5935 Hope Center
3400 Elizabeth St
Denver, CO 80205-4801
303-388-4801
Fax: 303-388-0249
gghope@comcast.net
www.hopecenterinc.org

Charlse T. Smith, Chairperson
Sid Davidson, Vice Chairperson
John Hanson, Treasurer
Barbara Batey, Secretary
Provides educational and vocational opportunities for spe-
cial-needs and at-risk children and adults from 2 1/2 to adulthood.

**5936 Imagine: Innovative Resources for Cognitive & Physical
Challenges**
1400 Dixon St
Lafayette, CO 80026-2790
303-665-7789
Fax: 303-665-2648
caroline@imaginecolorado.org
www.imaginecolorado.org

Mark Emery, Executive Director
Judy James-Anderson, Behavioral Health Services Dir
Provides support services to more than 2,600 people of all ages
with developmental delays and cognitive disabilities including
autism, cerebral palsy and Down syndrome.

5937 Las Animas County Rehabilitation Center
P.O.Box 781
Trinidad, CO 81082-781
719-846-3388
Fax: 719-846-4543
www.scdds.com

Duane Roy, Executive Director
Bernice Whalen, Human Resources Manager
Jeannette Vialobos, SPCC Director
Leslie Lark, Finance Director
Job placement programs, remunerative work services and work
adjustment training programs.

5938 NORESCO Workshop
903 E Burlington Ave
Fort Morgan, CO 80701-3637
970-867-5702
Ramona Proctor, Executive Director
Nancy Study, Manager
Provides remunerative work.

5939 Regional Assessment and Training Center
1145 Gayley Avenue
Suite 304
Los Angeles, CA 90024-3108
303-866-7253
Russell Porter, Executive Director
Work adjustment and renumerative work programs.

5940 Sedgwick County Workshop
7001 W. 21 st St.
North Wichita, KN 67205-1759
316-660-0100
Fax: 316-722-1432
sedgwickinfo@k-state.edu
www.sedgwick.ksu.edu

Maria Contreras, Manager
Provides remunerative work.

5941 Vocational and Rehabilitation Agency
Unit B
2 Peachtree Street, NW
Atlanta, GA 30303-3855
404-232-1998
866-489-0001
Fax: 404-232-1800
TTY: 303-866-3980
GVRAcustomer-service@gvra.ga.gov
https://gvra.georgia.gov

Diana Huerta, Director
James N. Defoor, Chair
Louise Hill, Vice Chair
Purpose is to assist eligible individuals with disabilities to be-
come productive members of the Colorado workforce and to live
independently.

5942 **Yuma County Workshop**
710 E 2nd Ave
Yuma, CO 80759
970-848-2874
www.yellowpages.com/yuma-co

Robert Stephens
Andrea Anderson, Manager
Provides remunerative work.

Connecticut

5943 **Abilities Without Boundaries**
615 W Johnson Avenue
Cheshire, CT 06410
203-272-5607
Fax: 203-272-4284
cconway@abilitieswithoutboundaries.org
www.abilitieswithoutboundaries.or g
Charlie Conway, Executive Director
Christopher Fanelli, Business Manager
Nancy Knapp, Office Manager
Richard Ambro Jr., Employment Specialist
Formerly known as Cheshire Occupational & Career Opportunities (COCO), provides opportunities in the community through employment and social experiences for people with developmental disabilities.

5944 **Allied Community Services**
Six Craftsman Road
East Windsor, CT 06088
860-741-3701
Fax: 860-741-6870
TTY:860-741-3701
www.alliedgroup.org

Dean M Wern, President/CEO
Provides individuals with disabilities or other challenges the opportunity to live and enjoy a productive, independent, and fulfilling life

5945 **Area Cooperative Educational Services(ACES)**
350 State St
North Haven, CT 06473
203-498-6800
acesinfo@aces.org
www.aces.org
Craig W Edmondson EdD, Executive Director
Claudette J. Beamon, Human Resources Director
Carolyn McNally, Program Development Director
Exists to improve public education through high quality, cost effective programs and services.

5946 **CW Resources**
200 Myrtle Street
New Britain, CT 06053
860-229-7700
Fax: 860-229-6847
info@cwresources.org
www.cwresources.org
Ronald H Buccilli, President
CW Resources is dedicated to serving the needs of persons with disabilities through the creation of integrated vocational training and employment opportunities for those individuals who are physically, developmentally, emotionally and/or socio-economically challenged.

5947 **Central Connecticut Association For Retarted Citizens**
950 Slater Rd
New Britain, CT 06053-1658
860-229-6665
Fax: 860-826-6883
ccarc@ccarc.com
www.ccarc.com
Anne Ruwet, CEO
Julie Erickson, Senior Vice President
William allyn, Vice President of Residential Services
Anna Cardona, Vice President
Empowerment through Employment

5948 **Community Enterprises**
441 Pleasant Street
Northampton, MA 01060
413-584-1460
www.communityenterprises.com
Dick Venne, President/CEO
William Donohue, Chairman
Donald Milner, Vice Chairman
Joanne Carlisle, Clerk
Support self-determination for individuals with disabilities and/or other challenges to actively live, learn, and work in the community.

5949 **Connecticut Governor's Committee on Employment of People With Disabilities**
200 Folly Brook Boulevard
Wethersfield, CT 06109-1153
860-263-6000
Fax: 860-263-6039
dol.webhelp@ct.gov
http://www.ctdol.state.ct.us
Dennis Murphy, Acting Commissioner
Dannel P. Malloy, Governor
Work adjustment and remunerative work programs.

5950 **Fotheringhay Farms**
84 Waterhole Rd
Colchester, CT 06415-2323
860-267-4463
Fax: 860-267-7628
http://caringcommunityct.org
Wesley Martins, Executive Director
Job placement programs, remunerative work services and work adjustment training programs.

5951 **George Hegyi Industrial Training Center**
5 Coon Hollow Rd
Derby, CT 06418-1149
203-735-8727
Fax: 203-735-2204
bob.wood@snet.net
http://www.varcainc.com
Joan Bucci, Executive Director
Robert Wood, President
Cecelia Staiano-Hayes, Program Manager
Work adjustment and remunerative work programs.

5952 **Kennedy Center**
2440 Reservoir Ave
Trumbull, CT 06611-4757
203-365-8522
Fax: 203-365-8533
info@kennedyctr.org
www.thekennedycenterinc.org
Martin D. Schwartz, President & CEO
Stuart Gordon, Vice President of Finance
Lynn Pellegrino, Vice President of HR
Marie Farina, HR Generalist
Provides vocational rehabilitation, job training and job placement services to 1,000 adults with disabilities including mental retardation, traumatic brain injury, psychiatric disabilities and more. Residential services, well integrated within the community, serve 97 individuals on a daily basis. Children's programs provide support to 85 children age birth to three, in addition to after hours and recreation programs to appromxately 100 school age children. Staff size is presently 450 employees.

5953 **Quaezar**
285 Riverside Avenue
Suite 300
Westport, CT 06880-4806
203-226-8711
Fax: 203-454-5780
sterlinglp.com
William J Sedarweck, President
Agency for adult mentally retarded/autistic people providing residential care in a group home or apartment setting. Also provides placement in community employment.

5954 Valley Memorial Health Center
435 E Main St
Ansonia, CT 06401-1964   203-736-2601
                                   Fax: 203-736-2641
                                   info@bghealth.org
                                   www.bghealth.org

Marilyn Cormack, CEO
Provides innovative, exceptional behavioral health care through
quality services and programs that focus on, and respect the
consumer.

5955 Vocational and Rehabilitation Agency
2 Peachtree Street, NW
Atlanta, GA 30303-4536   404-232-1998
                                       866-489-0001
                                  Fax: 404-232-1800
                                  TTY: 860-602-4221
                   GVRAcustomer-service@gvra.ga.gov
                                https://gvra.georgia.gov

Keith Maynard, Deputy Director
Brian Sigman, Executive Director
Alan Sylvestre, Chairman
Mission is to provide quality educational and rehabilitative services to all people who are legally blind or deaf/blind and children who are visually impaired at no cost to our clients or their
families.

**5956 Vocational and Rehabilitation Agency: State Department of
Social Services**
Department of Social Services
25 Sigourney St
11th Floor
Hartford, CT 06106-5041   860-424-4844
                                       800-537-2549
                                  Fax: 860-424-4850
                                  TTY: 860-424-4839
                                  brs.dss@po.state.ct.us
                                       www.ct.gov/brs

Amy L Porter, Director
Roderick L Bremby, Commissioner
Provides a broad range of services to the elderly, disabled, families, and individuals who need assistance in maintaining or
achieving their full potential for self-direction, self-reliance and
independent living.

Delaware

5957 Delaware Division of Vocational Rehabilitation
Delaware Department of Labor
4425 N Market Street
Wilmington, DE 19802   302-761-8085
                                       www.delawareworks.com

John McMahon, Secretary of Labor
The state's public program that helps people with physical and
mental disabilities obtain or retain employment. Also, and Independent Living Program helps people with disabilities function
in the community. DVR's commitment is to help people with disabilities increase independence through employment.

5958 Delaware Job Training Program Liaison
Division of Employment & Training
P.O.Box 9828
820 N. French Street
Wilmington, DE 19801- 828   302-577-8977
                                  Fax: 302-577-3996
                                       www.jobaps.com

Harold Stafford, Manager
Work adjustment and remunerative work programs. Also offers
career guidance, supported employment, work readiness and job
placement.

5959 Service Source
3030 Bowers St
Wilmington, DE 19802   302-762-0300
                                       800-738-1733
                                  Fax: 302-762-8797
                                       www.servicesource.org

Michelle Lee, President/CEO
Rhonda VanLowe, Legal Counsel
Joseph J. Sorota, President
Marilynn Bersoff, BTG
ServiceSource is a leading nonprofit disability resource organization with regional offices and programs located in eight states
and the District of Columbia. We serve more than 14,000 individuals with disabilities annually through a range of innovative and
valued employment, training, habilitation, housing and other
support services. ServiceSource directly employs more than
1,500 individuals on government and commercial affirmative
employment contracts.

District of Columbia

5960 District of Columbia Department of Employment Services
4058 Minnesota Avenue NE
Washington, DC 20019   202-724-7000
                                  Fax: 202-673-6993
                                       does@dc.gov
                                       does.dc.gov

**5961 District of Columbia Dept. of Employment Services: Office
of Workforce Development**
4058 Minnesota Avenue, NE
Washington, DC 20019   202-671-1633
                                       877-319-7346
                                  Fax: 202-673-6993
                                  TTY: 202-673-6994
                                       does@dc.gov
                                       www.does.dc.gov

Diana C Johnson, Public Information Officer
Marianna Lourenco, Specialist/ADA Coordinator
To foster economic development and growth in the District of Columbia by providing workforce training, bringing together job
seekers and employers, compensating unemployed and injured
workers and promoting safe and healthy workplaces.

5962 District of Columbia Fair Employment Practice Agencies
D C Office of Human Rights
Ste 570n
441 4th Street NW
Washington, DC 20001-2714   202-727-3400
                                  Fax: 202-347-8922
                                  TTY: 202-727-3400
                                       oag@dc.gov
                                       http://oag.dc.gov

Elizabeth Noel, Executive Director
Irvin B. Nathan, Attorney General
Ariel B. Levinson-Waldman, Senior Counsel to the Attorney G
Victor Bonett, Legislative Director FOIA Office
Investigations and discrimination complaints.

5963 Goodwill of Greater Washington
2200 South Dakota Ave NE
Washington, DC 20018-1622   202-636-4225
                                       888-817-4323
                                  Fax: 202-526-3994
                                       info@dcgoodwill.org
                                       dcgoodwill.org

Catherine Meloy, CEO
Brendan Hurley, Vice President Marketing & Commu
Judy Sklar, Regional Director Retail Operati
Colleen Paletta, Vice President Workforce Develop
Offers vocational training, job training, sheltered employment
and work experience.

5964 Green Door
1221 Taylor Street, NW
Washington, DC 20011-3063 202-464-9200
Fax: 202-464-5730
info@greendoor.org
www.greendoor.org

Judith Johnson, Executive Director
Brenda Randall, Assistant Director
Richard R. Bebout, Ph.D., President and CEO
Linda Wheeler Banton, Chair
Green Door is a community program which prepares people with a severe and persistent mental illness to live and work independently. Since 1976, Green Door has provided comprehensive services to mentally ill people, including housing, job training, job placement, education, homeless outreach, case management, support for people with substance abuse problems, family support,and specialized help for people who have had repeated hospitalizations.

5965 Operation Job Match
National Multiple Sclerosis Society
Suite 750 South
1800 M St NW
Washington, DC 20036-5802 202-887-0136
Fax: 202-296-3425
OJM@nmss.org
operationjobmatch.org

Steven Nissen, Manager
Jeanne Angulo, Executive Director
Job readiness program for individuals with adult-onset physical disabilities.

5966 Rehabilitation Services Administration
10th Floor
810 First Street NE
Washington, DC 20002-4227 202-442-8663
Fax: 202-442-8742
dds@dc.gov

Elizabeth Parker, Administrator
Mark D. Back, FOIA Officer
Laura L. Nuss, Director, Department on Disabili
State Rehabilitation Agency providing services to eligible persons with disabilities.

5967 WAVE Work, Achievement, Value, & Education
Suite 500
525 School St SW
Washington, DC 20024-2762 202-484-0103
800-274-2005
Fax: 202-488-7595
wave4kids@aol.com
www.waveinc.org

Dr. Steven W Edwards, President & CEO
Arthur Griffin, Senior Vice President
Dr. Beth P. Reynolds, Executive Director
Dr. Sandy Addis, Associate Director
Job placement programs, remunerative work services and work adjustment training programs for 18 and 21 years of age in many cities across the country including Drop-Out Recovery Programs and Drop-Out Prevention Programs. Programs also available for youth ages 12-18. Youth Professionals Development and Training and key aspects of WAVE services, as well.

Florida

5968 Abilities of Florida: An Affiliate of Service Source
2735 Whitney Road
Clearwater, FL 33760-1610 727-538-7370
Fax: 727-538-7387
abilities@ourpeoplework.org
servicesource.org

Janet Samuelson, President & CEO
Mark Hall, Executive Vice President, Corpor
David Hodge, Executive Vice President & Chief
Bruce Patterson, Executive Vice President & Chief

Provides a full range of employment services including work evaulation, training, job coaching, job placement, advocacy and education. Also provides housing assistance and specialized to adults with cystic fibrosis.

5969 Able Trust, The
3320 Thomasville Road
Suite 200
Tallahassee, FL 32308 850-224-4493
888-838-2253
888-838-2253
Fax: 850-224-4496
TTY:850-224-4493
info@abletrust.org
www.abletrust.org

Susanne Homant, President & CEO
Guenevere Crum, Senior Vice President
Ray Ford, Assistant Director of Communicat
Jessica Taylor, Assistant to the President & CEO
Provides grant funds for employment-related programs for non-profit agencies in Florida. Assists families, individuals and agencies through educational conferences, and youth training programs. Provides businesses free resources for hiring people with disabilities.

5970 Career Assessment & Planning Services
Goodwill Industries - Suncoast Incorporated
10596 Gandy Blvd
St Petersburg, FL 33702-1422 727-523-1512
888-279-1988
Fax: 727-563-9300
TTY: 727-579-1068
www.goodwill-suncoast.org

Oscar J. Horton, Chair
Martin W. Gladysz, Sr. Vice Chair
Heather Ceresoli, Vice Chair
Deborah A. Passerini, President
Career assessment and planning services help determine how prepared an individual is for employment, training, or future education. It is a comprehensive assessment that can predict current and future employment and potential adjustment factors for physically, emotionally or developmentally disabled persons who may be unemployed or underemployed.

5971 Choices to Work Program
Goodwill Industries-Suncoast
10596 Gandy Blvd
St Petersburg, FL 33702-1422 727-523-1512
888-279-1988
Fax: 727-563-9300
TTY: 727-579-1068
gw.marketing@goodwill-suncoast.com
goodwill-suncoast.org

Oscar J. Horton, Chair
Martin W. Gladysz, Sr. Vice Chair
Heather Ceresoli, Vice Chair
Deborah A. Passerini, President
Assisting individuals currently eligible for Workman's Compensation, this program allows those recovering from injury on the job to prepare to return to independent employment, either through increasing ability and confidence in using adaptive behaviors and/or equipment to return to related employment, or adjusting to a more compatible employment environment.

5972 Florida Division of Vocational Rehabilitation
Bldg A
4070 Esplanade Way
Tallahassee, FL 32399-7016 800-451-4327
800-451-4327
Fax: 850-245-3316
TTY: 866-515-3692
ombudsman@vr.fldoe.org
rehabworks.org

Bill Palmer, Manager
Debra Thompson, Florida Rehabilitation Council C
Roy Cosgrove, Administrator
Andrea Schwendinger, Government Analyst

Rehabilitation services are important when a physical or mental handicap interferes with your ability to work. Our purpose is to help prepare for, and return to, gainful employment.

5973 Florida Fair Employment Practice Agency
Florida Commission on Human Relations
4075 Esplanade Way
Suite 110
Tallahassee, FL 32301-4830 850-488-7082
800-342-8170
Fax: 850-487-1007
fchrinfo@fchr.myflorida.com
fchr.state.fl.us

Michelle Wilson, Executive Director
Cheyanne Costilla, General Counsel
Francisco Penela III, Communications Director
The Commission is the state agency charged with enforcing the state's civil rights laws and serves as a resource on human relations for the people of Florida.

5974 Goodwill Industries-Suncoast Adult Day Training
10596 Gandy Blvd N
St Petersburg, FL 33702-1422 727-523-1512
888-279-1988
Fax: 727-563-9300
gw.marketing@goodwill-suncoast.com
goodwill-suncoast.org

Lee Waits, President
Goodwill's adult day training programs enable people with developmental disabilities to set and achieve personal goals within a work-like setting. Participants work at various jobs throughout Goodwill and engage in a variety of activities that will allow them to become more self-sufficients.

5975 Goodwill Industries-Suncoast Inc. Adult Day Training
10596 Gandy Blvd.
St. Petersburg, FL 33702-3305 727-523-1512
888-279-1988
Fax: 727-563-9300
TTY: 727-579-1068
gw.marketing@goodwill-suncoast.com
www.goodwill-suncoast.org

Oscar J. Horton, Chair
Martin W. Gladysz, Sr. Vice Chair
Heather Ceresoli, Vice Chair
Deborah A. Passerini, President
Goodwill's adult day training programs enable people with developmental disabilities to set and achieve personal goals within a work-like setting. Participants work at various jobs throughout Goodwill and engage in a variety of activities that will allow them to become more self-sufficients.

5976 Goodwill Industries-Suncoast Inc. Adult Day Training
10596 Gandy Blvd.
St. Petersburg, FL 33702-3704 727-523-1512
888-279-1988
Fax: 727-563-9300
TTY: 727-579-1068
gw.marketing@goodwill-suncoast.com
www.goodwill-suncoast.org

Oscar J. Horton, Chair
Martin W. Gladysz, Sr. Vice Chair
Heather Ceresoli, Vice Chair
Deborah A. Passerini, President
Goodwill's adult day training programs enable people with developmental disabilities to set and achieve personal goals within a work-like setting. Participants work at various jobs throughout Goodwill and engage in a variety of activities that will allow them to become more self-sufficients.

5977 Goodwill Industries-Suncoast Non-Residential Supports And Services Program
10596 Gandy Blvd N
St Petersburg, FL 33702-1422 727-523-1512
888-279-1988
Fax: 727-563-9300
TTY: 727-579-1068
gw.marketing@goodwill-suncoast.com
goodwill-suncoast.org

Lee Waits, President
Jean-Marie Moore, Director Of Operations
Goodwill's adult day training programs enable people with developmental disabilities to set and achieve personal goals within a work-like setting. Participants earn paychecks working at various jobs throughout Goodwill and engage in a variety of activities that will allow them to become more self-sufficients.

5978 Goodwill Industries-Suncoast Supported Living
10596 Gandy Blvd
St Petersburg, FL 33702-1422 727-523-1512
888-279-1988
Fax: 727-563-9300
TTY: 727-579-1068
gw.marketing@goodwill-suncoast.com
goodwill-suncoast.org

Oscar J. Horton, Chair
Martin W. Gladysz, Sr. Vice Chair
Heather Ceresoli, Vice Chair
Deborah A. Passerini, President
Goodwill's supported living program helps people with developmental disabilities expand their skills so they can lead increasingly independentlives. Individuals receive training and assistance with daily living activities while living in the community. Additional support includes assistance with legal issues, adocacy, community resources, banking, safety procedures, self-medication, household management, meal preparation, interpersonal relationships and parenting training.

5979 Goodwill Industries-Suncoast, Adult Day Training
10596 Gandy Blvd
St Petersburg, FL 33702-5654 727-523-1512
888-279-1988
Fax: 727-563-9300
TTY: 727-579-1068
gw.marketing@goodwill-suncoast.com
goodwill-suncoast.org

Oscar J. Horton, Chair
Martin W. Gladysz, Sr. Vice Chair
Heather Ceresoli, Vice Chair
Deborah A. Passerini, President
Goodwill's adult day training programs enable people with developmental disabilities to set and achieve personal goals within a work-like setting. Participants work at various jobs throughout Goodwill and engage in a variety of activities that will allow them to become more self-sufficients.

5980 Goodwill Temporary Staffing
Goodwill Industries- Suncoast
10596 Gandy Blvd
St Petersburg, FL 33702-1422 727-523-1512
888-279-1988
Fax: 727-576-1314
TTY: 727-579-1068
gw.marketing@goodwill-suncoast.com
goodwill-suncoast.org

Oscar J. Horton, Chair
Martin W. Gladysz, Sr. Vice Chair
Heather Ceresoli, Vice Chair
Deborah A. Passerini, President
Provides employment links from potential employees, both disabled and non-disabled alike to employers with immediate employment opportunities seeking qualified candidates. Pre-screening on all applicants include: Employment history, personal references, law enforcement background checks and substance screening.

5981 Impact: Ocala Vocational Services
Goodwill Industries- Suncoast
10596 Gandy Blvd
St Petersburg, FL 33702-1422
727-523-1512
888-279-1988
Fax: 727-563-9300
TTY: 727-579-1068
gw.marketing@goodwill-suncoast.com
goodwill-suncoast.org

Oscar J. Horton, Chair
Martin W. Gladysz, Sr. Vice Chair
Heather Ceresoli, Vice Chair
Deborah A. Passerini, President
Designed to enable individuals with disabilities to work in inte-
grated settings in the community, receiving wages and benefits
matching those of non-handicapped workers.

5982 JobWorks NISH Food Service
Goodwill Industries- Suncoast
10596 Gandy Blvd
St Petersburg, FL 33702-1422
727-523-1512
888-279-1988
Fax: 727-563-9300
TTY: 727-579-1068
gw.marketing@goodwill-suncoast.com
goodwill-suncoast.org

Oscar J. Horton, Chair
Martin W. Gladysz, Sr. Vice Chair
Heather Ceresoli, Vice Chair
Deborah A. Passerini, President
An enclave style (or group) supported employment program de-
signed to give consumers additional supports that allow and en-
courage increasingly independent employment opportunities
within a food services environment.

5983 JobWorks NISH Postal Service
Goodwill Industries - Suncoast
10596 Gandy Blvd
St Petersburg, FL 33702-1422
727-523-1512
888-279-1988
Fax: 727-563-9300
TTY: 727-579-1068
gw.marketing@goodwill-suncoast.com
goodwill-suncoast.org

Oscar J. Horton, Chair
Martin W. Gladysz, Sr. Vice Chair
Heather Ceresoli, Vice Chair
Deborah A. Passerini, President
An enclave style (or group) supported employment program de-
signed to give consumers additional supports that allow and en-
courage increasingly independent employment opportunities
within a mailroom environment.

5984 Lighthouse Central Florida
215 East New Hampshire Street
Orlando, FL 32804-6403
407-898-2483
888-898-2483
Fax: 407-898-0236
lvancepoel@lcf-fl.org
lighthousecentralflorida.com

Lee Nasehi, Executive Director
Lee Van Eepoel, Program Service Director
Donna Esbensen, Vice President, Chief Financial
Kimberly Pawling, Director of Education & Rehabili
Lighthouse Central Florida (LCF) is the only non-profit organi-
zation offering comprehensive, professional, vision rehabilita-
tion services to Central Floridians of all ages with low vision or
blindness.

5985 MAClown Vocational Rehabilitation Workshop
6390 NE 2nd Ave
Miami, FL 33138-6036
305-759-0212
Sabrina Shelton, Manager
Provides remunerative work.

5986 One-Stop Service
Goodwill Industries- Suncoast
10596 Gandy Blvd.
St Petersburg, FL 33702-1422
727-523-1512
888-279-1988
Fax: 727-563-9300
TTY: 727-579-1068
gw.marketing@goodwill-suncoast.com
goodwill-suncoast.org

R. Lee Waits, President and CEO
Deborah A. Passerini, Executive Vice President and Chi
Gary Hebert, Corporate Treasurer and Chief Fi
Lee C. Zeh, Corporate Secretary and Vice Pre
Provides universal job search and placement related services are
available to any person entering the service center. Each
One-Stop Services Center provides on-site representation from a
variety of employment-related service providers. All One-Stops
host and/or facilitate local employment fairs and provides access
to computerized job-postings.

5987 Palm Beach Habilation Center
4522 South Congress Avenue
Lake Worth, FL 33461-4797
561-965-8500
Fax: 561-433-8816
postman@pbhab.com
pbhab.com

Jeffrey Chapman, Chief Financial Officer
David Lin, Vice President of Programs & Services
Roxanne Jacobs, Director of Developmen
Tina Philips, President/CEO
Providing work evaluation, work adjustment, job placement, em-
ployment, residential and retirement services for mentally, emo-
tionally and physically disabled adults.

5988 Primrose Supported Employment Programs
2733 South Ferncreek Ave
Orlando, FL 32806-5538
407-898-7201
Fax: 407-898-2120
www.primrosecenter.org

Mary Vanburen, Executive Director
Leslie North, Chairman
Helen Galloway, Board Director
Faye Scott-Evans, Board Director
Mission is to transform the lives of people with developmental
disabilities by providing opportunities to achieve their fullest
potential.

5989 Quest
500 E. Colonial Drive
Orlando, FL 32803-4504
407-218-4300
888-807-8378
Fax: 407-218-4301
contact@questinc.org
questinc.org

John Gill, President / CEO
Todd Thrasher, Chief Financial Officer
Eb Blakely, Vice President, Behavioral Services
Karenne Levy, Chief Operating Officer
Quest has built communities where people with disabilities have
achieved their goals for nearly 50 years. Through a variety of resi-
dential and employment options, behavioral therapy, therapeutic
day programs, charter schools and even a recreational summer
camp, Quest serves more than 1000 individuals each day in the
Orlando and Tampa areas.

5990 Quest - Tampa Area
1404 Tech Blvd
Tampa, FL 33619
813-423-7700
888-807-8378
Fax: 813-423-7701
contact@questinc.org
www.questinc.org

John Gill, President / CEO
Todd Thrasher, Chief Financial Officer
Eb Blakely, Vice President, Behavioral Services
Karenne Levy, Chief Operating Officer
Quest has built communities where people with disabilities have
achieved their goals for nearly 50 years. Through a variety of resi-

dential and employment options, behavioral therapy, therapeutic day programs, charter schools and even a recreational summer camp, Quest serves more than 1000 individuals each day in the Orlando and Tampa areas.

5991   SCARC, Inc Evaluation, Training + Emploment Center
213 West McCollum Avenue
Bushnell, FL 33513-5916   352-793-5156
                                              Fax: 352-793-6545
                                              http://scarcinc.com

Marsha Perkins, Administrator
Training and employment program for adults with disabilities. SCARC offers vocational evaluation, training, work services, transportation, supported independent living and community based training.

5992   Seagull Industries for the Disabled
3879 Byron Drive
West Palm Beach, FL 33404-3311   561-842-5814
                                              Fax: 561-881-3554
                                              main@seagull.org
                                              www.seagull.org

Fred Eisinger, Executive Director
Linda Moore, Assistant Executive Director, Se
Joyce Hambrick, Director of Program Services
Ellen Hoffacker, Director of Finance
Dedicated to improving the quality of life of mentally, physically and emotionally challenged adults in Palm Beach County, Florida through advocacy and the provision of a variety of social service, vocational training and residential programs designed to encourage self reliance and independence.

5993   Supported Employment Program
Goodwill Industries - Suncoast
10596 Gandy Blvd.
St Petersburg, FL 33702-1422   727-523-1512
                                                    888-279-1988
                                              Fax: 727-563-9300
                                              TTY: 727-579-1068
                                              gw.marketing@goodwill-suncoast.com
                                              www.goodwill-suncoast.org

R. Lee Waits, President and CEO
Deborah A. Passerini, Executive Vice President and Chi
Gary Hebert, Corporate Treasurer and Chief Fi
Lee C. Zeh, Corporate Secretary and Vice Pre
Goodwill's supported employment program enables people with developmental disabilities to work in the community, earning wages and benefits marching those of non-disabled workers. Participants receive intensive on-the-job training at job sites that have been carefully chosen for their suitability. A support facilitator provides follow-up job coaching to ensure success. Serving people in Pinellas, Hillsborough and Pasco counties.

5994   Vocational and Rehabilitation Agency Department of Education
Bldg A
4070 Esplanade Way
Tallahassee, FL 32399-7016   850-245-3399
                                                    800-451-4327
                                              Fax: 850-245-3316
                                              TTY: 850-488-0867
                                              speaker@vr.fldoe.org
                                              rehabworks.org

Bill Palmer, Manager
Aleisa McKinlay, Director
Work adjustment and remunerative work programs.

5995   Vocational and Rehabilitation Agency: Division of Blind Services
401 Platt Street
Daytona Beach, FL 32114-2803   386-254-3856
                                                    800-522-5078
                                              Fax: 386-252-3800

Bill Palmer, Manager
Carl Augusto, President and CEO
Kelly Bleach, Chief Administrative Officer
Rick Bozeman, Chief Financial Officer

Mission is to ensure blind and visually impaired Floridians have the tools, support, and opportunity to achieve success.

5996   Work Exploration Center
3000 N West 83rd Street i 40
Gainesville, FL 32606   352-395-5265
                                              Fax: 352-395-5271

Karla Wooten, Coordinator
The Work Exploration Center embraces a holistic approach to Comprehensive Vocational Evaluation and Community Employment services, encouraging individual understanding, hope and growth for a productive and fulfilling future.

Georgia

5997   Employment and Training Division, Region B
Goodwill Industries of North Georgia
1123 Progress Rd
Ellijay, GA 30540-5504   706-276-4722
                                                    888-514-8112
                                              Fax: 706-276-4732

Linda Rau, Director Programs/Services
Employment training, assessment and job placement for people who have disabilities and/or are disadvantaged. Serving 15 counties in Northern Georgia.

5998   Fair Housing and Equal Employment
Georgia Commission on Equal Opportunity
7 Martin Luther King, Jr. Drive, S.
3rd Floor
Atlanta, GA 30334-9000   404-656-1736
                                                    800-473-6736
                                              Fax: 404-656-4399
                                              gceo@gceo.state.ga.us
                                              www.gceo.state.ga.us

Teresa Chappell, Fair Housing Division Director
Stephanie Randolph, Intake Coordinator/Housing
Abdul Wali Khadeem, Equal Employment Division Director
Melvin J. Everson, Executive Director/Administrator
To investigate housing and employment discrimination in the state of Georgia.

5999   Griffin Area Resource Center Griffin Community Workshop Division
931 Hamilton Boulevard
Post Office Box 83
Griffin, GA 30224   770-229-4212
                                              Fax: 770-229-4212
                                              united_way@bellsouth.net
                                              http://www.gscunitedway.org

Cary Grubbs, Executive Director
Charles Cary Grubbs, Garc Executive Director
Rodney Shurman, President
Dr. Curtis Jones, Vice-President
A CARF (The Rehabilitation Accreditation Commission) accredited Employment and Community Support organization providing daily services to participants with disabilities from 16 years of age and up in a 5 county area.

6000   IBM National Support Center
Special Needs Systems
P.O.Box 2150
Atlanta, GA 30301-2150   404-577-7995
                                                    800-426-2133
                                              Fax: 561-982-6059
                                              TTY: 800-284-9482
                                              www.skepticfiles.org/md001/mobility.htm

6001   Kelley Diversified
P.O.Box 967
Athens, GA 30603-967   706-549-4398
                                              Fax: 706-549-4479

Mary Patton, Executive Director
Sherry Burns, Rehabilitation Services Director
Jenny Taylor, Business Operations Manager
Patricia Horne, Bookkeeper

Work adjustment and remunerative work programs.

6002 **New Ventures**
306 Fort Dr
Lagrange, GA 30240-5900
706-882-7723
Fax: 706-882-5401
customersvc@newventures.org
newventures.org

Dave Miller, CEO
Kelly Anderson, Quality Director
Jeff Chamberlain, Director of Business Services
Mike Wilson, Director of Industrial Marketing
A rehabilitation and work training facility for individuals with barriers to employability. The program utilizes community based industrial work of varying levels of difficulty. A return to work conditioning program for the industrially injured is offered which features: first-day contact, workers compensation rehabilitation team management, and light-duty work conditioning. A training stipend is paid to defray costs associated with training.

Hawaii

6003 **Assets School**
One Ohana Nui Way
Honolulu, HI 96818-4497
808-423-1356
Fax: 808-422-1920
info@assets-school.net
assets-school.net

John F. Morton, Chairman
Kristi L. Maynard, Vice Chairman
Robert W. Wo, Secretary
Russell J. Lau, Treasurer
ASSETS is an independent school for gifted and or dyslexic children that provides an individualized, integrated learning enviroment. ASSETS' enviroment empowers these children to maximize their potential and to find their place as lifelong learners in school and society.

6004 **Hawaii Fair Employment Practice Agency**
Room 411
830 Punchbowl St
Honolulu, HI 96813-5080
808-586-8636
800-586-8800
Fax: 808-586-8655
TTY: 808-586-8692
DLIR.HCRC.INFOR@hawaii.gov
http://hawaii.gov/labor/hcrc

Michael O Yamamoto
William Hoshijo, Executive Director
HCRC enforces state laws prohibiting discrimination in employment.

6005 **Hawaii Vocational Rehabilitation Division**
1901 Bachelot St.
Honolulu, HI 96817
808-586-9744
Fax: 808-586-9755
TTY:808-586-9744
info@hawaiivr.org
hawaiivr.org

Jonathan Chun, Chair
Albert Perez, Administrator
Susan Foard, Assistant Administrator
Katie Keim, Staff Specialist
Mission is our committed staff strive, day-in day-out, to provide timely efficient and effective programs, services and benefits, for the purpose of achieving the outcome of empowering those who are the most vulnerable in our state to expand thier capacity for self sufficiency , self-determination, independence, healthy choices, quality of life and personal dignity.

6006 **Lanakila Rehabilitation Center**
1809 Bachelot St
Honolulu, HI 96817-2430
808-531-0555
Fax: 808-533-7264
TTY:808-531-0555
info@lanakilahawaii.org
www.lanakilahawaii.org

Marian Tsuji, President
Wayne Fujishige, Vice President
Dwayne MASUTANI, Director Budget & Finance
Rachael Young, Director Human Resources
Lanakila is a private nonprofit organization whose mission is to provide services and supports that assist individuals with physical, mental, or age-related challenges to live as independently as possible within our community. A broad range of services are offered which include meal/senior services, community based adult day programming for individuals with disabilities, work training opportunities, and extended/supported employment for individuals with special needs.

6007 **Vocational and Rehabilitation Agency**
P.O.Box 339
601 Kamokila Boulevard, Room 515
Kapolei, HI 96707-339
808-692-7719
Fax: 808-692-7727
TTY:808-692-7715
sfoard@dhs.hawaii.gov
http://www.hawaiivr.org/

Albert Perez, Manager
Work adjustment and remunerative work programs.

6008 **Wahiawa Family**
302 California Ave
#204
Wahiawa, HI 96786-1883
808-621-7407
wpf-dentalcare.com/

Leslie Chinna
Work adjustment and remunerative work programs.

Idaho

6009 **Idaho Employment Service and Job Training Program Liaison**
Idaho Department of Employment
317 W Main St
Boise, ID 83735-1
208-332-3578
Fax: 208-327-7470
idahocis@labor.idaho.gov
http://labor.idaho.gov

Roger Madsen, Manager
C.L Butch Otter, Governor
Roger B. Madson, Director
Renee Cox, Program Manager
Work adjustment and remunerative work programs.

6010 **Idaho Fair Employment Practice Agency**
Idaho Human Rights Commission
P.O.Box 83720
450 West State Street
Boise, ID 83720-3
208-334-2873
Fax: 208-334-2664

David Rogers, Administrator
Mission is to adminnister state and federal anti-discrimination laws in Idaho in a mannner that is fair, accurate, and timely; and to work towards ensuring that all people withink the state are treated with dignity and respect in their places of employment, housing, education, and public accomodations.

6011 **Idaho Governor's Committee on Employment of People with Disabilities**
317 W Main St
Boise, ID 83735-1
208-332-3750
Fax: 208-327-7331
www.dol.gov

6012 Idaho Vocational Rehabilitation Agency
Room 150
650 W. State St.
Boise, ID 83704-8780 208-334-3390
Fax: 208-327-7417
TTY:208-327-7040
department.info@vr.idaho.gov
vr.idaho.gov

Darrell Quist, Manager
Janet Thaldorf, Supervisor
Vocational Rehabilitation assists many individuals with disabilities to go to work. With VR assistance, these individuals have overcome numerous obstacles and disability related barriers to achieve employment.

6013 Vocational and Rehabilitation Agency
Idaho Commission for the Blind & Visually Impaired
341 W Washington St
PO Box 83720
Boise, ID 83720-0012 208-334-3220
800-542-8688
Fax: 208-334-2963

Angela Roan, Manager
Raelene Thomas, Management Assistant
Bruce Christopherson, Rehabilitation Services Chief
Dana Ard, Vocational Rehabilitation Counse
Vocational rehabilitation, independent living training, medical intervention, adaptive technology and devices and employer advocacy.

Illinois

6014 Ada S McKinley Vocational Services
1359 W Washington Blvd
Chicago, IL 60607-4577 312-554-0600
Fax: 312-554-0292
TTY:312-697-9794
info@adasmckinley.org
adasmckinley.org

George Jones, Jr., Executive Director
Marion G. Sleet, Chief Operating Officer
Hans J. Schuster, Chief Financial Officer
Kathleen D. Chappell, Chief Development Officer
Mission is to serve those who, because of disabilities or other limiting conditions, need help in finding and pursuing paths leading to healthy, productive, and fulfilling lives.

6015 Anixter Center
2001 N. Clybourn Ave.
3rd Floor
Chicago, IL 60614 773-973-7900
Fax: 773-973-5268
TTY:773-973-2180
AskAnixter@anixter.org
anixter.org

Kevin Limbeck, President and CEO
Stacy Brown, Executive Vice President
Lauren K. Hill, Managing Director
Dan Sabol, Vice President and Business Deve
A Chicago-based human services agency that assists people with disabilities to live and work successfully in the community. Anixter Center provides vocational training, employment services, residences, special education, prevention programs, community services and health care. In addition, Anixter Center offers Illinois' only substance abuse treatment programs specifically for people with disabilities including Addiction Recovery of the Deaf.

6016 C-4 Work Center
4740 North Clark St.
Chicago, IL 60640 773-769-0205
infoc4@c4chicago.org
www.c4chicago.org

Eileen Durkin, President and CEO
Bruce Seitzer, LCPC, Senior Vice President
John Troy, MBA, CPA, Vice President of Finance
Danielle Byron, MS, Vice President of Information Systems
Aftercare, case finding, information and referrals, vocational training and work activities offered to mentally ill persons.

6017 Clearbrook
1835 W Central Rd
Arlington Heights, IL 60005-2410 847-870-7711
Fax: 847-870-7741
TTY:847-870-2239
info@clearbrook.org
www.clearbrook.org

Carl M La Mell, President
Tracy Martin, Admissions Director
Bernie Andersen, Assistant to the President
Rosa Baez-Lopez, Vice President of Human Resource
Offers educational, employment and residential services to the developmentally disabled children and adults.

6018 Cornerstone Services
777 Joyce Rd
Joliet, IL 60436-1876 815-741-7600
Fax: 815-723-1177
jhogan@cornerstoneservices.org
cornerstoneservices.org

James A Hogan, CEO
Susan Murphy, Coordinator Public Relations
Ben Stortz, President/Chief Executive Officer
Don Hespell, Vice-President/Chief Operating Officer
Cornerstone Services provides progressive, comprehensive services for people with disabilities, promoting choice, dignity and the opportunity to live and work in the community. Established in 1969, the agency provides developmental, vocational, employment, residential and behavioral health services at various community-based locations. The nonprofit social service agency helps approximately 750 people each day.

6019 Fulton County Rehab Center
500 N Main St
Canton, IL 61520-1844 309-647-6510
Fax: 309-647-7965
www.fultoncountyrehabilitationcenter.com

Rex L. Lewis, Executive Director
John C. Harmon, Public Relations / Marketing
Rhonda S. Dawson, Production Director
Residential rehab center with health care incidental; manufactures wood pallets and skids; job training and vocational rehabilitation services.

6020 Glenkirk
3504 Commercial Ave
Northbrook, IL 60062-1863 847-272-5111
Fax: 847-272-7350
info@glenkirk.org
glenkirk.org

Allan G. Spector, CEO
Helps infants, children and adults with developmental disabilities reach higher levels of independence. A non-profit organization serving people in north and northwest Chicago suburbs. Glenkirk's residential, vocational, educational and support programs include services which provide individual evaluation, therapeutic treatment and training.

6021 Illinois Employment Service
Department of Employment Security
Fl 4
401 S State St
Chicago, IL 60605-1293 312-793-4880
800-247-4984
www2.illinois.gov

6022 Jewish Vocational Services
216 West Jackson Blvd.
Suite 700
Chicago, IL   60606-4602   312-673-3400
                                      Fax: 312-553-5544
                                jvschgo@jvschicago.org
                                http://jvschicago.org/

H. Debra Levin, President
Alan S. Crane, Vice President
Marc Jacobs, Vice President
Benn Feltheimer, Secretary
Occupational training and job placement for handicapped persons of all religions.

6023 JoDavies Workshop
P.O.Box 6087
706 West Street
Galena, IL   61036-6087   815-777-2211
                                      Fax: 815-777-3386
                          theworkshopgalena@theworkshopgalena.org
                                         www.jdwi.org

Jean Muchow, Treasurer
Peg Tonne, Chairperson
Dale Gereau, Plant Manager
Lynn Berning, Vice Chairperson
Intake and referral, early intervention for children only, vocational evaluation and work adjustment training services offered.

6024 Kennedy Job Training Center
18350 Crossing Drive
Tinley Park, IL   60487-6122   708-342-5246
                                      Fax: 708-594-7156
                               Information@stcolettail.org
                                http://www.stcolettail.org

Robin Mertes, Placement Manager
Kandy Stamer, QMRP/Intake Coordinator
Bob Loquercio, Board of Director
Wayne A. Kottmeyer, Executive Director
Offers vocational evaluation, vocational training work adjustment training, and job placement services for developmentally disabled and hearing impaired persons.

6025 Knox County Council for Developmental Disabilities
2015 Windish Dr
Galesburg, IL   61401-9774   309-344-2600
                                      Fax: 309-344-1754
                                 mcrittenden@kccdd.com
                                         kccdd.com

Mary Crittenden, Executive Director
Pam Green, Director of Operations
Jeff Gomer, Director of Finance
Lynndel Messmore, Director of Rehabilitation
Developmental training, vocational evaluation, work adjustment training, extended training, placement, supported employment.

6026 Kreider Services
500 Anchor Road
Dixon, IL   61021-366   815-288-6691
                                      Fax: 815-288-1636
                                   TTY:815-288-5931
                                info@kreiderservices.org
                                    kreiderservices.org

Dr. Richard Piller, President
Dr. Vernon Brickley, Vice President
Cheryl Ebens, Director
Mike Hickey, Director
Offers day service programs, vocational training programs, job placement, supported employment, respite care, residential and family support for ages birth to three years.

6027 Lambs Farm
14245 W Rockland Rd
Libertyville, IL   60048-9745   847-362-4636
                                      Fax: 847-362-9688
                                   info@lambsfarm.org
                                       lambsfarm.org

Dianne Yaconetti, President & CEO
Kathy Buresch, Director, Operations, Marketing
Nikki Bonamarte, Director, Development
Jose Martinez, Director, Quality Assurance
Person-centered, comprehensive program of residential, vocational and social support service for adults with developmental disabilities.

6028 Land of Lincoln Goodwill Industries
1220 Outer Park Drive
Springfield, IL   62704   217-789-0400
                                      Fax: 217-789-0540
                                      info@llgi.org
                                       www.llgi.org

Sharon Durbin, CEO and President
Valerie Ausmus, VP of Finance
Deborah Clark, VP of Retail Operations
Kim Wonnell, VP of Human Resources
Empowers people with special needs to become self-sufficient through the power od work.

6029 Orchard Village
7660 Gross Point Road
Skokie, IL   60077-2628   847-967-1800
                                      Fax: 847-967-9543
                                 info@orchardvillage.org
                                   www.orchardvillage.org

Joy Decker, President & CEO
Sally Ruecking, Vice President, Development
Allison Stark, Vice President, Programs
Jennifer Burgess, Director, Residential Services
Vocational program and counseling, respite services and community living group homes for the disabled and cognitively impaired. Orchard village also operates a private hope school especially devoted to teaching young adults independent living and skills necessary to flourish in the community.

6030 President's Committee on Employment of Employment of the Disabled
1331 F Street, NW,
Suite 300
Washington, DC   20004-1614   202-376-6200
                                       800-ASK-DORI
                                      Fax: 202-376-6219
                                    TTY: 202-376-6205
                       www.usccr.gov/pubs/crd/federal/pcepd.htm

Carol Adams, President
John Lancaster, Executive Director
Work adjustment and remunerative work programs.

6031 Sertoma Centre
4343 W 123rd St
Alsip, IL   60803-1807   708-371-9700
                                      Fax: 708-371-9747
                                 info@sertomacentre.org
                                    sertomacentre.org

Gus Vanden Brink, Executive Director
Paula Phillips, Assistant Director
A nationally accredited, not-for-profit agency that provides services to students and adults with developmental disabilities and mental illness. MIssion is to provide opportunities that empower individuals with disabilities to achieve success.

6032 Shore Training Center
Shore Community Services
8350 Laramie Ave.
Skokie, IL   60077   847-982-2030
                                      Fax: 847-982-2039
                                   TTY:847-581-0076
                                 info@shoreservices.org

India Alexia Ehioba, CEO

605

Mission is to improve the quality of life for citizens with developmental disabilities through community based services providing education/training.

6033 Skills Inc.
44 Morris Street
Webster, MA 01570-1233   508-943-0700
                                       Fax: 508-949-6129
                                  life-skills@life-skillsinc.org

Robert Miller, President
Pamela Guanci, Vice President
Raymond Bembenek, Treasurer
Janice Smith, Secretary
Accredited through the Commission on Accreditation of Rehabilitation Facilities; offers job training partnership act and vocational evaluation services offered.

6034 Thresholds AMISS
12145 Western Ave
Blue Island, IL 60406-1387   708-597-7997
                                       Fax: 708-597-8073

Julia Rupp, Executive Director
Camille Rucks, Team Leader
Services offered include psychosocial, vocational and residential programs for ages 18 or older with a primary diagnosis of mental illness. Facility is wheelchair accessible.

6035 Vocational and Rehabilitation Agency
207 Staehouse
Springfield, IL 62706-1   217-782-0244
                                            800-843-6154
                                       Fax: 217-524-6262
                                       TTY: 888-261-3336
                                  ITTF.Web@illinois.gov
                                       www2.illinois.gov

Pat Quinn, Governor
Provides work adjustment and remunerative skills.

6036 Washington County Vocational Workshop
781 E Holzhauer Dr
Nashville, IL 62263-2055   618-327-4461
                                       Fax: 618-327-4477
                                       www.mapquest.com

Keith Curran, Executive Director
Provides job training and related services and vocational rehabilitation services.

6037 Westside Parents Work Activity Center
3395 Mottman Road SW
Olympia, WA 98512   360-339-7297
                         blackhillsgym.com/family-activity-center
Theresa McKenzieSullivan, General Manager
Offers developmental training programs providing basic skills in self care for multiply and physically handicapped persons.

Indiana

6038 ADEC Resources for Independence
19670 State Road 120
Bristol, IN 46507-9162   574-848-7451
                                            877-342-8954
                                       Fax: 574-848-5917
                                  shivelyp@adecinc.com
                                            adecinc.com

Donna Belusar, President & CEO
Mitch Walorski, CFO
Sally Russell, Vice President
Joe Blocher, Vice President of Human Relation
Serves Elkhart County and surrounding area.

6039 Arc Bridges
2650 W 35th Ave
Gary, IN 46408-1416   219-985-6562
                                       Fax: 219-980-7315
                                  mailbox@thearcnwindiana.com
                                  www.thearcnwindiana.com

Brian Davis, Contact
Kris Prohl, Executive Director
Mission is to improve the welfare of people with intellectual and development disabilities and their families.

6040 BI-County Services
425 East Harrison Rd
Bluffton, IN 46714-9013   260-824-1253
                                       Fax: 260-824-1892
                                  info@adifferentlight.com
                                  bi-countyservices.com

John Whicker, President
Serves Wells and Adam Counties. Infant services, Medicaid waivers, music therapy, ICF, MR, group homes, sheltered employment, pay program and supported employment services available.

6041 Balance Centers of America
3831 Hughes Ave.
Ste 504B
Culver, CA 90232-2630   310-625-5657
                                  americanbalancecenters.com/

Jane Labar, Contact
Offers developmental training programs providing basic skills in self care for physically handicapped persons.

6042 Bridge Pointe Services & Goodwill of Southern Indiana, Inc
Goodwill International
1329 Applegate Lane
P.O. Box 2488
Clarksville, IN 47131-2488   812-283-7908
                                            800-660-3355
                                       Fax: 812-283-6248
                                  http://www.goodwillsi.org/

Candice C. Barksdale, Chief Executive Director
Joel Henderson, PHR, Vice President of Human Resource
Bonnie Davis, Vice President of Donated Goods
Michelle Dayvault, Vice President of Development an
Career assesment, job readiness and placement, office skills training. Pediatric family support services. Childrens Academy, a developmental preschool.

6043 Carey Services
2724 S Carey St
Marion, IN 46953-3515   765-668-8961
                                       Fax: 765-664-6747
                                       www.careyservices.com

Bonnie Smith, Human Resources Manager
James Allbaugh, Chief Executive Officer
Gary Hendricks, Corporate Compliance
David Sprowl, Intake Coordinator
The mission of Carey Services is to create pathways towards self-sufficiency with personal satisfaction.

6044 Evansville Association for the Blind
500 North 2nd Avenue
Evansville, IN 47710-2355   812-422-1181
                                       Fax: 812-424-3154
                                  http://www.evansvilleblind.org/

Karla Horrell, Executive Director
Daniel Dana, President
Larry Arp, Vice President
Pam Doerter, Vice President
An community rehabilitation facility untilizing individual goals to assist persons with disabilities achieve or maintain potenial

6045   **Four Rivers Resource Services**
P.O.Box 249
Hwy. 59 South
Linton, IN 47441-249

812-847-2231
Fax: 812-847-8836
fourrivers@frrs.org
frrs.org

Kenton Barnes, President
Mary Lou Chapman, Vice-President
Ray Hart, Treasurer
Kathy Pennington, Secretary
Employment, community living, connections, follow-along, early intervention, preschool, healthy families, child care resource and referral and child care voucher program, impact, and transpotation services.

6046   **Gateway Services/JCARC**
P.O.Box 216
3500 North Morton Street
Franklin, IN 46131-216

317-738-5500
888-494-8069
Fax: 317-738-5522
www.gatewayarc.com

Karen Luehmann, Executive Director
Utilizes individual goals to assist persons with disabilities achieve or maintain potential.

6047   **Goodwill Industries of Central Indiana**
1635 West Michigan St
Indianapolis, IN 46222-3852

317-524-4313
Fax: 317-524-4336
TTY:317-524-4309
goodwill@goodwillindy.org
goodwillindy.org

James M. Mc Clelland, President & CEO
Nicki Washburn, Disability Services Coordinator
Kent A. Kramer, Senior Vice President and Chief Operating Officer
Daniel J. Riley, Senior Vice President, Administration and Chief Financial Of
Goodwill is in the business of helping people find jobs and provides programs and services for people who want to work. Goodwill is a community resource committed to deploying our assets and leveraging our resources with those of others in the community to create more opportunities for people who need assistance to improve their ability to earn a living.

6048   **Indiana Civil Rights Commission**
100 North Senate Avenue
Suite N103
Indianapolis, IN 46204-2208

317-232-2600
800-628-2909
Fax: 317-232-6580
TTY: 800-743-3333
info@icrc.in.gov
www.in.gov/icrc

Jamal Smith, Executive Director
Works to develop public policies that ensure equal opportunity in education to all.

6049   **Indiana Employment Services and Job Training Program Liaison**
10 North Senate Avenue
Indianapolis, IN 46204-2201

317-232-6702
Fax: 317-233-5499
www.in.gov/dwd/

6050   **Michigan Resources**
4315 East Michigan Blvd
Michigan City, IN 46360-3151

219-874-4288
Fax: 219-874-2689
TTY:219-873-2245
michiana@michianaresources.org
michianaresources.org

Nancy J Matela, Board Member
Matt Hollander, Chair
Gretchen Kalk, Treasurer
Andie Wolfinsohn, Secretary

Vocational training center for persons 16 and older with disabilities.

6051   **New Hope Services**
725 Wall Street
Jeffersonville, IN 47130-3616

812-288-8248
800-237-6604
Fax: 812-288-1206
info@newhopeservices.org
newhopeservices.org

James A. Bosley, President and CEO
John Broady, Senior Vice President and CFO
Bonnie Long, Senior Vice President, CAO
Jody Kitch, Chief Operating Officer
Mission is to provide hope through services which are responsive to individual needs.

6052   **New Horizons Rehabilitation**
P.O.Box 98
237 Six Pine Ranch Road
Batesville, IN 47006-98

812-934-4528
Fax: 812-934-2522
mdausch@nhrinc.org
www.nhrehab.org

Marie Dausch, Executive Director
Serves Ripley, Franklin, Ohio, Switzerland Dearborn, and Decatur. Provides training and services to adults with mental/physical disabilities and infants birth to age 3 with developmental delays or conditions of risk which could result in a developmental delay.

6053   **Noble Of Indiana**
Noble, Inc.
7701 East 21st Street
Indianapolis, IN 46219-2406

317-375-2700
Fax: 317-375-2719
rita.davis@nobleofindiana.org
www.nobleofindiana.org

Julia Huffman, President & CEO
Rita Davis, Director, Community Relations
Julie Brown, Director of Human Resources
Jeanine Coleman, Director of Community Living
Since 1953, Noble of Indiana has been dedicated to its mission: to create opportunities for people with developmental disabilities to live meaningful lives.

6054   **Office of State Coordinator of Vocational Education for Students with Disability**
Rm 212
10 N Senate Ave
Indianapolis, IN 46204-2201

317-232-1829
800-891-6499
www.state.in.us/dwd/techd

Scott B. Sanders, Commissioner
Randy Gillespie, Chief Financial Officer
Jeff Gill, General Counsel
Michelle Marshel, Deputy Commissioner of Communica
Manages and impliments innovative employment programs, unemployment insurance systems, and facilitates regional economic growth initiatives for Indiana.

6055   **Putnam County Comprehensive Services**
630 Tennessee St
Greencastle, IN 46135-2102

765-653-9763
877-653-9763
Fax: 765-653-3646
cns_pccs@yahoo.com
www.pccsinc.org

Chuck Schroeder, CEO
Charles Schroeder, Executive Director
Teresa Human, Community Living Services Director
Josi Blunton, Residential Director
A not-for-profit organization serving individuals with disabilities and similar characteristics in Indiana. Their mission is to provide services to individuals with disabilities in order for them to reach their optimum potential in attitudes, habits, and skills through training and integration, making them contributing mem-

bers of their community, and to promote community awareness and acceptance of people with different abilities.

6056 Southern Indiana Resource Solutions
1579 S Folsomville Rd
Boonville, IN 47601-9465   812-897-4840
                                         Fax: 812-897-0123
                                         kelly@sirs.org
                                         www.sirs.org

Kelly Mitchell, CEO/President
Don Critchlow, Chairperson
Larry Oathout, Vice-Chairperson
Jeff Hagedorn, Board Member
Adult services including jobs, community connections, and residential, childrens services, including service coordination and all therapies.

6057 Sycamore Rehabilitation Services
1001 Sycamore Lane
Danville, IN 46122-1474   317-745-4715
                                         888-573-0817
                                         Fax: 317-745-8271
                                         info@sycamoreservices.com
                                         sycamoreservices.com

Ralph Dunkin, President
Terry Kessinger, Vice President
Steve Patterson, Treasurer
Peg Murphy, Secretary
Provides individuals training and services for persons with disabilities that enhance independence in all areas of life.

6058 Vocational and Rehabilitation Agency
P.O.Box 7083
2 Peachtree Street, NW
Atlanta, GA 30303- 7083   404-232-1998
                                         800-545-7763
                                         Fax: 404-232-1800
                                         GVRAcustomer-service@gvra.ga.gov
                                         gvra.georgia.gov

Mike Hedden, Executive Director
James N. Defoor, Chair
Louise Hill, Vice Chair
Vocational training center for persons with disabilities.

6059 Wabash/Employability Center
201 I.U. Willets Road
S C6395 Earl Ave
Albertson, NY 11507   516-465-1400
                                         Fax: 765-447-6456
                                         info@viscardicenter.org
                                         http://www.nbdc.com

Bill Carmichael, Contact
John D. Kemp, Esq., President & CEO
Kenneth J. Kunken, Esq., County Court Deputy Bureau Chief
Constantina Petallides-Markou, Human Resources Manager
Serves Tippecanoe County.

Iowa

6060 ACT Assessment Test Preparation Reference Manual
American College Testing Program
P.O.Box 168
500 ACT Drive
Iowa City, IA 52243-168   319-337-1000
                                         Fax: 319-339-3021
                                         act.org

Jon Whitmore, Chief Executive Officer
Janet E. Godwin, Chief of Staff and Accountability Officer
Jon L. Erickson, President, Education and Career Solutions
Martin L. Scaglione, President, Workforce Development
This reference manual was developed as a resource for high school teachers and counselors in assisting students with test preparation.

6061 Franklin County Work Activity Center
20 5th St NW
Hampton, IA 50441-1908   641-456-2532
                                         Fax: 641-456-4682

Harry Jacoby, Executive Director
Jim Koenen, Owner
Nonprofit organization providing residential and vocational services in Franklin and Hardin counties in the state of Iowa. Residential Services include RCF/MR services, Supported Community Living Services and Community Supervised Apartment Living Arrangement Services. Vocational Services include Work Services and Supported Employment Services. Accredited by the Commission on Accreditation of rehabilitation Facilities since 1984, and serves individuals with a wide range of needs.

6062 Innovative Industries
405 E Madison St
Box 41205
Cleveland, OH 44141-2402   330- 46- 260
                                         800-THE-M IR
                                         Fax: 330- 46- 260
                                         info@innovativeindustries.com
                                         www.innovativeindustries.com

Duane Nelson, Program Manager

6063 Iowa Civil Rights Commission
400 E 14th Street
Des Moines, IA 50319-201   515-281-4121
                                         800-457-4416
                                         Fax: 515-242-5840
                                         don.grove@iowa.gov
                                         www.state.ia.us/government/crc

Ralph Rosenberg, Executive Director
Ron Pothast, Acting Executive Director
Corlis Moody, Executive Director
Beth Townsend, Executive Director
A neutral, fact-finding administrative agency that enforces the 'Iowa Civi Rights Act of 1965,' Iowa's anti-discrimination law. The commission doesn not provide legal representation. The commission's vision is a state free of discrimination.

6064 Iowa Employment Service
1000 East Grand Ave
Suite 140
Des Moines, IA 50309   515-282-5823
                                         Fax: 515-288-2184
                                         fering@iowacareerconnection.com
                                         www.iowacareerconnection.com

L.M. (Al) Fering, SPHR, FLMI, President
Miles Morrow, CPC
Specializes in accounting and human resources talent aquisition in the Upper-Midwest.

6065 Iowa Job Training Program Liaison
Iowa Department of Economic Development
200 East Grand Ave
Des Moines, IA 50309-1856   515-725-3000
                                         Fax: 515-725-3010
                                         info@iowa.gov
                                         iowalifechanging.com

David Lyons, President
Debi Durham, Director
Kathy Anderson, Director, Communications Team
Jody Benz, Director, Iowa Commission on Vol
To engender and promote economic development policies and practices which stimulate and sustain Iowa's economic growth and climate and that integrate efforts across public and private sectors.

6066   Iowa Valley Community College
3700 S. Center St.
Marshalltown, IA   50158-4783   641-752-7106
                                             866-622-4748
                                        Fax: 641-752-5909
                                        http://www.iavalley.edu/

Dr. Chris Wynes, Chancellor
Robin Anctil, Director of Marketing
Dr. Lisa Breja, Institutional Researcher/AQIP Li
Nate Chua, MCC Director of Retention & Lear
Offers two levels of specialized vocational preparatory programming for adults with disabilities. The Career Development Center serves dependent adults. The goal of the program is to maintain or improve skills to enable persons served to enter sheltered or supported employment. The IRP/CBVT programs are non-credit specialized vocational programs for independent adults served by Vocational Rehabilitation and our programs. The goals are for competitive placements in jobs. CARF accredited.

6067   Iowa Vocational Rehabilitation Services
510 East 12th Street
Jessie Parker Building
Des Moines, IA   50319-0240   515-281-4211
                                        Fax: 515-281-7645
                                        TTY:515-281-4211
                                        Victoria.Carrington@iowa.gov
                                        www.ivrs.iowa.gov

David Mitchell, Administrator
Matthew Coulter, Chief Financial Officer
Kenda Jochimsen, Bureau Chief
Charlie Levine, Assistant Bureau Chief
The mission is to work for and with individuals who have disabilities to achieve their employment, independence and economic goals.

6068   New Focus
102 W Washington St
Centerville, IA   52544-1550   641-437-1722
                                        Fax: 641-437-1028

Peggy Oden, Executive Director
Provides vocational services for adults with disabilities. Includes work activity, supported employment and supported community living.

6069   Second Time Around
560 Harrison Ave
Suite 501
Boston, MA   02118-1709   641-437-7355
                                        www.secondtimearound.net/

Monica Blizeck, Manager
Debbie Steen, Store Supervisor
Deana Edwards, Manager
Work training site for adults with disabilities.

Kansas

6070   Clay Center Adult Training Center
40 Beech Street
Port Chester, NY   10573-2903   914-937-2047
                                        Fax: 914-935-1205
                                        mail@clayartcenter.org
                                        www.clayartcenter.org

Michael Spielman, Manager
Robert Rattet, President
Bruce Fern, Vice President
Reena Kashyap, Treasurer
Work training site for adults with disabilities.

6071   Kansas Fair Employment Practice Agency
Suite 568-South
900 SW Jackson St
Topeka, KS   66612-2818   785-296-3206
                                        Fax: 785-296-0589

Mostafa Kamal, Manager
William V. Minner, Executive Director
Melvin Neufeld, Chair
Terry Crowder, Vice Chair

6072   Kansas Vocational Rehabilitation Agency
915 SW Harrison
8th Floor West
Topeka, KS   66612-1995   785-368-7471
                                             866-213-9079
                                        Fax: 785-368-7467
                                        TTY: 785-368-7478

Michael Donnelly, Director
Helps people with disabilities achieve employment and self-sufficiency. Also links employers with qualified and productive individuals to meet thier work force needs.

Kentucky

6073   Kentucky Committee on Employment of Peoplewith Disabilities
2nd Floor
275 East Main St
Frankfort, KY   40601-2321   502-564-7456
                                             800-648-6057
                                        Fax: 502-564-7459
                                        VivianL.Bettis@ky.gov
                                        www.oet.ky.gov

Greg Higgins, Manager
Tom Bowell, Manager
Shane Smith, Manager
Terri Bradshaw, Communications Director
Provides qualified people for jobs, quality jobs for people, temporary financial support for the unemployed, comprehensive labor market information, and preserve the integrity and viability of the Unemployment Insurance Trust Fund.

6074   Kentucky Department for Employment Serviceand Job Training Program Liaison
275 E Main Street 2-W
Frankfort, KY   40621-1   502-564-5331
                                        Fax: 502-564-7452
                                        http://www.oet.ky.gov

Gina Oney, Assistant Director
Linda Prewitt, Acting Division Director/ Assist
Linda Pierce, Compliance Support Branch Manage
Gregory Higgins, Acting Unemployment Insurance Di
Provides qualified people for jobs, quality jobs for people, temporary financial support for the unemployed.

6075   Kentucky Office for the Blind
275 East Main Street
Frankfort, KY   40621   502-564-7456
                                             800-321-6668
                                        Fax: 502-564-2951
                                        TTY: 502-564-2929
                                        JenniferN.Wright@ky.gov
                                        blind.ky.gov

Christopher Smith, Executive Director
Michelle McElmurray, Executive Assistant
Allison Jessee, Director of Consumer Services
Cora McNabb, VR Administrator, Training and H
Our mission is to provide opportunities for employment and independence to individuals with visual impairments.

6076 **Kentucky Vocational Rehabilitation Agency**
275 East Main Street
Frankfort, KY 40621
502-564-4440
800-372-7172
Fax: 502-564-6745
WFD.VOCREHAB@ky.gov
http://ovr.ky.gov

Dr. David Beach, Executive Director
Holly Hendricks, Assistant Director of Program Se
Jason Jones, Director of Community Relations
Mindy Yates, Administrative Services Branch M
Assists eligible individuals with disabilities achieve their employment goals.

6077 **Office for the Blind**
275 E Main St
Frankfort, KY 40621
502-564-4754
800-321-6668
Fax: 502-564-2951
TTY: 502-564-2929
amy.mefford@ky.gov
blind.ky.gov

Cora McNabb, Executive Director
Deanna Doll, Vocational Rehabilitation Counselor
Tonisha Everhart, Vocational Rehabilitation Counselor
Provides career services and assistance to adults with severe visual handicaps who want to become productive in the home or work force. The office also runs a Client Assistance Program established to provide advice, assistance and information available from rehabilitation programs to persons with handicaps.

6078 **Pioneer Vocational/Industrial Services**
150 Corporate Drive
P.O Box 1396
Danville, KY 40422-1396
859-236-8413
800-527-4198
Fax: 859-238-7115
TTY: 859-236-1251
pioneer@pioneerservices.org

Mike Pittman, Chief Executive Officer / Executive Director
Danny Rigney, Director of Marketing and Operations
Dot Carman, Office Administration Director / Safety / Compliance Officer
Mike Fayne, Director of Services Assistant
Mission is to provide vocational development and extended employment programs to people who are disabled and or disadvantaged to assist them in obtaining employment and maximizing independent living skills.

6079 **Work Enhancement Center of Western Kentucky**
1906 College Heights Blvd.
Bowling Green, KY 42101-3576
270-745-0111
Fax: 502-767-3600
wku@wku.edu
www.wku.edu

Steve Passmore, Director
John O'Shaughnessy, Chief Executive Officer
J. David Porter, Chair
Frederick A. Higdon, Vice Chair
The center has been established in order to service industry in the three state area surrounding Kentucky. This service includes job/skill evaluation, job design consultation, pre-employment employee evaluations and economic evaluation.

Louisiana

6080 **Community Opportunities of East Ascension**
1121 E Ascension Complex Blvd
Gonzales, LA 70737
225-621-2000
Fax: 225-621-2022
http://coea.homestead.com

Mark Thomas, Director
Committed to affording individuals the opportunities that reflect and support choices, dignity, individuality, self-determination, community, coherency and commen sense. Programs incloude Respite, Personal Care Attendant, Support Living, Support Environment, Adult Day Training, and Elderly/Adult Waiver Services.

6081 **Louisiana Employment Service and Job Training Program Liaison**
1001 North 23rd Street
Post Office Box 94094
Baton Rouge, LA 70804-9094
225-342-3111
800-259-5154
Fax: 225-342-7960
owd@lwc.la.gov
http://www.laworks.net

Curt Eysink, Executive Directo
Carey Foy, Deputy Executive Director
Jay Augustine, Executive Counsel
Renee Ellender Roberie, Chief Financial Officer
Provides services for job seekers and job training programs.

6082 **Louisiana Vocational Rehabilitation Agency**
950 N 22nd St
Baton Rouge, LA 70802-6109
225-219-2225
800-737-2958
Fax: 225-219-4993
www.dss.state.la.us/departments/lrs

James Gaston, Manager
Ed Barras, Manager
Mark Martin, Director
Offers individuals with disabilities a wide range of services designed to provide them with skills, resources, attitudes, and expectations needed to compete in the interview process, get the job, keep the job, and develop a lifetime career.

6083 **St. James Association for Retarded Citizens**
29150 Health Unit St
Vacherie, LA 70090-4221
225-265-2181
Fax: 225-265-7427
info@brightscope.com
www.brightscope.com

Judy Bastian, Manager
Bruce Hansen, Chairman
John Sarkisian, Board of Directors
A private sheltered work program for mentally retarded and developmentally disabled adults.

6084 **Westbank Sheltered Workshop**
606 OPELOUSAS AVE
New Orleans, LA 70114-4344
504-362-1311
www.taxexemptworld.com

Maine

6085 **Addison Point Specialized Services**
P.O.Box 207
Addison, ME 04606-207
207-483-6500
Fax: 207-483-2817
www.faqs.org

Paula Chartrand, Owner
Provides services to individuals who are deaf/blind, mentally retarded, autistic, behaviorally challenged and/or dual diagnosed. Training services to place these individuals in community employment.

6086 **Bangor Veteran Center: Veterans Outreach Center**
Veteran's Administration
368 Harlow St
Bangor, ME 04491
207-947-3391
Fax: 207-941-8195
Patricia.Albert-Dehetre@va.gov
http://www.maine.va.gov

Joseph A Degrasse, Team Leader
Robert L Daisey LCSW, Clinical Coordinator
Eric K. Shinseki, Secretary
W. Scott Gould, Deputy Secretary
Readjustment counseling services for veterans of Vietnam, Vietnam Era, Persian Gulf, Panama, Grenada, Lebanon, Somalia,

WWII and Korean conflicts, as well as Iraq, Afganistan, and military sexual trauma.

6087   Creative Work Systems
619 Brighton Ave
Portland, ME   04102
207-879-1140
Fax: 207-879-1146
kraye@creativeworks.com
creativeworksystems.com

Susan Percy, Executive Director
Edward McGeachey, President
Jim Houle, Vice President
Provides residential, day habilitation and supported emploment in Central and Southern Maine.

6088   Maine Department Of Labor
45 Commerce Drive
Augusta, ME   04330
207-623-7900
Fax: 207-287-3042
mdol@maine.gov
www.state.me.us/labor

Patrick Fleming, Executive
Jeanne Shorey Paquette, Commissioner
Provides a wide range of services such as employment, labor market information, rehabilitation/disability and others.

6089   Maine Governor's Committee on Employment of the Disabled
45 Commerce Drive
Augusta, ME   04330-7880
207-621-5087
800-794-1110
Fax: 207-624-5302
www.maine.gov

6090   Maine Human Rights Commission
Maine Human Rights Commission
51 State House Station
Augusta, ME   04333-51
207-624-6290
Fax: 207-624-8729
Amy.Sneirson@maine.gov
www.maine.gov/mhrc

Amy Sneirson, Executive Director
Barbara Archer Hirsch, Commission Counsel
Victoria Ternig, Chief Investigator
Jill Duson, Compliance Manager
State agency with the responsibility of enforcing Maine's anti-discrimination laws. The commission investigates complaints of unlawful discrimination in employment, housing, education, access to public accommodations, extension of credit and offensive names.

6091   Northeast Occupational Exchange
29 Franklin Street
Bangor, ME   04401-3857
207-942-3685
800-857-0500
Fax: 207-561-4725
TTY: 207-992-2298
www.noemaine.org

Charles O Tingley, Executive Director
A fully licensed, comprehensive mental health and substance abuse treatment and rehabilitation facility.

6092   Vocational and Rehabilitation Agency
Division for the Blind and Visually Impaired
55 State House Station
Augusta, ME   04333-55
207-623-7981
888-457-8883
Fax: 207-624-5980
TTY: 800-794-1110
jobbank.careercenter@maine.gov
www.mainecareercenter.com

Jill Busond, Bureau Director
The Maine CareerCenter provides a variety of employment and training services at no charge for Maine workers and businesses. Whether you are looking to improve your job qualifications, explore a different profession, find a new career or hire an employee, the CareerCenter can help.

Maryland

6093   Ardmore Developmental Center
3000 Lottsford Vista Road
Bowie, MD   20721-4001
301-577-2575
Fax: 301-306-9799
grow@ArdmoreEnterprises.org
www.ardmoreenterprises.org

Patrick L. Carter, President
Eileen Baker, Vice-President
Marilynn W. Riley, Secretary
Daphne Pallozzi, Chief Executive Officer
Offers supported employment programs and vocational education for persons who are mentally retarded as well as residential services and Emergency Respite Care.

6094   Job Opportunities for the Blind
National Federation of the Blind
200 East Wells Street at Jernigan P
Baltimore, MD   21230- 4914
410-659-9315
Fax: 410-685-5653
nfb@nfb.org
www.nfb.org

Marc Mauer, President
John Berggren, Executive Director for Operation
John G. Paré Jr., Executive Director for Strategic
Mark Riccobono, Executive Director, NFB Jernigan
This free service allows individuals touch-tone telephone access to the thousands of jobs listed in America's Job Bank, and internet service run by the Department of Labor. Any person registered with either a state rehabilitation agency or a state employment service can search across the country for jobs by either type of work or location.

6095   Mainstream
9800 Mt. Pyramid Ct.
Suite 360
Englewood, CO   80112-6301
303-268-1920
Fax: 303-268-1926
investigativerisk.com

Patricia M Jackson, Executive Director
Charles Moster
Nonprofit organization dedicated to improving competitive employment opportunities for persons with disabilities. Provides specialized services and acts as a bridge that links service providers, employers and persons with disabilties. Provides training, educational publications, and videos on disablityemployment issues. Educationa materials include a magazine, brochures, and audio-visual aids.

6096   Maryland Employment Services and Job Training Program Liaison
500 North Calvert Street
#401
Baltimore, MD   21202-2201
410-230-6001
det@dllr.state.md.us
http://www.dllr.state.md.us

Maria Simms
Maureen O'Connor, Communications and Media Relatio
Jill Porter, Director of Legislative Services
Kathleen Spencer, Human Resources
Provides job development and placement and services

6097   Maryland Fair Employment Practice Agency
9th Fl
6 Saint Paul St
Baltimore, MD   21202-6806
410-767-8600
800-637-6247
Fax: 410-333-1841
TTY: 410-333-1737

Adrienne Jones, Executive Director
James Neil Bell, Deputy Director
Glendora Hughes, General Counsel
Benny F. Short, Assistant Director
Mission is to ensure equal opportunity to all through the enforcement of Maryland's laws against discrimination in employment, housing, and public accomodations; to provide educational and

outreach services related to the provisions of this law: and to promote and improve human relations in Maryland.

6098 Maryland State Department of Education
Division of Rehabilitation Services (DI RS)
200 West Baltimore Street
Baltimore, MD 21218-1628
            410-767-0100
            888-246-0016
            Fax: 410-554-9412
            TTY: 410-333-6442
            http://www.marylandpublicschools.org
Robert Burns, Manager
The Vocational Rehabilitation Program delivers to eligible individuals with physical and/or mental disabilities to enable them to become employed. The Independent Living Program's goal is to assist people in remaining in their homes and communities. The Division operates the Maryland Rehabilitation Center, a comprehensive evaluation and training center that has dormitory space. There are field offices located statewide with counselors to advise and manage the provision of services offered.

6099 Melwood
5606 Dower House Road
Upper Marlboro, MD 20772-3432
            301-599-8000
            Fax: 301-599-0180
            services@melwood.org
            www.melwood.org
Donald A. Donahue, DHEd, MBA, FA, Chair
Richard Mahan, CPA, Vice Chair
George Watkins, CPA, Treasurer
Shelly Gardeniers, Secretary
Melwood is a dynamic nonprofit that creates jobs and opportunities to improve the lives of people with disabilities. Melwood serves more than 1900 people with disabilities in the greater Washington DC area.

6100 PWI Profile
Projects W Industry Goodwill Industries of America
16120 W Bernardo Dr
San Diego, CA 92127
            858-673-6050
            Fax: 858-673-0085

6101 Project LINK
Mainstream
Suite 700
3 Bethesda Metro Ctr
Bethesda, MD 20814-6301
            301-215-9100
            800-247-1380
            Fax: 301-891-8778
            cosmoscorp.com
Charles Moster
Provides job development and placement in services to dislocated workers with disabilities in the Washington, DC and Dallas, TX areas.

6102 Treatment and Learning Centers (TLC)
14901 Dufief Mill Road
Suite 100
North Potomac, MD 20878
            301-738-6424
            Fax: 301-340-6082
            TTY:301-424-5203
            www.ttlc.org
Dr Patricia Ritter, Executive Director
Suellyn Sherwood, Operations Director
Rhona Schwartz, High School Program Director
Janet Graves-Wright, Outpatient Services Director
A non-profit organization that specializes in educational, therapeutic and vocational services for invididuals with special needs. Programs include speech-language and occupational therapy, psycho-educational testing, tutoring, audiology, employment opportunities and the Katherine Thomas School for students with moderate to severe language and learning disabilities and/or high-functioning autism.
Preschool-12

Massachusetts

6103 Department Of Workforce Development
State of Massachusetts
Rm 2112
1 Ashburton Pl
Boston, MA 02108-1518
            617-626-7100
            800-439-0183
            TTY:800-439-2370
            Dhurley@detma.org
            www.massworkforce.org
Suzanne M. Bump, Secretary
Deval L. Patrick, Governor
Timothy P. Murray, Lt. Governor
Serves as the Governor's principal advisory board on workforce development.

6104 Gateway Arts Center: Studio, Craft Store& Gallery
Vinsen Corporation
60-62 Harvard St
Brookline, MA 02445-7993
            617-734-1577
            Fax: 617-734-3199
            gateway@vinfen.org
            www.gatewayarts.org
Rae Edelson, Director
Stephanie Schmidt, Program Director
Mona Thaler, Marketing Director
Stephen De Fronzo, Artistic Director
Award winning, nationally recoginized Arts based rehabilitation service with over 100 talented adults with disabilities.

6105 Massachusetts Fair Employment Practice Agency
Rm 601
1 Ashburton Pl
Boston, MA 02108-1524
            617-994-6000
            Fax: 617-720-6053
            TTY:617-994-6196
            Barbara.Green@massmail.state.ma.us
            www.state.ma.us/mcad
Julian T. Tynes, Chairman
Sunila Thomas George, Commissioner
Jamie R. Williamson, Commissioner
Joel Berner, Esq., Chief of Enforcement
The commission works to eliminate discrimination on a variety of bases and areas, and strives to advance the civil rights of the people of commonwealth through law enforcement, outreach and training.

6106 Massachusetts Governor's Commission on Employment of Disabled Persons
11th Floor
One Ashburton Place
Boston, MA 02108-2502
            617-573-1600
            appointments.state.ma.us
Theodore Schipani, Owner
John Polanowicz, Secretary
Kathleen Betts, Assistant Secretary
Claudia Henderson, Chief of Staff
State vocational rehabilitation agency.

6107 Vocational Rehabilitation Agency
2 Peachtree Street, NW
Atlanta, GA 30303-1616
            404-232-1998
            866-489-0001
            Fax: 404-232-1800
            TTY: 800-764-0200
            elmer.bartels@mrc.state.ma.us
            disabilitycompendium.org
Charles Carr, Commissioner of Rehabilitation
Kasper M. Goshgarian, Deputy Commissioner
Debra Kamen, Assistant Commissioner, Communit
Barbara Kinney, Assistant Commissioner, Disabili
Provides residential, day habilitation and supported employment

6108 Vocational and Rehabilitation Agency Massachusetts Commission for the Blind
600 Washington Street
Boston, MA 02111-4718
617-727-5550
800-392-6450
Fax: 617-626-7685
TTY: 800-392-6556
Ronald.Gallagher@MassMail.State.MA.US
www.mass.gov/eohhs/gov/departments/mcb/
Charles Carr, Commissioner of Rehabilitation
Kasper M. Goshgarian, Deputy Commissioner
Debra Kamen, Assistant Commissioner, Communit
Barbara Kinney, Assistant Commissioner, Disabili
Provides residentail, habilitation, and supported employment

6109 Work Inc.
25 Beach Street
Dorchester, MA 02122-2734
617-691-1500
Fax: 617-691-1595
workinc.org
James Cassetta, CEO
James R. Flanagan, Chairman
Philip Dould, Vice Chairman
David Anderson, Treasurer (CFO)
Mission is all individuals have the ability to grow, the right to make choices and to participate in community life. It is the mission of WORK inc. to join with others in creating the conditions under which all persons with disablilities will experience.

Michigan

6110 Department Of Human Services
P.O.Box 30037
235 S. Grand Ave.
Lansing, MI 48909-8152
517-887-9400
800-292-4200
Fax: 517-335-5140
TTY: 5173734025
Maura D. Corrigan, Director
Duane Berger, Chief Deputy Director/Chief Oper
Terrence Beurer, Director, Field Operations
Susan Kangas, Deputy Director, Financial Servi
The DHS is Michigan's public assistance, child and family welfare agency. DHS directs the operations of public assistance and service programs through a network of over 100 county department of human service offices around the state.

6111 Lamplighter's Work Center
1320 W State St
Cheboygan, MI 49721-1402
231-627-4319
www.usa.com/frs/lamplighters-work-center.html
Robert Spinella, Executive Director
Offers small business counseling and training to individuals with disabilities

6112 Michigan Department of Civil Rights
3054 W Grand Blvd
Ste 3-600
Detroit, MI 48202-6054
313-456-3700
800-482-3604
Fax: 313-456-3791
TTY: 877-878-8464
MDCR-INFO@michigan.gov
www.michigan.gov/mdcr
Daniel H. Krichbaum, Director
Investigates and resolves discrimination complaints and works to prevent discrimination through educational programs that promote voluntary compliance with civil rights laws

6113 Michigan Employment Service
201 N. Washington Square
Lansing, MI 48913-3165
517-335-5858
888-605-6722
Fax: 517-241-8217
TTY: 888-605-6722
www.michigan.gov/mdcd
Christine Quinn, Director, Michigan Rehabilitatio
Job development and placement in services to dislocated workers with disabilities

6114 Michigan Rehabilitation Services: Dept of Labor & Regulatory Affairs
235 S Grand Ave
PO Box 30037
Lansing, MI 48909-7510
517-373-3390
800-605-6722
Fax: 517-335-7277
TTY: 888-605-6722
porterj3@michigan.gov
www.michigan.gov/mrs
Jaye N Porter, Director
Laurie Eggers, Administrative Assistant
State vocational rehabilitation agency.

6115 Small Business Development Center
Ann Arbor Center for Independent Living
409 3rd St, SW
Washington, DC 20416-6832
800-827-5722
Fax: 313-971-0826
answerdesk@sba.gov
www.sba.gov
Sarah Bard, Director
Phil Zepeda, Manager
Maria Contreras-Sweet, SBA Administrator
Fred Baldassaro, Assistant Administrator
Offers small business counseling and training to individuals with disabilities in the state of Michigan.

Minnesota

6116 Jewish Vocational Service of Jewish Familyand Children's Services
401 N 3rd St
Suite 605
Minneapolis, MN 55401-1388
612-692-8920
Fax: 612-692-8921
jfcs@jfcsmpls.org
http://www.jfcsmpls.org
Nancy Rhein, Vice President of Board Development
Howard Zack, President
Sherri Feuer, Vice President of Fund Development
Eileen Kohn, Vice President of Marketing
The mission of JVS is to be a recognized leader in delivering employment, training, and career development services that positively impact individuals of all backgrounds, business and society.

6117 Minnesota Department of Employment and Economic Development - Vocational Rehab Services
332 Minnesota St
1st National Bank Bldg #E-200
Saint Paul, MN 55101-1314
651-259-7114
800-657-3858
Fax: 651-296-3900
TTY: 800657397373
DEED.CustomerService@state.mn.us
www.positivelyminnesota.com
Kim Peck, Director
Service for people with disabilities who need skills to prepare for work, or to find and keep a job.

6118 Minnesota Employment Practice Agency
Minnesota Dept. Of Human Rights
Freeman Building
625 Robert Street North
Saint Paul, MN 55155
651-539-1100
800-657-3704
Fax: 651-296-9042
TTY: 651-296-1283
Info.MDHR@state.mn.us
Kevin Lindsey, Commissioner
Denise Romero-Zasada, Executive Assistant to the Commi
Ytmar Santiago, Deputy Commisioner
Gregory Torrence, Assistant Commisiner
Mission and vision is to make Minnesota discrimination free.

6119 PWI Forum
Multi Resource Centers
1900 Chicago Ave
Minneapolis, MN 55404-1903
612-752-8138
pwi-forum.perfectworld.com/

6120 Vocational and Rehabilitation Agency
332 Minnesota Street
Suite E200
Saint Paul, MN 55101-1351
651-259-7114
800-657-3858
Fax: 651-649-5927
TTY: 612-642-0506
info@ngwmail.des.state.mn.us
www.mnssb.org
Richard Strong, Executive Director
People seeking work, businesses seeking employees, students, and those looking for a first job or returning to the workforce, will find services to meet their needs.

Mississippi

6121 Allied Enterprises of Tupelo
Ability Works Incorporated
1281 Highway 51
Madison, MS 39110
800-443-1000
Fax: 662-287-1463
mdrs.state.ms.us
Michael Byrd, Manager
Jack Virden, Chairman
Jean Massey, Associate State Superintendentof Education
Carey Wright, Superintendentof Education
Vocational evaluation, work adjustment and job placement of disabled persons in a rehabilitation workshop.

6122 Mississippi Department of Rehabilitation Services
1281 Highway 51
Madison, MS 39110-1698
601-853-5100
800-443-1000
Fax: 601-359-1695
TTY: 800-443-1000
Ed LeGrand, Executive Director
Shelia Browning, Deputy Director
Chris Howard, Deputy Director
Richard Sorey, Director
Offers low vision aids and appliances, counseling, social work, educational and professional training, residential services, recreational services, computer training and employment opportunities for the handicapped.

6123 Mississippi Employment Secutity Commission
P.O.Box 1699
1235 Echelon Parkway
Jackson, MS 39215-1699
601-321-6000
Fax: 601-961-7405
www.mdes.ms.gov
Mark Henry, Executive Director
Phil Bryant, Governor
A federally funded state agency. The programs of MDES, under direction of the governor of Mississippi, report to the federal government.

6124 Worksight
Mississippi State University
PO Drawer 6189
108 Herbert - South, Room 150
Mississippi State, MS 39762-6189
662-325-2001
800-675-7782
Fax: 662-325-8989
TTY: 662-325-2694
nrtc@colled.msstate.edu
www.blind.msstate.edu
Michele Capella McDonnall, Research Professor and Interim D
Jacqui Bybee, Research Associate II
Jessica Thornton, Business Manager
Angela Shelton, Coordinator of Instructional Mat
Discusses news, activities, research projects and training programs of the Center.

Missouri

6125 Missouri Commission on Human Rights
421 EastDunklinSt.
P.O. Box 59
Jefferson City, MO 65102-0059
573-751-3215
800-320-2519
Fax: 573-751-4945
mchr@labor.mo.gov
http://www.labor.mo.gov
Alisa Warren, Executive Director
Tracey Allan, Intake Officer
Nia Ray, Director
The Missouri Commission on Human Rights enforces the state's anti-discrimination law that prohibits discrimination in housing, employment and places of public accommodations. It prohibits discrimination due to race, color, religion, national origin, ancestry, sex, disability, age and familial status. Complaints must be filed within 180 days of the alleged discrimination. If discrimination is found after investigation, the Commission can hold hearings to enforce the law.

6126 Missouri Governor's Council on Disability
P.O. Box 687
1706 East Elm
Jefferson City, MO 65102-1668
573-751-8676
800-877-8249
Fax: 573-526-4109
TTY: 573-751-2600
gcd@oa.mo.gov
Douglas E. Nelson, Acting Commissioner
James Trout, Acting Chair and Council Members
Linda Baker, Executive Director Governor's Co
Dawn Evans, Disability Program Specialist
Advocate training, civil rights, community education services, community resource referral, conferences, consumer education, disability awareness program, educational information and resources, information and education services, information and referral, newsletter, policy issues and services, publications, resource directory, seminars, technical assistance, training and seminars.

6127 Missouri Job Training Program Liaison
221 Metro Dr
Jefferson City, MO 65109-4412
573-634-2321
Joe Jerkins, Manager
Services for individuals with disabilities who want to become employed.

6128 Missouri Vocational Rehabilitation Agency
205 Jefferson St.
Jefferson Cty, MO 65101-6188
573-751-4212
877-222-8963
Fax: 573-751-1441
TTY: 573-751-0881
info@vr.dese.mo.gov
Jeanne Loyd, Assistant Commissioner
Michelle Scherer, Administrator

A team of decicated individuals working for the continuous improvement of education and services for all citizens.

6129 WX: Work Capacities
Suite 103
17331 E 40th Hwy
Independence, MO 64055
816-478-2333
Fax: 816-478-2335

Chris Walters, Manager
Mike Heinz, Manager
Services for individuals with disabilities who want to become employed.

Montana

6130 Montana Fair Employment Practice Agency
1805 Prospect Avenue
PO Box 1728
Helena, MT 59624-1728
406-444-2840
800-542-0807
Fax: 406-444-2978
TTY: 406-444-9696
erdquestions@mt.gov
www.erd.dli.mt.gov

Marieke Chief, Bureau Chief
Kathleen Hel , Case Manager
Advocate training, civil rights, community education services, community resource referral and conferences

6131 Montana Governor's Committee on Employment of Disabled People
PO Box 200801
Helena, MT 59620-127
406-444-4405
800-243-4091
Fax: 406-444-4151
Boards@mt.gov
svc.mt.gov/gov/boards/

Nebraska

6132 Nebraska Employment Services
Department of Labor
140 S 27th St Ste C
Lincoln, NE 68510-2601
402-474-9675
www.yellowpages.com

6133 Nebraska Fair Employment Practice Agency
301 Centennial Mall South, 5th Floo
PO Box 94934
Lincoln, NE 68509-4394
402-471-2024
800-642-6112
Fax: 402-471-4059
www.nol.org/home/neoc

Royce Jeffries, Chairperson
Kristin Yates, Vice-Chairman
Ms.Barbara Albers, Executive Director
he Nebraska Equal Opportunity Commission is a neutral administrative agency created by statute in 1965 to enforce the public policy of the state against discrimination. The principal function of the NEOC is to receive, investigate and pass upon charges of unlawful discrimination occurring anywhere within the State of Nebraska in the areas of Employment, Housing, and Public Accommodations.

6134 Nebraska Vocational Rehabilitation Agency
3901 N 27th St, Ste 6
Lincoln, NE 68521-2529
402-471-3231
800-472-3382
Fax: 402-471-0788

Cheryl Ferree, Manager
Rod Armstrong, Vice President of Strategic Part
Mitch Arnolds, President
Amanda Jedlicka, Executive Director

Services for individuals with disabilities who want to become employed. Services are free to those who qualify.

Nevada

6135 Nevada Equal Rights Commission - Dept. of Employment, Training & Rehabilitation
1820 E Sahara Ave
Ste 314
Las Vegas, NV 89104-6512
702-486-7161
800-326-6868
Fax: 702-486-7054
http://detr.state.nv.us/nerc

6136 Nevada Governor's Committee on Employment of Persons with Disabilities
Suite#202
896 W. Nye Lane
Carson City, NV 89703-5062
775-684-8619
Fax: 775-684-8626
www.nevadaddcouncil.org

Sherry Manning, Executive Director
Kari Horn, Projects Manager
Diana Peachay, Executive Assistant
Services for individuals with disabilities who want to become employed.

6137 Vocational and Rehabilitation Agency
State of Nevada
Ste 502
1933 N. Carson Street
Carson City, NV 89701-3705
775-684-0400
Fax: 775-684-4186
TTY:775-684-0360
detr.state.nv.us

Frank Woodbeck, Director
Dennis Perea, Deputy Director
Renee Olson, Administrator for the Employment
William Anderson, Chief Economist for the Research

New Hampshire

6138 Fit for Work at Exeter Hospital
5 Alumni Drive
Exeter, NH 03833-2160
603-778-7311
Fax: 603-580-6592
http://www.exeterhospital.com

Kevin Calahan, President
Staffed by a team of allied health professionals, our outpatient rehabilitation program offers functional restoration, work therapy, diagnostic testing and physical therapy.

6139 New Hampshire Employment Security
32 S Main St
Concord, NH 03301-4857
603-224-3311
800-852-3400
Fax: 603-228-4010
TTY: 800-735-2964
webmaster@nhes.state.nh.us
www.nh.gov/nhes

George Copadis, Commissioner
Darrell Gates, Deputy Commissioner
Zandy L. Dezonie, Administrative Assistant
Operates a free public employment service and provides assisted and self directed employment and career related services and labor market information for employers and the general public.

6140   New Hampshire Fair Employment Practice Agency
2 Chenell Dr Unit 2
Concord, NH   03301-8501
603-271-2767
Fax: 603-271-6339
humanrights@nhsa.state.nh.us
www.nh.gov/hrc

Joni N. Esperian, Esquire, Executive Director
Roxanne Juliano, Assistant Director
Deborah M Evans, Administrative Secretary
Nancy Rodgers, Secretary
Established for the purpose of eliminating discrimination in employment, public accomodations and the sale or rental of housing or commercial property.

6141   New Hampshire Job Training Program Liaison
26 College Drive
Concord, NH   03301-7317
603-230-3500
Fax: 603-271-2725
info@ccsnh.edu
www.ccsnh.edu/

Dr. Ross Gittell, Chancellor
Ron Rioux, Vice Chancellor
Michael Marr, Director of Financial Operations
Sara Sawyer, Director of Human Resources
Services for individuals with disabilities who want to become employed.

6142   Vocational and Rehabilitation Agency
Department of Education
101 Pleasant Street
Concord, NH   03301-3860
603-271-3494
Fax: 603-271-1953
TTY:603-271-3471
Lori.Temple@doe.nh.gov
www.ed.state.nh.us

Paul K Leather, Manager
Virginia Barry, Commissioner
Trisha Allen, Administrative Assistant
Steven Aylward, Rehabilitation Counselor
Offers services for the totally blind, legally blind, visually impaired, mentally retarded blind and more with health, counseling, educational, recreational, rehabilitation, computer training and professional training services.

New Jersey

6143   ARC of Gloucester County
1555 Gateway Blvd
West Deptford, NJ   08096-1018
856-629-9061
Fax: 856-848-7753
www.thearcgloucester.org

Robert.H Weir, President
Charles Funk, VP
Ethel Lucas, Board Member
Ralph Sundy, Board Member
Non-profit organization serving people with intellectual and related developmental disabilities and their families through education, advocacy and direct services.

6144   ARC of Hunterdon County, The
1465 Route 31 South
Suite 23
Annandale, NJ   08801-3127
908-730-7827
Fax: 908-730-7726
jeff@archunterdon.org
www.archunterdon.org

Jeffrey Mattison, Executive Director
Colleen Dennis, Deputy Executive Director
Gail Stepka, Executive Assistant
Our mission is to support, training and opportunities to individuals with intellectual & developmental disabilities to achieve the greatest degree of independence and productivity to become contributing, responsible, and proud members of society.

6145   ARC of Mercer County
180 Ewingville Road
Ewing, NJ   08638-2425
609-406-0181
Fax: 609-406-9258
arc@arcmercer.org
www.arcmercer.org

Geoffrey Morris, President
Rick Koreyva, 1st Vice President
Ethel Lucas, Board Member
Ralph Sundy, Board Member
Committed to securing for all people with disabilities mental retardation and developmental disabilities the opportunity to choose and realize their goals.

6146   ARC of Monmouth
1158 Wayside Road
Tinton Falls, NJ   7712-3148
732-493-1919
Fax: 732-493-3604
info@arcofmonmouth.org
www.arcofmonmouth.org

Joyce Quarles, President
Roger Trendowski, Immediate Past President
Rachel Weiss, First Vice-President
Bill Mirkin, Treasurer
A non-profit organization providing services and supports for individuals who have cognitive and developmental disabilities and for their families.

6147   Abilities Center of New Jersey
1208 Delsea Drive
Westville, NJ   08093-2227
856-848-1025
Fax: 856-848-8429
info@abilities4work.com
abilities4work.com

Susan Spies Perron, President/CEO
Sharon Kneubuehl, VP
Karen Weitzman, Director of Finance and Adminidt
Bill Urie, Director of Operations
A non-profit organization dedicated to developing employment opportunities for people with disabilities or other disadvantages through education, training and job placement.

6148   Abilities of Northwest New Jersey
264 Rt 31 North
Washington, NJ   07882
908-689-1118
info@abilitiesnw.com
abilities-nw.com

a.B Wildermuth, CEO
Private not-for-profit community rehabilitation program providing vocational training and employment services since 1974 to the disabled and disadvantaged population.

6149   Alliance Center for Independence (ACI)
629 Amboy Ave.
First Floor
Edison, NJ   08837-3579
732-738-4388
Fax: 732-738-4416
ctonks@adacil.org
www.adacil.org

Carole Tonks, Executive Director
Luke Koppisch, Deputy Director
ACI is a non-profit, Center for Independent Living, that provides information and referral services and develops and implements educational programs and innovative activities that promote activism, peer support, health and wellness, employment and independent living skills for people with disabilities.

6150   Alternatives for Growth: New Jersey
137 W. Hanover St.
Trenton, NJ   08618
609-393-0008
Fax: 609-393-1189
experts@afg-lca.com
www.njfuture.org

Donna Flannery, Contact
Peter Kasabach, Executive Director
Elaine Clisham, Director of Communications and Development
Nicholas Dickerson, Planning and Policy Analyst

Serves all New Jersey.

6151   Arc of Bergen and Passaic Counties
223 Moore Street
Hackensack, NJ   7601-7402   201-343-0322
                                          Fax: 201-343-0401
                                          arc@arcbp.com
                                          arcbergenpassaic.org

Kathy Walsh, President/CEO
Alice Siegel, Senior VP
Olga Podolsky, Director of Family Support Servi
Anne Gallucci, Vocational Services Director
Serving persons with disabilities and their families in Bergen and
Passaic Counties, NJ.

6152   Career Opportunity Development of New Jersey
901 Atlantic Avenue
Egg Harbor City, NJ   08215-1810   609-965-6871
                                          Fax: 609-965-3099
                                          njcodi.org

Linda L. Carney, President & CEO
Ellen Loughney, Vice Chairperson
Joe Silipena, Board Chairperson
Joe Cella, Secretary
Serves Bergen and Passaic Counties. Provides services to indi-
viduals with varying forms of physical, mental and economic dis-
abilities and disadvantages. Provides services to more than 1,000
unduplicated consumers annually.

6153   Center for Educational Advancement New Jersey
11 Minneakoning Road
Flemington, NJ   08822-5726   908-782-1480
                                          Fax: 908-782-5370

Michael Skoczek, President & CEO
John Reardon, Secretary
Michael Collins, Treasurer
Nancy Vargas, Employee Relations
Serves Somerset and Hunterdon Counties. Skills training in of-
fice technology and food service. Job placement and job coaching
services are available. Employer Network for Ticket to Work.

6154   Cerebral Palsy Association of Middlesex County
10 Oak Drive
Edison, NJ   08837-2313   732-549-6187
                                          800-852-7897
                                          Fax: 732-549-0629
                                          Info@cpamc.org
                                          cpamc.org

Dominic M. Ursino, President
Robert Ferrara, Executive Director
Rob Gross, MBA, Controller
Debra Gilbert, M.S.I.L.R, Director of Human Resources
Dedicated to the provision of comprehensive, superior,
multi-faceted programs of service to individuals with develop-
mental and related disabilities

6155   Easter Seal Society of New Jersey Highlands Workshop
Easter Seals
133 Main St
Franklin, NJ   7416-1542   973-827-9066
                                          Fax: 973-827-3828
                                          pskipp@nj.easterseals.com
                                          www.nj.easterseals.com

Peggy Skipp, Manager
Enabling indidividuals with special needs or disabilities and their
families to learn, live, work and play in their communities with
equality, dignity and independence.

6156   Easter Seal of Ocean County
25 Kennedy Blvd.
Suite 600
East Brunswick, NJ   08816   732-257-6662
                                          Fax: 732-257-7373
                                          http://nj.easterseals.com

Brian.J Fitzgerald, President/CEO

Helping people and families with disabilities and special needs
live, work, and play in their communities with equality, dignity
and independence.

6157   Easter Seals New Jersey
25 Kennedy Blvd
Ste 600
E Brunswick, NJ   08816-2035   732-257-6662
                                          Fax: 732-257-7373
                                          TTY:732-545-1317
                                          www.eastersealsnj.org

Brian Fitzgerald, CEO
Cheryl Young, CFO
Helen Drobnis, VP Corporate Affairs
To enable individuals with disabilities or special needs and their
families to live, work and play in their communities with equality,
dignity, and independence.

6158   Eden Acres Administrative Services
2 Merwick Road
Princeton, NJ   08540-5711   609-987-0099
                                          Fax: 609-734-0069
                                          www.nj.com/mercer/index.ssf/

Peter H. Bell, President & CEO
Jennifer Bizub, Chief Operating Officer
Carol Markowitz, M.A., M.Ed, Chief Program Officer
Melinda Gorny McAleer, Chief Development Officer
Provides services for the disabilitated.

6159   Edison Sheltered Workshop
328 Plainfield Avenue
Edison, NJ   08817-3117   732-985-8834
                                          Fax: 732-985-2216
                                          info@eswnj.org
                                          http://www.eswnj.org

Veronica Valez, Executive Director
Robert.A Ellymer, President
John J. Hogan, First Vice President
Pat Colletto, Treasurer
Serves Middlesex County. Vocational training and job placement
services.

6160   First Occupational Center of New Jersey
861 Asbury Avenue
Ocean City, NJ   08226-2809   609-399-6111
                                          800-894-6265
                                          Fax: 973-672-0065
                                          ocnj@idt.net
                                          www.ocnj.org

Rocco Meola, CEO
Tanya M. Edghill, VP Of Program Services
A private, nonprofit multi-service community rehabilitation program. Services are offered to all people, such as developmentally
disabled, visually impaired, hearing impaired and welfare recipients. Services include vocational evaluation and training, respite
care, basic and remedial education and job placement and
community support services.

6161   Goodwill Industries of Southern New Jersey
2835 Route 73
Maple Shade, NJ   08052-1620   856-439-0200
                                          Fax: 856-439-0843
                                          esmith@goodwillnj.org
                                          goodwillnj.org

Mark B Boyd, President and CEO
Michael Shaw, Chief Operating Officer
Stephen Castro, Chief Financial Officer
*Deb Eckenhoff, Vice President of Goodwill Home Medical
Equipment*
A non profit, community-based organization governed by a vol-
unteer bard of trustees.

6162   Hausmann Industries
130 Union Street
Northvale, NJ   7647-2290   201-767-0255
                                               888-428-7626
                                          Fax: 201-767-1369
                                          info@hausmann.com
                                               hausmann.com

David Hausmann, CEO
George Batchelor, Director Sales & Marketing
Michelle Riley, Mail order Sales
Julie Skoda, Sales and Marketing Adminitrator
Wheelchair acessible exam tables, treatment tables and mat platforms.

6163   Jersey Cape Diagnostic Training & Opportunity Center
152 Crest Haven Road
Cape May Court House, NJ   08210-1651   609-465-4117
                                          Fax: 609-465-3899
                                            www.sjworks.org/

George J Plewa, Executive Director
George Plewa, Executive Director
Serves Cape May County. Employment training services. A vocational rehabilitation center that serves individuals with disabilities, the disabled, and the handicapped or others having barriers to work.

6164   New Jersey Commission for the Blind and Visually Impaired
Department of Human Services
153 Halsey St
6th Floor, PO Box 47017
Newark, NJ   07101- 8004   973-648-3333
                                             877-685-8878
                                          Fax: 973-648-3388
                                             www.state.nj.us

Vito J Desantis, Executive Director
Bernice Davis, Executive Assistant
Marcus Stabile Esq., Manager Human Resources
Frank Scheik, Fiscal Operations
The Commission for the Blind and Visually Impaired (CBVI) promotes and provides services in the areas of education, employment, independence and eye health for persons who are blind or visually impaired, their families and the community. It seeks to provide or ensure access to services that will enable consumers to obtain their fullest measure of self-reliance and quality of life and fully integrated into their community.

6165   New Jersey Employment Service and Job Training Program Services
Department of Labor
John Fitch Plaza
Trenton, NJ   08625   609-292-1040
                                            wd.dol.state.nj.us/

Roland Machold, Manager
Harold J. Wirths, Commissioner
Aaron R. Fichtner, Ph.D., Deputy Commissioner
Frederick J. Zavaglia, Chief of Staff
Services for individuals with disabilities who want to become employed.

6166   Occupational Center of Hudson County
68-70 Tuers Avenue
Jersey City, NJ   07306   201-434-3303
                                          Fax: 201-434-3660
                                       info@hudsoncommunity.org
                                     http://www.hudsoncommunity.org

Christine Remler, Executive Director
Services for individuals with disabilities who want to become employed.

6167   Occupational Center of Union County
301 Cox St
Roselle, NJ   07203-1797   908-241-7200
                                          Fax: 908-241-2025
                                          ocuc@OCUCNJ.com
                                      www.occupationalcenter.org

Michele Ford, VP

The Occupational Center is the only agency in the State of New Jersey which offers a unique combination of individualized training leading to long term employment for people with disabilities in the competitive job market or in our on-site industrial work center. This comprehensive package helps ensure on-the-job success and a productive, dignified life for those with disabilities.

6168   Occupational Training Center of Burlington County
2 Manhattan Drive
Burlington, NJ   08016-4408   609-267-6677
                                                 otcbc.org

Joseph S Bender, CEO
Mission is to assist individuals with disabilities in reaching their maximum potential.

6169   Occupational Training Center of Camden County, New Jersey
520 Market Street
Suite 306
Camden, NJ   08102-1300   866-226-3362
                                          Fax: 856-767-1378
                                      camcofreeholders@gmail.com
                                        www.camdencounty.com

Matt Treihart, President
Serves Camden County.

6170   Pathways to Independence, Inc.
60 Kingsland Ave
Kearny, NJ   07032-3305   201-997-6155
                                          Fax: 201-997-7070
                                          PTI450@aol.com
                                        www.pathwaysnj.org

Alvin Cox, Executive Director
Tessa Farrell, Program Director
Marie Yakabofski, Financial Director
Lisa M. Johnson, Qualilty Assurance Director
Pre-vocational and vocational programming for people with disabilities. Specializing in Developmental Disabilities, Learning Disabilities and Mental Health issues. Serving over 100 people in Hudson, South Bergen, Passaic and East Essex counties. CARF accredited.

6171   Somerset Training and Employment Program
900 Hamilton Street
Somerset, NJ   08873-3206   732-846-8888
                                          Fax: 732-246-7257
                                        www.somersetcap.org/

Laurie Falka, Executive Director
Courtney Throckmorton, Owner
Services for individuals with disabilities who want to become employed.

6172   St. John of God Community Services Vocational Rehabilitation
1145 Delsea Dr
Westville, NJ   8093-2252   856-848-4700
                                          Fax: 856-848-3965
                                       devctr@stjohnofgod.org

Dr. Jerome Knast, Manager
Serves Gloucester and Camden Counties providing exemplary special education, vocational and habilitative services to residents of southern New Jersey since 1967.

6173   United Cerebral Palsy Associations of New Jersey
Suite 1
1005 Whitehead Road Ext
Ewing, NJ   08638-2424   609-882-4182
                                             888-322-1918
                                          Fax: 609-882-4054
                                          TTY: 609-882-0620
                                                 cpofnj.org

Warren Kelemen, President
Jim Bartolomei, CPA, Vice President
Elizabeth R. Faircloth, Secretary
Michael Yarrow, Treasurer
Dedicated to changing lives and bringing independence to people with all types of disabilities.

6174 **Vocational and Rehabilitation Agency**
P.O.Box 398
Trenton, NJ 08625   609-659-3045
Fax: 609-292-8347
TTY:609-292-2919
http://lwd.dol.state.nj.us

Brian Fitzgibbons, Manager
Frederick J. Zavaglia, Chief of Staff
Harold J. Wirths, Commissioner
Programs and services for people with disabilities.

6175 **West Essex Rehab Center**
83 Walnut St
C
Montclair, NJ 07042-4088   973-744-7733
Fax: 973-744-3744
businessfinder.nj.com

Eugene Sefanelli, Executive Director
Shannon Williams, Contact
Eugene Stefanelli, Executive Director
Services and programs for individuals with disabilities who want
to become employed.

New Mexico

6176 **Adelante Development Center**
3900 Osuna Rd Ne
Albuquerque, NM 87109   505-341-2000
Fax: 505-341-2001
info@GoAdelante.org
www.goadelante.org

Mike Kivitz, President
Pamela Sullivan, Board Chair
Mike Lowrimore, Borad Treasurer
Richard Cronin, Physician
Serves Albuquerque and Belen.

6177 **Goodwill Industries of New Mexico**
5000 San Mateo Blvd NE
Albuquerque, NM 87109-2499   505-881-6401
866-376-0182
Fax: 505-884-3157
goodwillnm.org

Mary Best, President/CEO
Michael P. Keoghan, Chief Operating Officer
Roberta Valesquez, Finance Director
Ricky Sanchez, Facilities Logistics Director
Serves Albuquerque, Santa Fe and Rio Rancho.

6178 **New Mexico Employment Services and Job Training Liaison**
P.O.Box 1928
Albuquerque, NM 87103-1928   505-898-3599
Fax: 505-827-6812
http://www.dws.state.nm.us

Reese Suliten, Director
Celina Bussey, Secretary
Provides employment to improve economic progress.

6179 **RCI**
1111 Menaul Blvd NE
Albuquerque, NM 87107-1614   505-255-5501
Fax: 505-255-9971
info@LifeROOTSnm.org
www.liferootsnm.org

Kathleen Cates, President/CEO
Serves Bernalillo County. Mission is to improve the abilities, interests, and choices of children and adults with physical, developmental or behavioral challenges toward achieving their highest
levels of self-sufficiency.

6180 **Tohatchi Area of Opportunity & Services**
100 Manuelita Drive, P.O.Box 49
Tohatchi, NM 87325   505-733-2027
Fax: 505-733-2161
patkeptner@yahoo.com
http://taos-inc.org

Patrick Keptner, CEO
Carol Charles, Administrative Assistant
Judith Woodie, Accounting Clerk
Melinda Golden, Program Manager
Serves McKinley County, San Jose County and the Havanjo Na-
tion.

6181 **Vocational Rehabilitation Agency**
Ste D
435 Saint Michaels Dr
Santa Fe, NM 87505-7679   505-954-8500
800-224-7005
Fax: 505-954-8562
TTY: 877-954-8583
www.dvrgetsjobs.com

Gary Beene, Manager
Purpose is to help people with disabilities achieve a suitable employment outcome.

6182 **Vocational and Rehabilitation Agency**
Bldg 4
2905 Rodeo Park Dr E
Santa Fe, NM 87505-6342   505-827-4479
888-513-7968
greg.trapp@state.nm.us
www.state.nm.us

Greg Trapp, Executive Director
James Salas, Deputy Director
Adelmo Vigil, Deputy Director-IL/OB
Catherine Cross-Maple, Manager
The Commission for the Blind provides vocational rehabilitation
and independent living services designed to enable persons who
are blind to become more participating and contributing members
of society. Blind people lead normal lives, have families, raise
children, participate in community activities, and work in a wide
range of jobs. They are secretaries, lawyers, teachers, engineers,
machinists, scientists, supervisors and business owners.

New York

6183 **JOBS VI and SAGE**
P ES CO International
21 Paulding St
Pleasantville, NY 10570-3108   914-769-4266
800-431-2016
Fax: 914-769-2970
pesco@pesco.org
www.pesco.org

Joseph Kass, President
A computerized matching system matching people to occupations, training, local jobs, local employers and giving job out-
looks for the year 2005. Computerized Sage is online
computerized testing with the ability for system to read all questions, and job descriptions. Manual Sage is a hands on-computer
scored test battery with various adaptation. Braille, large print,
bi-lingual and special devices.

6184 **Just One Break (JOBS)**
6th Floor
570 Seventh Aveune
New York, NY 10018-1653   212-785-7300
Fax: 212-785-4513
TTY:212-785-4515
jobs@justonebreak.com
www.justonebreak.com

Orin Lehman, Founder
John D Kemp, President
Angela Burgess, Board of Director
C.Jeffrey Knittel, Board of Director

A not-for-profit organization that is dedicated to supporting and increasing the employment of people with disabilities.

6185 New York State Department of Labor
Building 12
State Office Campus
Albany, NY 12240
518-457-9000
888-469-7365
TTY:800-662-1220

James J Mcgowan, Commissioner
Fredda Peritz, Employment Service Division Dire
Thomas Malone, Unemployment Insur Div Dir
The missin of the New York State Department of Labor is to help New York work by preparing individuals for the jobs of today and tomorrow. Provides direct job search and counseling services to job seekers, and can refer people who have disabilities for training opportunities. Provides unemployment insurance for those out of work through no fault of their own.

6186 Rational Effectiveness Training Systems
IRET Corporate Services Division
45 E 65th St
New York, NY 10021-6508
212-535-0822
Fax: 212-249-3582

Michael Broder, Owner
Offers advanced training for employee assistance professionals, full service outpatient counseling, consulting services and on-site workshops for the disabled.

6187 Special Education and Vocational Rehabilitation Agency: New York
Room 580 EBA
89 Washington Ave.
Albany, NY 12234
518-474-2925
800-222-5627
accesadm@mail.nysed.gov

Richard Mills, Manager
Mission is to promote educational equity and excellence for students with disabilitites while ensuring that they receive the rights and protection to which they are entitled.

North Carolina

6188 Division Of Workforce Development
NC Department Of Commerce
313 Chapanoke Road
Suite 120
Raleigh, NC 27603
919-814-0400
800-562-6333
Fax: 919-662-4770
http://www.nccommerce.com

Sherry Allen, Accountant
Delores Amogida, Program Assistant V
Barbara Barner, Business & Technology Applicatio
Robbin Broome, Training Manager
Offers vocational assessment and training, adult developmental activities.

6189 Iredell Vocational Workshop
200 Clanton Rd
Charlotte, NC 28217-1446
704-944-5100
www.lifespanservices.org

John Cervantes, Secretary
Davan Cloninger, President & CEO
Robert L. Mendenhall, Vice Chairperson
Jeff Hay, Chairperson
Mission of lifespan is to transform the lives of children and adults with developmental disabilities by providing education, employment, and enrichment programs that promote inclusion, choice, family supports, and other best practices.

6190 North Carolina Division of Services for the Blind
Department of Health and Human Services
2601 Mail Service Center
Raleigh, NC 27699-2601
919-733-9822
800-222-1546
Fax: 919-715-8711
TTY: 919-733-9700
VRStatePlan2015@dhhs.nc.gov
www.dhhs.state.nc.us/dsb

Eddie Weaver, Director
Carla Parker, Executive Assistant
Mary Flanagan, Assistant Director
Marvin Gilmore, LAN Administrator
Since 1935, the mission of the North Carolina Division of Services for the Blind has been to enable people who are blind or visually impaired to reach their goals of independence and employment.

6191 Rowan County Vocational Workshop
2728 Old Concord Rd
Salisbury, NC 28146-1338
704-637-9592
Fax: 704-633-6224

Carl Rapsher, Executive Director
Offers vocational assessment and training, adult developmental activities.

6192 Rutherford Vocational Workshop
230 Fairground Rd
Spindale, NC 28160
828-286-4352
Fax: 828-287-3295
rutherfordlifeservices.com

Amanda Freeman, Program Supervisor
Christy Beddinfield, Staff
Larry Brown, Executive Director
John Jarrett, Human Resource Director
Offers vocational assessment and training, adult developmental activities.

6193 Transylvania Vocational Services
11 Mountain Industrial Drive
P.O. Drawer 1115
Brevard, NC 28712-6723
828-884-3195
info@tvsinc.org
tvsinc.org

Nancy Stricker, Executive Director
A private non-profit corporation with the mission to provide skills development, career opportunities and related services in a supportive environment for people with barriers to employment.

6194 Vocational and Rehabilitation Agency
2001 Mail Service Center
Raleigh, NC 27699-2001
919-855-4800
800-689-9090
Fax: 919-733-7968
TTY: 919-733-9700
dvr.WebInfoRequest@dhhs.nc.gov
http://www.ncdhhs.gov

Albert Delia, Acting Secretary
Beth Melcher, PhD, Chief Deputy Secretary for Healt
Maria. F Spaulding, Deputy Secretary for Long-Term C
Steven Cline, DDS, Assistant Secretary for Health I
Mission statement is to promote employment and independence for people with disabilities through customer partnership and community leadership.

6195 Vocational and Rehabilitation Agency: Department of Health and Human Services
2001 Mail Service Center
Raleigh, NC 27699-2001

919-855-4800
800-689-9090
Fax: 919-733-7968
TTY: 919-733-5924
dvr.WebInfoRequest@dhhs.nc.gov
dvr.dhhs.state.nc.us

Albert Delia, Acting Secretary
Beth Melcher, PhD, Chief Deputy Secretary for Healt
Maria. F Spaulding, Deputy Secretary for Long-Term C
Steven Cline, DDS, Assistant Secretary for Health I
Mission statement is to promote employment and independence for people with disabilities through customer partnership and community leadership.

6196 Webster Enterprises Inc.
140 Little Savannah Rd
Sylvia, NC 28779-220

828-586-8981
800-978-2681
Fax: 828-586-8125
grobinson@websterenterprises.org
www.websterenterprises.org

Gene Robinson, Executive Director
Wendy Cagle, Vice-Chair
Bob Cochran, Secretary/Treasurer
Tom Stovall, Chair
A community based employment and training program for people with disabilities. A full service program which includes a youth transitional program for life beyond high school, job coaching, vocational assessment and job placement.

6197 Western Regional Vocational Rehabilitation Facility Clifford File, Jr.
P.O.Box 1443
200 Enola Rd.
Morganton, NC 28655

828-433-2423
dvr.dhhs.state.nc.us

Connie Barnette, Facility Director
Elizabeth Watson, Executive Director
Frances Battle, Director of Training
Karen Romito, Program Assistant
Vocational Evaluation, Work Adjustment, Job Placement, On-site Work Services Program. Serves most disability groups including CMI, DD, Deaf and Physically impaired.

North Dakota

6198 North Dakota Department of Labor, and Human Rights
Dept 406
600 East Boulevard Avenue
Bismarck, ND 58505- 0340

701-328-2660
800-582-8032
800-366-6888
Fax: 701-328-2031
labor@nd.gov
www.nd.gov/labor

Mark Nelson, Manager
Kathy Kulesa, Human Rights Director
Michelle Kommer, Labor Commissioner
Through a work-sharing agreement with the Equal Employment Opportunity Commission (EEOC), the North Dakota Department of Labor's Human Rights Division enforces the Americans with Disabilities Act (ADA) as related to employment discrimination.

6199 North Dakota Employment Service and Job Training Program Liaison
Job Service North Dakota
1601 E. Century Avenue
PO Box 5507
Bismarck, ND 58506- 5507

701-328-2825
Fax: 701-328-4000
TTY:800-366-6888
www.jobsnd.com/

Leslie Weiss, Manager

Offers vocational assessment and training, adult developmental activities.

6200 North Dakota Vocational Rehabilitation Agency
1237 W Divide Ave
Suite 1B
Bismarck, ND 58501-1208

701-328-8950
800-755-2745
Fax: 701-328-8969
dhsvr@nd.gov
www.nd.gov/dhs/dvr/

Russ Cusack, State Director
LouAnn Nider, Chief of Field Services
Patty Wanner, Operations Administrator
Robyn Throlson, Planning & Evaluation Administrator
The North Dakota Vocational Rehabilitation Agency offers services for blind and visually impaired people such as health, counseling, educational, recreational, rehabilitation, computer training and professional training services.

Ohio

6201 Cornucopia
18120 Sloane Ave
Lakewood, OH 44107-3108

216-521-4600
Fax: 216-521-9460
Ronda.mohammad@cornucopia-inc.org
www.cornucopia-inc.org

Wm. Scott Duennes, Executive Director
Anthony Rospert, President
Judy DeFrancesco, 1st Vice President
David Westerfield, Treasurer
Provides work adjustment training for people with and developmental disabilities in a unique community based setting; Nature's Bin, a natural fresh foods market. Consumers learn through participation in retail operations in produce, grocery, bakery, deli, maintenance and customer service areas. Retail revenues help offset the cost of the program. Job search skills training and placement assistance available to program graduates.

6202 Great Oaks Joint Vocational School
3254 E Kemper Rd
Cincinnati, OH 45241-1581

513-771-8881
800-441-6257
Fax: 513-771-4932
http://www.greatoaks.com/

Harold Carr, Medical Director
Deb Graw, Manager
Jim Perdue, Chair
Sue Steele, Vice Chair
Offers vocational assessment and training, adult developmental activities.

6203 Hearth Day Treatment and Vocational Services
8301 Detroit Ave
Cleveland, OH 44102-1805

216-281-2660
Don Cook, Manager
Hearth offers time-limited, paid work adjustment experiences to consumers with mental illness. The goal of Hearth Programs is to prepare the consumer for success in the competitive workforce.

6204 Highland Unlimited Business Enterprises of CRI
1501 Madison Road
Cincinnati, OH 45206-2223

513-354-5200
Fax: 513-354-7115
gcbhs.com

Tony Datillo, CEO
Debbie Dutton Lambert, Director Employment Programs
Tony Carter, Chairman of GCB Board
Adrienne Russ, Secretary
Offers vocational assessment and training, adult developmental activities.

6205   Ohio Civil Rights Commission
Rhodes State Office Tower
30 East Broad Street, 5th Floor
Columbus, OH   43215-3414   614-466-5928
                                        TTY:614-753-2391
                                        http://crc.ohio.gov

Leonard Hubert, Chairman
Eddie Harrell, Jr, Commissioner
Rashmi Yajnik, Commissioner
Stephanie Mercado, Commissioner
Primary function is to enforce state laws against discrimination.

6206   Ohio Commission On Minority Health
77 S High Street
18th Floor
Columbus, OH   43215-6108   614-466-4000
                                        Fax: 614-752-9049
                                        minhealth@mih.ohio.gov
                                        www.mih.ohio.gov

Angela C Dawson, Executive Director
Sheronda Whitner, Executive Assistant
Reina M. Sims, MSA, Program Manager
Venita O'Bannon, Fiscal Specialist
Offers vocational assessment and training, adult developmental
activities.

6207   Vocational and Rehabilitation Agency
400 East Campus View Boulevard
Columbus, OH   43235-4604   614-438-1210
                                        800-282-4536
                                        Fax: 614-438-1257
                                        TTY: 614-438-1334
                                        www.state.oh.us

John M Connelly, Administrator
Rose Reed, Manager
State agency that provides vocational rehabilitation services to
help people with disabilities become employed and independent.

Oklahoma

6208   Oklahoma Department of Rehabilitation Services
3535 NW 58th St.
Suite 500
Oklahoma City, OK   73112-4824   405-424-4932
                                        800-845-8476
                                        Fax: 405-951-3529
                                        info@okdrs.gov
                                        www.okrehab.org

Noel Tyler, Director
The Oklahoma Department of Rehabilitation Services (DRS)
provides assistance to Oklahomans with disabilities through vocational rehabilitation, employment, independent living, residential and outreach programs, and the determination of medical
eligibility for disability benefits.

**6209   Oklahoma Employment Services and Job Training Program
Liaison**
2401 North Lincoln Boulevard
Oklahoma City, OK   73105-4409   405-557-7100
                                        Fax: 405-557-5368
                                        TTY:800-722-0353
                                        http://www.ok.gov

Richard McPherson, Executive Director
Teresa Keller, Deputy Director
Mike Evans, Chief Information Technology Officer
*Lisa Graven, Reemployment Services/Customer Service Division
Director*
As the primary agency dedicated to disability services in
Oklahoma, we offer a wide range of programs for many individu-
als each year.

**6210   Oklahoma Governor's Committee on Employment of People
with Disabilities**
Ste 90
2401 NW 23rd
Oklahoma City, OK   73107-2423   405-521-3756
                                        800-522-8224
                                        Fax: 405-522-6695
                                        www.odc.ok.gov

Steve Stokes, Executive Director
Doug MacMillan, Director
William Ginn, Disability Program Specialist
Dalene Barton, Office Manager
Mission is to promote the employment of people with disabilities.
The vision of the committee is to facilitate partnerships with com-
mitment to full, high quality employment of people with
disabilities.

Oregon

6211   Bend Work Activity Center
P.O. Box 430 835 E Hwy 126
Redmond, OR   97756   541-548-2611
                                        Fax: 541-548-9573
                                        info@ofco.org
                                        www.ofco.org

James Booth, Chairperson
Bill Schertzinger, Vice Chairperson
Cam Chambers, Manager
Seth Johnson, Executive Director
Offers vocational assessment and training, adult developmental
activities and programs.

6212   Oregon Fair Employment Practice Agency
Oregon Bureau of Labor & Industry
Suite 1045
800 NE Oregon St
Portland, OR   97232-2180   971-673-0761
                                        Fax: 971-673-0762
                                        mailb@boli.state.or.us
                                        www.boli.state.or.us/civil

6213   State of Oregon Office of Vocational Rehabilitation Service
Ste 500
3165 10th St
Baker City, OR   97814-1480   541-524-1800
                                        800-578-9990
                                        Fax: 541-523-5667
                                        wendy.m.wall@state.or.us
                                        www.oregon.gov/dhs/vr

Wendy Wall, Voc Rehab Counselor
Allan McCandless, Voc Rehab Counselor
Offers vocational assessments and training, adult developmental
activities, and helps remove disability related barriers to
employment.

6214   Vocational and Rehabilitation Agency
500 Summer St NE E-87
Salem, OR   97301-1063   503-945-5880
                                        877-277-0513
                                        Fax: 503-947-5010
                                        vr.info@state.or.us
                                        www.oregon.gov/dhs/vr/index.shtml
Stephanie Taylor, Administrator
Offers vocational assessments and training, adult developmental
activities and programs.

6215 Vocational and Rehabilitation Agency: Oregon Commission for the Blind
535 SE 12th Avenue
Portland, OR 97214-2408
971-673-1588
888-202-5463
Fax: 503-234-7468
TTY: 971-673-1577
ocb.mail@state.or.us
www.oregon.gov/Blind

Linda Mock, Administrator
Frank Armstrong, Representative
Pat MacDonell, Director
Jodi.C Roth, Chair
A resource for visually impaired Oregonians, as well as their families, friends, and employers. Nationally recognized programs and staff that make a difference in people's lives every day.

Pennsylvania

6216 ACLD/An Association for Children and Adults with Learning Disabilities: Greater Pittsburgh
4900 Girard Rd
Pittsburgh, PA 15227-1440
412-881-2253
info@acldonline.org
acldonline.org

Thomas Fogarty, Administrator
Kathleen Donahoe, Director ACLD Tillotson School
Jackie Lulich, Director Business Services
Dedicated to helping children, adolescents, and adults with Specific Learning Disabilities and related disorders succeed in school, employment and life.

6217 Office of Vocational Rehabilitation
7th and Forester St
Harrisburg, PA 17120-1
717-787-4746
Fax: 717-783-5221
www.dli.state.pa.us

Barry Brandt, Rehabilitation Specialist
Information in vocational counseling and the governor's committee on Employment of People with Disabilities. Also serves persons with disabilities that present a substantial handicap to employment and independence. Services are provided when there is a reasonable expectation that employment is possible as a result of those services.

6218 Pennsylvania Employment Services and Job Training
P A Department of Labor and Industry
Room 1700
7th and Forster St
Harrisburg, PA 17120-1
717-787-2500
Fax: 717-772-8284
www.dli.state.pa.us

Edward G Rendell, Manager
Stephen Schmerin, Manager
Administers benefits to unemployed individuals, oversees the administration of worker's compensation benefits to individuals with job related injuries, and provides vocational rehabilitation to individuals with disabilities.

6219 Pennsylvania Governor's Committee on Employment of Disabled Persons
121 N Sixth Street
Harrisburg, PA 17120-1
717-772-6382
Fax: 717-783-5221
www.dli.state.pa.us/landi/cwp

6220 Pennsylvania Human Relations Commission Agency
8th Floor
333 Market St.
Harrisburg, PA 17101-2210
717-787-4410
Fax: 717-772-4340
TTY:717-787-7279
phrc@pa.gov
phrc.state.pa.us

JoAnn. L Edwards, Executive Director
Gerald.S Robinson, Chairman
Tom Corbett, Governor
Dr. Raquel O Yiengst, Vice Chairperson
Mission is to administer and enforce the PHRAct and the PFEOA of the Commonwealth of Pennsylvania for the identification and elimination of discrimination and the providing of equal opportunity for all persons.

6221 US Healthworks
25124 Springfield Court
Suite 200
Valencia, CA 91355- 3333
661-678-2600
800-720-2432
Fax: 610-926-6225
www.ushealthworks.com

Beverly Shaeff, Manager
Stephanie Makovsky, Sales Consultant
Daniel D. Crowley, President & Chief Executive Officer
Joseph T. Mallas, Chief Operating Officer
Offers employers comprehensive occupational health services and state-of-the-art physical and occupational therapy. Staff works as a team to produce the best possible patient care while delivering cost savings through workers compensation disability management programs.

6222 Vocational and Rehabilitation Agency
1521 North Sixth Street
Harrisburg, PA 17102-1100
717-787-5244
800-442-6351
Fax: 717-783-5221
TTY: 717-787-4885
ovr@dli.state.pa.us
dli.state.pa.us

William Gannon, Manager
Thomas Washic, Manager
Mission is to assist with disabilities, to secure and maintain employment and independence.

6223 Vocational and Rehabilitation Agency: Department of Labor and Industry
909 Green St
Harrisburg, PA 17102-2913
717-236-6211
800-622-2842
Fax: 717-236-3390
TTY: 717-787-6176
cboone@state.pa.us

Thomas Carlock, CEO
Mission is to assist people with disabilities, to serve and maintain employment and independence.

Rhode Island

6224 Goodwill Industries of RI
100 Houghton Street
Providence, RI 02904-1013
401-861-2080
Fax: 401-454-0889
TTY:401-331-2830
www.goodwillri.org

Jeffrey D. Machado, President/CEO
Justine Beatini, Transitional Resource Specialist
Shirl Berger, Employee Development & Program
Daniel Burgess, Finance Director
The mission of Goodwill Industries of Rhode Island is to provide training, education and other services which result in employment and expanded opportunities for people with disabilities and other barriers to employment in order to enhance their capacity for independent living, increased quality of life and work.

6225 Groden Center
86 Mount Hope Avenue
Providence, RI 02906-1648 401-274-6310
grodencenter.org

Helen Morcos, Chief Executive Officer
Jane I Carlson, Ph.D., BCBA, Vice President Day & Residential Programs
Cooper Woodard, Ph.D., Vice President Clinical Services
Peggy H. Stocker, Admissions Coordinator

The Groden Center is a school and residential treatment center in Rhode Island enhancing the lives of children and youth with autism, behavioral disorders, and developmental disabilities by providing early autism intervention services, an early childhood education program as well as providing functional and social development instruction to school-age children with learning disabilities.

6226 Newport County Chapter of Retarded Citizens
P.O.Box 4390
906 Aquidneck Avenue
Middletown, RI 02842 401-846-0340
Fax: 401-847-9459
danam@mahercenter.org
mahercenter.org

John Maher, Executive Director
Daniel J Oakley, VP
Barbara Burns, Secretary
Walter Jachna, Chairman

Vocational training and job placement services.

6227 Office of Rehabilitation Services
40 Fountain Street
Providence, RI 02903-1898 401-421-7005
Fax: 401-222-3574
TTY:401-421-7016
garyw@ors.ri.gov
ors.ri.gov

Ron Racine, Deputy Administrator
Steve Brunero, Acting Deputy Administrator-ORS
John Microulis, Deputy Administrator-Disability
Walter Jachna, Chairman Board of Directors

Their goal is to help individuals with physical and mental disabilities prepare for and obtain appropriate employment.

6228 Vocational and Rehabilitation Agency: Department of Human Services
RI Services for the Blind and Visually Impaired
40 Fountain St
Providence, RI 02903-1830 401-421-7005
Fax: 401-222-3574
TTY:401-421-7016
garyw@ors.ri.gov

Ron Racine, Deputy Administrator
Steve Brunero, Acting Deputy Administrator-ORS
John Microulis, Deputy Administrator-Disability
Walter Jachna, Chairman Board of Directors

Their goal is to help individuals with physical and mental disabilities prepare for and obtain appropriate employment.

South Carolina

6229 South Carolina Employment Security Commission South Carolina Center
P.O.Box 567
Columbia, SC 29201 803-777-2400
800-436-8190
www.sces.org

Camille Fallow, Disability Program Navigator
Regina Ratterros, Program Coordinator/State Office

Public agency taht offers job search assistance. Unemployment Benefits and WIA program. Also offered is Disability Program Navigator who helps persons with disabilities to find needed resources

6230 South Carolina Governor's Committee on Employment of the Handicapped
1410 Boston Avenue
P.O.Box 15
West Columbia, SC 29171-15 803-896-6500
800-832-7526
Fax: 803-896-1224
TTY: 806-896-6553
http://www.scvrd.net/

Barbara G. Hollis, Executive Director
Derle A. Lowder Sr., Agency Board Chairman
Dr. Roxzanne Breland, Vice Chair
Joseph A. Thomas, Vice Chair

Goal is to help individuals with physical and mental disabilities prepare for and obtain appropriate employment.

6231 South Carolina Vocational Rehabilitation Department
P.O.Box 15
1410 Boston Avenue
West Columbia, SC 29171-15 803-896-6500
800-832-7526
TTY:806-896-6553
info@scvrd.state.sc.us
www.scvrd.net

Larry C Bryant, Commissioner
Barbara G Hollis, Executive Director
Dr. Roxzanne Breland, Vice Chair
Derle A Lowder Sr., Agency Board Chairman

The SCVRD's mission is to enable eligible South Carolinians with disabilities to prepare for, achieve and maintain competitive employment.

6232 Vocational and Rehabilitation Agency: Commission for the Blind
Vocational and Rehabilitation Agency
P.O.Box 79
1430 Confederate Avenue
Columbia, SC 29201-79 803-898-8764
800-922-2222
Fax: 803- 89- 879
publicinfo@sccb.sc.gov
http://www.sccb.state.sc.us/

Zertie Johnson, Manager
James Kirby, Commissioner
Don Bradley, Director Consumer Affairs
Rhonda Thompson, Director, Prevention & Older Blind

Goal is to help individuals with physical and mental disabilities prepare for and obtain appropriate employment.

South Dakota

6233 South Dakota Governor's Advisory Committeeon Employment of the Disabled
700 Governors Drive
Pierre, SD 57501-2291 605-773-3101
Fax: 605-773-6184
http://dlr.sd.gov

Patrick Keating, Manager
Marcia Hultman, Secretary of Labor and Regulation
Lyle Harter, Director of Administrative Services
Bret Afdahl, Director of the Division of Banking

Goal is to help individuals with physical and mental disabilities prepare for and obtain appropriate employment.

6234 South Dakota State Vocational Rehabilitation
Department of Human Services
3800 E Highway 34 Hillview Plz
Pierre, SD 57501 605-773-3195
Fax: 605-773-5483
eric.weiss@state.sd.us
www.state.sd.us

Jeff Pierce, Manager
Bernie Grimme, Assistant Director, DRS
Eric Weiss, Director

South Dakota State Vocational Rehabilitation consists of two agencies; Rehab Services and service to the Blind and Visually

Impaired. There mission is the same to provide individualized rehabilitation services that result in optimal employment and independent living outcomes for individuals with disabilities.

6235 South Dakota Workforce Investment Act Training Programs
700 Governors Dr
Pierre, SD 57501-2291

605-773-3101
800-952-3216
Fax: 605-773-6184
www.sdjobs.org

Michael Ryan, Administrator
Patrick Keating, Manager
Marcia Hultman, Secretary of Labor and Regulation
Lyle Harter, Director of Administrative Services
Mission is to enhance the South Dakota workforce by providing business with employment-related solutions and helping people with job placement and career transition services

6236 Vocational and Rehabilitation Agency: Division of Services to the Blind/Visually Impaired
3800 E Highway 34 Hillview Plz
Pierre, SD 57501

605-773-3195
Fax: 605-773-5483
gaye.mattke@state.sd.us
www.state.sd.us

Dawn Backer, Manager, Rehabilitation Center for the Blind
Eric Weiss, Director
Gaye Mattke, Division Director, Service to the Blind and Visually Impaire
Nancy Hoyme, Program Specialist
To provide individualized rehabilitation services that result in optimal employment and independent living outcomes for people with disabilities.

Tennessee

6237 Division of Rehabilitative Services
Tennessee Department Human Services
400 Deaderick Street
15th Floor
Nashville, TN 37243-1403

615-313-4700
Fax: 615-741-4165
mandy.johnson@tn.gov
www.state.tn.us/humanserv/rehabilitation.htm
Raquel Hatter, Commisioner

6238 Tennessee Department of Labor: Job Training Program Liaison
220 French Landing Drive
Nashville, TN 37243-1712

615-741-6642
Fax: 615-741-5078
www.tn.gov

Ruth S Letson, Manager
Burns Phillips, Commissioner
Dustin Swayne, Deputy Commissioner
Stephanie Mitchell, Mitchell
Goal is to help individuals with physical and mental disabilities prepare for and obtain appropriate employment.

6239 Tennessee Fair Employment Practice Agency
Human Rights Commission
23rd floor
312 Rosa L Parks Ave
Nashville, TN 37243-1

615-741-5825
800-251-3589
Fax: 615-253-1886
www.state.tn.us/humanrights

Tricia Crawford, Manager
Beverly L. Watts, Executive Director
Sabrina Hooper, Deputy Director
Shalini Rose, General Counsel
An independent state agency charged with preventing and eradicating discrimination in employment, public accomodations, and housing.

Texas

6240 C-CAD Center of United Cerebral Palsy of Metropolitan Dallas
8802 Harry Hines Blvd.
Dallas, TX 75235

800-999-1898
www.ucpdallas.org

Mark Denzin, President/Chief Operating Officer
Frank Pickens, CPA, Chief Financial Officer
April Allen, Chief Program Officer
Shea Needham, Regional Director
Offers a wide range of technology opportunities for persons with all types of disabilities, their families and the professionals who serve them. Services include assesments, traiing, technology access showroom, and workshops for rehabilitation and educational personnel.

6241 Handbook of Career Planning for Students with Special Needs
Pro- Ed Publications
8700 Shoal Creek Boulevard
Austin, TX 78757-6897

512-451-3246
800-897-3202
Fax: 512-451-8542
general@proedinc.com
www.proedinc.com

Donald D Hammill, Owner
Courtney King, Marketing Coordinator
Thomas F. Harrington, Editor
The practitioner's guide will show you how to help special needs adolescents and young adults overcome barriers to employment by identifying goals and problems, assessing interests and aptitudes, involving client families and developing communication skills. *$42.00*
358 pages

6242 Texas Employment Services and Job Training Program Liaison
Texas Workforce Commission
101 E 15th St
Rm 665
Austin, TX 78778-0001

512-463-2236
866-938-4444
TTY:700-735-2989
ombudsman@twc.state.tx.us
http://www.twc.state.tx.us

Larry Temple, Executive Director
Lasha Lenzy, Division Director
Reagan Miller, Division Director
Tom McCarty, Division Director
State government agency charged with overseeing and providing workforce development services to employers and job seekers of Texas. Offers career development information, job search resources, training programs, and, as appropriate, unemployment benefits.

6243 Vocational and Rehabilitation Agency: State Rehabilitation Commission
Vocational and Rehabilitation Agency
4800 N Lamar Blvd
Austin, TX 78756-3106

512-383-7000
800-628-5115
Fax: 512-424-4730
TTY: 800-628-5115
www.dars.state.tx.us

Marilyn Hancock, Executive Director
Michelle Crain, Executive Director
Veronda L. Durden, Commissioner
Glenn Neal, Deputy Commissioner
Helps people with disabilities prepare for, find and keep jobs. Work related services are individualized and may include counseling, training, medical treatment, assistive devices, jon placement assistance and other services.

Utah

6244 Utah Employment Services
P.O. Box 45249
2292 South Redwood Road
West Valley, UT 84119-0249
801-978-0378
Fax: 801-978-0374
info@utahemploy.com
www.utahemploy.com

Kristen Cox, Executive Director
To help individuals prepare and obtain appropriate employment.

6245 Utah Governor's Committee on Employment ofthe Handicapped
195 North 1950 West
Salt Lake City, UT 84116-5238
801-538-4200
800-837-6811
Fax: 801-538-4279
dspd@utah.gov
dspd.utah.gov

George Kelner, Executive Director
Promotes opportunities and provide support for persons with disabilities to lead self-determined lives.

6246 Utah Veterans Centers
Ste 105
200 South Central Campus Drive
Salt Lake City, UT 84112-1686
801-587-7722
800-246-1197
Fax: 801-377-0227
www.military.com/benefits/veteran-benefits

Dennis Stevens, Executive Director
Brent Price, Manager
Roger Perkins, Director of Veterans Support
Sylvia O'Hara, Executive Assistant
Readjustment counseling services to veterans.

6247 Utah Vocational Rehabilitation Agency
Utah State Office of Rehabilitation
P.O.Box 144200
1501 M Street, NW Seventh Floor
Washington, DC 20005-4200
202-466-6550
800-473-7530
Fax: 202-785-1756
www.ppsv.com/

Donald Uchida, Executive Director
Heidi Kubbe, Executive Assistant
Jennifer Smart, Training Coordinator
Coy Jackson, Program Specialist
Vocational Rehabilitation Services for individuals with disabilities. To assist individuals with disabilities to prepare for and obtain employment and increase their independence.

6248 Vocational and Rehabilitation Agency: Division of Services for the Blind/Visually Imp.
1st Floor
160 E 300 S
Salt Lake City, UT 84111-7902
801-530-4849
877-526-3994
Fax: 801-530-6438
utah.gov

Willam G Gibson, Executive Director
Cheryl Ritchie, Administrative Secretary
LuWana Martin, Network Specialist
Sharon Pipkin, Office Specialist
Mission is to assist individuals who are blind or visually impaired to obtain employment or increase their independence.

Vermont

6249 State of Vermont Department of Disabilities, Aging and Independent Living
Agency of Human Services
103 South Main Street
Weeks IC
Waterbury, VT 05671-2304
802-241-2210
888-405-5005
Fax: 802-241-2128

Fred Jones, Director
Stacy Rollins, Executive Administrative Assistant
Carl Augusto, President and CEO
Rick Bozeman, Chief Financial Officer
Mission is to support the efforts of Vermonters who ar blind and visually impaired to achieve or sustain their economic independence, self reliance, and social integration to a level consistent with thier interests, abilities and informed choices.

6250 Vermont Employment Services and Job Training
5 Green Mountain Drive P.O.Box 488
Montpelier, VT 05601- 488
802-828-4000
Fax: 802-828-4022
TTY:802-828-4203
tdouse@labor.state.vt.us
www.labor.vermont.gov

Annie Noonan, Commissioner
Deborah Bruce, Human Resource Administrator
Richard Gray, State Director
Tracy Phillips, Director, Unemployment Insurance & Wages
The primary focus is to help support the efforts to make Vermont a more competitive place to do business and create good jobs.

6251 Vermont Governor's Committee on Employmentof People with Disabilities
103 South Main Steet
Weeks 1A
Waterbury, VT 05671-2303
802-241-6757
866-879-6757
Fax: 802-241-3359
www.vocrehabvermont.org

Diane Dalmasse, Manager
Melita DeBeliss, Staff
Committed to facilitating successful, long-term relationships between employers and people with disabilities in Vermont.

Virginia

6252 Alexandria Community Y Head Start
418 S Washington St
Alexandria, VA 22314-3673
703-549-0111
Fax: 703-549-2097
www.campagnacenter.org/

Tammy.L Mann, Ph.D, President and CEO
Raj Kapur, Chief Financial Officer
Karla Kelley, Senior Director of Out-of-School
Chrystal Starr Brown, Senior Director, Early Childhood
Offers social services, on-the-job-training for parents, play therapy, physical therapy, speech therapy and any other specialized services.

6253 Department Of Rehabilitative Services
8004 Franklin Farms Drive
Henrico, VA 23229-5019
804-662-7000
Fax: 804-662-9532
dars@dars.virginia.gov

Jay Windsor, Contact Pers
Jim Rothrock, Commissioner
Helps people with disabilities get ready for,find, and keep a job.

6254 Didlake
8641 Breeden Ave
Manassas, VA 20110-8431

703-361-4195
866-361-4195
Fax: 703-369-7141
www.didlake.com

Rex Parr, CEO
John S Craig, VP Rehabilitation Services
Tammara L. Hoover, Treasurer
Patty Tracy, Secretary
Offers situational assessments, work training, employment and job placement services to people with disabilities.

6255 Learning Services: Shenandoah
204 Howe Hall
1460 University Drive
Winchester, VA 22601-5829

540-665-4928
Fax: 540-665-3470
www.su.edu/academic

Peter Patrick, Administrator
Michelle Shenk, Director of Learning Resources and Services
Jeremai Santiago, M.S., Assistant Director & Learning Enrichment Coach
Erin Beaupre, Learning Services Specialist
Postacute rehabilitation program.

6256 NISH
8401 Old Courthouse Road
Vienna, VA 22182-3820

571-226-4660
Fax: 703-849-8916
nish.org

E. Robert Chamberlin, President and CEO
Dennis.A Fields, Chief Operating Officer
Elizabeth W. Goodman, Chief Financial Officer
Paul W. Plattner, Vice President of Operations
A nonprofit agency desigated by the Committee for Purchase from People Who Are Blind or Severely Disabled to provide technical assistance to rehabilitation programs interested in obtaining federal contracts under Public Law 92-28, the Javits-Wagner-O'Day Act. NISH's primary objective is to assist community rehabilitation programs in providing jobs for people with severe disabilities.

6257 Richmond Research Training Center
P.O.Box 842011
1314 West Main Street
Richmond, VA 23284-2011

804-828-1851
Fax: 804-828-2193
TTY:804-828-2494
RRTC@vcu.edu
http://www.worksupport.com

Paul Wehman Ph.D., Professor and Director
Dolores Taylor, Executive Director
John Kregel, Ed.D, Associate Director
Vicki Brooke, M. Ed., Director of Training and Knowledge Translation
Research and training center report on the supported employment of persons with developmental and other disabilities.

6258 ServiceSource
Suite 175
6295 Edsall Rd
Alexandria, VA 22312-2670

703-461-6000
800-244-0817
Fax: 703-461-3906

Janet Samuelson, President & CEO
Edie Castner, Assistant Director
Mark Hall, Executive Vice President, Corporate Development
David Hodge, Executive Vice President & Chief Financial Officer
Provides training, job placement and employment services in private sector and government contract employment.

6259 Sheltered Occupational Center of Virginia
750 23rd St
Arlington, VA 22202-2452

703-521-4441
Fax: 703-521-3443
socent.org

Perla Ni, CEO
Hayley Gefell, Chief Business Development Offic
Marshall Henson, Chief Operating Officer
Donnell Karimah, Chief Administrative Officer
Assists, empowers and supports people with disabilities to achieve employment, independence and integration in the workplace and community. Our services include: printing, copying, hand work, mail shop, fulfillment and distribution.

6260 Vocational and Rehabilitation Agency: Department for the Blind/Visually Impaired
397 Azalea Avenue
Richmond, VA 23227-3623

804-371-3140
800-622-2155
Fax: 804-371-3154
Kimberley.Jennings@dbvi.virginia.gov
www.vdbvi.org

Raymond E. Hopkins, Commissioner
James A Taylor, Chief Deputy
Kimberley Jennings, Contact Person
Dr. Rick L. Mitchell, Deputy Commissioner, Services Delivery
DBVI envisions a world in which blind, vision impaired and deafblind people can access all that society has to offer and can, in turn, contribute to the greater community. We believe this is achievable.

Washington

6261 Career Connections
P.O.Box 141806
431 East Colfax Ave.
South Bend, IN 46617-1806

574-232-5400
866-404-5867
Fax: 574-245-5822

Susan Warwick, Executive Director
Teresa Antosyn, Program Coordinator
Dan Moody, CFO
Sadie Takila, Production Manager
Offers structured work sites at several locations. Production work at various skill levels, with training as needed.

6262 Department of Services for the Blind National Business & Disability Council
Department of Services for the Blind
P.O.Box 40933
4565 7th Avenue SE
Olympia, WA 98504-933

360-725-3830
Fax: 360-407-0679
info@dsb.wa.gov
www.dsb.wa.gov

Louana Durand, Executive Director
A state rehabilitation agency that offers assistance to persons who are blind or visually impaired. Also provides various services for employers interested in accomodating or hiring workers with vision loss.

6263 Division of Developmental Disabilities: Department of Social & Health Services
P.O.Box 45310
Olympia, WA 98504-5310

360-725-3413
800-737-0617
Fax: 360-407-0955
dddcoreception@dshs.wa.gov
www.dshs.wa.gov/dda

Robin Arnold-Williams, Secretary
Colleen Cawston, Senior Director
Steve Lowe, Senior Director
Tracy Guerin, Chief of Staff
The Division of Developmental Disabilities offers persons with developmental disabilities quality supports and services that are

individual/family driven, stable and flexible, satisfying to the person and their family, and able to meet individual needs.

6264   SL Start and Associates
901 N Monroe St.
Suite 200
Spokane, WA 99201-4800   509-328-2740
                                            888-355-7155
                                       Fax: 509-326-9207
                                         info@slstart.com
                                            slstart.com

Stephen L Start, Owner
A diversified and innovative human and health services company focused on a wide range of social, employment and long-term services.

6265   School of Piano Technology for the Blind
2510 E Evergreen Blvd
Vancouver, WA 98661-4323   360-693-1511
                                       Fax: 360-693-6891
                                 info@pianotuningschool.org
                                     pianotuningschool.org

Len Leger, Executive Director
Jeff Lane, Executive Director
Donald L. Mitchell, Director of Instructional Operat
Les Fitzpatrick, Technician/Instructor
Teaches piano tuning and repair to blind and visually impaired menand women, leading to employment and/or self-employment in the piano service industry. Licensed by Washington State and accredited by the Accrediting Commission of Career Schools and Colleges of Technology (ACCSCT). 20-month course.

6266   Vocational and Rehabilitation Agency: Division of Vocational Rehabilitation
Department of Social and Health
P.O.Box 45340
Olympia, WA 98504-5340   360-704-3560
                                            800-637-5627
                                       Fax: 360-570-6941
                                       TTY: 360-438-8000
                                         krulik@dshs.wa.gov
                                      www1.dshs.wa.gov/dvr

Patrick Raines, Manager
Andres , Director
Mission is to empower individuals with disabilities to achieve a greater quality of life by obtaining and maintaining employment.

West Virginia

6267   West Virginia Division of Rehabilitation Services
P.O.Box 50890
107 Capitol Street
Charleston, WV 25301- 2609   304-356-2060
                                            800-642-8207
                                       Fax: 304-766-4905
                                       TTY: 304-766-4809
                                            www.wvdrs.org

Deborah Lovely, Director
Donna Ashworth, Assistant Director
DRS specializes in helping people with disabilities who want to find a job or maintain current employment. Rehabilitation counselors at more than 30 field offices help with applications. Once eligibility is determined, counselors & clients work as a team to develop a plan to meet the individuals employment goal. Services may include work-related counseling/guidance, evaluation/assessment, job development & placement assistance, vocational training, college assistance & assistive technology.

6268   West Virginia Employment Services and Job Training Programs Liaison
112 California Ave
Charleston, WV 25305-12   304-558-2660
                                       Fax: 304-558-1343
                                         workforcelmi@wv.gov
                                       http://workforcewv.org

Valerie Comer, Director
Allan Galloway, Manager
Workforce West Virginia, a division of the Department of Commerce, effectively coordinates all availiable state and federal resources by orchestrating the efforts of state agencies and local organizations.

6269   West Virginia Vocational Rehabilitation
P.O.Box 1004
107 Capitol Street
Charleston, WV 25301- 2609   304-356-2060
                                            800-642-8207
                                            www.wvdrs.org

Earl Wolfe, Director
Offers services for the totally blind, legally blind, visually impaired, mentally retarded blind and more with health, counseling, educational, recreational, rehabilitation, computer training and professional training services.

Wisconsin

6270   Vocational and Rehabilitation: State of Wisconsin
201 E Washington Ave
Madison, WI 53702-1   608-266-0050
                                            800-442-3477
                                       Fax: 608-266-3131
                                       TTY: 888-877-5939
                                       dvr@dwd.wisconsin.gov

Tamara Monsees, Office Manager/Admin. Support
Offers vocational rehabilitation services for the totally blind, legally blind, visually impaired, mentally retarded blind and more with health, counseling, educational, rehabilitation, computer training and professional training services, and displaced worker.

Wyoming

6271   Division of Vocational Rehabilitation of Wyoming
Wyoming Department of Workforce Services
1100 Herschler Buiding
Cheyenne, WY 82002-1   307-777-7364
                                       wyomingworkforce.org

Jim Mcintosh, Administrator
Kathy Emmones, Director Workforce Services
Provides only those services which are necessary for eligible individuals to reach the employment goal agreed to in the Individualized Plan for Employment.

6272   Vocational Rehabilitation, Division of Department of Workforce Services
Suite 1e
1510 East Pershing Blvd.
Cheyenne, WY 82002-1   307-777-7364
                                            866-804-3678
                                       Fax: 307-777-3759
                                       TTY: 307-777-7386
                                         jmcint@state.wy.us
                                       wyomingworkforce.org

Jim McIntosh, Administrator
Joan K. Evans, Director
Lisa M. Osvold, Deputy Director
Provides only those services which are necessary for eligible individuals to reach the employment goal agreed to in the individualized plan for employment.

6273   Wyoming Department of Employment Unemployment Insurance

P.O.Box 2760
100 West Midwest
Casper, WY 82602-2760

307-235-3264
Fax: 307-235-3277
doe.state.wy.us

Randy Hopper, Manager

A combined state/federally funded agency of the state of Wyoming, headed by a Department Director who is appointed by the Governor.

6274   Wyoming Governor's Committee on Employment of the Handicapped

Room 1126
1510 East Pershing Blvd.
Cheyenne, WY 82002-1

307-777-3700
Fax: 307-777-5870
workforceservices@state.wy.us
doe.state.wy.us/Inetclaims

Brenda Oswald, Manager
Joan K. Evans, Director
Lisa M. Osvold, Deputy Director

Assists, empowers and supports people with disabilities to achieve employment, independence and intergration in the workplace and community.

Rehabilitation Facilities, Acute

Alabama

6275 HealthSouth Lakeshore Rehabilitation Hospital
3800 Ridgeway Dr
Birmingham, AL 35209-5599   205-868-2000
                                        Fax: 205-868-2029
                          www.healthsouthlakeshorerehab.com
Vickie Demers, Chief Executive Officer
April Cobb, Chief Nursing Officer
Al Rayburn, Director, Therapy Operations
A 100 bed facility whos key services is physical rehabilitation.
Also specialized services (inpatient) infection isolation room. In
addition, also has outpatient physical rehabilitation and sports
medicine. Patient family support services include patient repre-
sentative, transportation for elderly/handicapped and patient
support groups. Imaging services(diagnostic & theraputic) include ct scanner, diagnostic diagnostic radioisotope facility,
MRI, and ultrasound.

6276 HealthSouth Rehabilitation Hospital of North Alabama
107 Governors Dr
Huntsville, AL 35801   256-535-2300
                                        Fax: 256-428-2608
                              www.healthsouthhuntsville.com
Douglas H. Beverly, Chief Executive Officer
Susan Creekmore, Director, Therapy Operations
Risha Hoover, Director, Marketing Operations
Joy McMinn, Director, Nursing
A comprehensive 50 bed rehabilitation hospital serving the need
of patients in the North Alabama area. Guides patients with physically disabling conditions along an individualized treatment
pathway so they can reach their highest level of physical, social
and emotional well-being. A wide range of medical and
theraputic services are delivered by qualified and experienced
professionals.

6277 J.L. Bedsole/Rotary Rehabilitation Hospital
Infirmary Health
5 Mobile Infirmary Circle
Mobile, AL 36607-3513   251-435-3417
                                         www.infirmaryhealth.org
D. Mark Nix, President & CEO
Kenneth C. Brewington, Chief Medical Office, Mobile Infirmary
Jennifer Eslinger, President, Mobile Infirmary
Provides rehabilitation for patients affected by stroke, spinal
cord injury, brain injury or other neurological illnesses.

6278 More Than Just a Job
Institute On Disability/UCED
60 5th Avenue
Suite 101
New York, NY 10011   212-366-8900
                                        Fax: 603-862-0555
                                            www.forbes.com

6279 Rocky Mountain Resource & Training Institute
3630 Sinton Road
Suite 103
Colorado Springs, CO 80907- 5072   719-444-0268
                                              800-949-4262
                                        Fax: 719-444-0269
                                        TTY: 800-949-4232
                                         www.adainformation.org
Jana Copeland, Principal Investigator
Patrick Going, Senior Advisor
Serves people with disabilities and provides training to the agencies that assist them. Facilitates disabled individuals' transition
from school to adult life; provides information and resources concerning assistive technology, devices, and services; promotes
and ensures compliance with the federal Americans with Disabi-
ities Act (ADA) and other legislation promoting the rights and inclusion of people with disabilities; promotes supported
employment, strategic planning and development.

Arkansas

6280 Central Arkansas Rehab Hospital
2201 Wildwood Ave
Sherwood, AR 72120-5074   501-834-1800
                                        Fax: 501-834-2227
                               www.stvincentrehabhospital.com
Lee Frazier, MPH, Dr, CEO
Dr. Sean Foley, Medical Director
Debbie Taylor, Director of Marketing Operations
Stacy Sawyer, Director Of Therapy Operations
A nonprofit hospital licensed for 69 acute care beds with all private rooms. Opened in 1999the hospital offers a full range of outpatient diagnostic services, including MRI,CT,PET along with
surgical procedures, cardiology, neurology, neurosurgery,
othopedic, rehab and a 24 hour emergency department staffed
with board certified emergency room physicians. Includes an outpatient surgery center, rehabilitation hospital, senior health program, diabetic program and physician offices.

6281 HealthSouth Rehabilitation Hospital
1401 South J St
Fort Smith, AR 72901-5158   479-785-3300
                                        Fax: 479-785-8599
                                          www.healthsouth.com
Juli Stec, CEO
Provides physical rehabilitation as its key services. Also provides other services such as end-of-life services, pain management and an infection isolation room.

6282 Northwest Arkansas Rehabilitation Hospital
153 E Monte Painter Dr
Fayetteville, AR 72703-4002   479-444-2233
                                        Fax: 479-444-2390
                             www.healthsouthfayetteville.com
Marty Hurlbut, Medical Director
Denise Wilson, Director Of Clinical Services
A 60-bed acute medical rehabilitation hospital that offers com-
prehensive inpatient and outpatient rehabilitation services.

6283 Rebsamen Rehabilitation Center
P.O.Box 159
Jacksonville, AR 72078-159   501-985-7000
                                        Fax: 501-985-7384
                             www.rebsamenmedicalcenter.com
Mack McAlister, Chairperson
Murice Green, Vice Chairman
Tommy Swaim, Secretary
Mission is to provide personal healthcare for your family. Vision
is to develop a family of caregivers to become your community
hospital. A 113 bed acute care facility operated by a volunteer
Board of Directors made up of community leaders. Rebsamen
Medical Center is accredited by the Joint Commission on
Accredidation of Healthcare Organizations as well as the Arkan-
sas Department of Health. Through JCAHO we voluntary sumbit
to evaluations of our compliance with nationwide hospital
standards.

Arizona

6284 Barrow Neurological Institute Rehab Center
350 W Thomas Rd
Phoenix, AZ 85013-4409   602-406-3000
                                        Fax: 602-406-4104
                                        www.stjosephs-phx.org
Jackie Aragon, VP Care Management
Linda Hunt, President
Dedicated resources to delivering compassionate, high-quality,
affordable health services; serving and advocating for our sisters
and brothers who are poor and disenfranchised; and partnering
with others in the community to improve the quality of life. Our
vision:a growing and diversified health care ministry distinguished by excellent quality and committed to expanding access
to those in need.

6285 HealthSouth Sports Medicine Center
5111 N Scottsdale Rd
Ste 100
Scottsdale, AZ 85250-7076   480-990-1379
                                          Fax: 480-423-8458
                                          www.healthsouth.com
Troy Meiners, Manager
An out patient facility specialising in sports medicine and treatment of sports injuries.

6286 Healthsouth Rehab Institute of Tucson
2650 N Wyatt Dr
Tucson, AZ 85712-6108   520-325-1300
                                               800-333-8628
                                          Fax: 520-327-4045
                                          www.rehabinstituteoftucson.com
Lee Sanford, Plant Manager
Jon Larson, Medical Director
An accredited member of the Joint Commission On Accreditation of Health Care Organizaions (JCAHO) An 80 bed facility specializing in rehabilitation

6287 Scottsdale Healthcare
9630 E Shea Blvd
Scottsdale, AZ 85260-6285   480-551-5400
                                          Fax: 480-551-5401
                                          preiley@shc.org
                                          www.shc.org
Thomas Sadvary, CEO
Pegg Reiley, Chief Nursing Officer
Kathy Zarubi, Associate VP of Nursing Practice
Lisa Sandoval, Director fo Marketing
A 343 bed full-service hospital providing medical/surgical, critical care, obstetrics, pediatrics, surgery, cardiovascular, and oncology services, as well as the Sleep Disorder Center. All patient rooms are private. Emergency department is a level II Trauma Center. The Radiology Department offers state-of-the-art diagnostic equipment, including MRI, PET/CT scanning, nuclear medicine and ultrasound. Also located are the Piper Surgery Center, Cancer Center, and several medical office plazas.

6288 St. Joseph Hospital and Medical Center
350 W Thomas Rd
Phoenix, AZ 85013-4496   602-406-3000
                                          Fax: 602-406-4190
                                          http://hospitals.dignityhealth.org/stjosephs/
Linda Hunt, President
Rehabilitation programs offered by the clinic assists clients with rehabilitation health needs in the comfort of their own home. The home care rehabilitation team of professionals focuses on correcting deficiencies in self-care, mobility skills and communication. Services offered include physical therapy, occupational therapy, speech pathology, rehabilitative nursing and restorative nursing assistants.

California

6289 Bakersfield Regional Rehabilitation Hospital
5001 Commerce Dr
Bakersfield, CA 93309-648   661-323-5500
                                               800-288-9829
                                          Fax: 661-633-5254
                                          www.healthsouthbakersfield.com
Chris Yoon, Medical Director
Sandra Hegland, Chief Executive Officer
A specialty hospital that treats an array of physical disabilities. It has 60 beds and offers physical rehabilitation services including support groups and education classes on illnesses such as arthritis, asthma and strokes. No surgery facilities on site.

6290 Brotman Medical Center: RehabCare Unit
3828 Delmas Ter
Culver City, CA 90232-6806   310-836-7001
                                          Fax: 310-202-4141
                                          info@brotmanmed.com
Howard Levine, CEO

The mission of Brotman Medical Center is to deliver innovative, quality health care to our patients and their families in an environment of compassion, respect, patient saftey, education, and fiscal responsibility.

6291 Casa Colinas Centers for Rehabilitation
255 E Bonita Ave
Pomona, CA 91767-1923   909-596-7733
                                               866-724-4127
                                          Fax: 909-593-0153
                                          TTY: 909-596-3646
                                          rehab@casacolina.org
                                          www.casacolina.org
Felice Loverso, CEO/President
Steve Norin, Chairman
Stephen W. Graeber, Vice Chairman
Mary Lou Jensen, Secretary
Casa Colina will provide individuals the opportunity to maximize their medical recovery and rehabilitation potential efficiently in an environment that recognizes their uniqueness, dignity and self esteem. The vision is to strategically reposition themselves at the forefront of the post-acute continuum by becoming the center of excellence in the provision of services to persons who can benefit from rehabilitation care.

6292 Community Hospital of Los Gatos Rehabilitation Services
815 Pollard Rd
Los Gatos, CA 95032-1400   408-378-6131
                                          Fax: 408-866-4003
                                          communityhospitallosgatos.com
Ned Borgstrom, CEO
Rehabilitation Services provide individualized treatment programs for inpatient/outpatient care. The team is supervised by a Physiatrist and may include Nurses, Physical Therapists, Occupational Therapists, Speech/Language Therapists, Psychologists, Case Managers, Dietitians, Respiratory Therapists, Recreation Therapists and/or Prosthetists/Orthotists.

6293 Garfield Medical Center
525 N Garfield Ave
Monterey Park, CA 91754-1205   626-573-2222
                                          Fax: 626-571-8972
                                          www.garfieldmedicalcenter.com
Philip Cohen, CEO
Provides quality care to all citizens of all ages. We are foreward looking to meet the changing health care needs of Forsyth and the surrounding area. At the same time, we are a stable organization that is financially sound. We involve all of our medical staff through good communication. We support them by trying to meet their professional needs in training, equipment and services. We emphasize good communication with all county citizens who support us financially and through the use of services

6294 Grossmont Hospital Rehabilition Center
5555 Grossmont Center
La Mesa, CA 91942   619-740-6000
                                               800-827-4277
                                          Fax: 619-644-4159
                                          www.sharp.com
Michael Murphy, President/CEO
Daniel Gross, EVP
It is our mission to improve the health of those we serve with a commitment to excellence in all that we do. Our goal is to offer quality care and programs that set community standards, exceed patients' expectations and are provided in a caring, convenient, cost-effective and accessible manner.

6295 Health South Tustin Rehabilitation Hospita
14851 Yorba St
Tustin, CA 92780-2925   714-832-9200
                                          Fax: 714-508-4550
                                          www.healthsouth.com
Sandra Yule, CEO

6296   Holy Cross Comprehensive Rehabilitation Center
15031 Rinaldi St
Mission Hills, CA   91345-1207   818-365-8051
                                                  888-432-5464
                                             Fax: 818-898-4472
                                             www.providence.org

Larry Bowe, CEO
Derek Berz, COO
Known for providing exceptional treatment through its Cancer
Centers, Heart Center, Orthopedics, Neurosciences and Rehabilitation Services, as well as Woman's and Children's Services. As a
254-bed, not-for-profit facility, Providence offers a full continuum of health services, from outpatient to inpatient to home
health care. Providence operates one of the only round-the-clock
trauma centers in the San Fernando Valley and surrounding
communities.

6297   Job Hunting Tips for the So-Called Handicapped
Special Needs Project
324 State St
Ste H
Santa Barbara, CA   93101-2364   805-962-8087
                                                  800-333-6867
                                             Fax: 805-962-5087
                                             editor@specialneeds.com
                                             www.specialneeds.com
Hod Gray, Owner
This nifty booklet from the guru of job hunting himself is sincere,
useful and brief. *$4.95*

6298   Kentfield Rehabilitation Hospital & Outpatient Center
1125 Sir Francis Drake Blvd
Kentfield, CA   94904-1418   415-456-9680
                                             Fax: 415-485-3563
                                             info@kentfieldrehab.com
                                             www.kentfieldrehab.com
Deborah Doherty, MD
Provides specialized inpatient and outpatient programs. We provide quality services that are patient centered and family-oriented. Under the medical direction of board-certified hospitalists
and other physician specialists, our dedicated interdisciplinary
teams provide a coordinated, comprehensive treatment approach
to a wide range of neurological, orthopedic, pulmonary and
complex medical problems.

6299   Laurel Grove Hospital: Rehab Care Unit
20103 Lake Chabot Rd
Castro Valley, CA   94546-4093   510-537-1234
                                             Fax: 510-727-2778
                                             nissims@sutterhealth.org
                                             www.edenmedcenter.org
George Bischalaney, CEO & President
Kent Myers, Treasurer
Jeffrey Randall, Secretary
David Davini, CPA Chairman
The mission of Eden Medical Center is carried out by our Board
of Directors, employees, physicians and volunteers who are committed to providing our patients and their families with the highest quality medical care and customer service. Creating standards
of excellence to ensure quality and value for our patients. Maintaining a financially sound organization through effective clinical and administrative support. Encouraging a culture that
supports employees and physicians in development.

6300   Lodi Memorial Hospital West
Lodi Memorial Hospital
975 S Fairmont Ave
Lodi, CA   95240   209-334-3411
                                                  800-323-3360
                                             Fax: 209-333-7131
                                             lmh@lodihealth.org
                                             www.lodihealth.org
Joseph Harrington, President
Ron Kreutner, Vice President And CFO
Judy Begley RN, MSN, Chief Nursing Officer
Our vision is to provide a system of health-care services which is
clinically effective, quality driven and community focused in an
environment that supports and encourages excellence. In partner-

ship with our medical staff, we will assume accountability for the
health of our community, be responsible for illness and injury
prevention and provide care for the ill and injured. We will measure our success on quality outcomes and customer satisfaction.

**6301   Long Beach Memorial Medical Center Memorial
         Rehabilitation Hospital**
2801 Atlantic Ave
Long Beach, CA   90806-1701   562-933-2000
                                             Fax: 562-933-9018
                                             www.memorialcare.org
Nissar Syed, Administrator
Barry Arbuckle, President
The hospital offers rehabilitation after catastrophic injury of disabling disease to give patients the opportunity for maximum recovery. The Hospital offers many of the area's finest
rehabilitation specialists and most advanced technology, making
it one of Southern California's most respected rehabilitation
centers.

6302   North Coast Rehabilitation Center
1165 Montgomery Drive
Santa Rosa, CA   95405-4869   707-546-3210
                                             Fax: 707-525-8413
                                             www.santarosamemorial.org
Joyce Cavagnaro, Admissions
Combines state-of-the-art medicine, compassionate care, and the
widest array of resources to enhance your health and promote
healthy communities. Dedicated to continually introducing new
programs and services that help you live life to the fullest.

6303   Northridge Hospital Medical Center
18300 Roscoe Blvd
Northridge, CA   91328   818-885-8500
                                             Fax: 818-885-5435
                                             www.northridgehospital.org
Mike Wall, CEO
dedicating resources to delivering compassionate, high-quality,
affordable health services; serving and advocating for our sisters
and brothers who are poor and disinfranchised; and partnering
with others in the community to improve the quality of life.

6304   PEERS Program
8912 W Olympic Blvd
Beverly Hills, CA   90211-3514   310-553-4833
                                             Fax: 310-553-4833
Paul Berns, Medical Director
Offers a new approach for wheelchair users. PEERS uses a combination of modern physical therapy, the DOUGLAS Reciprocat-
ing Gait System and when necessary, functional electrical
stimulation to assist selected individuals to walk with recently
patented specially made lightweight braces.

6305   PIRS Hotsheet
Placer Independent Resource Services
11768 Atwood Rd
Ste 29
Auburn, CA   95603   530-885-6100
                                                  800-833-8453
                                             Fax: 530-885-3032
                                             TTY: 530-885-0326
                                             lbrewer@pirs.org
                                             pirs.org
Susan Miller, Executive Director
Harry Powell, President
Paul Opper, Vice President
Dawn Davidson, Secretary
Monthly newletter to customers and other constituents.
6 pages Monthly

6306   Providence Holy Cross Medical Center
Providence Health System
15031 Rinaldi St
Mission Hills, CA   91345-1285   818-365-8051
                                                818-898-4603
                                        Fax: 818-365-4472
                                        www.providence.org
Kerry Carmody, CEO
Physicains and nurses are among the best and are recognized nationally for clinical excellence. We are committed to improving your health and wellness as you journey through life. Our services span beyond the latest advancements in medical procedures, equipment and medication to also include education and wellness services-all provided with compassion and respect. We help our patients understand and use some of the healthiest tools at their disposal, including nutrition & excercise.

6307   Queen of Angels/Hollywood Presbyterian Medical Center
1300 N Vermont Ave
Los Angeles, CA   90027-6005   213-413-3000
                                        Fax: 213-413-3500
                                        www.hollywoodpresbyterian.com
Kathy Wong, Manager
A 434 bed acute-care facility that has been caring for the Hollywood community and surrounding areas since 1924. The hospital is committed to serving local multicultural communities with quality medical and nursing care. With more then 500 physicians representing virtually every speciality. Ready to serve your medical needs and those of your loved ones and strive to distinguish itself as a leading healthcare provider, recognized for providing quality, innovative care in a compassionate manner.

6308   Queen of the Valley Hospital
1000 Trancas St
Napa, CA   94558-2941   707-252-4411
                                        Fax: 707-257-4032
                                        www.thequeen.org
Walt Mickens, President
Vincent Morgese, Vice President
For more then 40 years, Queen of the Valley Hospital has been the premiere medical facility in the Napa Valley. Our long history of providing high quality and caring service is founded on 4 core values:Dignity, Service, Excellence and Justice. These central principals inspire us to reach out to those in need and to help heal the whole person-mind, body and spirit.They are the driving force behind our mission to improve the health and quality of life of people in the community we serve.

6309   Rancho Los Amigos National Rehabilitation Center
7601 E Imperial Hwy
Downey, CA   90242-3496   562-401-7111
                                                877-726-2461
                                                888-RAN-CHO1
                                        Fax: 562-401-6690
                                        TTY:562-401-8450
                                        inquiry@rancho.org
                        dhs.lacounty.gov/wps/portal/dhs/rancho
Jorge Orozco, CEO
Mindy Lipson Aisen, Chief Medical Officer
Michelle Sterling, Interim Chief Nursing Officer
Robin Bayus, CFO
Internationally renowned in the field of medical rehabilitation, consistently ranked in the top Rehabilitation Hospitals in the United States by U.S. News and World Report. It is one of the largest comprehensive rehabilitaion centers in the United States. Licensed for 395 beds, providing service through over 20 centers of excellence.

6310   San Joaquin Valley Rehabilitation Hospital
7173 N Sharon Ave
Fresno, CA   93720-3329   559-436-3600
                                        Fax: 559-436-3606
                                        sjvrehab.com
Edward Palacios, CEO
Complete comprehensive rehabilitation services from acute rehab, outpatient and community fitness services.

6311   Santa Clara Valley Medical Center
County of Santa Clara
751 S Bascom Ave
San Jose, CA   95128-2699   408-885-5000
                                        www.scvmed.org
Paul E. Lorenz, CEO
Jeffrey Arnold, Medical Officer
Trudy Johnson, Director of Patient Care Services & Nursing
Carolyn Brown, Director of Quality & Patient Safety
The mission of the medical center is to provide high-quality, cost-effective medical care to all residence of Santa Clara County regardless of their ability to pay. Make availiable a wide range of inpatient, outpatient, emergency services within resource constraints. Maintain an environment within which the needs of our patients are paramount and where patients, their families and all our visitors are treated in a compassionate, supportive, friendly, and dignified manner.

6312   Scripps Memorial Hospital at La Jolla
9888 Genesee Ave
La Jolla, CA   92037-1205   858-626-4123
                                                800-727-4777
                                        Fax: 858-626-6122
                                        www.scripps.org
Sean A Deitch, President/CEO
Gary Fybel, Executive Director/Administrator
One of the county's 6 designated trauma centers, offers a wide range of clinical and surgical services including 24-hour emergency services; intensive care; interventional cardiology and radiology; radiation oncology; cardiothoracic and orthopedic services; neurology; ophthalmology; and mental health and psychology services.

6313   South Coast Medical Center
12 Mason
Ste A
Irvine, CA   92618-2733   714-669-4446
                                        Fax: 714-669-4448
                                        info@southcoastmedcenter.com
Leigh Erin Connealy, Manager
Bruce Christian, President
A 208 bed acute care hospital. Services include maternity, surgical, subacute care, psychiatric program, eating disorder treatment, chemical dependency treatment, radiology, ICU/CCU, comprehensive rehabilitation services, bariatric surgery and movement disorders program..

6314   St. Joseph Rehabilitation Center
St. Joseph Health System
2200 Harrison Ave
Eureka, CA   95501-3215   707-441-4414
                                        Fax: 707-441-4429
                                        www.stjosepheureka.org

6315   St. Jude Brain Injury Network
St. Jude Hospital
130 W Bastanchury Rd
Fullerton, CA   92835-1058   714-446-5626
                                                866-785-8332
                                        Fax: 714-446-5979
                                        ocrcuser@stjoe.org
                                        www.tbioc.org
Jana Gable, Program Coordinator
David Bogdan, Service Coordinator
Lina Marroquin, Servicer Coordinator
Provides comprehensive planning, program referral, assists with funding possibilities, and interagency coordination of services. Areas of emphasis include day treatment, vocational and housing options, and the requirements are adults who have suffered a brain injury from an external force.

6316   St. Jude Medical Center
101 E Valencia Mesa Dr
Fullerton, CA   92835-3809   714-871-3280
                                                800-627-8106
                                        Fax: 714-992-3029
                                        stjudemedicalcenter.org
Robert Fraschetti, President

633

We are one of Southern California's most respected and technologically advanced hospitals, and our four core values: dignity, excellence, service and justice are the guiding principles for everything we do. St. Jude is synonymous with exceptional care that extends beyond good medicine to a commitment to caring for you - mind, body and spirit.

6317 St. Mary Medical Center
1050 Linden Ave
Long Beach, CA 90813-3393   562-491-9000
Fax: 562-491-9053
www.stmarymedicalcenter.org
Chris Desicco, CEO

6318 Sunnyside Nursing Center
22617 S Vermont Ave
Torrance, CA 90502-2595   310-320-4130
Fax: 310-212-3232
businessdevelopment@sunnysidenursing.com
www.sunnysidenursing.com
Shane Dahl, Administrator
Manny Cordero, Director of Nursing
El Sayad, Medical Director
Skilled nursing care facility; residential care facility; intermediate care facility; specialty hospital.

6319 UCLA Medical Center: Department of Anesthesiology, Acute Pain Services
U CL A Medical Center
1245 16th Street Medical Plz
Ste 225
Santa Monica, CA 90404   310-794-1841
Fax: 310-794-1511
access@mednet.ucla.edu
Michael Ferrante, Clinical Director
A 337-bed acute-care medical center, has been serving the healthcare needs of West Los Angeles and Santa Monica since 1926. Highly regarded for its primary and specialty care, the medical center features many outstanding clinical programs, including its women's and children's services, emergency services, and family medicine programs.

Colorado

6320 Children's Hospital Rehabilitation Center
University of Colorado Health Sciences Center
1056 E 19th Ave
Denver, CO 80218-1007   303-861-8888
800-624-6553
chipteam.org
Lou Blankenship, CEO
Michael J Farrell, Chief Operating Officer
Helen Martinez, Manager
Private not-for-profit pediatric healthcare network, the hospital is 100 percent dedicated to caring for kids of all ages and stages of growth. That dedication is evident in more then 1000 pediatric specialists and more then 2400 employees. It is also our continual dedication that has placed us at the forefront of research in childhood disease with several nationally and internationally recognized medical programs.

6321 Craig Hospital
3425 S Clarkson St
Englewood, CO 80113-2899   303-789-8000
Fax: 303-789-8214
khosack@craighospital.org
www.craighospital.org
Michael Fordyce, President
Thomas Balazy, Medical Director
Julie Keegan, VP of Finance
Dona Polonsky, VP of Clinical Services
A 93-bed, private, not-for-profit, free-standing, acute care and rehabilitation hospital that provides a comprehensive system of inpatient and outpatient medical care, rehabilitation, neurosurgical rehabilitative care, an equipment company, and long-term follow up services.

6322 HealthSouth Rehabilitation Hospital of Colorado Springs
HealthSouth Corporation
325 S Parkside Dr
Colorado Springs, CO 80910-3134   719-630-8000
Fax: 719-520-0387
www.healthsouthcoloradosprings.com
Steve Schaefer, CEO
A 56 bed rehabilitation hospital, its key services are: cardiology department, physical rehabilitation, and orthopedics department. Accredidted to the Joint Commission on Accreditation of Health Care Organizations (JCAHO)

6323 Mapleton Center
North Broadway & Balsam
Boulder, CO 80301-9130   303-440-2273
Fax: 303-441-0536
pr@bch.org
www.bch.org
David Gehant, President/CEO
Comprehensive inpatient and outpatient rehabilitation services for all age groups. Treatment provided by interdisciplinary teams and staff physicians. CARF accredited in brain injury rehabilitation, pediatric rehabilitation, pain management, work hardening and inpatient rehabilitation.

6324 Mediplex Rehab: Denver
Vibra Health Care
8451 Pearl St
Thornton, CO 80229-4804   303-288-3000
Fax: 303-496-1120
info@vhdenver.com
www.northvalleyrehab.com
Walter Sacckett, CEO
Encompasses the broadest mix of professional talent, the finest technology and a total commitment by our people to deliver the highest quality care today, and well into the future. The services can be divided into 4 main categories: long term Acute Care and rehab. Skilled nursing facility and residential ventilator program. Outpatient services and pain management. Adult and Geriatric inpatient psychiatric services.

Connecticut

6325 Mariner Health Care: Connecticut
23 Liberty Way
Niantic, CT 06357   860-739-4007
Fax: 860-701-2202

District of Columbia

6326 National Rehabilitation Hospital
102 Irving St NW
Washington, DC 20010-2949   202-877-1760
Fax: 202-829-2789
www.nrhrehab.org
Edward Healton, Medical Director
Robert Bunning, Associate Medical Director
A private facility dedicated solely to medical rehabilitation. The hospital offers intensive inpatient programs and full-service outpatient programs.

Florida

6327 Florida Hospital Rehabilitation Center
601 E Rollins St
Orlando, FL 32803-1248   407-303-1527
855-303-3627
Fax: 407-303-7566
fh.web@flhosp.org
www.flhosp.org
Rex Alleyne, President

Florida Hospital Orlando uses the latest technology to treat over 32,000 inpatients and 53,600 outpatients annually. This 881-bed, acute-carecommunity hospital also serves as a major tertiary facility for much of the Southeast, the Caribbean and South America

6328 HealthSouth Regional Rehab Center/Florida
20601 Old Cutler Rd
Miami, FL 33189-2441   305-251-3800
                                        Fax: 305-259-0498
                                        www.healthsouth.com
Murray Rolnick, Medical Director
Elizabeth Izquierdo, Chief Executive Officer
HealthSouth Rehabilitation Hospital of Miami is a member of the HealthSouth Corporation, the nation's largest healthcare services provider. The hospital is accredited by the Joint Commission on Accreditation of Healthcare Organizations (JCAHO) and Commission on Accreditaion of Rehabilitation Facilities (CARF). Services offered include dietary services, occupational therapy, and respitory care.

6329 HealthSouth Rehab Hospital: Largo
901 Clearwater Largo Rd N
Largo, FL 33770-4121   727-586-2999
                                        Fax: 727-588-3404
                                        www.healthsouthlargo.com
Elaine Ebaugh, CEO
Linda Russo, Director, Therapies
A specialty hospital devoted to providing comprehensive medical rehabilitation services. The hospital is licensed as a Comprehensive Medical Rehabilitation Hospital by the state of Florida, and accredited by the Joint Commission on Accreditation of Healthcare Organizations (JCAHO). HealthSouth of Largo is the only free standing Rehabilitation Hospital in the Tampa Bay region, and serves patients of all ages. Provides inpatient medical rehabilitation services as well as outpatient programs.

6330 HealthSouth Sports Medicine & Rehabilitation Center
3280 Ponce De Leon Blvd
Coral Gables, FL 33134-7252   305-444-0909
                                        Fax: 305-444-5760
                                        www.healthsouth.com
Jay Greeney, President
Ray Jaffet, Administrator
Provides specialized medical and therapeutic services designated to help physically disabled individuals reach their optimum level of independence and function by providing inpatient and outpatient comprehensive medical rehabilitation services.

6331 HealthSouth Sports Medicine and Rehabilitation Center
2141 South Highway A1A Alt
Jupiter, FL 33477   561-743-8890
                                        Fax: 561-743-8795
Diane Reiley, Manager
Outpatient orthopedic and sports medicine/physical therapy.

6332 HealthSouth Treasure Coast Rehabilitation Hospital
Health South Corporation of Alabama
1600 37th St
Vero Beach, FL 32960-4863   772-778-2100
                                        Fax: 772-567-7041
                                        www.healthsouthtreasurecoast.com
Jimmy Lockhart, Medical Director
HealthSouth Treasure Coast Rehabilitation Hospital is a 90-bed inpatient comprehensive rehabilitation hospital serving Indian River, St. Lucie, Martin and Okeechobee counties. Outpatient services are available at the hospital and at four other clinics. Therapies include physical, occupational, speech and psychology services.

6333 Manatee Springs Care & Rehabilitation Center
5627 9th St E
Bradenton, FL 34203-6105   941-753-8941
                                        Fax: 941-739-4409
                                        info@manateespringsrehab.com
                                        www.manateespringsrehab.com
Donna Steiermann, Administrator

Skilled rehabilitation facility specializing in PT, OT, speech therapy, aquatic therapy and an indoor pool. Piped oxygen bed for specialized respiratory care. Compassionate end of life care. Some Medicare, private insurance, and Medicaid.

6334 Perry Health Facility
207 Marshall Dr
Perry, FL 32347-1897   850-584-6334
                                        Fax: 850-838-1801
Rebkah Hatch, Administrator
Full rehabilitation team available, Physiatrist, DOR, Psychiatrist, Psychologist, RD, Geriatric Nursing, PT/OT/ST/RT, Orthotiet/Prosthetist. Provider for PPO's & HMO's as well as medicare, private insurance and medicare/medicaid.

6335 Pinecrest Rehabilitation Hospital and Outpatient Centers
Tenet South Florida
5352 Linton Blvd
Delray Beach, FL 33484-6514   561-498-4440
                                            800-283-8326
                                        Fax: 561-495-3103
                                        www.pinecrestrehab.com
Mark Bryan, CEO
Pinecrest Rehabilitation Hospital is a 90 bed, accredited hospital and is comprised of a Specialty Unit, a Neuro Trauma Unit and Joint Replacement Unit. Additional services at Pincrest include six outpatient rehab centers throughout Palm Beach County. The Outpatient Centers each focus on various specialties such as orthopedic and neurological rehab, pain management, cardiac and pulmonary rehab, occupational medicine, Hearing Institute, dizziness and balance and wellness.

6336 Rehabilitation Institute of Sarasota
3251 Proctor Rd
Sarasota, FL 34231-8538   941-921-8796
                                        Fax: 941-922-6228
Stacy Shepherd, Director Clinical Services
a 75-bed hospital that offers individualized medical and theraputic services tailored to patients and clinics for those affected with stroke, multiple sclerosis, Parkinson's, muscular dystrophy and Lou Gehrig's disease (ALS)

6337 Sea Pines Rehabilitation Hospital
101 E Florida Ave
Melbourne, FL 32901-8398   321-984-4600
                                        Fax: 321-727-7440
                                        ellen.lyons-olski@healthsouth.com
                                        www.healthsouthseapines.com
Stuart Miller, Medical Director
Donna Bohdal, Director of Therapy Operations
Denise McGrath, Administrator
A 90-bed facility specializing in rehabilitation of brain and spinal injuries.

6338 Shriners Hospitals for Children: Tampa
12502 USF Pine Dr
Tampa, FL 33612-9411   813-972-2250
                                            813-281-0300
                                        Fax: 813-975-7125
                                        aargiz-lyons@shrinenet.org
                                        www.shrinershq.org/hospitals/tampa
David Ferrell, FACHE
Maureen Maciel, Chief of Staff
Alicia Argis-Lyons, Develpoment Officer
Recognizing that the family plays a vital role in a child's ability to overcome an illness or injury, Shriners Hospitals helps the family provide the support the child needs by involving the family in all aspects of the child's care and recovery. The purpose of all Shriners Hospitals for Children is to provide care to children with orthopedic problems and burn injuries to help them lead fuller, more productive lives.

6339   South Miami Hospital
6200 SW 73rd St
South Miami, FL 33143-4679   786-662-4000
Fax: 786-662-5302
www.baptisthealth.net

Brian E. Keely, CEO
The mission is to improve the health and well-being of individuals, and to promote the sanctity and preservation of life, in the communities we serve. We are committed to maintaining the highest standards of clinical and service excellence, rooted in utmost integrity and moral practice.

6340   St. Anne's Nursing Center
11855 Quail Roost Dr
Miami, FL 33177-3956   305-252-4000
Fax: 305-969-6752
www.catholichealthservices.org

Tony Farinella, Executive Director
Francisco Cruz, Medical Director
Julia Shillingford, Director of Nursing
Provides spacious, comfortable accommodations with ample recreational areas in a beautifully landscaped setting.

6341   St. Anthony's Hospital
1200 7th Ave N
St Petersburg, FL 33705-1388   727-825-1100
www.stanthonys.com

William Ulbricht, President
James McClint, VP
Ron Colaguori, VP Operations
Mary McNally, VP Mission
A not-for-profit, 395-bed hospital established in 1931. St. Anthony's is dedicated to improving the health of the community through community-owned health care that sets the standard for high-quality, compassionate care.

6342   St. Anthony's Rehabilitation Hospital
3487 NW 35th Ave
Lauderdale Lakes, FL 33311-1107   954-485-4023
                                          954-739-6233
www.catholichealthservices.org

Linda Motte, Hospital Administrator
Kathy Torbertsonn, Dir. Rehab.
Provides spacious, comfortable accommodations with ample recreational areas in a beautifully landscaped setting.

6343   St. Catherine's Rehabilitation Hospital and Villa Maria Nursing Center
1050 NE 125th St
North Miami, FL 33161-5805   305-357-1735
                                     305-891-3361
www.catholichealthservices.org

Virginia Irving, Hospital Administrator
Jim Reiss, Executive Director
Greg Hartley, Director Rehab
St. Catherine's Rehabilitation Hospital is a CARF accredited, 60 bed facility offering inpatient and outpatient rehabilitation and medical clinics; including physical, occupational, and speech therapy, neurology, neurodiagnostics, wound care, and hyperbaric medicine. Villa Maria Nursing center is a JCAHO accredited, 212 bed skilled nursing center providing short term nursing and rehabilitation , as well as long term care.

6344   St. John's Nursing Center
3075 NW 35th Ave
Lauderdale Lakes, FL 33311-1107   954-739-6233
Fax: 954-733-9579
www.catholichealthservices.org

Ralph E. Lawson, Chairman
Elizabeth Worley, Vice Chairman
Thomas Marin, Assistant Secretary
Provides spacious, comfortable accommodations with ample recreational areas in a beautifully landscaped setting.

6345   Successful Job Accommodation Strategies
LRP Publications
36- Hiatt Dr
Palm Beach Gardens, FL 33418   561-622-6520
                                        800-341-7874
Fax: 561-622-0757
webmaster@lrp.com
www.lrp.com

Honora McDowell, Product Group Manager
Kenneth Kahn, Chief Executive Officer
This monthly newsletter provides you with quick tips, new accommodation ideas and innovative workplace solutions. You learn the outcomes of the latest cases involving workplace accommodations. *$ 140.00*
12 pages Monthly

6346   Tampa General Rehabilitation Center
1 Tampa General Circle
Tampa, FL 33601-1289   813-844-7000
Fax: 813-844-1477
jstone@tgh.org
tgh.org

Ron Hytoff, President/CEO
Devanand Mangar MD, Vice Chief of Staff
Thomas L. Bernasek MD, Chief of Staff
Offers a full range of inpatient and outpatient programs all aimed at helping patients achieve their full potentials. JCAHO and CARF accredited and V.R. designated center. A wide range of inpatient and outpatient programs are available such as Brain and Spinal Cord Injury Programs, Comprehensive Medical Rehabilitation, Pain Management, Cardiac Rehab, Pediatric Therapy Service, Sleep Disorders, Epilepsy, and Wheelchair Seating.Hosts the Florida Alliance for Assistive Services and Technolgy.

6347   University of Miami: Jackson Memorial Rehabilitation Center
University of Miami
1611 NW 12th Ave
Miami, FL 33136-1005   305-585-6970
Fax: 305-585-6092
info@jhsmiami.org
www.jhsmiami.org

Michael Butler, Chief Medical Officer
An accredited, non-profit, tertiary care hospital and the major teaching facility for the University of Miami School of Medicine. With more then 1,550 beds, Jackson Memorial is a referral center, a magnet for medical research, and home to the Ryder Trauma Center- the only adult and pediatric level 1 trauma center in Miami-Dade County.

6348   Winter Park Memorial Hospital
Florida Hospital
200 N Lakemont Ave
Winter Park, FL 32792-3273   407-646-7000
Fax: 407-646-7639
healthcare@winterparkhospital.com
www.winterparkhospital.com

Ken Bradley, CEO
Offers Acute Rehabilitation.

Georgia

6349   Candler General Hospital: Rehabilitation Unit
5353 Reynolds St
Savannah, GA 31405-6015   912-819-6000
Fax: 912-819-8829
www.sjchs.org/body.cfm?id=383

Paul Hinchey, President/CEO
Special Physical Therapy Services at Candler Outpatient Center: Aquatic therapy, pediatric services, outpaitient neurological rehabilitation program, woman's health therapy, orthotics, and spine specialty

6350 Children's Healthcare of Atlanta at Egleston
1405 Clifton Rd NE
Atlanta, GA 30322-1060   404-785-6000
                                      Fax: 404-315-2158
                                         www.choa.org

Donna Hyland, President/CEO
Ruth Fowler, CFO
Patrick Friars, Chief Children's Physician
Ron Frieson, Chief Public Policy Officer

Rehabilitation Center at Egleston accepts children from birth to age 18 with acute or chronic problems. The length of rehab stay varies for each child according to the determined program of care. The center offers inpatient, outpatient & day rehab programs for comprehensive evaluation & treatment. The program emphasizes the development of the child's abilities & concentrates on helping the family & child compensate for any long-term disabilities. Short term stays require one or two weeks.

6351 Cobb Hospital and Medical Center: Rehab Care Center
3950 Austell Rd
Austell, GA 30106-1121   770-732-5126
                                  generalinfo@wellstar.org
                                        www.wellstar.org

David Anderson, Executive VP
Michael Andrews, Chief Cancer Network Officer
Avril Beckford, Chief Pediatrics Officer

To deliver world class healthcare we equip our healthcare facilities and employees with the best technology, resources and education availiable. To deliver world class healthcare we keep seeking ways to improve the way we deliver care knowing each day holds more miracles, more life, more chances, more compassion, and more opportunities.

6352 HealthSouth Central Georgia Rehabilitation Hospital
3351 Northside Dr
Macon, GA 31210-2587   478-201-6500
                                      Fax: 478-471-6536
                                    www.centralgarehab.com

6353 Specialty Hospital
Floyd Healthcare Resources
304 Turner McCall Blvd SW
Rome, GA 30165-5621   706-509-5000
                                      Fax: 706-802-4175
                                     contactus@floyd.org
                                        www.floyd.org

Kurt Stuenkel, CEO
Dee Russell, Chief Medical Officer

Our mission is to be responsive to the communities we serve with a comprehensive and technologically advanced heal care system commited to the delivery of care that is characterized by continually improving quality, accessability, affordability and personal dignity.

Hawaii

6354 Shriners Hospital for Children: Honolulu
1310 Punahou St
Honolulu, HI 96826-1099   808-941-4466
                                            888-888-6314
                                      Fax: 808-942-8573
                                      jburda@shrinenet.org
                             www.shrinershospitalsforchildren.org
Kenneth Guidera, Chief Medical Officer
Eugene D'Amore, Vice President
Kathy A. Dean, Vice President Human Resources
Sharon Russell, VP Finance & Accounting

One of 22 hospitals across North America that provide excellent, no-cost medical care to children with orthopedic problems and burn industries.

Idaho

6355 Pocatello Regional Medical Center
777 Hospital Way
Pocatello, ID 83201-2797   208-234-6154
                                      Fax: 208-239-3719
                                    robbieo@portmed.org
                                        www.portmed.org

Mark Bukalew, Chairman
John Abreu, VP Finance
Stephen Weeg, Vice-Chairman
David Swindell, Treasurer

Pocatello Regional Medical Center offers 24-hour emergency care, specialized heart services, a dialysis center, a full service rehabilitation unit including transition care, and the Woman's Center For Health including obstetrics.

Illinois

6356 Builders of Skills
515 Busse Hwy
Park Ridge, IL 60068-3154   847-318-0870
                                      Fax: 847-292-0873
                             www.avenuestoindependence.org

Jacqueline Kinmel, Chair
Peg O'herron, Vice Chair
Eric Johnson, Treasurer
Bob Healy, Secretary

Residential setting for hearing-impaired, developmentally disabled adults who are assisted with daily living skills.

6357 Center for Learning
National-Louis University
2840 Sheridan Rd
Evanston, IL 60201-1730   847-256-5150
                                      Fax: 845-256-1057
                                         kadamle@nl.edu

Jerry Dachs, Manager

Psycho-educational evaluations for children, adolescents, and adults. Individualized remedial academic programs, individual counseling

6358 DBTAC-Great Lakes ADA Center
1640 W Roosevelt Road
Room 405
Chicago, IL 60608-1316   312-413-1407
                                            800-949-4232
                                      Fax: 312-413-1856
                                    www.adagreatlakes.org

Robin Jones, Project Director
Glenn Fujiura, PhD, Director of Research and Co-Inve
Claudia Diaz, Associate Project Director
Peter Berg, Project Coordinator for Technica

Provides training, technical assistance and consultation on the rights and resposibilities of indiviualsand entities covered by the ADA. Toll free number for technical assistance and materials provided electronically or via mail at no cost.

6359 Institute of Physical Medicine and Rehabilitation
6501 N Sheridan Rd
Peoria, IL 61614-2932   309-692-8110
                                            800-957-4767
                                      Fax: 309-692-8673
                                            ipmr.org

Lisa Snyder, Medical Director

Comprehensive CARF accredited programs in outpatient medical rehabilitation services. Eight outpatient locations, specialty programs include adult day services, driving evaluations, balance and visual rehabilitation board certified physiatrists.

6360 LaRabida Children's Hospital and Research Center
E 65th At Lake Michigan
Chicago, IL 60649   773-363-6700
                                          Fax: 773-363-9554
                                          pr@larabida.org
                                          www.larabida.org

Brenda Wolf, President/CEO
Dedicated to excellence in caring for children with chronic illness, disabilitiesm or who have been abused, allowing them to achieve their fullest potential through expertise and innovation within the health care and academic communities.

6361 Marianjoy Rehabilitation Hospital and Clinics
26W171 Roosevelt Rd
Wheaton, IL 60187-6078   630-909-8000
                                                 800-462-2366
                                          Fax: 630-909-8001
                                          www.marianjoy.org

Maureen Beal, Chairperson
John Oliverio, Vice Chairman
Kathleen Dvorakk, Treasurer
Thomas A. Keiser, Secretary
Goal at Marianjoy Rehabilitation Hospital is to help you and your family return to the lifestyle you enjoyed before your illness or injury. To meet this goal, we provide you with a dedicated team of experienced professionals to assist you every step of the way.

6362 Rush Copley Medical Center-Rehab Neuro Physical Unit
2040 Ogden Ave
Ste 303
Aurora, IL 60504-7222   630-898-3700
                                                 866-426-7539
                                          Fax: 630-898-3681
                                          clord@rsh.net
                                          www.rushcopley.com

Barry Finn, CEO
Mary Shilkaitis, VP, Patient Care Services
The mission of the medical center and the medical staff is to work together to serve your healthcare needs through excellence in education, technology and a caring touch. Rush-Copley Medical Center will be the leading healthcare provider of the greater Fox Valley area. At Rush-Copley we pride ourselves on providing everyone with extrodinary service.

Indiana

6363 ATTAIN
U S Department of Education/ NI DR R
32 E Washington St
Ste 1400
Indianapolis, IN 46204-3552   317-534-0236
                                                 800-528-8246
Gary Hand, Executive Director
The mission of Attain is to create solutions that enable people with functional limitations to live, learn, work and play in the community of their choice. All will have access to assistive devices. We will do this in partnership with people with functional limitations, families and members of the community through training, system change, services and support, research, dissemination and consumer advocacy.

6364 About Special Kids
7172 Graham Rd
Suite 100
Indianapolis, IN 46250-2879   317-257-8683
                                                 800-964-4746
                                          Fax: 317-251-7488
                                          FamilyNetw@aboutspecialkids.org
                                          www.aboutspecialkids.org

Joe Brubaker, Executive Director
Jane Scott, Director Of Information
Nancy Stone, Project Director
A Parent to Parent organization that works throughout the state of Indiana to answer questions and provide support, information and resources. We are parents and family members of children with special needs and we help other families and professionals

understand the various systems that are encountered related to special needs. Our central office is where parents from the entire state can access information, resources and support.

6365 Clark Memorial Hospital: RehabCare Unit
1220 Missouri Ave
Jeffersonville, IN 47130-3743   812-282-6631
                                          Fax: 812-283-2656
                                          humanresources@clarkmemorial.org
                                          clarkmemorial.org

Martin Padgett, CEO
The mission of Clark Memorial Hospital is to provide superior health services to the people and communities we serve. The vision of Clark Memorial Hospital is to be the best community healh care provider in the United States. We value each individual and work together to explore new ways to improve the quality of life of all. We persue excellence in all we do. We treat all individuals with the same compassion, dignity, and privacy that we want in ourselves.

6366 Developmental Disabilities Planning Council
402 W Washington St
Indianapolis, IN 46204-2855   317-232-7770
                                          Fax: 317-233-3712
                                          gpcpd@gpcpd.org
                                          www.state.in.us/gpcpd

Suellen Jackson-Boner, Executive Director
Christine Dahlberg, Associate Director
Jim Geswein, CFO
Betty Jones, Secretary
The mission of the Indiana Governor's Council is to promote public policy which leads to the independence, productivity and inclusion of people with disabilities in all aspects of society. This mission is accomplished through planning, evaluation, collaboration, education, research and advocacy. The Council is consumer-driven and is charged with determining how the service delivery system in both the public and private sectors can be most responsible to the people with disabilities.

6367 Easter Seals Wayne/Union Counties
P.O.Box 86
Centerville, IN 47330-86   765-855-2482
                                          Fax: 756-855-2482
                                          eastersealswu@comcast.net
                                          eastersealswu.tripod.com

Kathy Stephen, Treasurer
Vickey Allen, President
Leslie Mayl Whitney, Secretary
Helps people discover nature and much more at camps equipped to offer physcial, social and emotional support and fun for campers with physical and/or developmental disabilities.

6368 IN-SOURCE
Indiana Resource Center for Families with Special
1703 S Ironwood Dr
South Bend, IN 46613-3414   574-234-7101
                                                 800-332-4433
                                          Fax: 574-234-7279
                                          insource@insource.org
                                          insource.org

Richard Burden, Executive Director
Scott Carson, Assistant Director
Dory Lawrence, Project Director
Sally Hamburg, Project Director
The mission of IN*SOURCE is to provide parents, families and service providers in Indiana the information and training necessary to assure effective educational programs and appropriate services for children and young adults with disabilities.

6369   Indiana Congress of Parent and Teachers
2525 N Shadeland Ave
Ste D4
Indianapolis, IN   46219-1770   317-357-5881
                                         Fax: 317-357-3751
                                         info@indianapta.org
                                         www.indianapta.org

Sharon Wise, President
Theresa Distelrath, VP
Job Wise, Secretary
Julie Klingenberger, Treasurer
The mission of the Indiana PTA is three-fold: to support and
speak on behalf of children and youth in the schools, community
and before governmental agencies and other organizations that
make decisions affecting children; to assist parents in developing
the skills they need to raise and protect their children; and, to
encorage parent and community involvement in the public
schools of this state and nation.

6370   Indiana Protection and Advocacy Services Commission
4701 N Keystone Ave
Ste 222
Indianapolis, IN   46205-1561   317-722-5555
                                              800-838-1131
                                         Fax: 317-722-5564
                                         dward@ipas.IN.gov
                                         www.in.gov/ipas
Karen Pedevilla, Education and Training Director
IPAS was created in 1977 by state law to protect and advocate the
rights of people with disabilities and its Indiana's federally designated Protection (P&A) system and client assist program. It is an
independent state agency, with receives no state funding and is
independent from all service providers, as required by federal and
state law.

6371   Kokomo Rehabilitation Hospital
829 N Dixon Rd
Kokomo, IN   46901-7709   765-452-6700
                                         Fax: 765-452-7470

Brenda Harry, Admissions Director
a 60 bed facility specializing in rehabilitation services to the people of Indiana.

6372   Memorial Regional Rehabilitation Center
615 N Michigan St
South Bend, IN   46601-1033   574-647-1000
                                         www.qualityoflife.org

6373   Methodist Hospital Rehabilitation Institute
8701 Broadway
Merrillville, IN   46410-7035   219-738-5500
                                         Fax: 219-755-0448
                                         methodisthospitals.org

Ian McFadden, President/CEO
Matthew Doyle, VP & CFO
Wright Alcorn, VP Operations
Michael Davenport, Vp Medical Affairs
Methodist Hospitals, of all the hospitals in Northwest Indiana, attracts the most complex cases across a range of specialties, including stroke, brain tumor, cancer, trauma and high-risk
pregnancy. This is the result of our commitment to providing the
expertise and technology needed to offer the most advanced
clinical care.

6374   NAMI Indiana
P.O.Box 22697
Indianapolis, IN   46222-697   317-925-9399
                                              800-677-6442
                                         Fax: 317-925-9398
                                         info@namiindiana.org
                                         www.namiindiana.org

Marilynn Walker, President
Joshua Sprunger, Executive Director
Linda Williams, Program Coooridnator
Leslie Gay, Office Manager
NAMI Indiana is a non-profit grassroots organization dedicated
to improving the lives of people afflicted by serious and

persistant mental illness. We are dedicated to helping families
through a network of support, education, advocacy, and promotion of research. NAMI's goal is to help establish a system of care
that provides community based services for persons with serious
mental illness, as well as support for them and their families.

6375   Parkview Regional Rehabilitation Center
2200 Randallia Dr
Fort Wayne, IN   46805-4638   260-373-4000
                                              888-480-5151
                                         Fax: 260-373-4288
                                         www.parkview.com

Mike Packnett, President & CEO
Mike Browning, CFO
Rick Henvey, Chief Administrative Officer
Sue Ehinger, President (Parkview & Affiliates)
Provides a full range of inpatient, theraputic services and pro-
grams for patients as young as 3 years of age to the very elderly.
Our accute care rehabilitation center, is well equipped to care for
patients with neurological and orthopedic injuries and diseases.

6376   Programs for Children with Disabilities: Ages 3 through 5
Indiana Department of Education
151 W Ohio St
Indianapolis, IN   46204-1905   317-232-0570
                                              877-851-4106
                                         Fax: 317-232-0589
                                         specialed@doe.in.gov
                                         www.doe.in.gov
Heather Neal, Chief of Staff
The division provides leadership and state-level support for public school gifted and talented (grades K-12) programs and for students with disabilities from ages 3-21. The division ensures that
Indiana, in its compliance with the federal Individuals With Disabilities Education Act, through monitoring of special education
programs, oversight of community and residential programs, provision of mediation and due process rights, and sound fiscal
management.

6377   Programs for Children with Special Health Care Needs
Indiana State Department of Health
2 N Meridian St
Indianapolis, IN   46204-3021   317-233-1325
                                         www.in.gov/isdh/

Sean Keefer, Chief of Staff
The Children's Special Health Care Services (CSHCS) program
provides financial assistance for needed medical treatment to
children with serious and chronic medical conditions to reduce
complications and promote maximum quality of life.

**6378   Programs for Infants and Toddlers with Disabilities: Ages
Birth through 2**
402 W Washington St
Indianapolis, IN   46204-2773   317-232-1144
                                              800-441-7837

6379   Riley Child Development Center
705 Riley Hospital Drive
Rm 5837
Indianapolis, IN 46202-5128   317-274-7819
                                         Fax: 317-944-9760
                                         info@child-dev.com

Cristy James, Communication Coordinator
Riley Hospital for Children is Indiana's only comprehensive children's hospital, with pediatric specialists in evry field of medicine and surgery. Riley is committed to providing the highest
quality health care to children in a compassionate, family-centered environment. Riley is a national leader in cutting edge research and medical education, ensuring health care excellence for
children for generations to come. Riley provides medical care to
all children, regardless of family's ability to pay.

6380 St. Anthony Memorial Hospital: Rehab Unit
301 W Homer St
Michigan City, IN 46360-4358   219-879-8511
                                      Fax: 219-877-1409
                                www.saintanthonymemorial.org
Joseph Allegreti, Board of Directors
Calvin Bellamy, Board of Directors
Saint Anthony Memorial is an acute care hospital located in
Michigan City, primary serving La Porte and Porter Counties in
Indiana as well as Berrien County Michigan.

6381 State Division of Vocational Rehabilitation
402 W Washington St
P O Box 7083
Indianapolis, IN 46207-7083   317-233-4475
                                     800-545-7763
                                Fax: 317-232-6478
                                vrcommission@fssa.in.gov
                                www.state.in.us/fssa
Megan Ornellas, Chief of Staff
Susie Howard, Deputy Chief of Staff

6382 VSA Indiana
Harrison Center for the Arts
1505 N Delaware St
Indianapolis, IN 46202-4466   317-974-4123
                                Fax: 317-974-4124
                                     info@vsai.org
                                     www.vsai.org
Gayle Holtman, President
Linda Wisler, Vice President
Ron Lenz, Chairman of the Board
Bruce Westpahl, Vice Chairman
For over 25 years VSA arts of Indiana has led the movement to
make the arts accessable to people with disabilitites. VSA arts of
Indiana offers a variety of opportunities for people with disabilities of all ages to engage the power of the arts as a means of education, creative self-expression, and personal and professional
growth. As a result, VSA promotes change in public perceptions
and raises public awareness, and advocates for increased
accessability in providing art experiences for all.

Iowa

**6383 Younker Rehabilitation Center of Iowa Methodist Medical
Center**
1776 W Lakes Pkwy
Des Moines, IA 50266   515-241-6161
                                     888-584-6311
                                Fax: 515-241-5137
                                     www.ihs.org
Bill Leaver, President
Kevin Vermeer, EVP
Danny Drake, VP
Kara Dunham, VP Finance
Iowa Health System is the state's first and largest integrated
healthcare system. We are physicians, hospitals, civic leaders and
local volunteers committed to providing the highest possible
quality and the lowest possible cost. We serve over 70 communi-
ties in Iowa, Western Illinois, and Eastern Nebraska.

Kansas

6384 Kansas Rehabilitation Hospital
1504 SW 8th Ave
Topeka, KS 66606-2714   785-235-6600
                                Fax: 785-232-8545
                                www.kansasrehabhospital.com
Mark LeNeave, CEO
Mindy Mitchell, Chief Nursing Officer
A free standing physical rehabilitation hospital located in Topeka
Kansas. Designated to provide a barrier-free access to all treat-
ment and patient service areas. This 79-bed facility offers a total

rehabilitation environment in a warm, caring setting that encourages patient, family and staff interaction.

6385 Mid-America Rehabilitation Hospital HealthSouth
Health South Corporation
5701 W 110th St
Overland Park, KS 66211-2503   913-491-2400
                                Fax: 913-491-1097
                                tiffany.kiehl@healthsouth.com
                                www.midamericarehabhospital.com
Kristen De Hart, CEO
Tiffany Kiehl, Director Marketing/Operations
Paul Matlack, Director Therapy Operations
Damon Parker, Chief Nursing Officer
97 bed Acute Rehab hospital offering full continuum from in-pa-
tient, day treatment and outpatient services for individuals with
physical limitations due to CVA, TBI, SCI, other traumas, joint
replacement, etc.

Kentucky

6386 Cardinal Hill Rehabilitation Hospital
2050 Versailles Rd
Lexington, KY 40504-1499   859-254-5701
                                     800-233-3260
                                Fax: 859-231-1365
                                webmaster@cardinalhill.org
                                www.cardinalhill.org
Kerry Gillihan, CEO
William J. Lester, Medical Director
Russell Travis, Assistant Medical Director
CARF-accredited rehab center provides comprehensive inpatient
and outpatient services in two locations to people with physical
and cognitive disabilities. We provide diagnosis-specific pro-
grams to 100 inpatients, outpatient clinics, outpatient therapies,
pain management and therapeutic pool services. The Pediatric
Center serves children from birth to age 18 years of age.

6387 HealthSouth Rehabilitation of Louisville
1227 Goss Ave
Louisville, KY 40217-1287   270-769-3100
                                Fax: 502-636-0351
                                www.healthsouth.com
Tim Nichol, Manager
Regina Durbin, Administrator
HealthSouth Rehabilitation Hospitals lead the way, consistently
outperforming peers with a unique, intensive approach to rehabilitative care, partnering with every patient to find a treatment plan
that works for them. We offer a wide range of comprehensive rehabilitation programsfor a wide variety of diagnoses. At
HealthSouth, we provide access to independent private practice
physicians, specializing in physical medicine and rehabilitation,
who work in conjunction with HealthSouth's highly qual

6388 Lakeview Rehabilitation Hospital
134 Heartland Dr
Elizabethtown, KY 42701-2778   270-769-3100
                                Fax: 270-769-6870
                                www.healthsouthlakeview.com
Lori Jarboes, CEO
Chris Koford, Medical Director
HealthSouth Rehabilitation Hospitals lead the way, consistently
outperforming peers with a unique, intensive approach to rehabilitative care, partnering with every patient to find a treatment plan
that works for them. We offer a wide range of comprehensive rehabilitation programsfor a wide variety of diagnoses. At
HealthSouth, we provide access to independent private practice
physicians, specializing in physical medicine and rehabilitation,
who work in conjunction with HealthSouth's highly qual

6389 Shriners Hospitals for Children, Lexington
1900 Richmond Rd
Lexington, KY 40502-1204   859-266-2101
                                       800-444-8314
                                  Fax: 859-268-5636
                         Dwallenius@shrinenet.org
                www.shrinershq.org/hospitals/lexington

Warren E. Hopkins, Chairman
Kirk E. Carter, Vice Chairman
Ken R. Dougherty, Treasurer
David E. Hager, Secretary
Shriners Hospitals for Childrenr - Lexington, is a 50-bed pediatric orthopaedic hospital. Our family-centered approach to care is designed to support the whole family during the acute and reconstructive phases of a child's injury. Located in Lexington, Ky., our hospital treats children from all over the country and around the world, and has unique relationships with some of the top hospitals and universities in the world.

Louisiana

6390 HealthSouth Specialty Hospital Of North Louisiana
1401 Ezelle St
Ruston, LA 71270-7218   318-251-3126
                                       800-548-9157
                                  Fax: 318-251-1594
                        mark.rice@lifecare-hospitals.com
                              www.healthsouth.com

Mark Rice, CEO
A 90-bed specialty hospital offering both inpatient and outpatient services. Acute long term care.

6391 Our Lady of Lourdes Rehabilitation Center
4801 Ambassador Caffery Pkwy
Lafayette, LA 70508   337-470-2000
                                  Fax: 318-289-2681
                             info@lourdesrmc.com
                              www.lourdesrmc.com

William Barrow, CEO
Gerald R. Boudreaux, Chairman of the Board
D. Wayne Elmore, Secretary
Our Lady of Lourdes outpatient physical medicine and rehabilitation department is comprprised of a multi-disciplinary team of physical therapists, oppcuptational therapists and speech languare pathologists.

6392 Rehabilitation Center of Lake Charles Memorial Hospital
1701 Oak Park Boulevard
Lake Charles, LA 70601-8911   337-494-3000
                                  Fax: 337-494-2656
                             webmaster@lcmh.com
                                  www.lcmh.com

Dale Shearer, Director
Larry Graham, President/CEO
Ben F. Thompson, MD, Medical Staff President
Ronald Lewis, Jr., Medical Staff President - Elect
Rehabilitation center offering intensive physical, occupational, speech, neuropsychology, recreational therapies along with rehabilitation nursing.

6393 Shriners Hospital for Children-Shreveport
3100 Samford Ave
Shreveport, LA 71103-4239   318-222-5704
                                  Fax: 318-424-7610
                              jburda@shrinenet.org
                www.shrinershospitalsforchildren.org

Richard McCall, Chief of Staff
Phillip Gates, Assistant Chief
An interdisciplinary approach is used in patient care programs to ensure comprehensive care for each patient. The staff includes orthopaedists, pediatricians, nurses, therapists, social workers, child life specialists, and more. The Shreveport Hospital is equipped and staffed to provide care for virtually all pediatric orthopaedic problems, with the exception of acute trauma.

6394 South Louisiana Rehabilitation Hospital
715 W Worthy Rd
Gonzales, LA 70737-3844   225-647-8277
                                  Fax: 225-647-2446
                        sober@powerhouseprograms.com
                          www.powerhouseprograms.com

Cody Gautreux, Executive Director
Tonja Randolph, President
Power House Programs is a male only facility for the treatment of Chemical Dependency/Dual Diagnosis, located in Gonzales, Louisiana. Applicants must have participated in a primary treatment program for substance abuse prior to acceptance. Our program is divided into 3 phases and is staffed by Board Certified Social Workers and Board Certified Substance Abuse Counselors. We provide individual, group and family therapy; plus 12 step meetings in a community setting.

6395 St. Frances Cabrini Hospital: Rehab Unit
St Frances Cabrini Hospital
3330 Masonic Dr
Alexandria, LA 71301-3899   318-487-1122
                                  Fax: 318-448-6822
                          www.christusstfrancescabrini.org

Curman Gaines, Chairperson
Dallas Hixson, Vice Chairperson
CHRISTUS St. Frances Cabrini Hospital is a 265-bed facility located in Alexandria, Louisiana. Employing approximately 1,400 Associates and with a staff of neary 320 physicians, CHRISTUS St. Frances Cabrini Hospital offers a comprehensive array of services providing the highest quality patient care in a compassionate setting.

6396 St. Patrick Hospital: Rehab Unit
524 Doctor Michael Debakey Dr
Lake Charles, LA 70601-5725   337-491-7577
                                       888-722-9355
                                  Fax: 337-430-4284
                              www.christusstpatrick.org

Ellen Jones, CEO
Committed to providing care and service of the highest quality for children and adults, and to ensuring that the basic human rights of expression, decision making and personal dignity are preseved. We are also committed to treating our patients with respect, understanding and Christian love. We realize that this committment involves much more then attending to your medical needs.

6397 Thibodaux Regional Medical Center
602 N Acadia Rd
PO Box 1118
Thibodaux, LA 70301-4847   985-447-5500
                                       800-822-8442
                                  Fax: 985-449-4600
                             info@thibodaux.com
                              www.thibodaux.com

Greg Stock, CEO
Jacob Giardina, Chairman
Andrew Hoffman, Chief of Staff
Mission is to provide the highest quality, most cost effective health care services possible to the people of Thibodaux and surrounding areas. The vision is to be the regional medical center of choice for health care services in the southeast Louisiana by recognizing the value of physicians and employees, committing to quality improvement, partnering with other health care providers, and remaining financially viable in a competitive environment.

Maine

6398 Brewer Rehab and Living Center
74 Parkway S
Brewer, ME 04412-1628   207-989-7300
                                       800-359-7412
                                  Fax: 207-989-4240
                              www.brewerrehab.com

Janet Hope, Executive Director

Brewer Rehab and Living Center accomodates 106 residents. We are located in Brewer, Maine. We have a 24-hour nursing staff and experienced dedicated on-site physical therapists, occupational therapists and speech language pathologists. We have a specialized inpatient program for individuals with brain injury resulting from a traumatic injury or neurological event such as a stroke. We also have a specialized care unit for individuals with Alzheimer's disease and other dementias.

6399   New England Rehabilitation Hospital of Portland
335 Brighton Ave
Portland, ME   04102-2363   207-662-8000
                                        Fax: 207-879-8168
                                   jaye.sewall@healthsouth.com
                                              www.nerhp.org

Elissa Charbonneau, Medical Director
Amy Morse, CEO
Mission is to provide individuals with guidance, education, support, and motivation while helping them achieve maximum independence and function. Our professionals work with the patient and family through a team approach, to establish and implement an individualized rehabilitation plan designed to meet specific patient goals.

Maryland

6400   Mt. Washington Pediatric Hospital
1708 W Rogers Ave
Baltimore, MD   21209-4596   410-578-8600
                                        Fax: 410-466-1715
                                              www.mwph.org

Sheldon Stein, President
Richard Katz, VP, Medical Affairs
Provides inpatient, outpatient and day programs for infants and children with rehabilitation and/or complex medical needs. We are dedicated to maximizing the rehabilitation and development of our patients through the delivery of interdisciplinary services and programs and providing every resource availiable to enable our patients to attain the highest quality of life within their families and their communities.

Massachusetts

6401   New Bedford Rehabilitation Hospital
4499 Acushnet Ave
New Bedford, MA   02745-4707   508-995-6900
                                        Fax: 508-998-8131
                                      www.newbedfordrehab.com

6402   New England Rehabilitation Hospital: Massachusetts
2 Rehabilitation Way
Woburn, MA   01801-6098   781-939-5050
                                        Fax: 781-933-9257
                                      www.newenglandrehab.com

Deniz Ozel, Medical Director
A 168-bed comprehensive inpatient rehabilitation hospital, which includes 2 off-campus satellite units. Offers an array of area outpatient rehabilitation centers. New England Rehabilitation Hospital remains committed to a personal caring approach. The vision is to provide the communities with a complete continuum of acute rehabilitative programs and services.

6403   Shriners Burns Hospital: Boston
51 Blossom St
Boston, MA   02114-2623   617-722-3000
                                              800-255-1916
                                        Fax: 617-523-1684
                                       sberkowitz@shrinenet.org
                               www.shrinershospitalsforchildren.org
Thomas D'Esmond, Administrator
Matthias Donelan, Chief of Staff
Provides treatment for children to their 18th birthday with acute, fresh burns, plastic reconstructive surgery for patients with healed burns, severe scarring and facial deformity. Some

non-burn conditions such as Scalded Skin Syndrome, Cleft Lip, Cleft Palate and purpura fulminians are also treated. Call the Hospital for information. All medical treatment is without cost to the patient, parents, or any third party.

6404   Shriners Hospital Springfield Unit Springfield Unit for Crippled Children
516 Carew St
Springfield, MA   01104-2330   413-787-2000
                                              800-237-5055
                                        Fax: 413-787-2009
                               www.shrinershospitalsforchildren.org
Kenneth Guidera, Chief Medical Officer
Eugene D'Amore, Vice President
Kathy A. Dean, Vice President Human Resources
Sharon Russell, VP Finance & Accounting
Shriners Hospital for Children is fully equipped and staffed to provide care for pediatric orthopaedic conditions and disorders.

Michigan

6405   Covenant Healthcare Rehabilitation Program
1447 N Harrison
Saginaw, MI   48602-4316   989-583-2930
                                        Fax: 989-583-0000
                                      www.covenanthealthcare.com
Spence Maidlow, President
Juli Martin, Program Director
Offers a broad spectrum of programs and services ranging from obstetrics, neonatal and pediatric care, to acute care including cardiology, oncology, surgery and many other services on the leading edge of medicine. All our programs and services exemplify our commitment to providing quality, compassionate care. As a medical facility with more then 700 beds, and a complete range of medical services, Covenant stands ready to meet the healthcare needs of the 15 counties in Michigan we serve.

6406   Farmington Health Care Center
34225 Grand River Ave
Farmington, MI   48335-3440   248-477-7373
                                        Fax: 248-477-2888
Brian Garavaglia, Administrator
Skilled nursing facility specializing in ventilator dependent residents.

6407   Flint Osteopathic Hospital: RehabCare Unit
3921 Beecher Rd
Flint, MI   48532-3602   810-606-5000
                                        Fax: 810-762-2153
                                        TTY:888-633-2368
                                              www.genesys.org
Susan Malone, Program Manager
Joy Finkenbiner, Executive Director
Genesys Health System takes great pride in the fact that we strive to deliver the highest quality health care, in a model healing environment, for the entire continuum of care needed throughout one's life. From birth to the twilight years, and everywhere in between, Genesys is there to get you back to the things you love to do.

6408   Integrated Health Services of Michigan at Clarkston
4800 Clintonville Rd
Clarkston, MI   48346-4297   248-674-0903
                                        Fax: 248-674-3359
                                     donna.cook@fundltc.com
Carol Doll, Admissions Director
Margaret Canny, Administrator
At Clarkston Specialty Healthcare Center, our mission is to deliver personalized care to the members of our community at a time when our support is most needed. We strive to maximize and enhance the quality of life in a compassionate and professional environment.

6409 **St. John Hospital: North Shore**
Ascension Health
26755 Ballard St
Harrison Township, MI 48045-2419   586-465-5501
                                           866-501-3627
                                      Fax: 586-466-5352
                                      webcenter@stjohn.org
                                      www.stjohnprovidence.org

David Sessions, CEO
A 96-bed specialty hospital that provides comprehensive physical medicine and rehabilitation, along with a wide range of medical and surgical services. St. John North Shores Hospital also provides emergency and urgent care, extensive outpatient rehabilitation services, and most ancillary diagnostic services.

Minnesota

6410 **Alinna Health**
800 E 28th St
Minneapolis, MN 55407-3798   612-863-4200
                                     866-880-3550
                                Fax: 612-863-5698
                                sisterkenny@allina.com
                                www.allinahealth.org/ahs/ski.nsf/

Helen Kettner, Nurse-Liaison
Courage Kenny Rehabilitation Institute provides a continuum of rehabilitation services for people with short- and long-term conditions and disabilities in communities throughout Minnesota and western Wisconsin. Our goal is to improve health outcomes, make it easier for clients and families to get the right services for their needs, and reduce costs by preventing complications.

Missouri

6411 **Columbia Regional Hospital: RehabCare Unit**
404 N Keene St
Columbia, MO 65201-6698   573-882-2501
                             Fax: 573-449-7588
                                  www.muhealth.org

James Ross, CEO
Anita Larsen, COO
A medical and physical rehabilitation program serving patients throughout Mid-Missouri with functional deficits due to neurologic, orthopaedic or other medical conditions.

6412 **Jewish Hospital of St. Louis: Department of Rehabilitation**
1 Barnes Jewish Hospital Plz
Saint Louis, MO 63110-1003   314-747-3000
                                     855-925-0631
                                Fax: 314-454-5277
                                     www.barnesjewish.org

Richard Liedweg, President
Mark Krieger, VP/CFO
John Lynch, Chief Medical Officer
Craig D. Schnuck, Chairman
We take exceptional care of people by providing world-class healthcare, delivering care in a compassionate, respectful and responsive way. By advancing medical knowledge and continously improving our practices. By educating current and future generations of healthcare professionals.

6413 **St. Mary's Regional Rehabilitation Center**
201 NW R D Mize Rd
Blue Springs, MO 64014-2513   816-228-5900
                                 Fax: 816-655-5348

Fleury Yelvington, President/CEO
Amy McKay, Executive Director of Nursing
A 143-bed inpatient physical rehabilitation unit offering PT, OT, ST, recreational therapy, psychiatry and all other ancillary services of a full-service hospital. Specialize in orthopedic and neurologic disabilities.

6414 **Three Rivers Health Care**
2620 N Westwood Blvd
Poplar Bluff, MO 63901-3396   573-785-7721
                                      800-582-9533
                                 Fax: 573-686-5388
                                 info@pbrmc.hma-corp.com
                                 www.poplarbluffregional.com

Charles Stewart, Market CEO
Gerald Faircloth, Administrator
Melissa Samuelson, Chief Nursing Officer
Kevin Fowler, CFO
Poplar Bluff Regional Medical Center is a regional medical center with 2 hospital campuses and more then 100 active physicians. The 423-bed facility is the largest medical center in Southeast Missouri and is located in ButlerCounty. With outreach clinics in Bloomfield, Dexter, Malden, Piedmont, and Puxico, Poplar Bluff Regional Medical Center is committed to serving its 6 county region.

Montana

6415 **St. Vincent Hospital and Health Center**
1233 N 30th St
Billings, MT 59101-165   406-657-7000
                            Fax: 406-657-8817
                                 www.svhhc.org

Jason Barker, CEO
Steve Loveless, COO
Joan Thullberry, Chief Nursing Officer
Ron Oldfield, VP Finance
Vision is to be recognized for our vitality, best in class performance and providing easy access to compassionate and trust-worthy healthcare. The healthcare we offer is based on community need. We strive to improve the health status of the community, with a special concern for the poor and those who have limited access to healthcare.

Nebraska

6416 **Madonna Rehabilitation Hospital**
5401 South St
Lincoln, NE 68506-2150   402-489-7102
                                 800-676-5448
                            Fax: 402-483-9406
                                 info@madonna.org
                                 www.madonna.org

Marsha Lommel, CEO
Provides a complete range of inpatient and outpatient rehabilitation for patients of all ages and abilities. Through highly specialized programs and services, Madona offers individualized treatment and support to help every patient.

Nevada

6417 **University Medical Center**
1800 W Charleston Blvd
Las Vegas, NV 89102-2386   702-383-2000
                              Fax: 702-383-2536
                                   feedback@umcsn.com
                                   www.umcsn.com

Brian Brannman, CEO
Lawrence Barnard, Chief Operating Officer
Joan Brookhyser, Chief Medical Officer
Stephanie Merril, Chief Financial Officer
University Medical Center is dedicated to providing the highest level of health care possible by maintaining its ongoing commitment to personal, individualized care for each patient.Through the latest treatment techniques, comfortable surroundings and a dedicated staff, that commitment is expressed every day, in every area of the hospital.

New Hampshire

6418 Head Injury Treatment Program at Dover
307 Plaza Dr
Dover, NH 03820-2455

603-742-2676
Fax: 603-749-5375
www.doverrehab.com

Sue Mills, Program Rep
Jill Bosa, Administrator

A provider of postacute services in the greater New Hampshire Seacost area. We accomodate 112 residents and are licensed by the state of New Hampshire. We employ nearly 150 licensed nurses, therapists, and other healthcare professionals, who strive to provide quality care. The goal of our patient service model is to bridge the gap between hospitalization and home so that recovery and physical functioning are maximized and hospital re-admission is minimized.

6419 Lakeview NeuroRehabilitation Center
244 Highwatch Road
Effingham, NH 03882

603-539-7451
800-473-4221
Fax: 603-539-8815
www.lakeviewsystem.com

Anton Merka, Chairman
Carolyn McDermott, President
Christopher Slover,, Chief Executive Officer
Tina M. Trudel, PhD,, Chief Operating Officer

Residential treatment center serving individuals with neurologic/behavioral disorders. Lakeview serves both children and adults in functionally based program environment. Transistional programs in various group homes also available to clients as they progress in their treatment.

6420 Northeast Rehabilitation Hospital
70 Butler St
Salem, NH 03079-3974

603-893-2900
800-825-7292
Fax: 603-893-1638
TTY: 800-439-2370
webmaster@northeastrehab.com
www.northeastrehab.com

John Prochilo, CEO

NRHN is an organization characterized by the positive and proactive commitment to the delivery of customer centered care. Our employees exemplify our organizational commitment to providing quality rehabilitation services throughout the continuum. NRHN will be prudent with all resources and will take individual and collective responsibility for fiscal health. NRHN will remain a model by which other rehabilitation and post acute networks seek to emulate.

6421 St. Joseph Hospital Rehabilitation
172 Kinsley St
Nashua, NH 03060-3688

603-595-3076
800-210-9000
Fax: 603-595-3635
www.stjosephhospital.com

Judy Grilli, Medical Staff Officer

A comprehensive healthcare system that serves the Greater Nashua area, western New Hampshire and Northern Massachusetts. Our hospital is licensed for 208 beds and includes a Level 2 Trauma Center. In addition to the hospital, St. Joseph Healthcare system also includes a satellite emergency center in Milford, 5 family medical centers, a large network of primary care and specialty physician practices.

New Jersey

6422 Betty Bacharach Rehabilitation Hospital
61 W Jimmie Leeds Rd
Pomona, NJ 08240-9102

609-652-7000
Fax: 609-652-7487
www.bacharach.org

Philip J. Perskie, Esq., Chairman
Roy Goldberg, Vice Chairman
Craig Anmuth, Medical Director
Ross Berlin, Medical Director

Therapists, nurses and other specialists, led by physiatrists - doctors specially trained in the medical practice of physical medicine and rehabilitation.

6423 Children's Specialized Hospital
150 New Providence Rd
Mountainside, NJ 07092-2590

908-259-3330
888-344-5373
Fax: 908-233-4176
jbrooks@childrens-specialized.org
www.childrens-specialized.org

Robin A. Walton, Chairwoman
Margaret M. Pego, First Vice Chairwoman
Steven M. Rosenberg, Esq, Second Vice Chairman
Victoria Wicks, Treasurer

New Jersey's largest comprehensive pediatric rehabilitation hospital, treats children and adolescents from birth through 21 years of age. Programs include spinal dysfunction, brain injury, respiratory, burn, Day Hospital, early intervention, preschool, and cognitive rehabilitation. Locations in Fairwood, Roselle Park, Newark, Toms River and Hamilton

6424 HealthSouth Rehabilitation Hospital
14 Hospital Dr
Toms River, NJ 08755-6402

732-244-3100
Fax: 732-244-7790
www.rehabnj.com/tomsriver/

Patty Ostaszewski, CEO
Joseph Stillo, Medical Director

A comprehensive 131-bed medical rehabilitation hospital dedicated to treating individuals with a variety of physical disabilities resulting from injury and illness. We serve all of New Jersey, Manhattan, and Philiadelphia. Accredited by the Joint Commission on Accredidation of Healthcare Organizations (JCAHO). The mission of the hospital is to get people back to work, to play, to living.

6425 JFK Johnson Rehab Institute
65 James St
Edison, NJ 08820-3947

732-321-7070
Fax: 732-321-0994
jfkjri@solarishs.org
www.njrehab.org

Krishna Urs, Physician
David Brown, Physician

JRI has developed programs in such specialties as stroke rehabilitation, orthopedic programs, fitness, cardiac rehabilitation, women's health, pediatrics and brain injury rehabilitation. We also offer the most sophisticated diagnostic services available.

6426 Kessler Institute for Rehabilitation, Welkind Facility
201 Pleasant Hill Rd
Chester, NJ 07930-2141

973-252-6300
Fax: 973-252-6343
jkment@kessler-rehab.com
kessler-rehab.com

Sue Kida, CEO
Sam Bayoumy, Director of Rehabilitation
Bruce Pomeranz, MD, Medical Director
Norma Glennon, Associate Director of Outpatient Rehabilitation

Set in the rolling hills of Morris County, this 72 bed facility provides specialized services to brain injury patients, including our unique Cognitive Redmediation Program, as well as a full range of stroke, amputee and orthopedic services. Kessler's team of dedicated rehabilitation professionals, including physicians, nurses and therapists, work with each patient to build physical strength, optimize movement, maximize independence, increase cognitive skills and address any other issues.

6427   Mediplex Rehab: Camden
1 Cooper Plz
Camden, NJ   08103-1461   856-342-2300
                                             Fax: 856-342-7979
                                             www.cooperhealth.org

John P. Sheridan, Jr. President/CEO
Adrienne Kirby, Phd, President/CEO
Raymond L. Baraldi, Interim Chief Medical Officer
Celeste Johnson, Administrator
Cooper University Hospital is the leading provider of comprehensive health services, medical education and clinical research in Southern New Jersey and the Delaware Valley. With over 550 physicians in over 75 specialties, Cooper is uniquely equipped to provide an almost unlimited number of medical services. The hospital is committed to excellence in medical education, patient care, and research. Offers training programs to medical students, residents, and nurses in a variety of specialties.

6428   Universal Institute Rehabilitation & Fitness Center
15 Microlab Rd
Ste 101
Livingston, NJ   07039   973-992-8181
                                             800-468-5440
                                             Fax: 973-992-7178
                                             www.uirehab.com

Adam Steinberg, President
Lisa Lasso, Vice President, Chief Financial Officer
Universal institute is a 15,000 square foot, state of the art rehabilitation facility that specializes in neurological disorders such as brain injuries, spinal cord injury, strokes, etc. Services include PT, OT, speech patholgy, cognitive remediation, aqua therapy and EMG biofeedback.

New Mexico

6429   HealthSouth Rehabilitation Center: New Mexico
7000 Jefferson St NE
Albuquerque, NM   87109-4357   505-344-9478
                                             800-293-7226
                                             Fax: 505-345-6722
                                             www.healthsouthnewmexico.com

Sylvia Kelly, CEO
Rocky BigCrane, Director of Plant Operations
Lisa Brower, Director of Therapy Operations
Angela Eaton-Walker, M.D, Medical Director
Our hospital offers highly specialized inpatient rehabilitation services. From hip fractures to joint replacements and stroke to Parkinson's disease - our hospital has the experts, technology and experience to meet your rehabilitation needs.

6430   St. Joseph Rehabilitation Hospital and Outpatient Center
Ardence
505 Elm St NE
Albuquerque, NM   87102-2500   505-727-4700
                                             Fax: 505-727-4793
Janelle Raborn, Administrator/CEO
Sherrie Peterson, Director
A member of the four hospital, St. Joseph healthcare system, this facility provides inpatient and outpatient care for those requiring physical medicine and rehabilitation. Specialty programs include brain injury, stroke, spinal cord, orthopedics, occupational and physical therapies, clinical psychology, speech/language pathology, hand clinic and functional capacity evaluations. The only facility in New Mexico accredited in four areas by the commission on accreditation of rehab facilities.

New York

6431   Burke Rehabilitation Hospital
785 Mamaroneck Ave
White Plains, NY   10605-2523   914-597-2500
                                             888-99 -URKE
                                             Fax: 914-946-0866
                                             web@burke.org
                                             www.burke.org
John Ryan, Executive Director
Mary Beth Walsh, M.D., Executive Medical Director/CEO
Brett Langley, Physician
We provide inpatient and outpatient care for a broad range of neurological, musculoskeletal, cardiac, and pulmonary disabilities caused by disease or injury. Burke treats patients who have suffered a stroke, spinal cord injury, brain injury, amputation, joint replacement, complicated fracture, arthritis, cardiac and pulmonary disease, and neurological disorders. Patients are most frequently transferred to Burke from acute care hospitals once their condition is stable and they are able to partici

6432   Occupational Therapy Strategies and Adaptations for Independent Daily Living
Haworth Press
10 Alice St
Binghamton, NY   13904-1503   607-722-5857
                                             800-429-6784
                                             Fax: 607-722-6362
                                             orders@haworthpress.com
                                             www.tandf.co.uk
186 pages Softcover
ISBN 0-866563-50-4

6433   Rusk Institute of Rehabilitation Medicine
301 East 17th Street
Second Avenue (in the Hospital for
New York, NY   10016-4901   212-263-6034
                                             Fax: 212-263-8510
                                             DevelopmentOffice@nyumc.org
                                             www.med.nyu.edu/rusk
Steven Flanagan, Chairman
Operates under the auspices of the Dept. Of Rehabilitation Medicine of New York University School of Medicine, one of the nations foremost medical schools. The relationship between Rusk and other clinical and research units within the medical center contributes to an environment which provides the optimal rehabilitation setting for patients. Rusk provides patients with access to treatment across a continuum of care depending on their individual medical needs.

6434   Silvercrest Center for Nursing & Rehabilitation
144-45 87th Ave
Briarwood, NY   11435-3109   718-480-4000
                                             800-645-9806
                                             Fax: 718-658-2367
                                             admissions@silvercrest.org
                                             www.silvercrest.org
Andrea Gibbon, Clinical Care Coordinator
Penny Blakely, Unit Manager
The Silvercrest Center for Nursing and Rehabilitation has earned a wide-spread reputatiopn for combing the best in clinical care with the best in nursing care and for making available to its communities the broadest menu of services to ease a patients' path to recovery from hospital to home. The Center is for the treatment of medically complex patients beginning their recovery, for the rehabilitation of patients who need restorative therapy before going home and much more.

6435   Vocational Rehabilitation and Employment
Books on Special Children
PO Box 305
Congers, NY   10920-305   845-638-1236
                                             Fax: 845-638-0847
                                             www.vba.va.gov/bln/vre/
372 pages Hardcover

North Carolina

6436 Horizon Rehabilitation Center
Trans Health Incorporated
3100 Erwin Rd
Durham, NC 27705-4505   919-383-1546
                                          800-541-7750
                                     Fax: 919-383-0862

6437 Integrated Health Services of Durham
Duke University Medical Center
3100 Erwin Rd
Durham, NC 27705-4505   919-383-1546
                                     Fax: 919-383-0862
Aaron Lony, Administrator

6438 Learning Services Corporation
Corporate Office
10 Speen St
Ste 4
Framingham, MA 01701-4661   508-626-3671
                                          888-419-9955
                                     Fax: 866-491-7396
                                     www.learningservices.com
Susan Snow, Director of Admissions
Deb. Braunling-McMorrow, Ph, President and CEO
A licensed postacute rehabilitation program for adults who have
an acquired brain injury. Individuals who are enrolled in the program participate in active, intensive rehabilitation carried out by
a team of neuropsychology, speech/language therapy, physical
therapy, occupational therapy, vocational services, family services and life skills training. Services include residential rehabilitation, home based treatment, day treatment, subacute
rehabilitation and supported living.

Ohio

6439 Columbus Rehab & Subactute
44 S Souder Ave
Columbus, OH 43222-1539   614-228-5900
                                     Fax: 614-228-3989
                                     columbusrehab@extendicare.com
                                     www.columbusrehabskillednursing.com
Kelly Fligor, Administrator
Columbus Rehabilitation and Subacute Institute is a leading provider of long-term skilled nursing care and short-term rehabilitation solutions. Our 120 bed facility offers a full continuum of
services and care focused around each individual in today's
ever-changing healthcare environment.

6440 Great Lakes Regional Rehabilitation Center
3700 Kolbe Rd
Lorain, OH 44053-1611   440-960-3470
                                     Fax: 440-960-4636
Julie Jones, Manager
Provides excellent, innovative and comprehensive rehabilitation
programs to people in our community. Committed to a better quality of life for all individuals, the Rehabilitation Center has grown
to become a regional resource for individuals needing all types of
rehabilitation services.

6441 HCR Health Care Services
1 Seagate
Toledo, OH 43604-1541   419-321-5470
                                          800-736-4427
                                     Fax: 419-252-5543
                                     www.harborfund.net

6442 Heather Hill Rehabilitation Hospital
Heather Hill
12340 Bass Lake Rd
Chardon, OH 44024-8327   440-285-4040
                                          800-423-2972
                                     Fax: 440-285-0946
                                     info@heatherhill.org
Ed Davis, Operations
Donald Goddard, Chief Medical Officer
Individualized treatment programs for adults and adolescents can
participate in and benefit from three-plus hours a day of active
therapy.

**6443 Parma Community General Hospital Acute Rehabilitation
Center**
7007 Powers Blvd
Parma, OH 44129-5437   440-743-3000
                                     Fax: 440-843-4387
                                     www.parmahospital.org
David Nedrich, Chairman
Thomas P. O'Donnell, First Vice Chairman
Nancy E. Hatgas, Second Assistant Treasurer
Alex I. Koler, First Assistant Treasurer
Parma Hospital offers acute and subacute inpatient care includ-
ing specialty centers for heart, cancer, robotic surgery, orthope-
dics, pain management, acute rehabilitation and bariatric care.

6444 Rehabilitation Institute of Ohio at Miami Valley Hospital
1 Wyoming St
Dayton, OH 45409-2793   937-208-8000
                                     TTY: 937-208-2006
                                     www.miamivalleyhospital.com
Vanessa Sandarusi, Executive Director
Anita Marie Greer, Program Manager, Acute Therapy Services
Jessica Hallum, Nurse Manager of the Inpatient Rehabilitation Unit
*Phillip Boarman, Clinical Coordinator for Acute Care Occupa-
tional Therapy and*
The Miami Valley Hospital Rehabilitation Institute of Ohio
(RIO) is one of the largest and most comprehensive rehabilitation
services providers in the United States. RIO offers a full spectrum
of specialized rehabilitation programs delivered by the region's
most experienced rehabilitation experts.

6445 Shriners Burn Institute: Cincinnati Unit
Shriners Hospitals for Children Cincinnati
3229 Burnet Ave
Cincinnati, OH 45229-3095   513-872-6000
                                          800-875-8580
                                     Fax: 513-872-6999
                                     www.shrinershospitalsforchildren.org
Richard Kagan, Chief of Staff
Petra Warner, Assistant Chief of Staff
Tony Lewgood, Interim Administrator
Vanessa Mosley, Development Officer
All the attention and resources are focused on just one kind of pa-
tient-the burn-injured child. Shriners combine excellent clinical
skill, compassionate care, and innovative research, providing
comprehensive pediatric burn care and reconstructive rehabilitation to achieve the best possible outcome for a child that has suffered a burn injury. There is never a charge to the patient or family
for any of the medical care or services provided by the Shriners
Hospitals throughout North America.

6446 St. Francis Health Care Centre
401 N Broadway St
Green Springs, OH 44836-9653   419-639-2626
                                          800-248-2552
                                     Fax: 419-639-6225
                                     www.sfhcc.org
Kim Eicher, CEO
Jane Holmer, Admissions Coordinator
Provides compassionate care for the elderly and physically chal-
lenged. We are a healthcare ministry under the sponsorship of the
Franciscan Sisters of Our Lady of Perpetual Help. As a Catholic
facility. we respectfully offer those we serve, care hope and dig-
nity in a joyful and compassionate manner.

6447 **St. Rita's Medical Center Rehabilitation Services**
730 W Market St
Lima, OH   45801-4602   419-227-3361
                                           800-232-7762
                                     Fax: 419-226-9750

James Reber, CEO
The St. Rita's Inpatient Acute Care Rehabilitation service provides individualized service to you or your family member 7 days a week, wherever you might stay in the hospital. Acute rehabilitation care includes physical, occupational, and speech therapy services. Our goal is to make you as independent as possible before your discarge to home or, when necessary to extended services in other parts of the hospital.

6448 **University of Cincinnati Hospital**
Health Alliance
234 Goodman St
Cincinnati, OH   45219-2316   513-584-1000
                                    Fax: 513-584-7712
                          universityhospital.uchealth.com/

James Kingsbury, President/CEO
University Hospital has an international reputation, bringing thousands of people, from the region and around the world to Cincinnati to receive care from world renowned physicians in state-of-the-art medical facilities.

6449 **Upper Valley Medical/Rehab Services**
3130 N County Road
25-A
Troy, OH   45373-1309   937-440-4000
                                    Fax: 937-440-7337
                                         info@uvmc.com
                                          www.uvmc.com

Rafay Atiq, Director Rehab Services
A not-for-profit health care system serving the health care needs of Miami County and the surrounding area. The health care system features a state-of-the-art acute care hospital which opened in 1998. Comprehensive inpatient and outpatient services are provided with a full compliment of diagnostic and treatment services and behavioral health care programs.

Oklahoma

6450 **Hilcrest Medical Center: Kaiser Rehab Center**
1125 S Trenton Ave
Tulsa, OK   74120-5498   918-579-7100
                                    Fax: 918-579-7110
                                       www.hillcrest.com

Perri Craven, Medical Director
Kaiser Rehabilitation Center offers a wide range of services to help people regain functionality and independence after a debilitating injury or illness. Our approach to rehabilitation is a team approach, bringing the expertise of physicians, therapists, nurses and other health professionals together with patient family to achieve the best possible outcome. Each patient is given an individualized treatment plan that stimulates and challenges them to achieve their maximum potential.

6451 **Jane Phillips Medical Center**
Jane Phillips Medical Center
3500 E Frank Phillips Blvd
Bartlesville, OK   74006-2464   918-333-7200
                                    Fax: 918-331-1360
                                     webmaster@jpmc.org
                                          www.jpmc.org

David Stire, CEO
Mike Moore, CFO
Jane Phillips Health System is sponsored by St. John Health System. This partnership helps our patients by ensuing access to the most sophisticated levels of care availiable in this area. It offers a wide range of services, including general medicine, surgery, cardiopulmonary care, maternal and infant care, cancer treatment, geriatric care, orthopedics, and physical medicine.

6452 **Jim Thorpe Rehabilitation Center at Southwest Medical Center**
Southwest Medical Center
4100 S. Douglas Ave.
Oklahoma City, OK   73109   405-644-5445
                                          800-677-1238
                                    Fax: 405-644-5384
                                    www.integris-health.com

Al Moorad, Medical Director
Provides inpatient rehabilitation for people with head injuries, spinal cord injuries, orthopedic conditions, pain management, neurological diseases, strokes and a variety of diagnoses that stop individuals from being able to take care of themselves independently. Services available include medical direction, physical therapy, social work, occupational therapy, speech therapy, recreational therapy, and aftercare follow-up.

6453 **Mercy Memorial Health Center-Rehab Center**
1011 14th Ave NW
Ardmore, OK   73401-1828   580-223-5400
                                          800-572-1182
                                    Fax: 580-220-6463
                                          www.mercy.net

Jan Shores, Manager
Lynn Britton Britton, President/CEO
Randy Combs, Executive Vice President Strategic Growth
Michael McCurry, Executive Vice President/Chief Operating Officer
A full service tertiary hospital with 176 licensed beds, 913 co-workers and 100 physicians. Four primary care clinics

6454 **St. Anthony Hospital: Rehabilitation Unit**
St. Anthony Hospital
1000 N Lee Ave
Oklahoma City, OK   73102-1036   405-272-7000
                                          800-851-0888
                                    Fax: 405-272-7075
                                    st_anthony@ssmhc.com
                                         www.saintsok.com

S Beaver, President
18 spacious private rooms, each with bathroom, and furnishings designed with patient safety in mind. Horticulture room where patients can work with plants and flowers as part of their rehabilitation. And a residential-style training apartment with fully equipped kitchen, bathroom, and bedroom to make the patient feel more at home.

6455 **Valir Health**
700 NW 7th St
Oklahoma City, OK   73102-1212   405-609-3600
                                          888-898-2080
                                    Fax: 405-605-8638
                                          info@valir.com
                                           www.valir.com

Dirk O'Hara, Principal
Tonya Purvine, Corporate Compliance Officer
Inpatient Rehab Facility including all therapy services serving people who have been injured and had an illness resulting in a decreased level of independence.

Oregon

6456 **Shriners Hospitals for Children: Portland**
3101 SW Sam Jackson Park Rd
Portland, OR   97239-3095   503-241-5090
                                          800-237-5055
                                    Fax: 503-221-3701
                              www.shrinershospitalsforchildren.org

Michael Aiona, Chief of Staff
Craig Patchin, Administrator
Mark Thoreson, Development Officer
Joslyn Davidson, M.D, Anesthesiology
Pediatric orthopedic and plastic surgery; inpatient and outpatient services. No charge for any services provided at the Hospital. Diagnosis, rehabilitation, surgery, sports and recreation for ages 0-18 for people with physical disabilities involving bones, mus-

cles or joints or in need of plastic surgery for burn scars or cleft lip/palate.

Pennsylvania

6457 Allied Services John Heinz Institute of Rehabilitation Medicine
150 Mundy St
MAC III Building, 1st Floor
Wilkes Barre, PA 18702-6830   570-826-3900
Fax: 570-830-2027
tpugh@allied-services.org
www.allied-services.org

Gerald Franceski, Chairman
Thomas Speicher, Vice-Chairman
William Conaboy, CEO
Gregory Basting, VP Medical Affairs
John Heinz Rehab is one of the foremost providers of rehabilitation in the country. Under the supervision of board-certified psychiatrists, a team of highly qualified professionals provides a broad range of specialized services and therapies for inpatients, with speacialized programs in the areas of brain injury, injured worker recovery and pediatrics. John Heinz Rehab is the only CARF accredited program in northeastern Pennsylvania for treatment of brain injury rehabilitation.

6458 Allied Services Rehabilitation Hospital
475 Morgan Hwy
Scranton, PA 18508-2656   570-348-1359
Fax: 570-341-4548
www.allied-services.org

Gerald Franceski, Chairman
Thomas Speicher, Vice-Chairman
William Conaboy, CEO
Gregory Basting, VP Medical Affairs
We are committed to the people of our commuinity, to help them overcome challenges and reach their greatest potential by providing quality care, people-oriented services and comfort. Our approach is a hands-on, people-oriented style which places the physical and emotional needs of those in our care at the center of all we do. Whether in our rehabilitation hospitals, our skilled nursing facilities, or mental health/mental retardation program, we strive to help people reach their potential.

6459 Brighten Place
131 North Main St
Chalfont, PA 18914-245   215-997-7746
Fax: 215-997-2517
brightenplace@enter.net

William Koffros, CEO
A residential brain injury program with the mission to encourage growth and foster independence on an individual level for each resident. We are CARF accredited and provide additional services which include a day program and respite care.

6460 Chestnut Hill Rehabilitation Hospital
8601 Stenton Ave
Wyndmoor, PA 19038-8312   215-233-6200
Fax: 215-233-6879
www.extendedcare.com

Cammi Lubking, Administrator
Chestnut Hill Rehab Hospital is dedicated to meeting patients' physical, emotional, social, and vocational goals. Through innovative programs, sophisticated equipment, and support by specially trained staff members committed to the progress of every patient, Chestnut Hill achieves results.

6461 Doylestown Hospital Rehabilitation Center
595 W State St
Doylestown, PA 18901-2597   215-345-2200
Fax: 215-345-2512
www.dh.org

James Brexler, President and Chief Executive Officer
Eleanor Wilson, RN, MSN, MHA, Vice President, Patient Services/Chief Operating Officer
Dan Upton, Vice President, Chief Financial Officer
Scott S. Levy, MD, Vice President, Chief Medical Officer
The mission of Doylestown Hospital is to provide a responsive healing environment for patients and their families, and to improve the quality of life for all members of our community. We combine the creative energies of Medical Staff, Board, Associates and Volunteers to make Doylestown Hospital a place where each patient and family feels healed and whole, even when disease cannot be cured.

6462 Health Care Solutions
500 Abbott Dr
Ste B
Broomall, PA 19008-4301   610-544-6023
800-451-1671
Fax: 610-544-6035
www.lincare.com

John Byrnes, CEO
Shawn Schabel, President/COO
Develops unique containment programs, offers equipment set-up, patient instruction, patient assessment and equipment usage. Offers clinical services that include oxygen systems, ventilators, aerosol therapy, suction equipment, T.E.N.S. programs, compression pumps, custom orthotics, enteral feeding.

6463 HealthSouth Harmarville Rehabilitation Hospital
P.O.Box 11460
320 Guys Run Road
Pittsburgh, PA 15238-460   412-828-1300
877-937-7342
Fax: 412-828-7705
www.healthsouthharmarville.com

Ken Anthony, Chief Executive Officer
Thomas Franz, M.D., Medical Director
Catherine M. Birk, M.D., Staff Physiatrist
Brian Cicuto, D.O., Staff Physiatrist
A 202-bed facility providing inpatient and outpatient physical medicine and rehabilitation to adults and adolescents in Pennsylvania, West Virginia, Ohio and Maryland.

6464 HealthSouth Nittany Valley Rehabilitation Hospital
Health South of Nittany Valley
550 W College Ave
Pleasant Gap, PA 16823-7401   814-359-3421
800-842-6026
Fax: 814-359-5898
www.nittanyvalleyrehab.com

Richard Allatt, Medical Director
Susan Hartman, CEO
Sara Godwin, CNO
Ann Foster, Therapy Operations Director
Comprehensive inpatient and outpatient facilities. Treatment for symptoms relating to: stroke, head injury, pulmonary disease, orthopedic conditions, neurological disorders, cardiac illnesses and spinal cord injuries. Healthsouth Nittany Valley Rehabilitation Hospital is a part of Healthsouth's national network of more than 2,000 facilities in 50 states.

6465 HealthSouth Rehab Hospital Of Erie
143 E 2nd St
Erie, PA 16507-1501   814-878-1200
800-234-4574
Fax: 814-878-1399
www.healthsoutherie.com

Douglas Grisier, Medical Director
Shelly Mayes, Director of Therapy Operations
An acute inpatient rehabilitation hospital that was founded in 1986. HealthSouth Erie is one of the only rehabilitation hospitals in the country to hold a triple-certification by the Joint Commis-

sion in the areas of Brain Injury, Stroke and Parkinson's disease Rehabilitation.

6466 **HealthSouth Rehabilitation Hospital of Altoona**
2005 Valley View Blvd
Altoona, PA 16602-4548 814-944-3535
800-873-4220
Fax: 814-944-6160
www.healthsouthaltoona.com

Scott Filler, Chief Executive Officer
Paul Sutton, Director Of Clinical Services
Rakesh (Rock Patel, D.O., Medical Director
Mary Gen Boyles, Director of Nursing Services
Inpatient and outpatient physical rehabilitation programs and services.

6467 **Healthsouth Rehabilitation Hospital of Greater Pittsburgh**
2380 McGinley Rd
Monroeville, PA 15146-4400 412-856-2400
Fax: 412-856-9320
www.lifecare-hospitals.com

Mary Lee Dadey, Administrator
Rehabilitation and long-term acute care hospital that treats brain injury, stroke, multiple sclerosis, Parkinson's disease, back and spinal cord injuries, cancer, pulmonary disease, cardiac disease, traumatic and work injuries.

6468 **Healthsouth Rehabilitation Hospital of Mechanicsburg**
175 Lancaster Blvd
Mechanicsburg, PA 17055-3562 717-691-3700
800-933-3831
Fax: 717-697-6524
annette.bates@healthsouth.com
www.healthsouthpa.com

Mark Freeburn, CEO
Annette Bates, Director of Marketing Operations
Jeff Brandenburg, MPT, Director of Therapy Operations
Michael F. Lupinacci, M.D, Medical Director
HealthSouth provides comprehensive rehabilitation and recovery services to patients with stroke, brain injury, hip fracture, medically complex, pulmonary, wound, spinal cord injury, amputation, and other neuro-muscular, and orthopedic impairments. Our primary goal is to provide individualized treatment programs to people requiring physical rehabilitation and medical recovery in order to help patients get back to work, to play, to living.

6469 **Healthsouth Rehabilitation Hospital of York**
1850 Normandie Dr
York, PA 17408-1552 717-767-6941
Fax: 717-767-8776
www.healthsouthyork.com

Sally Arthur, Director of Human Resources
Bruce Sicilia, Medical Director
Elaine Charest, Director of Therapy Operations
Daniel C. DeFalcis, M.D., Associate Medical Director
A 120-bed rehabilitation hospital dedicated to providing advanced, comprehensive services to patients who have suffered head injury, spinal cord injury, stroke, burns, amputation, chronic pain and other neurological and musculoskeletal disorders. HRH of York provides outpatient services in seven locations. Healthsouth is located in York, Pennsylvania, approximately 50 miles north of Baltimore and 25 miles south of Harrisburg.

6470 **Magee Rehabilitation Hospital**
1513 Race St
Philadelphia, PA 19102-1177 215-587-3000
800-966-2433
Fax: 215-568-3736
hskoczen@mageerehab.org
www.mageerehab.org

Jack Carroll, CEO
A not-for-profit health organization which is the home to the nation's first brain injury rehabilitation program to be accredited by the Commission on the Accreditation of Rehabilitation Facilities (CARF) and is one of 14 federally designated Regional Spinal Cord Injury Centers. Our staff and management are committed to restoring the highest level of independence possible to individuals with disabilities.

6471 **Moss Rehabilitation Hospital**
1200 W Tabor Rd
Philadelphia, PA 19141-3099 215-456-9800
Fax: 215-456-9381
www.mossrehab.com

Alberto Esquenazi, Plant Manager
Alberto Esquenazi, MD, Director
Carmen Angles, MD, Director
Cynthia Farrell, DO, Director
The Philadelphia region's major resource for medical rehabilitation since 1959. This 152 bed facility offers comprehensive care to people with broad ranges of conditions, diagnostic laboratories and a multidisciplinary team of rehabilitation professionals.

6472 **Shriners Hospitals for Children, Philadelphia**
Shriners Hospitals for Children
3551 N Broad St
Philadelphia, PA 19140-4131 215-430-4000
800-281-4051
Fax: 215-430-4126
www.shrinershq.org

Alan W. Madsen, Chairman of the Board
John A. Cinotto, 1st Vice President
Dale W. Stauss, 2nd Vice President
Ernest Perilli, Administrator
At Shriners Hospitals for Childrenr - Philadelphia, we provide state-of-the-art medical care for children with spinal cord injuries, as well as a host of orthopaedic and neuromusculoskeletal disorders and diseases

6473 **Shriners Hospitals for Children, Erie**
1645 W 8th St
Erie, PA 16505-5007 814-875-8700
Fax: 814-875-8756
www.shrinershq.org

John Lubahn, Chief of Staff
Charles Walczak, Administrator
The Shriners Hospitals for Children, Erie, is a 30-bed pediatric orthopaedic hospital providing comprehensive orthopaedic care to children at no charge. The hospital is one of 22 Shriners Hospitals throughout North America. The Erie Hospital accepts and treats children with routine and complex orthopaedic and neuromuscular problems, utilizing the latest treatments and technology available in pediatric orthopaedics, resulting in early ambulation and reduced length of stay.

6474 **Shriners Hospitals, Philadelphia Unit, for Crippled Children**
3551 N Broad St
Philadelphia, PA 19140-4105 215-430-4000
Fax: 215-430-4079
www.shrinershq.org/hospitals/philadelphia

Randal Betz, Chief of Staff
Ernest Perilli, Administrator
Provides comprehensive medical, surgical and rehabilitative care for children with orthopaedic conditions and spinal cord injuries. All services are provided at no charge. The hospital is one of 22 located throughout North America. In addition to treating children with routine and complex orthopaedic problems, the Philadelphia hospital provides a comprehensive and individualized rehabilitation program for children and adolescents who have sustained a traumatic injury to their spine.

South Carolina

6475 **Colleton Regional Hospital: RehabCare Unit**
501 Robertson Blvd
Walterboro, SC 29488-5714 843-782-2000
Fax: 843-549-7562
www.colletonmedical.com

Mitchell Mongel, CEO
Colleton Medical Center's 8-bed physical and mental rehabilitation department is the oldest in the Lowcountry and has been serving the community for nearly 20 years. Strives to provide patient-centered care in a family atmosphere. The team includes nurses, physical therapists, occupational therapists, speech therapists, and nutritionists. The typical patient requires rehabilita-

tion following a stroke, spinal injury, close head injury, and orthopedic rehabilitation.

6476 HealthSouth Rehab Hospital: South Carolina
2935 Colonial Dr
Columbia, SC 29203-6811   803-254-7777
                                        Fax: 803-414-1414
                                www.healthsouthcolumbia.com
W. Anthony Jackson, CEO
Lydia Carpenter, Director of Therapy Operations
Devin Troyer, M.D., Medical Director
Luanne Burton, Director of Human Resources
Offers a wide range of specialized medical and therapeutic services designed to help physically disabled individuals reach their optimum level of function and independence.

6477 Shriners Hospitals for Children, Greenville
950 W Faris Rd
Greenville, SC 29605-4255   864-271-3444
                                            866-459-0013
                                        Fax: 864-271-4471
                                    tmcreynolds@shrinenet.org
                            www.shrinershq.org/hospitals/greenville
Randall Romberger, Administrator
Peter Stasikelis, Chief of Staff
Tracy McReynolds,, Development Officer
A 50-bed pediatric orthopaedic hospital providing comprehensive orthopaedic care to children at no charge to their families. The hospital is one of 22 Shriners Hospitals throughout North America. The hospital accepts and treats children with routine and complex orthopaedic problems, utilizing the latest tretments and technology availiable in pediatric orthopaedics, resulting in early ambulatory and reduced length of stay.

Tennessee

6478 Health South Cane Creek Rehabilitation Center
Health South Corporation
180 Mount Pelia Rd
Martin, TN 38237-3812   731-587-4231
                                        Fax: 731-588-1454
                                dayle.unger@healthsouth.com
                            www.healthsouthcanecreek.com
Eric Garrard, CEO
William Eason, Medical Director
Lindsey Box-Rotger, BSN, RN, C, Director of Quality and Risk Management
Cindy Cooper, RN, Director of Case Management
Offers a wide variety of programs and services for patients in need of acute rehabilitation. Programs and services are availiable through inpatient and outpaitent. Thereapy services availiable are physical, occupational, speech, and respiratory.

6479 HealthSouth Chattanooga Rehabilitation Hospital
2412 McCallie Ave
Chattanooga, TN 37404-3398   423-697-9129
                                             800-763-5189
                                        Fax: 423-697-9124
                                www.healthsouthchattanooga.com
Scott Rowe, CEO
Amjad Munir, Medical Director
Karen Jonakin, Director Clinical Services
Offers orthopaedic rehabilitation, stroke rehabilitation, amputee rehabilitation, brain injury program, pain management, ventilator weaning, carpal tunnel screening, low intensity program, oncology program, aquatic therapy, day treatment, burn program and outpatient services.

6480 HealthSouth Rehabilitation Cntr/Tennessee
1282 Union Ave
Memphis, TN 38104-3414   901-722-2000
                                        Fax: 901-729-5171
                                      healthsouthmemphis.com
Tracy Willis, CEO
Toni Wackerfuss, Director of Therapy Operation

An 80-bed acute medical rehabilitation hospital that offers comprehensive inpatient and outpatient rehabilitation services.

6481 James H And Cecile C Quillen Rehabilitation Hospital
2511 Wesley St
Johnson City, TN 37601-1723   423-952-1700
                                             800-235-1994
                                        Fax: 423-283-0906
                                            www.msha.com
Tammy Bishop, Manager
A 60-bed, freestanding comprehensive medical rehabilitation hospital. Full range of outpatient and day treatment, 14-bed traumatic brain injury unit, in ground therapeutic pool, transitional living apartment, outdoor ambulation course. All inpatient and outpatient programs utilize an interdisciplinary team approach designed to improve a patient's physical and cognitive functioning.

6482 Nashville Rehabilitation Hospital
610 Gallatin Ave
Nashville, TN 37206-3225   615-650-2600
                                             800-227-3108
                                        Fax: 615-650-2562
Alan Miller, CEO
Marc Miller, President
A free-standing physical rehabilitation facility offering services to patients on an inpatient and outpatient basis. Programs include CVA, orthopedic, neuromuscular, traumatic brain injury, spinal cord injury, general rehabilitation and Bridges - geriatric psychiatric unit. Intra-disciplinary team approach is utilized to assist patients in obtaining their maximum fuctional level.

6483 Patricia Neal Rehab Center : Ft. Sanders Regional Medical Center
Covenant Health
1901 W Clinch Ave
Knoxville, TN 37916-2307   865-541-1111
                                             800-728-6325
                                        Fax: 865-541-2247
                                          www.patneal.org
J.E. Henry, Co-Chair
David Kugley, Co-Chair
Mary Dillon, M.D., Medical Director, Patricia Neal Rehabilitation Center
Sharon E. Glass, M.D., Stroke Program Director, Patricia Neal Rehabilitation Center
A CARF accredited 73-bed facility, it offers a comprehensive team approach to care. Physical, occupational, recreational, behavioral medicine and speech language therapists work with physiatrists to develop individual plans of care designed to return patients to a normal lifestyle as quickly as possible. In addition, rehabilitation nurses collaborate with specialists to teach self-care techniques and provide education to help patients reach optimal functionality.

6484 Rehabilitation Center Baptist Hospital
137 E Blount Ave
Suite 6-B
Knoxville, TN 37920-1643   865-632-5520

6485 Rehabilitation Center at McFarland Hospital
University Medical Center
500 Park Ave
Lebanon, TN 37087-3721   615-449-0500
                                        Fax: 615-453-7405
                                www.universitymedicalcenter.com
Saad Ehtisham, CEO
Matt Caldwell, Chief Executive Officer
Michael Cherry, Chief Financial Officer
Greg Carda, Chief Operating Officer
An Acute Inpatient Rehab, located on the hospital's second floor. The center has 26 patient rooms, three therapy treatment rooms, a patient dining area, and an 'activities of daily living' area which includes a kitchen/laundry area and a patient apartment, for those individuals who will be returning home.

6486 St. Mary's Medical Center: RehabCare Center
900 E Oak Hill Ave
Knoxville, TN 37917-4505   865-545-7962
                                        Fax: 865-545-8133
                                        www.tennova.com

Jeffrey Ashin, President
Committed to providing individualized and flexable treatment programs designed for individuals who have been disabled by an injury or illness. The primary mission of the RehabCare Center is to help patients achieve basic skills that may allow independent living and working.

6487 Sumner Regional Medical Center
555 Hartsville Pike
Gallatin, TN 37066-2400   615-328-8888
                                        Fax: 615-328-3903
                                        www.mysumnermedical.com

Susan Peach, BSN, MBA, CEO
Kevin Rinks, Chief Financial Officer
Michael S. Herman, Chief Operating Officer
Anne Melton, RN, MSN, Chief Nursing Officer
SRMC operates as a 155-bed healthcare facility and provides quality Gallatin hospital and medical care services in numerous areas, including cancer treatment, cardiac care, same- day surgery, orthopaedics, diagnostics, women's health and rehabilitation services. As the community grows, SRMC strives to continually improve its services and programs to meet the changing needs of its service area.

Texas

6488 Bayshore Medical Center: Rehab
4000 Spencer Hwy
Pasadena, TX 77504-1202   713-359-2000
                                        Fax: 713-359-1283
                                        www.bayshoremedical.com

Dr. Charles Bessire, Board
Jeanna Barnard, FACHE,, CEO
Alice Hopkins Adams, Board
Wilfred J. Broussard, Board
A 345-bed facility, providing the award-winning care for which we have been nationally recoginzed. Members are here to care for the physical and emotional well-being of those who arrive at Bayshore Medical Center often frightned, in pain and perhaps even alone. We offer patients solace and security through constant communication and compassionate listening in the midst of their medical emergencies and surgical or diagnostic procedures. Kindness, empathy & quality are triats that patients trust.

6489 Cecil R Bomhr Rehabilitation Center of Nacogdoches Memorial Hospital
1204 N Mound St
Nacogdoches, TX 75961-4027   936-564-4611
                                        Fax: 936-564-4616
                                        info@nacmem.org
                                        www.nacmem.org
Jerry Whitaker, Chairperson
Larry Walker, M.D., Vice-Chairperson
Lisa King, Secretary
Walter Scott, Board Member
The goal of Nacogdoches Memorial Hospital's rehabilitation services is to assist patients in attaining their highest potential activity level for independent daily living, thereby reducing the number of necessary hospitalizations. Keeping folks healthy and in their homes lowers healthcare costs for all of us.

6490 Covenant Health Systems Owens White Outpatient Rehab Center
9812 Slide Rd
Lubbock, TX 79424-1116   806-725-5627
                                        Fax: 806-723-6009
                                        www.covenanthealth.org

Walt Cathey, Manager
A comprehensive rehabilitation program designed to help patients attain their maximum level of independence following a debilitating stroke, illness or injury. Our fully accredited program features outpatient physical, occupational and speech language therapies, as well as certified athletic trainers and a certified strength and conditioning specialist.

6491 Gonzales Warm Springs Rehabilitation Hospital
200 Memorial Dr
Luling, TX 78648-3213   830-875-8400
                                        Fax: 830-875-5029
                                        www.warmsprings.org

Anthony Misitano, President/CEO
Vonnie Cromwell, Operations Manager
Statewide not-for-profit system of inpatient and outpatient rehabilitation speciality centers. Throughout the communities we serve, the Warm Springs Rehabilitation System offers hope and acts as a catalyst for achieving an optimal quality of life by providing comprehensive physical and/or cogenitive care. Investing resources in educational and recreational programs. Supporting research efforts.

6492 Harris Methodist Fort Worth Hospital Mabee Rehabilitation Center
1301 Pennsylvania Ave
Fort Worth, TX 76104-2122   817-250-2760
                                        866-847-7342
                                        Fax: 814-250-6846
                                        www.texashealth.org

Lillie Biggins, B.S.N., M.S.N, CEO/President
Elaine Nelson, R.N., M.S.N., Chief Nursing Officer
Joseph Prosser, M.D., M.B.A., Chief Medical Officer
Professionals at the Harris Methodist Fort Worth Hospital's Mabee Rehabilitation Center work closely with each patient to develop a specialzed treatment plan for personal achievement. The center offers highly trained clinical staff members and spacious facilities An incredibly wide range of treatment programs and educational services are provided for both inpatient and outpatient needs.

6493 HealthSouth Plano Rehabilitation Hospital
6701 Oakmont Blvd.
Fort Worth, TX 76132-7526   817-370-4700
                                        Fax: 972-423-4293
                                        www.healthsouth.com

Jon F. Hanson, Chairman
John W. Chidsey, Board of director
Donald L. Correll, Board of director
Yvonne M. Curl, Board of director
A 62-bed medical reahabilitation facility serving inpatient and out patient needs in the Northern Dallas area. The team coordinate all aspects of the patient's rehabilitation to maximize results. The overall effort is directed by board-certified physical medicine and rehabilitation physicians who specialize in medical rehabilitation. Whatever the cause of the disability, our services can benefit patients who have functional limitations in such areas as mobility, communication and self care.

6494 HealthSouth Rehab Hospital Of Arlington
3200 Matlock Rd
Arlington, TX 76015-2911   817-468-4000
                                        Fax: 817-468-3055
                                        www.healthsouth.com

Jon F. Hanson, Chairman
John W. Chidsey, Board of director
Donald L. Correll, Board of director
Yvonne M. Curl, Board of director
A modern 65-bed hospital dedicated to providng inpatient programs in a general rehabilitation setting for persons recovering for a disabling injury or illness. As part of our continuum of care, we also offer outpatient therapy, a day program, and individual therapy services. Our goal is to help our patients resume a productive and more meaningful life through appropriate rehabilitative care and restorative nursing in a wellness-oriented environment that promotes healing and functional recovery.

6495 HealthSouth Rehab Hospital Of Austin
1215 Red River St
Austin, TX 78701-1921   512-474-5700
                                     Fax: 512-479-3765
                                     www.healthsouthaustin.com
Duke Saldiver, CEO
Corey Helm Swartz, Director of Therapy Operations
Maria Arizmendez, M.D., Medical Director
Debbie Belcher, Human Resource Director
A comprehensive 83 bed medical rehabilitation hospital serving
the needs of patients in the Central Texas area. The mission is to
promote recovery for persons with disabling conditions by pro-
viding individualized treatment so they can reach the highest
level of physical, social and emotional well-being.

6496 HealthSouth Rehabilitation Center of Humble Texas
19002 McKay Blvd
Humble, TX 77338   281-446-6148
                                     Fax: 281-446-5616
                                     www.healthsouthhumble.com
Angie Simmons, CEO
Mikael Simpson, Director of Therapy Operations
Emile Mathurin, Jr., M.D., Medical Director
Christy Dixon, Human Resources Director
Offers comprehensive rehabilitation services for patients with di-
verse diagnoses. Rehabilitation can be defined as
multidisciplinary therapy designed to increase patient's overall
functioning to a level that meets or exceeds where the patient was
prior to illness or injury or to maximize current level of ability.
The benefits of these services to patients and their families is
invaluable.

6497 HealthSouth Rehabilitation Hospital
6701 Oakmont Blvd
Fort Worth, TX 76132-2957   817-370-4700
                                     Fax: 817-370-4977
                                     www.healthsouthcityview.com
Deborah Hopps, CEO
Mark Bussell, Medical Director
Mark Bussell, M.D., Medical Director
Kenneth Akwar, PharmD, Director of Pharmacy
A 62-bed acute medical rehabilitation hospital that offers com-
prehensive inpatient and outpatient rehabilitation services.

6498 HealthSouth Rehabilitation Hospital of Beaumont
3340 Plaza 10 Dr
Beaumont, TX 77707-2551   409-835-0835
                                     Fax: 409-835-0898
Sam Coco, Director of Therapy Operations
HJ Gaspard, CEO
Linda Smith, M.D., Medical Director
Sam Coco, PT, Director of Therapy Operations
A state of the art freestanding 61-bed comprehensive physical rehabilitation hospital. The hospital is specifically designed to
meet the needs of individuals and their families who have experienced a disabling injury or illness or are recovering from a surgery. An experienced team of physicians, nurses, therapists, treat
conditions and other disorders.

6499 HealthSouth Rehabilitation Institute Of San Antonio (RIOSA)
9119 Cinnamon Hill
San Antonio, TX 78240-5401   210-691-0737
                                     Fax: 210-558-1297
                                     www.hsriosa.com
Scott Butcher, CEO
Richard Senelick, Medical Director
Christine Chesnut, OTR, MPH, Director of Therapy Operations
Linda Hart, LVN, Director of Marketing
HealthSouth Rehabilitation Institute of San Antonio is the largest
free-standing physical rehabilitation hospital in San Antonio and
is proud to enter our 11th year of delivering quality, comprehensive medical rehabilitation in a pristine environment.
HealthSouth annually serves over 1,500 inpatients and more then
20,000 outpatient visits from throughout San Antonio and Mexico. 108-bed hospital has more then 300 personell on staff
providing extensive experience.

6500 Hillcrest Baptist Medical Center: Rehab Care Unit
100 Hillcrest Medical Blvd
Waco, TX 76712-3239   254-202-2000
                                     Fax: 254-202-8975
Fred Walters, President
Jon Ellis, Secretary
A fully accredited 393-bed acute care facility in Waco including a
Level II Trauma Center, Hillcrest Family Health Center, a net-
work of family medicine clinics; and many key services. Hillcrest
is a ministry of Texas Baptists and is one of 7 health care institu-
tions affiliated with the Baptist General Convention of Texas.

6501 Institute for Rehabilitation & Research
1333 Moursund St
Houston, TX 77030-3405   713-942-6159
                                     800-447-3422
                                     Fax: 713-942-5289
                                     tirr.referrals@memorialhermann.org
                                     www.memorialhermann.org
Jeffrey Berliner, Physician
Michelle Pu, Physician
A national center for information, training, research, and technical assistance in independent living. The goal is to extend the
body of knowledge in independent living and to improve the utilization of results of research programs and demonstration projects
in this field. It has developed a variety of strategies for collecting,
synthesizing, and disseminating information related to the field
of independent living.

6502 Midland Memorial Hospital & Medical Center
400 Rosalind Redfern Grover Parkway
Midland, TX 79701-9980   432-685-1111
                                     800-833-2916
                                     russell.meyers@midland-memorial.com
                                     www.midland-memorial.com
J.T. Lent Jr., President
Russell Meyers, CEO
Greg Wright, Board of Directors
Pete Hulder, Board of Directors
The Occupational and Physical Therapy Center is a specialzed
outpatient clinic. The clinic provides a wide variety of rehabilita-
tion services designed to adequately assist you in returning back
to your normal duties. Our highly trained professionals are here
to help you with all your rehabilitation needs.

6503 Navarro Regional Hospital: RehabCare Unit
Navarro Hospital
3201 W State Highway 22
Corsicana, TX 75110-2469   903-654-6800
                                     Fax: 903-654-6955
                                     www.navarrohospital.com
Xavier Villarreal, CEO
Glenda Teri, Chief Nursing Officer
The rehab unit is located on the 4th floor and is designed for individuals who require intense rehab for an injury or disease process
where the goal would be to return home. Our team is committed to
helping individuals return to the highest level of functioning. Our
team consists of physicians, nurses, physical therapist, occupational therapist, speech therapist, social workers, dieticians and
other professionals as needed.

6504 Rebound: Northeast Methodist Hospital
12412 Judson Rd
Live Oak, TX 78233-3255   210-757-7000
                                     Fax: 210-757-5072
Joe Hernandez, Manager
Methodist Healthcare provides quality, comprehensive rehabilitation services for children and adults. Working as a team, rehabilitation professionals help patients define and achieve
individual goals in restoring function and productivity.

6505 Rio Vista Rehabilitation Hospital
1740 Curie Dr
El Paso, TX 79902-2900   915-544-8336
                                     800-999-8392
                                     Fax: 915-544-4838
Gene Miller, Administrator

6506 San Antonio Warm Springs Rehabilitation Hospital
5101 Medical Dr
San Antonio, TX 78229-4801 210-595-2380
Fax: 210-614-0649
www.warmsprings.org

Kurt Meyer, SVP Operations
Rick Marek, VP Post Acute Medical

A statewide not-for-profit system of inpatient and outpatient rehabilitation specialty centers. Warm Springs Rehabilitation System offers hope and acts as a catalyst for achieving an optimal quality of life by providing comprehensive physical and/or cognitive rehabilitative care. Investing resources in educational and recreational programs. Supporting research efforts.

6507 Shannon Medical Center: RehabCare Unit
120 E Harris Ave
San Angelo, TX 76903-5904 325-653-6741
Fax: 325-657-5706
www.shannonhealth.com

Bryan Horner, CEO
Irv Zeitler, VP Medical Affairs
Shane Plymell, Chief financial officer
Gary Gibian, Executive director

Committed to improving the health of our community, using the latest technologies available in the spirit of caring and integrity. Strives to create an environment committed to the values of accountability, service, pride, integrity, respect and excellence. We foster growth toward the highest quality care and customer service and strive for excellent financial performance. We hire and develop the best people to accomplish these tasks.

6508 Shriners Burn Institute: Galveston Unit
815 Market St
Galveston, TX 77550-2725 409-770-6600
Fax: 409-770-6919
www.totalburncare.com

David Herndon, Chief Of Staff
David Ferrell, F.A.C.H.E., Administrator

Providing expert, orthopaedic and burn care to children under 18 regardless of ability to pay.

6509 Shriners Hospitals for Children, Houston
6977 Main St
Houston, TX 77030-3701 713-797-1616
800-853-1240
Fax: 713-797-1029
www.shrinershq.org

David Ferrell, Administrator
Douglas Barnes, Chief of Staff
Melanie Lux, M.D.,, Director
Gloria Gogola, M.D., Doctor

Shriners Hospitals provides at no charge quality pediatric orthopedic serivces to children ages newborn to 18 years old. These services include both outpatient and inpatient needs. Specialties include cerebrel palsy, spina bifida, scoliosis, hand, hip and feet problems. An application is required and may be completed by phone.

6510 South Arlington Medical Center: Rehab Care Unit
3301 Matlock Rd
Arlington, TX 76015-2908 817-472-4849
Fax: 817-472-4946
mca@hcahealthcare.com
www.medicalcenterarlington.com

Patrice Oliver, Manaager

Above all else, we are committed to the care and improvement of human life. In recognition of this committment, we strive to deliver high-quality, cost-effective healthcare in the communities we serve.

6511 South Texas Rehabilitation Hospital
Ernest Health
425 E Alton Gloor Blvd
Brownsville, TX 78526-3361 956-554-6000
Fax: 956-350-6150
www.strh.ernesthealth.com

Christopher Wilson, Medical Director
Jessie Eason, CEO
Mary Valdez, Director of Marketing

STRH was designed for the provision of specialized rehabilitative care, in the only freestanding acute rehabilitation hospital serving Brownsville and the Rio Grande Valley. The hospital provides rehabilitative services for patients with functional deficits as a result of debilitating illnesses or injuries.

6512 St. David's Rehabilitation Center
St. David s Medical Center
621 Radam Lane
Suite 200
Austin, TX 78745-4237 512-447-1083
Fax: 512-447-1338
www.stdavids.com

Anisa Godinez, Medical Director
Everett Heinze, MD Neurology, Medical Director
Tom Hill, MD, Medical Director
Albert Horn, MD, Medical Director

Mission is to provide exceptional care to every patient every day with a spirit of warmth, friendliness and personal pride. Values are integrity, compassion, accountability, respect and excellence.

6513 Texas NeuroRehab Center
1106 W Dittmar Rd
Austin, TX 78745-6328 512-444-4835
800-252-5151
Fax: 512-462-6749

Alison Crawford Sinsky, Inpatient and Outpatient Manager
Ed Varando, Occupational Therapy Manager

Internationally recognized provider in brain injury/neurobehavioral treatment for children, adolescents, and adults with complex medical, physical and/or behavioral issues. Medical rehabilitation, neurobehavioral, and neuropsychiatric programs combine traditional therapies with education, vocational, substance abuse, and sensory integration services.

6514 Texas Specialty Hospital at Dallas
7955 Harry Hines Blvd
Dallas, TX 75235-3305 214-637-0000
Robin Burns, CEO
66 beds offering active/acute rehabilitation, brain injury day treatment, cognitive rehabilitation, complex care, extended rehabilitation and short term evaluation.

6515 Touchstone Neurorecovery Center
Nexus Health Systems
9297 Wahrenberger Rd
Conroe, TX 77304-2441 936-788-7770
800-414-4824
Fax: 936-788-7785
tncinfo@nhsltd.com
www.touchstoneneuro.com

John W. Cassidy, MD, Executive Medical Director
Jude Theriot, MD, Medical Director
Ron Tintner, MD, Associate Clinical Director
Nelson Valena, MD, Director of Physical Medicine and Rehabilitation

Touchstone provides treatment and rehabilitation in a residential environment on a tranquil, wooded 26-acre site just north of Houston in Conroe, TX. Touchstone offers customized treatment programs designed to help individuals with known or suspected brain injury or neurological deficits progress to their highest functional level possible. Touchstone offers both on-campus and off-campus housing in home-like settings for residents based on their needs.

6516   Valley Regional Medical Center: RehabCare Unit
100A E Alton Gloor Blvd
Brownsville, TX   78526-3328   956-350-7000
                                            Fax: 956-350-7111
                                    www.valleyregionalmedicalcenter.com
Billy Bradford Jr.,, Chair
Francisco Javier Del Castillo, M, Vice Chair
Subramaniam Anandasivam, MD, Board
Christopher Olson, MD, Board
Our mission is to treat our community as family by providing quality compassionate care.

Utah

6517   HealthSouth Rehab Hospital Of Utah
8074 S 1300 E
Sandy, UT   84094-743   801-561-3400
                                                 801-565-6666
                                            Fax: 801-565-6576
                                        www.healthsouthutah.com
Phil Eaton, CEO
William McNutt, Director of Therapy Operations
Mark Rada, M.D., Interim Medical Director
Richard Ashby, Western Regional Director of Plant Operations/Safety Officer
A full spectrum of services, including inpatient, outpatient, day hospital and home health. Holistic patient care, education and community assimilation are the hallmarks of our programs, and evidence of our leadership in the field of rehabilitation. Working together as a team, we are able to tailor the needs of our patients and provide the highest quality services. We believe that education and involvement of family and friends, will assist them in maintaining independence after discharge.

6518   LDS Hospital Rehabilitation Center
8th Ave & C Street
Salt Lake City, UT   84143-0001   801-408-1100
                                                 800-527-1118
                                            Fax: 801-408-5610
                                    contactus@intermountainmail.org
                                    www.intermountainhealthcare.org
Lizz Daley, Administrator
Jim Sheets, Administrator
Located within a Trauma I Center, this facility provides comprehensive inpatient and outpatient rehabilitation to people with physical disabilities. CARF/JCAHO accredited. Low cost family housing is available and Medicaid/Medicare is accepted.

6519   Primary Children's Medical Center
100 Mario Capecchi Dr
Salt Lake City, UT   84113-1100   801-662-1000
                                            Fax: 801-588-2318
                                    www.intermountainhealthcare.org
Scott Parker, President
Kevin Jones, Manager
Ore-Ofe O. Adesina, MD, Ophthalmology
Zeinab A. Afify, MD, Pediatric Hematology Oncology
Primary Children's Medical Center is the pediatric center serving 5 states in the Intermountain West Utah, Idaho, Wyoming, Nevada and Montana. The 289-bed facility is equipped and staffed to treat children with complex illness and injury. PCMC is owned by Intermountain Healthcare, a non-profit health care system. In addition, it is affiliated with the Dept. of Pediatrics, University of Utah, integrating pediatric programs. The hospital is designed to meet the needs of children & their families.

6520   Shriners Hospitals for Children: Intermountain
Fairfax Road at Virginia St
Salt Lake City, UT   84103   801-536-3500
                                                 800-313-3745
                                            Fax: 801-536-3782
                                        www.shrinershq.org
Kevin Martin, Administrator
Jacques D'Astous, Chief of Staff
One of nineteen hospitals in North America specializing in pediatric orthopedics (plus four hospitals providing pediatric burn

treatment). This hospital serves the Intermountain region. All services provided in the hospital are at no cost to family, insurance company, nor state/federal agency regardless of ability to pay.

6521   Stewart Rehabilitation Center: McKay Dee Hospital
4401 Harrison Blvd
Ogden, UT   84403-3195   801-387-2080
                                            Fax: 801-387-7720
                                    www.intermountainhealthcare.org
Corey Anden, Nurse Coordinator
Judy Grover, Manager
With 10 affiliated clinics, McKay-Dee serves northern Utah, and portions of southeast Idaho and western Wyoming. A part of Intermountain Healthcare's system of 21 hospitals, McKay-Dee Hospital Center offers nationally ranked programs such as the Heart & Vascular Institute, the Newborn ICU and a new Cancer Treatment Center.

6522   University Healthcare-Rehabilitation Center
50 N Medical Dr
Salt Lake City, UT   84132-1   801-587-3422
                                                 801-58 -EHAB
                                            Fax: 801-581-2111
                                    www.healthcare.utah.edu/rehab/
David Entwistle, Administrator
Trish Jensen, Program Coordinator
Provides quality, comprehensive, rehabilitation services to persons with complex rehabilitation needs, including spinal cord injuries, head trauma, stroke, and other disabling conditions. Rehabilitation Services has been serving physicians, their patients, and the community since 1965. Rehabilitation Services has been an established leader in comprehensive inpatient, outpatient and home/community rehabilitation programs. Accredited by CARF and JCAHO.

Vermont

6523   Vermont Achievement Center
88 Park St
Rutland, VT   05701-4715   802-775-2395
                                            Fax: 802-773-9656
                                        www.vac-rutland.com
Kiki Mc Shane, CEO
Rebecca Wisell, Administrator
Vermont Achievement Center is recognized as a catalyst in building a community where all people are capable of change. Individuals flourish because they are nutured, valued and treated with respect. Education is empowering. The family is the primary influence in a person's life. Children belong in a family. Families are enhanced by support of the community. Children and family services are flexible and responsive to changing needs.

Virginia

6524   Inova Mount Vernon Hospital Rehabilitation Program
Inova Rehabilitation Center
2501 Parkers Ln
Alexandria, VA   22306-3209   703-664-7000
                                                 800-554-7342
                                            Fax: 703-664-7423
                                        www.inova.com
Barbara Doyle, CEO
Inova Mount Vernon Hospital is a 237-bed hospital offering patients convenience and state-of-the-art care in a community environment. Our hospital sits on 26 acres of beautifully landscaped open space, where patients can find moments of serenity in our specially designed gardens..

6525 Kluge Children's Rehabilitation Center
University of Virginia
2270 Ivy Rd
Charlottesville, VA 22903-4977   434-924-5161
                                        800-627-8596
                                  Fax: 434-924-5559
                          www.healthsystem.virginia.edu
Janet Allaire, Administrator
Richard Stevenson, Research Director
The Kluge Childrens's Rehabilitation Center (KCRC) is a place
dedicated to serving children with special needs. Children be-
tween the ages of birth and 21 come to the KCRC from all over
Virginia, the United States, and even overseas for many reasons.
Some need specific therapy or rehabilitation after injuries, accidents, or surgery. Others have chronic illness such as diabetes,
and cystic fibrosis. Many families come to find out why their
child is experiencing behavior problems.

Washington

**6526 Good Samaritan Healthcare Physical Medicine and
Rehabilitation**
Good Samaritan Hospital
407 14th Ave SE
Puyallup, WA 98372-3770   253-697-4000
                                  Fax: 253-697-5157
                             info@goodsamhealth.org
                                   www.multicare.org
Glenn Kassman, President
Vince Schmitz, CFO
Good Samaritan is part of the Multi-Care Health System, a
non-for-profit medical system serving the growing populations
of Pierce and King Counties in the greater Puget Sound region of
Washington. Our medical staff includes 1,600 of the regions most
respected primary care physicians and specialists.

6527 Northwest Hospital Center for Medical Rehabilitation
1550 N 115th St
Seattle, WA 98133-9733   206-364-0500
                                  Fax: 206-364-0500
                                  TTY:877-694-4677
                                   www.nwhospital.org
Peter Evans, Chairman
Scott L. Hardman, Vice Chairman
James K. Anderson, Board
C W Schneider, CEO
Provides complete medical and surgical services in both inpatient
and outpatient settings. Services across multiple specialties include: 24hr emergency services, critical care, cardiac care, stroke
program, cancer care, childbirth center, rehabilitation center, diagnostic imaging and education and wellness services. Mission is
to raise the long-term health status of our community by providing personalized, quality care with compassion dignity, and
respect.

6528 Providence Medical Center
500 17th Ave
Seattle, WA 98122-5711   206-000-1111
                                  Fax: 206-320-3387
                                   www.providence.org

6529 Providence Rehabilitation Services
Providence Rehabilitation Services
1321 Colby Ave
Everett, WA 98201-1665   425-261-3825
                                  Fax: 425-261-3823
                                   www.providence.org
Jim Phillips, Manager
Leslie Baumgarten, Manager
Continuum of care available: Acute Care, Inpatient Rehabilita-
tion Unit, Transitional Care, Outpatient therapies, and In-home
services.

6530 Shriners Hospitals for Children: Spokane
Shriners Hospitals
911 W 5th Ave
Spokane, WA 99204-2901   509-455-7844
                                  Fax: 509-744-1223
                          www.shrinershq.org/hospitals/spokane
Kristin Monasmith, Public Relations Director
Craig Patchin, Administrator
Paul M. Caskey, M.D., Chief of Staff
Provides pediatric orthopedic services plus burn scar revision to
children birth to 18. All services at no charge to the family.

West Virginia

6531 HealthSouth Mountain View Regional Rehab Hospital
1160 Van Voorhis Rd
Morgantown, WV 26505-3437   304-598-1100
                                        800-388-2451
                                  Fax: 304-598-1103
                          www.healthsouthmountainview.com/
Vicki Demers, Chief Executive Officer
Govind Patel, M.D., Medical Director
Robbin Butler, OTR/L, Director of Therapy Operations
Ginger Dearth, RN, Director of Marketing Operations
A 96-bed inpatient accute rehabilitation hospital. Outpatient ser-
vices, physical, occupational and speech therapy, and interior
therapy pool. Programs include neuro/stroke, brain injury, spinal
cord injury and pediatric.

6532 HealthSouth Western Hills Regional Rehab Hospital
3 Western Hills Dr
Parkersburg, WV 26105-8122   304-420-1392
                                  Fax: 304-420-1374
                             www.healthsouthwesternhills.com
Kalapala Rao, Medical Director
Candace Ross, Director of Human Resources
Greg Holland, Director of Marketing Operations
Michelle Lowers, MS, LSW, Director of Care Management
A 40-bed medical rehabilitation hospital serving inpatient and
outpatient needs in the western West Virginia area. Our hospital is
accredited by the Joint Commission on Accreditation of
Healthcare Organizations (JCAHO) Our mission is to guide patients whtih physically disabling conditions along an individualized treatment pathway so they can reach the highest level of
physical, social and emotional well-being. We strive to provide
the highest quality care for you and your family.

Wisconsin

6533 Extendicare Health Services, Inc.
3540 South 43rd Street
Milwaukee, WI 53220-2903   414-541-1000
                                        800-395-5000
                                  Fax: 414-541-1942
                                   www.extendicare.com
Timothy Lukenda, CEO
Douglas Harris, SVP
David Pearce, Vice President, General Counsel
Sunrise Care Center is a leading provider of long-term skilled
nursing care and short-term rehabilitation solutions. Our 99 bed
facility offers a full continuum of services and care focused
around each individual in today's ever-changing healthcare environment. Our facility is Medicare and Medicaid certified.

6534 St. Catherine's Hospital
9555 76th St
Pleasant Prairie, WI 53158   262-577-8000
                                  Fax: 262-653-5795
                                   www.uhsi.org
Vicki Lewis, Manager
Committed to living out the healing ministries of the
Judeo-Christian faiths by providing exceptional and compas-
sionate healthcare service that promotes the dignity and well-be-
ing of the people we serve.

6535   St. Joseph Hospital
611 Saint Joseph Ave
Marshfield, WI 54449-1898

715-387-1713
Fax: 715-389-3939
sjhweb@stjosephs-marshfield.org
www.ministryhealth.org

Michael Schmidt, CEO
Catherine Olson, Director

A values-driven healthcare delivery network of aligned hospitals, clinics, long-term care facilities, home care agencies, dialysis centers and many other programs and services in Wisconsin and Minnesota.

Wyoming

6536   Spalding Rehabilitation Hospital at Memorial Hospital of Laramie
2301 House Ave
Suite 300
Cheyenne, WY 82001-3748

307-635-4141
800-374-7687
Fax: 307-638-2656
www.imgwy.com

Mitchell Schwarzbach, Executive Director
Tanya Boerkircher, Wyoming Endoscopy Center Manager
Andrea Bailey, Charge Entry Supervisor
Michelle Flanagan, Front Office Supervisor

We are a professional corporation of physicians trained in various medical specialties and subspecialties including Internal Medicine, Gastroenterology and Chest Diseases.It is our mission to provide the highest quality, cost-effective primary and subspecialty medical care, and education to the people of southern Wyoming, western Nebraska, and northern Colorado.

Rehabilitation Facilities, Post-Acute

Alabama

6537 Alabama Department of Rehabilitation Services
602 S Lawrence St
Montgomery, AL 36104-4787
334-293-7500
800-441-7607
Fax: 334-293-7383
www.rehab.alabama.gov

Cary F. Boswell, Commissioner
Anna Taylor
State agency which provides services and assistance to Alabama's children and adults with disabilities.

6538 Briarcliff Nursing Home & Rehab Facility
3201 North Ware Road
McAllen, TX 78501
956-631-5542
Fax: 956-631-5777
http://www.briarcliffnursingcenter.com

6539 Butler Adult Training Center
South Central Alabama Mental Health
680 Hardscramble Rd
Greenville, AL 36037
334-382-2353
Fax: 334-382-9518
www.scamhc.org

6540 Centers for The Developmentally Disabled - North Central Alabama
1602 Church St SE
P.O. Box 2091
Decatur, AL 35602
256-350-1458
Fax: 256-350-1485
info@cddnca.org
www.cddnca.org

Earl Brightwell, Executive Director
CDD NCA provides services and programs for individuals who are mentally and/or physically challenged, or developmentally delayed. These services range from early intervention services for infants and toddlers to residential and employment programs for adults. All services are typically provided at no cost to the individual or their family, regardless of income. Funding sources for the CDD NCA include DMH, United Way, and ADRS.

6541 Cheaha Regional Mental Health Center
351 W 3rd St
Sylacauga, AL 35150
256-245-1340
Fax: 256-245-1343
crmhc.org

Cynthia L. Atkinson, Executive Director
Dr. Shakil Khan, Medical Director
Karen McKinney, Clinical Director, Mental Health Services
Ann Cunningham, Director, Intellectual Disabilities Services
CRMHC provides a continuum of services for persons with intellectual disabilities, serious mental illness and substance abuse in a four county area in east Alabama, which includes Clay, Coosa, Randolph, and Talladega Counties.

6542 Children's Rehabilitation Service - District Office, Montgomery
Alabama Department of Rehabilitation Services
602 S. Lawrence St.
Montgomery, AL 36104
334-293-7500
800-568-9034
Fax: 334-293-7374
www.rehab.alabama.gov

6543 Chilton-Shelby Mental Health Center
110 Medical Center Dr
Calera, AL 35045
205-755-8800
Fax: 205-668-4957
chiltonshelby.org

Melodie D. Crawford, Chief Executive Officer
Vicki M. Potts, Chief Financial Officer
Kathryn T. Crouthers, Chief Operations Officer
Dena Smitherman, Intellectual Disabilities Division Director
Mental health rehabilitation services and more for the recovery of mentally disabled adults. Serves Chilton and Shelby counties.
Business Office Location

6544 Darden Rehabilitation Center
1001 E Broad Street
Ste C
Gadsden, AL 35903-2400
256-547-5751
Fax: 256-547-5761
darden@dardenrehab.org
dardenrehab.org

Lynn Curry, Executive Director
Derek Coburn, Operations Manager
Dana Johnson, Program Coordinator
Lisa Wilson, Executive Assistant
Work adjustment and job placement programs. Serves the counties of Etawah, Marshall, Dekalb, Clair and Cherokee.

6545 Easter Seals Central Alabama
2125 E. South Blvd
Montgomery, AL 36116-2409
334-288-0240
Fax: 334-288-7171
info@eastersealsca.org
www.eastersealscentralalabama.org

Debbie Lynn, Executive Director
Ed Collier, Director, Programs
Sharis LeMay, CNA Instructor
Frankie Thomas, Senior Employment Program
A private, nonprofit organization offering services audiology, physical, occupational, lymphedema and speech therapy, psychological counseling, vocational evaluation and assessment, person, social and work adjustment training, GED preparation, computer service training, job placement and follow-up, and special learning disabilities service and supported employment service.

6546 Easter Seals Northwest Alabama
1450 Avalon Ave
Muscle Shoals, AL 35660-3110
256-391-1110
Fax: 256-314-5105
www.eastersealsnwal.org

Danny Prince, Administrator
John Ives, Chairman
Tommy Hester, Treasurer
Susie White, Secretary
Easter Seals has been helping individuals with disabilities and special needs, and their families live better lives for more then 80 years. From child development centers to physical rehabilitation and job training for people with disabilities, Easter Seals offers a variety of services to help people with disabilities address life's challenges and achieve personal goals.

6547 Easter Seals West Alabama
1110 Dr. Edward Hillard Drive
Tuscaloosa, AL 35401-7446
205-759-1211
800-726-1216
Fax: 205-349-1162
eswa@eswaweb.org
eswaweb.org

Ronny Johnston, Executive Director
Dusty Beam, Administrative Coordinator
Holly Hillard, Director, Development
Leading organization in helping children and adults with disabilities to live with equality, dignity and independence. Rehabilitation services are provided in two divisions: outpatient rehabilitation division (physical therapy, occupational therapy, speech therapy, hearing evaluation, sell and service hearind aids) and vocational division (vocational evaluation and vocational

development). Services are rendered regardless of age, race, sex, color, creed, national origin, veteran's status.

6548   **Easter Seals West Central Alabama Rehabilitation Center**
2906 Citizens Pkwy
P.O. Box 750
Selma, AL   36702-0750   334-872-8421
                                          800-801-4776
                              Fax: 334-872-3907
                              wcarcdw@tomnet.com
                              www.eswcarc.us

6549   **Geer Adult Training Center**
P.O.Box 419
83 South Canaan Road
Canaan, CT   06018-419   860-824-7067
                              Fax: 205-367-8032
                              geercares.org/content/about-geer
Yvonne Williams, Program Coordinator

6550   **Goodwill Easter Seals of the Gulf Coast**
2440 Gordon Smith Dr.
Mobile, AL   36617-2319   251-471-1581
                              info@al.easterseals.com
                              www.gesgc.org
Peter D'Olive, Chairman
Frank Harkins, President & CEO
Bill Dillman, Vice President, Marketing & Development
Vocational, medical, pre-school education, day care, recreation and other support services.

6551   **HealthSouth Corporation**
3660 Grandview Parkway
Ste 200
Birmingham, AL   35243-3332   205-967-7116
                                          800-765-4772
                              Fax: 225-928-0317
                              healthsouth.com
Jacque Shadle, CEO
Derrick Landreneau, Director of Nursing services
Dedicated to one field of medicine - physical rehabilitation medicine - and are committed to one goal, helping patients achieve the highest level of functioning possible after a debilitating injury or illness.

6552   **Indian Rivers Mental Health Center - Bibb**
2439 Main St
Brent, AL   35034   205-926-4681
                              Fax: 205-296-6016
                              www.irmhc.org

6553   **Indian Rivers Mental Health Center - Pickens**
890 Reform St.
Carrollton, AL   35447   205-367-8032
                              Fax: 205-367-9291
                              www.irmhc.org

6554   **Indian Rivers Mental Health Center - Tuscaloosa**
2209 - 9th St
Tuscaloosa, AL   35401   205-391-3131
                              Fax: 205-391-3135
                              http://www.irmhc.org
Barbara Friedman, President
Elizabeth Rice, First Vice President
Services are available to adults who have serious mental illness resulting in personal, family or work-related problems. Counseling may take place in either individual or group settings, identification, evaluation and treatment services are available to persons who experience problems related to alcohol and drug abuse and counseling services are available for children and adolescents who have a severe emotional disturbance causing discipline problems at home and school.

6555   **Mobile ARC**
2424 Gordon Smith Dr
Mobile, AL   36617-2397   251-479-7409
                              Fax: 251-473-7649
                              jzoghby@mobilearc.org
                              mobilearc.org
Jeff Zoghby, Executive Director
Amy Odom, Public Relations and Development Director
Mobile Arc, Inc. (MARC) offers a wide range of services for persons with intellectual and developmental disabilities.

6556   **Southeastern Blind Rehabilitation Center**
U.S. Department of Veteran Affairs
700 S 19th St
Birmingham, AL   35233-1927   205-558-4706
                              Fax: 205-933-4484
                              george.sands@med.va.gov
                              www.rehab.va.gov/blindrehab/

6557   **UAB Eye Care**
University Of Alabama at Birmingham
1716 University Blvd
Birmingham, AL   35233   205-975-2020
                              Fax: 205-934-6755
                              www.uab.edu/optometry/home/eyecare
Rodney W. Nowakowski, Dean
Dr. Marsha Snow, Chief, Low Vision Patient Care
Brittney Bolen, Optometric Technician
Joseph Fleming, D.D., Chief Of Staff
Complete eye services, including low vision services and materials.

6558   **Vaughn-Blumberg Services**
2715 Flynn Rd
P.O. Box 8646
Dothan, AL   36304   334-793-3102
                              Fax: 334-793-7740
                              www.vaughnblumbergservices.com
Ed Dorsey, Executive Director
Linda Cunningham, Director of Human Resources
Billy McCarthy, Director of Finance
Karen Amos, Director of Nursing
Provides comprehensive services for people with intellectual disabilities that reside in Houston County as well as assist in facilitating their participation in society to the fullest extent of their individual capabilities. Offers early intervention services for the mentally handicapped adult including diagnosis and evaluation and physical, speech, and occupational therapies. They also offer counseling, day training,employment assistance and residental homes.

Alaska

6559   **Alaska Center for the Blind and Visually Impaired**
3903 Taft Drive
Anchorage, AK   99517-3069   907-248-7770
                                          800-770-7517
                              Fax: 907-248-7517
                              info@alaskabvi.org
                              www.alaskabvi.org
Regan Mattingly, Executive Director
Robert Tasso, Program Manager
Caren Ailleo, Development & Communications Director
Bonnie Lucas, Visually Impaired Senior Coordinator
Services to help the adult residential or community-based student become independent and self-sufficient by offering independent travel, Braille reading and writing, use of assiative technology such as talking computers, manual skills and personal, as well as home management. There is a special program for those 55 years of age and older who are experiencing a vision loss and another program for rural Alaska Native youth who are visually impaired.

Arizona

6560 Arizona Center for the Blind and Visually Impaired
3100 E Roosevelt St
Phoenix, AZ 85008-5036   602-273-7411
                                          Fax: 602-273-7410
                                          jlamay@acbvi.org
                                          acbvi.org

James La May, CEO
Frank Vance, Director
Christine Boisen, Chair
Alexia Matek, Secretary
A private, nonprofit organization that provides comprehensive
rehabilitation services and more for the blind and visually handi-
capped. The staff includes 20 instructional and adminstrative
professionals.

6561 Arizona Industries for the Blind
Suite 130
515 N 51st Avenue
Phoenix, AZ 85043-2711   602-771-9100
                                          Fax: 602-353-5701
                                          DanielMartinez@azdes.gov
                                          www.azdes.gov/aib

Richard Monaco, General Manager
Daniel Martinez, Community Services Liaison
Offers rehabilitation services, vocational/pre-vocational evaluation and training, work adjustment, job development and employment and training opportunities for individuals who are blind.

6562 Banner Good Samaritan Medical Center
1111 E McDowell Road
Phoenix, AZ 85006-2666   602-839-2000
                                          Fax: 602-239-5868
                                          www.bannerhealth.com

Steve Narang, MD, Chief Executive Officer
Lorraine Hudspeth, Controller
Letty Cerpa, Senior Accountant
Larry Mann, IT Manager
Nearly 1,700 physicians representing more than 50 specialties
work with Banner Good Samaritan staff to care for more then
36,000 inpatients a year. Houses more then 650 licensed patient
care beds. A teaching hospital that trains more then 220 physicians annually and a premier medical center in Arizona and the
Southwest. Provides a comprehensive foundation of major programs and an equally impressive offering of highly specialized
programs not availiable in most hospitals.

6563 Beacon Foundation for the Mentally Retarded
308 W. Glenn St.
Tucson, AZ 85703   520-622-4874
                                          Fax: 520-620-6620
                                          sking@beacongroup.org
                                          http://beacongroup.org

Steven R King, President
Chuck Tiller, Vice President Rehabilitation Se
Greg Natvig, Vice President of Business Opera
Michelle Kroeger, CFO
Committed to effectively assisting adults with disabilities to
maximize their personal, social, vocational and educational skills
in order to attain a successful and meaningful independence
within the Tucson community.

**6564 Carondelet Brain Injury Programs and Services (Bridges
Now)**
2202 N. Forbes Blvd.
Tucson, AZ 85745-2602   520-872-7324
                                          Fax: 520-873-3743
                                          comments@carondelet.org
                                          carondelet.org

Daisy M Jenkins, Executive VP, Chief HR/Administr
James K Beckmann, President/Chief Executive Officer
Alan Strauss, Executive VP, Finance and Chief Financial Officer
Christen Castellano, MBA, Executive VP and Chief Strategy Officer
Comprehensive outpatient rehabilitation program. PT, OT, ST,
Psychology and Rehab Counseling Services.

6565 Desert Life Rehabilitation & Care Center
1919 W Medical St
Tucson, AZ 85704-1133   520-369-9620
                                          Fax: 520-867-6612
                                          www.desertlifecc.com

Amad Nazifi, Executive Director
Accomodates 240 residents. Provides skilled and intermediate
nursing with occupational, physical, speech and respiratory therapy services. Offers special programs including an Alzheimer's
Unit and a Young Adult program

6566 Devereux Advanced Behavioral Health Arizona - Scottsdale
Scottsdale Administrative Office
2025 N 3rd St
Suite 250
Phoenix, AZ 85004   602-283-1573
                                          Fax: 480-443-5587
                                          azadmissions@devereux.org
                                          www.devereuxaz.org

Lane Barker, Executive Director
Yvette Jackson, Director of Operations
Donovan S Carman, MBA, Director of Finance
Janelle Westfall, Clinical Director
Engages in the treatment of behavioral health issues through services such as residential treatment centers, day school, outpatient
services, prevention programs, adult foster care, and foster care
for children. Also offered are evidence-based interventions to
improve lives.

6567 Devereux Arizona - Tucson
Tuscon Administrative Office
6141 E Grant Rd
Tucson, AZ 85712   520-296-5551
                                          Fax: 520-296-8244
                                          azadmissions@devereux.org
                                          www.devereuxaz.org

Lane Barker, Executive Director
Yvette Jackson, Director of Operations
Donovan S Carman, MBA, Director of Finance
Janelle Westfall, Clinical Director
Organization offering culturally competent care for individuals
with emotional and behavioral health disorders. Some of the pro-
grams offered include Adult Foster Care, kinship program, Ther-
apeutic Foster Care Program, Parent Aide and more.

6568 Freestone Rehabilitation Center
10617 E Oasis Drive
Mesa, AZ 85208   480-986-1531
                                          Fax: 480-986-1538
                                          www.manta.com

Randy Gray, Executive Director
Cherie Vance, Manager

6569 HealthSouth Valley Of The Sun Rehabilitation Hospital
13460 N 67th Ave
Glendale, AZ 85304-1000   623-878-8800
                                          Fax: 623-878-5254
                                          healthsouth.com

Beth Bacher, Manager
A 60-bed free-standing hospital that offers acute physical rehabilitation, outpatient therapy services and day hospital treatment.
Works in cooperation with local, regional and national managed
care organizations and other sources to maximise patient recovery while conserving financial resources.

6570 Institute for Human Development
Northern Arizona University
912 Riordan Rd. P.O.Box 5630
Flagstaff, AZ 86011-5630   928-523-4791
                                          Fax: 928-523-9127
                                          TTY:928-523-1695
                                          ihd@nau.edu
                                          www.nau.edu/ihd

Levi Esguerra, Director
Lisa Andrew, Advisory Commitee
Lynn Black, Advisory Commitee
Maria Bravo, Advisory Commitee

The Institute values and supports the independence, productivity and inclusion of Arizona's citizens with disabilities. Based on the values and beliefs, the Institute conducts training, research and services that further these goals.

6571 John C Lincoln Hospital North Mountain
250 E Dunlap Ave
Phoenix, AZ 85020-2871   602-943-2381
                                        Fax: 602-944-8062
                                      webmaster@jcl.com
                   www.jcl.com/content/northmountain/default.htm
Rhonda Forsyth, President
Bruce Pearson, FACHE, Senior Vice President
Maggi Griffin, RN, MS, Vice President & Chief Executive Officer
Jessica Rivas, RN, MSN, Vice President and Chief Nursing Officer
Mission is to assist each person entrusted to our care to enjoy the fullest gift of health possible, and work with others to build a community where a helping hand is available for our most vulnerable members.

6572 La Frontera Center
504 W 29th St
Tucson, AZ   85713-3394   520-884-9920
                                        Fax: 520-792-0654
                                       www.lafronteraaz.org
Kevin Heath, Board Chair
Frank Valenzuela, Vice Chair
Celestino Fernandez, Treasurer
Susan Agrillo, Recording Secretary
A nonprofit community-based behavioral health agency that has been helping southern Arizona children, adults, and families since 1968.

6573 Manor Care Nursing and Rehab Center: Tucson
3705 N Swan Rd
Tucson, AZ   85718-6939   520-299-7088
                                        Fax: 520-529-0038
                                      www.hcr-manorcare.com
Clifton J. Porter II, Vice President - Government Rela
Martin Allen, Vice President
A leading provider of short-term post-acute medical care and rehabilitation and long-term skilled nursing care. High quality medical care is provided through registered (RN) and licensed practical (LPN) nurses and certified nursing assistants (CNA) in concert with physical , occupational and speech rehabilitation therapists. Our more then 275 skilled nursing centers are Medicare-and Medicaid-certified.

6574 Nova Care
Second Floor
680 American Avenue
King of Prussia, PA 19406-2607   800-331-8840
                                        Fax: 602-256-7292
                                           novacare.com
Scott Lusted, General Manager
Brian Beal, Market Manager
NovaCare Rehabilitation's highly respected clinical team provides preventative and rehabilitative services that maximize functionality and promote well-being. NovaCare Rehabilitation also provides physical therapy and athletic training services to more then 20 professional sports teams and 300 universities, colleges, and highschools thoughout the nation.

6575 Perry Rehabilitation Center
3146 E Windsor Avenue
Phoenix, AZ 85008-1199   602-956-0400
                                        Fax: 602-957-7610
                                      perrycenter@qwest.net
                                          www.azafh.com
Diana Casillas, Human Resources Director
Jim Musick, President
Provides services for people with disabilities, cognitive disabilities including residential services, day treatment, job training and job placement.

6576 Phoenix Veterans Center
Ste 100
1544 W. Grant St.
Phoenix, AZ   85004-1554   602-358-8494
                                        Fax: 602-379-4130
                                   www.azcremationcenter.com/?
Ken Benckwitz, Manager
Veterans medical clinic offering disabled veterans medical treatments.

6577 Progress Valley: Phoenix
10505 North 69th Street
Suite 1100
Paradise Valley, AZ 85253-6106   480-922-9427
                                        Fax: 602-274-5473
                                   recovery@progressvalley.org
                                      alcoholism.about.com
Susanne Lambert, Executive Director
Jennifer White, Director of Programs
Cathie Scott, Sober Housing Manager
Kristine Peltier, Finance Director
Residential aftercare for alcoholism and chemical dependency. Certified chemical dependency counselors provide individual treatment.

6578 Rehabilitation Services Administration
Suite 102
3425 East Van Buren
Phoenix, AZ   85008-3202   602-771-9100
                                           800-563-1221
                                        Fax: 602-250-8584
                                        TTY: 855-475-8194
                                         azrsa@azdes.gov
Katharine Levandowsky, Administrator
Provides a variety of specialized services to assist in removing barriers to employment and/or independent living for individuals with physical or mental disabilities. RSA offers 3 major service programs and several specialized programs/services.

6579 Southern Arizona Association For The Visually Impaired
3767 East Grant Rd
Tucson, AZ   85716-2935   520-795-1331
                                           800-563-1221
                                        Fax: 520-795-1336
                                       reception@saavi.us
                                           www.saavi.us
Michael Gordon, Executive Director
Amy Murillo, Associate Director
Carol Lopez, Finance Director
Lenetta Lefko, Tucson Services Manager
Offers health services, counseling, social work, home and personal management, computer training, low vision aids and more for the visually handicapped 18 years or older.

6580 Toyei Industries
Hc 58 Box 55
Ganado, AZ   86505-55   928-736-2417
                                           888-45T-OYEI
                                        Fax: 928-736-2495
Anthony Lincoln, CEO
Serves the needs of developmentally disabled and the severely mentally impaired adult citizens of the Navajo Nation and other Indian Nations. Staff of 60+ serves the needs of all the Navajo adults. Services include day treatment programs, and residential and group home services.

6581 Yuma Center for the Visually Impaired
328 W. Spears Street
Yuma, AZ   85365-6580   928-247-8890
                                        Fax: 928-344-1863
                                      https://www.azdes.gov
Calvin Roberts, Executive Director
Kathy Lucero, Store Manager
Dana Clayton, Human Resources Specialist
Lorraine Hudspeth, Controller
A private nonprofit agency offering services for totally blind and legally blind children and adults in the Arizona area.

Arkansas

6582 **Arkansas Lighthouse for the Blind**
P.O.Box 192666
6818 Murray St.
Little Rock, AR 72209- 2666

501-562-2222
Fax: 501-568-5275
info@arkansaslighthouse.org
arkansaslighthouse.org

Bill Johnson, Chief Executive Officer
Danny Novielli, COO
John McAtee, Chief Financial Officer
Ronnie Cates, Director of Communications & Procurement
Manufacturer of textiles, apparel and paper products and employs blind and legally blind individuals.

6583 **Beverly Enterprises Network**
1 Thousand Beverly
Fort Smith, AR 72901-2629

479-201-2000
800-666-9996
Fax: 479-452-5131

Randy Churchey, CEO
Offers a progressive approach to subacute care. The goal of this organization is to assist injured and disabled individuals regain the level of independence to which they have been accustomed. Provides support and training programs, patient and family services and specialty programs for patients.

6584 **Easter Seals: Arkansas**
3920 Woodland Heights Rd
Little Rock, AR 72212-2495

501-227-3600
877-533-3700
Fax: 501-227-4021
TTY: 501-227-3686
lrogers@ar.easterseals.com
www.eastersealsar.com

Sharon Moone-Jochums, President/ CEO
Linda Rogers, VP Programs
Michael E. Stock, Treasurer
Cindy Nash, Secretary
Their mission is to provide exceptional services to ensure that all people with disabilities or special needs have equal opportunities to live, learn, work and play in their communitites.

6585 **HealthSouth Rehabilitation Hospital Of Fort Smith**
1401 South J. Street
Fort Smith, AR 72901-5158

479-785-3300
Fax: 479-785-8599
healthsouth.com

Ryan Cassedy, CEO
Cygnet Schroeder, M.D., Medical Director
Donna Beallis, D.O., Director of Medical Management
Brandi Denham, Director of Human Resources
A free-standing 80-bed comprehensive physical medicine and rehabilitation hospital offering inpatient and outpatient services. Provides specialized medical and therapy services, designed to assist physically challenged persons to reach their highest level of independent function.

6586 **Lions World Services for the Blind**
2811 Fair Park Blvd
Little Rock, AR 72204-5044

501-664-7100
800-248-0734
Fax: 501-664-2743
training@lwsb.org
www.wsblind.org/

Larry Dickerson, President/ CEO
Tony Woodell, President & Chief Executive Officer
Bill Smith, Director of Development
Melanie Jones, Marketing & Communications Director
Offers services in the areas of health education, recreation, rehabilitation, counseling, employment, computer training and more for all legally blind residents of the U.S. The staff includes 56 full time employees.

6587 **Little Rock Vet Center #0713**
Department of Veterans Affairs of Washington DC
Suite A
201 W Broadway St
North Little Rock, AR 72114- 5505

501-324-6395
877-927-8387
Fax: 501-324-6928

Elizabeth N Ruggiero, Team Leader
Ida L Fogle, Counselor
Van A Hall, Counselor
Darryl A Lasker, Office Manager
Vet Center provides PTSD counseling to veterans of a combat zone. No medical care provided.

6588 **Timber Ridge Ranch NeuroRestorative Services**
4500 W Commerce Dr
North Little Rock, AR 72116

501-758-8799
800-743-6802
Fax: 501-758-8778
neuroinfo@thementornetwork.com
www.neurorestorative.com

Bill Duffy, Chief Operating Officer
Michael E. Hofmeister, MS, MBA, Vice President of Operations
Sean Byrne, MBA, Chief Financial Officer
Roger P. Carrillo, M.Ed, Vice President of Business Development
Comprehensive, individualized services from a transdisciplinary team of licensed professionals assist clients along a course to greater independence. A separate team is dedicated to the needs of children, adolescents, and their families. A clinical team may include professionals from the disciplines of: behavior analysis, neuropsychology, physiatry, psychology, speech-language pathology, occupational therapy, physical therapy, social work, couseling, education, nursing, and case management.

California

6589 **ARC Fresno-Kelso Activity Center**
4567 N Marty Ave
Fresno, CA 93722-7810

559-226-6268
Fax: 559-226-6269
arcfresno@arcfresno.org
arcfresno.org

Lori Ramirez, Executive Director
Catherine Wooliever, Director of Human Resources
Jamie Marrash, Director of Program Services
Pamela Wirth, Director of Finance
The Arc Fresno is a private, non-profit 501(c)(3) organization who was founded in 1953. They provide services and supports for over 550 individuals with developmental disabilities throughout Fresno County. They currently offer eight (8) programs, and do so with the help of 145 employees.

6590 **ARC Of San Diego-ARROW Center, The**
3030 Market Street
San Diego, CA 92102-3297

619-685-1175
Fax: 619-234-3759
arc-sd.com

Dwight Stratton, Chair
Jerry Wechsler, 1st Vice Chairman
David W. Schneider, President & CEO
Anthony J. DeSalis, Executive Vice President & COO
The ARC of San Diego will be the premier provider of services to persons with disabilities. Arc-SD will be an advocate for diversity of opportunities, enhancing individual life choices as a member of the communuity. Our values: Everyone will be treated equally, without prejudice and with respect. Will provide Quality Services and Supports with a well trained and caring staff. State of the art equipment and methods. A willingness to innovate and collaborate.

6591   ARC Of San Diego-East County Training Center, The
1374 E Lexington Ave
El Cajon, CA   92019-2312   619-444-9417
                                          Fax: 619-234-3759
                                               arc-sd.com

Dwight Stratton, Chair
Jerry Wechsler, 1st Vice Chairman
David W. Schneider, President & CEO
Anthony J. DeSalis, Executive Vice President & COO
Work adjustment and remunerative work programs.

6592   ARC Of San Diego-Rex Industries, The
9575 Aero Dr
San Diego, CA   92123-1803   858-571-4369
                                               800-748-5575
                                          Fax: 858-715-3788
                                               arc-sd.com

Dwight Stratton, Chair
Jerry Wechsler, 1st Vice Chairman
David W. Schneider, President & CEO
Anthony J. DeSalis, Executive Vice President & COO
Offers many different programs including: North County Parent/Infant Program which is an educational program for children, birth to three years who are showing delays in development or who are at risk for developmental delays. The Adult Development Center is a program for adults, eighteen and over, with a developmental disability in the severe to profound range. The program focuses on self-help, communication, daily living and pre-vocational skills. Other programs are available..

6593   ARC Of San-Diego-South Bay
1280 Nolan Avenue
Chula Vista, CA   91911-3738   619-427-7524
                                          Fax: 619-427-4657
                                            info@arc-sd.com
                                          www.arc-sd.com/locations

Becky Thaller, Director
Steve Hojsan, Arc Enterprises Director
Michael Bruce, Workshop Manager
David W. Schneider, President & CEO
Provides remunerative work.

6594   ARC Of Southeast Los Angeles-Southeast Industries
9501 Washburn Rd
Downey, CA   90242-2913   562-803-1556
                                          Fax: 562-803-4080
                                            www.arcselac.org/

6595   ARC: VC Community Connections West
5103 Walker Street
Ventura, CA   93003-7358   805-650-8611
                                          Fax: 805-644-7308
                                               www.arcvc.org

Robert Hogan, President
Gene West, First Vice President
Eve Liebman, Recording Secretary
Kathy Raffaelli, Treasurer
Caring and experienced staff is dedicated to serving participants with a variety of physical, mental and social disabilities who require a higher level of support and supervision. Using a person-centered planning approach, Arc Ventura County promotes self-directed services for all clients and families served. Adult development centers serve individuals with physical and mental disabilities, as well as people with challenging behaviors, who require assistance with basic skills such as self care.

6596   ARC: VC Ventura
5103 Walker Street
Ventura, CA   93003-7358   806-650-8611
                                          Fax: 806-644-7308
                                               www.arcvc.org

Robert Hogan, President
Gene West, First Vice President
Eve Liebman, Recording Secretary
Kathy Raffaelli, Treasurer
Arc Ventura County is a private, nonprofit organization that provides educational, vocational and residential services for people with developmental disabilities. Informed decisions, positive changes, and integration in the community are fundamental principals in all programs. As evidence of our programming excellence, Arc Ventura County has been accredited by CARF (The Rehabilitation Accreditation Commission.

6597   AbilityFirst
1300 E Green Street
Pasadena, CA   91106-2606   626-396-1010
                                               877-768-4600
                                          Fax: 626-396-1021
                                             info@abilityfirst.org
                                             www.abilityfirst.org

Lori E. Gangemi, President
Steve S. Schultz, Chief Financial Officer
Keri Castaneda, Chief Program Officer
Syed Kazmi, Controller
AbilityFirst serves children and adults with special needs through 24 locations in Southern California.

6598   Accentcare
17855 North Dallas Pkwy
Dallas, TX   75287-2468   972-201-3800
                                               800-834-3059
                                            info@accentcare.com
                                               accentcare.com

Mark Pacala, Chairman of the Board and CEO (i
Vincent E. Cook, EVP and Chief Financial Officer
Melvin Warriner, SVP and Chief Culture Officer
Mel Deutsch, General Counsel
Postacute rehabilitation program: home care aides follow through with rehabilitation instructions given by physical, occupational and speech therapists. Other home care services are available, serving special needs for Alzheimer's, blind, brain injury, MS, ostomies, parkinsonism, spinal injury and stroke.

6599   Anaheim Veterans Center
859, South Harbor Blvd
Anaheim, CA   92805-4680   714-776-0161
                                               800-225-8387
                                          Fax: 714-776-8904
                                       anaheimvetcenter@yahoo.com
                                  www.longbeach.va.gov/visitors/vet_center.asp

6600   Association for Retarded Citizens: Alameda County
1101 Walpert St
Hayward, CA   94541-3721   510-582-8151
                                          Fax: 510-639-4684
                                               www.sbn.com

Ram Sirck, Director
Offers the Right Track program in which selected workers are grouped together on a contract basis to maximize work productivity. Provides a full benefit package, as well as a permanent supervisor. A worker is matched to a job of at least 20 hours per week and then trained by the staff of The Right Track.

6601   Azure Acres Recovery Center
5777 Madison Avenue
Suite 1210
Sacramento, CA   95841-9034   877-977-3755
                                               877-762-3735
                                          Fax: 707-823-8972
                                             info@azureacres.com
                                               azureacres.com

Joe Tinervin, MSW, Executive Director
Michael Roeske, Psy.D., Clinical Director
Christie Splitstone, MA, Counselor/Case Manager
James Canter, CATC, Counselor/Case Manager
Offers rehabilitation services and residential care for the person with an alcohol or drug abuse related problems.

6602 Back in the Saddle
2 BITS Trail
P.O. Box 3336
Chelmsford, MA   01824-0936   800-865-2478
                                     877-756-5068
                              Fax: 800-866-3235
                              help@BackInTheSaddle.com
                                     www.thesaddle.com

Richard Smith PhD, Owner
Erika Reed, Co-Director
A long term community residential facility for head injured adults. House parents live on-site; and oversee a variety of programs which are individually designed and might include classes in community college, placement in a workshop or on a workstation, volunteer positions and home skills assignments. Recreational outing range from horseback riding to weekend camping. Apartment programs available as set-up. Price: $2800-$3000 per month.

6603 Ballard Rehabilitation Hospital
1760 W 16th St
San Bernardino, CA   92411-1150   909-473-1200
                                      800-761-1226
                               Fax: 909-473-1276
                                      www.ballardrehab.com

Edward C. Palacios, RN,MPH, Administrator
Mary Hunt, Chief Operating Officer
Patty Meinhardt, Director Marketing/Admissions
Ballard Rehab Hospital is a free standing specialty hospital and provides the complete continuum of acute rehabilitation and outpatient rehabilitation, dedicated to providing rehab care to adults and children. The following inpatient and outpatient programs are available: CNA (Stroke) Rehab; Spinal Cord Injury Rehab; Brain Injury Rehab; Pain Management Rehab; Bariatric program, pulmonary program, injured Worker Programs; and Post Amputation Rehab.

6604 Bayview Nursing and Rehabilitation
516 Willow Street
Alameda, CA   94501-6132   510-521-5600
                              Fax: 510-865-6441
                              TTY:800-735-2922
                              http://www.bayviewnursing.com/

Richard S Espinoza, Administrator
Offers a full range of medical services to meet the individual needs of our residents, including short-term rehabilitative services and long termed skilled care. Working with the resident's physician, our staff-including medical specialists, nurses, nutritionists, dietitians, and social workers-establishes a comprehensive treatment plan intended to restore you or your loved one to the highest practicable potential.

6605 Belden Center
606 Humboldt St
Santa Rosa, CA   95404-4219   707-579-2735
                               Fax: 707-579-4145

Casey Harding, Owner
Pamela Fadden, Owner
Postacute rehabilitation program.

6606 Blind Babies Foundation
Suite 300
1814 Franklin St
Oakland, CA   94612-3487   510-446-2229
                               Fax: 510-446-2262
                              bbfinfo@blindbabies.org
                                     blindbabies.org

Dottie Bridge, President
Aben Hill, 1st Vice President
Clare Friedman, PhD, 2nd Vice President
Beverly Libaire, Treasurer
Mission: when an infant or pre school child is identified as blind or visually impaired, provides family-centered services to support the child's optimal development and access to the world.

6607 Brotman Medical Center: RehabCare Unit
Brotman Medical Center
3828 Delmas Terrace
Culver City, CA   90232-2713   310-836-7000
                                      800-677-1238
                               Fax: 310-202-4105
                              info@brotmanmed.com
                                     phvc.com

Jennifer Cortez, Program Manager
Kevin O'Connor, CEO
Scott Leonard, CTO
Ben Taylor, Senior Editor
Culver City is centrally located within the city of Los Angeles. These are two programs offering inpatient rehabilitation. The acute rehab program is designed for patients who need physical rehabilitation due to injury or medical disability. This program requires patients to participate in 3 hours therapy per day. The sub-acute program is designed especially for patients who need rehab but cannot tolerate the intensity of the acute rehab program..

6608 Build Rehabilitation Industries
12432 Foothill Blvd
Sylmar, CA   91342   818-898-0020
                               Fax: 818-898-1949
                                     buildindustries.com

6609 California Elwyn
18325 Mt. Baldy Circle
Fountain Valley, CA   92708-6115   714-557-6313
                               Fax: 714-963-2961
                              info@elwyn.org
                                     elwyn.org

Sandra S. Cornelius, President of Elwyn
Daniel M. Reardon, Senior Vice President and Chief Operating Officer
Stan H. Retif, Vice President for Development a
Richard T. Smith, Vice President for Information Technology
Provides opportunities for people challenged by physical and mental disabilities who are 18 or older. California Elwyn develops an Individual Rehabilitation Plan for all consumers. Contract work, shrinkwrap, janitorial are just some of the types of jobs done. Supported Employment Services are available and over 100 consumers currently are employed. Funded by the State Department of Rehabilitation and Vocational Rehabilitation.

6610 California Eye Institute
1360 E Herndon Ave
Fresno, CA   93720-3326   559-449-5000
                                     www.samc.com

Nancy Hollingsworth, President and CEO
Michael W. Martinez, EVP/Chief Operating and Financial Officer
Stephen Soldo, Chief Medical Officer
Christine Sarrico, Chief Financial Officer
A private, nonprofit agency offering services such as health, educational, recreational, rehabilitation and employment counseling to the totally blind, legally blind and visually impaired. The staff includes two full time workers.

6611 Camp Recovery Center
3192 Glen Canyon Rd
Scotts Valley, CA   95066-4916   877-557-6237
                               Fax: 831-438-2789
                                     camprecovery.com

Michael Johnson, Ph.D, Executive Director
Tim Sinnott, Clinical Director
Zoe R., Case Manager
Jeff Geiger, Clinical Tech Director
A free-standing social model recovery center for chemical dependency located on 25 wooded acres in the Santa Cruz Mountains. The services include: medical detoxification, complete medical evaluation, psychiatric evaluation and counseling, psychological testing, individual counseling and more. Helps the recovery from chemical dependency in a easier, warm and caring environment.

6612   Campobello Chemical Dependency Recovery Center
2448 Guerneville Road
Suite 400
Santa Rosa, CA   95402- 4030   707-546-1547
                                                800-805-1833
                                          Fax: 707-579-1603
                                                campobello.org

6613   Casa Colina Centers for Rehabilitation
P.O.Box 6001
255 East Bonita Avenue
Pomona, CA   91767- 6001   909-596-7733
                                                866-724-4127
                                          Fax: 909-593-0153
                                            TTY: 909-596-3646
                                                casacolina.org

Steve Norin, Chairman
Felice L Loverso, President
Chandrahas Agarwal, Medical Director
Elmer B. Pineda, M.D., Chief Of Medical Staff
Casa Colina, has pioneered effective programs to create opportunity for health, productivity and self-esteem for persons with disability since 1936. Through medical rehabilitation, transitional living, residential, community, and prevention and wellness programs. Casa Colina serves more than 7,000 persons annually. Casa Colina, a non-profit organization, offers a unique spectrum of opportunities, achievement and results to patients and their families.

6614   Casa Colina Padua Village
P.O.Box 6001
255 East Bonita Avenue
Pomona, CA   91767- 6001   909-596-7733
                                                866-724-4127
                                          Fax: 909-593-0153
                                            TTY: 909-596-3646
                                                casacolina.org

Steve Norin, Chairman
Chandrahas Agarwal, Medical Director
Felice L Loverso, President
Elmer B. Pineda, M.D., Chief Of Medical Staff
Long term residential services for adults with developmental disability. Residences include Malmquist House, Woodbend House, and Hillsdale House, all located in Claremont, California.

6615   Casa Colina Residential Services: Rancho Pino Verde
Casa Colina Center for Rehabilitation
P.O.Box 6001
255 East Bonita Avenue
Pomona, CA   91767- 7517   909-596-7733
                                                866-724-4127
                                          Fax: 909-593-0153
                                            TTY: 909-596-3646
                                            www.casacolina.org

Steve Norin, Chairman
Randy Blackman, Vice Chairman
Felice L. Loverso, President
Elmer B. Pineda, M.D., Chief Of Medical Staff
Long term residential services in rural environment for adults with brain injury.

6616   Casa Colina Transitional Living Center
255 East Bonita Avenue
P.O.Box 6001
Pomona, CA   91767- 1923   909-596-7733
                                                866-724-4127
                                          Fax: 909-593-0153
                                            TTY: 909-596-3646
                                                casacolina.org

Steve Norin, Chairman
Felice L Loverso, President
Chandrahas Agarwal, Medical Director
Elmer B. Pineda, M.D., Chief Of Medical Staff
Postacute rehabilitation program.

6617   Casa Colina Transitional Living Center: Pomona
P.O.Box 6001
255 East Bonita Avenue
Pomona, CA   91767- 6001   909-596-7733
                                                866-724-4127
                                          Fax: 909-593-0153
                                            TTY: 909-596-3646
                                                casacolina.org

Steve Norin, Chairman
Felice L Loverso, President
Chandrahas Agarwal, Medical Director
Elmer B. Pineda, M.D., Chief Of Medical Staff
Post acute short term residential program for persons with brain injury. In a home-like setting, therapy promotes successful re-entry to home and community living.

6618   Cedars of Marin
PO Box 947
Ross, CA   94957-947   415-454-5310
                                          Fax: 415-454-0573
                                      lauren@thecedarsofmarin.org
                                            thecedarsofmarin.org

Jefferson Rice, Board Chair
James Brentano, Board Vice President
Andrew Hinkelman, Board Treasurer
Chuck Greene, Executive Director
The Cedars of Marin has provided residential and day programs for adults with developmental disabilities for over 91 years. Our award-winning programs help our clients to live creative, productive, joyous lives.

6619   Center for Neuro Skills
5215 Ashe Rd.
Bakersfield, CA   93313-2988   661-872-3408
                                                800-922-4994
                                          Fax: 661-872-5150
                                        skatomski@neuroskills.com
                                                neuroskills.com

Mark J Ashley, President/CEO and Co-Founder
A comprehensive, post-acute, community based head-injury rehabilitation program serving over 100 clients per year. Since 1980, CNS has effectively treated the entire spectrum of head-injured clients, including those with severe behavioral disorders, cognitive/perceptual impairments, speech/language problems, physical disabilities and post-concussion syndrome.

6620   Center for the Partially Sighted
Suite 150
6101 W. Centinela Ave.
Culver City, CA   90230   310-988-1970
                                          Fax: 310-988-1980
                                            info@low-vision.org
                                                low-vision.org

La Donna S. Ringering, Ph.D, President/CEO
Pam Thompson, Director of Psychological Servic
Phyllis Amaral, Clinical Director
Laura Valencia, Psychosocial Services Coordinato
Services for partially sighted and legally blind people include low vision evaluations, the design and prescription of low vision devices and adaptive technology, as well as counseling and rehabilitation training (independent living skills and orientation/mobility training). Special programs include children's program, diabetes and vision loss program, Technology demonstrations. Store carries low vision aids. Catalog available.

6621   Central Coast Neurobehavioral Center OPTIONS
P.O.Box 877
800 Quintana Road Suite 2C
Morro Bay, CA 93442-877   805-772-6066
                                          Fax: 805-772-6067

Michael Mamot, CEO
Ole von Frausing-Borch, COO
Serves adults with developmental disabilities, traumatic head injuries, or other neurological impairments. OPTIONS operates two transitional living centers, eight licensed residential facilities, two licensed community integration day programs and a licensed short term stabilization center. Services offered include: supported and independent living services, group and individual

vocational services, neuropsychological assessment, occupational therapy, cognitive therapy, speech therapy and more.

6622 Cerebral Palsy: North County Center
#209
8525 Gibbs Drive
San Diego, CA 92123-1758   858-571-7803
                                        Fax: 858-571-0919
                                        info@ucpsd.org
                                        www.ucpsd.org
David Carucci, Executive Director
Mary Krieger, Associate Executive Director
Bruce Neufeld, Chief Financial Officer
Sophia Williams, Director of Human Resources
The mission of UCP San Diego County is to advance the independence, productivity and full citizenship of people affected by cerebral palsy and other disabilities. By making solid steps, UCP can build a better community for all in the process.

6623 Children's Hospital Central California Rehabilitation Center
9300 Valley Childrens Place
Madera, CA 93636-8762   559-353-3000
                                        www.valleychildrens.org
Todd Suntrapak, President & Chief Executive Officer
David Christensen, MD, SVP Medical Affairs & Chief Medical Officer
Beverly Hayden-Pugh, Vice President & Chief Nursing Officer
Kirk Larson, Vice President & Chief Informati
A 297-bed pediatric medical center on a 50-acre campus. We now have more then 500 doctors practicing in over 40 pediatric subspecialties with clinics and services throughout the state.

6624 Children's Hospital Los Angeles Rehabilitation Program
4650 W Sunset Blvd
Los Angeles, CA 90027-6062   323-361-4155
                                             888-631-2452
                                        Fax: 323-361-8101
                                        webmaster@chla.usc.edu
                                        www.childrenshospitalla.org
Richard D. Cordova, President & CEO
Rodney B. Hanners, Senior Vice President and Chief
Henri R. Ford, M.D.
Lawrence L. Foust, J.D.,, Secretary
Designated as a Level I Pediatric Trauma Canter by the Los Angeles County EMS Agency, the hospital treats more then 1,500 pediatric trauma patients per year. Performs more then 13,900 pediatric surgeries a year, including more complex surgical procedures then any other hospital in Southern California

6625 Children's Therapy Center
Ste 120
770 Paseo Camarillo
Camarillo, CA 93010-6092   805-383-1501
                                        Fax: 805-383-1504
Beth Maulhardt, Owner
Provides individual occupational therapy, speech/language therapy, family/child consulting, education services and physical therapy consultation for children. Evaluations and treatment are on an individual basis and special emphasis is placed on a multidisciplinary approach with information sharing, and often team treatment.

6626 Clausen House
88 Vernon Street
Oakland, CA 94610-4217   510-839-0050
                                        clausenhouse.org
Deborah Levy, Interim Executive Director
Michael A. Scott, Director of Development
Stan Nicholson, Director of Human Resources
Jaynette Underhill, Director of Program Services
Residential, supported employment, independent and supported living, adult education, and social recreation activities. Serving the developmentally disabled since 1967.

6627 Community Gatepath
350 Twin Dolphin Dr
Suite 123
Redwood City, CA 94065   650-259-8500
                                        Fax: 650-697-5010
                                        info@gatepath.org
                                        gatepath.org
Bryan Neider, CEO
Steve D'Eredita, Chief Financial Officer
Tracey Fecher, Vice President of Programs
Erin Montgomery, Vice President of Human Resources
Gatepath is a non-profit organization serving children, youth and adults with special needs and developmental disabilities and their families in the greater San Francisco Bay Area. The organization partners with various local non-profits, businesses, government agencies and third party providers to better serve this community.

6628 Community Hospital and Rehabilitation Center of Los Gatos-Saratoga
815 Pollard Rd
Los Gatos, CA 95032-1438   408-378-6131
                                        Fax: 408-866-4003
Gary Honts, CEO
Offers rehabilitation services, inpatient and outpatient care, physical therapy, occupational therapy and more for the physically challenged adult. We have a commitment to health care excellence. It is in this commitment that we have dedicated ourselves to provide personal and professional service to our patients. Our goal is to work closely with staff, physicians and the community to attain shared goals and positive changes, now and in the future..

6629 Contra Costa ARC
1340 Arnold Drive
Suite 127
Martinez, CA 94553-4189   925-370-1818
                                        Fax: 925-370-2048
                                        feedback@arcofcc.org
                                        www.ContraCostaARC.com
Barbara Maizie, Executive Director
Diana Jorgensen, Program Coordinator
Andrey George, Administrative Coordinator
A private nonprofit membership-based organization dedicated to enhancing the quality of life of individuals with mental retardation and other developmental disabilities.

6630 Corona Regional Medical Center- Rehabiltation Center
800 S. Main St.
Corona, CA 92882-3117   951-737-4343
                                        Fax: 951-736-7276
                                        www.coronaregional.com
Diane Mc Donald, Manager
Mark Uffer, Chief Executive Officer
Doreen Dann, Chief Nursing Officer
Douglas Crouse, Chairman of the Board
Offers inpatient and outpatient rehabilitation services. The Center consists of an acute rehab unit, a subacute rehab unit containing modules for long-term ventilator care, respiratory rehab, coma intervention and orthopedics. In addition to inpatient therapies, the Center's outpatient programs include sports and industrial medicine.

6631 Critical Air Medicine
Montgomery Field
8775 Aero Drive
Suite 235
San Diego, CA 92123-1705   858-300-0224
                                             800-247-8326
                                        Fax: 858-300-0228
                                        criticalair.ops@criticalair.com
                                        www.aircharterguide.com
Frank Craven, Publisher of the Air Charter Guide
Offers emergency medical care by air medical transport carriers. These carriers are fully equipped with medical equipment and supplies for cardiovascular emergencies, respiratory supplies, orthopedic supplies and medications..

6632   Crutcher's Serenity House
P.O.Box D
50 Hillcrest Drive
Deer Park, CA   94576-504   707-963-3192
                                        Fax: 707-963-2309
                                        www.crutcherssh.com

Robert Crutcher, Owner/CEO
Lu Crutcher, Executive Director
A privately owned and operated facility that introduces to residents a new lifestyle free of all chemicals, and a new awareness of their total being. The length of the program is four weeks and is within five minutes of an acute care hospital. The Center is licensed for 19 beds, male and female located in a home-like setting with an emphasis on maintaining a family atmosphere.

6633   Daniel Freeman Rehabilitation Centers
333 N Prairie Ave
PO Box 28990
Santa Ana, CA   92799-4501   714-230-3150
                                        Fax: 714-850-0153
                               advertising@acupuncturetoday.com
                                        www.acupuncturetoday.com

H Arndt, Associate Administrator
Gabrielle Lindsley, Business Development Manager
Evelyn Petersen, Human Resources / Payroll Manager
Andrea Weeks, Accountant
Comprehensive rehabilitation services which address needs and issues of the physically diabled and their families. We offer accute input rehabilitation, outpatient and short term skilled nursing rehabilitaion. Specialty areas include: brain injury, stroke, spinal chord injury, chronic pain, arthritis..

6634   Delano Regional Medical Center
1401 Garces Highway
Delano, CA   93215-3690   661-725-4800
                                        info@drmc.com
                                        drmc.com

Bahram Ghaffari, President
Jeremy Klemm, HealthStream Regional Director
Robert A. Frist, HealthStream CEO
Delano Regional Medical Center (DRMC) is proud to be known throughout California & beyond as an innovative regional hospital, deeply rooted in the local communities and committed to providing an exceptional patient experience. A non-profit acute-care facility serving a region of 10 rural central Californiatowns. With over 100 physicians on our active medical staff and additional courtesy or consulting physicians, patients are assured of receiving high-quality care in multiple specialties.

6635   Desert Regional Medical Center
1150 N Indian Canyon Dr
Palm Springs, CA   92262   760-323-6511
                                        800-491-4990
                                        www.desertmedctr.com

Carolyn Caldwell, Chief Executive Officer
Tracey Cowles, Physician Relations Manager
Jeanne Stanton, RN, Chair
Lee Bledsoe, Physician Relations Manager
Our dedicated physicians and caregivers provide a broad array of quality programs and services, including comprehensive cancer care, women's health services, heart care, surgical weight loss reduction and orthopedics.

6636   Devereux Advanced Behavioral Health California
P.O. Box 6784
Santa Barbara, CA   93160   805-968-2525
                                        Fax: 805-968-3247
                                        rpopke@devereux.org
                                        www.devereuxca.org

Amy Evans, Executive Director
Rebecca Popke, Marketing & Admissions Manager
Wendy Cooper, Manager of External Affairs
Veronica Arenas-Soto, Human Resources Director
Serves adults age 18 through 85 who have intellectual and developmental disabilities such as emotional disturbances, neurological impairments, autism, dementia and more. Devereux California currently provides a continuum of services, including on-campus residential, day programs, behavior management and supported living services in the community.

6637   Division of Physical Medicine and Rehabilitation
San Joaquin General Hospital
500 W Hospital Rd
French Camp, CA   95231-9693   209-468-6000
                                        Fax: 209-468-6501
                                        www.sjphysicalmedicine.com

**6638   Dr. Karen H Chao Developmental Optometry Karen H.
Chao. O.D.**
Suite A
121 S Del Mar Ave
San Gabriel, CA   91776-1345   626-287-0401
                                        Fax: 626-287-1457
                                        drkhchao@yahoo.com
                                        www.healthgrades.com

Karen Chao, Owner
Karen Chao OD, Owner
Roger C. Holstein, Chief Executive Officer
Jeff Surges, President
Developmental optometrist specializing in the testing and treatment of vision problems and the enhancement of visual performance. Performs visual perceptual testing and training for children and adults. Undetected vision problems interfere with the ability to achieve and are highly correlated with learning difficulties and developmental problems. Provides the opportunity to overcome vision and visual-perceptual dysfunctions..

6639   Early Childhood Services
Desert Area Resources and Training
201 E Ridgecrest Blvd
Ridgecrest, CA   93555-3919   760-375-9787
                                        Fax: 760-375-1288
                                        www.dartontarget.org/

Peter V. Berns, Chief Executive Officer
Cris Bridges, Chief of Client Services
Bob Beecroft, Chief Operations Officer
Jeannie Luke, Human Resources Director/Risk Ma
Provides early intervention services to children who have disabilities or are experiencing delays in development. Provides developmental activities to promote the attainment of developmental milestones so that each child may reach his/her maximum potential. The program also provides therapeutic and educational intervention and offers support and guidance to families.

6640   East Los Angeles Doctors Hospital
4060 Whittier Boulevard
Los Angeles, CA   90023-2526   323-268-5514
                                        www.elalax.com

Hector Hernandez, Chief Executive Officer
Kamlesh Dhawan, Chief Of Staff
Michael Austerlitz, Vice-Chief Of Staff
Horacio Fleischman, Secretary Treasurer
Postacute rehabilitation program.

6641   Easter Seals Disability Svcs: Bay Area
Suite 250
391 Taylor Boulevard
Pleasant Hill, CA   94523- 4851   925-849-8999
                                        800-221-6827
                                        Fax: 312-726-1494
                                        info@easterseals.com
                                        www.bayarea.easterseals.com

6642   Easter Seals Superior California
Sacramento Center & Regional Offices
2617 A & B Alta Arden Expy.
Sacramento, CA   95825-1306   916-679-3113
                                        888-877-3257
                                        Fax: 916-485-2653
                                        www.superiorca.easterseals.com

Harry Johns, President and CEO
Kathie Wright, Program Director
Terry Colborn, VP Programs/Government Affairs
Joanne Budge, Chief Financial Officer

Provides outpatient rehabilitation services including day training programs for adults with disabilities and traumatic brain injuries, warm water therapy, non-public agency services to children including pediatric OT and PT services, work training/employment services, medical equipment loans, early intervention services for infants and toddlers. Serving the counties of Alpine, Calaveras, El Dorado, Sacramento, San Joaquin, Sutter, Tuolumne, Yolo, Yuba, Amador, Stanislaus, Nevada and Placer, CA.

6643 Exceed: A Division of Valley Resource Center
P.O.Box 1773
1285 N. Santa Fe
Hemet, CA 92543-1773   951-766-8659
800-423-1227
Fax: 951-929-9758
vrctwohip@aol.com
Pattie Robert, Business Development Specialist
Mary Morse, Marketing Director
Kathy Cooke, Manager
Our vision is an environment where each client is valued as an individual and is provided the opportunity to reach his/her maximum potential. Our mission is to provide service and advocacy, which creates choices and opportunities, for adults with disabilities to reach their maximum potential..

6644 Eye Medical Center of Fresno
Eye Medical Center
1360 E. Herndon Avenue
Suite 301 & 210
Fresno, CA 93720-1498   559-486-5000
emcfresno.com

6645 Fontana Rehabilitation Workshop
Industrial Support Systems
8333 Almeria Ave
Fontana, CA 92335-3283   909-428-3883
800-755-4755
Fax: 909-428-3835
www.industrial-support.org
Silvia Anderson, Executive Director
U. Jones, CFO
C.Steven Bowen Plant, Operations manager
Bonnie Edwards, Operations Manager
The Fontana Rehabilitation Workshop, Inc., through its business divisions is committed to maintaining a stable environment wherein people with disabilities are provided with those services and supports that enable them to overcome barriers to employment and empower them to maximize their employment potential.

6646 Foothill Vocational Opportunities
789 North Fair Oaks Avenue
Pasadena, CA 91103-3045   626-449-0218
Fax: 626-449-0218
info@foothillvoc.org
foothillvoc.org

6647 Fred Finch Youth Center
3800 Coolidge Ave
Oakland, CA 94602-3399   510-482-2244
Fax: 510-488-1960
receptionist@fredfinch.org
fredfinch.org
Thomas N. Alexander, President/CEO
FFYC seeks to provide a continuum of high quality programs for the care and treatment of children, youth, young adults, and their families, whose changing needs can best be met by a variety of mental health and support services. The goal is for the program participants to receive the most effective services in the least restrictive environment appropriate to their needs so that they may function at their highest potential.

6648 Gateway Center of Monterey County
850 Congress Ave
Pacific Grove, CA 93950-4898   831-372-8002
Fax: 831-372-2411
info@gatewaycenter.org
gatewaycenter.org
Stephanie Lyon, Executive Director
Mike Price, Chief Financial Officer
Desiree Boller, Accounting Assistant
Heidy Welch, Human Resources
Our mission is to be a caring and stimulating environment for the Developmentally Disabled where all people can achieve their individual goals safely and with dignity. Our goal is to continue our programs and to find new and innovative ways of assisting the developmentally disabled to live in our community in surroundings compatable with their ability to live and work at the highest level possible.

6649 Gateway Industries: Castroville
7055 Veterans Blvd
Unit A
Burr Ridge, IL 60527   630-321-1333
888-473-3744
Fax: 630-321-1321
www.redshift.com

6650 Gilroy Workshop
7471 Monterey Street
Gilroy, CA 95020-3629   408-430-2810
Fax: 408-842-6770
info@leadershipgilroy.org
www.leadershipgilroy.org/
Kristi Alarid, Manager
Sally French, Manager
Denise Martin, Executive Director
Andrea Gamble, Administrative Director
Work adjustment and remunerative work programs..

6651 Glendale Adventist Medical Center
1509 Wilson Ter
Glendale, CA 91206-4098   818-409-8000
Fax: 818-546-5609
www.glendaleadventist.com/services/rehab
Kevin Roberts, President/CEO
Warren Tetz, Sr. Vice President and COO
Kelly Turner, Sr. Vice President and CFO
Judy Blair, Sr. Vice President and CNO
Rehabilitative team is made up of physician specialists, as well as professional and certified staff nurses, thereapists and others who meet regularly to ensure tht each patients progress is carefully planned and closely monitored.

6652 Glendale Memorial Hospital and Health Center Rehabilitation Unit
Glendale Memorial Hospital and Health Center
1420 South Central Ave
Glendale, CA 91204-2508   818-502-1900
Fax: 818-409-7688
www.glendalememorialhospital.org
Catherine M. Pelley, President
Offers rehabilitation services, occupational therapy, physical therapy, residential services and more for the disabled.

6653 Goleta Valley Cottage Hospital
Cottage Health System
351 S Patterson Ave
Santa Barbara, CA 93111-2496   805-967-3411
Fax: 805-681-6437
cverkiak@cottagehealthsystem.org
www.sbch.org
Ronald C. Wreft, President & CEO
Rosemary Bray, Clinical Manager
Diana Gray Miller, Administrator
Betty Jane Petrich, Manager
A 122-bed acute care hospital was founded in 1966 to serve the growing community of Goleta Valley. Today, we admit more then 2,000 patients a year, see more then 17,000 emergency visits, and

welcome nearly 400 newborns to our designated 'Baby Friendly' Birth Center each year. We are also recognized for our Level IV trauma designation. We take great pride in fulfilling our goal of providing each patient with comfortable, personalized care.

6654 HealthSouth Tustin Rehabilitation Hospital
Health South Corporation
14851 Yorba St
Tustin, CA 92780-2925
714-832-9200
www.tustinrehab.com/

Diana Hanyak, Chief Executive Officer
Rodric Bell, Medical Director
Lindsey Barrett, Director of Case Management
Maryam Jouharzadeh, Pharm.D., Director, Pharmacy
HealthSouth Tustin Rehabilitation Hospital is part of the HealthSouth Corportation, the nation's largest provider of rehabilitative healthcare services, we are the only facility of its kind in Orange County. Fully accredited by the Joint Commission on Accreditation of Healthcare Organizations (JACHO) we provide inpatient and outpatient care designed to meed individual needs of patients and their families.

6655 Hi-Desert Medical Center
6601 White Feather Road
Joshua Tree, CA 92252-760
760-366-3711
hdmc.org

Lionel Chadwick, Chief Executive Officer
Tom Duda, Chief Financial Officer
Judy Austin, Chief Operating Officer & Chief
Barbara Staresinic, Director, Human Resources
Postacute rehabilitation program.

6656 Home of the Guiding Hands
Suite 200
1825 Gillespie Way
El Cajon, CA 92020-0501
619-938-2850
Fax: 619-938-3055
info@guidinghands.org
guidinghands.org

Mary Miller, President
Debby McNeil, Vice President
Michael Harris, Treasurer
Mark Klaus, Executive Director
The mission of Home og the Guiding Hands is to provide quality services, training and advocacy for people with developmental disabilities, their families, and others who will benefit.

6657 Hospital of the Good Samaritan Acute Rehabilitation Unit
1225 Wilshire Blvd
Los Angeles, CA 90017-1901
213-977-2121
800-366-8338
Fax: 213-482-2770
info@goodsam.org
goodsam.org

Andrew B Leeka, President and CEO
Charles T. Munger, Chairman
Physicians, researchers and staff are united by a common mission: to foster growth into one of the most comprehensive medical centers in the West. Services offered include: cardiology and cardiovascular services, neurosciences, movement disorders and Parkinsons disorder, wound care center and transfusion-medicine and surgery center.

6658 Innovative Rehabilitation Services
Hacienda La Puente Unified School District
15959 E. Gale Ave
City Of Industry, CA 91745
626-933-1000
Fax: 626-934-2900
info@hlpusd.k12.ca.us
www.hlpusd.k12.ca.us

Matthew Smith, Site Administrator
George Stransky, Counselor
Crystal Ontiveros, Counselor
Provides innovative student-centered learning opportunities and support services to a diverse population that enable individuals to achieve thier goals as lifelong learners, productive workers and effective communicators.

6659 Janus of Santa Cruz
Suite 150
200 7th Ave
Santa Cruz, CA 95062-4669
831-462-1060
866-526-8772
janussc.org

Rod Libbey, Executive Director
Bill Morris, Medical Director
Margie Storms, Clinical Director
Chris Storms, Intake Manager
A private not-for-profit corporation, licensed by the state of California. The Janus Clinic has a 3 year accreditation by the Council on Accreditation for Health Care Facilities.

6660 John Muir Medical Center Rehabilitation Services, Therapy Center
1601 Ygnacio Valley Rd
Walnut Creek, CA 94598-3122
925-939-3000
Fax: 925-308-8944
www.johnmuirhealth.com

Calvin Knight, President and CEO
Helen Doughty, Librarian
A 324-bed acute care facility that is designated as the only trauma center for Contra Costa County and portions of Solano County. Recognized as one of the region's premier healthcare providers, areas of specialty include high-and low-risk obstetrics, orthopedics, neurosciences, cardiac care and cancer care. The campus is accredited by the Joint Commission on Accreditation of Healthcare Organizations (JCAHO), a national surveyor of quality patient care.

6661 Kindred Hospital-La Mirada
14900 E. Imperial Hwy
La Mirada, CA 90638-2172
562-944-1900
Fax: 562-906-3455
TTY:800-735-2922
www.kindredlamirada.com

April Myers, Administrator
Adam Darvish, Executive Director
Committed to the delivery of high quality care in a cost-effective manner to enable us to become 'a model of excellence' in Long-Term Acute Care. Committed to treat our patients and families with dignity and respect, in the same manner we would want to be treated.

6662 King's View Work Experience Center- Atwater
559 East Bardsley Avenue
P. O. Box 688
Tulare, CA 93275-0688
559-688-7531
Fax: 559-688-3509
info@kingsview.org
www.kingsview.org

Leon Hoover, Chief Executive Officer
Vida Jalali, Chief Financial Officer Interim
Sue Essman, Director of Human Resources
Jeff Gorski, Director of Business Development
The primary mission of the Kings View Work Experience Center (KVWEC) is to serve people who have developmental disabilities. We believe in the dignity and worth of each person and in their right to rehabilitation, education and community integration. It is Kings View's aim to provide quality services to people who need assistance in the development of social, vocational and independent living skills.

6663 LaPalma Intercommunity Hospital
7901 Walker St
La Palma, CA 90623-1764
714-670-7400
LPIHInfo@primehealthcare.com
www.lapalmaintercommunityhospital.com

Virg Narbutas, Regional CEO
Sami Shoukair, Chief Medical Officer
Linda Gonzaba, Medical Staff Office Director
Hilda Manzo-Luna, Chief Nursing Officer
Lapalma Intercommunity Hospital endeavors to provide comprehensive, quality healthcare in a convenient, compassionate and cost effective manner. Lapalma is consistenly at the forefront of evolving national healthcare reform. Our organization provides an innovative and integrated healthcare delivery system. We re-

main ever cognizant of our patient's needs and desires for high quality affordable healthcare.

6664 Learning Services of Northern California
131 Langley Drive
Suite B
Lawrenceville, GA 30046-9315
408-848-4379
888-419-9955
Fax: 866-491-7396
www.learningservices.com
Dr. Debra Braunling-McMorrow, President and CEO
Jeanne Mack, Chief Financial Officer and Vice President of Operations
Michael Weaver, Chief Development Officer
Susan Snow, Director of Admissions
Located on 10 acres of ranchland in rural Santa Clara Valley, our Gilroy Program offers treatment, structure, and support in a spacious, campus-based living environment. Sharing living residences are complimented by a treatment and recreation facility for individuals who require intensive support.

6665 Learning Services: Morgan Hill
131 Langley Drive
Suite B
Lawrenceville, GA 30046-9315
408-848-4379
888-419-9955
Fax: 866-491-7396
www.learningservices.com
Dr. Debra Braunling-McMorrow, President and CEO
Jeanne Mack, Chief Financial Officer and Vice President of Operations
Michael Weaver, Chief Development Officer
Susan Snow, Director of Admissions
Located in the quaint rural town within walking distance from the old main street of Morgan Hill. Our Morgan Hill program offers the convenience and amenities of small-town living within the supportive community of Morgan Hill.

6666 Learning Services: Supported Living Programs
131 Langley Drive
Suite B
Lawrenceville, GA 30046-9315
408-848-4379
888-419-9955
Fax: 866-491-7396
www.learningservices.com
Dr. Debra Braunling-McMorrow, President and CEO
Jeanne Mack, Chief Financial Officer and Vice President of Operations
Michael Weaver, Chief Development Officer
Susan Snow, Director of Admissions
We offer a variety of diverse and stimulating environments for people with different needs, capabilities and personal goals. Within comfortable, homelike, age-appropriate settings we provide the structure and support necessary to ensure the richest possible quality of life. Program offered in both Northern and Southern facilities of California

6667 Leon S Peters Rehabilitation Center
2823 Fresno St
Fresno, CA 93721-1324
559-459-6000
www.communitymedical.org
Florence Dunn, Chairwoman
John McGregor, Esquire, Secretary
Tim A. Joslin, President, Chief Executive Officer
Patrick Rafferty, Executive Vice President, Chief Operating Officer
Community's flagship hospital that offers world class specialized critical care with the area's only stroke unit with 24-hour vascular neurology and neurosurgery coverage and a team of specially trained stroke nurses. The world's first G4 CyberKnife. The table Mountain Rancheraia Level 1 Trauma Center. The Leon S. Peters burn center. The region's only perinatology program for high rish pregnancies and deliveries. The Da-Vinci robotic surgical system, and 3 helicopeter landing pads.

6668 Lion's Blind Center of Diablo Valley, Inc. Lions Center For The Visually Impaired
175 Alvarado Ave
Pittsburg, CA 94565-4862
925-432-3013
800-750-3937
Fax: 925-432-7014
edward.329@comcast.net
www.seniorvision.org
Edward Schroth, Executive Director
Barbara Cronin, President
Charles Dunham, First Vice President
Phillis Neitling, Secretary
A private, nonprofit agency offering services such as health, educational, recreational, rehabilitation, employment and counseling to the totally blind, legally blind and visually impaired. The staff includes two full time workers..

6669 Lion's Blind Center of Oakland
2115 Broadway
Oakland, CA 94612-2698
510-450-1580
Fax: 510-654-3603
lbcenter.org
Michelle Taylor Lagunas, Executive Director/ CEO
Christina Easiley, Administrative Manager
Scott Blanks, Director of Rehabilitation Servi
Danette Davis, Orientation & Mobility Instructor
A private nonprofit organization offering services for the totally blind, legally blind, deaf-blind and multihandicapped blind. Services include: professional training, rehabilitation, education, counseling, social work, self help and more. The staff includes 12 full time and 1 part time worker.

6670 Living Skills Center for the Visually Impaired
2430 Road 20
#B112
San Pablo, CA 94806-5005
510-234-4984
Fax: 510-234-4986
info@hcblind.org
www.hcblind.org
Patricia Williams, Executive Director
Patricia Maffei, Program Director
Ronald Hideshima, Adaptive Technology Instructor
Lee Staub, Orientation and Mobility Instruc
A private, nonprofit agency offering services such as independent living skills training, recreational, employment and accessible technology training to the totally blind, legally blind and visually impaired. The staff includes six full time teachers.

6671 Loma Linda University Orthopedic and Rehabilitation Institute
25333 Barton Rd
Loma Linda, CA 92354-3123
909-558-1000
Fax: 909-558-0308
www.llu.edu
Richard H. Hart, MD, DrPH, President & Chief Executive Officer
Ronald L. Carter, PhD, Senior Vice President, Educational Affairs
Cari Dominguez, DHS, Senior Vice President, Human Resources
Mark L. Hubbard, Senior Vice President, Risk Management
Offers a full range of clinical programs for both inpatients and outpatient. The specific diagnosis leading to patient admission includes stroke, spinal cord injury, traumatic or anoxic brain damage, amputation, post neurosurgery, chronic neurological disease, Guillain-Barre syndrome, arthritis, multiple trauma or other complex orthopedic problems. The facilities and professional services are comprehensive and ensure that the best care is provided to pediatric and adult patients..

6672 Manor Care Health Services- Citrus Heights
7807 Uplands Way
Citrus Heights, CA 95610-7500
916-967-2929
Fax: 916-965-8439
hcr-manorcare.com
Steven M. Cavanaugh, Chief Financial Officer
Paul A. Ormond, Chairman, President and Chief Ex
The nations leader in skilled nursing and rehabilitation care. Our facility has been serving the Sacramento area for more then 12 years. We are known for our beautiful decor, outstanding rehabilitation staff and loving nursing care. We offer short term rehabili-

tation, long term skilled nursing care, respite care and post hospital surgical care.

6673 Manor Care Health Services- Palm Desert
74-350 Country Club Dr
Palm Desert, CA 92260-1608

760-341-0261
Fax: 760-779-1563
hcr-manorcare.com

Steven M. Cavanaugh, Chief Financial Officer
Paul A. Ormond, Chairman, President and Chief Ex

Centrally located in the Coachella Valley, specializing in skilled nursing whith an emphasis on rehabilitation, post surgery recovery, hospice, alzheimer's care and long term care. In addition, we offer 2 unique service options for the discriminating consumer. Our Arcadia unit offers a specialized Alzheimer's care program in a dedicated secure wing. ManorCare offers rehabilitation services including physical, occupational and speech therapies for those recovering from illness injury or surgery.

6674 Manor Care Health Services-Fountain Valley
11680 Warner Ave
Fountain Valley, CA 92708-2513

714-241-9800
Fax: 714-966-1654
hcr-manorcare.com

Steven M. Cavanaugh, Chief Financial Officer
Paul A. Ormond, Chairman, President and Chief Ex

Provides 24-hour skilled nursing, rehabilitative therapies and specialized Alzheimer's care. Our in-house therapists provide physical, occupational and speech therapies in our rehabilitation area. Our team is goal oriented and focuses on producing positive outcomes for those recovering from illness, injury or surgery. Our respite care program provides a full range of services for a few days, a week or even a season.

6675 Manor Care Health Services-Hemet
1717 W Stetson Ave
Hemet, CA 92545-6882

951-925-9171
Fax: 951-925-8186
hcr-manorcare.com

Steven M. Cavanaugh, Chief Financial Officer
Paul A. Ormond, Chairman, President and Chief Ex

Provides skilled nursing, Rehabilitation services, and specialized Alzheimer's care. In addition we offer short term respite stays for family caregivers that simply need a break from the stress of daily care. Our Arcadia unit staff is specially trained in the care of residents with Alzheimer's disease. The secured unit is designed to provide a soothing and homelike environment while enhancing each resident's remaining abilities.

6676 Manor Care Health Services-Sunnyvale
1150 Tilton Dr
Sunnyvale, CA 94087-2440

408-735-7200
Fax: 408-736-8629
hcr-manorcare.com

Steven M. Cavanaugh, Chief Financial Officer
Paul A. Ormond, Chairman, President and Chief Ex

Our in-house therapists provide physical, occupational and speech therapies in our rehabilitation area. Our team is goal oriented and focuses on producing positive outcomes for those recovering from illness, injury or surgery. Our skilled nursing staff works with our therapy department and dietary department to provide positive wound care programs for patients requiring skin management care.

6677 Manor Care Health Services-Walnut Creek
1226 Rossmoor Pkwy
Walnut Creek, CA 94595-2538

925-975-5000
Fax: 925-937-1132
hcr-manorcare.com

Steven M. Cavanaugh, Chief Financial Officer
Paul A. Ormond, Chairman, President and Chief Ex

Provides luxurious long term care and rehabilitation services. In house therapists provide, physical, occupational and speech therapies in our rehabilitation area. Our team is goal oriented and focuses on producing positive outcomes for those recovering from illness, injury or surgery. Our years of combined management experience add value to our resident's quality of life.

6678 Maynord's Chemical Dependency Recovery Centers
19325 Cherokee Road
Tuolumne, CA 95379-1657

209-928-3737
800-228-8208
Fax: 209-928-1152
maynords.com

James Berry, Director

Maynord's Recovery Centers has always been dedicated to the recovery of good people whose lives are being destroyed by alcohol and drugs. Since 1978, Maynord's residential program has helped thousands of people put their lives back together after addiction has taken its toll. Today, Maynord's offers a treatment system over much of the San Joaquin Valley and the San Francisco Bay Area.

6679 Maynord's Ranch for Men
19325 Cherokee Road
Tuolumne, CA 95379-1657

209-928-3737
800-228-8208
Fax: 209-928-1152
maynords.com

James Berry, Director

Provides treatment for chemical dependency problems to men. The treatment addresses their recovery through a comprehensive plan created for their individual needs. Also offers a program for women called the Meadows.

6680 Meadowbrook Manor
431 West Remington Boulevard
Bolingbrook, IL 60440

630-759-1112
Fax: 630-759-6925
jmolen@meadowbrookmanor.com
www.meadowbrookmanor.com

6681 Meadowview Manor
41 Crestview Terrace
Bridgeport, WV 26330

304-842-7101
Fax: 304-842-7104
info@meadowviewmanor.com
www.meadowviewmanor.com

6682 Memorial Hospital of Gardenia
1145 West Redondo Beach Blvd
Gardena, CA 90247-3528

310-532-4200
800-782-2288
www.avantihospitals.com

Edward Mirzabegian, Corporate Chief Executive Officer

Postacute rehabilitation program.

6683 Mercy Medical Group
Mercy Hospital
3000 Q Street
Sacramento, CA 95816

916-733-3333
www.mymercymedicalgroup.org

6684 Napa County Mental Health Department
2344 Old Sonoma Road
Bldg. D
Napa, CA 94559-3708

707-259-8151
800-648-8650
www.countyofnapa.org/MentalHealth/

6685 Napa Valley Support Systems
1700 Second Street Suite 212
Napa, CA 94559-1344

707-253-7490
Fax: 707-253-0115
napavalleysupportservices.org

Beth Kahiga, Executive Director
Heather Jump, Administrative Manager
Katy Vanzant, Program Director
Emmy Lesko, Program Supervisor

Work hardening and disciplinary programs.

6686 North Valley Services
1040 Washington
Red Bluff, CA 96080-4509
530-527-0407
Fax: 530-527-7091
www.northvalleyservices.org

Joe Brown, President
Larry Donnelley, Vice President
Lynn DeFreece, CEO
Delbert Brownfield, COO
Provides vocational rehabilitation services, such as job counseling, job training, and work experience, to unemployed and underemployed persons, persons with disabilities.

6687 Northridge Hospital Medical Center Rehabiltation Medicine
18300 Roscoe Blvd
Northridge, CA 91328-4167
818-885-8500
Fax: 818-701-7367
www.northridgehospital.org/index.htm

Mike L. Wall, President
Thomas L. Hedge, Medical Director
Joel S. Rosen, Associate Medical Director
Alex L. Lin, Managing Director
A full service, comprehensive rehabilitation program suited to treat patients of all ages who have suffered catastrophic or debilitating injury or illness. The goal of the program is to deliver exceptional patient care to maximise each individual's skills and independence.

6688 Northridge Hospital Medical Center: Centerfor Rehabilitation Medicine
18300 Roscoe Blvd
Northridge, CA 91328-4167
818-885-8500
Fax: 818-701-7367
www.northridgehospital.com

Mike L. Wall, President
Thomas L. Hedge, Medical Director
Joel S. Rosen, Associate Medical Director
Alex L. Lin, Managing Director
Committed to serving the health needs of our communities with particular attention to the needs of the poor, the disadvantaged, and vulneralbe, and the comfort of the suffering and dying. Catholic Healthcare West has a commitment to quality-quality healthcare services and the promotion of optimal quality of life for all of life.

6689 Old Adobe Developmental Services
1301A Rand Street
Suite A
Petaluma, CA 94954-5697
707-763-9807
Fax: 707-763-7708
www.oadsinc.org

Elizabeth Clary, Executive Director
Marie Padgett, Controller
The mission of Old Adobe to provide opportunities for individuals with developmental challenges to reach thier fullest potentials. Our job at OADS is to find ways for these individuals to find full expression in all parts of their lives. We have a partnership with the Adult Education Department of the Petaluma School District in providing services to persons with developmental challenges. We are funded by the Dept. of Rehabilitation and the Dept. Of Developmental services.

6690 Old Adobe Developmental Services-Rohnert Park Services (Behavioral)
5401 Snyder Ln.
Rohnert Park, CA 94928-3124
707-584-5859
Fax: 707-664-8057
www.oadsinc.org

Elizabeth Clary, Executive Director
Helen Gunderson, Administrative Assistant
The program services are designed to assist individuals who demonstrate basic work skills, to develop social skills and work habits necessary to succeed in supported or competitive employment. Most often individual program services involve working with the client to replace those behavioral excesses that have been a barrier to vocational placement.

6691 PRIDE Industries
10030 Foothills Blvd
Roseville, CA 95747-7102
916-788-2100
800-550-6005
Fax: 800-888-0447
info@prideindustries.com
prideindustries.com

Michael Ziegler, President & CEO
Bob Selvester, Vice Chair
Mike Snegg, Treasurer
Tim Yamauchi, Executive Vice President and Chi
To provide opportunities through employment, training, evaluation and placement maximizing community access, independence and quality of life for people with barriers to employment.

6692 Pacific Hospital Of Long Beach-Neuro Care Unit
2776 Pacific Ave
Long Beach, CA 90806-2613
562-997-2000
webmaster@phlb.org

Michael D. Drobot, CEO
Clark Todd, President
Teri Plemmons, Administrative Assistant
Our mission is to heal with compassion and to perform with distinction. Our vision: to improve the hospital's orthopedic and Spine Center of Excellence. Achieve exceptional financial performance to enhance hospital services. Improve the vertically integrated ancillary, outpatient and inpatient surgery system. Develop a professionally challenging work environment that reflects an agile, peak performance culture.

6693 Paradise Valley Hospital-South Bay Rehabilitation Center
2400 East 4th St
National City, CA 91950-2026
619-470-4321
paradisevalleyhospital.net

Prem Reddy, Chairman
Neerav Jadeja, Administrator
Luis Leon, President
Gemma Rama-Banaag, Chief Nursing Officer
South Bay Rehabilitation Center, offers a complete range of treatment for patients with physical disabilities. Our specialized inpatient and outpatient programs are designed to meet each person's individual needs or injuries, with the goal of restoring as much independence as possible and significantly improving their lives.

6694 Parents and Friends
350 South Main Street
Fort Bragg, CA 95437-5408
707-964-4940
parentsandfriends.org

Rick Moon, Executive Director
Jessica Dickey, Administrative Assistant
Kristy Tanguay, Manager
Kathy Connell, Bookkeeper
Parents and Friends provides opportunities for persons with developmental challenges and similar needs to participate fully in our community.

6695 People Services
4195 Lakeshore Blvd
Lakeport, CA 95453-6411
707-263-3810
peopleservices.org

Ilene Dumont, Executive Director
Martin Diesman, Director
Vicki Cole, Director
Kathy Ryan, Director
Providing an array of services for adults with developmental disabilities and other people with disabilities. Services include supported employment, work services, supported living, personal, social and community training, transportation, specialized individual services and much more.

6696 Petaluma Recycling Center
Old Adobe Developmental Services
315 2nd St
Petaluma, CA 94952-4230
707-763-4761
Fax: 707-763-4921

Elizabeth Clary, Executive Director

Began in 1974; has been one of the major employers of persons with developmental challenges for 26 years; is the primary recycling facility in the growing city of 52,000; accepts over 20 different kinds of recyclables; employs 20-25 persons a day.

6697   Pomerado Rehabilitation Outpatient Service
15615 Pomerado Rd
Poway, CA 92064-2405   858-485-6511
                                               Fax: 858-613-4248

Bob Blake, Director Rehab Services
Jonathan Pee, Manager
A 107-bed acute care hospital. In addition to a round-the-clock Emergency Department, Pomerado offers the area's finest outpaient surgery center and general medical/surgical services. Pomerado Hospital also is home to a world-class Birth Center and a Level II NICU. Fully JCAHO-accredidted, Pomerado is well-known for offering only private rooms, each with a scenic view of the North Countryside, which enhances the healing atmosphere..

6698   Pride Industries: Grass Valley
12451 Loma Rica Dr
Grass Valley, CA 95945-9059   530-477-1832
                                                      800-550-6005
                                                 Fax: 530-477-8038
                                            info@prideindustries.com
                                             www.prideindustries.com

Bob Olsen, Chairman
Bob Selvester, Vice Chairman
Walt Payne, President/CEO
Mike Snegg, Treasurer
Work adjustment and remunerative work programs. We offer an adult day program as well.

6699   Rancho Adult Day Care Center
Rancho Los Amigos Medical Center
7601 Imperial Hwy
Downey, CA 90242-3456   562-401-7111
                                                 Fax: 562-401-7991
                                                  TTY:562-401-8450
                                dhs.lacounty.gov/wps/portal/dhs/rancho
Valerie Orange, CEO
Margaret L Campbell, Research Director
Provides personal care, social services and a therapeutic program to older adults in order to improve their quality of life. Offers a Clinical Gerontology Service, an Alzheimer's Disease Diagnostic and Treatment Center and a Geriatric Assessment and Rehabilitation Unit..

6700   Regional Center for Rehabilitation
2288 Auburn Blvd
Sacramento, CA 95821-1618   916-421-4167
                                                 Fax: 916-925-1586

6701   Rehabilitation Institute of Santa Barbara
2415 De La Vina St
Santa Barbara, CA 93105-3819   805-569-8999
                                                 Fax: 805-687-3707
                                                          risb.org

Ralph Pollock, President
Scott Silic MBA, Vice President Of Operations
Cheryl Ellis MD, MHA, VP Medical Services
A regional rehabilitation system with an acute care hospital at the center, the Institute provides specialized inpatient and outpatient programs for brain injury, spinal cord injury, stroke, work-related injury, chronic pain, orthopedic problems and more. Offers a 46-bed acute-care rehabilitation hospital, a free-standing outpatient center, the brain injury continuum, chronic pain program..

6702   Rehabilitation Institute of Southern California
1800 E La Veta Ave
Orange, CA 92866-2902   714-633-7400
                                                 Fax: 714-633-4586
                                              adults@rio-rehab.com
                                                       riorehab.org

Praim S. Singh, Executive Director
Carol Reese, Executive Assistant
Grace Lee, Administrative Assistant
Dana Patton, Personnel Officer
Outpatient rehabilitation serving physically and disabled children and adults. Child development programs, adult day care for disabled seniors, child care for disabled and non-disabled children, outpatient therapy, aquatics, adult day healthcare, independent living, vocational services, social services, and housing.

6703   Rubicon Programs
2500 Bissell Avenue
Richmond, CA 94804-1815   510-235-1516
                                                 Fax: 510-235-2025
                                            rubicon@rubiconpgms.org
                                             www.rubiconprograms.org

Rob Hope, Chief Program Officer
Jane Fischberg, President and Executive Director
Roger Contreras, CFO
Kelly Dunn, General Counsel and Director of Legal Services
Rubicon Programs Inc. helps people and communities build assets to achieve greater independence. Since 1973, Rubicon has built and operated affordable housing and provided employment, job training, mental health, and other supportive services to individuals who have disabilities, are homeless, or are otherwise economically disadvantaged.

6704   San Bernardino Valley Lighthouse for the Blind
762 North Sierra Way
San Bernardino, CA 92410-4438   909-884-3121
                                                 Fax: 909-884-2964
                                                        www.afb.org

Robert Mc Bay, Executive Director
Sandra Wood, Administrative Assistant
Provides training in independent living skills - cooking, mobility and orientation, sewing, Braille and typing. Also, we have classes in macrame, ceramics and basket weaving. Weekly support group and Bible study..

6705   Santa Clara Valley Blind Center, Inc.
101 N Bascom Ave
San Jose, CA 95128-1805   408-295-4016
                                                 Fax: 408-295-1398
                                            info@visionbeyondsight.org
                                                visionbeyondsight.org

Arnold Chew, President
John Glass, Vice President
Arlene Holmes, Secretary
Sue Szucs, Treasurer
SCVBC's mission is to increase the confidence, independence, and quality of life of the blind and visually impaired through educational, recreational, and rehabilitative programs.

6706   Scripps Memorial Hospital: Pain Center
4275 Campus Point Ct.
San Diego, CA 92121-1205   858-626-4123
                                                      800-727-4777
                                           clinicalresearch@scrippshealth.com
                                                      www.scripps.org

Chris Van Gorder, President and CEO
Richard K Rothberger, Vice President, Chief Financial Officer
Robin B Brown, Chief Executive
Richard R Sheridan, Corporate Senior Vice President
Offers both inpatient and outpatient programs including: physical activity management, individual pain management, group therapy, medication adjustment, pain control classes, occupational therapy, biofeedback training, family counseling, vocational and leisure counseling and recreational therapy.

6707   Sharp Coronado Hospital
250 Prospect Place
Coronado, CA   92118-1999   619-522-3600
                                              erica.carlson@sharp.com
                                                      sharp.com

Marcia Hall, CEO
Mark Tamsen, Chairman
Tom Smisek, Vice Chairman
Dan Gensler, Secretary
Providing medical and surgical care, intensive care, sub-acute
and long-term care, rehabilitation therapies and emergency services in a peaceful setting is part of our live+heal+grow philosophy. We are one of the county's few community-owned hospitals
and are proud of our history of providing convenient, award-winning heath care to Coronado and San Diego.

6708   Shriners Hospitals For Children-Northern California
2425 Stockton Blvd.
Sacramento, CA   95817   916-453-2000
                                         patientreferrals@shrinenet.org
                                   www.shrinershospitalsforchildren.org
John McCabe, Executive Vice President
Dale W Stauss, Chairman
Jerry G Gantt, 1st Vice President
Chris L Smith, 2nd Vice President
The only hospital in the Shriners system that houses facilities for
treatment of all 3 Shriner specialties -spinal cord injuries, ortho-
paedic, and burns. The hospital features 80 patient beds, 9 parent
apartments, 5 state-of-the-art operating rooms, a high-tech Mo-
tion Analysis lab, and an entire floor devoted to research.

6709   Shriners Hospitals for Children: Los Angeles
3160 Geneva Street
Los Angeles, CA   90020-1199   213-388-3151
                                         patientreferrals@shrinenet.org
                                   www.shrinershospitalsforchildren.org
John McCabe, Executive Vice President
Dale W Stauss, Chairman
Jerry G Gantt, 1st Vice President
Chris L Smith, 2nd Vice President
Shriners Hospitals for Children: Los Angeles, treats children un-
der age 18 with burn scars, orthopedic conditions, cleft lip and
palate and limb deficiencies at no cost to the patient or their
families.

6710   Society for the Blind
1238 S St.
Sacramento, CA   95811-3256   916-452-8271
                                         Fax: 916-492-2483
                                        info@societyfortheblind.org
                                            societyfortheblind.org
Shari Roesler, Executive Director
Shane Snyder, Director of Programs
A private, local nonprofit organization providing blind and visually impaired people with the training supplies and support they
need to live independent, productive and fulfilled lives with limited vision. Services include the Low Vision Clinic, Braille
classes, computer training, support groups, living skills instruction, mobility training and the Products for Independence Store.

6711   Solutions at Santa Barbara: Transitional Living Center
1135 N Patterson Ave
Santa Barbara, CA   93111-1113   805-683-1995
                                         Fax: 805-683-4793
                                            sol1135@aol.com
                                       solutionsatsantabarbara.com
Sue Hannigan, Director
Postacute rehabilitation program. Short-term transitional living
program for individuals with traumatic brain injury, stroke, aneurysm and other neurological disorders.

6712   St. John's Pleasant Valley Hospital Neuro Care Unit
2309 Antonio Ave
Camarillo, CA   93010-1414   805-389-5800
                                                      shw.org
Jerry Conway, President
Maureen M. Malone, Administrator
Raye Burkhardt, Vice President and Chief Nursing
Houses 82 acute-care beds, a 99-bed extended care unit, and the
only hyperbaric medicine unit in Ventura County. Employ's
1,800 people and count 250 active medical staff.

**6713   St. John's Regional Medica Center- Industrial Therapy
Center**
1600 North Rose Ave
Oxnard, CA   93030-3723   805-988-2500
                                            www.stjohnshealth.org
Gudrun Moll, Vice President and Chief Nursing
Laurie Harting, President & CEO
Kim Wilson, Vice President
Chris Champlin, Senior Vice President
A non-profit health care facility offering multi-disciplinary pro-
grams for pain management and work hardening, as well as physi-
cal and occupational therapy.

6714   Sub-Acute Saratoga Hospital
13425 Sousa Lane
Saratoga, CA   95070-4663   408-378-8875
                                         Fax: 408-378-7419
                                            subacutesaratoga.com
Jack Stephens, President & CEO
Paul Quintana, Medical Director
Gary Vernon, NHA Administrator
Lindsay Zarcone, Marketing Manager
Dedicated to the fulfillment of human needs, desires, and wishes
in illness and in health. The cohesiveness of caring in a family
community of staff, patients, and their loved ones. The celebration of each unique life through their therapeutic journey, while
preserving their individual spirit. The achievement of advanced
medical expertise, knowledge, and skill given with the human
touch of caring toward the ultimate goal: enhancing the healing
process from acute illness to the joy of going home.

6715   Synergos Neurological Center: Hayward
27200 Calaroga Avenue
Hayward, CA   94545-4383   510-264-4000
                                         Fax: 510-264-4007
                                               strosehospital.org
Richard C. Hardwig, Chair
Alan McIntosh, Vice Chair
Lex Reddy, President and CEO
Roger Krissman, Chief Financial Officer
Postacute rehabilitation program.

6716   Synergos Neurological Center: Mission Hills
27200 Calaroga Avenue
Hayward, CA   94545-4383   510-264-4000
                                         Fax: 510-264-4007
                                            www.strosehospital.org
Richard C. Hardwig, Chair
Alan McIntosh, Vice Chair
Lex Reddy, President and CEO
Roger Krissman, Chief Financial Officer
For over 30 years, St. Rose Hospital Rehabilitation Services De-
partment has helped thousands of patients recover from illness
and injury through the help of our specially trained therapists.
These therapists have been trained in specific rehabilitative areas
such as physical, occupational, and speech therapies.

6717   Temple Community Hospital
235 N Hoover St
Los Angeles, CA   90004-3672   213-382-7252
                                         Fax: 213-382-1874
                                          templecommunityhospital.com

6718 Tunnell Center for Rehab
680 South Fourth Street
Louisville, CA   40202-4807   502-596-7300
                                      Fax: 800-545-0749
                        web_administrator@kindred.com
                                 kindredhealthcare.com

Mary R., Activities Assistant
Kristen W., Health and Rehabilitation Center
The Tunnell Center for Rehabilitation and Healthcare
accomodates 178 residents. We are dedicated to short-term complex medical and rehabilitative care. Using a holistic care management approach we work with residents who have suffered
debilitating injury or illness, and who need comprehensive nursing and rehabilitation services to achieve their highest practicable level of functional ability and independence.

6719 Ukiah Valley Association for Habilitation
Ukiah, CA   95482-689   707-468-8824
                                 Fax: 707-468-9149
                                 TTY:800-735-2929
                                 www.uvah.org

Pamela Jensen, Executive Director
Kris Vipond, Business Manager
Sharrae Elston, Director
Suzanne Warner, Employment Training Specialist
Work adjustment and suppoted employment and social and com-
munity services.

6720 Valley Center for the Blind
2491 W Shaw Avenue
Suite 124
Fresno, CA   93711-3331   559-222-4088
                                 Fax: 559-222-4844

Bud Breslin, Executive Director
Millie Marshall, Marriage Family Therapist
Saramarie Katich, Office Mngr/Program Director
Connie Parrick, Secretary
A private, nonprofit organization that offers educational, health,
recreational and professional training services to the totally
blind, legally blind or severely visually impaired.

6721 Villa Esperanza Services
2060 East Villa Street
Pasadena, CA   91107   626-449-2919
                                 Fax: 626-449-2850
                        info@villaesperanzaservices.org
                        www.villaesperanzaservices.org

Candice Rogers, Chairman
Richard Hubinger, President
Vicky Castillo, CFO
Kelly White, Chief Executive Officer
Serving disabled infants to seniors in a school, adult day pro-
gram, adult work program and residences and adult day health
care program and care management program.

6722 Village Square Nursing And Rehabilitation Center
Kindred Healthcare, Inc.
1586 West San Marcos Blvd
San Marcos, CA   92078-4019   760-471-2986
                                 www.villagesquarerehab.com

6723 Vista Center for the Blind & Visually Impaired
2500 El Camino Real,
Suite 100
Palo Alto, CA   94306   650-858-0202
                                 800-660-2009
                                 Fax: 650-858-0214
                                 info@vistacenter.org
                                 www.vistacenter.org

Pam Brandin, Executive Director
Nacole Barth-Ellis, Co-Director of Development
Terry Kurfess, Co-Director of Development
Meg Faville, Administrative Services Manager
Private nonprofit agency that serves the visually impaired in the
San Mateo, Santa Clara, San Benito and Santa Cruz Counties with
offices in Palo Alto and Santa Cruz. Offers Low Vision Evalua-
tions, mobility training, daily living skills training, social ser-

vices, counseling, support groups, computer training, other rehabilitation services, and a store.

6724 Winways at Orange County
7732 E Santiago Canyon Rd
Orange, CA   92869-1829   714-771-5276
                                 Fax: 714-771-1452
                                 winwaysrehab.com

Pamela Kauss, Director
The program offers clients highly personalized, comprehensive
programs to meet the needs of individuals with traumatic brain injury, stroke, tumors, aneurysm, post concussive syndrome or
other neurological disorders. Winways also has a special program
that provides services to Spanish speaking clients, called Contigo
Adelante with materials in Spanish, and Spanish speaking interpreters to assist in the therapy process.

Colorado

6725 Capron Rehabilitation Center
Penrose Hospital/ St. Francis Healthcare System
2222 N Nevada Ave
Colorado Springs, CO   80907-6819   719-776-5000
                                 penrosestfrancis.org
Margaret Sabin, President & CEO
Nate Olson, Chief Executive Officer
Jameson Smith, Senior VP & Chief Admnistrative Officer
Gil Porat, Chief Medical Officer
Southern Colorado's most complete inpatient and outpatient re-
habilitation center.

6726 Cerebral Palsy of Colorado
801 Yosemite Street
Denver, CO   80230   303-691-9339
                                 Fax: 303-691-0846
                                 abilityconnectioncolorado.org
Judith I Ham, CEO
James Reuter, Chairman of the Board
Penfield Tate, Vice Chairman
Kathy Higgins, Treasurer
Provides services for children birth-5 years, employment ser-
vices for adults, information and referral, donation pickup and
cell phone/ink cartridge recycling services.

6727 Cherry Hills Health Care Center
Kindred
3575 S Washington St
Englewood, CO   80110-3807   303-789-2265

6728 Community Hospital Back and Conditioning Clinic
1060 Orchard Ave
Grand Junction, CO   81501-2997   970-243-3400
                                 800-621-0926
                                 Fax: 970-856-6510
Amy Hibberd, Executive Director
David Scherman, Manager
Post-accute rehabilitation program .

6729 Devereux Advanced Behavioral Health Colorado
8405 Church Ranch Blvd.
Westminster, CO   80021   303-466-7391
                                 800-456-2536
                                 agorman@devereux.org
                                 www.devereuxco.org
Lisa Gaudia, Interim Clinical Director
A non-profit partner for individuals, families, schools and communities, serving people in the areas of autism, intellectual and
developmental disabilities, mental health issues, and child welfare. Programs offered include residential services, community
based services, educational programs, employment supports and
more.

6730 **Laradon Hall Society for Exceptional Children and Adults**
5100 Lincoln St
Denver, CO 80216-2056

303-296-2400
866-381-2163
Fax: 303-296-4012
laradon.org

William Mitchell, Chair
Suzanne Bradeen, Vice Chair
Jason Adams, Treasurer
Nancy Hodges, Secretary
Laradon provides educational, vocational and residential services to children and adults with developmental disabilities and other special needs. Laradon was founded in 1948. It is among the largest and most comprehensive service providers in Colorado.

6731 **Learning Services: Bear Creek**
7201 W Hampden Ave
Lakewood, CO 80227-5305

303-989-6660
888-419-9955
Fax: 866-491-7396
lengland@learningservices.com
learningservices.com

Susan Snow, Director of Admissions
Dr. Debra Braunling-McMorrow, President and CEO
Jeanne Mack, Chief Financial Officer
Michael Weaver, Chief Development Officer
Supported living program for persons with acquired brain injury.

6732 **MOSAIC In Colorado Springs**
888 W. Garden of the Gods Road
Ste 100
Colorado Springs, CO 80907-6251

719-380-0451
Fax: 719-380-7055
mosaic_cosprings@mosaicinfo.org
www.mosaicincoloradosprings.org

Tom Maltais, Executive Director
Mosaic in Colorado Springs provides a variety of services to assist adults and families in achieving positive goals. Services to persons with intellectual disabilities include community living options, vocational training and supported employment, spiritual growth and personal development options, and day programs habilitation and community participation.

6733 **Manor Care Nursing and Rehabilitation Center: Boulder**
Manor Care Ohio
2800 Palo Pkwy
Boulder, CO 80301-1540

303-440-9100
Fax: 303-440-9251
www.hcr-manorcare.com

Steven M. Cavanaugh, Chief Financial Officer
Paul A. Ormond, Chairman, President and Chief Ex
150 bed center offers a full spectrum of nursing care and rehabilitation. This includes our Arcadia Special Care Unit for Alzheimer's patients. Specialized unit for post acute skilled nursing care. Physical and massage therapies. And a 48 bed upscale Heritage unit offering additional amenities and furnishings.

6734 **Manor Care Nursing: Denver**
290 S Monaco Pkwy
Denver, CO 80224-1105

303-355-2525
Fax: 303-333-6960
www.hcr-manorcare.com

Steven M. Cavanaugh, Chief Financial Officer
Paul A. Ormond, Chairman, President and Chief Ex
Our center has delveloped a reputation for its luxurious environment, comprehensive rehabilitation service and focus on quality care. A wide range of individual and group activities and many gracious amenities create the finest combination of elegance and professional skilled nursing care. Arcadia, our special care unit for persons with Alzheimer's disease and related memory impairments, promotes independence and preserves dignity within a safe and secure environment.

6735 **Mediplex of Colorado**
8451 Pearl St
Thornton, CO 80229-4804

303-288-3000
Fax: 303-286-5136
info@vhdenver.com
www.northvalleyrehab.com

Jan Eyer, Chief Executive Officer
Our programs and services help each patient along the road to recovery toward our ultimate aim; the greatest possible restoration of the individual's self-esteem, ability to set goals, and self-sufficiency. Also offer specialized acute inpatient rehabilitative services, including special programs in Trauma Rehabilitation.

6736 **Platte River Industries**
490 Bryant St
Denver, CO 80204-4808

303-825-0041
Fax: 303-825-0564

Bob Smith, Executive Director
Postacute rehabilitation facility and program..

6737 **Pueblo Diversified Industries**
2828 Granada Blvd
Pueblo, CO 81005-3198

800-466-8393
Fax: 719-564-3407
info@pdipueblo.org
www.pdipueblo.net

Karen K Lillie, President & CEO
Robin Forbes, Director Human Services
Tom Drolshagen, Chief Operating Officer
Tom Denslow, Manager, Human Resources
A place where people can turn limitations into opportunities. People can experience the independence, pride and self worth of securing and maintaining a job.

6738 **SHALOM Denver**
2498 W 2nd Ave
Denver, CO 80223-1007

303-623-0251
Fax: 303-620-9584
akover@jewishfamilyservice.org
shalomdenver.com

Arnie Kover, Disability and Employment Servic
Sara Leeper, Coordinator of Client Services
Vicky Brittain, Mailing Business Manager
Bari Belinsky, Work Services Manager
SHALOM Denver provides employment, training, and job placement opportunities to people with disabilities, resettled immigrants, and people moving from welfare to work.

6739 **SPIN Early Childhood Care & Education Cntr**
1333 Elm Ave
Canon City, CO 81212-4431

719-275-0550
www.starpointco.com/spin

Diane Trujillo, Manager
SPIN center is a fully inclusive non-discriminating community early childhood program, offering a variety of schedule choices for families. The philosophy of the SPIN program is to promote each child's growth and development. Special attention is given to cognitive, physical, speech language and social-emotional growth. Staff is specifically trained to facilitate and prepare environments that promote exploration, key experiences, creativity and self-expression..

6740 **Schaefer Enterprises**
500 26th Street
P.O. Box 200009
Greeley, CO 80631-8427

970-353-0662
Fax: 970-353-2779
schaefenterprises@comcast.net
www.schaeferenterprises.com

Valorie Randall, Executive Director
Alex Witt, Executive Assistant
Veronica Griego, Production Director
Schaefer Enterprises, Inc., located in Greely, Colorado, is a vaulable community resource that has been fulfilling the outsourcing needs of businesses in Weld County and outlying areas since 1952.

6741 Spalding Rehab Hospital West Unit
150 Spring St
Morrison, CO 80465
303-697-4334
Fax: 303-697-0570

Connecticut

6742 ACES/ACCESS Inclusion Program
350 State Street
North Haven, CT 06473-3218
203-498-6800
Fax: 203-234-1369
acesinfo@aces.org
www.aces.org

Thomas M Danehy, Executive Director
Erika Forte, Assistant Executive Director
Evelyn Rossetti, Manager
Provides a person centered planning approach for integrated employment, volunteer community based opportunities for adults who have developmental disabilities..

6743 Apria Healthcare
26220 Enterprise Court
Lake Forest, CA 92630-1015
800-277-4288
contact_us@apria.com
www.apria.com

Lisa M. Getson, Executive Vice President, Govern
Nichola Denney, Executive Vice President, Revenue Management
Dan Stark, Chief Executive Officer
Debra L Morris, Chief Financial Officer
Provides a broad range of high quality and cost effective specialty infusion therapies and related services to patients in their homes throughout the Northeastern United States. Offer home infusion antibiotic therapy, quality pharmacy services, skilled nursing services and related support services.

6744 Arc Of Meriden-Wallingford, Inc.
200 Research Parkway
Meriden, CT 06450
203-237-9975
Fax: 203-639-0946
www.arcmw.org

Pamela Fields, Executive Director
Joseph Palfini, Board President
Becky Blazejowski, Financial Director
Maritza Dell, Director of Program Services
A membership agency that provides comprehensive, full-service, community-based opportunities for people with disabilities. Guided by over 120 community members and an active Board of Directors, the Arc always has its focus on improving the lives of people with disabilities. The Arc of Meriden-Wallingford offers advocacy and assistance to our members along with advocating for the rights and choices of people with disabilities in our community.

6745 Arc of the Farmington Valley
225 Commerce Drive
Canton, CT 06019-2478
860-693-6662
Fax: 860-693-8662
rcipolla@favarh.org
favarh.org

George Kral, President
Ernest E Mack, Vice President
Larry Pollock, Treasurer
Robin Dinicola, Secretary
Serving over 300 mentally retarded adults through a comprehensive program of residential and support services. These include three group homes, three apartments, competitive and supported employment options, a day program for mentally retarded seniors, community experience day services for severe and profoundly disabled adults, recreation and leisure services, advocacy, transportation, case management, in-home respite and other support services.

6746 Connecticut Subacute Corporation
19 Tuttle Pl
Middletown, CT 06457-1881
860-347-6300
Fax: 860-347-2446

Evan K Lyle, Managed Care Director
Cheri Kauset, Corporate Rep.
Specializes in subacute medical and rehabilitation programming. The strength of our system is in its' ability to service a broad range of clinical and psychosocial needs which enable each individual to attain his/her optimal potential. Programming includes neurological and orthopedic rehabilitation, post-surgical and wound care management, intravenous therapy, pulmonary rehabilitation including ventilator services, and long term care..

6747 Datahr Rehabilitation Institute
4 Berkshire Blvd
Bethel, CT 06801-1001
203-775-4700
888-8DA-TAHR
Fax: 203-775-4688
abilitybeyonddisability.com

Thomas Fanning, CEO
Providers of comprehensive rehabilitation services with a history of nearly 5 decades of service. This institute is recognized as a leading resource in meeting the needs of those disabled by illness, injury or developmental disorders in Connecticut and New York. A team of rehabilitation and health care professionals offering career development, residential services, supported employment, volunteer services, occupational therapy, day activities and more.

6748 Eastern Blind Rehabilitation Center
810 Vermont Avenue
Washington, DC 20420
202-461-7600
800-273-8255

Eric K. Shinseki, Secretary of Veterans Affairs
W. Scott Gould, Deputy Secretary of Veterans Aff
Jose D Riojas, Chief of Staff
Richard J Griffin, Acting Inspector General
Provides residential rehabilitation services to eligible legally blind veterans in the Northeast and Middle Atlantic portions of the country. Referral applications by Veterans Administration Medical Centers and Outpatient Clinics in the geographical area served by the Blind Rehabilitation Center.

6749 FAVRAH Senior Adult Enrichment Program
23 W Avon Rd
Avon, CT 06001
860-674-8839
Fax: 860-676-0275

Nancy Ralston, Manager
Provides remunerative work. Post acute rehabilitation programs and facility.

6750 Gaylord Hospital
Gaylord Farm Road
P.O.Box 400
Wallingford, CT 06492-7048
203-284-2800
866-429-5673
Fax: 203-284-2894
TTY: 203-284-2700
lcrispino@gaylord.org
www.gaylord.org

James Cullen, President
Works to restore ability and build courage. Offers rehabilitation care with one goal in mind: to help patients return to their homes, communities and jobs.

6751 Hockanum Greenhouse
Hockanum Industry
290 Middle Tpke
Storrs Mansfield, CT 06268-2908
860-429-6697
Fax: 860-429-7496

Christopher Campbell, Manager
Beth Chaty, Director
Betsy Treiber, Director
A non profit agency that strives to provide gainful employment, training, support and retirement services for developmentally

disabled individuals through the dignity of work, community interaction and structured activities.

6752   Kuhn Employment Oppurtunities
1630 North Colony Road
P.O.Box 941
Meriden, CT   06450   203-235-2583
                                                    860-347-5843
                                                    www.kuhngroup.org

Paul O'Sullivan, Chairperson
Mark DuPuis, Vice Chairperson
John J. Ausanka III, Treasurer
James Anderson, Secretary
Kuhn is committed to developing quality skill enhancement programs which provide meaningful employment for persons with disabilities so that they will become independentm gain self-esteem, and be accepted by the community. Our vision is that all individuals have the ability to fully participate in the community through work. Kuhn believes that all participants have a right to integrated community employment.

6753   Norwalk Hospital Section Of Physical Medicine And Rehabilitation
34 Maple Street
Norwalk, CT   06856   203-852-2000
                                              Fax: 800-789-4584
                                        marketing@norwalkhealth.org

Diane M. Allison, Chair
Edward A. Kangas, Vice Chair
Andrew J. Whittingham, Treasurer
Barbara Butler, Secretary
A 25 bed inpatient Rehabilitation Unit. This CARF and JCAHO accredidted rehab unit is located on the 8th floor of Norwalk Hospital. The focus of the rehab unit is to restore lost function and assist patients in returning to the community. Who have recently experienced a life changing medical event. The progam is tailored to meet individual therapy needs and address activities of daily living. Family and caregiver participation in the program is welcomed and encouraged.

6754   Rehabilitation Associates, Inc.
1931 Black Rock Tpke
Fairfield, CT   06825-3506   203-384-8681
                                              Fax: 203-384-0956
                                        info@rehabassocinc.com
                                www.rehabilitationassociatesinc.com
Carol Landsman, Director
A comprehensive outpatient rehabilitation facility offering physical therapy, occupational therapy, speech-language pathology, clinical social work services and nutritional services to all age groups. Facility locations in Fairfield, Stratford, Milford, Shelton and Westport.

6755   Reliance House
40 Broadway
Norwich, CT   06360-5702   860-887-6536
                                              Fax: 860-885-1970
                                                    reliancehouse.org
Jack Malone, President
Jackie Falman, Vice President
Sam Bliven, Secretary
Raul Walker, Treasurer
A residential vocational and recreational support network. An active and productive clubhouse where people with mental illness can gain skills, strength and self-esteem.

6756   Yale New Haven Health System-Bridgeport Hospital
789 Howard Avenue
New Haven, CT   06519   203-384-3000
                                              www.yalenewhavenhealth.org
Marna P. Borgstrom, President and CEO
Richard D'Aquila, Executive Vice President
Peter N. Herbert, MD, Senior VP, Medical Affairs
Kevin Myatt, Senior VP of Human Resources
Medical services are provided by physicians who are specialists in physical medicine and rehabilitation. The physical therapy department provides a variety of services and utilizes sophisticated modalities to restore and reinforce physical abilities.

6757   Alfred I DuPont Hospital for Children
Division of Rehabilitation
1600 Rockland Road,
PO Box 269
Wilmington, DE   19803-269   302-651-4000
                                                    888-533-3543
                                              Fax: 302-651-4055
                                        infodupont@nemours.org
                                                    www.nemours.org
William G. Mackenzie, MD, Chair
David J. Bailey, President and Chief Executive Officer
Robert D. Bridges, Executive Vice President, Enterprise Services/Chief Financia
Roy Proujansky, Executive Vice President, Health Operations and Chief Operat
The hospital is a division of Nemours, which operates one of the nations largest subspecialty group practices devoted to pediatric patient care, teaching, and research. A 180-bed hospital that offers all the specialties of pediatric medicine, surgery, and dentistry in a spacious, comfortable, and family focused facility.

6758   Community Systems Inc.
2 Penns Way
Suite 301
New Castle, DE   19720   302-325-1500
                                              Fax: 302-325-1505
                                                    communitysystems.org
David Paige, Executive Director
Amy Yento, Chair
A 4 state family of non-profit, tax exempt corporations whose mission is helping persons with disabilities to find happiness in their own homes, in their personal relationships, and as contributing members of their community.

6759   DDDS/Georgetown Center
5 Academy St
Georgetown, DE   19947-1915   302-856-5366
                                              Fax: 302-856-5305
                                                    dhss.delaware.gov/dhss

6760   Delaware Association for the Blind
2915 Newport Gap Pike
Landis Lodge Building
Wilmington, DE   19808   302-998-5913
                                                    888-777-3925
                                              Fax: 302-691-5810
                                              contact@dabdel.org
                                                    dabdel.org
Janet L. Berry, Executive Director
Ken Rolph, President
Jennifer Smith, Secretary
Robert Mosch, Treasurer
A private, nonprofit organization that offers adjustment to blindness counseling, recreation activities, summer camps and financial assistance for the legally blind. The staff includes five full time, nine part time and twelve seasonal. Operates a store selling items for the blind.

6761   Delaware Veterans Center
810 Vermont Avenue
Washington, DC   20420   302-994-2511
                                                    800-273-8255
                                              Fax: 302-633-5591
Slaon D Gibson, Acting Secretary of Veterans Affairs
Jose D Riojas, Chief of Staff
Richard J Griffin, Acting Inspector General
A 60-bed hospital and 60-bed NHCU, both accredited by the Joint Commission on Accreditation of Healthcare Organizations with a VBA Regional Office and 2 Vet Centers (one on campus) offering veterans the unique opportunity to obtain heathcare, benefits services, and Readjustment Counseling at one location. The center provides a wide spectrum of primary and tertiary acute and extended care inpatient and outpatient activities an an academic setting..

6762   Easter Seals Delaware & Maryland's Eastern Shore
233 South Wacker Drive
Suite 2400
Chicago, IL   60606   302-324-4444
                                              800-221-6827
                                         Fax: 302-324-4441
                                         TTY: 302-324-4442
                                              easterseals.com

Richard W. Davidson, Chairman
Sandy Tuttle, President
Ralph F. Boyd, Treasurer
Eileen Howard Boone, Secretary
Provides exceptional services to ensure that all people with disabilities or special needs and their families have equal opportunities to live, learn, work and play in their communities.

6763   Edgemoor Day Program
500 Duncan Rd
Wilmington, DE   19809-2369   302-762-9077
                                         Fax: 302-762-1652
           www.dhss.delaware.gov/dhss/main/maps/other/ed
Scott Borino, Executive Director
Carol Koyste, Manager, Finance & Administratio
Brandon Furrowh, Director, Recreation & Youth Pro
Avani Patel, Administrative Assistant
Our mission is providing affordable and accessible services which help improve the quality of life for community members of all ages through a broad range of educational, recreational, self-enrichment, and family support services. ECC is a not-for-profit, community-based, multi-service agency located just north of Wilmington. We provide a broad range of educational, recreational, self-enrichment, and family support services.

6764   Elwyn Delaware
321 E 11th St
Wilmington, DE   19801-3422   302-658-8860
                                         Fax: 302-654-5815
                                              info@elwyn.org
                                              www.elwyn.org
Sandra S. Cornelius, President of Elwyn
Daniel M. Reardon, Senior Vice President and Chief
H. Scott Campbell, Vice President
Richard T. Smith, Vice President for Information T
A non-profit human services organization recognized nationally and internationally as experts in the education and care of individuals with special challenges and disadvantages. Today Elwyn is a leading provider of services for people with special needs of all ages.

6765   First State Senior Center
291a N Rehoboth Blvd
Milford, DE   19963-1303   302-422-1510
           dhss.delaware.gov/dhss/main/maps/other/dddssr

6766   Woodside Day Program
941 Walnut Shade Rd
Dover, DE   19901-7765   302-739-4494
                                         Fax: 302-697-4490
Connie Grace, Supervisor
Joyce Oliver, Manager

District of Columbia

6767   Barbara Chambers Children's Center
1470 Irving St NW
Washington, DC   20010-2804   202-387-6755
                                         Fax: 202-319-9066
                                              barbarachambers.org
Barbara Chambers, Founder
Mission is to provide comprehensive, quality child care services to the community at large, by offering a variety of opportunities for childrens's intellectual, emotional, social and physical development in a clean, safe, and nurturing environment. Our philosophy is to provide a supportive environment in which children can

be children..allowing each child to learn at his/her pace and most of all allowing the child to learn through his/her daily play.

6768   District of Columbia General Hospital Physical Medicine & Rehab Services
Room 1358
19th and Mass Ave
Washington, DC   20003   202-727-6055
                                         Fax: 202-675-7819
Dr. Maribel Bieberach, Chairperson PM&R
Dr. Raman Kapur, Staff Physiatrist
Offers comprehensive physical medicine and rehabilitation services including in and outpatient consultations and electrodiagnostic testing; in and outpatient physical and occupational therapy; inpatient recreational therapy, and a multidisciplinary prosthetic clinic which meets once a month..

6769   George Washington University Medical Center
George Washington University Medical Center
2150 Pennsylvania Ave NW
Washington, DC   20037-3201   202-741-3000
                                         Fax: 202-741-3183
                                              www.gwdocs.com

6770   HSC Pediatric Center, The
1731 Bunker Hill Rd NE
Washington, DC   20017-3026   202-832-4400
                                              800-226-4444
                                         Fax: 202-467-0978
                                              efowler@cscn.org
                                              www.hscpediatriccenter.org
Debbie Zients, CEO
Dr Murry M Pollack, VP, Medical Affairs
Eva Fowler, Media Contact
Provides the highest quality rehabilitative and transitional care for infants, children, adolescents, and young adults with special health care needs and their families in a supportive environment that respects their needs, strengths, vslues and priorities..

6771   Howard University Child Development Center
1911 5th St NW
Washington, DC   20001-2314   202-797-8134
                                         Fax: 202-986-6580
Connie Siler, Manager
Offers children with developmental problems diagnosis, treatment, evaluation and follow along visits..

6772   Psychiatric Institute of Washington
4228 Wisconsin Ave NW
Washington, DC   20016-2138   202-885-5600
                                              800-369-2273
                                         Fax: 202-885-5614
Ken Courage, Chairman
Carol Desjuns, Chief Operations Officer
Howard Hoffman, Executive Medical Director
Aarti Subramanian, VP/Chief Financial Off
Psychiatric intensive care, crisis intervention, adult day treatment, drug treatment and other services to children and adults who have psychiatric and chemical dependency problems.

6773   Spina Bifida Program of DC Children's Hospital
Department of Physical Medicine and Rehabilitation
111 Michigan Ave NW
Washington, DC   20010-2916   202-476-5000
                                         Fax: 202-476-2270
                                              childrensnational.org
Kurt Newman, President and Chief Executive Of
Elizabeth Flury, Chief Strategy Officer
Kathleen E. Chavanu Gorman, Chief Operating Officer
Mary Anne Hilliard, Chief Risk Counsel
Offers neurosurgery, orthopedics,physical medicine, social work, urology and nursing. Mission is to improve health outcomes for children regionally, nationally, and internationally. Be a leader in creating innovative solutions to pediatric healthcare problems. Excel in Care, Advocacy, Research, and Education to meet the unique needs of children, adolescents and their families.

Florida

6774 Bayfront Rehabilitation Center
Bayfront Medical Center
701 6th St S
St Petersburg, FL   33701-4814   727-823-1234
www.bayfrontstpete.com
Kathryn Gillette, President and CEO
Eric Smith, Chief Financial Officer
Lavah Lowe, Chief Operating Officer
Karen Long, Chief Nursing Executive
Bayfront Medical Center has an Inpatient Rehabilitation Hospital and two outpatient rehabilitation clinics that each provide progressive, comprehensive, individualized treatment. Specialized care in Physiatry (physical medicine), rehab nursing, occupational therapy, speech language pathology, recreational therapy, patient/family services and psychology is tailored to each patient from admission to community and/or school reintegration.

6775 Brain Injury Rehabilitation Center Dr. P. Phillips Hospital
Brain Injury Rehabilitation Center Dr. P. Phillips
9400 Turkey Lake Rd
Orlando, FL   32819-8001   407-351-8580
www.orlandohealth.com/drpphillipshospital/ind
Shannon Elswick, President
Linda Chapin, Chairman
Mark Swanson, Chief Quality Officer
John Hillenmeyer, CEO Emeritus, Orlando Health
Dedicated to restoring brain injured patients with rehabilitation potential to their highest level of functioning. This is accomplished through an interdisciplinary team demonstrating personal responsibility to the patient, their family and each other.

6776 Brooks Memorial Hospital Rehabilitation Center
3599 University Blvd. South
Jacksonville, FL   32207-6215   904-858-7600
Fax: 904-858-7619
louise.spierre@brookshealth.org
www.brookshealth.org
Douglas Baer, Chief Executive Officer/ Preside
Holly Morris, Director, Brooks Rehabilitation
Louise Spierre, Medical Director
Floris Singletary, Research Manager, Clinical Resea
An entire care facility featuring five day inpatient evaluation, pre-operative evaluation programs, five week pain management program, referral criteria and treatment goals, therapy services, psychological services and more to the physically challenged.

6777 Center for Pain Control and Rehabilitation
Ste 607
2780 Cleveland Ave
Fort Myers, FL   33901-5858   239-337-4332
Mary Bonnette, Owner
.

6778 Comprehensive Rehabilitation Center at Lee Memorial Hospital
2776 Cleveland Ave
Fort Myers, FL   33901-5864   239-343-2000
leememorial.org
James R. Nathan, Chief Executive Officer System P
Larry Antonucci, Chief Operating Officer
Jon Cecil, Chief Human Resources Officer
Mike German, Chief Financial Officer
Lee Memorial hospital has achieved national recognition as one of the top 100 hospitals for stroke, orthopedics, and Intensive Care Unit (ICU) It is a 367 bed hospital that provides 24-hour emergency and trauma care, inpatient rehabilitation, orthopedics, neuroscience, trauma, cancer, diabetes, digestive, general surgery, urology, endocrinology, gastroenterology, opthamology, and many others.

6779 Comprehensive Rehabilitation Center of Naples Community Hospital
350 7th Street North
Naples, FL   34102   239-436-5000
Fax: 239-436-5250
www.nchmd.org
Allen S. Weiss, CEO
Mariann MacDonald, Chairman
Thomas Gazdic, Chairman/Treasurer
John Lewis, Secretary
Offers rehabilitation services, inpatient and outpatient care at 5 locations in the county and more for the benefit of the disabled.

6780 Conklin Center for the Blind
405 White St
Daytona Beach, FL   32114-2999   386-258-3441
Fax: 386-258-1155
info@conklincenter.org
www.conklincenter.org
Robert T Kelly, Executive Director
The Conklin Center's mission is to empower children and adults who are blind and have one or more additional disabilities to develop their potential to be able to obtain competitive employment, live independently and fully participate in community life.

6781 Davis Center for Rehabilitation Baptist Hospital of Miami
8900 N Kendall Dr
Miami, FL   33176-2118   786-596-1960
corporatepr@baptisthealth.net
www.baptisthealth.net/bhs
Brian E. Keeley, President and Chief Executive Of
Calvin Babcock, Chairman
A full-service, nonprofit community hospital providing a full range of inpatient and outpatient rehabilitation services. The overall commitment to excellence has extended to this specialized field. Access to medical expertise and services ensures that the best in medical resources are available should an unforeseen medical problem arise.

6782 Devereux Advanced Behavioral Health Florida - Titusville Campus
1850 S. Deleon Ave.
Titusville, FL   32780   407-473-5238
800-338-3738
referral@devereux.org
www.devereuxfl.org
Gwendolyn B Skinner, Vice President of Operations
Dave Detro, Human Resource Director
Carlos F Pozzi-Montero, Psy.D, Clinical Director
Lindsey Phillips, Director of External Affairs
The Devereux Florida Titusville Campus offers a variety of residential, foster care and community support services for youth with behavioral and intellectual/developmental disabilities. Services include a residential group home with private rooms and a therapeutic group home.

6783 Devereux Advanced Behavioral Health - Florida
Devereux Florida Corporate Office
5850 T.G. Lee Blvd.
Suite 400
Orlando, FL   32822   407-362-9210
800-338-3738
referral@devereux.org
www.devereuxfl.org
Gwendolyn B Skinner, Vice President of Operations
Dave Detro, Human Resource Director
Carlos F Pozzi-Montero, Psy.D, Clinical Director
Lindsey Phillips, Director of External Affairs
Offering care for children with mental health, behavioral, intellectual and developmental disabilities and challenges. Some services offered include a psychiatric program, community based group homes, foster care, counseling centers, case management, abuse and neglect prevention services, community-based care and outreach programs.

6784 Devereux Florida - Orlando Campus
Devereux Orlando Campus
6147 Christian Way
Orlando, FL 32808
407-296-5300
800-338-3738
referral@devereux.org
www.devereuxfl.org

Gwendolyn B Skinner, Vice President of Operations
Dave Detro, Human Resource Director
Carlos F Pozzi-Montero, Psy.D, Clinical Director
Lindsey Phillips, Director of External Affairs

The Orlando Campus provides intensive residential services for children and adolescents who suffer from emotional, behavioral and psychological problems. Programs offered include Devereux's Statewide Inpatient Psychiatric Program (SIPP), Residential Group Care and the Residential Treatment Center.

6785 Devereux Florida - Viera Campus
Devereux Viera Campus
8000 Devereux Dr.
Viera, FL 32940
321-242-9100
800-338-3738
Fax: 321-259-0786
vischool@devereux.org
www.devereuxfl.org

Gwendolyn B Skinner, Vice President of Operations
Dave Detro, Human Resource Director
Carlos F Pozzi-Montero, Psy.D, Clinical Director
Lindsey Phillips, Director of External Affairs

The campus offers two residential programs for youth with developmental or behavioral challenges: the Intensive Residential Treatment Center (IRTC) and the Intellectual/Developmental Disabilities (I/DD) Program. The Viera Campus also offers six residential units and the Devereux School.

6786 Devereux Threshold Center for Autism
Threshold Center For Autism
3550 N Goldenrod Rd
Winter Park, FL 32792
407-671-7060
800-338-3738
Fax: 407-671-6005
referral@devereux.org
www.devereuxfl.org

Gwendolyn B Skinner, Vice President of Operations
Dave Detro, Human Resource Director
Carlos F Pozzi-Montero, Psy.D., Clinical Director
Lindsey Phillips, Director of External Affairs

The Devereux Threshold Center for Autism includes a therapeutic residential program and an adult day treatment program for people with intellectual/developmental disabilities.

6787 Division of Blind Services
325 West Gaines Street
Suite 1114
Turlington Building, FL 32399-0400
850-245-0300
800-342-1828
Fax: 850-245-0386
ana.saint-ford@dbs.fldoe.com
dbs.myflorida.com

Aleisa McKinlay, Interim Director
Phyllis Vaughn, Bureau Chief, Administrative Services
William Findley, Bureau Chief, Business Enterprise Program
Edward Hudson, Bureau Chief of the Rehabilitation Center for the Blind and

Serves the totally blind, legally blind, visually impaired, deaf-blind, learning disabled, mentally retarded and other multiply handicapped by offering health, counseling, educational, recreational and computer training services.

6788 Easter Seals Broward County
1475 N.W. 14th Ave.
Miami, FL 33125
305-325-0470
Fax: 305-325-0578
www.easterseals.com/southflorida

Loreen Chant, President and Chief Executive Officer

ESBC provides direct services to children and adults with physical, neurological and communications disabilities and their families.

6789 Easter Seals South Florida
1475 NW 14th Avenue
Miami, FL 33125-1616
305-325-0470
Fax: 305-325-0578
www.southflorida.easterseals.com

Luanne Welch, President

The mission of Easter Seals South Florida is to provide exceptional services to ensure that all children and adults with disabilities or special needs and their families have equal opportunities to live, learn, work and play in their communities.

6790 Easter Seals Southwest Flordia
Sarasota, FL 34243-2001
941-355-7637
themeadowscup.com

6791 Easter Seals: Volusia and Flagler Counties, FL
Easter Seals National
233 South Wacker Drive
Suite 2400
Chicago, IL 60606-2405
800-221-6827
easterseals.com

Richard W. Davidson, Chairman
Ralph F. Boyd, Jr., Treasurer
Eileen Howard Boone, Secretary
James E. Williams, Jr., Assistant Secretary

Provides early intervention services: inclusive pre-school, aquatherapy and sensory processing therapy, OT, PT, ST and parenting programs, audiology services, equipment loan program, assistive technology information and referral. Residential summer camp and respite.

6792 Florida CORF
Columbia Medical Center: Peninsula
www.memorial-health.com

John Feore, Executive VP
Sandra Trovato, Executive Director

Offers Medicare authorized therapy programs for seniors, disabled and others who need rehabilitation. CORF can provide coordinated and extended services in the home after a hospital stay, or when physical status changes. Patients who are treated at CORF, include amputations, arthritis, chronic/acute pain, depression/anxiety, nerve injury, sports injury, stroke and swallowing problems.

6793 Florida Institute Of Rehabilitation Education (FIRE)
3071 Highland Oaks Terrace
Tallahassee, FL 32301-4876
850-942-3658
888-827-6033
Fax: 850-942-4518
info@lighthousebigbend.org
www.firesight.org

Barbara Ross, Executive Director
Evelyn Worley, Assistant Director
Wayne Warner, Vocational Program Director
Toni King, Independent Living Specialist

Provides independent living and vocational rehabilitation services to Florida residents who are legally blind. Services include instruction in orientation and mobility, accessible technology, daily living skills and employability skills. Information, referral and counseling services are also offered. All services are provided without charge.

6794 Florida Institute for Neurologic Rehabilitation, Inc
1962 Vandolah Road
P O Box 1348
Wauchula, FL 33873-1348
863-773-2857
800-697-5390
Fax: 863-773-0867
finr.net

John Richards, Administrator
Stephanie Ortiz, RN, Director of Nursing
Kevin E. O'Keefe, Program Director
Dana Lucas, Director of Nursing

A residential rehabilitation facility providing a therapeutic environment in which children, adolescents and adults who have survived head-injury can develop the independence and skills necessary to re-enter the community.

6795   Fort Lauderdale Veterans Medical Center
713 NE 3rd Ave
Fort Lauderdale, FL 33304-2619   954-356-7926
                                                          Fax: 954-356-7609
                                             www.va.gov/directory/guide/
Robert White, Executive Director
Sloan D Gibson, Acting Secretary
Jose D Riojas, Chief of Staff
Richard J Griffin, Acting Inspector General
Veterans medical clinic offering disabled veterans medical treatments.

6796   Halifax Hospital Medical Center Eye Clinic Professional Center
308 Farmington Avenue
Farmington, CT 06032   860-658-4388
                                              888-444-3598
                                     webmaster@evariant.com
                                            www.evariant.com
Bill Moschella, CEO
Rob Grant, Executive Vice President
Michael Clark, Chief Operating Officer
James Orsillo, Chief Financial Officer
Offers services for the totally blind, legally blind, visually impaired, mentally retarded blind and more with health, counseling, educational, recreational, rehabilitation, computer training and professional training services.

6797   HealthQuest Subacute and Rehabilitation Programs
Regenta Park
8700 a C Skinner Pkwy
Jacksonville, FL 32256-836   *Fax: 904-641-7896*

6798   HealthSouth Emeral Coast Sports & Rehabilitation Center
1847 Florida Avenue
Panama City, FL 32405-3730   850-784-4878
                                                   Fax: 850-769-7566
                                     www.healthsouthpanamacity.com
Tony Bennett, CEO
Michelle Miller, Manager
Outpatient sports medicine and rehabilitation center providing physical therapy, occupational therapy, industrial rehab, work hardening/work simulation, worksite and ergonomic analysis, FCE's, work assessment and pre-employment goals of returning the clients back to work, and returning to all recreational, sports and functional activities safely..

6799   HealthSouth Rehabilitation Hospital of Tallahassee
Healthsouth Corporation
1675 Riggins Rd
Tallahassee, FL 32308-5315   850-656-4800
                                     www.healthsouthtallahassee.com
Heath Phillips, Chief Executive Officer
Robert Robert Rowland, Medical Director
Tom Abbruscato, Controller
Deborah Baird, Director of Quality and Risk Man
North Florida's sole acute rehabilitation hospital between Jacksonville \, Panama City, and Gainesville. With 250 employees providing a full continuum of care form its 70 bed facility, the hospital is accredited by JCAHO, CARF and state designated and certified by Vocational Rehabilitation for traumatic brain injury, as well as a wide variety of other diagnoses. With the addition of our outpatients, the facility has served the greater community by touching the lives of over 50,000 patients.

6800   HealthSouth Rehabilitation Hospital Of Miami
20601 Old Cutler Rd
Miami, FL 33189-2441   305-251-3800
                                     www.healthsouthmiami.com
Elizabeth Izquierdo, Chief Executive Officer
Angelo Appio, Director of Marketing Operations
Reyna M. Hernandez, Chief Financial Officer
Paige Keil, Director of Quality and Risk Man

A comprehensive source of medical rehabilitation services for Pinellas County, Florida area residents, their families and their physicians. Offers the people of Florida all the clinical, technical and professional resources of the nation's leading provider of comprehensive rehabilitation care.

6801   HealthSouth Rehabilitation Hospital of Sarasota
Health South Corporation in Burmingham Alabama
6400 Edgelake Drive
Sarasota, FL 34240-8813   941-921-8600
                                              866-330-5822
                                     www.healthsouthsarasota.com
Marcus Braz, Chief Executive Officer
Alexander DeJesus, Medical Director
Nancy Arnold, Director of Marketing Operations
Brenda Benner, Director of Human Resources
HealthSouth Rehabilitation Hospital of Sarasota is a 96-bed inpatient rehabilitation hospital that offers comprehensive inpatient rehabilitation services designed to return patients to leading active and independent lives.

6802   HealthSouth Sea Pines Rehabilitation Hospital
Sea Pines Rehabilitation Hospital
101 E Florida Ave
Melbourne, FL 32901-8398   321-984-4600
                                                   Fax: 321-952-6532
                                     www.healthsouthseapines.com
Stuart Miller, Medical Director
Denise McGrath, Chief Executive Officer
Donna Anderson, Director of Human Resources
Jerry Bishop, Director of Quality and Risk Man
Designed to return patients to leading active, independent lives, HealthSouth Sea Pines Rehabilitation Hospital is a 90-bed rehabilitation hospital that provides a higher level of comprehensive rehabilitation services.

6803   Holy Cross Hospital
Catholic Southwest
4725 North Federal Hwy
Fort Lauderdale, FL 33308-4668   954-771-8000
                                              www.holy-cross.com
Patrick Taylor, President & Chief Executive Offi
Luisa Gutman, Senior Vice President & Chief Op
Linda Wilford, Senior Vice President & Chief Fi
Kenneth Homer, Chief Medical Officer & Medical
Holy Cross Hospital in Fort Lauderdale is a full-service, non-profit Catholic hospital, sponsored by the Sisters of Mercy. Holy Cross is a US News & World Report 'Best Hospital' and HealthGrades Distinguished Hospital for Clinical Excellence, 2004 and 2005

6804   Lee Memorial Hospital
2776 Cleveland Ave
Fort Myers, FL 33901-5855   239-343-2000
                                              www.leememorial.org
Sanford Cohen, Chairman
Chris Hansen, Vice Chairman
David Collins, Treasurer
Diane Champion, Secretary
Offers a complete inpatient program of intensive rehabilitation designed to restore a patient to a more independent level of functioning. The comprehensive care includes medical rehabilitation and training for spinal cord injury, brain injury, stroke and neurological disorders.

6805   Lighthouse for the Blind of Palm Beach
1710 Tiffany Drive East
West Palm Beach, FL 33407-3224   561-586-5600
                                                   Fax: 561-84- 80
                                     lighthousepalmbeaches.org
Marvin A. Tanck, President and CEO
Dont, Mickens, Chair
John R. Banister, Vice Chairman
David B. Cano, MD
A private, non-profit rehabilitation and education agency in its 55th year of service. Offers programs to assist persons who areblind or visually impaired, an on-site Industrial Center, a technology training center, an Aids and appliances Store, special

equipment grant programs, outreach services for children and adults, Early Intervention and Preschool Services, and a variety of support groups. These programs provide services and education for blind children and their parents.

6806 Lighthouse for the Visually Impaired and Blind
8610 Galen Wilson Blvd
Port Richey, FL 34668-5974
727-815-0303
866-962-5254
Fax: 727-815-0203
lighthouse@lvib.org
www.lvib.org

Sylvia Stinson-Perez, Executive Director
Dr. John Mann, President
Melissa M. Suess, Orientation and Mobility Instruc
Peter James, Business Development Specialist
The Lighthouse offers services for visually impaired or blind adults and children ages 0-5 years old. Counseling, educational services, recreational services, rehabilitation, computer training and support groups.

6807 MacDonald Training Center
5420 W Cypress Street
Tampa, FL 33607-1706
813-870-1300
866-948-6184
Fax: 813-872-6010
TTY: 813-873-7631
jfreyvogel@macdonaldcenter.org
macdonaldcenter.org

Jim Freyvogel, President/CEO
Judith DeStasio, CFO
Debi Hamilton, Director of Services
Joe Donato, COO
A private, non-profit, community-based human services organization serving adults with disabilities (since 1953). Persons are provided the opportunity to achieve their highest potential through the Center's various programs that include day training, employment, community living and various support services.

6808 Medicenter of Tampa
4411 North Habana Avenue
Tampa, FL 33614-7211
813-872-2771
Fax: 813-871-2831
rehabilitationandhealthcarecenteroftampa.com

Dan Davis, President
Mariluz G, Social Services Director
Brenda Pace, Secretary
Hilda B, Medicaid Coordinator
Postacute rehabilitation program. A 174 bed non-profit facility with postacute reahbilitation programs..

6809 Miami Heart Institute Adams Building
4300 Alton Rd
Miami Beach, FL 33140-2997
305-674-2121
www.msmc.com

Steven D. Sonenreich, President/CEO
The mission is to provide high quality health care to our diverse community enhanced through teaching, research, charity care and financial responsibility.

6810 Miami Lighthouse for the Blind
601 SW 8th Ave
Miami, FL 33130-3200
305-856-2288
Fax: 305-285-6967
info@miamilighthouse.org
miamilighthouse.org

Virginia A. Jacko, President & Chief Executive Officer
Sharon Caughill, Special Projects Manager
Jeannie Reinoso, Executive Assistant
Arnie Paniagua, Chief Financial Officer
Offers services for the legally blind and severely visually impaired (including those who are developmentally delayed) of all ages in the areas of counseling and educational, recreational, rehabilitation, computer and vocational training services.

6811 Mount Sinai Medical Center Rehabilitation Unit
4300 Alton Rd
Miami Beach, FL 33140-2997
305-674-2121
www.msmc.com

Steven D. Sonenreich, President/CEO
A comprehensive inpatient and outpatient rehabilitation programs have been helping patients recover for more then 20 years. Fully customized treatment plans based on the needs of each patient is 1 reason why our services are among the best in South Florida. Our team approach takes into account the medical, physical, psychological, social, spiritual, cultural and economic needs of patients and their families.

6812 Neurobehavioral Medicine Center
Ste 1
4821 Us Highway 19
New Port Richey, FL 34652-4259
727-849-2005
Fax: 727-849-2087

Otsenre Matos, Medical Director
Gerard Taylor PhD, Counseling/Stress Management
Donna Taylor RN, Manager
Joyce Park Matos ARNP, Clinical Specialist
A multidisciplinary outpatient program for the evaluation and treatment of chronic pain. Consultation services for hospitalized patients are also provided upon request. Comprehensive treatment of individuals with closed traumatic brain injuries..

6813 North Broward Rehab Unit
North Broward Medical Center
201 E Sample Rd
Deerfield Beach, FL 33064-3596
954-941-8300
www.browardhealth.org

Douglas Ford, Chiefs of Staff
Pauline Grant, Chief Executive Officer
CARF accredited, 30-bed inpatient rehabilitation unit treating adults with brain injuries, spinal cord injuries, stroke, orthopedic and neurologic injuries.

6814 Northwest Medical Center
Health Care Corporation of America
2801 North State Road 7
Margate, FL 33063-5727
954-974-0400
866-256-7720
northwestmed.com

Mark Rader, CEO
Above all else, we are committed to the care and improvement of human life. In recognition of this commitment, we strive to deliver high quality, cost effective healthcare in the communities we serve. We recognize and affirm the unique and intrinsic work of each individual. We treat all those we serve with compassion and kindness. We act with absolute honesty, integrity, and fairness in the way we conduct our business and the way we live our lives.

6815 Pain Institute of Tampa
4178 N Armenia Ave
Tampa, FL 33607-6429
813-875-5913
John E Barsa, Founder & MD
Offers a comprehensive and multidisciplinary approach to pain controll and management. Most services are provided on-site but other services may require you to be referred elswhere. We will monitor and coordinate your care in a manner to provide optimal recovery potential.

6816 Pain Treatment Center, Baptist Hospital of Miami
8900 N Kendall Dr
Miami, FL 33176-2118
786-596-1960
corporatepr@baptisthealth.net
www.baptisthealth.net

Calvin Babcock, Chairman
Brian E. Keeley, President and Chief Executive Of
Since 1960, Baptist Hospital of Miami has been one of the most respected medical centers in South Florida. The hospitals full range of medical and technological services is the natural choice for a growing number of people throughout the world.

6817   Pine Castle
4911 Spring Park Rd
Jacksonville, FL 32207-7496   904-733-2650
                                      Fax: 904-733-2681
                                      info@pinecastle.org
                                      pinecastle.org

Jonathan May, Executive Director
Randall Duncan, Associate Executive Director
Leigh Griffin, Director of Finance
Cliff Evans, Director of Development
Provides remunerative work, training, community employment
and community living options for adults with developmental
disabilities.

6818   Polk County Association for Handicapped Citizens
1038 Sunshine Dr E
Lakeland, FL 33801-6338   863-858-2252
                                      Fax: 863-665-2330

Kecia Howell, Owner
Anthony J. Senzamici Jr., 1st Vice Chairman
Carol N. Asbill, 2nd Vice Chairman
A private non-profit organization that provides an adult day
training program to people with developmental disabilities and is
under the direction of a volunteer board of directors. The primary
goal for our services is to provide people with knowledge and
practical experience to be independent adults so they can become
contributing members of their community..

6819   Quest
500 E Colonial Drive
P O Box 531125
Orlando, FL 32853- 4504   407-218-4300
                                           888-807-8378
                                      Fax: 407-218-4301
                                           questinc.org

David Canora, Chair
James Gallagher, Vice-Chair
Suzanne Bennett, Treasurer
Ruth Bresnick, Secretary
Quest has built communities where people with disabilities have
achieved their goals for nearly 50 years. Through a variety of resi-
dential and employment options, behavioral therapy, therapeutic
day programs, charter schools and even a recreational summer
camp, Quest serves more than 1000 individuals each day in the
Orlando and Tampa areas.

6820   Quest - Tampa Area
1404 Tech Blvd
Tampa, FL 33619   813-423-7700
                                           888-807-8378
                                      Fax: 813-423-7701
                                      contact@questinc.org
                                           www.questinc.org

David Canora, Chair
James Gallagher, Vice-Chair
Suzanne Bennett, Treasurer
Ruth Bresnick, Secretary
Quest has built communities where people with disabilities have
achieved their goals for nearly 50 years. Through a variety of resi-
dential and employment options, behavioral therapy, therapeutic
day programs, charter schools and even a recreational summer

6821   Rehabilitation Center for Children and Adults
300 Royal Palm Way
Palm Beach, FL 33480-4305   561-655-7266
                                      Fax: 561-655-3269
                                           info@rcca.org
                                           rcca.org

John C. Whelton, Chairman
Jacob L. Lochner, Co-Chairman
Christopher Adams, MD
A private, nonprofit organization whose purpose is to improve
physical function, independence and communication of people
with physical disabilities. Any child or adult with a physical or
speech disability is eligible for services.

6822   Renaissance Center
3599 University Blvd
Suite 604
Jacksonville, FL 32216- 9249   904-399-0905
                                      Fax: 904-743-5109
                           www.obiplasticsurgery.com/index.php
Lewis Obi, MD

6823   Rosomoff Comprehensive Pain Center, The
5200 NE 2nd Avenue
Miami, FL 33137-2706   305-532-7246
                                      Fax: 305-534-3974
                           painrelief@rosomoffpaincenter.com
                           www.rosomoffpaincenter.com
Elsayed Abdel-Moty, Director
Hubert Rossomoff, Owner
A state-of-the-art Center of Excellence offering inpatient, outpa-
tient, outpatient rehabilitation services and seniors programs.
The Center became an internationally renowned model for the
evalutation and treatment of all persons seeking pain relief.

**6824   Sarasota Memorial Hospital/Comprehensive Rehabilitation
          Unit**
1700 S Tamiami Trail
Sarasota, FL 34239-3509   941-917-9000
                                      Fax: 941-917-2211
                                           www.smh.com

Marguerite G Malone, Chair
Gregory Carter, First Vice Chair
Alex Miller, Second Vice Chair
Joseph J. DeVirgilio, Jt. Treasurer
The goal of the 34-bed Comprehensive Rehabilitation Unit
(CRU) is to increase patient functional independence, adjust to
illness or disability and successfully return to the community.
The unit is dedicated to patients who have experienced
conditions such

6825   Strive Physical Therapy Centers
2620 SE Maricamp RD
Ocala, FL 34471-4517   352-732-8868
                                      Fax: 352-732-8890
                                           www.striverehab.com

R W Shutes, Owner
Johanna Solbato, Administrator
R.W. Shutes, President and CEO
Certified as an Outpatient Rehabilitation Agency, providing a
comprehensive approach to patient evaluation and treatment. Our
objective is to return our patients back to a productive life as
quickly as possible and safely as possible.

6826   Sunbridge Care and Rehabilitation
101 East State Street,
Kennett Square, FL 19348-6105   610-444-6350
                                      Fax: 610-925-4000
                                      info@genesishcc.com
                                           www.genesishcc.com

Dan Hirschfeld, President
George V Hager, Chief Executive Officer
Robert A Reitz, Executive Vice President & Chief Operating Officer
Michael Sherman, Senior VP
A comprehensive medical rehabilitation facility that is commit-
ted to helping individuals with disabilities improve their quality
of life. This is a 120-bed facility offering a full range of acute and
sub-acute inpatient programs as well as community-based

6827   Tampa Bay Academy
12012 Boyette Rd
Riverview, FL 33569-5631   813-677-6700
                                           800-678-3838
                                      Fax: 813-671-3145
                                      tlamb@tampahope.org
                                           www.tampahope.org

Renee Scott, Chair
Amy McClure, Vice-Chair
Titania Lamb, Executive Director
A psychiatric residential treatment center and partial hospitaliza-
tion program for ages 7 to 17.

6828   Tampa General Rehabilitation Center
1 Tampa General Circle
P.O.Box 1289
Tampa, FL 33606-3571   813-844-7700
                                           866-844-1411
                                     Fax: 813-844-1477
                                        jstone@tgh.org
                                              tgh.org

James R. Burkhart, President & CEO
Bruce Zwiebel, Chief Of Staff
Deana L. Nelson, Chief Operating Officer
Steve Short, Cheif Financial Officer
Offers a full range of programs all aimed at helping patients achieve their full potentials. It is one of three centers in the state that provides Driver Training and Evaluation Programs for persons with disabilities, and also an Assisted Reproduction Pro

6829   Tampa Lighthouse for the Blind
1106 West Platt Street
Tampa, FL 33606-2142   813-251-2407
                                     Fax: 813-254-4305
                                       tampalighthouse.org
Sheryl Brown, Executive Director
Offers services for the totally blind, legally blind, visually impaired, mentally retarded blind and more with health, counseling, educational, recreational, rehabilitation, computer training and professional training services.

6830   Upper Pinellas Association for Retarded Citizens
1501 N Belcher Rd
Suite 249
Clearwater, FL 33765-1300   727-799-3330
                                     Fax: 727-799-4632
                                          www.uparc.com
Karen Crown, Executive Director
Offers services to more than 500 persons with mental retardation and other developmental disabilities. Services include two early intervention pre-schools, physical, speech and occupational therapies, homebound education and family support for children, b

6831   Visually Impaired Persons of Southwest Florida
35 W Mariana Ave
North Fort Myers, FL 33903-5515   239-997-7797
                                     Fax: 239-997-8462
                                       mmcgrael@vipcenter.org
                                           vipcenter.org
Doug Fowler, Executive Director
Margaret Ruhe Lincoln, Director of operations
Provides training in independent living skills, orientation and mobility, counseling, computer and other communication skills, family support groups, peer counseling, socialization and a low vision clinic. Second location in Charlotte County. Phone: 941-6

6832   West Florida Hospital: The Rehabilitation Institute
8383 North Davis Hwy
Pensacola, FL 32514-6039   850-494-4000
                                           800-342-1123
                                     Fax: 850-494-4881
                                      www.westfloridahospital.com
Roman S Bautista, President/CEO
Carol Saxton, Senior VP Patient Care Services
A 58-bed comprehensive rehabilitation facility offering inpatient and outpatient services. JCAHO and CARF accredited and a State designed head and spinal cord injury center. CARF accredited programs include: comprehensive inpatient rehab, spinal cord inju

6833   West Gables Health Care Center
2525 SW 75th Ave
Miami, FL 33155-2800   305-262-6800
                                     Fax: 888-453-1928
                                    www.westgablesrehabhospital.com
Jose Vargas, Medical Director
Walter Concepcion, Chief Executive Officer
Cesar Sepulveda, Materials Manager
Zely Santos, Admissions Director

Services provide by West Gables Health Center: activities services are provided onsite to residents. Clinical laboratory services are provided, dental, dietary, housekeeping, mental health services, nursing services, occupational therapy, pharmacy, physic

6834   Willough at Naples
9001 Tamiami Trail East
Naples, FL 34113-3397   239-775-4500
                                           800-722-0100
                                     Fax: 239-793-0534
                                    info@thewilloughatnaples.com
                                      thewilloughatnaples.com

James O'Shea, President
A licensed psychiatric hospital in Southwest Florida which provides quality management and treatment for eating disorders and chemical dependency in adults.

Georgia

6835   Annandale Village
3500 Annandale Ln
Suwanee, GA 30024-2150   770-945-8381
                                     Fax: 770-945-8693
                                          annandale.org
Adam Pomeranz, Chief Executive Officer
Melissa Burton, Chief Financial Officer
Keith Fenton, Chief Development & Marketing Officer
Nancy Trujillo, Chief Operating Officer
Private nonprofit residential facility for adults with developmental disabilities. Located on 124 acres just north of Atlanta. Annandale provides full program and 24 hour residential services, pay program services, respite care and skilled nursing services.

6836   Atlanta Institute of Medicine and Rehabilitation
Ste E
2911 Piedmont Rd NE
Atlanta, GA 30305-2782   404-365-0160
                                     Fax: 404-365-0751
Lawrence E Eppelbaum, Founder
Galina Vayner, MD
One of the most famous medical centers in the state of Georgia. The Institute employs more then 40 highly qualified medical professionals and fully equipped with the latest medical equipment. It has gathered recognition and respect from the people of Atla

6837   Bobby Dodd Institute (BDI)
2120 Marietta Blvd NW
Atlanta, GA 30318-2122   678-365-0071
                                     Fax: 678-365-0098
                                      TTY:678-365-0099
                                          bobbydodd.org

Rodney Hall, Chair
Christopher Rosselli, Vice Chair
Wayne McMillan, President & CEO
John Ralls, Treasurer
BDI annually serves approximately 400 clients in Atlanta, GA. BDI works primarily with people with developmental disabilities such as autism, down syndrome or mental retardation, but includes clients with physical or acquired disabilities. Client age va

6838   Cave Spring Rehabilitation Center
Georgia Department of Labor
7 Georgia Ave
P.O.Box 303
Cave Spring, GA 30124-2718   706-777-2341
                                     Fax: 706-777-2366
                             gvra.georgia.gov/cave-spring-center-contacts-
Russell Fleming, Director
Karen Hulsey, Administrative Operations Coordinator
Renee Lambert, Rehabilitation Assistant
Renaultha Houston, Residential Program Supervisor

6839   Center for Assistive Technology and Environmental Access
490 10th St
Atlanta, GA   30332-0156   404-894-4960
                                             800-726-9119
                                        Fax: 404-894-9320
                                        catea@coa.gatech.edu
                                             www.catea.org

Carrie Bruce, Research Scientist
Charlie Drummond, Administrative Assistant
Summer Ienuso, Wen Developer
Trin Intra, Financial Administrator
The Center for Assistive Technology and Environmental Access
(CATEA) promotes maximum function, activity and access of
persons with disabilities through the use of technology. The foci
of the Center includes the development, evaluation and
utilization of

6840   Center for the Visually Impaired
739 West Peachtree St NW
Atlanta, GA   30308-1137   404-875-9011
                                        Fax: 404-607-0062
                                        info@cviatlanta.org
                                             cviga.org
Susan Hoy, Chair
Fontaine M. Huey, President
Doreen Zaksheske, Vice President of Finance & Operations
Anisio Correia, Vice President for Programs
Offers services to people of all ages who are blind or visually im-
paired with training in orientation and mobility, computer tech-
nology, activities of daily living, communication skills and
employment readiness. Aso offers two children's programs, a
comm

6841   Devereux Advanced Behavioral Health Georgia
Devereux Georgia Treatment Network
1291 Stanley Rd.
Kennesaw, GA   30152   770-427-0147
                                             800-342-3357
                                        Fax: 770-427-4030
                                        info@devereux.org
                                             www.devereuxga.org
Gwendolyn B Skinner, Vice President of Operations
Dave Detro, Human Resource Director
Carlos F Pozzi-Montero, Psy.D, Clinical Director
Lindsey Phillips, Director of External Affairs
Facility offering services to youth with emotional and behavioral
health challenges. Services include Intensive Residential Treat-
ment, Foster Care Program, Group Homes, and educational
programs.

6842   Easter Seals East Georgia
1500 Wrightsboro Road
Augusta, GA   30904-2441   706-667-9695
                                             866-667-9695
                                        Fax: 706-667-8831
                                        sthomas@esega.org
                                        www.easterseals.com/eastgeorgia
Sheila H. Thomas, CEO
Patrick Clayton, Chairman
Easter Seals East Georgia assists people with disabilities and
other special needs to maximize opportunities for employment,
independence and full inclusion into society.

6843   Georgia Industries for the Blind
700 Faceville Highway
Bainbridge, GA   39819-218   229-248-2666
                                        Fax: 229-248-2669
                                        gvra.georgia.gov/gib/about-us
James Hughes, Executive Director
Offers services for the totally blind, legally blind, visually impaired, mentally retarded blind and more with health, counseling,
educational, recreational, rehabilitation, computer training and
professional training services.

6844   Hillhaven Rehabilitation
26 Tower Rd NE
Marietta, GA   30060-6947   770-422-8913
                                             800-526-5782
                                        Fax: 770-425-2085
Leslie Ann Marie Parrish, Case Manager
Valerie Hamilton, Administrator
Routine skilled and subacute medical and rehabilitation care including physical therapy, occupational therapy, speech pathology and therapeutic recreation. Programs include stroke and head
injury rehab; orthopedic rehab; complex IV therapy; woundcare;
can.

6845   In-Home Medical Care
Care Master Medical Services
240 Odell Rd
P.O.Box 278
Griffin, GA   30223-4787   770-227-1264
                                             800-542-8889
                                        Fax: 770-412-0014
                                        caremaster@accesunited.com
                                        caremastermedical.com
Nancy Frederick, VP
Eddie Grogan, Chief Executive Officer
Offers the devoted attention of a professional nurse, the use of
I.V. therapies, pain management and provision of medical equip-
ment and supplies right where the patient wants to be.

6846   Learning Services: Harris House Program
131 Langley Drive
Suite B
Lawrenceville, GA   30046-4446   404-298-0144
                                             888-419-9955
                                        Fax: 866-491-7396
                                             learningservices.com
Dr. Debra Braunling-McMorrow, President and CEO
Susan Snow, Director of Admissions
Michael Weaver, Chief Development Officer
Jeanne Mack, Chief Financial Officer
Situated in the small, historic district of Stone Mountain, just out-
side of Atlanta, this 6 bed program is designed to encourage inde-
pendence while providing appropriate support for each
individuals needs. Community-based productive activities are
customi

6847   Pain Control & Rehabilitation Institute of Georgia
Ste 120
2784 N Decatur Rd
Decatur, GA   30033-5993   404-297-1400
                                        Fax: 404-297-1427
Shulim Spektor, CEO
Anna Britman, Office Manager
Provides pain management for chronic and acute pain resulted
from injuries, diseases of muscles and nerve, Reflex Sympathetic
Dystrophy, perform disabilities and impairment ratings.

6848   Savannah Association for the Blind
214 Drayton Street
Savannah, GA   31401-4021   912-236-4473
                                        Fax: 912-234-9286
                                             www.sabinc.org
Gregory Hodges, President
Robert Falligant, Vice-president
Gary Sadowski, Treasurer
Lula Baker, Secretary
Offers services for the totally blind, legally blind, visually im-
paired, mentally retarded blind and more with health, counseling,
educational, recreational, rehabilitation, computer training and
professional training services.

6849   Shepherd Center for Treatment of Spinal Injuries
2020 Peachtree Rd NW
Atlanta, GA   30309-1465   404-352-2020
                                                  Fax: 404-350-7479
                                             admissions@shepherd.org
                                                    www.shepherd.org

Gary R. Ulicny, President & CEO
David F. Apple, Jr., M.D., Medical Director
Angela Beninga, D.O., Staff Physiatrist
ChiChi Berhane, M.D., MBA, Director, Reconstructive Surgery
Dedicated exclusively to the care of patients with spinal cord injuries and other paralyzing spinal disorders. It serves predominately residents of Georgia and neighboring states as one of the only 14 hospitals designated by the U.S. Department of Educati

6850   Transitional Hospitals Corporation
Ste 1000
7000 Central Pkwy NE
Atlanta, GA   30328-4592   770-821-5328
                                                       800-683-6868
                                                  Fax: 770-913-0015
                                                    staff@csins.com
                                                         csins.com

Dean Kozee, Owner
Carolyn Norton, Special Projects Consultant/Broker
Amaury Rentas, Event Insurance/Broker
A national network of intensive care hospitals providing care for patients who suffer from a chronic illness and/or catastrophic accident. The mission is founded on providing quality health care to patients who require highly skilled nursing care and acce.

6851   Walton Rehabilitation Health System
1355 Independence Dr
Augusta, GA   30901-1037   706-823-8584
                                                       866-492-5866
                                                  Fax: 706-724-5752
                                           vickig@waltonfoundation.net
                                             www.waltonfoundation.net

Robert Taylor, Chair
Dennis Skelley, President/CEO
David Dugan, Treasurer
Brent Smith, Secretary
A 58-bed comprehensive physical rehabilitation hospital offering inpatient and outpatient services. Services offered include: stroke recovery, orthopedic injury, pediatrics, head injury, pain management for chronic pain syndrome, TMJ/Craniofacial pain and

Hawaii

6852   Rehabilitation Hospital of the Pacific
226 N Kuakini St
Honolulu, HI   96817-2498   808-531-3511
                                                  Fax: 808-566-3411
                                         rehabfoundation@rehabhospital.org
                                                www.rehabhospital.org

John Komeiji, Chair
Glenn O. Sexton, Vice Chair
E. Lynne Madden, Secretary/Treasurer
Timothy J. Roe, President & Chief Executive Officer
The only acute care medical rehabilitation organization serving both Hawaii and the Pacific. For over 52 years, the hospital and its 7 outpatient clinics on Oahu, and Maui and Hawaii have been dedicated to providing comprehensive, cost effective rehabilit

Idaho

6853   Ashton Memorial Nursing Home and Chemical Dependency Center
700 N 2nd
Ashton, ID   83420   208-652-7461
                                                  Fax: 208-652-7595
                                                   ashtonmemorial.com

Sheila Kellogg, Administrator

6854   Easter Seals-Goodwill Northern Rocky Mountains
Easter Seals National
1465 S Vinnell Way
Boise, ID   83709-1659   208-378-9924
                                                       800-374-1910
                                                  Fax: 208-378-9965
                                                  www.easterseals.org

Richard W. Davidson, Chairman
Ralph F. Boyd, Jr., Treasurer
Eileen Howard Boone, Secretary
James E. Williams, Jr., Assistant Secretary
Provides services for children and adults with disabilities and other special needs, and support to their families

6855   Idaho Elks Rehabilitation Hospital
600 N Robbins Rd
Boise, ID   83702   208-489-4444
                                                  Fax: 208-344-8883
                                                   info@elksrehab.org
                                                    www.elksrehab.org

Joseph P. Caroselli, CEO
Doug Lewis, Chief Financial Officer
Mellisa Honsinger, Chief Operating Officer
A nonprofit hospital serving Idaho and the Pacific Northwest. All inpatient and outpatient programs and services are supervised by the hospital's full-time medical directors whose specialty is physical rehabilitative medicine. Services include: occupation

6856   Portneuf Medical Center Rehabilitation
777 Hospital Way
Pocatello, ID   83201-4004   208-239-1000
                                                  charlesa@portmed.org
                                                     www.portmed.org

Mark Buckalew, Chairman
Michael Nosacka, MD
Dan Ordyna, CEO
John Abreu, Vice President
Provides compassionate, quality health care services needed by the people of eastern Idaho in collaboration with other providers and community resources.

Illinois

6857   Advocate Christ Hospital and Medical Center
4440 W 95th St
Oak Lawn, IL   60453-2600   708-684-8000
                                                  Fax: 708-684-4440
                                                   advocatehealth.com

Jim Skogsbergh, CEO
Bill Santulli, COO
Kate K, Director
A 665-bed, not-for-profit teaching, research and referral medical center in Oak Lawn, Illinois. It also is home to the Advocate Hope Childrens's Hospital, one of the most comprehensive providers of pediatric care in the state. The medical center is a lead

6858   Advocate Christ Medical Center & Advocate Hope Children's Hospital
4440 W 95th St
Oak Lawn, IL   60453-2600   708-684-8000
                                                  Fax: 708-684-4440
                                                   advocatehealth.com

Kenneth Lukhard, CEO
Darcie Brazel, Market Chief Nurse Executive
Jan McCrea, Rehab Services Director
William Adair MD, Medical Director/Rehab Services
The largest fully integrated not-for-profit health care delivery system in metropolitan Chicago and is recognized as one of the top 10 systems in the country. The mission of Advocate Health Care is to serve the health needs of individuals, families and co

6859 Advocate Illinois Masonic Medical Center
836 W Wellington Ave
Chicago, IL 60657-5147 773-975-1600
www.advocatehealth.com/immc
Jim Skogsbergh, CEO
Ajay V. Maker, MD
Consultation, education, family counseling, parent training in behavior modification techniques offered to developmentally disabled adults.

6860 Alexian Brothers Medical Center
800 Biesterfield Rd
Elk Grove Village, IL 60007-3396 847-437-5500
www.alexian.org
Mark Frey, President/CEO
Tracy Rogers, Senior Vice President and Chief Operating Officer
Paul Belter, Senior Vice President and Chief Financial Officer
Patricia Cassidy, Senior Vice President and Chief Strategy Officer
A threefold mission: Works toward maximizing physical function, enhance independent social skills and optimize communication skills consistent with an individual's ability. The Center helps those disabled by accident or illness achieve a new personal best

6861 Back in the Saddle Hippotherapy Program
Corcoran Physical Therapy
4200 W Peterson Ave
Chicago, IL 60646-6074 312-286-2266
847-604-4145
Fax: 847-673-8895
Julie Naughton, Program Coordinator
Maureen Corcoran, Physical Therapist
Tom Corcoran, Owner
A direct medical treatment used by licensed physical therapists who have a strong treatment background in posture and movement, neuromotor function and sensory processing. The benefits of Hippotherapy are available to individuals with just about any disab

6862 Barbara Olson Center of Hope
3206 N Central Ave
Rockford, IL 61101-1797 815-964-9275
Fax: 815-964-9607
info@b-olsoncenterofhope.org
b-olsoncenterofhope.org
Carm Herman, Executive Director
Pam Sondell, Director of Programs and Services
Pam Carey, Director of Human Resources
Mike Marvell, Director of Business Development
We provide vocational employment, educational and social opportunities for adults with developmental disabilities.

6863 Bartolucci Center, The- ILC Enterprises
6415 Stanley Ave
Berwyn, IL 60402-3130 708-745-5277
Fax: 708-698-5090
www.pillarscommunity.org
Zada Clarke, Chairman
Ann Schreiner, President & CEO
Jennifer Hogberg, Vice Chair
Sheila Eswaran, Secretary
A nonprofit tax exempt private social service agency serving suburban Chicago offering day treatment and vocational counseling to individuals who encountered a pattern of job loss due to emotional problems.

6864 Baxter Healthcare Corporation
1 Baxter Pkwy
Deerfield, IL 60015-4625 224-948-2000
800-422-9837
224-948-1812
Fax: 800-568-5020
Phillip L. Batchelor, Corporate Vice President - Quality and Regulatory Affairs
Jean-Luc Butel, Corporate Vice President - President, International
Robert M. Davis, Corporate Vice President - President, Medical Products
Robert Parkinson Jr, Chairman of the Board and Chief Executive Officer
Baxter International Inc. is a global healthcare company that, through its subsidiaries assists healthcare professionals and their patients with treatment of complex medical conditions including hemophelia, immune disorders, kidney disease, cancer, trauma and other conditions. Baxter applies its expertise in medical devices, pharmaceuticals, and biotechnology to make a meaningful difference in patient's lives.

6865 Beacon Therapeutic Diagnostic and Treatment Center
10650 S Longwood Dr
Chicago, IL 60643-2617 773-881-1005
Fax: 773-881-1164
Susan Reyha-Guerrero, President & CEO
Cheryl Thompson, Deputy CEO
Paul Morley, Chief Operating Officer
Offers community day treatment, education, diagnostic services, family counseling, learning disabled, speech and hearing and psychiatric services.

6866 Blind Service Association
17 N State St
Ste 1050
Chicago, IL 60602-3510 312-236-0808
blindserviceassociation.org
Ann Lousin, President
Linda Schwartz, Executive Vice President
Arthur M. Shapiro, Secretary
John Powen, Treasurer
Offers services for the totally blind, legally blind and visually impaired with reading and recording low vision network, social services, referrals and support groups.

6867 Brandecker Rehabilitation Center
1939 West 13th Street
Suite 300
Chicago, IL 60643-6316 312-491-4110
Fax: 312-733-0247
www.easterseals.com/chicago
Richard W. Davidson, Chairman
Ralph F. Boyd, Jr., Treasurer
Eileen Howard Boone, Secretary
James E. Williams, Jr., Assistant Secretary
We offer early intervention services for infants and toddlers with developmental delays and disabilities. Our outpatient Medical Rehabilitation Program offers direct therapy services for children from age birth-16.

6868 Brentwood Subacute Healthcare Center
T HI Brentwood
5400 W 87th St
Burbank, IL 60459-2913 866-300-3257
www.savaseniorcare.com
Audrey Protrowski, Director Business Development
Jill Sattersield, Administrator
John Walton, CEO
Seeks to help patients and their families through what can be a very emotional decision-making process. We provide guidance and consultation on everything from how to properly choose the facility to providing resources that help you cope with the nature of the decision itself.

6869 Caremark Healthcare Services
2211 Sanders Rd
Northbrook, IL 60062-6128   847-559-4700
                                          800-423-1411
                                          Fax: 847-559-3905
                                          www.caremark.com

Larry J. Merlo, President & CEO
Mark Cosby, Executive Vice President
An 80-service-center network providing services anywhere in
the U.S. Offers 24 hour access to nursing and pharmacy services,
case management resource centers, HIV/AIDS services,
women's health services, transplant care services, nutrition
support services

6870 Centegra Northern Illinois Medical Center
4209 West Shamrock Lane
Suite B
McHenry, IL 60050-8499   815-759-8017
                                          877-236-8347
                                          Fax: 815-759-8062
                                          www.centegra.org

Michael S. Eesley, CEO
Jason Sciarro, President
David L. Tomlinson, Executive Vice President
Kumar Nathan, MD
Providing rehabilitation services in Lake and McHenry Counties,
the Rehabilitation Unit is a complete living environment for up to
15 patients after a debilitating illness of trauma. Various loca-
tions offering a multitude of services: PT, OT, speech, HT,

6871 Center for Comprehensive Services
Mentor Network
P.O.Box 2825
Carbondale, IL 62902-2825   618-457-4008
                                          800-582-4227
                                          Fax: 618-457-5372
                                          dayna.foreman@thementornetwork.com
                                          mentorabi.com

Bill Duffy, Chief Operating Officer
Michael E. Hofmeister, Vice President
Sean Byrne, Chief Financial Officer
Post-acute rehabilitation services for adults and adolescents with
acquired brain injuries. Residential, day-treatment and out-pa-
tient services tailored to individual needs.

**6872 Center for Rehabilitation at Rush Presbyterian: Johnston R
Bowman Health Center**
1653 W Congress Parkway
Chicago, IL 60612-3833   312-942-5000
                                          Fax: 312-942-3601
                                          TTY:312-942-2207
                                          teri_sommerfeld@rush.edu
                                          www.rush.edu

Larry J. Goodman, CEO
A 613-bed hospital serving adults and children, the John R. Bowman Health Center and Rush University is home to one of the first
medical colleges in the Midwest and one of the nation's
top-ranked nursing colleges, as well as graduate programs in
allied he

6873 Center for Spine, Sports & Occupational Rehabilitation
345 E Superior St
Chicago, IL 60611-2654   312-238-7767
                                          800-354-7342
                                          Fax: 312-238-7709
                                          webmaster@ric.org
                                          www.rehabchicago.org

Joanne C. Smith, President & CEO
Edward B. Case, Executive Vice President
M. Jude Reyes, Chair
Offers evaluation and treatment of patients with acute and sub-
acute musculoskeletal and sports injuries. RIC offers different
levels of care, including inpatient, day rehabilitation, and outpatients services, according to the special needs of each patient

6874 Children's Home and Aid Society of Illinois
125 South Wacker Drive
14th Floor
Chicago, IL 60606-4448   312-424-0200
                                          contact@chasi.org
                                          www.childrenshomeandaid.org

Beverley Sibblies, Chairman
Chris Leahy, Vice-Chairman
Mark Tresnowski, Secretary
David Gookin, Treasurer
Private state-wide. Multi-service, racially integrated staff and
client populations. Provides educational, placement and commu-
nity services for children-at-risk and their families. Advocacy,
consultation and follow-up services provided according to our ph

6875 Clinton County Rehabilitation Center
1665 North Fourth Street
P O Box 157
Breese, IL 62230- 1791   618-526-8800
                                          Fax: 618-526-2021
                                          info@commlink.org
                                          commlink.org

Wesley A. Gozia, President
Judge Joseph L. Heimann, Vice President
John L. Lengerman, Treasurer
Jerry Albers, Secretary
Provides Adult Day Programs (developmental training, work
training, job readiness and job placements); Residentail Pro-
grams (CILA Intermittent Care, CILA 24 hour care); Infant Pro-
grams (early interventions, early head start); Community
Services (specializ

6876 Continucare, A Service of the Rehab Institute of Chicago
West Suburban Hospital Medical Center
3 Erie Ct
Oak Park, IL 60302-2519   708-383-6200
                                          800-354-7342
                                          Fax: 312-908-1369

Heidi Asbury MD
We respond to the needs of the whole person: body, mind and
spirit. We foster a climate of care, hospitality and a spirit of community. We develop systems and structures that attend to the
needs of those at risk of discrimination because of age, gender,
lifestyle, ethnic background, religious beliefs or socioeconomic
status.

6877 Delta Center
1400 Commercial Ave
Cairo, IL 62914-1978   618-734-2665
                                          800-471-7213
                                          Fax: 618-734-1999
                                          deltacenter.org

Lisa Tolbert, Executive Director
Lisa Tholbert, Assistant Executive Director
The Delta Center is a non-profit mental health center, substance
abuse counseling facility, and also provides various community
services to Alexander and Pulaski County, Illinois. The purpose
and mission is to promote, encourage, foster and engage exclusi

**6878 Division of Rehabilitation-Education Services, University of
Illinois**
Beckwith Hall
201 E. John Street
Champaign, IL 61820- 6901   217-333-4603
                                          Fax: 217-333-0248
                                          disability@uiuc.edu

Ann Fredricksen, Disability Specialist
Jon Gunderson, Coordinator
Pat Malik, Director
Dennis Cable, Accountant
Offers services for the totally blind, legally blind, visually im-
paired, mentally retarded blind and more with health, counseling,
educational, recreational, rehabilitation, computer training and
professional training services.

6879 Easter Seals
Easter Seals Joliet Region
233 South Wacker Drive
Suite 2400
Chicago, IL 60606-5272

312-726-6200
800-221-6827
Fax: 312-726-1494
www.easterseals.com

Richard W. Davidson, Chairman
Sandra L. Bouwman, 1st Vice Chairman
Joseph G. Kern, 2nd Vice Chairman
Ralph F. Boyd, Treasurer
Services for children and adults with disabilities and their families. Pediatric outpatient medical rehabilitation, inclusive childcare, fostercare, residential homes, clinics.

6880 Easter Seals DuPage and Fox Valley
830 S Addison Ave
Villa Park, IL 60181-1153

630-620-4433
Fax: 630-620-1148
info@eastersealsdfvr.org
www.easterseals.com/dfv

Theresa Forthofer, President & CEO
Erik Johnson, Vice President of Development
Kathy Schrock, MS, Vice President of Clinical Services
Jim Alviti, BS, Director of Physical Therapy
The mission of Easter Seals DuPage & the Fox Valley Region is to enable infants, children & adults with disabilities to achieve maximum independence and to provide support to the families who love and care for them. Key services provided include: physical, occupational, speech-language, nutrition and assistive technology therapies and audiology services for all ages.

6881 Easter Seals Gilchrist-Marchman Rehab Center
1939 West 13th Street
Suite 300
Chicago, IL 60608-1226

312-491-4110
Fax: 312-733-0247
Mcancel@eastersealschicago.org
www.easterseals.com/chicago

David A. Pearre, Chairman
Jeff Buchanan, Vice Chairman
Mark O'Toole, Secretary
John G. Anos, Treasurer
Provides comprehensive services for individuals with disabilities or other special needs and their families to improve quality of life and maximize independence.

6882 Easter Seals Jayne Shover Center
799 S McLean Blvd
Elgin, IL 60123-6704

847-742-3264
Fax: 847-742-9436
dfvr.easterseals.com

Dr. Haydee Muse, Chair
Kelly N. Taira, Vice Chairman
Karen Janousek, Secretary
Roger McDougal, Treasurer
A free-standing, comprehensive outpatient rehabilitation center serving children and adults with physical and developmental disabilities.

6883 El Valor
Main Office & Developmental Training Center
1850 W 21st St
Chicago, IL 60608

312-666-4511
Fax: 312-666-6677
TTY:312-666-3361
info@elvalor.net
elvalor.org

Rafael Malpica, Chairman
Rey B Gonzalez, President & CEO
Carmen Ziegler, Chief Financial Officer
Eduardo Moreno, Director of Employment & Facilities Services
El Valor's mission is to serve people with disabilities and their families, by offering programs in the areas of early childhood education, adult services and parental and community engagement.

6884 Elgin Training Center
Association For Individual Development Elgin Area
1135 Bowes Road
Elgin, IL 60123-1321

847-931-6200
Fax: 847-888-6079
www.the-association.org

Chuck Miles, Chairmen
Patrick Flaherty, Vice Chairmen
Walter Dwyer, Treasurer
Lynn O'Shea, Executive Director
Day training services to develop work habits and attitudes while providing training in small product assembly, sorting, packaging, collating, & material handling. Instruction also offered in job related knowledge & in personal, social and independent living skills. There is also an on-site specialized Autism Program. Additionally, residential programs (group homes & apartments) are also available for people with developmental disabilities.

6885 Family Counseling Center
PO Box 759
Golconda, IL 62938

618-683-2461
Fax: 618-683-2066
fccinconline.org

Larry Mizell, Executive Director
Connie Duncan, Director
Nora Beth Hacker, Financial Director
Provides counseling, developmental training, evaluations, assisted living services, referrals, psychosocial rehabilitation, and a variety of work services.

6886 Family Matters
A RC Community Support Systems
1901 S. 4th St
Ste 209
Effingham, IL 62401-4123

217-347-5428
866-436-7842
Fax: 217-347-5119
deinhorn@arc-css.org
www.fmptic.org

Debbie Einhorn, Executive Director
Debbie Einhorn, Director Family Support
Nancy Mader, Project Coordinator
Barbara Utz, Vice President
Parent Training and Information Center and family support programs for families of children who have disabilities from the ages of birth through 21. Services include: Parent support and training, school advocacy, home visits, information and referral, pa

6887 Five Star Industries
1308 Wells Street Road
P O Box 60
Du Quoin, IL 62832-60

618-542-5421
Fax: 618-542-5556
fivestarinc@5starind.com
5starind.com

Susan Engelhardt, Executive Director
Incorporated as a private, non-profit corporation under the laws of the State of Illinois, is an equal opportunity employer and provides equal opportunity in compliance with the Civil Rights Act of 1964 and all other appropriate laws, rules and regulation

6888 HSI Austin Center For Development
1819 S Kedzie Ave
Chicago, IL 60623-2623

773-854-1676
Fax: 773-854-8300

6889 Hyde Park-Woodlawn
950 E 61st St
Chicago, IL 60637-2623

773-324-0280
Fax: 773-324-0285

Clarissa Williams, Manager

6890   Illinois Center for Autism
548 South Ruby Lane
Fairview Heights, IL   62208-2614   618-398-7500
Fax: 618-394-9869
info@illinoiscenterforautism.org
illinoiscenterforautism.org
Hardy Ware, Chairperson
Thomas E. Berry, Vice Chairperson
Gary Guthrie, Secretary
Joy Rick, Treasurer
A community-based mental health/educational treatment center
dedicated to serving autistic clients.

6891   Julius and Betty Levinson Center
1825 K Street NW
Suite 600
Washington, DC   60304-1557   202-776-0406
800-872-5827
Fax: 708-383-9025
www.ucp.org

Woody Connette, Chair
Ian Ridlon, Vice Chair
Mark Boles, Treasurer
Pamela Talkin, Secretary
Houses one of its three adult developmental training programs for
substantially physically disabled men and women.

6892   Lake County Health Department
18 N. County Street
Waukegan, IL   60085   847-377-2000
Fax: 847-336-1517
www.lakecountyil.gov
Aaron Lawlor, Chairman
Stevenson Mountsier, Vice Chairman
Barry Burton, Administrator
Includes counseling, crisis intervention, emergency manage-
ment, psychotherapy and chemotherapy management for individ-
uals and families.

6893   Little Friends, Inc.
140 N Wright Street
Naperville, IL   60540-4799   630-355-6533
Fax: 630-355-3176
info@lilfriends.com
www.littlefriendsinc.com
Dan Casey, Chairman
Matt Johanson, Vice Chairman
Michele Calbi, Treasurer
Kathy West, Secretary
Little Friends has been serving children and adults with autism
and other developmental disabilities for over 40 years. Based in
Naperville, Little Friends operates three schools, vocational
training programs, community-based residential services and the

6894   MAP Training Center
7th and Mc Kinley St
Karnak, IL   62956   618-634-9401
Fax: 618-634-9090
Larry Earnhart, President
Cindy Earnhart, Community Liaison
Training, employment, residential and support services, targeted
for adults with developmental disabilities.

6895   Macon Resources
2121 Hubbard Ave.
P O Box 2760
Decatur, IL   62524-2760   217-875-1910
Fax: 217-875-8899
TTY:217-875-8898
jpatterson@maconresources.org
maconresources.org
Tom Hill, President
Michael Breheny, Vice President
Barb Nadler, Secretary
Chris Funk, Treasurer
The purpose is to provide a comprehensive array of
habilitative/rehabilitative training programs and support ser-

vices to assist individuals and/or family units of an individual
with a developmental disability, mental illness, or other
handicapping conditi

6896   Mary Bryant Home for the Blind
2960 Stanton
Springfield, IL   62703-4385   217-529-1611
888-529-1611
Fax: 217-529-6975
mbha@marybryanthome.org
marybryanthome.org
Jerry Curry, Executive Director
Robert E. Maxey, President
Allan J. Rupel, Vice President
Gary Rapaport, Secretary
Supportive living facility for blind or visually impaired adults
over the age of 22. A supportive living facility remodeled to foster the move to increased independence for residents. The new
apartment style housing combined with personal care and other a

6897   Northern Illinois Special Recreation Association (NISRA)
285 Memorial Drive
Crystal Lake, IL   60014-3650   815-459-0737
Fax: 815-459-0388
info@nisra.org
www.nisra.org
Brian Shahinian, Executive Director
Carol Amoroso, Manager of Finance and Personnel
Kerri Ruddy, Manager of Office Services
Sarah Holcombe, Manager of Communications & Marketing
Leisure and recreation services to those with disabilities who are
unable to participate successfully in park district and city recre-
ation programs.

6898   Oak Forest Hospital of Cook County
15900 Cicero Ave
Oak Forest, IL   60452   708-687-7200
Fax: 708-687-7979
TTY:708-687-4794
http://www.cchil.org
Robert Weinstein, Department Chair
Suja Mathew, Associate Chair
A 654 bed health care center devoted to the diagnosis, rehabilita-
tion and long-term care of adults suffering from chronic illnesses,
diseases and physical impairments.

6899   PARC
1913 W. Townline Road
P.O.Box 3418
Peoria, IL   61615-3418   309-691-3800
Fax: 309-689-3613
parcway.org
Pat Kawczynski, Chair
Heyl Royster, Vice Chair
Terry Waters, Treasurer
Alexis Duhon, Secretary
Serves all ages that are diagnosed with mental retardation and
other developmental and physical disabilities. Programs include
early intervention, family support, respite care, vocational train-
ing, supported employment, adult day programs and residential

6900   Peoria Area Blind People's Center
2905 W Garden St
Peoria, IL   61605-1316   309-637-3693
Fax: 309-637-3693
info@cicbvi.org
cicbvi.org
Carol Warren, President
Cora Quinn, Vice President
Prasad Parupalli, Treasurer
Offers services for the totally blind, legally blind, visually impaired, mentally retarded blind and more with health, counseling,
educational, recreational, rehabilitation, computer training and
professional training services.

6901 Pioneer Center for Human Services
4031 W Dayton St
McHenry, IL 60050
815-344-1230
Fax: 815-344-3815
TTY:815-344-6243
gethelp@pioneercenter.org
www.pioneercenter.org

Dan McCaleb, Chairman
Sam Tenuto, Co-CEO
Frank Samuel, Co-CEO
DJ Newport, MS, Director of Developmental Disability Services
Pioneer Center is a non-profit agency in McHenry County delivering services to more than 4,000 people annually. Pioneer Center provides developmental disability services, youth and family behavioral health services and homeless services (McHenry County PADS).

6902 Prosthetics and Orthotics Center in Blue Island
2310 York St
Blue Island, IL 60406-2411
708-597-2611
800-354-7342
Fax: 800-908-1932
www.rehabchicago.org/about/blue_island.php

6903 RB King Counseling Center
2300 N Edward St
Decatur, IL 62526-4163
217-877-8121
Fax: 217-875-0966

Gordon Cross MD
Offers outpatient, individual, group, divorce and meditation, family and re-adjustment counseling.

6904 REHAB Products and Services
3715 N Vermilion St
Danville, IL 61832-1130
217-446-1146
Fax: 217-446-1191
rehab@soltec.net
workse.org

Frank L. Brunacci, President/CEO
Crystal Meece, Vice President Production
Todd Seabaugh, VP Programs
Scott Rudy, VP Operations
janitorial, lawn care, distribution services.

6905 RIC Northshore
Rehabilitation Institute of Chicago
345 E Superior St
Chicago, IL 60611-2654
312-238-1000
800-354-7342
webmaster@ric.org
www.rehabchicago.org

Joanne C. Smith, President/CEO
Edward B. Case, Vice President
Provides rehabilitation for sports-related injuries, musculoskeletal conditions, neurological conditions, stroke, arthritis, amputation, burns, and general deconditioning.

6906 RIC Prosthetics and Orthotics Center
Rehabilitation Institute of Chicago
345 E. Superior Street
Suite 101
Chicago, IL 60611-4615
312-238-1000
800-345-7342
Fax: 708-957-8353
webmaster@rehabchicago.org
ric.org

Martin Buckner, CPO, Inpatient Coordinator
Nicole T. Soltys, CP, Clinical Coordinator
Robert D. Lipschutz, CP, Director of Prosthetic and Orthotic Education
Walter Afable, CP, Clinical Operations Manager
Offers almost all the prosthetics and orthotics services provided at RIC's main hospital in downtown Chicago, including consultations, fittings and training.

6907 RIC Windermere House
5548 S Hyde Park Blvd
Chicago, IL 60637-1909
773-256-5050
800-354-7342
Fax: 773-256-5060
www.rehabchicago.org

Meghan Scalise, Manager
Evaluation, therapeutic services and patient education are offered in the areas of arthritis, multiple sclerosis, musculoskeletal conditions, orthopedics, stroke, spinal cord injury, brain injury and sports medicine.

6908 Ray Graham Association for People with Disabilities
901 Warrenville Road
Suite 500
Lisle, IL 60532-1038
630-620-2222
Fax: 630-628-2350
TTY:630-628-2352
cathyfickerterill@yahoo.com
ray-graham.org

Michael Komoll, Chairperson
Neville Bilimoria, Vice Chairperson
Kim zoeller, President & CEO
Jeff Park, Secretary/Treasurer
Provides developmental services at 15 sites to infants, children and adults with disabilities. Services range from 1 hr/wk respite to full-time residential.

6909 Reach Rehabilitation Program: Americana Healthcare
9401 S Kostner Ave
Oak Lawn, IL 60453-2697
708-423-1505
Fax: 708-423-3822

Jean M Roche, Owner
Postacute rehabilitation program.

6910 Rehabilitation Achievement Center
345 E Superior St
Chicago, IL 60611-4805
312-238-1000
800-354-7342
www.ric.org

M. Jude Reyes, Chair
Mike P. Krasny, Vice Chair
Joanne C. Smith, President & CEO
Ed Case, Treasurer
Rehabilitation Institute of Chicago (RIC) has aquired the assets of the Rehabilitation Achievement Center (RAC).

6911 Rehabilitation Institute of Chicago: Alexian Brothers Medical Center
800 Biesterfield Rd
Elk Grove Village, IL 60007-3361
847-437-5500
866-253-9426
Fax: 847-631-5663
TTY: 847-956-5116
www.alexianbrothershealth.org

Mark Frey, President and Chief Executive Officer
Tracy Rogers, Senior Vice President and Chief Operating Officer
Paul Belter, Senior Vice President and Chief Financial Officer
Janice Jastrowski, Manager
A 32-bed rehabilitation unit under the medical direction and supervision of the Rehabilitation Institute of Chicago.

6912 Riverside Medical Center
Mental Health Unit
350 N Wall St
Kankakee, IL 60901-2991
815-933-1671
Fax: 815-935-8160
rhuber@rsh.net
riversidehealthcare.org

Phillip Kambic, CEO
Bill W. Douglas, Vice President
Offers recreation, parenting therapy, emergency services, psychological testing and inpatient treatment programs. Riverside is nationally recognized for its specialty programs in heart care, obstetrics, trauma, oncology, rehabilitation, geriatrics, occupa

6913 Robert Young Mental Health Center Division of Trinity Regional Haelth System
Trinity Health Foundation
2701 17th St
Rock Island, IL 61201-5351 309-779-2800
800-322-1431
Fax: 309-779-2027
www.unitypoint.org

Rick Seidler, President & CEO
Jim Hayes, CFO
Tamara Byram, VP, Legal/Compliance
Matt Behrens, Regional VP, UnityPoint Clinic

Services include comprehensive inpatient rehabilitation, chronic pain management programs, outpatient medical rehabilitation, work hardening programs, vocational evaluation, alcohol and other drug dependency rehabilitation programs, Burn Center, and menta

6914 Sampson-Katz Center
216 West Jackson Blvd
Suite 700
Chicago, IL 60606-2104 312-673-3400
Fax: 312-553-5544
TTY:773-761-6672
jvsskc@jvschicago.org
www.jvschicago.org

Andrew M. Glick, Chair
John L. Daniels, Vice Chair
H. Debra Levin, President
Benn Feltheimer, Secretary

6915 Shelby County Community Services
160 North Main Street
Memphis, TN 38103-650 901-222-2300
Fax: 912-222-2090
www.shelbycountytn.gov

Dottie Jones, Director
Primary focus is substance abuse treatment.

6916 Streator Unlimited
305 N Sterling St
P O Box 706
Streator, IL 61364-2369 815-673-5574
Fax: 815-673-1714
contact@streatorunlimited.org
www.streatorunlimited.org

Jeffrey Dean, Executive Director
Lynn Fukar, Director of Day Services
Julie Caestens, Director Residential Services

Vocational and personal skills training, residential services, client and family support, supported and computerized employment. Serves adults with intellectual disabilities with the goal of enabling them to reach their fullest potential, live as independ

6917 Swedish Covenant Hospital Rehabilitation Services
5145 N California Ave
Chicago, IL 60625-3661 773-878-8200
Fax: 773-561-0490
ask_us@schosp.org

Mark Newton, President & CEO

Provides acute rehabilitation services, subacute care and outpatient services for many types of disabling injuries and conditions, including amputation, arthritis, brain injury, general deconditioning, multiple sclerosis, musculoskeletal injuries, stroke,

6918 TCRC Sight Center
21310 Route 9
Tremont, IL 61568-2558 309-347-7148
Fax: 309-925-4241
info@tcrcorg.com
www.tcrcorg.com

Jamie Durdel, President & CEO
Molly Anderson, Vice President
Offers services for persons who are totally blind, legally blind, partially sighted or visually impaired along with other disabili-

ties. Have support group, rehabilitation classes, orientation and mobility services, counseling services, low vision clinic,

6919 Tazewell County Resource Center
Box 12
Rr 1
Tremont, IL 61568 309-347-7148
Fax: 309-925-4241
info@tcrcorg.com
http://www.tcrcorg.com

Jamie Durdel, President & CEO
Molly Anderson, Vice President
A private, nonprofit agency providing programs for the special needs of infants, adults, children and their families residing in Tazewell County. Services offered include: birth-three infant/parent program, adult day care services, family support, residen

6920 Thresholds Bridge Deaf North Program
Thresholds Psychiatric Rehabilitation Centers
4101 N. Ravenswood Ave
Chicago, IL 60613 773-572-5500
Fax: 773-989-1075
thresholds@thresholds.org
www.thresholds.org

Jana Barbe, President
Marianne Doan, Vice President
Harold E. D'Orazio, Treasurer
Kathy Graham, Secretary
A private, nonprofit psychosocial rehabilitation center that serves the deaf mental health consumers at the highest risk of hospitalization, those with serious and persistent mental illness. The program provides residential case management services focuse

6921 Thresholds South Suburbs
4101 N. Ravenswood Ave
Chicago, IL 60613 773-572-5500
Fax: 708-597-8053
thresholds@thresholds.org
www.thresholds.org

Jana Barbe, President
Marianne Doan, Vice President
Harold E. D'Orazio, Treasurer
Kathy Graham, Secretary
Services offered include psychosocial, vocational and residential programs for ages 18 or older with a primary diagnosis of mental illness. Facility is wheelchair accessible.

6922 Trumbull Park
10530 S Oglesby Ave
Chicago, IL 60617-6140 773-375-7022
Fax: 773-375-5528

Gregory Terry, Director
Diana Moore, Site Supervisor
Ada McKinley, Manager
Offers consultation, education, general counseling, recreation, self-help and social services for children and adults.

6923 University of Illinois Medical Center
1740 West Taylor Street
Chicago, IL 60612-7232 312-355-4000
866-600-2273
Fax: 312-996-7770
hospital.uillinois.edu

Rajiv Pai, Chief
Marilyn Plomann, Manager
Offers services for the totally blind, legally blind, visually impaired, mentally retarded blind and more with health, counseling, educational, recreational, rehabilitation, computer training and professional training services.

6924 VanMatre Rehabilitation Center
950 S Mulford Rd
Rockford, IL 61108-4274 815-381-8500
866-754-3347
Fax: 815-484-9953
webcontentcoordinator@rhsnet.org
www.vanmatrerehab.com
Gary E. Kaatz, President and Chief Executive Officer
Scott Craig, Medical Director
A CARF-accredited comprehensive rehabilitation center based
within the Rockford Memorial Hospital providing inpatient and
outpatient services for physically and cognitively challenged
persons with debilitating illness and injuries.

6925 Warren Achievement Center
1220 E 2nd Ave
Monmouth, IL 61546-2404 309-734-3131
Fax: 309-734-7114
info@warrenachievement.com
warrenachievement.com
Rick Barnhill, President
Jim Kesse, Vice President
Sherry Waite, Chief Operations Officer
Linda Baker, Chief Financial Officer
For developmentally disabled children and adults. Parent-infant
education programs are for parents of infants with disabilities or
developmental delays; Children's Group Homes which serve
children on a fulltime basis and can serve additional children on a

Indiana

6926 Ball Memorial Hospital
2401 W University Ave
Muncie, IN 47303-3499 765-747-3111
Fax: 765-747-3313
iuhealth.org/ball-memorial
Mike Haley, CEO
Offers rehabilitation services, occupational therapy, physical
therapy and more for the physically challenged child or adult.

6927 Community Health Network
1500 N Ritter Ave
Indianapolis, IN 46219-3027 317-355-4275
800-775-7775
Fax: 317-351-7723
www.ecommunity.com
Keith Thompson, Manager
Anita Harden, President
A leading not-for-profit health system offering convenient access
to expert physicians, advanced treatments and leading edge technology, all focused on getting patients well and back to their
lives. With caring compassion, Community's 5 hospitals and 70 +
sites of care continually strive to improve the health and well being of those individuals in central Indiana who entrust care to us.

6928 Crossroads Industrial Services
8302 E 33rd Street
Indianapolis, IN 46226 317-897-7320
Fax: 317-897-9763
info@crossroadsindustrialservices.com
www.crossroadsindustrialservices.c om
Anne Shupe, Finance Executive
Curtiss Quirin, CEO
Assisting customers with short-term, seasonal, and long-term
outsourcing needs. Many consider Crossroads an extension of
their company

6929 Department of Veterans Affairs Vet Center #418
302 W. Washington St
Room E120
Indianapolis, IN 46204- 2738 317-232-3910
800-490-4520
Fax: 317-232-7721
www.in.gov/veteran/sso/fac
Charles T. Applegate, Director

Provides readjustment counseling to combat veterans. Onsite assistance for employment problems, vocational rehabilitation and
sexual trauma counsel.

**6930 Frasier Rehabilitation Center Division of Clark Memorial
Hospital**
2201 Greentree N
Clarksville, IN 47129-8957 812-218-6590
Fax: 812-218-6597
http://www.jhsmh.org/Frazier-Rehab-Institute-
Catherine Lucas Spalding, Administrator
Designed to help patients in their adjustment to a physically limiting condition, both psychologically and physically, by helping to
maximize each patient's abilities so he or she can function as independently as possible. The program treats patients whos

6931 HealthSouth Deaconess Rehabilitation Hospital
4100 Covert Ave
Evansville, IN 47714-5559 812-476-9983
800-677-3422
Fax: 812-476-4270
www.healthsouthdeaconess.com
Barbara Butler, Chief Executive Officer
Ashok . Dhingra, M.D, Medical Director
Brett Hirt, Director, Therapy Operations
Doron Finn, M.D., Wound Care Program Director
AHealthSouth Deaconess Rehabilitation Hospital is a joint venture partner with Deaconess Health System. Our hospital is an
80-bed inpatient rehabilitation hospital that offers comprehensive inpatient and outpatient rehabilitation services designed to
return patients to leading active and independent lives. - See more
a t :
http://www.healthsouthdeaconess.com/en/our-hospital#sthash.
RCsNTk1u.dpuf

6932 Healthwin Specialized Care
20531 Darden Rd
South Bend, IN 46637-2999 574-272-0100
Fax: 574-277-3233
info@healthwin.org
healthwin.org
Connie McCahill, President
Lauren Davis, Vice President
John Cergnul, Treasurer
Stephen J. Gazdick, Chief Financial Officer
No other facility in the area has a homelike environment like ours.
Its simply part of our culture. Rehabilitation therapy that includes
physical, occupational, speech, respiratory and a full time
in-house therapist. Other services include a wound special

6933 Memorial Regional Rehabilitation Center
615 N Michigan St
South Bend, IN 46601-1033 574-647-1000
877-282-0964
www.qualityoflife.org/rehab
Johan Kuitse, MSA, PT, Outpatient Clinical Manager
Anne Clifford, DPT, Physical Therapists
Shanti Shrestha Dalson, DPT, Physical Therapists
Brandi DeMont, DPT, Physical Therapists
20-bed CARF accredited inpatient rehabilitation, outpatient orthopedic clinic and work performance program, head injury
clinic. Outpatient neuro rehab and a driver education and training
program are provided.

6934 Saint Joseph Regional Medical Center- South Bend
5215 Holy Cross Parkway
Mishawaka, IN 46545-2814 574-335-5000
Fax: 574-237-7312
thefoundation@sjrmc.com
sjmed.com
Albert Gutierrez, President & CEO
Steven Gable, Vice President
Janice Dunn, CFO
Christopher Karam, Chief Operating Officer
Continuum of rehabilitation services offered. Included are: acute
rehabilitation, a 26 bed CARF accredited comprehensive inpa-
tient unit, a CARF certified inpatient brain injury program, a

CARF outpatient day treatment brain injury program, comprehensive o

Iowa

6935 Crossroads of Western Iowa
1 Crossroads Pl
Missouri Valley, IA 51555-6069
712-642-4114
Fax: 712-642-4115
info@cwiowa.org
explorecrossroads.com
Brent Dillinger, CEO
Pat Kocour, President
Steven Van Riper, Vice President
Darci Tierney, Secretary
CWI provides services in Missouri Valley, Onawa and Council Bluffs, Iowa. An array of services for people with mental illness, mental retardation and brain injury are provided in each location.

6936 Des Moines Division-VA Central Iowa Health Care System
3600 30th St
Des Moines, IA 50310-5753
515-699-5999
800-294-8387
Fax: 515-699-5862
www.centraliowa.va.gov
Judith Johnson-Mekota, Director
Fredrick Bahls, Chief Of Staff
Susan A. Martin, Associate Director
Alton C. Alexander, Associate Director
VA Cental Iowa Health Care System is the result of the 1997 merger of the Des Moines and Knoxville, Iowa, VA Medical Centers. This integrated healthcare system brings 2 previously separate organizational structures, located 40 miles apart, into one cohesi

6937 Easter Seals Iowa
Easter Seals National
401 N.E. 66th Avenue
Des Moines, IA 50313-4002
515-289-1933
Fax: 515-289-1281
TTY:515-289-4069
ia.easterseals.com
Steve Niebuhr, Chair
Rochelle Burnett, Vice Chair
Sherri Nielsen, President & CEO
David Lester, Treasurer
Easter Seals is a leading nonprofit provider of services to Iowans with disabilities. Services include vocational and employment training, camping recreation and respite services, craft training and sales, home and farm adaptations, transportation, schola

6938 Genesis Regional Rehabilitation Center
Genesis Health System
1227 E.Rusholme Street
Davenport, IA 52803-3396
563-421-1000
Fax: 563-421-3499
genesishealth.com
Doug Cropper, President & CEO
Kenneth Croken, Vice President
Joseph Lohmuller, Chief Medical Officer
Karen Bolton, Vice President
Serves persons of all ages experiencing a disability, whether acquired at birth or following a serious interdisciplinary service. Rehabilitation programs include acute rehabilitation; adult rehabilitation, pediatric rehabilitation, outpatient orthopaedics

6939 Homelink
Van G Miller & Associates
1101 W S Marnan Drive
Waterloo, IA 50701-2817
319-235-7173
866-575-8483
Fax: 319-235-7822
homelinkprivacyofficer@vgm.com
www.vgmhomelink.com
Dave Kazynski, President
Rick Hibben, Coordinator

A national network of home medical equipment, respiratory therapy, rehabilitation and infusion therapy service providers with over 2,500 locations serving all fifty states.

6940 Iowa Central Industries
127 Avenue M
Fort Dodge, IA 50501-5797
515-576-2126
Fax: 515-576-2251
Tom Eckman, Executive Director
Services include evaluation and training in pre-vocational and vocational skills, personal behavior management, cognitive skills, communication skills, self-care skills and social skills. Services arranged include: independent living training, medical ser

6941 Life Skills Laundry Division
1510 Industrial Rd SW
Le Mars, IA 51031-3009
712-546-4785
Fax: 712-546-4985
Don Nore, Executive Director

6942 MIW
909 S 14th Ave
Marshalltown, IA 50158-3610
641-752-3697
Fax: 641-752-1614
Rich Byers, President/CEO
Vocational services for adults with disabilities. Includes organizational employment services, supported employment, job placement.

6943 Mercy Dubuque Physical Rehabilitation Unit
250 Mercy Drive
Dubuque, IA 52001-7320
563-589-8000
Fax: 563-589-8162
www.mercydubuque.com
Russel M. Knight, CEO
Provides services which open the door to improved communication, offering the opportunity to enrich the quality of life. Mercy offers many other branches of services including, rehabilitation services for children and a pulmonary rehabilitation program.

6944 Mercy Medical Center-Pain Services
1111 6th Ave
Des Moines, IA 50314-2611
515-247-3121
Fax: 515-248-8867
webmaster@mercydesmoines.org
Dana L. Simon, MD
Dave Vellinga, President & CEO
Laurie Conner, Vice President
An outpatient program dedicated to helping people with chronic pain live more productive, satisfying lives. The program is not designed for conditions that are surgically curable, but rather approaches the problem using a comprehensive, holistic treatment.

6945 Nishna Productions-Shenandoah Work Center
902 Day Street
Shenandoah, IA 51601-70
712-246-1242
Fax: 712-246-1243
nci@nishna.org
Mary Rolf, President
Sherri Clark, Executive Director
Melissa Mueller, Program Manager
Barb Hammer, Team Leader
Shelter, workshop and job training for the disabled. Some of the services we provide are Work Activity, Adult Day Activity Program, Personal & Social Adjustment, Residential Services, Home & Community Based Services & Employment Resources.

6946 Northstar Community Services
3420 University Avenue
Waterloo, IA 50701-2050
319-236-0901
888-879-1365
Fax: 319-236-3701
www.northstarcs.org

Mark Witmar, Executive Director
Jeff Conrey, President
Kathy Folkerts, Vice President
Mary Wankowicz, Director of operations
Provides adult day services, employment services and supported community living so people with disabilities can live and work in the community.

6947 Options of Linn County
935 2nd street
SW
Cedar Rapids, IA 52404-3100
319-892-5000
Fax: 319-892-5849
linncounty.org

Joel D. Miller, Auditor
Sharon Gonzalez, Treasurer
Options of Linn County works with community businesses in providing employment services to adults with disabilities. Options is a publicly operated service provider within the Linn County Community Services department.

6948 RISE
106 Rainbow Dr
Elkader, IA 52043-9075
563-245-1868
Fax: 563-245-2859
Ed Josten, Manager

6949 Ragtime Industries
116 N 2nd St
Albia, IA 52531-1624
641-932-7813
Fax: 641-932-7814
Lisa Glenn, Executive Director
A work-oriented rehabilitation organization which provides training for mentally and physically disabled adults in Monroe County. A variety of programs which help to develop each person's individual potential are offered.

6950 Sunshine Services
1106 East 9th St
Spencer, IA 51301-225
712-262-7805
Fax: 712-262-8369
Ann Vandehar, Executive Director

6951 Tenco Industries
710 Gateway Dr
Ottumwa, IA 52501-2204
641-682-8114
Fax: 641-684-4223
clogan@tenco.org
www.tenco.org

Ben Wright, Executive Director
Dixie Merritt, Vocational Director
Brenda Miller, Marketing and Development DirectoR
Joanie Lundy, Human Resources Director
To advocate and provide opportunities for people with disabilities, or conditions that limit their abilities, to develop and maintain the skills necessary for personal dignity and independence in all areas of life. Provide a wide array of services to individuals with disabilities. By looking at each person as individuals, we are able to work with them to maximize their skills. Residentials services, including HCBS and CSALA are also provided in all communities.

6952 Arrowhead West
1100 E Wyatt Earp Blvd
Dodge City, KS 67801-5337
620-227-8803
Fax: 620-227-8812
web@arrowheadwest.org
www.arrowheadwest.org

Kelly Mason, Chairperson
Michael Stein, Vice Chairperson
Lori Pendergast, President
Anita Allard, Treasurer
Services and programs offered include: developmental and therapy services for children birth to age 3; adult center-based work services and community integrated employment options; adult life skills and retirement programs; and adult residential services.

6953 Big Lakes Developmental Center
1416 Hayes Dr
Manhattan, KS 66502-5066
785-776-9201
Fax: 785-776-9830
biglakes@biglakes.org
biglakes.org

Lori Feldkamp, President
Shawn Funk, Community Education Director
A private nonprofit Community Developmental Disability Organization (CDDO) serving individuals with developmental disabilities in Riley, Geary, Clay and Pottawatome counties in Kansas. Big lakes is supported by county mill levy and federal and state fundi

6954 Developmental Services of Northwest Kansas
2703 Hall St
Suite 10
Hays, KS 67601-1964
785-625-5678
800-637-2229
Fax: 785-625-8204
Jerry Michaud, President
Ruth Lang, Administrative Assistant
A private nonprofit organization serving both children and adults with disabilities. Offers services to children ages birth to three years, youth and adults through a network of community-based and outreach programs and inter-agency agreements with other

6955 ENVISION
2301 S Water St
Wichita, KS 67213-4819
316-267-2244
Fax: 316-267-4312
Info@envisionus.com
www.envisionus.com

Sam Williams, Chair
Jon Rosell, PhD, Vice-Chair
Michael Monteferrante, President and CEO
Greg Unruh, Vice President, CFO
Provides jobs, job training and vision rehabilitation services to people who are blind or low vision. A private not-for-profit agency uniquely combining employment opportunitites with rehabilitation services and public education.

6956 Heartspring
8700 E 29th St N
Wichita, KS 67226-2169
316-634-8700
800-835-1043
Fax: 316-634-0555
kgrover@heartspring.org
www.heartspring.org

Gary W. Singleton, President and CEO
Paul Faber, Executive Vice President, Operations
Katie Grover, Director Of Marketing
David Dorf, CPA, Chief Financial Officer
Heartspring provides outpatient therapies, evaluations and consultations for children with special needs through Heartspring Pediatric Services. The Heartspring School is a residential and day school for children ages 5-21 with multiple disabilities. Children with autism and their families receive resources through the Heartspring CARE program. The Heartspring Hearing Center provides services to individuals of all ages.

6957 Indian Creek Nursing Center
6515 W 103rd St
Overland Park, KS 66212-1798
913-633-7000
Fax: 913-642-3982
www.savaseniorcare.com

Randy Sutterfield, Administrator
Postacute rehabilitation program. A 120-bed nursing home facility.

6958 Johnson County Developmental Supports
111 South Cherry Street
Olathe, KS 66061-1223
913-715-5000
Fax: 913-715-0800
info@jocogov.org
www.jocogov.org

Ed Eilert, Chairman
Michael Lally, Vice Chair
Scott Tschudy, Treasurer
Jessica Dain, Secretary
JCDS is the community Developmental Disability Organization for Johnson County, Kansas. Provides supports in the form of direct services to people on a daily basis. Through a person-centered process and within availiable resources services are shaped to f

6959 Ketch Industries
1006 E Waterman St
Wichita, KS 67211-1525
316-383-8700
800-766-3777
Fax: 316-383-8715
webmaster@ketch.org
ketch.org

Fred Badders, Chairman
Carla Bienhoff, Chairman
Loren Anthony, Secretary
Dan Crug, Treasurer
The mission of Ketch is to promote independence for persons with disabilities through innovative learning experiences that support individuals choices for working, living and playing in their community.

6960 Lakemary Center
100 Lakemary Dr
Paola, KS 66071-1855
913-557-4000
Fax: 913-557-4910
lakemaryctr.org

William Craig, President
Paul Sokoloff, Chair
Gayle Richardson, Vice Chair
Lydia Marien, Secretary
A private, not-for-profit day and residential training facility which provides for the assessment, education, training, therapy and social development of children and adults, moderate and severe mental retardation. The Center is based 28 miles southwest o

6961 Northview Developmental Services
700 E 14th St
Newton, KS 67117-5702
316-283-5170
Fax: 316-283-5196
http://northviewdev.mennonite.net/

Mary Holloway, CEO
The mission is to provide quality supportive and coordinating services to persons with developmental disabilities, assisting them to grow as they integrate into the community. Further, our mission is to improve the quality of their lives by providing acce

Kentucky

6962 Cardinal Hill Rehabilitation Hospital
Cadinal Hill Medical Center
2050 Versailles Rd
Lexington, KY 40504-1499
859-254-5701
800-233-3260
Fax: 859-231-1365
www.cardinalhill.org

Gary R. Payne, CEO

Provides occupational health services, therapy services and urgent medical treatment of injured workers.

6963 Frazier Rehab Institute
220 Abraham Flexner Way
Louisville, KY 40202-1887
502-582-7400
Fax: 502-582-7477

Jamie Ochsner, Manager
Steve Ahr, VP Frazier Rehab/Neurscience
Frazier Rehab Institute is a regional healthcare system dedicated entirely to rehabilitation. Through an expansive network of inpatient and outpatient facilites in Kentucky and southern Indiana, Frazier offers a wide array of services based on one common

6964 HealthSouth Northern Kentucky Rehabilitation Hospital
201 Medical Village Dr
Edgewood, KY 41017-3407
859-341-2044
800-860-6004
Fax: 859-341-2813
www.healthsouthkentucky.com

Richard Evans, CEO
Mary Pfeffer, Director Therapy Operations
Neal Moser, M.D., Medical Director
Mary Beth Bauer, RD, CSG, LD, Director of Quality and Risk Management
Offers all types of inpatient and outpatient rehabilitation services such as occupational therapy, physical therapy, speech therapy. Respiratory therpay, Psychology, Aquatics, Case Managemenet/Social Work and Nutritional Services.

6965 King's Daughter's Medical Center's Rehab Unit/Work Hardening Program
2201 Lexington Ave
Ashland, KY 41101-2843
606-408-4000
888-377-5362
Fax: 606-327-7542
info@kdmc.net
www.kdmc.com

Kristie Whitlatch, President & CEO
Matt Ebaugh, VP / Chief Strategy and Information Officer
Philip Fioret, M.D., VP / Chief Medical Officer
Howard Harrison, Vice President, Facilities
Offers a 27-bed, inpatient rehabilitation services unit treating physical disabilities related to accident or illness. The program provides an interdisciplinary inpatient program designed to restore the individual to the highest level of independence. It

6966 LifeSkills Industries
380 Suwannee Trail St
Bowling Green, KY 42103-6499
270-901-5000
800-223-8913
Fax: 270-782-0058
sbell@lifeskills.com
lifeskills.com

Alice Simpson, CEO
LifeSkills will be the reliable advocate, dependable safety net and provider of choice, for high quality, accessable services and supports for the citizens of south-central Kentucky whos lives are affected by mental illness, developmental disablilities or

6967 Low Vision Services of Kentucky
120 N. Eagle Creek Drive
Suite 500
Lexington, KY 40509-1827
859-263-3900
800-627-2020
Fax: 859-977-1136
jvanarsdall@retinaky.com
www.lowvisionky.com

Regina Callihan-May, O.D.
Jeanne Van Arsdall, Co-ordinator
Maryanne Inman, Practice Administrator
William J. Wood, MD, Physician
Offers educational, recreational and rehabilitational services and devices for the visually impaired, legally blind, totally blind.

6968 **Muhlenberg County Opportunity Center**
PO Box 511
Greenville, KY   42345-1416   270-754-5590
                                          Fax: 270-338-5977
                                               muhlon.com

Chuck Hammonds, Manager
Charles Hamonds, Director
Post-acute rehabilitation facility with programs including a
workshop with hand packaging of manufactured goods.

6969 **New Vision Enterprises**
1900 Brownsboro Rd
Louisville, KY   40206-2102   502-893-0211
                                               800-405-9135
                                          Fax: 502-893-3885
Larry Sherman, Plant Manager
Offers employment training and services for the blind and legally
blind.

6970 **Park DuValle Community Health Center, Inc.**
3015 Wilson Ave
Louisville, KY   40211-1969   502-774-4401
                                          Fax: 502-775-6195
                                            rjones@pdchc.org
                                               www.pdchc.org

Richard K Jones, President
John Howard MD, Medical Director
Dave Gerwig, CFO
Ann Hagan, Administrator
Offers services for the totally blind, legally blind, visually im-
paired, mentally retarded blind and more with health, counseling,
educational, recreational, rehabilitation, computer training and
professional training services.

Louisiana

6971 **Alliance House**
427 S Foster Drive
Baton Rouge, LA   70806-2723   225-987-0013
                                          Fax: 225-346-0857

6972 **Assumption Activity Center**
4201 Highway 1
Napoleonville, LA   70390-8628   985-369-2907
                                          Fax: 985-369-2657
Warren Gonzales, Manager
A community work center providing prevocational training and
extended employment for adults with disabilities. Services include: social services, work activities, specialized training and
supported employment.

6973 **Bancroft Rehabilitation Living Centers**
425 Kings Highway East
P.O. Box 20
Haddonfield, NJ 08033-0018   504-482-3075
                                               800-774-5516
                                          Fax: 504-483-2135
                                      lynn.tomaio@bancroft.org
                                               www.bancroft.org
Dr. Robert Voogt, Owner
Toni Pergolin, President & CEO
Cynthia Boyer, Executive Director
Thomas J. Burke, MBA, Chief Financial Officer
Mission is to nurture abilities and independence of people with
neurological challenges by providing a broad spectrum of ad-
vanced therapeutic and educational programs and by fostering
the development of best practices in the field through research
and pro

6974 **Caddo-Bossier Association for Retarded Citizens**
4103 Lakeshore Dr
Shreveport, LA   71109-1998   318-636-0258
                                          Fax: 318-221-4262
Janet Parker, Director

A community operated workshop for male and female mentally
retarded individuals. It provides work evaluation and transitional
and extended employment.

6975 **Deaf Action Center Of Greater New Orleans**
Catholic Charities
1000 Howard Ave
Suite 200
New Orleans, LA   70113-1903   504-523-3755
                                               866-891-2210
                                          Fax: 504-523-2789
                                          TTY: 504-615-4944
                                               www.ccano.org

Tommie A. Vassel, Chairman
Sr.Marjorie Hebert, MSC, President & CEO
This community service and resource center serves deaf,
deaf-blind, hard of hearing and speech-impaired persons in the
greater New Orleans area regardless of age, religion, race or secondary disability. DAC provides interpreting services,
equipment distri

6976 **Donaldsville Association for Retarded Citizens**
1030 Clay St
Donaldsonville, LA   70346-3518   225-473-4516
                                          Fax: 225-473-4517
                                            daarc@eatel.net
Marlene Domingue, Executive Director
A private, nonprofit sheltered work program working with the
mentally retarded and developmentally disabled adults.

6977 **East Jefferson General Hospital Rehab Center**
4200 Houma Blvd
Metairie, LA   70006-2996   504-454-4000
                                               www.ejgh.org
Newell D. Normand, Chairman
Ashton J. Ryan, Jr., Vice Chairman
Mark J, Peters, President & CEO
*Judy Brown, CPA, MHA, FACHE, Executive Vice President / Chief
Operating Officer*
Provides the highest quality, compassionate healthcare to the
people we serve. East Jefferson General Hospital will be the re-
gion's healthcare leader providing the highest quality care
through innovation and collaboration with our team members,
medical st

6978 **Family Service Society**
2515 Canal Street
Suite 201
New Orleans, LA   70119-6489   504-822-0800
                                          Fax: 504-822-0831
                                           family@fsgno.org
                                               www.fsgno.org
L. Blake Jones, Chair
Jackie Sullivan, 1st Vice Chair
Kathleen Vogt, 2nd Vice Chair
Ronald P McClain JD, President & CEO
Offers services for the totally blind, legally blind, visually im-
paired, mentally retarded blind and more with health, counseling,
educational, recreational, rehabilitation, computer training and
professional training services.

6979 **Foundation Industries**
9995 Highway 64
Zachary, LA   70791   225-654-6288
                                          Fax: 225-654-3988
Jim Lambert-Oswald, President
Jim Oswald, General Manager
A private, nonprofit sheltered workshop providing extended employment and work activities for the mentally retarded and developmentally disabled clients. Objectives are to build work skills
through supervision, develop social interaction and manifest
basi

6980 **Handi-Works Productions**
2700 Lee St
Alexandria, LA   71301-4358   318-442-3377
                                          Fax: 318-473-0858

6981 Iberville Association for Retarded Citizens
24615 J.Gerald Berret Blvd
Plaquemine, LA 70764-201   225-687-4062
                                       Fax: 225-687-3272
                                          arci@eatel.net

Paul Rhorer, Executive Director
A private sheltered work program operating out of one facility
and providing transitional, extended employment and work activities for mentally and developmentally ill adults.

6982 Lighthouse for the Blind in New Orleans
123 State St
New Orleans, LA 70118-5793   504-899-4501
                                            888-792-0163
                                       Fax: 504-895-4162
                                       lighthouselouisiana.org

Curtis Eustis, Chair
Paul Masinter, Chair Elect
Tabatha George, Secretary
Peyton Bush, Treasurer
Offers services for the totally blind, legally blind, visually im-
paired, mentally retarded blind and more with health, counseling,
educational, recreational, rehabilitation, computer training and
professional training services.

6983 Louisiana Center for the Blind
101 South Trenton Street
Ruston, LA 71270-4431   318-251-2891
                                             800-234-4166
                                        Fax: 318-251-0109
                                        pallen@lcb-ruston.com
                                        www.louisianacenter.org

Pam Allen, Executive Director
Neita Ghrigsby, Office Manager
Janette Woodard, Residential Manager
Jack Mendez, Director of Technology
A new kind of orientation and training center for blind persons.
The center is privately operated and provides quality instruction
in the skills of blindness. Offers employment assistance, com-
puter literacy training, summer training and employment project

6984 Louisiana State University Eye Center
Lousiana State University
433 Bolivar Street
New Orleans, LA 70112-2272   504-568-4808
                                       Fax: 504-412-1315
                                            www.lsuhsc.edu

Jayne S. Weiss, Director
Kelli McMichael, Manager
The LSU Eye Center is part of the LSU Medical Center complex
in downtown New Orleans. It is in the LSU-Lions Building at
2020 Gravier Street between South Bolivar and South Prieur
streets.

6985 New Orleans Speech and Hearing Center
1636 Toledano St
New Orleans, LA 70115-4598   504-897-2606
                                       Fax: 504-891-6048

Mary Beth Green, President
Jessica Vinturella, Treasurer
Kindall James, Secretary
This non-residential facility serves male and female clients for
purposes of evaluating speech and hearing problems and providing speech therapy, hearing aids and other assistive technology
for speech and hearing.

6986 Port City Enterprises
836 North Seventh Street
Port Allen, LA 70767-113   225-344-1142
                                             877-344-1142
                                        Fax: 225-344-1192
                                        www.portcityenterprises.org

William Kleinpeter, President
Mark Graffeo, Vice President
L.J. Treuil Jr, Secretary
Philip Bourgoyne, Treasurer

Offers supported employment, sheltered work and supervised
programs for the mentally retarded, ages 22 and over.

6987 Rehabilitation Center at Thibodeaux Regional
Rehab Care
602 N Acadia Rd
Thibodaux, LA 70301-4847   985-493-4731
                                            800-822-8442
                                       Fax: 985-449-4600
                                       www.thibodaux.com/rehabilitation.html

Jan Torres, Program Manager
Rose Pipes, Clinical Coordinator
Designed to help patients in their adjustment to a physically limiting condition, both physically and psychologically, by helping to
maximize each patients abilities so he or she can function as independently as possible.

6988 St. Patrick RehabCare Unit
RehabCare
524 Doctor Michael Debakey Dr
Lake Charles, LA 70601-5725   337-491-7590
                                            888-722-9355
                                       Fax: 337-491-7157

Larry A Hauskins, Manager
Ruth Thornton, Admissions
A comprehensive physical and cognitive rehabilitation program
designed to help individuals who have experienced a disabling
injury or illness.

**6989 Touro Rehabilitation Center - LCMC (Louisiana Children's
       Medical Center)**
1401 Foucher St
New Orleans, LA 70115-3515   504-897-8565
                                       Fax: 504-897-8393
                                       GeneralRehabilitationProgram@touro.com
                                       www.touro.com/rehab

Jeanette Ray, VP of Rehab and Post Acute Srv
Janet Clark, Director of Inpatient Rehabilitation Programs
Marylee Pontillas, Director of Outpatient Rehab Srv
Lynn Drake, Patient Care Manager
Located in New Orleans' Garden District, Touro Rehabilitation is
a comprehensive rehabilitation facility dedicated to the restora-
tion of function and independence for individuals with disabili-
ties. The scope of rehabilitation services is broad, with 3 CARF
accreditations for Brain Injury, Spinal Cord Injury and General
Rehabilitation. TRC opened in 1984 and offers 69 rehab beds.
TRC is part of Touro Infirmary which has a proud 150 year history
as a nonprofit teaching hospital.

6990 Training, Resource & Assistive-Technology
2000 Lakeshore Drive
New Orleans, LA 70148-1   504-280-6000
                                            888-514-4275
                                       Fax: 504-280-5707
                                            ggaglian@uno.edu
                                            www.uno.edu

Ken Zangla, Director
Naomi Moore, Assistant Director
Connie Lanier, Coordinator
Peter J. Fos, President
Provides quality services to persons with disabilities, rehabilita-
tion professionals, educators and employers. Built a solid reputa-
tion for its innovative training programs and community outreach
efforts. The Center is recognized as a valuable resource st

Maine

6991   Charlotte White Center
572 Bangor Rd
Dover Foxcroft, ME   04426-3373   207-564-2426
                                                        888-440-4158
                                                   Fax: 207-564-2404
                                             info@charlottewhite.org
                                             charlottewhitecenter.com

Richard M. Brown, CEO
Charles G. Clemons, COO
Dale Shaw, CFO
Mary Louis McEwen, President

A nonprofit agency, devoted to assisting adults and children with
mental retardation, mental health, physical handicaps, and elder
age related issues. With headquarters in Dover-Foxcroft Maine,
the agency provides multiple levels of social services, inclu

6992   Iris Network for the Blind
189 Park Avenue
Portland, ME   04102-2909   207-774-6273
                                                  Fax: 207-774-0679
                                                     ashah@theiris.org
                                                         theiris.org

Leonard Cole, Chairman
Katharine Ray, 1st Vice Chairman
Bruce Roullard, 2nd Vice Chairman
James E. Phipps MBA/JD, Executive Director

A statewide resource and catalyst for people who are visually impaired or blind so they can attain their determined level of independence and integration into the community.

6993   Roger Randall Center
45 School St
Houlton, ME   04730-2010   207-532-4068
                                                  Fax: 207-532-7334
                                                      www.cla-maine.org

Rob Moran, Executive Director
Tom Moakler, President
Vicki Moody, Vice President
Peter Crovo, Treasurer

The Roger Randall Cneter is one of five Day Habilitation Programs adminsitered by Community Living Association, a private,
non-profit agency. These programs may provide a supportive environment that allows the individual to achieve their maximum
growth po

6994   Sebasticook Farms-Great Bay Foundation
P.O.Box 65
Saint Albans, ME   04971   207-487-4399
                                                  Fax: 207-938-5670

Tom Davis, Executive Director
Pam Erskin, Program Coordinator

Provides residential, educational and vocational services to
adults who are developmentally disabled in order to maximize independent living and to provide assistance in obtaining an earned
income.

6995   Social Learning Center
10 Shelton McMurphey Blvd
Eugene, OR   97401-3363   541-485-2711
                                                        877-208-6134
                                                  Fax: 541-485-7087
                                                          www.oslc.org

Sam Vuchinich, Ph.D, Chair
Gordon Naga Hall, Ph.D., Vice President
Susan Miller, J.D., Secretary/Treasurer
Sally Guyer, Staff Representative

Post accute rehabilitation program.

Maryland

6996   Blind Industries and Services of Maryland
3345 Washington Blvd
Baltimore, MD   21227-1602   410-737-2600
                                                        888-322-4567
                                                  Fax: 410-737-2665
                                                        info@bism.org
                                                             bism.org

Donald J. Morris, Chairperson
Walter A. Brown, Vice Chairperson
Fredrick J. Puente, President
James R. Berens, Treasurer

Offers a comprehensive residential rehabilitation training program for people who are blind. Areas of instruction: braille, cane
travel, independent living, computer, adjustment and blindness
seminars.

6997   Center for Neuro-Rehabilitation
2340238 N Cary St
Annapolis, MD   21223   410-263-1704
                                                        410-462-4711

Jeanne Fryer
Laurent Pierre-Philippe

Provide community-based inpatient and outpatient acute rehabilitation, vocational services and long-term care. Specializing in
treating complex neurological conditions including spinal cord
injuries, multiple sclerosis, strokes, and other brain injuries resulting from trauma, anoxia, tumors, genetic malformations and
other related conditions. Locations in Annapolis, Bethesda, Frederick, Towson, MD and Fairfax, Va. CNR is licensed, a Medicare
provider and CARF accredited.

**6998   Child Find/Early Childhood Disabilities Unit Montgomery
County Public Schools**
Ste A4
10731 Saint Margarets Way
Kensington, MD   20895- 2831   301-929-2224
                                                  Fax: 301-929-2223

Julie Bader, Supervisor

Offers free developmental screening for children ages 3 years until eligible for kindergarten, evaluation and placement services.

6999   Greater Baltimore Medical Center
6701 N Charles St
Baltimore, MD   21204-6881   443-849-2000
                                                        800-597-9142
                                                  Fax: 443-849-2631
                                                          www.gbmc.org

John B. Chessare MD, President & CEO
Harold J. Tucker MD, Chief Of Staff
Eric L. Melchoir, Vice President & CFO
Keith Poisson, Executive VP & COO

Offers services for the visually impaired and blind with low vision exams. Rehabilitation teaching and orientation and mobility
in the home or workplace. Also offers a bimonthly newsletter for
$12/yr for Hoover patients and monthly share group.

7000   James Lawrence Kernan Hospital
2200 Kernan Drive
Baltimore, MD   21207-6697   410-285-6566
                                                        888-453-7626
                                                  Fax: 410-448-6854
                                                  www.umrehabortho.org

Michael Jablonover MD,MBA, President & CEO
John P. Straumanis MD, FAAP, Vice President
*W. Walter x Augustin, III, CPA, Vice President of Financial Ser-
vices*
*Cheryl D. Lee, RN, MSN, CRRN, Vice President, Patient Care
Services*

Kernan reigns as Maryland's origional orthopaedic hospital with
a staff which consists of a support team of orthopaedic physician
assistants and dedicated nurses in the Post Anesthesia Care Unit
and on the Medical/Surgical Unit, guaranteeing the highest q

7001 Levindale Hebrew Geriatric Center
2401 W. Belvedere Ave.
Baltimore, MD 21215-5267
410-601-9000
Fax: 410-601-2700
www.lifebridgehealth.org

Jason A. Blavatt, Chair
David Uhlfelder, Vice Chair
Edward L. Morris, Treasurer
Sharon Caplan, Secretary
a 292-licensed bed facility, which includes 172-comprehensive care beds, 20 subacute beds, and a 26-bed dementia care unit. Levindale's 120-bed specialty hospital consists of 20 gerospychiatric beds, 80 complex medical beds, some with ventilator capacity

7002 Meridan Medical Center For Subacute Care
770 York Rd
Towson, MD 21204
410-821-5500
Fax: 410-821-6735

Yvette Caldwell, Administrator
Patients receive around-the-clock professional nursing care; physical and occupational, speech and respiratory therapists also assist patients. Each patient's individualized plan of care is reviewed and updated as patient needs change. Careful discharge p.

7003 Rehabilitation Opportunities
5100 Philadelphia Way
Lanham, MD 20706-4412
301-731-4242
Fax: 301-731-4191
roiworks.org

Tom Purcell, President
Bruce Shapiro, Vice President
David Fierst, Secretary
Henry Neloms, Treasurer
Organization offering day programs, evaluation, work adjustments and sheltered workshops for persons who are mentally retarded or developmentally disabled.

7004 Rosewood Center
410-951-5000
888-300-7071
Fax: 410-581-6157
www.dhmh.state.md.us/dda/rosewood

Leslie Smith, Program Director
James Anzalone, Director
Rosewood Center is a State residential Center that supports adults with mental retardation from the central Maryland region. Rosewood will provide comprehensive supports to Maryland citizens with developmental disabilities and their families in a setting .

7005 TLC: Treatment and Learning Centers
2092 Gaither Road
Suite 100
Rockville, MD 20850-3316
301-424-5200
Fax: 301-424-8063
www.ttlc.org

Patricia Ritter Ph.D., CCC-SLP, Executive Director
Cathleen Burgess Ms Ed, CCC-SLP, Director
Bill McDonald, President
Michael Cogan, Vice President
Provides audiological evaluations, testing and hearing aids, physical and occupational therapy and evaluation; speech-language evaluation and therapy, psycho-educational testing and tutoring services for learning disabled students, head injury services an

7006 Workforce and Technology Center
Division of Rehabilitation Services
2301 Argonne Drive
Baltimore, MD 21218-1628
410-554-9442
888-554-0334
Fax: 410-554-9112
www.dors.state.md.us

Dan Frye, Chairperson
Josie Thomas, Vice Chairperson

Is one of nine state operated comprehensive rehabilitation facilities in the country providing a wide range of services to individuals with disabilities. The Maryland Division of Rehabilitation Services operates the Workforce and Technology Program. Avail

Massachusetts

7007 Baroco Corporation
136 West Street
Northampton, MA 01060-2711
413-534-9978
Fax: 413-585-9019
www.baroco.com

Rick Barnard, President/Owner
Suzanne Darby, Executive Administrator
Julia McLaughlin, Executive Administrator
Janet Lawlor, Executive Administrator
Provides training and therapeutic support for its recipients with developmental disabilities in order to aid them in securing and maintaining placement in a less-restrictive setting.

7008 Berkshire Meadows
160 Gould Street
Suite 300
Needham, MA 02494-2300
781-559-4900
Fax: 413-528-0293
lkelly@jri.org
berkshiremeadows.org

Andy Pond, President
Gregory Canfield, Vice President
Deborah Reuman, CFO
Stephen H. Webster, Executive Advisor
Private, non profit school for children, adolescents, young adults who are severely, developmentally disabled. Approved special education learning center, work site program and foster care. Physical therapy, speech and language development, behavioral pro *$8200.00*

7009 Blueberry Hill Healthcare
75 Brimbal Ave
Beverly, MA 01915-6009
978-927-2020
Fax: 978-922-5213
admissions@BlueberryHillRehab.com
www.blueberryhillrehab.com

Ralph Epstein, Medical Director
Accomodates 146 residents. We are centrally located close to Route 128 and Route 1A in Beverly Massachusetts. We offer short-term rehab care, long term care and Alzheimer's Special Care Programs. Our interdisciplinary team designs individual care plans fo

7010 Boston University Hospital Vision Rehabilitation Services
One Boston Medical Center Place
Boston, MA 02118-2371
617-638-8000
Fax: 617-638-7769
www.bmc.org/rehab.htm

Simona Manasian, Medical Director
Karen Mattie, Director
Jenn Blake, Clinical Outpatient Supervisor
Kara Schworm, Clinical In-patient Supervisor
Offers services for the totally blind, legally blind, visually impaired, mentally retarded blind and more with health, counseling, educational, recreational, rehabilitation, computer training and professional training services.

7011 Burbank Rehabilitation Center
275 Nichols Rd
Fitchburg, MA 01420-1919
978-343-5000
888-840-3627
Fax: 978-343-5342
www.umassmemorialhealthcare.org

David Bennett, Chair
Eric Dickson, President & CEO
The largest community hospital and regional referral center in the area. Offers the most extensive high quality, cost-effective healthcare services in the region. The hospital provides outstanding hospital-based services such as case management of high ri

7012   Carl and Ruth Shapiro Family National Center for Accessible Media
WGBH Educational Foundation
1 Guest St.
Boston, MA   02135-2016
617-300-3400
Fax: 617-300-1035
TTY:617-300-2489
ncam@wgbh.org
ncam.wgbh.org

Donna Danielewski, Director
Madeleine Rothberg, Senior Subject Matter Expert
Geoff Freed, Director of Technology
Bryan Gould, Director of Accessible Learning and Assessment Technologies
The Carl and Ruth Shapiro Family National Center for Accessible Media (NCAM) is a research and development facility dedicated to addressing barriers to media and emerging technologies for people with disabilities in their homes, schools, workplaces, and communities.

7013   Carroll Center for the Blind
770 Centre St
Newton, MA   02458-2597
617-969-6200
800-852-3131
Fax: 617-969-6204
www.carroll.org

Josepth Abely, President
Arthur O'Neill, Vice President
Brian Charlson, Director of Computer Training Services
Robert McGillivray, Director of Low Vision Services
Offers services for the totally blind, legally blind, visually impaired, mentally retarded blind and more with health, counseling, educational, in dependent living, tronell skills, computer traing, recreational, rehabilitation, computer training and professional training services.

7014   Center for Psychiatric Rehabilitation
Boston University
940 Commonwealth Ave
West
Boston, MA   02215-1203
617-353-3549
Fax: 617-353-7700
psyrehab@bu.edu
cpr.bu.edu

Kim T. Mueser, Executive Director
Deborah Dolan, Director of operations
Larry Kohn, Director of Development
E. Sally Rogers, Director of Research
The mission of the Center is to increase knowledge, to train treatment personnel, to develop effective rehabilitation programs and to assist in organizing both personnel and programs into efficient and coordinated service delivery systems for people with

7015   Clark House Nursing Center At Foxhill Village
Kindred Healthcare
30 Longwood Dr
Westwood, MA   02090-1132
781-326-5652
800-359-7412
Fax: 781-326-4034
www.clarkhousefhv.com

Chris Wasel, Administrator
Clark House At Fox Hill Village accomodates 70 residents. We are part of the Fox Hill Village Assisted Living and Retirement Center campus. Clark House Nursing center has been named a recipient of a 2005 step II quality Award from the American Health Care

7016   College Internship Program at the Berkshire Center
18 Park St
Lee, MA   01238-1702
413-243-2576
Fax: 413-243-3351
admissions@berkshirecenter.org
berkshirecenter.org

Lucy Gosselin, Program Director
Laina Hubbard, Admissions Coordinator
Charles D. Houff, Head Therapist
A highly individualized postsecondary program for learning disabled young adults 18-30. Provides job placement services and follow-ups; college support; money management and social skills. Residential students share an apartment and have their own room. T

7017   Devereux Advanced Behavioral Health Massachusetts & Rhode Island
Devereux School
60 Miles Rd.
P.O. Box 219
Rutland, MA   01543
508-886-4746
800-338-3738
Fax: 508-886-4773
tbeauvai@devereux.org
www.devereuxma.org

Stephen Yerdon, Executive Director
Bonnie Byer, Business Development Director
Evans Chiyombwe, Quality Management Director
Sandy Fleek, Executive Assistant
Serving children and youth with emotional, behavioral, intellectual and developmental disorders. Services include residential treatment, community-based group homes, therapeutic foster care, special needs day school, substance abuse and autism spectrum programs, diagnostic services and in-home services.

7018   Eagle Pond Rehabilitation and Living Center
1 Love Lane
P.O.Box 208
South Dennis, MA   02660-3445
508-385-6034
Fax: 508-385-7064
www.eaglepond.com

Paul Marchwat, Executive Director
Ellen Reil, Marketing Director
Eagle Pond accomodates 142 residents. Medicare and Medicaid certified as well as being accredited by the Joint Comission (formerly (JCAHO) which enables us to contract with many insurance companies.

7019   FOR Community Services
75 Litwin Ln
Chicopee, MA   01020-4817
413-592-6142
Fax: 413-598-0478
ggolash1@aol.com

Gina Golash, Executive Director
Providing a world of meaning for individuals with developmental disabilities throughout Western Massachusetts since 1967.

7020   Fairlawn Rehabilitation Hospital
189 May Street
Worcester, MA   01602-4399
508-791-6351
Fax: 508-831-1277
www.fairlawnrehab.org

Dave Richer, CEO
Peter Bagley MD, Medical Director
Matthew Akulonis, Director Of Support Operations
Judy Chuli, Chief Nursing Officer
Offers comprehensive rehabilitation on both an inpatient and outpatient basis. Specialty programs include: head injury, spinal cord injury, young/senior stroke, oncology, geriatrics and orthopedics.

7021   Greenery Extended Care Center: Worcester
59 Acton Street
Worcester, MA   01604-4899
508-791-3147
800-633-0887
Fax: 508-753-6267
worcester@wingatehealthcare.com
wingatehealthcare.com

Scott Schuster, Founder & President
Brian Callahan, CFO
Michael Benjamin, Vice President
Trent Guthrie, Senior Director
173 beds offering complex care, extended rehabilitation and neurobehavioral intervention. Offering life care homes and Nursing home services. Specialties include life events and physical care, long term and home health care, and nursing homes and nursing

7022 Greenery Rehabilitation & Skilled Nursing Center
P.O.Box 1330
Middleboro, MA 02346-4330   508-947-9295
                                          Fax: 508-947-7974

7023 Harrington House Nursing And Rehabilitation Center
160 Main Street
Walpole, MA 02081-4037   508-660-3080
                                          Fax: 508-660-1634
                                        www.harringtonrehab.com

Joseph Haron, Medical Director
Accomodates 90 residents. Our state-of-the-art center offers
post-accute services including rehabilitation and medical management. Our center also provides a long term care program including hospice services.

**7024 HealthSouth Rehabilitation Hospital Of Western
Massachusetts**
222 State Street
Ludlow, MA 01056-3478   413-308-3300
                                          Fax: 413-547-2738
                                        www.healthsouthrehab.org

Victoria Healy, CEO
Adnan Dahdul, M.D., Medical Director
Deborah Cabanas, Chief Nursing Officer
AnnMaria Elder, M.D., Medical Staff President
A 53-bed acute Rehabilitation Hospital. The facility has been op-
erating for 14 years and has provided rehabilitative care to pa-
tients and families in the greater Springfield area with an
outstanding reputation for attention to detail and compassion.
Becau

7025 Holiday Inn Boxborough Woods
242 Adams Pl
Boxborough, MA 01719-1735   978-263-8701
                                               800-465-4329
                                          Fax: 978-263-0518
                                       box_sales@fine-hotels.com
                                        www.ihg.com/holidayinn

Kevin Murray, Manager
Marcel Girard, Manager
Nancy Ellen Hurley, Chief Marketing Officer
Located on 35 acres of wooded countryside just off I-495 at exit
#28. Minutes from the Mass Turnpike, Route 2, 290 and 9. Con-
ference center located on main level with 30,000 square feet of
meeting space. Guest rooms feature two-line telephones, voice
mail
$129 - $159

7026 Lifeworks Employment Services
1400 Providence Highway
Suite 2300
Norwood, MA 02062- 4551   781-769-3298
                                          Fax: 781-551-0045
                                         www.lifeworksma.org
Dan Burke, President & CEO
Chris Page, Vice President
Brenda Calder, CFO
Mary Hagen, Controller
Providing homes, jobs, education and supportive living for peo-
ple with developmental disabilities.

**7027 Massachusetts Eye and Ear Infirmary & Vision
Rehabilitation Center**
243 Charles Street
Boston, MA 02114-3002   617-523-7900
                                          Fax: 617-573-4178
                                          TTY:617-523-5498
                                        www.masseyeandear.org

Wycliffe Grousbeck, Chairman
John Fernandaz, President & CEO
Lily H. Bentas, Secretary
Jonathan Uhrig, Treasurer
Visual rehabilitation encompasses a low vision rehabilitation
evaluation, occupational therapy evaluation (with home visit if
necessary), and social service evaluation.

7028 New England Center for Children
260 Tremont Street
Boston, MA 02116-2108   617-636-4600
                                          Fax: 617-636-4866
                                           cwelch@necc.org
                                               necc.org

Lisel Macenka, Chair
James C. Burling, Vice Chair
L.Vincent Strully, President
Michael F. Downey, Treasurer
A comprehensive year-round program for students with autism
and PDD who require a highly specialized educational and behavior management program. Students are from all over the country
and receive intensive, positive, behavioral counseling and social
skil

7029 New England Eye Center - Tufts Medical Center
Tufts Medical Center
260 Tremont St
Boston, MA 02116   617-636-4600
                                               800-231-3316
                                          Fax: 617-636-4866
                                       eli_peli@meei.harvard.edu
                                             www.necc.com

Jeannette Spillane, Executive Director
Shana Bellus, Director, Admitting Operations
Linnea Olsson, Special Projects Consultant
ChiHae Kwan, Optometrist
The New England Eye Center offers services for the legally blind
and visually impaired, as well as for health care providers. Services include health care, counseling, education, vision research
and professional training. Emphasis is on mobility related vision
enhancement, including devices for driving and safe walking.

**7030 New Medico Rehabilitation and Skilled Nursing Center at
Lewis Bay**
89 Lewis Bay Rd
Hyannis, MA 02601-5207   508-775-7601
                                          Fax: 508-790-4239

Edmund Steinle, Executive Director
Post acute rehabilitation services.

7031 Protestant Guild Learning Center
411 Waverley Oaks Rd
Suite 104
Waltham, MA 02452-8449   781-893-6000
                                          Fax: 781-893-1171
                                        www.theguildschool.org

Eric H. Rosenberger, President
Thomas P. Corcoran, Vice President & Treasurer
Thomas Belski, Chief Executive Officer
Sandra L. Skinner, Clerk
Offers services for the diagnostically disabled children and ado-
lescents with ages 6-22 years with health, counseling, educa-
tional, recreational, rehabilitation, computer training and
professional training services.

7032 Shaughnessy-Kaplan Rehabilitation Hospital
1 Dove Ave
Salem, MA 01970   978-745-9000
                                          Fax: 978-740-4730
                                         skrhinfo@partners.org
                                          spauldingrehab.org

Anthony Sciola, CEO
Maureen Banks, RN, MS, MBA, CN, President
Mary Beth DiFilippo, Vice President
Charles Pu, MD, Chief Medical Officer
A 160-bed private, non-profit hospital. We have been providing
care for residents of greater North Shore communities since 1975.
Shaughnessy has 120 long-term care hospital beds and a 40-bed
transitional care unit sometimes referred to as a skilled nursin

7033 Son-Rise Program
2080 South Undermountain Road
Sheffield, MA 01257-9643
413-229-2100
877-766-7473
Fax: 413-229-3202
correspondence@option.org
www.autismtreatmentcenter.org

Barry Neil Kaufman, Co Founder
Samahria Lyte Kaufman, Co Founder
THe Son-Rise Program is a powerful, effective and totally unique treatment for children and adults challengedby Autism, Autuism Spectrum Disorders, Pervasive Developmental Disorder (PDD), Asperger's Syndrome and other developmental difficulties.

7034 Southern Worcester County Rehabilitation Inc. D/B/A
Life-Skills, Inc.
44 Morris St
Webster, MA 01570-1812
508-943-0700
Fax: 508-949-6129
www.life-skillsinc.org

J Thomas Amick, Executive Director
Kristin Nelson, Board President
Barbara Butrym, Board Vice President
Janice Smith, Board Secretary
Life-Skills, Inc. assists mentally and developmentally challenged adults with meeting their individual needs, and empowering them to take full advantage of meaningful opportunities in their communities. We provide residential, employment, transportation, behavior, and theraputic day habilitation services to 350 adults in MA. We operate thrift & consignment stores, a small cafe, an ice cream shop, mini golf & arcade center, vending and greenhouse businesses, bank courier service, and others.

7035 Vinfen Corporation
950 Cambridge Street
Cambridge, MA 02141-1001
617-441-1800
877-284-6336
Fax: 617-441-1858
TTY: 617-225-2000
info@vinfen.org
www.vinfen.org

Philip A. Mason, Ph.D., Chairperson
Bruce L. Bird, Ph.D., CEO/ President
Elizabeth K. Glaser, Chief Operations Officer
Glen Mattera, Chief Financial Officer
A private, nonprofit company, Vinfen Corporation is the largest human services provider in Massachusetts. Vinfen offers clinical, educational, residential and support services to individuals of all ages with mental illness and or mental retardation, who also may have another disability (e.g. substance abuse, homelessness, AIDS). The company also trains professionals in the mental health field and helps consumers to learn to live in community-based settings at the highest levels.

7036 Visiting Nurse Association of North Shore
5 Federal St
Danvers, MA 01923-3687
508-751-6926
800-728-1862
Fax: 978-777-0308
www.vnacarenetwork.org

Mary Ann O'Connor, CEO/ President
Stephanie Jackman-Havey, Chief Operating Officer/Chief Financial Officer
David Rose, Vice President of Human Resources
Jane Woodbury, Vice President of Fund Development
Home health services including nurses, physical, occupational and speech therapy, home health aides and more. Special programs include nutrition counseling, IV care, pediatric therapy, HIV/AIDS services and wound management. Provides services 7 days a week, 365 days a year and we accept Medicare, Medicaid and most HMO's and health insurers.

7037 Weldon Center for Rehabilitation
233 Carew St
Springfield, MA 01104-2377
413-748-6800
Fax: 413-748-6806
mercycares.com

Barbara Haswell, Manager

One of the most vital, necessary health resources in the region by helping thousands of people toward restored health and independence. A comprehensive, integrated, non-profit facility offering inpatient, outpatient, day rehabilitation and pediatric services on one site.

7038 Youville Hospital & Rehab Center
1575 Cambridge St
Cambridge, MA 02138-4398
617-876-4344
Fax: 617-547-5501
www.youville.org

Michigan

7039 Botsford Center For Rehabilitation & Health
Improvement-Redford
28050 Grand River Ave.
Farmington Hills, MI 48336-5919
248-471-8000
877-442-7900
Fax: 313-387-3838
www.botsford.org

John Darin, Manager
A 20 bed inpatient physical rehabilitation unit, servicing individuals who have experienced a stroke, amputation, orthopedic fracture, or other neurological impairment.

7040 Chelsea Community Hospital Rehabilitation Unit
775 South Main Street
Chelsea, MI 48118-1383
734-593-6000
800-231-2211
Fax: 734-475-4191
www.stjoeschelsea.org

Nancy K. Graebner, CEO/ President
Kathy Brubaker, RN, Vice President and Chief Nursing Officer
Randall Forsch, MD, Chief Medical Officer
Barbara Fielder, VP Finance
A private, non-profit, acute care facility that combines the best of small town values with national standards of healthcare excellance. The hospital has a 19-bed acute care inpatient rehabilitation unit with comprehensive outpatient programs, including a coordinated brain injury program.

7041 Clare Branch
790 Industrial Dr
Clare, MI 48617-9224
989-386-7707
888-773-7664
Fax: 989-386-2199
mail@mmionline.com
www.mmionline.org

Cris Zeigler, Executive Director
MMI will strive to be the premier provider of person-centered services to people with barriers to employment. We will connect individuals with community resources that provide mutual benefit to them and to the community. MMI will be known for excellence in service provision, ethical business practices, a quality work environment, and for providing services that enhance the dignity and value of the people we serve.

7042 Clarkston Spec Healthcare Center
4800 Clintonville Rd
Clarkston, MI 48346-4297
800-454-5909
fundltc.com

Margaret Canny, Administrator
120 beds offering active/acute rehabilitation, complex care, day treatment, extended rehabilitation, neurobehavioral intervention and short-term evaluation.

7043   DMC Health Care Center-Novi
42005 W 12 Mile Rd
Novi, MI 48377-3113   248-305-7575
                                                   Fax: 425-201-1450
                                                   novi@patch.com
                                                   novi.patch.com

Bud Rosenthal, CEO
Leigh Zareli Lewis, COO
Andreas Turanski, CTO
Melanie Pereira, VP of Finance
The Detroit Medical Center's record of service has provided medical excellence throughout the history of the Metropolitan Detroit area. From the founding of the Children's Hospital in 1886, to the creation of the first mechanical heart at Harpers Hospital 50 years ago, to our compassion for the underdeserved, our legacy of caring is unmatched.

7044   Eight CAP, Inc. Head Start
904 Oak Drive
Greenville, MI 48838-9277   616-754-9315
                                                   Fax: 616-754-9310
                                                   laurelm@8cap.org
                                                   www.8cap.org

Ralph Loeschner, Executive Director
Nancy Secor, Contact
Post accute rehabilitation programs.

7045   Greater Detroit Agency for the Blind and Visually Impaired
16625 Grand River Ave
Detroit, MI 48227-1419   313-272-3900
                                                   Fax: 313-272-6893
                                                   Information@gdabvi.org
                                                   gdabvi.org

Frederick J Simpson, Board Chairman
Charles L. Cone, Vice Chairman
Leonard W Robinson, Board Secretary
John W. Rhinesmith, CPA, Board Treasurer
Offers services for seniors 60 and over who are legally blind. Also provides eye health information, counseling, education and rehabilitation services.

7046   Hope Network Neuro Rehabilitation
1490 E Beltline SE
Grand Rapids, MI 49506   616-940-0040
                                                      855-407-7575
                                                   Fax: 616-942-7130
                                                   rehabreferral@hopenetwork.org
                                                   www.hopenetworkrehab.org

Jeffrey Bennett, Chair
Phil Weaver, President & CEO
Richard Fabbrini, Chief Financial Officer
Jill Szyszko, Executive Administrator
Neuro Rehabilitation serves those with brain injuries and other neurological conditions by offering them treatments and person-centered care towards recovery.

7047   Lakeland Center
26900 Franklin Rd
Southfield, MI 48033-5312   248-350-8070
                                                   Fax: 248-350-8078
                                                   peggys@thelakelandcenter.net
                                                   thelakelandcenter.net

Irving Shapiro, CEO
Santhosh Madhavan, Director Physical Medicine
Gary Yashinsky, Associate Medical Director
Subacute rehabilitation program directed toward those with severe neurologic diagnoses, ie: TBI, cerebral aneurysm, anoxic encephalopathy, CVA and cerebral hemorrhage, orthopedic injuries, and spinal cord injury. Subacute rehabilitation is provided for those who recover slowly and require individualized treatment plans. Residential program available as well.

7048   Mary Free Bed Rehabilitation Hospital
235 Wealthy St SE
Grand Rapids, MI 49503-5247   616-493-9657
                                                      800-528-8989
                                                   Fax: 616-454-3939
                                                   info@maryfreebed.com
                                                   maryfreebed.com

Kent Riddle, CEO
John Butzer, MD, Medical Director
Randy DeNeff, Vice President of Finance
Founded more than 100 years ago, Mary Free Bed Rehabilitation Hospital is and 80-bed, not-for-profit, acute rehabilitation center. Its mission is to restore hope and freedom through rehabilitation to people with disabilities. Mary Free Bed offers comprehensive inpatient and outpatient rehabilitationfor children and adults using an interdisciplinary approach. Also available are numerous specialty programs designed to increase the quality of life and independence of people with disabilities.

7049   Michigan Career And Technical Institute
11611 Pine Lake Rd
Plainwell, MI 49080-9225   269-664-4461
                                                      877-901-7360
                                                   Fax: 269-664-5850

Dennis Hart, Executive Director
A residential vocational training center for adults with physical, mental or emotional disabilities.

7050   Michigan Commission for the Blind Training Center
1541 Oakland Dr
Kalamazoo, MI 49008   269-337-3848
                                                      800-292-4200
                                                   Fax: 269-337-3872
                                                   mossc@michigan.gov

Christine Boone, Director
Bruce Schultz, Assistant Director
Residential facility that provides instruction to legally blind adults in braille, computer operation and assistive technology, handwriting, cane travel, cooking, personal management, industrial arts and also crafts. During training students will develop career plans which may include work experience, internships, volunteer opprtunities and even part-time paid employment.

7051   Mid-Michigan Industries
2426 Parkway Dr
Mt Pleasant, MI 48858-4723   989-773-6918
                                                      888-773-7664
                                                      888-773-7664
                                                   Fax: 989-773-1317
                                                   mail@mmionline.com
                                                   mmionline.com

Alan Schilling, President
Andrea Christopher, Director Admissions
Linda Wagner, Branch Director
Sheri Alexander, Director of Community Employment
Providing jobs and training for persons with barriers to employment. Services include vocational evaluation, job placement, supported employment, work services, prevocational training and case management

7052   New Medico Community Re-Entry Service
216 St Marys Lake Rd
Battle Creek, MI 49017-9710   *Fax:* 269-962-2241
James Rekshan, Executive Director

7053   Sanilac County Community Mental Health
171 Dawson St
Sandusky, MI 48471-1062   810-648-0330
                                                      888-225-4447
                                                      888-225-4447
                                                   Fax: 810-648-0319

Roger Dean, Executive Director
Post-acute rehabilitation facility and programs.

7054 Special Tree Rehabilitation System
600 Stephenson Highway
Troy, MI 48083-1110

248-616-0950
800-648-6885
Fax: 248-616-0957
info@specialtree.com
www.specialtree.com

Joseph Richart, CEO
Special Tree exists to provide hope, encouragement, and expertise for people who have experienced life-altering changes. Our team approach to rehabilitation, custom designed for each person's needs and goals, offers these individuals the best opportunity for healing and recovery.

7055 Thumb Industries
1263 Sand Beach Rd
Bad Axe, MI 48413-8817

989-269-9229
Fax: 989-269-2587
thumbindustries@hotmail.com
www.thumbindustries.com

Rhonda Wisenbaugh, Executive Director
Provides job training and employment for disabled persons. Vocational rehabilitation agency, manufactures household furnishings, direct mail advertising service.

7056 Visually Impaired Center
1422 W Court St
Flint, MI 48503-5008

810-767-4014
Fax: 810-767-0020
info@vicflint.org
www.vicflint.org

a pages

7057 Welcome Homes Retirement Community for the Visually Impaired
1953 Monroe Ave NW
Grand Rapids, MI 49505-6242

616-447-7837
888-939-9292
888-939-9292
Fax: 616-447-9891

Beth Lucksted, Manager
Offers services for the totally blind, legally blind, visually impaired, mentally retarded blind and more with health, counseling, educational, recreational, rehabilitation, computer training and professional training services.

7058 William H Honor Rehabilitation Center Henry Ford Wyanclotte Hospital
Henry Ford Health System
2333 Biddle Ave
Wyandotte, MI 48192-4668

734-246-6000
Fax: 734-246-6926
www.henryfordwyandotte.com
Denise Dailing, Administration Leader/rehabilita
James Sexton, Chief Executive Officer
Henry Ford, Owner
Henry Ford Wyandotte Hospital offers an array of educational programs, health screenings, and support groups. The hospital is CARF accredited and has a CARF certified stroke specialty unit.

Minnesota

7059 Industries: Cambridge
601 Cleveland St S
Cambridge, MN 55008-1752

763-689-5434
Fax: 763-552-1281
jspicer@industriesinc.org
www.industriesinc.org

Daryl Peterson, Board Chair
Bruce Montgomery, Vice Chair
Marilyn Bachman, Secretary
Kevin Troupe, Treasurer
Nonprofit organization that does vocational assessment and training for people with disabilities.

7060 Industries: Mora
500 Walnut St S
Mora, MN 55051-1936

320-679-2354
Fax: 320-679-2355
jspicer@industriesinc.org
www.industriesinc.org

Daryl Peterson, Board Chair
Bruce Montgomery, Vice Chair
Marilyn Bachman, Secretary
Kevin Troupe, Treasurer
Nonprofit organization that does vocational assessment and training for people with disabilities.

7061 Shriners Hospitals for Children: Twin Cities
2025 E River Pkwy
Minneapolis, MN 55414-3696

612-596-6100
888-293-2832
888-293-2832
Fax: 612-339-5954
www.shrinershospitalsforchildren.org

Charles C. Lobeck, Administrator
Cary Mielke, M.D, Interim Chief of Staff
Don Engel, Development Officer
Shriners Hospital for Children-Twin Cities offers quality orthopedic medical care regardless of the patients' ability to pay. Shriners Hospitals provide inpatient and outpatient services, surgery, casts, braces, artificial limbs, x-rays and physical and occupational therapy to any child under the age of 18 who may benefit from treatment.

7062 Vision Loss Resources
1936 Lyndale Ave S
Minneapolis, MN 55403-3101

612-871-2222
Fax: 612-872-0189
TTY:612-382-8422
info@vlrw.org
www.visionlossresources.org

Barry Shear, Chair
Lisa David, Vice Chair
Mary McDougall, Secretary
Jackie Peichel, Treasurer
Offers services for the totally blind, legally blind, visually impaired, and more with health, counseling, educational, recreational, rehabilitation, computer training and professional training services.

Mississippi

7063 Addie McBryde Rehabilitation Center for the Blind
PO Box 5314
Jackson, MS 39296-5314

601-364-2700
800-443-1000
Fax: 601-364-2677

H. S. McMillan, Executive Director
Shelia Browning, Deputy Director Non-Vocational P
Offers services for the totally blind, legally blind, visually impaired, mentally retarded blind and more with health, counseling, educational, recreational, rehabilitation, computer training services and orientation and mobility.

7064 Mississippi Methodist Rehabilitation Center
1350 E Woodrow Wilson Ave
Jackson, MS 39216-5198

601-981-2611
800-223-6672
Fax: 601-364-3571
www.methodistonline.org

Mark A. Adams, President/ CEO
Matthew L. Holleman, III, Chair
Mike P. Sturdivant Jr, Vice Chairman
David L. McMillin, Secretary
Rebuild lives that have been broken by disabilities and impairments from serious illness or severe injury. The challenge is to help patients regain abilities, restore function and movement, and renew emotionally. It features personal rehabilitation treatment plans administered by specialized teams of health care profes-

sionals through a variety of outpatient programs, treatments and other services.

Missouri

7065   Alpine North Nursing and Rehabilitation Center
4700 NW Cliff View Dr
Kansas City, MO   64150-1237
816-741-5105
Fax: 816-746-1301

Mike Stacks, Executive Director
Bob Richard, Administrator
Postacute rehabilitation program.

7066   Christian Hospital Northeast
11133 Dunn Rd
Saint Louis, MO   63136-6119
314-653-5000
877-747-9355
Fax: 314-653-4130
christianhospital.org

Ron McMullen, President
Bryan Hartwick, Vice President Human Resources
Sebastian Rueckert, MD, Vice President and Chief Medical Officer
Jennifer Cordia, Vice President and Chief Nurse Executive
A non-profit organization, a 493 bed acute care facility on 28 acres. Christian Hospital has more then 600 physicians on staff and a diverse workforce of more then 2,5000 health-care professionals who are dedicated to providing the absolute best care with the latest technology and medical advances.

7067   Integrated Health Services of St. Louis at Gravois
10954 Kennerly Rd
Saint Louis, MO   63128-2018
314-843-4242
Fax: 314-843-4031

Lisa Niehaus, Administrator
Subacute, skilled and intermediate care; ventilator/tracheostomy management program; wound management program and complex rehabilitation program.

7068   Metropolitan Employment & Rehabilitation Service
M ER S Goodwill
1727 Locust St
Saint Louis, MO   63103-1703
314-241-3464
Fax: 314-241-9348
www.mersgoodwill.org

Lewis C. Chartock, Ph.D., President/ CEO
Dawayne Barnett, CFO
Mark Arens, Executive Vice President, Chief of Program Services
Mark Kahrs, Executive Vice President, Retail Services
Vocational rehabilitation, primarily with the disabled, skills training and placement services.

7069   Missouri Easter Seal Society: Southeast Region
233 South Wacker Drive
Suite 2400
Chicago, IL   60606
312-726-6200
800-221-6827
Fax: 312-726-1494
easterseals.com

Richard W. Davidson, Chairman
Sandra L. Bouwman, 1st Vice Chairman
Ralph F. Boyd, Jr., Treasurer
Eileen Howard Boone, Secretary
The mission of the Easter Seal Society is to work with individuals, their families and the community to enhance the independence and quality of life for persons with disabilities.

7070   Poplar Bluff RehabCare Program
Lucy Lee Hospital
2620 N Westwood Blvd
Poplar Bluff, MO   63901-3396
573-785-7721
Fax: 573-686-5987

Jim Martin, Program Manager
Chris Murray, Care Coordinator
Darlene Hill, Care Admissions Coordinator

Provides physical medicine and rehabilitation to individuals with a physically limiting condition. The program is designed to help individuals function as independently as possible by maximizing their strength and abilities.

7071   Shriners Hospitals for Children St. Louis
2001 S Lindbergh Blvd
Saint Louis, MO   63131-3597
314-432-3600
800-850-2960
Fax: 314-432-2930
www.shrinershq.org/hospitals/st.louis

John McCabe, Executive Vice President
Kenneth Guidera, M.D., Chief Medical Officer
Eugene R. D'Amore, Vice President, Hospital Operations
Kathy A. Dean, Vice President, Human Resources
Medical care is provided free of charge for children 18 and under with orthopaedic conditions.

7072   St. Louis Society for the Blind and Visually Impaired
8770 Manchester Rd
Saint Louis, MO   63144-2724
314-960-9000
Fax: 314-968-9003
www.slsbvi.org

David Ekin, President
Chris Pickel, Chair
Ann Shapiro, Vice Chair
Sherine Apte, Secretary
Offers vision rehabilitation services for the totally blind, legally blind, visually impaired, including counseling, educational, recreational, rehabilitation, computer training and professional training services. Low vision aids and appliance available through low vision clinic by appointment.

7073   Truman Medical Center Low Vision Rehabilitation Program
Eye Foundation of Kansas City
2300 Holmes St.
Kansas City, MO   64108
816-404-1780
Fax: 816-404-1786

Nelson R. Sabates, M.D., Chairman
Monika Malecha, MD, Residency Program Director
Abraham Poulose, MD, Director of Clinics
Our program is designed to maximize daily tasks for a person with low vision. We are able to evaluate a person's home and provide recommendations as needed.

7074   Truman Neurological Center
12404 E. US 40 Highway
Independence, MO   64055-1354
816-373-5060
Fax: 816-373-5787
tnccommunity.com

James Landrum, Executive Director
Ann Johnson, Finance Director
Terri Boyce, Office Assistant
Mary Beth Johnson, Compliance Director
A licensed habilitation center established for the purpose of assisting persons with developmental disabilities and/or mental retardation. The minimum age is 18. Residential care is provided in four group homes in the community licensed by the DMH and CARF accredited.

Montana

7075   Benefis Healthcare
1101 26th St S
Great Falls, MT   59405-5104
406-455-5000
Fax: 406-455-2110
benefis@benefis.org
www.benefis.org

John Goodnow, CEO
Laura Goldhahn-Konen, President
Forrest Ehlinger, Chief Financial & Treasury Officer
Paul Dolan, MD, Chief Medical Information Officer
Benefis Healthcare is a not-for-profit community asses governed by a 15-member local board of directors. Benefis is locally owned and controlled. Benefis is a Level II trauma center- one of only 4 in the state and 107 in the country.

7076 Disability Services Division of Montana
Department of Public Health
Helena, MT 59604
406-444-7734
Fax: 406-444-3465

Keith Messmer, Manager
Sandi Gory, Administrative Assistant
Janice Frisch, Chief Management Operations
Responsible for coordinating, developing and implementing comprehensive programs to assist Montanans with disabilities with activities of daily living, community base services and coordinated programs of habilitation, rehabilitation and independent living.

Nebraska

7077 Las Vegas Healthcare And Rehabilitation Center
680 South Fourth Street
Louisville, KY 40202
502-596-7300
TTY:800-545-0749
web_administrator@kindredhealthcare.com
kindredhealthcare.com
Paul J. Diaz, President/ CEO
Accomodates 79 residents. Serving the community for approximately 40 years. Located in close proximity to local hospitals and surrounded by medical complexes, out center offers both short-term rehabilitation and long term.care.

7078 Sierra Pain Institute
265 Golden Ln
Reno, NV 89502-1205
775-323-7092
Fax: 775-323-5259

Lyle Smith, Owner
The program consists of a medically supervised outpatient program managed by an interdisciplinary team with input from specialties of Pain Medicine, Physical Therapy and Occupational Science. The format insures that each patient receives the full range of behavioral techniques in a well-integrated, individually tailored therapeutic regimen.

New Hampshire

7079 Department of Physical Medicine and Rehabilitation
Exeter Hospital
5 Alumni Dr
Exeter, NH 03833-2128
603-778-7311
Fax: 603-580-6592
www.exeterhospital.com

Kevin Calahan, President
Offers patient treatment, committed to enhancing the lives of individuals with short and long term physically disabling conditions.

7080 Farnum Rehabilitation Center
580 Court St
Keene, NH 03431-1718
603-354-6630
Fax: 603-355-2078

Susan Loughrey, Program Director
Judy Bell, Manager
Offers rehabilitation services, occupational therapy, physical therapy and more for the physically challenged individual.

7081 Hackett Hill Nursing Center and Integrated Care
191 Hackett Hill Rd
Manchester, NH 03102-8993
603-668-8161
Fax: 603-622-2584

Daniele Peckham, Administrator
Brett Lennerton, Administrator
A 68-bed certified nursing home.Postacute rehabilitation program.

7082 Mental Health Center: Riverside Courtyard, The
3 Twelfth St
Berlin, NH 03570-3860
603-752-7404
Fax: 603-752-5194

Eileen Theriault, Manager
A center to help people that have mental disabilities.

7083 New Hampshire Rehabilitation and Sports Medicine
Catholic Medical Center
Ste 201
769 S Main St
Manchester, NH 03102-5166
603-647-1899
800-437-9666
Fax: 603-668-5348

Stuart Draper, Owner
Victor Carbone, Manager
A specialized facility for comprehensive rehabilitation for individuals who have been injured or have a disability.

7084 New Medico, Highwatch Rehabilitation Center
Highwatch Rd
Center Ossipee, NH 03814
Fax: 603-539-8888
William Burke, Executive Director
Post-acute rehabilitation service.

7085 Northern New Hampshire Mental Health and Developmental Services
87 Washington St
Conway, NH 03818-6044
603-447-3347
Fax: 603-447-8893
www.northernhs.org

Dennis Mackay, CEO
Provides mental health and developmental services to northern New Hampshire, including early intervention, elderly services, residential program, outpatient services, employee assistance programs, inpatient services, etc.

New Jersey

7086 All Garden State Physical Therapy
44 Ridge Road
North Arlington, NJ 07031
201-998-6300
Fax: 201-998-6344

7087 Bancroft
425 Kings Highway East
PO Box 20
Haddonfield, NJ 08033- 1284
856-429-0010
800-774-5516
Fax: 856-429-1613
TTY: 856-428-2697
inquiry@bancroft.org
www.bancroft.org

Cynthia Boyer, PhD, Executive Director, Brain Injury Services
Toni Pergolin, President and Chief Executive
Clair Rohrer, Med, Executive Director, Programs for Adults
Dennis . Morgan, M.Ed, Executive Director of Bancroft Special Education Programs
Private, not-for-profit organization serving people with disabilities since 1883. Based in Haddonfield, New Jersey, help more than 1000 children and adults with autism, developmental disabilities, brain injuries, and other neurological impairments. Operates more than 140 sites throughout the U.S. and abroad.

7088 Daughters of Miriam Center/The Gallen Institute
155 Hazel St
Clifton, NJ 07011-3423
973-772-3700
Fax: 973-253-5389
administration@daughtersofmiriamcenter.org
www.daughtersofmiriamcenter.o rg
Fred Feinstein, Executive Director
Dedicated to providing the highest quality care, the Center has far exceeded a stereotypical nursing home by offering a continuum of care environment, making us a leader in Jewish eldercare.

7089 Devereux Advanced Behavioral Health New Jersey
Devereux New Jersey
286 Mantua Grove Rd.
Building 4
West Deptford, NJ   08066   856-599-6400
                                        Fax: 856-423-8916
                                        drenner@devereux.org
                                        www.devereuxnj.org

Brian Hancock, Executive Director
Christine DiGiampaolo, Human Resources Department
Kelly McGhee, Quality Improvement Department
Donna Marie Renner, Development & External Affairs Department
Serves people of all ages who have special needs. Individuals
with emotional, behavioral, and developmental disabilities are
offered services such as community-based homes and apartments, vocational training programs, family care homes, and consulting services. Devereux New Jersey also has a
residential/educational center for individuals with autism.

7090 Ladacain Network
Schroth School & Technical Education Center
1701 Kneeley Blvd
Wanamassa, NJ   07712-7622   732-493-5900
                                        Fax: 732-493-5980
                                        ladacin.org

Patricia Carlesimo, Executive Director
Provides an array of services and programs specifically for children and adults with developmental and physical disabilities.
Services include approved Department of Education school programs; adult education and training; vocational training, personal care assistance services, in-home and Saturday respite;
child care programs, housing opportunities, and more.

7091 Lourdes Regional Rehabilitation Center
Our Lady of Lourdes Medical Center
1600 Haddon Ave
Camden, NJ   08103-3101   856-757-3864
                                            856-757-3500
                                        Fax: 856-968-2511
                                        info@lourdesnet.org
                                        www.lourdesnet.org

Alexander J. Hatala, President
Kimberly D. Barnes, Vice President, Planning and Development
Michael Hammond, Chief Financial Officer
Maureen Hetu, Chief Information Officer
The only comprehensive rehabilitation facility located within an
acute care hospital in Southern New Jersey. Patients benefit from
the proximity to the full range of state of the art medical and surgi-
cal services should the need arise.

7092 Mt. Carmel Guild
1160 Raymond Blvd
Newark, NJ   07102-4168   973-596-4100
                                        Fax: 973-639-6583

Anita Holland, Manager
Offers services for the totally blind, legally blind, visually impaired, mentally retarded blind and more with health, counseling,
educational, recreational, rehabilitation, computer training and
professional training services.

7093 Pediatric Rehabilitation Department, JFK Medical Center
65 James St
Edison, NJ   08818-3947   732-321-7362
                                            732-321-7000
                                        Fax: 732-548-7751
                                        www.jfkmc.org

Michael A. Kleiman, DMD, Chair
Douglas A. Nordstrom, Vice Chair
John L. Kolaya, PE, Secretary
Leonard Sendelsky, Treasurer
Comprehensive interdisciplinary, family focused outpatient pe-
diatric rehabilitation services including evaluation and individ-
ual and group treatment programs for children birth-21.

**7094 REACH Rehabilitation Program: Leader Nursing and
Rehabilitation Center**
550 Jessup Rd
West Deptford, NJ   08066-1921   856-848-9551
Karen Fattore, Case Manager
Anthony Stenson, Administrator
Postacute rehabilitation program.

7095 REACH Rehabilitation and Catastrophic Long-Term Care
1180 Us Highway 22
Mountainside, NJ   07092-2810   908-654-0020
                                        Fax: 908-654-8661

Allen Swanson, Manager
Archie Ordana, Manager
Postacute rehabilitation program.

7096 Rehabilitation Specialists
18-01 Pollitt Drive
Ste 1A
Fair Lawn, NJ   07410-2815   201-478-4200
                                            800-441-7488
                                        Fax: 201-478-4201
                                        program@rehab-specialists.com
                                        www.rehab-specialists.com

Virgilio Caraballo, President/CEO
Dustin Gordon, Director of Neuropsychological and Clinical Ser-
vices
Dr. Brian Greenwald, Medical Director
Cindy Dittfield, Director of Marketing & Public Relations
Rehabilitation Specialists, founded in 1983, is a quality, cost effective community re-entry center treating individuals with acquired brain injury. A non clinical environment based in the
community is utilized that offers professional services enabling
participants to learn skills they need to return to a productive life.
Both our Day and Residential programming emphases focus on
Functional Life Skills, Work Skills and Learning Skills. Each
participant's program is tailored to meet their needs.

7097 Somerset Valley Rehabilitation and Nursing Center
Care-One
11300 Cornell Park Drive
Suite 360
Cincinnati, OH   45242   513-469-7222
                                        Fax: 513-469-7230
                                        info@healthbridge.org
Trudi Matthews, Director of Policy and Public Re
Subacute rehabilitation program, long term care, respite care.

7098 Summit Ridge Center
101 East State Street
Kennett Square, PA   19348   973-736-2000
                                        Fax: 973-736-2764
                                        genesishcc.com

New Mexico

7099 SJR Rehabilitation Hospital
525 S Schwartz Ave
Farmington, NM   87401-5955   505-609-2625
                                        Fax: 505-327-6562
                                        eniemand@sjrmc.net
                                        www.sjrrh.com

Ena M Niemand, Executive Director
Sue Clay, Program Director
Jill Morgan, Nursing Director
Uses a team of professionals to provide a comprehensive rehabilitation program. Accomplishing the best possible physical and
cognitive improvement is the aim of the following treatment
members: nurses, physical therapists, physicians, speech and occupational therapists, therapeutic recreation specialist. Providing inpatient and out patient services.

7100 Southwest Communication Resource
P.O.Box 788
Bernalillo, NM 87004-788
505-867-3396
Fax: 505-867-3398
info@abrazosnm.org
swcr.org

New York

7101 Aspire of Western New York
2356 N Forest Rd
Getzville, NY 14068-1224
716-838-0047
Fax: 716-894-8257
info@aspirewny.org
aspirewny.org

Thomas A. Sy, Executive Director
Janet Hansen, Chief Operating Officer
Mary Anne Coombe, V.P. of Service Coordination & Fiscal Management Services
Helen Trowbridge Hanes, Vice President of Community Living
Provides comprehensive services to individuals with disabilities from infancy through adulthood. Also serves people with all types of developmental disabilities as well as providing clinical services to persons with other types of disabilities such as: spinal cord injury, head trauma and others. Aspire employs 1500 people.

7102 Bronx Continuing Treatment Day Program
1527 Southern Blvd
Bronx, NY 10460-5619
718-893-1414
Fax: 718-893-0707

Mary Jane Purcell, Manager
Post-acute rehabilitation program.

7103 Brooklyn Bureau of Community Service
285 Schermerhorn St
Brooklyn, NY 11217-1098
718-310-5600
Fax: 718-855-1517
info@WeAreBCS.org
www.wearebcs.org

Marla Simpson, Executive Director
Anthony B. Edwards, MBA, CCF, MFM, CFO
Janelle Farris, Chief Operating Officer
Sonya Shields, Chief Officer for External Relations and Advancement
Offers independent living skills, counseling, work readiness, vocational trianing, job placement and job follow-up services to individuals with disabilities (to include individuals with psychiatric, physical, and developmental disabilities). Special programs to move disabled welfare recipients from welfare to work. Publishes a bi-annual newsletter.

7104 Buffalo Hearing and Speech Center
50 E North St
Buffalo, NY 14203-1002
716-885-8318
Fax: 716-885-4229
askbhsc.org

Frank J. Polino, Chairman
Dennis J. Szefel, First Vice Chairman
Kenneth J. Wilson, Treasurer
Gerald Chiari, Esq., Secretary
Assists individuals with speech, language and/or hearing impairments to achieve maximum communication potential.

7105 Cora Hoffman Center Day Program
2324 Forest Ave
Staten Island, NY 10303-1506
718-447-8205
Fax: 718-815-2182
Kevin Kenney, Manager
Post-acute rehabilitation program specializing in Cerebral Palsy. Part of the Cerebral Palsey Association of New York State.

7106 Devereux Advanced Behavioral Health New York
Devereux New York
40 Devereux Way
Red Hook, NY 12571
845-758-1899
Fax: 845-758-1817
www.devereuxny.org

John Lopez, Executive Director
Arthur Roberts, Director of Human Resources
Jeffrey Obiekwe, Program Supervisor
Devereux New York provides a wide range of educational, clinical, residential, and community-based programs and services to people of all ages with intellectual disabilities, Autism Spectrum Disorder, and dual diagnoses. Some services include psychotherapy, life skills development, physical therapies, residential programs, case management, self advocacy and more.

7107 Elmhurst Hospital Center
7901 Broadway
Elmhurst, NY 11373-1368
718-334-4000
www.nyc.gov/html/hhc/ehc/html/home/home.shtml
Chris D Constantino, Executive Director
Hospital is comprised of 525 beds and is a Level I Trauma Center, and Emergency Heart Care Stattion and a 911 recieving hospital. It is the premiere health care organization for key areas such as Surgery, Cardiology, Women's health, Pediatrics, Rehabilitation Medicine, Renal and Mental Health Services.

7108 Federation Employment And Guidance Service(F-E-G-S)
315 Hudson St
New York, NY 10013-1086
212-366-8400
Fax: 212-366-8441
info@fegs.org
www.fegs.org

Gail Magaliff, CEO
Ira Machowsky, Executive Vice President
Thomas M. Higgins, CFO
Kristin M. Woodlock, Chief Operating Officer
The largest and most diversified private, not-for-profit health related and human service organization in the United States. With operations in over 258 facilities, residences, and off-site locations, F-E-G-S has served more then 2 million people since its inception.

7109 Flushing Hospital
4500 Parsons Blvd
Flushing, NY 11355-2205
718-670-5000
Fax: 718-670-3082
flushinghospital.org

Robert V. Levine, Executive Vice President and COO
Bruce J. Flanz, President/ CEO
Mounir Doss, Executive Vice President/CFO
Offers services for the totally blind, legally blind, visually impaired, mentally retarded blind and more with health, counseling, educational, recreational, rehabilitation, computer training and professional training services.

7110 Gateway Community Industries Inc.,
1 Amy Kay Pkwy
Kingston, NY 12401-6444
845-331-1261
800-454-9395
Fax: 845-331-4920
info@gatewayindustries.org
gatewayindustries.org

Francoise C. Gunefsky, President/ CEO
Eva Graham, CFO
Ralph Smith, Chief Information Officer
Mary Ann Hildebrandt, Chief Quality and Compliance Officer
Gateway Community Industries, Inc., founded in 1957, is one of the leading independent not-for-profit vocational rehabilitation and training centers for people with mental and/or physical disabilities. The agency provides comprehensive services in vocational evaluation, job training, job placement, vocational work center employment, supported employment, psychiatric rehabilitation, continuing day treatment, and residential habilitation/rehabilitation.

7111 Henkind Eye Institute Division of Montefiore Hospital
111 East 210th Street
Bronx, NY 10467-2404   718-920-4321
                                        www.montefiore.org
Philip O. Ozuah, MD, PhD, Executive Vice President/ COO
Steven M. Safyer, MD, President/ CEO
Joel A. Perlman, Executive Vice President, Chief Financial Officer
Alfredo Cabrera, Senior Vice President & Chief Human Resources Officer
Offers services for the totally blind, legally blind, visually impaired, mentally retarded blind and more with health, counseling, educational, recreational, rehabilitation, computer training and professional training services. Low vision services offered.

7112 Industries for the Blind of New York State
194 Washington Ave
Ste 300
Albany, NY 12210-6314   518-456-8671
                                        800-421-9010
                                        Fax: 518-456-3587
                                        customercare@nyspsp.org
                                        www.abilityone.com
Richard Healey, CEO
Offers services for the totally blind, legally blind, visually impaired, mentally retarded blind and more with health, counseling, educational, recreational, rehabilitation, computer training and professional training services.

7113 Inpatient Pain Rehabilitation Program
550 First Avenue
New York, NY 10016   212-263-7300
                                        Fax: 212-598-6468
                                        www.med.nyu.edu
William Pinter Phd, Administrative Director
The Inpatient Rehabilitation Program, established in 1983 specializes in the treatment of chronic pain. Our inpatient program is one of the oldest and well established pain programs in the country. It is the only interdisciplinary inpatient pain program in the tri-state area and one of only 20 pain programs in the entire US to have CARF accreditation. Upon completion of an extensive evaluation, patients are admitted for an 18-day inpatient stay.

7114 Koicheff Health Care Center
2324 Forest Ave
Staten Island, NY 10303-1506   718-447-0200
                                        Fax: 718-981-1431
Paul Castello, Clinic Director
Post-accute rehabilitation programs.

7115 New York-Presbyterian Hospital
622 W 168th St
New York, NY 10032-3796   212-305-4600
                                        Fax: 212-305-1017
                                        www.nyp.org
Steven J. Corwin, MD, CEO
Robert E. Kelly, MD, President
New York Presbyterian Hospital is internationally recognized for its outstanding comprehensive services. Its medical, surgical, and emergency care services provide each patient with the highest possible level of care. In addition, as part of the Hospital's commitment to the total well-being of each patient, it offers a range of specialized services, as well as special healthcare programs for neighboring communities.

7116 Norman Marcus Pain Institute
30 E 40th St
Ste 1100
New York, NY 10016   212-532-7999
                                        Fax: 212-532-5957
                                        support@nmpi.com
                                        backpainusa.com
Norman J Marcus, Medical Director
We focus on muscles as the cause of most common pains, i.e. back, neck, shoulders, and headaches. We make specific muscle diagnoses and have specific treatments that in many cases will eliminate the need for surgery or relieve the pain. Patients diagnosed with herniated disc, spinal stenosis, rotator cuff tear, impingement syndrome, sciatica, fibromyalgia and headache will generally find relief.

7117 Pain Alleviation Center
Comprehensive Pain Management Associates
125 S Service Rd
Jericho, NY 11753-1038   516-997-7246
                                        Fax: 516-997-7281
                                        www.paincenter.com
Alex Weingarten, Director
Phillip Fyman, Director
Marisa French, Manager
One of the first pain clinics to gain national accreditation from the Commission on Accreditation of Rehabilitation Facilities. This is due largely to a patient-centered program based on the latest research.

7118 Pathfinder Village
3 Chenango Rd
Edmeston, NY 13335-2314   607-965-8377
                                        Fax: 607-965-8655
                                        info@pathfindervillage.org
                                        www.pathfindervillage.org
Paul Landers, CEO
Caprice S. Eckert, Chief Financial Officer
Kelly A. Meyers, Director of Admissions
Paula B. Schaeffer, Director of Enrichment Programs
Pathfinder Village is a warm, friendly community in the rolling hills of Central New York. Here children and adults with Down Syndrome gain independence, build lasting friendships, become partners in the world and take in all that life has to offer.

7119 Pilot Industries: Ellenville
845-331-4300
48 Canal St
Ellenville, NY 12428-1327   845-647-7711
                                        Fax: 845-647-7711
Peter Pierri, Executive Director
Betty Marks, Plant Manager
Post-accute rehabilitation services.

7120 Skills Unlimited
405 Locust Ave
Oakdale, NY 11769-1695   631-567-3320
                                        Fax: 631-567-3285
                                        info@skillsunlimited.org
                                        skillsunlimited.org
Richard Kassnove, Executive Director
Our basic goals is to offer persons with disabilities the opportunity to explore and develop their full vocational potential. Our programs are unique in that by offering comprehensive services, individuals are able to deal with many different issues that could potentially affect their vocational success. Any individual that has an impairment that interferes with their ability to work is entitles to the services that we offer.

North Carolina

7121 Center for Vision Rehabilitation
Academy Eye Associates
3115 Academy Rd
Durham, NC 27707-2652   919-493-7456
                                        800-942-1499
                                        Fax: 919-493-1718
                                        henry.greene@academyeye.com
                                        academyeye.com
Henry A Greene, Owner
Vision rehabilitation and low-vision care for the visually impaired, post-stroke, head trauma and for neuro-oncology vision complications.

7122 Diversified Opportunities
1010 Herring Ave E
Wilson, NC 27893-3311 252-291-0378
Fax: 252-291-1402
www.diversifiedopportunitiesinc.com
Cindy Dixon, Executive Director
Carlton Goff, Business Manager
Ericka Simmons, QP Program Manager
Ken Jones, Chairman
Vocational rehabilitation agency, better outcomes, lower cost, guaranteed performance standards.

7123 Forsyth Medical Center
3333 Silas Creek Pkwy
Winston Salem, NC 27103-3090 336-718-5000
Fax: 336-718-9250
www.novanthealth.org
Jeffrey T. Lindsay, President
Denise Mihal, Chief Operating Officer
Stephen J. Motew, MD, Senior Vice President
Bruce D. Walley, MD, Senior Vice President
Provides care that is state-of-the-art and second to none, both because of advanced treatments availiable through our clinical research and technology to the academic excellence-and caring nature-of our doctors and nurses.

7124 Industries of the Blind
914-920 W Lee St
Greensboro, NC 27403-2803 336-274-1591
800-909-7086
Fax: 336-544-3739
customerservice@iob-gso.com
industriesoftheblind.com
David Thompson, Chairperson
Scott Thornhill, 1st Vice Chairperson
Ashley S. James, Jr., 2nd Vice Chairperson
Chi Anyansi-Archibong, Secretary
Offers services for the totally blind, legally blind, visually impaired, mentally retarded blind and more with health, counseling, educational, recreational, rehabilitation, computer training and professional training services.

7125 Johnston County Industries
1100 East Preston Street
Selma, NC 27576-3162 919-743-8700
Fax: 919-965-8023
jcindustries.com
John Shallcross, Jr., President
Durwood Woodall, Vice President
Lina Sanders-Johnson, Secretary/Treasurer
JCI is an entrepreneurial not-for-profit corporation dedicated to empowering people with disabilities or disadvantages to succeed through training and employment

7126 Learning Services: Carolina
707 Morehead Ave
Durham, NC 27707-1319 919-688-4444
888-419-9955
Fax: 919-419-9966
learningservices.com
Debra Braunling-McMorrow, President and CEO
Jeanne Mack, Chief Financial Officer and Vice President of Operations
Michael Weaver, Chief Development Officer
Terri Dorman, V.P. of Customer Service and Care Management
Located in an historic neighborhood in the heart of Durham, this campus-style setting offers easy access to resources at 3 outstanding facilities: Duke University, The University of North Carolina at Chapel Hill, and Research Triangle Park. This program provides a range of services and activities that draw upon the many resources availiable in the community.

7127 LifeSpan
200 Clanton Road
Charlotte, NC 28217 704-944-5100
lifespanservices.org
Davan Cloninger, President & CEO
Ralph Adams, Treasurer & CFO
Christopher White, Vice President of Operations & Business Development
Lori Avery, Senior Development Director
Provide vocational and enrichment program for adults with developmental disabilities.

7128 Lions Club Industries for the Blind
4500 Emperor Blvd.
Durham, NC 27703 919-596-8277
800-526-1562
Fax: 919-598-1179
inquire@buylci.com
Bill Hudson, President
Offers services for the totally blind, legally blind, visually impaired, mentally retarded blind and more with health, counseling, educational, recreational, rehabilitation, computer training and professional training services.

7129 Lions Services Inc.
5 Penn Plaza
New York, NY 10001 21 -62 -210
lsisale@aol.com
Jimmy R Cranford, President
Jimmy Cranford, President
Offers services for the totally blind, legally blind, visually impaired, mentally retarded blind and more with health, counseling, educational, recreational, rehabilitation, computer training and professional training services.

7130 Regional Rehabilitation Center Pitt County Memorial Hospital
2100 Stantonsburg Rd
Greenville, NC 27834-2818 252-847-4448
Fax: 252-816-7552
mdixon@pcmh.com
Martha M Dixon, VP General Services
An accredited, comprehensive rehabilitation center-part of a statewide network- and we're the largest such facility in eastern North Carolina. Our service area covers 29 counties, and we offer a complete array of rehabilitation services for patients of all ages. Because the Regional Rehabilitation Center is associated with both Pitt County Memorial Hospital And the Brody School of Medicine at East Carolina University, patients have access to a full range of state of the art medical services.

7131 Rehab Home Care
2660 Yonkers Rd
Raleigh, NC 27604-3384 800-447-8692
Fax: 919-831-2211
Alan Silver, CEO
Janis Hansen, Chief Operating Officer
A Medicare/Medicaid certified, state-licensed home health agency with emphasis on rehabilitation.

7132 Thoms Rehabilitation Hospital
Thoms Rehabilitation Hospital
68 Sweeten Creek Rd
Asheville, NC 28803-2318 828-277-4800
Fax: 828-277-4812
TTY:800-735-2962
www.carepartners.org
Tracy Buchanan, President & CEO
Gary Bowers, COO
Freestanding physical rehabilitation hospital, founded 1938 - 100 beds, including 90 acute and 10 transitional - JCAHO accredited.

7133 Winston-Salem Industries for the Blind
7730 N Point Blvd
Winston Salem, NC 27106-3310
336-759-0551
800-242-7726
Fax: 336-759-0990
info@wsifb.com
www.wsifb.com

Mike Faircloth, Chairman
Karen Carey, Vice Chairman, Secretary
W. Robert Newell, Treasurer
David Horton, Executive Director
Offers services for the totally blind, legally blind, visually impaired, mentally retarded blind and more with health, counseling, educational, recreational, rehabilitation, computer training and professional training services.

Ohio

7134 Bellefaire Jewish Children's Bureau
22001 Fairmount Blvd
Cleveland, OH 44118-4819
216-932-2800
800-879-2522
Fax: 216-932-6704
info@bellefairejcb.org
www.bellefairejcb.org

Adam Jacobs, CEO
Adam G. Jacobs PhD, Executive Vice President
Residential treatment for ages 12 to 17 1/2 at time of admission offering individualized psychotherapy, special education, and group living for severaly emotionally disturbed children and adolescents. Also offers a variety of other programs including specialized and therapuetic foster care, partial hospitalization, outpatient counseling, home-based intensive counseling and adoption services.

7135 Christ Hospital Rehabilitation Unit
2139 Auburn Ave
Cincinnati, OH 45219-2906
513-585-2737
Fax: 513-585-4353
www.thechristhospital.com

Mike Keating, President and CEO
Chris Bergman, Vice President and Chief Financial Officer
Berc Gawne, MD, Vice President and Chief Medical Officer
Peter Greis, Vice President and Chief Information Officer
Patients of this 555-bed, not-for-profit acute care facility receive personalized health care provided by trained specialists using the most sophisticated medical technology available, including state-of-the-art intensive care units, surgical facilities, cardiac catheterization labs, three new electrophysiology labs, and the tristates first positron emission tomography (PET) scanning capabilities.

7136 Cleveland Society for the Blind
Cleveland Sight Center
P.O.Box 1988
1909 East 101st Street
Cleveland, OH 44106-8696
216-791-8118
Fax: 216-696-2582
jcarey@clevelandsightcenter.org
www.clevelandsightcenter.org

William L. Spring, Chair
Thomas J. Gibbons, Vice Chair
Gary W. Poth, Treasurer
Sheryl King Benford, Secretary
Social, rehabilitation, education and support services for blind and visually impaired children and adults, early intervention program for children birth to age 6, low vision clinic, aid and appliance shop, Braille and taping transcription, training for rehabilitation, orientation, mobility and computer access, employment services and job placement, recreation program, resident camping, talking books, radio reading services, food service training and snack bar employment. Free screening.

7137 Columbus Speech and Hearing Center
510 E North Broadway St
Columbus, OH 43214-4114
614-263-5151
Fax: 614-263-5365
columbusspeech.org

Dawn Gleason, Au.D., President/ CEO
Karen Deeter, Director of Operations
Serves persons who have speech-language and hearing challenges. Provides vocational rehabilitation services for individuals who are deaf, hard-of-hearing or deaf-blind.

7138 CommuniCare of Clifton Nursing and Rehabilitation Center
Communi Care Health Services
4700 Ashwood Drive
Cincinnati, OH 45241
513-489-7100
Fax: 513-281-2559
communicarehealth.com

Stephen L. Rosedale, Founder/ CEO
A long term care facility which specializes in rehabilitation. Offers a full range of rehabilitative services including physical therapy, occupational therapy and speech therapy.

7139 Doctors Hospital
5100 W Broad St
Columbus, OH 43228-1672
614-544-1000
800-837-7555
Fax: 614-544-1844
www.ohiohealth.com/homedoctors

David Blom, President/ CEO
Michael Bernstein, Senior Vice President and Chief
We believe our first responsibility is to the patients we serve. We respect the physical, emotional and spiritual needs of our patients and find that compassion is essential to fostering healing and wholeness.

7140 Dodd Hall at the Ohio State University Hospitals
410 W 10th Ave
Columbus, OH 43210-1240
614-293-3300
800-293-5123
OSUCareConnection@osumc.edu
www.medicalcenter.osu.edu

Steven G. Gabbe, MD, Senior Vice President / CEO
Larry Anstine, CEO
Gail Marsh, Chief Strategy Officer
Phyllis Teater, Chief Information Officer
Dodd Hall is a full service medical rehabilitation hospital offering comprehensive inpatient and outpatient rehabilitation.

7141 Easter Seal Society of Mahoning
National Easter Seals Chicago
299 Edwards Street
Youngstown, OH 44502-1599
330-743-1168
800-221-6827
Fax: 330-743-1616
www.easterseals.com/mtc

7142 Four Oaks Center
245 N. Valley Road
Xenia, OH 45385-2605
937-562-6500
Fax: 937-562-6520
www.greenedd.org

Todd McManus, President
Jill A. LaRock, Director
Dr. Vijay Gupta, Vice President
Melinda Mays, Recording Secretary
Starts children on the road to discovery by providing a learning environment rich in opportunities and encouragement. The program was designed to give children with delays or disabilities, or those at-risk the extra help needed to develop fully. Any child under the age of six who exhibits developmental delays, handicapping conditions, or is considered at risk may qualify to participate.

7143 Genesis Healthcare System
Rehabilitation Services
800 Forest Ave
Zanesville, OH 43701-2881
740-454-5000
800-322-4762
Fax: 740-455-7527
llynn@genesishcs.org
www.genesishcs.org

Matt Perry, President/ CEO
Paul Masterson, CFO
Richard Helsper, COO
A CARF and JACHO accredited 19-bed rehabilitation facility located within Genesis Healthcare System, a 732 bed, non-profit hospital system, located in Zanesville, Ohio. Freestanding outpatient services, including work hardening, pain management, vocational services, audiology, lymphedema, vestibular rehab, off-the-road driving evals, aquatic therpay, womens health and sports enhancement.

7144 George A Martin Center
3603 Washington Ave
Cincinnati, OH 45229-2009
513-221-1017
Fax: 513-221-3817

Karen Doggett, Executive Director
Offers services for the totally blind, legally blind, visually impaired, mentally retarded blind and more with health, counseling, educational, recreational, rehabilitation, computer training and professional training services.

7145 Grady Memorial Hospital
561 W Central Ave
Delaware, OH 43015-1489
740-615-1000
800-487-1115
Fax: 740-368-5114
ohiohealth.com

Bruce Hagen, Regional Executive and President
As a progressive healthcare leader, Grady Memorial Hospital is committed to excellence while providing the Deleware community with comprehensive quality service delivered with compassionate, personal care. Our membership in Ohio's largest healthcare system, Ohio Health, enables us to improve access to a broader range of healthcare services, enhance development of new programs and services, and provide a complete continuum of care for patients in the deleware area.

7146 Hamilton Adult Center
3400 Symmes Rd
Hamilton, OH 45015-1359
513-867-5970
Fax: 513-874-2977

Donald Musnuff, Executive Director

7147 Holzer Clinic
100 Jackson Pike
Gallipolis, OH 45631-1560
740-446-5000
Fax: 740-446-5532
info@holzer.org
www.holzer.org

T. Wayne Munro, MD, CEO
Brent A. Saunders, Chair
Christopher Meyer, Chief Medical Officer
John Cunningham, Chief Administrative Officer
Serves medical needs of patients in an 8 county area, including counties in Ohio and West Virginia.

7148 Holzer Clinic Sycamore
Holzer Medical Center
4th Avenue & Sycamore St
Gallipolis, OH 45631-1560
740-446-5244
Fax: 740-446-5448
info@holzer.org
www.holzer.org

T. Wayne Munro, MD, CEO
Brent A. Saunders, Chair
Christopher Meyer, Chief Medical Officer
John Cunningham, Chief Administrative Officer
Offers an individualized quality comprehensive rehabilitation program for people with disabilities by an interdisciplinary team including physical therapy, occupational, speech, nursing and social services to restore the patient to the highest degree of rehab outcomes attainable.

7149 IKRON Institute for Rehabilitative and Psychological Services
2347 Vine St
Cincinnati, OH 45213-1745
513-621-1117
Fax: 513-621-2350
ikron@ikron.org
ikron.org

Randy Strunk, MA, LPCC-S, Executive Director
Ken Carbonell, BBA, Fiscal Director
Melissa Harmeling, MA, PCC-S, Program Director
Jake Striker, President
An accredited mental health facility and a certified rehabilitation center. Through a variety of creative treatment and rehabilitation services, IKRON assists adults with mental health and/or substance abuse problems to attain greater independence, to lead lives of sobriety, to obtain competitive work and live more satisfying lives. IKRON places a strong emphasis on respect and support for persons with problems of adjustment. Special contracts to persons desiring job placement.

7150 Integrated Health Services at Waterford Commons
955 Garden Lake Pkwy
Toledo, OH 43614-2777
419-382-2200
Fax: 419-381-8508

Nicole Giesige, Executive Director
A subacute and rehabilitation program specializing in ventilator weaning and management, I.V. therapeutics and pain management, wound management and subacute rehabilitation.

7151 Lester H Higgins Adult Center
3041 Cleveland Ave SW
Canton, OH 44707-3625
330-484-4814
Fax: 330-484-9416
http://www.theworkshopsinc.com/
Margalie Belazaire, Manager
Ed Allar, Manager
Post-accute rehabilitation service

7152 Live Oaks Career Development Campus
5936 Buckwheat Rd
Milford, OH 45150
513-575-1906
Fax: 513-575-0805

Harold Carr MD, Superintendent
Robin White, President/CEO
Jim Dixon, Principal
Post-accute rehabilitation facility and services.

7153 Metro Health: St. Luke's Medical Center Pain Management Program
2500 Metrohealth Dr
Cleveland, OH 44109-1900
216-778-7800
www.metrohealth.org

Mark Moran, President
CARF accredited comprehensive multidisciplinary pain management program.

7154 MetroHealth Medical Center
2500 Metrohealth Dr
Cleveland, OH 44109-1900
216-778-7800
www.metrohealth.org

Mark Moran, President
Located on the near west side of Cleveland, is a leader in trauma, emergency, and critical care; women's and childrens's services, including high risk obstetrical care and neonatal intensive care; comprehensive medical and surgical subspecialties.

7155 Middletown Regional Hospital: Inpatient Rehabilitation Unit
105 McKnight Dr
Middletown, OH 45044-4838 513-422-1401
800-338-4057
Fax: 513-422-1520
www.middletownhospital.org
C N Reddy, Owner
Douglas McNeill, Chief Executive Officer
Our mission is to serve and help people, improving the status of their health and the quality of thier lives. Our vision is to be the premier integrated delivery system in Southwest Ohio. Our Values are quality, respect, service and teamwork

7156 Newark Healthcare Center
680 South Fourth Street
Louisville, KY 40202 502-596-7300
TTY:800-545-0749
web_administrator@kindred.com
kindredhealthcare.com
Paul J. Diaz, President/ CEO
Accomodates 300 residents. We are located in the heart of Newark, Ohio. Newark Healthcare is a 2004 recipient of the American Health Care Association's Quality Award.

7157 Parma Community General Hospital Acute Rehabilitation Center
7007 Powers Blvd
Parma, OH 44129-5495 440-743-3000
Fax: 440-843-4387
www.parmahospital.org
David Nedrich, Chairman
Thomas P. O'Donnell, First Vice Chairman
Alex I. Koler, First Assistant Treasurer
Sharon Martin, Assistant Secretary
The mission of this CARF accredited unit is to provide the most comprehensive, cost-effective, acute rehabilitation program possible in order for every patient and family to adjust to his/her disability and to achieve the maximum potential of independent functioning when returning to community living.

7158 Peter A Towne Physical Therapy Center
Ste 10
447 Nilles Rd
Fairfield, OH 45014-2626 513-829-7726
Fax: 513-829-7726
Debbie Wilkerson, Office Manager
Outpatient, private practice physical and occupational therapy. Three other offices in Hamilton, Monroe and West Chester.

7159 Philomatheon Society of the Blind
2701 Tuscarawas St W
Canton, OH 44708-4638 330-453-9157
www.philomatheon.com
David Miller, President
Denise Dessecker, Vice President
Angela Randall, Secretary
Paul Williams, Treasurer
Offers services for the totally blind, legally blind, visually impaired, mentally retarded blind and more with health, counseling, educational, recreational, rehabilitation, computer training and professional training services.

7160 Providence Hospital Work
2270 Banning Rd
Cincinnati, OH 45239-6621 513-591-5600
Fax: 513-591-5604
Kay Brogle, Executive Director
Post-acute rehabilitation services.

7161 Six County, Inc.
2845 Bell St
Zanesville, OH 43701-1794 740-454-9766
800-344-5818
Fax: 740-588-6452
www.sixcounty.org
John A Creek, President
Tim Llewellyn, Senior VP/Community Intervention
Robert Santos, Ex Vp & Coo
Mary Denoble, Vp Qip
Six County, Inc., is a private, not-for-profit corporation under contract with the Mental Health and Recovery Services Board. Six County, Inc., provides comprehensive community mental health services to people of all ages in each of the six Southeastern Ohio counties served: Coshocton, Guernsey, Morgan, Muskingum, Noble, and Perry. SCI's counseling centers provide a full range of services including outpatient counseling; diagnostic assessment, referrals, and psychological testing.

7162 Society for Rehabilitation
9290 Lake Shore Blvd
Mentor, OH 44060-1664 440-352-8993
800-344-3159
Fax: 440-352-6632
info@societyhelps.org
www.societyhelps.org
Richard Kessler, Executive Director
Vision is to provide individuals with comprehensive services to improve their quality of life. Our mission is to meet the needs of individuals and their families by delivering a wide range of affordable accessible and personalized services, providing treatment by a team of highly qualified, caring professionals. Collaborating with other agencies to meet community needs.

7163 Southeast Ohio Sight Center
425 E. Alvarado Street
Suite E
Fallbrook, CA 92028 800-677-4180
www.charityadvantage.com

7164 St. Francis Rehabilitation Hospital
401 N Broadway St
Green Springs, OH 44836-9638 419-639-2626
800-248-2552
Fax: 419-639-6225
Kim Eicher, CEO
Dan Schwanke, Chief Executive Officer
Program offers specialized treatment for patients who have suffered a head injury, spinal cord injury, or stroke, or who have an orthopedic injury. The Head Injury Program provides a continuum of care from coma stimulation through transitional living. Their physicians, nurses, counselors and therapists are dedicated to helping our patients develop the motivation, strength and skills needed to overcome or adapt to their disability.

7165 TAC Enterprises
2160 Old Selma Rd
Springfield, OH 45505-4600 937-525-7400
Fax: 937-525-7401
info@tacind.com
www.tacind.com
Clifford Meyer, CEO
TAC Enterprises provides employment opportunities for individuals to develop marketable skills by completing contract work in partnership with other industries. Work and self-help skills, social adjustment, and a variety of daily living experiences are offered to the workers by our specialized staff.

Oklahoma

7166 Dean A McGee Eye Institute
608 Stanton L Young Blvd
Oklahoma City, OK 73104-5065   405-271-6060
                                                                    800-787-9012
                                                      Fax: 405-271-4442
                                                                    www.mei.org

Gregory L. Skuta, M.D., President/CEO
Matthew D. Brown, Executive Vice President
Lana G. Ivy, Vice President of Development
Kimberly A. Howard, Chief Financial Officer and Vice President of Finance
Offers services for the totally blind, legally blind, visually impaired, mentally retarded blind and more with health, counseling, educational, recreational, rehabilitation, computer training and professional training services.

7167 Jane Phillips Medical Center
Rehab Care
3500 E Frank Phillips Blvd
Bartlesville, OK 74006-2464   918-333-7200
                                                      Fax: 918-333-7801
                                                      webmaster@jpmc.org
                                                                    jpmc.org

David Stire, President/ COO
Mike Moore, Chief Financial Officer/Vice President Fiscal Services
Susan Herron, RN, Vice President Nursing Services
Paul W. McQuillen, MD, Chief Medical Officer
Comprehensive inpatient rehabilitation services are provided to patients with orthopedic, neurologic, and other medical conditions of recent onset or regression, who have experienced a loss of function in activities of daily living, mobility, cognition and communication.

7168 McAlester Regional Health Center RehabCare Unit
1 E Clark Bass Blvd
McAlester, OK 74501-4255   918-426-1800
                                                      Fax: 918-421-6832
                                                      nbrinlee@mrhcok.com
                                                                    www.mrhcok.com

David Keith, President/ CEO
Cara Bland, Chairman
Evans McBride, Vice-Chairman
A 19-bed inpatient physical rehabilitation unit serving the Southeast Oklahoma area. Offers physical therapy, occupational therapy, social work, speech and psychological services in an interdisciplinary framework.

7169 Oklahoma League for the Blind
501 N Douglas Ave
Oklahoma City, OK 73106-5085   405-232-4644
                                                                    888-522-4644
                                                      Fax: 405-236-5438
                                                      info@newviewoklahoma.org
                                                      www.newviewoklahoma.org

Lauren White, President/ CEO
Carol Campbell, Executive Assistant
John Wilson, Chief Financial Officer
Randy Hearn, Chief Operations Officer
Offers services for the blind and visually impaired, counseling, educational, recreational, rehabilitation, computer training and professional training services.

7170 Valley View Regional Hospital-RehabCare Unit
430 N Monte Vista St
Ada, OK 74820-4657   580-332-2323
                                                      Fax: 580-421-1395
W. Kent Rogers, President/ CEO
Comprehensive physical medicine and rehabilitation services designed to help patients in their adjustment to a physically limiting condition.

Oregon

7171 Garten Services
PO Box 13970
Salem, OR 97309   503-581-1984
                                          Fax: 503-581-4497
                                          garten@garten.org
                                                      garten.org

Tim Rocak, CEO
Pamela Best, CFO
Steve Babcock, Mail Services Manager
Stacie Braun, Custodial Services Manager
Garten's mission is to support people with disabilities in their effort to contribute to the community through employment, career, and retirement opportunities. Our actions increase society's awareness of human potential. Garten's vision is to be recognized as an organization positively demonstrating to the community that people with disabilities can be contributing and valued employees of a thriving business.

7172 Legacy Emanuel Rehabilitation Center
2801 N. Gantenbein
Portland, OR 97227-1542   503-413-2200
                                                      Fax: 503-413-1501
                                                      www.legacyhealth.org
Gary Guidetta, Executive Director
Gail Weisgerber, Manager
A non-profit tax-exempt corporation that includes 5 full-service hospitals and a children's hospital. The Legacy system provides an integrated network of healthcare services, including acute and critical care, inpatient and outpatient treatment, community health education and a variety of specialty services.

7173 Oakcrest Care Center
2933 Center St NE
Salem, OR 97301-4527   503-585-5850
                                                      Fax: 503-585-8781

7174 Oakhill-Senior Program
1190 Oakhill Ave SE
Salem, OR 97302-3496   503-364-9086
                                                      Fax: 503-365-2879

Jan Dillon, Senior Services Manager
Garten Senior Services provides an adult day service program to seniors with and without developmental disabilities. The program will provide community opportunities, college classes and a wide variety of leisure activities in group and individual settings.

7175 Pacific Spine and Pain Center
1801 Highway 99 N
Ashland, OR 97520-9152   541-488-2255
                                                                    866-482-5515
                                                      Fax: 541-482-2433

Janel R Guyette, Manager

7176 Vision Northwest
9225 SW Hall Blvd
Portland, OR 97223-6794   503-684-8389
                                                                    800-448-2232
                                                      Fax: 503-684-9359
                                                                    visionnw.com

Evelyn Maizels, Executive Director
Offers services for the totally blind, legally blind, visually impaired, mentally retarded blind and more with health, counseling, educational, recreational, rehabilitation, computer training and professional training services.

7177 Willamette Valley Rehabilitation Center
1853 W Airway Rd
Lebanon, OR 97355-1233   541-258-8121
                                                      Fax: 541-451-1762
                                                                    wvrc.org

Martin Baughman, Executive Director
Provides the best professional vocational services to those adults in the community who, by virtue of their physical or mental limi-

tations, are negatively impacted by their ability to attain or maintain employment.

Pennsylvania

7178 Alpine Nursing and Rehabilitation Center of Hershey
Pennstate
405 Martin Ter
State College, PA   16803-3426   814-865-1710
                                                 Fax: 814-863-9423

Melissa A Hardy, Director
Anna Shuey, Administrative Assistant
Postacute rehabilitation program.

**7179 Beechwood Rehabilitation Services A Community
        Integrated Brain Injury Program**
469 E Maple Ave
Langhorne, PA   19047-1600   215-750-4299
                                                  800-782-3299
                                             Fax: 215-750-4327
                                             beechwoodrehab.com

Thomas Felicetti, President
Services include residential, day treatment and community based support services. Individuals with brain injury are served. The facility is Care Accredited.

7180 Blind & Vision Rehabilitation Services Of Pittsburgh
1800 West St
Homestead, PA   15120-2578   412-368-4400
                                                  800-706-5050
                                             Fax: 412-368-4090
                                             www.bvrspittsburgh.org

Erika M. Arbogast, President
Brian Glass, Director of Information Services and Facilities
Leslie Montgomery, Director of Development and Public Relations
Barbara Peterson, Director of Client Services
Offers services for the totally blind, legally blind, visually impaired, mentally retarded blind and more with health, counseling, educational, recreational, rehabilitation, computer training and professional training services.

7181 Bradford Regional Medical Center
116 Interstate Pkwy
Bradford, PA   16701-1036   814-368-4143
                                             Fax: 814-368-4130
                                             www.brmc.com

Marek Dzionara, Owner
Andrew Lehman, Executive Director
Timothy J. Finan, President and CEO
Offers rehabilitation services to individuals with an alcohol or drug related problem.

7182 Bryn Mawr Rehabilitation Hospital
414 Paoli Pike
Malvern, PA   19355-3311   610-251-5400
                                                  888-734-2241
                                                  888-734-2241
                                             Fax: 610-647-3648
                                             www.mainlinehealth.org

Donna M. Phillips, President
We are dedicated to serving individuals and their families whose lives can be enhanced through physical or cognitive rehabilitation. We continually strive for excellence by providing care and services which are valued by those we serve and by contributing to the community through education, research and prevention of disability.

7183 Devereux Advanced Behavioral Health - National Office
National Headquarters
444 Devereux Dr
Villanova, PA   19085   800-345-1292
                                             devereuxhr@devereux.org
                                             www.devereux.org

Samuel G Coppersmith, Esq, Chairman
Robert Q Kreider, President & CEO
*Marilyn B Benoit, MD, Senior Vice President, Chief Clinical &
Medical Officer*
Carl E Clark, Senior Vice President & Chief Operations Officer
Devereux is a behavioral health organization supporting people with autism, intellectual and developmental disabilities, and specialty mental health needs. Some of the services offered by Devereux include diagnostics, special education, professional training, research and advocacy.

7184 Devereux Pennsylvania
444 Devereux Dr
Villanova, PA   19085   610-788-6565
                                                  800-345-1292
                                             Fax: 610-430-0567
                                             lhender4@devereux.org
                                             www.devereuxpa.org

Carol Oliver, MS, State Director & Vice President of Operations
Melanie Beidler, MS, Executive Director, Intellectual/Developmental Disabilities
Stephen Bruce, M.Ed, BCBA, Executive Director, Adult Services
*Rhea Fernandes, Psy.D., Executive Director, Children's Behavioral
Health Services*
Devereux Pennsylvania provides educational and residential programs, therapeutic foster care, case management, customized employment and community-based behavioral health programs to children and adults with intellectual and behavioral challenges.

7185 Fox Subacute Center
2644 Bristol Rd
Warrington, PA   18976-1404   800-782-2288
James Foulke, CEO
Vic Costenko, COO
Walter Dunsmore, CFO
Fox subacute recognizes the great need for alternative programs for today's medically compromised patients. Fox has developed Models of Care and offers subacute programs fore the management of ventilator-dependent patients. We recognize that the best road to recovery for these patients is an environment with special care in an alternative setting. We believe that setting should be outside the hospital, in facilities where the focus is on the management of individual patients.

7186 Fox Subacute at Clara Burke
251 Stenton Ave
Plymouth Meeting, PA   19462-1220   610-828-2272
                                                  800-424-7201
                                             Fax: 610-828-7939
                                             admissions@foxsubacute.com
                                             www.foxsubacute.com

Terri Herd, Director of Marketing
Amy Swartley, RN,, Director of Admissions
Kathy Palladino, Director of Human Resources
Erik I. Soiferman, DO, FACOI, Chief Medical Officer
Fox Subacute at Clara Burke in Plymouth Meeting, PA offers attentive, nurturing management of ventilator dependent, medically compromised patients in the PA, NJ, DE, Tri-State area. This sixty-bed facility, with its picturesque setting on 16 acres in historic Plymouth Meeting, is ideal for the specialized services and programs offered by Fox. With a team of highly motivated professionals, we offer the discharge alternative to prolonged lengths of stay in more costly acute care settings.

7187 Good Samaritan Health System
4th & Walnut Sts
P.O.Box 1281
Lebanon, PA   17042-1281   717-270-7500
                                             www.gshleb.org

Robin Weiler, Manager
Frederick Davis, VP Clinical Services

Offers services for the totally blind, legally blind, visually impaired, mentally retarded blind and more with health, counseling, educational, recreational, rehabilitation, computer training and professional training services.

7188 Good Samaritan Hospital-Health System Center
Good Samaritan Hospital
4th & Walnut Sts
P.O.Box 1281
Lebanon, PA 17042-1281   717-270-7500
                               www.gshleb.org

June Nafziger-Eberl, Manager
Stuart Hartman, Medical Director
Comprehensive inpatient rehab unit for adults regarding general physical rehabilitation. Specific programs include orthopedic, neurological, stroke, amputee, etc.

7189 Pediatric Center at Plymouth Meeting Integrated Health Services
491 Allendale Rd
King of Prussia, PA 19406-1426   610-265-9290
                                    800-220-7337

Fran Currick, Manager
Subacute programs such as intensive respiratory care, stressing ventilator dependent children, pre and post transplant care, total parenteral nutrition, IV therapy, intensive/behavioral oral feeding programs. Provides extensive discharge planning including teaching or review for all the above programs with an emphasis on development and accessing community resources.

7190 Penn State Milton S. Hershey Medical Center College Of Medicine
500 University Dr
Hershey, PA 17033-2360   717-531-8521
                               800-243-1455
                          Fax: 717-531-4558
                       www.pennstatehershey.org

Harold L Paz, CEO
Alan L. Brechbill, Executive Director
Wayne Zolko, Associate Vice President for Finance and Business
Andrew S. Resnick, Chief Quality Officer
a non-sectarian, not-for-profit community hospital whose purpose is to provide high quality acute, rehabilitative and preventive health services for the entire community, regardless of creed, race, nationality, or ability to pay.

7191 Pennsylvania Pain Rehabilitation Center
Ste 2
252 W Swamp Rd
Doylestown, PA 18901-2465   215-230-9707
                          Fax: 215-348-5106

Kenneth Lefkowitz, Manager
Post acute rehabilitation facility and programs.

7192 Rehabilitation & Nursing Center at Greater Pittsburgh, The
890 Weatherwood Ln
Greensburg, PA 15601-5777   724-837-8076
                          Fax: 724-837-7456
                    www.healthbridgemanagement.com
Nancy Flenner, Administrator
Marsha Echard, Admissions Coordinator
Craig Stepien, Admissions Director
Subacute care, ventilator and pulmonary managment, comprehensive rehabilitation.

Rhode Island

7193 In-Sight
43 Jefferson Blvd
Warwick, RI 02888-6400   401-941-3322
                          Fax: 401-941-3356
                          cbutler@in-sight.org
                               in-sight.org
Chris Butler, Executive Director
Lucille Gaboriault, Director of Community Resources
Paul Hopkins, Director of First Impressions
Richard Andrade, Director of Vision Rehabilitation
Offers services for the totally blind, legally blind, visually impaired, mentally retarded blind and more with health, counseling, educational, recreational, rehabilitation, computer training and professional training services.

7194 Vanderbilt Rehabilitation Center
Newport Hospital
167 Point Street
Providence, RI 02903   401-444-3500
                             www.lifespan.org

Timothy J. Babineau, President/CEO
Kenneth E. Arnold, SVP, General Counsel
Carole M. Cotter, SVP, Chief Information Officer
Cathy Duquette, EVP, Nursing Affairs
The Vanderbilt Rehabilitation Center at Newport Hospital has been providing comprehensive rehabilitation sercices for more than 40 years and is known throughout the region for its unique programs and high-quality, patient focused care.

South Carolina

7195 Association for the Blind
One Carriage Lane
Building A
Charleston, SC 29407   843-723-6915
                          Fax: 843-577-4312
                             www.abvisc.org

J. Douglas Hazelton, President
Capers A. Grimball, Vice President
Lea B. Kerrison, Secretary
Mary Morrison, Executive Director
Offers services for people who are blind, or are visually impaired with health, counseling, educational, recreational, rehabilitation, computer training and professional training services.

7196 Hitchcock Rehabilitation Center
690 Medical Park Dr
Aiken, SC 29801-6348   803-648-8344
                             800-207-6924
                        Fax: 803-648-1631
                  mail@hitchcockhealthcare.org

Karen Bowlen, Administrator
Dan Hillman, Case Manager
Carrie Morgan, Finance Director
Comprehensive outpatient rehabilitation for adults, children, geriatrics, pediatric therapy, special needs preschool, sports medicine, home health and hospice.

7197 Mentor Network, The
3600 Forest Drive
Suite 100
Columbia, SC 29204-1891   803-799-9025
                               800-297-8043
                          Fax: 803-931-8959
                          thementornetwork.com

Edward Murphy, Executive Chairman
Bruce Nardella, President and CEO
Denis Holler, Chief Financial Officer
Jeffrey Cohen, Chief Information Officer
Mentor provides a full network of individually tailored services for people with development disabilities and their families. Individuals may be served in their homes, shared living home, or in a host home.

Tennessee

7198   Humana Hospital: Morristown RehabCare
726 McFarland St
Morristown, TN 37814-3989   423-522-6000
www.lakewayregionalhospital.com
James Perry, Program Director
Designed to help patients in their adjustment to a physically limiting condition by helping to maximize each patient's abilities so he or she can function as independently as possible.

7199   Opportunity East Rehabilitation Services for the Blind
758 W Morris Blvd
Morristown, TN 37813-2136   423-586-3922
800-278-6274
Fax: 423-586-1479
volblind.org

Fred Overbay, CEO
Vic Mende, Director Rehabilitation Services
Offers services for the totally blind, legally blind, visually impaired, mentally retarded blind and more with health, counseling, educational, recreational, rehabilitation, computer training and professional training services.

7200   Patrick Rehab Wellness Center
Lincoln County Health System
106 Medical Center Blvd
Fayetteville, TN 37334-2684   931-433-0273
Fax: 931-433-0378
Gloria Meadows, Administrator
Jim Stewart, Principal
Provides rehabilitation services of physical, occupational, and speech therapy. Also, wellness memberships are available to the public.

7201   PharmaThera
1785 Nonconnah Blvd
Memphis, TN 38132-2104   901-348-8100
800-767-6714
Fax: 901-348-8270

7202   Siskin Hospital For Physical Rehabilitation
1 Siskin Plz
Chattanooga, TN 37403-1306   423-634-1200
info@siskinrehab.org
siskinrehab.org
Bob Main, CEO
Robert P. Main, President
Dedicated exclusively to physical rehabilitation and offers specialized treatment programs in brain injury, amputation, stroke, spinal cord injury, orthopedics, and major multiple trauma. The hospital also provides treatment for neurological disorders and loss of muscle strength and controll following illness or surgery.

7203   St. Mary's RehabCare Center
900 E Oak Hill Ave
Knoxville, TN 37917-4556   865-545-7962
Fax: 865-545-8133
Debbie Keeton, Director
Beth Greco, Executive Director
Provides comprehensive rehabilitation services for patients experiencing CVA, head trauma, orthopedic conditions, spinal cord injury or neurological impairment.

Texas

7204   Alpine Ridge and Brandywood
444 Devereux Drive
Victoria, TX 19085-2666   361-575-8271
800-345-1292
Fax: 361-575-6520
devereux.org

Robert Q. Kreider, President and CEO
Margaret McGill, SVP, Chief Operations Officer
Robert C. Dunne, SVP & Chief Financial Officer, Treasurer
Marilyn B. Benoit, M.D., SVP, Chief Clinical Officer, Chief Medical Officer

7205   Amity Lodge
Devereux Foundation
444 Devereux Drive
Victoria, TX 19085-2666   361-575-8271
800-345-1292
Fax: 361-575-6520
devereux.org

Robert Q. Kreider, President and CEO
Margaret McGill, SVP, Chief Operations Officer
Robert C. Dunne, SVP & Chief Financial Officer, Treasurer
Marilyn B. Benoit, M.D., SVP, Chief Clinical Officer, Chief Medical Officer
Offers residents a continuum of services ranging from minimal care and supervision to total physical and medical care.

7206   Baylor Institute for Rehabilitation
3500 Gaston Avenue
Dallas, TX 75246-2017   214-820-9300
800-4BA-YLOR
Fax: 214-841-2679
www.baylorhealth.com
Joel T. Allison, Chief Executive Officer
Gary Brock, President and Chief Operating Officer
LaVone Arthur, Vice President of Business Development
Wm. Stephen Boyd, Chief Legal Officer
A 92-bed specialty hospital offering comprehensive rehabilitation services for persons with spinal cord injury, traumatic brain injury, stroke, amputation, and other orthopedic and neurological disorders.

7207   Beneto Center
Devereux Foundation
444 Devereux Drive
Victoria, TX 19085-2666   361-575-8271
800-345-1292
Fax: 361-575-6520
devereux.org

Robert Q. Kreider, President and CEO
Margaret McGill, SVP, Chief Operations Officer
Robert C. Dunne, SVP & Chief Financial Officer, Treasurer
Marilyn B. Benoit, M.D., SVP, Chief Clinical Officer, Chief Medical Officer
Offers a continuum of services for residents requiring services ranging from minimal care and supervision to total physical and medical care.

7208   CORE Health Care
E&J Health Care
400 Highway 290
Bldg B, Suite. 205,
Dripping Springs, TX 78620   512-894-0801
866-683-1007
Fax: 512-858-4627
info@corehealth.com
www.corehealth.com

Eric Makowski, CEO
Kristi Jones, Marketing/Admissions Director
Erika Mountz, MBA, OTR/L, Director of Rehabilitation
Annie Freeman, MBA, PHR, Director of Huma Resources
Post acute and transitional rehabilitation, long-term care, community re-entry, for brain injury and complex psychiatric disorders.

7209 Center for Neuro Skills
1320 W Walnut Hill Ln
Irving, TX 75038-3007   972-580-8500
                                       800-544-5448
                              Fax: 972-255-3162
                              srobinson@neuroskills.com
                                       neuroskills.com

John Schultz, Administrator
Mark J. Ashley, President
Centre for Neuro Skills (CNS) seeks to provide medical rehabilitation programs, lifecare programs, advocacy, and research for people with brain injury in order to achieve a maximum quality of life.

7210 Dallas Services
4242 Office Pkwy
Dallas, TX 75204-3629   214-828-9900
                              Fax: 214-828-9901
                                       www.dallasservices.org
Thomas . Turnage, Ph.D, Executive Director
Clark Thomas, Ph.D., Chair
Melissa Malonson, Vice-Chair
Cynthia O'Brien Robinson, Secretary
Offers four programs:1) an early education for children(6weeks-6yrs)with and without special needs.2)low vision clinic-provides low cost eye examsand glasses to low-income families as well as assistance to individuals who vision problems which cannot be corrected with glasses/surgery.3)mesquite day school- an early head start program for infants and toddlers of low-income families.4)special needs advocacy and inclusion program that offers families of special need children guidance and education.

7211 Daman Villa
Devereux Foundation
444 Devereux Drive
Victoria, TX 19085-2666   361-575-8271
                                       800-345-1292
                              Fax: 361-575-6520
                                       devereux.org
Robert Q. Kreider, President and CEO
Margaret McGill, SVP, Chief Operations Officer
Robert C. Dunne, SVP & Chief Financial Officer, Treasurer
Marilyn B. Benoit, M.D., SVP, Chief Clinical Officer, Chief Medical Officer
Offers residents a continuum of services ranging from minimal care and supervision to total physical and medical care.

7212 Devereux Advanced Behavioral Health - Texas Victoria Campus
Texas Victoria Campus
120 David Wade Dr.
P.O. Box 2666
Victoria, TX 77902   361-574-7208
                                       800-383-5000
                              Fax: 361-575-6250
                                       www.devereuxtx.org
Pam Reed, Executive Director
Offering residential services for people of all ages with emotional, behavioral, developmental, and psychiatric disorders. Services include community based living and vocational programs, residential programs and foster care.

7213 Devereux Advanced Behavioral Health Texas - League City Campus
Texas League City Campus
1150 Devereux Dr
League City, TX 77573   281-335-1000
                                       800-373-0011
                              Fax: 281-554-6290
                                       www.devereuxtx.org
Gail Atkinson, Vice President of Operations & Marketing
Offering long-term hospitalization and intensive residential services for adolescents and young adults with emotional, behavioral, developmental and psychiatric disorders.

7214 El Paso Lighthouse for the Blind
200 Washington St
El Paso, TX 79905-3897   915-532-4495
                              Fax: 915-532-6338
                                       www.lighthouse-elpaso.com
Craig Hays, President
Lea Cochran, Vice President
Lola Dawkins, Secretary
Rusty Hooten, Chief Financial Officer
Enables people of all ages to embody blindness and vision impairment through training, rehabilitation, employment opportunity, advocacy and research. Provides access to opportunities and quality of life so that the blind and visually impaired can reach their fullest potential for self-sufficiency and independence.

7215 Harris Methodist Fort Worth/Mabee Rehabilitation Center
612 E. Lamar Boulevard
Arlington, TX 76011-2122   877-847-9355
                              Fax: 817-882-2753
                                       www.texashealth.org
Louise Baldwin, President
Peggyo Ehrlich, Rehab Manager
Karen Mallett, Executive Director
Douglas D. Hawthorne, Chief Executive Officer
A hospital based inpatient rehab program and outpatient day programs in chronic pain management, work hardening and brain injury transitional services.

7216 HealthSouth Hospital of Cypress
13031 Wortham Center Dr
Houston, TX 77065   832-280-2500
                              feedback@healthsouth.com
                                       healthsouthcypress.com
Jerome Lengel, Executive Officer
Dewitt Hilton, Owner
Offers an individualized approach to the process of rehabilitation for severely injured or disabled individuals. The process begins with a pre-admissions assessment of each referred patient. The Center combines state-of-the-art technology and equipment with multi-disciplinary therapy and education in a cheerful, secure environment.

7217 Heights Hospital Rehab Unit
1917 Ashland St
Houston, TX 77008-3994   713-861-6161
                              Fax: 713-802-8660
                                       www.selectmedical.com
Theresa Davis, CEO
Robert A. Ortenzio, Executive Chairman and Co-Founder
Rocco A. Ortenzio, Vice Chairman and Co-Founder
David S. Chernow, President and Chief Executive Officer
This program is designed to assist patients with physical disabilities achieve their maximum functional abilities.

7218 Hillcrest Baptist Medical Center
100 Hillcrest Medical Blvd
Waco, TX 76712   254-202-2000
                              Fax: 254-202-5105
                                       www.sw.org
Anne Hott Kimberly, Program Director
Ann Gammel, Nurse Manager
Debbie Meurer, Manager
Designed to assist patients in adjustment to a physically limiting condition, utilizing interdisciplinary strategies to maximize each patient's ability and capability.

7219 Institute for Rehabilitation & Research
1333 Moursund St
Houston, TX 77030-3405   713-799-5000
                                       800-447-3422
                              Fax: 713-797-5289
                                       tirr.memorialhermann.org
Carl Josehart, CEO
Jean Herzog, President
Gerard E. Francisco, M.D., Chief Medical Officer
Mary Ann Euliarte, CNO/COO

A national center for information, training, research, and technical assistance in independent living. The goal is to extend the body of knowledge in independent living and to improve the utilization of results of research programs and demonstration projects in this field. It has developed a variety of strategies for collecting, synthesizing, and disseminating information related to the field of independent living.

7220   Integrated Health Services of Amarillo
6141 Amarillo Blvd. West
Amarillo, TX   79106   806-356-0488
                                          Fax: 806-356-8074
Mary Bearden, Chairman
Jay L. Barrett, President
Marvin Franz, Executive Director & CEO
Provides acute, post acute, residential and outpatient health care services. IHS of Amarillo is a 153-bed facility with 120 beds licensed by The Texas Department of Health and Human Services, and is accredited by JCAHO. We serve urban and rural populations of over 500,000, drawing from a 5-state region.

7221   Kanner Center
Devereax Foundation
444 Devereux Drive
Victoria, TX   19085-2666   361-575-8271
                                              800-345-1292
                                          Fax: 361-575-6520
                                              devereux.org
Robert Q. Kreider, President and CEO
Margaret McGill, SVP, Chief Operations Officer
Robert C. Dunne, SVP & Chief Financial Officer, Treasurer
Marilyn B. Benoit, M.D., SVP, Chief Clinical Officer, Chief Medical Officer
A private nonprofit nationwide network of treatment services for individuals of all ages with emotional and/or developmental disabilities.

7222   Lighthouse of Houston
3602 W Dallas St
Houston, TX   77019-1704   713-527-9561
                                          Fax: 713-284-8451
                                  custserv@houstonlighthouse.org
                                      houstonlighthouse.org
Gibson DuTerroil, President
Shelagh Moran, VP/COO
Chelean Zander, VP Community Programs
Serves the blind, visually impaired, deaf-blind and multihandicapped blind. Provides workshops, vocational training and placement, low vision clinic, orientation and mobility, housing, Braille, volunteer services, senior center, visual aid sales, counseling and support, diabetic education and day health activity services and day summer camp, Summer Transition for Youth.

7223   Mainland Center Hospital RehabCare Unit
6801 Emmett F Lowry Expy
Texas City, TX   77591-2500   409-938-5000
                                          Fax: 409-938-5501
                                      www.mainlandmedical.com
Michael Ehrat, CEO
The RehabCare program is designed and staffed to assist functionally impaired patients improve to their maximum potential. The opportunities for improvement and adjustments are provided in a pleasant, supportive inpatient environment by therapists from the occupational, physical, recreational and speech therapy disciplines.

7224   North Texas Rehabilitation Center
1005 Midwestern Pkwy
Wichita Falls, TX   76302-2211   940-322-0771
                                          Fax: 940-766-4943
                                              ntrehab.org
Mike Castles, President/ CEO
Provides outpatient rehabilitation services to maximize independence or promote development to children and adults with disabilities. Programs include: physical, occupational, speech therapy, closed head injury, infant/child development, support

groups, aquatics and wellness program and a child achievement program.

7225   South Texas Lighthouse for the Blind
PO BOX 9697
Corpus Christi, TX   78469-3321   361-883-6553
                                              888-255-8011
                                          Fax: 361-883-1041
                                  Customer.service@stlb.net
                                              www.stlb.net
Regis Barber, President
Nicky Ooi, Chief Operations Officer
Alana Manrow, Public Affairs Director
Their mission is to Employ, Educate and Empower their neighbors who are blind and visually impaired. They offer job opportunities in manufacturing, retail and administration, as well as orientation and mobility and adaptive technology training.

7226   Texas Specialty Hospital at Dallas
7955 Harry Hines Blvd
Dallas, TX   75235-3305   214-637-0000
                                          Fax: 214-637-6512
                                  Mary.Alexander@fundltc.com
Mary Alexander, CEO
Cathy Campbell, Chief Executive Officer
66 beds offering active/acute rehabilitation, brain injury day treatment, cognitive rehabilitation, complex care, extended rehabilitation and short term evaluation.

7227   Transitional Learning Center at Gavelston and Lubbock
1528 Post Office St
Galveston, TX   77550   409-762-6661
                                          Fax: 409-763-3930
                                              www.tlcrehab.org
Brent Masel, MD, President and Medical Director
Gary Seale, Ph.D., VP Clinical Programs
Jim Lovelace, MBA, VP of Operations
Shelley Kessler, CPA, Chief Financial Officer
Specializes solely in post-acute brain injury. A nationally known pioneer in the field and a not for profit with a three fold mission: treatment, research and education. Offers 6 hours of therapy a day from licensed/certified staff, on site physician and nursing services and long-term living for brian injured adults at Tideway on Gavelston Island. Accredited by CARF.
1982

7228   Treemont Nursing And Rehabilitation Center
5550 Harvest Hill Rd
Dallas, TX   75230-1684   972-661-1862
                                          Fax: 972-788-1543
Bob Barker, Administrator
Postacute rehabilitation program.

7229   West Texas Lighthouse for the Blind
2001 Austin St
San Angelo, TX   76903-8796   325-653-4231
                                          Fax: 325-657-9367
                          customerservice@lighthousefortheblind.org
                              www.lighthousefortheblind.org
David Wells, Executive Director
Stephen Horton, Operations Manager
Fonda V. Galindo, Finance & Human Resources Manager
Vickie Sanders, Sales & Marketing Manager
Offers services for the totally blind, legally blind, visually impaired, mentally retarded blind and more with health, counseling, educational, recreational, rehabilitation, computer training and professional training services.

Utah

7230   Quincy Rehabilitation Institute of Holy Cross Hospital
1050 E South Temple
Salt Lake City, UT   84102-1507   801-350-8140
                                          Fax: 801-350-4791
Dave Jenson, President

Postacute rehabilitation program.

7231   Wasatch Vision Clinic
849 E 400 S
Salt Lake City, UT   84102-2928   ·   801-328-2020
Fax: 801-363-2201
email@wasatchvision.com
eyeappointment.com

Craig Cutler, Owner
Camron Bateman OD, Doctor
Postacute rehabilitation program.

Vermont

7232   Rutland Mental Health Services
78 S Main St
Rutland, VT   05701-4594   802-775-2381
Fax: 802-775-4020
rmhsccn.org

Dan Quinn, President/ CEO
Scott Dikeman, Vice Chairman
Ron Holm, Secretary
Tom Pour, Treasurer
A private, non-profit comprehensive community mental health center. It provides services to individuals and families for mental health and substance abuse related problems and also to persons who are mentally retarded.

Virginia

7233   Bay Pine-Virginia Beach
680 South Fourth Street
Louisville, KY   40202   502-596-7300
TTY:800-545-0749
web_administrator@kindred.com
kindredhealthcare.com

Paul J. Diaz, President/ CEO
Postacute rehabilitation program.

7234   Carilion Rehabilitation: New River Valley
2013 S Jefferson Street
Roanoke, VA   24014   540-981-7377
Fax: 540-981-8233
www.carilionclinic.org

Nancy Howell Agee, President/ CEO
James A. Hartley, Chair
Briggs W. Andrews, Corporate Secretary
G. Robert Vaughan, Jr., Treasurer, SVP
CARF-accredited pain management program, work hardening program and comprehensive outpatient therapy clinic, massage therapy, outpatient programs and more. Program emphasis is on interdisiplinary behavioral rehab based pain management and functional restoration in conjunction with medical treatment. Work hardening is a transdisciplinary work simulation program taylored to the individual. Comprehensive outpatient program is multi-disciplinary with emphasis on manual treatment.

7235   Faith Mission Home
3540 Mission Home Ln
Free Union, VA   22940-1505   434-985-2294
Fax: 434-985-7633
www.beachyam.org

Paul Beiler, Manager
Reuben Yoder, Director
A Christian residential center that serves 60 mentally retarded children, including individuals with Down Syndrome, Cerebral palsy and other similar conditions. Children may be admitted from the time they are ambulatory until they reach 15 years of age. He or she may stay as long as it is in the child's best interests. The training program stresses the following areas: self-care, social, academic, vocational, crafts, speech and physical development.

7236   ManorCare Health Services-Arlington
333 N. Summit St.
Toledo, OH   43604   800-366-1232
CareLine@hcr-manorcare.com
hcr-manorcare.com

Marcia K Jarrell, Administrator
Ric Birch, Marketing Director
ManorCare-Arlington offers residents a full Continuum of Care in a caring environment. ManorCare's wide range of services includes subacute medical and rehabilitation programs for short term patients transitioning from hospital to home and Skilled Nursing Care.

7237   Pines Residential Treatment Center
825 Crawford Pkwy
Portsmouth, VA   23704-2301   757-393-0061
Fax: 757-393-1029

Lenard J Lexier, Medical Director
Judy Kemp, Admissions Director
A 310-bed residential treatment center in Portsmouth Virginia, providing a therapeutic environment for severely emotionally disturbed children and youth. Five unique programs meet behavioral, educational and emotional needs of males and females, five to twenty-two years of age. Multi-disciplinary teams devise individual service plans to enhance strengths and reverse self-defeating behavior. A highly effective positive reinforcement program with a proven track record.

7238   Roanoke Memorial Hospital
Carilion Health System
2013 S Jefferson Street
Roanoke, VA   24014   540-981-7377
Fax: 540-981-8233
www.carilionclinic.org

Nancy Howell Agee, President/ CEO
James A. Hartley, Chair
Briggs W. Andrews, Corporate Secretary
G. Robert Vaughan, Jr., Treasurer, SVP
Carilion Health System exists to improve the health of the communities it serves. The vision is to assure accessible, affordable, high quality healthcare that meets the needs of the community. Motivate and educate individuals to improve their health. Champion community initiatives to reduce health risk

7239   Southside Virginia Training Center
P.O.Box 4030
Petersburg, VA   23803-30   804-524-7000
Fax: 804-524-7228
www.svtc.dbhds.virginia.gov
Bob Kaufman, Director, Administrative Service
Offers residential, vocational, occupational, physical, and speech therapies.

7240   Woodrow Wilson Rehabilitation Center
P.O.Box 1500
Fishersville, VA   22939-1500   540-332-7000
800-345-9972
Fax: 540-332-7132
www.wwrc.net

Rick Sizemore, Executive Director
Amy Blalock, Admissions and Marketing Director
Comprehensive residential rehabilitation center offering complete medical and vocational rehabilitation services including: vocation evaluation, vocational training, transition from school to work, occupational therapy, physical therapy, speech, language and audiology, assistive technology, rehabilitation engineering, counseling/case management, behavioral health services, nursing and physician services, etc.

Washington

7241 Arden Rehabilitation And Healthcare Center
680 South Fourth Street
Louisville, KY   40202
502-596-7300
TTY:800-545-0749
web_administrator@kindred.com
kindredhealthcare.com
Paul J. Diaz, President/ CEO
Arden can accomodate 90 residents- post-acute/rehabilitation patients as well as long term residents. Medicare certified, the center also takes most managed healthcare insurance plans, as well as VA, respite and hospice patients.

7242 Bellingham Care Center
680 South Fourth Street
Louisville, KY   40202
502-596-7300
TTY:800-545-0749
web_administrator@kindred.com
kindredhealthcare.com
Paul J. Diaz, President/ CEO
Postacute rehabilitation program.

7243 Division of Vocational Rehabilitation Department of Social and Health Services
P.O.Box 45130
Olympia, WA   98504-5130
360-704-3560
800-737-0617
Fax: 360-570-6941
krulik@dshs.wa.gov
www1.dshs.wa.gov/dvr
Patrick Raines, Manager
Lynnea Ruttledge, Manager
Information on computers, supported employment, marketing rehabilitation facilities and transition.

7244 First Hill Care Center
1334 Terry Ave
Seattle, WA   98101
206-682-2661
Fax: 206-624-0188
www.khseattlefirsthill.com

7245 Harborview Medical Center, Low Vision Aid Clinic
Harborview Medical Center
325 9th Ave
Seattle, WA   98104-2499
206-744-3300
TTY:206-744-3246
comment@u.washington.edu
www.uwmedicine.org
Eileen Whalen, Executive director
J. Richard Goss, M.D.,, Medical director
Darcy Jaffe, Chief nursing officer and senior associate for patient care
Elise Chayet, Associate administrator, clinical support services and plan
Harborview Medical Center is the only designated Level 1 adult and pediatric trauma and burn center in the state of Washington and serves as the regional trauma and burn referral center for Alaska, Montana and Idaho. UW Medicine physicians and staff based at Harborview provide highly specialized services for vascular, orthopedics, neurosciences, ophthalmology, behavioral health, HIV/AIDS and complex critical care.

7246 Integrated Health Services of Seattle
820 NW 95th St
Seattle, WA   98117-2207
206-783-7649
Fax: 206-781-1448
Jerry Harvey, Administrator
Marlette Basada, Director Nursing
Flavia Lagrange, Director Admissions
Postacute rehabilitation program. IHS provides 24 hour subacute and long-term care. We can handle vent/trach/hemo andritoneal dialysis and provide a full scope of rehabilitation services.

7247 Lakeside Milam Recovery Centers (LMRC)
3315 S. 23rd Street
Ste 102
Tacoma, WA   98405
253-272-2242
800-231-4303
Fax: 253-272-0171
help@lakesidemilam.com
www.lakesidemilam.com
Michael Kinder, Administrator
LMRC was established in 1983 with a single mission, to help victims and families recover from the pain of drug/alcohol addiction. Enlightned by the work of Dr. James Milam in the 1960's and 70's, the founders of LMRC created a treatment system based on a bedrock set of principals.

7248 Lakewood Health Care Center
11411 Bridgeport Way SW
Lakewood, WA   98499-3047
253-581-9002
800-359-7412
Fax: 253-581-7016
www.lakewoodhc.com
Gwynn Rucker, Executive Director
Patty Wood, Administrator
Linda Doll, Social Services
Dr. Mian , Medical Director
Accomodates 80 residents. We offer 24 hour skilled nursing services, long-term care and rehab services which include Physical, Occupational and Speech Therapy.

7249 Manor Care Health Services-Tacoma
5601 S Orchard St
Tacoma, WA   98409-1371
253-474-8421
Fax: 253-471-8857
www.hcr-manorcare.com
Tina Irwin, Administrator
124-bed skilled nursing and rehabilitation center provides services for those seeking long term Skilled Nursing Care, short term subacute care, hospice services, Alzheimer's and respite care. Our Acadia Wing, a specialized Alzheimer's care unit, provides specialized programming and trained staff that truly makes us the leader in Alzheimers Services.

7250 ManorCare Health Services-Lynnwood
3701 188th St SW
Lynnwood, WA   98037-7626
425-775-9222
Fax: 425-712-3685
www.hcr-manorcare.com
Liza Loyet, Administrator
Our in-house therapists provide physical, occupational and speech therapies in our state-of-the-art therapy gym. Our team is goal oriented and focuses on producing positive outcomes for those recovering from illness, injury or surgery.

7251 ManorCare Health Services-Spokane
6025 N Assembly St
Spokane, WA   99205-7674
509-326-8282
Fax: 509-326-4790
www.hcrmanorcare.com
Cheri Kubu, Administrator
Sandra Hayes, Administrator
Provides skilled nursing and respite stays for those needing a break from care giving. We specialize in Rehabilitation Services provided by our in-house occupational, physical and speech therapists.

7252 Northwest Continuum Care Center
Kindred Health Care
128 Old Beacon Hill Dr
Longview, WA   98632-5859
360-423-4060
Fax: 360-636-0958
Steve M. Ross, Executive Director
Tami Wilson, Director of Nursing
Mary R., Activities Assistant
Kristen W., Health and Rehabilitation Center
Accomodates 69 residents. Employs the Angel Care Program designed to address any special needs that may arise during a resident's stay in our facility. The program focuses extra attention on

residents and, in some cases, family members. The goal is to meet the special needs of the people we provide care to every day.

7253   Park Manor Convalescent Center
1710 Plaza Way
Walla Walla, WA 99362-4362   509-529-4218
                                        Fax: 509-522-1729
                                    egines@ensigngroup.net
                                    www.parkmanorcare.com
Jed Gines, Administrator
Krista Maiuri, Directr Of Nursing
Sonya Taylor, Director of Rehabilitation
Mike Henckel, Admissions & Marketing Director
Residents of Park Manor enjoy a range of activities, developed to meet their needs, including excercise programs, social and recreational activities, arts and crafts, shopping trips and other excursions. We also offer religious services.

7254   Queen Anne Health Care
Queen Anne Health Care
2717 Dexter Ave N
Seattle, WA 98109-1914   206-284-7012
                                        Fax: 206-283-3936
                                    www.queenannehealthcare.com
Heather Eacker, Executive Director
Mary R., Activities Assistant
Kristen W., Health and Rehabilitation Center
Becky D., Activity Director
Our goal is to provide quality, compassionate care. Our cozy building accomodates 120 residents. We offer semi private rooms with space to add items from home for a special personalized touch

7255   Rainier Vista Care Center
920 12th Ave SE
Puyallup, WA 98372-4920   253-841-3422
                                        Fax: 253-848-3937
Linda Larson, Administrator
Nancy L. Erckenbrack, Executive Director
Kristen W., Health and Rehabilitation Center
Becky D., Activity Director
Accomodates 120 residents. We are certified for Medicare and Medicaid and we offer a continuum of healthcare services from short-term or outpatient rehabilitation to long-term care. We offer semi-private and private rooms as well as rehabilitation and hospice suites. Rainier Vista Care Center is a recipient of the American Health Care Association Quality Award.

7256   Rehabilitation Enterprises of Washington
430 E Lauridsen Blvd
Port Angeles, WA 98362-7978   360-452-9789
                                        Fax: 360-452-9700
Brett White, President
REW is the professional trade association representing community rehabilitation programs before government and other publics. These organizations provide a wide array of employment and training services for people with disabilities. The goal is to assist member organizations to provide the highest quality rehabilitative and employment services to their customers.

7257   Seattle Medical and Rehabilitation Center
Evergreen Healthcare
12040 NE 128th St
Kirkland, WA 98034-3013   425-899-3000
                                          877-601-2271
                                      TTY:425-899-2007
                                comment@evergreenhealthcare.org
                                    evergreenhealthcare.org
Al DeYoung, Chair
Robert H. Malte, Chief Executive Officer
Neil Johnson, RN, MSA, Senior Vice President & Chief Operating Officer
Nancee Hofmeister, Vice President, Chief Nursing Officer
103 beds offering subacute rehabilitation, complex care, subacute treatment and short-term evaluation. Pulmonary unit offering long and short term care for ventilator dependent patients.

7258   Slingerland Institute for Literacy
Educators Publishing Service
12729 Northup Way
Suite 1
Bellevue, WA 98005   425-453-1190
                                        Fax: 425-635-7762
                                      mail@slingerland.org
                                      www.slingerland.org
Bonnie Meyer, Executive Director
Elyce Newton, Program Support
A nonprofit public corporation founded in 1977 to carry on the work of Beth H. Slingerland in providing classroom teachers with the techniques, knowledge and understanding necessary for identifying and teaching children with Specific Language Disability. The main objective is to educate teachers in successful methods of identifying, diagnosing and instructing children and adults with SLD and to promote literacy through reading, writing and oral expression.

7259   Timberland Opportunities Association
400 W Curtis St
Aberdeen, WA 98520-7698   360-533-5823
                                        Fax: 360-533-5848
                                      jimeddy@techline.com
Jim Eddy, Executive Director
Provides training and employment for disabled people.

7260   Vancouver Health and Rehabilitation Center
400 E 33rd St
Vancouver, WA 98663-2238   360-696-2561
                                        Fax: 360-696-9275
                                    www.vancouverhealthcare.com
Jody Wigen, Human Resources
Joe Joy, Executive Director
Kristen W., Health and Rehabilitation Center
Becky D., Activity Director
Postacute rehabilitation program.

Wisconsin

7261   Colonial Manor Medical And Rehabilitation Center
1010 E Wausau Ave
Wausau, WI 54403-3101   715-842-2028
                                        Fax: 715-848-0510
                                    www.colonialmanormrc.com
Ericca Ylitalo, Administrator
Shelley Solberg, Executive Director
Colonial Manor Medical and Rehabilitation Center is part of the Kindred Community and is located in Wausau, Wisconsin. The corporate headquarters are based in Louisville Kentucky. Our facility accomodates 150 residents.

7262   Waushers Industries
210 E Chicago Rd
Wautoma, WI 54982-6932   920-787-4696
                                        Fax: 920-787-4698
Richard King, Human Resources
Provides various programming for individuals with disabilities in waushara county.

7263   Woodstock Health and Rehabilitation Center
3415 Sheridan Rd
Kenosha, WI 53140-1924   262-657-6175
                                        Fax: 262-657-5756
Debra Lamb, Administrator
Darlene Einerson, Executive Director
Kristen W., Health and Rehabilitation Center
Becky D., Activity Director
Offers a full range of medical services to meet the individual needs of our residents, including short term rehabilitative services and long-tern skilled care.

Rehabilitation Facilities, Sub-Acute

Alabama

7264 UAB Spain Rehabilitation Center
1717 6th Ave S
Birmingham, AL 35233-7330   205-934-3450
www.uab.edu/medicine/physicalmedicine/
Tracy L Brewer, Administrative Manager
A 49-bed rehabilitation hospital featuring advanced, individualized care for adolescents and adult patients recovering from a
broad variety of health problems. Patient care teams include
physiatrists (doctors who specialized in rehabilitation medicine),
nurses, nurse practitioners, physical therapists, occupational
therapists, speech/language pathologists, psychologists, social
workers, rehabilitation professionals and other health care
professionals from all areas of the UAB Health System.

Alaska

7265 Fairbanks Memorial Hospital & Denali Center
1650 Cowles St
Fairbanks, AK 99701-5998   907-452-8181
Fax: 907-458-5324
www.fmhdc.com
Sheldon Stadnyk, MD, Interim Chief Executive Officer
The Denali Center offers the following rehabilitation services:
Physical Therapy, Occupational Therapy, Speech Therapy,
Sub-Acute Rehab.

Arizona

7266 Desert Life Rehabilitation & Care Center
Kindred Healthcare
1919 W Medical St
Tucson, AZ 85704-1133   520-297-8311
Fax: 520-544-0930
Amad Nazifi, Executive Director
Jane Olmstead, Director of Nursing
Accomodates 240 residents. We provide skilled and intermediate
nursing with occupational, physical, speech and respiratory ther-
apy services. We offer special programs including an Alzhei-
mer's Unit and a Young Adult Program, and are located in
beautiful Southern Arizona where there is plenty of sunshine,
mountains and desert views. Desert Life is a 2005 recipient of the
American Health Care Association Quality Award.

7267 Hacienda Rehabilitation and Care Center
660 S Coronado Dr
Sierra Vista, AZ 85635-3386   520-459-4900
Fax: 520-458-4082
www.haciendarcc.com
Monica Vandivort, Medical Director
Kristen W., Health and Rehabilitation Center Executive Director
Becky D., Activity Director
Mary R., Activities Assistant
Accomodates 100 residents. We are located in Sierra Vista, near
Kartchner Caverns, Fort Huachuca, Coronado National Forest
and historic Tombstone. Serving the medical needs of the com-
munity since 1983, we strive to provide care with quality, com-
passion and integrity.

7268 Kachina Point Health Care & Rehabilitation Center
505 Jacks Canyon Rd
Sedona, AZ 86351-7856   928-284-1000
Fax: 928-284-0626
Michael Amadei, Medical Director
Accomodates 120 residents. We have met the healthcare needs of
the community since 1984. Kachina Point is a 2004 recipient of
the American Health Care Association's Quality Award.

7269 Mayo Clinic Scottsdale
13400 E Shea Blvd
Scottsdale, AZ 85259-5499   480-301-8000
800-446-2279
Fax: 480-301-9310
www.mayoclinic.org/arizona
Neena S. Abraham, Gastroenterology/ Hepatology
Roberta H. Adams, Hematology/Oncology
*Charles H. Adler, Parkinson's Disease and Movement Disorders
Center*
Neera Agarwal, Hospital Internal Medicine
Mayo clinic is a not-for-profit medical practice dedicated to the
diagnosis and treatment of virtually every type of complex illness. Mayo clinic staff members work together to meet your
needs. You will see as many doctors, specialists, and other health
care professionals as needed to provide comprehensive diagnosis, understandable answers and effective treatment.

7270 Sonoran Rehabilitation and Care Center
Kindred
4202 N 20th Ave
Phoenix, AZ 85015-5101   602-264-3824
Fax: 602-279-6234
Jeffrey Barrett, Executive Director
Offers the following rehabilitation services: Respiratory Ther-
apy, Physical Therapy, Speech Therapy, Occupational Therapy,
Restorative Therapy, Sub-Acute Rehabilitation, Wound Care.

7271 Valley Health Care and Rehabilitation Center
Kindred Health Care Center
5545 E Lee St
Tucson, AZ 85712-4205   520-296-2306
Fax: 520-296-4072
Dale Pelton, Executive Director
Sandra Lewis, Administrator
Offers the following rehabilitation services: Physical Therapy,
Occupational Therapy, Speech Therapy, Sub-Acute Rehab.

California

7272 Alamitos-Belmont Rehab Hospital
3901 E 4th St
Long Beach, CA 90814-1699   562-434-8421
Fax: 562-433-6732
www.alamitosbelmont.com
John L. Sorensen, Chairman of the Board of Directors.
Jonathan Sloey, Administrator
Offers the following rehabilitation services: Speech Therapy,
Occupational Therapy, Physical Therapy, Sub-Acute Rehab.

7273 Bay View Nursing and Rehabilitation Center
Kindred Health Care
516 Willow St
Alameda, CA 94501-6132   510-521-5600
Fax: 510-865-9035
www.kindredhealthcare.com
Richard S Espinoza, Administrator
Say Silva, Assistant Executive Director
Accomodates 180 residents. Bay View is a 2004 recipient of the
American Health Care Association's Quality Award. We provide
short-term rehabilitative care, traditional long-term skilled care
and Alzheimer's/dementia special care. Our combination of clin-
ical skill and comprehensive rehabilitation services enables us to
care for a variety of complex medical conditions.

7274 Foothill Nursing and Rehab Center
401 W Ada Ave
Glendora, CA 91741-4241   626-335-9810
Fax: 626-963-0720
www.foothillnursing.com
Arnie Shafer, Executive Director
Marianne Schultz, Administrator
Offers the following rehabilitation services: Physical Therapy,
Occupational Therapy, Speech Therapy, In and Out Patient
Rehab.

7275   Long Beach Memorial Medical Center Memorial Rehabilitation Hospital
2801 Atlantic Ave
Ground Floor
Long Beach, CA 90806-1701   562-933-9001
                                          Fax: 562-933-9019
                                      www.memorialcare.org/long_beach
Barry Arbuckle, President/CEO
The goal of the MemorialCare Rehabilitation Institute is to help persons with disabilities regain independence and rebuild their lives in an environment where loved ones are involved in the rehabilitation process. We are dedicated to the pursuit of our mission, vision and values.

7276   Mercy Medical Center Mt. Shasta
914 Pine St
Mount Shasta, CA 96067-2143   530-926-6111
                                          Fax: 530-926-0517
                                          www.mercymtshasta.org
Greg Lippert, Senior Director of Support and Information Services
Scott Foster, Director of Hospital Finance
Sister Anne Chester, Director of Mission Integration
Joyce Zwanziger, Director Marketing, Community Relations & Volunteer Services
Mercy Medical Center is committed to furthering the healing ministry of Jesus, and to provide high-quality, affordable healthcare to the communities we serve.

7277   Northridge Hospital Medical Center
18300 Roscoe Blvd
Northridge, CA 91328-4167   818-885-8500
                                      www.northridgehospital.org
Michael Wall, CEO
Offers the following rehabilitation services: Physical Therapy, Occupational Therapy, Speech Therapy, Sub-Acute Rehab. As a member of the Catholic Heathcare West Northridge Hospital Medical Center is committed to serving the health needs of our communities with particular attention to the needs of the poor, the disadvantaged and vulnerable, and the comfort of the suffering and dying.

7278   Riverside Community Hospital
4445 Magnolia Ave
Riverside, CA 92501   951-788-3000
                                          Fax: 630-792-5636
                                      complaint@jointcommission.org
                                  www.riversidecommunityhospital.com
Jaime Wesolowski, President/CEO
Patrick Brilliant, CEO
At Riverside Community Hospital, we are able to provide the healthcare services that you and your family will need through the many stages of your life. Services like Emergency/Trauma, Labor and Delivery, Cardiac Care, Orthopedics and Transplant are among our many Centers of Excellence.

7279   Saint Jude Medical Center
101 E Valencia Mesa Dr
Fullerton, CA 92835-3809   714-871-3280
                                              800-870-7537
                                          Fax: 714-992-3029
                                      www.stjudemedicalcenter.org
April De Cou, Wellness Educator
Jane Wang, Wellness Programs Supervisor
Offers the following rehabilitation services: Out-patient Rehab, Sub-Acute Rehab, Occupational Therapy, Physical Therapy, Speech and Audiology Therapy, Pain Management Program.

7280   South Coast Medical Center
12 Mason
Suite A
Irvine, CA 92618-2733   714-669-4446
                                          Fax: 714-669-4448
                                      info@southcoastmedcenter.com
                                          www.mission4health.com
Leigh Erin Connealy, Manager
Bruce Christian, President

Offers the following services: physical therapy, occupational therapy, speech therapy, cardica rehabilitation, incontinence program, sub-acute rehabilitation.

7281   Valley Garden Health Care and Rehabilitation Center
1517 Knickerbocker Dr
Stockton, CA 95210-3119   209-957-4539
                                          Fax: 209-957-5831
                                      www.valleygardenshealth.com
Dr. Alexande Chan, Medical Director
Accomodates 120 residents. Our center provides short-term nursing and rehabilitative care as well as traditional long-term skilled care. Our combination of clinical skill and comprehensive rehabilitation services enables us to care for a variety of complex medical conditions. Rehabilitative therapies are provided as needed by physical, occupational and speech therapists.

Colorado

7282   Boulder Community Hospital Mapleton Center
1100 Balsam
PO Box 9019
Boulder, CO 80301-9019   303-440-2273
                                              info@bch.org
                                              www.bch.org
Lou DellaCava, Chairman
Ric Porreca, Vice Chairman
Jean Dubofsky, Secretary
R. David Hoover, Treasurer
159-bed acute care hospital and 24-hour emergency department.

7283   Fairacres Manor
1700 18th Ave
Greeley, CO 80631-5152   970-353-3370
                                          Fax: 970-353-9347
Kathy Gardner, Admissions/Marketing Director
Marla Trujillo, Director of Nursing
Ben Gonzales, Admissions/Marketing Assistant Director
Kathleen Mekelburg, Administrator
Offers the following rehabilitation services: Physical Therapy, Occupational Therapy, Speech Therapy, Restorative Therapy, Skilled Nursing, and Sub-Acute Rehabilitation.

7284   Rowan Community
4601 E Asbury Cir
Denver, CO 80222-4722   303-757-1228
                                          Fax: 303-759-3390
                                      tgleisner@pinonmgt.com
Tammy Gleisner, Director/Admissions/Marketing Director
Jeff Jerebker, President/CEO
Bruce Odenthal, VP Operations
John D. Brammeier, CPA, FHFMA,, Chief Financial Officer
Rowan is a 70-bed community, small enough to support personal relationships between residents and caregivers. Our residents vary in age, reflecting the diversity of a much larger community. Rowan's focus is on a psycho-social model of care with a dynamic activities and social service program. Our staff is specially trained in behavior management and many are certified Eden AlternativeT associates and certifid Elder Care Specialists.

Connecticut

7285   Hamilton Rehabilitation and Healthcare Center
89 Viets St
New London, CT 6320-3355   860-447-1471
                                          Fax: 860-439-0107
Steve Roizen, Executive Director
Offers the following rehabilitation services: Sub-Acute, Occupational Therapy, Speech Therapy, Physical Therapy.

7286 Hospital For Special Care (HSC)
2150 Corbin Ave
New Britain, CT   06053-2298
860-223-2761
Fax: 860-827-4849
www.hfsc.org

John J. Votto, President/CEO
Paul J. Scalise, M.D., F.C.C.P, Senior Vice President
Thomas J. Soltis, M.D., M.P.H., Chief of Geriatrics
HSC is a private, not-for-profit 200-bed rehabilitation long-term acute and chronic care hospital, widely-known and respected for its expertise in physical rehabilitation, respiratory care, and medically-complex pediatrics. Special programs for spinal cord injuries, pulmonary rehabilitation, acquired brain injuries, stroke, ventilator management and geriatrics, make HSC an important regional resource for patients with special healthcare needs.

7287 Masonic Healthcare Center
MasoniCare Corporation
22 Masonic Ave
PO Box 70
Wallingford, CT   06492-3048
203-679-5900
877-424-3537
Fax: 203-679-6459
info@masonicare.org
www.masonicare.org

Stephen B. McPherson, President
Arthur Santilli, President
The states leading provider of healthcare and retirement living communities for seniors. We are not-for-profit and have more then 100 years of experience behind us. We're recognized for the quality, compassionate care and steadfast support we provide to our residents and patients.

7288 Stamford Hospital
30 Shelburne Rd
Stamford, CT   06904-3628
203-276-1000
Fax: 203-325-7905
info@stamhealth.org
www.stamfordhospital.org

Brian Grissler, President/CEO
Kathleen Silard, EVP/Chief Operating Officer
Kevin Gage, Senior Vice President, Finance/Chief Financial Officer
Sharon Kiely, MD, Senior Vice President, Medical Affairs/Chief Medical Officer
A not-for-profit, community teaching hospital that has been serving Stamford and surrounding communities for more then 100 years. We have 305 inpatient beds in medicine, surgery, obstetrics/gynecology, psychiatry, and medical and surgical critical care units and maintain an educational partnership with Columbia University College of Physicians and Surgeons for its teaching program in the internal medicine, family practice, obstetrics/gynecology and surgery

7289 Windsor Rehabilitation and Healthcare Center
581 Poquonock Ave
Windsor, CT   06095-2202
860-688-7211
Fax: 860-688-6715
www.windsorrehab.com

Jeffrey Robbins, Medical Director
Accomodates 116 residents. We offer private and semi-private rooms with access to private telephones and cable television. Our goal is to be a comprehensive, leading care center viewed by our community as an excellent resource for patients, families, and professionals.

Delaware

7290 Arbors at New Castle
32 Buena Vista Dr
New Castle, DE   19720-4660
302-328-2580
Fax: 302-326-4132
newcastle@extendicare.com
www.extendicareus.com/newcastle

Annette Moore, Administrator
A subacute and rehabilitation center offering skilled medical services, infusion therapies, cardiac recovery services, renal disease services, cancer services and digestive disease services. Skilled rehabilitation services include physical therapy, occupational therapy and speech therapy. Also provides case management and discharge planning, general nursing and restorative care and respite care.

Florida

7291 Avon Oaks Skilled Care Nursing Facility
37800 French Creek Rd
Avon, OH   44011-1763
440-934-5204
800-589-5204
jreidy@avonoaks.net
www.avonoaks.net

Natalie McIntyre, Human Resources Director
Stephanie Auvil, RN, BC, Director of Nursing
Joan Reidy, Administrator
Richard J. Reidy, Technologies & Information Manager
Oaks at Avon provides a full range of skilled nursing services including infusion therapy, enteral therapy, wound care, tracheotomy care, and portable diagnostics.

7292 Boca Raton Rehabilitation Center
755 Meadows Rd
Boca Raton, FL   33486-2384
561-391-5200
Fax: 561-391-0685

Stanley Mucinic, Administrator
Tracey Dougherty, Administrator
Offers the following rehabilitation services: Occupational Therapy, Speech Therapy, Physical Therapy, Sub-Acute Rehabilitation

7293 Cape Coral Hospital
636 Del Prado Blvd
Cape Coral, FL   33990
239-424-2000
Fax: 239-574-1935
www.leememorial.org

Richard Akin, Chairman
Sanford Cohen, MD, Vice Chairman
Marilyn Stout, Treasurer
Diane Champion, Secretary
A 291-bed acute care facility, Cape Coral Hospital features all private rooms. The hospital currently is undergoing a complete renovation, expansion and modernization of the Weigner-Taeni Center for Emergency Services, which will make the emergency department the largest in Lee County.

7294 Evergreen Woods Health and Rehabilitation Center
7045 Evergreen Woods Trl
Spring Hill, FL   34608-1306
352-596-8371
Fax: 352-596-8032

Janet Hanciles, Administrator
Offers the following rehabilitation services: Sub-Acute rehabilitation, Occupational therapy, Speech pathology therapy, Physical therapy.

7295 Healthcare and Rehabilitation Center of Sanford
950 Mellonville Avenue
Sanford, FL   32771-2237
407-322-8566
Fax: 407-322-0121
www.healthcareandrehabofsanford.com

Dr. S. Joshi, Medical Director
Kate Hilgar, Administrator
Vicky Smith, Director Admissions
We provide post-acute services, rehabilitative services, skilled nursing, short and long term care through Physical, Occupational, and Speech Therapists; Registered and Licensed Practical Nurses; and Certified Nursing Assistants. This is complemented by Social Services, Activities, Nutritional Services, Housekeeping and Laundry Services. With over 224 years of combined experience, our staff of professionals is here to meet the needs of each and every patient and resident.

7296 Highland Pines Rehabilitation Center
1111 S Highland Ave
Clearwater, FL 33756-4432   727-446-0581
                                    Fax: 727-442-9425
Paula Anthony, Administrator
Offers the following rehabilitation services: Sub-Acute rehabilitation, Occupational Therapy, Speech Therapy, Physical Therapy.

7297 Jupiter Medical Center-Pavilion
1210 S Old Dixie Hwy
Jupiter, FL 33458-7205   561-747-2234
                                    Fax: 561-744-4467
                                    JCouris@jupitermed.com
                                    www.jupitermed.com
John D. Couris, President/Chief Executive Officer
Dale Hocking, Vice President, Finance/Chief Financial Officer
Mike Fehr, Vice President, Information Services/Chief Information Offic
Steven Seeley, Vice President, Chief Operating Officer/Chief Nursing Office
Offers the following rehabilitation services: Sub-Acute Rehabilitation, Occupational Therapy, Speech Therapy, Physical Therapy.

7298 North Broward Medical Center
201 E Sample Rd
Deerfield Beach, FL 33064-4441   954-941-8300
                                    Fax: 954-941-4233
                                    www.browardhealth.org
Pauline Grant, CEO
Douglas Ford, Chief of Staff
Offers the following rehabilitation services: Sub-Acute rehabilitation, Physical Therapy, Occupational Therapy, Speech Therapy, Respiratory Therapy.

7299 Pompano Rehabilitation and Nursing Center
Senior Health Care Management
51 W Sample Rd
Pompano Beach, FL 33064-3542   954-942-5530
                                    Fax: 954-942-0941
Jeff Nusbusn, Administrator
Offers the following rehabilitation services: Sub-Acute Rehabilitation, Physical Therapy, Occupational Therapy, Speech Therapy

7300 Rehabilitation Center of Palm Beach
300 Royal Palm Way
Palm Beach, FL 33480-4385   561-655-7266
                                    Fax: 561-655-3269
                                    info@rcca.org
                                    www.rcca.org
Ellen O'Bannon, Manager
Pamela Henderson, Executive Director
Our mission is to improve the physical function, communication & independence of people with disabilities.

7301 Rehabilitation and Healthcare Center of Tampa
4411 N Habana Ave
Tampa, FL 33614-7211   813-872-2771
                                    Fax: 813-871-2831
Dr. Gustavo Barrazuetta, Medical Director
We provide post-acute services, rehabilitative services, skilled nursing, short and long term care through Physical, Occupational, and Speech Therapists; Registered and Licensed Practical Nurses; and Certified Nursing Assistants. This is complemented by Social Services, Activities, Nutritional Services, Housekeeping and Laundry Services. With over 60 years of combined experience, our staff of professionals is here to meet the needs of each and every patient and resident.

7302 Shands Rehab Hospital
4101 NW 89th Blvd
Gainesville, FL 32606-3813   352-265-8938
                                    Fax: 352-265-5420
                                    www.ufhealth.org/shands-rehab-hospital
Tim Goldfarb,M.S., Chief Executive Officer
David S. Guzick, M.D., Ph.D., Senior Vice President
Ed . Jimenez, M.B.A, Senior Vice President/Chief Operating Officer
James Roberts, J.D., Senior Vice President/General Counsel
UF Health Shands Rehab Hospital is a 40-bed acute rehab hospital for patients who have suffered strokes, traumatic brain and spinal cord injuries, amputations, burns or major joint replacements.

7303 St. Anthony's Hospital
1200 7th Ave N
St Petersburg, FL 33705-1388   727-825-1100
                                    www.stanthonys.com
William Ulbricht, President
Ron Colaguori, VP Operations
James McClintic, M.D., Vice President, Medical Affairs
Sr. Mary McNally, OSF, Vice President, Mission
We offer outstanding diagnostic and treatment options of all types of cancer. Our Susan Sheppard McGillicuddy Breast Center is unmatched in the community in diagnostic services and helping patients navigate their treatment options should they find a cancer diagnosis.

7304 Winkler Court
3250 Winkler Avenue Ext
Fort Myers, FL 33916-9414   239-939-4993
                                    Fax: 239-939-1743
                                    www.winklercourt.com
Michael Collier, Medical Director
Michael Stens, Medical Director
We provide post-acute services, rehabilitative services, skilled nursing, short and long term care through Physical, Occupational, and Speech Therapists; Registered and Licensed Practical Nurses; and Certified Nursing Assistants. This is complemented by Social Services, Activities, Nutritional Services, Housekeeping and Laundry Services. With over 100 years of combined experience, our staff of professionals is here to meet the needs of each and every patient and resident.

7305 Winter Park Memorial Hospital
Florida Hospital
200 N Lakemont Ave
Winter Park, FL 32792-3273   407-646-7000
                                    Fax: 407-646-7639
                                    healthcare@winterparkhospital.com
                                    www.winterparkhospital.com
Ken Bradley, CEO
Nestled among the oak-shaded, brick-paved streets of one of the most picturesque hometowns in the country, Winter Park Memorial Hospital has continuously served the residents of Winter Park and its surrounding communities for more than 50 years.

Georgia

7306 Athena Rehab of Clayton
2055 Rex Rd
Lake City, GA 30260-3944   404-361-5144
                                    Fax: 404-363-6366
Reginald Washington, Administrator
Offers the following rehabilitation services: Sub-Acute rehabilitation, Occupational therapy, Speech therapy, Physical therapy, Restorative care.

7307 Lafayette Nursing and Rehabilitation Center
110 Brandywine Blvd
Fayetteville, GA 30214-1500   770-461-2928
                                    Fax: 770-461-8507
                                    www.lafayetterehab.com
Wendy Goza, Medical Director
Lafayette Nursing and Rehab Center accomodates 179 residents. We are Medicare certified and our center also features a 25-bed

postacute rehab unit and a 24-bed dementia unit. We have RN's LPN's and CNA's 24 hours a day. We also have physician services availiable seven days a week.

7308   Savannah Rehabilitation and Nursing Center
815 E 63rd St
Savannah, GA 31405-4499   912-352-8615
                                                  Fax: 912-355-4642
Sandra Casper, Executive Director
At our facility, we provide quality care with modern rehabilitation and restorative nursing techniques. We aim to provide an atmosphere which encourages family involvement in the care-planning process, with the right mix of activities addressing the social, spiritual and intellectual needs of our residents.

7309   Specialty Hospital
PO Box 1566
Rome, GA 30162-1566   706-509-4100
                                                  Fax: 706-509-4159

7310   Walton Rehabilitation Health System
523 13th St.
Augusta, GA 30901-1037   706-823-8505
                                                  866-492-5866
                                                  Fax: 706-724-5752
                                                  postmaster@wrh.org
                                                  www.wrh.org
Dennis Skelley, President/CEO
Has Centers of Excellence in Stroke Brain Injury, Complex Orthopedics, Spinal Cord Injury and Pain Management. 58-bed nonprofit facility.

7311   Warner Robins Rehabilitation and Nursing Center
1601 Elberta Rd
Warner Robins, GA 31093-1393   478-922-2241
                                                  Fax: 478-328-1984
www.warnerrobinsrehabilitation.com
Laura Fergason, Administrator
Offers the following rehabilitation services: Sub-Acute rehabilitation, Physical Therapy, Occupational Therapy, Speech Therapy.

Hawaii

7312   Aloha Nursing and Rehab Center
45-545 Kamehameha Hwy
Kaneohe, HI 96744-1943   808-247-2220
                                                  Fax: 808-235-3676
                                                  info@alohanursing.com
                                                  alohanursing.com
Charles Harris, Executive Director
Amy Lee, Administrator
Our unique nursing care facility is nestled in the picturesque town of Kaneohe, Oahu, amid the towering Koolau Mountains and the panoramic vistas of Kaneohe Bay. In this tranquil setting, our 141-bed facility offers both long and short term care to residents who meet intermediate or skilled level of care criteria.

Idaho

7313   Boise Health And Rehabilitation Center
1001 S Hilton St
Boise, ID 83705-1925   208-345-4464
                                                  Fax: 208-345-2998
Jason Ludwig, Medical Director
Aaron Moorhouse, Medical Director
Debbie Mills, Executive Director
Offers the following rehabilitation services: Sub-acute rehabilitation, occupational therapy, speech therapy, physical therapy.

7314   Eastern Idaho Regional Medical Center
3100 Channing Way
Idaho Falls, ID 83404-7533   208-529-6111
                                                  Fax: 208-529-7021
                                                  www.eirmc.com
Cindy Smith-Putnam, Executive Director of Business Development, Marketing & Comm
Lou Fatkin, Executive Director of Risk Management, Physician Relations,
Matt Campbell, Director of Human Resources
Jared Rickabaugh, Director of Quality Management
The largest medical facility in the region, Eastern Idaho Regional Medical Center (EIRMC) is a modern, JCAHO-accredidted, full-service hospital. EIRMC serves as the region's healthcare hub, offering specialty services including open-heart surgery, leading-edge cancer treatment, trauma, neurosurgery, intensive care for adults and infants, and a helicopeter service.

7315   Kindred Transitional Care and Rehabilitation
3315 8th St
Lewiston, ID 83501-4966   208-743-9543
                                                  Fax: 208-746-8662
                                                  www.lewistonrehab.com
Debbie Freeze, Administrator
Lewiston Rehabilitation and Care Center has years of experience providing diversified healthcare services. We have our own staff of physical, occupational and speech therapists. Our therapy gym and rehab kitchen are a lovely atmosphere in which to work toward your therapy goals. We are an Eden Alternative Certified facility.

7316   Mountain Valley Care and Rehabilitation Center
601 West Cameron Avenue
PO Box 689
Kellogg, ID 83837- 2004   208-784-1283
                                                  Fax: 208-784-0151
                                                  www.mountainvalleycare.com
Maryruth Butler, Executive Director
Mountain Valley Care and Rehabilitation Center accomodates 68 residents. We are conveniently located in the heart of Kellogg Idaho. We strive to offer quality care and superior customer service in a home-like environment. Upon admission, you or your loved one is looked after by an assigned staff member. We call this our 'Angel Care' program. Our rehabilitation program focuses on meething the individual needs of the resident so you or your loved one can see how they are going to progress.

7317   River's Edge Rehabilitation and Healthcare
Kindred Healthcare
714 N Butte Ave
Emmett, ID 83617-2799   208-365-4425
                                                  Fax: 208-365-6989
                                                  GDecker@ensigngroup.net
                                                  www.riversedgerehab.com
Janis Shields, Executive Director
Steve Balle, MPT, Director of Rehabilitation
Margaret Williams RN, BSN, Director of Nursing
Patty Alsup, Business Office Manager
Emmett Rehab & healthcare accomodates 95 residents. We are located in Emmett, Idaho, a rural community located an easy 30 minute drive from Boise. Emmett Rehab &' healthcare has served the area for more then 40 years by providing healthcare for residents of Gem County.

Illinois

7318   Chevy Chase Nursing and Rehabilitation Center
3400 S Indiana Ave
Chicago, IL 60616-3841   312-842-5000
                                                  Fax: 312-842-3790
Tony Prather, Administrator
Our approach to care is multidisciplinary; our medical staff members work together as a team in a proactive fashion, challenging residents each and every day, in order to motivate them to rehabilitate and achieve their ultimate potential.

7319 Glenview Terrace Nursing Center
1511 Greenwood Rd
Glenview, IL 60026-1513 847-729-9090
Fax: 847-729-9135
www.glenviewterrace.com
Ian Crook, Administrator
We're best known as the industry leader in post-hospital rehabilitation, including orthopedic rehabilitation and stroke recovery. Our highly effective rehabilitation services feature one-on-one physical, occupational, speech and respiratory therapies up to seven days a week.

7320 Halsted Terrace Nursing Center
10935 S Halsted St
Chicago, IL 60628-3189 773-928-2000
Fax: 773-928-9154
Ted O'Brien, Administrator
Offers the following rehabilitation services: Sub-acute rehabilitation, physical therapy, occupational therapy, speech therapy, cardiac rehabilitation.

7321 Harmony Nursing and Rehabilitation Center
3919 W Foster Ave
Chicago, IL 60625-6056 773-588-9500
Fax: 773-588-9533
www.harmonychicago.com
John Sianghio, Administrator
Offers a friendly healthcare experience. You'll find compassionate experts who provide short-term rehabilitation and therapy, wound care, Alzheimer's and memory loss care, long-term nursing care and more.

7322 Imperial
1366 W Fullerton Ave
Chicago, IL 60614-2199 773-248-9300
Fax: 773-935-0036
www.imperialpavilion.com
David Hartman, Administrator
Mary Bangayan, M.D., Pulmonary Care Programme
Sanjay Gill, M.D., Cardiac Management Program
We offer a comprehensive approach to post acute care. One that takes into consideration our guests' unique needs, and utilizes a progressive healthcare model to provide them with a personalized rehabilitation program designed to offer them the fullest possible recovery.

7323 Jackson Square Nursing and Rehabilitation Center
5130 W Jackson Blvd
Chicago, IL 60644-4332 773-921-8000
Fax: 773-287-9302
www.jacksonsquarecare.com
Rick Walworth, Administrator
At Jackson Square, there is one primary goal: to help guests regain maximum independence and functioning so that they can safely, comfortably, and happily get their life back. Our physicians, therapists, and nurses use their experience, compassion, and skill-combined with the latest and best technology-to provide comprehensive rehabilitation for a wide range of physical disabilities and medical conditions.

7324 Renaissance at 87th Street
2940 W 87th St
Chicago, IL 60652-3832 773-434-8787
Fax: 773-434-8717
www.renaissanceat87.com
Juli Foy, Administrator
At Renaissance at 87th, there is one primary goal: to help guests regain maximum independence and functioning so that they can safely, comfortably, and happily get their life back. Our physicians, therapists, and nurses use their experience, compassion, and skill-combined with the latest and best technology-to provide comprehensive rehabilitation for a wide range of physical disabilities and medical conditions.

7325 Renaissance at Hillside
4600 N. Frontage Rd.
Hillside, IL 60162-1761 708-544-9933
Fax: 708-544-9966
www.ariapostacute.com
John Stare, Administrator
Utilizing a progressive healthcare model that takes into account each patient's individual needs, Aria Post Acute Care designs a personalized rehabilitation program offering guests the best chance at the fullest possible recovery.

7326 Renaissance at Midway
4437 S Cicero Ave
Chicago, IL 60632-4333 773-884-0484
Fax: 773-884-0485
www.renaissanceatmidway.com
Jeff Baker, Executive Director
At Renaissance at Midway, there is one primary goal: to help guests regain maximum independence and functioning so that they can safely, comfortably, and happily get their life back. Our physicians, therapists, and nurses use their experience, compassion, and skill-combined with the latest and best technology-to provide comprehensive rehabilitation for a wide range of physical disabilities and medical conditions.

7327 Renaissance at South Shore
2425 E 71st St
Chicago, IL 60649-2612 773-721-5000
Fax: 773-721-6850
www.rensouthshore.com
Dave Schechter, Administrator
The Renaissance at South Shore is a 248 bed skilled nursing facility with multiple services that include short-term rehabilitation, specialized dementia care and long-term care and hospice care. Our highly trained nursing professionals provide loving care in a home-like atmosphere.

7328 Schwab Rehabilitation Hospital
Mt. Sinai
1401 S California Ave
Chicago, IL 60608-1858 773-522-2010
www.schwabrehab.org
Suzan Rayner, Medical Director
Lisa Thornton, Medical Staff President
Alan Channing, President/ Chief Executive Officer
Anita Halvorsen, Vice President of Schwab Rehabilitation Hospital
Schwab Rehabilitation Hospital is a freestanding, not-for-profit, 102-bed rehabilitation hospital located on Chicago's west side. It offers a therapeutic environment of comprehensive inpatient and outpatient rehabilitation, both for adults and children.

Indiana

7329 Angel River Health and Rehabilitation
5233 Rosebud Ln
Newburgh, IN 47630-9283 812-473-4761
Fax: 812-473-5190
Kay Congleton, Executive Director
Our wide array of services enables our patients and residents to receive the medical care they need, the restorative therapy they require, and the support they and their families deserve. We serve many types of patient and resident needs - from short-term rehabilitation to traditional long-term care. Our resident council meets regularly to ensure that our residents' needs are being met to their satisfaction.

7330 Chalet Village Health and Rehabilitation Center
Magnolia Health Systems
1065 Parkway St
Berne, IN 46711-2366 260-589-2127
Fax: 260-589-3521
www.chalet-village.net
Vicki Shepherd, Administrator
We provide dedicated, community-centered healthcare which was founded in Indiana, operates in Indiana, for people who live in Indiana.

7331 Columbus Health and Rehabilitation Center
2100 Midway St
Columbus, IN 47201-3722   812-372-8447
                                        Fax: 812-375-5117
                                        www.columbushrc.com

Sherry Harrison, Executive Director
William Lustig, Medical Director
Accomodates 235 residents. We offer a continuum of healthcare
services. Our center also provides a Special Care Alzheimer's
Unit. We are licensed by the Stat of Indiana and are Medicare and
Medicaid approved provider. We are proud to offer a friendly
home-like atmosphere while providing comprehensive
healthcare services. These services include short-term medical
and rehabilitation treatment, which is designed to address the individual needs of our residents and patients.

7332 Harrison Health and Rehabilitation Centre
150 Beechmont Drive
Corydon, IN 47112-1717   812-738-0550
                                        Fax: 812-738-6273
                                 HSDED0131@kindredhealthcare.com
                                        www.harrisonrehab.com

Sheila Bieker, Executive Director
Bruce Burton, Medical Director
We serve many types of patient and resident needs - from
short-term rehabilitation to traditional long-term care. Working
with your physician, our staff - including medical specialists,
nurses, nutritionists, therapists, dietitians and social workers - establishes a comprehensive treatment plan intended to restore you
or your loved one to the fullest practicable potential.

7333 Indian Creek Health and Rehabilitation Center
240 Beechmont Dr
Corydon, IN 47112-1718   812-738-8127
                                             877-380-7211
                                        Fax: 812-738-2917
                                 HSDED0288@kindredhealthcare.com
                                        www.indiancreekhrc.com

Bonnie Fallin, Executive Director
Bruce Burton, Medical Director
140 bed facility offering the following rehabilitation services:
Sub-Acute rehabilitation, Physical therapy, Occupational Ther-
apy, Speech Therapy, pain management, Wound rehabilitation.
Short and long term skilled nursing care certified for Medicare,
Medicaid, Private Pay and Private Insurance. Hospice and respite
care rated #1 in clinical care in southern Indiana district for 2002.

7334 Meadowvale Health and Rehabilitation Center
Kindred Health Care
1529 Lancaster St
Bluffton, IN 46714-1507   260-824-4320
                                             800-743-3333
                                        Fax: 260-824-4689

Todd Beaulieu, Executive Director
Yadagiri Jonna, Medical Director
Working with your physician, our staff - including medical specialists, nurses, nutritionists, therapists, dietitians and social
workers - establishes a comprehensive treatment plan intended to
restore you or your loved one to the fullest practicable potential.

7335 Muncie Health Care and Rehabilitation
680 South Fourth Street
Louisville, KY 40202   502-596-7300
                                             800-545-0749
                                   web_administrator@kindred.com
                                        www.kindredhealthcare.com

Dee Harrold, Executive Director
Dr. Jeffery Hiltz, Medical Director
Offers the following rehabilitation services: Sub-Acute rehabili-
tation, physical therapy, occupational therapy, speech therapy.

7336 Rehabilitation Hospital of Indiana
4141 Shore Dr
Indianapolis, IN 46254-2607   317-329-2000
                                        Fax: 317-329-2104
                                        www.rhin.com

Ian Worden, MHA, MBA, CPA, RHI Board Chair
James G. Terwilliger, MPH, Vice Chair/Secretary
*Kyle Netter, MBA, PT, Executive Director of Corporate and Affili-
ate Relations*
Larissa Swan, MS, OTR, Executive Director of Therapies
We approach every patient understanding that every diagnosis,
every illness, and every injury are different. It's the collective effort of trained and compassionate team members who value the
quality of life of every patient and their caregivers. It's the right
kind of treatment- inpatient, outpatient, and follow-up services-
provided under the same roof. It's one step closer to home. It's a
continuum of care

7337 Sellersburg Health and Rehabilitation Centre
7823 Old State Road 60
Sellersburg, IN 47172-1858   812-246-4272
                                        Fax: 812-246-8160
                                        www.sellersburgrehab.com

Dave Powell, Administrator
Chris Hansen, Executive Director
Sellersburg is a modern healthcare center conveniently located
on the edge of the community. Our center accomodates 110 residents and includes a rehabilitative program with a goal of returning residents home as quickly as possible. Sellersburg is a 2006
recipient of the American Health Care Association Quality
Award.

7338 Westpark Rehabilitation Center
1316 N Tibbs Ave
Indianapolis, IN 46222-3024   317-634-8330
                                        Fax: 317-263-9442
                                        www.westparkhealthcare.com

Dave Mc Carroll, Owner
Offers the following rehabilitation services: Sub-acute rehabilitation, occupational therapy, physical therapy, speech therapy,
respiratory therapy.

7339 Westview Nursing and Rehabilitation Center
1510 Clinic Dr
Bedford, IN 47421-3530   812-279-4494
                                        Fax: 812-275-8313
                          www.ascseniorcare.com/westview-nursing—rehab
Sholin Montgomery, Executive Director
Mike Spencer, Executive Director
Offers the following rehabilitation services: Sub-acute rehabili-
tation, physical therapy, occupational therapy, speech therapy.

7340 Windsor Estates Health and Rehab Center
429 W Lincoln Rd
Kokomo, IN 46902-3508   765-453-5600
                                        Fax: 765-455-0110
                                 HSDED0294@kindredhealthcare.com
                                        www.kindredkokomo.com
Brenda Alfrey, Administrator
Monica Martin, Executive Director
Our wide array of services enables our patients and residents to
receive the medical care they need, the restorative therapy they
require, and the support they and their families deserve. We serve
many types of patient and resident needs - from short-term rehabilitation to traditional long-term care.

Iowa

7341 Madison County Rehab Services
Madison County Hospital
300 W Hutchings St
Winterset, IA 50273-2109   515-462-2373
                                        Fax: 515-462-4492

Marcia Harris, CEO
Panndee Stebbins, Director

Offers the following rehabilitation services: Sub-acute rehabilitation, occupational therapy, physical therapy, speech therapy, home health rehab, wellness programs.

7342 Mercy Subacute Care
603 E 12th St
Des Moines, IA 50309-5515
515-247-4400
Fax: 515-643-0945

Bonnie Mc Coy, Manager
Pam Nelson, Intake Coordinator
Offers the following rehabilitation services: Sub-acute rehabilitation, physical therapy, speech therapy, occupational therapy.

Kentucky

7343 Danville Centre for Health and Rehabilitation
642 N 3rd St
Danville, KY 40422-1125
859-236-3972
Fax: 859-236-0703
HSDED0782@kindredhealthcare.com
www.danvillecentre.com

Debbie Gibson, Executive Director
We offer short-term rehabilitative care as well as long-term care. Our emphasis is on service excellence - providing quality care in a home-like environment to allow for independence and to enable our patients and residents to receive the medical care they need, the restorative therapy they require, and the support they and their families deserve.

7344 Fountain Circle Health & Rehabilitation
Kindred Healthcare
200 Glenway Rd
Winchester, KY 40391
859-744-1800
Fax: 859-744-0285

William Whited, Executive Director
Kathryn Jones, Medical Director
Offers the following rehabilitation services: Sub-acute rehabilitation, speech therapy, physical therapy, occupational therapy.

7345 Lexington Center for Health and Rehabilitation
353 Waller Ave
Lexington, KY 40504-2974
859-252-3558
Fax: 859-233-0192

Karole Ward, Administrator
Offers the following rehabilitation services: Sub-acute rehabilitation, speech therapy, occupational therapy, physical therapy.

7346 Paducah Centre For Health and Rehabilitation
Wellsouth Health Systems
501 N 3rd St
Paducah, KY 42001-0749
270-444-9661
Fax: 270-443-9407

Jean Glisson, RN, Director of Nursing
Elizabeth Kay Chilton, Admissions Director
Tracy Summers, Rehab/Specialty Program Director
Cathy Ortega, Administrator
Paducah Center is an 86-bed skilled and long-term care facility with a 28-bed Alzheimer's secure unit. This unit has a private courtyard and structured activities throughout the day, and is the only true Alzheimer's secure unit in the area.

7347 Pathways Brain Injury Program
4200 Browns Ln
Louisville, KY 40220-1523
502-459-8900
Fax: 502-459-5026
www.hcr-manorcare.com

Pam Pearson, Manager
Offers the following rehabilitation services: Sub-acute rehabilitation, speech therapy, occupational therapy, physical therapy, recreational therapy.

Louisiana

7348 Guest House of Slidell Sub-Acute and Rehab Center
1051 Robert Blvd
Slidell, LA 70458-2011
985-643-5630
800-303-9872
Fax: 985-649-6065

Brandy Wheat, Administrator
116 bed healthcare center offering the following subacute services within the skilled nursing setting: physical, occupational, and speech therapies, infusion therapy, respiratory care, wound care, neurological rehabilitation, cardiac reconditioning, pain management, post surgical recovery, orthopedic rehabilitation.

7349 Irving Place Rehabilitation and Nursing Center
1736 Irving Pl
Shreveport, LA 71101-4606
318-631-9121
Fax: 318-222-2095

Webster Johnson, Administrator
Offers the following rehabilitation services: sub-acute rehabilitation, speech therapy, occupational therapy, physical therapy

Maine

7350 Augusta Rehabilitation Center
188 Eastern Ave
Augusta, ME 04330-5928
207-622-3121
800-457-1220
Fax: 207-623-7666
HSDED0544@kindredhealthcare.com
www.augustarehabcenter.com

Malcolm Dean, Executive Director
Cathleen O'Connor
From intensive short term rehabilitation therapy to longer-term restorative care, our Nursing and Rehabilitation Centers provide a full range of nursing care and social services to treat and support each of our patients and residents. Our clinical capabilities allow us to accept patients with greater medical complexity than a traditional nursing home. This is increasingly important as many patients require transitional care before they are ready to return home.

7351 Brentwood Rehabilitation and Nursing Center
370 Portland St
Yarmouth, ME 04096-8101
207-846-9021
800-457-1220
Fax: 207-846-1497
HSDED0555@kindredhealthcare.com

Malcolm Dean, Executive Director
Daniel M. Pierce, Medical Director
Brentwood accomodates 82 residents. We are located at 370 Portland Street in Yarmouth, Maine. We strive to meet the healthcare needs of the greater Yarmouth community, including Portland and Brunswick, which are located within 10 miles of the center. In addition to Brentwood's rehabilitation and skilled nursing services, we also offer Alzheimer's specialty care in a comfortable setting.

7352 Den-Mar Rehabilitation and Nursing Center
44 South St
Rockport, MA 01966-1800
978-546-6311
800-439-2370
Fax: 978-546-9185
HSDED0542@kindredhealthcare.com
www.denmarrnc.com

Christine Marek, Executive Director
Den-Mar nursing and Rehab center accomodates 80 residents. We provide skilled nursing and rehabilitation services as well as long term care. We are certified for Medicare and Medicaid as well as many insurance carriers. We offer semi-private and private rooms, with many common areas for socializing.

7353 Eastside Rehabilitation and Living Center
516 Mount Hope Ave
Bangor, ME   04401-4215   207-947-6131
                                                               800-457-1220
                                              Fax: 207-942-0884
                          HSDED0545@kindredhealthcare.com
                                              www.eastsiderehab.com
Ryan Kelley, Executive Director
From intensive short term rehabilitation therapy to longer-term
restorative care, our Nursing and Rehabilitation Centers provide
a full range of nursing care and social services to treat and support
each of our patients and residents. Our clinical capabilities allow
us to accept patients with greater medical complexity than a traditional nursing home. This is increasingly important as many patients require transitional care before they are ready to return
home.

7354 Kennebunk Nursing & Rehabilitation Center
158 Ross Rd
Kennebunk, ME   04043-6532   207-985-7141
                                                               800-457-1220
                                              Fax: 207-985-0961
                          HSDED0549@kindredhealthcare.com
Stephen Alaimo, Executive Director
We treat a variety of conditions and provide an array of services
including, but not limited to:Respiratory conditions such as
pneumonia and post-acute COPD episodes Cardiac conditions
and post surgical care (grafts, valves, stints) Wound Stroke Orthopedic Neurological illnesses Diabetes

7355 Norway Rehabilitation and Living Center
29 Marion Ave
Norway, ME   04268-5601   207-743-7075
                                                               800-457-1220
                                              Fax: 207-743-9269
Carolyn Farley, Administrator
Norway Rehabilitation and Living Center has been a fixture in
the Norway community since 1976. We are a 70-bed facility offering short-term rehabilitation, skilled nursing services, long
term care and residential care services. Utilizing an interdisciplinary team led by a physician and consisting of qualified health
care specialists, we develop individualized plans of care for each
patient that are designed to restore maximum health and optimize
functional abilities and independence

7356 Shore Village Rehabilitation & Nursing Center
201 Camden St
\, ME   04841-2534   207-596-6423
                                                               800-457-1220
                                              Fax: 207-596-7235
Phyllis Nickerson, Administrator
Shore Village accomodates 60 residents and is located in the
mid-coast region of the state of Maine. We have a cozy size and a
primary goal for the staff is to ensure a home-like atmosphere for
all the residents. Shore Village provides skilled nursing and rehabilitation, respite care, and long term care. The facility is dually
certified for Medicare and Medicaid and accepts many commercial insurance plans.

Maryland

7357 Greater Baltimore Medical Center
6701 N Charles St
Baltimore, MD   21204-6881   443-849-2000
                                              Fax: 443-849-3024
                                              TTY:800-735-2258
                                              www.gbmc.org
John B. Chessare, M.D., President/Chief Executive Officer
Eric L. Melchior, Executive Vice President/Chief Financial Officer
Keith Poisson, Executive Vice President/Chief Operating Officer
John W. Ellis, Senior Vice President/Corporate Strategy & Business
Developm
The 281-bed medical center (acute and sub-acute care) is located
on a beautiful suburban campus and handles more than 26,700 in-
patient cases and approximately 60,000 emergency room visits
annually.

Massachusetts

7358 Bolton Manor Nursing Home
400 Bolton St
Marlborough, MA   01752-3912   508-481-6123
                                                               800-439-2370
                                              Fax: 508-481-6130
Michele Ricard, Medical Director
Thomas Sullivan, Executive Director
Bolton Manor accomodates 157 residents. We are located in
Marlboro, Massachusetts. We provide medical management and
long-term care through comprehensive skilled and post-acute
nursing services. We also provide physical, occupational, and
speech therapy services from an onsite dedicated staff of therapists. The facility is Joint Commission (formerly JCAHO) accredited and has an excellent survey history with the State
Department of Public Health.

7359 Brigham Manor Nursing and Rehabilitation Center
77 High St
Newburyport, MA   01950-3071   978-462-4221
                                                               800-439-2370
                                              Fax: 978-463-3297
Stephen Cynewski, Executive Director
Brigham Manor accomodates 64 residents. We are a
Medicare-certified facility offering private, semi-private and
multi-bed suites. Our bright, formal dining room, with French
doors that open to a shaded courtyard, provides a warm atmosphere for entertaining family and friends. Each resident's personal tastes and medical needs are considered in the planning of
our weekly menus.

7360 Country Gardens Skilled Nursing and Rehabilitation Center
2045 Grand Army Hwy
Swansea, MA   02777-3932   508-379-9700
                                                               800-439-2370
                                              Fax: 508-379-0723
                          HSDED0534@kindredhealthcare.com
Sandy Sarza, Executive Director
Country Gardens Skilled Nursing and Rehabilitation Center
accomodates 86 residents. We are located in a beautiful rural setting conveniently located about 15 minutes east of Providence
and 10 minutes west of Fall River. We have provided healthcare
service to the greater Swansea area for over 34 years.

7361 Country Manor Rehabilitation and Nursing Center
180 Low St
Newburyport, MA   01950-3519   978-465-5361
                                                               800-439-2370
                                              Fax: 978-463-9366
                                              www.countryrehab.com
Stephen Doyle, Executive Director
Country Rehabilitation and Nursing Center accomodates 123 residents. We are located in the quaint seaport town of Newburyport,
Massachusetts. We provide medical management and long-term
care through comprehensive skilled and intermediate nursing services. We also provide physical, occupational, and speech therapy services from an onsite dedicated staff of therapists. The
center offers an Alzheimer's special care unit with staff trained in
dimentia care and dementia specific programs.

7362 Franklin Skilled Nursing and Rehabilitation Center
130 Chestnut St
Franklin, MA   02038-3903   508-528-4600
                                                               800-439-2370
                                              Fax: 508-528-7976
                          HSDED0584@kindredhealthcare.com
Paula Topijan, Executive Director
We treat a variety of conditions and provide an array of services
including, but not limited to :Respiratory conditions such as
pneumonia and post-acute COPD episodes,Cardiac conditions
and post surgical care (grafts, valves, stints),Wound,Stroke,Or-
thopedic,Neurological illnesses,Diabetes

7363 Great Barrington Rehabilitation and Nursing Center
148 Maple Ave
Great Barrington, MA 01230-1906
413-528-3320
800-439-2370
Fax: 413-528-2302
HSDED0585@kindredhealthcare.com
www.greatbarringtonrnc.com

William Kittler, Executive Director
Andrew Potler, Medical Director

Great Barrington Rehabilitation and Nursing Center accomodates 106 residents. As part of a national network of long-term healthcare centers, we have the expertise and resources to provide care appropriate to the individual needs of each and every one of our residents. We provide personal care with minimal daily living assistance to the most skilled treatment for medically complex patients.

7364 Ledgewood Rehabilitation and Skilled Nursing Center
87 Herrick St
Beverly, MA 01915-2773
978-921-1392
800-439-2370
Fax: 978-927-8627
www.ledgewoodrehab.com

Frank Silvia, Executive Director

Ledgewood Rehabilitation and Skilled Nursing Center is a unique provider of healthcare services. We are part of a continuum of services that includes acute care services at Beverly Hospital, subacute care at Ledgewood, and care after discharge through Northeast Homecare. We believe this partnership offers the highest quality post-acute services north of Boston.

7365 Leo P La Chance Center for Rehabilitation and Nursing
59 Eastwood Cir
Gardner, MA 01440-3901
978-632-8776
Fax: 978-632-5048

Mark Alinger, Administrator
Leo P. LaChance, Founder

A privately owned facility, combines the best of medical technology with the ultimate in healing, compassionate rehabilitation and nursing care. Our goal is to help each client reach that ultimate goal of living life to the fullest.

7366 Oakwood Rehabilitation and Nursing Center
11 Pontiac Ave
Webster, MA 01570-1629
508-943-3889
800-439-2370
Fax: 508-949-6125
www.oakwoodrehab.com

Thomas Sullivan, Executive Director

Oakwood Rehabilitation and Nursing Center accomodates 81 residents. We offer 24-hour skilled nursing, inpatient rehabilitation, respite care, and hospice services. Our center has been successfully serving the greater Webster, Massachusetts, community for 35 years. We have a dedicated and caring staff and our common goal is to promote recovery and enhance quality of live whether your needs are short or long term.

7367 Walden Rehabilitation and Nursing Center
785 Main St
Concord, MA 01742-3310
978-369-6889
800-439-2370
Fax: 978-369-8392
HSDED0588@kindredhealthcare.com
www.waldenrehab.com

Ladan Azarm, Executive Director

Walden Rehabilitation and Nursing Center accomodates 123 residents. We are located in the quaint town of Concord, Massachusetts, across the street from Emerson Hospital and a short drive from the town center. Walden provides medical management and long-term care through comprehensive skilled and intermediate nursing services. We also provide physical, occupational, and speech therapy services from an onsite dedicated staff of therapists.

Michigan

7368 Boulder Park Terrace
14676 W Upright St
Charlevoix, MI 49720-1201
231-547-1005
Fax: 231-547-1039

Reezie DeVet, President/CEO
Mary-Anne Ponti, COO

A partnership formed with Charlevoix Area Hospital, Boulder Park Terrace is a long-term care facility and Sub-acute Rehabilitation Center located in Chalrevoix near the shores of Lake Michigan. The Sub-acute Rehabilitation Center was created as a transition between an acute care hospital and home. Patients enter into the program to increase their strength, endurance and over-all functioning before returning home.

Minnesota

7369 Park Health And Rehabilitation Center
4415 W 36 1/2 St
St Louis Park, MN 55416-4890
952-927-9717
Fax: 952-927-7687
park@extendicare.com
www.extendicare.com

Jennifer Kuhn, Administrator

Park Health & Rehabilitation Center is a leading provider of long-term skilled nursing care and short-term rehabilitation solutions. Our 93 bed facility offers a full continuum of services and care focused around each individual in today's ever-changing healthcare environment.

Missouri

7370 Barnes-Jewish Hospital Washington University Medical Center
1 Barnes Jewish Hospital Plz
Saint Louis, MO 63110-1003
314-747-3000
866-867-3627
Fax: 314-362-8877
www.barnesjewish.org

Richard Liekweg, President
John Beatty, Vice President of Human Resources
John Lynch, MD, Chief Medical Officer
David Jaques, MD, Vice President for Surgical Services

Barnes-Jewish Hospital at Washington University Medical Center is the largest hospital in Missouri and the largest private employer in the St. Louis region. An affiliated teaching hospital of Washington University School of Medicine, Barnes-Jewish Hospital has a 1,700 member medical staff with many who are recognized in the 'Best Doctors in America.'

Montana

7371 Parkview Acres Care and Rehabilitation Center
200 N Oregon St
Dillon, MT 59725-3624
406-683-5105
866-253-4090
Fax: 406-683-6388
HSDED0433@kindredhealthcare.com
www.parkviewacres.com

Claire Miller, Executive Director

We are Medicare and Medicaid certified skilled nursing facility which accomodates 108 residents serving scenic Dillon and surrounding Montana communities.

Nebraska

7372   Homestead Healthcare and Rehabilitation Center
4735 S 54th St
Lincoln, NE   68516-1335

402-488-0977
800-833-0920
Fax: 402-488-4507
www.homesteadrehab.com

Matt Romshek, Executive Director
Gay Bate, RN, Director of Nursing
James Murray, Administrator
James Murray,LPN, Clinical Liaison/Admissions
Homestead Healthcare and Rehabilitation Center is one of the area's oldest providers of skilled nursing and rehabilitation services. We are a 163-bed skilled nursing and rehabilitation center nestled in a lovely, quiet established neighborhood in South Lincoln.

7373   Madonna Rehabilitation Hospital
5401 South St
Lincoln, NE   68506-2150

402-413-3000
800-676-5448
Fax: 402-486-5448
info@madonna.org
www.madonna.org

Marsha Lommel, CEO
Tom Stalder, VP Medical Affairs
Madonna provides intensive rehabilitation and expertise for a wide variety of conditions, such as: orthopedic injuries, work injuries, arthritis, amputation, neuromuscular diseases, cardiac conditions, pulmonary disease and conditions including those dependent upon a ventilator, cancer, lymphedema, osteoporosis, wounds, renal disorders, burns, fibromyalgia, multiple sclerosis, parkinson's disease and degenerative diseases.

7374   Mary Lanning Memorial Hospital
715 N Saint Joseph Ave
Hastings, NE   68901-4497

402-463-4521
866-460-5884
tanderson@mlmh.org
www.mlmh.org

Beth Schlichtman, Compensation/Benefit Services - Director
Lisa Brandt, Public Relations & Marketing Services - Director
Carrie Edwards, Home Care Services - Director
Chris Page, Ancillary Services - Director
Mary Lanning Healthcare is in its 95th year of providing quality healthcare for residents of the central Nebraska area. We continue to grow and expand, working to provide patient-centered care in a positive environment, while implementing some of the newest technologies available.

Nevada

7375   Las Vegas Healthcare and Rehabilitation Center
2832 S Maryland Pkwy
Las Vegas, NV   89109-1502

702-735-5848
800-326-6888
Fax: 702-735-6218
www.lasvegaskindred.com

Randall Fuller, Executive Director
Las Vegas Healthcare accomodates 79 residents. We have been serving the community for approximately 40 years. Located in close proximity to local hospitals and surrounded by medical complexes, our center offers both short-term rehabilitation and long-term care.

New Hampshire

7376   Dover Rehabilitation and Living Center
307 Plaza Dr
Dover, NH   03820-2455

603-742-2676
800-735-2964
Fax: 603-749-5375
www.doverrehab.com

Daniel Estee, Executive Director
Dover Rehab is a provider of postacute services in the greater New Hampshire Seacost area. We accomodate 112 residents and are licensed by the state of New Hampshire. We employ nearly 150 licensed nurses, therapists and other healthcare professionals, who strive to provide quality care. The goal of our patient service model is to bridge the gap between hospitalization and home so that recovery and physical functioning are maximized and hospital readmission is minimized.

7377   Northeast Rehabilitation Clinic
70 Butler St
Salem, NH   03079-3925

603-893-2900
800-825-7292
Fax: 603-893-1638
TTY: 800-439-2370
www.northeastrehab.com

John Prochilo, CEO/Administrator
Subacute rehabilitation at NRH was designed for people who have experienced an acutely disabling orthopedic, medical, or neurologic condition but who either do not require or are unable to participate in a full acute inpatient program. Impairment groups pertinent to this level of care include brain injury, spinal cord injury (traumatic/non-traumatic), stroke, orthopedic injury, amputation, and neurologic disorder.

New Jersey

7378   Atlantic Coast Rehabilitation & Healthcare Center
485 River Ave
Lakewood, NJ   08701-4720

732-364-7100
Fax: 732-364-2442
abby@atlanticcoastrehab.com
www.atlanticcoastrehab.com

Simon Shain, Administrator
Sharon Sckbower, Director of Nursing
Atlantic Coast is family owned and operated. It's a warm, friendly place where caregivers and patients know each other by first name. But it's also an innovative and energetic place, where the most advanced therapies and cutting edge techniques are offered. It's a comprehensive health care center that provides three distinct areas of care:Rehabilitative Therapy & Sub Acute Care, Long Term Care ,Alzheimer's/Memory Impaired Care.

7379   Crestwood Nursing & Rehabilitation Center
101 Whippany Rd
Whippany, NJ   7981-1407

973-887-0311
Fax: 973-887-8355

Carol Shepard, Administrator
Sub-acute rehabilitation facility.

7380   Lakeview Subacute Care Center
130 Terhune Dr
Wayne, NJ   7470-7104

973-839-4500
87 -UBA-UTE
Fax: 973-839-2729
www.lakeviewsubacute.com

Richard Grosso, Jr, Director
Sue Ahlers, Director of Admission
Kerry Iamurri, Director of Rehab
Nicole Iacolina, Director Social Services
Our comprehensive medical, nursing and rehabilitation services cater to a diverse patient population. In addition to long-term care, we offer exceptional inpatient subacute programs. We're proud to report that our average length of stay for subacute patients is a brief 14 days.

7381   Merwick Rehabilitation and Sub-Acute Care
79 Bayard Ln
Princeton, NJ   8540-3045   609-497-3000
                                            Fax: 609-497-3024

Ryan Wismer, Administrator
76-bed skilled nursing and residential center as well as a separate
17-bed comprehensive rehabilitation center. Offers rehabilitation, physiatry, occupational therapy, respite care, speech/hear-
ing therapy, sub-acute care.

7382   Seacrest Village Nursing Center
1001 Center St
Little Egg Harbor Twp, NJ   8087-1364   609-296-9292
                                            Fax: 609-296-0508
                                      info@seacrestvillagenj.com
                                           seacrestvillagenj.com

Brian T Holloway, Administrator
Seacrest Village Nursing and Rehabilitation Center has specialized in quality rehabilitation, transitional and restorative care for
more then a decade and is a perfect alternative for bridging the
gap between hospital and home.

7383   St. Lawrence Rehabilitation Center
2381 Lawrenceville Rd
Lawrenceville, NJ   08648-2098   609-896-9500
                                            Fax: 609-895-0242
                                            epiechota@slrc.org
                                                www.slrc.org

Kevin McGuigan, MD, Medical Director
Robyn F. Agri, MD, Doctor
Dr. Madhu Jain, Doctor
Charles Terry MD, Doctor
St. Lawrence Rehabilitation Center, a non-profit facility sponsored by the Roman Catholic Diocese of Trenton, is committed to
maximizing the quality of human life by providing comprehensive physical rehabilitation and related programs to meet the
healthcare needs of our communities.

7384   Summit Ridge Center Genesis Eldercare
20 Summit St
West Orange, NJ   07052-1501   973-736-2000
                                                 800-699-1520
                                            Fax: 973-736-2764
                                          info@genesishcc.com
                                           www.genesishcc.com

Michele Cartagena, Director of Admissions
Elizabeth (L Orlando, Rehabilitation Program Director
Tsega Asefaha, LNHA, BS, MHA, Administrator
Elizabeth Martin, Customer Relations Manager
Summit Ridge Center provides skilled nursing, medical and reha-
bilitative care for patients requiring post-hospital, short stay re-
habilitation and for longer term residents. Our Clinical Care
Teams are focused on implementing your personalized care pro-
gram to facilitate your recovery and improve your well-being.

New York

7385   Beth Abraham Health Services
612 Allerton Ave
Bronx, NY   10467-7495   718-519-4037
                                                 888-238-4223
                                            Fax: 718-547-1366
                                               info@bethabe.org
                                  www.bethabrahamhealthservices.org

Maria Provenzano, Program Director
Yolanda Lester, Director of Admissions
Rosalie Bernard, Director of Nursing Services
Vincent Bonadies, Director of Therapeutic Recreation
Offers the following rehabilitation services: Sub-Acute rehabilitation, brain injury rehabilitation, pain management, post-opera-
tive recovery. Home visits and a network of community-based
programs help patients and their families with a successful
transition home.

7386   Central Island Healthcare
825 Old Country Rd
Plainview, NY   11803-4913   516-433-0600
                                            Fax: 516-868-7251

Michael Ostreicher, Administrator
Serving the community for over 33 years, Central Island
Healthcare is Long Island's largest and most active sub-acute
care provider. We offer comprehensive programs focused on restoring our patients to their maximum potential and returning
home. Central Island's 202-bed facility provides top notch professionals and the latest in rehabilitation and therapeutic equipment in a beautiful and comfortable setting.

7387   Clove Lakes Health Care and Rehabilitation Center
25 Fanning St
Staten Island, NY   10314-5307   718-289-7900
                                            Fax: 718-761-8701
                                           info@clovelakes.com
                                            www.clovelakes.com

Helene Demisay, CEO
Clove Lakes seeks to rehabilitate those who have sustained injury
or illness to the highest level of independence possible and support those with disabling conditions to live meaningful and
productive lives.

7388   Dr. William O Benenson Rehabilitation Pavilion
36-17 Parsons Blvd
Flushing, NY   11354-5931   718-961-4300
                                            Fax: 718-939-5032
                                          www.flushingmanors.com

Esther Benenson, Executive Director
Liza Marie Dowd, Director of Nursing
Erika Rossi, Director of Social Services
Diane Marron, Director of Admissions
The Dr. William O Benson Reahbilitation Pavilion is a subacute
short-term rehabilitation center committed to the excellence of
elevated health care for our patients. Through the use of the most
comprehensive and specialized services available, our staff of
dedicated professionals are devoted to putting patients back to
the road to full recovery 24 hours a day.

7389   Flushing Manor Nursing and Rehab
35-15 Parsons Blvd
Flushing, NY   11354-4297   718-961-3500
                                            Fax: 718-461-1784

Esther Benenson, Executive Director
Dr. Ion Oltean, Medical Director
Myung Chung, Director of Nursing
Bridgett Brown, Director of Admissions
At the Flusing Manor Nursing and Rehabilitation, we stress the
importance of family involvement because it is the true source of
strength and stability in ones life...a tie that brings us all together
as a team, enhancing the quality of life of the patients in our care.

7390   Glengariff Health Care Center
141 Dosoris Ln
Glen Cove, NY   11542   516-676-1100
                                            Fax: 516-759-0216
                                          info@glengariffcare.com
                                             www.glenhaven.org

Jean Campo, Director Admissions
Michael Miness, President
Licensed skilled nursing and subacute medical and rehabilitation
facility.

7391   Haym Salomon Home for The Aged
2340 Cropsey Ave
Brooklyn, NY   11214-5706   718-266-4063
                                            Fax: 718-372-4781

Chain Lipschitz, Administrator
Religious nonmedical health care institution.

7392 Kings Harbor Multicare Center
2000 E Gun Hill Rd
Bronx, NY   10469-6016   718-320-0400
Fax: 718-671-5022
info@kingsharbor.com
www.kingsharbor.com

Morris Tenenbaum, Owner
Octavio Marin, Vice President
Kings Harbor Multicare Center provides long-term and short-term skilled nursing care for more then 700 residents. Kings Harbor is located in the Pelham Gardens neighborhood of Northeast Bronx, easily accessible to major highways and near public transportation. A 3 building campus facility with surrounding gardens ensures that residents with similar capabilities are grouped together.

7393 Northwoods of Cortland
28 Kellogg Rd
Cortland, NY   13045-3155   607-753-9631
Fax: 607-756-2968

Lawrence Mennig, Administrator
Subacute rehabilitation facility.

7394 Port Jefferson Health Care Facility
141 Dosoris Lane
Glen Cove, NY   11542   631-676-1100
Fax: 631-759-0216
www.glengariffcare.com

Ellen Harte, Administrator
Subacute medical and rehabilitative care and long term residential skilled nursing care.

7395 Rehab Institute at Florence Nightingale Health Center
1760 3rd Ave
New York, NY   10029-6810   212-410-8760
800-786-8968
Fax: 212-410-8792

7396 Schnurmacher Center for Rehabilitation and Nursing
Beth Abraham of Family Health Services
12 Tibbits Ave
White Plains, NY   10606-2438   914-287-7200
888-238-4223
Fax: 914-428-1824
info@schnurmacher.org
www.schnurmacher.org

Linda Murray, Executive Director
Thomas Camisa, Medical Director
Iryn Obaldo Fontanosa, Director of Rehabilitation
Filomena Cristo, Director of Therapeutic Recreation
The environment at Schnurmacher is tailored to the needs of patients who require medical and nursing services but who do not need the complexity of services associated with an acute-care hospital. And Schnurmacher Subacute Medical patients are out of bed more quickly and as often as possible, which helps them maintain functional status while recovery progresses.

7397 South Shore Healthcare
275 W Merrick Rd
Freeport, NY   11520-3346   516-623-4000
Fax: 516-223-4599
Winnie Mack, RN, BSN, MPA, Regional Executive Director
Gene Tangney, Senior Vice President/ Regional Executive Director
Michael J. Dowling, President/ CEO
David L. Battinelli, MD, Senior Vice President/Chief Medical Officer
North Shore-LIJ Health System includes 16 award-winning hospitals and nearly 400 physician practice locations throughout New York, including Long Island, Manhattan, Queens and Staten Island. Proudly serving an area of seven million people, North Shore-LIJ delivers world-class services designed for every step of your health and wellness journey.

7398 St. Camillus Health and Rehabilitation Center
813 Fay Rd
Syracuse, NY   13219-3009   315-488-2951
Fax: 315-488-3255
info@st-camillus.org
www.st-camillus.org

Aileen Balitz, President
Patrick VanBeveren, PT, DPT, M, Supervisor of Physical Therapy
Nancy , Pirro, RN, Case Manager
Kathy Walsh,PT, DPT, NCS, Designer/Facilitator
Since our founding in 1969, St. Camillus' mission has been to provide high-quality services and facilities emphasizing the rehabilitation of individuals to their maximum potential. The importance of the human spirit drives all we do. We are dedicated to caring for life and helping individuals achieve their highest possible level of independence.

North Carolina

7399 Chapel Hill Rehabilitation and Healthcare Center
1602 E Franklin St
Chapel Hill, NC   27514-2892   919-967-1418
800-735-8262
Fax: 919-918-3811

Turner Prichett, Executive Director
Chapel Hill Rehabilitation and Healthcare Center accomodates 120 residents. We are located in downtown Chapel Hill on Franklin Street and we provide roud the clock nursing care 365 days a year. Intensive rehabilitation services are administered by our licensed speech, occupational and physical therapists. Our staff is trained to care for medically complex patients such as those requiring intensive wound care, dialysis, and artificial nutrition.

7400 Cypress Pointe Rehabilitation and Healthcare Center
2006 S 16th St
Wilmington, NC   28401-6613   910-763-6271
800-735-8262
Fax: 910-251-9803
www.cypresspointehc.com

Sara Deiter, Executive Director
Dr. Jose Gonzalez, Medical Director
Cypress Pointe offers comprehensive physical, occupational, speech and respiratory therapy services. Following a physician's referral, patients are evaluated to determine their needs. Recommendations are then made for the appropriate interventions and rehabilitation. If therapy is required, a personalized care plan is developed.

7401 Pettigrew Rehabilitation and Healthcare Center
1551 W Pettigrew St
Durham, NC   27705-4821   919-286-0751
800-735-8262
Fax: 919-286-5992

La'Ticia Beatty, Executive Director
Pettigrew Rehabilitation and Healthcare Center accomodates 107 residents. Our healthcare center is certified by Medicare and Medicaid. We have experienced staff members who care for our residents. We strive to improve the quality of life our residents experience as a result of the services they receive from our nursing and therapy departments.

7402 Raleigh Rehabilitation and Healthcare Center
616 Wade Ave
Raleigh, NC   27605-1237   919-828-6251
800-735-8262
Fax: 919-828-3294
www.raleighrehabhc.com

Steven Jones, Executive Director
Raleigh Rehabilitation and Healthcare Center accomodates 172 residents. We provide short-term rehabilitation-including, physical, occupational, and speech therapies-as well as long-term nursing services. We specialize in neurological disorders, complex diabetes treatment, amputation recovery and pain management. We welcome short stays (respite care). Transportation services are availiable for physician appointments and dialysis treatments.

7403 Rehabilitation and Healthcare Center of Monroe
1212 E Sunset Dr
Monroe, NC 28112-4318   704-283-8548
                                          800-735-8262
                                    Fax: 704-283-4664
                    HSDED0707@kindredhealthcare.com
Judy Olson, Executive Director
We accomodate 159 residents and are certified for Medicare and
Medicaid. We specialize in short-term rehabilitation as well as
long-term care. Our therapists, wound nurse and dietician work
closely to administer wound care. We hav 2 dialysis centers
within a 10-block radius and gladly accpet their patients. We have
an on-staff medical director as well as a psychiatrist.

7404 Winston-Salem Rehabilitation and Healthcare Center
1900 W 1st St
Winston Salem, NC 27104-4220   336-724-2821
                                          800-735-8262
                                    Fax: 336-725-8314
Tom Bauer, Administrator
We accommodate 230 residents and we have approximately 250
employees. Our staffing ratio averages 1 licensed nurse for every
20 residents and 1 Certified Nursing Assistant for every 10 residents. We offer a wide range of services including but not limited
to respiratory care, tracheotomy care and gastric tube feeding and
we also feature an in house licensed therapy program.

Ohio

7405 Arbors East Subacute and Rehabilitation Center
5500 E Broad St
Columbus, OH 43213-1476   614-575-9003
                                    Fax: 614-575-9101
                           arborseast@extendicare.com
                       www.arborseastskillednursing.com

7406 Arbors at Canton Subacute And Rehabilitation Center
2714 13th St NW
Canton, OH 44708-3121   330-456-2842
                                    Fax: 330-456-5343
                              www.laurelsofcanton.com
Amy McDermand, Director of Marketing
Beth Jones, PT, DPT, Rehabilitation Services Director
Cindy Shingler, RN,, Director of Nursing
Jennifer Fess, Administrator
We provide individualized, quality care to guests staying
short-term for rehabilitation services or long-term for extended
care services. The highest level of independence for our guests is
the creed of The Laurels of Canton.

7407 Arbors at Dayton
320 Albany St
Dayton, OH 45408-1402   937-496-6200
                                    Fax: 937-496-1990
                             dayton@extendicare.com
                        www.extendicareus.com/dayton
Dave Maxwell, Administrator
Carlisa Pedalino, Administrator
Arbors at Dayton is a leading provider of long-term skilled nursing care and short-term rehabilitation solutions. Our 106 bed facility offers a full continuum of services and care focused around
each individual in today's ever-changing healthcare
environment.

7408 Arbors at Marietta
400 N 7th St
Marietta, OH 45750-2024   740-373-3597
                                    Fax: 740-376-0004
                            marietta@extendicare.com
                       www.extendicareus.com/marietta
Joan Florence, Director of Nursing
Kenneth Leopold, Medical Director
Arbors at Marietta is a leading provider of long-term skilled nurs-
ing care and short-term rehabilitation solutions. Our 150 bed fa-
cility offers a full continuum of services and care focused around

each individual in today's ever-changing healthcare
environment.

7409 Arbors at Milford
5900 Meadow Creek Dr
Milford, OH 45150-5641   513-248-1655
                                    Fax: 513-248-7340
                             milford@extendicare.com
                        www.extendicareus.com/milford
Bruce Yarwood, President/CEO
Mark Ostendorf, Administrator
Arbors at Milford is a leading provider of long-term skilled nursing care and short-term rehabilitation solutions. Our 139 bed facility offers a full continuum of services and care focused around
each individual in today's ever-changing healthcare
environment.

7410 Arbors at Sylvania
7120 Port Sylvania Dr
Toledo, OH 43617-1158   419-841-2200
                                    Fax: 419-841-2822
                            sylvania@extendicare.com
                       www.extendicareus.com/sylvania
Sheril Flowers, Administrator
Graig Hopple, Medical Director
Arbors at Sylvania is a leading provider of long-term skilled nursing care and short-term rehabilitation solutions. Our 79 bed facility offers a full continuum of services and care focused around
each individual in today's ever-changing healthcare
environment.

7411 Arbors at Toledo Subacute and Rehab Centre
2920 Cherry St
Toledo, OH 43608-1716   419-242-7458
                                    Fax: 419-242-6514
                                    www.extendicare.com
Jill Schlievert, Administrator
Subacute rehabilitation services and facility.

7412 Bridgepark Center for Rehabilitation and Nursing Services
145 Olive St
Akron, OH 44310-3236   330-762-0901
                                          800-750-0750
                                    Fax: 330-762-0905
Joseph Burick, Medical Director
A skilled nursing and rehabilitation center located in Akron,
Ohio, across the street from St. Thomas Hospital with a beautiful
view of the Akron skyline. Access to Interstate 77 and State Route
8 is just minutes away. Our entire staff is committed to providing
caring, customer-focused skilled nursing and rehabilitation. For
your convenience, we accept Medicare, Medicaid and most managed care and private insurance.

7413 Broadview Multi-Care Center
5520 Broadview Rd
Parma, OH 44134-1605   216-749-4010
                                    Fax: 216-749-0141
                          info@broadviewmulticare.com
                            www.broadviewmulticare.com
Harold Shachter, Owner
Mike Flank, VP
Broadview Multi-Care Center is a family run business with more
than 40 years of experience providing quality care to the community. We are committed to meeting your needs and providing you
with a warm, home-like environment. Our family is on-site and
our doors are always open for your suggestions or to drop in and
say hello. We always try to take and honor requests, whether it's a
favorite food, an exciting activity or a particular room.

7414 Caprice Care Center
9184 Market St
North Lima, OH 44452-9558
330-965-9200
Fax: 330-726-6097
capriceadm@chcccompanies.com
www.chcccompanies.com

Lori Crowl, Owner
Becky Berger, Director of Nursin
Stacey Howell, Administrator
Valerie Conzett, Admission Liaison
A 106-bed skilled nursing, subacute and rehabilitation facility. Our goal is to provide comfortable living to all who are in our care. Caprice Health Care Center is a contemporary Medicare and Medicaid approved facility specializing in short-term rehabilitation services. The inpatient/outpatient rehab department includes physical, occupational, speech therapies, indoor aquatic therapy pool, as well as complimentary van transportation for outpatient services.

7415 Cleveland Clinic
9500 Euclid Ave
Cleveland, OH 44195-2
216-444-2200
800-801-2273
Fax: 216-444-7021
my.clevelandclinic.org/default.aspx

Gene Altus, Executive Director
Delos M. Cosgrove, MD, Chief Executive Officer, Preside
Joseph F. Hahn, MD, Chief of Staff, Vice Chairman of
David Bronson, MD, Chief Executive Officer, Clevela
A not-for-profit, multispecialty academic medical center that integrates clinical and hospital care with research and education. Cleveland clinic was founded in 1921 by 4 renowned physicians with a vision of providing outstanding patient care based upon the principals of cooperation, compassion and innovation. Today, Cleveland Clinic is one of the largest and most respected hospitals in the country.

7416 Columbus Rehabilitation And Subacute Institute
111 West Michigan Street
Milwaukee, WI 53203-2903
800-395-5000
kschaewe@extendicare.com
www.extendicareus.com

Kelly Fligor, Administrator
Jillian Fountain, Secretary
Subacute rehabilitation programs and facility.

7417 LakeMed Nursing and Rehabilitation Center
70 Normandy Dr
Painesville, OH 44077-1616
440-357-1311
800-750-0750
Fax: 440-352-9977
www.lakemednursing.com

Connie Eyman, Administrator
Vesta Jones, Executive Director
Our goal is to provide you with quality care and we are known for our successful short-term rehab and care of the clinically complex. We also offer respite services to give caregivers a rest, and hospice services through our local hospice care provider. Our interdisciplinary team works together as they strive to deliver quality care and responsive service to our residents.

7418 Oregon Nursing And Rehabilitation Center
904 Isaac Streets Dr
Oregon, OH 43616-3204
419-691-2483
Fax: 419-697-5401
www.extendicareus.com/oregon

Mark Rogers, Administrator
Subacute rehabilitation facility and services.

7419 Sunset View Castle Nursing Homes Castle Nursing Homes
434 N Washington St
Millersburg, OH 44654-1188
330-674-0015
Fax: 330-763-2238

Becky Snyder, Admissions Coordinator
Kathy Edwards, Admissions And Marketing
310 licensed, certified beds. Subacute rehabilitation facility and programs.

Oregon

7420 Care Center East Health & Specialty Care Center
Expendicare
11325 NE Weidler St
Portland, OR 97220-1950
503-253-1181
Fax: 503-253-1871
www.extendicareus.com

Glydon Kimbrough, Administrator
Subacute rehabilitation facility and programs

7421 Medford Rehabilitation and Healthcare Center
Kindred Healthcare
625 Stevens St
Medford, OR 97504-6719
541-779-3551
800-735-1232
Fax: 541-779-3658

Grant Gloor, Administrator
Dane Reeves, Executive Director
Kristen W., Health and Rehabilitation Center
Becky D., Activity Director
We strive to provide quality, compassionate care. Our cozy building accomodates 110 residents. Our smaller size creates an inviting and homelike environment. We offer semi-private rooms with space to add items from home for a special personalized touch.

Pennsylvania

7422 Dresher Hill Health and Rehabilitation Center
1390 Camp Hill Rd
Dresher, PA 19034-2805
215-643-0600
Fax: 215-641-0628
www.dresherhillskillednursing.com

Earl Kimble, Administrator
Subacute rehabilitation facility and programs: physical/speech.

7423 Good Shepherd Rehabilitation
850 S 5th St
Allentown, PA 18103-3295
610-776-3586
888-447-3422
Fax: 610-776-8336
goodshepherdrehab.org

John Kristel, MBA, MPT, President & CEO
Mike Bonner, MBA, Vice President, Neurosciences
Ronald J. Petula, CPA, Senior Vice President, Finance and Chief Financial Officer
Joseph Shadid, Administrator, Good Shepherd Home-Bethlehem
A world class rehabilitation network, Good Shepherd provides comprehensive inpatient and outpatient services throughout Pennsylvania's Lehigh Valley. Founded in 1908, Good Shepherd has steadily expanded over last 95 years. Good Shepherd is one of the most comprehensive rehabilitation institutes in the world.

7424 Statesman Health and Rehabilitation Center
2629 Trenton Rd
Levittown, PA 19056-1428
215-943-7777
Fax: 215-943-1240
www.statesmanskillednursing.com

Jamie Tanner, Administrator
Subacute rehabilitation facility and programs.

7425 UPMC Braddock
200 Lothrop St.
Pittsburgh, PA 15213-2582
412-647-8762
800-533-8762
Fax: 412-636-5398
hospitalbill@upmc.edu
upmc.com

Mark Sevco, Administrator
Rodney Jones, Vice President
With a team of more then 43,000 employees, UPMC serves the health needs of more then 4 million people each year, improving lives in western Pennsylvania-and beyond-through redefined models of health care delivery and superb clinical outcomes.

7426 UPMC McKeesport
Presby
1500 5th Ave
McKeesport, PA 15132-2422   412-664-2000
Fax: 412-664-2309
fisherpj@upmc.edu
upmc.com

Ronald H Ott, CEO
Offers 56 beds for patients who need skilled nursing care. Offers ongoing rehabilitation and educational programs to patients with cardiac, neurologic, and orthopaedic diagnosis.

7427 UPMC Passavant
9100 Babcock Blvd
Pittsburgh, PA 15237-5842   412-367-6700
800-533-8762
gloordc@ph.upmc.edu
upmc.com

William Kristan, Dir Inpatient Physical Therapy
Teresa Petrick, Chief Executive Officer
Patients who have had an acute illness, injury, or exacerbation of a disease and no longer need the intensity of services in the acute care setting, but still require some complex medical care or supervision and rehabilitation services, may be appropriate to be transferred into the Subacute Unit.

Rhode Island

7428 Kindred Heights Nursing & Rehabilitation Center
Kindred Healthcare
680 South Fourth Street
Louisville, KY 40202   502-596-7300
800-545-0749
web_administrator@kindred.com
www.kindredheights.com

Sandra Sarza, Manager
Jean Aubin, Director
Kindred Heights Nursing and Rehabilitation Center accomodates 58 residents and serves the needs of elders in the greater East Bay and Providence area. We are conveniently located on Wampanoag Trail in East Providence. Kindred Heights provides skilled nursing, short-term rehab and long-term care in a family environment, but we are large enough to manage the complex nursing and rehab care needs our residents may have.

7429 Oak Hill Nursing and Rehabilitation Center
Kindered Health Care
544 Pleasant St
Pawtucket, RI 02860-5776   401-725-8888
800-745-6575
Fax: 401-723-5720
www.oakhillrehab.com

Scott M. Sandborn, Executive Director
Heidi Capela, Director Nursing
Amybeth Almeida, Director Admissions
Aman Nanda, Medical Director
Accomodates 143 residents. Throughout our 40 year history, Oak Hill has developed a reputation as one of the finest healthcare centers in Rhode Island. Our center consists of 3 separate units. A 34-bed post-acute unit provides care to the medically complex and those in need of extensive rehabilitative services. A 20-bed Alzheimer's Special Care Unit provides a unique style of care utilizing habilitative therapy in comfortable, home-like surroundings.

7430 Southern New England Rehab Center
200 High Service Avenue
North Providence, RI 02904   401-456-3801
888-456-4501
Fax: 401-456-3784
www.snerc.com

Vivian Hagstrom, Manager
The Center's skilled staff of over 100 professionals provides a full range of coordinated rehabilitative care. Our clinical expertise and compassion make a big difference as we develop first-rate plans of care for the unique needs of each patient. Our medical staff is comprised of physicians board-certified in rehabilitation medicine and internal medicine.

South Carolina

7431 Tuomey Healthcare System
129 N Washington St
Sumter, SC 29150-4949   803-774-9000
Fax: 803-774-8737
www.tuomey.com

R Jay Cox, CEO
Here to anticipte the needs of the communities we serve, responding with proactive healthcare initiatives, providing expert rehabilitative services and delivering life-saving acute care.

Tennessee

7432 Camden Healthcare and Rehabilitation Center
680 South Fourth Street
Louisville, KY 40202   502-596-7300
800-545-0749
web_administrator@kindred.com
kindredhealthcare.com

Mark Walker, Administrator
Subacute rehabilitation products and services, nursing and life care homes.

7433 Centennial Medical Center Tri Star Health System
2300 Patterson St
Nashville, TN 37203-1538   615-342-1000
800-242-5662
Fax: 615-342-1045
Laurel.Haskamp@HCAHealthcare.com
tristarcentennial.com

Thomas L Herron, President/Chief Executive Office
Above all else we are committed to the care and improvement of human life by caring for those we serve with integrity, compassion, a positive attitude, respect and exceptional quality.

7434 Cordova Rehabilitation and Nursing Center
955 N Germantown Pkwy
Cordova, TN 38018-6215   901-754-1393
800-848-0299
Fax: 901-754-3332
cdadmi@gracehc.com
www.gracehccordova.com

John Palmer, Administrator
Renee Tutor, Executive Director
Our professional staff can help you make an informed decision. Upon admission, our interdisciplinary team develops a comprehensive care plan to meet not only physical and rehabilitative goals, but also social and emotional needs. We understand the importance of family and resident involvement and encourage participation in the development of a personalized plan of care.

7435 Erlanger Medical Center Baronness Campus
975 E 3rd St
Chattanooga, TN 37403-2147   423-778-7000
Fax: 423-778-7615
guestrelations@erlanger.org
www.erlanger.org

Kevin M. Spiegel, FACHE, President and CEO
James Creel, MD, Chief Medical Officer
Gregg T. Gentry, Chief Administrative Officer
Robert M. Brooks, FACHE, Executive Vice President and Chief Operating Officer
Our mission is to improve the health of the people we touch. Our vision is to be recognized locally, regionally, and and nationally, as a premiere healthcare system.

7436 Huntington Health and Rehabilitation Center
635 High St
Huntingdon, TN 38344-1703 731-986-8943
Fax: 731-986-3188
w.summers@huntingdonhealth.com
huntingdonhealth.com

Heidi Hawkins, Administrator
Windi Summers, Admissions Director
Subacute rehabilitation facility and programs.

7437 Madison Healthcare and Rehabilitation Center
431 Larkin Springs Rd
Madison, TN 37115-5005 615-865-8520
800-848-0299
Fax: 615-868-4455
Phyllis Cherry, Executive Director
At our facility, we provide quality care with modern rehabilitation and restorative nursing techniques. We aim to provide an atmosphere which encourages family involvement in the care-planning process, with the right mix of activities addressing the social, spiritual and intellectual needs of our residents.

7438 Mariner Health of Nashville
3939 Hillsboro Cir
Nashville, TN 37215-2708 615-297-2100
Fax: 615-297-2197

David Reeves, Administrator
Amy Artrip, Director of Nursing
Religious nonmedical health care institution. 150-bed subacute rehabilitation facility

7439 Pine Meadows Healthcare and Rehabilitation Center
700 Nuckolls Rd
Bolivar, TN 38008-1531 731-658-4707
Fax: 731-658-4769
s.mckeen@pinemeadowshc.com
www.pinemeadowshc.com
Larry Shrader, Administrator
Sharon McKeen, Admissions Director
Our goal is to take care of your loved ones. Our professional team works with skilled hands, is directed by creative minds and is guided by compassionate hearts. Upon your admission, our interdisciplinary team develops a comprehensive care plan designed with a goal of meeting not only physical and rehabilitative objectives, but also social and emotional needs. We understand the importance of family and resident involvement and encourage participation in the development of a plan of care.

7440 Primacy Healthcare and Rehabilitation Center
Kindred Health Care
6025 Primacy Pkwy
Memphis, TN 38119-5763 901-767-1040
800-848-0299
Fax: 901-685-7362
Donnie Dubert, Executive Director
Dr. Mark Hammond, Medical Director
Kristen W., Health and Rehabilitation Center
Becky D., Activity Director
Upon a resident's admission, our interdisciplinary team develops a comprehensive care plan with a goal of meeting not only physical and rehabilitative objectives but also social and emotional needs. We understand the importance of family and resident involvement and encourage participation in the development of a personalized plan of care.

7441 Ripley Healthcare and Rehabilitation Center
118 Halliburton St
Ripley, TN 38063-2011 731-635-5180
Fax: 731-635-0663
j.hodge@ripleyhc.com
www.ripleyhc.com
Johnny Rea, Executive Director
Brandon Whiteside, Executive Director
Jan Hodge, Admissions Directo
Jennifer Pitts, Administrator
Upon admission, our interdisciplinary team develops a comprehensive care plan to meet not only physical and rehabilitative goals, but also social and emotional needs. We understand the importance of family and resident involvement and encourage participation in the development of a personalized care plan. Our goal is to take care of your loved ones.

7442 Shelby Pines Rehabilitation and Healthcare Center
3909 Covington Pike
Memphis, TN 38135-2281 901-377-1011
Fax: 901-377-0032
Rene Tutor, Executive Director
Subacute rehabiltation facility and programs.

7443 Siskin Hospital for Physical Rehabilitation
1 Siskin Plz
Chattanooga, TN 37403-1306 423-634-1200
Fax: 423-634-4538
TTY:423-634-1201
info@siskinrehab.org
siskinrehab.org
Robert Main, CEO
Lindsay Wyatt, Media Coordinator, Marketing Co
Dedicated exclusively to physical rehabilitation and offers specialized treatment programs in brain injury, amputation, stroke, spinal cord injury, orthopeadics, and major multiple trauma.

Texas

7444 North Hills Hospital
4401 Booth Calloway Rd
North Richland Hills, TX 76180-7399 817-255-1000
Fax: 817-255-1991
northhillshospital.com
Randy Moresi, CEO
North Hills Hospital's services include a wide range of cardiovascular services, surgical services, emergency services, radiology, a rehabilitation unit, a senior health center, therapy services, and women's services.

7445 Valley Regional Medical Center
100 E Alton Gloor Blvd
Brownsville, TX 78526-3328 956-350-7000
Fax: 956-350-7111
valleyregionalmedicalcenter.com
Susan Andrews, CEO
Francisco Javier Del Castillo, MD
Subramaniam Anandasivam, MD
Christopher Olson, MD
Above all else, we are committed to the care and improvement of human life. In recognition of this committment, we strive to deliver high quality, cost effective healthcare in the communities we serve. In persuit of our mission, we recognize and affirm the unique and intrinsic worth of each individual. We treat all those we serve with compassion and kindness. We act with absolute honesty and integrity and fairness in the way we conduct our business and the way we live our lives.

Utah

7446 Crosslands Rehabilitation and Healthcare Center
680 South Fourth Street
Louisville, KY 40202 502-596-7300
800-545-0749
web_administrator@kindred.com
www.kindredhealthcare.com
John Williams, Executive Director
Lyle Black, Manager
Crossroads Rehabilitation and Healthcare accomodates 120 residents. We are fully Medicare and Medicaid certified. We are proud of our reputation for providing quality, compassionate care. Services availiable include in-house physical, occupational and speech therapies, as well as 24-hour licensed nursing staff coverage. We offer therapeutic recreation, in-house social services and registered dietician services, among many other professional services.

7447 Federal Heights Rehabilitation and Nursing Center
Kindred Health Care
680 South Fourth Street
Louisville, KY 40202
502-596-7300
800-545-0749
web_administrator@kindred.com
www.kindredhealthcare.com

Pete Zeigler, Executive Director
Dr. Charles Canfield, Medical Director
Federal Heights accomodates 120 residents. We are located near three major hospitals in the Salt Lake Valley. We specialize in providing nursing services for complex medical and rehabilitation conditions. Our discharge planning works jointly with the family and resident in determining the future needs and goals upon discharge.

7448 St. George Care and Rehabilitation Center
Kindred Health Care Publications
1032 E 100 S
Saint George, UT 84770-3005
435-628-0488
800-346-4128
Fax: 435-628-7362
www.stgeorgecare.com

John Larson, Plant Manager
Erin Hammon, Director of Nursing
Derrick Glum, Executive Director
St. George Care and Rehabilitation accomodates 95 residents. We offer a 4,000 square foot rehabilitation gym with an indoor therapy pool for inpatient and outpatient services. Therapy is provided to meet specific needs seven days a week. There is a dietitian on staff for individualized nutritional needs. We offer an Alzheimer's unit with specialized staff. We provide compassionate health services including physicians, nurses, physical therapists, and occupational therapist and licensed aides.

7449 St. Mark's Hospital
1200 E 3900 S
Salt Lake City, UT 84124-1390
801-268-7111
Fax: 801-270-3489
www.stmarkshospital.com

Steve B. Bateman, CEO
Above all else we are committed to the care and improvement of human life. In recognition of this commitment, we strive to deliver high quality, cost effective healthcare in the communities we serve. We define quality as 'caring people with the commitment to a continuous process of improvement in the services provided, that will better enable the hospital to meet or exceed our customer's needs and expectations.

7450 Wasatch Valley Rehabilitation
Kindred Healthcare
680 South Fourth Street
Louisville, KY 40202
502-596-7300
800-545-0749
web_administrator@kindred.com
www.kindredhealthcare.com

Alex Stevenson, Executive Director
Ric Toomer, Executive Director
Wasatch Valley accomodates 110 residents. We are licensed for Medicare and Medicaid and we are conveniently located in the heart of Salt Lake City with easy access from I-15 and I-215. We are known by the area hospitals as a specialist in wound care and for the care we provide to those with complex medical conditions.

Virginia

7451 Nansemond Pointe Rehabilitation and Healthcare Center
200 Constance Rd
Suffolk, VA 23434-4960
757-539-8744
800-828-1140
Fax: 757-539-6128
www.nansemondhc.com

Mel Epelle, Executive Director
Mary R, Activities Assistant
Kristen W., Health and Rehabilitation Center
Becky D., Activity Director

Nansemond Pointe Rehabilitation and Healthcare Center accomodates 160 residents in private and semi-private rooms. We have been serving the needs of Suffolk, Virginia and the surrounding areas for over 38 years. We offer an entire continuum of care from assisted living apartments to skilled nursing to long-term care. Our licensed therapists, working with our dedicated nursing staff, share a common goal- to help our residents improve their level of recovery and independence.

7452 Rehabilitation and Research Center Virginia Commonwealth University
1250 East Marshall Street
Richmond, VA 23298
804-828-9000
Fax: 804-828-5074
www.vcuhealth.org

Michael Rao, Ph.D., VCU President & VCUHS President,
Sheldon M. Retchin, M.D., VP Health Sciences & CEO, VCUHS
John Duval, Chief Executive Officer MCV Hosp
Dominic J. Puleo, Executive VP Finance and CFO, VC
The Rehabilitation and Research Center is a collaborative effort between the Department of Physical Medicine and Rehabilitation and the Medical College of Virginia Hospitals. The goals of the Rehabilitation and Research Center at the Medical College of Virginia Hospitals (MCVH) are to provide highly-skilled, interdisciplinary, inpatient rehabilitative care to adults with complex needs; to be an advocate and educator for patients and people with disabilities.

7453 Warren Memorial Hospital
1000 N Shenandoah Ave
Front Royal, VA 22630-3598
540-636-0300
800-994-6610
Fax: 540-636-0258
complaint@jointcommission.org
www.valleyhealthlink.com

Mark H. Merrill, President & Chief Executive Officer
Tonya Smith, Vice President of Operations
Pete Gallagher, Senior Vice President & CFO
Joan Roscoe, Vice President of Information Sy
A nonprofit organization of health care providers, Valley Health offers a full spectrum of services in acute care, rehabilitation and extended care facilities, and outpatient and community settings to help the people of the region manage their health and enjoy a high quality of life. Valley Health has the resources to diagnose, treat and help patients manage virtually any medical problem that may be encountered.

7454 Winchester Rehabilitation Center
333 W Cork St
Suite 230
Winchester, VA 22601-3870
540-536-5114
800-994-6610
Fax: 540-536-1122
complaint@jointcommission.org
www.valleyhealthlink.com

Mark H. Merrill, President & Chief Executive Officer
Tonya Smith, Vice President of Operations
Pete Gallagher, Senior Vice President & CFO
Joan Roscoe, Vice President of Information Sy
Offers the following rehabilitation services: Sub-Acute inpatient rehabilitation, Speech therapy, Physical therapy, Occupational therapy, Disability evaluations. 30-bed inpatient center.

Washington

7455 Aldercrest Health and Rehabilitation Center
21400 72nd Ave W
Edmonds, WA 98026-7702
425-775-1961
Fax: 425-771-0116
aldercrest@extendicare.com
www.aldercrestskillednursing.com

Rick Milsow, Administrator
Aldercrest Health & Rehabilitation Center is a leading provider of long-term skilled nursing care and short-term rehabilitation solutions. Our 124 bed facility offers a full continuum of services

and care focused around each individual in today's ever-changing healthcare environment.

7456   Arden Rehabilitation and Healthcare Center
16357 Aurora Ave N
Seattle, WA 98133-5651
206-542-3103
800-833-6384
Fax: 206-542-7192
www.ardenrehab.com

Matthew Preston, Administrator
Ann Zell, Executive Director
Kristen W., Health and Rehabilitation Center
Becky D., Activity Director
Arden Rehabilitation has been an integral part of the Shoreline community since 1953. It is a one-level building set on mature grounds with several beautiful courtyards for the residents to enjoy. Arden can accomodate 90 residents-post acute/rehabilitation patients as well as long-term residents. Medicare certified, the center also takes most managed healthcare insurance plans, as well as VA, respite and hospice patients.

7457   Bellingham Health Care and Rehabilitation Services
1200 Birchwood Ave
Bellingham, WA 98225-1302
360-734-9295
800-833-6384
Fax: 360-671-4368
www.avamererehabofbellingham.com

Melissa Nelson, Executive Director
Dr. Richard McClenahan, Medical Director
Kristen W., Health and Rehabilitation Center
Becky D., Activity Director
At Bellingham Health Care and Rehab, we strive to provide quality, compassionate care. Our cozy building accomodates 84 residents. Our smaller size creates an inviting and homelike environment for your loved one. We offer semi-private rooms with space to add items from home for a special personalized touch. Provides meals served restaurant style in our dinning room overlooking our beautiful grounds.

7458   Bremerton Convalescent and Rehabilitation Center
2701 Clare Ave
Bremerton, WA 98310-3313
360-377-3951
Fax: 360-377-5443
bremertonskillednursing.com
Stephanie Bonanzino, Administrator
Subacute rehabilitation facility and programs.

7459   Edmonds Rehabilitation & Healthcare Centerer
Kindred Healthcare
21008 76th Ave W
Edmonds, WA 98026-7104
425-778-0107
800-833-6384
Fax: 425-776-9532
Jane Davis, Executive Director
At Edmonds Rehabilitation and Healthcare, we strive to provide quality, compassionate care. Our center accomodates 91 residents. Our smaller size creates an inviting and homelike environment. We offer semi-private rooms with space to add items from home for a special personalized touch. Edmonds Rehabilitation and Healthcare provides delicious meals served restaurant style in our dinning room.

7460   Heritage Health and Rehabilitation Center
Kindred Health Care
3605 Y St
Vancouver, WA 98663-2647
360-693-5839
800-833-6384
Fax: 360-693-3991
www.heritagerehab.com
Michael Moses, Executive Director
Su Patchett, Director of Nursing
Heritage Health & Rehabilitation Center is the smallest free-standing healthcare center in southwest Washington with accomodations of 49, enabling more personal care and a more home-like environment. Heritage has licensed nursing staff, restorative aides, and certified nurses assistants, trained and experienced in providing Alzheimer's care, end of life/hospice care, psychiatric care, rehabilitative care, and respite care.

7461   North Auburn Rehabilitation And Health Center
111 West Michigan Street
Milwaukee, WI 53203-2903
800-395-5000
kschaewe@extendicare.com
extendicare.com
Allyson Jenkins, Administrator
Subacute rehabilitation facility and programs.

7462   Northwoods Lodge
2321 NW Schold Pl
Silverdale, WA 98383-9504
360-698-3930
Fax: 360-692-2169
mhalverson@encorecommunities.com
www.encorecommunities.com
Leslie Krueger, Owner
Debbie Griffin, Director of Rehab Services
Silverdale Campus, Executive Director
Provides you with a full-range of services from weekly housekeeping and laudry services, to grounds keeping and maintenance. Our monthy fee inculdes utilities and hot, delicious, nutritious meals served table side every day. We offer transportation services, full-time activities directors, and numerous amenities to add to your comfort and enjoyment.

7463   Pacific Specialty & Rehabilitation Center r
1015 N Garrison Rd
Vancouver, WA 98664-1313
360-694-7501
Fax: 360-694-8148
www.pacificskillednursing.com
Rebecca Pruett, Administrator
Subacute rehabilitation facility and programs.

7464   Puget Sound Healthcare Center
4001 Capitol Mall Dr SW
Olympia, WA 98502-8657
360-754-9792
Fax: 360-754-2455
www.pugetsoundskillednursing.com
Sheila Oberg, Administrator
Our goal is to provide excellence in patient care, veteran's benefits and customer satisfaction. We have reformed our department internally and are striving for high quality, prompt and seamless service to veterans. Our department employees continue to offer their dedication and commitment to help veterans get the services they have earned.

7465   Vancouver Health & Rhabilitation Center
400 E 33rd St
Vancouver, WA 98663-2238
360-696-2561
800-833-6384
Fax: 360-696-9275
www.vancouverhealthcare.com
Jody Wigen, Human Resources
Joe Joy, Executive Director
Kristen W., Health and Rehabilitation Center
Becky D., Activity Director
At Vancouver Health and Rehab Center we strive to provide quality, compassionate care. Our cozy building accomodates 98 residents. Our smaller size creates an inviting and homelike environment. We offer semi-private rooms with space to add items from home for a special personalized touch. Provides delicious meals served restaurant style in our dining room.

West Virginia

7466   War Memorial Hospital
1 Healthy Way
Berkeley Springs, WV 25411-1743
304-258-1234
Fax: 304-258-5618
complaint@jointcommission.org
www.valleyhealthlink.com
Mark H. Merrill, President & Chief Executive Officer
Tonya Smith, Vice President of Operations
Pete Gallagher, Senior Vice President & Chief Financial Officer
Joan Roscoe, Vice President of Information Systems
Offers physical therapy, occupational therapy, speech therapy, social services, and patient/family education for individuals who

have experienced a recent physical disability due to disease, dysfunction, or general debilitation. Helps patients to maximize their abilities through activities of daily living, mobility, self-medication, and self-care and restore their ability to return to their previous lifestyle.

Wisconsin

7467 Cedar Spring Health and Rehabilitation Center
N27w5707 Lincoln Blvd
Cedarburg, WI 53012-2852   262-376-7676
                                           Fax: 262-376-7808
                              www.cedarspringsskillednursing.com
Mary Wirth, Executive Director
Subacute rehabilitation facility and programs.

7468 Clearview-Brain Injury Center
198 Home Rd
Juneau, WI   53039-1401   920-386-3400
                                               877-386-3400
                                           Fax: 920-386-3800
Jane E. Hooper, Administrator
Jacqueline Kuhl, Household Coordinator
Laura Bertagnoli
Kathy Lorenz, AFH Manager
A 30-bed, state certified, subacute neuro-rehabilitation program in Juneau, WI. We are located just 45 minutes northeast of Madison WI and 10 minutes east of Beaver Dam, WI. We are the first and longest standing of only 2 community re-entry programs in the state of Wisconsin providing subacute neuro-rehabilitation to teens and adults who have experienced a brain injury.

7469 Colonial Manor Medical and Rehabilitation Center
1010 E Wausau Ave
Wausau, WI   54403-3101   715-842-2028
                                               800-947-6644
                                           Fax: 715-848-0510
                                  www.colonialmanormrc.com
Ericca Ylitalo, Administrator
Shelley Solberg, Executive Director
Kristen W., Health and Rehabilitation Center
Becky D., Activity Director
Colonial Manor Medical and Rehabilitation Center is part of the Kindred Community and is located in Wausau, Wisconsin. The corporate headquarters are based in Louisville Kentucky. Our facility accomodates 150 residents.

7470 Eastview Medical and Rehabilitation Center
729 Park St
Antigo, WI   54409-2745   715-623-2356
                                               800-947-6644
                                           Fax: 715-623-6345
Wanda Hose, Administrator
Wanda Hose, Executive Director
Kristen W., Health and Rehabilitation Center
Becky D., Activity Director
Eastview Medical Center and Rehabilitation Center accomodates 165 residents. We are Medicare and Medicaid certified, as well as being Joint Commission accredited. Our 'TEAM' approach means specially trained staff work around the clock to assist in meeting rehabilitative goals established by our team of professionals. We encourage family involvement in our rehabilitative process. The support of loved ones is a major key to a speedy recovery.

7471 Hospitality Nursing Rehabilitation Center
8633 32nd Ave
Kenosha, WI   53142-5187   262-694-8300
                                           Fax: 262-694-3622
                              www.hospitalityskillednursing.com
Marla Benson, Administrator
LaRae Nelson, President
Lisa Behling, Secretary
Scott Miller, Treasurer
Subacute rehabilitation facility and programs.

7472 Kennedy Park Medical Rehabilitation Center
Kindred Healthcare
6001 Alderson St
Schofield, WI 54476-3614   715-359-4257
                                               800-947-6644
                                           Fax: 715-355-4867
                              info@kennedyparkrehab.com
                              www.kennedyparkrehab.com
Judy Kowalski, Manager
Jim Torgerson, Executive Director
Kristen W., Health and Rehabilitation Center
Becky D., Activity Director
Kennedy Park Medical & Rehabilitation Center accomodates 154 residents. We are located in Schofield, WI. At Kennedy Park, we specialize in dementia care, with our Reflections and Passages Units. Short-term rehabilitation and sub-acute care are provided in a setting conducive to meeting the individual needs of our residents and patients. We also provide general nursing care for persons with long-term care needs.

7473 Middleton Village Nursing & Rehabilitation
Kindred
6201 Elmwood Ave
Middleton, WI 53562-3319   608-831-8300
                                               800-947-6644
                                           Fax: 608-831-4253
                                  www.middletonvillage.com
Nicholas Stamatas, Manager
Ashley Ostrowski, Executive Director
Kristen W., Health and Rehabilitation Center
Becky D., Activity Director
Middleton Village accomodates 97 residents. We specialize in post-surgical and post-acute rehabilitation and long-term care services.

7474 Mount Carmel Health & Rehabilitation Center
5700 W Layton Ave
Milwaukee, WI 53220-4099   414-281-7200
                                           Fax: 414-281-4620
Mike Berry, Administrator
Darrin Hull, Executive Director
Kristen W., Health and Rehabilitation Center
Becky D., Activity Director
Subacute rehabilitation facility and programs.

7475 Mount Carmel Medical and Rehabilitation Center
680 South Fourth Street
Louisville, KY   40202   502-596-7300
                                               800-545-0749
                              web_administrator@kindred.com
                                  kindredhealthcare.com
Randy Nitschke, Administrator
Jeanne Piccioni, Executive Director
Mount Carmel Medical and Rehabilitation Center accomodates 155 residents. We are located in Burlington Wisconsin. Mount Carmel Medical and Rehabilitation center is a recipient of the American Health Care Association Quality Award.

7476 North Ridge Medical and Rehabilitation Center
1445 N 7th St
Manitowoc, WI 54220-2011   920-682-0314
                                               800-947-6644
                                           Fax: 920-682-0553
Jane Conway, Interim ED
Mary Ann Hamer, Executive Director
North Ridge Medical and Rehabiliation Center accomodates 110 residents. We have been serving the Manitowoc, Wisconsin area for over 25 years. Our goal is to provide services in a warm, homey environment. Many of our staff in all departments have a long history with North Ridge and have worked here for more then 20 years. We also take pride in the fact that we have all in-house staff. Our therapy team is availiable to provide physical, occupational and speech therapy 7 days a week.

7477 Oshkosh Medical and Rehabilitation Center
1580 Bowen St
Oshkosh, WI 54901
920-233-4011
Fax: 920-233-5177
www.northpointmedicalandrehab.com

Tom Wagner, President
Subacute rehabilitation facility and programs.

7478 San Luis Medical and Rehabilitation Center
680 South Fourth Street
Louisville, KY 40202
502-596-7300
800-545-0749
web_administrator@kindred.com
www.kindredhealthcare.com

Heather Dreier, Administrator
Tim Dietzen, Executive Director
Dr. John T. Warren, Medical Director
Kristen W., Health and Rehabilitation Center
San Luis Medical and Rehabilitation Center accomodates 126 residents. We are located in Green bay, WI. At San Luis, we strive to meet the needs of our residents and we specialize in dementia care, with our Reflections Unit. Our goal is to provide short-term rehabilitation and sub-acute care in a setting conducive to assisting the needs of our residents.

7479 Strawberry Lane Nursing & Rehabilitation Center
130 Strawberry Lane
Wisconsin Rapids, WI 54494-2156
715-424-1600
Fax: 715-424-4817
www.strawberrylanenursing.com

Cyndi Glodoski, Admissions Director
Carrie Russert, Administrator
Skilled nursing facility that provides both long term and short term care. Offer Alzheimer's and Dementia care units, as well as Hospice Care. Medicare and Medicaid certified.

Wyoming

7480 Mountain Towers Healthcare & Rehabilitation Center
3128 Boxelder Dr
Cheyenne, WY 82001-5808
307-634-7901
800-877-9975
Fax: 307-634-7910
www.mttowersrehab.com

Dan Stackis, Administrator
Toni Wyenn, Director of Nursing
Daniel G. Stackis, Executive Director
Dr. Kent Britton, Medical Director
Mountain Towers Healthcare and Rehabilitation Center accomodates 170 residents, including a 16-bed acute secure unit. We offer a full range of nursing and medical care to meet individual needs. We have a full staff to meet the needs of our residents.

7481 South Central Wyoming Healthcare and Rehabilitation
Kindred Healthcare
542 16th St
Rawlins, WY 82301-5241
307-324-2759
800-877-9975
Fax: 307-324-7579
www.kindredrawlins.com

Chris Tanner, Executive Director
Anthony Janusz, Administrator
Kristen W., Health and Rehabilitation Center
Becky D., Activity Director
South Central Wyoming Healthcare and Rehabilitation accomodates 52 residents. We are located in Rawlings, in south central Wyoming. We are Medicare and Medicaid certified by the State of Wyoming. We strive to provide quality personal services, long-term care or short-term rehabilitation to our residents in a comfortable home-like environment.

7482 Wind River Healthcare and Rehabilitation Center
Kindred Health Care
1002 Forest Dr
Riverton, WY 82501-2918
307-856-9471
800-877-9975
Fax: 307-856-1665
www.windriverhealthcare.com

Jo Ann Aldrich, Executive Director
Amelia Asay, Business Office Manager
Kristen W., Health and Rehabilitation Center
Becky D., Activity Director
Offers a full range of medical services to meet the individual needs of our residents, including short-term rehabilitative services and long-term skilled care. Working with the residents physician, our staff-including medical specialists, nurses, nutritionists, dietitians and social workers-establishes a comprehensive treatment plan intended to restore you or your loved one to the highest practicable potential.

Aging

Associations

7483 Aging Life Care Association
3275 W Ina Road
Suite 130
Tucson, AZ 85741-2198 520-881-8008
Fax: 520-325-7925
info@aginglifecare.org
www.aginglifecare.org

Kaaren Boothroyd, CEO
Amanda Mizell, Member Relations
Julie Wagner, Director of Administration
Joseph Lutovsky, Manager of Technology

A nonprofit association providing geriatric care for aging individuals through sharing of knowledge in 8 areas: health and disability, financial matters, housing, planning, local resources, advocacy, legal and crisis intervention.

7484 Aging Services of Michigan
201 North Washington Square
Suite 920
Lansing, MI 48933 517-323-3687
Fax: 517-323-4569
info@leadingagemi.org
www.leadingagemi.org

David Herbel, President & CEO
Deanna Mitchell, Senior Vice President for Performance & Education

Aging Services of Michigan represents and supports organizations that provide services to the elderly and disabled adults. Types of supports offered by Aging Services include advocacy, education and other programs that enhance an organization's ability to serve their constituencies.

7485 Aging Services of South Carolina
2711 Middleburg Dr
Suite 309-A
Columbia, SC 29204 803-988-0005
Fax: 803-988-1017
www.leadingagesc.org

Frazier Jackson, Chair
Vickie Moody, President

Aging Services of South Carolina represents non-profit organizations dedicated to providing high-quality health care, housing and services to the seniors of South Carolina. Supports include public policy initiatives and education.

7486 Aging Services of Washington
1102 Broadway
Suite 201
Tacoma, WA 98402 253-964-8870
Fax: 253-964-8876
info@leadingagewa.org
leadingagewa.org

Jay Woolford, Chair
Deb Murphy, CEO
Laura Hofmann, Director, Clinical & Nursing Facility Services
LeighBeth Merrick, Director, Senior Living & Community Services

LeadingAge Washington is a state association supporting non-profit organizations that specialize in housing and long term care for the elderly. Supports offered include advocacy, education and more.

7487 Aging and Disability Services
2100 Washington Blvd
4th Floor
Arlington, VA 22204 703-228-1700
TTY:703-228-1788
arlaaa@arlingtonva.us
aging-disability.arlingtonva.us
Anita Friedman, Director, Department of Human Services
The Aging and Disability Services Division offers care coordination, home care, and supportive services to the aging residents of Arlington. Services are provided to adults over 60, adults with developmental disabilities and their caregivers.

7488 Aging in America
2975 Westchester Ave
Suite 301
Purchase, NY 10577 914-205-5030
Fax: 718-824-4242
contact@aginginamerica.org
aginginamerica.org

Katharine Weiss, Chair
William T Smith, President & CEO
Dina Nejman, Service Coordinator
Kathleen Bufano, Executive Assistant

Non-profit organization providing services for individuals and caregivers to assist them with the challenges of aging. One strategy employed towards this goal is collaboration with other organizations with experience in senior housing and community based services.

7489 Alliance for Aging Research
1700 K St., NW
Suite 740
Washington, DC 20006 202-293-2856
Fax: 202-955-8394
info@agingresearch.org
www.agingresearch.org

James E Eden, Chair
James G Scott, Vice Chair
Sue Peschin, President & CEO
Kelsey Allcorn, Health Programs Coordinator

A nonprofit organization dedicated to accelerating the pace of scientific discoveries and their application to improve the human experience of aging. This is accomplished through policies, initiatives and research that promote health and quality of care.

7490 Alliance for Retired Americans
815 16th St, NW
4th Floor
Washington, DC 20006 202-637-5399
Fax: 202-637-5398
retiredamericans.org

Robert Roach, President
Joe Peters, Secretary-Treasurer
Joe Etta Brown, Executive Vice President
Liz Shuler, Executive Vice President

An alliance made up of community members advocating for social and economic justice and civil rights for all citizens so that they may enjoy lives of dignity, security and fulfillment. Some of the topics covered in their advocacy include Medicare, the Affordable Care Act, fair trade, pensions, social security, prescription drugs and more.

7491 American Aging Association
2885 Sanford Ave SW
Suite 39542
Grandville, MI 49418 contact@americanagingassociation.org
www.americanagingassociation.org

Janko Nikolich-Zugich, Chair & CEO
Christian Sell, President
Dudley Lamming, Secretary

A group of experts dedicated to understanding the basic mechanisms of aging and the development of interventions in age-related diseases to increase human lifespans. This is accomplished through biomedical aging studies and public education.

7492 American Association of Retired Persons
AARP
601 E St NW
Washington, DC 20049 888-687-2277
TTY:877-342-2277
member@aarp.org
www.aarp.org

Jo Ann Jenkins, CEO
Sarah Shaw, SVP & Senior Associate General Counsel
Cindy Lewin, Executive Vice President & General Counsel
Karen L Mercer, Senior Vice President & Treasurer

A nonprofit membership organization dedicated to addressing the needs and interests of people 50 and older in the areas of social security, financial planning and health care.

7493 American Geriatrics Society
40 Fulton St.
18th Floor
New York, NY 10038   212-308-1414
                                        Fax: 212-832-8646
                    info.amger@americangeriatrics.org
                         www.americangeriatrics.org

Debra Saliba, President
Nancy E Lundebjerg, CEO
Elvy Ickowicz, Senior Vice President of Operations
Alanna Goldstein, Director of Public Affairs & Advocacy
A non-profit organization consisting of geriatrics healthcare professionals dedicated to improving health, independence and quality of life for older people. The society advocates for programming in health care, research, professional and public education, and public policy.

7494 American Planning Association
205 N Michigan Ave
Suite 1200
Chicago, IL 60601   312-431-9100
                                        Fax: 312-786-6700
                         foundation@planning.org
                    www.planning.org/ontheradar/aging/

Mary Kay Peck, FAICP, Chair
James Drinan, CEO
Ann Simms, Chief Operating Officer
Harriet Bogdanowicz, Chief Communications Officer
An association supporting planners to develop communities that would be more livable for aging people. The association offers membership, a knowledge center, publications, conferences and meetings, certification, policy and advocacy services, community outreach and more.

7495 American Society on Aging
575 Market St
Suite 2100
San Francisco, CA 94105-2869   415-974-9600
                                             800-537-9728
                                        Fax: 415-974-0300
                                         info@asaging.org
                                         www.asaging.org

Robert Blancato, Chair
Robert Stein, President & CEO
Robert R Lowe, Chief Operating Officer
Carole Anderson, Vice President of Education
A membership organization of colleges and universities offering education, training, and research programs for those involved in caring for aging people. Some subjects covered include disability, gerontology, chronic conditions, abuse resources, mental health and more.

7496 Association for Gerontology in Higher Education
1220 L St NW
Suite 901
Washington, DC 20005   202-289-9806
                                        Fax: 202-289-9824
                                          geron@geron.org
                                           www.aghe.org

Nina M Silverstein, President
Judith L Howe, President-Elect
Dana B Bradley, Treasurer
Karen Kopera-Frye, Secretary
Membership association of colleges and universities offering gerontology education, training, and research programs on the subject of aging. The association seeks to enhance the knowledge and skills of those who work with older adults and their families.

7497 Association of Jewish Aging Services
2519 Connecticut Ave NW
Washington, DC 20008   202-543-7500
                                        Fax: 202-543-4090
                                            info@ajas.org
                                            www.ajas.org

Daniel Reingold, Chair
Don Shulman, President & CEO
Rachel Stevens, Director of Operations
Michael l Sattell, Treasurer
The Association of Jewish Aging Services is a non-profit community-based organization offering support services for the aging population. Inspired by Jewish values, the organization offers resources, conferences, education, professional development and advocacy to its members so they could better serve their communities.

7498 Association on Aging with Developmental Disabilities
2385 Hampton Ave.
St. Louis, MO 63139   314-647-8100
                                        Fax: 314-647-8105
                                      agingwithdd@msn.com
                                          agingwithdd.org

Pamela Merkle, Executive Director
Michelle Darden, Program Development Coordinator
Erika Donaldson, Department Director
The organization offers services to accommodate the complex needs of older adults with developmental disabilities such as mental retardation, cerebral palsy, epilepsy, autism, severe learning disabilities and head injuries.

7499 Center for Positive Aging
1440 Dutch Valley PL NE
Suite 120
Atlanta, GA 30324-5367   404-872-9191
                                        Fax: 404-872-1737
                               www.centerforpositiveaging.org

Connie White, Chair
Walter Coffey, President & CEO
Jacque Thornton, Sr. Vice President
Susan Watkins, Director of Member Services
The Center for Positive Aging provides education to assist consumers in aging well. Resources offered cover areas such as adult day care, assisted living, community services, subsidized housing, nursing homes and more.

7500 Children of Aging Parents
PO Box 167
Richboro, PA 18954-0167   800-227-7294
                                        Fax: 215-945-8720
                                    info@caps4caregivers.org

Louise Fradkin, Co-Founder
Mirca Liberti, Co-Founder
A non-profit clearinghouse for caregivers of the elderly, providing information, referral, educational programs and materials to caregivers.

7501 Colorado Association of Homes and Services for the Aging
1888 Sherman St
Suite 610
Denver, CO 80203   303-837-8834
                                        Fax: 303-837-8836
                                        Karen@CAHSA.org
                                           www.cahsa.org

Maureen Hewitt, President
Lynn O'Connor, President-Elect
Laura Landwirth, Executive Director
Karen Simmering, Director of Operations
The association represents nonprofit organizations dedicated to providing health care and housing services to Colorado's elderly. Some services provided by the association include information and education to assist in developing programs for long term care.

7502 Healthy Aging Association
3500 Coffee Rd
Suite 19
Modesto, CA 95355   209-523-2800
                                        Fax: 209-523-2800
                              healthy.aging2000@gmail.com
                              www.healthyagingassociation.org

Mike Mallory, Board President
Dianna L Olsen, Executive Director
Samantha Borba, MA, Fitness Program Manager
Erlinda Bourcier, BA, Health Educator & Senior Coalition
Coordinator

A non-profit organization whose mission is to help older Americans live longer, healthier, more independent lives by promoting increased physical activity through fitness programs.

7503 Justice in Aging
1444 Eye St NW
Suite 1100
Washington, DC 20005   202-289-6976
                                        Fax: 202-289-7224
                              info@justiceinaging.org
                              www.justiceinaging.org

Phyllis J Holmen, Esq., Chair
Kevin Prindiville, Executive Director
Jennifer Goldberg, Directing Attorney
Tom Smith, Finance & Administration Director

Justice in Aging is a non-profit legal organization whose principal mission is to protect the rights of low-income older adults and vulnerable groups in society. Through advocacy, litigation, and training of local advocates, Justice in Aging seeks to ensure the health and economic security of those they serve.

7504 LeadingAge
2519 Connecticut Ave NW
Washington, DC 20008   202-783-2242
                                        Fax: 202-783-2255
                              info@leadingage.org
                              www.leadingage.org

Kathryn Roberts, Chair
Katie Smith Sloan, President & CEO
Robyn I Stone, Senior Vice President, Research
Cheryl Phillips, Senior Vice President, Public Policy and Health

LeadingAge represents non-profit organizations dedicated to providing high-quality health care, housing and services to the nation's elderly. Supports offered by LeadingAge include advocy, education and events.

7505 LeadingAge Arizona
3877 N 7th St
Suite 240
Phoenix, AZ 85014   602-230-0026
                                        Fax: 602-230-0563
                              pkoester@leadingageaz.org
                              www.arizonaleadingage.org

Steven Kolnacki, President
Pam Koester, CEO
Donald G Isaacson, Lobbyist
Cheyenne Walsh, Lobbyist

LeadingAge Arizona is a non-profit association representing organizations that provide health care, housing and services to the elderly citizens of Arizona. The association supports these organizations by offering them leadership, education and advocacy services.

7506 LeadingAge California
1315 I Street
Suite 100
Sacramento, CA 95814   916-392-5111
                                        Fax: 916-428-4250
                              info@leadingageca.org
                              www.aging.org

Kathryn Roberts, Chair
Jeannee Parker Martin, President & CEO
Jan Guiliano, Vice President of Education
Felicia Price, Director of Meetings & Events

LeadingAge California advocates for non-profit organizations that provide health care, housing and community services to older adults. Services offered by LeadingAge include advocacy, public education and advertising.

7507 LeadingAge Connecticut
110 Barnes Rd
Wallingford, CT 06492   203-678-4477
                                        Fax: 203-678-4650
                              leadingagect@leadingagect.org
                              www.leadingagect.org

William Fiocchetta, Chair
Mag Morelli, President
Nurka Carrero, Office Manager
Andrea Bellofiore, Director of Member Programs & Services

LeadingAge Connecticut is a provider of support services to non-profit organizations serving elderly and chronically ill individuals. Supports include advocacy and information provided to members of skilled nursing facilities, intermediate care facilities, residential care homes, chronic disease hospitals, adult day centers, senior housing communities and more.

7508 LeadingAge Gulf States
P.O. Box 1748
Marrero, LA 70073   504-442-0483
                                        Fax: 504-689-3982
                              kcontrenchis@leadingagegulfstates.org
                              www.leadingagegulfstates.org

Dennis Adams, Chair
Karen Contrenchis, NFA, CASP, President
Scott Crabtree, Vice Chair
Joe Townsend, Treasurer

Organization offering educational and advocacy supports to long term care organizations working in the areas of senior housing, nursing homes, adult day care, assisted living, retirement communities, Alzheimer programs and home and community based services.

7509 LeadingAge Illinois
1001 Warrenville Rd
Suite 150
Lisle, IL 60532   630-325-6170
                                        Fax: 630-325-0749
                              info@leadingageil.org
                              www.leadingageil.org

Deb Reardanz, Chair
Karen Messer, President & CEO
Angela Schnepf, Executive Vice President
Ruta Prasauskas, Vice President of Health Services

LeadingAge Illinois represents organizations specializing in the field of senior care services, offering them advocacy, networking, public policy and employment resources to help them thrive in their missions.

7510 LeadingAge Indiana
PO Box 68829
Indianapolis, IN 46268-0829   317-733-2380
                                        Fax: 317-733-2385
                              mrinebold@leadingageindiana.org
                              www.leadingageindiana.org

Mike Rinebold, President
Susan Darwent, Vice President of Operations
Kathy Johnson, RN, WCC, Vice President of Clinical & Regulatory
Services
Jennifer Clark, Marketing & Membership

LeadingAge Indiana is an association representing non-profit organizations that provide health care, services and housing for seniors throughout Indiana. LeadingAge offers education, advocacy and networking opportunities to their members.

7511 LeadingAge Iowa
4200 University Ave
Suite 305
West Des Moines, IA   50266   515-440-4630
                                      888-440-4630
                                  Fax: 515-440-4631
                          info@leadingageiowa.org
                          www.leadingageiowa.org

Bert Vigen, Chair
Shannon Strickler, President & CEO
Matt Blake, Director, Government Relations & Member Services
Liz Davidson, Director of Clinical Services
LeadingAge Iowa serves non-profit and missiondriven organizations dedicated to providing quality housing, health, community, and related services to Iowa's seniors. Supports provided include advocacy, education and collaboration.

7512 LeadingAge Kentucky
2501 Nelson Miller Pkwy
Suite 101
Louisville, KY   40223   502-992-4380
                                Fax: 502-992-4390
                            info@leadingageky.org
                            leadingageky.org

Timothy Veno, President & CEO
LeadingAge Kentucky represents non-profit organizations that offer services for the elderly and the disabled. LeadingAge offers advocacy and educational services and resources to their members.

7513 LeadingAge Maine & New Hampshire
55 Main St
Suite 316
Newmarket, NH   03857   603-292-6441
                      lhenderson@leadingagemenh.org
                          www.leadingagemenh.org

Rebecca Smith, Chair
Deb Riddell, Vice Chair
Lisa Henderson, Executive Director
Katie Sweet, Communications & Education Manager
LeadingAge Maine & New Hampshire aims to promote the interests of its non-profit members which provide healthy, affordable and ethical long-term care to the older citizens of Maine and New Hampshire. LeadingAge offers this support through education, advocacy, representation and collaboration.

7514 LeadingAge Massachusetts
246 Walnut St
Suite 203
Newton, MA   02460   617-244-2999
                                Fax: 617-244-2995
                          office@LeadingAgeMA.org
                            www.leadingagema.org

Jered Stewart, Chairperson
Elissa Sherman, President
Lynn Monaghan, Events & Education Manager
Rita Kostiuk, Member Engagement Manager
LeadingAge Massachusetts represents non-profit providers of health care, housing, and services for seniors in Massachusetts. Some services offered by LeadingAge include education and events, webinars, networking opportunities, technology resources, advocacy and consumer resources.

7515 LeadingAge Missouri
3412 Knipp Dr
Suite 102
Jefferson City, MO   65109   573-635-6244
                                Fax: 573-635-6618
                  debbiecheshire@leadingagemissouri.org
                          www.leadingagemissouri.org

Chris Crouch, Chair
Bill Bates, CEO
Nancie McAnaugh, Chief Operating Officer
Debbie Cheshire, Administrative Assistant
LeadingAge Missouri's work is dedicated to assisting its members to be leaders in the delivery of quality long-term health care, housing, and services for older adults in Missouri. Some services

provided by LeadingAge include advocacy, public education, consumer resources and more.

7516 LeadingAge Nebraska
900 N 90th St
Suite 940
Omaha, NE   68114   402-326-2790
                            jeremy@leadingagene.org
                            www.leadingagene.org

Julie Sebastian, Board Chair
Jeremy Hohlen, CEO
Cheryl Wichman, Director of Professional Development
Melissa Bergoch, Administrative Support
LeadingAge Nebraska represents the full continuum of mission-driven, non-profit providers of health care, housing and services for older adults in Nebraska. Some supports offered by LeadingAge include educational conferences, webinars, workshops and advocacy.

7517 LeadingAge New Jersey
3705 Quakerbridge Rd
Suite 102
Hamilton, NJ   08619   609-452-1161
                                Fax: 609-452-2907
                            mkent@leadingagenj.org
                            www.leadingagenj.org

Toni Lynn Davis, Chairperson
Michele M Kent, President & CEO
Diane Borgstrom, Finance Coordinator
Hillary Critelli, Membership & Engagement Specialist
LeadingAge New Jersey represents non-profit nursing homes, assisted living residences, residential health care centers, independent senior housing, and continuing care retirement communities throughout New Jersey. Members are supported through advocacy, education, and fellowship.

7518 LeadingAge New York
13 British American Blvd
Suite 2
Latham, NY   12110-1431   518-867-8383
                                Fax: 518-867-8384
                            info@leadingageny.org
                            www.leadingageny.org

James W Clyne, President & CEO
Daniel J Heim, Executive Vice President
Ellen Quinn, SPHR, Vice President of Human Resources
Ami Schnauber, Vice President of Advocacy & Public Policy
LeadingAge New York represents non-profit, mission-driven and public continuing care providers, including nursing homes, senior housing, adult care facilities, continuing care retirement communities, assisted living and community service providers. LeadingAge provides its members with education, publications, conferences and consultation services to help them better serve their communities.

7519 LeadingAge North Carolina
222 N Person St
Raleigh, NC   27601   919-571-8333
                                Fax: 919-571-1297
                            info@leadingagenc.org
                            www.leadingagenc.org

Robert Wernet, Chair
Tom Akins, President & CEO
Leslie Roseboro, Vice President
Jennifer Gill, Director of Strategic Communications
LeadingAge North Carolina represents non-profit providers of care, housing, health, community and related services to the elderly. One of its primary goals is to advance policies, practices and research to empower the aging population.

7520   **LeadingAge Ohio**
2233 N Bank Dr
Columbus, OH   43220   614-444-2882
                                          Fax: 614-444-2974
                                       info@leadingageohio.org
                                       www.leadingageohio.org

Judy Budi, Chair
Kenneth Daniel, Vice Chair
Kathryn Brod, President & CEO
Stephanie DeWees, Quality & Regulatory Specialist

LeadingAge Ohio represents long-term care organizations. Service providers supported include those working in the fields of senior housing, adult day care, home- and community-based services, assisted living and nursing. Some supports offered by LeadingAge Ohio include policy advocacy, education, employment support and resources for families.

7521   **LeadingAge Oklahoma**
P.O. Box 1383
El Reno, OK   73036   405-640-8040
                                       inquiry@leadingageok.org
                                       leadingageok.org

Lindsay Fick, President
Mary Brinkley, Executive Director
Mark Gray, Public Policy Congress
Lauren Cantu, Director

LeadingAge Oklahoma represents non-profit organizations that serve the aging people of Oklahoma. LeadingAge assists these organizations through advocacy, consumer services, directories, education, a job bank and more.

7522   **LeadingAge Oregon**
7340 SW Hunziker
Suite 104
Tigard, OR   97223   503-684-3788
                                          Fax: 503-624-0870
                                       info@leadingageoregon.org
                                       www.leadingageoregon.org

Greg Franks, President
Ruth Gulyas, MHA, CEO
Margaret Cervenka, Deputy Director
Denise Wetzel, Manager Membership Services

LeadingAge Oregon represents non-profits that provide housing, health care, community and related services to the elderly and disabled of Oregon. LeadingAge offers its members advocacy, networking events and education to help them succeed in their missions.

7523   **LeadingAge PA**
1100 Bent Creek Blvd
Mechanicsburg, PA   17050   717-763-5724
                                               800-545-2270
                                          Fax: 717-763-1057
                                       info@leadingagepa.org
                                       www.leadingagepa.org

Susan Drabic, Chair
Ronald Barth, President & CEO
Heidie Dolan, Office Manager & Executive Assistant
Brandie Karpew, Manager, Policy Analytics

LeadingAge PA's mission is to promote the interests of its members through education, advocacy, community forums and events. Member organizations include adult day care services, assisted living residences, home care services, skilled nursing facilities and other non-profits that serve the aging population of Pennsylvania.

7524   **LeadingAge RI**
1 Virginia Ave
Providence, RI   02905   401-490-7612
                                          Fax: 401-490-7614
                                       TTY:401-383-6578
                                       info@leadingageri.org
                                       www.leadingageri.org

Sandra Cullen, President
Stephanie Igoe, Vice President
James Nyberg, MPA, Director
Adderlin Bailey, MPH, Special Projects Assistant

LeadingAge RI seeks to advance excellence in the field of aging services by fostering innovation, collaboration, and ethical leadership through advocacy for public policy, education and professional development.

7525   **LeadingAge Texas**
2205 Hancock Dr
Austin, TX   78756   512-467-2242
                                          Fax: 512-467-2275
                                       info@leadingagetexas.org
                                       www.leadingagetexas.org

Roque Christensen, Chair
George Linial, President & CEO
Melanie Harrison, Director of Education
Alyse Meyer, Director of Public Policy

LeadingAge Texas provides leadership, advocacy, and education for non-profit retirement housing and nursing home communities that serve the needs of Texas retirees.

7526   **LeadingAge Wisconsin**
204 S Hamilton St
Madison, WI   53703   608-255-7060
                                          Fax: 608-255-7064
                                       info@leadingagewi.org
                                       www.leadingagewi.org

Fran Petrick, Chair
John Sauer, President & CEO
Jim Williams, Director of Member Enrichment
Denise May, Director of Business Development

LeadingAge Wisconsin is committed to advancing the fields of long-term care, assisted living and retirement living. Towards this purpose, LeadingAge offers advocacy, education and collaborative strategies to its members so they could better serve aging people.

7527   **LeadingAge Wyoming**
2005 Warren Ave
Cheyenne, WY   82001   307-632-9344
                                          Fax: 307-632-9347
                                       eric@wyohospitals.com
                                       www.leadingagewyoming.org

7528   **LifeSpan Network**
10280 Old Columbia Rd
Suite 220
Columbia, MD   21044   410-381-1176
                                          Fax: 410-381-0240
                                       ifirth@lifespan-network.org
                                       www.lifespan-network.org

Dennis Hunter, Chair
Kevin Heffner, President
Danna Kauffman, Public Policy Consultant
Kathy Bernetti, CPA, Senior Vice President of Finance

Senior care provider representing more than 330 senior care provider organizations in Maryland and the District of Columbia. Lifespan members include non-profit and proprietary independent living, assisted living, continuing care retirement communities, nursing facilities, subsidized senior housing and community and hospital based services. LifeSpan provides education, advocacy, products and services to its members.

7529   **National Association for Home Care and Hospice**
228 Seventh St, SE
Washington, DC   20003   202-547-7424
                                          Fax: 202-547-3540
                                       www.nahc.org

Denise Schrader, Chair
Val J Halamandaris, President
Lucy Andrews, Vice Chair
Karen M Thompson, Secretary

Professional association representing the interests of chronically ill, disabled, and dying Americans and their caregivers. The association offers advocacy services on policy, resources related to hospice and home care, research sponsorships, education for the public on hospice services and more.

7530 **National Association of Area Agencies on Aging**
1730 Rhode Island Ave, NW
Suite 1200
Washington, DC 20036 202-872-0888
Fax: 202-872-0057
info@n4a.org
www.n4a.org

Kathryn Boles, President
Doug McKenzie, Chief, Finance & Administration
Martin Kleffner, Director of Operations
Joellen Leavelle, Director of Communications

The National Association of Area Agencies on Aging (n4a) is the
leading voice on aging issues for Area Agencies on Aging and a
champion for Title VI Native American aging programs. n4a provides advocacy, training and technical assistance, employment
support and information resources to these agencies.

7531 **National Association of Counties**
660 N Capitol St NW
Suite 400
Washington, DC 20001 202-393-6226
888-407-6226
Fax: 202-393-2630
nacomeetings@naco.org
www.naco.org

Bryan Desloge, President
Matthew Chase, Executive Director
Deborah Stoutamire, Director of Operations
Alicia Dorsey, Finance Director

NACO brings together elected officials and aging administrators
who are interested in providing quality programs and beter policies for their older constituents. NACO members work with Congress, the Administration on Aging, and other federal agencies to
ensure that the nation maintains an effective and efficient safety
net of services for the elderly and their families.

7532 **National Association of Nutrition and Aging Services
Programs (NANASP)**
1612 K St NW
Suite 200
Washington, DC 20006 202-682-6899
Fax: 202-223-2099
pcarlson@nanasp.org
www.nanasp.org

Tony Sarmiento, Chair
Robert Blancato, Executive Director
Pam Carlson, Membership & Education
Scott Carlson, Finance & Operations

A national membership organization supporting those working to
provide older adults with healthy food and nutrition through community-based services. NANASP engages in advocacy on issues
such as nutrition, Medicare and Medicaid, elder justice, social security and other retirement security, transportation, and older
workers' issues.

7533 **National Association of States United for Aging and
Disabilities**
1201 15th St NW
Suite 350
Washington, DC 20005 202-898-2578
Fax: 202-898-2583
info@nasuad.org
www.nasuad.org

Gary Jessee, President
Martha Roherty, Executive Director
Camille Dobson, Deputy Executive Director
Robert Alonso, Finance Director

The National Association of States United for Aging and Disabilities (NASUAD) represents the nation's agencies serving in the
areas of aging and disabilitie. NASUAD supports state leadership
as well as national policies that support home and community
based services for seniors and individuals with disabilities.

7534 **National Council on Aging**
251 18th St S
Suite 500
Arlington, VA 22202 571-527-3900
Fax: 202-479-0735
TTY:202-479-6674
newsletters@ncoa.org
www.ncoa.org

Carol Zernial, Chair
James Firman, EdD, President & CEO
Donna Whitt, Senior Vice President & Chief Financial Officer
Howard Bedlin, Vice President, Public Policy & Advocacy

The National Council on Aging (NCOA) is an organization supporting older Americans and the community organizations that
serve them. Services offered by NCOA cover the areas of health
and nutrition resources, policy and advocacy, elder justice, economic security, resources for caregivers and more.

7535 **National Gerontological Nursing Association**
121 W State St
Geneva, IL 60134 630-748-4616
ngna@affinity-strategies.com
www.ngna.org

Joanne Alderman, President
Sandra Kuebler, Treasurer
Elizabeth Tanner, Secretary

An association providing clinical care for older adults. Their
member organizations include clinicians, educators, and researchers specializing in different areas of senior care services.

7536 **National Hispanic Council on Aging**
734 15th St NW
Suite 1050
Washington, DC 20005 202-347-9733
Fax: 202-347-9735
nhcoa@nhcoa.org
www.nhcoa.org

Octavio Martinez, Ph.D, Chair
Yanira Cruz, Ph.D, President & CEO
Maria Eugenia Hernandez-Lane, Vice President
Amina Ferreira, Communications Specialist

The National Hispanic Council on Aging (NHCOA) works to improve quality of life for Hispanic seniors. With a Hispanic Aging
Network of community-based organizations across the U.S., the
District of Columbia and Puerto Rico, NHCOA aims to provide
public education and adovocacy in areas such as economic security, health, and housing.

7537 **National Indian Council on Aging, Inc.**
8500 Menaul Blvd. NE
Suite B470
Albuquerque, NM 87112 505-292-2001
Fax: 505-292-1922
info@nicoa.org
www.nicoa.org

Randella Bluehoose, Executive Director

A non-profit organization was founded by members of the National Tribal Chairmen's Association that called for a national organization to advocate for improved, comprehensive health and
social services to American Indian and Alaska Native Elders.

7538 **Senior Service America**
8403 Colesville Rd
Suite 200
Silver Spring, MD 20910 301-578-8900
Fax: 301-578-8947
contact@ssa-i.org
www.seniorserviceamerica.org

Spence Limbocker, Chair
Gary A Officer, Executive Director
Donna Satterthwaite, Director, Workforce Development
Lynn Woo, Director of Finance

Senior Service America offers employment programs for seniors
in America.

7539 Tennessee Hospital Association
5201 Virginia Way
Brentwood, TN 37027   615-256-8240
                          Fax: 615-242-4803
                          yjames@tha.com
                          tha.com

Alan Watson, Chairman
Craig Becker, President & CEO
Mary Layne Van Cleave, Executive Vice President & Chief Operating Officer
Beth Atwood, Senior Director, Communications & Marketing
The Tennessee Hospital Association provides education and information to its members in the health care field so that organizations may serve their constituencies more effectively. The association also offers professional development programs in the areas of insurance, administration and operations, project management, financial services and human resources.

7540 The Gerontological Society of America
1220 L St NW
Suite 901
Washington, DC 20005   202-842-1275
                          geron@geron.org
                          www.geron.org

Barbara Resnick, PhD, CRNP, President
James Appleby, Executive Director & CEO
Patricia M D'Antonio, Senior Director, Professional Affairs & Membership
Judie Lieu, Senior Director, Publications & Marketing
The organization seeks to advance the study of aging by supporting gerontology research. This is accomplished through encouraging communication among professionals, promoting research publications, expanding gerontology education programs and more.

Print: Books

7541 Activities in Action
Routledge (Taylor & Francis Group)
270 Madison Ave
Fl 4 #4
New York, NY 10016-0601   212-695-6599
                          800-634-7064
                          Fax: 212-563-2269
                          www.routledgementalhealth.com

Jeffrey Lim, Director
Francis Chua, Manager
Tamaryn Anderson, Marketing Manager
An invaluable resource which serves as a catalyst for professional and personal growth and provides a national forum on geriatric and activity issues. *$30.00*
116 pages Hardcover
ISBN 1-560241-32-4

7542 Activities with Developmentally Disabled Elderly and Older Adults
Routledge (Taylor & Francis Group)
270 Madison Ave
Fl 4 #4
New York, NY 10016-601   212-695-6599
                          800-637-7064
                          Fax: 212-563-2269
                          www.routledgementalhealth.com

Jeffrey Lim, Director
Francis Chua, Manager
Tamaryn Anderson, Marketing Manager
Learn how to effectively plan and deliver activities for a growing number of older people with developmental disabilities. It aims to stimulate interest and continued support for recreation program development and implementation among developmental disability and aging service systems. *$42.00*
164 pages Hardcover
ISBN 1-560241-74-4

7543 Aging and Developmental Disability: Current Research, Programming, and Practice
Routledge (Taylor & Francis Group)
270 Madison Ave
Fl 4 #4
New York, NY 10016-601   212-695-6599
                          800-634-7064
                          Fax: 212-563-2269
                          www.routledgementalhealth.com

Joy Hammel, Author
Susan Nochajski, Co-Author
Explores research findings and their implications for practice in relation to normative and disability-related aging experiences and issues. It discusses the effectiveness of specific intervention targeted toward aging adults with developmental disabilities such as Down's Syndrome, cerebral palsy, autism, and epilepsy, and offers suggestions for practice and future research in this area. *$48.00*
112 pages Hardcover
ISBN 0-789010-39-1

7544 Aging and Family Therapy: Practitioner Perspectives on Golden Pond
Routledge (Taylor & Francis Group)
270 Madison Ave
Fl 4 #4
New York, NY 10016-601   212-695-6599
                          800-634-7064
                          Fax: 212-563-2269
                          www.routledgementalhealth.com

George Hughston, Author
Victor Christopherson, Co-Author
Marilyn Bojean, Co-Author
Here are creative strategies for use in therapy with older adults and their families. This significant new book provides practitioners with information, insight, reference tools, and other sources that will contribute to more effective intervention with the elderly and their families. *$48.00*
260 pages Hardcover
ISBN 0-866567-78-7

7545 Aging in Stride
IlluminAge Communications Partners
2200 1st Ave South
Suite 400
Seattle, WA 98134-1408   206-269-6363
                          888-620-8816
                          Fax: 206-269-6350
                          www.cobaltgroup.com

Dennis Kenny, Owner
Elizabeth N Oettinger, Co-Author
Dennis E Kenny JD, Co-Author
Guide to aging, the special needs of older adults, and the demands of providing care and support. Experts explain potential conflicts, planning opportunities and strategies for success. Six guides. *$24.95*
Paperback

7546 Aging in the Designed Environment
Routledge (Taylor & Francis Group)
270 Madison Ave
Fl 4 #4
New York, NY 10016-601   212-216-7800
                          800-634-7064
                          Fax: 212-563-2269
                          www.routledgementalhealth.com

Margaret Christenson, Author
Ellen D Taira, Co-Author
The key sourcebook for physical and occupational therapists developing and implementing environmental designs for the aging. *$30.00*
146 pages Hardcover
ISBN 1-560240-31-0

7547   Aging with a Disability
Special Needs Project
1405 Anderson Lane
Santa Barbara, CA   93111-2946   805-962-8087
                                      800-333-6867
                              Fax: 805-962-5087
                              www.specialneeds.com
Hod Gray, Owner
Laura Mosqueda, Co-Author
Aging with a Disability provides clinicians with a complete guide
to the care and treatment of persons aging with a disability. Divided into five parts, this book first addresses the perspective of
the person with a disability and his or her family. *$ 24.95*
328 pages Paperback

7548   Assistive Technology for Older Persons: A Handbook
Idaho Assistive Technology Project
University of Idaho
1187 Altiras Dr.
Moscow, ID   83843   208-885-3557
                                      800-432-8324
                              Fax: 208-885-6102
                              idahoat@uidaho.edu
                              www.idahoat.org
Ron Seiler, Project Director
This handbook is designed as a guide for Idaho's older citizens
who, as they age, wish to preserve their independence, autonomy,
productivity, and dignity. It is intended to provide information
about assistive technology, home modifications, and the many
service options available to older people in the mcomunities
across the state.

**7549   Caring for Those You Love: A Guide to Compassionate Care
for the Aged**
Horizon Publishers & Distributors
191 N 650 E
Bountiful, UT   84010-3628   801-295-9451
                                      866-818-6277
                              Fax: 801-298-1305
                              www.duanescrowther.com
Duane S. Crowther, Author/President
Jean Crowther, Vice President/Sec
David Crowther, Vice President
This book is a practical guide to coping with special problems of
the aged and infirm, and examines the many challenges of caring
for the elderly on a personal and family level. *$12.98*
108 pages
ISBN 0-882902-70-9

7550   Chronically Disabled Elderly in Society
Greenwood Publishing Group
88 Post Rd W
Westport, CT   06880-4208   203-226-3571
                                      800-225-5800
                              Fax: 877-231-6980
                              customer-service@greenwood.com
                              www.greenwood.com
Merna J Alpert, Author
Lisa Scott, President
Herman Bruggink, CEO
This timely work increases awareness of and knowledge about
problems of societal living among the chronically disabled el-
derly, with implications for policy makers, educational institu-
tions, advocacy groups, families and individuals. *$76.95*
160 pages Hardcover
ISBN 0-313291-09-8

7551   Coping and Caring: Living with Alzheimer's Disease
AARP Fulfillment
601 E St NW
Washington, DC   20049   800-687-2277
                              TTY:877-434-7589
                              member@aarp.org
                              www.aarp.org
Charles Leroux, Author
Steve Cone, Executive Vice President of Inte
Lorraine Cortes-Vazquez, Executive Vice President, Multic

Addresses the questions: What is Alzheimer's? How does the disease progress? How long does it last? How can families cope?
24 pages

7552   Elder Abuse and Mistreatment
Routledge (Taylor & Francis Group)
270 Madison Ave
Fl 4 #4
New York, NY   10016-601   212-695-6599
                                      800-634-7064
                              Fax: 212-563-2269
                              www.routledgementalhealth.com
Joanna Mellor, Author
Patricia Brownell, Co-Author
Elder Abuse and Mistreatment is a comprehensive overview of
current policy issues, new practice models, and up-to-date research on elder abuse and neglect. Experts in the field provide insight into elder abuse with newly examined populations to create
an understanding of how to design service plans for victims of
abuse and family mistreatment. The book addresses all forms of
abuse and neglect, examining the value issues and ethical dilemmas that social workers face in providing service to elderl
$120.00
284 pages Paperback
ISBN 0-789030-22-1

7553   Explore Your Options
Kansas Department on Aging
503 S Kansas Ave
New England Building
Topeka, KS   66603- 3404   785-296-4986
                                      800-432-3535
                              Fax: 785-296-0256
                              TTY: 785-291-3167
                              wwwmail@kdads.ks.gov
                              www.agingKansas.org
Maria Russo, President
This book will help you through the maze of services available to
Kansas seniors. It is designed to help you take an active role in
making decisions that affect your health care and living situation.

7554   Falling in Old Age
Springer Publishing Company
11 W 42nd St
Fl 15 #15
New York, NY   10036-8002   212-431-4370
                                      877-687-7476
                              Fax: 212-941-7842
                              cs@springerpub.com
                              www.springerjournals.com
Ursula Springer, President
Ted Nardin, CEO
Edie Lambiase, CFO
Presented are practical techniques for the prevention of falls and
for determining and correcting the causes. *$60.00*
412 pages Hardcover
ISBN 0-826152-91-6

7555   Family Intervention Guide to Mental Illness
New Harbinger Publications
5674 Shattuck Ave
Oakland, CA   94609-1662   510-652-0215
                                      800-748-6273
                              Fax: 800-652-1613
                              customerservice@newharbinger.com
                              www.newharbinger.com
Matthew McKay, Owner
Kim T Mueser, Co-Author
Kirk Johnson, CFO
Bodie Morey, Co-Author
The Family Intervention Guide to Mental Illness outlines the nine
fundamental steps to recognizing, managing, and recovering
from mental illness. It provides both diagnostic information and
details about therapy options and useful medications. With the

right advice, determined effort, and a lot of love, you can make a difference. *$17.95*
240 pages
ISBN 1-572245-06-8

7556 Handbook of Assistive Devices for the Handicapped Elderly
Routledge (Taylor & Francis Group)
270 Madison Ave
Fl 4 #4
New York, NY   10016-601
212-695-6599
800-634-7064
Fax: 212-563-2269
www.routledgementalhealth.com

Joseph A Breuer, Author
Jeffrey Lin, Director
Francis Chua, Manager
Tamaryn Anderson, Marketing Manager
Concise yet comprehensive reference of assistive devices for handicapped elders. *$42.00*
77 pages Hardcover
ISBN 0-866561-52-5

7557 Handbook on Ethnicity, Aging and Mental Health
Greenwood Publishing Group
88 Post Rd W
Westport, CT   6880-4208
203-226-3571
800-225-5800
Fax: 877-231-6980
customer-service@greenwood.com
www.greenwood.com

Deborah K Padgett, Author
Lisa Scott, President
Herman Bruggink, CEO
State-of-the-art reference by leading experts and first book-length appraisal of research, practices and policies concerning mental health needs of the ethnic elderly in America. *$141.95*
376 pages Hardcover
ISBN 0-313282-04-8

7558 Health Care of the Aged: Needs, Policies, and Services
Routledge (Taylor & Francis Group)
270 Madison Ave
Fl 4 #4
New York, NY   10016-601
212-695-6599
800-634-7064
Fax: 212-563-2269
www.routledgementalhealth.com

Abraham Monk, Author
Jeffrey Lim, Director
Francis Chua, Manager
Tamaryn Anderson, Marketing Manager
Focusing on the need for developing new service delivery models for the aged, this book examines fiscal, political, and social criteria influencing this challenge of the 1990's. The aged are caught in the sweeping changes currently occurring in the financing, organizing and delivery of human health care services. *$36.00*
800 pages Hardcover
ISBN 1-560240-65-5

7559 Health Promotion and Disease Prevention in Clinical Practice
Lippincott, Williams & Wilkins
2001 Market Street
Two Commerce Square
Philadelphia, PA 19103-3603
215-521-8300
800-638-3030
Fax: 215-521-8902
customerservice@lww.com
www.lww.com

Steven H Woolf MD, Co-Author
Steven Jonas MD, Co-Author
Evonne Kaplan-Liss, Co-Author
Rick Perry, CEO
Incorporating the latest guidelines from major organizations, including the U.S. Preventive Services Task Force, this book offers the clinician a complete overview of how to help patients adopt healthy behaviors and to deliver recommended screening tests and immunizations. *$52.95*
218 pages Softcover
ISBN 0-781775-99-1

7560 Life Planning for Adults with Developmental Disabilities
New Harbinger Publications
5674 Shattuck Ave
Oakland, CA   94609-1662
510-652-0215
800-748-6273
Fax: 800-652-1613
customerservice@newharbinger.com
www.newharbinger.com

Matthew McKay, Publisher
Kirk Johnson, CFO
Judith Greenbaum PhD, Author
The book begins by assessing the quality of life of the adult with a disability. It offers a wealth of suggestions for making that person's life even better. The book then focuses on long-term planning for the individual with a disability and helps answer the question, Who will take care of my child after I'm gone? *$19.95*
208 pages
ISBN 1-572244-51-1

7561 Long-Term Care: How to Plan and Pay for It
NOLO
950 Parker St
Berkeley, CA   94710-2524
510-549-1976
800-728-3555
Fax: 800-645-0895
www.nolo.com

Joseph L Matthews, Author
Ralph Warner, Chariman/CEO
Ann Heron, COO
Bob Dubow, CFO
This book helps you choose a nursing home, or find a viable alternative. Covers how to get the most out of Medicare and other benefit programs.
384 pages Paperback
ISBN 1-413305-21-0

7562 Mentally Impaired Elderly: Strategies and Interventions to Maintain Function
Routledge (Taylor & Francis Group)
270 Madison Ave
Fl 4 #4
New York, NY   10016-601
212-695-6599
800-634-7064
Fax: 212-653-2269
www.routledgementalhealth.com

Ellen D Taira, Author
Jeffrey Lim, Director
Francis Chua, Manager
Tamaryn Anderson, Marketing Manager
Provides effective support and sensitive care for the most vulnerable segment of the elderly population, those with mental impairment. *$34.00*
171 pages Hardcover
ISBN 1-560241-68-3

7563 Mirrored Lives: Aging Children and Elderly Parents
Praeger Publishers
88 Post Rd W
Westport, CT   06880-4208
203-226-3571
800-225-5800
Fax: 877-231-6980
www.greenwood.com

Tom Koch, Author
Lisa Scott, President
Herman Bruggink, CEO
Discusses geriatric decline connected to nonterminal illness in old age. Koch takes a sensitive but thorough look at the declining years of his father. *$117.95*
240 pages Hardcover
ISBN 0-275936-71-6

7564 Physical & Mental Issues in Aging Sourcebook
Omnigraphics
155 W Congree St
Suite 200 #200
Detroit, MI 48226-3261

313-961-1340
800-234-1340
Fax: 313-961-1383
info@omnigraphics.com
www.omnigraphics.com

Jennifer Swanson, Editor
Frederic Ruffner, Chairman
Kay Gill, Vice President
Laurie Harris, Manager

Basic information about maintaining health through the post-reproductive years. Includes stats, recommendations for lifestyle modifications, a glossary and resrouce information $84.00
660 pages Hard cover
ISBN 0-780802-33-9

7565 Prescriptions for Independence: Working with Older People Who are Visually Impaired
American Foundation for the Blind/AFB Press
11 Penn Plz
Suite 300
New York, NY 10001-2006

212-502-7600
800-232-3044
Fax: 212-502-7777
www.afb.org

Carl Augusto, President
Gerda Groff, Co-Author
Richard Obnen, Chairman of the Board
Alan Lindroth, Principal

Easy-to-read manual on how older visually impaired persons can pursue their interests and activities in community residences, senior centers, long-term care facilities and other community settings. Paperback.
99 pages Paperback
ISBN 0-891282-44-0

7566 Sharing the Burden
Brookings Institution
1775 Massachusetts Ave NW
Washington, DC 20036-2188

202-797-6000
Fax: 202-797-6004
www.brookings.edu

Joshua N Weiner, Author
Laurel Hixon Illston, Co-Author
Raymond J Hanley, Co-Author
Strobe Talbott, President

The authors examine the cost of public and private initiatives and who would pay for them. Their answers emerge from a large computer simulation model that the authors developed. $42.95
342 pages Cloth
ISBN 0-815793-78-2

7567 Social Security, Medicare, and Government Pensions
NOLO
950 Parker St
Berkeley, CA 94710-2524

510-549-1976
800-728-3555
Fax: 800-645-0895
www.nolo.com

Joseph L Matthews, Author
Dorothy Matthews Berman, Co-Author
Ralph Warner, Chairman/CEO
Ann Heron, COO

Social Security, Medicare, SSI and more explained in this all-in-one resource that gets you the most out of your retirement benefits. $24.95
480 pages Paperback
ISBN 1-413307-53-5

7568 Successful Models of Community Long Term Care Services for the Elderly
Routledge (Taylor & Francis Group)
270 Madison Ave
Fl 4 #4
New York, NY 10016-601

212-695-6599
800-637-7064
Fax: 212-563-2269
www.routledgementalhealth.com

Eloise Killeffer, Author
Ruth Bennett, Co-Author
Jeffrey Lim, Director
Francis Chua, Manager

Experienced practitioners provide examples of successful community-based long term care service programs for the elderly. $72.00
174 pages Hardcover
ISBN 0-866569-87-3

7569 Therapeutic Activities with Persons Disabled by Alzheimer's Disease
Sage Publications
804 Anacapa Stree
Sanat Barbara, CA 93101-2212

805-899-8620
info@sagepub.com
www.sagepub.com

Sara Miller McCune, Founder, Publisher, Chairperson
Blaise Simqu, CEO
Tracey Ozmina, COO
Stephen Barr, Managing Director

A program of functional skills for activities of daily living. Hardcover. $86.00
432 pages
ISBN 0-834211-62-9

7570 Visually Impaired Seniors as Senior Companions: A Reference Guide
American Foundation for the Blind/AFB Press
11 Penn Plz
Suite 300
New York, NY 10001-2006

212-502-7600
800-232-3044
Fax: 212-502-7777
afborders@abdintl.com
www.afb.org

Carl Augusto, President
Alan Lindroth, Principal
Richard Obnen, Chairman of the Board
Michael Gilliam, Vice Chairman

This useful guide describes the Senior Companion Program that is intended to broaden opportunities for older persons with disabilities. Appendix includes training materials, evaluation forms, recruitment and public relations information. $15.00
108 pages Paperback
ISBN 0-891282-38-6

7571 Work, Health and Income Among the Elderly
Brookings Institution
1775 Massachusetts Ave NW
Washington, DC 20036-2188

202-797-6000
Fax: 202-797-6004
www.brookings.edu

Gary Burtless, Author
Strobe Talbott, President
Steven Bennett, Vice President/COO
Stewart Uretsky, Vice President/CFO

Employment, health and financial information for the elderly. $26.95
276 pages Cloth
ISBN 0-815711-76-6

Print: Journals

7572   ATS Journals
25 Broadway
New York, NY   10004   212-315-8600
                                        atsjournals.org
Marc Moss, President
Polly E. Parsons, President Elect
Juan C. Celed¢N, Secretary/Treasurer
Stephen C. Crane, Executive Director
The American Thoracic Society publishes medical research journals with a focus on respiratory issues. Publications include: Respiratory and Critical Care Medicine, Respiratory Cell and Molecular Biology, and Annals of the American Thoracic Society.

7573   Gerontology: Abstracts in Social Gerontology
National Council on the Aging
1901 L St NW
4th Floor
Washington, DC   20036-3506   202-479-1200
                                        Fax: 202-479-0735
                                        TTY:202-479-6674
                                        info@ncoa.org
                                        www.ncoa.org
James Firman, President/CEO
Jay Greenberg, ScD, Senior Vice President, Social Enterprise
Richard Birkel, PhD, MPA, Senior Vice President, Center for Healthy Aging and Director
Nora Dowd Eisenhower, JD, Senior Vice President, Economic Security and Director
Detailed abstracts are provided for recent major journal articles, books, reports and other materials on many facets of aging, including: adult education, demography, family relations, institutional care and work attitudes. Item No. AB100; Journals $114.00; Member Discount: $94.00.
Quarterly

7574   Physical & Occupational Therapy in Geriatrics
Taylor & Francis Group, LLC
325 Chestnut Street
Suite 800 #800
Philadelphia, PA 19106-2608   215-625-8900
                                        800-354-1420
                                        Fax: 215-625-2940
                                        haworthpress@taylorandfrancis.com
                                        www.tandf.co.uk
Ellen Dunleavey Taira, Editor
Barbara Pucher, CFO
Focuses on current practices and emerging issues in the care of the older client, including long-term care in institutional and community settings, crisis intervention, and innovative programming; the entire range of problems experienced by the elderly; and the current skills needed for working with older clients.
$99.00
Quarterly

Print: Magazines

7575   AARP Magazine
American Association of Retired Persons
601 E St NW
Washington, DC   20049-3   202-434-7700
                                        888-687-2277
                                        Fax: 202-434-7710
                                        TTY: 877-434-7598
                                        member@aarp.org
                                        www.aarp.org
A Barry Rand, President/CEO
Hop Backus, Executive Vice President, State
Steve Cone, Executive Vice President of Integrated Value
Lorraine Cort,s-V zquez, Executive Vice President, Multicultural Markets
A nonprofit membership organization of persons 50 and older dedicated to addressing their needs and interests.

Print: Newsletters

7576   Aging & Vision News
Lighthouse International
111 E 59th St
New York, NY   10022-1202   212-821-9216
                                        800-829-0500
                                        Fax: 212-821-9707
                                        info@lighthouse.org
                                        www.lightfair.com
Laurie A Silbersweig, Editorial Director
Intended for professionals engaged in research, education or service delivery in the field of vision and aging.
6-12 pages Newsletter

7577   Aging News Alert
C D Publications
8204 Fenton St
Silver Spring, MD   20910-4502   301-588-6380
                                        800-666-6380
                                        Fax: 301-588-6385
                                        subscription@cdpublications.com
Michael Gerecht, President
Ash Gerecht, Co-Owner
Reports on successful senior programs, funding opportunities, and federal actions that effect the elderly. Available in 6, 12 or 24 month subscriptions online and online/print combinations.
$192.00
8 pages Monthly

7578   Aging and Vision News
Lighthouse International
111 E 59th St
New York, NY   10022-1202   212-821-9384
                                        800-829-0500
                                        Fax: 212-821-9707
                                        TTY: 212-821-9713
                                        info@lighthouse.org
                                        www.lighthouse.org
Robert Rosenberg, Editor
Mark G. Ackermann, President/ Chief Executive Officer
Maura J. Sweeney, Senior Vice President/Chief Operating Officer
John Vlachos, Senior Vice President/Chief Financial Officer
Newsletter

7579   Enabling News
Access II Independent Living Centers
101 Industrial Parkway
Gallatin, MO   64640-1280   660-663-2423
                                        888-663-2423
                                        Fax: 660-663-2517
                                        TTY: 660-663-2663
                                        access@accessii.org
                                        www.accessii.org
Debra Hawman, Executive Director
Gary Matticks, Owner
Debra Hawman, Executive Director
It is a newsletter published by Access II.
8 pages Quarterly

7580   Part B News
DecisionHealth
9737 Washingtonian Blvd
Two Washingtonian Center, Suite. 20
Gaithersburg, MD   20878-7364   301-287-2682
                                        855-225-5341
                                        Fax: 301-287-2535
                                        customer@decisionhealth.com
                                        www.decisionhealth.com
Scott Kraft, Editor
Scott Kraft, Director, Content Management
Steve Greenberg, President
Tonya Nevin, Vice President, New Business Development
Each week Part B News brings you comprehensive Medicare Part B regulatory coverage, plain-English interpretive guidance, Fee Schedule updates, claims filing strategies, coding, documenta-

tion and payment best practices, and the latest on Congressional health care deliberations and how they affect your practice. *$519.00*
Yearly

7581   Social Security Bulletin
US Social Security Administration
2100 M Street NW
Suite 829 #829
Washington, DC   20037- 0002   202-358-6066
                                       800-772-1213
                                  Fax: 202-282-7219
                                  TTY: 800-325-0778
                                  www.ssa.gov/policy

Karyn Tucker, Managing Editor
Richard Balkus, Assoc. Comm. Office Of Dis
Carolyn W. Colvin, Commissioner
James A. Kissko, Chief of Staff
Reports on results of research and analysis pertinent to the Social Security and SSI programs. *$16.00*
Monthly

Non Print: Newsletters

7582   AGRAM
Assoc of Ohio Philanthropic Homes, Housing/Service
855 S Wall St
Columbus, OH   43206-1921   614-444-2882
                                  Fax: 614-444-2974
                                       info@aopha.org
                                       www.aopha.org

John Alfano, CEO
Tim White, Executive Director
P Alfano, President/CEO
Weekly

7583   Aging News Alert
C D Publications
8204 Fenton Street
Silver Spring, MD   20910-4502   301-588-6380
                                       800-666-6380
                                  Fax: 301-588-6385
                                  www.cdpublications.com

Ash Gerecht, Co-Owner
Sharon Livermore, Businesss Manager
Reports on successful senior programs, funding opportunities, and federal actions that effect the elderly. Available in 6, 12 or 24 month subscriptions online and online/print combinations. *$192.00*
8 pages Monthly

7584   CAHSA Connecting
Colorado Assoc of Homes and Services for the Aging
1888 Sherman St
Suite 610
Denver, CO   80203-1160   303-837-8834
                                  Fax: 303-837-8836
                                       info@cahsa.org
                                  www.leadingagecolorado.org

Laura Landwirth, Executive Director
Elisabeth Borden, Director
Maureen Hewitt, President
Vennita Jenkins, Secretary
CAHSA Connecting is published monthly by the Colorado Association of Homes and Services for the Aging (CAHSA)

7585   CANPFA-Line
CT Assoc of Not-for-Profit Providers of the Aging
1340 Wilmington Rdg
Berlin, CT   6037   860-828-2903
                                  Fax: 860-828-8694
                            leadingagect@leadingagect.org
                                  www.leadingagect.org

Mag Morelli, President
Nurka Carrero, Office Manager
Andrea Bellofiore, Director of Member Programs & Se
Beth Ricker, Finance Manager & Membership Dir
LeadingAge Connecticut promotes and advocates for a vision of the world in which every community offers an integrated and co-ordinated continuum of high quality, affordable health care, housing and community based services.
Bi-Monthly

7586   Capitol Focus
Colorado Assoc of Homes and Services for the Aging
1888 Sherman St
Suite 610
Denver, CO   80203-1160   303-837-8834
                                  Fax: 303-837-8836
                                       info@cahsa.org
                                  www.leadingagecolorado.org

Laura Landwirth, Executive Director
Elisabeth Borden, Director
Maureen Hewitt, President
Vennita Jenkins, Secretary
Capitol Focus is a weekly activities summary of the Colorado Legislature for CAHSA members, provided by staff of the Colorado Association of Homes and Services for the Aging.

7587   Capsule
Children of Aging Parents
P.O.Box 167
Richboro, PA   18954-167   215-945-6900
                                       800-227-7294
                                  Fax: 215-945-8720
                            info@caps4caregivers.org
                            www.caps4caregivers.org

Karen Rosenberg, Director
An informative newsletter for caregivers.
Quarterly

7588   Communique
Iowa Association of Homes & Services for the Aging
Bi-weekly

7589   Elder Visions Newsletter
National Indian Council on Aging
8500 Menaul Blvd. NE
Suite B470
Albuquerque, NM   87112   505-292-2001
                                  Fax: 505-292-1922
                                       info@nicoa.org
                                       www.nicoa.org

Randella Bluehouse, Executive Director
Provides information on issues affecting American Indian and Alaska Native Elders.
Quarterly

7590   Innovations
National Council on Aging
1901 L Street NW
4th Floor
Washington, DC   20036-3506   202-479-1200
                                  Fax: 202-479-0735
                                  TTY:202-479-6674
                                       info@ncoa.org
                                       www.ncoa.org

Austin Han, Manager
James Firman, President/CEO
Donna Whitt, SVP/CFO
Nancy Whitelaw, SVP/Director

Explores significant developments in the field of aging, keeping individuals informed on a broad range of topics.
Quarterly

7591 NASUA News
National Association of State Units on Aging
1201 15th Street NW
Suite 350
Washington, DC 20005-2842 202-898-2578
Fax: 202-898-2583
info@nasua.org
www.nasuad.org

Martha Roherty, Executive Director
Peggie Rice, Director of Policy and Legislative Affairs
Eric Risteen, Chief Operating Officer
Kimberly Fletcher, Conference and Outreach Coordinator
It is the newsletter of the National Association of State Units on Aging
Monthly

7592 NCOA Week
National Council on Aging
1901 L Street NW
4th Floor
Washington, DC 20036-3540 202-479-1200
Fax: 202-479-0735
TTY:202-479-6674
info@ncoa.org
www.ncoa.org

James P Firman, President/CEO
Donna Whitt, SVP/CFO
Nancy Whitelaw, SVP/Director
A concise e-newsletters focused on the issues you care about, including policies that affect funding, grants and awards you can apply for, and best practices you can adapt for your center.
Weekly

7593 NNEAHSA
Northn New England Assoc of Homes & Svcs for Aging
PO Box 1428
Standish, ME 04084-1428 207-773-4822
Fax: 207-773-0101
www.agingservicesmenh.org
Sheila Deringis, Editor
Providing healthy, affordable and ethical long-term care to older citizens throughout Maine, New Hampshire and Vermont.

7594 NSCLC Washington Weekly
National Senior Citizens Law Center
1444 Eye St NW
Suite 1100
Washington, DC 20005-6547 202-289-6976
Fax: 202-289-7224
www.nsclc.org

Paul Nathanson, Executive Director
Edward King, Executive Director
Edward Spurgeon, Executive Director
Provides the latest case information, administration and congressional developments of importance for the elderly.

7595 Quality First
American Assoc of Homes and Services for the Aging
2519 Connecticut Ave NW
Washington, DC 20008-1520 202-783-2242
Fax: 202-783-2255
www.leadingage.org
William L Minnix Jr, President
Features helpful tips for marketing services and earning the public's trust through the web site.
Quarterly

7596 Senior Focus
National Council on Aging
1901 L Street
4th Floor
Washington, DC 20036-3540 202-479-1200
Fax: 202-479-0735
TTY:202-479-6674
info@ncoa.org
www.ncoa.org

Austin Han, Manager
James Firman, President/CEO
Donna Whit, SVP/CFO
Nancy Whitelaw, SVP/Director
Contains health, financial, lifestyle tips written for seniors
Quarterly

Support Groups

7597 Area Agency on Aging of Southwest Arkansas
600 Columbia Road 11 East
PO Box 1863
Magnolia, AR 71753 870-234-7410
800-272-2127
Fax: 870-234-6804
www.agewithdignity.com
Janet Morrison, Executive Director
The Area Agency on Aging of Southwest Arkansas, Inc. is a non-profit organization serving adults age 60 or older, family caregivers, agencies and organizations working with seniors. It is part of a national network of more than 650 Area Agencies on Aging throughout the United States.

7598 Area Agency on Aging: Region One
1366 E Thomas Rd
Suite 108
Phoenix, AZ 85014-5739 602-264-2255
888-783-7500
Fax: 602-230-9132
www.aaaphx.org

Mary Lynn Kasunic, President
Jeannine Berg, Vice Chairman
Bobbie Garland, Vice Chairman
Richard Peitzmeier, Vice Chairman
We have a vast variety of programs and services to enhance the quality of life for residents of Maricopa County, Arizona. If you would like more information about services mentioned within the website please call.

7599 High Country Council of Governments Area Agency on Aging
468 New Market Blvd
Boone, NC 28607-1820 828-265-5434
Fax: 828-265-5439
breece@regiond.org
www.regiond.org
Robert L. Johnson, Chairman
Gary D. Blevins, Vice Chair
Brenda Lyerly, Secretary
Danny McIntosh, Treasurer
High Country Council of Governments is the multi-county planning and development agency for the seven northwestern North Carolina counties of Alleghany, Ashe, Avery, Mitchell, Watauga, Wilkes, and Yancey. The High Country region is a voluntary association of towns and counties located in the northern mountains of North Carolina.

7600   **Institute on Aging**
3575 Geary Blvd
San Francisco, CA   94118-3212   415-750-4111
                                              877-750-4111
                                         Fax: 415-750-5337
                                         info@ioaging.org
                                         www.ioaging.org

J. Thomas Briody, MHSc, President
Dustin Harper, Vice President, Community Living Services
Cindy Kauffman, MS, COO
Roxana Tsougarakis, MBA, Chief Financial Officer
Support Services for Elders (SSE) provides care coordination, household management, personal support, bookkeeping, and other assistance to help protect your financial affairs.

7601   **Land-of-Sky Regional Council Area Agency on Aging**
339 New Leicester Hwy
Suite 140
Asheville, NC   28806-2087   828-251-6622
                                         Fax: 828-251-6353
                                         info@landofsky.org
                                         www.landofsky.org

LeeAnne Tucker, Aging & Volunteer Services Director
Terry Albrecht, Program Director
Joan Tuttle, Director
Joe Mc Kinney, Manager
Is the designated regional organization to meet the needs of persons over 60 in Buncombe, Henderson, Madison, and Transylvania counties, by the North Carolina Division of Aging and Adult Services.

7602   **Lumber River Council of Governments Area Agency on Aging**
30 Cj Walker Rd
COMtech Park
Pembroke, NC   28372-7340   910-618-5533
                                         Fax: 910-521-7556
                                         lrcog@mail.lrcog.dst.nc.us
                                         www.lumberrivercog.org

Michelle Gaitley, Nutrition Program Director
Renee Cooper, Nutrition Program Assistant
Kristen Elk Maynor, Aging Program Coordinator
Margaret Lennon, Division Administrator
The Family Caregiver Support Program was created to assist family members, neighbors, and friends who help care for a person over the age of 60, or minor grandchildren being reared by a grandparent over 60.

7603   **Mid-America Regional Council - Aging and Adult Services**
600 Broadway
Suite 200
Kansas City, MO   64105-1659   816-474-4240
                                         Fax: 816-421-7758
                                         marcinfo@marc.org
                                         www.marc.org/Community/Aging/
James Stowe, Director of Aging & Adult Services
Bob Hogan, Manager of Aging Administrative Services
Shannon Halvorsen, Information & Referral Coordinator
Toni Bartram, Administrative Assistant
The Department of Aging and Adult Services offers community-based services to aging people in the Cass, Clay, Jackson, Platte and Ray counties. Services include home care, transportation, legal aid, breaks for caregivers and meal delivery.

7604   **Mid-Carolina Area Agency on Aging**
130 Gillespie Street
3rd Floor, Post Office Drawer 1510
Fayetteville, NC   28301-1510   910-323-4191
                                         Fax: 910-323-9330
                                         gdye@mccog.org
                                         www.mccog.org

James Caldwell, COG Executive Director
Glenda Dye, Aging Director
Lynda Barnett, Aging Care Manager
Carla Smith, Aging Program Specialist
The Mid-Carolina Area Agency on Aging is designated for planning, administration, and advocacy of services for persons aged

60 and older and their spouses who need assistance in order to remain as independent as possible.

7605   **Piedmont Triad Council of Governments Area Agency on Aging**
2216 W Meadowview Rd
Suite 201
Greensboro, NC   27407-3480   336-294-4950
                                         Fax: 336-632-0457
                                         acalhoun@ptcog.org
                                         www.ptcog.org

Blair Barton-Percival, Director
Adrienne Calhoun, Assistant Director
Bob Cleveland, Aging Program Planner
Joe Dzugan, Aging Systems Coordinator
Responsible for planning, developing, implementing, and coordinating aging services for seven counties in the Piedmont Triad (Alamance, Caswell, Davidson, Guilford, Montgomery, Randolph, and Rockingham) and their 185,00 residents age 60 and older.

7606   **Southwestern Commission Area Agency on Aging**
125 Bonnie Ln
Sylva, NC   28779-8552   828-586-1962
                                         Fax: 828-586-1968
                                         www.regiona.org

Ryan Sherby, Executive Director
Beth Cook, Workforce Development Director
Janne Mathews, Aging Program Coordinator
Sarajane Melton, Area Agency on Aging Administrator
The Area Agency on Aging (AAA) works on behalf of older adults and their caregivers in the seven southwestern counties of North Carolina. The Southwestern Commission Area Agency on Aging was established in 1980 as mandated by the 1977 Amendments of the Older Americans Act in order for a Planning and Service Area (PSA) to receive funds from the Act.

7607   **Tompkins County Office for the Aging**
214 W. Martin Luther King Jr./State
Ithaca, NY   14850-4299   607-274-5482
                                         Fax: 607-274-5495
                                         lholmes@tompkins-co.org

Lisa Holmes, Director
Lisa Lunas, Aging Services Planner
Katrina Schickel, Aging Services Specialist
David Stoyell, Aging Services Specialist
We provide objective and unbiased information regarding the array of services available for older adults and their caregivers. Established in 1975, our mission is to assist the senior population of Tompkins County to remain independent in their homes as long as is possible and appropriate, and with a decent quality of life and human dignity.

7608   **Triangle J Council of Governments Area Agency on Aging**
4307 Emperor Blvd
Suite 110
Durham, NC   27703   919-549-0551
                                         Fax: 919-549-9390
                                         ejones@tjcog.org
                                         www.tjaaa.org

Kristen Jackson, Aging Program Coordinator
Mary Warren, Director
Ashley Price, Program Specialist
Jennifer Link, Regional Ombudsman for Long-Term Care
The Triangle J Council of Governments serves to facilitate and support the development of programs addressing the needs of older adults and to support investment in their talents and interests.

7609 University of California Memory and Aging Center
675 Nelson Rising Lane
Suite 190
San Francisco, CA 94143-1207   415-353-2057
Fax: 415-476-5591
webmaster@memory.ucsf.edu
www.memory.ucsf.edu

Bruce L Miller, Director
Mary Koestler, Project Administrator
Carrie Cheung, Clinic Coordinator
Ken Edwards, Administrative Assistant
Provides support for patients and families affected by
neurodegenerative diseases. In addition to our established sup-
port groups, we continue to develop new support groups.

**7610 Upper Coastal Plain Council of Governments Area Agency
on Aging**
PO Box 9
Wilson, NC 27894-9   252-234-5952
Fax: 252-234-5971
www.ucpcog.org

Greg Godard, Executive Director
Jody Riddle, AAA Program Director
Helen Page, Aging Programs Specialist
Abigail W. Harper, Regional Ombudsman
The Upper Coastal Plain Area Agency On Aging is one of 16 Area
Agencies on Aging across the state of NC, serving Region L.
Counties include Edgecombe, Halifax, Nash, Northampton, and
Wilson. The mission of the Area Agency on Aging is to empower
senior adults, family caregivers, and individuals with disabilities
residing in Edgecombe, Halifax, Nash, Northampton, and Wilson
Counties to live independent, meaningful, healthy, and dignified
lives.

Blind & Deaf

Associations

7611 American Association of the Deaf-Blind
3825 LaVista Rd, W-2
Tucker, GA 30084

301-495-4403
Fax: 301-495-4404
TTY:301-495-4402
aadb-info@aadb.org
www.aadb.org

Jenee Alleman-Goodman, President
Rene Pellerin, Vice President
Chris Woodfill, Secretary
Mark Gasaway, Treasurer

The American Association of the Deaf-Blind (AADB) is a non-profit national consumer organization run by and for deaf-blind Americans and their supporters. Deaf-Blind includes all types and degrees of dual vision and hearing loss. The association offers an information clearinghouse, service provider summit, deaf-blind technology summit, research projects, interpretation services, conferences and more.
Membership dues

7612 American Society for Deaf Children
800 Florida Ave NE
Suite 2047
Washington, DC 20002-3695

800-942-2732
Fax: 410-795-0965
asdc@deafchildren.org
deafchildren.org

Avonne Brooker-Rutowski, Ed.S, President
Lisalee Egbert, Ph.D, Vice President
Timothy Frelich, M.A., Treasurer
Gina A Oliva, Ph.D, Secretary

The American Society for Deaf Children provides information for the caretakers of deaf children so children can have full communication access in their home, school and community. The society covers areas such as visual language, audiologists, healthcare providers, assistive technology and more.

7613 Arena Stage
1101 Sixth St, SW
Washington, DC 20024

202-554-9066
Fax: 202-488-4056
TTY:202-484-0247
arena@arenastage.org
www.arenastage.org

Judith N Batty, Chair
Joseph Berardelli, CEO
Khady Kamara, Associate Executive Director
Anita Maynard-Losh, Director of Community Engagement

A pioneer in providing access to theater for people with disabilities and the birthplace of Audio Description. Arena Stage offers infrared assistive listening devices (both loop and headset), program books in Braille and large print and wheelchair accessible seating with adjacent companion seating. Audio cassette format is available upon request. Sign interpretation and audio description are offered at selected performances.

7614 Association of Late-Deafened Adults
8038 Macintosh Ln
Suite 2
Rockford, IL 61107

815-332-1515
866-402-2532
Fax: 877-907-1738
TTY: 866-402-2532
info@alda.org
www.alda.org

Sharaine Rawlinson Roberts, President
Paul Wummer, Vice President
Eleanor Shafer, Region I Director
Carol Postulka, Region II Director

The Association of Late-Deafened Adults supports the empowerment of late-deafened people by offering programs and information resources on a variety of topics: technology, disability laws, airline travel and more.

7615 Canadian Deafblind Association
1860 Appleby Line
Unit 14
Burlington, ON, Canada L7L-7H7

866-229-5832
Fax: 905-319-2027
info@cdbanational.com
www.cdbanational.com

Carolyn Monaco, President
Tom McFadden, National Executive Director
Cathy Proll, Executive Director, Ontario Chapter

The mission of the Canadian Deafblind Association is to promote and enhance the well-being of people who are deafblind by offering them advocacy, developing and dissemination information, and supporting members and community partners who also serve deafblind people.

7616 Foundation Fighting Blindness
7168 Columbia Gateway Dr.
Suite 100
Columbia, MD 21046

410-423-0600
800-683-5555
TTY:410363713951
info@FightBlindness.org
www.blindness.org

William T. Schmidt, Chief Executive Officer
Valerie Navy-Daniels, Chief Development Officer
Stephen M. Rose, PhD, Chief Research Officer

The Foundation Fighting Blindness (FFB) works to promote research in order to prevent, treat and restore vision. FFB is currently the world's leading private funder of retinal disease research, funding over 100 research grants and 150 researchers.

7617 Hearing Loss Association of America
7910 Woodmont Ave
Suite 1200
Bethesda, MD 20814

301-657-2248
Fax: 301-913-9413
TTY:301-657-2249
inquiry@hearingloss.org
www.hearingloss.org

Barbara Kelley, Executive Director
Lise Hamlin, Director of Public Policy
Nancy Macklin, Director of External Affairs & Events
Erin Mirante, National Chapter Coordinator

The mission of the Hearing Loss Association of America is to open the world of communication to people with hearing loss by offering information, education, resources, advocacy and training.

7618 Helen Keller National Center for Deaf- Blind Youths and Adults
141 Middle Neck Rd
Sands Point, NY 11050

516-944-8900
Fax: 516-944-7302
TTY:516-944-8637
hkncinfo@hknc.org
www.helenkeller.org

Joseph F Bruno, President & CEO
Marc Feldman, CPA, Chief Financial Officer
Chris Mastrangelo, Director of Facilities
Mia Murro, Chief Human Resources Officer

The center serves deafblind people by offering them assistive technology, vocational services, education, case management, interpretation, medical and mental health services, professional training and other supports that would empower them to work and live independently within their communities.

7619   Idaho Commission for the Blind and Visually Impaired
341 W. Washington St
PO Box 83720
Boise, ID 83720-0012   208-334-3220
                                          800-542-8688
                                     Fax: 208-334-2963
                                     kgrant@icbvi.idaho.gov
                                     www.icbvi.state.id.us

Britt Raubenheimer, Chair
Beth Cunningham, Administrator
Raelene Thomas, Management Assistant
Mike Walsh, Rehabilitation Services Chief
The Idaho Commission for the Blind and Visually Impaired
works to empower persons who are blind or visually impaired by
providing vocational rehabilitation training, skills training and
educational opportunities to achieve self fulfillment ang gain employment. The Commission also strives to serve as a resource to
families and employers and to expand public awareness regarding the potential of all persons who are blind or visually impaired.

7620   International Hearing Society
16880 Middlebelt Rd
Suite 4
Livonia, MI 48154   734-522-7200
                                     Fax: 734-522-0200
                                     amarkey@ihsinfo.org
                                          ihsinfo.org

Richard Giles, ACA, BC-HIS, President
Kathleen Mennillo, MBA, Executive Director
Ted Annis, Senior Marketing Specialist
Tara Douglass, Business Development Manager
The International Hearing Society (IHS) represents hearing
healthcare professionals worldwide. Members include professionals engaged in the practice of testing human hearing and selecting, fitting and dispensing hearing instruments. IHS offers
accreditation programs, advocacy, education and training in
support of these services.

7621   Lilac Services for the Blind
1212 N Howard St
Spokane, WA 99201   509-328-9116
                                          800-422-7893
                                     Fax: 509-328-8965
                                     contact@lilacblind.org
                                          lilacblind.org

Eddie Eugenio, President
Cheryl L Martin, Executive Director
Robin Waller, Development Director
Raychel Callary, Certified Orientation & Mobility Specialist
Lilac Services for the Blind provides independent living instruc-
tion, adaptive aids, counseling, low-vision evaluations, support
groups, Braille transcription services and more for 14 counties in
the inland Northwest.

7622   National Center on Deaf-Blindness
345 N. Monmouth Ave
Monmouth, OR 97361   503-838-8754
                                     Fax: 503-838-8150
                                     info@nationaldb.org
                                          nationaldb.org

Linda McDowell, Executive Director
Gail Leslie, Project Specialist & Website Management
Betsy McGinnity, Senior Advisor
Shelby Morgan, Project Specialist
Promotes academic achievement and results for children and
youth who are deaf-blind by offering them technical assistance
and information dissemination activities. National intiatives
cover the areas of early identification, family engagement,
training, literacy and more.

7623   National Family Association for Deaf-Blind
141 Middle Neck Rd
Sands Point, NY 11050   516-944-8900
                                          800-255-0411
                                     Fax: 516-883-9060
                                     TTY: 516-944-8637
                                     nfadbinfo@gmail.com
                                          nfadb.org

Clara Berg, President
Diana Griffen, Vice President
Jacqueline Izaguirre, Treasurer
Patti McGowan, Secretary
The National Family Association for Deaf-Blind (NFADB) is a
non-profit, volunteer-based family association. The association
offers advocacy, education and family supports to help create em-
powerment opportunities for deaf-blind people.

7624   National Federation of the Blind
200 E Wells St.
Baltimore, MD 21230   410-659-9314
                                     Fax: 410-685-5653
                                     nfb@nfb.org
                                          nfb.org

Mark Riccobono, President
John Berggren, Executive Director, Operations
Mya Jones, Executive Assistant
Ficarro Paul, Director of Program Facilities
The National Federation of the Blind (NFB) works to help blind
people achieve self-confidence, self-respect and self-determination and to achieve complete integration into society on a basis of
equality. The Federation provides public educations, information
and referral services, scholarships, literature and publications,
adaptive equipment, advocacy services, legal services,
employment assistance and more.

Camps

7625   Florida Lions Camp
Lions of Multiple District 35
2819 Tiger Lake Road
Lake Wales, FL 33898-9582   863-696-1948
                                     Fax: 863-696-2398
                                     bjcage@hotmail.com
                                     www.lionscampfl.org

Barbara Cage, Executive Director
Liz Cage, Program Director
Carissa Moen, Bookkeeping/Registrar
One-week sessions June-August for youths and adults with visual impairments and other challenging disabilities. Coed, ages 5
and up. A variety of traditional summer camp activities which include: swimming, canoeing, fishing, hiking, camping out and
cooking over a fire, games, arts & crafts, singing & dancing,
hay-wagon rides, challenge course and much more. Activities are
adapted to the age and ability of each camper to ensure maximum
participation, safety and fun.

7626   Florida School for the Deaf and Blind
207 San Marco Ave
St Augustine, FL 32084-2799   904-827-2200
                                          800-344-3732
                                     Fax: 904-827-2325
                                     info@fsdb.k12.fl.us
                                     www.fsdb.k12.fl.us

Dr. Jeanne Glidden Prickett, EdD, Shelter Administrator
Debbie Schuler, Administrator of Instructional S
Cindy Day, Executive Director of Parent Ser
Terri Wiseman, Administrator of Business Servic
Statewide public boarding school for eligible students who are
deaf/hard-of-hearing or blind/visually impaired. FSDB serves
children who are pre-k through high school.

Print: Books

7627   A Handbook for Writing Effective Psychoeducational Reports (2nd Edition)
PRO-ED Inc.
8700 Shoal Creek Blvd.
Austin, TX   78757-6897
512-451-3246
800-897-3202
Fax: 800-397-7633
general@proedinc.com
www.proedinc.com

Sharon Bradley-Johnson, Author
C. Merle Johnson, Author
This comprehensive book shows how to write useful reports once assessment information has been attained. It is a valuable resource for professionals working in school systems, as well as for those graduate students who are just learning to write reports. *$32.00*
134 pages Paperback
ISBN 1-416401-40-7

7628   Communicating with People Who Have Trouble Hearing & Seeing: A Primer
National Association for Visually Handicapped
22 W 21st St
Fl 6
New York, NY   10010-6943
212-255-2804
Fax: 212-727-2931
www.lighthouse.org
Roger O Goldman, Chairman Of The Board
Line drawings that depict problems for those with both deficiencies. *$2.00*

7629   Helen and Teacher: The Story of Helen & Anne Sullivan Macy
American Foundation for the Blind/AFB Press
11 Penn Plz
Suite 300
New York, NY   10001-2006
212-502-7600
800-232-5463
Fax: 212-502-7777
afbinf@afb.net
www.afb.org

Carl Augusto, President
Richard Obnen, Chairman Of The Board
Michael Gilliam, Vice Chairman
Alan Lindroth, Principal
A pictorial biography emphasizing Hellen Keller's accomplishments in public life over a period of more than 60 years. Traces Anne Sullivan's early years and her meeting with Helen Keller, and goes on to recount the joint events of their lives. A definitive biography. *$29.95.*
Paperback
ISBN 0-891282-89-0

7630   Independence Without Sight and Sound: Suggestions for Practitioners
American Foundation for the Blind/AFB Press
11 Penn Plz
Suite 300
New York, NY   10001-2006
212-502-7600
800-232-8463
Fax: 212-502-7777
afbinfo@afb.net
www.afb.org

Carl Augusto, President
Richard Obnen, Chairman Of The Board
Michael Gilliam, Vice Chairman
Alan Lindroth, Principal
This practical guidebook covers the essential aspects of communicating and working with deaf-blind persons. Includes useful information on how to talk with deaf-blind people, and adapt orientation and mobility techniques for deaf-blind travelers. *$39.95*
193 pages Paperback
ISBN 0-891282-46-7

7631   Reclaiming Independence: Staying in the Drivers Seat When You Are no Longer Drive.
American Printing House for the Blind
1839 Frankfort Ave
Louisville, KY   40206-3148
502-895-2405
800-223-1839
Fax: 502-899-2274
info@aph.org
www.aph.org

Tuck Tinsley, President
Joseph Paradis, Chairman
Kathleen Huebner, Vice Chairman
Jane Thompson, Executive Director
Useful for both individuals and professionals, this video/resource guide will help you successfuly use rehabilitation and transportation resources. *$60.00*

7632   Verbal View of the Web & Net
American Printing House for the Blind
1839 Frankfort Ave
Louisville, KY   40206-3148
502-895-2405
800-223-1839
Fax: 502-899-2274
info@aph.org
www.aph.org

Tuck Tinsley, President
Joseph Paradis, Chairman
Kathleen Huebner, Vice Chairman
Jane Thompson, Executive Director
One of a series of Verbal View titles, Verbal View of the Net & Web explains how to access information on the internet and teaches accessability features of Internet Explorer. *$50.00*

Print: Magazines

7633   Braille Montior
National Federation of the Blind Senior Division
200 E Wells St
Baltimore, MD   21230-4914
410-659-9314
Fax: 410-685-5653
nfbpublications@nfb.org
www.nfb.org

Barbara Pierce, Editor
The Braille Monitor is the leading publication of the National Federation of the Blind. It covers the events and activities of the NFB and addresses the many issues and concerns of the blind.
11 times a year

7634   Deaf-Blind American
American Association of the Deaf-Blind (AADB)
8630 Fenton Street
PO Box 2831, Suite 121
Kensington, MD 20891-3803
301-495-4403
Fax: 301-495-4404
TTY:301-495-4402
aadb-info@aadb.org
www.aadb.org

Jamie Pope, Executive Director
Elizabeth Spiers, Information Services Director
Timothy Jackson, President
We are a consumer membership organization of, by and for people who have dual vision and hearing loss. Services we provide include an information clearinghouse on deaf blindness, a quarterly magazine (The Deaf Blind American), a newsletter, AADB news, a task force to improve interpreting for deaf-blind people, a listen for members, a partnership with the American Red Cross, and national conferences. *$5.00*
Quartlery

7635 Hearing Loss Magazine
HearingLoss Association of America
7910 Woodmont Ave
Ste 1200
Bethesda, MD   20814-7022   301-657-2248
                                        Fax: 301-913-9413
                                        www.hearingloss.org

Brenda Battat, Executive Director
Barbara Kelley, Editor-in-Chief/Deputy Executive Director of
HLAA
Lisa Hamlin, Director Of Public Policy
Cindy Dyer, Graphic Design
Readers look to Hearing Loss Magazine to provide them with the
latest information on products, services, research, and technol-
ogy in the hearing health care field. They also look for personal
stories of hard of hearing people to find encouragement, and give
them the feeling that they're not alone in living with a hearing
loss. They look for practical and useful information. Hearing
Loss Magazine readers view the magazine as a lifeline to help
them help themselves and live well with hearing loss.
Bi-Monthly

7636 Hearing Professional Magazine
International Hearing Society
Ste 4
16880 Middlebelt Rd
Livonia, MI   48154-3374   734-522-7200
                                        Fax: 734-522-0200
                                        knacarato@ihsinfo.org
                                        www.ihsinfo.org

Scott Beall, Treasurer Director
Alan Lowell, President
Kathleen Mennillo, Executive Director
The Hearing Professional magazine is the official publication of
the International Hearing Society. This quarterly publication includes industry news, membership highlights and best practices,
hearing healthcare legislation, and other information and tools
for hearing healthcare professionals.

Print: Newsletters

7637 Deaf-Blind Perspective
National Consortium on Deaf-Blindness
345 Monmouth Ave
Monmouth, OR   97361   503-838-8391
                                        800-438-9376
                                        Fax: 503-838-8150
                                        TTY: 800-854-7013
                                        dbp@wou.edu
                                        www.tr.wou.edu/dblink

John Reiman PhD, Director
Peggy Malloy, Managing Editor
A free publication with articles, essays, and announcements
about topics related to people who are deaf-blind. The primary fo-
cus is on the education of children and youth with deaf-blindness.
Published two times a year (Spring and Fall) by the national con-
sortium on Deaf-blindness at the Teaching Research Institute at
Western Oregon University.

7638 InFocus
7168 Columbia Gateway Dri
Suite 100
Columbia, MD   21046   410-423-0600
                                        800-683-5555
                                        Fax: 410-363-2393
                                        TTY: 800-683-5551
                                        www.blindness.org

Gordon Gund, Chairman
Edward H. Gollob, President
David Brint, VP
Haynes Lea, VP & Treasurer
Presents articles on coping, research updates, and Foundation
news.
3x/year

7639 News from Advocates for Deaf-Blind
National Family Association for Deaf-Blind
141 Middle Neck Rd
Sands Point, NY   11050-1218   516-944-8900
                                        800-225-0411
                                        Fax: 516-883-9060
                                        TTY: 516-944-8637
                                        NFADB@gmail.com
                                        www.NFADB.org

Clara Berg, President
Edgenie Bellah, Affiliate Coordinator
Paddi Davies, Treasurer
Patti McGowan, Secretary
A membership organization which provide resources, education,
advocacy, referrals and support for families with children who
are deaf-blind; professionals in the field; and individuals who are
deaf-blind.
20 pages TriAnnual

Non Print: Newsletters

7640 AADB E-News
American Association of the Deaf-Blind
8630 Fenton Street
Suite 121
Silver Spring, MD   20910- 3803   301-495-4403
                                        Fax: 301-495-4404
                                        aadb-info@aadb.org
                                        www.aadb.org

Jill Gaus, President
Lynn Jansen, VP
Debby Lieberman, Secretary
Mike Reese, Vice Treasurer
Contains information about the latest events occurring within
AADB and in the deaf-blind community.

7641 ALDA Newsletter
ALDA
8038 Macintosh Ln
Suite 2
Rockford, IL   61107-5336   815-332-1515
                                        866-402-2532
                                        Fax: 877-907-1738
                                        TTY: 815-332-1515
                                        info@alda.org
                                        www.alda.org

Mary Lou Mistretta, President
Dave Litman, President Elect
Brenda Estes, Past President
Articles, stories and poems by and about late-deafened adults.

7642 Beam
1850 W Roosevelt Rd
Chicago, IL   60608-1298   312-666-1331
                                        Fax: 312-243-8539
                                        TTY:312-666-8874
                                        www.chicagolighthouse.org

James Kesteloot, President
Terrence Longo, Assistant Director
Quarterly newsletter of the organization offering progressive
programs for the blind, visually impaired, deaf-blind and
multi-disabled children and adults, including vocational programs, computer and office skills training, job placement, independent living skills, orientation and mobility training,
counseling and a low vision clinic.

7643 Endeavor
American Society for Deaf Children
800 Florida Ave NE
Washington, PA 20002-3695 717-703-0073
800-942-2732
Fax: 717-909-5599
TTY: 202-664-9204
asdc@deafchildren.org
www.deafchildren.org

Robert B Wells, Editor
Tami Hossler, Editor
ASDC's qurterly publication featuring committee reports, stories, and fun.
Quarterly

7644 HKNC Newsletter
Helen Keller National Center
141 Middle Neck Rd
Sands Point, NY 11050-1218 516-944-8900
Fax: 516-944-7302
TTY:516-944-8637
hkncinfo@hknc.org
www.hknc.org

Joseph McNulty, Executive Director
Highlights recent activities at the national center.

7645 NAT-CENT
Helen Keller National Center
141 Middle Neck Rd
Sands Point, NY 11050-1218 516-944-8900
Fax: 516-944-7302
TTY:516-944-8637
hkncinfo@hknc.org
www.hknc.org

Joseph McNulty, Executive Director
Contains articles on legislation, services, aids and devices, human interest and issues related to deaf-blindness.

Non Print: Software

7646 Braille + Mobile Manager
American Printing House for the Blind
1839 Frankfort Ave
Louisville, KY 40206-0085 502-895-2405
800-223-1839
Fax: 502-899-2284
info@aph.org
aph.org

Tuck Tinsley, President
Joseph Paradis, Chairman
Kathleen Huebner, Vice Chairman
Jane Thompson, Executive Director
Use it like a hand-held PDA or like a laptop. *$1395.00*

7647 MaximEyes
American Printing House for the Blind
1839 Frankfort Ave
Louisville, KY 40206-0085 502-895-2405
800-223-1839
Fax: 502-899-2284
info@aph.org
aph.org

Tuck Tinsley, President
Joseph Paradis, Chairman
Kathleen Huebner, Vice Chairman
Jane Thompson, Executive Director
MaximEyes is a plug-in for Internet Explorer that adds a toolbar that allows you to controll the size of website text and images. *$59.95*

Non Print: Video

7648 Getting in Touch
2612 N Mattis Ave
PO Box 7886
Champaign, IL 61826-1053 217-352-3273
800-519-2707
Fax: 217-352-1221
orders@researchpress.com
www.researchpress.com

Russell Pence, President
David Parkinson, Chairman
Cynthia Martin, Principal
Ann Parkinson, Principal

7649 Journey
Landmark Media
3450 Slade Run Dr
Falls Church, VA 22042-3940 703-241-2030
800-342-4336
Fax: 703-536-9540
info@landmarkmedia.com
landmarkmedia.com

Michael Hartogs, President
Richard Hartogs, VP Acquisitions
Peter Hartogs, VP New Business & Development
Eric Miller, Sales Representative
A moving portrayal of the extraordinary journey to Japan of 74-year-old Billie Sinclair, who is deaf, blind and mute. He funds his travels by weaving and selling baskets. In Japan he rides a roller coaster, tries judo and visits a deaf and blind acupuncturist. He demonstrates how it is possible to communicate by touch alone. *$195.00*
Video

Sports

7650 ASD Athletics
Alabama Institute for Deaf and Blind
205 South St E
Talladega, AL 35160-2411 256-761-3222
Fax: 256-761-3278
Ripley.Walter@aidb.state.al.us
aidb.org/alabama-school-for-the-deaf/athl etic
John Jernigan, Director, Student Development (ASD)
Walter Ripley, Director, Athletics & After-School Programs
Offers students opportunities to participate in a number of organizzed sports including basketball, volleyball, baseball, football, and cheerleading. Student athletes compete at national and international levels.

Support Groups

7651 Aurora of Central New York
518 James Street
Suite 100
Syracuse, NY 13203-2282 315-422-7263
Fax: 315-422-4792
TTY:315-422-9746
auroraofcny.org

John Scala, President
John McCormick, President
Ryan Emery, Treasurer
Leslie Rapson, Secretary
Professional counseling services to assist individuals and their families deal with the trauma of hearing or vision loss.

7652   Wendell Johnson Speech And Hearing Clinic
University Of Iowa
250 Hawkins Dr
Iowa City, IA   52242-1025   319-335-8736
                                          Fax: 319-335-8851
                              kathy-miller@uiowa.edu
                  www.clas.uiowa.edu/comsci/clinical-services
Linda Souke, Clinic Director
Kathy Miller, Clinic Assistant
The clinic offers assessment and remediation for communication disorders in adults and children. The clinic also offers services during the Summer for school age children needing intervention services because of speech, language, hearing and/or reading problems.

Cognitive

Associations

7653 Academy of Cognitive Therapy
245 N. 15th St
Suite 403
Philadelphia, PA   19102   Fax: 215-537-1789
info@academyofct.org
www.academyofct.org

Lata K McGinn, Ph.D, President
Troy Thompson, Executive Director
Allen Miller, Ph.D, MBA, Treasurer
Elaine Elliott-Moskwa, Ph.D, Secretary
The Academy of Cognitive Therapy is a non-profit organization that supports continuing education and research in cognitive therapy, provides resources for professionals and the public, and offers certification for those skilled in the field.

7654 American Academy of Child & Adolescent Psychiatry
3615 Wisconsin Ave NW
Washington, DC   20016-3007   202-966-7300
Fax: 202-464-0131
communications@aacap.org
www.aacap.org

Gregory K Fritz, MD, President
Heidi B Fordi, CAE, Executive Director
Karen Ferguson, Deputy Director of Clinical Practice
Rob Grant, Communications Director
The American Academy of Child & Adolescent Psychiatry is a non-profit organization engaged in research, education and advocacy specific to child and adolescent psychiatry. The academy's mission is to provide resources and knowledge beneficial to patients, their families and psychiatric professionals.

7655 American Delirium Society
1183 University Dr
Suite 105 - 106
Burlington, NC   27215   410-955-2343
info@americandeliriumsociety.org
www.americandeliriumsociety.org
Rakesh C Arora MD, Ph.D, Director
Noll Campbell, PharmD, MS, Director
John W Devlin, PharmD, Director
Ann Gruber-Baldini, Ph.D, Director
The American Delirium Society fosters research, education, quality improvement, advocacy and science to minimize the impact of delirium on short- and long-term health and well being and the effects of delirium on the health care system as a whole. The organization offers educational resources including videos and publications on the subject.

7656 American Psychiatric Association
1000 Wilson Blvd
Suite 1825
Arlington, VA   22209-3901   703-907-7300
703-907-7300
888-357-7924
Fax: 703-907-1085
apa@psych.org
www.psychiatry.org

Anita Everett, MD, President
Saul M Levin, MD, MPA, CEO & Medical Director
Mark Myers, Director, Administrative Services
Christie Couture, Associate Director of Marketing
The American Psychiatric Association is a medical specialty society with over 37,000 member physicians engaged in the field of psychiatric practice, research, and academia. The association's mission is to ensure humane care and effective treatment of all persons with mental disorders, including substance use disorders. Services offered by them include collegial support, advocacy, publications and more.

7657 Anxiety and Depression Association of America
8701 Georgia Ave
Suite 412
Silver Spring, MD   20910   240-485-1001
Fax: 240-485-1035
information@adaa.org
adaa.org
Karen Cassiday, PhD, President
Susan K Gurley, Executive Director
Lise Bram, Director of Communications & Marketing
Sarah Gerfen, Director of Finance & Operations
The Anxiety and Depression Association of America (ADAA) is a non-profit organization focusing on the treatment of anxiety, depressive and obsessive-compulsive disorders through education and research.

7658 Association for Behavioral and Cognitive Therapies (ABCT)
305 7th Ave
16th Floor
New York, NY   10001   212-647-1890
Fax: 212-647-1865
www.abct.org
Gail Steketee, Ph.D, President
Barbara Kamholz, Ph.D, Convention & Continuing Education Issues
Shireen Rizvi, Ph.D, Academic & Professional Issues
Hilary Vidair, Ph.D, Membership
The ABCT is an organization committed to the advancement of scientific approaches to address the issues of soldiers with PTSD. The association offers information in a number of areas: combat related stress, military posttraumatic stress disorder, military suicide and veterans' health.

7659 Association for Contextual Behavioral Science
1880 Pinegrove Dr
P.O. Box 655
Jenison, MI   49429   225-302-8688
staff@contextualscience.org
contextualscience.org
Emily Rodrigues, Executive Director
Courtney Zirkle, CMP, Administrative & Social Media Manager
The Association for Contextual Behavioral Science specializes in helping people through research and practice based in contextual behavioral science (including RFT and CBS). The association offers learning resources, training, internships, events, consultations, conferences, continuing education opportunities and more.

7660 Autism Research Institute
4182 Adams Ave.
San Diego, CA   92116-2599   866-366-3361
www.autism.com
Stephen Edelson, Ph.D, Executive Director
Anthony Morgali, Producer, ARI Media
Denise Fulton, Administrative Director
Rebecca McKenney, Office Manager
Conducts research on the causes, diagnosis and treatment of autism. The institute also offers a quarterly newsletter that reviews worldwide research, referrals to health care professionals and clinics serving autistic people, advocacy, continuing education and more.

7661 Autism Services Center
929 4th Ave.
P.O. Box 507
Huntington, WV   25701-0507   304-525-8014
Fax: 304-525-8026
www.autismservicescenter.org
Ralph N Bentley, President
Jimmie Beirne, Ph.D, CEO
The Autism Services Center assists families and agencies to meet the needs of individuals with autism and other developmental disabilities by offering services such as technical assistance in designing treatment programs, a hotline providing informational packets to callers, supported employment, day programs, residential services and more.

7662 Autism Society of Minnesota
Autism Society of Minnesota
2380 Wycliff St.
#102
St. Paul, MN 55114

651-647-1083
camp@ausm.org
www.ausm.org

Jean Bender, President
Paul D'Arco, Vice President
Katie Knutson, Secretary
Paul Schmidt, Treasurer
The Autism Society of Minnesota (AuSM) is a nonprofit, membership organization dedicated to the education, advocacy, and support of individuals and families who have been affected by autism.

7663 Autism Treatment Center of America
2080 S Undermountain Rd
Sheffield, MA 01257-9643

413-229-2100
877-766-7473
Fax: 413-229-8931
correspondence@option.org
www.autismtreatmentcenter.org

Barry Neil Kaufman, Founder & CEO
Clyde Haberman, Senior Teacher & Director of Development
Blair Borgeson, Developmental Therapist
Emily Vitale Aronow, Program Advisor & Client Support Coordinator
The Autism Treatment Center of America provides innovative training programs for parents and professionals caring for children challenged by Autism, Autism Spectrum Disorders, Pervasive Developmental Disorders (PDD) and other development difficulties. The center's Son-Rise Program teaches a comprehensive system of treatment and education designed to help families and caregivers enable their children to improve in all areas of learning.

7664 Beck Institute for Cognitive Behavior Therapy
1 Belmont Ave
Suite 700
Bala Cynwyd, PA 19004

610-664-3020
Fax: 610-709-5336
info@beckinstitute.org
www.beckinstitute.org

Aaron T Beck, Ph.D, President Emeritus
Judith S Beck, Ph.D, President
Lisa Pote, Executive Director
Quethelyn Blake, Finance Manager
The Beck Institute for Cognitive Behavior Therapy serves as a training ground for cognitive therapists and cognitive behavior therapists. The institute provides online resources, training workshops and CBT therapy for the public and mental health professionals.

7665 Best Buddies
907-1243 Islington Ave
Toronto, ON, Canada M8X-1Y9

416-531-0003
888-779-0061
Fax: 416-531-0325
info@bestbuddies.ca
bestbuddies.ca

Daniel J Greenglass, Co-Chair
Sarah McCarthy, Program Coordinator
Kimberly Janohan, Program Support
Best Buddies offers programs for people with intellectual or developmental disabilities including those with Down syndrome, autism, cerebral palsy, traumatic brain injury and other undiagnosed disabilities. Programs include schooling, transition programs, sports, scholarships and more.

7666 Biologically Inspired Cognitive Architectures Society
4450 Rivanna River Way
Suite 3707
Fairfax, VA 22030-4441

703-910-3014
Fax: 877-532-0197
info@bicasociety.org
bicasociety.org

Alexei V Samsonovich, President-Treasurer
Antonio Chella, Chair
Kamilla R Johannsdottir, Secretary
The Biologically Inspired Cognitive Architectures Society brings together researchers from disjointed fields and communities in order to combine their knowledge into forming a larger, unifying framework for the study of cognitive architectures.

7667 Brain Injury Alliance of Texas
9050 N Capital of Texas Hwy
Building 3, Suite 130
Austin, TX 78759

512-326-1212
800-392-0040
Fax: 512-478-3370
info@texasbia.com
www.texasbia.org

Kelly Ramsey, President
Greg Walton, Vice President
Mendi West, Secretary-Treasurer
The Brain Injury Alliance of Texas is a community of people with brain injuries, their families and the professionals that serve them. The alliance offers information, support groups, prevention strategies, educational opportunities, public policy advocacy, a resource library and more.

7668 Brain Injury Association of America
1608 Spring Hill Rd
Suite 110
Vienna, VA 22182

703-761-0750
800-444-6443
Fax: 703-761-0755
braininjuryinfo@biausa.org
www.biausa.org

Bud Elkind, MS, CBIST, Chairman
Susan Connors, President & CEO
Dianna Fahel, Marketing & Communications Coordinator
Amy Colberg, Director of Government Affairs
The Brain Injury Association of America specializes in brain injury prevention, research, education and advocacy.

7669 Brain Injury Association of New York State
4 Pine W Plaza
Suite 402
Albany, NY 12205

518-459-7911
800-444-6443
Fax: 518-482-5285
info@bianys.org
bianys.org

Barry Dain, President
Eileen Reardon, Executive Director
Debbie Berenda-Chilandese, Director of Finance & Administration
Victoria Clingan, Director of Engagement & Advocacy
The Brain Injury Association of New York State is a statewide non-profit membership organization that provides education, advocacy and community support services leading to improved outcomes for children and adults with brain injuries and their families. The association also offers chapters and support groups throughout the state, prevention programs, mentoring programs, speakers bureau and publications library.

7670 BroadFutures
National Youth Transitions Center
2013 H St, NW
5th Floor
Washington, DC 20006

202-521-4304
info@broadfutures.org
broadfutures.org

Bradley P Holmes, Chairman
Carolyn K Jeppsen, CEO & President
Diana Eisenstat, Secretary
John Sheffield, Treasurer

BroadFutures offers transitional programs for youth with learning disabilities. The mission of the organization is to assit these youth in overcoming barriers to employment.

7671 Center Academy
6710 86th Ave N
Pinellas Park, FL 33782 727-541-5716
Fax: 727-544-8186
infopp@centeracademy.com
centeracademy.com

Mack R Hicks, Ph.D, Founder & Chairman
Andrew P Hicks, Ph.D, CEO & Clinical Director
Eric V Larson, Ph.D, President & Chief Operating Officer
Lisa Hartmann, Director of Education
Center Academy assists children with learning disabilities, difficulties in concentration and underdeveloped social skills. Programs offered include high impact learning, community involvement opportunities, ADHD schools, autism and asperger's schools, dyslexia treatment, special education schools and more.

7672 Cerebral Palsy Associations of New York State
Central Office & Metropolitan Services
330 W 34th St
15th Floor
New York, NY 10001-2488 212-947-5770
information@cpofnys.org
www.cpofnys.org

Stephen C Lipinski, Chairman
Susan Constantino, President & CEO
Michael A Alvaro, Executive Vice President
Cheryl Bradway, Office Manager
The Cerebral Palsy Associations of New York is a multi-service organization that provides services and programs for individuals with cerebral palsy and developmental disabilities, as well as resources for families.

7673 Child Neurology Society
1000 W County Rd E
Suite 290
Saint Paul, MN 55126 651-486-9447
Fax: 651-486-9436
nationaloffice@childneurologysociety.org
www.childneurologysociety.org

Kenneth Mack, President
Roger Larson, Executive Director
Sue Hussman, Associate Director
Emily McConnell, Professional Development Manager
The Child Neurology Society is designed for patiens, parents, and professionals alike, with the aim of promoting continued research, providing support, and offering informational resources and guidance on the subject of child neurology. Members include child neurologists and related medical professionals.

7674 Children and Adults with Attention-Deficit Hyperactivity Disorder
CHADD
4601 Presidents Dr
Suite 300
Lanham, MD 20706 301-306-7070
Fax: 301-306-7090
affiliate-services@chadd.org
www.chadd.org

Michael MacKay, President
Leslie Kain, MBA, Executive Director
Robyn Maggio, MSW, Education & Training Coordinator
April Gower, Chief Operating Officer
The Children and Adults with Attention-Deficit/Hyperactivity Disorder (CHADD) is a non-profit organization providing supports to people with ADHD. Some services offered include advocacy, education, employment, a resource directory, training programs, publications on research and more.

7675 Cognitive Neuroscience Society
267 Cousteau Place
Davis, CA 95618 916-850-0837
cnsinfo@cogneurosociety.org
www.cogneurosociety.org

Roberto Cabeza, Ph.D, Board Member
Marta Kutas, Ph.D, Board Member
Kate Tretheway, Executive Director
Sangay Wangmo, Administrative Assistant
The Cognitive Neuroscience Society is committed to investigating the psychological, computational, and neuroscientific bases of cognition through research.

7676 Cognitive Science Society
108 E Dean Keeton
Stop A8000
Austin, TX 78712-1043 512-471-2030
Fax: 512-471-3053
cogsci@austin.utexas.edu
www.cognitivesciencesociety.org

Susan Gelman, Chair
Terry Regier, Chair Elect
Anna Drummey, Executive Officer
Jessica Wong, Conference Officer
The Cognitive Science Society brings together researchers from around the world who desire to understand the workings of the human mind. The society's mission is to promote the study of cognitive science and build connections between researchers in various areas of study (including Artificial Intelligence, Linguistics, Anthropology, Psychology, Neuroscience, Philosophy, and Education).

7677 Cognitive Science Student Association
University of California
Berkeley, CA cssa.berkeley@gmail.com
cssa.berkeley.edu

Timothy Guan, President
Harshali Wadge, Internal Vice President
Connor Brown, Outreach Coordinator
James Wang, Marketing Director
The Cognitive Science Student Association supports and enriches the academic life of anyone interested in the interdisciplinary field of cognitive science. Some programs offered by the association include guest lectures and information sessions, professor-student dinners, academic outreach program and California Cognitive Science Conference.

7678 Dementia Society of America
PO Box 600
Doylestown, PA 18901 800-336-3684
knowdementia@dementiasociety.org
www.dementiasociety.org

Kevin Jameson, President & Founder
The Dementia Society of America (DSA) is a nonprofit volunteer-run organization providing resources and information about dementia to individuals, corporations and organizations.

7679 Depression and Bipolar Support Alliance
55 E Jackson Blvd
Suite 490
Chicago, IL 60604 800-826-3632
Fax: 312-642-7243
dbsasocial@gmail.com
www.dbsalliance.org

William Gilmer, MD, Chair
Allen Doederlein, President
Cindy Specht, Executive Vice President
Brittany Telander, Development Director
The Depression and Bipolar Support Alliance is a peer-directed national organization dedicated to offering supports to those living with depression or bipolar disorder. Some services they offer include peer support, education, advocacy and research.

7680 Epilepsy Foundation
8301 Professional Place E
Suite 200
Landover, MD 20785- 2353

800-332-1000
Fax: 301-459-1569
ContactUs@efa.org
www.epilepsy.com

Robert W Smith, Chair
Phillip M. Gattone, M.Ed, President & CEO
M. Vaneeda Bennett, Chief Development Officer
May J. Liang, Secretary

The Epilepsy Foundation is the national voluntary health agency dedicated to the welfare of people with epilepsy in the U.S. and their families. The organization works to ensure that people with seizures are able to participate in all life experiences; to improve how people with epilepsy are perceived, accepted and valued in society; and to promote research for a cure.

7681 Focus Center for Autism
126 Dowd Ave
PO Box 452
Canton, CT 06019

860-693-8809
Fax: 860-693-0141
info@focuscenterforautism.org
focuscenterforautism.org

Patricia A Cables, President
Donna Swanson, Executive Director
Fred Evans, Associate Director
Jenee Hepp, Finance Manager

A non-profit learning center specialized in the treatment of children and young adults with autism spectrum disorder. Some of their programs include schools, mentorship, residential programs, consulting services, festivals and more.

7682 International OCD Foundation
18 Tremont St
Suite 308
Boston, MA 02108

617-973-5801
Fax: 617-973-5803
info@iocdf.org
iocdf.org

Shannon A Shy, Esq, President
Jeff Szymanski, PhD, Executive Director
Pamela Layne, Director of Operations
Meghan Buco, Communications Manager

The International OCD Foundation aims to provide resources for those living with OCD and their families. The foundation offers a research grant program, public education and a forum for professional networking.

7683 Lewy Body Dementia Association
912 Killian Hill Rd, SW
Lilburn, GA 30047

404-975-2322
Fax: 480-422-5434
lbda@lbda.org
www.lbda.org

Christina M Christie, President
Mike Koehler, CEO
Mark Wall, Vice President
Angela Taylor, Director of Programs

The Lewy Body Dementia Association is a non-profit organization dedicated to raising awareness of the Lewy body dementias (LBD). The association offers services and information to people with LBD, their families and caregivers and works to promote research in the area.

7684 Life Development Institute
18001 N 79th Ave
Suite B-42
Glendale, AZ 85308

866-736-7811
Fax: 623-773-2788
info@life-development-inst.org
discoverldi.com

Robert Crawford, M.Ed, CEO
Veronica Lieb (Crawford), MA, President
Justin Coller, BS, Director of Operations
Estelle Esposito, Manager of Administrative Services

The Life Development Institute serves older adolescents and adults with learning disabilities, ADD and related disorders. The Institute's mission is to help program participants pursue responsible independent living, enhance academic/workplace literacy skills and facilitate employment or educational placements.

7685 Life Unlimited
Life Unlimited, Inc.
2135 Manor Way
Liberty, MO 64068

816-781-4332
www.lifeunlimitedinc.org

Erin Lankford, President
Scott Wingerson, Vice President
Jessie Smith, Secretary
Dan Jurgensen, Treasurer

Life Unlimited is a nonprofit working to provide support and services to individuals with developmental disabilities in the Kansas City Northland. Services include community living, day services, employment services, and recreation programs.

7686 Mental Health America
500 Montgomery St.
Suite 820
Alexandria, VA 22314

703-684-7722
800-969-6642
Fax: 703-684-5968
info@mentalhealthamerica.net
www.mentalhealthamerica.net

Reginald D Williams, Chair
Paul Gionfriddo, President & CEO
Jennifer Cheang, Digital Marketing Manager
Nathaniel Counts, Senior Policy Director

Mental Health America is a non-profit organization addressing all issues related to mental health and mental illness. Some programs offered include advocacy, education and outreach, research and services. Issues covered include anxiety, bipolar disorder, depression, PTSD, psychosis and more.

7687 Multiple Sclerosis Association of America
375 Kings Hwy N
Cherry Hill, NJ 08034

800-532-7667
Fax: 856-661-9797
msaa@mymsaa.org
mymsaa.org

John McCorry, Chair
Gina Murdoch, President & CEO
Lauren Hooper, Northeast Regional Director
Emily MacHenry, Communications Coordinator

The Multiple Sclerosis Association of America is an organization dedicated to providing the most up-to-date resources for those affected by Multiple Sclerosis, including research, publications, assistive equipment, public education, and best practices and policy for professionals working with patients.

7688 NLP Comprehensive
PO Box 348
Indian Hills, CO 80454-0348

303-987-2224
800-233-1657
Fax: 303-987-2228
learn@nlpco.com
www.nlpco.com

Tom Dotz, President
Sharon DeBault, Director of Community Relations
Jamie Reaser, PhD, Director of Professional Relations
Christian Miller, Publishing Manager

NLP Comprehensive provides a body of publications by Steve and Connirae Andreas on the subject of NLP (Neuro-linguistic programming), as well as training.

7689 NLP University - Dynamic Learning Center
NLP University
PO Box 1112
Ben Lomond, CA 95005 831-336-3457
Fax: 503-738-9546
teresanlp@aol.com
www.nlpu.com

Robert B Dilts, Founder & Director of Training
Teresa Epstein, Coordinator
Deborah Bacon Dilts, Trainer
Judith DeLozier, Trainer
NLP (neuro-lingusitic programming) University seeks to create a context in which professionals of different backgrounds can develop fundamental and advanced NLP skills for applications relevant to their profession. The University provides guidance, training, certification, culture, and community support to those interested in exploring the global potential of Systemic NLP.

7690 National Alliance on Mental Illness (NAMI)
3803 N Fairfax Dr
Suite 100
Arlington, VA 22203 703-524-7600
800-950-6264
888-999-6264
Fax: 703-524-9094
info@nami.org
www.nami.org

Steve Pitman, J.D., President
Mary Giliberti, J.D., CEO
Cheri Villa, M.P.A, Chief Operating Officer
David Levy, Chief Financial Officer
NAMI is a grassroots mental health organization working to provide people with mental health issues the technical assistance, tools and referrals to resources they need in order to manage the challenges they face.

7691 National Association for Developmental Disabilities (NADD)
The NADD
132 Fair St
Kingston, NY 12401 845-331-4336
800-331-5362
Fax: 845-331-4569
info@thenadd.org
thenadd.org

Donna McNelis, Ph.D, President
Robert J Fletcher, Ph.D, Founder & CEO
Michelle Jordan, Office Manager
Terrence McNelis, MPA, Treasurer
NADD is a non-profit membership association established for professionals, care providers and families to promote understanding of and services for individuals who have developmental disabilities and mental health needs. The mission of NADD is to advance mental wellness for persons with developmental disabilities through the promotion of excellence in mental health care.

7692 National Association for Down Syndrome
1460 Renaissance Dr
Suite 405
Park Ridge, IL 60068 630-325-9112
Fax: 847-376-8908
info@nads.org
www.nads.org

Steve Connors, President
Diane Urhausen, Executive Director
Debbie Taus-Barth, Development Coordinator
Ann Garcia, Family Support Coordinator
The National Association for Down Syndrome provides services and information to those with Down Syndrome and their families. The association's mission is to maintain a strong network of support systems within their own organization and with medical, educational and school service professionals who work with children and adults with Down Syndrome.

7693 National Association of Cognitive- Behavioral Therapists
102 Gilson Ave
Weirton, WV 26062 304-224-2534
800-253-0167
nacbt@nacbt.org
www.nacbt.org

Aldo R Pucci, Ph.D, President
The association's mission is to promote the teaching and practice of cognitive-behavioral psychotherapy and to support those professionals and students seeking to practice it. Some services offered by the association include educational videos, membership, CBT certification, workshops and more.

7694 National Association of Epilepsy Centers
600 Maryland Ave SW
Suite 835W
Washington, DC 20024 202-524-6767
888-525-6232
Fax: 202-484-1244
info@naec-epilepsy.org
www.naec-epilepsy.org

Nathan B Fountain, MD, President
Ellen Riker, MHA, Executive Director
Johanna Gray, MPA, Deputy Director
Jennifer McCrindle, MPA, Accreditation & Programs Manager
The National Association of Epilepsy Centers educates public and private policy makers and regulators about appropriate patient care standards, reimbursement and medical services policies. The association is designed to complement the efforts of existing scientific and charitable epilepsy organizations.

7695 National Ataxia Foundation
600 Hwy 169 S
Suite 1725
Minneapolis, MN 55426 763-553-0020
Fax: 763-553-0167
naf@ataxia.org
www.ataxia.org

William P Sweeney, President
Charlene Danielson, Treasurer
Joel Sutherland, Executive Director
Susan Hagen, Patient & Research Services Director
The National Ataxia Foundation is a non-profit, membership-supported organization established to help improve the lives of persons affected by ataxia and their families through support, education, and research.

7696 National Autism Association
1 Park Ave
Suite 1
Portsmouth, RI 02871 401-293-5551
877-622-2884
Fax: 401-293-5342
naa@nationalautism.org
nationalautismassociation.org

Lori McIlwain, Board Chairperson
Wendy Fournier, President
Kelly Vanicek, Executive Director
Katie Wright, Vice President
The mission of the National Autism Association is to educate and empower families affected by autism and other neurological disorders, while advocating on behalf of those who cannot fight for their own rights. The association offers programs as well as educational resources.

7697 National Down Syndrome Congress
30 Mansell Ct
Suite 108
Roswell, GA 30076 770-604-9500
800-232-6372
Fax: 770-604-9898
info@ndsccenter.org
www.ndsccenter.org

Kishore Vellody, MD, President
David Tolleson, Executive Director
MaryKate Vandemark, Office Manager
Kathy Edwards, Development Director

The National Down Syndrome Congress provides information, advocacy and support concerning all aspects of life for individuals with Down syndrome. It is the purpose of the Congress to create a national climate in which all people will recognize and embrace the value and dignity of people with Down syndrome.

7698 National Down Syndrome Society
8 E 41st St
8th Floor
New York, NY 10017   212-460-9330
                                                   800-221-4602
                                              Fax: 212-979-2873
                                                   info@ndss.org
                                                   www.ndss.org
Sara Weir, MS, President
Josh Hill, Executive Assistant
Ashley Helsing, Director of Government Relations
Melissa Robertson, Office Manager
Non-profit organization dedicated to increasing public awareness about Down syndrome as well as engaging in research, education and advocacy. The organization distributes informative materials, encourages and supports the activities of local parent support groups, sponsors conferences and scientific symposiums and undertakes major advocacy efforts.

7699 National Hydrocephalus Foundation
12413 Centralia Rd
Lakewood, CA 90715-1653   562-924-6666
                                                   888-857-3434
                                              Fax: 562-924-6666
                                                   info@nhfonline.org
                                                   www.nhfonline.org
Michael Fields, President & Treasurer
Debbi Fields, Executive Director
Sarah Dunn, Junior Director
Jaynie Dunn, Secretary
The National Hydrocephalus Foundation assembles and disseminates information pertaining to hydrocephalus, its treatments and outcomes. The foundation also establishes and facilitates a communication network among affected families and individuals.

7700 Oak-Leyden Developmental Services
411 Chicago Ave
Oak Park, IL 60302   708-524-1050
                                              Fax: 708-524-2469
                                                   info@oak-leyden.org
                                                   www.oak-leyden.org
Melissa Wyatt, President
Bertha Magana, Executive Director
Nancy Thomas, Director of Human Resources
Lori Malinski, Director of Fund Development
Oak-Leyden Developmental Services works to help people with developmental disabilities meet life's challenges and reach their highest potential. Services offered by the organization include Early Intervention Program, Vocational Evaluation, Developmental Training Program, Supported Employment Program, Community Integrated Living Arrangements and Multi-disciplinary Clinic.

7701 Ontario Federation for Cerebral Palsy
104-1630 Lawrence Ave W
Toronto, ON, Canada M6L-1C5   416-244-9686
                                                   877-244-9686
                                              Fax: 416-244-6543
                                                   info@ofcp.ca
                                                   www.ofcp.ca
Victor Gascon, President
Nilu Alizadeh, Supervisor
Cindy DeGraaff, Planning Services Manager
Deborah Grosdanis, Treasurer
The Ontario Federation for Cerebral Palsy is dedicated to assisting individuals with cerebral palsy through research, financial resources, education, recreation programs, housing and life planning.

7702 Society for Cognitive Rehabilitation
668 Exton Commons
Exton, PA 19341   127-647-2369
                                      www.societyforcognitiverehab.org
Kit Malia, President
Rita Carroll, Secretary
Pat Benfield, Treasurer
Ron Savage, Board Member
The Society for Cognitive Rehabilitation is a non-profit organization committed to the advancement of cognitive rehabilitation therapy across the globe.

7703 St. John Valley Associates
291 Newberry Dr
Suite 105
Madawaska, ME 04756   207-728-7197
                                                   800-339-9502
                                              Fax: 207-728-3825
Robin Jackson-Eldridge, Program Director
A non-profit association with the mission of empowering adult citizens with intellectual disabilities. The association offers center-based community supports and residential supports to help members develop a sense of independence. *$75.00*

7704 TEACCH Autism Program
100 Renee Lynne Ct
Carrboro, NC 27510   919-966-2174
                                              Fax: 919-966-4127
                                                   teacch@unc.edu
                                                   teacch.com
Laura G Klinger, Ph.D, Executive Director
Lauren Turner-Brown, Ph.D, Assistant Director
Rebecca Mabe, Assistant Director, Business & Operations
TEACCH Autism Program offers community-based services, training programs and research to help those with Autism Spectrum Disorder. Some programs offered by TEACCH include clinical evaluations, intervention, consultation and training, living and learning centers, supported employment and more.

7705 The Arc of North Carolina
343 E Six Forks Rd
Suite 320
Raleigh, NC 27609   919-782-4632
                                                   800-662-8706
                                              Fax: 919-782-4634
                                                   info@arcnc.org
                                                   www.arcnc.org
John Nash, Executive Director
Melinda Plue, Director of Advocacy & Chapter Development
Nicole Kiefer, Housing Resources Coordinator
Foresa Walker, Director of Human Resources
The Arc of North Carolina is committed to providing services for people with intellectual and developmental disabilities. Services include advocacy, housing, supported employment and other supports.

7706 The Arc of the United States
1825 K St NW
Suite 1200
Washington, DC 20006   202-534-3700
                                                   800-433-5255
                                              Fax: 202-534-3731
                                                   info@thearc.org
                                                   www.thearc.org
Elise McMillan, President
Peter V Berns, CEO
Dawn Cooper, Manager, Diversity & Cultural Competence
Karen Wolf-Branigin, Senior Executive Officer
The Arc promotes and protects the rights of people with intellectual and developmental disabilities and actively supports their inclusion and participation in the community throughout their lifetimes. The Arc's clients include people with autism, Down syndrome, Fragile X syndrome, and various other developmental disabilities. Some services offered by The Arc include public policy advocacy, education and vocational services.

7707 The Hemispherectomy Foundation
8235 Lethbridge Rd
Millersville, MD 21108 410-987-5221
lynn@hemifoundation.org
hemifoundation.homestead.com
Kristi Hall, President, CEO & Co-Founder
Cris A Hall, Executive Director & Co-Founder
Jane Stefanik, Vice President & Chief Financial Officer
Lindy Shelton, Director of Accounting & Office Manager
The Hemispherectomy Foundation is a non-profit organization dedicated to providing emotional, financial and educational support to individuals and their families who have undergone, or will undergo, a hemispherectomy or similar brain surgery.

7708 Tourette Association of America
42-40 Bell Blvd
Suite 205
Bayside, NY 11361 718-224-2999
Fax: 718-279-9596
support@tourette.org
www.tourette.org
John Miller, President & CEO
Sonja Mason-Vidal, MBA, VP, Finance & Administration
Amanda Talty, VP, Resource Development & Marketing
Diana Felner, VP, Public Policy
Non-profit organization with the mission of researching and controlling the effects of Tourette syndrome. Some services they offer include seminars, conferences and support groups. The association publishes brochures, flyers, educational materials and papers on treatment and research.

7709 United Cerebral Palsy
1825 K St NW
Suite 600
Washington, DC 20006 202-776-0406
800-872-5827
Fax: 202-776-0414
info@ucp.org
ucp.org
Diane Wilush, Chair
Armando Contreras, President & CEO
Ellie Collinson, Chief Program Officer
Tanneka Jones, Director of Finance
United Cerebral Palsy educates, advocates, and provides support services to ensure a life without limits for people with cerebral palsy and other disabilities. Some services offered include networking, educational information, assistive technology information, research, public policy resources and more.

Camps

7710 Adventure Learning Center at Eagle Village
4507 170th Ave
Hersey, MI 49639-8785 231-832-2234
800-748-0061
Fax: 231-832-1468
alcinfo@eaglevillage.org
www.eaglevillage.org
Cathey Prudhomme, President/CEO
Jim McCain, Director of Support Services/CFO
Craig Weidner, Director of Advancement
Offers a variety of fun camp experiences with a low staff-to-camper ratio and exciting, challenging activities. This program accepts youth, ages 5-17, who are high risk or special needs - behavioral problems, emotionally unstable or Attention Deficit. The camping experience includes canoeing, hiking, swimming and high adventure activities. Half-week, one-week, and two-week sessions June-August. Coed.

7711 CNS Camp New Connections
Mclean Hospital Child/Adolescent Program
115 Mill St
Mailstop115
Belmont, MA 02478-1064 617-855-2000
800-333-0338
Fax: 617-855-2833
mcleaninfo@mclean.harvard.edu
www.mcleanhospital.org
Roya Ostovar PhD, Center Director
Scott L. Rauch, MD., President and Psychiatrist in Ch
Joseph Gold MD, Clinical Director
Cynthia Kaplan, CAP Administrative Director
Four-week summer day camp for children ages 7-17 who have pervasive developmental disorders, Asperger's Syndrome, autism spectrum disorders and non-verbal learning disabilities. The camp is designed to help children develop social skills through fun activities including: communication games, swimming, field trips, drama, and arts and crafts. *$4500.00*

7712 Camp Baker
Greater Richmond ARC
7600 Beach Rd
Chesterfield, VA 23838-6513 804-748-4789
Fax: 804-796-6880
campbaker@RichmondARC.org
richmondarc.org
Robert L. Sommerville, Chair - Officer
Thomas G. Haskins, Vice Chair - Officer
Chriss Mumford, Secretary Officer
Marshall W. Butler Jr., President
An organization created by families, for families that has grown to provide a continuum of programs and services for individuals with developmental disablities acroos the lifespan, helping each person achieve his or her potential and improving the quality of life for everyone in the community.

7713 Camp Buckskin
4124 Quebec Ave N
Suite 300, PO Box 389
Ely, MN 55731- 389 763-208-4805
Fax: 218-365-2880
info@campbuckskin.com
www.campbuckskin.com
Thomas R Bauer CCD, Camp Director
Mary Bauer, Co-Director
Jared Griffin, Program Director
Camp is located in Ely, Minnesota. Buckskin assists LD, AD/HD, Asperger's, and adopted individuals to realize and develop the potentials and abilities which they possess. Teaches a combination of traditional camp, academic activities and social skills so the campers experience success in many areas. Ages 6-18.

7714 Camp Candlelight
Epilepsy Foundation Arizona
3033A N. 7th Ave
Ste 104
Phoenix, AZ 85013 602-406-3581
800-332-1000
info@epilepsyaz.org
epilepsyaz.org/programs/camp-candlelight/
Suzanne Matsumori, Executive Director
Min Skivington, Program Manager
Camp Candlelight provides children ages 8 to 15 a unique camp experience that mixes traditional summer camp with special sessions that teach campers about their seizures and gives them resources to manage the challenges that the seizures represent. Staff includes a neurologist, several nurses and a school psychologist, in addition to traditional camp staff who are given specialized training in responding appropriately to the needs of kids with epilepsy.

7715   Camp Evoked Potential @ Camp ASCCA
Epilepsy Foundation of Alabama
310-273 Azalea Rd
Office Park 3
Mobile, AL   36609-1970   251-341-0170
                                                 800-626-1582
                                         ddodson@efala.org
                            www.efala.org/camp-evoked-potential/
Donna Dodson, Executive Director
Paige Norris, Outreach/Program Director
Camp Evoked Potential is a 5-day overnight camp for children
and teens aged 6 to 18 years old living with epilepsy. The camp
provides a great opportunity for kids to experience the fun of
camp activities—swimming, fishing, sports, hiking and
more—in a safe, medically monitored setting. Camp activities are
designed to be accessible and adapted to campers' individual
needs and abilities.

7716   Camp Horizons
127 Babcock Hill Rd
PO Box 323
South Windham, CT   06266- 323   860-456-1032
                                            Fax: 860-456-4721
                                         www.camphorizons.org
Adam Milne, Chairman
L. Sanford Rice, Treasurer
Kathleen McNAboe, VP
Deirdhre Delaney, Board Secretary
Bordering Lake Probus, the facilities at the camp are equipped to
accomodate a wide range of activities and programs for campers
with developmental disabilities, or other challenging emotional
and social needs. There is a 5:1 camper-counselor ratio with a
schedule of three programs in the morning and four in the
afternoon.

7717   Camp Huntington
56 Bruceville St
High Falls, NY   12440   845-687-7840
                                                 855-707-2267
                                            Fax: 855-707-2267
                                         www.camphuntington.com
Alex Mellor, Camp Director
Daniel Falk, Camp Owner
Margaret Short, Health Director
Cathy Crowley, Program Supervisor
A co-ed residential summer camp specifically designed to focus
on Adaptive and Therapeutic Recreation. Campers include those
with learning and developmental disabilities, ADD/HD, Autism
Spectrum Disorders, Asperger's, PDD, and other special needs.
Three programs are offered that focus on: recreation and social
skills; independence; and participation.

7718   Camp Nissokone
YMCA Camping Services
1401 Broadway
Suite A
Detroit, MI   48226-8929   313-267-5300
                                         www.ymcadetroit.org
Doug Grimm, Vice President Camping Services
David Marks, Director
A six week summer resident camp program for boys and girls
whose learning and behavior styles have made successful participation in the traditional camp program difficult. All camp activities have a special emphasis on building self-esteem and peer
relationships. Strong in waterfront, nature, campcrafts and a
special arts program.

7719   Camp Northwood
132 State Route 365
Remsen, NY   13438-5700   315-831-3621
                                      northwoodprograms@hotmail.com
                                         www.nwood.com
Gordon Felt, Camp Director
Donna Felt, Director
Camp Northwood is an overnight camp for children with
non-agressive learning issues such as Asperger's Syndrome, Attention Deficits, HFA, and other learning issues. The camp is
co-ed and accepts children ages 8-18. The camp has a strong focus on developing age appropriate skills, as well as traditional
camping activities.

7720   Camp Nuhop
Nuhop Corporate Office
404 Hillcrest Dr
Ashland, OH   44805   419-289-2227
                                         nuhop.org
Trevor Dunlap, Executive Director, CEO
Nate Holton, Summer Camp Director
Chris Clyde, Associate Director
Ben King, Director of Outdoor Education
A summer residential program for any youngster from 6 to 18
with a learning disability, behavior disorder or Attention Deficit
Disorder. 84 campers and 41 staff members live on site in groups
of to seven campers to every three counselors. Activities focus on
positive self-concept and behaviors and teaches children to learn
how to find their strengths, abilities and talents from a positive,
yet realistic viewpoint. Each program is around 6 weeks long.

7721   Camp Ramapo
22 Camp Ramapo Rd
Rhinebeck, NY   12572   845-876-8403
                                            Fax: 845-876-8414
                                    office@ramapoforchildren.org
                                         ramapoforchildren.org
Adam Weiss, CEO
Teri Golberg Horowitz, President
David Ross, Vice President
Bob Dean, Treasurer
Ramapo's specific focus is adventure-based, experiential learn-
ing programs that promote positive character values in children
and teens with special needs.

7722   Camp Royall
250 Bill Ash Rd
Moncure, NC   27559   919-542-1033
                                            Fax: 919-542-6343
                                camproyall@autismsociety-nc.org
                            www.autismsociety-nc.org/camp-royall/
Lesley Fraser, Program Director, Camp Royall
Cindy Lodestro, Administrative Assistant
Sara Gage, Director, Soecial Recreation Services
Curtis Sobie, Fellow
A week-long overnight and day camp for children and adults with
autism. Campers will participate in traditional camp activities in
a structured environment that helps them develop confidence, in-
dependence, and a willingness totry new things.

7723   Camp Ruggles
PO Box 353
Chepachet, RI   02814   401-567-8914
                                         campruggles@gmail.com
                                         www.campruggles.org
Gregory Gauthier, President
Jim Field, Camp Director
Brandon Ruotolo, Vice President
Ethan Roe, Assistant Director
Camp Ruggles is located in Glocester, RI, and is a summer day
camp for emotionally and behaviourally handicapped children.
The Camp offers a 6 week co-ed summer session for 60 children
ages 6-12.

7724   Camp Sisol
Jewish Community Center of Greater Rochester/JCC
1200 Edgewood Ave
Rochester, NY   14618   585-461-2000
                                            Fax: 585-461-0805
                                         www.jccrochester.org
Ricchard Gray, President
Daniel Goldstein, Vice President
Arnie Sohinki, Executive Director
Howard Cohen, Treasurer
Camp is located in Honeoye Falls, New York. Coed, ages 5-16.
Camp Sisol accomodates children with special needs.

7725 Camp World Light
Florida Baptist Convention
1230 Hendricks Ave
Jacksonville, FL 32207-8619   904-396-2351
                                          800-226-8584
                                     Fax: 904-396-6470
                                     www.campworldlight.com

Anne Wilson, Camp Director
Delicia Garland, Ministry Assistant to Director
Camp is located in Marianna, Florida. One-week sessions
June-July for girls with ADD. Ages 3-12. Activities include
arts/crafts, challenge/rope courses, clowning, community service, dance, drama, drawing/painting, leadership development,
performing arts and sailing.

7726 Camp-A-Lot And Leisure Express (PALS Program)
Arc of San Diego
3030 Market Street
San Diego, CA 92102   619-685-1175
                                     Fax: 619-234-3759
                                          pals@arc-sd.com
                                          www.arc-sd.com

Lin Taylor, Camp Director
David W Schneider, President/CEO
Anthony J Desalis, Esq, Executive Vice President
Rich Coppa, Vice President Of Infrastructure
Offers one-week sessions for children and adults with attention
deficit disorder, autism, mobility limitation and developmental
disabilities.

7727 Casowasco Camp, Conference and Retreat Center
158 Casowasco Dr
Moravia, NY 13118-3498   315-364-8756
                                     Fax: 315-364-7636
                                          info@casowasco.org

Mike Huber, Executive Director
Shelly Sherboneau, CRM Coordinating Registrar
Kevin Dunn, Casowasco Assistant Director
Roger Marshall, Property Manager
Camp is located in Moravia, New York. Summer sessions for chil-
dren with ADD. Coed, ages 6-18 and families.

7728 Center Academy at Pinellas Park
6710 86th Ave North
Pinellas Park, FL 33782-4502   727-541-5716
                                     Fax: 727-544-8186
                                          infopp@centeracademy.com
                                          www.centeracademy.com

Patricia Lambert, Principal
Mack R Hicks PhD, Founder/Chairman of the Board
Andrew P Hicks PhD, CEO/Clinical Director
Lisa Hartmann, Director Education
Specifically designed for the learning disabled child and other
children with difficulties in concentration, strategy, social skills,
impulsivity, distractibility and study strategies. Programs offered
include: attention training, visual-motor remediation, socialization skills training, relaxation training, horseback riding and
more. The day camp meets weekdays from 9-3 for 3,4 or 5 week
sessions.

7729 Council for Extended Care of Mentally Retarded Citizens
11140 So. Towne Square
Ste. 101
Saint Louis, MO 63123   314-845-3900
                                     Fax: 314-845-3901
                                          info@sunnyhillinc.org
Derrick Good, Chairman of the Board
Wes Burns, Vice Chairman
Vicky James, President/CEO
Sean King, Secretary
Services are provided to adults and children with developmental
disabilities. Supported living arrangements are located in St.
Louis city, St. Louis county and St. Charles County. Group home
and camp services are located in Dittmer, MO. Travel program
also available.

7730 Dallas Academy
950 Tiffany Way
Dallas, TX 75218   214-324-1481
                                     Fax: 214-327-8537
                                          www.dallas-academy.com

Terrence S. Welch, Chair
Jim Lucius, Vice Chair
Chris Bellew, Secretary
Redonna Higgins, Treasurer
Dallas Academy is a school for children with diagnosed learning
differences such as autism, ADD/ADHD, dyslexia, and more.
The academy offers a number of academic or athletic summer
school programs.

7731 Eagle Hill School: Summer Program
242 Old Petersham Road
P.O. Box 116
Hardwick, MA 01037- 0116   413-477-6000
                                     Fax: 413-477-6837
                                          admission@ehs1.org
                                          www.ehs1.org

Peter J. Mc Donald, Headmaster
Marilyn Waller, President
Alden Bianchi, Vice President
Arthur Langhaus, Treasurer
For children ages 9-19 with specific learning (dis)abilities and/or
Attention Deficit Disorder, this summer program is designed to
remediate academic and social deficits while maintaining prog-
ress achieved during the school year. Electives and sports activi-
ties are combined with the academic courses to address the needs
of the whole person in a camp-like atmosphere.

7732 Easter Seals Oklahoma
701 NE 13th St
Oklahoma City, OK 73104   405-239-2525
                                          info@eastersealsoklahoma.org
                                          eastersealsok.org/

Keither McCombs, Chairman
Krista Massad, Chairman-Elect
Cassie Wilson, Secretary
Matt Vance, Treasurer
Offers an Adult Day Health Center, and Child Development Cen-
ter.The Child Development Center offers developmentally appropriate learning activities and services to meet the unique
needs of each child, and the adult center provides solutions to
meet the physical, social and emotional needs of adults from the
ages of 21 to 100+.

7733 Englishton Park Academic Remediation
Englishton Park Presbyterian
P.O.Box 228
Lexington, IN 47138-228   812-889-2046
                                          ThomasLisaBarnett@etczone.com
                                          www.englishtonpark.org

Lisa Barnett, Director
Thomas Barnett, Co-Director
Camp is located in Lexington, Indiana. Two-week sessions for
children with ADD. Boys and girls, ages 7-12.

7734 Florida Sheriffs Caruth Camp
Florida Sheriffs Youth Ranches
2486 Cecil Webb Place
Boys Ranch, FL 32060   386-842-5501
                                          800-765-3797
                                     Fax: 386-842-2429
                                          fsyr@youthranches.org
                                          www.youthranches.org

Roger Bouchard, President
Bill Frye, Executive Vice President
Janet Bass, Vice President of Operations
Maria Knapp, Vice President of Donor Relation
Camp is located in Inglis, Florida. One-week sessions for chil-
dren with ADD. Coed, ages 10-15.

7735 Gow School Summer Programs
2491 Emery Road
South Wales, NY 14139   716-652-3450
                                     Fax: 716-652-3457
                                     summer@gow.org
                                     www.gow.org

Douglas B. Cotter, Director of Admissions
Bradley Rogers Jr., Headmaster
Jon Chafin, Assistant Summer Program Director
Joseph Cendrowski, Summer Program Administer
Co-ed summer programs for students ages 8-16 with dyslexia or
similar learning disabilities offer a balanced blend of morning academics, afternoon/evening traditional camp activities and
weekend overnights. The primary purpose of these programs is to
provide a positive experience while balancing these three elements. Committed to the creation of a positive and enjoyable experience for each participant by defining and merging the goals of
the camp and the school, with those of camper students.

7736 Hill School of Fort Worth
4817 Odessa Ave
Fort Worth, TX 76133   817-923-9482
                                     Fax: 817-923-4894
                                     hillschool@hillschool.org
                                     www.hillschool.org

Roxann Breyer, Principal
Joanna Gant, Business Manager
John W. Wright, Chairman
Randall Connelly, Vice Chair
Provides an alternative learning environment for students who
have average or above-average intelligence with learning differ-
ences. Hill School caters to individuals with disabilities by offer-
ing smaller class sizes and individualized learning programs.
Offers and academic summer program during the month of June.

7737 Indian Acres Camp for Boys
1712 Main St
Fryeburg, ME 04037-4327   207-935-2300
                                     Fax: 954-349-7812
                                     geoff@indianacres.com
                                     www.indianacres.com

Michael Burness, Assistant Director
Mary Beth 'Bert' Wiig, Head Counselor, Camp Forest Acre
Lisa Newman, Director
Geoff Newman, Director
Camp is located in Fryeburg, Florida. Four and seven-week ses-
sions June-August for boys with ADD ages 7-16.

7738 Lab School of Washington
4759 Reservoir Rd NW
Washington, DC 20007-1921   200-965-6600
                                     www.labschool.org

Katherine Schantz, Head of School
Diana Meltzer, Associate Head of School
Laurelle Sheedy McCready, Associate Head of School for Fin
Bob Lane, Director of Admissions
The Lab School six week summer session includes individualized
reading, spelling, writing, study skills and math programs. A
multisensory approach addresses the needs of bright learning disabled children. Related services such as speech/language therapy
and occupational therapy are integrated into the curriculum. Ele-
mentary/Intermediate; Junior High/High School.

7739 Lions Den Outdoor Learning Center
600 Kiwanis Dr
Eureka, MO 63025-2212   636-938-5245
                                     Fax: 636-938-5289
                                     info@wymancenter.org
                                     www.wymancenter.org

David Hilliard, President
Theresa Mayberry, Executive VP
Kristine Ramsey, Sr. VP
Tony Etzkorn, VP
Varied programs for mentally retarded children, ages 6 and up, in-
cludes daily living, socialization and language skills. Sports, tent
camping, crafts, and nature study are also offered. Sliding scale
tuition for 2 weeks.

7740 Maplebrook School
5142 Route 22
Amenia, NY 12501   845-373-9511
                                     Fax: 845-373-7029
                                     admissions@maplebrookschool.org
                                     www.maplebrookschool.org

Donna Konkolics, Head of School
Roger Fazzone, President
Jennifer Scully, Assistant Head, Postsecondary Studies
Lori Hale, Executive Director
A coeducational boarding school which offers a six week camp for
children with learning differences and ADD.

7741 Marvelwood Summer
Marvelwood School
476 Skiff Mountain Road
PO Box 3001
Kent, CT 06757-3001   860-927-0047
                                     Fax: 860-927-0021
                                     www.marvelwood.org

Alfred C Brooks, President
Arthur F Goodearl, Jr, Head Of School
The emphasis in this summer program is on diagnosis and
remediation of individual reading, spelling, writing, mathematics and study problems. Offered to ages 12-16.

7742 New Horisons Summer Day Camp
YMCA
13821 Newport Avenue
Suite 200
Tustin, CA 92780-7803   714-549-9622
                                     Fax: 714-838-5976
                                     www.ymcaoc.org

Jeff Black, Vice Chair
Tom Reyes, Director
Christian Buell, Director
John Rochford, Director
One-week sessions for children with ADD and speech/communi-
cation impairment. Coed, ages 5-14.

7743 New Jersey YMHA/YWHA Camps Milford
21 Plymouth St
Fairfield, NJ 07004-1686   973-575-3333
                                     800-776-5657
                                     Fax: 973-575-4188
                                     info@njycamps.org
                                     www.njycamps.org

Leonard Robinson, President
Bruce Nussman, President
Camp is located in Milford, Pennsylvania. Summer sessions for
children with ADD. Coed, ages 6-17 and families.

7744 Oakland School & Camp
128 Oakland Farm Way
Troy, VA 22974   434-293-9059
                                     Fax: 434-296-8930
                                     information@oaklandschool.net
                                     www.oaklandschool.net

Carol Williams, Head of School
Abby Sprague, Admissions Director
Amanda Baber, Admissions Director
Pete Cormons, Operations Director
A highly individualized program that stresses improving reading
ability. Subjects taught are reading, English composition, math
and word analysis. Recreational activities include horseback riding, sports, swimming, tennis, crafts, archery and camping. For
girls and boys, ages 8-14. Students who attend the summer camp
often have a variety of learning disabilities, such as ADHD, dyslexia, visual/auditory processing disorders, and more.

7745 Outside In School Of Experiential Education, Inc.
P.O.Box 639
Greensburg, PA 15601   724-837-1518
                                     Fax: 724-837-0801
                                     myoutsidein.org

Michael C. Henkel, Executive Director

Camp programs primarily focus on substance abuse, but some services are available for special needs related to school'work. Programs are for boys ages 13-18.

7746 Phelps School Academic Support Program
583 Sugartown Rd
Malvern, PA 19355
610-644-1754
Fax: 610-540-0156
admis@thephelpsschool.org
www.thephelpsschool.org

Stephany Phelps Fahey, President
Daniel E. Knopp, Head of School
Gerald D. Fahey, Treasurer
Andrew Wilmerding, Secretary
The Phelps School is a day and boarding school for grades 6-12. They run an Academic Support Program for English, Reading, Mathematics, and Study Skills for students who have diagnosed learning differences.

7747 Quest Camp
2355 San Ramon Valley Blvd.
Suite 208
San Ramon, CA 94583-1763
925-743-2900
800-313-9733
Fax: 925-820-9761
www.questcamps.com

Robert Field, Founder/Executive Director
Debra Forrester-Field, M.A., Administrative Director
Adam Berman, Psy.D., Director
Aprilyn Artz, MA, Director
Camp is located in Alamo, California. Day camp offering three to eight-week sessions including psychological treatment for children with ADD and other mild to moderate psychological disorders. Coed, ages 6-15.

7748 Raven Rock Lutheran Camp
17912 Harbaugh Valley Road
P.O.Box 136
Sabillasville, MD 21780-136
410-303-2108
800-321-5824
ravenrock@innernet.net

Brenda Minnich, Executive Director
Christ-centered program for youth and mentally retarded adults.

7749 Rimland Services for Autistic Citizens
1265 Hartrey Ave
Evanston, IL 60202-1056
847-328-4090
877-395-6937
Fax: 847-328-8364
pwatson@rimland.org
www.rimland.org

Pamela Watson, CEO
Dave Work, Assoc Executive Director Program
Brendy Sims, Chief Operating Officer
Terrance Wimberly, Associate Executive Director of
An accessible camp facility that can be utilized by groups for day use or overnight camping experiences. Six winterized cabins, a meeting facility, indoor pool, full food service, and an excellent staff are available. Educational programs can be arranged or you can utilize the facility to manage your own programs.

7750 Rolling Hills Country Day Camp
P.O.Box 172
Marlboro, NJ 07746
732-308-0405
Fax: 732-780-4726
info@rollinghillsdaycamp.com
www.rollinghillsdaycamp.com

Billy Breitner, Director
Summer sessions for children with ADD. Coed, ages 3-12.

7751 SOAR Summer Adventures
NC Base Camp
226 SOAR Lane
P.O.Box 388
Balsam, NC 28707
828-456-3435
Fax: 801-820-3050
admissions@soarnc.org
www.soarnc.org

John Willson, Executive Director
Catey Terry, Chief Financial Officer
Laura Pate, Director of Operations
Lynne Neaves, Admissions Director
A nonprofit adventure program working with disadvantaged youth diagnosed with learning disabilities in an outdoor, challenge based environment. Focuses on esteem building and social skills development through rock climbing, backpacking, whitewater rafting, mountaineering, sailing, snorkeling, and much more. Offers two week, one month, and semester programs. SOAR programs utilize North Carolina, Florida, Colorado, American Southwest, Alaska, and Jamaica as program areas.

7752 Sherman Lake YMCA Outdoor Center
6225 N 39th St
Augusta, MI 49012-9722
269-731-3000
Fax: 269-731-3020
shermanlakeymca@ymcasl.org
www.shermanlakeymca.org

Luke Austenfeld, Executive Director
Jean Henderson, Business Manager
Lorrie Syverson, Director of Camping, Education &
Mark VanDaff, Facility Manager
Summer camping sessions for campers with ADD and spina bifida. Coed, ages 6-15 and families, seniors.

7753 Squirrel Hollow Summer Camp
The Bedford School
5665 Milam Rd
Fairburn, GA 30213-2851
770-774-8001
Fax: 770-774-8005
bbox@thebedfordschool.org
www.thebedfordschool.org

Betsy Box, Executive Director
Jeff James, Headmaster/Athletic Director./MS
Allisom DaY, Asst. Headmaster/MS Admin./ MS
Susan Blake, Art/After-School Care Coordinato
A remedial summer program for children with academic needs held on the campus of The Bedford School in Fairburn, Georgia. It is a five week day camp held from June 19 to July 21 and serves ages 6-16. For mor information contact Betsy Box at (770) 774-8001.

7754 Summer@Carroll
25 Baker Bridge Rd.
Lincoln, MA 01773-3199
781-259-8342
Fax: 781-259-8842
gsummers@carrollschool.org
carrollschool.org

Steve Wilkins, Head of School
Greely Summers, Director
Donna Brown, Assistant Director
Summer@Carroll is a unique educational experience designed for children with language-based learning disabilities entering grades 1-9 in the Fall. Carroll's five-week, full-day program provides specialized reading support as well as writing and math classes. Classes are formed according to age and skill level, typically with eight or fewer students in a class.

7755 Summit Camp
322 Route 46 West
Suite 210
Parsippany, NJ 07054
973-732-3230
Fax: 973-732-3226
info@summitcamp.com
www.summitcamp.com

Eugene Bell, Senior Director
Leah Love, Assistant Director
Thea Mullis, Travel Director
Maryann Santora, Clinical Social Worker/Admission

The camp is located in Honesdale, Pennsylvania, and is for children, ages 8-19, who have a variety of developmental, social, or learning issues. In addition to regular camp activities like swimming, sports, and arts and crafts, Summit Camp has a strong focus on social skills development and interpersonal growth.

7756 Sunnyhill Adventure Center
Council for Extended Care
6555 Sunlit Way
Dittmer, MO 63023-3306   636-274-9044
                                           314-781-4950
                                Fax: 636-285-1305
                                dropin4fun@aol.com
                                sunnyhilladventures.org

Victoria James, President/CEO
Kathleen Branson, Director of Finance
Donald Mitchell, Director of ISLA
Rob Darroch, Director of Sunnyhill Adventures
Camp is located in Dittmer, Missouri. Summer sessions for campers with developmental disabilities and autism. Coed, ages 8-99. Sunnyhill Adventures is program that offers campers fun, exciting, educational experiences in a beautiful outdoor setting. Our residential summer camp combines traditional camping activities plus specially selected and adapted events to meet the needs of each camper group.

7757 Talisman Summer Camp
64 Gap Creek Rd
Zirconia, NC 28790   828-697-6313
                                info@talismancamps.com
                                www.talismancamps.com
Linda Tatsapaugh, Operations Director & Owner
Robiyn Mims, Admissions Director
Doug Smathers, Camp Director & Owner
Lee Kisselburg, Facilities Manager
Talisman Summer Camp is located 40 minutes south of Asheville, North Carolina. Offers a program of hiking, rafting, climbing, and caving for learning disabled ADD/ADHD and autistic young people. Coed, ages 6-22.

7758 Timbertop Nature Adventure Camp
YMCA Camp Glacier Hollow
1000 Division St
Stevens Point, WI 54481   715-342-2980
                                Fax: 715-342-2987
                                pmatthai@spymca.org
                        www.glacierhollow.com/timbertop-camp/
Pete Matthai, Camp Director
Tiffany Praeger, Summer Camp Program Director
For children who can benefit from an individualized program of learning in a non-competitive outdoor setting under the skilled leadership of people who understand the environment and the unique potential of these children. Timbertop combines traditional camp programs with extra reading practice and special group activities. The camp lasts 7 days, and activities include stargazing, canoeing, archery, and more.

7759 Triangle Y Ranch YMCA
YMCA of Southern Arizona
PO Box 1111
Tucson, AZ 85702   520-623-5511
                                Fax: 520-624-1518
                                www.tucsonymca.org
Dane Woll, President and CEO
Kerry Dufour, V.P. Chief Development Officer
Cathy Scheirman, Chief Financial Officer
Amanda Thomas, Director of Communications and Special Projects
Summer camp programs for children and young adults ages 6-17. Camp offers horseback riding, sports, story telling, arts & crafts, swimming, archery and nature programs.

7760 Wendell Johnson Speech And Hearing Clinic
University Of Iowa
250 Hawkins Dr
Iowa City, IA 52242-1025   319-335-3500
                                Fax: 319-335-8851
                                dorothy-albright@uiowa.edu
                                www.uiowa.edu
Dorothy Albright, Department Administration
Lauren Eldridge, Undergraduate Academic Programs
Mary Jo Yotty, Graduate Programs
Lauren Eldridge, Clinic Appointments
The clinic offers assessment and remediation for communication disorders in adults and children. The clinic also offers a Intensive Summer Residential Clinic for school age children needing intervention services because of speech, language, hearing and/or reading problems.

Print: Books

7761 A Miracle to Believe In
Option Indigo Press
2080 S Undermountain Rd
Sheffield, MA 01257-9643   413-229-8727
                                           800-714-2779
                                Fax: 413-229-8727
Barry Neil Kaufman, Author
A group of people from all walks of life come together and are transformed as they reach out, under the direction of the Kaufmans, to help a little boy the medical world had given up as hopeless. This heartwarming journey of loving a child back to life will not only inspire you, the reader, but presents a compelling new way to deal with life's traumas and difficulties.
379 pages
ISBN 0-449201-08-2

7762 ADD: Helping Your Child
Warner Books
1271 Avenue of the Americas
New York, NY 10020-1300   212-522-7200
                                Fax: 212-522-7989
Barbara Smalley, Author
Bruce Paonessa, Vice President
Elizabeth Nunuz, Manager
The definitive guide to helping children with AD/HD *$ 12.95*
224 pages Paperback
ISBN 0-446670-13-8

7763 ADHD Book of Lists: A Practical Guide for Helping Children and Teens with ADDs
Jossey-Bass
111 River St
Hoboken, NJ 7030-5773   201-748-6000
                                Fax: 201-748-6008
                                info@wiley.com
                                www.wiley.com
Sandra F Rief, Author
Information about Attention Deficit/Hyperactivity Disorder including strategies, supports, and interventions that have been found to be the most effective. For teachers, parents, and counselors. *$29.95*
320 pages
ISBN 0-787965-91-X

7764 ADHD in the Schools: Assessment and Intervention Strategies
Guilford Press
72 Spring St
New York, NY 10012-4019   212-431-9800
                                           800-365-7006
                                Fax: 212-966-6708
                                info@guilford.com
                                www.guilford.com
George J DuPaul, Author
Gary Stoner, Co-Author

This landmark volume emphasizes the need for a team effort among parents, community-based professionals, and educators. Provides practical information for educators that is based on empirical findings. Chapters focus on: how to identify and assess students who might have ADHD; the relationship between ADHD and learning disabilities; how to develop and implement classroom-based programs; communication strategies to assist physicians; and the need for community-based treatments. *$ 36.00*

269 pages Hardcover
ISBN 0-898622-45-X

7765 ADHD with Comorbid Disorders: Clinical Assessment and Management
Guilford Press
72 Spring St
New York, NY 10012-4019 212-431-9800
800-365-7006
Fax: 212-966-6708
info@guilford.com
www.guilford.com

Steven R Pliszka, MD, Author
Caryn Leigh Carlson, Co-Author
James M Swanson, Co-Author
$44.00
Cloth
ISBN 1-572304-78-2

7766 Adolescents with Down Syndrome: Toward a More Fulfilling Life
Brookes Publishing
P.O.Box 10624
Baltimore, MD 21285-624 410-337-9580
800-638-3775
Fax: 410-337-8539
custserv@brookespublishing.com
www.brookespublishing.com

Maria Sustrova, Author
Lauren Smith, Western Region Sales Representat
Jeannine Blimline, Central Region Sales Representat
Kevin Warg, Northeastern Region Sales Repres
Written for health care professionals, psychologists, other developmental disabilities practitioners, educators, and parents, it covers biomedical concerns; behavioral, psychological, and psychiatric challenges; and education, employment, recreation, community, and legal concerns. *$35.95*
416 pages Paperback
ISBN 1-55766 -81-9

7767 Adult ADD: The Complete Handbook: Everything You Need to Know About How to Cope with ADD
Prima Publishing
P.O.Box 1260
Rocklin, CA 95677-1260 916-787-7000
800-632-8676
Fax: 916-787-7001

David B Sudderth, Author
In simple and friendly terms, the authors offer help to those leading frustrating lives. They provide coping mechanisms, both psychological and an up-to-date guide to the latest technology *$14.95*
272 pages
ISBN 0-761507-96-5

7768 All About Attention Deficit Disorders, Revised
Parent Magic
800 Roosevelt Rd
Glen Ellyn, IL 60137-5839 630-208-0031
800-442-4453
Fax: 630-208-7366
custcare@parentmagic.com
www.parentmagic.com

Thomas Phelan, Owner
A psychologist and expert on ADD outlines the symptoms, diagnosis and treatment of this neurological disorder. *$12.95*
248 pages Paperback
ISBN 1-889140-11-2

7769 Assistive Technology for Individuals with Cognitive Impairments Handbook
Idaho Assistive Technology Project
University of Idaho
1187 Alturas Dr.
Moscow, ID 83843- 2268 208-885-3557
800-432-8324
Fax: 208-885-6102
idahoat@uidaho.edu
www.idahoat.org

Ron Seiler, Project Director
A handbook designed to provide resources and information on finding and acquiring assistive technology for individuals with cognitive impairments.

7770 Attention Deficit Disorder
Sage Publications
2455 Teller Road
Thousand Oaks, CA 91320 800-818-7243
Fax: 800-583-2665
info@sagepub.com
www.sagepub.com

Sara Miller McCune, Founder, Publisher, Chairperson
Blaise R Simqu, President & CEO
A book providing helpful suggestions for both home and classroom management of students with attention deficit disorder.

7771 Attention Deficit Disorder and Learning Disabilities
Books on Special Children
P.O.Box 305
Congers, NY 10920-305 845-638-1236
Fax: 845-638-0847

Barbara Ingersoll, Author
Introduces ADD and learning disabilities. This is an easy reading book. Gives definitions and discusses some effective and controverial medication, dietary, biofeedback, cognitive therapy, and many more issues. *$15.95*
246 pages Softcover
ISBN 0-385469-31-4

7772 Attention Deficit Disorder in Adults Workbook
Taylor Publishing Company
7211 Circle S. Road
Austin, TX 78745-5007 214-637-2800
800-225-3687
Fax: 214-819-8220
Rings@balfour.com
www.balfour.com

Don Percenti, CEO
Workbook for adults with ADD. *$17.99*
192 pages Paperback
ISBN 0-878338-50-0

7773 Attention Deficit Disorder: A Different Perception
Underwood Books
PO Box 1919
Nevada City, CA 95959-1919 800-788-3123
www.underwoodbooks.com

Thorn Hartmann, Author
Supports theory linking ADD to the genetic makeup of men and women who hunted for their food in prehestoric times. Also links second hand smoke to disruptive behavior. *$9.95*
180 pages Paperback
ISBN 0-887331-56-4

7774 Attention Deficit Disorders: Assessment & Teaching
Brooks/Cole Publishing Company
10650 Toebben Drive
Independence, KY 41051 859-525-2230
Fax: 859-282-5700
www.brookscole.com

Janet W Lerner, Author
A handy resource that offers teachers, school psychologists, councelors, social workers, administrators, and parents practical

advice for working with children who have attention deficit disorders. *$18.95*
258 pages Paperback
ISBN 0-534250-44-0

7775   Attention-Deficit Hyperactivity Disorder: Symptoms and Suggestons for Treatment
Slosson Educational Publications Inc.
538 Buffalo Rd
East Aurora, NY   14052-280   716-652-0930
                                                      888-756-7766
                                              Fax: 800-655-3840
                                              slosson@slosson.com
                                              www.slosson.com

Thomas W Phelan, Author
Steven Slosson, President
John Slosson, Vice President
David Slossan, Vice President
An exhaustive review of current research and decades of experience as practicing school-based professionals, as well as being a parent of an ADHD child, have culminated in this brief, to-the-point, and yet informed ADHD package which has recieved tremendous reviews. Well-grounded answers and suggestions which would facillitate behavior, learning, social-emotional functioning, and other factors in preschool and adolesence are discussed. Answers most commonly asked questions about ADHD/ADD. *$60.00*
61 pages

7776   Attention-Deficit/Hyperactivity Disorder, What Every Parent Wants to Know
Brookes Publishing
P.O.Box 10624
Baltimore, MD   21285-0624   410-337-9580
                                                      800-638-3775
                                              Fax: 410-337-8539
                                              custserv@brookespublishing.com
                                              www.brookespublishing.com

Lauren Rohe, Regional Sales Consultant
Jeff Stickler, Educational Sales Representative
Sam Schissler, Educational Sales Representative
Dant Washington, Account Sales Manager
New easy-to-understand, non-technical edition helps teachers and parents get accessible answers to their ADHD. *$21.95*
304 pages Paperback
ISBN 1-557663-98-X

7777   Augmenting Basic Communciation in Natural Contexts
Brookes Publishing
P.O.Box 10624
Baltimore, MD   21285-0624   410-337-9580
                                                      800-638-3775
                                              Fax: 410-337-8539
                                              custserv@brookespublishing.com
                                              www.brookespublishing.com

Lauren Rohe, Regional Sales Consultant
Jeff Stickler, Educational Sales Representative
Sam Schissler, Educational Sales Representative
Dant Washington, Account Sales Manager
Here you will find the techniques needed to establish a basic communication system for people of all ages with cognitive disabilities or motor sensory impairments. *$41.95*
304 pages Paperback
ISBN 1-55766-43-6

7778   Autism 24/7: A Family Guide to Learning at Home & in the Community
Autism Society of North Carolina Bookstore
505 Oberlin Rd
Suite 230
Raleigh, NC   27605-1345   919-743-0204
                                                      800-442-2762
                                              Fax: 919-743-0208
                                              info@autismsociety-nc.org
                                              www.autismsociety-nc.org

David Lax, Manager
Martina Ballen, Chair
Beverly Moore, Vice Chair
Elizabeth Phillippi, Secretary
Parents are encouraged to focus on skill sets and behaviors that most negatively affect family functioning, and replacing these behaviors with acceptable alternatives. *$19.95*

7779   Autism Handbook: Understanding & Treating Autism & Prevention Development
Oxford University Press
2001 Evans Rd
Cary, NC   27513-2010   919-677-0977
                                                      800-445-9714
                                              Fax: 919-677-1303
                                              custserv.us@oup.com
                                              www.oup-usa.org

Thomas Carty, Senior Vice President
Simon Li, Regional Director
Adam Glazer, Director
Thomas McCarty, Manager/VP Operations
$25.00
320 pages
ISBN 0-195076-67-2

7780   Autism and Learning
Taylor & Francis
7625 Empire Dr
Florence, KY   41042-2919   212-695-6599
                                                      800-634-7064
                                              Fax: 212-563-2269
                                              orders@taylorandfrancis.com
                                              www.taylorandfrancis.com

Rita Jordan, Author
Stuart Powell, Co-Author
This book is about how a cognitive perception on the way in which individuals with autism think and learn may be applied to particular curriculum areas.
160 pages Paperback
ISBN 1-853464-21-X

7781   Autism in Adolescents and Adults
Springer Publishing
11 W 42nd St
Floor 15
New York, NY   10036-8002   212-431-4370
                                              Fax: 212-460-1575
                                              service-ny@springer.com
                                              www.springerjournals.com

Eric Schopler, Editor
$63.00
456 pages
ISBN 0-306410-57-5

7782   Autism...Nature, Diagnosis and Treatment
Autism Society of North Carolina Bookstore
505 Oberlin Rd
Suite 230
Raleigh, NC   27605-1345   919-743-0204
                                                      800-442-2762
                                              Fax: 919-743-0208
                                              jchampion@autismsociety-nc.com
                                              www.autismbookstore.com

David Lax, Manager
Covers perspectives, issues, neurobiological issues and new directions in diagnosis and treatment. *$49.00*

7783 Autism: Explaining the Enigma
Wiley Publishers
111 River St
Suite 2000
Hoboken, NJ 7030-5773   201-748-6000
                              Fax: 201-748-6088
                                info@wiley.com
                                www.wiley.com

Uta Firth, Author
Explains the nature of autism. *$27.95*

7784 Autism: From Tragedy to Triumph
Branden Books
Po Box 812094
Wellesley, MA 02482   617-734-2045
                              Fax: 781-790-1056
                              www.brandenbooks.com

Carol Johnson, Author
Julia Crowder, Co-Author
A new book that deals with the Lovaas method and includes a
foreward by Dr. Ivar Lovaas. The book is broken down into two
parts — the long road to diagnosis and then treatment. *$12.95*

7785 Autism: Identification, Education and Treatment
Routledge (Taylor & Francis Group)
7625 Empire Dr
Florence, KY 41042-2919   212-695-6599
                               800-634-7064
                              Fax: 212-563-2269
                         orders@taylorandfrancis.com
                                www.routledge.com

Dianne Zager, Editor
Jeffrey Lin, Director
Francis Chua, Manager
Tamaryn Anderson, Marketing Manager
Chapters include medical treatments, early intervention and com-
munication development in autism. *$36.00*
ISBN 0-805820-44-7

7786 Autism: The Facts
Oxford University Press
2001 Evans Rd
Cary, NC 27513-2010   919-677-0977
                               800-445-9714
                              Fax: 919-677-1303
                           custserv.us@oup.com
                                www.oup-usa.org

Simon Cohen, Author
Patrick Bolton, Co-Author
$22.50
128 pages
ISBN 0-192623-27-3

7787 Autistic Adults at Bittersweet Farms
Routledge (Taylor & Francis Group)
7625 Empire Dr
Florence, KY 41042-2919   212-695-6599
                               800-634-7064
                              Fax: 212-563-2269
                         orders@taylorandfrancis.com
                                www.routledge.com

Norman Giddan PhD, Author
Jane Giddan MA, Co-Author
Jefferey Lin, Director
Francis Chua, Manager
A touching view of an inspirational residential care program for
autistic adolescents and adults. Also available in softcover.
$94.95
Hardcover
ISBN 1-560240-42-3

7788 Be Quiet, Marina!
Star Bright Books
13 Landsdowne St
Cambridge, MA 02139   617-354-1300
                              Fax: 617-354-1399
                         orders@starbrightbooks.com
                              www.starbrightbooks.com

Kirsten Debear, Author
A noisy little girl with cerebral palsy and a quiet little girl with
Down Syndrome learn to play together and eventually become
best friends. *$16.95*
40 pages Hardcover
ISBN 1-887734-79-1

7789 Breakthroughs: How to Reach Students with Autism
Aquarius Health Care Media
30 Forest Road
PO Box 249
Millis, MA 02054   508-376-1244
                              Fax: 508-376-1245
                                aqvideos@tiac.net
                              www.aquariusproductions.com

Leslie Krussman, President/Producer
Joseph Wellington, Distribution Coordinator
Anne Baker, Billing & Accounting
Jane Hutchinson, Associate Director William Patte
A hands-on, how-to program for reaching students with autism,
featuring Karen Sewell, Autism Society of America's teacher of
the year. Here Sewell demonstrates the successful techniques
she's developed over a 20-year career. A separate 250 page manual ($59) is also available which covers math, reading, fine mo-
tor, self help, social adaptive, vocational and self help skills as
well as providing numerous plan reproducibles and an exhaustive
listing of equipment and materials resources. Video. *$99.00*

7790 Bus Girl: Selected Poems
Brookline Books
8 Trumbull Rd
Suite B-001
Northampton, MA 01060   617-734-6772
                               800-666-2665
                              Fax: 617-734-3952
                                brbooks@yahoo.com
                              www.brooklinebooks.com

Gretchen Josephson, Author
Lula O Lubchenco, Editor
Poems written over several decades by a young woman with
Down Syndrome. *$14.95*
144 pages Paperback
ISBN 1-57129-41-9

7791 Change Your Brain, Change Your Life: The Breakthrough
Program for Conquering Depression
Three Rivers Press
3rd Floor
175 Broadway
New York, NY 10019   212-782-9000
                              Fax: 212-940-7860
                              www.randomhouse.com

Daniel G Amen MD, Author
Clinical neuroscientist and psychiatrist Amen uses nuclear brain
imaging to diagnose and treat behavioral problems. He explains
how the brain works, what happens when things go wrong, and
how to optimize brain function. Five sections of the brain are discussed, and case studies clearly illustrate possible problems.
$15.00
352 pages
ISBN 0-812929-98-5

7792 Child and Adolescent Therapy: Cognitive-Behavioral Procedures, Third Edition
Guilford Press
72 Spring Street
New York, NY   10012-4019
212-431-9800
800-365-7006
Fax: 212-966-6708
info@guilford.com
www.guilford.com

Chris Jennison, Publisher Emeritus, Education
Seymour Weingarten, Editor-in-Chief
Jody Falco, Managing Editor: Periodicals
Natalie Graham, Editor: School Psychology, Liter
Incorporating significant developments in treatment procedures, theory and clinical research, new chapters in this second edition examine the current status of empirically supported interventions and developmental issues specific to work with adolescents. *$45.00*
432 pages Cloth
ISBN 1-572305-56-8

7793 Children with Mental Retardation
Woodbine House
6510 Bells Mill Rd
Bethesda, MD   20817-1636
301-897-3570
800-843-7323
Fax: 301-897-5838
info@woodbinehouse.com
www.woodbinehouse.com

Irv Shapell, Owner
A book for parents of children with mild to moderate mental retardation, whether or not they have a diagnosed syndrome or condition. It provides a complete and compassionate introduction to their child's medical, therapeutic, and educational needs, and discusses the emotional impact on the family. New parents can rely on Children with Mental Retardation to provide that solid foundation and confidence they need to help their child reach his or her highest potential. *$14.95*
437 pages Paperback
ISBN 0-933149-39-5

7794 Cognitive Behavioral Therapy for Adult Asperger Syndrome
Autism Society of North Carolina Bookstore
505 Oberlin Rd
Ste 230
Raleigh, NC   27605-1345
919-743-0204
800-442-2762
Fax: 919-743-0208
jchampion@autismsociety-nc.org
www.autismbookstore.com

David Lax, Manager
Text is prepared with case studies and examples from the author's own experiences working as a cognitive-behavioral therapist specializing in adults and adolescents with dual diagnosis, autism spectrum disorders, mood disorders, and anxiety disorders.

7795 Communication Development in Children with Down Syndrome
Brookes Publishing
P.O.Box 10624
Baltimore, MD   21285-0624
410-337-9580
800-638-3775
Fax: 410-337-8539
custserv@brookespublishing.com
www.brookespublishing.com

Lauren Rohe, Regional Sales Consultant
Jeff Stickler, Educational Sales Representative
Sam Schissler, Educational Sales Representative
Dant Washington, Account Sales Manager
This book offers an extensive, detailed explanation of communication development in children with Down syndrome relative to their advancing cognitive skills. It introduces a critical framework for assessing and treating hearing, speech, and language problems and provides explicit intervention methods and tested clinical protocols.
Paperback
ISBN 1-55766 -50-5

7796 Comprehensive Guide to ADD in Adults: Research, Diagnosis & Treatment
ADD Warehouse
300 NW 70th Ave
Suite 102
Plantation, FL   33317-2360
954-792-8100
800-233-9273
Fax: 954-792-8545
websales@addwarehouse.com
www.addwarehouse.com

Harvey C Parker, Owner
The first to provide broad coverage of the burgeoning field. Written for professionals who diagnose and treat adults with ADD, it provides information from psychologists and physicians on the most current research and treatment issues *$50.95*
426 pages
ISBN 0-876307-60-8

7797 Concentration Cockpit: Explaining Attention Deficits
Educators Publishing Service
P.O.Box 9031
Cambridge, MA   02139-9031
617-367-2700
800-225-5750
Fax: 617-547-0412
CustomerService.EPS@schoolspecialty.com
eps.schoolspecialty.com

Rick Holden, President
Melvin D Levine, Author
This eight-page pamphlet explains the administration of The Concentration Cockpit, a newly revised poster that helps children with attention deficits gain insight into their problems and monitor their progress in grappling with these problems. *$64.50*
ISBN 0-838820-59-X

7798 Coping with ADD/ADHD
Rosen Publishing Group
29 E 21st St
New York, NY   10010-6209
212-420-1600
800-237-9932
Fax: 888-436-4643
www.rosenpublishing.com

Jaydene Morrison, Author
At least 3.5 million American youngsters suffer from attention deficit disorder. This book defines the syndrome and provides specific information about treatment and counseling. *$16.95*
ISBN 0-823920-70-4

7799 Count Us In
Exceptional Parent Library
P.O.Box 1807
Englewood Cliffs, NJ   7632-1207
201-947-6000
800-535-1910
Fax: 201-947-9376

Jason Kingsley, Author
Mitchell Levitz, Co-Author
Offers information on growing up with Downs Syndrome. *$9.95*

7800 Culture and the Restructuring of Community Mental Health
Greenwood Publishing Group
130 Cremona Drive
Santa Barbara, CA   93117
805-968-1911
800-368-6868
Fax: 866-270-3856
CustomerService@abc-clio.com
www.greenwood.com

William A Vega, Author
John W Murphy, Co-Author
Michael Millman, Editor, American History
Hilary Clagget, Editor, Business, Economics & Finance
Examines treatment, organizational planning and research issues and offers a critique of the theoretical and programmatic aspects of providing mental health services to traditionally underserved populations. $45.00-$52.95. *$95.00*
168 pages Hardcover
ISBN 0-313268-87-8

7801 Difficult Child
Bantam Books
1745 Broadway, 10th Floor
New York, NY 10019 212-782-9000
Fax: 212-302-7985
BBDPublicity@randomhouse.com
www.randomhouse.com/bantamdell
Stanley Turecki, Author
Leslie Tonner, Co-Author
The classic and definitive work on parenting hard-to-raise children with new sections on ADHD and the latest medications for childhood disorders. *$15.95*
302 pages Paperback
ISBN 0-553380-36-2

7802 Disability Culture Perspective on Early Intervention
Through the Looking Glass
3075 Adeline Street
Suite 120
Berkeley, CA 94703-2212 510-848-1112
800-644-2666
Fax: 510-848-4445
TTY: 510-848-1005
TLG@lookingglass.org
www.lookingglass.org
Megan Kirshbaum PhD, Author
For parents with physical or cognitive disabilities and their families. Available in braille, large print or cassette. *$2.00*
12 pages

7803 Down Syndrome
Aquarius Health Care Media
30 Forest Road
PO Box 249
Millis, MA 02054-1066 508-376-1244
888-440-2963
Fax: 508-376-1245
aqvideos@tiac.net
www.aquariusproductions.com
Lesile Kussmann, Owner
This is an excellent video for families who have just had a baby with Down Syndrome as well as professionals in the field of genetics and nursing. Through honest and open discussion, parents of children with Down Syndrome express the feelings and concerns they had during the early years of their child's life. Preview option available. *$150.00*
Video

7804 Driven to Distraction
Simon & Schuster/Touchstone Publishing
1230 Avenue of the Americas
Fl 11
New York, NY 10020- 1513 212-698-7000
Fax: 212-698-7009
www.simonsays.com
Edward M Hallowell, MD, Author
John J Ratey, MD, Co-Author
A practical book discussing adult as well as child attention deficit disorder (ADD). Non-technical, realistic and optimistic, it is an informative how-to manual for parents and consumers. *$23.00*

7805 Dyslexia over the Lifespan
Educators Publishing Service
PO Box 9031
Cambridge, MA 02139-9031 617-367-2700
800-225-5750
Fax: 617-547-0412
eps@schoolspecialty.com
www.epsbooks.com
Margaret B Rawston, Author
Discusses the educational and career development of 56 dyslexic boys from a private school that was one of the first to have a program to detect and treat developmental language disabilities. *$18.00*
224 pages
ISBN 0-838816-70-3

7806 Embracing the Monster: Overcoming the Challenges of Hidden Disabilities
Paul H Brookes Publishing Company
PO Box 10624
Baltimore, MD 21285-624 410-337-9580
800-638-3775
Fax: 410-337-8539
www.brookespublishing.com
Veronica Crawford M.A., Author
Larry B Silver, MD, Foreword/Commentary
The author shares her experience of living with LD, ADHD and bipolar disorder to give readers an awareness of the challenges of living with hidden disabilities and what can be done to help *$24.95*
272 pages paperback
ISBN 1-557665-22-2

7807 Encounters with Autistic States
Jason Aronson
400 Keystone Industrial Park
Dunmore, PA 18512-1507 800-782-0015
Fax: 201-840-7242
Theodore Mitrani, Author
This book explores and explands the work of the late Frances Tustin, which was devoted to the psychoanalytic understanding of the bewildering elemental world of the autistic child. *$50.00*
448 pages Hardcover
ISBN 0-765700-62-

7808 Equal Treatment for People With Mental Retardation: Having and Raising Children
Harvard University Press
79 Garden St
Cambridge, MA 02138-1423 617-495-1000
800-405-1619
Fax: 617-495-5898
www.hup.harvard.edu
William Sisler, President
Valerie A Sanchez, Co-Author
Martha A Field, co-Author
A Harvard law professor and civil liberties practitioner provide a comprehensive examination of the reproductive and parental rights of mentally retarded citizens. *$19.95*
464 pages Paperback
ISBN 0-674006-97-6

7809 Families of Adults With Autism: Stories & Advice For the Next Generation
Autism Society of North Carolina Bookstore
505 Oberlin Road
Suite 230
Raleigh, NC 27605-1345 919-743-0204
800-442-2762
Fax: 919-743-0208
books@autismsociety-nc.org
www.autismbookstore.com
Tracey Sheriff, Chief Executive Officer
Paul Wendler, Chief Financial Officer
David Laxton, Director of Communications
Kristy White, Director of Development
This book's unique point of view is that of a parent who's been there and done that and is now willing to tell the reader what it was like. *$19.95*

7810 Family Therapy for ADHD: Treating Children, Adolescents and Adults
Guilford Press
72 Spring St
New York, NY 10012-4019 800-365-7006
www.guilford.com
Craig A Everett, Author
Sandra Volgy Everett, Co-Author
Presents an innovative approach to assesing and treating ADHD in the family context. *$29.00*
Paperback
ISBN 1-572304-38-3

7811 Fighting for Darla: Challenges for Family Care & Professional Responsibility
Teachers College Press
1234 Amsterdam Ave
New York, NY 10027-6602
212-678-3929
Fax: 212-678-4149
tcpress@tc.columbia.edu
Mary Lynch, Manager
Susan M Klein, Co-Author
Samuel Guskin, Co-Author
Samuel Guskin, Co-Author
Follows the story of Darla, a pregnant adolescent with autism.
$18.95
161 pages
ISBN 0-807733-56-3

7812 Fragile Success
Brookes Publishing
PO Box 10624
Baltimore, MD 21285-624
410-337-9580
800-638-3775
Fax: 410-337-8539
www.brookespublishing.com
Virginia Walker Sperry, Author
A book about the lives of autistic children, whom the author has followed from their early years at the Elizabeth Ives School in New Haven, CT, through to adulthood. *$27.50*
ISBN 1-557664-58-7

7813 Getting Our Heads Together
Thoms Rehabilitation Hospital
68 Sweeten Creek Rd
Asheville, NC 28803-2318
828-274-2400
Fax: 828-274-9452
Kathi Petersen, Director Planning/Communication
Edgardo Diez MD, Medical Director Brain Injury
Kathy Price, Director Admissions
Chat Norvell, CEO
A handbook for families of head injured patients - available in Spanish as well as English. *$4.00*
40 pages Paperback

7814 Getting a Grip on ADD: A Kid's Guide to Understanding & Coping with ADD
Educational Media Corporation
1443 Old York Rd
Warmister, PA 18794
763-781-0088
800-448-9041
Fax: 215-956-9041
www.educationalmedia.com
Kim Frank Ed.S., Author
Susan Smith-Rex Ed.D., Co-Author
Free catalog of resources.
64 pages Yearly

7815 Getting the Best for Your Child with Autism
Autism Society of North Carolina Bookstore
505 Oberlin Road
Suite 230
Raleigh, NC 27605-1345
919-743-0204
800-442-2762
Fax: 919-743-0208
books@autismsociety-nc.org
www.autismbookstore.com
Tracey Sheriff, Chief Executive Officer
Paul Wendler, Chief Financial Officer
David Laxton, Director of Communications
Kristy White, Director of Development
This treatment guide helps parents navigate the complex and overwhelming world of Autism. *$16.95*

7816 Group Activity for Adults with Brain Injury
Sage Publications
2455 Teller Road
Thousand Oaks, CA 91320
805-499-0721
800-818-7243
Fax: 805-499-0871
info@sagepub.com
www.sagepub.com
Sara Miller McCune, Founder, Publisher, Executive Chairman
Blaise R Simqu, President & CEO
Tracey A. Ozmina, Executive Vice President & Chief Operating Officer
Chris Hickok, Senior Vice President & Chief Financial Officer
This manual addresses attention, memory, reasoning, and language skills in group settings. *$53.00*

7817 Guide to Successful Employment for Individuals with Autism
Brookes Publishing
P.O.Box 10624
Baltimore, MD 21285-0624
410-337-9580
800-638-3775
Fax: 410-337-8539
custserv@brookespublishing.com
www.brookespublishing.com
Marcia Daltow Smith, Author
Ronald G Belcher, Co-Author
Patricia D Juhrs, Co-Author
Lauren Smith, Western Region Sales Representat
Describing all aspects of job placement, this book details strategies for assessing workers, networking for job opportunities, and tailoring job supports to each individual. Also illustrates how to help individuals with autism become productive workers, and with detailed descriptions of specific jobs help provide ideas for employment. *$ 32.95*
336 pages Paperback
ISBN 1-55766 -71-5

7818 Handbook of Autism and Pervasive Developmental Disorders
Autism Society of North Carolina Bookstore
505 Oberlin Road
Suite 230
Raleigh, NC 27605-1345
919-743-0204
800-442-2762
Fax: 919-743-0208
books@autismsociety-nc.org
www.autismbookstore.com
David Laxton, Director of Communications
Paul Wendler, Chief Financial Officer
Tracey Sheriff, Chief Executive Officer
Kristy White, Director of Development
A list of contributors address such topics as characteristics of autistic syndromes and interventions. *$125.00*

7819 Helping People with Autism Manage Their Behavior
Indiana Resource Center For Autism
2853 E 10th St
Bloomington, IN 47408-2696
812-855-6508
Fax: 812-855-9630
prattc@indiana.edu
www.iidc.indiana.edu
David Mank, Executive Director
Scott Bellini, Assistant Director
Covers the broad topic of helping people with autism manage their behavior. *$7.00*

7820 Helping Your Hyperactive: Attention Deficit Child
Crown Publishing Company (Random House)
1745 Broadway
New York, NY 10019-4305
212-782-9000
800-632-8676
Fax: 212-572-6066
crownpublishing.com
John Taylor, Author
$19.95
ISBN 1-559584-23-8

7821 Hidden Child: The Linwood Method for Reaching the Autistic Child
Woodbine House
6510 Bells Mill Road
Bethesda, MD 20817-1636
301-897-3570
800-843-7323
Fax: 301-897-5838
info@woodbinehouse.com
www.woodbinehouse.com

Irv Shapell, Owner
Sabine Oishi, Co-Author
Chronicle of the Linwood Children's Center's successful treatment program for autistic children. *$17.95*
286 pages Paperback
ISBN 0-933149-06-9

7822 How To Reach and Teach Children and Teens with Dyslexia
Jossey-Bass
111 River St
Hoboken, NJ 7030-5773
201-748-6000
Fax: 201-748-6008
info@wiley.com
www.wiley.com

Cynthia M Stowe, Author
This practical resource gives educators at all levels essential information, techniques, and tolls for understanding dyslexia and adapting teaching methods in all subject areas to meet the learning style, social, and emotional needs of students who have dyslexia. *$ 22.95*
340 pages
ISBN 0-130320-18-8

7823 How to Own and Operate an Attention Deficit Disorder
Learning Disabilities Association of America
4156 Library Rd.
Pittsburgh, PA 15234-1349
412-341-1515
Fax: 412-344-0224
info@ldaamerica.org
www.ldaamerica.org

Mary-Clare Reynolds, Executive Director
Stephanie Fedro-Byrom, Operations Manager
Joyce Kraemer, Conference Coordinator
Ericka Pardun, Communications Coordinator
LDA's mission is to create opportunities for success for all individuals affected by learning disabilities and to reduce the incidence of learning disabilities in future generations. *$8.95*
43 pages

7824 Hyperactive Child, Adolescent, and Adult: ADD Through the Lifespan
Oxford University Press
198 Madison Ave
New York, NY 10016-4308
212-726-6000
www.us.oup.com/us

Paul H Wender, Author
Comprehensive general review. Update on previous research by the author, offering a basic text. Published by Connecticut Association for Children & Adults with Learning Disabilities (CACLD). *$8.75*
162 pages
ISBN 0-195113-49-7

7825 Hyperactivity, Attention Deficits, and School Failure: Better Ways
Learning Disabilities Association of America
4156 Library Rd.
Pittsburgh, PA 15234-1349
412-341-1515
Fax: 412-344-0224
info@ldaamerica.org
www.ldaamerica.org

Mary-Clare Reynolds, Executive Director
Stephanie Fedro-Byrom, Operations Manager
Joyce Kraemer, Conference Coordinator
Ericka Pardun, Communications Coordinator
LDA's mission is to create opportunities for success for all individuals affected by learning disabilities and to reduce the incidence of learning disabilities in future generations.

7826 Identifying and Treating Attention Deficit Hyperactivity Disorder
Learning Disabilities Association of America
4156 Library Rd.
Pittsburgh, PA 15234-1349
412-341-1515
Fax: 412-344-0224
info@ldaamerica.org
www.ldaamerica.org

Mary-Clare Reynolds, Executive Director
Stephanie Fredo-Byrom, Operations Manager
Joyce Kraemer, Conference Coordinator
Ericka Pardun, Communications Coordinator
LDA's mission is to create opportunities for success for all individuals affected by learning disabilities and to reduce the incidence of learning disabilities in future generations.

7827 In Search of Wings: A Journey Back from Traumatic Brain Injury
Lash & Associates Publishing/Training
100 Boardwalk Drive, Suite 150
Youngsville, NC 27596
919-556-0300
Fax: 919-556-0900
orders@lapublishing.com
www.lapublishing.com

Marilyn Lash, President
Bob Cluett, CEO
Bill Herrin, Director of Graphics & Design
Nick Vidal, Director of IT
The true story of one woman coping with traumatic brain injury after a car accident that affected her cognitive skills and memory
$14.95
233 pages
ISBN 1-882332-00-8

7828 In Their Own Way
Alliance for Parental Involvement in Education
375 Hudson Street
New York, NY 10014
212-366-2000
Fax: 212-366-2933
ecommerce@us.penguingroup.com
http://us.penguingroup.com

Thomas Armstrong, Author
John Makinson, Chairman and Chief Executive
Coram Williams, CFO
David Shanks, CEO
For the parents whose children are not thriving in school, Armstrong offers insight into individual learning styles. *$11.95*

7829 Increasing and Decreasing Behaviors of Persons with Severe Retardation and Autism
Research Press
PO Box 9177
Champaign, IL 61826-9177
217-352-3273
800-519-2707
Fax: 217-352-1221
rp@researchpress.com
www.researchpress.com

Dennis Wiziecki, Marketing
Richard M Fox, Author
These well-organized manuals are written for teachers, aides and persons responsible for designing or evaluating behavioral programs. Offers specific guidelines for arranging and managing the learning environment as well as standards for evaluating and maintaining success. In Volume Two of this series, chapters address more restrictive procedures including physical restraing, punishment, time-out and overcorrection. Set of two volumes. *$39.50*
230 pages Paperback
ISBN 0-878222-63-4

7830   Jumpin' Johnny Get Back to Work, A Child's Guide to ADHD/Hyperactivity
Ste 15-5
25 Van Zant St
Norwalk, CT 6855-1729   203-838-5010
                                            Fax: 203-866-6108
                                    CACLD@optonline.net
                                        www.CACLD.org
Beryl Kaufman, Executive Director
Written primarily for elementary age youngsters with ADHD to help them understand their disability. Also valuable as an educational tool for parents, siblings, friends and classmates. Includes two pages on medication. *$12.50*
24 pages

7831   Keys to Parenting a Child with Attention Deficit Disorder
Barron's Educational Series
250 Wireless Blvd
Hauppauge, NY 11788-3924   631-434-3311
                                                 800-645-3476
                                            Fax: 631-434-3723
                                    barrons@barronseduc.com
                                        barronseduc.com
Manuel H Barron, CEO
Francine McNamara MSW CSW, Co/Author
This book shows how to work with the child's school, effectively manage the child's behavior and act as the child's advocate. *$6.95*
160 pages Paperback
ISBN 0-812014-59-6

7832   Keys to Parenting a Child with Downs Syndrome
Barron's Educational Series
250 Wireless Blvd
Hauppauge, NY 11788-3924   631-434-3311
                                                 800-645-3476
                                            Fax: 631-434-3723
                                    barrons@barronseduc.com
                                        barronseduc.com
Manuel H Barron, CEO
Lucy Guarino
Down Syndrome poses many challenges for children and their families. This book prepares parents and guardians to raise a child with Down Syndrome by discussing adjustment, advocacy, health and behavior, education and planning for greater independence. *$5.95*
160 pages Paperback
ISBN 0-812014-58-8

7833   Keys to Parenting the Child with Autism
Barron's Educational Series
250 Wireless Blvd
Hauppauge, NY 11788-3924   631-434-3311
                                                 800-645-3476
                                            Fax: 631-434-3723
                                    barrons@barronseduc.com
                                        barronseduc.com
Manuel H Barron, CEO
Parents of children with autism will find a solid balance between home and practical information in this book. It explains what autism is and how it is diagnosed, then advises parents on how to adjust to their child and give the best care. *$6.95*
208 pages Paperback
ISBN 0-812016-79-3

7834   LD Child and the ADHD Child: Ways Parents & Professionals Can Help
1406 Plaza Dr
Winston Salem, NC 27103-1470   336-768-1374
                                                 800-222-9796
                                            Fax: 336-768-9194
                                    southern@blairpub.com
                                        www.blairpub.com
Carolyn Sakowski, President
Susan H Stevens, Author
Book about learning disabilities available to parents. Stevens cuts through the jargon and complex theories which usually characterize books on the subject to present effective and practical

techniques that parents can employ to help their child succeed at home and at school. New edition adds information about ADHD children. *$12.95*
201 pages Paperback
ISBN 0-895871-42-4

7835   Labeling the Mentally Retarded
University of California Press
2120 Berkeley Way
Berkeley, CA 94704-1012   510-642-4247
                                            Fax: 510-643-7127
                                        www.ucpress.edu
Lynne Whity, Executive Director
Jane R Mercer, Author
Clinical and social system perspectives on mental retardation. *$12.95*
333 pages Paper

7836   Let Community Employment be the Goal for Individuals with Autism
Indiana Resource Center For Autism
2853 E 10th St
Bloomington, IN 47408-2601   812-855-9396
                                                 800-825-4733
                                            Fax: 812-855-9630
                                    prattc@indiana.edu
                                        www.iidc.indiana.edu
David Mank, Executive Director
Scott Bellini, Assistant Director
A guide designed for people who are responsible for preparing individuals with autism to enter the work force. *$7.00*

7837   Making the Writing Process Work
Brookline Books
8 Trumbull Rd
Suite B-001
Northampton, MA 01060   617-734-6772
                                                 800-666-2665
                                            Fax: 617-734-3952
                                    brbooks@yahoo.com
                                        www.brooklinebooks.com
Karen R Harris, Author
Steve Grahm, Co-Author
Making the Writing Process Work: Strategies for Composition and Self-Regulation is geared toward students who have difficulty organizing their thoughts and developing their writing. The specific strategies teach students how to approach, organize, and produce a final written product. *$24.95*
240 pages Paperback
ISBN 1-57129 -10-9

7838   Management of Autistic Behavior
Sage Publications
2455 Teller Road
Thousand Oaks, CA 91320   805-499-0721
                                                 800-818-7243
                                            Fax: 800-583-2665
                                    info@sagepub.com
                                        www.sagepub.com
Sara Miller McCune, Founder, Publisher, Executive Chairman
Blaise R Simqu, President & CEO
Tracey A. Ozmina, Executive Vice President & Chief Operating Officer
Stephen Barr, Managing Director/SAGE London
This excellent reference is a comprehensive and practical book that tells what works best with specific problems. *$41.00*
450 pages

785

7839 Management of Children and Adolescents with ADHD
Learning Disabilities Association of America
4156 Library Rd.
Pittsburgh, PA 15234-1349 412-341-1515
Fax: 412-344-0224
info@ldaamerica.org
www.ldaamerica.org

Mary-Clare Reynolds, Executive Director
Stephanie Fedro-Byrom, Operations Manager
Joyce Kraemer, Conference Coordinator
Ericka Pardun, Communications Coordinator
LDA's mission is to create opportunities for success for all individuals affected by learning disabilities and to reduce the incidence of learning disabilities in future generations.

7840 Managing Attention Deficit Hyperactivity in Children: A Guide for Practitioners
John Wiley & Sons Inc
111 River St
Hoboken, NJ 07030-5774 201-748-6000
800-825-7550
Fax: 201-748-6088
info@wiley.com
www.wiley.com

Warren J Baker, President
Michael Goldstein, Co-Author
Matthe S Kissner, CEO
Offers information about human personality, structure and dynamics, assessment and adjustment. *$27.50*
214 pages Hardcover
ISBN 0-471121-58-9

7841 Mental Retardation
McGraw-Hill, School Publishing
PO Box 182605
Columbus, OH 43218 800-338-3987
Fax: 609-308-4480
customer.service@mheducation.com
mcgraw-hill.com

David Levin, President and CEO
Patrick Milano, Chief Administrative Officer & CFO
Stephen Laster, Chief Digital Officer
David Stafford, SVP & General Counsel
Combines significant findings from the most current research, focusing on a unique relationship between the special educator and the learner with mental retardation.
656 pages Casebound

7842 Mental Retardation: A Life-Cycle Approach
Pearson Publishing
200 Old Tappan Rd
Old Tappan, NJ 07675-7033 201-785-2721
800-922-0579
Fax: 201-797-2993
www.pearsonhighered.com

Clifford J Drew, Author
Michael L Hardman, Co/Author
This text considers the needs of the retarded individual at every stage of life.
512 pages

7843 Neurobiology of Autism
Johns Hopkins University Press
2715 N Charles St
Baltimore, MD 21218-4363 410-516-6900
Fax: 410-516-6968
www.press.jhu.edu

William Brody, President
Thomas L Kemper, Co-Author
Margaret L Bauman, M.D., Co-Author
Thomas L Kemper, M.D., Co-Author
This book discusses recent advances in scientific research that point to a neurobiological basis for autism and examines the clinical implications of this research. *$28.00*
272 pages
ISBN 0-801880-47-5

7844 Out of the Fog: Treatment Options and Coping Strategies for ADD
Hyperion
1500 Broadway
3rd Floor
New York, NY 10036 212-563-6500
800-331-3761
Fax: 212-456-0176
www.hyperionbooks.com

Robert Miller, President
Suzanne Levert, Co-Author
Discusses the recent recognition of attention deficit disorder as a problem that is not outgrown in adolescence, and cogently summarizes the stumbling blocks this affliction creates in the pursuit of a career or attainment of a healthy family life *$14.95*
300 pages
ISBN 0-786880-87-2

7845 Overcoming Dyslexia
Vintage-Random House
3rd Fl
1745 Broadway
New York, NY 10019-4305 212-782-9000
Fax: 212-302-7985
www.randomhouse.com/vintage

Markus Dohle, CEO
Sally Shawitz, M.D., Author
Yale neuroscientist Shaywitz demystifies the roots of dyslexia (a neurologically based reading difficulty affecting one in five children) and offers parents and educators hope that children with reading problems can be helped. *$15.00*
432 pages
ISBN 0-679781-59-5

7846 Parent Survival Manual
Springer Publishing Company
11 W 42nd St
15th Floor
New York, NY 10036 212-431-4370
877-687-7476
Fax: 212-941-7842
cs@springerpub.com
www.springerpub.com

Ursula Springer, President
Ted Nardin, CEO
Edie Lambiase, CFO
A guide to crises resolution in autism and related developmental disorders. *$39.95*

7847 Parent's Guide to Down Syndrome: Toward a Brighter Future
Brookes Publishing
PO Box 10624
Baltimore, MD 21285-0624 410-337-9580
800-638-3775
Fax: 410-337-8539
custserv@brookespublishing.com
www.brookespublishing.com

Siegfried Pueschel MD PhD, Author
Highlights developmental stages and shows the advances that improve a child's quality of life. Includes discussions on easing the transition from home to school and choosing integration and curricular priorities, as well as guidelines for confronting adolescent and adult issues such as social and sexual needs and independent living and vocational options. *$21.95*
352 pages
ISBN 1-557664-52-8

7848 Parenting Attention Deficit Disordered Teens
CACLD
25 Van Zant Street
Norwalk, CT 06855-1729 203-838-5010
Fax: 203-866-6108
CACLD@optonline.net
cacld.org

Beryl Kaufman, Executive Director

Detailed outline of the various problems of adolescents with ADHD. Published by Connecticut Association for Children & Adults with Learning Disabilities (CACLD). *$3.25*
14 pages

7849 Parents Helping Parents: A Directory of Support Groups for ADD
Novartis Pharmaceuticals Division
59 State Route 10
East Hanover, NJ 7936-1005   862-778-7500
                                     800-742-2422
Paulo Costa, CEO

7850 Please Don't Say Hello
Human Sciences Press
233 Spring St
New York, NY 10013-1522   212-229-2859
                                     800-221-9369
                                Fax: 212-463-0742
                                     http://isbndb.com
Charles Stenken, Author
Jaroslav Chobot, Author
Zirul Evany, Author
Bill Feldmaier, Author
Paul and his family moved into a new neighborhood. Paul's brother was autistic. The children thought that Eddie was retarded until they learned that there were skills that he could do better than they could. *$10.95*
47 pages Paperback
ISBN 0-89885-99-8

7851 Preventable Brain Damage
Springer Publishing Company
11 W 42nd St
15th Floor
New York, NY 10036   212-431-4370
                                     877-687-7476
                                Fax: 212-941-7842
                                     cs@springerpub.com
                                     www.springerpub.com
Donald L Templer, Author
Lawrence C Hartlage, Co-Author
Ursula Springer, President
Ted Nardin, CEO
Offers information on brain injuries from motor vehicle accidents, contact sports and injuries of children. *$35.95*
256 pages

7852 Reading, Writing and Speech Problems in Children
International Dyslexia Association
40 York Rd.
4th Floor
Baltimore, MD 21204   410-296-0232
                                Fax: 410-321-5069
                                     info@idamd.org
                                     www.interdys.org
Samuel Orton, Author
Rick Smith, Chief Executive Officer
This book provides reading, reading and speech excercises for educating people with dyslexia. *$27.00*
ISBN 0-89079-79-1

7853 Reality of Dyslexia
Brookline Books
8 Trumbull Rd
Suite B-001
Northampton, MA 01060   617-734-6772
                                     800-666-2665
                                Fax: 617-734-3952
                                     brbooks@yahoo.com
                                     www.brooklinebooks.com
John Osmond, Author
An informative and sensitive study of living with dyslexia which affects one in 25. He introduces the reader to the subject by sharing the difficulties of his dyslexic son. He then uses the personal

accounts of other children and adult dyslexics, even entire dyslexic families, to illuminate the problems they encounter. *$14.95*
150 pages Paperback
ISBN 1-57129-17-6

7854 Relationship Development Intervention with Young Children
Jessica Kingsley Publishers
400 Market St
Suite 400
Philadelphia, PA 19106   215-922-1161
                                Fax: 215-992-1417
                                     orders@jkp.com
                                     www.jkp.com
Steven E Gustein, Author
Rachelle Sheely, Co-Author
Social and emotional development activities for Asperger Syndrome, Autism, PDD and NLD. Comprehensive set of activities emphasizes foundation skills for younger children between the ages of two and eight. Covers skills such as social referencing, regulating behvior, conversational reciprocity, and synchronized actions. For use in therapeutic settings as well as schools and parents. *$22.95*
256 pages
ISBN 1-843107-14-7

7855 Retarded Isn't Stupid, Mom!
Brookes Publishing
4501 Forbes Blvd
Suite 200
Lanham, MD 20706   301-459-3366
                                     800-638-3775
                                Fax: 301-429-5748
                                     custserv@brookespublishing.com
Sandra Z Kaufman, Author
Sandra Kaufman reveals the feelings of denial, guilt, frustration and eventual acceptance that resulted in a determination to help her daughter, Nicole, live an independent life. This edition, revised on the 10th anniversary of the book's original publication, adds a progress report that updates readers on Nicole's adult years and reflects on the revolutionary changes in society's attitudes toward people with disabilities since Nicole's birth. *$22.95*
272 pages Paperback
ISBN 1-557663-78-5

7856 Rethinking Attention Deficit Disorder
Brookline Books
8 Trumbull Rd
Suite B-001
Northampton, MA 01060-4533   617-734-6772
                                     800-666-2665
                                Fax: 617-734-3952
                                     brbooks@yahoo.com
                                     www.brooklinebooks.com
Miriam Cherkes-Julkowski, Author
In contrast to the common focus on behavioral symptoms of attention disorders, this book emphasizes internal factors that make attention regulation difficult. In-depth discussions of social, emotional, and academic consequences and appropriate interventions are provided. *$27.95*
250 pages Paperback
ISBN 1-571290-30-7

7857 Riddle of Autism: A Psychological Analysis
Jason Aronson
4501 Forbes Blvd
Suite 200
Lanham, MD 20706-4346   301-459-3366
                                     800-782-0015
                                Fax: 301-429-5746
                                     www.rowmanlittlefield.com
Jason Aronson, Author
James Lyons, President/CEO
Stanley Plotnick, Chairman

Dr. Victor examines the myths that cloud an understanding of this disorder and describes the meanings of its specific behavioral symptoms. *$30.00*
356 pages Paperback
ISBN 1-568215-73-8

7858   SCATBI: Scales Of Cognitive Ability for Traumatic Brain Injury
Sage Publications
2455 Teller Road
Thousand Oaks, CA   91320   805-499-0721
                                              800-818-7243
                                         Fax: 805-499-0871
                                      happiness@option.org
                                          www.sagepub.com
Sara Miller McCune, Founder, Publisher, Executive Chairman
Blaise R Simqu, President & CEO
Tracey A. Ozmina, Executive Vice President & Chief Operating Officer
Stephen Barr, Managing Director/SAGE London
Assesses cognitive and linguistic abilities of adolescent and adult parents with head injuries. *$287.00*

7859   Sex Education: Issues for the Person with Autism
Indiana Resource Center For Autism
2853 E 10th St
Bloomington, IN   47408-2696   812-855-6508
                                              800-825-4733
                                         Fax: 812-855-9630
                                        iidc@indiana.edu
                                         www.iidc.indiana.edu
David Mank, Executive Director
Scott Bellini, Assistant Director
Discusses issues of sexuality and provides methods of instruction for people with autism. *$4.00*

7860   Son-Rise: The Miracle Continues
2080 S Undermountain Rd.
Sheffield, MA   01257   413-229-2100
                                              800-562-7171
                                     correspondence@option.org
                                    www.autismtreatmentcenter.org
Barry Neil Kaufman, Founder & CEO
Clyde Haberman, Senior Teacher & Director of Development
Blair Borgeson, Developmental Therapist
Emily Vitale Aronow, Program Advisor & Client Support Coordinator
The center's Son-Rise Program teaches a comprehensive system of treatment and education designed to help families and caregivers enable their children to dramatically improve in all areas of learning. *$12.95*
343 pages
ISBN 0-915811-53-7

7861   Soon Will Come the Light
Future Horizons Inc
721 W Abram St
Arlington, TX   76013-6995   817-277-0727
                                              800-479-0727
                                         Fax: 817-277-2270
                                          www.fhautism.com
Wayne Gilpin, Owner
Jennifer Gilpin, Vice President
Annette Vick, Manager
Offers new perspectives on the perplexing disability of autism. *$19.95*

7862   Successful Job Search Strategies for the Disabled: Understanding the ADA
Wiley Publishing
605 3rd Ave
New York, NY   10158-180   212-850-6000
                                         Fax: 212-850-6088
                                             www.wiley.com

Jeffrey G Allen, Author
Following a concise overview of the Americans with Disabilities Act (ADA), covers such topics as job identification, self-assess-
ment, job leads, resumes, disability disclosure, interviewing, and accommodating specific disabilities. Includes dozen of relevant and instructive situation analyses, case examples, and answers to commonly asked questions. *$165.00*
229 pages

7863   Taking Charge of ADHD Complete Authoritative Guide for Parents
Guilford Press
72 Spring St
New York, NY   10012-4019   212-431-9800
                                              800-365-7006
                                         Fax: 212-966-6708
                                        info@guilford.com
                                          www.guilford.com
Russell A Barkley, Author
Revised and updated to incorporate the most current information on ADHD and its treatment. Provides parents with the knowledge, guidance and confidence they need to ensure that their child receives the best care possible. Also in cloth at $40.00 (ISBN# 1-57230-600-9 *$18.95*
331 pages Paperback
ISBN 1-572305-60-1

7864   Teaching Children with Autism: Strategies for Initiating Positive Interactions
Brookes Publishing
P.O. Box 10624
Baltimore, MD   21285-0624   410-337-9580
                                              800-638-3775
                                         Fax: 410-337-8539
                                custserv@brookespublishing.com
                                   www.brookespublishing.com
Robert L. Koegel, Author
Lynn Kern Koegel, Co-Author
Robert Miller, Sales Director
Offers strategies for initiating positive interactions and improving learning opportunities. This guide begins with an overview of characteristics and long-term strategies and proceeds through discussions that detail specific techniques for normalizing environments, reducing disruptive behavior, improving language and social skills, and enhancing generalization. *$39.95*
256 pages Paperback
ISBN 1-557661-80-4

7865   Teaching and Mainstreaming Autistic Children
Love Publishing Company
9101 E Kenyon Ave
Suite 2200
Denver, CO   80237-1854   303-221-7333
                                         Fax: 303-221-7444
                                       lpc@lovepublishing.com
                                        www.lovepublishing.com
Stan Love, Owner
Peter Knoblock, Author
Dr. Knoblock advocates a highly organized, structured environment for autistic children, with teachers and parents working together. His premise is that the learning and social needs of autistic children must be analyzed and a daily program designed with interventions that respond to this functional analysis of their behavior. *$24.95*
ISBN 0-89108 -11-9

7866   Techniques for Aphasia Rehab: (TARGET) Generating Effective Treatment
Speech Bin
1965 25th Ave
Vero Beach, FL   32960-3062   772-770-0007
                                              800-477-3324
                                         Fax: 772-770-0006
                                        store.schoolspecialty.com
Mary Jo Santo Pietro, Co-Author
Robert Goldfarb, Co-Author
TARGET is the kind of resource aphasia clinicians beg for. A practical resource that answers not only the what and how questions of treatment, but also the why. It describes dozens of treatment methods and gives you practical exercises and activities to

implement each technique. It shows you how to treat all components of the disability, language disorder, overall impairment, communication problems, and the needs of the person with aphasia. *$45.00*
384 pages
ISBN 0-93785-50-5

7867 Teenagers with ADD
Woodbine House
6510 Bells Mill Rd
Bethesda, MD 20817-1636   301-897-3570
800-843-7323
Fax: 301-897-5838
info@woodbinehouse.com
www.woodbinehouse.com

Irv Shapell, Owner
Chris A Ziegler Dendy, M.S., Author
This best selling guide to understanding and coping with teenagers with attention deficit disorder (ADD) provides complete coverage of the special issues and challenges faced by these teens. Based on current diagnostic criteria and the latest literature and research in the field, the book discusses diagnosis, medical treatment, family and school life, intervention, advocacy, legal rights, and options after high school. Parents find strategies for dealing with their teen's difficult behaviors. *$18.95*
370 pages Paperback
ISBN 0-933149-69-7

7868 Understanding Down Syndrome: An Introduction for Parents
Brookline Books
8 Trumbull Rd
Suite B-001
Northampton, MA 01060-4533   617-734-6772
800-666-2665
Fax: 617-734-3952
brbooks@yahoo.com
www.brooklinebooks.com

Cliff Cunningham, Author
Using positive and readable language, this book helps parents understand Down Syndrome. Medical details are explained in lay terms, and advice is given on working with professionals, obtaining services, and treatment techniques that help the child. Cunningham alerts families to potential problems, the prospects for the child in schooling and the passage to adulthood. Revised 1996. *$14.95*
Softcover
ISBN 1-57129-09-5

7869 Valley News Dispatch
New York Families For Autistic Children
95-16 Pitkin Avenue
Ozone Park, NY 11417-2834   718-641-3441
Fax: 718-641-2228
www.nyfac.org

Cheryl L. Marsh, Chairperson
Robert Burt, Treasurer
Education, recreation and support services for families and children with developmental disabilities.

7870 Verbal Behavior Approach: How to Teach Children with Autism & Related Disorders
Autism Society of North Carolina Bookstore
505 Oberlin Road
Suite 230
Raleigh, NC 27605-1345   919-743-0204
800-442-2762
Fax: 919-743-0208
books@autismsociety-nc.org
www.autismbookstore.com

David Laxton, Director of Communications
Paul Wendler, Chief Financial Officer
Tracey Sheriff, Chief Executive Officer
Kristy White, Director of Development
Provides full descriptions of how to teach the verbal operants that make up expressive languate which include: manding, tacting, echoing and intraverbal skills. *$19.95*

7871 Without Reason: A Family Copes with two Generations of Autism
Books on Special Children
721 W Abram St
Arlington, TX 76013-6995   817-277-0727
800-489-0727
Fax: 817-277-2270
www.futurehorizons-autism.com

Wayne Tilton, President
The author discovers his son has autism. He delves into problems of the autistic person and explains reasons for their actions. *$20.95*
292 pages Hardcover

7872 Women with Attention Deficit Disorder: Embracing Disorganization at Home and Work
Underwood-Miller
708 Westover Dr
Silver Spring, MD 20901-1242
ISBN 1-887424-057

7873 You Mean I'm Not Lazy, Stupid or Crazy?!: A Self-Help Book for Adults with ADD
Simon & Schuster
1230 Avenue Of The Americas
11th Floor
New York, NY 10020-1513   212-698-7000
Fax: 212-698-7099
www.simonsays.com

Kate Kelly, Author
Peggy Ramundo, Co-Author
Practical advice on controlling adult ADD, a straightforward guide explains how to get along in groups, become organized, improve memory, and pursue professional help. *$15.00*
464 pages
ISBN 0-684815-31-1

7874 You and Your ADD Child
Nelson Publications
1 Gateway Plz
Port Chester, NY 10573-4674   914-481-5490
Fax: 914-937-8950

Paul Warren MD, Author
Jody Capehart M.Ed., Co-Author
$12.99
252 pages Paperback
ISBN 0-785278-95-8

Print: Journals

7875 American Journal on Mental Retardation
American Association on Mental Retardation
501 3rd Street NW
Suite 200
Washington, DC 20001   202-387-1968
800-424-3688
Fax: 202-387-2193
www.aamr.org

Leonard Abbeduto, Editor
Articles cover biological, behavioral, and educational research: theory papers; and reviews of research literature on specific aspects of mental retardation. *$142.00*
112 pages BiMonthly

7876 Annals of Dyslexia
International Dyslexia Association
40 York Road
4th Floor
Baltimore, MD 21204   410-296-0232
800-ABC-D123
Fax: 410-321-5069
www.interdys.org

Hal Malchow, President
Ben Shifrin, Vice President
Elsa C. Hagen, Vice President
Suzanne Carreker, Secretary

IDA is a clearinghouse of scientific data and practice-based information related to dyslexia. Provides community-based referrals and information fact sheets in response to thousands of emails, calls & letters. Our annual conference attracts thousands of outstanding researchers, clinicians, parents, teachers, psychologists, educational therapists and people with dyslexia. *$15.00*
Paper

7877 **Journal of Cognitive Rehabilitation**
Neuroscience Publishers
6555 Carrollton Ave
Indianapolis, IN 46220-1664

317-257-9672
Fax: 317-257-9674
neuroscience.cnter.com

Odie L Bracy, Executive Director
Publication for therapists, family and patient, designed to provide information relevant to the rehabilitation of impairment resulting from brain injury. *$50.00*
36-48 pages Quarterly

Print: Magazines

7878 **AWARE**
National Fibromyalgia Association
1000 Bristol Street North
Suite 17-247
Irvine, CA 92660

714-921-0150
Fax: 714-921-6920
www.fmaware.org

Lynne Matallana, President/Founder
Mark Dobrilovic, Board of Director
John Fry, PhD, Board of Director
Michael Seffinger, DO, FAAFP, Board of Director
Magazine published three times a year with membership only.

7879 **Attention**
Children & Adults with ADHD
8181 Professional Place
Suite 150
Landover, MD 20785- 2264

301-306-7070
800-233-4050
Fax: 301-306-7090
webmaster@chadd.org
www.chadd.org

Bryan Goodman, Director
A bi-monthly publication from CHADD. Free with membership.
Bi-monthly

Print: Newsletters

7880 **ADHD Report**
Guilford Press
72 Spring St
New York, NY 10012-4019

212-431-9800
800-365-7006
Fax: 212-966-6708
info@guilford.com
www.guilford.com

Russell A Barkley PhD, Editor
Presents the most up-to-date information on the evaluation, diagnosis and management of ADHD in children, adolescents and adults. This important newsletter is an invaluable resource for all professionals interested in ADHD. *$49.95*
16 pages BiMonthly
ISSN 1065-8025

7881 **Arc Connection Newsletter**
Arc of Tennessee
151 Athens Way
Suite 100
Nashville, TN 37228

615-248-5878
800-835-7077
Fax: 615-248-5879
info@thearctn.org
thearctn.org

John Lewis, President
John H. Shouse, VP,Planning & Rules committee Chair
Donna Lankford, Secretary
Ann Curl, Treasurer,Budget/Finance Committee Chair
Quarterly publication from the ARC of Tennessee. *$10.00*
12 pages Quarterly

7882 **Autism Research Review International**
Autism Research Institute
4182 Adams Ave
San Diego, CA 92116-2599

619-281-7165
Fax: 619-563-6840
br@autismresearchinstitute.com
autism.com

Steve Edelson, Executive Director
The Autism Research Institute has pubished this quarterly newsletter, Autism Research Review International (ARRI), since 1987. The ARRI has received worldwide praise for it's thoroughness and objectivity in reporting the current developments in biomedical and educational research. The latest findings are gleaned from a computer search of the 25,000 scientific and medical articles published every week. *$18.00*
8 pages Quarterly

7883 **Chadder**
Children & Adults with Attention Deficit Disorder
4601 Presidents Drive
Suite 300
Lanham, MD 20706

301-306-7070
Fax: 301-306-7090
www.chadd.org

Michael MacKay, President
Ruth Hughes, CEO
Susan Buningh, Executive Editor
Christine hoch, Director of Development
Quarterly newsletter
Quarterly

7884 **Down Syndrome News**
National Down Syndrome Congress
30 Mansell Court
Suite 108
Roswell, GA 30076

770-604-9500
800-232-6372
Fax: 770-604-9898
info@ndsccenter.org
www.ndsccenter.org

Jim Faber, President
Marilyn Tolbert, 1st VP
Carole J. Guess, 2nd Vice President
Lori Mckee, Treasurer
Must become a member to receive the newsletter.

7885 **Farmington Valley ARC**
225 Commerce Dr
Canton, CT 06019-1099

860-693-6662
Fax: 860-693-8662
favarh.org

Diane Brown, President
Stephen Morris, Executive Director
The official newsletter containing information, new ideas, progress and more on the Farmington Valley Association for Retarded and Handicapped Citizens.

7886 Imagine!
Imagine!
1400 Dixon St
Lafayette, CO   80026-2790
303-665-7789
Fax: 303-665-2648
imaginecolorado.org

John Taylor, President
Mark Emery, Executive Director
John Nevins, CFO
Susan LaHoda, Foundation Executive Director
For people of all ages with cognitive, developmental, physical &
health related needs, so they may live lives of independence &
quality in their homes and communities.
12-16 pages quarterly

7887 Pure Facts
Feingold Association of the US
11849 Suncatcher Dr
Fishers, IN   46037
631-369-9340
800-321-3287
Fax: 631-369-2988
help@feingold.org
www.feingold.org

Debbie Lehner, Manager
Relationship between foods, food additives and behavior/learn-
ing problems, including Attention Deficit Disorder (ADD) and
hyperactivity. *$38.00*
10+ pages Monthly

7888 Rettsyndrome.org
4600 Devitt Dr
Cincinnati, OH   45246
513-874-3020
800-818-7388
Fax: 513-874-2520
admin@rettsyndrome.org
www.rettsyndrome.org

Peter White, Chair
Gordon Rich, Chief Operating Officer
Steven Kaminsky, Ph.D, Chief Science Officer
Mary Woods, Director of Marketing & Communications
Rettsyndrome.org offers informational resources and programs
for those affected by Rett syndrome as well as their families.

Non Print: Newsletters

7889 Arc Light
Arc of Arizona
5610 S Central Ave
Phoenix, AZ   85040-3090
602-268-6101
800-252-9054
Fax: 602-268-7483
thearcaz@gmail.com

Cindy Waymire, Editor
For people with intellectual and developmental disabilities.
Quarterly

7890 BIATX Newsletter
Brain Injury Association of Texas
316 W 12th Street
Suite 405
Austin, TX   78701-1845
512-326-1212
800-392-0040
Fax: 512-478-3370
www.texasbia.org

Judith Abner, Director
Penny Phillips, President
Donna Kuhlmann, Chairman
Kelly Ramsay, CFO
A online quarterly e-newsletter, as well as news and updates on
the Brain Injury Association of Texas.

7891 BIAWV Newsletter
Brain Injury Association of America
PO Box 574
Institute, WV   25112-0574
304-766-4892
800-356-6443
Fax: 304-766-4940
biawv@aol.com

Peggy Brown, Director
Mike Davis, President

7892 Best Buddies Times
Best Buddies Times
907-1243 Islington Ave
Toronto, ON, Canada
416-531-0003
888-779-0061
Fax: 416-531-0325
info@bestbuddies.ca
www.bestbuddies.ca

Steven Pinnock, Director
Emily Bolyea-Kyere, Regional Program Manager
Bi-annual newsletter.

7893 Cognitive Therapy Today
Beck Institute for Cognitive Therapy & Research
One Belmont Avenue
Ste 700
Bala Cynwyd, PA   19004-1610
610-664-3020
Fax: 610-709-5336
info@beckinstitute.org
www.beckinstitute.org

Judith S Beck, Director
Aaron T Beck, President
Cognitive Therapy TodayT features articles on a wide range of
topics in CBT by leading clinicians from around the world. Articles have addressed evaluating psychotherapies; CBT and special populations, such as soldiers, the elderly, or diagnoses such
as schizophrenia; conceptualizing emotions; cross-cultural issues and many other issues of interest to clinicians. You will also
find information on workshops, speaking engagements by Beck
Institute faculty and more.

7894 Focus Times Newsletter
Focus Alternative Learning Center
126 Dowd Avenue
PO Box 452
Canton, CT   06019-0452
860-693-8809
Fax: 860-693-0141
info@focuscenterforautism.org
www.focus-alternative.org

Marcia Bok, President
Claudia Godburn, Secretary
Rita Barredo, Treasurer
Monthly online newsletter on autism.

7895 NAMI Advocate
National Alliance on Mental Illness
3803 N Fairfax Dr
Suite 100
Arlington, VA   22203-3080
703-524-7600
800-950-6264
Fax: 703-524-9094
www.nami.org

Suzanne Vogel-Scibilia, President
Our mission is to provide you with the technical assistance, tools
and referrals to resources you need to build organizational capacity and achieve the goals of the NAMI Standards of Excellence.

7896 NLP News
NLP Comprehensive
PO.Box 348
Indian Hills, CO 80454-648 303-987-2224
800-233-1657
Fax: 303-987-2228
learn@nlpco.com
www.nlpco.com

Christian Miller, Editor
Tom Dotz, President
Tom Hoobyar, Director Of Planning
Sharon DeBault, Director Of Community Relations
An online e-newsletter on Neuro-linguistic programming.

7897 REACH
TEACCH
100 Renee Lynn Ct
Carrboro, NC 27510 919-966-2174
Fax: 919-966-4127
teacch@unc.edu
www.teacch.com

Dr. Laura Klinger, Director
Walter Kelly, Business Officer
Rebecca Mabe, Assistant Director of Business
Mark Klinger, Director of Research
Free online newsletter.

7898 Weekly Wisdom
Autism Treatment Center of America
2080 S Undermountain Rd
Sheffield, MA 01257-9643 413-229-2100
877-766-7473
Fax: 413-229-3202
www.son-rise.org
Barry Kausman, Owner
Weekly Wisdom is available through a free email subscription.

Non Print: Software

7899 Cogrehab
Life Science Associates
1 Fenimore Rd
Bayport, NY 11705-2115 631-472-2111
Fax: 631-472-8146
lifesciassoc.home.pipeline.com
Joann Mandriota, President
Divided into six groups for diagnosis and treatment of attention, memory and perceptual disorders to be used by and under the guidance of a professional. $95.-$1,950

Non Print: Video

7900 ADD, Stepping Out of the Dark
Child Development Media
5632 Van Nuys Blvd
Suite 286
Van Nuys, CA 91401-4602 818-989-7221
800-405-8942
Fax: 818-989-7826
info@childdevelopmentmedia.com
www.childdevelopmentmedia.com

Margie Wagner, Owner
A powerful, effective video, ideal for health professionals, educators and parents providing a visual montage designed to promote an understanding and awareness of attention deficit disorder. Based on actual accounts of those who have ADD, including a neurologist, an office worker, and parents of children with ADD. The DVD allows the viewer to feel the frustration and lack of attention that ADD brings to many. *$52.95*
Video

7901 ADHD in Adults
Guilford Press
72 Spring St
New York, NY 10012-4019 212-431-9800
800-365-7006
Fax: 212-966-6708
info@guilford.com
www.guilford.com

Russell A Barkley, Editor
This program integrates information on ADHD with the actual experiences of four adults who suffer from the disorder. Representing a range of professions, from a lawyer to a mother working at home, each candidly discusses the impact of ADHD on his or her daily life. These interviews are augmented by comments from family members and other clinicians who treat adults with ADHD. *$99.00*
DVD 1906
ISBN 0-898629-86-1

7902 ADHD: What Can We Do?
Guilford Press
72 Spring St
New York, NY 10012-4019 212-431-9800
800-365-7006
Fax: 212-966-6708
info@guilford.com
Russell A Barkley, Editor
A video program that introduces teachers and parents to a variety of the most effective technologies for managing ADHD in the classroom, at home, and on family outings. *$99.00*
DVD 1906
ISBN 0-898629-72-1

7903 ADHD: What Do We Know?
Guilford Press
72 Spring St
New York, NY 10012-4019 212-431-9800
800-365-7006
Fax: 212-966-6708
info@guilford.com
www.guilford.com

Bob Matloff, President
Russell A Barkley, Editor
An introduction for teachers and special education practitioners, school psychologists and parents of ADHD children. Topics outlined in this video include the causes and prevalence of ADHD, ways children with ADHD behave, other conditions that may accompany ADHD and long-term prospects for children with ADHD. *$99.00*
DVD 1906
ISBN 0-898629-71-3

7904 Around the Clock: Parenting the Delayed AD HD Child
Guilford Press
72 Spring St
New York, NY 10012-4019 212-431-9800
800-365-7006
Fax: 212-966-6708
info@guilford.com

Joan F Goodman, Editor
Susan Hoban, Editor
This videotape provides both professionals and parents a helpful look at how the difficulties facing parents of ADHD children can be handled. Video. *$150.00*
VHS 1994
ISBN 0-898629-68-3

7905   Attention Deficit Disorder: Adults
Aquarius Health Care Media
30 Forest Road
Millis, MA   02054   508-376-1244
                                                            888-440-2963
                                                    Fax: 508-376-1245
                                                    aqvideos@tiac.net
                                            www.aquariusproductions.com

Lesile Kussmann, President/Owner
Joseph Wellington, Distribution Coordinator
Anne Baker, Billing & Accounting
Adults with ADD talk about how the disorder that went
undiagnosed for so many years has affected their choice of
spouses and work, and what they have found to help them. Biofeedback, which is growing as a treatment, is explained and demonstrated by its founder, Dr. Joel Lubar. Medical treatments like
antidepressants and stimulants are also discussed, along with behavioral changes that can help the person with ADD and his or her
spouse and family. *$149.00*
Video

7906   Attention Deficit Disorder: Children
Aquarius Health Care Media
30 Forest Rd
PO Box 249
Millisrn, MA   02054-7159   508-376-1244
                                                            888-440-2963
                                                    Fax: 508-376-1245
                                                    aqvideos@tiac.net
                                            www.aquariusproductions.com

Lesile Kussmann, President/Owner
Everyone has been impulsive or easily distracted for different periods of time, so these symptoms that are hallmarks of Attention
Deficit Disorder (ADD) have also led to criticism that too many
people are being diagnosed with this biochemical brain disorder.
This program examines who is being diagnosed, and what treatments are working. An innovative private school specializing in
alternative education is profiled, and tips on structuring the
school and home environment are included. *$149.00*
Video

7907   Autism: A World Apart
Fanlight Productions C/O Icarus Films
32 Court Street
Brooklyn, NY   11201-1731   718-488-8900
                                                            800-876-1710
                                                    Fax: 718-488-8642
                                                    info@fanlight.com
                                                    www.fanlight.com

Ben Achtenberg, Owner
Nicole Johnson, Publicity Coordinator
Anthony Sweeney, Marketing Director
In this documentary, three families show us what the textbooks
and studies cannot: what it's like to live with autism day after day;
to raise and love children who may be withdrawn and violent and
unable to make personal connections with their families. 29 min-
utes. *$195.00*
VHS/DVD 1988
ISBN 1-572950-39-0

7908   Autism: the Unfolding Mystery
Aquarius Health Care Media
30 Forest Road
PO Box 249
Millis, MA   02054   508-376-1244
                                                    Fax: 508-376-1245
                                            lkussmann@aquariusproductions.com
                                            www.aquariusproductions.com

Lesile Kussmann, Owner
Explore what it means to be autistic, how you can recognize the
signs of autism in your child, and hear about new treatments and
programs to help children learn to deal with the disorder. *$145.00*
DVD 1905

7909   Biology Concepts Through Discovery
Educational Activities Software
5600 W 83rd Street
Suite 300, 8200 Tower
Bloomington, MN 55437   800-447-5286
                                                    Fax: 239-225-9299
                                                    info@cdmentum.com
                                            http://www.ea-software.com

Vin Riera, President/CEO
Rob Rueckel, CFO
Dave Adams, Chief Academic Officer
Paul Johansen, Chief Technology Officer
These videos, available in English and Spanish versions, encour-
age learning by presenting interactive problem solving in an ef-
fective VISUAL/AUDITORY style. *$89.00*
Video

7910   Concentration Video
Learning disAbilities Resources
6 E Eagle Road
Havertown, PA   19083   610-446-6126
                                                            800-869-8336
                                                    Fax: 610-525-8337
                                                    rcooper-ldr@comcast.net
Video

7911   Educating Inattentive Children
ADD Warehouse
300 Northwest 70th Avenue
Suite 102
Plantation, FL 33317-2360   954-792-8100
                                                            800-233-9273
                                                    Fax: 954-792-8545
                                            websales@addwarehouse.com
                                                    www.addwarehouse.com

Harvey C Parker, Owner
Ideal for in-service to regular and special educators concerning
the problems inattentive, elementarty and secondary students experience. *$49.00*
Video

7912   Getting Started with Facilitated Communication
Facilitated Communication Institute, Syracuse Univ
230 Huntington Hal
Syracuse, NY   13244-1   315-443-4752
                                                    Fax: 315-443-2258
                                                    http://thefci.syr.edu

Annegret Schubert, Director
Describes in detail how to help individuals with autism and/or severe communication difficulties to get started with facilitated
communication.
Video

7913   How to Cope with ADHD: Diagnosis, Treatment & Myths
Aquarius Health Care Media
30 Forest Road
PO Box 249
Millis, MA   02054   508-376-1244
                                                    Fax: 508-376-1245
                                            lkussmann@aquariusproductions.com
                                            www.aquariusproductions.com

Lesile Kussmann, President/Owner
Learn how ADHD is diagnosed, clear up some of the myths, explain the treatmens that are availiable, and give you tips on how
you can help your child at home. *$145.00*
DVD 1905

7914 **I Just Want My Little Boy Back**
Autism Treatment Center Of America
2080 South Undermountain Road
Sheffield, MA   01257   413-229-2100
                                                         800-714-2779
                                                 happiness@option.org
                                                     www.option.org

Samahria Lyt Kaufman, Co-Founder and Co-Director
Dane Griffith, Director of Administrative Services
Bears Kaufman, Co-Founder and Co-Director
Raun Kaufman, Director of Global Education
A great video for parents and professionals caring for children
with special needs. Join one British family and their autistic son
before, during and after their journey to America to attend The
Son-Rise Program at The Autism Treatment Center of America.
This informative, inspirational and deeply moving story not only
captures the joy, tears, challenges and triumps of this amazing little boy and his family, but also serves as a powerful introduction
to the attitude and principles of the program. *$25.00*

7915 **It's Just Attention Disorder**
Western Psychological Services
625 Alaska Avenue
Torrance, CA   90503-5124   424-201-8800
                                                         800-648-8857
                                                    Fax: 424-201-6950
                                        customerservice@wpspublish.com
                                                        wpspublish.com

Gregg Gillmar, VP
This ground-breaking videotape takes the critical first steps in
treating attention-deficit disorder; it enlists the inattentive or hyperactive child as an active participant in his or her treatment.
$99.50
Video

7916 **Understanding ADHD**
Aquarius Health Care Videos
30 Forest Road
PO Box
Millis, MA   02054   508-376-1244
                                                    Fax: 508-376-1245
                                           www.aquariusproductions.com

Leslie Kussmann, President/Owner
A look at some of the controversies surrounding Attention Deficit
Hyperactivity Disorder. This video shows how the disorder is diagnosed and presents strategies for living with a child with the
disorder. Diverse and candid opinions from teachers, social
workers, a behavior specialist, a pediatrician and a parent with
ADHD twins. Recommended for child development students, social workers, and caregivers. Preview option available. *$120.00*
Video

7917 **Understanding Attention Deficit Disorder**
CACLD
25 Van Zant Street
Norwalk, CT   6855-1713   203-838-5010
                                                    Fax: 203-866-6108
                                               CACLD@optonline.net
                                                      www.CACLD.org

Beryl Kaufman, Executive Director
Helen Bosch, President
A video in an interview format for parents and professionals providing the history, symptoms, methods of diagnosis and three approaches used to ease the effects of attention deficit disorder.
Published by Connecticut Association for Children & Adults
with Learning Disabilities (CACLD). *$20.00*
45 Minutes VHS

7918 **Understanding Autism**
Fanlight Productions C/O Icarus Films
32 Court Street
Brooklyn, NY   11201   718-488-8900
                                                         800-876-1710
                                                    Fax: 718-488-8642
                                                      info@fanlight.com
                                                      www.fanlight.com

Ben Achtenberg, Owner
Susan Newman, Editor

Parents of children with autism discuss the nature and symptoms
of this lifelong disability and outline a treatment program based
on behavior modification principles. 19 minutes *$199.00*
VHS/DVD 1993
ISBN 1-572951-00-1

7919 **We're Not Stupid**
Media Projects Inc
5215 Homer St
Dallas, TX   75206-6623   214-826-3863
                                                    Fax: 214-826-3919
                                               mail@mediaprojects.org
                                                 www.mediaprojects.org

Fonya Naomi Mondell, Producer
We're Not Stupid is an insightful and very personal video that
gives a voice to people who are struggling with learning disabilities. It was made by filmmaker Fonya Naomi Mondell, who is also
living with learning differences. The filmmaker camptures the
personal stories of young people from all walks of life who discuss what it's like to live with Attention Deficit Disorder and
Dyslexia. Their comments are open, honest and direct, and their
determination to manage their condition shines through. *$125.00*
Video

7920 **Why Won't My Child Pay Attention?**
ADD Warehouse
300 Northwest 70th Avenue
Suite 102
Plantation, FL 33317-2360   954-792-8100
                                                        800-233-9273
                                                   Fax: 954-792-8545
                                                 www.addwarehouse.com

Sam Goldstein, Ph.D, Author
Michael Goldstein, M.D., Co-Author
Practical and reassuring videotape, noted child psychologist tells
parents about two of the most common and complex problems of
childhood: inattention and hyperactivity. *$49.50*
224 pages Hardcover 1992
ISBN 0-471530-77-8

Support Groups

7921 **Autism Society of America**
4340 East-West Highway
Suite 350
Bethesda, MD   20814   301-657-0881
                                                         800-328-8476
                                                    Fax: 301-657-0869
                                               info@autism-society.org
                                                 www.autism-society.org

Scott Badesch, President/CEO
Jennifer Repella, VP Programs
John Dabrowski, CFO
Doreen Allen, Marketing Manager
ASA is the largest and oldest grassroots organization within the
autism community, with more than 200 chapters and over 20,000
members and supporters nationwide. ASA is the leading source of
education, information and referral about autism and has been the
leader in advocacy and legislative initiatives for more than three
decades.

7922 **National Autism Hotline**
Autism Services Center
929 4th Ave
PO Box 507
Huntington, WV   25701-1408   304-525-8014
                                                   Fax: 304-525-8026
                                             www.autismservicescenter.org

Mike Grady, CEO
Jimmie Beirne, COO
Nathel Lewis, ASC Training Coordinator
Service agency for individuals with autism and developmental
disabilities, and their families. Assists families and agencies attempting to meet the needs of individuals with autism and other
developmental disabilities. Makes available technical assistance
in designing treatment programs and more. The hotline provides

informational packets to callers and assists via telephone when possible.

7923   National Health Information Center
Office Of Disease Prevention And Health Promotion
P.O.Box 1133
Washington, DC   20013-1133

301-565-4167
800-336-4797
301-468-7394
Fax: 301-984-4256
info@nhic.org
www.health.gov/nhic

Jessica Rowden, Sec Dept. Health Human Services
William Corr, J.D., Deputy Secretary

National health information center provides information referral and support. NHIC links consumers and health professionals to organizations that are best able to provide reliable health information.

Dexterity

Associations

7924 American Amputee Foundation
1805 Wewoka Dr
North Little Rock, AR 72116   501-835-9290
                                           Fax: 501-835-9292
                                    info@americanamputee.org
                                     www.americanamputee.org

Catherine J Walden, Executive Director
Serves primarily as a national information clearinghouse and referral center assisting amputees and their families. The foundation researches and gathers information including studies,
product information, services, self-help publications and review
articles written within the field.

**7925 American Board for Certification in Orthotics, Prosthetics
& Pedorthics**
330 John Carlyle St
Suite 210
Alexandria, VA 22314   703-836-7114
                                           Fax: 703-836-0838
                                              info@abcop.org
                                              www.abcop.org

Eric Ramcharran, CPO, President
Catherine Carter, Executive Director
Samlane Ketevong, Director, Certification Services
Debbie Ayres, Director, Marketing & Public Relations
The American Board for Certification in Orthotics, Prosthetics
and Pedorthics is the national certifying and accrediting body for
the orthotic and prosthetic professions.

7926 American Physical Therapy Association
1111 N Fairfax St
Alexandria, VA 22314-1488   703-684-2782
                                                800-999-2782
                                           Fax: 703-684-7343
                                           TTY: 703-683-6748
                                               web@apta.org
                                               www.apta.org

Justin Moore, PT, DPT, CEO
Mandy Frohlich, Chief Operations Officer & Strategic Affairs
Rob Batarla, MBA, CPA, Chief Financial Officer & Business Affairs
*William Boissonnault, Executive Vice President, Professional
Affairs*
The American Physical Therapy Association fosters advance-
ments in physical therapy practice, research and education. The
association offers courses, career counceling, advocacy,
publications and more.

7927 American Stroke Association
7272 Greenville Ave
Dallas, TX 75231   888-478-7653
                                    strokeconnection@heart.org
                        www.strokeassociation.org/STROKEORG

John Warner, Presiednt
James Postl, Chairman
Nancy Brown, Chief Executive Officer
Raymond Vara, Jr., Treasurer
The American Stroke Association offers educational materials,
seminars, conferences and transportation for those effected by
strokes as well as their families, caregivers and interested
professionals.

7928 Charcot-Marie-Tooth Association
PO Box 105
Glenolden, PA 19036   610-499-9264
                                                800-606-2682
                                           Fax: 610-499-9267
                                              info@cmtausa.org
                                              www.cmtausa.org

Gilles Bouchard, Chairman
Amy J Gray, CEO
Kim Magee, Director of Finance
Susan Ruediger, Director of Development
The Charcot-Marie-Tooth Association supports the development
of new drugs to treat CMT, to improve the quality of life for people with CMT and to search for a cure. The association also offers
a resource center, emotional support group, treatment options,
genetic testing, medication and more.

7929 Dyspraxia Foundation USA
1012 Windsor Rd
Highland Park, IL 60035   847-780-3311
                               foundation@mail.dyspraxiausa.org
                                        www.dyspraxiausa.org

Warren Fried, President & Founder
Theresa A Bidwell, Vice President
Dyspraxia Foundation USA is a non-profit organization centered
on understanding, accepting and educating on issues connected
to Developmental Dyspraxia.

7930 Epilepsy Foundation
8301 Professional Place E
Suite 200
Landover, MD 20785- 2353   800-332-1000
                                           Fax: 301-459-1569
                                           ContactUs@efa.org
                                             www.epilepsy.com

Robert W Smith, Chair
Philip M Gattone, M.Ed, President & CEO
M. Vaneeda Bennett, Chief Development Officer
*Ellen Hobby, Chief Financial Officer & VP, Finance & Administra-
tion*
The Epilepsy Foundation is the national voluntary agency dedicated to the welfare of people with epilepsy in the U.S. and their
families. The organization works to ensure that people with seizures are able to participate in all life experiences and to prevent,
control and cure epilepsy through research, education, advocacy
and services.

7931 International Parkinson and Movement Disorder Society
555 East Wells Street
Suite 1100
Milwaukee, WI 53202- 3823   414-276-2145
                                           Fax: 414-276-3349
                                    info@movementdisorders.org
                                     www.movementdisorders.org

Christopher Goetz, MD, President
Susan Fox, PhD, Secretary
Victor Fung, MBBS, PhD, FRACP, Treasurer
A professional society of clinicians, scientists, and other
healthcare professionals who are interested in Parkinson's disease, related neurodegenerative and neurodevelopmental disorders, hyperkinetic movement disorders, and abnormalities in
muscle tone and motor control.

7932 Lewy Body Dementia Association
912 Killian Hill Road S.W.
Lilburn, GA 30047   404-975-2322
                                           Fax: 480-422-5434
                                                 www.lbda.org

Mike Koehler, CEO
Shannon McCarty-Caplan, Vice President
Christina M. Christie, President
Angela Taylor, Director of Programs
A nonprofit organization dedicated to raising awareness of the
Lewy body dementias (LBD), supporting people with LBD, their
families and caregivers and promoting scientific advances.

7933 Multilingual Children's Association
20 Woodside Ave
San Francisco, CA 94127   415-690-0026
Fax: 415-341-1137
www.multilingualchildren.org

7934 National Amputation Foundation
40 Church St
Malverne, NY 11565-1735   516-887-3600
516-887-3600
Fax: 516-887-3667
amps76@aol.com
www.nationalamputation.org
Paul Bernacchio, President
William Sturges, 1st Vice President
Al Pennacchia, 2nd Vice President
Doanld A. Sioss, Executive Secretary
Information & resources for amputees. Scholarship programs for
college students with major limb amputation. Free donated dura-
ble medical equipment open to anyone in need locally-as items
need to be picked up.
Quarterly

7935 National Commission on Orthotic and Prosthetic Education
330 John Carlyle Street
Suite 200
Alexandria, VA 22314- 5760   703-836-7114
Fax: 703-836-0838
info@ncope.org
www.ncope.org
Robin C Seabrook, Executive Director
Jonathan D. Day, CPO
Dominique Mungo, Residency Program Manager
Joan M. Dallas, Accreditation Assistant
The mission of NCOPE is to be recognized authority for the development and accreditation of O&P education and residency
standards leading to competent patient care in the changing
healthcare environment. NCOPE develops, applies, and assures
standards for orthotic and prosthetic education through accreditation and approval to promote exemplary patient care.

**7936 National Institute of Neurological Disorde Disorders &
Stroke**
PO Box 5801
Bethesda, MD 20824-5801   301-496-5751
800-352-9424
Fax: 301-402-2186
www.ninds.nih.gov
Samahria Lyt Landis, Executive Director
Walter J Koroshetz MD, Deputy Director
Caroline Lewis, Executive Officer
Alfred W. Gordon, Ph.D., Associate Director for Special P
The mission of the National Institute of Neurological Disorders
and Stroke is to reduce the burden of neurological disease.

7937 National Stroke Association
9707 E Easter Ln
Suite B
Centennial, CO 80112-3754   303-649-9299
800-787-6537
Fax: 303-649-1328
info@stroke.org
www.stroke.org
James Baranski, CEO
Sharon Jaunchowski, Executive VP
Teran Nash, Customer Relations
Carol Griffin, Development Manager
The only national health organization solely committed to stroke
prevention, treatment, rehabilitation and community reintegration. Provides packaged training programs, on-site assistance,
physician, patient and family education materials to acute and
rehab hospitals. Develops workshops; operates the Stroke Information & Referral Center and produces professional publications
such as Stroke: Clinical Updates and the Journal of Stroke and
Cerebrovascular Diseases.

7938 World Chiropractic Alliance
2950 N Dobson Rd
Suite 3
Chandler, AZ 85224-1819   480-786-9235
800-347-1011
Fax: 480-732-9313
comments@worldchiropracticalliance.org
www.worldchiropracticalliance.org
Terry A Rondberg, Founder/CEO
Richard Barwell, President
Dedicated to protecting and strengthening chiropractic around
the world. Serving as a watchdog and advocacy organization, we
place our emphasis on education and political action.

Print: Books

7939 Carpal Tunnel Syndrome
Arthritis Foundation
1330 W Peachtree St
Suite 100
Atlanta, GA 30309   404-872-7100
800-283-7800
Fax: 404-872-0457
help@arthritis.org
www.arthritis.org
John H Klippel, President/CEO
Daniel T. McGowan, Chairman Of The Board
Rowland W. Chang, Vice Chair
Patricia Nov Nelson, Vice Chair
The Arthritis Foundation is committed to raising awareness and
reducing the unacceptable impact of arthritis, a disease which
must be taken as seriously as other chronic diseases because of its
devastatng consequences.

7940 Don't Feel Sorry for Paul
Harper Collins Publishing
76 Ninth Ave
New York, NY 10011   800-843-2665
www.barnesandnoble.com
Bernard Wolf, Author
Ann Ledden, Vice President
Lorna Metzler, Manager
Paul is seven but was born with deformities of both hands and
feet. Paul must wear a prosthesis on both feet so that he can walk.
He has a third prosthesis for his right hand. The third prosthesis
has a pair of hooks Paul uses as fingers.
94 pages Hardcover
ISBN 0-39731 -88-0

**7941 Functional Restoration of Adults and Children with Upper
Extremity Amputation**
Demos Medical Publishing
11 West 42nd Street
15th Floor
New York, NY 10036-8804   212-683-0072
800-532-8663
Fax: 212-683-0118
www.demosmedpub.com
Robert Meier III, Author
Diane Atkins, OTR, Co-Author
Provides a comprehensive reference to the surgery, prosthetic fitting, and rehabilitation of individuals sustaining an arm amputation. Covers the recent advancements in prosthetics and
rehabilitation. *$165.00*
384 pages
ISBN 1-888799-73-0

Print: Magazines

7942   ABC Mark of Merit Newsletter
Amer Board for Cert in Otthotics & Prosthetics
330 John Carlyle St
Suite 210
Alexandria, VA   22314-5760
703-836-7114
Fax: 703-836-0838
info@abcop.org
www.abcop.org

Timothy E. Miller, CPO
Curt A. Bertram, President Elect
James H. Wynne, CPO
Donald D. Virostek, CPO/Past President
An online bi-monthly newsletter.

7943   Active Living Magazine
American Amputee Foundation
PO Box 94227
North Little Rock, AR   72190
501-835-9290
Fax: 501-835-9292
info@americanamputee.org
www.americanamputee.org

Catherine J Walden, Executive Director
A print magazine published four times a year.

7944   Stroke Connection Magazine
American Heart Association
7272 Greenville Ave
Dallas, TX   75231-5129
214-373-6300
888-478-7653
Fax: 214-706-5231
www.strokeassociation.org/STROKEORG/

John Caswell, Editor
Debra Lockwood, Chairman
Nancy Brown, CEO
Ralph Sacco, President/Director
Free magazine for stroke survivors and their family caregivers.

Print: Newsletters

7945   NINDS Notes
Ntn'l Institute of Neurological Disorders & Stroke
P.O.Box 5801
Bethesda, MD   20284
301-496-5751
800-352-9424
Fax: 202-944-3295
sbaa@sbaa.org

Caroline Lewis, Executive Officer
Story C. Landis, Director
Denise Dorsey, Chief Administrative Officer
Maryann Sofranko, Deputy Executive Officer
A print newsletter published three times a year.

Non Print: Newsletters

7946   Advocacy Pulse
American Stroke Association
7272 Greenville Ave
Dallas, TX   75231-5129
214-373-6300
888-478-7653
Fax: 214-706-5231
www.strokeassociation.org/STROKEORG/
Ralph Sacco, President/Director
Debra Lockwood, Chairman
Nancy Brown, CEO

7947   Noteworthy Newsletter
Ntn'l Comm on Orthotic & Prosthetic Education
330 John Carlyle Street
Suite 200
Alexandria, VA   22314- 5760
703-836-7114
Fax: 703-836-0838
info@ncope.org
www.ncope.org

Robin C Seabrook, Executive Director
Jonathan D. Day, CPO
Dominique Mungo, Residency Program Manager
Joan M. Dallas, Accreditation Assistant
The mission of NCOPE is to be recognized authority for the development and accreditation of O&P education and residency standards leading to competent patient care in the changing healthcare environment. NCOPE develops, applies, and assures standards for orthotic and prosthetic education through accreditation and approval to promote exemplary patient care.

7948   Stroke Smart Magazine
National Stroke Association
9707 E Easter Ln
Suite B
Centennial, CO   80112-3754
303-649-9299
800-787-6537
Fax: 303-649-1328
info@stroke.org
www.stroke.org

James Baranski, CEO
Sharon Jaunchowski, Executive VP
Teran Nash, Customer Relations
Carol Griffin, Development Manager
The only national health organization solely committed to stroke prevention, treatment, rehabilitation and community reintegration. Provides packaged training programs, on-site assistance, physician, patient and family education materials to acute and rehab hospitals. Develops workshops; operates the Stroke Information & Referral Center and produces professional publications such as Stroke: Clinical Updates and the Journal of Stroke and Cerebrovascular Diseases.

Hearing

Associations

7949 Alexander Graham Bell Association for the Deaf and Hard of Hearing
3417 Volta Pl. NW
Washington, DC 20007
202-337-5220
Fax: 202-337-8314
info@agbell.org
agbell.org

Ted A. Meyer, Chair
Catharine McNally, Chair-Elect
Susan Lenihan, Secretary
Emilio Alonso Mendoza, Cheief Executive Officer
The Alexander Graham Bell Association for the Deaf and Hard of Hearing (AG Bell) is the world's oldest and largest membership organization promoting the use of spoken language by children and adults who are hearing impaired. Members include parents of children with hearing loss, adults who are deaf or hard of hearing, educators, audiologists, speech-language pathologists, physicians and other professionals in fields related to hearing loss and deafness.

7950 American Association of People with Disabilities
2013 H St, NW
5th Floor
Washington, DC 20006
202-521-4316
800-840-8844
Fax: 866-536-4461
communications@aapd.com
www.aapd.com

Helena Berger, President & CEO
Jason Mida, Director of Development
Lisa Ekman, Policy Consultant
Amy Naoum, Director of Finance
The American Association of People with Disabilities is dedicated to ensuring economic self-sufficiency and political empowerment for Americans with disabilities.

7951 American Cochlear Implant Alliance
P.O. Box 103
McLEAN, VA 22101-103
703-534-6146
info@acialliance.org
www.acialliance.org

Craig A. Buchman, Chair
Teresa A. Zwolan, Vice Chair
Nancy M. Young, Secretary
Jill B. Firszt, Treasurer
A not-for-profit membership organization created with the purpose of eliminating barriers to cochlear implantation by sponsoring research, driving heightened awareness and advocating for improved access to cochlear implants for patients of all ages across the US.

7952 American Society for Deaf Children
800 Florida Ave NE
Suite 2047
Washington, DC 20002-3695
800-942-2732
Fax: 410-795-0965
www.deafchildren.org

Avonne Brooker-Rutowski, Ed.S, President
Lisalee Egbert, Ph.D, Vice President
Timothy Frelich, M.A., Treasurer
Gina A Oliva, Ph.D, Secretary
Supports and educates families of deaf and hard of hearing children and advocates for high quality programs and services.

7953 American Speech-Language-Hearing Association
2200 Research Blvd
Rockville, MD 20850-3289
301-296-5700
800-638-8255
actioncenter@asha.org
www.asha.org

Gail J. Richard, President
Elise Davis-Mcfaland, President-Elect
Margot L. Beckerman, Chair
Arlene A. Pietranton, CEO
Provides information for both the general public and physicians in an easy-to-access manner. The subjects of focus are speech, hearing and language disorders.

7954 American Tinnitus Association
522 S W 5th Ave
Suite 825
Portland, OR 97204-2143
503-248-9985
800-634-8978
Fax: 503-248-0024
tinnitus@ata.org
www.ata.org

LaGuinn Sherlock, Chair
Randy E. Philips, Vice Chair
Scott C. Mitchell, Secretary
Gary P. Reul, Treasurer
The American Tinnitus Association (ATA) is the national champion of tinnitus awareness, prevention, and treatment. The ATA offers prevention programs in schools, urges governmental and private organizations to support hearing conservation, funds research, and facilitates self-help groups around the country.

7955 Association of Adult Musicians with Hearing Loss
AAMHL, Inc.
P.O. Box 522
Rockville, MD 20848
301-838-0443
info@musicianswithhearingloss.org
www.musicianswithhearingloss.org

Wendy Cheng, President
Jennifer Castellano, Secretary
Janice Rosen, Treasurer
Marshall Chasin, Board Member
The Association of Adult Musicians with Hearing Loss creates a space for adult musicians with hearing loss to discuss the challenges they face in making and listening to music. The association also offers opportunities for public performance.

7956 Association of Late-Deafened Adults
8038 Macintosh Ln
Suite 2
Rockford, IL 61107
815-332-1515
866-402-2532
Fax: 877-907-1738
TTY: 866-402-2532
info@alda.org
www.alda.org

Sharaine Rawlinson Roberts, President
Paul Wummer, Vice President
Eleanor Shafer, Region I Director
Carol Postulka, Region II Director
The Association of Late-Deafened Adults supports the empowerment of late-deafened people by offering programs and information resources on a variety of topics: technology, disability laws, airline travel and more.

7957 Better Hearing Institute
1444 I St NW
Suite 700
Washington, DC 20005
202-449-1100
800-327-9355
Fax: 202-216-9646
mail@betterhearing.org
www.betterhearing.org

Sergei Kochkin, Ph.D, Executive Director
The Better Hearing Institute is a non-profit corporation that educates the public about the neglected problem of hearing loss and what can be done about it. Its mission is to erase the stigma and

end the embarassment that prevents millions of people from seeking help for hearing loss.

7958   Center for Hearing and Communication
50 Broadway
6th Floor
New York, NY 10004   917-305-7700
                                              Fax: 917-305-7888
                                              TTY:917-305-7999
                                              info@chchearing.org
                                              chchearing.org

Laurie Hanin, Executive Director
Ellen Lafargue, Co-Director Speech & Hearing Services
Kshitija Sarpotdar, Director of Finance
Nancy Nadler, Deputy Executive Director & Development Director
The Center for Hearing and Communication provides hearing health services to people of all ages who have hearing loss. Some of its services include free hearing screenings, complete hearing evaluations, pediatric services and more.

7959   Communication Service for the Deaf
3520 Gateway Lane
Sioux Falls, SD 57106   866-642-6410
                                              Fax: 605-362-2806
                                              TTY:866-273-3323
                                              inquiry@c-s-d.org
                                              www.c-s-d.org

Dr. Benjamin Soukup, Founder, Chairman & CEO
Christopher Soukup, President
Brad Hermes, CFO
Ann Marie Mickleson, VP, CSD Interpreting
CSD's mission is to create greater opportunities for Deaf and hard of hearing individuals to reach their full potential. Through global leadership and the development of innovative technologies, CSD provides tools conducive to a positive and fully integrated life.

7960   Conference of Educational Administrators of Schools and Programs for the Deaf
PO Box 1778
St Augustine, FL 32085-1778   904-810-5200
                                                   866-697-8805
                                              Fax: 904-810-5525
                                              nationaloffice@ceasd.org
                                              www.ceasd.org

Joseph Finnegan, Executive Director
Ronald Stern, President
Nancy Hlibok Amann, Secretary
Peter L. Bailey, Treasurer
CEASD provides an opportunity for professional educators to work together for the improvement of schools and educational programs for individuals who are deaf or hard of hearing. The organization brings together a rich composite of resources and reaches out to both enhance educational programs and influence educational policy makers.

7961   Council of American Instructors of the Deaf (CAID)
PO Box 377
Bedford, TX 76095-0377   817-354-8414
                                              Fax: 817-354-8414
                                              caid@swbell.net
                                              www.caid.org

Keith Mousley, President
Helen Lovato, Office Manager
The CAID continues to follow the tradition begun in 1850 and recognizes the value of bringing fellow teaching professionals together to share experiences and ideas for the purpose of improving learning opportunities for deaf and hard of hearing children, adolescents and young adults.

7962   Davis Center
110 Wesley St.
P.O. Box 508
Manlius, NY 13104   862-251-4637
                                              Fax: 862-251-4642
                                              ddavis@thedaviscenter.com
                                              www.thedaviscenter.com

Dorinne S. Davis MA CCC-A FAAA, Director

The Davis Center's Sound Therapy Programs make positive changes for children and adults with autism, ADD/ADHD, auditory processing issues, Dyslexia, learning disabilities, and other learning and wellness challenges. Programs address issues such as phonics, spelling, writing, reading comprehension, hearing only parts of words, following directions, discriminating between sounds, sound sensitivity, behavioral responses, focus, attention, and more.

7963   Deaf REACH
3521 12th St NE
Washington, DC 20017-2545   202-832-6681
                                              Fax: 202-832-8454
                                              deaf-reach.org

Sarah E. Brown, Executive Director
Annette Reichman, President
Jonathan Tomar, Vice-President
Myrene Sargent, Director of Administration
The psychosocial rehabilitation approach, ulitzed by all Deaf-REACH programs, provides the solid foundation to member's success. Participants are activly involved in establishing the format and level of highly individualized service delivery that they receive. The concept, which has achieved national acclaim, involves teaching members necessary life skills, thus minimizing the need for assistance from a service professional. This is part of what distinguishes the approach at Deaf-REACH.

7964   Deaf Women United
PO Box 61
South Barre, VT 5670   info@dwu.org
                                              www.dwu.org

Alana Beal, President
Keri Darling, Vice President
Caroline Koo, Secretary
Amanda Tuite, Treasurer
It is committed to continuing a community of support of Deaf women from all walks of life.

7965   Deafness Research Foundation
363 Seventh Avenue,
10th Floor
New York, NY 10001-3904   212-257-6140
                                                   866-454-3924
                                              Fax: 212-257-6139
                                              TTY: 888-435-6104
                                              info@hearinghealthfoundation.org
                                              www.drf.org

Shari Eberts, Chairman
Mark Angelo, President
Robert Boucai, Principal
Judy R. Dubno, Dept. of Otolaryngology-Head and Neck Surgery
Founded in 1958, the Deafness Research Foundation is the leading source of private funding for basic and clinical research in the hearing science. The DRF is committed to making lifelong hearing health a national priority by funding research and implementing education projects in both the government and private sectors.

7966   Dogs for the Deaf
10175 Wheeler Rd
Central Point, OR 97502-9360   541-826-9220
                                                   800-990-3647
                                              Fax: 541-826-6696
                                              TTY: 541-826-9220
                                              info@dogsforthedeaf.org
                                              dogsforthedeaf.org

Robin Dickson, CEO
Vaughan Maurice, General Manager
Janine Bol, Finance Director
John Drach, Training Dept. Manager
Rescues dogs from shelters and professionally trains them for people with special needs such as: deafness, autism for children, seniors, stroke victims, cerebral palsy, etc.

7967 Ear Foundation
1817 Patterson St
Nashville, TN 37203-2110   615-329-7849
                                             800-545-4327
                                        Fax: 615-329-7935
                                        info@earfoundation.org
                                        www.earfoundation.org

Suzanne Wyatt, Executive Director
National, nonprofit organization committed to integrating the
hearing and balance impaired into the mainstream of society
through public awareness and medical education. Also administers The Meniere's Network, a national network of patient support groups providing people with the opportunity to share
experiences and coping strategies.

7968 Georgiana Institute
736 Harmony Street
New Orleans, LA 70115   203-994-8215
                                        georgianainstitute@snet.net
                                        www.georgianainstitute.org

Annabel Stehli, President
The information source for Auditory Integration Training
(AIT)/Digital Auditory Aerobics (DAA).

7969 HEAR Center
301 E Del Mar Blvd
Pasadena, CA 91101-2714   626-796-2016
                                        Fax: 626-796-2320
                                        info@hearcenter.org
                                        hearcenter.org

Ellen Simon, Executive Director
Deborah Lorino, Office Manager
Berenice Castro, Accounting Supervisor
Maline Medina, Accounts Receivable/Billing Cle
Auditory and verbal program designed to help hearing impaired
children, infants and adults lead normal and productive lives.
Seeks to develop auditory techniques to aid people who have
communication problems due to deafness. Offers diagnostic
evaluations for speech and hearing. Individual auditory, verbal
training and speech-language therapy.

7970 Hearing Education and Awareness for Rockers
1405 Lyon St
San Francisco, CA 94115-2914   415-409-3277
                                        Fax: 415-409-5683
                                        info@hearnet.com
                                        www.hearnet.com

Kathy Peck, Executive Director
Joseph Monatano, Chief of Audiology
Flash Gordon, Primary Care Physician
John Doyle, Secretary of the Board
H.E.A.R.'s mission is the prevention of hearing loss and tinnitus
among musicians and music fans (especially teens) through edu-
cation awareness and grassroots outreach advocacy.

7971 Hearing Industries Association
1444 I Street, N.W.
Suite 700
Washington, DC 20005   202-449-1090
                                        Fax: 202-216-9646
                                        mjones@bostrom.com
                                        www.hearing.org

7972 Hearing Loss Association of America
7910 Woodmont Ave
Suite 1200
Bethesda, MD 20814-7022   301-657-2248
                                        Fax: 301-913-9413
                                        TTY:301-657-2248
                                        hearingloss.org

Brenda Battat, Executive Director
Barbara Kelley, Dep Exec Dir, Editor-In-Chief
Nancy Macklin, Director of Events & Marketing
Lisa Hamlin, Director of Public Policy
The mission of the Hearing Loss Association of America is to
open the world of communication to people with hearing loss
through information, education, advocacy and support.

7973 Hearing, Speech and Deafness Center (HSDC)
1625 19th Ave.
Seattle, WA 98122-2848   206-323-5770
                                             888-222-5036
                                        Fax: 206-328-6871
                                        seattle@hsdc.org
                                        www.hsdc.org

Lindsay Klarman, Executive Director
Michelle Coleman, Operations Director
Hearing, Speech & Deaf Center (HSDC) is a nonprofit for clients
who are deaf, hard of hearing, or who face other communication
barriers such as speech challenges. Their mission is to foster inclusive and accessible communities through communication, advocacy, and education.

7974 House Ear Institute
2100 W 3rd St
Los Angeles, CA 90057-1944   213-483-4431
                                             800-388-8612
                                        Fax: 213-484-8789
                                        TTY: 213-484-2642
                                        info@hei.org
                                        www.hei.org

James Boswell, CEO
John.W House, M.D, President
Daniel. M Graham, Executive Vice President Develop
Neil Segil, Ph.D, Executive Vice President
Offers pediatric hearing tests, otologic and audiologic evaluation
and treatment, rehabilitation, hearing aid dispensing, and co-
chlear implant services. Outreach programs focus on families
with hearing impaired children.

7975 International Catholic Deaf Association
7202 Buchanan St
Landover Hills, MD 20784-2236   301-429-0697
                                        Fax: 301-429-0698
                                        homeoffice@icda-us.org
                                        icda-us.org

Jean Cox, President
Kate Slosar, Vice President
T.K Hill, Secretary
Jimmy Kelly, Treasurer
An organization of Catholic deaf people and hearing people in the
church working with the deaf in the united states of America.

7976 International Hearing Dog
5901 E 89th Ave.
Henderson, CO 80640-8315   303-287-3277
                                        Fax: 303-287-3425
                                        info@hearingdog.org
                                        www.hearingdog.org

Valerie Foss-Brugger, President
Robert Cooley, Field Representative
Andrea Paul, Vetinary Technician
Larry Norby, Accounting/HR
Trains and places Hearing dogs with deaf or hard-of-hearing per-
sons, with or without multiple disabilities, nationwide, free of
charge to the recipient.

7977 International Hearing Society
1688 Middlebelt Rd
Suite 4
Livonia, MI 48154-3374   734-522-7200
                                             800-521-5247
                                        Fax: 734-522-0200
                                        chelms@ihsinfo.org
                                        ihsinfo.org

Kathleen Mennillo, Executive Director
Joy Wilkins, Director of Education
Fran Vincent, Marketing Manager
Alissa Parady, Manager of Government Affairs
The IHS is the professional association that represents Hearing
Instrument Specialists worldwide. IHS members are engaged in
the practice of testing human hearing and selecting, fitting and
dispensing hearing instruments. Founded in 1951, the Society
continues to recognize the need for promoting and maintaining
the highest possible standards for its members in the best
interestof the hearing impaired it serves.

7978 League for the Hard of Hearing
50 Broadway
6th Fl
New York, NY   10004-3810   917-305-7700
                                        TTY:917-305-7999
                                             www.lhh.org

Laurie Hanin, Executive Director
Ellen Pfeffer Lafargue, Au.D, Director
Dorene Watkins, Coordinator
Anita Stein-Meyers, Au.D, C, Assistant Director
The Center for Hearing and Communication is a leading hearing center offering state-of-the-art hearing testing, hearing aid fitting, speech therapy and full range of services for people of all ages with hearing loss. Visit our offices in New York City and Florida for services that meet all of your hearing and communication needs.

7979 Lexington School for the Deaf: Center for the Deaf
30th Avenue and 75th St
Jackson Heights, NY   11370   718-350-3300
                                        Fax: 718-899-9846
                                        TTY:718-350-3056
                                   generalinfo@lexnyc.org
                                             www.lexnyc.org

Regina Carroll PhD, CEO/Executive Director
Philip W. Bravin, President
Gregory Hlibok, Vice President
Seth Bravin, Treasurer
Offers a comprehensive range of services to deaf, hard of hearing and speech impaired persons from infancy to elderly through its affiliate agencies: The Center for Mental Health Services; The Lexington Hearing and Speech Center, Lexington Vocational Services, and the Lexington School for the Deaf. The Lexington Center also provides services through its research division which houses the only federally funded Rehabilitation Engineering Center.

7980 Michigan Association for Deaf and Hard of Hearing
5236 Dumond Court
Suite C
Lansing, MI   48917-6001   517-487-0066
                                             800-968-7327
                                        Fax: 517-487-0202
                                        info@madhh.org
                                             www.madhh.org

Nancy Asher, Executive Director
Pat Walton, Office Manager
MADHH is a statewide collaboration agency dedicated to improving the lives of people who are deaf or hard of hearing through leadership in education, advocacy and services.

7981 Mississippi Speech-Language-Hearing Association
PO Box 22664
Jackson, MS   39225   800-664-6742
                                        Fax: 601-510-7833
                                        admin@mshausa.org
                                             www.mshausa.org

Claudette Edwards, President
Ricki Garrett, Executive Director
The Mississippi Speech-Language-Hearing Association is the statewide organization supporting audiologists and speech-language pathologists in Mississippi by offering them resources, information, and professional development opportunities so they could better serve their clients.

7982 National Alliance of Black Interpreters
P.O. Box 90532
Washington, DC   20090-532   202-810-4451
                                             www.naobidc.org

7983 National Association of Hearing Officials
PO Box 4999
Midlothian, VA   23112-17   www.naho.org
Bonny M Fetch CALJ, President
The mission of the National Association of Hearing Officials is to improve the administrative hearing process and thereby benefit hearing officials, their employing agencies, and the individuals they serve through promoting professionalism and by providing traininf, continuing education, a national forum for discussion of issues, and leadership concerning administrative harings.

7984 National Association of Parents with Children in Special Education
3642 E Sunnydale Dr.
Chandler Heights, AZ   85142   800-754-4421
                                        Fax: 800-424-0371
                                        contact@napcse.org
                                             www.napcse.org
George Giuliani, President
NAPCSE is a national membership organization dedicated to rendering all possible support and assistance to parents whose children receive special education services, both in and outside of school.

7985 National Association of Special Education Teachers
1250 Connecticut Ave., NW
Suite 200
Washington, DC 20036-2643   800-754-4421
                                        Fax: 800-754-4421
                                        contactus@naset.org
                                             www.naset.org

Roger Pierangelo, Executive Director
George Giuliani, Executive Director
The National Association of Special Education Teachers (NASET) is a national membership organization dedicated to rendering all possible support and assistance to those preparing for or teaching in the field of special education. NASET was founded to promote the profession of special education teachers and to provide a national forum for their ideas.

7986 National Association of the Deaf
8630 Fenton Street
Suite 820
Silver Spring, MD   20910- 3819   301-587-1788
                                        Fax: 301-587-1791
                                        TTY:301-587-1789
                                        nadinfo@nad.org
                                             www.nad.org

Howard A. Rosenblum, CEO
Shane H. Feldman, COO
Marc P. Charmatz, Staff Attorney
Lizzie Sorkin, Director of Communications
Nation's largest organization safeguarding the accessability and civil rights of 28 million deaf and hard of hearing Americans in education, employment, health care, and telecommunications. Focuses on grassroots advocacy and empowerment, captioned media deafness-related information and publications, legal assistance, and policy development.

7987 National Black Association for Speech Language and Hearing
P.O. Box 779
Pennsville, NJ   08070   877-936-6235
                                        Fax: 877-936-6235
                                        nbaslh@nbaslh.org
                                             www.nbaslh.org

Cathy Runnels, Interim
Kia N. Johnson, Parliamentarian
Martine Elie, Treasurer
The mission of the National Black Association of Speech-Language and Hearing is to maintain a viable mechanism through which the needs of black professionals, students and individuals with communication disorders can be met.

7988 National Black Deaf Advocates
PO Box 32
Frankfort, KY   40602   585-475-2411
                                             800-421-1220
                                        Fax: 585-475-6500
                                        president@nbda.org
                                             www.nbda.org

Benro Ogunyipe, President
Cory Parker, VP
Sharon.D White, Secretary
Betty Henderson, Treasurer

The Mission of the National Black Deaf Advocate is to promote the leadership development, economic and educational opportunities, social equality, and to safeguard the general health and welfare of Black deaf and hard of hearing people.

7989 National Catholic Office of the Deaf
7202 Buchanan St
Landover Hills, MD   20784-2299   301-577-1684
                                         Fax: 301-577-1684
                                         TTY:301-577-4184
                                         info@ncod.org
                                         www.ncod.org
Consuelo Martinez Wild, Executive Director
Helps coordinate efforts of deaf or hard of hearing people who are involved in the ministry, acts as a resource center, assists bishops and pastors become available to the deaf and hard of hearing.

7990 National Cued Speech Association
1300 Pennsylvania Ave, NW
Suite 190-713
Washington, DC 20004   917-439-5126
                                         800-459-3529
                                         Fax: 866-269-9877
                                         info@cuedspeech.org
                                         www.cuedspeech.org
Anne Huffman, President
Sarina Roffe, Executive Director
Ben Lachman, Director of Development
Brian Kelly, Treasurer
Champions effective communication, language development and literacy through the use of cued speech.

7991 National Deaf Women's Bowling Association
9244 E Mansfield Ave
Denver, CO   80237-1915   303-771-9018
                                         ndwbast@gmail.com
Gayle Willingham, President
Ali Martinez, VP
Holds world Deaf Bowling Torunament annually in July. Also holds Las Vegas Scratch Classic annually in October.

7992 National Hearing Conservation Association
3030 W 81st Ave
Westminster, CO   80031   303-224-9022
                                         Fax: 303-458-0002
                                         nhcaoffice@hearingconservation.org
                                         www.hearingconservation.org
Jennifer Tufts, President
Beth Cooper, President Elect
Nancy Wojcik, Secretary/Treasurer
Cory Portnuff, Director of Communications
The mission of the NHCA is to prevent hearing loss due to noise and other environmental factors in all sectors of society.

7993 National Institute on Deafness and Other Communication Disorders
31 Center Dr
MSC 2320
Bethesda, MD   20892-2320   301-827-8183
                                         800-241-1044
                                         Fax: 301-402-0018
                                         TTY: 800-241-1055
                                         nidcdinfo@nidcd.nih.gov
                                         www.nidcd.nih.gov
James F Battey Jr., MD, Ph.D, Director
Timothy J Wheeles, Executive Officer
Chad Wysong, Deputy Executive Officer
Mark Lucano, Ethics Coordinator
The National Institute on Deafness and Other Communication Disorders (NIDCD) supports and conducts research to help prevent, detect and diagnose disabilities that affect hearing, balance, taste, smell, voice, speech, and communication.

7994 National Student Speech Language Hearing Association
2200 Research Blvd
Suite 450
Rockville, MD   20850-3289   301-296-5650
                                         800-498-2071
                                         Fax: 301-296-8580
                                         TTY: 301-296-5650
                                         nsslha@asha.org
                                         www.nsslha.org
Patricia A. Prelock, PhD, President
Elizabeth S. McCrea, President-Elect
Shelly S. Chabon, Immediate Past President
Donna Fisher Smiley, Vice President for Audiology Practice
The American Speech-Language-Hearing Association is committed to ensuring that all people with speech, language, and hearing disorders receive services to help them communicate effectively.

7995 Registry of Interpreters for the Deaf
333 Commerce St
Alexandria, VA   22314-2801   703-838-0030
                                         Fax: 703-838-0454
                                         TTY:7038380459
                                         ridinfo@rid.org
                                         rid.org
Brenda Walke Prudhomme, President
Kelly L. Flores, VP
Dawn Whitcher, Secretary
Chris Grooms, Treasurer
The Registry of Interpreters for the Deaf, Inc. (RID), a national membership organization, plays a leading role in advocating for excellence in the delivery of interpretation and transliteration services between people who use sign language and people who use spoken language. In collaboration with the Deaf community, RID supports our members and encourages the growth of the profession through the establishment of a national standard for qualified sign language interpreters and transliterators, o

7996 Sight & Hearing Association
1246 University Ave. W.,
Suite #226
St. Paul, MN   55104- 4125   651-645-2546
                                         800-992-0424
                                         Fax: 651-645-2742
                                         mail@sightandhearing.org
                                         www.sightandhearing.org
Kathy Webb, Executive Director
Karen Klevar, Screening Director
Bernice Burgy, Program Assistant
Charles F. Barer, President
It is a nonprofit organization with a mission to enable lifetime learning by identifying preventable loss of vision and hearing in children.

7997 Spring Dell Center
6040 Radio Station Rd
La Plata, MD   20646-3368   301-934-4561
                                         Fax: 301-870-2439
                                         info@springdellcenter.org
                                         www.springdellcenter.org
Patsy Finch, President
Badgley CPA, Treasurer
Jean Hubbard, Secretary
Donna Rretzlaff, Executive Director
Since 1967, Spring Dell center has been, bridging the gap to enhance the lives of developmentally disabled people. Spring Dell's goal is to empower people in every aspect of their lives through the implementation of two programs, employment/vocational services and residential services including transportation. Spring Dell offers transportation door-to-door for persons with developmental disabilities, including day care programs, supportive environment, residential and any other transportation.

7998 Starkey Hearing Foundation
6700 Washington Ave S
Eden Prairie, MN 55344   952-941-6401
                                866-354-3254
                                Fax: 952-828-6900
                                info@starkeyfoundation.org
                                www.starkeyhearingfoundation.org

Richard S Brown, President
Brady Forseth, Executive Director
Keith Becker, Senior Director of Operations
Bruce Schmaltz, Chief Financial Officer
The Starkey Hearing Foundation works to assist those with hearing impairments by offering hearing aids and aftercare services.

7999 Telecommunications for the Deaf and Hard of Hearing
8630 Fenton St
Suite 121
Silver Spring, MD 20910-3803   301-563-9122
                                      Fax: 301-589-3797
                                      TTY:301-589-3006
                                      info@tdi-online.org
                                      tdiforaccess.org

Claude L Stout, Executive Director
James House, Director of Public Relations
John Skjeveland, Business Manager
Promoting equal access to telecommunications and media for people who are deaf, late-deafened, hard of hearing or deaf-blind through consumer education and involvement; technical assistance and consulting; applications of exisiting and emerging technologies; networking and collaboration; uniformity of standards; and national policy development and advocacy.

8000 United States Deaf Ski & Snowboard Association
76 Kings Gate N
Rochester, NY 14617   585-286-2780
                            info@usdssa.org
                            usdssa.org

Anthony Di Giovani, Officer
It provides means for deaf people to get together to share their love for skiing and sponsor races for deaf skiers.

8001 Vestibular Disorders Association
5018 NE 15th Ave
Portland, OR 97213-305   503-229-7705
                                800-837-8428
                                Fax: 503-229-8064
                                veda@vestibular.org
                                www.vestibular.org

Sue Hickey, President
Cynthia Ryan, MBA, Executive Director
Kerrie Denner, Outreach Coordinator
Karen Ilari, Administrative Support Coordinator
The mission of the Vestibular Disorders Association is to serve people with vestibular disorders by providing access to information, offering a support network, and elevating awareness of the challenges associated with these disorders.

Camps

8002 ASD Summer Camp
Alabama Institute for Deaf & Blind
205 E South St
P.O. Box 698
Talladega, AL 35160   256-761-3214
                            Fax: 256-761-3278
                            TTY:256-761-3215
                            wiggins.lavina@aidb.state.al.us
                            www.aidb.org

Paul Millard, Principal
The Alabama School for the Deaf Summer Enrichment Camp is designed especially for deaf and hard of hearing children ages 6-15. Recreation activities include swimming, skating, outdoor games, horseback riding, field trips, arts and craft. Tuition is free.

8003 Aspen Camp School for the Deafearing
PO Box 1494
Aspen, CO 81612-1494   970-923-2511
                              Fax: 970-923-0643
                              info@aspencamp.org
                              www.aspencamp.org

Lesa Thompson, Camp Director
DJ Monahan, Program Coordinator
Katie Murch, Outreach Coordinator
Chelsea Bridges, Advocacy Coordinator
Aspen Camp's mission is to enrich the lives of Deaf and Hard of Hearing individuals by providing experiential educational and recreational activities which increase self-esteem, confidence, and individual skills.

8004 Aspen Camp of the Deaf & Hard of Hearing
PO Box 1494
Aspen, CO 81612   970-923-2511
                        Fax: 970-923-0643
                        info@aspencamp.org
                        www.aspencamp.org

Lesa Thompson, Camp Director
Aspen Camp's mission is to enrich the lives of Deaf and Hard of Hearing individuals by providing experiential educational and recreational activities which increase self-esteem, confidence, and individual skills.

8005 CHAMP Camp
1116 East Market St
Suite B-210
Indianapolis, IN 46202- 5629   317-679-1860
                                      Fax: 317-245-2291
                                      admin@champcamp.org
                                      www.champcamp.org

Dave Carter, Co-Camp Director/Founder
Jamie Mitchell, Co-Camp Director
Nancy McCurdy, Camp Consultant/Founder
Kristina Watkins, Program Coordinator
We are an ACA accredited camp.

8006 Camp Alexander Mack
Indiana Deaf Camps Foundation
P.O.Box 158
Milford, IN 46542   574-658-4831
                          www.campmack.org

Galen Jay, Interim Executive Director
Lauren Carrick, Director of Development/Facility Manager
Amber Barrett, Food Service
Norma Miller, Ordained Minister
Our program is intentionally designed to provide campers with life changing experiences that lead to a formation of personal faith within a safe faith community.

8007 Camp Bishopswood
Diocese of Maine Episcopal
143 State St
Portland, ME 04101   207-772-1953
                            800-244-6062
                            Fax: 207-773-0095
                            mike@bishopswood.org
                            www.bishopswood.org

Laurie Kazilionis, President
Robert Johnston, VP
Jeff Mansir, Treasurer
Pam Waite, Secretary
Camp is located in Hope, Maine. One to seven-week sessions for hearing impaired children June-August. Coed, ages 7-16.

8008 Camp Capella
8 Pearl Point Road
Dedham, ME 04429   207-843-5104
                          www.campcapella.org

Dana Mosher, Religious Leader
Provides an opportunity for children with disabilities to engage in various recreational and social experiences.

8009 **Camp Chris Williams**
Lions 11 B-2 and MADHH
5236 Dumond Court
Suite C
Lansing, MI 48917-6001 Fax: 586-778-4188
Fax: 586-285-1842
TTY:586-285-1842
info@madhh.org
www.madhh.org

Nancy Asher, Executive Director
An exciting summer camp experience for deaf and hard of hearing youth and their siblings ages 8-14.

8010 **Camp Comeca & Retreat Center**
United Methodist Church
75670 Road 417
Conzad, NE 69130 308-784-2808
www.campcomeca.com

John , Asst. Director
Camp is located in Cozad, Nebraska. Summer sessions for campers with diabetes and hearing impairment. Coed, ages 6-19, families, seniors, single adults.

8011 **Camp Emanuel**
P.O. Box 752343
Dayton, OH 45475 937-477-5504
www.campemanuel.org

Stephanie Ackner, Vice President
Brian Demarke, President
Nan Crawford, Executive Director
Mary Foreman, Secretary
Camp Emanuel is a camp for hearing impaired and normal hearing youth. There are day sessions for children 5-14, and overnight resident sessions for children and teens 9-17. The camp aims to promote descision making, self-esteem, and acceptance by integrating non-hearing children with hearing children.

8012 **Camp Grizzly**
NorCal Services For Deaf & Hard Of Hearing, Inc.
4708 Roseville Road
Suite 112
North Highlands, CA 95660-5172 916-349-7500
Fax: 916-349-7580
www.norcalcenter.org

Cheryl Bella, Chair
Sheri Farinah, CEO
Yim Orsi, Secretary
Andrew Metz, Treasurer
This camp is designed the deaf and hard of hearing youth or hearing youth with deaf or hard of hearing parent. The camp helps with social interaction, building self esteem, leadership skills while enriching the lives of the deaf and hard of hearing.

8013 **Camp Isola Bella On Twin Lakes, Salisbury, Ct.**
American School for the Deaf
139 N Main St
West Hartford, CT 06107-1264 860-570-2300
Fax: 860-570-2301
TTY:860-570-2222
Steve.Borsotti@asd-1817.org
www.asd-1817.org

Alyssa Pecorino, Director
Edward Peltier, Executive Director
Steve Borsotti, Reunion Chairperson
Jenilee Terry, Camp Registrar
Hearing-impaired children, ages 6-19, blend educational instruction in communications with recreational activities. Qualified deaf and hearing staff members with experience in education, child care and counseling are employed at the camp.

8014 **Camp Joy**
3325 Swamp Creek Rd
Schwenksville, PA 19473-1518 610-754-6878
Fax: 610-754-7880
campjoy@fast.net
www.campjoy.com

Angus Murray, Camp Director

A special needs camp for kids and adults (ages 4-80+) with developmental disabilities such as: mental retardation, autism, brain injury, neurological disorder, visual and/or hearing impairments, Angelman and Down syndromes, and other developmental disabilities.

8015 **Camp Juliena**
Georgia Center for the Deaf and Hard of Hearing
4151 Memorial Dr
Suite 103-B
Decatur, GA 30032 404-292-5312
Fax: 404-299-3642
TTY:800-541-0710
gachiboard@gachi.org
www.gcdhh.org/gcdhh-programs/camp-juliena

Meredith Albert, President
Jimmy Peterson, Executive Director
LaQuanda Jackson, Executive Assistant
Kathy Keeter, Employment Support Coordinator
A weeklong residential summer camp for youths and teens who are deaf or hard of hearing. Through challenging, team-oriented activities, campers form lasting friendships and acquire valuable leadership, social and communication skills.

8016 **Camp Mark Seven**
Mark Seven Deaf Foundation
144 Mohawk Hotel Rd
Old Forge, NY 13420 315-207-5706
TTY:315-357-6089
registrar@campmark7.org
www.campmark7.org

Dave Staehle, Camp Director
Adirondack Mountain camp for hard-of-hearing, deaf and hearing people. Coed, ages 1-99, families, seniors and single adults.

8017 **Camp Meadowood Springs**
122 SE Court Ave
P.O. Box 1025
Pendleton, OR 97801 541-276-2752
Fax: 541-276-7227
info@meadowoodsprings.org
www.meadowoodsprings.org

8018 **Camp Pacifica, Inc.**
California Lions Camp
45895 California Hwy. 49
Ahwahnee, CA 93601 559-683-4660
Fax: 209-543-9418
www.camppacifica.org/

Ann Tognetti, President
Bob Ransom, Treasurer
Russ Custer, VP
Jill Loving, Secretary
Camp Pacifica is a camp for special needs children ages 7-15 years old. The camp offers outdoor recreational activities, along with promoting greater independence and self confidence among the children, and provides opportunities for social interaction, and further development of social skills.

8019 **Camp Shocco for the Deaf**
AL Baptist State Board of Missions
P.O. Box 6569
Talladega, AL 35161-886 256-761-1100
800-264-1225
Fax: 256-761-1270
www.campshocco.org

Chad Fleming, Director
Matthew Dixon, Co-Director
Linnea Elliott, Assistant Director
Camp Shocco gives each child and teenager attending camp the opportunity to have an unforgettable one week of fun, games, and spiritual growth. Each camper also learns essence of teamwork, while developing their own unique abilities and talents that can often be overlooked.

8020 Camp Taloali
Lions Club of Oregon and Washington
15934 N Santiam Hwy
PO Box 32
Stayton, OR   97383   971-239-8153
                                             camp@taloali.org
                                             www.taloali.org

8021 Camp Tekoa UMC
United Methodist Camp Tekoa
P.O. Box 160
Hendersonville, NC   28793-0160   828-692-6516
                                         Fax: 828-697-3288
                                             www.camptekoa.org

James Johnson, Executive Director
John Isley, Assistant Director
Melisa Coates, Administrative Assistant
Karen Rohrer, Business Manager
Camping for children with developmental disabilities. Day
camps available for children aged 8-12, and overnight programs
for adults aged 18 and up.

8022 Deaf Kid's Kamp
Sproul Ranch, Inc.
42263 50th Street West
Suite 610
Quartz Hill, CA   93536   661-675-3323
                                             877-399-5449
                                             www.deafkidskamp.com

Buffy Sproul, Executive Director
Our purpose is to meet the needs of deaf children outside of the
classroom setting. These needs, as we have defined them, would
include but are not limited to: social contact with peers; contact
with the culture of the Deaf Community; educational and recreational programs not available in most school settings.

8023 Easter Seals Oklahoma
701 NE 13th St
Oklahoma City, OK   73104   405-239-2525
                                             info@eastersealsoklahoma.org
                                             eastersealsok.org/

Keith McCombs, Chairman
Krista Massad, Chairmain-Elect
Matt Vance, Treasurer
Cassie Wilson, Secretary
Offers an Adult Day Health Center, and Child Development Center. The Child Development Center offers developmentally appropriate learning activities and services to meet the unique
needs of each child, and the adult center provides solutions to
meet the physical, social and emotional needs of adults from the
ages of 21 to 100+.

8024 Father Drumgoole Connelly Summer Camp
MIV: Mount Loretto
6581 Hylan Blvd
Staten Island, NY   10309-3830   718-317-2600
                                         Fax: 718-317-2830
                                             www.mountloretto.org

Stephen Rynn, Executive Director
Maryann Virga, Executive Assistant
Loretta Polanish, Executive Secretary
Ed Gani, Facilities Manager
Summer sessions for children with epilepsy, hearing impairment
and developmental disabilities. Coed, ages 5-13.

8025 Lions Camp Crescendo, Inc.
1480 Pine Tavern Road
P.O. Box 607
Lebanon Junction, KY 40150   502-833-3554
                                             888-879-8884
                                         Fax: 502-833-4427
                                             www.lions-campcrescendo.org

Major Wheat, Chairperson
Barbara Walker, Vice Chairperson
Billie J. Flannery, Administrator
Melinda Gilbert, Secretary

The enhancement of the quality of life for youth, especially those
with disabilities, through the delivery of a traditional camp experience by caring individuals and to enable others to use our camping and retreat facilities to serve the larger communities
humanitarian needs.

8026 Lions Camp Kirby
1735 Narrows Hill Rd
Upper Black Eddy, PA   18972   610-982-5731
                                             info@lionscampkirby.org
                                             www.lionscampkirby.org

Alice Breon, Camp Director
Offers 2-week camps for deaf and hearing impaired children and
their siblings in eastern Pennsylvania.

8027 Lions Camp Merrick
Lions Clubs of District 22-C
P.O. Box 56
Nanjemoy, MD   20662   301-870-5858
                                         Fax: 301-246-9108
                                             info@LionsCampMerrick.org
                                             lionscampmerrick.org

Wayne Magoon, President
Ray Shumaker, Vice President
Julie Andrew, Board Member
Frank Culhane, Treasurer
This recreational camp for special needs children offers a complete waterfront program including swimming, canoeing and
fishing for ages 6-16. Designed for children who are deaf and
hard of hearing, children of deaf parents, and children with diabetes. Also helps children to learn to deal with their special
conditions.

8028 Lions Wilderness Camp for Deaf Children, Inc.
Lions Clubs of California and Nevada
P.O.Box 195
Knightsen, CA   94548   877-896-1598
                                             888-613-1557
                                             campdirector@lionswildcamp.org
                                             www.lionswildcamp.org

Richard A. Wilmot, President
Rachel Mix, Camp Program Director
Robin L. Nichol, Camp Manager
Dana Johnson, Secretary
A camp experience where a deaf child age 7 to 15 can learn out-
door skills and enjoy the wonder and beauty of nature to the full-
est extent.

8029 Ramah in the Poconos
2618 Upper Woods Road
Suite 734
Lakewood, PA   18439-3725   570-798-2504
                                         Fax: 570-798-2049
                                             info@ramahpoconos.org
                                             www.ramahpoconos.org

Todd Zeff, Executive Director
Rabbi Joel Seltzer, Director
Bruce Lipton, Director of Finance & Operations
Deborah Jo Essrog, Development Director
Camp is located in Lake Como, Pennsylvania. Summer sessions
for children and adults with hearing impairment. Coed, ages
10-16, families and seniors.

8030 Sandcastle Day Camp
Children's Beach House
1800 Bay Ave
Lewes, DE   19958   302-645-9184
                                         Fax: 302-645-9467
                                             www.cbhinc.org

Martha P. Tschantz, President
Maryann Helms, Vice President
Linda M. Fischer, Secretary
Charles H. Sterner, Treasurer
Camp is located in Lewes, Delaware. Four-week sessions
June-August for Delaware children with hearing impairment or
speech/communication impairment. Coed, ages 6-12.

8031 Sertoma Camp Endeavor
Sertoma Camp Endeavor
P.O.Box 910
Dundee, FL   33838-0910   863-439-1300
                                      Fax: 863-439-1300

Jeff Nunemaker, Executive Director
The intergration of deaf, hard of hearing and hearing youngsters
is a unique characteristic of our camping program. Both hearing,
deaf and hard of hearing children have the opportunity to learn
about themselves and each other in an informal and empowering
setting.

8032 Texas Lions Camp
Lions Club of Texas
P.O.Box 290247
Kerrville, TX   78029   830-896-8500
                                      Fax: 830-896-3666
                                      www.lionscamp.com

Stephen Mabry, Executive Director
Steven King, Director of Operations
Patty Rodriguez, Program Supervisor
Bailey Carter, Program Supervisor
Texas Lions Camp is a camp dedicated to seving children in Texas
with physical diabilities, ages 7-16. While at camp, campers will
participate in a variety of acitvties and they will be encouraged to
become more independent and self-confident.

8033 YMCA Camp Fitch
The YMCA's Camp Fitch on Lake Erie
12600 Abels Rd
North Springfield, PA   16430   814-922-3219
                                           877-863-4824
                                      Fax: 814-922-7000
                                      hannahkight@campfitchymca.org
                                      campfitchymca.org

Matt Pose, Executive Director
Tom Parker, Associate Executive Director
Hannah Kight, Office Manager
Jon Tully, Program Director
Camp is located in North Springfield, Pennsylvania. Camping
sessions for children and adults with diabetes or epilepsy. Ages
8-16, families and seniors.

8034 Youth Leadership Camp
National Association of the Deaf
8630 Fenton Street
Suite 820
Silver Spring, MD   20910   301-587-1788
                                      Fax: 301-587-1791
                                      www.nad.org

Christopher Wagnor, President
Melissa S. Draganac-Hawk, VP
Howard A. Rosenblum, CEO
Joshua Beckman, Secretary
Sponsored by the National Association of the Deaf, this camp em-
phasizes leadership training for deaf teenagers and young adults.
In addition to many recreational activities and sports, there are
academic offerings and camp projects.

Print: Books

8035 A Basic Course in American Sign Language
TJ Publishers
2544 Tarpley Rd
Suite 108
Carrollton, TX   75006-2288   972-416-0800
                                          800-999-1168
                                      Fax: 972-416-0944
                                      customerservice@tjpublishers.com
                                      www.tjpublishers.com

Tom Humphries, Author
Carol Padden, Co-Author
Terrence J O'Rouke, Co-Author
Tanner Beach, Director
The first three DVDs in this series are designed to illustrate and
demonstrate each of the exercises and dialogues presented in A

Basic Course in American Sign Language. Four Deaf teachers
and three hearing students provide a variety of models for the exercises. *$35.95*
288 pages Spiral Bound
ISBN 0-932666-42-6

8036 A Basic Course in Manual Communication
Gallaudet University Bookstore
800 Florida Ave NE
Washington, DC   20002-3600   202-651-5855
                                           866-204-0504
                                      Fax: 773-660-2235
                                      TTY: 202-651-5855
                                      gupress@gallaudet.edu
                                      www.clerccenter.gallaudet.edu

Terrence J O'Rourke, Author
T. Alan Hurwitz, President
Paul Kelly, Vice President Adm and Finance
Teach your students manual communication - that living, chang-
ing, growing language of signs.
161 pages Softcover

**8037 A Basic Vocabulary: American Sign Languagefor Parents
and Children**
TJ Publishers
2544 Tarpley Rd
Suite 108
Carrollton, TX   75006-2288   972-416-0800
                                           800-999-1168
                                      Fax: 972-416-0944
                                      customerservice@tjpublishers.com
                                      www.tjpublishers.com

Terrence J O'Rouke, Author
Tanner Beach, Director
Carefully selected words and signs include those that children
use every day. Alphabetically organized vocabulary incorporates
developmental lists helpful to both deaf and hearing children and
over 1000 clear sign language illustrations. *$9.95*
240 pages Softcover
ISBN 0-932666-00-0

8038 A Loss for Words
HarperCollins Publishers
10 E 53rd St
New York, NY   10022-5244   212-207-7901
                                           800-242-7737
                                      Fax: 212-702-2586
                                      spsales@harpercollins.com
                                      www.harpercollins.com

Lou Ann Walker, Author
From the time she was a toddler, Lou Ann Walker was the ears and
voice for her deaf parents. Their family life was warm and loving,
but outside the home, they faced a world that misunderstood and
often rejected them. *$13.00*
224 pages Paperback 1987
ISBN 0-060914-25-4

**8039 Access for All: Integrating Deaf, Hard of Hearing and
Hearing Preschoolers**
Gallaudet University Bookstore
800 Florida Avenue NorthEast
Washington, DC   20002-3600   202-651-5530
                                      Fax: 202-651-5489
                                      gupress@gallaudet.edu
                                      http://www.gallaudet.edu

Stephanie Cawthon, Ph.D., Book Review Editor
Peter V. Paul, Ph.D., Editor, Literary Issues
Ye Wang, Ph.D., Senior Associate Editor
Feifei Ye, Ph.D., Associate Editor for Research Methodology
This exciting new 90 minute videotape and manual describes a
model program for integrating deaf and hard of hearing children
in early education.
169 pages Book & Video

8040   Advanced Sign Language Vocabulary: A Resource Text for Educators
Charles C. Thomas
2600 S First St
Springfield, IL   62704-4730   217-789-8980
                                              800-258-8980
                                          Fax: 217-789-9130
                                       books@ccthomas.com
                                         www.ccthomas.com

Michael P. Thomas, President
Elizabeth E Wolf, Co-Author
A resource text for educators, interpreters, parents and sign language instructors. $53.95
202 pages Spiral Paper
ISBN 0-398057-22-0

8041   American Sign Language Handshape Dictionary
Gallaudet University Press
800 Florida Ave NE
Washington, DC   20002-3600   773-568-1550
                                              800-621-2736
                                          Fax: 773-660-2235
                                       TTY: 888-630-9347
                                   gupress@gallaudet.edu
                                 www.gupress.gallaudet.edu

Richard A Tennant, Author
Marianne Gluszak Brown, Co-Author
Valerie Nelson-Metlay, Illustrator
T. Alan Hurwitz, President
The new DVD shows how each sign is formed from beginning to end. Users can watch a sign at various speeds to learn precisely how to master it themselves. Together, the new edition of The American Sign Language Handshape Dictionary and its accompanying DVD presents students, sign language teachers, and deaf and hearing people alike with the perfect combination for enhancing communication skills in both ASL and English. $45.00
408 pages Hardcover
ISBN 1-563680-43-2

8042   American Sign Language Phrase Book
TJ Publishers
2544 Tarpley Rd
Suite 108
Carrollton, TX   75006-2288   972-416-0800
                                              800-999-1168
                                          Fax: 972-416-0944
                               customerservice@tjpublishers.com
                                      www.tjpublishers.com
Lou Fant, Author
Terrence O'Rourke, Principal
Tanner Beach, Director
The author provides interesting, realistic and meaningful situations. Sign language is learned through novel remarks cleverly organized around everyday topics. $18.95
362 pages Softcover
ISBN 0-809235-00-5

8043   American Sign Language: A Look at Its History, Structure & Community
TJ Publishers
2544 Tarpley Rd
Suite 108
Carrollton, TX   75006-2288   972-416-0800
                                              800-999-1168
                                          Fax: 972-416-0944
                               customerservice@tjpublishers.com
                                      www.tjpublishers.com
Charlotte Baker-Shenk, Author
Carol Padden, Co-Author
Terrence O'Rourke, Principal
Tanner Beach, Director
Answers basic questions about American Sign Language. What is it? What is its history? Who uses it? What is the Deaf community? Why is ASL important? What are the building blocks of ASL?

What is the relationship between ASL and body language? What are examples of ASL -grammar? $4.95
22 pages Softcover
ISBN 0-93266 -01-9

8044   At Home Among Strangers
Gallaudet University Press
800 Florida Ave NE
Washington, DC   20002-3600   773-568-1550
                                              800-621-2736
                                          Fax: 773-660-2235
                                       TTY: 888-630-9347
                                   gupress@gallaudet.edu
                                 www.gupress.gallaudet.edu

Jerome D Schein, Author
T. Alan Hurwitz, President
Paul Kelly, Vice President Adm And Finance
At Home Among Strangers presents an engrossing portrait of the Deaf community as a complex, nationwide social network that offers unique kinship to deaf people across the country. $36.95
264 pages Paperback
ISBN 1-563681-41-2

8045   BPPV: What You Need to Know
Vestibular Disorders Association
5018 NE 15th Ave
Portland, OR   97211-5331   503-229-7705
                                              800-837-8428
                                          Fax: 503-229-8064
                                       veda@vestibular.org
                                         www.vestibular.org

P J Haybach, Author
Lisa Haven, Executive Director
Jerry Underwood, Managing Director
Vincente Honrubia, Director
The aim of this book is to present basic information about benign paroxysmal positional vertigo (BPPV) including what it is, causes, how it is diagnosed, various treatments currently in use, and strategies for coping with the symptoms associated with BPPV. $29.95
207 pages Hardcover
ISBN 0-963261-14-2

8046   Ben's Story: A Deaf Child's Right to Sign
Gallaudet University Bookstore
800 Florida Avenue NorthEast
Washington, DC   20002-3600   202-651-5530
                                          Fax: 202-651-5489
                                   gupress@gallaudet.edu
                                 http://www.gallaudet.edu
Stephanie Cawthon, Ph.D., Book Review Editor
Peter V. Paul, Ph.D., Editor, Literary Issues
Ye Wang, Ph.D., Senior Associate Editor
Feifei Ye, Ph.D., Associate Editor for Research Methodology
This is a mother's story of how she responded to the diagnosis of her son's deafness and how she struggled to have her son educated using sign language.
267 pages Softcover
ISBN 0-930323-47-5

8047   Book of Name Signs: Naming in American Sign Language
DawnSign Press
6130 Nancy Ridge Dr
San Diego, CA   92121-3223   858-625-0600
                                              800-549-5350
                                          Fax: 858-625-2336
                                       info@dawnsign.com
                                         www.dawnsign.com
Joe Dannis, President
Sam Supalla, Author
To explain how a name sign is chosen in the Deaf community, professor and researcher Sam Supalla wrote this valuable resource book. Revealing fascinating insights about the origins of ASL name signs, Supalla shows how they serve the same function as given names used in the hearing community. He also details how the history of the name sign system dates back to the early years of

deaf education in America. Included for reference is a list of more than 500 name signs available for selection. *$12.95*
120 pages Paperback 1992
ISBN 0-915035-30-4

8048   Chelsea: The Story of a Signal Dog
Gallaudet University Bookstore
800 Florida Ave NE
Washington, DC   20002-3600   202-651-5855
                                                               866-204-0504
                                                     Fax: 773-660-2235
                                                   TTY: 202-651-5855
                                             gupress@gallaudet.edu
                                          www.clerccenter.gallaudet.edu
Paul Ogden, Author
T. Alan Hurwitz, President
Paul Kelly, Vice President Adm. And Finance
This is a story of a young deaf couple and their Belgian sheepdog, who acts as their ears. It explains how these dogs are trained and paired with their new owners.
169 pages

8049   Children of a Lesser God
Gallaudet University Bookstore
800 Florida Ave NE
Washington, DC   20002-3600   202-651-5855
                                                               866-204-0504
                                                     Fax: 773-660-2235
                                                   TTY: 202-651-5855
                                             gupress@gallaudet.edu
                                          www.clerccenter.gallaudet.edu
Mark Medoff, Author
T. Alan Hurwitz, President
Paul Kelly, Vice President Adm. And Finance
The movie that won the hearts of thousands. This is a story of a deaf woman who refuses to succumb to the hearing people's image of what a deaf person should be.
91 pages Softcover
ISBN 0-822202-03-4

8050   Choices in Deafness: A Parent's Guide to Communication Options
Woodbine House
6510 Bells Mill Rd
Bethesda, MD   20817-1636   301-897-3570
                                                               800-843-7323
                                                     Fax: 301-897-5838
                                             info@woodbinehouse.com
                                               www.woodbinehouse.com
Irv Shapell, Owner
Sue Schwartz, PhD., Editor
A useful aid in choosing the appropriate communication option for a child with a hearing loss. Experts present the following communication options: Auditory-Verbal Approach, Bilingual-Bicultural Approach, Cued Speech, Oral Approach, and Total Communication. This new edition explains medical causes of hearing loss, the diagnostic process, audiological assessment, and cochlear implants. Children and parents also offer their personal experiences. *$24.95*
400 pages Paperback
ISBN 1-890627-73-7

8051   Cochlear Implants for Kids
Alexander Graham Bell Association
3417 Volta Pl NW
Washington, DC   20007-2737   202-337-5220
                                                     Fax: 202-337-8314
                                                    info@agbell.org
                                          www.listeningandspokenlanguage.org
Warren Estabrooks MEd, Editor
Alexander T. Graham, Executive Director
Susan Boswell, Director of Communications and Marketing
Judy Harrison, Director of Programs

Designed to educate readers about cochlear implants, including surgery, the importance of rehabilitation and the significance of parents' and professionals' roles. *$12.49*
404 pages Paperback
ISBN 0-882002-08-2

8052   Cognition, Education and Deafness: Directions for Research and Instruction
Gallaudet University Press
800 Florida Ave NE
Washington, DC   20002-3600   773-568-1550
                                                               800-621-2736
                                                     Fax: 773-660-2235
                                                   TTY: 888-630-9347
                                             gupress@gallaudet.edu
David S Martin, Editor
T. Alan Hurwitz, President
Paul Kelly, Vice President Adm. And Finance
This groundbreaking book integrates the work of 54 contributors to the 1984 symposium on cognition, education, and deafness. It focuses on cognition and deaf students' growth and development, problem-solving strategies, thinking processes, language development, reading methodology, measurement of potential, and intervention programs. *$50.00*
248 pages Paperback
ISBN I-563681-49-8

8053   College and University Programs for Deaf and Hard of Hearing Students
Gallaudet & NTID
800 Florida Avenue NE
Gallaudet University
Washington, DC 20002   202-651-5000
                                                               800-451-8834
                                                     Fax: 202-651-5508
                                                        www.lulu.com
S. Benaissa, & L. Dunning, Co-Authors
J. DeCaro, M. Karchmer, Co-Authors
J Hochgesang , Co-Author
T. Alan Hurwitz, President
Compiled by Gallaudet University and the National Technical Institute for the Deaf, this publication is a guide to accessibility for deaf and hard of hearing students in American colleges and universities. Available through LuLu Publishing. *$11.50*
240 pages Paperback
ISBN 9-998242-81-9

8054   Come Sign with Us
Gallaudet University Press
800 Florida Ave NE
Washington, DC   20002-3600   773-568-1550
                                                               800-621-2736
                                                     Fax: 773-660-2235
                                                   TTY: 888-630-9347
                                             gupress@gallaudet.edu
                                            www.gupress.gallaudet.edu
Jan C Hafer, Author
Robert M Wilson, Co-Author
T. Alan Hurwitz, President
Paul Kelly, Vice President Adm. And Finance
This fun guide for parents and educators on teaching hearing children how to sign has been thoroughly revised with completely new activities that provide contexts for practice. *$39.95*
160 pages Paperback
ISBN 1-563680-51-3

8055   Comprehensive Reference Manual for Signers and Interpreters
Charles C. Thomas
2600 S First St
Springfield, IL   62704-4730   217-789-8980
                                                               800-258-8980
                                                     Fax: 217-789-9130
                                             books@ccthomas.com
                                                 www.ccthomas.com
Michael P. Thomas, President
Cheryl M. Hoffman, Author

A classic in sign language literature since its introduction over two decades ago, this updated and expanded sixth edition of Comprehensive Reference Manual for Signers and Interpreters contains almost seven thousand entries, including vocabulary and idioms, with cross-references and sign descriptions. It is intended primarily for interpreters, but it can also be used effectively by signers who have at least a working knowledge of sign language. *$59.95*
404 pages Spiral Paper 1909
ISBN 0-398078-58-4

8056 **Comprehensive Signed English Dictionary**
Gallaudet University Press
800 Florida Ave NE
Washington, DC 20002-3600   773-568-1550
                                  800-621-2736
                            Fax: 773-660-2235
                            TTY: 888-630-9347
                            gupress@gallaudet.edu
                            www.gupress.gallaudet.edu
Harry Bornstein, Editor
Karen L. Saulnier, Editor
Lillian B. Hamilton, Editor
T. Paul Hurwitz, President
The Comprehensive Signed English Dictionary is the premier volume of the Signed English series. This complete dictionary more than 3,100 signs, including signs reflecting lively, contemporary vocabulary. *$45.00*
464 pages Casebound
ISBN 0-913580-81-3

8057 **Conversational Sign Language II: An Intermediate Advanced Manual**
Gallaudet University Press
800 Florida Ave NE
Washington, DC 20002-3600   773-568-1550
                                  800-621-2736
                            Fax: 773-660-2235
                            TTY: 888-630-9347
                            gupress@gallaudet.edu
                            www.gupress.gallaudet.edu
William J Madsen, Author
T. Alan Hurwitz, President
Paul Kelly, Vice President Adm. And Finance
This book presents English words and their American Sign Language (ASL) equivalents in 63 lessons. Part one covers 750 words and their signs. Part two deals with the interpretation of 220 English idioms (which have over 300 usages in ASL). Part three presents over 300 ASL idioms and colloquialisms prevalent in informal conversations. *$17.95*
236 pages Paperback
ISBN 0-913580-00-7

8058 **Deaf Empowerment: Emergence, Struggle and Rhetoric**
Gallaudet University Press
800 Florida Ave NE
Washington, DC 20002-3600   773-568-1550
                                  800-621-2736
                            Fax: 773-660-2235
                            TTY: 888-630-9347
                            gupress@gallaudet.edu
                            www.gupress.gallaudet.edu
Katherine A Jankowski, Author
T. Alan Hurwitz, President
Paul Kelly, Vice President Adm. And Finance
Employing the methodology successfully used to explore other social movements in America, this meticulous study examines the rhetorical foundation that motivated Deaf people to work for social change during the past two centuries. *$49.95*
192 pages Hardcover
ISBN 1-563680-61-0

8059 **Deaf History Unveiled: Interpretations from the New Scholarship**
Gallaudet University Press
800 Florida Ave NE
Washington, DC 20002-3600   773-568-1550
                                  800-621-2736
                            Fax: 773-660-2235
                            TTY: 888-630-9347
                            gupress@gallaudet.edu
                            www.gallaudet.edu
John Vickrey Van Cleve, Editor
T. Alan Hurwitz, President
Paul Kelly, Vice President Adm. And Finance
Deaf History Unveiled features 16 essays, including work by Harlan Lane, Renate Fischer, Margret Winzer, William McCagg, and other noted historians in this field. Readers will discover the new themes driving Deaf history, including a telling comparison of the similar experiences of Deaf people and African Americans, both minorities with identifying characteristics that cannot be hidden to thwart bias. *$ 36.95*
316 pages Paperback
ISBN 1-563680-87-4

8060 **Deaf Like Me**
Gallaudet University Press
800 Florida Ave NE
Washington, DC 20002-3600   773-568-1550
                                  800-621-2736
                            Fax: 773-660-2235
                            TTY: 888-630-9347
                            gupress@gallaudet.edu
                            www.gupress.gallaudet.edu
Thomas S Spradley, Author
James P Spradley, Co-Author
T. Alan Hurwitz, President
Paul Kelly, Vice President Adm. And Finance
Deaf Like Me is the moving account of parents coming to terms with their baby girl's profound deafness. The love, hope, and anxieties of all hearing parents of deaf children are expressed here with power and simplicity. *$16.95*
292 pages Paperback
ISBN 0-930323-11-4

8061 **Deaf Parents and Their Hearing Children**
Through the Looking Glass
3075 Adeline Street
Suite 120
Berkeley, CA 94703   510-848-1112
                           800-644-2666
                     Fax: 510-848-4445
                     tlg@lookingglass.org
                     www.lookingglass.org
Maureen Block, J.D., President
Thomas Spalding, Treasurer
Alice Nemon, Secretary
Mega Kirshbaum, Author
The focus of this review article is on families with Deaf parents and hearing children. We provide a brief description of the Deaf community, their language, and culture; describe communication patterns and parenting issues in Deaf-parented families, examine the role of the hearing child in a Deaf family and how that experience affects their functioning in the hearing world; and discuss important considerations and resources for families, educators, and health care and service providers. *$2.00*
8 pages

8062   Deaf in America: Voices from a Culture
TJ Publishers
2544 Tarpley Rd
Suite 108
Carrollton, TX   75006-2288   972-416-0800
                                               800-999-1168
                                          Fax: 972-416-0944
                           customerservice@tjpublishers.com
                                      www.tjpublishers.com

Carol Padden, Author
Tom Humphries, Co-Author
Terrence O'Rourke, Principal
Tanner Beach, Director
Now available in paperback, this book opens deaf culture to outsiders, inviting readers to imagine and understand a world of silence. This book shares the joy and satisfaction many people have
with their lives and shows that deafness may not be the handicap
most hearing people think. *$15.95*
134 pages Softcover
ISBN 0-674194-24-1

8063   EASE Program: Emergency Access Self Evaluation
Telecommunications for the Deaf (TDI)
8630 Fenton St
Suite 604
Silver Spring, MD   20910-3822   301-589-3786
                                          Fax: 301-589-3797
                                         info@tdi-online.org
                                              tdi-online.org

Claude L Stout, Executive Director
Gloria Carter, Executive Secretary
James House, Public Relations Director
Robert McConnell, Advertising Manager
A complete training, testing, maintenance and self evaluation
program that helps emergency service providers prepare for
emergency calls from TTY users and to comply with the American with Disabilities Act. *$35.00*
48 pages

8064   Encyclopedia of Deafness and Hearing Disorders
Powell's Books
1005 W Burnside St
Portland, OR   97209-3114   503-228-4651
                                               800-873-7323
                                          help@powells.com
                                            www.powells.com

Carol Turkington, Author
Michael Powell, Owner
Presents the most current information on deafness and hearing
disorders in an authoritative A-to-Z compendium. *$7.50*
294 pages Hardcover
ISBN 0-816056-15-3

8065   Expressive and Receptive Fingerspelling for Hearing Adults
Gallaudet University Bookstore
800 Florida Ave NE
Washington, DC   20002-3600   202-651-5855
                                               866-204-0504
                                          Fax: 773-660-2235
                                          TTY: 202-651-5855
                                      gupress@gallaudet.edu
                              www.clerccenter.gallaudet.edu
LaVera M Guillory, Author
T. Alan Hurwitz, President
Paul Kelly, Vice President Adm. And Finance
Here is a new and meaningful way for adults to increase their
comfort with fingerspelling. The system is based on the princi-
ples of phonetics rather than letters of the English alphabet.
42 pages Softcover
ISBN 0-875110-55-X

8066   Eye-Centered: A Study of Spirituality of Deaf People
National Catholic Office for the Deaf
7202 Buchanan St
Hyattsville, MD   20784-2236   301-577-1684
                                          Fax: 301-577-1684
                                              info@ncod.org
                                               www.ncod.org
Bill Key, Author
Arvilla Rank, Executive Director
Deacon Patrick Graybill, Vice President
Gregory Schott, Member at Large
The findings of the five-year De Sales Project conducted by The
National Catholic Office for the Deaf. *$16.70*
167 pages

8067   For Hearing People Only
Harris Communications
15155 Technology Dr
Eden Prairie, MN   55344-2273   952-388-2152
                                               800-825-6758
                                          Fax: 952-906-1099
                                          TTY: 800-825-9187
                                       info@harriscomm.com
                                         www.harriscomm.com
Robert Harris, Owner
Linda Levitan, Co-Author
Matthew S. Moore, Co-Author
Harlan Lane, Foreword
For Hearing People Only answers some of the most common
questions hearing people ask about Deaf culture and how Deaf
people communicate and live. *$35.95*
724 pages Paperback
ISBN 0-963401-63-7

8068   From Gesture to Language in Hearing and Deaf Children
Gallaudet University Press
800 Florida Ave NE
Washington, DC   20002-3600   773-568-1550
                                               800-621-2736
                                          Fax: 773-660-2235
                                          TTY: 888-630-9347
                                      gupress@gallaudet.edu
                                   www.gupress.gallaudet.edu
Virginia Volterra, Editor
Carol J. Erting, Editor
In 21 essays on communicative gesturing in the first two years of
life, this vital collection demonstrates the importance of gesture
in a child's transition to a linguistic system. *$45.95*
358 pages Paperback
ISBN 1-563680-78-5

8069   From Mime to Sign Package
TJ Publishers
2544 Tarpley Rd
Suite 108
Carrollton, TX   75006-2288   972-416-0800
                                               800-999-1168
                                          Fax: 972-416-0944
                           customerservice@tjpublishers.com
                                      www.tjpublishers.com
Gilbert C Eastman, Author
Terrence O'Rourke, Principal
Tanner Beach, Director
More than 1,000 photographs illustrate how natural gestures,
mime and facial expressions used every day can become the basis
for learning sign language. *$27.95*
183 pages Softcover
ISBN 0-932666-34-5

8070   GA and SK Etiquette
Telecommunications for the Deaf
8630 Fenton Street
Suite 604
Silver Spring, MD   20910- 3822

301-589-3786
Fax: 301-589-3797
info@tdi-online.org
www.tdi-online.org

Claude L Stout, Executive Director
Keith Cagle, Co-Author
Roy Miller, President
Gloria Carter, Administrator
Promoting equal access to telecommunications and media for people who are deaf, late-deafened, hard-of-hearing or deaf-blind through consumer education and involvement; technical assistance and consulting; applications of exisiting and emerging technologies; networking and collaboration; uniformity of standards; and national policy development and advocacy. *$11.95*
54 pages Paperback
ISBN 0-961462-17-5

8071   Gallaudet Survival Guide to Signing
Gallaudet University Press
800 Florida Ave NE
Washington, DC   20002-3600

773-568-1550
800-621-2736
Fax: 773-660-2235
TTY: 888-630-9347
gupress@gallaudet.edu
www.gallaudet.edu

Jon Mitchiner, Manager
Leonard G. Lane, Author
Jan Skrobisz, Illustrator
T. Alan Hurwitz, President
Features 500 of the most frequently used signs with clear illustrations and descriptions for each one. *$9.95*
218 pages Paperback
ISBN 0-930323-67-X

8072   Goldilocks and the Three Bears: Told in Signed English
Gallaudet University Press
800 Florida Ave NE
Washington, DC   20002-3600

773-568-1550
800-621-2736
Fax: 773-660-2235
TTY: 888-630-9347
gupress@gallaudet.edu
www.gupress.gallaudet.edu

Harry Bornstein, Author
Karen L Saulnier, Co-Author
T. Alan Hurwitz, President
Paul Kelly, Vice President Adm. And Finance
Goldilocks and the Three Bears offers children ages 3 - 8 all of the fun their parents had when they first read about the little girl with the golden curls who turned the Bears' house upside down. *$ 21.95*
48 pages Hardcover
ISBN 1-563680-57-2

8073   Hearing Impaired Children and Youth with Developmental Disabilities
Gallaudet University Bookstore
800 Florida Ave NE
Washington, DC   20002-3600

202-651-5855
866-204-0504
Fax: 773-660-2235
TTY: 202-651-5855
gupress@gallaudet.edu
www.clerccenter.gallaudet.edu

Evelyn Cherow, Editor
T. Alan Hurwitz, President
Paul Kelly, Vice President Adm. And Finance
The insights of 24 experts help clarify relationships between hearing impairment and developmental difficulties and propose interdisciplinary cooperation as an approach to the problems created. *$29.95*
394 pages Hardcover
ISBN 0-913580-97-X

8074   Hollywood Speaks: Deafness and the Film Entertainment Industry
University of Illinois Press
1325 S Oak St
MC-566
Champaign, IL   61820-6903

217-333-0950
Fax: 217-244-8082
uipress@uillinois.edu
www.press.uillinois.edu

Willis G. Regier, Director
John S. Schuchman, Author
Kathy O'Neill, Assistant To The Director
Laurie Matheson, Editor-in-Chief
How deafness has been treated in movies and how it provides yet another window onto social history in addition to a fresh angle from which to view Hollywood. *$27.00*
200 pages Paperback 1999
ISBN 0-252068-50-8

8075   I Have a Sister, My Sister is Deaf
HarperCollins Publishers
10 E 53rd St
New York, NY   10022-5244

212-207-7901
800-242-7737
Fax: 212-702-2586
spsales@harpercollins.com
www.harpercollins.com

Jeanne Whitehouse Peterson, Author
Deborah Kogan Ray, Illustrator
Ann Ledden, Vice President
Lorna Metzler, Manager
An emphatic, affirmative look at the relationship between siblings, as a young deaf child is affectionately described by her older sister. This Coretta Scott King Honor Award winner helps young children develop an understanding that deaf children share the same interests as hearing children. *$6.99*
32 pages Paperback 1984
ISBN 0-064430-59-6

8076   Independence Without Sight or Sound
AFB Press
2 Penn Plaza
Suite 1102
New York, NY   10121-2006

212-502-7600
800-232-5463
Fax: 888-545-8331
afbweb@afb.net
www.afb.org

Richard Obnen, Chairman Of The Board
Carl Augusto, President and CEO
Rick Bozeman, Chief Financial Officer
Kelly Bleach, Chief Administrative Officer
This practical guidebook covers the essential aspects of communicating and working with deaf-blind persons. Full of valuable information on subjects such as how to talk with deaf-blind people, adapt orientation and mobility techniques for deaf-blind travelers, and interact with deaf-blind individuals socially, this useful manual also contains a substantial resource section detailing sources of information and adapted equipment. *$39.95*
193 pages Paperback
ISBN 0-891282-46-4

8077 **Innovative Practices for Teaching Sign Language Interpreters**
Gallaudet University Press
800 Florida Ave NE
Washington, DC 20002-3600

773-568-1550
800-621-2736
Fax: 773-660-2235
TTY: 888-630-9347
gupress@gallaudet.edu
www.gupress.gallaudet.edu

Cynthia B Roy, Editor
Researchers now understand interpreting as an active process between two languages and cultures, with social interaction, sociolinguistics, and discourse analysis as more appropriate theoretical frameworks. Roy's penetrating new book acts upon these new insights by presenting six dynamic teaching practices to help interpreters achieve the highest level of skill. *$45.95*
200 pages Hardcover
ISBN 1-563680-88-2

8078 **Intermediate Conversational Sign Language**
Gallaudet University Press
800 Florida Ave NE
Washington, DC 20002-3600

773-568-1550
800-621-2736
Fax: 773-660-2235
TTY: 888-630-9347
gupress@gallaudet.edu
www.gupress.gallaudet.edu

Willard J Madsen, Author
This fully illustrated text offers a unique approach to using American Sign Language (ASL) and English in a bilingual setting. Each of the 25 lessons involve sign language conversation using colloquialisms that are prevalent in informal conversations. *$31.50*
400 pages Softcover
ISBN 0-913580-79-1

8079 **Interpretation: A Sociolinguistic Model**
Sign Media
4020 Blackburn Ln
Burtonsville, MD 20866-1167

301-421-0268
800-475-4756
Fax: 301-421-0270
info@signmedia.com
www.signmedia.com

Verden Ness, President
Dennis Cokely, Author
This text presents a sociolinguistically sensitive model of the interpretation process. The model applies to interpretation in any two languages although this one focuses on ASL and English. *$22.95*
199 pages
ISBN 0-932130-10-0

8080 **Interpreting: An Introduction**
Registry of Interpreters for the Deaf
333 Commerce St
Alexandria, VA 22314-2801

703-838-0030
Fax: 703-838-0454
TTY:703-838-0459
ridinfo@rid.org
www.rid.org

Nancy J Frishberg, Author
Shane Feldman, Executive Director
Don Roose, Director
Emil Ladner, Director
This text is written by a practicing interpreter and includes information on history, terminology, research, competence, setting and a comprehensive bibliography. *$24.95*
249 pages Softcover
ISBN 0-916883-07-8

8081 **Joy of Signing**
Gospel Publishing House
1445 N Boonville Ave
Springfield, MO 65802-1894

417-862-8000
800-641-4310
Fax: 417-862-5881
CustSrvOrders@ag.org
www.gospelpublishing.com

Lottie L Riekehof, Author
This manual on signing includes illustrations, information on sign origins, practice sentences, and step-by-step descriptions of hand positions and movements. *$23.99*
352 pages Hardcover
ISBN 0-882435-20-5

8082 **Joy of Signing Puzzle Book**
Harris Communications
15155 Technology Dr
Eden Prairie, MN 55344-2273

952-388-2152
800-825-6758
Fax: 952-906-1099
TTY: 800-825-9187
info@harriscomm.com
www.harriscomm.com

Robert Harris, Owner
Lottie L Riekehof, Co-Author
Whether you are learning sign language to communicate with a family member, co-worker, student or friend, this puzzle book makes the learning fun and interesting. *$4.50*
57 pages Softcover
ISBN 0-882436-76-7

8083 **Kid-Friendly Parenting with Deaf and Hard of Hearing Children**
Gallaudet University Press
800 Florida Ave NE
Washington, DC 20002-3600

773-568-1550
800-621-2736
Fax: 773-660-2235
TTY: 888-630-9347
gupress@gallaudet.edu
www.gupress.gallaudet.edu

Daria Medwid, Author
Denise Chapman Weston, Co-Author
At each chapter's beginning, experts (some deaf, some hearing), including I. King Jordan, Jack Gannon, Merv Garretson, and others, offer their insights on the subject discussed. Designed for parents with various styles, Kid-Friendly Parenting is a complete, step-by-step guide and reference to raising a deaf or hard of hearing child. *$35.95*
320 pages Paperback
ISBN 1-563680-31-9

8084 **Laurent Clerc: The Story of His Early Years**
Gallaudet University Press
800 Florida Ave NE
Washington, DC 20002-3600

773-568-1550
800-621-2736
Fax: 773-660-2235
TTY: 888-630-9347
gupress@gallaudet.edu
www.gupress.gallaudet.edu

Cathryn Carroll, Author
T. Alan Hurwitz, President
Paul Kelly, Vice President Adm. And Finance
In his own voice, Clerc vividly relates the experiences that led to his later progressive teaching methods. Especially influential was his long stay at the Royal National Institute for the Deaf in Paris, where he encountered sharply distinct personalities - the saintly, inspiring deaf teacher Massieu, the vicious Dr. Itard and his heartless experiments on deaf boys, and the Father of the Deaf, Abbe Sicard, who could hardly sign. *$13.95*
208 pages Paperback
ISBN 0-930323-23-8

8085   Linguistics of American Sign Language: An Introduction
Gallaudet University Press
800 Florida Ave NE
Washington, DC   20002-3600   773-568-1550
                                           800-621-2736
                                      Fax: 773-660-2235
                                      TTY: 888-630-9347
                                      gupress@gallaudet.edu
                                      www.gupress.gallaudet.edu

Clayton Valli, Author
Ceil Lucas, Co-Author
Kristin J Mulrooney, Co-Author
Miako Villanueva, President
Completely reorganized to reflect the growing intricacy of the
study of ASL linguistics, the 5th edition presents 26 units in
seven parts. Part One: Introduction presents a revision of Defin-
ing Language and an entirely new unit, Defining Linguistics. Part
Two: Phonology has been completely updated with new terminol-
ogy and examples. *$75.00*
560 pages Hardcover
ISBN 1-563682-83-4

8086   Literacy & Your Deaf Child: What Every Parent Should
Know
Gallaudet University Press
800 Florida Ave NE
Washington, DC   20002-3600   773-568-1550
                                           800-621-2736
                                      Fax: 773-660-2235
                                      TTY: 888-630-9347
                                      gupress@gallaudet.edu
                                      www.gupress.gallaudet.edu

David A Stewart, Author
Bryan R Clarke, Co-Author
T. Alan Hurwitz, President
Paul Kelly, Vice President Adm. And Finance
Literacy and Your Deaf Child begins by introducing some com-
mon concepts, among them the importance of parental involve-
ment in a deaf child's education. It outlines how children acquire
language and describes the auditory and visual links to literacy.
$24.95
240 pages Paperback
ISBN 1-563681-36-6

8087   Mask of Benevolence: Disabling the Deaf Community, The
DawnSign Press
6130 Nancy Ridge Dr
San Diego, CA   92121-3223   858-625-0600
                                           800-549-5350
                                      Fax: 858-625-2336
                                      info@dawnsign.com
                                      www.dawnsign.com
Joe Dannis, President
Harlan Lane, Author
Dr. Harlan Lane does not view deafness as a handicap but rather a
different state from hearing. Deaf people are a societal minority
and should be treasured, not eradicated. *$12.95*
360 pages Paperback 1992
ISBN 1-581210-09-5

8088   Mother Father Deaf: Living Between Sound and Silence
Harvard University Press
79 Garden St
Cambridge, MA   02138-1423   617-495-2600
                                           800-405-1619
                                      Fax: 617- 49- 589
                                      contact_hup@harvard.edu
                                      www.hup.harvard.edu
William Sisler, President
Paul Preston, Author
The book explores the intimate intersection of families like his
own - families which embody the conflicts and resolutions of two
often opposing world views, the Deaf and the Hearing. Although
I have normal hearing, both of my parents are profoundly deaf.
$19.50
278 pages Paperback
ISBN 0-674587-48-0

8089   My First Book of Sign
Gallaudet University Press
800 Florida Ave NE
Washington, DC   20002-3600   773-568-1550
                                           800-621-2736
                                      Fax: 773-660-2235
                                      TTY: 888-630-9347
                                      gupress@gallaudet.edu
                                      www.gupress.gallaudet.edu

Pamela J Baker, Author
Patricia Bellan Gillen, Illustrator
T. Alan Hurwitz, President
Paul Kelly, Vice President Adm. And Finance
Full-color book gives alphabetically grouped signs for 150 words
most frequently used by young children. *$22.95*
80 pages Hardcover
ISBN 0-930323-20-3

8090   My Signing Book of Numbers
Gallaudet University Press
800 Florida Ave NE
Washington, DC   20002-3600   773-568-1550
                                           800-621-2736
                                      Fax: 773-660-2235
                                      TTY: 888-630-9347
                                      gupress@gallaudet.edu
                                      www.gupress.gallaudet.edu

Patricia Bellan Gillen, Author
This full-color book helps children learn their numbers in sign
language. Each two-page spread of this delightfully illustrated
book has the appropriate number of things or creatures for the
numbers 0 through 20. *$22.95*
56 pages Hardcover
ISBN 0-930323-37-8

8091   Nursery Rhymes from Mother Goose
Gallaudet University Press
800 Florida Ave NE
Washington, DC   20002-3600   773-568-1550
                                           800-621-2736
                                      Fax: 773-660-2235
                                      TTY: 888-630-9347
                                      gupress@gallaudet.edu
                                      www.gupress.gallaudet.edu

Harry Bornstein, Author
Karen L Saulnier, Co-Author
Patricia Peters, Illustrator
Linda Tom, Illustrator
Young readers, both hearing and deaf, will learn the special
charm of rhyme while also discovering new vocabulary and new
ways to experience English through signing. As they learn and
memorize their favorite verses, children will also strengthen their
language skills in a fun, entertaining way. *$21.95*
64 pages Hardcover
ISBN 0-930323-99-8

8092   Outsiders in a Hearing World: A Sociology of Deafness
Sage Publications
2455 Teller Rd
Thousand Oaks, CA   91320-2218   805-499-9774
                                           800-818-7243
                                      Fax: 805-499-0871
                                      www.sagepub.com
Paul C Higgins, Author
An introduction to the social world of deaf people. The author
gives a sociologists view of what it's like to be deaf. *$72.95*
208 pages Hardcover 1980
ISBN 0-803914-22-3

8093 **Perigee Visual Dictionary of Signing**
Harris Communications
15155 Technology Dr
Eden Prairie, MN 55344-2273   952-388-2152
                                     800-825-6758
                                Fax: 952-906-1099
                               TTY: 800-825-9187
                               info@harriscomm.com
                               www.harriscomm.com

Robert Harris, Owner
Mickey Flodin, Co-Author
Rod R Butterworth, Co-Author
An A-to-Z guide to American Sign Language vocabulary. *$15.26*
450 pages Softcover
ISBN 0-399519-52-1

8094 **Phone of Our Own: The Deaf Insurrection Against Ma Bell**
Gallaudet University Press
800 Florida Ave NE
Washington, DC 20002-3600   773-568-1550
                                   800-621-2736
                              Fax: 773-660-2235
                             TTY: 888-630-9347
                             gupress@gallaudet.edu
                             www.gupress.gallaudet.edu

Harry G Lang, Author
T. Alan Hurwitz, President
Paul Kelly, Vice President Adm. And Finance
A recount of the history of the teletypewriter, from the three deaf engineers who developed the acoustic coupler that made mass communication on TTY's feasible, through the deaf community's twenty-year struggle against the government and AT&T to have TTY's produced and distributed. *$36.50*
256 pages Hardcover
ISBN 1-563680-90-4

8095 **Place of Their Own: Creating the Deaf Community in America**
Gallaudet University Press
800 Florida Ave NE
Washington, DC 20002-3600   773-568-1550
                                   800-621-2736
                              Fax: 773-660-2235
                             TTY: 888-630-9347
                             gupress@gallaudet.edu
                             www.gallaudet.edu

John V Van Cleve, Author
Barry A Crouch, Co-Author
T. Alan Hurwitz, President
Paul Kelly, Vice President Adm. And Finance
Traces development of American deaf society to show how deaf people developed a common language and sense of community. Views deafness as the distinguishing characteristic of a distinct culture. *$22.95*
224 pages Paperback
ISBN 0-930323-49-1

8096 **PreReading Strategies**
Gallaudet University Bookstore
800 Florida Ave NE
Washington, DC 20002-3600   202-651-5855
                                   866-204-0504
                              Fax: 773-660-2235
                             TTY: 202-651-5855
                             gupress@gallaudet.edu
                             www.clerccenter.gallaudet.edu

David R Schleper, Author
T. Alan Hurwitz, President
Paul Kelly, Vice President Adm. And Finance
Here is a wealth of good advice for preparing students to understand what they read, building comprehension and enjoyment. *$14.95*
65 pages

8097 **Quad City Deaf & Hard of Hearing Youth Group: Tomorrow's Leaders for our Community**
Independent Living Research Utilization ILRU
2323 S Shepherd Dr
Houston, TX 77019-7019   713-520-9058
                           Fax: 713-520-5785
                           ilru@ilru.org

Lex Frieden, Director
Rose Sheperd, Manager
IICIL staff see this program as a way to develop young leaders for the movement. Emphasis is given to providing oppportunities for members of the youth group to develop skills in planning and organizing activities.

8098 **Religious Signing: A Comprehensive Guide for All Faiths**
TJ Publishers
P.O. Box 702701
Dallas, TX 75370   972-416-0800
                          800-999-1168
                     Fax: 972-416-0944
                    TTY: 301-585-4440
                    TJPubinc@aol.com
                    www.tjpublishers.com

Elaine Costello, Author
Terrence O'Rourke, Principal
Tanner Beach, Director
Contains over 500 religious signs for all denominations and their meanings illustrated by clear upper torso illustrations that show movements of hand, body and face. Includes a section on signing favorite verses, prayers and blessings. *$18.95*
219 pages Softcover
ISBN 0-553342-44-4

8099 **Seeing Voices**
Vintage and Anchor Books
1745 Broadway
3rd Floor
New York, NY 10019   212-782-9000
                       Fax: 212-572-6066
                       vintageanchor@randomhouse.com
                       www.randomhouse.com

Oliver Sacks, Author
Madeline McIntosh, President/Sales/Operations
Markus Dohle, Chairman/CEO
Andrew Weber, SVP Operations And Technology
Well known for his exploration of how people respond to neurological impairments, Dr Sacks explores the world of the deaf and discovers how deaf people respond to their loss of hearing and how they develop language. A highly readable introduction to deaf people, deaf culture and American Sign Language. *$13.95*
240 pages Softcover 2000
ISBN 0-375704-07-8

8100 **Sign Language Interpreting and Interpreter Education**
Oxford University Press
2001 Evans Rd
Cary, NC 27513-2009   919-677-0977
                             800-445-9714
                        Fax: 919-677-1303
                        custserv.us@oup.com
                        www.oup.com

Marc Marschark, Editor
Rico Peterson, Editor
Elizabeth A Winston, Editor
Patricia Sapere, Contributing Editor
Provides a coherent picture of the field as a whole, including evaluation of the extent to which current practices are supported by validating research. The first comprehensive source, suitable as both a reference book and a textbook for interpreter training programs and a variety of courses on bilingual education, psycholinguistics and translation, and cross-linguistic studies. *$65.00*
328 pages Hardcover
ISBN 0-195176-94-4

8101   Signed English Starter, The
Gallaudet University Press
800 Florida Ave NE
Washington, DC   20002-3600   773-568-1550
                                                        800-621-2736
                                          Fax: 773-660-2235
                                          TTY: 888-630-9347
                                          gupress@gallaudet.edu
                                          www.gupress.gallaudet.edu

Harry Bornstein, Author
Karen L Saulnier, Co-Author
T. Alan Hurwitz, President
Paul Kelly, Vice President Adm. And Finance
A first course in Signed English for adults and children, the book
is fully illustrated (several figures per page), and it is organized in
a way that leads to rewarding learning quite rapidly. The authors
of this new and exciting text believe firmly that Signed English
must be made as easy as possible if it is going to be as useful (and
used) as it can and should be. The book explains the rationale for
the Signed English system and the conventions used to teach it.
$18.50
232 pages Paperback
ISBN 0-913580-82-1

**8102   Signing Family: What Every Parent Should Know About
Sign Communication, The**
Gallaudet University Press
800 Florida Ave NE
Washington, DC   20002-3600   773-568-1550
                                                        800-621-2736
                                          Fax: 773-660-2235
                                          TTY: 888-630-9347
                                          gupress@gallaudet.edu
                                          www.gupress.gallaudet.edu

David A Stewart, Author
Barbara Luetke-Stahlman, Co-Author
T. Alan Hurwitz, President
Paul Kelly, Vice President Adm. And Finance
This reader-friendly book shows parents how to create a set of
goals around the communication needs of their deaf child. De-
scribes in even-handed terms the major signing options available,
from American Sign Language to Signed English. *$29.95*
192 pages Paperback
ISBN 1-563680-69-6

8103   Signing for Reading Success
Gallaudet University Press
800 Florida Ave NE
Washington, DC   20002-3600   773-568-1550
                                                        800-621-2736
                                          Fax: 773-660-2235
                                          TTY: 888-630-9347
                                          gupress@gallaudet.edu
                                          www.gupress.gallaudet.edu

Jan C Hafer, Author
Robert M Wilson, Co-Author
T. Alan Hurwitz, President
Paul Kelly, Vice President Adm. And Finance
This booklet provides summaries of four research students on the
usefulness of signing for reading achievement. *$7.95*
24 pages Paperback
ISBN 0-930323-18-1

8104   Signing: How to Speak with Your Hands
TJ Publishers
2427 Bond Street
Suite 108
University Park, IL   60466- 2288   972-416-0800
                                                        800-999-1168
                                          Fax: 972-416-0944
                                          customerservice@tjpublishers.com
                                          www.tjpublishers.com

Elaine Costello, Author
Terrence O'Rourke, Principal
Tanner Beach, Director
Presents 1,200 basic signs with clear illustrations in logical topi-
cal groupings. Linguistic principles are described at the begin-
ning of each chapter, giving insight into the rules which govern
American Sign Language. *$19.95*
248 pages Softcover
ISBN 0-553375-39-3

8105   Signs Across America
Gallaudet University Press
800 Florida Ave NE
Washington, DC   20002-3600   773-568-1550
                                                        800-621-2736
                                          Fax: 773-660-2235
                                          TTY: 888-630-9347
                                          gupress@gallaudet.edu
                                          www.gupress.gallaudet.edu

Edgar H Shroyer, Author
Susan P Shroyer, Co-Author
T. Alan Hurwitz, President
Paul Kelly, Vice President Adm. And Finance
A look at regional variations in ASL. Signs for selected words
collected from 25 different states. More than 1,200 signs illus-
trated in the text. *$28.95*
304 pages Paperback
ISBN 0-913580-96-1

**8106   Signs for Me: Basic Sign Vocabulary for Children, Parents
& Teachers**
TJ Publishers
2427 Bond Street
Suite 108
University Park, IL   60466- 2288   972-416-0800
                                                        800-999-1168
                                          Fax: 972-416-0944
                                          www.tjpublishers.com

Ben Bahan, Author
Joe Dannis, Co-Author
Terrence O'Rourke, Principal
Tanner Beach, Director
Sign language vocabulary for preschool and elementary school
children introduces household items, animals, family members,
actions, emotions, safety concerns and other concepts. *$14.95*
112 pages Softcover
ISBN 0-915035-27-8

8107   Signs for Sexuality: A Resource Manual
Planned Parenthood of Western Washington
2001 E Madison St
Seattle, WA   98122-2959   206-328-7715
                                          Fax: 206-328-6810
                                          www.plannedparenthood.org

Marlyn Minken, Author
Laurie Rosen-Ritt, Co-Author
Cecile Richards, President
An important book for those who want to listen to and talk with
other people about feelings, loving and caring. *$40.00*
122 pages Softcover

8108   Signs of the Times
Gallaudet University Press
800 Florida Ave NE
Washington, DC   20002-3600   773-568-1550
                                                        800-621-2736
                                          Fax: 773-660-2235
                                          TTY: 888-630-9347
                                          gupress@gallaudet.edu
                                          www.gupress.gallaudet.edu

Edgar H Shroyer, Author
Susan P Shroyer, Illustrator
T. Alan Hurwitz, President
Paul Kelly, Vice President Adm. And Finance
An excellent beginner's contact signing book that fills the gap be-
tween sign language dictionaries and American Sign Language
text. Designed for use as a classroom text. *$34.95*
448 pages Softcover
ISBN 0-913580-76-7

8109 Silent Garden, The
Gallaudet University Press
800 Florida Ave NE
Washington, DC   20002-3600
773-568-1550
800-621-2736
Fax: 773-660-2235
TTY: 888-630-9347
gupress@gallaudet.edu
www.gupress.gallaudet.edu

Paul W Ogden, Author
T. Alan Hurwitz, President
Paul Kelly, Vice President Adm. And Finance
The author explain the broad range of hearing loss types, from minor to profound. Parents also are advised about what type of school their child should attend and what kinds of professional help will be best for the entire family. The book describes all forms of communication, including choices in signing from American Sign Language to the various manual systems based upon English. Technological alternatives are presented also, including when and when not to consider cochler implants. *$34.95*
304 pages
ISBN 1-563680-58-0

8110 Sing Praise Hymnal for the Deaf
LifeWay Christian Resources
1 Lifeway Plz
MSN 146
Nashville, TN   37234-1001
615-251-2000
800-458-2772
Fax: 615-251-3899
www.lifeway.com

Thom Rainer, President/CEO
Jerry Rhyne, CFO/ VP Finance And Buisness
Tim Vineyard, VP Technology And CIO
Designed to be used by interpreters to the deaf, sign-language students, and deaf members of the congregation, this special combined hymnal edition offers 234 of the most popular hymns. *$12.95*
Hardcover 2000
ISBN 0-767314-09-3

8111 TDI National Directory & Resource Guide: Blue Book
Telecommunications for the Deaf
8630 Fenton Street
Suite 604
Silver Spring, MD   20910- 3822
301-589-3786
Fax: 301-589-3797
www.tdi-online.org

Claude L Stout, Executive Director
Promoting Equal Access to Telecommunications and Media for People who are Deaf, Late-Deafened, Hard-of-Hearing or Deaf-Blind. *$ 20.00*
600 pages Annual

8112 Theoretical Issues in Sign Language Research
University of Chicago Press
1427 E 60th St
Chicago, IL   60637-2902
773-702-7700
Fax: 773-702-9756
sales@press.uchicago.edu
www.press.uchicago.edu

Donald A Collins, President
Susan D Fischer, Author
Patricia Siple, Co-Author
These volumes are an outgrowth of a conference held at the University of Rochester in 1986, dealing with the four traditional core areas of phonology, morphology, syntax and semantics. *$29.95*
348 pages Paperback 1990
ISBN 0-226251-52-7

8113 We CAN Hear and Speak
Alexander Graham Bell Association
3417 Volta Pl. NW
Washington, DC   20007
202-337-5220
Fax: 202-337-8314
info@agbell.org
www.agbell.org

Carol Flexer PhD, Author
Catherine Richards MA, Co-Author
Emilio Alonso Mendoza, Chief Executive Officer
Written by parents for families of children who are deaf or hard of hearing, this work describes auditory-verbal terminology and approaches and contains personal narratives written by parents and their children who are deaf or hard of hearing. *$6.98*
184 pages Softcover

8114 Week the World Heard Gallaudet, The
Gallaudet University Press
800 Florida Ave NE
Washington, DC   20002-3600
202-651-5000
800-621-2736
Fax: 202-651-5508
gupress@gallaudet.edu
www.gupress.gallaudet.edu

Jack R Gannon, Author
T. Alan Hurwitz, President
Paul Kelly, Vice President Adm. And Finance
This day-to-day description of the events surrounding the Deaf President Now movement at Gallaudet University includes full color and black and white photographs and interviews with people involved in the events of that week. *$49.95*
176 pages Hardcover
ISBN 0-930323-54-8

8115 What is Auditory Processing?
Abilitations - Speech Bin
P.O.Box 922668
Norcross, GA   30010-2668
770-449-5700
800-850-8602
Fax: 770-510-7290
info@speechbin.com
www.speechbin.com

Susan Bell, Author
What is Auditory Processing? It is and information-packed 16-page booklet created to explain auditory processing and it's disorders and offers practical suggestions for coping with this problem. It describes the listening process and tells how to help children with auditory processing problems. It shows what families and teachers can do to help children who have trouble remembering and understanding what they hear and offers easy-to-use activities and practical suggestions. *$ 22.69*
16 pages Softcover

8116 You and Your Deaf Child: A Self-Help Guidefor Parents of Deaf and Hard of Hearing Children
Gallaudet University Press
800 Florida Ave NE
Washington, DC   20002-3600
773-568-1550
800-621-2736
Fax: 773-660-2235
TTY: 888-630-9347
gupress@gallaudet.edu
www.gupress.gallaudet.edu

John W Adams, Author
T. Alan Hurwitz, President
Paul Kelly, Vice President Adm. And Finance
Eleven chapters focus on such topics as feelings about hearing loss, the importance of communication in the family, and effective behavior management. Many chapters contain practice activities and questions to help parents retain skills taught in the chapter and check their grasp of the material. Four appendices provide references, general resources, and guidelines for evaluating educational programs. *$29.95*
224 pages Paperback
ISBN 1-563680-60-2

Print: Journals

8117 ADARA
1022 7th St NE
Washington, DC 20002
301-293-8969
Fax: 301-293-9698
TTY:301-293-8969
adaraorg@gmail.com
www.adara.org

John Gournaris, Ph.D, President
Kathy Schwabeland, MA, Vice President
Denise Thew Hackett, Ph.D, JADARA Editor
Charles Sterling, MBA, Office Manager
ADARA's mission is to improve service excellence for those who are deaf or hard of hearing. The ADARA Update is a quarterly newsletter published by the association, offering information on events, resources, legislation, employment opportunities and other matters related to the field. JADARA is another publication by them presenting research results, articles on deafness, social services, mental health and other areas of interest.

8118 American Journal of Audiology
American Speech-Language-Hearing Association
2200 Research Blvd
Rockville, MD 20850-3289
240-632-2081
800-638-8255
Fax: 301-296-8580
actioncenter@asha.org
www.asha.org

Gary Dunham, Editor-in-Chief
Bridget Murray Law, Managing Editor
Carol Polovoy, Assistant Managing Editor
Kellie Rowden-Racette, Print and Online Writer/Editor
Articles concern screening, assesment, and treatment techniques; prevention; professional issues; supervision; administration. Includes clinical forums, clinical reviews, letters to the editor, or research reports that emphasize clinical practice.
2 x year

8119 Hearing Professional
International Hearing Society
16880 Middlebelt Rd
Ste 4
Livonia, MI 48154-3374
734-522-7200
800-521-5247
Fax: 734-522-0200
akovach@ihsinfo.org
www.ihsinfo.org

Kathleen Mennillo, MBA, Executive Director
Kara Nacarato, Editor & Mgr Of Strgc. Alliances
Scott Beall, Treasurer Director
Alan Lowell, President
Provides authoritative technical and business information that will help hearing aid specialists serve the hearing impaired.
bi-monthly

8120 Journal of Speech, Language and Hearing Research
American Speech-Language-Hearing Association
2200 Research Blvd
Rockville, MD 20850-3289
301-296-5700
800-638-8255
Fax: 301-296-8580
actioncenter@asha.org
www.asha.org

Gary Dunham, Editor-in-Chief
Bridget Murray Law, Managing Editor
Carol Polovoy, Assistant Managing Editor
Kellie Rowden-Racette, Print and Online Writer/Editor
Pertains broadly to studies of the processess and disorders of hearing, language, and speech diagnosis and treatment of such disorders.

8121 Journal of the Academy of Rehabilitative Audiology
Academy of Rehabilitative Audiology
PO Box 2323
Albany, NY 12220-0323
952-920-0484
Fax: 952-920-6098
ara@audrehab.org
www.audrehab.org

Linda Thibodeau, President
Laura A. Wilber, Parlamentarian
Kristin V. Dilaj, Secretary
Sherri Smith, Treasurer
A peer-reviewed journal published annually. *$25.00*

8122 Literature Journal, The
Gallaudet University
800 Florida Ave NE
Washington, DC 20002-3695
202-651-5488
800-621-2736
Fax: 202-651-5508
Oluyinka.Fakunle@gallaudet.edu

Charles C Welsh-Charrier, Author
T. Alan Hurwitz, President
Paul Kelly, Vice President Adm. And Finance
This book includes extensive examples of student and teacher entries taken from actual journals of deaf high school students.
$12.95
44 pages Spiral Bound

8123 Sign Language Studies
Gallaudet University Press
800 Florida Ave NE
Washington, DC 20002-3695
202-651-5488
800-621-2736
Fax: 202-651-5508
gupress@gallaudet.edu
www.gupress.gallaudet.edu

Ceil Lucas, Editor
T. Alan Hurwitz, President
Paul Kelly, Vice President Adm. And Finance
Presents a unique forum for revolutionary papers on signed languages and other related disciplines, including linguistics, anthropology, semiotics, and deaf studies, history, and literature. *$55.00*
Quarterly

8124 Volta Review
Alexander Graham Bell Association
3417 Volta Pl. NW
Washington, DC 20007
202-337-5220
Fax: 202-337-8314
info@agbell.org
www.agbell.org

Ted A. Meyer, Chair
Catharine McNally, Chair-Elect
Susan Lenihan, Secretary
Emilio Alonso Mendoza, Chief Executive Officer
Professionally refereed journal that publishes articles and research on education, rehabilitation and communicative development of people who have hearing impairments. Also includes subscription to Volta Voices, up-to-date magazine, bimonthly. *$60.00*
Quarterly

Print: Magazines

8125   Endeavor Magazine
American Society for Deaf Children
800 Florida Avenue NorthEast
#2047
Washington, Dc 20002-3695   717-703-0073
                                        866-942-2732
                                        800-942-ASDC
                                Fax: 410-795-0965
                                asdc@deafchildren.org
                                www.deafchildren.org

Beth Benedict, President
Avonne Rutowski, VP
Timothy Frelich, Treasurer
Tami Hossler, Executive Secretary

8126   Hearing Health Magazine
Deafness Research Foundation
363 Seventh Avenue
10th Floor
New York, NY   10001-3904   212-257-6140
                                        866-454-3924
                                Fax: 212-257-6139
                                        info@drf.org
                                        www.drf.org

Andrea Boidman, Executive Director
Andrea Delbanco, Senior Editor
Yishane Lee, Editor
Julie Grant, Art Director
Serves as a source of quality information and provides the tools
and resources to help people seek treatment for and manage hearing loss. Each issue features relevant and timely information on
the latest research, articles written by leading authorities in the
field, news about the latest technology, and human interest stories
about those living with hearing loss.

8127   Hearing Loss Magazine
Hearing Loss Association of America
7910 Woodmont Ave
Ste 1200
Bethesda, MD   20814-7022   301-657-2248
                                Fax: 301-913-9413
                                info@hearingloss.org
                                www.hearingloss.org
Barbara Kelley, Editor-In-Chief/Deputy Ex. Dir.
Cindy Dyer, Graphic Design
Provides the latest information on products, services, research,
and technology in the hearing health care field. *$35.00*
40 pages BiMonthly

8128   Tinnitus Today
American Tinnitus Association
PO Box 5
Portland, OR   97207-5   503-493-2550
                                        800-634-8978
                                Fax: 503-248-0024
                                        tinnitus@ata.org
                                        www.ata.org

Nina Rogozen, Editor
Michael Malusevic, Executive Director
The magazine contains up-to-date medical and research news,
feature articles on urgent tinnitus issues, questions and answers,
self-help suggestions and letters to the editor from others with
tinnitus. *$35.00*
28 pages 3 x year

Print: Newsletters

8129   AAPD Newsletter
American Association of People with Disabilities
1629 K Street NW
Suite 950
Washington, DC   20006-1634   202-457-0046
                                        800-840-8844
                                        www.aapd.com

Mark Perriello, President/CEO
Helena Berger, COO
Robin Shaffert, Senior Director
Provides latest information on a variety of national disability pol-
icies and issues.

8130   ASHA Leader, The
American Speech-Language-Hearing Association
2200 Research Blvd
Rockville, MD   20850-3289   301-215-6710
                                        800-638-8255
                                Fax: 301-296-8580
                                        leader@asha.org
                                        www.asha.org

Gary Dunham, Editor-in-Chief
Bridget Murray Law, Managing Editor
Carol Polovoy, Assistant Managing Editor
Kellie Rowden-Racette, Print and Online Writer/Editor
Association publication containing news, notices of events and
activities and information for members on issues facing the pro-
fession of audiology and speech-language pathology. *$80.00*
35 pages 2 x month

8131   American Annals of the Deaf
Gallaudet University Press
800 Florida Ave NE
Washington, DC   20002-3600   202-651-5000
                                        800-621-2736
                                Fax: 202-651-5508
                                        paul.3@osu.edu
                                www.gupress.gallaudet.edu
Peter V. Paul, Editor, Literary Issues
T. Alan Hurwitz, President
Paul Kelly, Vice President Adm. And Finance
Quarterly publication from the Conference of Educational Ad-
ministrators Serving the Deaf. *$55.00*
Quarterly

8132   Communique
Michigan Assoc for the Deaf and Hard of Hearing
Quarterly

8133   Connect - Commmunity News
Hearing, Speech & Deafness Center (HSDC)
1625 19th Ave.
Seattle, WA   98122-2848   206-323-5770
                                        888-222-5036
                                Fax: 206-328-6871
                                        www.hsdc.org
David Delmar, Editor
Connect is the quarterly eNews of the Hearing, Speech & Deafness Center. HSDC is is a nonprofit for clients who are deaf, hard
of hearing, or who face other communication barriers such as
speech challenges.
8 pages Annual

8134   Deaf Catholic
International Catholic Deaf Association
7202 Buchanan St
Landover Hills, MD   20784-2236   301-429-0697
                                Fax: 301-429-0698
                                homeoffice@icda-us.org
                                        www.icda-us.org

Jean Cox, President
Kate Slosar, Vice President
TK Hill, Treasurer
Aline Shaw, Secretary

Newsletter reporting the news of the Archdiocese, Deaf Apostolate and each of the Catholic Deaf Organizations. *$20.00*
16 pages Quarterly

8135 International Hearing Dog, Inc.
International Hearing Dog
5901 E 89th Ave.
Henderson, CO 80640-8315
303-287-3277
Fax: 303-287-3425
info@hearingdog.org
www.hearingdog.org

Valerie Foss-Brugger, Executive Director
Samuel Cheris, Chairman
Matt Bailey, Treasurer
Aspen Matthew, Office Manager
International Hearing Dog, Inc. trains rescued shelter dogs for people who are deaf or hard-of-hearing, with and without disabilities, all at no cost to the recipient. Since 1979, 1300 dogs have been placed throughout all 50 states and Canada.
4-8 pages Quarterly

8136 League Letter
Center for Hearing and Communication
50 Broadway
6th Floor
New York, NY 10004-3810
917-305-7700
Fax: 917-305-7888
TTY:917-305-7999
info@chchearing.org
www.lhh.org

Laurie Hanin, Executive Director
Ellen Lafargue, Au.D., CCC, Director, Hearing Technology
Lois Kam Heymann, M.A., CCC, Director, Communication
Linda Kessler, M.A., CCC-SLP, Assistant Director, Communication
Quarterly

8137 NAHO News
National Association of Hearing Officials
PO Box 4999
Midlothian, VA 23112-17
701-328-3260
www.naho.org

Joy Wezelman, Editor
Janice Deshais, Editor
National Association of Hearing Officials newsletter.

8138 On the Level
Vestibular Disorders Association
5018 NE 15th Ave
Portland, OR 97211-5331
503-229-7705
800-837-8428
Fax: 503-229-8064
veda@vestibular.org
www.vestibular.org

Lisa Haven PhD, Executive Director
Jerry Underwood, Director
Vincente Honrubia, Director
Contents of each issue include information about local support groups, a calendar of conferences and training opportunities for health professionals, a list of donors, and special items indexed below. *$5.00*
12 pages Quarterly

8139 Soundings Newsletter
American Hearing Research Foundation
8 South Michigan Avenue
Suite 1205
Chicago, IL 60603- 4539
312-726-9670
Fax: 312-726-9695
ahrf@american-hearing.org
www.american-hearing.org
Sharon Parmet, Executive Director
Promote, conduct and furnish financial assistance for medical research into the cause, prevention and cure of deafness, impaired hearing and balance disorders; encourage the collaboration of clinical and laboratory research; encourage and improve teaching in the medical aspects of hearing problems; and disseminate the

most reliable scientific knowledge to physicians, hearing professionals and the public.
Quarterly

8140 Spring Dell Center Newsletter
Spring Dell Center
6040 Radio Station Rd
La Plata, MD 20646-3368
301-934-4561
Fax: 301-870-2439
www.springdellcenter.org

Donna Retzlaff, Executive Director
Jody Loper, President
Brett Hamorsky, Vice President
Jeff Hubbard, Treasurer
Quarterly

Non Print: Newsletters

8141 Canine Listener
Dogs for the Deaf
10175 Wheeler Rd
Central Point, OR 97502
541-826-9220
800-990-3647
800-990-3647
Fax: 541-826-6696
TTY:541-826-9220
info@dogsforthedeaf.org
dogsforthedeaf.org

Marvin Rhodes, Chair
Susan Bahr, Vice Chair
Kelly Gonzales, Development Director
Janine Bol, Finance Director
Provides information on Hearing Dogs, placements, dog training, and other news about happenings at Dogs for the Deaf.
Quarterly

8142 Cochlear Implants In Children: Ethics and Choices
Gallaudet University Press
800 Florida Ave NE
Washington, DC 20002-3600
202-651-5000
800-621-2736
Fax: 202-651-5508
gupress@gallaudet.edu
www.gupress.gallaudet.edu

John B Christiansen, Author
Irene W Leigh, Co-Author
T. Alan Hurwitz, President
Paul Kelly, Vice President Adm. And Finance
Designed to educate readers about cochlear implants, including surgery, the importance of rehabilitation and the significance of parents' and professionals' roles. *$55.00*
340 pages Casebound
ISBN 1-563681-16-1

8143 Communique
Michigan Association for Deaf Hard of Hearing
5236 Dumond Court
Suite C
Lansing, MI 48917-6001
517-487-0066
800-968-7327
Fax: 517-487-2586
www.madhh.org

Nancy Asher, Executive Director
Pat Walton, Office Manager
Provides leadership through advocacy and education. The association conducts leadership training for youth, information and referral services, interpreter referral, legislative advocacy, and a variety of other services.
4-8 pages Bi-annually

8144 Listner
HEAR Center
301 E Del Mar Blvd
Pasadena, CA 91101-2714   626-796-2016
                                       Fax: 626-796-2320
                                       info@hearcenter.org
                                       www.hearcenter.org
Ellen Simon, Executive Director
Berenice Castro, Accounting Supervisro
Debbie Lorino, Office Manager
Chronicals current events, spotlights pediatric and adult clients
as well as community outreach events.
Semi-Quarterly

8145 NAD E-Zine
National Association of the Deaf
8630 Fenton Street
Suite 820
Silver Spring, MD 20910- 3819   301-587-1788
                                       Fax: 301-587-1791
                                       TTY:301-587-1789
                                       www.nad.org
Bobbie Beth Scoggins, President
Christopher Wagner, Vice President
Includes up-to-the-minute information about the NAD, including
Board news, advocacy, outreach and community activities, as
well as NAD Conference and other information.

8146 Pinnacle Newsletter
Academy of Rehabilitative Audiology
PO Box 26532
Minneapolis, MN 55426-532   952-920-0484
                                       Fax: 952-920-6098
                                       sherri.smith@va.gov
                                       www.audrehab.org
John Greer Clark, Editor
Diana Derry, Co-Editor
Sherri Smith, Ph.D.,, Content Editor
Academy of Rehabilitative Audiology newsletter.

8147 Vision Magazine
National Catholic Office of the Deaf
7202 Buchanan St
Hyattsville, MD 20784-2236   301-577-1684
                                       Fax: 301-577-1684
                                       info@ncod.org
                                       www.ncod.org
Arvilla Rank, Editor/Executive Director
Published as a pastoral service for the deaf and hard of hearing.
Provides information to members and others working in ministry.
$15.00
Quarterly

Non Print: Video

8148 Christmas Stories
Video Learning Library
15838 N 62nd St
Scottsdale, AZ 85254-1988   480-596-9970
                                       800-383-8811
                                       Fax: 480-596-9973
                                       www.videolearning.com
Jim Spencer, Owner
Told by popular deaf story-tellers, the stories included are A
Christmas Carol, Night Before Christmas, Story of the First
Christmas Tree, Birth of Christ, The Great Walled City, and Little
Match Girl. *$29.95*
Video/80 Mins 1986
ISBN 1-882257-02-2

8149 Fantastic Series Videotape Set
Gallaudet University Press
800 Florida Ave NE
Washington, DC 20002-3695   202-651-5488
                                       800-621-2736
                                       Fax: 202-651-5489
                                       gupress@gallaudet.edu
                                       www.gupress.gallaudet.edu
Rita Corey, Director
T. Alan Hurwitz, President
Paul Kelly, Vice President Adm. And Finance
These videotapes offer a blend of entertainment and information
to both deaf and hearing children ages 6-10. A total of eight tapes
in the series. *$254.00*
Video 8 VHS
ISBN 1-563680-12-2

8150 Fantastic: Colonial Times, Chocolate, and Cars
Gallaudet University Press
800 Florida Ave NE
Washington, DC 20002-3695   202-651-5488
                                       800-621-2736
                                       Fax: 202-651-5489
                                       gupress@gallaudet.edu
                                       www.gupress.gallaudet.edu
Rita Corey, Director
T. Alan Hurwitz, President
Paul Kelly, Vice President Adm. And Finance
Young viewers visit Colonial Williamsburg in Virginia to see var-
ious crafts. Other parts show chocolate being made, and films of
old cars. *$39.95*
Video
ISBN 1-563680-06-8

8151 Fantastic: Dogs at Work and Play
Gallaudet University Press
800 Florida Ave NE
Washington, DC 20002-3695   202-651-5488
                                       800-621-2736
                                       Fax: 202-651-5489
                                       gupress@gallaudet.edu
                                       www.gupress.gallaudet.edu
Rita Corey, Director
T. Alan Hurwitz, President
Paul Kelly, Vice President Adm. And Finance
See how dogs are trained, including Fantastic's own hearing-ear
dog, police dogs, plus puppies, and dogs in space? *$39.95*
Video
ISBN 1-563680-03-3

8152 Fantastic: Exciting People, Places and Things!
Gallaudet University Press
800 Florida Ave NE
Washington, DC 20002-3695   202-651-5488
                                       800-621-2736
                                       Fax: 202-651-5489
                                       gupress@gallaudet.edu
                                       www.gupress.gallaudet.edu
Rita Corey, Director
T. Alan Hurwitz, President
Paul Kelly, Vice President Adm. And Finance
Welcomes young viewers for a trip to a crayon factory, a jump
rope tournament, and mime by actor Bernard Bragg. *$39.95*
Video
ISBN 1-563680-01-7

8153 Fantastic: From Post Offices to Dairy Goats
Gallaudet University Press
800 Florida Ave NE
Washington, DC 20002-3695   202-651-5488
                                       800-621-2736
                                       Fax: 202-651-5489
                                       gupress@gallaudet.edu
                                       www.gupress.gallaudet.edu
Rita Corey, Director
T. Alan Hurwitz, President
Paul Kelly, Vice President Adm. And Finance

In this video children follow the route of a letter from the mailbox through the post office to its final destination. Also, they visit dairy goats and other animals. *$39.95*
Video
ISBN 1-563680-05-X

8154 Fantastic: Imagination, Actors, and 'Deaf Way'
Gallaudet University Press
800 Florida Ave NE
Washington, DC 20002-3695   202-651-5488
                                  800-621-2736
                                  202-651-5508
                             Fax: 202-651-5489
                        gupress@gallaudet.edu
                        www.gupress.gallaudet.edu

Rita Corey, Director
T. Alan Hurwitz, President
Paul Kelly, Vice President Adm. And Finance
Deaf clowns, mimes, and actors display the wonders of imagination, along with performances at the international cultural celebration 'Deaf Way.' *$39.95*
Video
ISBN 1-563680-04-1

8155 Fantastic: Roller Coasters, Maps, and Ice Cream!
Gallaudet University Press
800 Florida Ave NE
Washington, DC 20002-3695   202-651-5488
                                  800-621-2736
                             Fax: 202-651-5489
                        gupress@gallaudet.edu
                        www.gupress.gallaudet.edu

Rita Corey, Director
T. Alan Hurwitz, President
Paul Kelly, Vice President Adm. And Finance
In this program Mike Montangino leads the way on rides at Kings Dominion, and also to see how maps are drawn, and how ice cream is made. *$39.95*
Video
ISBN 1-563680-07-6

8156 Fantastic: Skiing, Factories, and Race Hores
Gallaudet University Press
800 Florida Ave NE
Washington, DC 20002-3695   202-651-5488
                                  800-621-2736
                             Fax: 202-651-5489
                        gupress@gallaudet.edu
                        www.gupress.gallaudet.edu

Rita Corey, Director
T. Alan Hurwitz, President
Paul Kelly, Vice President Adm. And Finance
Snow Skiing starts this program, which continues in a factory where 'who-knows-what' is made. Also, young viewers learn about horse care, and also about the making of Oreos. *$39.95*
Video
ISBN 1-563680-08-4

8157 Fantastic: Wonderful Worlds of Sports and Travel
Gallaudet University Press
800 Florida Ave NE
Washington, DC 20002-3695   202-651-5488
                                  800-621-2736
                             Fax: 202-651-5489
                        gupress@gallaudet.edu

Rita Corey, Director
T. Alan Hurwitz, President
Paul Kelly, Vice President Adm. And Finance
In this program, young viewers ride on a train, watch deaf athletes compete, and see actor Bernard Bragg perform 'The Lion and the Mouse.' *$39.95*
Video
ISBN 1-563680-02-5

8158 Fingerspelling: Expressive and Receptive Fluency
DawnSign Press
6130 Nancy Ridge Dr
San Diego, CA 92121-3223   858-625-0600
                                  800-549-5350
                             Fax: 858-625-2336
                        info@dawnsign.com
                        www.dawnsign.com

Joe Dannis, President
Joyce Linden Groode, Fingerspelling Teacher
Improve your fingerspelling with this new video guide. A 24-page instructional booklet is included with fingerspelling practice suggestions. *$29.95*
120 Minutes
ISBN 1-581210-46-9

8159 Getting Better
Vestibular Disorders Association
5018 NE 15th Ave
Portland, OR 97211-5331   503-229-7705
                                  800-837-8428
                             Fax: 503-229-8064
                        veda@vestibular.org
                        www.vestibular.org

Cynthia Ryan MBA, Executive Director
Tony Staser,, Development Director
Vicente Honrubia, Director
Joel A. Goebel, MD, FACS, Director, Vestibular & Oculomotor Laboratory
Interviews with physicians, physical therapists, psychologists, social workers, and patients on Managing Symptoms, Diagnosis & Treatment, and Cognitive/Psychological Impacts. *$24.95*
Video

8160 Helping the Family Understand
Vestibular Disorders Association
5018 NE 15th Ave
Portland, OR 97211-5331   503-229-7705
                                  800-837-8428
                             Fax: 503-229-8064
                        veda@vestibular.org
                        www.vestibular.org

Cynthia Ryan MBA, Executive Director
Tony Staser,, Development Director
Vicente Honrubia, Director
Joel A. Goebel, MD, FACS, Director, Vestibular & Oculomotor Laboratory
Interviews with physicians, physical therapists, psychologists, social workers, and patients on Managing Symptoms, Diagnosis & Treatment and Cognitive/Psychological Impacts. *$24.95*
Video

8161 Managing Your Symptoms
Vestibular Disorders Association
5018 NE 15th Ave
Portland, OR 97211-5331   503-229-7705
                                  800-837-8428
                             Fax: 503-229-8064
                        veda@vestibular.org
                        www.vestibular.org

Cynthia Ryan MBA, Executive Director
Tony Staser,, Development Director
Vicente Honrubia, Director
Joel A. Goebel, MD, FACS, Director, Vestibular & Oculomotor Laboratory
Interviews with physicians, physical therapists, psychologists, social workers, and patients. on Managing Symptoms, Diagnosis & Treatment, and Cognitive/Psychological Impacts. *$24.95*
Video

Sports

8162   American Hearing Impaired Hockey Association
4214 W. 77th Place
Chicago, IL   60652-1618   978-922-0955
Fax: 312-829-2098
kkmm2won@aol.com
www.ahiha.org

Stan Mikita, President
Cheryl Hager, General Manager
Helen Tovey, Registrar, USA Hockey Reg.
The American Hearing Impaired Hockey Association provides
deaf and hard of hearing hockey players the opportunity to learn
about and improve their hockey skills through our program. We
offer these hockey players the opportunity to be coached by a
coaching staff with college, national and international
experience.

8163   USA Deaf Sports Federation
102 N Krohn Pl
PO Box 910338
Lexington, KY   40591-0338   605-367-5760
Fax: 605-782-8441
TTY:605-367-5761
www.usdeafsports.org

Jack C Lamberton, President
Mark Apodaca, VP Of Financial Affairs
William J Bowman, VP Of International Affairs
Jeffrey L. Salit?, Vice-President of NSO Affairs
The USA Deaf Sports Federation's purpose was to foster and reg-
ulate uniform rules of competition and provide social outlets for
deaf members and their friends; serve as a parent organization for
regional sports organizations; conduct annual athletic competitions; and assist in the participation of U.S. teams in international
competition.

Support Groups

8164   Dial-a-Hearing Screening Test
Occupational Hearing Services Inc.
300 S Chester Rd
Suite 301
Swarthmore, PA   19081-1800   610-544-7700
800-622-3277
Fax: 610-543-2802

George Biddle, President/Owner
James Biddle, Vice President
Phyllis Biddle, Treasurer
A national telephone resource providing information about hearing impairments and deafness. Dial-A-Hearing Screening Test:
national test number for free telephone hearing test:
1-800-222-EARS, MON-FRI: 9:00 AM to 5:00 PM Eastern time.

Mobility

Associations

8165 Academy of Spinal Cord Injury Professionals
206 S. 6th St
Springfield, IL 62701
217-321-2488
Fax: 217-525-1271
www.academyscipro.org
Destiny Nance-Evans, Director Of Memebership Services
Kim Ruff, Director Of Education
An interdisciplinary organization dedicated to advancing the care of people with spinal cord injury/dysfunction, providing resources, research, and insights for SCI/D professionals.

8166 Academy of Spinal Cord Injury Professionals: Psychologists, Social Workers & Counselors
Academy of Spinal Cord Injury Professionals
206 S. 6th St.
Springfield, IL 62701
217-321-2488
Fax: 217-525-1271
www.academyscipro.org/
Heather Russell, President, PSWC Section
Lisa Beck, President, Academy of Spinal Cord Injury Professionals
Toby Huston, Vice President
Denny O'Malley, Executive Director
Organizes and operates for scientific and educational purposes to advance and improve the psychosocial care of persons with spinal cord impairment, develops and promotes education and research related to the psychosocial care of persons with spinal cord injury, recognizes psychologists and social workers whose careers are devoted to the problems of spinal cord impairment.

8167 Acid Maltase Deficiency Association
P.O. Box 700248
San Antonio, TX 78270-0248
210-494-6144
Fax: 210-490-7161
TiffanyLHouse@aol.com
www.amda-pompe.org
Tiffany House, President
The Acid Maltase Deficiency Association offers resource materials to help raise awareness and provide education and insight into Pompe disease (a.k.a. Acid Maltase Deficiency), a rare genetic disease derived from the family of Lysosomal Storage Disease. The association offers information for patients, their families, as well as medical professionals.

8168 American Academy of Osteopathy
The Pyramids
3500 DePauw Blvd.
Suite 1100
Indianapolis, IN 46268-1136
317-879-1881
Fax: 317-879-0563
info@academyofosteopathy.org
www.academyofosteopathy.org
Sherri Quarles, Interim Executive Director & Accountant
Michael P. Rowane, DO, MS, FAAO, President
The mission of the American Academy of Osteopathy is to teach, advocate, and research the science, art and philosophy of osteopathic medicine, emphasizing the integration of osteopathic principles, practice and manipulative treatment in patient care.

8169 American Association of Neuromuscular & Electrodiagnostic Medicine
2621 Superior Drive NW
Rochester, MN 55901
507-288-0100
Fax: 507-288-1225
aanem@aanem.org
www.aanem.org
Shirlyn A. Adkins, JD, Executive Director
Scott Gerdes, Finance Director
Lori Nierman, Office Manager
Karen Reilly, Education & Meeting Director
The American Association of Neuromuscular & Electrodiagnostic Medicine (AANEM) is a nonprofitmembership association dedicated to the advancement of neuromuscular (NM), musculoskeletal, and electrodiagnostic (EDX) medicine.

8170 American Back Society
St. Joseph's Professional Center
2647 E. 14th St.
Suite 401
Oakland, CA 94601
510-536-9929
Fax: 510-536-1812
www.chiroweb.com/hp/abs/index.html
Philip E. Greenman, D.O., FAAO, President
Alexander Hadjipavlou, MD, MSc, 1st Vice President
Stephen Esses, BSc, MD, 2nd Vice President
Aubrey A. Swartz, MD, PharmD, Treasurer/Secretary
The American Back Society is a non-profit organization dedicated to providing an interdisciplinary educational forum for healthcare professionals committed to relieving pain and diminishing impairment in patients suffering from neck and back conditions through proper diagnosis and treatment.

8171 American Parkinson Disease Association
135 Parkinson Avenue
Staten Island, NY 10305
800-223-2732
Fax: 718-981-4399
apda@apdaparkinson.org
www.apdaparkinson.org
Leslie A. Chambers, President & CEO
Stephanie Paul, Vice President, Development and Marketing
Robin Kornhaber, MSW, Vice President, Programs and Services
Eloise Caggiano, Senior Director of Development
APDA was founded in 1961 with the dual purpose to find the curefor Parkinson's disease, and to assist Americans living with Parkinson's disease live a quality life.

8172 American Stroke Association
7272 Greenville Ave
Dallas, TX 75231
888-478-7653
strokeconnection@heart.org
www.strokeassociation.org/STROKEORG
John Warner, President
James Postl, Chairman
Nancy Brown, Chief Executive Officer
Raymond Vara, Jr., Treasurer
The American Stroke Association offers educational materials, seminars, conferences and transportation for those effected by strokes as well as their families, caregivers and interested professionals.

8173 Amytrophic Lateral Sclerosis Association
1275 K Street NW
Suite 250
Washington, DC 20005
202-407-8580
Fax: 202-464-8869
alsinfo@alsa-national.org
www.alsa.org
Barbara Newhouse, President/CEO
Calaneet Balas, Executive Vice President, Strategy
Gregory L. Mitchell, Executive Vice President, Finance & Administration
Lance Slaughter, Executive Vice President, Chapter Relations & Governance
The ALS association is the only national not-for-profit health organization dedicated soley to lead the fight against ALS. The Association covers all the bases-research, patient and community services, public education, and advocacy-in providing help and hope to those facing the disease. The mission is to lead the fight to cure and treat ALS through global cutting edge research, and to empower people with Lou Gehrig's disease to live fuller lives & provide them with compassion, care and support.

8174 Arthritis Foundation
1355 Peachtree St NE
6th Floor
Atlanta, GA 30309
404-872-7100
800-283-7800
www.arthritis.org

Laurie Stewart, Secretary/Vice Chair
Rowland W. (Bing) Chang, Chair
Frank Longobardi, Treasurer
Ann M. Palmer, President/CEO
Offers information and referrals regarding educational materials and programs, fund-raising, support groups, seminars and conferences, and aids Americans with arthritis in accessing optimal care.

8175 Association for Neurologically Impaired Brain Injured Children
61-35 220th St
Oakland Gardens, NY 11364
718-423-9550
Fax: 718-423-9838
jdebiase@anibic.org
www.anibic.org

Vincent Tancredi, Chief Financial Officer
John F DeBiase, Executive Director
Rachel Plakstis, MSC Director
Gail Baquero, Residential Director
ANIBIc is a voluntary, multi-service organization that is dedicated to serving individuals with severe learning disabilities, neurological impairments and other developmental disabilities. Services include: residential, vocational, family support services, recreation (children and adults), respite (adult), in home support services, counseling and traumatic brain injury services (adults).

8176 Capital Area Parkinsons Society
PO Box 27565
Austin, TX 78755-2565
512-371-3373
www.capitalareaparkinsons.org

Tereasa Ford, President
Deborah Bryson, Vice President
Donna Hohm, Secretary
Tim Ebest, Treasurer
Founded in 1984, the Capital Area Parkinson's Society addresses the needs for those impacted by Parkinson's disease in central Texas. The organization offers a multitude of support groups, resources, monthly meetings, exercise programs and a community for people afflicted by Parkinson's and their care partners.

8177 Children's Hemiplegia & Stroke Association
4101 W. Green Oaks Blvd
Suite 305-149
Arlington, TX 76016
www.chasa.org
Nancy Atwood, Executive Director & Founder
Jana Smoot White, President
Patti Scrivano, Vice President
Jackie Haley, Treasurer
Founded in 1996, CHASA offers support and information to families of infants, children and young adults who have hemiplegia, hemiparesis or hemiplegic cerebral palsy.

8178 Christopher & Dana Reeve Paralysis Resource Center
636 Morris Turnpike
Suite 3A
Short Hills, NJ 07078
973-467-8270
800-225-0292
InfoSpecialist@ChristopherReeve.org
www.christopherreeve.org

John M Hughes, Chairman
John E McConnell, Vice Chairman
Peter Wilderotter, President & CEO
Matthew Reeve, Vice Chairman, International Development
The Paralysis Resource Center's goal is to provide support and information to those living with paralysis and their caregivers. Some programs offered include financial grants, a family support program, advocay programs, a lending library, rehabilitation centers, a veteran program and a resource guide about paralysis.

8179 Consortium of Multiple Sclerosis Centers
3 University Plaza Dr.
Suite 116
Hackensack, NJ 07601
201-487-1050
Fax: 862-772-7275
www.mscare.org

June Halper, Chief Executive Officer
Gary Cutter, PhD, President
Lisa Skutnik, Chief Operating Officer
Marguerite Herman, Executive Assistant
CMSC provides leadership in clinical research and education; develops vehicles to share information and knowledge among members; disseminates information to the health care community and to persons affected by Multiple Sclerosis; and develops and implements mechanisms to influence health care delivery.

8180 Cure SMA
Cure SMA
925 Busse Rd
Elk Grove Village, IL 60007
800-886-1762
info@curesma.org
www.curesma.org

Jill Jarecki, Chief Scientific Officer
Kenneth Hobby, President
Richard Rubenstein, Chair
Kelly Cole, Secretary
Cure SMA is the largest international organization dedicated solely to eradicating spinal muscular atrophy (SMA) by promoting and supporting research, helping families cope with SMA through informational programs and support, and educating the public and professional community about SMA.

8181 Dystonia Advocacy Network
One East Wacker Drive
Suite 2810
Chicago, IL 60601
dystonia-advocacy.org

8182 Epilepsy Foundation
8301 Professional Place E
Suite 200
Landover, MD 20785- 2353
800-332-1000
Fax: 301-459-1569
ContactUs@efa.com
www.epilepsy.com

Robert W Smith, Chair
Phillip M. Gattone, M.Ed, Preisdent & CEO
M. Vaneeda Bennett, Chief Development Officer
May J. Liang, Secretary
The organization works to ensure that people with epilepsy are able to participate in all life experiences; to improve how people with epilepsy are perceived and treated in society; and to promote research for a cure.

8183 Friends of Disabled Adults and Children
4900 Lewis Rd
Stone Mountain, GA 30083
770-491-9014
866-977-1204
www.fodac.org

Chris Brand, President
Pam Holley, Director of Administration
Betty Felder, DME Office Manager
Ron Hess, Vehicle Modification Coordinator
FODAC's mission is to provide durable medical equipment (DME) at lost cost to the disabled and their families, and to enhance the quality of life for individuals with disabilities or illnesses.

8184 **Head Injury Rehabilitation And Referral Service, Inc. (HIRRS)**
11 Taft Court
Suite 100
Rockville, MD   20850   301-309-2228
                                    Fax: 301-309-2278
                              tbi@headinjuryrehab.org
                              www.headinjuryrehab.org
Maggie Hunter, Director of Admissions and Quality Assurance
Robert Cousland, Director of Rehabilitation
Ricardo Hunter, President
Janet McCloskey, Director of Community Living Services
Head Injury Rehabilitation and Referral Services, Inc. (HIRRS) is a private not-for-profit agency that provides comprehensive brain injury support including long-term living, daily programs, vocational supports and services to individuals that live in the community. The agency is located in Rockville, MD, but serves the DC Metropolitan area.

8185 **International Parkinson and Movement Disorder Society**
555 East Wells St.
Suite 1100
Milwaukee, WI   53202-3823   414-276-2145
                                    Fax: 414-276-3349
                              info@movementdisorders.org
                              www.movementdisorders.org
Christopher Goetz, MD, President
Susan Fox, PhD, Secretary
Victor Fung, MBBS, PhD, FRACP, Treasurer
The International Parkinson and Movement Disorder Society (MDS) is a professional society of clinicians, scientists, and other healthcare professionals who are interested in Parkinson's disease, related neurodegenerative and neurodevelopmental disorders, hyperkinetic movement disorders, and abnormalities in muscle tone and motor control.

8186 **Lewy Body Dementia Association**
912 Killian Hill Road S.W.
Lilburn, GA   30047   404-975-2322
                                    Fax: 480-422-5434
                                        www.lbda.org
Christina M. Christie, President
Shannon McCarty-Caplan, Vice President
Mike Koehler, CEO
Angela Taylor, Director of Programs
The Lewy Body Dementia Association (LBDA) is a nonprofit organization dedicated to raising awareness of the Lewy body dementias (LBD), supporting people affected by LBD, and promoting scientific advances.

8187 **Mobility International USA**
132 E. Broadway
Suite 343
Eugene, OR   97401   541-343-1284
                                    Fax: 541-343-6812
                                      info@miusa.org
                                      www.miusa.org
Susan Sygall, CEO/Co-Founder
Susan Dunn, Program Manager
Monica Malhotra, Program Manager
Cindy Lewis, Director of Programs
A US based national nonprofit organization dedicated to empowering people with disabilities around the world through leadership development, training and international exchange to ensure inclusion of people with disabilities in international exchange and development programs. The National Clearinghouse on Disability & Exchange, a joint project managed by MIUSA provides free information and referrals.

8188 **Multiple Sclerosis Association of America**
375 Kings Hwy N
Cherry Hill, NJ   08034   800-532-7667
                                    Fax: 856-661-9797
                                      msaa@mymsaa.org
                                        mymsaa.org/
John McCorry, Chair
Monica Derbes Gibson, Vice Chair
Steve Bruneau, Treasurer
Ira M. Levee, Esq., Secretary
MSAA is a national non-profit organization dedicated to enriching the quality of life for evryone affected by Multiple Sclerosis through vital services and support.

8189 **Multiple Sclerosis Foundation**
6520 N. Andrews Ave
Fort Lauderdale, FL   33309-2132   954-776-6805
                                          800-225-6495
                                    Fax: 954-938-8708
                                      admin@msfocus.org
                                      www.msfocus.org
Jules Kuperberg, Executive Director
Alan Segaloff, Co- Executive Director
Kasey Minnis, Director, Operations & Communications
Natalie Blake, Director, Programs & Services
A national, nonprofit organization that provides free support services and public education for persons with Multiple Sclerosis, newsletters, toll-free phone support, information, referrals, home care, assitive technology, and support groups.

8190 **NBIA Disorders Association**
2082 Monaco Ct.
El Cajon, CA   92019-4235   619-588-2315
                                    Fax: 619-588-4093
                                      info@NBIAdisorders.org
                                      www.nbiadisorders.org
Patricia Wood, President
Coleen Lukoff, Development Director
Melissa Woods, Social Media Director
Mike Cohn, Director of Adult Programs
NBIA provides support to families, educates the public and accelerates research with collaborators from around the world.

8191 **National Association for Continence**
P.O. Box 1019
Charleston, SC   29402   800-252-3337
                                      sgregg@nafc.org
                                        www.nafc.org
Katherine F. Jeter, EdD, Founder
Steven G. Gregg, PhD, Executive Director
Donna Deng, Chairperson
Lori Lyons-Willams, Vice Chairperson
NAFC's mission is to educate the public about the causes, diagnosis, categories, treatment options and management alternatives for incontinence, voiding dysfunction and related pelvic floor disorders; to network with other organizations and agencies; to elevate the visibility and priority given to these areas; and to advocate on behalf of consumers who suffer from such symptoms as a result of disease or other illness.

8192 **National Coalition for Assistive and Rehab Technology**
54 Towhee Court
East Amhurst, NY   14051   716-839-9728
                                    Fax: 716-839-9624
                                      info@ncart.us
                                        www.ncart.us
Don Clayback, Executive Director
Doug Westerdahl, President
Greg Packer, Vice President
Seth Johnson, Secretary/Treasurer
The coalition's mission is to ensure proper and appropriate access to complex rehab and assistive technologies.

8193 National Council on Independent Living
2013 H St. NW
6th Fl
Washington, DC 20006   202-207-0334
                                      877-525-3400
                                 Fax: 202-207-0341
                                 TTY: 202-207-0340
                                      ncil@ncil.org
                                      www.ncil.org

Kelly Buckland, Executive Director
Bruce Darling, President
Sarah Launderville, Vice President
Derrel Christenson, Treasurer
NCIL advances independent living and the rights of people with disabilities through consumer-driven advocacy.

8194 National Fibromyalgia Association
3857 Birch St.
Suite 312
Newport Beach, CA 92660   nfa@fmaware.org
                                      www.fmaware.org

Lynne Matallana, President/Founder
National Fibromyalgia Association's mission is to develop and execute programs dedicated to improving the quality of life for people with fibromyalgia.

8195 National Mobility Equipment Dealers Association
3327 West Bearss Ave
Tampa, FL 33618   813-264-2697
                                      866-948-8341
                                 Fax: 813-962-8970
                                      info@nmeda.org
                                      www.nmeda.com

Chad Blake, President
Richard May, Vice President
Bill Koeblitz, Secretary
Jud DeMott, Treasurer
The National Mobility Equipment Dealers Association (NMEDA) is a non-profit trade association dedicated creating and expanding oppotunities of safe transportation for people with disabilities in vehicles modified to fit their specific needs.

8196 National Spasmodic Dysphonia Association
300 Park Blvd.
Suite 335
Itasca, IL 60143   800-795-6732
                                 Fax: 630-250-4505
                                      nsda@dysphonia.org
                                      www.dysphonia.org

Charlie Reavis, President
Marcia Sterling, Treasurer
Kimberly Kuman, Executive Director
The National Spasmodic Dysphonia Association (NSDA) is a not-for-profit organization dedicated to advancing medical research into the causes of and treatments for SD, promoting physician and public awareness of the disorder, and providing support to those affected by SD through symposiums, support groups, and on-line resources.

8197 National Spasmodic Torticollis Association
9920 Talbert Ave
Fountain Valley, CA 92708   714-378-9837
                                      800-487-8385
                                      NSTAmail@aol.com
                                      www.torticollis.org

Ken Price, President/Treasurer
Diane Truong, Vice President
Janelle Lazzo, Secretary
The mission of the National Spasmodic Torticollis Association is to support the needs and well being of individuals affected by Spasmodic Torticollis; to promote awareness and education; and to advance research for more treatments and a cure.

8198 Paralyzed Veterans of America
801 18th St NW
Washington, DC 20006-3517   800-424-8200
                                 TTY:800-795-4327
                                      info@pva.org
                                      www.pva.org

Sherman Gillums, Jr., Executive Director
Larry Dodson, National Secretary
David Zurfluh, National President
Ken Weas, Senior Vice President
A congressionally chartered veterans service organization for veterans of the armed forces who have experienced spinal cord injury or dysfunction. This organization advocates for quality healthcare, research and education addressing spinal cord injury/dysfunction, benefits available to veterans, and civil rights that maximize the independence of veterans.

8199 Parkinson's Disease Research Society
Northwestern Medicine Central DuPage Hospital
25 N. Winfield Rd
4 North Tower
Winfield, IL 60190   630-933-4384
                                 Fax: 630-933-3077
                            info@parkinsonsprogress.org
                               parkinsonsprogress.org

Carol A. Santi, President
Alex Katz, Vice President
Mitchell King, Treasurer
Cacilia Reich Masover, Secretary
The PDRS mandate is to mount a concerted effort to intensify the research, both in the basic science laboratory as well as with clinical trials, to advance the diagnosis, treatment and prevention of Parkinson's disease.

8200 Post-Polio Health International
4207 Lindell Blvd
Suite 110
Saint Louis, MO 63108-2930   314-534-0475
                                 Fax: 314-534-5070
                                      info@post-polio.org
                                      www.post-polio.org

Joan L Headley, Executive Director
Gayla Hoffman, Editor
Sheryl R. Rudy, Editor
Brian M. Tiburzi, Assistant to the Executive Director
Educates, advocates and networks the survivors of polio and the health professionals who treat them. Funds a research grant, publishes Post Polio Health (Quarterly, 12 page newsletter).

8201 Simon Foundation for Continence
P.O. Box 815
Wilmette, IL 60091   847-864-3913
                                      800-237-4666
                                 Fax: 847-864-9758
                         webmaster@simonfoundation.org
                              www.simonfoundation.org

Cheryl B. Gartley, Founder/President
Elizabeth A. LaGro, Vice President, Communications & Education Services
Twila Yednock, Director of Special Events
The Simon Foundation is known throughout the world for its innovative educational projects and tireless efforts on behalf of people with loss of bladder and bowel control. The mission of the foundation is to remove the stigma surrounding incontinence and to provide help for people with incontinence, their families, and the healthcare professionals who provide care for people with incontinence.

8202 **Society for Progressive Supranuclear Palsy**
30 E. Padonia Road,
Suite 201
Timonium, MD 21093 800-457-4777
Fax: 410-785-7009
info@curepsp.org
www.psp.org

Janet Edmunson, Med, Chair
Dan Johnson, Vice-Chair
George S. Jankiewicz, CPA, CFP,, Treasurer
John T. Burhoe, Secretary
Members of the Board of Directors of CurePSP accept the major
responsibility of implementing the mission of the Foundation for
PSP | CBD and Related Brain Diseases. Board members are ac-
tively involved in continually defining and redefining the mission and participating in strategic planning to review purposes,
programs, priorities, funding needs, and levels of achievement.

8203 **United Spinal Association**
120-34 Queens Blvd
Ste 320
Kew Gardens, NY 11415 718-803-3782
Fax: 718-803-0414
www.unitedspinal.org

8204 **Vermont Back Research Center**
1 S Prospect St
Burlington, VT 05405 802-656-3131
Fax: 802-660-9243
learn@uvm.edu
www.uvm.edu

8205 **World Chiropractic Alliance**
2683 Via De La Valle
Suite G 629
Del Mar, CA 92014 480-786-9235
866-789-8073
Fax: 480-732-9313
www.worldchiropracticalliance.org

Linda Bevel, Manager
Terry A Rondberg DC, Founder/CEO
The World Chiropractic Alliance was founded in 1989 as a
non-profit organization dedicated to protecting and strengthening chiropractic around the world. Since its inception, the WCA
has played an important role in the global chiropractic community. In 1998, it was granted status as a Non-Governmental Organization (NGO) associated with the United Nations Department
of Public Information.

Camps

8206 **Autism Day Camp**
Hillcroft Services: Isanogel
114 E. Streeter Avenue
Muncie, IN 47304 765-288-1073
Fax: 765-288-3101
TTY:765-288-1073
demcintosh@bsu.edu
www.hillcroft.org

Ted Baker, Chair
Brenda Llyod, Vice Chair
Bruce Baldwin, Director
Julie Bering, Secretary/ Treasurer
The camp is designed to improve the academic, social skills, and
behaviors of children with autism spectrum disorders. The day
camp is an 8-week intensive experience for children classified
with autism spectrum disorders.

8207 **Camp Esperanza**
Southern California Chapter
West 6th Street
Suite 1250
Los Angeles, CA 90017 323-954-5760
800-954-2873
Fax: 213-954-5790
jziegler@arthritis.org
www.arthritis.org

Jennifer Ziegler, Camp Director
Lindsey Gonzales, Regional Director, Human Resources
Manuel Loya, Chief Executive Officer
Teri Lim, Chief Marketing Officer
A one-week camp in August that allows children with arthritis to
participate in such activities as horseback riding, swimming, etc.
in a fun-filled environment.

8208 **Camp Oakhurst**
New York Service for the Handicapped
111 Monmouth Rd
Oakhurst, NJ 7755 732-531-0215
Fax: 732-531-0292
info@nysh.org
www.nysh.org

Robert Pacenza, Executive Director:
Charles Sutherland, Camp Director
Andy Arno, Board Member
Hope Bach, Board Member
Camp Oakhurst, established in 1906, is operated by New York
Service for the Handicapped (NYSH), an independent non-profit
social service agency with offices in New York City and Oakhurst, New Jersey. The camp is for adults and children with with
special needs, including autism and physical and intellectual disabilities. Campers will experience all the traditional camp activities while gaining skills for greater independence.

8209 **Easter Seals Camp Stand by Me**
Easter Seal Society of Washington
17809 S. Vaughn Rd KPN
PO Box 289
Vaughn, WA 98394 253-884-2722
jmayer@wa.easterseals.com
www.wa.easterseals.com

Jeff Pavey, Board Chair
Carol Basile, Vice Chair
Ellen Briggs, Treasurer
Joshua Mayer, Camp Director
Camp Stand By Me provides a safe, barrier-free environment for
children and adults with any disability to experience all aspects of
camp without limitations. Respite weekends offered throughout
the year. Activities include campfires, fishing, swimming, sports,
archery, and more.

8210 **Summer Wheelchair Sports Camp**
University of Illinois
1207 S Oak St
Champaign, IL 61820-6901 217-333-4606
Fax: 217-244-0014
TTY:217-244-9738
sportscamp@illinois.edu
www.disability.illinois.edu

Brian Walsh, Camp Director
Kim Collins, Asst. Dir., Academic Disability Support Services
Pat Malik, Asst. Dir., Non-Academic Disability Support Services
Angella Anderson, Disability Specialist, Accessible Media
Rigorous camps designed for individuals with lower extremity
physical disabilities. Camp attendees will spend an average of
8-9 hours a day, focusing on development and refinement of fitness, techniques and strategies. Strength training, nutrition and
mental training sessions will also be included in all camps. The
camp staff is comprised of athletic staff and faculty front, the Division of Rehabilitation Education Services and local wheelchair
athletes with coaching experience.

8211 Twin Lakes Camp
1451 E Twin Lakes Rd
Hillsboro, IN   47949-8004   765-798-4000
outdoors@twinlakescamp.com
www.twinlakescamp.com

Jon Beight, Executive Director
Duane Bush, Guest Service
Dan Daily, Program Director
Donna Beight, Secretary
Provides a summer camp program for special needs children and
young adults. Campers suffer from a wide range of maladies in-
cluding crippling accidents, Spina Bifida, epilepsy, Cerebral
Palsy, Muscular Dystrophy, Quadriplegia, Paraplegia, and other
disabling diseases. Campers range in age from 8 to 27.

8212 YMCA Camp Fitch
The YMCA's Camp Fitch on Lake Erie
12600 Abels Rd
North Springfield, PA   16430   814-922-3219
877-863-4824
Fax: 814-922-7000
hannahkight@campfitchymca.org
campfitchymca.org

Matt Pose, Executive Director
Tom Parker, Associate Executive Director
Hannah Kight, Office Manager
Jon Tully, Program Director
Camp is located in North Springfield, Pennsylvania. Camping
sessions for children and adults with diabetes or epilepsy. Ages
8-16, families and seniors.

Print: Books

8213 Adapted Physical Education and Sport
Human Kinetics, Inc.
1607 N Market Street
Champaign, IL   61820-2220   217-351-5076
800-747-4457
Fax: 217-351-1549
info@hkusa.com
www.naspem.org

Joseph P Winnick EdD, Author
Scott Kimberly, Owner
Rainer Martens, President/Treasurer
Jill Wikgren, COO
Designed as a resource for both present and future physical edu-
cation leaders, this book is an exceptional book for teaching ex-
ceptional children. It emphasizes the physical education of young
people with disabilities. *$68.00*
592 pages Hardcover
ISBN 0-736052-16-X

8214 Arthritis Bible
Inner Traditions - Bear & Company
PO Box 388
Rochester, VT   05767-0388   802-767-3174
800-246-8648
Fax: 802-767-3726
customerservice@innertraditions.com
www.innertraditions.com

Craig Weatherby, Author
Leonid Gordin MD, Co-Author
A comprehensive guide to the alternative therapies and conven-
tional treatments for Arthritic diseases including Osteoarthritis,
Rheumatoid Arthritis, Gout, Fibromyalgia and more. *$16.95*
272 pages Paperback 1999
ISBN 0-892818-25-5

**8215 Arthritis Helpbook: A Tested Self Management Program for
Coping with Arthritis**
Da Capo Press
44 Farnsworth Street,
Boston, MA   02210   617-252-5200
Fax: 617-252-5265
www.dacapopress.com

Kate Lorig, Author
James Fries, Co-Author
The Arthritis Helpbook is the world's leading guide to coping
with joint pain, and has been used by more than 600,000 readers
over its twenty years in print. It succeeds because of its tested advice, its hundreds of useful hints, and its emphasis on self-man-
agement-helping people with arthritis and fibromyalgia to
achieve their own health goals. *$18.95*
Paperback
ISBN 0-738210-38-2

8216 Arthritis Sourcebook
McGraw-Hill Professional
7500 Chavenelle Rd
Dubuque, IA   52002-9655   563-584-6000
877-833-5524
Fax: 614-759-3749
pbg.ecommerce_custserv@mcgraw-hill.com
www.mhprofessional.com

Earl J Brewer Jr MD, Author
Kathy Cochran Angel, Co-Author
A comprehensive guide to the latest information on treatments,
medications, and alternative therapies for arthritis. *$ 16.95*
272 pages Paperback
ISBN 0-737303-81-6

**8217 Arthritis, What Exercises Work: Breakthrough Relief for
the Rest of Your Life**
MacMillan - St. Martin's Press
175 5th Ave
New York, NY   10010-7703   646-307-5151
Fax: 212-420-9314
press.inquiries@macmillanusa.com
www.us.macmillan.com

Dava Sorbel, Author
Arthur C Klein, Co-Author
What is the most powerful arthritis treatment ever developed to
help restore you to a healthy, pain-free, and vigorous life—for the
rest of your life? It's exercise. Here are the right exercised for
your kind of arthritis, pain-level, age, occupation, and hobbies.
$14.99
200 pages Paperback 1995
ISBN 0-312130-25-2

8218 Arthritis: A Take Care of Yourself Health Guide
Da Capo Press
44 Farnsworth Street,
Boston, MA   02210   617-252-5200
Fax: 617-252-5265
www.dacapopress.com

James F Fries, Author
Donald M Vickery, Co-Author
In this updated book the author draws on new research to recom-
mend exercises and new pain medications for both arthritis and
fibromyalgia. *$18.95*
Paperback 1909
ISBN 0-738202-25-8

8219 Disability and Sport
Human Kinetics, Inc.
1607 N Market Street
Champaign, IL   61820-2220   217-351-5076
800-747-4457
Fax: 217-351-1549
info@hkusa.com
www.naspem.org

Karen P DePauw, Author
Susan J Gavron, Co-Author
Scott Kimberley, Owner
Rainer Martens, President/Treasurer

Provides a comprehensive and practical look at the past, present, and future of disability sport. Topics covered are inclusive of youth through adult participation with in-depth coverage of the essential issues involving athletes with disabilities. This new edition has updated references and new chapter-opening outlines that assist with individual study and class discussions. *$48.00*

408 pages Hardcover
ISBN 0-736046-38-0

8220 **Fitness Programming for Physical Disabilities**
Human Kinetics, Inc.
1607 N Market Street
Champaign, IL 61820-2220 217-351-5076
800-747-4457
Fax: 217-351-1549
info@hkusa.com
www.naspem.org

Patricia D Miller, Editor
Scott Kimberley, Owner
Rainer Martens, President/Treasurer
Jill Wikgren, COO

A book offering information for developing and conducting exercise programs for groups that included people with physical disabilities. A dozen authorities in exercise science and adapted exercise programming explain how to effectively and safely modify existing programs for individuals with physical disabilities. *$42.00*

232 pages Paperback
ISBN 0-873224-34-5

8221 **Freedom from Arthritis Through Nutrition**
Tree of Life Publications
PO Box 126
Joshua Tree, CA 92252-0126 760-366-2937
Fax: 760-366-2937
www.treelifebooks.com

Philip J Welsh DDS ND, Author
Bianca Leonardo ND, Co-Author

Reveals the results of 60 years of research on arthritis by noted nutritionist, Dr. Philip J. Welsh, D.D.S. N.D. Here you will find simple, natural, inexpensive, tested ways of coping with the various forms of arthritis, using only nutrition and other natural methods. There are no drugs or gadgets in this program. *$24.95*

255 pages Softcover

8222 **Functional Electrical Stimulation for Ambulation by Paraplegics**
Krieger Publishing Company
1725 Krieger Drive
PO Box 9542
Malabar, FL 32950 321-724-9542
800-724-0025
Fax: 321-951-3671
info@krieger-publishing.com
www.krieger-publishing.com

Daniel Graupe, Author
Kate H Kohn, Co-Author

FES is employed to enable spinal cord injury patients who are complete paraplegics to stand and ambulate without bracing. The text covers 12 years of amulation experience. *$49.50*

210 pages Paperback 1994
ISBN 0-894648-45-4

8223 **Guide to Managing Your Arthritis**
Arthritis Foundation
1330 W. Peachtree St
Suite 100
Atlanta, GA 30309 404-872-7100
800-283-7800
Fax: 404-237-8153
AFOrders@pbd.com
www.arthritis.org

Mary Anne Dunkin, Author
John Klippel, President/CEO
Cecile Perich, Chairman
William Brackney, Vice Chair

Expert reviewers answer questions about basic arthritis facts, treatments, research, surgery and more. Also, specific information about six common conditions: rheumatoid arthritis, osteoarthritis, osteoporosis, fibromyalgia, lupus and gout. *$9.95*

193 pages Paperback
ISBN 0-912423-28-5

8224 **How to Deal with Back Pain and Rheumatoid Joint Pain: A Preventive and Self Treatment Manua**
Global Health Solutions
2146 Kings Garden Way
Falls Church, VA 22043-2593 703-848-2333
800-759-3999
Fax: 703-848-0028
information@watercure.com
www.watercure.com

Fereydoon Batmanghelidj, Author
Xiaopo Batmanjhelidj, President
Kristin Swan, Administrator

The physiology of pain production and its direct relationship to chronic regional dehydration of some joint spaces is explained: Special movements that would create vacuum in the disc spaces and draw water and the displaced discs into the vertebral joints are demonstrated. *$14.95*

100 pages Paperback
ISBN 0-962994-20-0

8225 **Inclusive Games**
Human Kinetics
1607 N Market Street
PO Box 5076
Champaign, IL 61825- 5076 217-351-5076
800-747-4457
Fax: 217-351-1549
info@hkusa.com
www.humankinetics.com

Susan L Kasser, Author
Scott Kimberley, Owner
Rainer Martens, President/Treasurer
Jill Wikgren, COO

Features more than 50 games, helpful illustrations, and hundreds of game variations. The book shows how to adapt games so that children of every ability level can practice, play and improve their movement skills together. The game finder makes it easy to locate an appropriate game according to its name, approximate grade level, difficulty within the grade level, skills required/developed, and number of players. *$17.95*

120 pages Paperback
ISBN 0-873226-39-9

8226 **Inside The Halo and Beyond: The Anatomy of a Recovery**
WW Norton & Company
500 5th Ave
New York, NY 10110-2 212-354-5500
Fax: 212-869-0856
www.wwnorton.com

Maxine Kumin, Author
W Drake McFeely, Chairman/President
Stephen King, VP Finance/CFO
Robert Weil, VP/Executive Editor

A skilled horsewoman and lifelong athlete, poet Kumin was 73 when a riding accident left her with two broken vertebrac in her neck. Kumin survived in the face of overwhelming odds that she would be paralyzed for the rest of her life. Miraculously, however, she was walking again within weeks of the accident; now, though one hand and an arm remain partially immobilized, her life has largely resumed its normal course. Here is the journal of her first nine months of recovery. *$ 13.95*

192 pages Softcover
ISBN 0-393049-00-0

8227 **Life on Wheels: For the Active Wheelchair User**
Patient-Centered Guides
1005 Gravenstein Hwy North
Sebastopol, CA 95472-2811   707-827-7000
                                                    800-998-9938
                                              Fax: 707-829-0104
                                              order@oreilly.com
                                              www.oreilly.com

Gary Karp, Author
For 1.5 million Americans, life includes a wheelchair for mobility. Life on Wheels is for people who want to take charge of their life experience. Author Gary Karp describes medical issues (paralysis, circulation, rehab, cure research); day-to-day living (exercise, skin, bowel and bladder, sexuality, home access, maintaining a wheelchair); and social issues (self-image, adjustment, friends, family, cultural attitudes, activism). *$24.95*
565 pages Paperback 1999
ISBN 1-565922-53-0

8228 **Paralysis Resource Guide**
Christopher and Dana Reeve Paralysis Resource Ctr
636 Morris Turnpike
Suite 3A
Short Hills, NJ 07078   973-467-8270
                                                    800-539-7309
                                              Fax: 973-912-9433
                                 information@christopherreeve.org
                                              www.paralysis.org

John M. Hughes, Chairman
John E. McConnell, Vice Chair
Matthew Reeve, Vice Chair
Peter T. Wilderotter, President
A comprehensive information tool for people affected by paralysis and for those who care for them. English or Spanish.
336 pages

8229 **Primer on the Rheumatic Diseases**
Arthritis Foundation
1330 W. Peachtree St
Suite 100
Atlanta, GA 30309-2111   404-872-7100
                                                    800-933-7023
                                              Fax: 404-237-8153
                                              AFOrders@pbd.com
                                              www.arthritis.org

Rob Shaw, President
Patience White M.D., Editor
John H. Klippel, Editor
The leading professional book about arthritis and related diseases, the Primer is published by Springer and the Arthritis Foundation. *$79.95*
724 pages Softcover
ISBN 0-387356-64-8

8230 **Sport Science Review: Adapted Physical Activity**
Human Kinetics
1607 N Market Street
Champaign, IL 61820-2220   217-351-5076
                                                    800-747-4457
                                              Fax: 217-351-1549
                                              info@hkusa.com
                                              www.naspem.org

Rainer Martens, President/Treasurer
Scott Kimberley, Owner
Jill Wikgren, COO
This issue of Sport Science Review examines the newly emerging academic discipline of adapted physical activity. Researchers from diverse academic backgrounds and parts of the world review the issues and controversies surrounding inclusion in physical education and sport. *$15.00*
96 pages Paperback
ISBN -073602-07-9

8231 **Still Me**
Random House
1745 Broadway
3rd Floor
New York, NY 10019-4305   212-782-9000
                                              Fax: 212-572-6066
                                 vintageanchor@randomhouse.com
                                              www.randomhouse.com

Christopher Reeve, Author
Markus Dohle, Chairman/CEO
Madeline McIntosh, President
Andrew Weber, SVP Operations
The man who was Superman begins with his debilitating riding accident, then weaves back and forth between past and present, creating a thorough biography of Reeve's life. *$7.99*
336 pages Paperback 1999
ISBN 0-345432-41-4

8232 **When Your Student Has Arthritis**
Arthritis Foundation
2970 Peachtree Rd NW
PO Box 932915, Ste 200
Atlanta, GA 31193-2915   404-237-8771
                                                    800-933-7023
                                              Fax: 404-237-8153
                                              aforders@arthritis.org
                                              www.afstore.org

Rob Shaw, President
An overview of arthritis, including juvenile rhuematoid arthritis and treatment. Also includes a school activities checklist for students, education rights, and how teachers can help.
28 pages

8233 **Yoga for Fibromyalgia: Move, Breathe, and Relax to Improve Your Quality of Life**
Mobility Limited
PO Box 838
Morro Bay, CA 93443-0838   805-772-3560
                                                    800-366-6038
                                              Fax: 805-772-4717
                                              shsh@mobilityltd.com
                                              www.mobilityltd.com

Shoosh Lettick Crotzer, Director
The first book devoted exclusively to managing the symptoms of fibromyalgia; the comprehensive program of 26 illustrated poses, breathing techniques, and guided visualization and relaxation sessions can be practiced regardless of age or experience. The Living with Fibromyalgia section discusses lifestyle concerns. *$14.95*
128 pages 1908

Print: Magazines

8234 **Arthritis Today**
Arthritis Foundation
1330 W. Peachtree St.
Suite 100
Atlanta, GA 30309   404-872-7100
                                                    800-933-7023
                                              Fax: 404-237-8153
                                              info.ga@arthritis.org
                                              www.arthritis.org

Dan McGowan, Chairman
Rowland W. Chang, Vice Chair
Ann M. Palmer, President and CEO
Patricia N. Nelson, Secretary
Magazine for patients, physicians, public authorities and others with an interest in the field of arthritis. (Price noted paid for yearly subscription) *$12.95*
Bi-Monthly

8235 Fibromyalgia AWARE Magazine
National Fibromyalgia Association
2121 S Towne Centre Pl
suite 30
Orange, CA 92865-6124

714-921-0150
Fax: 714-921-6920
fmaware.org

Lynne Matallana, Editor In Chief
Malina Anderson, CFO
Eroll Landy, Treasurer
Addresses the needs and concerns of people affected by
fibromyalgia and overlapping conditions. *$35.00*
3 times a year

8236 New Mobility
Leonard Media Group
75-20 Astoria Blvd.
East Elmhurst, NY 11370-2068

215-675-9133
888-850-0344
Fax: 215-675-9376
jeff@leonardmedia.com
www.newmobility.com

Amy Blackmore, Vice President Sales
Jean Dobbs, Editorial Director
Tim Gilmer, Editor
Josie Byzek, Managing Editor
The full-service, full-color lifestyle magazine for the disability
community. The award-winning magazine is contemporary, witty
and candid. Produced by professional journalists and visual artists, the magazine's voice is uncompromising and unsentimental,
yet practical, knowing and friendly. The magazine covers issues
that matter to readers: medical news, and cure research; jobs, benefits and civil rights; sports, recreation and travel; product news,
technology and innovation. *$27.95*
Monthly

**8237 PALAESTRA: Forum of Sport, Physical Education and
Recreation for Those with Disabilities**
Challenge Publications Limited
1807 N. Federal Drive
Urbana, IL 61801

217-359-5940
800-327-5557
Fax: 217-359-5975
challpub@macomb.com
www.palaestra.com

David P Beaver EdD, Fonding Editor
Martin.E Block, Editor-in-Chief
Julian U. Stein, Associate Editor
Kathleen Stanton, Asst. Editors
The most comprehensive resource on sport, physical education
and recreation for individuals with disabilities, their parents and
professionals in the field of adapted physical activity. Published
in cooperation with US Paralympics and AAHPERD's Adapted
Physical Activity Council. Informative yet entertaining and delivers valuable insights for consumers, families and
professionals in the field. Published quarterly.

8238 PN/Paraplegia News
PVA Publications
2111 E Highland Ave
Suite 180
Phoenix, AZ 85016-4702

602-224-0500
888-888-2201
Fax: 602-224-0507
www.pn-magazine.com

Richard Hoover, Editor
Ann Santos, Assistant Editor
Packed with timely information on spinal-cord-injury research,
new products, legislation that impacts people with disabilities,
accessible travel, computer options, car/van adaptations, news
for veterans, housing, employment, health care and all issues affecting wheelers and caregivers around the world.

8239 Spirit Magazine
Special Olympics International
1133 19th St NW
Washington, DC 20036-3604

202-628-3630
Fax: 202-824-0200
info@specialolympics.org
www.specialolympics.org

Kathy Smallwood, Editor
Timothy P Shriver PhD, Chariman/CEO
J Brady Lum, President/COO
This magazine reflects the power of Special Olympics to build
bridges between people with and without intellectual disabilities
and spark personal insight, compassion and gratitude for life.
Quarterly

8240 Strides Magazine
North American Riding for the Handicapped Assoc
7475 Dakin Street
Suite 600
Denver, CO 80221-6920

303-452-1212
800-369-7433
Fax: 303-252-4610
narha@narha.org

Carol Nickell, CEO
Sheila Dietrich, Executive Director
William Scebbi, CEO
This engaging magazine is a non-technical, yet accurate journal
that focuses on the work of NARHA. Rider profiles, how-to articles, editorials and instructional columns seek to educate a general readership of the diverse aspects of equine facilitated therapy
and activities. Each seasonal issue carries a theme.
Quarterly

8241 Stroke Connection Magazine
American Stroke Association
7272 Greenville Ave
Dallas, TX 75231-5129

214-373-6300
888-478-7653
Fax: 214-706-1191
www.strokeassociation.org

Ralph Sacco, President/Director
Nancy Brown, CEO
Debra Lockwood, Chairman
From in-depth information on conditions such as aphasia, central
pain, high blood pressure and depression, to tips for daily living
from healthcare professionals and other stroke survivors. Stroke
Connection keeps you abreast of how to cope, how to reduce your
risk of stroke and how to make the most of each day.
6 issues

Print: Newsletters

8242 Arthritis Foundation Great West Region
Arthritis Foundation
115 N.E. 100th St
Suite 350
Seattle, WA 98125

206-547-2707
888-391-9389
Fax: 206-547-2805
tzuehl@arthritis.org
www.arthritis.org

Scott Weaver, CEO
Kelsey Birnbaum, Vice President, Development
Deborah Genge, Vice President, Development
Duane Hille, Development Coordinator
Offers regional updates, information on activities and events, re-
sources and medical research for members.
Newsletter

8243   Arthritis Update
Arthritis Foundation
1330 W. Peachtree St.
Suite 100
Atlanta, GA   30309
404-872-7100
info.uny@arthritis.org
www.arthritis.org

Dan McGowan, Chairman
Rowland W. Chang, Vice Chair
Ann M. Palmer, President and CEO
Patricia N. Nelson, Secretary
Offers chapter updates, information on activities and events, re-
sources and medical research for members.
Newsletter

8244   Focus
Arthritis Foundation
1330 W. Peachtree St.
Suite 100
Atlanta, GA   30309
404-872-7100
info.coh@arthritis.org
www.arthritis.org

Dan McGowan, Chairman
Rowland W. Chang, Vice Chair
Ann M. Palmer, President and CEO
Patricia N. Nelson, Secretary
Offers chapter updates, information on activities and events, re-
sources and medical research for members.
Newsletter

8245   Joint Efforts
Arthritis Foundation
1330 W. Peachtree St.
Suite 100
Atlanta, GA   30309
404-872-7100
800-464-6240
Fax: 415-356-1240
info.nca@arthritis.org
www.arthritis.org

Dan McGowan, Chairman
Rowland W. Chang, Vice Chair
Ann M. Palmer, President and CEO
Patricia N. Nelson, Secretary
Offers chapter updates, information on activities and events, re-
sources and medical research for members.
Newsletter

8246   Post-Polio Newsletter
Post-Polio Health International
4207 Lindell Blvd
Suite 110
Saint Louis, MO   63108-2930
314-534-0475
Fax: 314-534-5070
info@post-polio.org
www.post-polio.org

Joan Headley, Executive Director
Gayla Hoffman, Editor
Contains current information about the late effects of polio, updates about post-polio related and neuromuscular respiratory research, as well as articles that offer practical and useful advice by
experienced survivors and health care professionals. Available
with membership.
12 pages Quarterly

8247   SCILIFE
National Spinal Cord Injury Association
75-20 Astoria Blvd
East Elmhurst, NY   11370
718-803-3782
800-404-2898
Fax: 718-803-0414
info@spinalcord.org
www.unitedspinal.org

David C. Cooper, Chairman
Patrick W. Maher, Vice Chairman
Joseph Gaskins, President and CEO
Denise A. McQuade, Secretary

Filled with issue-driven articles, and news of interest to the SCI
community and the larger disability community.
Bi-monthly

Non Print: Newsletters

8248   A World Awaits You
Mobility International USA
132 E Broadway
Suite 343
Eugene, OR   97401-3155
541-343-1284
Fax: 541-343-6812
clearinghouse@miusa.org
www.miusa.org

Susan Sygall, Executive Director
Includes interviews with people with disabilities who have participated in a wide range of international exchange programs.

8249   ABS Newsletter
American Back Society
2648 International Blvd
Suite 502
Oakland, CA   94601-1547
510-536-9929
Fax: 510-536-1812
info@americanbacksoc.org
www.americanbacksoc.org

Scott Haldeman, President
Aubrey Swartz MD, Executive Director
Keeps subscribers current with timely topics on the diagnosis and
treatment of a wide spectrum of painful and disabling conditions
of the spine.

8250   CurePSP Magazine
Society for Progressive Supranuclear Palsy
2648 International Blvd
Suite 502
Hunt Valley, MD 21031-1002
410-785-7004
800-457-4777
Fax: 410-785-7009
info@curepsp.org
www.psp.org

Richard Gordon Dyne DMin, President
Janet Edmunson, Chair
Dan Johnson, Vice Chair
Informs readers of findings in the area of PSP.

8251   EpilepsyUSA Magazine
Epilepsy Foundation of America
8301 Professional Pl
Landover, MD   20785-2237
301-459-3700
Fax: 301-577-2684
www.epilepsyfoundation.org

Brien J Smith Md, Chair
Mark E Nini, Senior Vice Chair
Richard P Denness, President/CEO
Alexandra K Finucane Esq, Executive Vice President
The Epilepsy Foundation's award-winning magazine,
epilepsyUSA, is published online four times a year. The maga-
zine is one of the only publications of its kind devoted entirely to
news and up-to-the-minute information about epilepsy.

8252   Exchange
ALS Association
27001 Agoura Rd
Suite 250
Agoura Hills, CA   91301-5105
818-340-0182
800-782-4747
Fax: 818-880-9006
www.alsa.org

Gary A Leo, CEO
Morton Charlestein, Chairman
Andrew Soffel, Chairman
Julie Sharpe, Executive Director

Covers a broad range of subjects including stories about the lives of ALS patients, special events, research and public policy in the ALS community.
4-6 times/year

8253 Fibromyalgia Online
National Fibromyalgia Association
2121 S Towne Centre Pl
suite 300
Ornage, CA 92865-6124   714-921-0150
                                    Fax: 714-921-6920
                                    www.fmaware.org

Lynne Matallana, President/Editor In Chief
Malina Anderson, CFO
Eroll Landy, Treasurer
An educational resource for patients and healthcare professionals that brings the latest news on fibrmyalgia and overlapping conditions.
Monthly

8254 MIUSA's Global Impact Newsletter
Mobility International USA
132 E. Broadway
Suite 343
Eugene, OR 97401-2767   541-343-1284
                                    Fax: 541-343-6812
                                    info@miusa.org
                                    www.miusa.org

Susan Sygall, Executive Director
Cindy Lewis, Director
Olivia Hardin, Information Services Coordinator
Each issue features photos, alumni updates, highlights from recent activities, and new publications.
semi-annually

8255 Motivator
Multiple Sclerosis Association of America
706 Haddonfield Rd
Cherry Hill, NJ 8002-2652   856-488-4500
                                    800-532-7667
                                    Fax: 856-661-9797
                                    jmasino@mymsaa.org
                                    www.msassociation.org

Andrea L GriesS, Editor
Susan W Courtney, Sr Writer & Creative Director
Amanda Bednar, Contributing Writer
MSAA's 48-plus page magazine highlights and explains many vital issues of importance to our readers affected by MS. These include cover and feature stories about a variety of topics such as depression, assistive technology, the role of pets and service animals, parents with MS, and clinical trials, to name a few.
48 pages Quarterly

8256 New York Arthritis Reporter
New York Chapter of the Arthritis Foundation
122 East 42nd Street
New York, NY 10168-1898   212-984-8700
                                    Fax: 212-878-5960
                                    info.ny@arthritis.org
                                    www.arthritis.org

Phyllis Geraghty, Editor
Ross Alfieri, President
Daniel T. McGowan, Chair
Provides public access to current arthritis information and resources on important health issues.
Quarterly

8257 SCI Psychosocial Process
American Assoc of Spinal Cord Injury Psych/Soc Wor
75-20 Astoria Blvd
East Elmhurst, NY 11370   718-803-3782
                                    800-404-2898
                                    Fax: 718-803-0414
                                    info@unitedspinal.org
                                    www.unitedspinal.org

David C. Cooper, Chairman
Patrick W. Maher, Vice Chairman
Joseph Gaskins, President and CEO
Denise A. McQuade, Secretary
The purpose of this e journal is disseminating information of value to psychologists, social workers and other psychological caring for spinal cord injured persons.
2 time a year

Non Print: Video

8258 A Wheelchair for Petronilia
Fanlight Productions C/O Icarus Films
32 Court St.
21st Floor
Brooklyn, NY 11201-1731   718-488-8900
                                    800-876-1710
                                    Fax: 718-488-8642
                                    info@fanlight.com
                                    www.fanlight.com

Bob Gliner, Director
Jonathan Miller, President
Meredith Miller, Sales Manager
Anthony Sweeney, Acquisitions
Profiles a program, organized and run by Guatemalans with disabilities, which trains them to manufacture and repair cheap, sturdy wheelchairs designed for conditions in developing countries. 28 Minutes.
VHS/DVD
ISBN 1-572953-98-5

8259 Beyond the Barriers
Aquarius Health Care Videos
30 Forest Road
PO Box 249
Millis, MA 02054   508-376-1244
                                    888-440-2963
                                    Fax: 508-376-1245
                                    www.aquariusproductions.com

Mark Wellman, Director
Leslie Kussmann, President/Producer
For too many years, paraplegics, amputees, quadraplegics and the blind have felt trapped by their disabilities. No more! Mark Wellman and other disabled adventurers, rock climb the desert towers of Utah, sail in British Columbia, body-board the big waves of Pipeline and Waimea Bay, scuba dive with sea lions in Mexico and hand glide the California coast. This film delivers the simple message: Don't give up, and never give in. If you can't ever lose, then you can't ever win. Preview option.
Video/47 Mins

8260 Breathing Lessons: The Life and Work of Mark O'Brien
Fanlight Productions C/O Icarus Films
32 Court St.
21st Floor
Brooklyn, NY 11201-1731   718-488-8900
                                    800-876-1710
                                    Fax: 718-488-8642
                                    info@fanlight.com
                                    www.fanlight.com

Jessica Yu, Director
Jonathan Miller, President
Meredith Miller, Sales Manager
Anthony Sweeney, Acquisitions
Breathing Lessons breaks down barriers to understanding by presenting an honest and intimate portrait of a complex, intelligent,

beautiful and interesting person, who happens to be disabled. *$225.00*
Video/35 Mins 1996
ISBN 1-572958-41-3

8261 Complete Armchair Fitness
CC-M Productions
7755 16th St NW
Washington, DC 20012-1460 202-882-7432
800-453-6280
Fax: 202-882-7432
info@armchairfitness.com
www.armchairfitness.com
Robert Mason, Manager
Armchair Fitness video series. 4 DVDs: Armchair Fitness Aerobic, Armchair Fitness Gentle, Armchair Fitness Strength and Armchair Fitness Yoga. *$120.00*
Video

8262 How Come You Walk Funny?
Fanlight Productions C/O Icarus Films
32 Court St.
21st Floor
Brooklyn, NY 11201-1731 718-488-8900
800-876-1710
Fax: 718-488-8642
info@fanlight.com
www.fanlight.com
Tina Hahn, Director
Jonathan Miller, President
Meredith Miller, Sales Manager
Anthony Sweeney, Acquisitions
Profiles a unique experiment in reverse integration: a school where non disabled kids attend a kindergarten designed for children with physical disabilities. The kids and families tackle their differences and discover common ground through finding a way that all can play. *$179.00*
Video/47 Mins 2004
ISBN 1-572958-84-7

8263 Key Changes: A Portrait of Lisa Thorson
Fanlight Productions C/O Icarus Films
32 Court St.
21st Floor
Brooklyn, NY 11201-1731 718-488-8900
800-876-1710
Fax: 718-488-8642
info@fanlight.com
www.fanlight.com
Cindy Marshall, Director
Jonathan Miller, President
Meredith Miller, Sales Manager
Anthony Sweeney, Acquisitions
A documentary profiling Lisa Thorson, a gifted vocalist who uses a wheelchair. Ms. Thorson defines herself as a performer first, a person with a disability second, and this thoughtful portrait respects that distinction. Her work as a jazz singer is at the heart of the film, reflecting her philosophy that the biggest contribution that she can make to the struggle for the rights of people with disabilities is doing her art the best way she can. *$149.00*
Video/28 Mins 1993
ISBN 1-572959-30-4

8264 Wheelchair Bowling
American Wheelchair Bowling Association
PO Box 69
Clover, VA 24534-69 434-454-2269
Fax: 434-454-6276
garyryan210@gmail.com
www.awba.org
Dick Schaaf, Author
Dave Roberts, Executive Secretary Treasurer
In addition to providing historical background, it includes principles of the game from keeping score through ball drilling for the wheelchair bowler. Through profiles of wheelchair bowlers, the

text covers ball delivery, spare making techniques and special equipment that can be used. *$9.95*
96 pages

8265 Yoga for Arthritis
Mobility Limited
601 Morro Bay Blvd
Suite E
Morro Bay, CA 93442-2000 805-772-3560
800-366-6038
Fax: 805-772-4717
shsh@mobilityltd.com
www.mobilityltd.com
Shoosh Crotzer, Owner/Executive Director
A yoga-based program with five separate segments, which includes breathing and relaxation techniques, stretching and strengthening routines, and aerobic exercises. This 52-minute program can also be performed seated. Available on DVD or VHS; DVD includes Spanish version. *$19.95*
Video

8266 Yoga for MS and Related Conditions
Mobility Limited
601 Morro Bay Blvd
Suite E
Morro Bay, CA 93442-2000 805-772-3560
800-366-6038
Fax: 805-772-4717
shsh@mobilityltd.com
www.mobilityltd.com
Shoosh Crotzer, Owner/Executive Director
A yoga-based program. Shows assisted versions of each exercise for those who require it; is available with an optional Instructional Guidebook with illustrations, alternative positions, and hints. This 48-minute program can also be performed seated. Available on DVD or VHS; DVD includes Spanish version. *$19.95*
Video

Sports

8267 Access to Sailing
423 E Shoreline Village Drive
Long Beach, CA 90802 562-901-9999
www.accesstosailing.org
Duncan Milne, Founder/Executive Director
Cliff Larson, Director
Gaile Oslapas, Assistant Director
Provides therapeutic rehabilitation to disabled and disadvantaged children and adults, through interactive sailing outings.

8268 Achilles Track Club
42 West 38th Street
Suite 400
New York, NY 10018-6241 212-354-0300
Fax: 212-354-3978
info@achillestrackclub.org
Richard Traum PhD, President/Founder
Mary Bryant, Vice President
Kathleen Bateman, Director
Organization whose goal is to guide disabled athletes into the able-bodied community.

8269 Adaptive Sports Center
PO Box 1639
Crested Butte, CO 81224-1639 970-349-2296
866-349-2296
Fax: 970-349-2077
info@adaptivesports.org
www.adaptivesports.org
Christopher Hensley, Executive Director
Chris Read, CTRS Program Director
Ella Fahrlander, Development Director
Erin English, Marketing/Communications Dir.
Year round adaptive, adventure recreation program located at the base of Crested Butte Mountain Resort, Crested Butte ,CO. The

Adaptive Sports Centers provides adaptive downhill and cross country ski lessons, ski rentals and snowboarding lessons in the winter. Offers a variety of wilderness based programs in the summer including multi-day trips into the back country, extensive cycling programs, canoeing, and white water rafting.

8270 American Wheelchair Bowling Association
PO Box 69
Clover, VA 24534-69   434-454-2269
                                         Fax: 434-454-6276
                                  garyryan210@gmail.com
                                           www.awba.org

Joseph L. Fox, Chairman
Wayne Webber, Vice Chairperson
Paul Kenney, Treasurer
Gary Rayan, Secretary
A non-profit organization, composed of wheelchair bowlers, dedicated to encouraging, developing, and regulating wheelchair bowling and wheelchair bowling leagues.

8271 Chesapeake Region Accessible Boating
177 Defense Hwy
Suite 9
Annapolis, MD 21401   410-266-5722
                                     info@crabsailing.org
                                          crabsailing.org

Brad La Tour, President
Paul Bollinger, Jr, Executive Director
Sarah Winchester, Operations Manager
George Pappas, Co-Fleet Director
Chesapeake Region Accessible Boating (CRAB) provides opportunities for the disabled and their friends to sail the Chesapeake Bay. Programs include group sails for organizations representing special guests, sailing clinics and camps, SailFree Sundays for families, and regattas for those who wish to race.

8272 Disabled Sports Program Center
Disabled Sports USA Far West
PO Box 9780
Truckee, CA 96162-7780   530-581-4161
                                         Fax: 530-581-3127
                                  dsusa@disabledsports.net

Doug Pringle, President
Marilyn Cummings,, Office Manager
Haakon Lang-Ree, Manager
Founded in 1967, Disabled Sports USA Far West is dedicated to innovative programs that provide an environment with positive therapeutic and psychological outcomes. Individuals are empowered to reach their full potential. Our programs allow individuals of all abilities to discover their own strengths and interests.

8273 Disabled Sports USA
451 Hungerford Dr
Suite 100
Rockville, MD 20850-5102   301-217-0960
                                         Fax: 301-217-0968
                                     information@dusa.org
                                  www.disabledsportsusa.org
Kirk Bauer, Executive Director
Kathy Chandler, Executive Director
Kathy Celo, Operations
Kathy Laffey, Special Projects Manager
Provides year-round sports and recreation opportunities for people with physical disabilities, veterans and non-veterans alike, such as sanctioned regional and national events in alpine and Nordic skiing, cycling, shooting swimming, table tennis, track and field, volleyball, and weightlifting. The organization handles physical disabilities which restrict mobility, including amputations paraplegia, quadriplegia, cerebral palsy, head injury, mulitple sclerosis, muscular dystrophy, and more.

8274 Disabled Watersports Program
Mission Bay Aquatic Center
1001 Santa Clara Pl
San Diego, CA 92109   858-488-1000
                                         Fax: 858-488-9625
                                           mbac@sdsu.edu
                              www.missionbayaquaticcenter.com

Kevin Starw, Director
Kevin Waldick, Asst. director
Eric Fehrs, Maintenance Director
Amanda Burgess, Office Supervisor
Devoted to providing accessible water sports and recreational opportunities for individuals with disabilities. Specially designed equipment makes water skiing, wake boarding, keelboat sailing, windsurfing, rowing, surfing, and kayaking possible for people with varying levels of mobility and ability.

8275 Galvin Health and Fitness Center
Rehabilitation Institute of Chicago
345 East Suuperior St.
Chicago, IL 60611   312-238-1000
                                              800-354-7342
                                              800-354-REHA
                                         Fax: 312-238-5017
                                           sports@ric.org
                                        http://www.ric.org

Jude Reyes, Chair
Mike P. Kransy, Vice Chair
Thomas Reynolds III, Vice Chair
Joanne C. Smith, President & CEO
The RIC Sports and Fitness Program offers people with physical disabilities an on-site fitness center, specialized exercise classes and services, and adult and junior competitive and recreational sports opportunities, including the recreational/social Caring for Kids program for youth ages 7-17. Most programs are provided free of charge or for a nominal fee.

8276 Guide to Wheelchair Sports and Recreation
Paralyzed Veterans of America
801 18th St NW
Washington, DC 20006-3517   202-872-1300
                                              800-424-8200
                                              888-888-2201
                                         Fax: 202-785-4432
                                        TTY:800-795-4327
                                           info@pva.org
                                            www.pva.org

Homer S. Townsend, Jr., Executive Director
Larry Dodson, National Secretary
Bill Lawson, National President
Al Kovach, Jr, Natonal Senior Vice President
This guide is published to introduce and increase awareness of people with disabilities to the many sports and recreational opportunities available. It lists descriptions of adaptive sports and recreation, activity and equipment directories, and additional resources for people with disabilities.
28 pages Booklet

8277 Handicapped Scuba Association International
Handicapped Scuba Association
1104 El Prado
San Clemente, CA 92672-4637   949-498-4540
                                         Fax: 949-498-6128
                                         hsa@hsascuba.com
                                         www.hsascuba.com

Jim Gatacre, President
Patricia Derk, Vice President
A nonprofit volunteer organization dedicated to improving the physical and social well being of those with special needs through the exhilarating sport of scuba diving. An educational program for able bodied scuba instructors to learn to teach and certify people with special needs. Accessible travel opportunities.

8278 Lakeshore Foundation
4000 Ridgeway Dr
Birmingham, AL   35209-5563   205-313-7400
                                         Fax: 205-313-7475
                                         information@lakeshore.org
                                         www.lakeshore.org

Jeff Underwood, President & CEO
Beth Curry, Chief Program Officer
Jen Remick, Director, Communications & Membership
Damian Veazey, Associate Director, Communications
Promotes independence for persons with physically disabling
conditions and provides opportunities to pursue active, healthy
lifestyles.

8279 National Disability Sports Alliance
25 W Independence Way
Kingston, RI   02881-1124   401-792-7130
                                         Fax: 401-792-7132
                         http://nationaldisabilitysportsalliance.webs.
Jerry McCole, Executive Director
Serves to present disabled athletes with the opportunity to perform in many different sports. Participants range from the beginning athlete to the elite, international caliber athlete.

8280 National Skeet Shooting Association
5931 Roft Rd
San Antonio, TX   78253-9261   210-688-3371
                                              800-877-5338
                                         Fax: 210-688-3014
                                         nsca@nssa-nsca.com
                                         www.mynssa.com

Michael Hampton, Jr., Executive Director
Royce Graff, NSSA Director
Amber Schwarz, NSC Assistant Director
Linda Mayes, NSSA Director
Offers information on sporting clay targets for the disabled
hunter.

8281 National Sports Center for the Disabled
33 Parsenn Rd
PO Box 1290
Winter Park, CO   80482   970-726-1518
                                         Fax: 970-726-4112
                                         volunteer@nscd.org
                                         nscd.org

Kim Easton, President & CEO
Diane Eustace, Marketing Director
Beth Fox, Outreach & Education Director
Erica Mays, Human Resources Director
The center's mission is to provide quality outdoor sports and therapeutic recreation programs that positively impact the lives of
people with physical, cognitive, emotional, or behavioral challenges. Winter programming includes alpine skiing,
snowboarding, ski racing, show shoeing, and cross-country skiing. Summer sports include rafting, sailing, kayaking, camping,
hiking, horseback riding, fishing, and rock climbing.
6-8 pages Quarterly

8282 National Wheelchair Poolplayers Association
90 Flemons Dr
Somerville, AL   35670   256-778-0449
                                         Fax: 703-817-1215
                                         www.nwpainc.org

Jeffrey Dolezal, President
Bob Calderon, Secretary
Ken Force, Editor
Works together with other groups, organizations, and tourna-
ments to update rules to include wheelchair players.

8283 North American Riding for the Handicapped Association
7475 Dakin Street
Suite 600
Denver, CO   80221-6920   303-452-1212
                                              800-369-7433
                                         Fax: 303-252-4610
                                         www.pathintl.org
Sheila Dietrich, Executive Director
Carolyn Malcheski,, Director of Finance and Human Resources
Kaye Marks, Director of Marketing and Communications
Kay Green, Chief Executive Officer
Professional Association of Therapeutic Horsemanship Interna-
tional (PATH Intl.), a federally-registered 501(c3) nonprofit, was
formed in 1969 as the North American Riding for the Handicapped Association to promote equine-assisted activities and
therapies (EAAT) for individuals with special needs. *$35.00*
42 pages Quarterly

8284 Ontario Cerebral Palsy Sports Association
P.O. Box 60082
Ottawa, ON, Canada   K1T-0K9   613-723-1806
                                              866-286-2772
                                         Fax: 613-723-6742

Amanda Fader, Executive Director
Don Sinclair, President
Lorette Dupuis, Vice President
Sue Bartol, Development Director
Organization that provides, promotes and coordinates competitive opportunities as well as encourages individual excellence
through sport for athletes within the cerebral palsy family. To that
end, OCPSA recruits, develops and supports athletes, coaches
and volunteers.

8285 Special Olympics
1133 19th St NW
Washington, DC   20036-3604   202-393-1251
                                         Fax: 202-715-1146
                                         info@specialolympics.org
                                         www.specialolympics.org
Timothy P Shriver PhD, Chariman/CEO
J Brady Lum, President/COO
Stephen M Carter, Lead Director/CEO/Vice Chair
A year-round worldwide program that promotes physical fitness,
sports training and athletic competition for children and adults
with intellectual disabilities.

8286 Special Olympics International
1133 19th St NW
Washington, DC   20036-3604   202-393-1251
                                         Fax: 202-715-1146
                                         info@specialolympics.org
                                         www.specialolympics.org
Timothy P Shriver PhD, Chariman/CEO
J Brady Lum, President/COO
Stephen M Carter, Lead Director/CEO/Vice Chair
Provides year-round training and athletic competition in a variety
of well-coached, Olympic-type sparts for persons with mental retardation. Offers opportunities to develop physical fitness, prepare for entry into school and community sports programs.
Athletes express courage, experience joy and participate in gifts,
skills and friendship with their families and other Special Olympics athletes. Local information can be provided by regional
offices.

8287 US Paralympics
United States Olympic Committee
1 Olympic Plaza
Colorado Springs, CO   80909   719-866-2030
                                              888-222-2313
                                         Fax: 719-866-2029
                                         customerservice@donorsupportusoc.org
                                         www.teamusa.org/us-paralympics

Scott Blackmun, CEO
Alan Ashley, Chief of Sport Performance
Lisa Baird, Chief Marketing Officer
Morane Kerek, Chief Financial Officer

A division of the US Olympic Committee focused on enhancing programs, funding and opportunities for persons with physical disabilities to participate in Paralympic sports.

8288   United Foundation for Disabled Archers
20 NE 9th Ave. Glenwood,
PO Box 251
Glenwood, MN 56334- 251   320-634-3660
                                            info@uffdaclub.com
                                            www.uffdaclub.com

Daniel James Hendricks, President
Russ Kalk, Vice President
Debbie Kalk, Treasurer
It is the mission of the United Foundation for Disabled Archers to promote and provide a means to practice all forms of archery for any physically challenged person.

8289   Wheelchair Sports, USA
PO Box 5266
Kendall Park, NJ   08824-5266   732-266-2634
                                          Fax: 732-355-6500

Kelly Behlmann, Owner
Gregg Baumgraten, Chairperson
Denise Hutchins, Vice-Chairperson
Jessica Galli, Secretary
Initiates, stimulates and promotes the growth and development of wheelchair sports.

Support Groups

8290   Information Hotline
Arthritis Foundation, Southeast Region Inc
1330 W. Peachtree St.
Suite 100
Atlanta, GA   30309   404-872-7100
                                           800-933-7023
                                           Fax: 404-237-8153
                                           info.ga@arthritis.org
                                           www.arthritis.org

Dan McGowan, Chairman
Rowland W. Chang, Vice Chair
Ann M. Palmer, President and CEO
Patricia N. Nelson, Secretary
The mission of the Arthritis Foundation is to improve lives through leadership in the prevention, control and cure of arthritis and related diseases.

8291   Kids on the Block Programs
9385 Gerwig Lane
Suite C
Maryland, MD   21157-2893   410-290-9095
                                           800-368-5437
                                           Fax: 410-290-9358
                                           kob@kotb.com
                                           www.kotb.com

Aric Darroe, President
Jane Thuman, Vice President
Christina Grogan, Marketing Manager
Features life-size puppets in educational programs that enlighten children and adults on the issues of disability awareness, medical and educational differences, and social concerns.

General Disorders

Associations

8292 AIDS United
1424 K Street, N.W.
Ste 200
Washington, DC 20005-1511   202-408-4848
888-234-2437
Fax: 202-408-1818
info@aidsunited.org
www.aidsunited.org

Jesse Milan Jr., JD, Interim President & CEO
Matthew J. Kessler, Vice President, Operations
Cody Barnett, Commuications Coordinator
Monique Tula, Vice President, Programs
AIDS United advocates for people living with or affected by
HIV/AIDS and the organizations that serve them. AIDS United's
mission is to end the AIDS epidemic in the United States through
strategic grantmaking, capacity building, policy/advocacy, tech-
nical assistance and formative research.

8293 American Academy of Allergy, Asthma & Immunology
555 E Wells St.
Ste 1100
Milwaukee, WI 53202-3823   414-272-6071
Fax: 414-272-6070
info@aaaai.org
www.aaaai.org

Thomas A. Fleisher, M.D.; FAAAAI, President
An association of medical professionals and specialists that
places focus on research and treatment for allergic and immunologic diseases, as well as improved patient care.

**8294 American Academy of Otolaryngology - Head and Neck
Surgery**
1650 Diagonal Rd
Alexandria, VA 22314-2857   703-836-4444
Fax: 703-683-5100
TTY:703-519-1585
www.entnet.org

James c. Denneny III, M.D., Executive Vice President & CEO
Sujana S. Chandrasekhar, M.D., President
Carol R. Bradford, Director, Academic
Michael D. Seidman, Director, Academic
The American Academy of Otolaryngology-Head and Neck Sur-
gery (AAO-HNS) is an organization representing specialists who
treat the ear, nose, throat, and related structures of the head and
neck.

8295 American Academy of Physical Medicine and Rehabilitation
9700 W Bryn Mawr Ave
Ste 200
Rosemont, IL 60018-5701   847-737-6000
877-227-6799
Fax: 847-737-6001
info@aapmr.org
www.aapmr.org
*Thomas E. Stautzenbach, Executive Director & Chief Executive Of-
ficer*
Gregory M. Worsowicz, President
Darryl L. Kaelin, Vice President
This national medical specialty society represents more than
6,500 physical medicine and rehabilitation physicians, whose patients include people with physical disabilities and chronic, disabling illnesses. The academy's mission is to maximize quality of
life, minimize the incidence and prevalence of impairments and
disability, promote societal health and enhance the understanding and development of the specialty. The organization offers
information, referrals, and patient materials.

8296 American Association for Respiratory Care
9425 N. MacArthur Blvd.
Ste 100
Irving, TX 75063-4706   972-243-2272
Fax: 972-484-2720
info@aarc.org
www.aarc.org

Tom Kallstrom, Executive Director
Steve Bowden, IT, General Inquiries
AARC's mission is to advance the science, technology, ethics and
art of respiratory care through research and education for its
members and to teach the general public about pulmonary health
and disease prevention.

**8297 American Association of Cardiovascular and Pulmonary
Rehabilitation**
330 N. Wabash Avenue
Suite 2200
Chicago, IL 60611   312-321-5146
Fax: 312-673-6924
aacvpr@aacvpr.org
www.aacvpr.org

Adam T. deJong, President
Megan Cohen, Executive Director
Jessica Eustice, Director Of Corporate Relations
Abigail Lynn, Operations Senior Manager
The mission of American Association of Cardiovascular and Pulmonary Rehabilitation is to reduce morbidity, mortality, and disability from cardiovascular and pulmonary diseases through
education, prevention, rehabilitation, research, and aggressive
disease management.

8298 American Brain Tumor Association
8550 W. Bryn Mawr Ave
Ste 550
Chicago, IL 60631-4106   773-577-8750
800-886-2282
Fax: 773-577-8738
info@abta.org
www.abta.org

Elizabeth Wilson, President & CEO
Martha Carlos, Chief Communications Officer
Kerri Mink, Chief Operating Officer
Sandy Abraham, Director, Marketing & Communications
A non-profit organization founded in 1973 dedicated to the elimi-
nation of brain tumors through research and patient education
services.

8299 American Diabetes Association
1701 N Beauregard St
Alexandria, VA 22311-1733   703-549-1500
800-342-2383
Fax: 703-836-7439
askada@diabetes.org
www.diabetes.org

Kevin L. Hagan, Chief Executive Officer
*Margaret Powers, PhD; RD; CDE, President, Health Care & Edu-
cation*
Provides diabetes research, information and advocacy. The mission of the Association is to prevent and cure diabetes and to improve the lives of all people affected by diabetes.

8300 American Group Psychotherapy Association
25 E. 21st St.
6th Floor
New York, NY 10010-6207   212-477-2677
877-668-2472
Fax: 212-979-6627
info@agpa.org
www.agpa.org

Marsha S. Block, Chief Executive Officer
Eleanor F. Counselman, EdD; CGP, President
Nina Brown, Secretary
AGPA serves as the national voice specific to the interests of
group psychotherapy. Its 4,100 members and 31 affiliate societies
provide a wealth of professional, educational and social support
for group psychotherapists in the United States and around the
world.

8301 **American Head and Neck Society**
11300 W. Olympic Blvd
Ste 600
Los Angeles, CA 90064-1663   310-437-0559
Fax: 310-437-0585
www.ahns.info

Dennis Kraus, MD, President
Jonathan Irish, MD, Vice President
Brian B. Burkey, MD; MEd, Secretary
Ehab Hanna, Treasurer
AHNS is a professional organization, formed in 1998 to promote research and education in head and neck oncology. The AHNS offers clinical practice guidelines, details of events, grants, and patient information. It aims to promote and advance the knowledge of prevention, diagnosis, treatment, and rehabilitation of neoplasms and other diseases of the head and neck.

8302 **American Lung Association**
55 W. Wacker Dr.
Ste 1150
Chicago, IL 60601   312-781-1100
800-548-8252
Fax: 202-452-1085
info@lung.org
www.lung.org

Harold P. Wimmer, President & CEO
Sue . Swan, National Chief Development Officer
Sally Draper, National Vice President, Development
Kim Lacina, National Vice President, Marketing & Communications
The ALA is an organization dedicated to combating tobacco use, eliminating lung diseases, and improving air quality through research, education, and advocacy. The association provides knowledge beneficial to patients, patients' families, and medical professionals and specialists.

8303 **American SIDS Institute**
528 Raven Way
Naples, FL 34110   239-431-5425
Fax: 239-431-5536
prevent@sids.org
www.sids.org

Marc Peterzell, JD, Chairman
Betty McEntire, PhD, Executive Director & CEO
Nicole Dobson, MD, Board Member
Alfred Steinschneider, MD, President Emeritus
American SIDS Institute is a national nonprofit health care organization that is dedicated to the prevention of sudden infant death and the promotion of infant health through an aggressive, comprehensive nationwide program of research, clinical services, education and family support.

8304 **American Sexual Health Association**
P.O. Box 13827
Research Triangle Park, NC 27709-3827   919-361-8400
Fax: 919-361-8425
info@ashasexualhealth.org
www.ashastd.org

Lynn Barclay, President & CEO
Deborah Arrindell, Vice President, Health Policy
The American Sexual Health Association is a trusted source of information on sexual health, relationships, and measures to prevent adverse sexual health

8305 **American Society of Pediatric Hematology/Oncology**
8735 West Higgins Rd.
Ste. 300
Chicago, IL 60631   847-375-4716
Fax: 847-375-6483
info@aspho.org
www.aspho.org

Sally Weir, Executive Director
Steve Biddle, Education Consultant
Jackie Holcomb, Education Manager
Sergio Miranda, Memeber Services
ASPHO is multidisciplinary organization dedicated to promoting optimal care of children and adolescents with blood disorders and

cancer by advancing research, education, treatment and professional practice.

8306 **American Thoracic Society**
25 Broadway
18th Floor
New York, NY 10004-2755   212-315-8600
Fax: 212-315-6498
atsinfo@thoracic.org
www.thoracic.org

Steve Crane, Executive Director
Nicola Black, Associate Director, Governance Activities
Jennifer A. Ian, Director, Member Services & Chapter Relations
Eileen Larsson, Chief Program Officer
The American Thoracic Society is dedicated to research, public health education, and patient care in relation to pulmonary disease, critical illness, and sleep disorders.

8307 **Aplastic Anemia and MDS International Foundation**
100 Park Ave
Ste 108
Rockville, MD 20850   301-279-7202
800-747-2820
Fax: 301-279-7205
help@aamds.org
www.aamds.org

John Huber, Executive Director
Angie Onofre, Director of Patient Programs and Services
Leigh Clark, Patient Educator
Benita Marcus, Senior Director Of Operations
This organization, formerly known as Aplastic Anemia Foundation of America, provides a resource directory for patient assistance, produces educational material and supports research into AA and MDS.

8308 **Arizona Hemophilia Association**
826 North 5th Ave
Phoenix, AZ 85003   602-955-3947
info@hemophiliaz.org
www.arizonahemophilia.org

Cindy Komar, Chief Executive Officer
Chelsea Bolyard, Program Director
Yleana Highes, Director, Client Services
The Arizona Hemophilia Association (AHA) is a volunteer based nonprofit organization working to support, educate, and advocate for families affected by bleeding disorders in Arizona.

8309 **CPATH Cerebral Palsy Awareness Transition Hope**
5501A Balcones
Suite 160
Austin, TX 78731   866-742-7284
info@cpathtexas.com
www.cpathtexas.com

Victoria Polega, President
Marielle Deckard, Secretary
Jamie Eppele, Director of Development
Ilona McCauley, Public Relations
CPATH is a non-profit organization whose mission is to provide resources, support, and financial assistance to families and individuals living with cerebral palsy.

8310 **Canadian Cancer Society**
55 St. Clair Avenue W.
Ste 300
Toronto, ON, Canada M4V- 2Y7   416-961-7223
888-939-3333
Fax: 416-961-4189
TTY:866-786-3934
ccs@cancer.ca
www.cancer.ca

Anne V,zina, Interim President & CEO
Martin Kabat, Chief Executive Officer
Lesley Ring, Vice President, Development & Marketing
A national community-based organization of volunteers whose mission is the eradication of cancer and the enhancement of the quality of life for people living with cancer.

8311 Canadian Diabetes Association
1400-522 University Ave
Toronto, ON, Canada   M5G-2R5   416-363-3373
800-226-8464
Fax: 416-408-7015
info@diabetes.ca
www.diabetes.ca

Doug Macnamara, President & CEO
Paul Kilbertus, Senior Director, Strategic Communications
The mission of the Canadian Diabetes Association is to promote the health of Canadians through diabetes research, education, service and advocacy.

8312 Canadian Lung Association
1750 Courtwood Cres.
Ottawa, ON, Canada   K2C-2B5   613-569-6411
888-566-5864
Fax: 613-569-8860
info@lung.ca
www.lung.ca

Terry Dean, President & CEO
The Canadian Lung Association is a non-profit and volunteer-based health charity, dedicated to improving lung health in the Canadian community through research, education, prevention and advocacy.

8313 Childhood Cancer Canada Foundation
21 St. Clair Ave E
Ste 801
Toronto, ON, Canada   M4T-1L9   416-489-6440
800-363-1062
Fax: 416-489-9812
info@childhoodcancer.ca
www.childhoodcancer.ca

Clare Davenport, President & CEO
Natasha Bowes, Senior Manager, Fund Development
Patricia Zareba, Fund Development Manager
Jessica MacInnis, Manager of Marketing & Communications
A national, volunteer governed, charitable organization dedicated to improving the quality of life for children with cancer. The foundation raises funds to assist with cancer research undertakings across Canada.

8314 Childhood Leukemia Foundation
807 Mantoloking Rd
Brick, NJ 08723   732-920-8860
888-253-7109
www.clf4kids.org

Barbara Haramis, Executive Director & Founder
Barb Estelle, Chief Operating Officer
Kim Wetmore, Director, Development
Kate Booth, Program Services Coordinator
The CLF is a national, non-profit organization providing education, information, support, and advocacy for patients of cancer and their families. the foundation works closesly with health professionals, social workers, and specialists to offer a variety of programs that aim to enrich the lives of children living with cancer.

8315 Division for Physical, Health & Multiple Disabilities
Council for Exceptional Children
2900 Crystal Dr.
Ste 1000
Arlington, VA 22202   888-232-7733
Fax: 703-264-9494
TTY:866-915-5000
www.community.cec.sped.org/dphmd/home

Pat Kuntzler, President
Angie Juarez, Vice President
Mari Beth Coleman, Communications
Laura Clarke, Policy & Advocacy Committee
This division of the CEC advocates for the provision of quality education for individuals with physical disabilities, multiple disabilities, and special health care needs served in schools, hospitals, or home settings. DPHMD's members include classroom teachers, administrators, related service personnel, hospital/homebound teachers, and parents.

8316 Emphysema Foundation for Our Right to Survive
PO Box 20241
Kansas City, MO 64119-0241   866-363-2673
efforts-request@effortslist.org
www.emphysema.net

Linda Watson, President
Debbie Snodell, Secretary
EFFORTS is a non-profit organization that takes an active role in promoting research for more effective treatments and perhaps a cure for emphysema and related lung diseases. It also works to further education about the disease and provides a support mailing list for members.

8317 Environmental Health Center: Dallas
8345 Walnut Hill Lane
Ste 220
Dallas, TX 75231-4205   214-368-4132
Fax: 214-691-8432
contact@ehcd.com
www.ehcd.com

William J Rea, Director
Chris Rea, Business Manager
Yaqin Pan, M.D., Research Physician
Bertie Griffiths, Ph.D., Microbiologist/Immunologist
Clinic providing patient care in the areas of Immunotherapy, Nutrition, Physical Therapy, Chemical Depuration, Energy Balancing, Electromagnetic Sensitivity Testing, Psychological Support Services, Family Practice Medicine and Internal Medicine. Provides services for individuals whose diseases are caused by environmental factors.

8318 Epilepsy Foundation of Alabama
3929 Airport Blvd
Suite 3-310
Mobile, AL 36609-2235   251-341-0170
800-626-1582
info@efala.org
www.efala.org

Donna Dodson, Executive Director
Paige Norris, Outreach & Program Director
David Toenes, Director, Client Services
Kelly Morris, Board President
The Epilepsy Foundation of Alabama provides health service programs and public education on behalf of people with seizures and epilepsy. Some of their services include emergency medication assistance, information referral, training, employer education, and camping trips.

8319 Eunice Kennedy Shriver National Institute of Child Health and Human Development (NICHD)
National Institutes of Health (NIH)
31 Center Dr.
Bldg 31, Rm 2A32
Bethesda, MD 20892-2425   301-496-5097
800-370-2943
Fax: 866-760-5947
TTY: 888-320-6942
nichdinformationresourcecenter@mail.nih.gov
www.nichd.nih.gov

Diana W. Bianchi, Director
The Eunice Kennedy Shriver National Institute of Child Health and Human Development, part of the federal National Institutes of Health, conducts and supports basic, translational, and clinical research in the biomedical, behavioral, and social sciences related to child and maternal health, in medical rehabilitation, and in the reproductive sciences.

8320 Herpes Resource Center
American Social Health Association
P.O. Box 13827
Research Triangle Park, NC 27709-3827   919-361-8400
800-227-8922
Fax: 919-361-8425
customerservice@ashastd.org
www.ashastd.org/stdsstis/herpes/

Lynn Barclay, President & CEO

The Herpes Resource Center (HRC) focuses on increasing education, public awareness, and support to anyone concerned about herpes.

8321 IKUS Life Enrichment Services
O-1859 Lake Michigan Dr NW
Grand Rapids, MI 49534
616-677-5251
Fax: 616-677-2955
info@ikuslife.org
www.ikuslife.org

Tim Hileman, Executive Director
Mary Allis, Camp Director & Respite Coordinator
Amy DeMott, Director, Programs & Services
IKUS Life Enrichment Services helps individuals with disabilities learn new skills and experience greater freedom by providing support, recreation and educational services. IKUS also works to serve the natural support systems by offering respite services to caregivers and families.

8322 International Academy of Biological Dentistry and Medicine
19122 Camellia Bend Circle
Suite 101
Spring, TX 77379
281-651-1745
Fax: 281-651-1745
drdawn@drdawn.net
www.iabdm.org

Dr. Dawn Ewing, Executive Director
The IABDM promotes non-toxic diagnostic and therapeutic approaches in dentistry and hosts seminars on biological diagnosis and therapy.

8323 International Academy of Oral Medicine & Toxicology
8297 ChampionsGate Blvd
Ste 193
ChampionsGate, FL 33896-8387
863-420-6373
Fax: 863-419-8136
info@iaomt.org
www.iaomt.org

Mark Wisniewski, President
Tammy DeGregorio, Executive Vice President
Kym Smith, Executive Director
A non-profit organization dedicated to funding solid peer-reviewed scientific research in the area of toxic substances used in dentistry as well as providing continuing education and carefully reviewed procedures, protocols, and methodologies to reduce the risk for patients and professionals.

8324 International Association for Cancer Victors & Friends
P.O. Box 745
Lakeport, CA 95453
408-834-5300
Fax: 408-264-9659
contact@cancervictors.net
www.cancervictors.net

a.k.a. Cancer Victors & Friends

8325 International Association of Hygienic Physicians
4620 Euclid Blvd
Youngstown, OH 44512-1633
330-788-0526
Fax: 330-788-0093
www.iahp.net

Alec Burton, Co-Founder
Mark A. Huberman, Secretary/Treasurer
The International Association of Hygienic Physicians (IAHP) is a professional association for licensed, primary care physicians (Medical Doctors, Osteopaths, Chiropractors, and Naturopaths) who specialize in Therapeutic Fasting Supervision as an integral part of Hygienic Care.

8326 International Medical and Dental Hypnotherapy Association
8852 SR 3001
RR 2
Laceyville, PA 18623-9417
570-869-1021
800-553-6886
Fax: 570-869-1249
www.hypnosisalliance.com/imdha

Linda Otto, Executive Director
Robert Otto, President & CEO
Christie Boecker, Membership Services Coordinator
The association provides and encourages education programs to further, the knowledge, understanding, and application of hypnosis in complementary healthcare; encourages research and scientific publication in the field of hypnosis; and advocates for further recognition and acceptance of hypnosis as an important tool in healthcare and focus for scientific research.

8327 International Myeloma Foundation
12650 Riverside Dr
Ste 206
North Hollywood, CA 91607- 3421
818-487-7455
800-452-2873
Fax: 818-487-7454
theimf@myeloma.org
www.myeloma.org

David Girard, Executive Director
Susie Novis, President
Diane Moran, Senior Vice President, Strategic Planning
Selma Plascencia, Director of Operations
The IMF serves myeloma patients, family members, and the medical community, offering a wide range of programs in the areas of Research, Education, Support, and Advocacy.

8328 Leukemia & Lymphoma Society
3 International Dr
Ste 200
Rye Brook, NY 10573
914-949-5213
800-955-4572
Fax: 914-949-6691
supportservices@lls.org
www.lls.org

Louis DeGennaro, President & CEO
Piper Medcalf, Executive Director
Nancy Hallberg, Chief Marketing Officer
Marcie Klein, Senior Vice President, Communications
The Leukemia and Lymphoma Society is the world's largest voluntary health organization dedicated to funding blood cancer research, education and patient services. The society offers information and support for patients of various blood cancer types, including leukemia, lymphoma, Hodgkin's disease and myeloma. It also offers services and resources to help improve the quality of life of patients and their families.

8329 Little People of America
250 El Camino Real
Ste 218
Tustin, CA 92780
714-368-3689
888-572-2001
Fax: 714-368-3367
info@lpaonline.org
www.lpaonline.org

Joanna Campbell, Executive Director
Gary Arnold, President
April Brazier, Senior Vice President
Mark Povinelli, Membership Director
Little People of America is a national non-profit organization that provides support and information to people of short stature and their families. Short stature is generally caused by one of the more than 200 medical conditions known as dwarfism. LPA offers information on employment, education, disability rights, adoption, medical issues, clothing, adaptive products, and the many stages of parenting a short-statured child - from birth to adult.

8330 **Lymphoma Canada**
Formerly The Lymphoma Foundation Canada
6860 Century Ave
Ste 202
Mississauga, ON, Canada   L5N-2W5   905-858-5967
                                          866-659-5556
                                          info@lymphoma.ca
                                          www.lymphoma.ca

Robin Markowitz, Chief Executive Officer
Lorna Warwick, National Director, Education & Services
Charlene Ragin, Marketing & Communications
Anwar Knight, Director, Mississauga, ON
Lymphoma Canada provides, at no cost and in both official languages: electronic and print materials on the Hodgkin lymphoma, non-Hodgkin lymphoma and CLL, peer and caregiver support groups, educational forums and advocacy on behalf of patients. Lymphoma Canada also funds Canadian research.

8331 **Merrimack Hall Performing Arts Center**
3320 Triana Blvd SW.
Huntsville, AL   35805   256-534-6455
                                          info@merrimackhall.com
                                          www.merrimackhall.com

8332 **Myositis Association**
1737 King Street
Ste 600
Alexandria, VA   22314   703-299-4850
                                          800-821-7356
                                          Fax: 703-535-6752
                                          tma@myositis.org
                                          www.myositis.org

Bob Goldberg, Executive Director
Theresa Reynolds Curry, Communications Manager
Aisha Morrow, Operations Manager
Charlia Sanchez, Member Services Coordinator
The aim of TMA's programs and services is to provide information, support, advocacy and research for those concerned about myositis, as well as serving those affected by these diseases. Support groups offer members the chance to share and discuss their concerns with people in similar situations.

8333 **National Association for Children of Alcoholics**
10920 Connecticut Ave
Ste 100
Kensington, MD   20895-3007   301-468-0985
                                          888-554-2627
                                          Fax: 301-468-0987
                                          nacoa@nacoa.org
                                          www.nacoa.org

Sis Wenger, President & CEO
Steve Hornberger, Program Director
National non-profit membership and affiliate organization working on behalf of children of alcohol and drug dependent parents to help eliminate the adverse impact of drug use on children through public awareness, policy, advocacy, education, and support.

8334 **National Association for Home Care & Hospice**
228 7th St SE
Washington, DC   20003-4306   202-547-7424
                                          Fax: 202-547-3540
                                          webmaster@nahc.org
                                          www.nahc.org

Val J. Halamandris, President
Lucy Andrews, Vice Chair
Karen Marshall Thompson, Secretary
Thomas Moreland, Treasurer
This is a non-profit trade association representing various home care, hospice and health aid organizations. With services aimed at assiting the chronically ill and disabled, the NAHC offers information on how to choose a home care provider and a zip code driven locator for home care and hospice.

8335 **National Association for Medical Direction of Respiratory Care**
8618 Westwood Center Dr
Ste 210
Vienna, VA   22182-2273   703-752-4359
                                          Fax: 703-752-4360
                                          execoffice@namdrc.org
                                          www.namdrc.org

Phillip Porte, Executive Director
Vickie Parshall, Director, Member Services
Karen Lui, RN, Associate Executive Director
NAMDRC's primary mission is to improve access to quality care for patients with respiratory disease by removing regulatory and legislative barriers to appropriate treatment.

8336 **National Association for Proton Therapy**
1155 15th St NW
Ste 500
Washington, DC   20005   202-495-3133
                                          Fax: 202-530-0659
                                          info@proton-therapy.org
                                          www.proton-therapy.org

Leonard Arzt, Executive Director
The National Association for Proton Therapy (NAPT) is registered as an independent, non-profit, public benefit corporation providing education and awareness for the public, professional and governmental communities. It promotes the therapeutic benefits of proton therapy for cancer treatment in the U.S. and abroad.

8337 **National Association of Anorexia Nervosa and Associated Disorders**
750 E Diehl Road
Ste 127
Naperville, IL   60563   630-577-1333
                                          Fax: 847-433-4632
                                          anadhelp@anad.org
                                          www.anad.org

Laura Zinger, Executive Director
Deb Prinz, Director, Community Relations
A non-profit organization that seeks to alleviate the problems of eating disorders, especially anorexia nervosa and bulimia nervosa, by promoting eating disorder awareness, prevention and recovery through supporting, educating, and connecting individuals, families and professionals.

8338 **National Association of Chronic Disease Directors**
2200 Century Parkway
Ste 250
Atlanta, GA   30345   770-458-7400
                                          Fax: 770-458-7401
                                          jrobitscher@chronicdisease.org
                                          www.chronicdisease.org

John w. Robitscher, Chief Executive Officer
Namvar Zohoori, President
John Patton, Director, Communications
Margaret Gillan Ritchie, Communications & Member Services Coordinator
A national public health association founded in 1988 to link the chronic disease program directors of each state and U.S. territory to provide a national forum for chronic disease prevention and control efforts. NACDD aims to mobilize national efforts to reduce chronic diseases and the associated risk factors.

8339 **National Association to Advance Fat Acceptance**
P.O. Box 4662
Foster City, CA   94404-0662   916-558-6880
                                          Fax: 916-558-6881
                                          www.naafaonline.com

8340   National Cancer Institute
National Institutes Of Health
9609 Medical Center Drive
Ste 300
Rockville, MD   20850   301-496-0909
                                                      800-422-6237
                                                 TTY:800-332-8615
                                        cancergovstaff@mail.nih.gov
                                                    www.cancer.gov

Douglas R. Lowy, Acting Director
The National Cancer Institute coordinates the National Cancer Program, which conducts and supports research, training, health information dissemination, and other programs with respect to the cause, diagnosis, prevention, and treatment of cancer, rehabilitation from cancer, and the continuing care of cancer patients and the families of cancer patients.

8341   National Diabetes Information Clearinghouse
National Institutes of Health
1 Information Way
Bethesda, MD   20892-3560   800-860-8747
                                                  Fax: 703-738-4929
                                                 TTY:866-569-1162
                                           ndic@info.niddk.nih.gov
                                          www.diabetes.niddk.nih.gov

Griffin Rodgers, Director
Gregory Germino, Deputy Director
An information and referral service of the National Institute of Diabetes and Digestive and Kidney Diseases, one of the National Institutes of Health. The clearinghouse responds to written inquiries, develops and distributes publications about diabetes, and provides referrals to diabetes organizations, including support groups. The NDIC maintains a database of patient and professional education materials, from which literature searches are generated.

8342   National Digestive Diseases Information Clearinghouse
National Institutes of Health
2 Information Way
Bethesda, MD   20892-3570   301-654-3810
                                                      800-891-5389
                                                  Fax: 703-738-4929
                                                 TTY: 866-559-1162
                                           nddic@info.niddk.nih.gov
                                          www.digestive.niddk.nih.gov

Griffin Rodgers, Director
Information and referral service of the National Institute of Diabetes and Digestive and Kidney Diseases. A central information resource on the prevention and management of digestive diseases, the clearinghouse responds to written inquiries, develops and distributes publications about digestive diseases, provides referrals to digestive disease organizations and support groups, and maintains a database of patient and professional education materials from which literature searches are generated.

8343   National Fibromyalgia Association
3857 Birch St.
Suite 312
Newport Beach, CA   92660   nfa@fmaware.org
                                                    www.fmaware.org

Lynne Matallana, Founder
National Fibromyalgia Association's mission is to develop and execute programs dedicated to improving the quality of life for people with fibromyalgia.

8344   National Hemophilia Foundation
7 Penn Plaza
Ste 1204
New York, NY   10001   212-328-3700
                                                      800-424-2634
                                                  Fax: 212-328-3777
                                              handi@hemophilia.org
                                                  www.hemophilia.org

Val Bias, Chief Executive Officer
Neil Frick, Vice President, Research & Medical Information
Joseph Kleiber, Chief Strategy Officer
Mady J. Schuman, Vice President, Development

The National Hemophilia Foundation is dedicated to finding better treatments and cures for bleeding and clotting disorders and to preventing the complications of these disorders through education,advocacy and research. Established in 1948, The National Hemophilia Foundation has chapters throughout the country.

8345   National Kidney and Urologic Diseases Information Clearinghouse
National Institutes of Health
3 Information Way
Bethesda, MD   20892-3560   800-860-8747
                                                 TTY:866-569-1162
                                          www.kidney.niddk.nih.gov

Griffin Rodgers, Director
Gregory Germino, Deputy Director
NKUDIC was established in 1987 to increase knowledge and understanding about diseases of the kidneys and urologic system among people with these conditions and their families, health care professionals, and the general public.

8346   National Organization for Albinism and Hypopigmentation
P.O. Box 959
East Hampstead, NH   03826-0959   603-887-2310
                                                      800-473-2310
                                                  Fax: 800-648-2310
                                                  info@albinism.org
                                                     www.albinism.org

Michael McGowan, Executive Director
Diana McCown, Vice-chair
Kris Baker, Secretary
Kathi O'Donnell, Administration
Organization offering information and support to people with albinism, their families and the prodessionals who work with them.

8347   National Organization for Rare Disorders
55 Kenosia Ave
Danbury, CT   06810   203-744-0100
                                                  Fax: 203-263-9938
                                            orphan@rarediseases.org
                                                   rarediseases.org

Marshall Summar, MD, Chairman
Peter Saltonstall, President & CEO
Pamela Gavin, Chief Operating Officer
Alexa Moore, Vice President of Business Development
The National Organization for Rare Disorders (NORD) is an organization serving individuals with rare diseases and the organizations that serve them. NORD offers educational programs, advocacy, research and patient services.

8348   National Organization on Fetal Alcohol Syndrome
1200 Eton Ct NW
3rd Fl
Washington, DC   20007-3239   202-785-4585
                                                      800-666-6327
                                                  Fax: 202-466-6456
                                              information@nofas.org
                                                       www.nofas.org

Tom Donaldson, President
Kathleen Tavenner Mitchell, Vice President
Andy Kachor, Communications Director
Katelyn Reitz, Development Director
Dedicated to eliminating birth defects caused by alcohol consumption during pregnancy and improving the qualtiy of life for those individuals and families affected.

8349   Prader-Willi Syndrome Association USA
8588 Potter Park Dr
Ste 500
Sarasota, FL   34238   941-312-0400
                                                      800-926-4797
                                                  Fax: 941-312-0142
                                                     www.pwsausa.org

Ken Smith, Executive Director
Jack Hannings, Development Director
Donny Moore, Development & Communications Specialist
National, nonprofit public charity that works for the benefit of individuals with Prader-Willi syndrome and their families. Dedi-

cated to serving individuals affected by Prader-Willi syndrome (PWS) their families, and interested professionals, providing information, education, and support services to its members.

8350 Simonton Cancer Center
P.O. Box 6607
Malibu, CA 90264-6607   818-879-7904
                                                       800-459-3424
                                                  Fax: 310-457-0421
                                        simontoncancercenter@msn.com
                                              www.simontoncenter.com

Dr. O. Carl Simonton, Founder
Edward Gilbert, MD, Medical Director
Karen Smith Simonton, Executive / Program Director
Jessica Jedvaj, Administrative Assistant

The Simonton Cancer Center is a non-profit organization dedicated to improving the health and lives of cancer patients and their families through psycho-social oncology.

8351 Special Care Dentistry Association
330 N. Wabash Avenue
Ste 2000
Chicago, IL 60611-4245   312-527-6764
                                                  Fax: 312-673-6663
                                                  scda@scdaonline.org
                                                    www.scdaonline.org

Kristin Dee, Executive Director
Miriam Robbins, President
Jeffrey Hicks, President-Elect
Sam Zwetchkenbaum, Vice President

The Special Care Dentistry Association serves as a resource to all oral health care professionals who serve or are interested in serving patients with special needs through education and networking to increase access to oral healthcare for patients with special needs.

8352 Spina Bifida Association
1600 Wilson Blvd
Ste 800
Arlington, VA 22209   202-944-3285
                                                       800-621-3141
                                                  Fax: 202-944-3295
                                                      sbaa@sbaa.org
                                        www.spinabifidaassociation.org

Sara Struwe, President & CEO
Lee Towns, National Director, Communications & Outreach
Elizabeth Merck, National Director, Development
Nora Beierwaltes, Marketing Coordinator

Non-profit organization whose mission is to promote the prevention of spina bifida and to enhance the lives of all affected. Addresses the specific needs of the spina bifida community and serves as the national representative of almost 60 chapters. Services include Toll free 800 information and referral service, as well as legislative updates.

8353 Spina Bifida and Hydrocephalus Association of Canada
167 Lombard Ave
Ste 647
Winnipeg, MB, Canada R3B-0v3   204-925-3650
                                                       800-565-9488
                                                  Fax: 204-925-3654
                                                     info@sbhac.ca
                                                     www.sbhac.ca

Susana Scott, President
Linda Randall, Vice President
Bonnie Hidlebaugh, National Manager, Communications & Development Coordinator
Cindy Garofalo, Administrative Assistant

The Spina Bifida and Hydrocephalus Association of Canada has been working on behalf of people with spina bifida and/or hydrocephalus and their families.

8354 Sunburst Projects
Sunburst Projects United States Headquarters
2143 Hurley Way
Suite 240
Sacramento, CA 95825   916-440-0889
                                                  Fax: 916-440-1208
                                             admin@sunburstprojects.org
                                               www.sunburstprojects.org

Geri DeLaRosa , PhD, Founder & Executive Director
Samantha Voelkel, Camp Director

Sunburst Projects is a international organization that works to keep families together by providing services and support for youth who are infected or affected by HIV/AIDS.

8355 Taking Control of Your Diabetes (TCOYD)
990 Highland Dr
Suite 312
Solana Beach, CA 92075   858-755-5683
                                                       800-998-2693
                                                  Fax: 858-755-6854
                                                      info@tcoyd.org
                                                       www.tcoyd.org

Steven Edelman, MD, Founder & Director
Sandra Bourdette, Co-Founder & Executive Director Emeritus
Jennifer Braidwood, Director of Marketing & Special Projects
Jill Yapo, Director, Operations

Taking Control of Your Diabetes works to educate and motivate people with diabetes to take a more active role in managing their condition. The organization also offers continuing education programs for medical professionals caring for people with diabetes.

8356 United Brachial Plexus Network, Inc.
32 William Rd
Reading, MA 01867   781-315-6161
                                                       ubpn@ubpn.org
                                                        www.ubpn.org

Richard Looby, President
Dan Aldrich, Co- Vice President & Traumatic BPI Group

The United Brachial Plexus Network, Inc. provides education, information, and assistance for those affected by Brachial Plexus Palsy by offering information, contacts, resources, parent matching, and assistance developing chapters or support groups throughout the United States and the world.

8357 World Service Office of Overeaters Anonymous
6075 Zenith Crt NE
Rio Rancho, NM 87144-6424   505-891-2664
                                                  Fax: 505-891-4320
                                                       info@oa.org
                                                        www.oa.org

Sarah Armstrong, Managing Director

OA aims to provide physical, emotional, and practical support for those seeking to improve their dietary habits. OA encourages members to develop a food plan with a health care professional and a sponsor.

Camps

8358 ADA Camp Grenada
American Diabetes Association
1701 N. Beauregard St.
Alexandria, VA 22311   217-875-9011
                                                       800-DIA-ETES
                                                       800-342-2383
                                                  Fax: 217-726-2260
                                                       diabetes.org

Dwight Holing, Chair
Larry Hausner, CEO
Debbie Johnson, CFO
Greg Elfers, Chief Field Development Officer

Camp Granada is an American Diabetes Association resident Camp located in Monticello, Illinois at the 4H Memorial Camp owned by the University of Illinois. For children with diabetes, ages 8-16. Activities include swimming, canoeing, wall climbing, tie-dying shirts, arts & crafts and fun filled evening programs.

8359 ADA Camp Needlepoint
American Diabetes Association
YMCA Camp St. Croix
532 County Road F
Hudson, WI 54016   763-593-5333
                                   Fax: 952-582-9000
                                   rbarnett@diabetes.org
                                   www.diabetes.org

Becky Barnett, Camp Director
Carol Holton, Associate Manager
Camp Needlepoint is a summer camp for children who have type 1
diabetes. Coed, ages 8-16. The Camp takes place at the YMCA
Camp St. Croix. The aim of Camp Needlepoint is to provide a safe
camping expeience where children with diabetes can meet others
with type 1 diabetes.

8360 ADA Camp for Kids
American Diabetes Association
1701 N. Beauregard St.
Alexandria, VA 22311-3649   505-266-5716
                                        888-342-2383
                                        800-DIA-ETES
                                   Fax: 505-268-4533
                                   lbrown@diabetes.org
                                   www.diabetes.org

Dwight Holing, Chair
Larry Hausner, CEO
Debbie Johnson, CFO
Greg Elfers, Chief Field Development Officer
One-week camping session for children with diabetes. Coed,
ages 8-13. Camp will be held at Manzano Mountain Retreat, one
hour from Albuquerque, New Mexico. Please call for exact dates.

8361 ADA Teen Adventure Camp
American Diabetes Association
1701 N. Beauregard St.
Alexandria, VA 22311   312-346-1805
                                        888-342-2383
                                        800-DIA-ETES
                                   Fax: 312-346-5342
                                   mejohnson@diabetes.org
                                   www.diabetes.org/adacampteenadventure
Dwight Holing, Chair
Larry Hausner, CEO
Debbie Johnson, CFO
Greg Elfers, Chief Field Development Officer
Camping for teenagers with diabetes. Coed, ages 14 to 18. Camp
dates are early in August. Located at the YMCA Camp Duncan in
Ingleside, Illinois. Featured activities include archery and crafts,
singing, outdoor movie night, and roller skating.

8362 ADA Triangle D Camp
American Diabetes Association
1701 N. Beauregard St.
Alexandria, VA 22311   312-346-1805
                                        888-342-2383
                                        800-DIA-ETES
                                   Fax: 312-346-5342
                                   www.diabetes.org/adacamptriangled
Dwight Holing, Chair
Larry Hausner, CEO
Debbie Johnson, CFO
Greg Elfers, Chief Field Development Officer
Triangle D Camp is a resident camp program located at the YMCA
Camp Duncan in Ingleside, Illinois. Activities include swim-
ming, row boating, canoeing, high ropes (11-13 yr. olds), climb-
ing tower (9-10 yr. olds), Camp games, singing, archery,
campfires, soccer, basketball, volleyball and diabetes education.

8363 ASCCA
Alabama Easter Seal Society
5278 Camp Ascca Dr
P.O. Box 21
Jacksons Gap, AL 36861   256-825-9226
                                        800-843-2267
                                   Fax: 256-825-8332
                                   info@campascca.org
                                   www.campascca.org

John Stephenson, Administrator
Matt Rickman, Camp Director
Dana Rickman, Director, Marketing Communications
Allison Wetherbee, Director, Community Relations
Camp ASCCA is for children and adults with disabilities or health
impairements. Camp ASCCA strives to help these individuals
achieve equality, independence and dignity in a safe environ-
ment.

8364 Adventure Day Camp
3480 Commission Ct
Lake Ridge, VA 22192   703-491-1444
                                   office@princewilliamacademy.com
                                   www.princewilliamacademy.com
Dr. Samia Harris, Founder & Executive Director
Rebecca Nykwest, Communications Director
Lindsay Chickering, Office Manager
Shiree Slade, Principal
Camping for children with asthma/respiratory ailments and can-
cer. Coed, ages 2-13.

8365 Agassiz Village
238 Bedford St
Suite B
Lexington, MA 02420-3477   781-860-0200
                                   Fax: 781-860-0352
                                   csimmonds@agassizvillage.org
                                   www.agassizvillage.org

Cliff Simmonds, Executive Director
Thomas Semeta, Camp Director
Warren Soar, Facility Director
Warren H Burroughs, Honorary Chairman
Agassiz Village offers a variety of activities for all campers, boys
and girls, younger camper and teens, and programs for physically
challenged children and teens. By participating in daily activities, campers build a cooperative and positive community of different races, ages, ethnic and cultural backgrounds while
enhancing confidence and individuality. Camp is located in
Poland, Maine. For ages 8-17.

8366 Arizona Camp Sunrise
American Cancer Society
PO Box 27872
Tempe, AZ 85285   602-952-7550
                                        800-865-1582
                                   Fax: 602-404-1118
                                   barb.nicholas@cancer.org
                                   www.azcampsunrise.org

Barbara Nicholas, Director
Leigh Ansley, Manager
Melissa Lee, Camp Director
Jason Poulter, Technical Media Director
Provides one-week summer camping sessions to children aged
8-16 who have had, or currently have, cancer. The classes range
from sports and outdoor games to dance and drama, arts, crafts,
and cooking. Other activities planned for the campers include
horseback riding, a trip to a lake, a dance, and learning to make
friendship bracelets.

8367 Bearskin Meadow Camp
Diabetic Youth Foundation
5167 Clayton Road
Suite F
Concord, CA 94521   925-680-4994
                                       Fax: 925-680-4863
                                             info@dyf.org
                                             www.dyf.org

Mark McComb, President
Paula Gogin, Development Director
Janet Kramschuster, Interim Executive Director
Jennifer Goerzen, Resident Camp manager
Bearskin Meadow Campis is for children, teens and their families
who are affected by diabetes. Bearskin teaches skills for blook
glucose checking and techniques for adjusting insulin, food
choices and how to have a fun, active life while living with
diabetes.

**8368 Becket Chimney Corners YMCA Camps and Outdoor
Center**
748 Hamilton Rd
Becket, MA 01223   413-623-8991
                                       Fax: 413-623-5890
                                       cburke@bccymca.org
                                           www.bccymca.org

Drew Lipsher, Chair
David Smith, Vice Chair
Christine Kalakay, Chief Financial Officer
Phil Connor, CEO
Half-week and one-week sessions for campers with asthma/respi-
ratory ailments. Coed, ages 3 and up, families, seniors, single
adults.

8369 Bright Horizons Summer Camp
Sickle Cell Disease Association of Illinois
8100 S. Western Avenue
Chicago, IL 60620   773-526-5016
                                             866-798-1097
                                       Fax: 773-526-5012
                          sicklecelldisease-illinois@scdai.org
                              sicklecelldisease-illinois.org

Darryl H. Armstrong, Chair
TaLana Hughes, Executive Director
Anquineice Brown, Outreach Coordinator
Alana Burke, Case Manager
Camping for children with blood disorders, ages 7-13. The joys
of learning include instruction in first aid, swimming and
water safety, boating, horseback riding and bowling plus arts and crafts.
In addition, there is a traditional menu of camp pleasures, like
hayrides, cookouts, nature hikes and sing-a-longs.

8370 Camp Alpine
Alpine Alternatives
2518 E. Tudor Road
Ste 105
Anchorage, AK 99507-1105   907-561-6655
                                             800-361-4174
                                       Fax: 907-563-9232
                            alpinealternatives@arctic.net
                         www.alpinealternatives.org/programs.html
Margaret Webber, Executive Director
LaVerne Lee, Day Outings Director & Camp Alpine Director
Offers programs aimed at helping disabled youth expand their horizons, master new skills, make new friends, and increase motor
coordination. Most importantly, participants experience growth
in self-confidence and independence that affects all aspects of an
individual's life. Camp services are open to all, regardless of type
of disability or age. Activities include canoeing, hiking, swimming, outdoor games, sports, nature identification and much
more.

8371 Camp Anuenue
250 Williams St. NW
Atlanta, GA 30303   808-595-7500
                                             888-227-2345
                                       Fax: 808-595-7502
                             debra.glowik@cancer.org
                                            www.cancer.org
Pamela K. Meyerhoffer, Chair
Robert E. Youle, Vice Chairman
Douglas K. Kelsey, Board Scientific Officer
Daniel P. Heist, Secretary/Treasurer
(1 week) June, children with or recovered from cancer.

8372 Camp Boggy Creek
30500 Brantley Branch Rd
Eustis, FL 32736   352-483-4200
                                             866-462-6449
                                       Fax: 352-483-0589
                           info@campboggycreek.org
                                       www.boggycreek.org
J. Patterson Cooper, Chair
Wendy Durden, Vice Chair
June Clark, President/CEO
Paul Newman, Founder
Year-round sessions for children with a variety of chronic or
life-threatening illnesses including cancer, hemophila, epilepsy,
heart defects, HIV, spina bifida and asthma/respiratory ailments.
Coed, ages 7-16.

8373 Camp Bon Coeur
Bon Coeur, Inc.
405 West Main St.
Lafayette, LA 70505-3765   337-233-8437
                                       Fax: 337-233-4160
                                       info@heartcamp.com
                                           www.heartcamp.com
Susannah Craig, Executive Director
Antonio Conner, MBA, President
Susan Randol, RN, MSN, Vice-President
Martha Wyatt, CPA, Treasurer
Two-week sessions June-July for children with heart defects.
Coed, ages 8-16.

8374 Camp Breathe Easy
American Lung Association

                                            404-231-9887
                                       annie@camptwinlakes.org
                                       campbreatheeasy.com
Annie Garrett, Camp Director
Camp Breathe Easy is a seven-day, six-night overnight camp for
children, ages 7-13, with asthma who need medication and are
limited in summer camping opportunities. The children learn
asthma self-management techniques and coping strategies to
better handle their illness. Campers swim, repel off trees, fish, canoe, play soccer, basketball and miniature golf, and participate in
ceramics and arts and crafts.

8375 Camp Can Do
Administrative Office
3 Unami Trail
Chalfont, PA 18914   •   717-273-6525
                                       info@campcandoforever.com
                                       campcandoforever.org
Tom Prader, Board
Karen MacAinsh, Board
Stephanie Cole, Board
Amy McGonigal, Board
Camp Can Do is for children, ages 8-17, who have been diag-
nosed with cancer in the last 5 years. The camp also offers a ses-
sion for siblings of children with cancer.

8376 **Camp Carefree**
American Diabetes Association
1846 West Seventh Street
Piscataway, NJ 08850-1918 732-752-1715
director@campcarefreekids.org
www.campcarefreekids.org

Phyllis Woestemeyer, Director
Katie Nitchie, Camp Coordinator
Camp is located in Wolfeboro, New Hampshire. Sessions for campers with diabetes.

8377 **Camp Catch-a-Rainbow**
American Cancer Society
250 Williams St. NW
Atlanta, GA 30303 808-595-7500
888-227-2345
Fax: 808-595-7502
debra.glowik@cancer.org
www.cancer.org

Pamela K. Meyerhoffer, Chair
Robert E. Youle, Vice Chairman
Douglas K. Kelsey, Board Scientific Officer
Daniel P. Heist, Secretary/Treasurer
Camp Catch-a-Rainbow's programs are available completely free to any child in MI or IN who has or has had cancer, between the ages of 4 and 20, with their doctor's approval. Family Camp is reserved for those campers who have attended camp during that year's summer sessions and their families. Day, week, adult retreat, and family camp are available options.

8378 **Camp Cheerful**
Achievement Centers For Children
15000 Cheerful Ln
Strongsville, OH 44136-5420 440-238-6200
Fax: 440-238-1858
jennie.amodio@achievementctrs.org
www.achievementcenters.org

Julie Boland, Chairwoman
James Kacic, Vice Chairman
Nicole Hilbert, Treasurer
Jennifer Vergilli, Secretary
Camp Cheerful provides a number of day and overnight camping options for children and adults who have disabilities. The camp hosts traditional camp activities, as well as year-round Therapeutic Horseback Riding sessions and a handicap-accessible High Ropes challenge course during the summer. The focus of activities is to increase the quality of life while encouraging confidence and independence.

8379 **Camp Christmas Seal**
American Lung Association of Oregon
102 W McDowell Rd
Phoenix, AZ 85003-1213 602-258-7505
Fax: 202-452-1805
info@lungoregon.org
www.lungoregon.org

Kathryn A. Forbes, Chairman
John F. Emanuel, Vice Chair
Harold Wimmer, President/CEO
Penny J. Siewert, Secretary/Treasurer
Camp is located in Sisterhood, Oregon. Sessions for children with asthma/respiratory ailments. Coed, ages 8-15.

8380 **Camp Classen YMCA**
YMCA of Greater Oklahoma City
10840 Main Camp Rd
Davis, OK 73030 580-369-2272
Fax: 580-369-2284
www.itsmycamp.org

Ford C. Price, Chair
Tricia Everest, Vice Chairman
Mike Grady, President & CEO
Don Harris, Vice President & CFO
Camp is located in Davis, Oklahoma. Sessions for children and adults with diabetes. Coed, ages 8-17, families, seniors and single adults.

8381 **Camp Conrad-Chinnock**
Diabetic Youth Services
12045 E. Waterfront Drive
Playa Vista, CA 90094 310-751-3057
Fax: 888-800-4010
www.dys.org

Rocky Wilson, Executive and Camp Director
Dale Lissy, Camp Manager
Ryan Martz, Program Director
Tom Jenkins, Chief Operating Officer
Camp Conrad-Chinnock offers many recreational programs such as swimming, canoeing, arts & crafts to young adults and their families with diabetes. Dietary education programs and diabetes management are also available.

8382 **Camp Courage North**
Courage Center
3915 Golden Valley Rd
Golden Valley, MN 55422 763-588-0811
888-846-8253
Fax: 763-520-0577
www.couragecenter.org

Jan Malcolm, CEO
Pamela J. Lindemoen, Executive Vice President of Oper
Stephen Bariteau, Chief Development Officer
Alice Johnson, Chief Financial Officer
Courage Center Camps - Camp Courage & Camp Courage North - are part of Courage Center, a non-profit rehabilitation and resource center for people of all ages and abilities who are experiencing barriers to health & independence. For more than 50 years, Courage Center camps have served children and adults with physical disabilities and those who are deaf and hard of hearing. In 2008, more than 800 people attended a Courage Center camp session. For more information, visit our web-site.

8383 **Camp Del Corazon**
11615 Hesby St
North Hollywood, CA 91601-3620 818-754-0312
888-621-4800
Fax: 818-754-0842
information@campdelcorazon.org
www.campdelcorazon.org

Kevin Shannon, Co-Founder/President/Medical Director
Dan Levi, Board Member
Joel McHale, Board Member
Tom Arnold, Board Member
Active program for campers with heart disease, Camp del Corazon provides summer activities free of charge that include hiking and archery, arts and crafts, court and field games, waterfront activities and a beach barbecue.

8384 **Camp Discovery**
American Diabetes Association
1168 K-157 Hwy
Junction, KS 35804 316-684-6091
Fax: 316-941-5699
www.diabetes.org

Mark Moyer, President
Terry Ackley, Executive Director
Anne Bowman, Camp Director
Camp is located in Junction City, Kansas. Offers young people with diabetes a week of fun at rock springs 4-H Center. Special attention to diabetes makes Camp Discovery a safe environment for active youth while providing valuable diabetes managment education. Call the American Diabetes Association Kansas area office for more information. Coed, ages 8-17.

8385 **Camp Discovery - Illinois**
American Diabetes Association
875 Roosevelt Rd
Health Track
Glen Ellyn, IL 60137 312-346-1805
Fax: 312-346-5342
illinoiscamps@diabetes.org
diabetes.org/in-my-community/diabetes-camp
Kalina Gurovski, Camp Director
The purpose of the American Diabetes Association, Northern Illinois Area Day Camp is to provide a unique recreational and edu-

cational experience for children with diabetes. With guidance from the camp staff, day campers can to participate in various camping activities and develop independence and confidence in caring for their diabetes. Diabetes education sessions teach campers about nutrition, exercise, insulin, highs and lows and blood sugar testing.

8386 Camp Eden Wood
Friendship Ventures
10509 108th St NW
Annandale, MN 55302

952-852-0101
800-450-8376
Fax: 952-852-0123
info@friendshipventures.org

Floyd Adelman, Chair
Jeff Bangsberg, Board Member
Robert Harnett, Board Member
Jerry Caruso, Board Member
Camp is located in Eden Prairie, Minnesota. Offers resident camp programs for children, teenagers and adults with developmental, physical or multiple disabilities, Down Syndrome, special medical conditions, Williams Syndrome, autism and/or other conditions. Fishing, creative arts, golf, sports and other activities are available. Respite care weekend camps year round for children, teenagers and adults. Guided vacations for teens and adults with developmental disabilities or other unique needs.

8387 Camp Floyd Rogers
Floyd Rogers Foundation
P.O.Box 541058
Omaha, NE 68154

402-885-9022
director@campfloydrogers.com
www.campfloydrogers.com

Erin Hoffman, President
Greg Penny, Vice President
Ashley Moore, Treasurer
Mike German, Secretary
A camp for diabetic children. Coed, ages 8-18. 100 children come to Camp Floyd Rogers each summer. They come to enjoy activities, participate in special events, engage in innovative evening programs, and they meet other children their own age with diabetes. Camp Floyd Rogers offers young people an opportunity to share some of life's adventures with others who also happen to have diabetes.

8388 Camp Glengarra
Girl Scouts - Foothills Council
33 Jewett Pl
Utica, NY 13501-4715

315-733-1909
Fax: 315-733-1909

Natalie Brown, Executive Director
Karen Lubecki, Director
Camp Glengarra is located on 500+ acres of fields and forests, about eight miles west of Camden. This Girl Scout Camp hosts a myriad of programs throughout the year as well as summer day and resident camp. Summer sessions for girls 5-17 with ADD or asthma/respiratory ailments.

8389 Camp Glyndon
American Diabetes Association
800 Wyman Park Dr
Suite 110
Baltimore, MD 21211-2837

410-265-0075
800-342-2383
Fax: 410-235-4048
askada@diabetes.org
www.childrenwithdiabetes.com

Heather Magoon, Director
Camp is located in Nanjemoy, Maryland. One and two-week sessions July-August for children with diabetes and their families. Coed, ages 8-16.

8390 Camp Harkness
Arc of New London County
125 Sachem St
Norwich, CT 06360

860-889-4435
Fax: 860-889-4662
TTY:860-859-5493
info@thearcnlc.org
www.thearcnlc.org/

Enrico DeMatto, President
Linda Rhodse, VP
Alan Messier, Treasurer
Wendy Mis, Secretary
In 1991 a group of parents and adults with spina bifida, were brought together with the mission to educate the public about spina bifida and issues affecting people who have this disability in addition To providing support and information and promoting programs that will help people with spina bifida. Since then SBAC has worked hard to support parents, adults with spina bifida and families

8391 Camp Hertko Hollow
101 Locust St
Des Moines, IA 50309

515-471-8523
888-437-8652
Fax: 515-288-2531
www.camphertkohollow.com

Troy Norman, President
Brant Ausenhus, VP
Vicki Hertko, Treasurer
Steve Roy, Legal Counsel
Camp Hertko Hollow is a resident camp held at the Des Moines YMCA Camp site, located along the Des Moines River north of Boone, Iowa. Activities include horseback riding, swimming, canoeing, rappelling, crafts, ropes course, archery and riflery to name a few, plus special activities for different ages. Half-week and one-week sessions for children with diabetes. Coed, ages 6-16.

8392 Camp Hickory Hill
Central Missouri Diabetic Childrens Camp
P.O.Box 1942
Columbia, MO 65205

573-445-9146
CampHickoryHill@gmail.com
www.camphickoryhill.com

David Bernhardt, President
Lisa Bernhardt, Camp Director
Nate Wisdom, Program Director
Frank La Mantia, Development Director
Educates diabetic children concerning diabetes and its care. In addition to daily educational sessions on some aspects of diabetes, campers participate in swimming, sailing, arts and crafts and overnight camping. Coed, ages 8-17.

8393 Camp Ho Mita Koda
14040 Auburn Rd
Newbury, OH 44065

info@chmkfoundation.org
www.chmkfoundation.org/

Julia Blanchette, Health Director
Ted Rusinoff, Board Member
Kristin Warzocha, Board Member
Camp Ho Mita Koda is a summer camp for children with type 1 diabetes. The camp aims to provide fun outdoor activties, while also educating and building life skills for children with diabetes. Day camp available for ages 5-11, and two overnight sessions for children ages 8-11 and 12-15.

8394 Camp Hodia
1701 N 12th Street
Boise, ID 83702

208-891-1023
Fax: 208-891-1023
alan@hodia.org
www.hodia.org

Natalie B. DelRio, Chair
Richard Christensen, Vice Chair
lLisa Gier, Executice Director
Vicki Cutshall, R.N., Director, Hodia Kids Camp

Camp is located in Alturas Lake, Idaho. One-week sessions for children with diabetes. Coed, ages 8-18. Ski Camp in Sun Valley in January, ages 12-18.

8395 **Camp Honor**
Arizona Hemophilia Association
826 N. 5th Ave.
Phoenix, AZ   85003
602-955-3947
888-754-7017
Fax: 602-955-1962
info@hemophiliaz.org
www.hemophiliaz.org

Steven Helm, President
Jim Drurr, Vice President
Cindy Komar, CEO
Lindsey Bogard, Communications Director
Camp is located in Payson, Arizona at the Whispering Hope Ranch. One-week sessions for children with hemophilia or HIV and their siblings, as well as children of hemophiliacs. Coed, ages 7-17. Activities include swimming, canoeing, sports, archery and arts and crafts (to name a few fun things).

8396 **Camp Independence**
National Kidney Foundation
30 East 33rd Street
New York, NY   10016
770-452-1539
800-622-9010
Fax: 212-689-9261
info@kidney.org
www.kidneyga.org

Gregory W. Scott, Chair
Beth Piraino, President
Bruce Skyer, CEO
Joseph Vassalotti, Chief Medical Officer
Camp Independence is Georgia's a overnight, week-long summer camp providing essential medical care, treatment & fun for kids with kidney disease and transplants. Camp Independence recognizes that campers are normal children but have special needs providing these children with opportunities for development & individual growth, peer support & normal life experiences. Activities include swimming, arts & crafts, fishing and horsebackriding, in addition to archery, games and sports, and ceramics.

8397 **Camp Jened**
United Cerebral Palsy Association New York
P.O.Box 483
Rock Hill, NY   12775-483
845-434-2220
Fax: 845-434-2253
Michael Branam, Executive Director
Camp is located in Rock Hill, New York. Sessions for adults with severe developmental and physical disabilities. Coed, ages 18-99.

8398 **Camp John Warvel**
American Diabetes Association
1701 N. Beauregard St.
Alexandria, VA   22311
312-346-1805
888-342-2383
800-DIA-ETES
Fax: 317-594-0748
www.diabetes.org

Dwight Holing, Chair
Larry Hausner, CEO
Debbie Johnson, CFO
Greg Elfers, Chief Field Development Officer
Camp is located in North Webster, Indiana. Provides an enjoyable, safe and educational out-of-doors experience for children with insulin-dependent diabetes. A unique learning atmosphere for children to acquire new skills in caring for their disease. The camp experience instills confidence for the child's self-management of diabetes. Offers one-week sessions and can accommodate 200 campers, boys and girls aged 7-16.

8399 **Camp Joslin**
Barton Center for Diabetes Education
30 Ennis Road
PO Box 356
North Oxford, MA   01537-0356
508-987-2056
Fax: 508-987-2002
info@bartoncenter.org
www.bartoncenter.org

Thomas C. Lynch, Chair
John Peri-Okonny, 1st Vice chiar
Kristin Dyer, 2nd Vice Chair
Mark W. Fuller, Treasurer
Camp is located in Charlton, Massachusetts. For boys, ages 7-16, with diabetes. This program offers active summer sports and activities, supplemented by medical treatment and diabetes education. Coed Winter Camp and Coed Weekend Retreats are offered during the school year.

8400 **Camp Joy**
3325 Swamp Creek Rd
Schwenksville, PA   19473-1518
610-754-6878
Fax: 610-754-7880
www.campjoy.com
Robert G Griffith, President
A special needs camp for kids and adults (ages 4-80+) with developmental disabilities such as: mental retardation, autism, brain injury, neurological disorder, visual and/or hearing impairments, Angelman and Down syndromes, and other developmental disabilities.

8401 **Camp Ko-Man-She**
Diabetes Dayton
2555 S Dixie Drive
Suite 112
Dayton, OH   45409
937-220-6611
Fax: 937-224-0240
dada@diabetesdayton.org
www.diabetesdayton.org
Tyler Starline, President
Michael Martens, Vice President
Becky Roberts, Secretary
Sheila DeWeese, Treasurer
Camp Ko-Man-She is located in Bellefontaine, Ohio, and is held annually for children with type 1 diabetes. The camp's goal is for children to socialize with other children who also have diabetes and to have fun outdoors in a medically supervised setting. Co-ed, ages 8-17.

8402 **Camp Kweebec**
157 Game Farm Rd.
Schwenksville, PA   19473
610-667-2123
Fax: 610-667-6376
info@kweebec.com
www.kweebec.com
Les Weiser, Owner/Director
Maddy Weiser, Owner/Director
Rachel Weiser, Associate Director, Director of
Josh Weiser, Associate Director
Camp is located in Schwenksville, Pennsylvania. Sessions for children and adults with diabetes. Coed, ages 6-16, families, seniors and single adults.

8403 **Camp L-Kee-Ta**
940 Golden Valley Drive
Bettendorf, IA   52722
319-752-3639
800-798-0833
Fax: 319-753-1410
www.gseiwi.org
Teresa Colgan, Chair
Jill Dashner, 1st Vice chiar
Anna Gibney, Development Manager
Ann Hulett, Business Operations Coordinator
Camp is located in Danville, Iowa. Half-week and one-week sessions June-August for children with asthma/respiratory ailments. Girls, ages 7-18 and families.

8404 Camp Latgawa
Oregon-Idaho Conference Center
13250 S Fork Little Butte Creek Rd
Eagle Point, OR 97524- 5593 541-826-9699
camplatgawa@hotmail.com
latgawa.gocamping.org/
Eva LaBonty, Director
Camp Latgawa provides year round hospitality for groups up to 90 people. The bunk/dormitory style facilities are heated and have restrooms and showers either in the cabin or nearby.

8405 Camp Libbey
Maumee Valley Girl Scout Center
2244 Collingwood Blvd
Toledo, OH 43620-1147 419-243-8216
800-860-4516
Fax: 419-245-5357
www.girlscoutsofwesternohio.org
Jody Wainscott, Chair
Ellen Iobst, 1st Vice Chair
Susan Gantz Matz, 2nd Vice Chair
Jerry Brose, Secretary
Camp for girls 7-18 with asthma/respiratory ailments, diabetes, epilepsy and muscular dystrophy is located in Defiance, Ohio.

8406 Camp MITIOG
Share, Inc
7615 N. Platte Purchase Drive
Kansas City, MO 64118 816-221-4450
877-221-4450
Fax: 816-221-1420
midlands@midlandsmc.org
www.midlandsmc.org
Mike Hale, President/Financial Officer
Pam Mathena, Adm. Assistant to MMC Financial Officer
Donna Fletcher, Congregational Consultant
Don McLaughlin, Outreach Coordinator
Camp is located in Excelsior Springs, Missouri. One-week summer sessions for children with spina bifida. Coed, ages 6-16.

8407 Camp Magruder
Oregon-Idaho Conference Center
17450 Old Pacific Hwy
Rockaway Beach, OR 97136 503-355-2310
Fax: 503-355-8701
office@campmagruder.org
www.campmagruder.org
Troy Taylor, Camp Director
Rik Gutzke, Facilities Manager
Angie Nebeker, Reservations/ Guest Services
Hope Montgomery, Program Director
Camp is located in Rockaway Beach, Oregon. Sessions for teens and adults with developmental disabilities through Camp Hope.

8408 Camp Nejeda
Camp Nejeda Foundation
910 Saddlebrook Road
P.O. Box 156
Stillwater, NJ 07875 973-383-2611
Fax: 973-383-9891
info@campnejeda.org
Ernest Post, MD, Secretary
Scott Ross, President
Bill Vierbuchen, Executive Director
Jim Daschbach, Camp Director
For children with diabetes, ages 7-15. Provides an active and safe camping experience which enables the children to learn about and understand diabetes. Activities include boating, swimming, fishing, archery, as well as camping skills.

8409 Camp Not-A-Wheeze
American Lung Association In Arizona
102 W McDowell Rd
Phoenix, AZ 85003-1213 602-258-7505
Fax: 202-452-1805
info@lungoregon.org
www.lungarizona.org
Kathryn A. Forbes, Chairman
John F. Emanuel, Vice Chair
Harold Wimmer, President/CEO
Penny J. Siewert, Secretary/Treasurer
Camp Not-A-Wheeze is designed especially for kids ages 7-14 with moderate to severe asthma and was created to provide a traditional residential camp experience and teach children how to manage their asthma.

8410 Camp Okizu
Okizu Foundation
16 Digital Dr
Suite 130
Novato, CA 94949 415-382-9083
Fax: 415-382-8384
info@okizu.org
www.okizu.org
John H. Bell, Chair
Michael D. Amylon, Vice Chair
Suzie Randall, Executive Director/Camp Director
Beth Dekker, Assistant Camp Director
Camp Okizu offers a place where children struggling with a life threatening illness and thier families can come to explore and enjoy a normal life experience. The camp also provides peer support, respite, mentoring, and a variety of other programs designed to help members of families affected by childhood cancer. The camp is open from April through October

8411 Camp Pelican
Louisiana Lions Camp
P.O. Box 290247
Kerrville, TX 78029 830-896-8500
Fax: 830-896-3666
tlc@ktc.com
www.lionscamp.org
Tim Matakas, President
Kim Breaux, Vice President
Tessie Guillory, Treasurer
Autumn Gaspard, Secretary
Camp Pelican is an overnight residential camp for children with moderate to severe asthma or other pulmonary problems. Founded in 1977, Camp Pelican is jointly sponsored by the Louisiana Pulmonary Disease Camp Inc and the Louisiana Lions Camp. Over 100 children attend annually and participate in education, sports, arts and crafts, swimming and other camping activities. Medical staff including physicians, nurses, respiratory therapists and social workers participate in camp. Coed, ages 5-17.

8412 Camp Rainbow
Phoenix Childrens Hospital
1919 East Thomas Road
Phoenix, AZ 85016 602-933-1000
888-908-5437
888-908-KIDS
Fax: 602-546-0276
rlyddon@phoenixchildrens.com
www.phoenixchildrens.org/
Jon Hulburd, Chair
Jacque Sokolov, MD, Vice Chair
Robert Meyer, President/CEO
David Lenhardt, Director
Camp is located in Prescott, Arizona. Offers one-week sessions for children who have had, or currently have, cancer. Boys and girls ages 7-17. Camp activities include swimming, horseback riding, arts and crafts, canoeing, performing arts, archery, rollerskating, fishing, an overnight camping trip and much more! It's a week filled with laughter, new experiences and new friends.

8413   Camp Rap-A-Hope
2701 Airport Blvd
Mobile, AL 36606
251-476-9880
Fax: 251-476-9495
info@camprapahope.org
www.camprapahope.org

Melissa McNichol, Executive Director
Roz Dorsett, Assistant Director
Cecy Lowell, Development Director
Camp Rap-A-Hope is a one-week summer camp for children and teenagers who are battling cancer or have ever been diagnosed with cancer and are 7 to 17 years of age. It is free of charge. Camp Rap-A-Hope strives to make sure every camper gets the opportunity to develop new skills and self-confidence. Camp activities are appropriate for our campers' ages and abilities and include, but are not limited to: swimming, music, arts and crafts, archery, fishing, canoeing and horseback riding.

8414   Camp Ronald McDonald for Good Times
Ronald McDonald House For Charities-Southern Calif
1250 Lyman Place
Los Angeles, CA 90029
310-268-8488
800-625-7295
Fax: 310-473-3338
www.campronaldmcdonald.org

Edward Lodgen, President
Jodi Lesh, Vice President
Sarah Orth, Executive Director
Ken Teasdale, Treasurer
Free year-round residential camping for children with cancer and their families.

8415   Camp Sawtooth
Oregon-Idaho Conference Center
P.O.Box 68
Fairfield, ID 83327-68
800-593-7539
sawtooth@gocamping.org
www.gocamping.org

David Hargreaves, Director
Camp located 35 miles north of fairfield, centrally located for all of southern Idaho.

8416   Camp Seale Harris
Southeastern Diabetes Education Services
500 Chase Park S
Ste 104
Birmingham, AL 35244
205-402-0415
Fax: 205-402-0416
info@campsealeharris.org
www.campsealeharris.org

Tip McAlpin, Chair
David Jamieson, Vice Chair
Rhonda McDavid, Executive Director
John Latimer, Camp & Community Programs Director
Camp Seale Harris is a medically-supervised, fun camp experience and family connection to year-round support that helps them fight diabetes every day.

8417   Camp Setebaid
Setebaid Services, Inc.
PO Box 196
Winfield, PA 17889-0196
570-524-9090
866-738-3224
Fax: 570-523-0769
info@setebaidservices.org
setebaidservices.org

Mark A. Moyer, Executive Director
Linda Neyhart, Business Operations Manager
Camping sessions for children with diabetes. The camp is Coed, for ages 8-18 years, and also hosts family conferences for children with diabetes and their families.

8418   Camp Smile-A-Mile
1510 5th Ave S
P.O. Box 550155
Birmingham, AL 35255
205-323-8427
888-500-7920
Fax: 205-323-6220
info@campsam.org
www.campsam.org

Bruce Hooper, Executive Director
Jennifer Amundsen, Program Director
Savannah Lanler, Development Director
Katie Langley, Administrative & Development Assistant
Camp Smile-A-Mile is a non-profit organization for children in Alabama who have or had cancer. Camp Smile-A-Mile's mission is to provide challenging, unforgettable recreational and educational experiences for young cancer patients from across Alabama at no cost to their families. The camp provides these children with avenues for fellowship, to help them cope with their disease, and to prepare them for life.

8419   Camp Stix
Camp Stix Diabetes Programs
P.O. Box 8308
Spokane, WA 99203
509-484-1366
Fax: 888-958-5730
campstix@campstix.org
www.campstix.org/Default.aspx

Bill Martin, Medical Director
Lynn Sander, Education Director
Camp Stix is an independent summer camp for children and teens with diabetes. Coed, ages 9-18. The camp is help for one week at the Riverview Bible Camp on the Pend Oreille River.

8420   Camp Sunrise
Johns Hopkins Hospital
600 North Wolfe Street
CMSC 800
Baltimore, MD 21287-5904
410-955-5311
Sherryce Robinson, Mission Delivery Manager
Kira Elring, Regional Mission Director
Gloria Jetter, Regional Executive Director
Jack Shipkoski, CEO
Week long summer camp in White Hall, MD., for children ages 6-18 who have been diagnosed with or have survived cancer. Camp sunrise also has a 'day camp' program available for children ages 4-5. Camp activities include sports & games, swimming, arts & crafts, and nature hikes.

8421   Camp Sweeney
Camp Sweeney
P.O.Box 918
Gainesville, TX 76241
940-665-2011
Fax: 940-665-9467
info@campsweeney.org
www.campsweeney.org

T. Milton Dickson, Jr. DDS, Chair
Ernie Fernandez, Executive Director
Robert D. Vandermeer, MD, Vice Chair
Skip Rigsby, Program Director
Camp Sweeney teaches self-care and self-reliance to children ages 5-18 with type 1 diabetes. Campers participate in such activities such as swimming, fishing, horseback riding and arts and crafts while learning about how to self manage their diabetes.

8422   Camp Tall Turf
816 Madison SE
Grand Rapids, MI 49507
616-452-7906
Fax: 616-452-7907
info@tallturf.org
www.tallturf.org

Eric Brown, Chair
Ed Van Poolen, Vice Chair
Miriam DeJong, Director of Programs
Victoria P. Gibbs, Interim Executive Director
Camp is located in Walkerville, Michigan. Summer camping sessions for youth with asthma/respiratory ailments and ADD. Coed, ages 8-16.

8423   **Camp Taylor, Inc.**
8224 West Grayson Rd.
Modesto, CA   95358   209-545-4715
                                          Fax: 209-543-1861
                                     kimberlie@kidsheartcamp.org
                                        www.kidsheartcamp.org

Kimberlie Gamino, Board Member
Rollin A. Podwys, Board Member
Steven Barbieri, Board Member
Charlie Liamos, Board Member
Camp Taylor is a place where children and young adults with
heart disease and thier families can come for recreational activi-
ties and programs. The camp is open from May through Septem-
ber.

8424   **Camp Vacamas**
256 Macopin Rd
West Milford, NJ   07480   973-838-0942
                                               877-428-8222
                                            www.vacamas.org

Felix A. Urrutia, Executive Director
Kristin Short, Camp Director
Karen Wendolowski, Executive Secretary
Seth Friedman, MPA, Program Director
Disadvantaged children with asthma or sickle cell anemia, ages
8-16, are offered special programs in canoeing, backpacking,
camping, music and leadership training. Sliding scale tuition.
Year round programs for youth at risk groups. Conference center
facility open for group rentals.

8425   **Camp Waziyatah**
530 Mill Hill Rd
Waterford, ME   04088-4011   207-583-2267
                                          Fax: 509-357-2267
                                             info@wazi.com
                                                 wazi.com

Gregg Parker, Owner/Director
Mitch Parker, Owner/Director
Camp is located in Waterford, Massachusetts. Three, four and
seven-week sessions June-August for campers with cancer and
diabetes. Coed, ages 8-15 and families, single adults.

8426   **Camp WheezeAway**
YMCA Camp Chandler
1240 Jordan Dam Rd
Wetumpka, AL   36092   334-229-0035
                                     jreynolds@ymcamontgomery.org
                                  ymcamontgomery.org/camp/wheezeaway
Jeff Reynolds, Executive Director
Art Mason, Operations Director
Suzy Stewart, Program Director
Kids age 8-12 suffering from moderate to severe asthma can ap-
ply for this FREE summer camp program offered at YMCA Camp
Chandler. Kids experience all the fun of summer camp while
learning confidence building skills in asthma management from
medical professionals.

8427   **Camps for Children & Teens with Diabetes**
Diabetes Society
1165 Lincoln Ave
Suite 300
San Jose, CA   95125-3052   408-287-3785
                                               800-989-1165
                                          Fax: 408-287-2701
                                       info@diabetessociety.org
Sharon Ogbor, Executive Director
Thomas Smith, Director
Since 1974, sponsors up to 20 day camps, family camps and resident camps for children 4 through 17. These camps provide an opportunity for children with diabetes to go to camp, meet other
children and gain a better understanding of their diabetes. The total experience can help campers develop more confidence in their
abilities to control their diabetes effectively while enjoying the
traditional camp experience. Camps are located throughout CA
and parts of Nevada.

8428   **Cedar Ridge Camp**
4120 Old Routt Road
Louisville, KY   40299   502-267-5848
                                          Fax: 502-267-0116
                                       info@cedarridgecamp.com
                                        www.cedarridgecamp.com
Andrew Hartmans, Executive Director
Half-week, one and two-week sessions for children with diabetes, developmental disabilities and muscular dystrophy. Coed,
ages 6-17.

8429   **Champ Camp**
American Lung Association In Alaska
7420 SW Bridgeport Road
Suite 200
Tigard, OR   97224   503-294-4094
                                               800-586-4872
                                          Fax: 503-294-4120
                                       info@lungmtpacific.org
                                            www.aklung.org
Kathryn A. Forbes, Chairman
John F. Emanuel, Vice Chair
Harold Wimmer, President and CEO
Penny J. Siewert, Secretary/Treasurer
Champ Camp is a week long summer recreation and asthma edu-
cation program at Camp Kushtaka on the beautiful shores of
Kenai Lake. Campers are able to explore their skills in outdoor
activities including canoeing, hiking, swimming, archery, and
arts and crafts. More importantly, Champ Camp boosts self-confidence and instills a sense of responsibility. It teaches preventive
measures to improve asthma management, and avoid asthmatic
episodes as well as increases a camper's sense of independence.

8430   **Diabetes Camp**
Tanager Place
1614 W Mount Vernon Road
Mount Vernon, IA   52314   319-363-0681
                                          Fax: 319-365-6411
                                       dpirrie@tanagerplace.org
                                        www.camptanager.org
Donald Pirrie, Camp Director
Provides children and adolescents with Diabetes a safe and
healthy environment and healthy environment to enjoy a variety
of recreational activities designed for fun and fitness. The camp
held each July has an on-site 24-hour physician and nursing staff.
Ages 6-13.

8431   **Dr. Moises Simpser VACC Camp**
Miami Childrens Hospital
3200 W.W. 60 Ct.
Suite 203
Miami, FL   33155-4076   305-662-8222
                                          Fax: 786-268-1765
                                        bela.florentin@mch.com
                                          www.vacccamp.com
Bela Florentin, Camp Coordinator
Ivette Hidalgo, MSN, ARNP, Camp Clinical Coordinator
Rose Ann Farrell, LCSW, Volunteer Assistant Coordinator
Javier Hern ndez, RRT, Volunteer Respiratory Therapist
VACC Camp gives families a fun opportunity to socialize with
peers and enjoy activities not readily accessible to technology dependent children. The program includes sailing, swimming, field
trips to local attractions, campsite entertainment, structured
games, free play, and more - all to promote family growth and development while enhancing individual self-esteem and social
skills. Parents have formal and informal opportunities to network
among themselves.

8432   **EDI Camp**
Wyman Center
600 Kiwanis Dr
St. Louis, MO   63025-2212   636-938-5245
                                          Fax: 636-938-5289
                                       info@wymancenter.org
                                         www.wymancenter.org
David Hilliard, President
Theresa Mayberry, Senior Vice President

Youngsters with diabetes learn how to care for themselves while participating in a wide variety of outdoor activities and trips. The camp, managed and financed by the American Diabetes Association Greater St. Louis Affiliate, offers camperships to children from the Greater St. Louis area, ages 7-16, but nonresidents may also apply.

8433   Echoing Hills
36272 County Road 79
Warsaw, OH   43844   740-327-2311
                                                      800-419-6513
                                                 Fax: 740-327-6371
                                          info@echoinghillsvillage.org
                                             www.echoinghillsvillage.org

Buddy Busch, President/CEO
Summer camp for children and adults with cerebral palsy. Coed, ages 7-70.

8434   Edward J Madden Open Hearts Camp
250 Monument Valley Road
Great Barrington, MA   01230   413-528-2229
                                            hearts@openheartscamp.org
                                              www.openheartscamp.org

Rick Farrell, President
David Zaleon, Executive Director
Jacqueline Reasor, Counselor
Jill Helme, Asst. Director
Eight week program for children who have had and are fully recovered from open heart surgery or a heart transplant. Four two week sessions by age group. Small camp - 25 campers per session.

8435   FCYD Camp
Foundation for Children and Youth with Diabetes
1995 W 9000 S
West Jordan, UT   84084   801-566-6913
                                                   www.fcydcamp.org

Nathan Gedge, Chair
David Okubo, President/Co-Founder
Elizabeth Elmer, Vice President
Sherrie Hardy, Director
Camping for children with diabetes. Coed, ages 1-18 and families.

8436   Father Drumgoole Connelly Summer Camp
MIV Mount Loretto
6581 Hylan Blvd
Staten Island, NY   10309-3830   718-317-2600
                                                 Fax: 718-317-2830
                                                  www.mountloretto.org

Stephen Rynn, Executive Director
Maryann Virga, Executive Assistant
Loretta Polanish, Executive Secretary
Ed Gani, Facilities Manager
Summer sessions for children with epilepsy, hearing impairment and developmental disabilities. Coed, ages 5-13.

8437   Florida Diabetes Camp
P.O.Box 14136
Gainesville, FL   32604   352-334-1321
                                                 Fax: 352-334-1326
                                          fccyd@floridadiabetescamp.org
                                             www.floridadiabetescamp.org

Gary Cornwell, Executive Director
Chris Satkely, Assistant Director
Amy Soileau, Outreach Director
Robena Cornwell, Finance
Camp is located in Florida. One and two-week sessions June-August for children with diabetes. Coed, ages 6-18 and families. Camps throughout the year.

8438   Friends Academy Summer Camps
Duck Pond Rd
Locust Valley, NY   11560   516-393-4207
                                                 Fax: 516-465-1720
                                                        camp@fa.org
                                               www.fasummercamp.org

Rich Mack, Camp Director

Summer sessions for children with diabetes. Coed, ages 3-14, families.

8439   God's Camp
Episcopal Church of Hawaii
68-729 Farrington Hwy
Waialua, HI   96791-9314   808-637-6241
                                                      808-637-5505
                                                 Fax: 808-637-5505
                                             info@campmokuleia.com
                                               www.campmokuleia.org

Debbie Alemeda, Manager
Episcopal Church tent camping, 5 nights, July. Church groups, family reunions, weddings, other organizations.

8440   Growing Together Diabetes Camp
ETMC
1000 S. Beckham
Tyler, TX   75701   903-597-0351
                                                      800-232-8318
                                                     info@etmc.org
                                                      www.etmc.org

Marty Wiggins, Development Director
Vicki Jowell, Director
Elmer G. Ellis, President
Jerry Massey, Senior Vice President
A summer camp for youths ages 6 to 15 with Type 1 or Type 2 diabetes.

8441   Happiness Is Camping
62 Sunset Lake Rd
Hardwick, NJ   07825   908-362-6733
                                                 Fax: 908-362-5197
                                         rich@happinessiscamping.org
                                            www.happinessiscamping.org

Laura San Miguel, RN, PNP, President
Julie McMahon, RN, Secretary
Alexander Chou, MD, Medical Director
Paulette Kelly, RN, Nursing Director
Happiness Is Camping, for children with cancer, was founded in 1980. About 400 children, girls and boys aged 6-15 years, attend the overnight camp, staying from one to all of the sessions, depending on their health.

8442   Hemophilia Camp
Tanager Place
1614 W Mount Vernon Road
Mount Vernon, IA   52314   319-363-0681
                                                 Fax: 319-365-6411
                                            dpirrie@tanagerplace.org
                                               www.camptanager.org

Donald Pirrie, Camp Director
During the six-day camp children with Hemophilia and their siblings participate in individual and group activities designed for fun and fitness. The camp held each year in mid-June has a 24-hour physician and nursing staff. Ages 5-16.

8443   Hole in the Wall Gang Camp
565 Ashford Center Rd
Ashford, CT   06278   860-429-3444
                                                 Fax: 860-429-7295
                                         ashford@holeinthewallgang.org
                                            www.holeinthewallgang.org

Raymond Lamontagne, Chairman
Ken Alberti, Chief Development Officer
James H. Canton, Chief Executive Officer
Kevin M. Magee, Chief Financial Officer
Low-cost eight-week sessions June-August for children with cancer and HIV. Coed, ages 7-15.

8444   Kiwanis Camp Wyman
Wyman Center
600 Kiwanis Dr
Eureka, MO   63025-2212   636-938-5245
                                        Fax: 636-938-5289
                                        www.wymancenter.org

Keat Wilkins, Chairman
Dave Hilliard, President/CEO
Tom Etzkorn, VP, Executive Resource Officer

Mindy Sharp, MBA, SVP, Finance & Administration

Summer sessions for youth with diabetes. Coed, ages 8-16, run in
conjunction with the American Diabetes Association. Call for
program description.

8445   Makemie Woods Camp
Presbytery of Eastern Virginia
P.O.Box 39
Barhamsville, VA   23011   757-566-1496
                                            800-566-1496
                                        Fax: 757-566-8803
                                        makwoods@makwoods.org
                                        www.makwoods.org

Mike Burcher, Director
Sherri Egerton, Program Director
Karen Broughman, Office Manager
Anthony Burcher, Storyteller in Residence
Residential Christian camp that tailors each group and individual
goals. Counselors serve as teachers, friends and activity leaders.
For children 8-18 with diabetes.

8446   Makemie Woods Camp/Conference Retreat
Presbytery of Eastern Virginia
P.O.Box 39
Barhamsville, VA   23011   757-566-1496
                                            800-566-1496
                                        Fax: 757-566-8803
                                        makwoods@makwoods.org

Mike Burcher, Director
Sherri Egerton, Program Director
Karen Broughman, Office Manager
Anthony Burcher, Storyteller in Residence
Counselors serve as teachers, friends and activity leaders. The individual is important within the small group. No camper is lost in
the crowd, but is an integral partner in the group process. Residential Christian Camp and conference center. Summer camp for
children 8-18 and special camp for children with diabetes.

8447   Marist Brothers Mid-Hudson Valley Camp
PO Box 197
Esopus, NY   12429   845-384-6620
                                        info@maristbrotherscenter.org

Amy Reinwald-Earle, Camp Director, Special Children
Brother Owen Ormsby, Executive Director
Scott Kuhner, Director of Operations
Mike Trainor, Facilities Director
The camp provides week-long summer sessions for children who
have a variety of special needs/illnesses, such as cancer, HIV,
deaf or mental disabilities. Each session is specific to the special
need/illness.

8448   Med-Camps of Louisiana
102 Thomas Road
Suite 615
West Monroe, LA   71291   318-329-8405
                                            877-282-0802
                                        Fax: 318-329-8407
                                        infos@medcamps.com
                                        www.medcamps.com

Caleb Seney, Executive Director
Bethany Gerfers, Administrative Assistant
Kacie Hobson, Events & Volunteer Coordinator

Serves children with severe asthma and allergies and many more.

8449   Mountaineer Spina Bifida Camp
534 New Goff Mountain Rd
Charleston, WV   25313   304-776-7513
                                        info@drewsday.org
                                        www.drewsday.org/

Suzie Humphreys
A summer camp for individuals with spina bifida. Campers can
participate in activities such as swimming, wheelchair hockey,
baseball, and more.

8450   Muscular Dystrophy Association Free Camp
222 S. Riverside Plaza
Suite 1500
Chicago, IL   60606   907-276-2131
                                            800-572-1717
                                        Fax: 907-276-0946
                                        www.mdausa.org

R. Rodney Howell, MD, Chairman
Steven M. Derks, President/CEO
Julie Faber, EVP/CFO
Pete Morgan, EVP/COO
MDA Camp provides a wide range of activities for those who
have limited mobility or are in wheelchairs. The camp offers may
outdoor sporting activities, art's & crafts and talent shows.

8451   NeSoDak
Lutherans Outdoors in South Dakota
3285 Camp Dakota Dr.
Waubay, SD   57273-1   605-947-4440
                                            800-888-1464
                                        nesodak@losd.org
                                        www.losd.org

Jake Hanson, Director
Sharon Oliver, Officer Manager
Kris Mueller, Hospitality Director
NeSoDak provides a safe place for youth to build relationships,
develop new skills, and live in a grace-filled community as they
learn about Christ's love for them-all while enjoying time at the
lake with a caring, well trained, energetic, and fun loving staff.
Hosts Camp Gilbert, a summer camp program for children with
diabetes.

8452   Northwest Kiwanis Camp
Camp Beausite NW
P.O.Box 1227
Port Hadlock, WA   98339   360-732-7222
                                        campbeausitenw.org/

Dr. Claudia Edmondson, Director
Cheryl Smith, Director of Programs
Northwest Kiwanis Camp is also known as Camp Beausite NW,
and is located in Chimacum, Washington. Campers range from
6-65 in age, and includes those with developmental disabilities,
cerebral palsy, autism, downs syndrome, and other physical
and/or mental handicaps. The camp currently offers five
week-long overnight summer camp sessions for adults and
children.

8453   Phantom Lake YMCA Camp
S110 W30240 YMCA Camp Road
Mukwonago, WI   53149   262-363-4386
                                        Fax: 262-363-4351
                                        office@phantomlakeymca.org
                                        www.phantomlakeymca.org

James Scharine, Chair of the Board
Jay Wall, Vice Chair
Dr. Karen Mulrooney, Secretary
Jodi Jacobsen, Treasurer
Phantom Lake Camp offers day and residential camping sessions
for boys, girls, and a coed session. All programs are open to indi-
viduals with disabilities as the camp welcomes any child, ages
3-17, regardless of race, religon, disability, etc.

8454 Shady Oaks Camp
16300 Parker Road
Homer Glen, IL   60491   708-301-0816
                                    Fax: 708-301-5091
                                    soc16300@sbcglobal.net
                                    shadyoakscamp.org

Harry Burroughs, Chairman
Robert Szajkovics, President
Lori McAleavy, Vice President
Scott Steele, Executive Director
Shady Oaks Camp provides outdoor fun and recreation for children and adults with cerebral palsy and similar disabilities. Our camp is organized with the goal of providing stimulating life experiences that our campers may not have the opportunity to engage in elsewhere.

8455 Sherman Lake YMCA Summer Camp
Sherman Lake YMCA Outdoor Center
6225 N 39th St
Augusta, MI   49012   269-731-3000
                                    Fax: 269-731-3020
                                    shermanlakeymca@ymcasl.org
                                    www.shermanlakeymca.org

Luke Austenfeld, Executive Director
Jean Henderson, Business Manager
Lorrie Syverson, Director,Camping, Education & Retreat Services
Mark VanDaff, Facility Manager
Summer camping sessions for campers with ADD and spina bifida. Coed, ages 6-15 and families, seniors.

8456 Strength for the Journey
Oregon-Idaho Conference Center
1505 SW 18th Ave
Portland, OR   97201-2524   503-226-7931
                                    800-593-7539
                                    suttlelake@gocamping.org
                                    www.gocamping.org

Jane Petke, Suttle Lake Camp Director
Geneva Cook, Camping Registrar
Camp is located near Sisters, Oregon at Suttle Lake Camp. Strength for the Journey is a program for adults living with HIV/AIDS.

8457 Summer Camp for Children with Muscular Dystrophy
Muscular Dystrophy Association - USA
222 S. Riverside Plaza
Suite 1500
Chicago, IL   60606   520-529-2000
                                    800-572-1717
                                    Fax: 520-529-5300
                                    mda@mdausa.org
                                    www.mdausa.org

R. Rodney Howell, MD, Chairman
Steven M. Derks, President/CEO
Pete Morgan, EVP/COO
Julie Faber, EVP/CFO
Offers a wide range of activities such as adaptive sports, swimming, fishing, archery, scavenger hunts, dances & talent shows, art's & crafts, karaoke, and campfires.

8458 Summer Camp for Physically & Mentally Challenged Children & Adults
Kansas Jaycees' Cerebral Palsy Foundation
P.O.Box 267
Augusta, KS   67010   316-775-2421
                                    Fax: 316-775-2421
                                    www.cpranch.org

Cheryl Schmeidler, Executive Director
Sarah Walker, Camp Director
Our mission is to provide a program which will allow individuals to enjoy their highest level of functioning and independence, consistant with their abilities, in a summer camp setting.

8459 Suttle Lake Camp
29551 Suttle Lake Rd
Sisters, OR   97759   541-595-6663
                                    suttlelake@gocamping.org
                                    suttlelake.gocamping.org/

Jane Petke, Co-Director
Daniel Petke, Co-Director
Camp is located in Sisters, Oregon. Camping sessions for children and adults with AIDS/HIV. Coed, ages 6-18, families, seniors and single adults.

8460 TSA CT Kid's Summer Event
Tourette Syndrome Association of Connecticut (TSA)
c/o Massachusetts Chapter
39 Godfrey Street
Taunton, MA 02780   617-277-7589
                                    info@tsa-ma.org
                                    www.tsact.org

Tom Meehan, Chairman
Peter Tavolacci, Vice-Chairman
Paul Nazario, Treasurer
TSA of Connecticut sponsors summer events for children with TS/Tourette Syndrome activities of which include minature golf in addition to an Annual Conference. The kids' program at this annual conference provides children who have TS a unique opportunity to meet other children like them who also struggle with TS. Entertainment includes puppeteers, magicians, learning karate from the experts, getting face paintings and more.
uniqu pages

8461 Texas Lions Camp
Lions Club Of Texas
P.O.Box 290247
Kerrville, TX   78029   830-896-8500
                                    Fax: 830-896-3666
                                    www.lionscamp.com

Stephen Mabry, Executive Director
Steven King, Director of Operations
Patty Rodriguez, Program Supervisor
Bailey Carter, Program Supervisor
Texas Lions Camp is a camp dedicated to seving children in Texas with physical diabilities, ages 7-16. While at camp, campers will participate in a variety of acitivties and they will be encouraged to become more independent and self-confident.

8462 The Barton Center Clara Barton Camp
The Barton Center for Diabetes Education, Inc.
30 Ennis Road
PO Box 356
North Oxford, MA   01537-0356   508-987-2056
                                    Fax: 508-987-2002
                                    www.bartoncenter.org

Kevin Wilcoxen, Executive Director
Jesse Welch, Site & Facilities Director
Thomas Racine, Facilities Assistant
Brendan Duffy, Facilities Assistant
Girls, ages 3-17, with diabetes participate in a well-rounded camp program with special education in diabetes, health and safety. Activities include swimming, boating, sports, dance, music and arts and crafts. Two week adventure camp for high school girls offering camping, hiking, canoeing, etc. Also a minicamp (one week) for girls 6-12. Day camps are offered in Worcester, Boston, and New York City.

8463 Twin Lakes Camp
1451 E Twin Lakes Rd
Hillsboro, IN   47949-8004   765-798-4000
                                    outdoors@twinlakescamp.com
                                    www.twinlakescamp.com

Jon Beight, Executive Director
Dan Daily, Program Director
Duane Bush, Guest Service
Donna Beight, Secretary
Provides a summer camp program for special needs children and young adults. Campers suffer from a wide range of maladies including crippling accidents, Spina Bifida, epilepsy, Cerebral Palsy, Muscular Dystrophy, Quadriplegia, Paraplegia, and other disabling diseases. Campers range in age from 8 to 27.

8464   Wisconsin Lions Camp
Wisconsin Lions Foundation
3834 County Road A
Ro3holt, WI   54473

715-677-4969
877-463-6959
Fax: 715-677-4527
info@wisconsinlionscamp.com
wisconsinlionscamp.com

Evett J. Hartvig, Executive Director
Andrea Yenter, Camp Director
Summer Allen, Program Supervisor
Dale Schroeder, Facility Director
Serves children who have either a visual, hearing or mild cognitive disability, as well as diabetes types I and II. Program activities include sailing, ropes course, hiking and canoe trips, environmental education, swimming, camping, canoeing, outdoor living skills and handicrafts. ACA accredited, located in central Wisconsin, near Stevens Point.

8465   Y Camp
YMCA of Greater Des Moines
1192 166th Drive
Boone, IA   50036

515-432-7558
Fax: 515-432-5414
ycamp@dmymca.org
www.y-camp.org

David Sherry, Executive Director
Mike Havlik, Program Director- Environmental
Alex Kretzinger, Program Director- Summer Camp
Amy Joanning, Development Coordinator/Registrar
Camp is located in Boone, Iowa. Year-round one and two-week sessions for boys and girls with cancer, diabetes, asthma, cystic fibrosis, hearing impaired and other disabilities. Coed, ages 6-16 and families.

8466   YMCA Camp Fitch
The YMCA's Camp Fitch on Lake Erie
12600 Abels Rd
North Springfield, PA   16430

814-922-3219
877-863-4824
Fax: 814-922-7000
hannahkight@campfitchymca.org
campfitchymca.org

Matt Pose, Executive Director
Tom Parker, Associate Executive Director
Hannah Kight, Office Manager
Jon Tully, Program Director
Camp is located in North Springfield, Pennsylvania. Camping sessions for children and adults with diabetes or epilepsy. Ages 8-16, families and seniors.

8467   YMCA Camp Ihduhapi
Minneapolis YMCA Camping Services
15200 Hanson Blvd.
Andover, MN   55304

763-230-9622
info@campihduhapi.org
campihduhapi.org

Kerry Pioske, Camp Executive
Josh Cobb, Overnight Camp Director
Devin Hanson, Day Camp Director
Eric Wobschall, Building Superintendent
Camp is located in Loretto, Minnesota. Summer sessions for campers with asthma/respiratory ailments and epilepsy. Coed, ages 7-16.

8468   YMCA Camp Kitaki
Lincoln YMCA
570 Fallbrook Blvd.
Suite 210
Lincoln, NE   68521

402-434-9200
Fax: 402-434-9208
info@ymcalincoln.org
www.ymcalincoln.org

Barb Bettin, President/CEO
J.P. Lauterbach, COO
Misty Muff, Chief Administrative Officer
Renee Yost, CFO

Camp is located in Louisville, Nebraska. Summer sessions for children with cystic fibrosis. Coed, ages 7-17 and families.

8469   YMCA Camp Shady Brook
YMCA of the Pikes Peak Region (PPYMCA)
316 N. Tejon Street
Colorado Springs, CO   80903

719-329-7227
Fax: 719-272-7026
campinfo@ppymca.org
www.campshadybrook.org

Sonny Adkins, Executive Director
Laura Petersen, Program Director
Patrick Casey, Facility Director
Michaela Eddleston, Conference & Retreat Director
Camp is located in Sedalia, Colorado. One-week sessions for campers with HIV. Boys and girls 7-16. Also families, seniors and single adults.

8470   YMCA Camp Weona
YMCA of Greater Buffalo
301 Cayuga Rd
Suite 100
Buffalo, NY   14225

716-565-6000
Fax: 716-565-6007
www.ymcabuffaloniagara.org

John D. Murray, President/CEO
Camp is located in Gainesville, New York. Camping sessions for children and adults with epilepsy. Coed, ages 7-16, families and single adults. Nestled in 1,000 acres of hardwood and pine forests, Weona has miles of picturesque hiking trails, brooks, a heated outdoor pool and a world class adventure ropes course. Our indoor facilities include arts and crafts studios, environmental classrooms and a challenging rock climbing wall. It is the ideal setting for hands-on fun, adventure and learning.

8471   YMCA Camp jewell
YMCA of Greater Hartford
6 Prock Hill Road
P.O. Box 8
Colebrook, CT   06021

860-379-2782
888-412-2267
Fax: 860-379-8715
camp.jewell@ghymca.org
www.ghymca.org

Eric Tucker, Executive Director
Camp is located in Colebrook, Connecticut. Two-week sessions for children with cancer. Coed, ages 8-16. Also families.

8472   YMCA Camp of Maine
305 Winthrop Center Rd
P.O. Box 446
Winthrop, ME   04364

207-395-4200
Fax: 207-395-7230
info@maineycamp.org
www.maineycamp.org

Tom Christensen, CVO
Rebecca Henry, Vice CVO
Marty Allen, Treasurer
Heather Priest, Secretary
Activities include arts and crafts, nature study, hiking, and overnight camping, dancing, and singing. Summer session dates run from June through August; for ages 8-16.

8473   YMCA Outdoor Center Campbell Gard
4803 Augspurger Road
Hamilton, OH   45011

513-867-0600
Fax: 513-867-0127
camp@gmvymca.org
www.ccgymca.org

Pete Fasano, Executive Director
Katie Depew, Summer Program Director
Tom Andrews, Facilities and Properties Manager
Wendi Moore, Office Manager
Camp is located in Hamilton, Ohio. Camping sessions for children and young adults with developmental disabilities. Runs overnight and day sessions for ages 7-22 and families.

Print: Books

8474   A Woman's Guide to Living with HIV Infection
Johns Hopkins University Press
2715 N Charles St
Baltimore, MD   21218-4363   410-516-6900
                                               800-548-1784
                                          Fax: 410-516-6998
                                    jwehmueller@press.jhu.edu
                                            www.press.jhu.edu

Rebecca A Clark M.D., PhD, Author
Robert T Maupin Jr. M.D. FACOG, Co-Author
Jill Hayes Hammer PhD, Co-Author
A resource for women with HIV that discusses coping with the diagnosis, finding a physician, recognizing symptoms, and preventing complications. Explains the latest treatment options and
advice on coping with gynecologic infections. *$18.00*
328 pages Hardback

8475   ABC of Asthma, Allergies & Lupus
Global Health Solutions
2146 Kings Garden Way
PO Box 3189
Falls Church, VA 22043-2593   703-848-2333
                                               800-759-3999
                                          Fax: 703-848-0028
                                    information@watercure.com
                                            www.watercure.com

Fereydoon Batmanghelidj MD, Author
Xiaopo Batmanghelidj, President
Kristin Swan, Administrator
This book introduces new approaches in preventing and treating
asthma, allergies and lupus without toxic chemicals. It also offers
new insight on how to prevent and treat children's asthma. *$17.00*
240 pages
ISBN 0-962994-26-x

8476   AIDS Sourcebook
Omnigraphics, Inc.
PO Box 31-1640
Detroit, MI   48231-8002   610-461-3548
                                               800-234-1340
                                          Fax: 610-532-9001
                                       info@omnigraphics.com
                                           www.omnigraphics.com

Sandra J Judd, Editor
Basic consumer health information about the Human Immunodeficiency Virus (HIV) and Acquired Immunodeficiency Syndrome
(AIDS), including facts about its origins, stages, types, transmission, risk factors, and prevention, and featuring details about diagnostic testing, antiretroviral treatments, and co-occurring
infections. *$85.00*
600 pages 5th Edition 1911
ISBN 0-780811-47-8

8477   AIDS and Other Manifestations of HIV Infection
Elsevier Inc
30 Corporate Dr
Suite 400
Burlington, MA   01803-4252   781-313-4700
                                               800-545-2522
                                          Fax: 800-568-5136
                                       usbkinfo@elsevier.com
                                            www.elsevier.com

Gary Wormser MD, Editor
A comprehensive overview of the biological properties of this
etiologic viral agent, its clinicopathological manifestations, the
epidemiology of its infection, and present and future therapeutic
options. *$249.95*
1000 pages 2004
ISBN 0-127640-51-7

8478   AIDS in the Twenty-First Century: Disease and Globalization
Palgrav Macmillan
175 5th Ave
New York, NY   10010-7703   888-330-8477
                                          Fax: 800-672-2054
                                    onlinesupportusa@palgrave.com
                                           www.palgrave-usa.com

Gabriella Georgiades, Editor
Alan Whiteside, Author
Tony Barnett, Co-Author
The authors — exprets in the field for over 15 years — argue that
it is vital to not only look at AIDS in terms of prevention and treatment, but to also consider consequences which affect house-
holds, communities, companies, governments, and countries.
This is a major contribution toward understanding the global public health crisis, as well as the relationship between poverty, inequality, and infectious diseases. *$32.00*
464 pages
ISBN 1-403997-68-5

8479   Adult Leukemia: A Comprehensive Guide for Patients and Families
O'Reilly Media Inc
1005 Gravenstein Hwy N
Sebastopol, CA   95472-2811   707-827-7000
                                               800-998-9938
                                          Fax: 707-829-0104
                                           order@oreilly.com
                                             www.oreilly.com

Linda Lamb, Editor
Barb Lackritz, Author
For the tens of thousands of Americans with adult leukemia,
Adult Leukemia: A Comprehensive Guide for Patients and Families addresses diagnosis, medical tests, finding a good
oncologist, treatments, side effects, getting emotional and other
support, resources for further study, and much more. The book includes real-life stories from those who have battled leukemia
themselves. *$29.95*
536 pages Paperback
ISBN 0-596500-01-7

8480   Advanced Breast Cancer: A Guide to Living with Metastic Disease
O'Reilly Media Inc
1005 Gravenstein Hwy N
Sebastopol, CA   95472-2811   707-827-7000
                                               800-998-9938
                                          Fax: 707-829-0104
                                           order@oreilly.com
                                             www.oreilly.com

Linda Lamb, Editor
Musa Mayer, Author
This is the only book on breast cancer that deals honestly with the
realities of living with metastic disease, yet offers hope and comfort. All aspects of facing the disease are covered, including: coping with the shock of recurrence, seeking information and making
treatment decisions, communicating effectively with medical
personnel finding support, and handling disease progression and
end-of-life issues. A comprehensive guide, it also provides updated resources and treatment developments. *$24.95*
532 pages Paperback 1998
ISBN 1-565925-22-X

8481   Allergies & Asthma: What Every Parent Needs To Know (2nd Edition)
American Academy of Pediatrics
141 Northwest Point Blvd
Elk Grove Village, IL   60007-1019   847-434-4000
                                               800-433-9016
                                          Fax: 847-434-8000
                                             newpubs@aap.org
                                                www.aap.org

Bernard P. Dreyer, MD; FAAP, President
Karen Remley, MD; MBA; MPH, Executive Director & CEO
Consumer resource for parents who need answers and informa-
tion about their children's allergies and asthma. Covers advice on

identifying allergies and asthma, preventing attacks, minimizing triggers, understanding medications, explaining allergies to young children, and helping children manage symptoms. *$14.95*
174 pages Paperback; eBook available 1910
ISBN 1-581104-45-6

8482 Allergies Sourcebook
PO Box 31-1640
Detroit, MI 48231-8002   610-461-3548
                                                           800-234-1340
                                                   Fax: 610-532-9001
                                               info@omnigraphics.com
                                               www.omnigraphics.com
Amy L Sutton, Editor
Basic comsumer health information about the immune system and allergic disorders, including rhinitis (hay fever), sinusitis, conjunctivitis, asthma, atopic dermatitis, and anaphylaxis, and allergy triggers such as pollen, mold, dust mites, animal dander, chemicals, foods and additives, and medications; along with facts about allergy diagnosis and treatment, tips on avoiding triggers and preventing symptoms, a glossary of related terms, and directories of resources for additional help and info. *$95.00*
608 pages 4th Edition 1911

8483 Alternative Approach to Allergies
Harper Collins Publishers
10 E 53rd St
New York, NY 10022-5244   212-207-7901
                                                          800-242-7737
                                                  Fax: 212-702-2586
                                              spsales@harpercollins.com
                                              www.harpercollins.com
Theron G Randolph M.D., Author
Ralph W Moss PhD, Co-Author
Here is the book that revolutionized the way allergies and other common illnesses were diagnosed and treated.
ISBN 0-060916-93-1

8484 Alzheimer Disease Sourcebook
Omnigraphics
PO Box 8002
Aston, PA 19014-8002   800-234-1340
                                                  Fax: 800-875-1340
                                              info@omnigraphics.com
                                              www.omnigraphics.com
Amy L. Sutton, Editor
Alzheimer Disease Sourcebook, Fifth Edition provides updated information about causes, symptoms, and stages of AD and other forms of dementia, including mild cognitive impairment, corticobasal degeneration, dementia with Lewy bodies, frontotemporal dementia, Huntington disease, Parkinson disease, and dementia caused by infections. *$95.00*
600 pages 1911
ISBN 0-780811-50-8

8485 Alzheimer Disease Sourcebook, 4th Edition
Omnigraphics
PO Box 8002
Aston, PA 19014-8002   610-461-3548
                                                          800-234-1340
                                                  Fax: 800-875-1340
                                      customerservice@omnigraphics.com
                                              www.omnigraphics.com
Peter Ruffner, President, Co-Founder
Fred Ruffner, Founder
Basic consumer health information about alzheimer disease, other dementias, and related disorders, including multi-infarct dementia, dementia with lewy bodies, frontotemporal dementia (pick disease), Wernicke-Korsakoff syndrome (alcohol-related dementia), AIDS dementia complex, Huntington disease, Creutzfeldt-Jacob disease, and delirium. *$84.00*
603 pages
ISBN 0-780810-01-3

8486 Amyotrophic Lateral Sclerosis: A Guide for Patients and Families
Demos Medical Publishing
11 West 42nd Street
15th Floor
New York, NY 10036   212-683-0072
                                                          800-532-8663
                                                  Fax: 212-683-0118
                                           support@demosmedical.com
                                              www.demosmedpub.com
Richard Winters, Executive Editor
Beth Kaufman Barry, Publisher
Noreen Henson, Executive Director of Demos Heal
Reina Santana, Director of Special Sales & Righ
This comprehensive guide covers every aspect of the management of ALS. Beginning with discussions of its clinical features of the disease, diagnosis, and an overview of symptom management, major sections deal with medical and rehabilitative management, living with ALS, managing advanced disease and end-of-life issues, and reources that can provide support and assistance. *$29.95*
470 pages 2001
ISBN 1-888799-28-5

8487 Arthritis Sourcebook.
Omnigraphics
PO Box 31-1640
Detroit, MI 48231-8002   610-461-3548
                                                          800-234-1340
                                                  Fax: 610-532-9001
                                              info@omnigraphics.com
                                              www.omnigraphics.com
Amy L Sutton, Editor
Basic consumer health information about osteoarthritis, rheumatoid arthritis, other rheumatic disorders, infectious forms of arthritis, and diseases with symptoms linked to arthritis, and facts about diagnosis, pain management, and surgical therapies. *$84.00*
567 pages 2nd Edition
ISBN 0-780806-67-2

8488 Asthma Sourcebook.
Omnigraphics
PO Box 31-1640
Detroit, MI 48231-8002   610-461-3548
                                                          800-234-1340
                                                  Fax: 610-532-9001
                                              info@omnigraphics.com
                                              www.omnigraphics.com
Karen Bellenir, Editor
Provides information about asthma, including symptoms, remedies and research updates. *$84.00*
581 pages 2nd Edition
ISBN 0-780808-66-9

8489 Asthma and Allergy Answers: A Patient Education Library
Asthma and Allergy Foundation of America
8201 Corporate Dr
Suite 1000
Landover, MD 20785   202-466-7643
                                                          800-727-8462
                                                  Fax: 202-466-8940
                                                       info@aafa.org
                                                       www.aafa.org
Amy Patterson, Senior Director of Administration & Governance
Jacqui Vok, Director of Programs and Services
William McLin, M.Ed., President/CEO
This resource contains 50 reproducible fact sheets for patients on a variety of popular asthma and allergy topics. Information is written in a patient-friendly question and answer format and packaged in a durable binder for easy storage and use. *$50.00*

8490   Back & Neck Sourcebook.
Omnigraphics
PO Box 31-1640
Detroit, MI   48231-8002   610-461-3548
                                             800-234-1340
                                        Fax: 610-532-9001
                                      info@omnigraphics.com
                                        www.omnigraphics.com
Amy L Sutton, Editor
Basic consumer health information about back and neck pain, spinal cord injuries, and related disorders, such as degenerative disk disease, osteoarthritis, scoliosis, sciatica, spina bifida, and spinal stenosis, and featuring facts about maintaining spinal health, self-care, rehabilitative care, chiropractic care, spinal surgeries, and complementary therapies. *$84.00*
607 pages 2nd Edition
ISBN 0-780807-38-9

8491   Being Close
National Jewish Health
1400 Jackson St
Denver, CO   80206-2761   303-398-1002
                                             877-225-5654
                                        Fax: 303-398-1125
                                        allstetterw@njc.org
                                        www.nationaljewish.org
Michael Salem M.D., President/CEO
William Allstetter, Director Media/External Relation
A booklet offering information to patients suffering from a respiratory disorder such as emphysema, asthma or tuberculosis, that discusses sexual problems and feelings.

8492   Bittersweet Chances: A Personal Journey o f Living and Learning in the Face of Illness
PublishAmerica
PO Box 151
Frederick, MD   21705-151   301-695-1707
                                        Fax: 301-631-9073
                                    support@publishamerica.com
                                      www.publishamerica.com
Dana Selenke Broehl, Author
Recounts Doug and Dana Broehl's journey of growth through the darkness of cystic fibrosis and the renewed hope of a double lung transplant. *$24.95*
189 pages Softcover
ISBN 1-413713-24-6

8493   Blood and Circulatory Disorders Sourcebook
Omnigraphics
PO Box 31-1640
Detroit, MI   48231-8002   610-461-3548
                                             800-234-1340
                                        Fax: 610-532-9001
                                      info@omnigraphics.com
                                        www.omnigraphics.com
Amy L Sutton, Editor
Sandra J. Judd, Editor
Blood and Circulatory Disorders Sourcebook, Third Edition offers facts about blood function and composition, the maintenance of a healthy circulatory system, and the types of concerns that arise when processes go awry. It discusses the diagnosis and treatment of many common blood cell disorders, bleeding disorders, and circulatory disorders, including anemia, hemochromatosis, leukemia, lymphoma, hemophilia, hypercoagulation, thrombophilia, atherosclerosis, blood pressure irregularities, coronary *$84.00*
634 pages 2nd Edition
ISBN 0-780807-46-4

8494   Blooming Where You're Planted: Stories From The Heart
Meeting Life's Challenges
9042 Aspen Grove Lane
Madison, WI   53717-2700   608-824-0402
                                        Fax: 608-824-0403
                                help@MeetingLifesChallenges.com
                                      www.makinglifeeasier.com
Shelley Peterman Schwatz, Editor

Author Shelley Peterman Schwarz takes you on her journey of self-discovery and change following her diagnosis of multiple sclerosis in 1979. Her personal stories are warm and humorous, and insightful. This 138-page book will motivate and inspire you to rise above life's challenges and live life to its fullest. *$12.95*
138 pages 1998
ISBN 0-891854-01-1

8495   Brain Allergies: The Psychonutrient and Magnetic Connections
McGraw-Hill
William Philpott PhD, Author
Dwight Keating PhD, Author
Linus Pauling PhD, Author
A complete overview of the concept of brain allergies - the theory that exposure to certain foods and other substances triggers mental disorders in people so predisposed, and that such disturbances can be cured by eliminating these substances. *$16.95*
ISBN 0-658003-98-1

8496   Brain Disorders Sourcebook
Omnigraphics
PO Box 31-1640
Detroit, MI   48231-8002   610-461-3548
                                             800-234-1340
                                        Fax: 610-532-9001
                                      info@omnigraphics.com
                                        www.omnigraphics.com
Sandra J Judd, Editor
Joyce Brennfleck Shannon, Editor
Brain Disorders Sourcebook, Third Edition provides readers with updated information about brain function, neurological emergencies such as a brain attack (stroke) or seizure, and symptoms of brain disorders. It describes the diagnosis, treatment, and rehabilitation therapies for genetic and congenital brain disorders, brain infections, brain tumors, seizures, traumatic brain injuries, and degenerative neurological disorders such as Alzheimer disease and other dementias, Parkinson disease, and am *$84.00*
600 pages 2nd Edition
ISBN 0-780807-44-0

8497   Breast Cancer Sourcebook
Omnigraphics
PO Box 31-1640
Detroit, MI   48231-8002   610-461-3548
                                             800-234-1340
                                        Fax: 610-532-9001
                                      info@omnigraphics.com
                                        www.omnigraphics.com
Sandra J Judd, Editor
Amy L. Sutton, Editor
Breast Cancer Sourcebook, Fourth Edition, provides updated information about breast cancer and its causes, risk factors, diagnosis, and treatment. Readers will learn about the types of breast cancer, including ductal carcinoma in situ, lobular carcinoma in situ, invasive carcinoma, and inflammatory breast cancer, as well as common breast cancer treatment complications, such as pain, fatigue, lymphedema, hair loss, and sexuality and fertility issues. Information on preventive therapies, nutrition *$84.00*
600 pages 3rd Edition
ISBN 0-780810-30-3

8498   Breathe Free
Lotus Press
P.O.Box 325
Twin Lakes, WI   53181   262-889-8561
                                             800-824-6396
                                        Fax: 262-889-8591
                                     lotuspress@lotuspress.com
                                        www.lotuspress.com
D Gagnon, Author
A Morningstar, Co-Author
A nutritional and herbal medicine self-help guide to treating a full range of respiratory conditions, including colds and flu. *$14.95*
179 pages
ISBN 0-914955-07-1

8499 Cancer Sourcebook
Omnigraphics
PO Box 31-1640
Detroit, MI   48231-8002   610-461-3548
                                                   800-234-1340
                                              Fax: 610-532-9001
                                          info@omnigraphics.com
                                              www.omnigraphics.com
Karen Bellenir, Editor
Cancer Sourcebook, Sixth Edition provides updated information
about common types of cancer affecting the central nervous system, endocrine system, lungs, digestive and urinary tracts, blood
cells, immune system, skin, bones, and other body systems. It explains how people can reduce their risk of cancer by addressing
issues related to cancer risk and taking advantage of screening exams. *$84.00*
1105 pages 5th Edition
ISBN 0-780809-47-5

8500 Cancer Sourcebook for Women
Omnigraphics
PO Box 31-1640
Detroit, MI   48231-8002   610-461-3548
                                                   800-234-1340
                                              Fax: 610-532-9001
                                          info@omnigraphics.com
                                              www.omnigraphics.com
Amy L Sutton, Editor
Karen Bellenir, Editor
Cancer Sourcebook for Women, Fourth Edition offers updated information about gynecologic cancers and other cancers of special
concern to women, including breast cancer, cancers of the female
reproductive organs, and cancers responsible for the highest
number of deaths in women. It explains cancer risks-including
lifestyle factors, inherited genetic abnormalities, and hormonal
medications-and methods used to diagnose and treat cancer.
$84.00
687 pages 5th Edition
ISBN 0-780808-67-6

**8501 Cardiovascular Diseases and Disorders Sourcebook, 3rd
Edition**
Omnigraphics
PO Box 8002
Aston, PA   19014-8002   610-461-3548
                                                   800-234-1340
                                              Fax: 800-875-1340
                                     customerservice@omnigraphics.com
                                              www.omnigraphics.com
Peter Ruffner, President, Co-Founder
Fred Ruffner, Founder
Cardiovascular Diseases and Disorders Sourcebook, Third Edi-
tion, provides information about the symptoms, diagnosis, and
treatment heart diseases and vascular disorders. It includes demographic and statistical data, an overview of the cardiovascular
system, a discussion of risk factors and prevention techniques, a
look at cardiovascular concerns specific to women, and a report
on current research initiatives. *$84.00*
687 pages Hard cover
ISBN 0-780807-39-6

**8502 Childhood Cancer Survivors: A Practical Guide to Your
Future**
O'Reilly Media Inc
1005 Gravenstein Hwy N
Sebastopol, CA   95472-2811   707-827-7000
                                                   800-998-9938
                                              Fax: 707-829-0104
                                              order@oreilly.com
                                              www.oreilly.com
Linda Lamb, Editor
Nancy Keene, Author
Wendy Hobbie, Co-Author
Kathy Ruccione, Co-Author
More than 250,000 people have survived childhood cancer - a
cause for celebration. Authors Keene, Hobbie, and Ruccione
chart the territory of long-term survivorship: relationships; over-
coming employment or insurance discrimination; maximizing

health; follow-up schedules; medical late effects. The stories of
over sixty survivors - their challenges and triumphs - are told. Includes medical history record-keeper. *$27.95*
464 pages Paperback 1906
ISBN 0-596528-51-5

**8503 Childhood Cancer: A Parent's Guide to Solid Tumor
Cancers**
O'Reilly Media Inc
1005 Gravenstein Highway North
Sebastopol, CA   95472   707-827-7000
                                                   800-889-8969
                                              Fax: 707-829-0104
                                              order@oreilly.com
                                              www.oreilly.com
560 pages Paperback
ISBN 0-596500-14-9

8504 Childhood Diseases and Disorders Sourcebook, 2nd Edition
Omnigraphics
PO Box 8002
Aston, PA   19014-8002   610-461-3548
                                                   800-234-1340
                                              Fax: 800-875-1340
                                     customerservice@omnigraphics.com
                                              www.omnigraphics.com
Peter Ruffner, President, Co-Founder
Fred Ruffner, Founder
Sandra J Judd, Editor
Basic consumer health information about medical problems often
encountered in pre-adolescent children, including respiratory
tract ailments, ear infections, sore throats, disorders of the skin
and scalp, digestive and genitourinary diseases, infectious diseases, inflammatory disorders, chronic physical and developmental
disorders, allergies, and more. *$84.00*
600 pages Hard cover
ISBN 0-780810-31-0

**8505 Childhood Leukemia: A Guide for Families, Friends &
Caregivers**
O'Reilly Media Inc
1005 Gravenstein Hwy N
Sebastopol, CA   95472-2811   707-827-7000
                                                   800-998-9938
                                              Fax: 707-829-0104
                                              order@oreilly.com
                                              www.oreilly.com
Linda Lamb, Editor
Nancy Keene, Author
The second edition of this comprehensive guide offers detailed
and precise medical information for parents that includes
day-to-day practical advice on how to cope with procedures, hospitalization, family and friends, school, and social, emotional,
and financial issues. It features a wealth of tools for prents and
contains significant updates on treatments and procedures.
$29.95
528 pages 4th Edition 1910
ISBN 0-596500-15-7

8506 Children with Cerebral Palsy: A Parents' Guide
Woodbine House
6510 Bells Mill Road
Bethesda, MD   20817-1636   301-897-3570
                                                   800-843-7323
                                              Fax: 301-897-5838
                                          info@woodbinehouse.com
                                              www.woodbinehouse.com
Irvin Shapell, Owner
Beth Binns, Special Marketing Manager
Sarah Glenner, Office Receptionist;
Fran Marinaccio, Marketing Manager
A classic primer for parents that provides a complete spetrum of
information and compassionate advice about cerebral palsy and
its effect on their child's development and education. *$18.95*
481 pages
ISBN 0-933149-82-4

8507 **Chronic Fatigue Syndrome: Your Natural Gu ide to Healing with Diet, Herbs and Other Methods**
Random House Publishing
1745 Broadway
3rd Floor
New York, NY 10019-4305

212-782-9000
Fax: 212-572-6066
ecustomerservice@randomhouse.com
www.randomhouse.com

Susanna Porter, Editor
Michael T Murray N.D.
Explains specific measures sufferers can take to improve stamina, mental energy, and physical abilities. *$15.00*
208 pages
ISBN 1-559584-90-6

8508 **Coffee in the Cereal: The First Year with Multiple Sclerosis**
Pathfinder Publishing

520-647-0158
800-977-2282
bill@pathfinderpublishing.com
www.pathfinderpublishing.com

96 pages
ISBN 0-934793-07-7

8509 **Colon & Rectal Cancer: A Comprehensive Guide for Patients & Families**
O'Reilly Media Inc
1005 Gravenstein Hwy N
Sebastopol, CA 95472-2811

707-827-7000
800-998-9938
Fax: 707-829-0104
order@oreilly.com
www.oreilly.com

Linda Lamb, Editor
Lorraine Johnston, Author
The fourth most common cancer, colon and rectal cancer is diagnosed in 130,000 new cases in the United States each year. Patients and families need uo-to-date and in-depth information to participate wisely in treatment decisions (e.g., knowing what sexual and fertility issues to discuss with the doctor before surgery). This book covers coping with tests and treatment side effects, caring for ostomies, finding supportt, and other practical issues. *$24.95*
544 pages Paperback 1999
ISBN 1-565926-33-1

8510 **Colon Health: Key to a Vibrant Life**
Norwalk Press
P.O.Box 190526
Boise, ID 83719-526

928-445-5567
Fax: 928-445-5567
Norman Walker MD, Editor
Includes complete glossary of terms and index of referrals.

8511 **Complementary Alternative Medicine and Multiple Sclerosis**
Demos Medical Publishing
11 West 42nd Street
15th Floor
New York, NY 10036

212-683-0072
800-532-8663
Fax: 212-683-0118
support@demosmedical.com
www.demosmedpub.com

Richard Winters, Executive Editor
Beth Kaufman Barry, Publisher
Noreen Henson, Executive Director of Demos Heal
Reina Santana, Director of Special Sales & Righ
Offers reliable information on the relevance, safety, and effectiveness of various alternative therapies that are not typically considered in discussions of MS management, yet are in widespread use. *$24.95*
304 pages
ISBN 1-932603-54-9

8512 **Conquering the Darkness: One Story of Recovering from a Brain Injury**
Paragon House
1925 Oakcrest Avenue
Suite 7
Saint Paul, MN 55113-2619

651-644-3087
800-447-3709
Fax: 651-644-0997
info@paragonhouse.com
www.paragonhouse.com

Rosemary Yokoi, Publicity Director
Gordon Anderson, Executive Director
Deborah Quinn, Author
The course of recovery from a brain injury by a woman who lived through it. *$15.95*
276 pages 1998
ISBN 1-557787-63-8

8513 **Coping with Cerebral Palsy**
Rosen Publishing
29 East 21st Street
New York, NY 10010

800-237-9932
Fax: 888-436-4643
www.rosenpublishing.com

Laura Anne Gilman, Author
This second edition book provides parents of children and adults with cerebral palsy the answers to more than 300 questions that have been carefully researched. It represents 40 years of experience by the author and is presented in a highly readable, jargon-free manner. *$31.95*
ISBN 0-823931-50-1

8514 **Curing MS: How Science is Solving the Mysteries of Multiple Sclerosis**
Random House Publishing
1745 Broadway
3rd Floor
New York, NY 10019-4305

212-782-9000
Fax: 212-572-6066
ecustomerservice@randonhouse.com
www.randomhouse.com

Howard L Weiner M.D., Author
Founder-director of the Multiple Sclerosis Center at Mass General Hospital discusses what ends up as a deconstruction of the last 30 years of his own and general MS research and of experience in treating patients with the puzzling disorder. Weiner summarizes what is currently known about treatments and the potential for a cure. *$14.95*
352 pages 1905
ISBN 0-307236-04-8

8515 **Cystic Fibrosis: A Guide for Patient and Family**
Lippincott Williams & Wilkins
16522 Hunters Green Parkway
PO Box 1620
Hagerstown, MD 21741-1620

301-223-2300
800-638-3030
Fax: 301-223-2400
orders@lww.com
www.lww.com

David M Orenstein MD, Author
Text is designed specifically for patients with cystic fibrosis and their families. Explains the disease process, outlines the fundamentals of diagnosing and screening, and addresses the challenges of treatment for those living with CF. Includes new material on carrier testing, infection control, and more. *$51.50*
448 pages 3rd Edition
ISBN 0-781741-52-1

8516 **Diabetes Sourcebook.**
Omnigraphics
PO Box 31-1640
Detroit, MI   48231-8002   610-461-3548
                                             800-234-1340
                                        Fax: 610-532-9001
                                     info@omnigraphics.com
                                      www.omnigraphics.com
Karen Bellenir, Editor
Diabetes Sourcebook, Fourth Edition contains updated information for people seeking to understand the risk factors, complications, and management of diabetes. It discusses medical interventions, including the use of insulin and oral diabetes medications, self-monitoring of blood glucose, and complementary and alternative therapies. *$84.00*
627 pages 4th Edition
ISBN 0-780810-05-1

8517 **Digestive Diseases & Disorders Sourcebook**
Omnigraphics
PO Box 8002
Aston, PA   19014-8002   610-461-3548
                                             800-234-1340
                                        Fax: 800-875-1340
                                customerservice@omnigraphics.com
                                      www.omnigraphics.com
Peter Ruffner, President, Co-Founder
Fred Ruffner, Founder
Digestive Diseases and Disorders Sourcebook provides basic information for the layperson about common disorders of the upper and lower digestive tract. It also includes information about medications and recommendations for maintaining a healthy digestive tract in addition to a glossary of important terms and a directory of digestive diseases organizations are also provided.
$84.00
323 pages Hard cover
ISBN 0-780803-27-5

8518 **Duchenne Muscular Dystrophy**
Oxford University Press
198 Madison Ave
New York, NY   10016-4308   212-726-6000
                                             800-445-9714
                                        Fax: 919-677-1303
                                     custserv.us@oup.com
                                       www.global.oup.com
William Lamsback, Editor
Alan Emery, Author
Francesco Muntoni, Co-Author
Identification of the genetic defect responsible for Duchenne Muscular Dystrophy and isolation of the protein dystrophin have led to the development of new theories for the disease's pathogenesis. This title incorporates these advances from the field of molecular biology, and describes the resultant opportunities for screening, prenatal diagnosis, genetic counselling and management. *$135.00*
282 pages 3rd Edition 2003
ISBN 0-198515-31-6

8519 **Ear, Nose, and Throat Disorders Sourcebook**
Omnigraphics
PO Box 31-1640
Detroit, MI   48231-8002   610-461-3548
                                             800-234-1340
                                        Fax: 610-532-9001
                                     info@omnigraphics.com
                                      www.omnigraphics.com
Sandra J Judd, Editor
Ear, Nose and Throat Disorders Sourcebook, Second Edition, provides consumers with updated health information on the most common disorders of the ear, nose, and throat. The book also includes descriptions of current diagnostic tests, discussion of common surgical procedures, including cosmetic surgery on the nose and ears, a glossary of related medical terms, and a directory of sources for further help and information. *$84.00*
631 pages 2nd Edition
ISBN 0-780808-72-0

8520 **Eating Disorders Sourcebook.**
Omnigraphics
PO Box 31-1640
Detroit, MI   48231-8002   610-461-3548
                                             800-234-1340
                                        Fax: 610-532-9001
                                     info@omnigraphics.com
                                      www.omnigraphics.com
Joyce Brennfleck Shannon, Editor
Provides general imformation, causes and treatments of eating disorders. *$84.00*
557 pages 2nd Edition
ISBN 0-780809-48-2

8521 **Educational Issues Among Children with Spina Bifida**
Spina Bifida Association of America
1600 Wilson Boulevard
Suite 800
Arlington, VA   22209   202-944-3285
                                             800-621-3141
                                        Fax: 202-944-3295
                                          sbaa@sbaa.org
                                           www.sbaa.org
Ana Ximenes, Chair
Sara Struwe, President & CEO
Mark Bohay, National Web Initiatives & Development Manager
Elizabeth Merck, Development Manager
Children with spina bifida/ hydrocephalus often show unique learning strengths and weaknesses that affect their schoolwork. Parents and schools need to work together to help the young people meet their physical, social, emotional, and academic goals.

8522 **Epilepsy, 199 Answers: A Doctor Responds to His Patients' Questions**
Demos Medical Publishing
11 West 42nd Street
15th Floor
New York, NY   10036   212-683-0072
                                             800-532-8663
                                        Fax: 212-683-0118
                                   support@demosmedical.com
                                       www.demosmedpub.com
Richard Winters, Executive Editor
Beth Kaufman Barry, Publisher
Noreen Henson, Executive Director of Demos Heal
Andrew N. Wilner MD, FACP, FAAN, Author
An epilepsy specialist answers questions about the causes, diagnosis, and treatments, and how to live and work with this brain disorder. Includes an epilepsy history timeline, patient health record form, resources, and a glossary. *$19.95*
180 pages
ISBN 1-932603-35-2

8523 **Epilepsy: Patient and Family Guide**
Demos Medical Publishing
11 West 42nd Street
15th Floor
New York, NY   10036   212-683-0072
                                             800-532-8663
                                        Fax: 212-683-0118
                                   support@demosmedical.com
                                       www.demosmedpub.com
Richard Winters, Executive Editor
Beth Kaufman Barry, Publisher
Noreen Henson, Executive Director of Demos Heal
Orrin Devinsky, MD, Author
A guide for adults with epilepsy and for parents of children with the disorder explains the nature and diversity of seizures, the risks and benefits of the various antiepileptic drugs, and medical and surgical therapies. *$16.95*
408 pages
ISBN 1-932603-41-7

8524   Ethnic Diseases Sourcebook
Omnigraphics
PO Box 8002
Aston, PA   19014-8002   610-461-3548
                                          800-234-1340
                                     Fax: 800-875-1340
                      customerservice@omnigraphics.com
                                     www.omnigraphics.com
Peter Ruffner, President, Co-Founder
Fred Ruffner, Founder
Ethnic Diseases Sourcebook provides health information about
genetic and chronic diseases that affect ethnic and racial minorities in the United States. Information about mental health services, women's health, and tips for improving health are also
included, along with a glossary and a list of resources for additional help and informatio methods, treatment options, and current research initiatives. *$84.00*
648 pages Hard cover
ISBN 0-780803-36-7

8525   From Where I Sit: Making My Way with Cerebral Palsy
Scholastic
557 Broadway
New York, NY   10012-3962   124-484-2800
                                     Fax: 212-343-6934
                       contact@scholastic.co.in
                                    www.scholastic.com
Dick Robinson, Chairman & CEO
Maureen O'Connell, Executive Vice President, Chief
Kyle Good, Senior Vice President, Corporate
Shelley Nixon, Author
An autobiographical account of a young woman explores how it
feels to live with cerebral palsy while struggling to have a full life
despite the challenges facing her every day. *$13.00*
136 pages
ISBN 0-590395-84-X

8526   Genetics and Spina Bifida
Spina Bifida Association of America
1600 Wilson Boulevard
Suite 800
Arlington, VA   22209   202-944-3285
                                          800-621-3141
                                     Fax: 202-944-3295
                                          sbaa@sbaa.org
                                          www.sbaa.org
Ana Ximenes, Chair
Sara Struwe, President & CEO
Mark Bohay, National Web Initiatives & Development Manager
Elizabeth Merck, Development Manager
Spina bifida is a birth defect involving incomplete formation of
the spine.

8527   Growing Up with Epilepsy: A Pratical Guide for Parents
Demos Medical Publishing
11 West 42nd Street
15th Floor
New York, NY   10036   212-683-0072
                                          800-532-8663
                                     Fax: 212-683-0118
                         support@demosmedical.com
                                     www.demosmedpub.com
Richard Winters, Executive Editor
Beth Kaufman Barry, Publisher
Noreen Henson, Executive Director of Demos Heal
Lynn Bennett Blackburn, PhD, Author
Developed to help parents with the uniques challenges that this
disorder presents *$19.95*
168 pages
ISBN 1-888799-74-9

8528   Guide to Living with HIV Infection: Developed at the Johns Hopkins AIDS Clinic
Johns Hopkins Universty Press
2715 N Charles St
Baltimore, MD   21218-4363   410-516-6900
                                          800-548-1784
                                     Fax: 410-516-6998
                        webmaster@jhupress.jhu.edu
                                     www.press.jhu.edu
William Brody, President
John G Bartlett, M.D., Author
Ann K Finkbeiner, Co-Author
A handbook and reference for people living with HIV infection
and their families, friends, and caregivers. *$19.95*
408 pages 6th Edition
ISBN 0-801884-85-6

8529   Handbook of Chronic Fatigue Syndrome
John Wiley & Sons
1 Wiley Dr.
Somerset, NJ   08875-1272   732-469-4400
                                          800-225-5945
                                     Fax: 732-302-2300
                                          custserv@wiley.com
                                          onlinelibrary.wiley.com
Leonard A. Jason, Editor
Discusses diagnosis and treatment as well as the history, phenomenology, symptomatology, assessment, and pediatric and community issues. Introduces phase-based therapy and nutritional
approaches. *$ 110.00*
794 pages 2003
ISBN 0-471415-12-1

8530   Handbook of Epilepsy
Lippincott, Williams & Wilkins
Philadelphia, PA   19106-3713   215-521-8300
                                          800-777-2295
                                     Fax: 301-824-7390
                                          www.lpub.com
J Lippincott, CEO
Pocket-sized reference provides concise, up-to-date, clinically
oriented reviews of each of the major areas of diagnosis and man-
agement of epilepsy. *$42.95*
272 pages
ISBN 0-781743-52-4

8531   Healthy Breathing
National Jewish Health
1400 Jackson St
Denver, CO   80206-2761   303-270-2708
                                          877-225-5654
                                     Fax: 303-398-1125
                         physicianline@njhealth.org
                                     www.nationaljewish.org
Richard A. Schierburg, Chair
Robin Chotin, Vice Chair
Don Silversmith, Vice Chair
Michael Salem, CEO
Offers patients with lung or respiratory disorders information on
exercise and healthy breathing.

8532   Heart of the Mind
New World Library
14 Pamaron Way
Novato, CA   94949   415-884-2100
                                          800-972-6657
                                     Fax: 415-884-2199
                           ami@newworldlibrary.com
                                     www.newworldlibrary.com
208 pages
ISBN 1-577311-56-6

8533 **Hepatitis Sourcebook**
Omnigraphics
PO Box 8002
Aston, PA 19014-8002   610-461-3548
                                        800-234-1340
                                   Fax: 800-875-1340
                          customerservice@omnigraphics.com
                                  www.omnigraphics.com
Peter Ruffner, President, Co-Founder
Fred Ruffner, Founder
Hepatitis Sourcebook provides basic consumer health information about hepatitis A, hepatitis B, hepatitis C, and other types of hepatitis, including autoimmune hepatitis, alcoholic hepatitis, nonalcoholic steatohepatitis, and toxin-induced hepatitis. It gives the facts about risk factors, prevention, transmission, screening and diagnostic methods, treatment options, and current research initiatives. *$84.00*
570 pages Hard cover
ISBN 0-780807-49-5

8534 **Hip Function & Ambulation**
Spina Bifida Association of America
1600 Wilson Boulevard
Suite 800
Arlington, VA 22209   202-944-3285
                                        800-621-3141
                                   Fax: 202-944-3295
                                        sbaa@sbaa.org
                                        www.sbaa.org
Ana Ximenes, Chair
Sara Struwe, President & CEO
Mark Bohay, National Web Initiatives & Development Manager
Elizabeth Merck, Development Manager
The ability to walk is important in our society, despite recent advances in wheelchair design and wheelchair accessibility. It also is a desire of children with spina bifida.

8535 **Hydrocephalus: A Guide for Patients, Families & Friends**
O'Reilly Media Inc
1005 Gravenstein Hwy N
Sebastopol, CA 95472-2811   707-827-7000
                                        800-998-9938
                                   Fax: 707-829-0104
                                        order@oreilly.com
                                        www.oreilly.com
Linda Lamb, Editor
Chuck Toporek, Author
Kellie Robinson, Author
Hydrocephalus is a life-threatening condition often referred to as, water on the brain, that is treated by surgical placement of a shunt system. Hydrocephalus: A Guide for Patients, Families and Friends educates families so they can select a skilled neurosurgeon, understand treatments, participate in care, know what symptoms need attention, discover where to turn for support, keep records needed for follow-up treatments, and make wise lifestyle choices. *$19.95*
379 pages Paperback 1999
ISBN 1-565924-10-X

8536 **Hypertension Sourcebook**
Omnigraphics
PO Box 8002
Aston, PA 19014-8002   610-461-3548
                                        800-234-1340
                                   Fax: 800-875-1340
                          customerservice@omnigraphics.com
                                  www.omnigraphics.com
Peter Ruffner, President, Co-Founder
Fred Ruffner, Founder
This Sourcebook describes the known causes and risk factors associated with essential (or primary) hypertension, secondary hypertension, prehypertension, and other hypertensive disorders. The book also provides information about blood pressure management strategies, including dietary changes, weight loss, exercise, and medications. *$84.00*
588 pages Hard cover
ISBN 0-780806-74-0

8537 **Immune System Disorders Sourcebook.**
Omnigraphics
PO Box 31-1640
Detroit, MI 48231-8002   610-461-3548
                                        800-234-1340
                                   Fax: 610-532-9001
                                        info@omnigraphics.com
                                  www.omnigraphics.com
Joyce Brennfleck Shannon, Editor
Immune System Disorders Sourcebook provides information about inherited, acquired, and autoimmune diseases including primary immunodeficiency, acquired immunodeficiency syndrome (AIDS), lupus, multiple sclerosis, type one diabetes, rheumatoid arthritis, and Graves' disease. Tips for coping with an immune disorder, caregiving, and treatments are presented along with a glossary and directory of additional resourcesories of additional resources. *$84.00*
643 pages 2nd Edition
ISBN 0-780807-48-8

8538 **Informed Touch; A Clinician's Guide To The Evaluation Of Myofascial Disorders**
Inner Traditions/Bear And Company
One Park Street
PO Box 388
Rochester, VT 05767-0388   802-767-3174
                                        800-246-8648
                                   Fax: 802-767-3726
                          customerservice@innertraditions.com
                                  www.innertraditions.com
Rob Meadows, VP Sales/Marketing
Jessica Arsenault, Sales Associate
Donna Finando, LAc, LMT, Author
Steven Finando, PhD, LAc, Co-Author
A Clinician's guide to the evaluation and treatment of myofascial disorders. *$30.00*
224 pages
ISBN 0-892817-40-5

8539 **Injured Mind, Shattered Dreams: Brian's Survival from a Severe Head Injury**
Brookline Books
8 Trumbull Rd,
Northampton, MA 01060-4533   413-584-0184
                                        800-666-2665
                                   Fax: 413-584-6184
                                        brbooks@yahoo.com
                                  www.brooklinebooks.com
Paperback
ISBN 0-91479-95-6

8540 **Interdisciplinary Clinical Assessment of Young Children with Developmental Disabilities**
Brookes Publishing
P.O.Box 10624
Baltimore, MD 21285-0624   410-337-9580
                                        800-638-3775
                                   Fax: 410-337-8539
                          custserv@brookespublishing.com
                                  www.brookespublishing.com
Paul H. Brookes, Chairman
Jeffrey D. Brookes, President
Melissa A. Behm, Executive Vice President
George S. Stamathis, Vice President & Publisher
Offers insight from veteran team members on interdisciplinary team assessments. Professionals organizing a team as well as students preparing for practice will find advice on how practitioners gather information, approach assessment, make decisions, and face the challenges of their individual fields. Includes case studies and appendix of photocopiable questionnaires for clinicians and parents. *$44.95*
796 pages Hardcover
ISBN 1-557664-50-1

8541 **Introduction to Spina Bifida**
Spina Bifida Association of America
1600 Wilson Boulevard
Suite 800
Arlington, VA 22209   202-944-3285
                                        800-621-3141
                                   Fax: 202-944-3295
                                        sbaa@sbaa.org
                                        www.sbaa.org

Ana Ximenes, Chair
Sara Struwe, President & CEO
Mark Bohay, National Web Initiatives & Development Manager
Elizabeth Merck, Development Manager
An aid for parents, family and nonmedical people who care for a child with spina bifida. *$7.00*

8542 **It's All in Your Head: The Link Between Mercury Amalgams and Illness**
Avery Publishing Group
299 W. Houston Street
New York, NY 10014   212-859-1100
                                   Fax: 212-859-1150
                                        info@programexchange.com

208 pages

8543 **Joslin Guide to Diabetes: A Program for Managing Your Treatment**
Joslin Diabetes Center
1 Joslin Pl
Boston, MA 02215-5306   617-732-2400
                                   Fax: 617-732-2452
                                        www.joslin.org

Richard S Beaser, M.D., Author
Amy Campbell,Ms, RD, CDE, Co-Author
Ralph M. James, Chairperson of the Board
John L. Brooks III, President/CEO
Discusses the causes of diabetes, the role of diet and exercise, meal planning and complications. Also provide information on drawing blood, mixing and injecting insulin, special challenges, living with diabetes. *$16.95*
352 pages Revised Edition

8544 **Journey to Well: Learning to Live After Spinal Cord Injury**
Altarfire Publishing
Margo Williams, author
Newcastle, CA 95658
The author's close-up view of what life is like during and after such an incident, including her experience with institutional medicine and insurance companies (for better and for worse), and her determined - and ultimately successful - effort to rehabilitate herself and reconstruct her life. *$15.95*
251 pages
ISBN 0-965555-82-8

8545 **Ketogenic Diet: A Treatment for Children and Others with Epilepsy**
Demos Medical Publishing
11 West 42nd Street
15th Floor
New York, NY 10036   212-683-0072
                                        800-532-8663
                                   Fax: 212-683-0118
                                        support@demosmedical.com
                                        www.demosmedpub.com

Richard Winters, Executive Editor
Beth Kaufman Barry, Publisher
Noreen Henson, Executive Director of Demos Heal
John M. Freeman, MD, Co Author
Patient education reference on the use of the ketogenic diet to conrol epilepsy in children. *$24.95*
328 pages Paperback
ISBN 1-932603-18-2

8546 **Latex Allergy in Spina Bifida Patients**
Spina Bifida Association of America
1600 Wilson Boulevard
Suite 800
Arlington, VA 22209   202-944-3285
                                        800-621-3141
                                   Fax: 202-944-3295
                                        sbaa@sbaa.org
                                        www.sbaa.org

Ana Ximenes, Chair
Sara Struwe, President & CEO
Mark Bohay, National Web Initiatives & Development Manager
Elizabeth Merck, Development Manager
The Spina Bifida Association (SBA) serves adults and children who live with the challenges of Spina Bifida.

8547 **Learning Among Children with Spina Bifida**
Spina Bifida Association of America
1600 Wilson Boulevard
Suite 800
Arlington, VA 22209   202-944-3285
                                        800-621-3141
                                   Fax: 202-944-3295
                                        sbaa@sbaa.org
                                        www.sbaa.org

Ana Ximenes, Chair
Sara Struwe, President & CEO
Mark Bohay, National Web Initiatives & Development Manager
Elizabeth Merck, Development Manager
The Spina Bifida Association (SBA) serves adults and children who live with the challenges of Spina Bifida.

8548 **Let's Talk About Having Asthma**
Rosen Publishing
29 E 21st St
New York, NY 10010-6209   212-420-1600
                                        800-237-9932
                                   Fax: 888-436-4643
                                        www.rosenpublishing.com

Marianna Johnstone, Co-Author
Elizabeth Weitzman, Co-Author
Kelly Chambers, Marketing Assistant
Many kids suffer from asthma, which can overtake them suddenly, causing them terror as they struggle for breath. This book talks about the causes and treatments for asthma, as well as precautions sufferers should take. *$21.95*
ISBN 0-823950-32-8

8549 **Leukemia Sourcebook**
Omnigraphics
PO Box 8002
Aston, PA 19014-8002   610-461-3548
                                        800-234-1340
                                   Fax: 800-875-1340
                                        customerservice@omnigraphics.com
                                        www.omnigraphics.com

Peter Ruffner, President, Co-Founder
Fred Ruffner, Founder
This Sourcebook provides health information about adult and childhood leukemias focusing on the diagnosis and treatments for leukemia, including chemotherapy, radiation, drug therapy, and transplantation of peripheral blood stem cells or marrow. Also included are tips for nutrition, pain and fatigue control, and recognizing possible long-term and late effects of leukemia treatment, along with a glossary and directories of additional resources. *$84.00*
564 pages Hard cover
ISBN 0-780806-27-6

8550   Life After Trauma: A Workbook for Healing
Guilford Press
72 Spring St
New York, NY   10012-4019   212-431-9800
                                            800-365-7006
                                       Fax: 212-966-6708
                                       info@guilford.com
                                       www.guilford.com

Denaour Rosenbloom, Author
Mary Beth Williams, Co-Author
Barbar E Watkins, Co-Author
Laurie Anne Pearlman, Foreword
A self-help book on how to deal with trauma. *$19.95*
300 pages Paperback 1910
ISBN 1-606236-08-6

8551   Life Line
National Hydrocephalus Foundation
12413 Centralia St
Lakewood, CA   90715-1653   562-402-3523
                                            888-857-3434
                                            888-260-1789
                                       Fax: 562-924-6666
                              debbifields@nhfonline.org
                                       www.nhfonline.org

Debbi Fields, Executive Director
Michael Fields, President/Treasurer
Jaynie Dunn, Secretary
Sarah Dunn, Junior Director
National Hydrocephalus Foundation quarterly newsletter.
$35.00
12 pages Quarterly

8552   Lipomas & Lipomyelomeningocele
Spina Bifida Association of America
1600 Wilson Boulevard
Suite 800
Arlington, VA   22209   202-944-3285
                                            800-621-3141
                                       Fax: 202-944-3295
                                            sbaa@sbaa.org
                                            www.sbaa.org

Ana Ximenes, Chair
Sara Struwe, President & CEO
Mark Bohay, National Web Initiatives & Development Manager
Elizabeth Merck, Development Manager
The Spina Bifida Association (SBA) serves adults and children
who live with the challenges of Spina Bifida.

8553   Liver Disorders Sourcebook
Omnigraphics
PO Box 8002
Aston, PA   19014-8002   610-461-3548
                                            800-234-1340
                                       Fax: 800-875-1340
                        customerservice@omnigraphics.com
                                    www.omnigraphics.com

Peter Ruffner, President, Co-Founder
Fred Ruffner, Founder
Liver Disorders Sourcebook contains basic consumer health information about the liver, how it works, and how to keep it
healthy through diet, vaccination, and other preventive care measures. Readers will learn about the symptoms and treatment options for such diseases as hepatitis, primary biliary cirrhosis,
Wilson's disease, hemochromatosis, liver failure, cancer of the
liver, and disorders related to drugs and other toxins. *$84.00*
580 pages Hard cover
ISBN 0-780803-83-1

8554   Living Beyond Multiple Sclerosis: A Woman's Guide
Hunter House
PO Box 2914
Alameda, CA   94501-914   510-865-5282
                                            800-266-5592
                                       Fax: 510-865-4295
                               ordering@hunterhouse.com
                                      www.hunterhouse.com

Judith Lynn Nichols, Author
Lily Jung, Foreword
This collection of e-mail conversations provides anecdotal and
personal information contributed by women with multiple sclerosis. *$14.95*
256 pages
ISBN 0-897932-93-6

8555   Living Well with Asthma
Guilford Press
72 Spring St
New York, NY   10012-4019   212-431-9800
                                            800-365-7006
                                       Fax: 212-966-6708
                                       info@guilford.com
                                       www.guilford.com

Cynthia L Divino, Author
Michael R Freedman, Co-Author
Samuel J Rosenberg, Co-Author
James D Crapo, Foreword
Meeting the needs of a growing clinical population, this
reader-friendly, practical book offers a lifeline to asthma patients
attempting to understand and cope with the psychological ramifi-
cations of their illness and its treatment. *$15.95*
213 pages Paperback
ISBN 1-572300-51-4

8556   Living Well with Chronic Fatigue Syndrome and
Fibromyalgia
Harper Collins Publishers
10 E 53rd St
New York, NY   10022-5244   212-207-7901
                                            800-242-7737
                                       Fax: 212-702-2586
                              spsales@harpercollins.com
                                    www.harpercollins.com

Mary J Shomon, Author
From the author of Living Well With Hypothyroidism, a comprehensive guide to the diagnosis and treatment of chronic fatigue
syndrome and fibromyalgia—vital help for the millions of people
suffering from pain, fatigue, and sleep problems. *$14.95*
416 pages 2004
ISBN 0-060521-25-2

8557   Living Well with HIV and AIDS
Bull Publishing
PO Box 1377
Boulder, CO   80306-1377   303-545-6350
                                            800-676-2855
                                       Fax: 303-545-6354
                                          www.bullpub.com

David Sobel, MPH, Author
Virginia Gonzalez MPH, Co-Author
Daina Laurent MPH, Co-Author
Kate Lorig RN, Co-Author
New drugs and drug combinations have turned HIV/AIDS into a
long-term illness rather than a death sentence. Practical advice on
mental adjustments and physical vigilance is outlined. *$18.95*
245 pages 3rd Edition
ISBN 0-923521-52-6

8558 **Living With Spinal Cord Injury Series**
Fanlight Productions C/O Icarus Films
32 Court St.
21st Floor
Brooklyn, NY 11201
718-488-8900
800-876-1710
Fax: 718-488-8642
info@fanlight.com
www.fanlight.com

Barry Corbet, Producer
Jonathan Miller, President
Meredith Miller, Sales Manager
Anthony Sweeney, Acquisitions
The producer, himself injured in a helicopter crash, brings a unique perspective to this classic three-part series on coming to terms with spinal cord injury. These films offer enduring proof that a tough break doesn't have to mean a ruined life. *$210.00*
VHS 1973

8559 **Living with Brain Injury: A Guide for Families**
Delmar Cengage Learning
PO Box 6904
Florence, KY 41022-6904
800-354-9706
Fax: 800-487-8488
esales@cengage.com
www.cengagesites.com

Richard C Senelick MD, Author
Karla Dougherty, Co-Author
A consumer text to aid people living with brain-injured survivors, includes facts on neuroplasticity, experimental rehabilitation research, and the process of rehabilitation itself. *$19.95*
225 pages Softcover 2001
ISBN 1-891525-09-3

8560 **Living with Spina Bifida: A Guide for Families and Professionals**
University of North Carolina at Chapel Hill
116 S Boundary St
Chapel Hill, NC 27514-3808
919-966-3561
800-848-6224
Fax: 919-962-2704
uncpress@unc.edu
www.uncpress.unc.edu

Adrian Sandler MD, Author
A handbook that addresses patients' biopsychosocial and developmental needs from birth through adolescence and into adulthood. Sandler's holistic approach encourages families to focus more on the child and less on the disability while providing abundant information about this condition. *$20.95*
296 pages 2004
ISBN 0-807855-47-8

8561 **Lung Cancer: Making Sense of Diagnosis, Treatment, and Options**
O'Reilly Media Inc
1005 Gravenstein Hwy N
Sebastopol, CA 95472-2811
707-827-7000
800-998-9938
Fax: 707-829-0104
order@oreilly.com
www.oreilly.com

Linda Lamb, Editor
Lorraine Johnston, Author
Straightforward language and the words of patients and their families are the hallmarks of this book on the number one cancer killer in the US. Written by a widely respected author and patient advocate, Lung Cancer: Making Sense of Diagnosis, Treatment, & Options has been meticulously reviewed by top medical experts and physicians. Readers will find medical facts simply explained, advice to ease their daily life, and tools to be strong advocates for themselves or a family member. *$ 27.95*
530 pages Paperback 2001
ISBN 0-596500-02-5

8562 **Lung Disorders Sourcebook**
Omnigraphics
PO Box 8002
Aston, PA 19014-8002
610-461-3548
800-234-1340
Fax: 800-875-1340
customerservice@omnigraphics.com
www.omnigraphics.com

Peter Ruffner, President, Co-Founder
Fred Ruffner, Founder
Lung Disorders Sourcebook offers information about specific types of lung disorders, including diagnosis, treatment, and prevention issues. The book offers advice for preventing some types lung disorder that are acquired by asbestos, radon, and other environmental exposures. *$84.00*
657 pages Hard cover
ISBN 0-780803-39-8

8563 **Lupus: Alternative Therapies That Work**
Inner Traditions
PO Box 388
Rochester
VT, 05 0388-802-
800-246-8648
802-767-3726
TTY:customerserv
info@innertraditions.com
www.innertraditions.com

Sharon Moore, Author
A comprehensive guise to noninvasive, nontoxic therapies for lupus - written by a lupus survivor. *$14.95*
256 pages 2000
ISBN 0-892818-89-1

8564 **MAGIC Touch**
MAGIC Foundation for Children's Growth
6645 North Ave
Oak Park, IL 60302-1057
708-383-0808
800-362-4423
Fax: 708-383-0899
mary@magicfoundation.org
www.magicfoundation.org

Mary Andrews, CEO
Dianne Kremidas, Executive Director
Pam Pentaris, Office Manager
Jamie Harvey, Technical Education Teacher
Provides support and education regarding growth disorders in children and related adult disorders, including adult GHD. Dedicated to helping children whose physical growth is affected be a medical problem by assisting families of afflicted children through local support groups, public education/awareness, newsletters, specialty divisions and programs for the children.
36-40 pages Quarterly

8565 **Management of Autistic Behavior**
Sage Publications
2455 Teller Road
Thousand Oaks, CA 91320
805-499-0721
800-818-7243
Fax: 805-499-0871
info@sagepub.com
www.sagepub.com

Sara Miller McCune, Founder, Publisher, Executive Chairman
Blaise R Simqu, President & CEO
Tracey A. Ozmina, Executive Vice President & Chief Operating Officer
Stephen Barr, Managing Director/SAGE London, President of SAGE Internation
Comprehensive and practical book that tells what works best with specific problems. *$51.00*
450 pages Paperback
ISBN 0-890791-96-1

8566 Management of Genetic Syndromes
John Wiley & Sons
111 River St
Hoboken, NJ 07030-5774
201-748-6000
201-748-6088
info@wiley.com
www.as.wiley.com

Suzanne B Cassidy, Editor
Judith E Allanson, Editor
Edited by two of the field's most highly esteemed experts, this landmark volume provides: A precise reference of the physical manifestations of common genetic syndromes, clearly written for professionals and families, Extensive updates, particularly in sections on diagnostic criteria and diagnostic testing, pathogenesis, and management, A tried-and-tested, user-friendly format, with each chapter including information on incidence, etiology and pathogenesis, diagnostic criteria and testing, and d *$204.95*
720 pages 3rd Edition
ISBN 0-470191-41-5

8567 Managing Post Polio: A Guide to Living Well with Post Polio
ABI Professional Publications
PO Box 149
St Petersburg, FL 33731-149
727-556-0950
800-551-7776
Fax: 727-556-2560
webmaster@vandamere.com
www.abipropub.com

Lauro S Halstead MD, Editor
Edited by Lauro S. Halstead, M.D., Managing Post-Polio, 2nd Edition, provides a comprehensive overview dealing with the medical, psychological, vocational, and many other challenges of living with post-polio syndrome. With contributions from over 15 healthcare professionals, the majority of whom are polio survivors themselves, Managing Post-Polio distills and summarizes the wealth of information presented from over the past 20 plus years.
256 pages
ISBN 1-886236-17-8

8568 Meniere's Disease
Vestibular Disorders Association
5018 NE 15th Avenue
Portland, OR 97211
800-837-8428
Fax: 503-229-8064
info@vestibular.org
www.vestibular.org

P. Ashley Wackym, Chair
Cynthia Ryan MBA, Executive Director
Tony Staser, Development Director
Kerrie Denner, Outreach Coordinator
VEDA's website contains a wealth of information on the symptoms, diagnosis and treatment of various types of vestibular disorders. *$5.00*

8569 Menopause without Medicine
Hunter House
PO Box 2914
Alameda, CA 94501-914
510-865-5282
800-266-5592
Fax: 510-865-4295
ordering@hunterhouse.com
www.hunterhouse.com

Linda Ojeda PhD, Author
Menopause Without Medicine provides complete information on the symptoms of menopause - hot flashes, fatigue, sexual changes, depression and osteoporosis - and how to alleviate them. *$18.95*
304 pages 5th Edition
ISBN 0-897934-05-3

8570 Movement Disorders Sourcebook
Omnigraphics
PO Box 8002
Aston, PA 19014-8002
610-461-3548
800-234-1340
Fax: 800-875-1340
customerservice@omnigraphics.com
www.omnigraphics.com

Peter Ruffner, President, Co-Founder
Fred Ruffner, Founder
This Sourcebook provides health information about neurological movement disorders, their symptoms, causes, diagnostic tests, and treatments. Readers will learn about Essential Tremor, Parkinson's Disease, Dystonia, and many other early-onset and adult-onset movement disorders. Information about mobility and assistive technology aids is included, along with a glossary and a listing of additional resources. *$84.00*
600 pages Hard cover
ISBN 0-780810-34-1

8571 Multiple Sclerosis and Having a Baby
Inner Traditions
PO Box 388
Rochester, VT 05767-0388
802-767-3174
800-246-8648
Fax: 802-767-3726
customerservice@innertraditions.com
www.innertraditions.com

Judy Graham, Author
Everything you need to know about conception, pregnancy and parenthood. *$12.95*
160 pages 2001
ISBN 0-892817-88-7

8572 Multiple Sclerosis: 300 Tips for Making Life Easier
Demos Medical Publishing
11 West 42nd Street
15th Floor
New York, NY 10036
212-683-0072
800-532-8663
Fax: 212-683-0118
support@demosmedical.com
www.demosmedpub.com

Richard Winters, Executive Editor
Beth Kaufman Barry, Publisher
Noreen Henson, Executive Director of Demos Heal
Shelley Peterman Schwarz, Author
This latest book in the Making Life Easier series features tip, techniques and shortcuts for conserving time and energy so you can do more of the things you want to do. These tips should help increase the number of good days you have while encouraging you to develop your own techniques for making life easier. *$16.95*
128 pages
ISBN 1-932603-21-2

8573 Multiple Sclerosis: A Guide for Families
Demos Medical Publishing
11 West 42nd Street
15th Floor
New York, NY 10036
212-683-0072
800-532-8663
Fax: 212-683-0118
support@demosmedical.com
www.demosmedpub.com

Richard Winters, Executive Editor
Beth Kaufman Barry, Publisher
Noreen Henson, Executive Director of Demos Heal
Rosalind C. Kalb, Ph.D., Author
Guide for living and coping with multiple sclerosis. *$24.95*
256 pages
ISBN 1-932603-10-7

8574 Multiple Sclerosis: A Guide for the Newly Diagnosed
Demos Medical Publishing
11 West 42nd Street
15th Floor
New York, NY 10036
212-683-0072
800-532-8663
Fax: 212-683-0118
support@demosmedical.com
www.demosmedpub.com

Richard Winters, Executive Editor
Beth Kaufman Barry, Publisher
Noreen Henson, Executive Director of Demos Heal
Nancy J. Holland, RN, EdD,, Co Author
A must-have title for anyone who has recently been diagnosed
with MS and a good idea for family members and friends. *$19.95*
256 pages
ISBN 1-932603-27-1

**8575 Multiple Sclerosis: The Guide to Treatment and
Management**
Demos Medical Publishing
11 West 42nd Street
15th Floor
New York, NY 10036
212-683-0072
800-532-8663
Fax: 212-683-0118
support@demosmedical.com
www.demosmedpub.com

Richard Winters, Executive Editor
Beth Kaufman Barry, Publisher
Noreen Henson, Executive Director of Demos Heal
Chris H. Polman, MD, FRCP, Co Author
A current guide to modern therapies. *$24.95*
216 pages
ISBN 1-932603-15-4

8576 Muscular Dystrophies
Oxford University Press
198 Madison Avenue
New York, NY 10016
212-726-6000
800-445-9714
Fax: 919-677-1303
custserv.us@oup.com
www.oup.com

Alan E.H. Emery, Author
Describes the opportunities for management of more than 30
types of MD through respiratory care, physiotherapy and surgical
correction of contractures, and examines the potential for effective treatment utilizing the new techniques of gene and cell therapy *$165.00*
330 pages
ISBN 0-192632-91-4

8577 Muscular Dystrophy in Children: A Guide for Families
Demos Medical Publishing
11 West 42nd Street
15th Floor
New York, NY 10036
212-683-0072
800-532-8663
Fax: 212-683-0118
support@demosmedical.com
www.demosmedpub.com

Richard Winters, Executive Editor
Beth Kaufman Barry, Publisher
Noreen Henson, Executive Director of Demos Heal
Defines the available medical options at every stage of the disease and offers guidance even when it may seem that little or nothing can be done. Includes a glossary and suggestions for furhter
reading. *$19.95*
144 pages Paperback
ISBN 1-888799-33-1

8578 Muscular Dystrophy: The Facts
Oxford University Press
198 Madison Avenue
New York, NY 10016
212-726-6000
800-445-9714
Fax: 919-677-1303
custserv.us@oup.com
www.oup.com

Peter Harper, Author
A good first book for individuals and families faced with the like-
lihood or reality of a muscular dystrophy diagnosis. *$22.50*
178 pages
ISBN 0-192632-17-5

**8579 My House is Killing Me! The Home Guide for Families with
Allergies and Asthma**
Johns Hopkins University Press
2175 N Charles St
Baltimore, MD 21218-4363
410-516-6900
800-548-1784
Fax: 410-516-6968
webmaster@jhupress.jhu.edu
www.press.jhu.edu

Jeffrey C May, Author
Jonathan M Samet, M.D., Foreword
Kathleen Keane, Director
Chemical consultant May describes where and how the various
parts of a residence can cause temporary or chronic illness for
those with allergies or other sensitivities. *$20.95*
352 pages
ISBN 0-801867-30-9

8580 Neuropsychiatry of Epilepsy
Cambridge University Press
100 Brookhill Dr
West Nyack, NY 10994
845-353-7500
845-353-4141
www.cambridge.org

Michael R Trimble, Editor
Bettina Schmitz, Editor
Covers the practical implications of ongoing research, and offers
a diagnostic and management perspective. Topics include cognitive aspects, nonepileptic attacks, and clinical aspects. For professionals treating epileptic patients. *$104.00*
232 pages 2nd Edition 1911
ISBN 0-521154-69-7

8581 Nick Joins In
Spina Bifida Association of America
1600 Wilson Boulevard
Suite 800
Arlington, VA 22209
202-944-3285
800-621-3141
Fax: 202-944-3295
sbaa@sbaa.org
www.sbaa.org

Ana Ximenes, Chair
Sara Struwe, President & CEO
Mark Bohay, National Web Initiatives & Development Manager
Elizabeth Merck, Development Manager
When Nick, who is in a wheelchair, enters a regular classroom for
the first time, he realizes that he has much to contribute. *$17.00*

8582 No More Allergies
Random House
1745 Broadway
3rd Floor
New York, NY 10019-4305
212-782-9000
Fax: 212-572-6066
www.randomhouse.com

Markus Dohle, CEO
Gary Null PhD, Author
Null redefines a health problem that afflicts 40 million Ameri-
cans: More than mere hay fever, contemporary allergic reactions
include chronic fatigue syndrome, Alzheimer's disease, and even
HIV infection. These conditions, he explains, occur when our im-

mune systems break down. This ground-breaking book now pre-scribes effective solutions. *$23.00*
464 pages 1992
ISBN 0-679743-10-1

8583 **No Time for Jello: One Family's Experience**
Brookline Books
8 Trumbull Rd,
Northampton, MA   01060-4533   413-584-0184
                                            800-666-2665
                                        Fax: 413-584-6184
                                        brbooks@yahoo.com
                                        www.brooklinebooks.com

Softcover
ISBN 0-91479 -56-5

8584 **Nocturnal Asthma**
National Jewish Health
1400 Jackson Street
Denver, CO   80206   303-270-2708
                                            877-225-5654
                                        Fax: 303-398-1125
                                        allstetterw@njc.org
                                        nationaljewish.org

Rich Schierburg, Chair
Robin Chotin, Vice Chair
Michael Salem, M.D., President and CEO
Christine Forkner, CFO and Executive Vice President
Offers information to patients about how to understand and man-age asthma at night.

8585 **Obesity**
Spina Bifida Association of America
1600 Wilson Boulevard
Suite 800
Arlington, VA   22209   202-944-3285
                                            800-621-3141
                                        Fax: 202-944-3295
                                        sbaa@sbaa.org
                                        www.sbaa.org

Ana Ximenes, Chair
Sara Struwe, President & CEO
Mark Bohay, National Web Initiatives & Development Manager
Elizabeth Merck, Development Manager
The Spina Bifida Association (SBA) serves adults and children who live with the challenges of Spina Bifida. *$8.00*

8586 **Obesity Sourcebook**
Omnigraphics
PO Box 8002
Aston, PA   19014-8002   610-461-3548
                                            800-234-1340
                                        Fax: 800-875-1340
                                        customerservice@omnigraphics.com
                                        www.omnigraphics.com

Peter Ruffner, President, Co-Founder
Fred Ruffner, Founder
Discusses diseases and other problems associated with obesity. *$78.00*
376 pages
ISBN 0-780803-33-6

8587 **Occulta**
Spina Bifida Association of America
1600 Wilson Boulevard
Suite 800
Arlington, VA   22209   202-944-3285
                                            800-621-3141
                                        Fax: 202-944-3295
                                        sbaa@sbaa.org
                                        www.sbaa.org

Ana Ximenes, Chair
Sara Struwe, President & CEO
Mark Bohay, National Web Initiatives & Development Manager
Elizabeth Merck, Development Manager
The Spina Bifida Association (SBA) serves adults and children who live with the challenges of Spina Bifida. *$8.00*

8588 **Official Patient's Sourcebook on Bell's Palsy**
Icon Group International
9606 Tierra Grande Street
Suite 205
San Diego, CA   92126   *Fax:* 858-635-9414
                                        orders@icongroupbooks.com
                                        www.icongroupbooks.com

ISBN 0-597835-20-9

8589 **Official Patient's Sourcebook on Cystic Fibrosis**
Icon Group International
9606 Tierra Grande Street
Suite 205
San Diego, CA   92126   *Fax:* 858-635-9414
                                        orders@icongroupbooks.com
                                        icongroupbooks.com

356 pages
ISBN 0-597831-46-7

8590 **Official Patient's Sourcebook on Muscular Dystrophy**
Icon Group International
9606 Tierra Grande Street
Suite 205
San Diego, CA   92126   *Fax:* 858-635-9414
                                        orders@icongroupbooks.com
                                        icongroupbooks.com

268 pages
ISBN 0-597832-10-2

8591 **Official Patient's Sourcebook on Osteoporosis**
Icon Group International
9606 Tierra Grande Street
Suite 205
San Diego, CA   92126   *Fax:* 858-635-9414
                                        orders@icongroupbooks.com
                                        icongroupbooks.com

ISBN 0-597833-04-4

8592 **Official Patient's Sourcebook on Post-Polio Syndrome: A Revised and Updated Directory**
Icon Group International
9606 Tierra Grande Street
Suite 205
San Diego, CA   92126   *Fax:* 858-635-9414
                                        orders@icongroupbooks.com
                                        icongroupbooks.com

124 pages
ISBN 0-597835-31-4

8593 **Official Patient's Sourcebook on Primary Pulmonary Hypertension**
Icon Group International
9606 Tierra Grande Street
Suite 205
San Diego, CA   92126   *Fax:* 858-635-9414
                                        orders@icongroupbooks.com
                                        icongroupbooks.com

ISBN 0-597831-54-8

8594 **Official Patient's Sourcebook on Pulmonary Fibrosis**
Icon Group International
9606 Tierra Grande Street
Suite 205
San Diego, CA   92126   *Fax:* 858-635-9414
                                        orders@icongroupbooks.com
                                        icongroupbooks.com

ISBN 0-597831-65-3

8595 **Official Patient's Sourcebook on Scoliosis**
Icon Group International
9606 Tierra Grande Street
Suite 205
San Diego, CA   92126   *Fax:* 858-635-9414
                                        orders@icongroupbooks.com
                                        icongroupbooks.com

ISBN 0-597829-90-X

8596   Official Patient's Sourcebook on Sickle Cell Anemia
Icon Group International
9606 Tierra Grande Street
Suite 205
San Diego, CA   92126
Fax: 858-635-9414
orders@icongroupbooks.com
icongroupbooks.com
ISBN 0-597831-57-2

8597   Official Patient's Sourcebook on Ulcerative Colitis
Icon Group International
9606 Tierra Grande Street
Suite 205
San Diego, CA   92126
Fax: 858-635-9414
orders@icongroupbooks.com
icongroupbooks.com
ISBN 0-597834-09-1

8598   One Day at a Time: Children Living with Leukemia
Gareth Stevens Publishing
111 East 14th Street
Suite #349
New York, NY   10003
800-542-2595
Fax: 877-542-2596
customerservice@gspub.com
www.garethstevens.com
56 pages Hardcover
ISBN 1-55532 -13-6

8599   Options: Revolutionary Ideas in the War on Cancer
People Against Cancer
P.O.Box 10
604 East Street
Otho, IA   50569
515-972-4444
800-662-2623
Fax: 515-972-4415
info@PeopleAgainstCancer.org
www.peopleagainstcancer.com
Frank D. Wiewel, Executive Director/Founder
Publication of People Against Cancer, a nonprofit, grassroots public benefit organization dedicated to 'New Directions in the War on Cancer.' We help people to find the best cancer treatment. We are a democratic organization of people with cancer, their loved ones and citizens working together to protect and enhance medical freedom of choice.

8600   Osteoporosis Sourcebook
Omnigraphics
PO Box 8002
Aston, PA   19014-8002
313-961-1340
800-234-1340
Fax: 800-875-1340
customerservice@omnigraphics.com
www.omnigraphics.com
Peter Ruffner, President, Co-Founder
Fred Ruffner, Founder
Discusses causes, risk factors, treatments and traditional and non-traditional pain management issues concerning osteoporosis. *$ 84.00*
568 pages Hard cover
ISBN 0-780802-39-1

8601   Parent's Guide to Allergies and Asthma
Allergy & Asthma Network Mothers of Asthmatics
Ste 150
PO Box 7474
Fairfax Station, VA   22039-7474
703-323-9170
800-756-5525
Fax: 703-323-9173
custsvc@parent-institute.com
www.parent-institute.com
John H Wherry, Ed.D, President
A up-to-date, easy-to-read resource offering essential information on asthma and allergies.

8602   Partial Seizure Disorders: A Guide for Patients and Families
O'Reilly Media Inc
1005 Gravenstein Hwy N
Sebastopol, CA   95472-2811
707-827-7000
800-998-9938
Fax: 707-829-0104
order@oreilly.com
www.oreilly.com
Linda Lamb, Editor
Mitzi Waltz, Author
Partial Seizure Disorders helps patients and families get an accurate diagnosis of this condition, understand medications and their side effects, and learn coping skills and other adjuncts to medication. It walks readers through developmental and school issues for young children; adult issues such as employment and driving; working with an existing health plan; and getting further help through advocacy and support organizations, articles, and online resources. *$19.95*
288 pages Paperback
ISBN 0-596500-03-3

8603   Penitent, with Roses: An HIV+ Mother Reflects
University Press of New England
1 Court St
Ste 250
Lebanon, NH   03766-1358
603-448-1533
800-421-1561
Fax: 603-448-7006
www.upne.com
Paula W Peterson, Author
Peterson, a married, middle-class, Jewish mother, was diagnosed with full-blown AIDS four years into her marriage and 11 months after her son was born. In seven poignant autobiographical essays and a collection of letters to her uninfected, four-year-old son, the author maintains an upbeat tone and describes her unsuccessful attempts to find the source of her infection (her husband tested negative), her relationships with her doctors, and her work as an HIV activist. *$ 26.95*
256 pages 2001
ISBN 1-584651-28-4

8604   Plan Ahead: Do What You Can
Spina Bifida Association of America
1600 Wilson Boulevard
Suite 800
Arlington, VA   22209
202-944-3285
800-621-3141
Fax: 202-944-3295
sbaa@sbaa.org
www.sbaa.org
Ana Ximenes, Chair
Sara Struwe, President & CEO
Mark Bohay, National Web Initiatives & Development Manager
Elizabeth Merck, Development Manager
Folic aciid information for women at risk for recurrence. *$15.00*

8605   Post-Polio Syndrome: A Guide for Polio Survivors and Their Families
Yale University Press
PO Box 209040
New Haven, CT   6520-9040
203-432-0960
203-432-0948
language.yalepress@yale.edu
Julie K Silver M.D., Author
Laro S Halstead, M.D., Foreword
A guide for polio survivors, their families, and their health care providers offers expert advice on all aspects of post-polio syndrome. Based on the author's experience treating post-polio patients, Silver discusses issues of critical importance, including how to find the best medical care, deal with symptoms, sustain mobility, manage pain, approach insurance issues, and arrange a safe living environment. *$ 19.50*
304 pages 2002
ISBN 0-300088-08-3

8606   Prader-Willi Syndrome: Development and Manifestations
Cambridge University Press
32 Avenue of the Americas
New York, NY   10013-2473   212-924-3900
                                                                  212-691-3239
                                                         www.cambridge.org

Joyce Whittington, Author
Tony Holland, Co-Author
Seeks to identify and provide the latest findings about how best
to manage the complex medical, nutritional, psychological, educational, social and therapeutic needs of people with PWS.
$130.00
230 pages 2004
ISBN 0-521840-29-3

**8607   Preventing Secondary Conditions Associated with Spina
           Bifida or Cerebral Palsy**
Spina Bifida Association of America
1600 Wilson Boulevard
Suite 800
Arlington, VA   22209   202-944-3285
                                                         800-621-3141
                                                    Fax: 202-944-3295
                                                         sbaa@sbaa.org
                                                         www.sbaa.org

Ana Ximenes, Chair
Sara Struwe, President & CEO
Mark Bohay, National Web Initiatives & Development Manager
Elizabeth Merck, Development Manager
This report is for health professionals, parents and teachers.
$3.00

8608   Prostate and Urological Disorders Sourcebook
Omnigraphics
PO Box 8002
Aston, PA   19014-8002   313-961-1340
                                                         800-234-1340
                                                    Fax: 800-875-1340
                                         customerservice@omnigraphics.com
                                                    www.omnigraphics.com

Peter Ruffner, President, Co-Founder
Fred Ruffner, Founder
Peter Ruffner, Co-Founder
Prostate and Urological Disorders Sourcebook provides information about prostate cancer and other prostate problems, such as
prostatitis and benign prostatic hyperplasia. A glossary of
andrological terms and a directory of resources for additional
help and information are also included. *$84.00*
604 pages Hard cover
ISBN 0-780807-97-6

8609   Protecting Against Latex Allergy
Spina Bifida Association of America
1600 Wilson Boulevard
Suite 800
Arlington, VA   22209   202-944-3285
                                                         800-621-3141
                                                    Fax: 202-944-3295
                                                         sbaa@sbaa.org
                                                         www.sbaa.org

Ana Ximenes, Chair
Sara Struwe, President & CEO
Mark Bohay, National Web Initiatives & Development Manager
Elizabeth Merck, Development Manager
Because awareness and proper action may help prevent an aller-
gic reation, learning about latex allergy is especially important
for parents, health care workers and anyone who is exposed to la-
tex regulary. *$20.00*

**8610   Questions and Answers: The ADA and Personswith
           HIV/AIDS**
US Department of Justice
950 Pennsylvania Ave NW
Washington, DC   20530-9   202-307-0663
                                                         800-514-0301
                                                    Fax: 202-307-1197
                                                    TTY: 800-514-0383
                                                         www.ada.gov

Joanne Graham, Manager
Rebecca B. Bond, Chief
Zita Johnson Betts, Deputy Chief
James Bostrom, Deputy Chief
A 16-page publication explaining the requirements for employ-
ers, businesses and nonprofit agencies that serve the public, and
state and local governments to avoid discriminating against per-
sons with HIV/AIDS.

8611   Raynaud's Phenomenon
Arthritis Foundation
1330 W. Peachtree Street
Suite 100
Atlanta, GA   30309   404-872-7100
                                                         800-283-7800
                                                    Fax: 404-872-0457
                                                         arthritis.org

Daniel T. McGowan, Chair
Michael V. Ortman, Vice Chair
Ann M. Palmer, CEO/President
Peter W.C. Barnhart, Treasurer
The Arthritis Foundation is the largest national nonprofit organization that supports the more than 100 types of arthritis and related conditions. Founded in 1948, with headquarters in Atlanta,
the Arthritis Foundation has multiple service points located
throughout the country.

8612   Reaching the Autistic Child: A Parent Training Program
Brookline Books
8 Trumbull Rd,
Northampton, MA   01060-4533   413-584-0184
                                                         800-666-2665
                                                    Fax: 413-584-6184
                                                         brbooks@yahoo.com

Softcover
ISBN 1-571290-56-7

8613   Respiratory Disorders Sourcebook
Omnigraphics
PO Box 8002
Aston, PA   19014-8002   313-961-1340
                                                         800-234-1340
                                                    Fax: 800-875-1340
                                         customerservice@omnigraphics.com
                                                    www.omnigraphics.com

Peter Ruffner, President, Co-Founder
Fred Ruffner, Founder
Sandra J Judd, Editor
Respiratory Disorders Sourcebook provides up-to-date information about infectious, inflammatory, occupational, and other
types of respiratory disorders. Tips for managing chronic respiratory diseases and suggestions for ways to promote lung health are
presented, and the book concludes with a glossary of related
terms and a list of additional resources. *$84.00*
638 pages Hard cover
ISBN 0-780810-07-5

8614 SPINabilities: A Young Person's Guide to Spina Bifida
Spina Bifida Association of America
1600 Wilson Boulevard
Suite 800
Arlington, VA 22209
202-944-3285
800-621-3141
Fax: 202-944-3295
sbaa@sbaa.org
www.sbaa.org

Ana Ximenes, Chair
Sara Struwe, President & CEO
Mark Bohay, National Web Initiatives & Development Manager
Elizabeth Merck, Development Manager
A cool and practical book for young adults becoming independent. *$22.30*

8615 Seizures and Epilepsy in Childhood: A Guide
John Hopkins University Press
2715 N Charles St
Baltimore, MD 21218-4363
410-516-6900
800-548-1784
Fax: 410-516-6998
webmaster@jhupress.jhu.edu
www.press.jhu.edu

Kathleen Keane, Director
Eileen P G Vining MD, Co-Author
Diana J Pillas, Co-Author
John M Freeman, M.D., Co-Author
The award-winning Seizures and Epilepsy in Childhood is the standard resource for parents in need of comprehensive medical information about their child with epilepsy. *$54.00*
432 pages 3rd Edition
ISBN 0-801870-51-4

8616 Sexuality and the Person with Spina Bifida
Spina Bifida Association of America
1600 Wilson Boulevard
Suite 800
Arlington, VA 22209
202-944-3285
800-621-3141
Fax: 202-944-3295
sbaa@sbaa.org
www.sbaa.org

Ana Ximenes, Chair
Sara Struwe, President & CEO
Mark Bohay, National Web Initiatives & Development Manager
Elizabeth Merck, Development Manager
Dr Sloan foucuses on sexual development, sexual activity and other important issues. *$11.00*

8617 Sinus Survival: A Self-help Guide
Penguin Group
375 Hudson St
New York, NY 10014-3658
212-366-2372
Fax: 212-366-2933
insidesales@penguingroup.com
us.penguingroup.com

Robert S Ivker, Author
Self-help manual for sufferers of bronchitis, sinusitis, allergies, and colds. *$15.95*
336 pages Paperback 2000
ISBN 1-101798-02-6

8618 Social Development and the Person with Spina Bifida
Spina Bifida Association of America
1600 Wilson Boulevard
Suite 800
Arlington, VA 22209
202-944-3285
800-621-3141
Fax: 202-944-3295
sbaa@sbaa.org
www.sbaa.org

Ana Ximenes, Chair
Sara Struwe, President & CEO
Mark Bohay, National Web Initiatives & Development Manager
Elizabeth Merck, Development Manager

Examines how spina bifida and hydrocephalus may influence development and learning social skills.

8619 Solving the Puzzle of Chronic Fatigue
Essential Science Publishing
1216 S 1580 W
Ste A
Orem, UT 84058-4906
801-224-6228
800-336-6308
Fax: 801-224-6229
info@essentialscience.net
www.essentialsciencepublishing.com

Michael Rosenbaum, Author
Murray Susser, Co-Author
Although primarily a book about CFS, this comprehensive study also provides a detailed overview of candidiasis, including its causes and best approaches for treatment. *$14.95*
190 pages
ISBN 0-943685-11-7

8620 Son Rise: The Miracle Continues
New World Library
14 Pamaron Way
Novato, CA 94949
415-884-2100
800-972-6657
Fax: 415-884-2199
ami@newworldlibrary.com
www.newworldlibrary.com

Barry Neil Kaufman, Author
Documents Raun Kaufman's astonishing development from a lifeless, autistic, retarded child into a highly verbal, lovable youngster with no traces of his former condition. Details Raun's extraordinary progress from the age of four into young adulthood, also shares moving accounts of five families that successfully used the Son-Rise Program to reach their own special children. *$14.96*
372 pages
ISBN 0-915811-53-7

8621 Steps to Independence: Teaching Everyday Skills to Children with Special Needs
Spina Bifida Association of America
1600 Wilson Boulevard
Suite 800
Arlington, VA 22209
202-944-3285
800-621-3141
Fax: 202-944-3295
sbaa@sbaa.org
www.sbaa.org

Ana Ximenes, Chair
Sara Struwe, President & CEO
Mark Bohay, National Web Initiatives & Development Manager
Elizabeth Merck, Development Manager
A guide to help parents teach life skills to their disabled child. *$34.25*

8622 Stroke Sourcebook
PO Box 8002
Aston, PA 19014-8002
313-961-1340
800-234-1340
Fax: 800-875-1340
customerservice@omnigraphics.com
www.omnigraphics.com

Peter Ruffner, President, Co-Founder
Fred Ruffner, Founder
Peter Ruffner, Co-Founder
Basic Consumer Health Information about Stroke, Including Ischemic, Hemorrhagic, and Mini Strokes, as Well as Risk Factors, Prevention Guidelines, Diagnostic Tests, Medications and Surgical Treatments, and Complications of Stroke.

8623 Stroke Sourcebook, 2nd Edition
Omnigraphics
PO Box 8002
Aston, PA 19014-8002   313-961-1340
                                         800-234-1340
                               Fax: 800-875-1340
                    customerservice@omnigraphics.com
                               www.omnigraphics.com
Peter Ruffner, President, Co-Founder
Fred Ruffner, Founder
Peter Ruffner, Co-Founder
Stroke Sourcebook, Second Edition provides updated information about stroke, its causes, risk factors, diagnosis, acute and long-term treatment, and recent innovations in poststroke care. Information on rehabilitation therapies, prevention strategies, and tips on caring for a stroke survivor is also included, along with a glossary of related terms and a directory of organizations that offer additional information to stroke survivors and their families. *$84.00*
626 pages Hard cover
ISBN 0-780810-35-8

8624 Succeeding With Interventions For Asperger Syndrome Adolescents
Autsim Society of North Carolina Bookstore
505 Oberlin Road
Suite 230
Raleigh, NC 27605-1345   919-743-0204
                                         800-442-2762
                               Fax: 919-743-0208
                    books@autismsociety-nc.org
                               www.autismbookstore.com
Tracey Sheriff, Chief Executive Officer
David Laxton, Director of Communications
Paul Wendler, Chief Financial Officer
Kristy White, Director of Development
This book includes a very useful outline of all the therapy sessions, which can be used as a template by a practitioner for creating their own interaction therapy intervention for adolescents.

8625 Symptomatic Chiari Malformation
Spina Bifida Association of America
1600 Wilson Boulevard
Suite 800
Arlington, VA 22209   202-944-3285
                                         800-621-3141
                               Fax: 202-944-3295
                               sbaa@sbaa.org
                               www.sbaa.org
Ana Ximenes, Chair
Sara Struwe, President & CEO
Mark Bohay, National Web Initiatives & Development Manager
Elizabeth Merck, Development Manager
The Spina Bifida Association (SBA) serves adults and children who live with the challenges of Spina Bifida.

8626 Taking Charge
Spina Bifida Association of America
1600 Wilson Boulevard
Suite 800
Arlington, VA 22209   202-944-3285
                                         800-621-3141
                               Fax: 202-944-3295
                               sbaa@sbaa.org
                               www.sbaa.org
Ana Ximenes, Chair
Sara Struwe, President & CEO
Mark Bohay, National Web Initiatives & Development Manager
Elizabeth Merck, Development Manager
Teenagers talk about life and physical disabilities. *$7.95*

8627 Ten Things I Learned from Bill Porter
New World Library
14 Pamaron Way
Novato, CA 94949   415-884-2100
                                         800-972-6657
                               Fax: 415-884-2199
                    ami@newworldlibrary.com
                               www.newworldlibrary.com
Shelly Ackerman, Author
Bill Porter worked for the Watkins Corp, selling household products door-to-door in one of Portland's worst neighborhoods. Afflicted with cerebral palsy and burdened with continual pain, Porter was determined not to live on government disability and went on to become Watkin's top-grossing salesman in Portland, the Northwest, and the US. This book was written by the woman who worked as Porter's typist and driver and later became his friend and cospeaker. *$20.00*
192 pages
ISBN 1-577312-03-1

8628 Thyroid Disorders Sourcebook
Omnigraphics
PO Box 8002
Aston, PA 19014-8002   313-961-1340
                                         800-234-1340
                               Fax: 800-875-1340
                    customerservice@omnigraphics.com
                               www.omnigraphics.com
Peter Ruffner, President, Co-Founder
Fred Ruffner, Founder
Thyroid Disorders Sourcebook provides essential information about thyroid and parathyroid function, diseases, and treatments. Also presented are symptoms, risk factors, diagnosis, treatments, thyroid effects on the body, and the impact of environmental conditions on the thyroid. *$84.00*
573 pages Hard cover
ISBN 0-780807-45-7

8629 Tourette Syndrome: The Facts
Oxford University Press
198 Madison Avenue
New York, NY 10016   212-726-6000
                                         800-445-9714
                               Fax: 919-677-1303
                               custserv.us@oup.com
                               www.oup.com
Mary Robertson, Co-Editor
Andrea Cavanna, Co-Editor
Johnathan Keats, Author
Jim Cullen, Author
The causes of the syndrome, how it is diagnosed, and the ways in which it can be treated. *$35.00*
122 pages
ISBN 0-198523-98-X

8630 Tourette's Syndrome: Finding Answers and Getting Help
O'Reilly Media Inc
1005 Gravenstein Hwy N
Sebastopol, CA 95472-2811   707-827-7019
                                         800-889-8969
                               Fax: 707-824-8268
                               order@oreilly.com
                               www.oreilly.com
416 pages Paperback
ISBN 0-596500-07-6

8631 Tourette's Syndrome: Tics, Obsessions, Compulsions: Developmental Psychopathology
John Wiley & Sons
111 River Street
Hoboken, NJ 07030-5774
201-748-6000
Fax: 201-748-6088
info@wiley.com
www.wiley.com

Peter Booth Wiley, Chairman
Stephen M. Smith, President & CEO
John Kitzmacher, EVP, CFO
Ellis E. Cousens, Executive Vice President, COO
Contains 21 contributions compromising the work of researchers associated with the Yale Child Study Center, which has been at the forefront of research on Tourette's syndrome and associated disorders. *$85.00*
600 pages
ISBN 0-471113-75-1

8632 Treating Epilepsy Naturally: A Guide to Alternative and Adjunct Therapies
McGraw-Hill Company
P.O.Box 182605
Columbus, OH 43218
800-338-3987
Fax: 609-308-4480
customer.service@mheducation.com
www.mcgraw-hill.com

David Levin, President and CEO
Patrick Milano, Chief Administrative Officer & CFO
Stephen Laster, Chief Digital Officer
David Stafford, SVP & General Counsel
Offers alternative treatments to replace and to complement traditional therapies and sound advice to find the right health practitioner. *$15.95*
288 pages
ISBN 0-658013-79-3

8633 Understanding Asthma
National Jewish Health
1400 Jackson Street
Denver, CO 80206
303-270-2708
877-225-5654
Fax: 303-398-1125
allstetterw@njc.org
nationaljewish.org

Rich Schierburg, Chair
Robin Chotin, Vice Chair
Michael Salem, M.D., President and CEO
Christine Forkner, CFO and Executive Vice President
Offers a brief introduction to asthma and then goes into the physiology of asthma, the triggers of asthma, and diagnosis and monitoring of asthma.
27 pages

8634 Understanding Asthma: The Blueprint for Breathing
Allergy & Asthma Network Mothers of Asthmatics
8229 Boone Boulevard
Suite 260
Vienna, VA 22182
800-878-4403
Fax: 703-288-5271
www.aanma.org

Michael Amato, Chair
Tonya Winders, President & CEO
Brenda Silvia-Torma, Project Manager
Gary Fitzgerald, Managing Editor
A layman's guide to asthma facts based on a presentation from the first national asthma patient conference.

8635 Understanding Cystic Fibrosis
University Press of Mississippi
3825 Ridgewood Road
Jackson, MS 39211-6492
601-432-6205
800-737-7788
Fax: 601-432-6217
press@ihl.state.ms.us
www.upress.state.ms.us

Leila W. Salisbury, Director
Craig Gill, Assistant Director/Editor-in-Chief
Anne Stascavage, Managing Editor
Vijay Shah, Acquiring Editor
A reference for CF patients and their families. *$14.00*
128 pages
ISBN 0-878059-67-9

8636 Understanding Multiple Sclerosis
University Press of Mississippi
3825 Ridgewood Road
Jackson, MS 39211-6492
601-432-6205
800-737-7788
Fax: 601-432-6217
press@ihl.state.ms.us
www.upress.state.ms.us

Melissa Stauffer, Author
Craig Gill, Assistant Director/Editor-in-Chief
Anne Stascavage, Managing Editor
Vijay Shah, Acquiring Editor
Two psychologists discuss their roles with a member who has multiple sclerosis. Includes chapters on adolescents with multiple sclerosis, employment, and research. *$14.00*
136 pages
ISBN 1-578068-03-7

8637 Urologic Care of the Child with Spina Bifida
Spina Bifida Association of America
1600 Wilson Boulevard
Suite 800
Arlington, VA 22209
202-944-3285
800-621-3141
Fax: 202-944-3295
sbaa@sbaa.org
www.sbaa.org

Ana Ximenes, Chair
Sara Struwe, President & CEO
Mark Bohay, National Web Initiatives & Development Manager
Elizabeth Merck, Development Manager
The Spina Bifida Association (SBA) serves adults and children who live with the challenges of Spina Bifida.

8638 Usher Syndrome
National Institute on Deafness & Other Communicati
31 Center Drive MSC 2320
Bethesda, MD 20892-2320
301-496-7243
800-241-1044
Fax: 301-770-8977
nidcdinfo@nidcd.nih.gov
www.nidcd.nih.gov

James F Battey Jr MD PhD, Director
Judith A. Cooper, Deputy Director
Timothy J. Wheeles, Executive Officer
Tanya Brown, Executive Assistant
Explains what is Usher Syndrome, who is affected by Usher syndrome, what causes Usher syndrome, how is Usher syndrome treated, and what research is being conducted on Usher syndrome.

8639 What Everyone Needs to Know About Asthma
Allergy & Asthma Network Mothers of Asthmatics
8229 Boone Boulevard
Suite 260
Vienna, VA 22182
800-878-4403
Fax: 703-288-5271
www.aanma.org

Michael Amato, Chair
Tonya Winders, President & CEO
Brenda Silvia-Torma, Project Manager
Gary Fitzgerald, Managing Editor

Offers information and facts on gaining control of asthma, asthma triggers and monitoring asthma disorders.

8640 When the Road Turns: Inspirational Stories About People with MS
Health Communications
3201 SouthWest 15th Street
Deerfield Beach, FL 33442
954-360-0909
800-441-5569
Fax: 954-360-0034

300 pages
ISBN 1-558749-07-1

8641 Young Person's Guide to Spina Bifida
Spina Bifida Association of America
1600 Wilson Boulevard
Suite 800
Arlington, VA 22209
202-944-3285
800-621-3141
Fax: 202-944-3295
sbaa@sbaa.org

Ana Ximenes, Chair
Sara Struwe, President & CEO
Mark Bohay, National Web Initiatives & Development Manager
Elizabeth Merck, Development Manager
Gives practical tips and suggestions for becoming independent and managing your health. *$19.00*

8642 Your Child and Asthma
National Jewish Health
1400 Jackson Street
Denver, CO 80206
303-270-2708
877-225-5654
Fax: 303-398-1125
allstetterw@njc.org
nationaljewish.org

Rich Schierburg, Chair
Robin Chotin, Vice Chair
Michael Salem, M.D., President and CEO
Christine Forkner, CFO and Executive Vice President
A booklet offering information to parents and family about their child with asthma. Offers information on diagnosis, treatments, triggers and family concerns.

8643 Your Cleft Affected Child
Hunter House Inc. Publisher
PO Box 2914
Alameda, CA 94501-914
510-865-5282
800-266-5592
Fax: 510-865-4295
www.hunterhouse.com

Carrie T Gruman Trinker, Author
The book also provides in-depth information, guidance, and support on a wide variety of relevant topics, from feeding to surgery to helping a child cope until his/her cleft has been fully corrected.
$ 16.95
288 pages Paperback
ISBN 0-897931-85-4

8644 Your Guide to Bowel Cancer
Oxford University Press
2001 Evans Road
Cary, NC 27513
919-677-0977
800-445-9714
Fax: 919-677-1303
custserv.us@oup.co
www.us.oup.com

ISBN 0-340927-46-1

8645 AIDS: The Official Journal of the International AIDS Society
Lippincott Williams & Wilkins
2 Commerce Square
2001 Market St.
Philadelphia, PA 19103
215-521-8300
Fax: 215-521-8902
customerservice@lww.com
lww.com

JA Levy, Co Editor
B. Autran, Co Editor
R. A Coutinho, Co Editor
J. P Phair, Co Editor
The latest groundbreaking research on HIV and AIDS. *$433.00*
18 per year

8646 American Journal of Orthopsychiatry
American Psychological Association
750 1st Street NorthEast
Washington, DC 20002-4242
202-336-5500
800-374-2721
Fax: 202-336-5502
TTY: 202-336-6123
www.apa.org

Nadine J. Kaslow, President
Norman B. Anderson, PhD, CEO & EVP
Bonnie Markham, Treasurer
Jennifer F. Kelly, Recording Secretary
Mental health issues from multidisciplinary and interprofessionals perspectives: clinical, research and expository approaches. *$45.00*
160 pages Quarterly

8647 Annals of Otology, Rhinology and Laryngology
Annals Publishing Company
4507 Laclede Ave
Saint Louis, MO 63108-2103
314-367-4987
Fax: 314-367-4988
www.annals.com

Ken Cooper, President
Richard J. Smith, Editor
Monica L. Bergers, Editor's Assistant
Jim Cunningham, Advertising Representative
Original, peer-reviewed articles in the fields of otolaryngology - head and neck medicine and surgery, broncho-esophagology, audiology, speech, pathology, allery, and maxillofacial surgery. Official journal of the American Laryngological Association/American Broncho-Esophagological Association.
$170.00
112 pages Monthly

8648 Archives of Neurology
American Medical Association
P.O.Box 10946
Chicago, IL 60654
312-670-7827
800-262-2350
Fax: 312-464-4184
subscriptions@jamanetwork.com
jamanetwork.com

Margaret Vanner, Manager
Mission is to publish scientific information primarily important to those physicians caring for people with neurologic disorders, but also for those interested in the structure and function of the normal and diseased nervous system. *$235.00*
198 pages Monthly

8649 Cleft Palate-Craniofacial Journal
American Cleft Palate-Craniofacial Association
2455 Teller Rd.
Thousand Oaks, CA 91320
800-818-7243
Fax: 800-583-2665
journal@acpa-cpf.org
www.cpcjournal.org

Jack C. Yu, Editor

A peer-reviewed, interdisciplinary, international journal dedicated to current research on etiology, prevention, diagnosis, and treatment in all areas pertaining to craniofacial anomalies. Publishes 10 issues a year.

8650 Journal of Head Trauma Rehabilitation
Lippincott, Williams & Wilkins
P.O.Box 1620
Hagerstown, MD 21740

301-223-2300
800-638-3030
Fax: 301-223-2400
orders@lww.com
www.lww.com

John D Corrigan PhD, ABPP, Editor
Scholarly journal designed to provide information on clinical management and rehabilitation of the head-injured for the practicing professional. Published bimonthly. *$113.96*

Print: Magazines

8651 Coping with Cancer Magazine
Media America
P.O.Box 682268
Franklin, TN 37068-2268

615-790-2400
Fax: 615-794-0179
copingmag.com

53 pages 6 x year

8652 CurePSP Magazine
Society for Progressive Supranuclear Palsy
Suite 201
30 E. Padonia Road
Timonium, MD 21093

410-785-7004
800-457-4777
Fax: 410-785-7009
info@curepsp.org
www.psp.org

John T. Burhoe, Chair
Everett R. Cook, Vice Chair
Richard Gordon Zyne, President-CEO
Kathleen Matarazzo Speca, VP,Development & Donor Relations
Quarterly newsletter. The society's mission is to promote and fund research into finding the cause and cure for progressive supranuclear palsy (PSP). Provides information, support and advocacy to persons diagnosed with PSP, their families and caregivers. Educates physicians and allied health professionals on PSP and how to improve patient care.

8653 EpilepsyUSA
Epilepsy Foundation
8301 Professional Place
Landover, MD 20785-2353

301-459-3700
800-332-1000
Fax: 301-459-1569
ContactUs@efa.org
epilepsyfoundation.org

Warren Lammert, Chair
Phil Gattone, President and CEO
May J. Liang, Secretary
Roger Heldman, Treasurer
Magazine reporting on issues of interest to people with epilepsy and their families. *$15.00*
22 pages Bi-Monthly

8654 International Ventilator Users Network
International Ventilator Users Network
4207 Lindell Blvd
Suite 110
Saint Louis, MO 63108-2930

314-534-0475
Fax: 314-534-5070
info@ventusers.org
www.ventnews.org

William G. Stothers, President/Chairperson
Saul J. Morse, Vice President
Joan L. Headley,MS, Editor
Marny E. Eulberg, Secretary

To enhance the lives and independence of ventilator-assisted living by promoting education, networking, and advocacy among these individuals and healthcare providers. Ventilator-Assisted Living supports Post-Polio Health International's educational, research, and advocacy efforts. Offers information about relevant events.
Quarterly

8655 MSFOCUS Magazine
Multiple Sclerosis Foundation
6520 North Andrews Avenue
Fort Lauderdale, FL 33309-2130

954-776-6805
888-673-6287
Fax: 954-351-0630
support@msfocus.org
www.msfocus.org

Jules Kuperberg, Executive Director
Alan Segaloff, Executive Director
Natalie Blake, Program Services Director
Nathalie Sloane, Funds Development Director
Contemporary national, nonprofit organization that provides free support services and public education for persons with Multiple Sclerosis, newsletters, toll-free phone support, information, referrals, home care, assistive technology and support groups.
48 pages Quarterly

8656 Orthotics and Prosthetics Almanac
American Orthotic & Prosthetics Association
330 John Carlyle Street
Suite 200
Alexandria, VA 22314

571-431-0876
Fax: 571-431-0899
info@aopanet.org
www.aopanet.org

Anita L. Lampear, President
Charles H. Dankmeyer, Vice President
Thomas F. Fise, JD, Executive Director
Don DeBolt, Chief Operating Officer
Features articles covering current professional, patient care, government, business and National Office activities affecting the orthotics and prosthetics profession and industry. *$40.00*
80 pages Monthly
ISSN 1061-46 1

8657 PDF News
Parkinson's Disease Foundation
1359 Broadway
Suite 1509
New York, NY 10018

212-923-4700
800-457-6676
Fax: 212-923-4778
info@pdf.org
www.pdf.org

Howard D. Morgan, Chair
Woodruff Atwell, Ph.D., Vice Chair
Stephen Ackerman, Treasurer
Isobel Robins Konecky, Secretary
8-12 pages Quarterly

8658 POZ Magazine
212 W 35th St
New York, NY 10001

212-242-2163
800-973-2376
Fax: 212-675-8505
website@poz.com
poz.com

8659 SCI Life
National Spinal Cord Injury Association
11300 Rockville Pike
Suite 803
Rockville, MD 20852

301-468-3902
Fax: 301-468-3904
info@ilcreations.com
ilcreations.com

Quarterly/Free

8660 Spine
Lippincott, Williams & Wilkins
530 Walnut St
Philadelphia, PA 19106-3603
215-521-8300
Fax: 215-521-8411
customerservice@lww.com
lww.com

James N Weinstein DO MSc, Editor
Publishes original papers on theoretical issues and research concerning the spine and spinal cord injuries. *$9.00*
26 Issues Year

Print: Newsletters

8661 ACPOC News
Assoc of Children's Prosthetic-Orthotic Clinics
6300 N River Rd
Suite 727
Rosemont, IL 60018-4226
847-698-1637
Fax: 847-823-0536
acpoc@aaos.org
www.acpoc.org

David B. Rotter, CPO, President
Jorge A. Fabregas, Vice President
Hank White, PT, PhD, Secretary-Treasurer
Anna Cuomo, Director
Quarterly publication from the Association of Children's Prosthetic/Orthotic Clinics. Included with membership.
40 pages Quarterly

8662 AID Bulletin
Project AID Resource Center
P.O. Box 5190
Kent, OH 44242-0001
330-672-3000
Fax: 330-672-4724
info@kent.edu
www.kent.edu/

Beverly Warren, President
Todd A. Diacon, Provost & SVP
Gregg S. Floyd, Sr. Vice President
Greg Jarvie, Vice President
Has the latest news on upcoming conferences, literature, developments in programs and/or services for disabled persons who are substance abusers. Offers articles on their experiences, ideas and questions of others in this field which includes providers and consumers. *$7.50*

8663 AIDS Alert
AHC Media LLC
PO Box 550669
Atlanta, GA 30355
404-262-5436
800-688-2421
Fax: 404-262-5560
www.ahcpub.com/

Joy Daughtery Dickinson, Senior Managing Editor
Source of AIDS news and advice for health care professionals. Covers up-to-the-minute developments and guidance on the entire spectrum of AIDS challenges, including treatment, education, precautions, screening, diagnosis and policy. *$499.00*
Monthly

8664 Adaptive Tracks
Adaptive Sports Center
P.O. Box 1639
Crested Butte, CO 81224
970-349-2296
866-349-2296
Fax: 970-349-2077
info@adaptivesports.org
www.adaptivesports.org

Christopher Hensley, Executive Director
Chris Read, CTRS, Program Director
Ella Fahrlander, Development Director
Mike Neustedter, Marketing Director
The Adaptive Sports Center (ASC) of Crested Butte, Colorado is a non-profit organization that provides year-round recreation activities for people with disabilities and their families. The ASC

provides adaptive snowboarding downhill skiing, cross country skiing as well as backcountry trips. Summer activities include a variety of wilderness-based programs, multi-day trips into the back country, extensive cycling programs, canoeing, and white water rafting.
6 pages Quarterly

8665 Arthritis Self-Management
Rapaport Publishing, Inc.
150 W 22nd St
Ste 800
New York, NY 10011-2421
212-989-0200
Fax: 212-989-4786
ASMcustserv@cdsfulfillment.com
www.arthritisselfmanagement.com

Richard A Rapaport, President
Maryanne Schott Turner, Director of Manufacturing
Richard Boland, Art Director
James Moorehead, Circulation Director
Arthritis Self-Management publishes practical 'how-to' information for the growing number of people with arthritis who want to know more about managing their condition. We focus on the day-to-day and long-term aspects of arthritis in a positive and upbeat style, giving our subscribers up-to-date news, facts, and advice to help them make informed decisions about their health.
$9.97
BiMonthly

8666 Breaking Ground
Tennessee Council on Developmental Disabilities
404 James Robertson Pkwy
Suite 130
Nashville, TN 37243- 0228
615-532-6615
Fax: 615-532-6964
TTY:615-741-4562
tnddc@tn.gov
www.tn.gov/cdd

Stephanie Brewer cook, Chair
Roger D. Gibbens,, Vice Chair
Wanda Willis, Executive Director
Errol Elshtain, Director of Development
Newsletter
20 pages 6 x Year

8667 Breaking New Ground News Note
Purdue University
225 West University Street
West Lafayette, IN 47907
765-494-4600
800-825-4264
Fax: 765-496-1356
engineering.purdue.edu/

Paul Jones, Project Manager
Bill Field, Project Director
Denise Heath, Project Asst.
Robert Stuthridge, Project Ergonomist
News, practical ideas and success stories of and for farmers and other agricultural workers with physical disabilities.
2 pages Quarterly

8668 Diabetes Self-Management
Rapaport Publishing, Inc.
150 W 22nd St
Ste 800
New York, NY 10011-2421
212-989-0200
Fax: 212-989-4786
www.diabetesselfmanagement.com

Richard A Rapaport, President
Maryanne Schott Turner, Director of Manufacturing
Richard Boland, Art Director
James Moorehead, Circulation Director
Publishes practical how-to information, focusing on the day-to-day and long-term aspects of diabetes in a positive and upbeat style. Gives subscribers up-to-date news, facts and advice to help them maintain their wellness and make informed decisions regarding their health. *$9.97*
BiMonthly

8669 Directions
Families of Spinal Muscular Dystrophy
925 Busse Road
Elk Grove Village, IL 60007   847-367-7620
                                               800-886-1762
                                          Fax: 847-367-7623
                                               info@fsma.org
                                               www.fsma.org

Richard Rubenstein, Chair
Kenneth Hobby, President
Sue Kovach, Director of Finance
Megan Lenz, Communications Manager
$35.00
60-70 pages Quarterly

8670 IAL News
International Association of Laryngectomees
925B Peachtree Street NE
Suite 316
Atlanta, GA 30309   866-425-3678
                                               www.larynxlink.com

Wade Hampton, President
Susan Reeves, Administrative Manager
Jodi Knott, Director, Voice Institute
Charles Rusky, Treasurer
Focuses on rehabilitation and well-being of persons who have
had laryngectomy surgery.

8671 Informer
Simon Foundation
P.O.Box 815
Wilmette, IL 60091   847-864-3913
                                               800-237-4666
                                          Fax: 847-864-9758
                                           info@simonfoundation.org
                                               simonfoundation.org

Cheryle Gartley, President and Founder
Elizabeth T. LaGro, VP, Communications & Education
Twila Yednock, Director of Special Events
Monica Liebert, Scientific Liason
Publishes items of interest to people with bladder or bowel incon-
tinence, including medical articles, helpful devices, publications
and a pen pal list. Quarterly newsletter.
Quarterly

8672 Moisture Seekers
Sjogren's Syndrome Foundation
6707 Democracy Boulevard
Suite 325
Bethesda, MD 20817   301-530-4420
                                               800-475-6473
                                          Fax: 301-530-4415
                                               tms@sjogrens.org
                                               www.sjogrens.org

Kenneth Economou, Chair
Steven Taylor, CEO
Sheriese DeFruscio, VP of Development
Elizabeth Trocchio, Director of Marketing
Newsletter of the organization for lay people and professionals
interested in Sjogren's Syndrome. Contains medical news, cur-
rent research, and essential tips for daily living. *$25.00*
15-16 pages Monthly

8673 Momentum
National Multiple Sclerosis Society
Ste 6
421 New Karner Rd
Albany, NY 12205-3838   518-464-0850
                                               800-344-4867
                                          Fax: 518-464-1232
                                               nyr@nmss.org
                                               www.nationalmssociety.org

Eli Rubenstein, Chair
Cynthia Zagieboylo, President & CEO
Sherri Giger, EVP, Marketing
Jennifer Douglas, EVP, Technology

News and information on research progress, medical treatments,
patient services, therapeutic claims and activities.

8674 Options
People Against Cancer
P.O.Box 10
604 East Street
Otho, IA 50569   515-972-4444
                                               800-662-2623
                                          Fax: 515-972-4415
                                           info@PeopleAgainstCancer.org
                                               www.peopleagainstcancer.com
Frank D. Wiewel, Executive Director/Founder
Publication of People Against Cancer, a nonprofit, grassroots
public benefit organization dedicated to 'New Directions in the
War on Cancer.' We help people to find the best cancer treatment.
We are a democratic organization of people with cancer, their
loved ones and citizens working together to protect and enhance
medical freedom of choice.
8 pages Quarterly

8675 PDF Newsletter
Parkinson's Disease Foundation
1359 Broadway
Suite 1509
New York, NY 10018   212-923-4700
                                               800-457-6676
                                          Fax: 212-923-4778
                                               info@pdf.org
                                               www.pdf.org

Howard D. Morgan, Chair
Woodruff Atwell, Ph.D., Vice Chair
Stephen Ackerman, Treasurer
Isobel Robins Konecky, Secretary
The Parkinson's Disease Foundation (PDF) is a leading national
presence in Parkinson's disease research, education and public
advocacy.
12-16 pages Quarterly

8676 Parkinsons Report
National Parkinson Foundation
200 SE 1st Street
Suite 800
Miami, FL 33131   305-243-6666
                                               800-473-4636
                                               800-4PD-INFO
                                          Fax: 305-537-9901
                                               contact@parkinson.org
                                               www.parkinson.org

John W. Kozyak, Chairman
Andrew B. Albert, Vice Chairman
Joyce Oberdorf, President and CEO
Leilani Pearl, VP, Marketing & Communications
Articles, reports and news on Parkinson's disease and the activi-
ties of the National Parkinson Foundation.
32 pages Qarterly

8677 Post-Polio Health
Post-Polio Health International
Ste 110
4207 Lindell Blvd
Saint Louis, MO 63108-2930   314-534-0475
                                          Fax: 314-534-5070
                                               info@post-polio.org
                                               www.post-polio.org

William G. Stothers, President
Saul J. Morse, Vice President
Joan L. Headley, MS, Executive Director
Marny E. Eulberg, Secretary
To enhance the lives and independence of polio survivors by pro-
moting education, networking, and advocacy among these indi-
viduals and healthcare providers. Post-Polio Health supports
Post-Polio Health International's educational, research, and ad-
vocacy efforts. Offers information about relevant events. *$30.00*
12 pages quarterly

8678 **Prader-Willi Alliance of New York Newsletter**
244 5th Avenue
Suite D-110
New York, NY   10001   716-276-2211
                                     800-442-1655
                                Fax: 585-271-2782
                          alliance@prader-willi.org
                               www.prader-willi.org

Amy McDougall, President
Rachel Johnson, Vice President
Nancy Finegold, Vice President
Nina Roberto, Executive Director
The Prader-Willi Foundation is a national, nonprofit public charity that works for the benefit of individuals with Prader-Willi syndrome and their families. *$20.00*
Quarterly

8679 **Quality Care Newsletter**
National Association for Continence
P.O. Box 1019
Charleston, SC   29402-1019   843-352-2559
                                     800-BLA-DER
                                Fax: 843-352-2563
                            memberservices@nafc.org
                                   www.nafc.org

Donna Deng, Chairman
Nancy Hicks, Vice Chaiperson
Steven Gregg, Executive Director
Wendy Pokoski, Financial Administrator
Newsletter from NAFC. By donating $25 and becomming a Quality Care donor, you may receive our quarterly newsletter. *$25.00*
14-16 pages Quarterly

8680 **Rasmussen's Syndrome and Hemispherectomy Support Network Newsletter**
55 Kenosia Avenue
Danbury, CT   06810   203-744-0100
                                Fax: 203-798-2291
            http://www.rarediseases.org/rare-disease-info
Ronald J. Bartek, Chair
Sheldon M. Schuster, Vice Chair
Peter L. Saltonstall, President & CEO
Pamela Gavin, COO
National, not-for-profit organization dedicated to providing information and support to individuals affected by Rasmussen's Syndrome and hemispherectomy. Publishes a periodic newsletter and disseminates reprints of medical journal articles concerning Rasmussen's Syndrome and its treatments. Maintains a support network that provides encouragement and information to individuals affected by Rasmussen's Syndrome and their families.

8681 **SCI Psychosocial Process**
Amer Assn of Spinal Cord Injury Psych & Soc Wks
75-20 Astoria Blvd
East Elmhurst, NY   11370   718-803-3782
                                     800-404-2898
                                Fax: 718-803-0414
                               info@unitedspinal.org
                           http://www.unitedspinal.org/
David C. Cooper, Chairman
Patrick W. Maher, Vice Chairman
Joseph Gaskins, President and CEO
Denise A. McQuade, Secretary
Quarterly newsletter.

8682 **Special Care in Dentistry**
Blackwell Publishing
350 Main St
Malden, MA   02148   781-388-0200
                                Fax: 781-388-8210
                            www.blackwellpublishing.com

Peter Booth Wiley, Chairman
Stephen M. Smith, President & CEO
John Kitzmacher, EVP, CFO
Ellis E. Cousens, Executive Vice President, COO
  $125.00
48 pages BiMonthly

8683 **TSA Newsletter**
Tourette Syndrome Association
42-40 Bell Boulevard
Bayside, NY   11361   718-224-2999
                                     800-237-0717
                                Fax: 718-279-9596
                                   ts@tsa-usa.org
                                  www.tsa-usa.org

Stephen M. McCall, President
National non-profit membership organization whose mission is to identify the cause of, find the cure for, and control the effects of this disorder. A growing number of local chapters nationwide provide educational materials, seminars, conferences and support groups for over 35,000 members.
Quarterly

8684 **Tethering Cord**
Spina Bifida Association of America
PO Box 5801
Bethesda, MD   20284   301-496-5751
                                     800-352-9424
                                Fax: 202-944-3295
                                    sbaa@sbaa.org
                                 www.ninds.nih.gov/

Caroline Lewis, Executive Officer
Story C. Landis, Director
Denise Dorsey, Chief Administrative Officer
Maryann Sofranko, Deputy Executive Officer
Tethered spinal cord syndrome is a neurological disorder caused by tissue attachments that limit the movement of the spinal cord within the spinal column. Attachments may occur congenitally at the base of the spinal cord (conus medullaris) or they may develop near the site of an injury to the spinal cord.

8685 **Tourette Syndrome Association Children's Newsletter**
42-40 Bell Boulevard
Bayside, NY   11361   718-224-2999
                                     800-237-0717
                                Fax: 718-279-9596
                                   ts@tsa-usa.org
                                   tsa-usa.org

Stephen M. McCall, President
National, nonprofit membership organization. Mission is to identify the cause of, find the cure for, and control the effects of this disorder. A growing number of local chapters nationwide provide educational materials, seminars, conferences and support groups for over 35,000 members.

8686 **Voice of the Diabetic**
NFB Diabetes Action Network
200 East Wells Street
Baltimore, MD   21230-4914   410-659-9314
                                     888-581-4741
                                Fax: 410-685-5653
                                     www.nfb.org

Elizabeth Lunt, Editor
Marc Maurer, President
Fredric Schroeder, First Vice President
Ron Brown, Second Vice President
Newsletter containing personal stories and practical guidelines by blind diabetics and medical professionals, medical news, resource column and a recipe corner. We are a support and information network for all diabetics.
28 pages Quarterly

Non Print: Newsletters

8687 **Teens & Asthma**
American Lung Association
530 7th St SE
Washington, DC   20003   202-546-5864
                                Fax: 202-546-5607
                                     www.epa.gov/

Rolando E Bates Jr, CEO

Tips from other teens with asthma to help those having it get on with the serious business of having fun with the rest of their lives.
Online/Free

Non Print: Video

8688 **Fragile X Family**
Fanlight Productions
c/o Icarus Films
32 Court Street, 21st Floor
Brooklyn, NY 11201

718-488-8900
800-876-1710
Fax: 718-488-8642
info@fanlight.com
www.fanlight.com

Ben Achtenberg, Founder, Owner
Eric Kutner, Producer
Fragile X Family takes viewers inside the lives of a developmentally disabled family who are affected by Fragile X Syndrome, an inherited chromosomal disorder which is the second most common cause of mental retardation. *$149.00*
VHS/VIDEO
ISBN 1-572954-14-0

8689 **In the Middle**
Fanlight Productions
c/o Icarus Films
32 Court Street, 21st Floor
Brooklyn, NY 11201

718-488-8900
800-876-1710
Fax: 718-488-8642
info@fanlight.com
www.fanlight.com

Ben Achtenberg, Founder, Owner
Documents the problems and joys shared by Ryanna, who has Spina Bifida, and her parents, teachers and classmates during her first year of being mainstreamed in a Head Start Program. *$99.00*

8690 **Narcolepsy**
Fanlight Productions
c/o Icarus Films
32 Court Street, 21st Floor
Brooklyn, NY 11201

718-488-8900
800-876-1710
Fax: 718-488-8642
info@fanlight.com
www.fanlight.com

Ben Achtenberg, Founder, Owner
Jason Margolis, Producer
Presents the experiences of three individuals who lives and relationships have been disrupted by narcolepsy. Rental $50/day. *$199.00*
VHS/25 Minutes

8691 **Twitch and Shout**
Fanlight Productions
c/o Icarus Films
32 Court Street, 21st Floor
Brooklyn, NY 11201

718-488-8900
800-876-1710
Fax: 718-488-8642
info@fanlight.com
www.fanlight.com

Ben Achtenberg, Founder, Owner
Laurel Chitden, Producer
This documentary provides an intimate journey into the startling world of Tourette Syndrome (TS), a genetic disorder that can cause a bizarre range of involuntary movements, vocalizations, and compulsions. Through the eyes of a photojournalist with TS, the film introduces viewers to others who have this puzzling disorder. This is an emotionally absorbing, sometimes, unsettling, and finally uplifting program about people who must contend with a society that often sees them as crazy or bad. *$225.00*

Sports

8692 **National Sports Center for the Disabled**
33 Parsenn Rd
PO Box 1290
Winter Park, CO 80482

970-726-1518
Fax: 970-726-4112
volunteer@nscd.org
nscd.org

Kim Easton, President & CEO
Diane Eustace, Marketing Director
Beth Fox, Outreach & Education Director
Erica Mays, Human Resources Director
Organization providing year-round recreation for children and adults with disabilities. Winter programming includes alpine skiing, snowboarding, ski racing, show shoeing, and cross-country skiing. Summer sports include rafting, sailing, kayaking, camping, hiking, horseback riding, fishing, and rock climbing.

8693 **Rehabilitation Institute of Chicago's Virginia Wadsworth Sports Program**
345 East Suuperior St.
Chicago, IL 60611

312-238-1000
800-354-7342
800-354-REHA
Fax: 312-238-5017
sports@ric.org
www.ric.org

Jude Reyes, Chair
mike P. Kransy, Vice Chair
Thomas Reynolds III, Vice Chair
Joanne C. Smith, President & CEO
RIC's Center for Health and Fitness is a full service fitness center for individuals with disablilties and the administrative offices for RIC's Wirtz Sports Program. Eighteen different sport and recreation programs are offered free of charge. The facility is adjacent to RIC's main building and also is the location of a branch of The National Center for Physical Activity and Disability (NCPAD), a joint project operated by the University of Illinois-Chigcago.

Support Groups

8694 **AAN's Toll-Free Hotline**
Allergy and Asthma Network Mothers of Asthmatics
8229 Boone Boulevard
Suite 260
Vienna, VA 22182

800-878-4403
Fax: 703-288-5271
www.aanma.org

Michael Amato, Chair
Tonya Winders, President & CEO
Brenda Silvia-Torma, Project Manager
Gary Fitzgerald, Managing Editor
Offers answers to questions regarding allergies and asthma, provides referrals and support to assist the patient and his or her family.

8695 **Breaking New Ground Resource Center**
Purdue University
225 S University St
West Lafayette, IN 47907

765-494-5088
800-825-4264
Fax: 765-496-1356
bng@ecn.purdue.edu
engineering.purdue.edu/

Bill Field, Project Director
Paul Jones, Project Manager
Steve Swain, Rural Rehab Specialist
Robert Stuthridge, Project Ergonomist
A resource center devoted to helping farmers and ranchers with physical disabilities. Resource materials and a free newsletter are available to anyone.

8696 Cancer Information Service
National Cancer Institute
BG 9609 MSC 9760
9609 Medical Center Drive
Bethesda, MD 20892-9760 301-496-8531
800-422-6237
800-4 C-NCER
Fax: 304-402-0181
cancergovstaff@mail.nih.gov
www.cancer.gov

Barbara K. Rimer, Chairperson
Harold Varmus,MD, Director
Abby Sandler, Executive Secretary
Bruce A. Chabner, Chair
A nationwide network of 19 regional field offices supported by the National Cancer Institute which provides accurate, up-to-date information on cancer to patients and their families, health professionals and the general public. The CIS can provide specific information in understandable language about particular types of cancer, as well as information on second opinions and the availability of clinical trials.

8697 Clearinghouse on Disability Information: Office Special Education & Rehabilitative Service
U S Department of Education
400 Maryland Ave SW
Washington, DC 20202-1 202-245-7549
800-872-5327
Fax: 202-245-7614
www.ed.gov

Arne Duncan, Secretary Of Education
Tony Miller, Deputy Secretary
Martha Kanter, Under Secretary
Jo Anderson, Senior Advisor
Provides information to people with disabilities or anyone requesting information, by doing research and providing documents in response to inquiries. The information provided includes areas of federal funding for disability-related programs. Information provided may be useful to disabled individuals and their families, schools and universities, teacher's and/or school administrators, and organizations who have persons with disabilities as clients.

8698 Compassionate Friends, The
P.O.Box 3696
Oak Brook, IL 60522 630-990-0010
877-969-0010
Fax: 630-990-0246
nationaloffice@compassionatefriends.org
compassionatefriends.org

Patrick O'Donnell, President
Georgia Cockerham, Vice President
Lisa Corrao, COO
Alan Pedersen, Executive Director
Peer support for bereaved parents, grandparents and siblings, offering over 600 chapters in the United States. The organization also offers a quarterly magazine, We Need Not Walk Alone, and TCF resources of brochures, DVDs, and memorial wristbands for the bereaved parent, grandparent and sibling.

8699 Cornerstone Services
777 Joyce Rd
Joliet, IL 60436 815-741-7600
Fax: 815-723-1177
jhogan@cornerstoneservices.org
cornerstoneservices.org

John R. Rogers, Chair
Vincent A. Benigni, Vice Chairperson
Ben Stortz, President/CEO
Don Hospell, Vice President/COO
Cornerstone Services provides progressive, comprehensive services for people with disabilities, promoting choice, dignity and the opportunity to live and work in the community. Established in 1969, the agency provides developmental, vocational, residential and behavior health services.

8700 Disability Network
Ste 54
3600 S Dort Hwy
Flint, MI 48507 810-742-1800
Fax: 810-742-2400
TTY:810-742-7647
tdn@disnetwork.org
www.disnetwork.org

Bruce Chargo, Chairman
Diane Brown, Treasurer/ Vice Chairman
Mike Zelley, President & CEO
Linda F, Director, Finance, Operations
The Disability Network's mission is to realize consumer empowerment, self determination, full inclusion and participation of all people in the communities through independent living philosophy and the unequivocal implementation of the Americans with Disabilities Act

8701 Disability and Health: National Center for Birth Defects and Developmental Disabilities
Centers for Disease Control and Prevention
1600 Clifton Road
Atlanta, GA 30333 404-498-3012
800-232-4636
800-CDC-INFO
Fax: 404-498-3060
cdcinfo@cdc.gov
www.cdc.gov/ncbddd/dh

Dr. Tom Frieden, Director
Sherri A. Berger, COO
Carmen Villar, Chief of Staff
Ileana Arias, Principal Deputy Director
Located within the new CDC, National Center for Birth Defects and Developmental Disabilities, the Disability and Health section, operates a ralatively small program that primarily supports: data collection on the prevalence of people with disabilities & their health status and risk factors for poor health and well-being; research on measures of disability, functioning and health; health promotion intervention studies; and dissemination of health information.

8702 Easterseals
141 W. Jackson Blvd.
Suite 1400A
Chicago, IL 60604 312-726-6200
800-221-6827
Fax: 312-726-1494
info@easterseals.com
www.easterseals.com

Richard W. Davidson, Chairman
Sandra L Bouwman, 1st Vice Chairman
Joseph G. Kern, 2nd Vice Chairman
Eileen H. Boone, Secretary
Easterseals provides services, education, outreach, and advocacy so that people living with autism and other disabilities can live, learn, work and play in our communities.

8703 Epilepsy Foundation
8301 Professional Place E
Suite 200
Landover, MD 20785- 2353 800-332-1000
Fax: 301-459-1569
ContactUs@efa.org
www.epilepsy.com

Robert W Smith, Chair
Philip M Gattone, M.Ed, President & CEO
M. Vaneeda Bennett, Chief Development Officer
Ellen Hobby, Chief Financial Officer & VP, Finance & Administration
Offers information, referrals and support groups for those diagnosed with epilepsy.

8704 Family Support Project for the Developmentally Disabled
3424 Kossuth Ave
Bronx, NY 10467-2410   718-519-5000
                                                  Fax: 718-519-4902
                              www.nyc.gov/html/hhc/ncbh/home.html
William Walsh, Vice President
Sheldon McLeod, COO

8705 Head Injury Hotline
Brain Injury Resource Center
P.O.Box 84151
Seattle, WA 98124-5451   206-621-8558
                                                  Fax: 206-329-0912
                                                  brain@headinjury.com
                                                  www.headinjury.com
Hugh R. MacMahon, Neurology
Constance Miller, Founder
Paul M. Kuroiwa, Performance management consultant
B. Parker Lindner, Communications specialist
Disseminates head injury information and provides referrals to
facilitate adjustment to life following head injury. Organizes
seminars for professionals, head injury survivors, and their
families.

8706 International Braille and Technology Center for the Blind
National Federation of the Blind
200 East Wells Street
Baltimore, MD 21230-4914   410-659-9314
                                                  Fax: 410-685-5653
                                                  access@nfb.org
                                                  www.nfb.org
Marc Maurer, President
Fredric Schroeder, First Vice President
Ron Brown, Second Vice President
Marc Maurer, CEO
World's largest and most complete evaluation and demonstration
center of all assistive technology used by the blind from around
the world. Includes all braille, synthetic speech, print-to-speech
scanning, internet and portable devices and programs. Available
for tours by appointment to blind persons, employers, technology
manufacturers, teachers, parents and those working in the
assistive technology field.

8707 Lung Line Information Service
National Jewish Health
1400 Jackson Street
Denver, CO 80206   877-225-5654
                                                        877-225-5654
                                                  Fax: 303-398-1125
                                                  allstetterw@njc.org
                                                  nationaljewish.org
Rich Schierburg, Chair
Robin Chotin, Vice Chair
Michael Salem, M.D., President & CEO
Christine Forkner, CFO and Executive Vice President
A free information service answering questions, sending litera-
ture and giving advice to patients with immunologic or respira-
tory illnesses. The Line is an educational service and not a
substitute for medical care. Diagnosis or suggested treatment
will not be provided for a caller's specific condition.

8708 National AIDS Hotline
Centers for Disease Control and Prevention
1600 Clifton Road
Atlanta, GA 30333   404-639-3311
                                                        800-232-4636
                                                        800-CDC-INFO
                                                  Fax: 404-498-3060
                                                  cdcinfo@cdc.gov
                                                  www.cdc.gov
Dr. Tom Frieden, Director
Sherri A. Berger, COO
Carmen Villar, Chief of Staff
Ileana Arias, Principal Deputy Director
Offers free confidential information and publications on HIV in-
fection and AIDS.

8709 PALS Support Groups
Parent Professional Advocacy League
10th Fl
45 Bromfield St
Boston, MA 02108   866-815-8122
                                                  Fax: 617-542-7832
                                                  info@ppal.net
                                                  ppal.net
Earl N. Stuck, Chair
Lisa Lambert, Executive Director
Deborah A Fauntleroy, Associate Director
Meri Viano, Senior Regional Manager
Offers emotional support to parents and families of disabled chil-
dren.

8710 PXE International
Ste 404
4301 Connecticut Ave NW
Washington, DC 20008- 2369   202-362-9599
                                                  Fax: 202-966-8553
                                                  info@pxe.org
                                                  www.pxe.org
Patrick F. Terry, President
Sharon Terry, CEO
Terry M. Dermaid, Executive Director
Ian Terry, Webmaster
Provides support for individuals and families affected by
psukdoxanthoma elasticum (PXE), and resources for healthcare
professionals. PXE causes select elastic tissue to mineralize, and
effects the skin, eyes, cardiovascular, and GI systems.

8711 Parent Assistance Network
Good Samaritan Hospital
10 E. 31st Street
Kearney, NE 68847   308-865-7100
                                                        800-235-9905
                                                  Fax: 308-865-2924
                                                  sheilameyer@catholichealth.net
                                                  www.gshs.org
Randy DeFreece, President
Kent Barney, Chairman
Mary Henning, Vice Chairman
Julie Speirs, Secretary
Provides information and emotional support to all parents and es-
pecially to parents of children with disabilities in the central Ne-
braska area. Ongoing activities include parent support group
meetings, parent-to-parent networking and referrals and Respite
Care provider trainings.

8712 Post-Polio Support Group
Adventist Hinsdale Hospital
120 N Oak St
Hinsdale, IL 60521-3829   630-856-9000
                                                  Fax: 630-856-6000
                                                  www.keepingyouwell.com
David Crane, President
Information and support for polio patients and their families;
meets the fourth Wednesday of each month.

8713 Prevent Child Abuse America
288 South Wabash Avenue
10th floor
Chicago, IL 60604   312-663-3520
                                                        800-244-5373
                                                        800-CHI-DREN
                                                  Fax: 312-939-8962
                                                  mailbox@preventchildabuse.org
                                                  preventchildabuse.org
Fred M. Riley, Chair
David Rudd, Vice Chair
James Hmurovich, President & CEO
Robert Allen, Sr. Director, Administration
Through public education, community partnerships and support
services, PCAMW helps everyone play a role in prevention. We
share information on prevention stategies and effective parenting
at community forums and events and advocate for polices and services that keep children safe. We operate PhoneFriend, a telephone support line for children at home without adult supervision

and conduct personal safety workshops in schools, camps and libraries.

8714   Son-Rise Program
2080 S Undermountain Rd.
Sheffield, MA   01257-9643   413-229-2100
877-766-7473
Fax: 413-229-8931
www.autismtreatmentcenter.org
Barry Neil Kaufman, Founder & CEO
Clyde Haberman, Senior Teacher & Director of Development
Blair Borgeson, Developmental Therapist
Emily Vitale Aronow, Program Advisor & Client Support Coordinator
The center's Son-Rise Program teaches a comprehensive system of treatment and education designed to help families and caregivers enable their children to dramatically improve in all areas of learning.

8715   Special Children
1306 Wabash Ave
Belleville, IL   62220-3370   618-234-6876
Fax: 618-234-6150
specialchildren.net
Kathleen Cullen, Administrator
A nonprofit agency serving children with developmental disabilities ages birth to 6 years

8716   Support Works
1607 Dilworth Rd W
Charlotte, NC   28203-5213   704-331-9500
www.supportworks.org
Joel Fisher, Manager
SupportWorks helps people find and form support groups. An 8 page publication Power Tools, clearly walks new group leaders through steps of putting together a healthy self-help group. SupportWorks also has a telephone conference program which allows people with similar diseases or other nonprofit issues to meet by phone conference for free or at very low cost.

8717   Toll-Free Information Line
Asthma and Allergy Foundation of America
8201 Corporate Drive
Suite 1000
Landover, MD   20785   202-466-7643
800-727-8462
800-7 A-THMA
Fax: 202-466-8940
info@aafa.org
aafa.org
Lynn Hanessian, Chair
Yolanda Miller, SVP & COO
Lynda Mitchell, VP, Food Allergies
Nancy Kercher, Secretary
The Asthma and Allergy Foundation of America (AAFA) provides practical information, community based services and support through a national network of chapters and support groups. AAFA develops health education, organizes state and national advocacy efforts and funds research to find better treatments and cures.

8718   Visiting Nurse Association of America
2121 Crystal Drive
Suite 750
Arlington, VA   22202   571-527-1520
888-866-8773
Fax: 571-527-1527
webadmin@vnaa.org
vnaa.org
Mary B. DeVeau, Chair
Linnea Windel, Vice Chair
Tracey Moorhead, President & CEO
Magaret Terry, VP of Quality & Innovation
The VNAA is the official national association for not-for-profit, community based home health organizations known as the Visiting Nurse Associations (VNA's). They created the profession of home health care more then 100 years ag. They have a united mission to bring compassionate, high-quality and cost-effective home care to individuals in their communities.

Speech & Language

Associations

8719   Academic Language Therapy Association
14070 Proton Rd.
Suite 100
Dallas, TX   75244
                                    972-233-9107
                              Fax: 972-490-4219
                              office@altaread.org
                              www.altaread.org

Janna Curry-Dobbs, President
Jo Ann Handy, VP Membership
Susan Louchen, VP Public Relations
Tim Odegard, VP Programs
The Academic Language Therapy Associationr (ALTA) is a non-profit national professional organization with the purpose of establishing, maintaining, and promoting standards of education, practice and professional conduct for Certified Academic Language Therapists. Academic Language Therapy is an educational, structured, comprehensive, phonetic, multisensory approach for the remediation of dyslexia and/or written-language disorders.
1986

8720   American Speech-Language-Hearing Association
2200 Research Blvd.
Rockville, MD   20850-3289
                                    301-296-5700
                                    800-638-8255
                              actioncenter@asha.org
                              www.asha.org

Gail J. Richard, President
Elise Davis-Mcfaland, President-Elect
Margot L. Beckerman, Chair
Arlene A. Pietranton, Chief Executive Officer
The American Speech-Language Association is the professional, scientific, and credentialing association for members and affiliates who are speech-language pathologists, audiologists, and speech, language, and hearing scientists in the United States and internationally. ASHA provides information for the public, professionals, students, and the research community related to hearing, balance, speech, language and swallowing disorders.

8721   Aphasia Hope Foundation
P.O. Box 79701
Houston, TX   77279
                                    855-764-4673
                              jstradinger@comcast.net
                              www.aphasiahope.org

Sandy Caudell, Program Diretor
Judi Stradinger, Executive Director
Aphasia Hope Foundation is a nonprofit foundation whose mission is to promote research into the prevention and cure of aphasia and to ensure that all survivors of aphasia and their caregivers are aware of and have access to the best prossible tratments.

8722   Association of Language Companies
9707 Key West Ave.
Suite 100
Rockville, MD   20850
                                    240-404-6511
                              Fax: 301-990-9771
                              info@alcus.org
                              www.alcus.org

Christopher Carter, President
Rick Antezana, Vice President
Lenani P. Craig, Treasurer
Susan Amarino, Secretary
The Association of Language Companies (ALC) is a national trade association representing businesses that provide translation, interpretation, localization, and language training services.

8723   Autism Research Institute
4182 Adams Ave.
San Diego, CA   92116-2599
                                    866-366-3361
                              www.autism.com

Stephen Edelson, Executive Director
Rebecca McKenney, Office Manager
Christopher Flynn, Treasurer
Jane Johnson, Secretary
Conducts research on the causes, diagnosis, and treatment of autism and publishes a quarterly newsletter that reviews worldwide research. Literature on causes and treatment available. Refers patients and families to health care professionals and clinics.

8724   Autism Services Center
929 4th Ave.
P.O. Box 507
Huntington, WV   25701-0507
                                    304-525-8014
                              Fax: 304-525-8026
                              www.autismservicescenter.org

Jimmie Beirne, Chief Executive Officer
Jodi Fields, Director
Barbara Bragg, Director
David Finley, Chief Operations Officer
Provides developmental disabilities services with a specialty in autism. Services include case management, residential, personal care, assessments and evaluations, supported employment, independent living and family support.

8725   Autism Treatment Center of America
2080 S Undermountain Rd.
Sheffield, MA   01257-9643
                                    413-229-2100
                                    877-766-7473
                              Fax: 413-229-8931
                              correspondence@option.org
                              www.autismtreatmentcenter.org

Barry Neil Kaufman, Founder & CEO
Clyde Haberman, Senior Teacher & Director of Development
Blair Borgeson, Developmental Therapist
Emily Vitale Aronow, Program Advisor & Client Support Coordinator
The Autism Treatment Center of America provides innovative training programs for parents and professionals caring for children challenged by Autism, Autism Spectrum Disorders, Pervasive Developmental Disorders (PDD) and other development difficulties. The center's Son-Rise Program teaches a comprehensive system of treatment and education designed to help families and caregivers enable their children to dramatically improve in all areas of learning.

8726   Carl and Ruth Shapiro Family National Center for Accessible Media
WGBH Educational Foundation
1 Guest St.
Boston, MA   02135-2016
                                    617-300-3400
                              Fax: 617-300-1035
                              TTY:617-300-2489
                              ncam@wgbh.org
                              ncam.wgbh.org

Donna Danielewski, Director
Geoff Freed, Director of technology projects and Web media standards
Madeleine Rothberg, Senior Subject Matter Expert
Bryan Gould, Director of Accessible Learning and Assessment Technologies
The Carl and Ruth Shapiro Family National Center for Accessible Media (NCAM) is a research and development facility dedicated to addressing barriers to media and emerging technologies for people with disabilities in their homes, schools, workplaces, and communities.

8727 **Childhood Apraxia of Speech Association**
416 Lincoln Ave.
2nd Fl.
Pittsburgh, PA 15209 412-343-7102
www.apraxia-kids.org

Mary Sturm, President
Michele R. Atkins, Executive Director
Joshua Zellers, Treasurer
Sue Freidurger, Secretary
The Childhood Apraxia of Speech Association is a nonprofit publicly funded charity whose mission is to strengthen the support systems in the lives of children with apraxia so that each child is afforded their best opportunity to develop speech and communication.

8728 **Davis Center**
110 Wesley St.
P.O. Box 508
Manlius, NY 13104 862-251-4637
Fax: 862-251-4642
ddavis@thedaviscenter.com
www.thedaviscenter.com

Dorinne S Davis MA CCC-A FAAA, Director
The Davis Center's Sound Therapy Programs make positive changes for children and adults with autism, ADD/ADHD, auditory processing issues, Dyslexia, learning disabilities, and other learning and wellness challenges. Programs address issues such as phonics, spelling, writing, reading comprehension, hearing only parts of words, following directions, discriminating between sounds, sound sensitivity, behavioral responses, focus, attention, and more.

8729 **Deafness and Communicative Disorders Branch of Rehab Services Administration Office**
Special Education and Rehab Services
400 Maryland Ave., SW
Washington, DC 20202 800-872-5327
www.ed.gov

Kimberly Richey, Secretary Of Education
Promotes improved rehabilitation services for deaf and hard of hearing people and individuals with speech or language impairments. Provides technical assistance to public and private agencies and individuals.

8730 **Dysphagia Research Society**
2800 West Higgins Rd.
Suite 440
Hoffman Estates, IL 60169 888-775-7361
Fax: 847-885-8393
info@dysphagiaresearch.org
www.dysphagiaresearch.org

Gary H. McCullough, President
Sudarshan R. Jadcherla, President Elect
Susan Langmore, Secretary/Treasurer
Maggie-Lee Huckabee, Councilor
The Dysphagia Research Society is a nonprofit organization with the purpose of enhancing and encouraging research pertinent to normal and disordered swallowing, to promote the dissemination of knowledge related to normal and disordered swallowing, and to provide a multidisciplinary forum for presentation of research into normal and disordered swallowing.

8731 **Hearing, Speech and Deafness Center (HSDC)**
Hearing, Speech & Deafness Center (HSDC)
1625 19th Ave.
Seattle, WA 98122-2848 206-323-5770
888-222-5036
Fax: 206-328-6871
seattle@hsdc.org
www.hsdc.org

Lindsay Klarman, Executive Director
Michelle Coleman, Director of Operations
Hearing, Speech & Deaf Center (HSDC) is a nonprofit for clients who are deaf, hard of hearing, or who face other communication barriers such as speech challenges. Their mission is to foster inclusive and accessible communities through communication, advocacy, and education.

8732 **International Cluttering Association**
705 Tilbury Court
Sun City Center, FL 33573 elanouette@tampabay.rr.com
associations.missouristate.edu/ica

Charley Adams, Ph.D., Chair
Susanne Cook, Chair Elect
Katarzyna Wesierska, Secretary
Dan Hudock, Treasurer
They work to increase awareness of the communication disorder of cluttering worldwide among speech-language therapists/logopedists, healthcare professionals, people with cluttering, and the public.

8733 **International Fluency Association**
Northern Illinois University
Dept. of Communicative Disorders
DeKalb, IL 60115-2899 www.theifa.org
Elaine Kelman, President
Nan Bernstein Ratner, President Elect
Shelly Jo Kraft, Treasurer
Kurt Eggers, Secretary
The International Fluency Association is a not-for-profit, international, interdisciplinary organization devoted to the understanding and management of fluency disorders, and to the improvement in the quality of life for persons with fluency disorders.

8734 **Lindamood-Bell Home Learning Process**
CA 805-541-3836
800-233-1819
www.lindamoodbell.com

Nanci Bell, Founder/Director
Patricia C. Lindamood, Founder/Director
Lindamood-Bell Learning Process is dedicated to enhancing human learning. Lindamood-Belll programs teach children and adults to read, spell, comprehend, and express language.
1986

8735 **Myositis Association**
1940 Duke St.
Suite 200
Alexandria, VA 22314 703-553-2632
800-821-7356
Fax: 703-548-9446
TMA@myositis.org
www.myositis.org

Bob Goldberg, Executive Director
Linda Kobert, Communications Director
Aisha Morrow, Operations Manager
Ruthann Devine, Program Services Director
The Myositis Association is a nonprofit organization that supports patients of myisitis.

8736 **National Aphasia Association**
P.O. Box 87
Scarsdale, NY 10583 800-922-4622
naa@aphasia.org
www.aphasia.org

Darlene S. Williamson, President
Daniel Martin, Vice President Strategic Planning
Barbara Kessler, Vice President Community Outreach & Education
The National Aphasia Association (NAA) is a nonprofit organization that promotes public education, research, rehabilitation and support services to assist people with aphasia and their families.

8737 **National Association of Special Education Teachers**
1250 Connecticut Ave., NW
Suite 200
Washington, DC 20036-2643 800-754-4421
Fax: 800-754-4421
contactus@naset.org
www.naset.org

Roger Pierangelo, Executive Director
George Giuliani, Executive Director
The National Association of Special Education Teachers (NASET) is a national membership organization dedicated to ren-

dering all possible support and assistance to those preparing for or teaching in the field of special education. NASET was founded to promote the profession of special education teachers and to provide a national forum for their ideas.

8738 National Black Association for Speech-Language and Hearing
P.O. Box 779
Pennsville, NJ 08070

877-936-6235
Fax: 877-936-6235
nbaslh@nbaslh.org
www.nbaslh.org

Cathy Runnels, Interim Chair
Kia N. Johnson, Parliamentarian
Martine Elie, Treasurer
The mission of the National Black Association of Speech-Language and Hearing is to maintain a viable mechanism through which the needs of black professionals, students and individuals with communication disorders can be met.

8739 National Cued Speech Association
1300 Pennsylvania Ave, NW
Suite 190-713
Washington, DC 20004

917-439-5126
800-459-3529
Fax: 866-269-9877
info@cuedspeech.org
www.cuedspeech.org

Anne Huffman, President
Sarina Roffe, Executive Director
Ben Lachman, Director of Development
Brian Kelly, Treasurer
The association champions effective communication, language development and literacy through the use of cued speech. Families are informed about Cued Speech along with other communication options.

8740 National Fragile X Foundation
2100 M St., NW
Suite 170, P.O. Box 302
Washington, DC 20037-1233

800-688-8765
www.fragilex.org

Tony Ferlenda, Chief Executive Officer
Linda Sorensen, Chief Operating Officer
Jayne Dixon Weber, Director of Education & Support Services
Paula Lipford, Volunteer Program Director
Unites the fragile X community to enrich lives through educational and emotional support, promote public and professional awareness and advance research toward improvemed treatments and cure for fragile X syndrome.

8741 National Spasmodic Dysphonia Association
300 Park Blvd.
Suite 335
Itasca, IL 60143

800-795-6732
Fax: 630-250-4505
NSDA@dysphonia.org
www.dysphonia.org

Charlie Reavis, President
Marcia Sterling, Treasurer
Kimberly Kuman, Executive Director
The National Spasmodic Dysphonia Association (NSDA) is a not-for-profit organization dedicated to advancing medical research into the causes of and treatments for SD, promoting physician and public awareness of the disorder, and providing support to those affected by SD through symposiums, support groups, and on-line resources.

8742 National Stuttering Association
119 W. 40th St.
14th Fl.
New York, NY   10018

212-944-4050
800-937-8888
Fax: 212-944-8244
info@westutter.org
www.westutter.org

Gerald Maguire, Chairman
Evan Sherman, Vice Chairman
Bob Wellington, Treasurer
Sarah Onofri, Secretary
A nonprofit organization dedicated to bringing hope, dignity, support, education, and empowerment to children and adults who stutter and their families, and the professionals who serve them.

8743 National Tourette Syndrome Association
42-40 Bell Blvd.
Suite 205
Bayside, NY   11361

888-4TO-URET
www.tsa-usa.org

John Miller, President & CEO
Diana Felner, VP Public Policy
Sonji Mason-Vidal, VP Finance & Administration
The Tourette Association is dedicated to making life better for all people affected by Tourette and Tic Disorders.

8744 Providence Speech and Hearing Center
1301 Providence Ave.
Orange, CA 92868-3892

714-923-1521
855-901-7742
Fax: 714-639-2593
pshc@pshc.org
www.pshc.org

Bruce May, President
Kevin Timone, Vice President - Fund Development
Randy Free, Vice President - Finance
Casey Immel, Treasurer
Mission is to provide the highest quality services available in the identification, diagnosis, treatment and prevention of speech, language and hearing disorders for persons of all ages.

8745 Scottish Rite Center for Childhood Language Disorders
1733 16th St., NW
Washington, DC 20009-3103

202-323-3579
Fax: 202-464-0487
council@scottishrite.org
www.scottishrite.org

Bill Sizemore, Executive Director
Offers speech-language evaluations and treatment, hearing screening and consultations to children ages birth through adolescence. Bilingual services are also available.

8746 Stern Center for Language and Learning
183 Talcott Rd.
Suite 101
Williston, VT 05495-9209

802-878-2332
learning@sterncenter.org
www.sterncenter.org

Blanche Podhajski, President
Michael Shapiro, Chief Operating Officer
Moneer Greenbaum, Director of Development
The Stern Center is a nonprofit learning center dedicated to helping children and adults reach their full potential. Stern Center professionals evaluate and teach all kinds of learners, including those with learning disabilities such as dyslexia or attention deficit disorders.

8747 Stuttering Foundation of America
1805 Moriah Woods Blvd.
Suite 3
Memphis, TN 38117
901-761-0343
800-992-9392
Fax: 901-761-0484
info@stutteringhelp.org
www.stutteringhelp.org

Jane Fraser, President
Dennis Drayna, Director
Joseph R. G. Fulcher, Director
Frances Cook, Director

Provides resources, services, and support to those who stutter and their families, as well as support for research into the causes of stuttering.

8748 Texas Speech-Language-Hearing Association
2025 M St., NW
Suite 800
Washington, DC 20036-2342
855-330-8742
888-729-8742
Fax: 512-463-9468
staff@txsha.org
www.txsha.org

Judy Rudebusch Rich, President
Erin Bellue, VP of Educational & Scientific Affairs
Shannon Butkus, VP of Social & Governmental Policy
Rebecca Linke, VP of Research & Development

Mission is to encourage and promote the role of the speech-language pathologist and audiologist as a professional in the delivery of clinical services to persons with communications disorders. Encourages basic scientific study of processes of individual human communication with reference to speech, hearing and language.

8749 The Cherab Foundation
P.O. Box 8524
Port St. Lucie, FL 34952-8524
772-335-5135
cherabfoundation.org

Lisa Geng, Founder/President
Jolie Abreu, Vice President

The Cherab Foundation is a world-wide nonprofit organization working to improve the communication skills and education of all children with speech and language delays and disorders. Their area of emphasis is verbal and oral apraxia, severe neurologically-based speech and language disorders that hinder children's ability to speak.

8750 Wendell Johnson Speech And Hearing Clinic
University Of Iowa
Iowa City, IA 52242-1025
319-335-8736
Fax: 319-335-8851
TTY: 319-335-8736
speech-path-aud@uiowa.edu
clas.uiowa.edu/comsci/clinical-services

Ann Fennell, Clinical Coordinator

The clinic offers assessment and remediation for communication disorders in adults and children. The clinic also offers a Intensive Summer Residential Clinic for school age children needing intervention services because of speech, language, hearing and/or reading problems.

Camps

8751 CNS Camp New Connections
Mclean Hospital Child/Adolescent Program
Mailstop115
115 Mill Street
Belmont, MA 02478
617-855-2000
800-333-0338
Fax: 617-855-2833
mcleaninfo@partners.org
mcleanhospital.org

Scott L. Rauch, MD, President & Chief Psychiatrist
Blaise Aguirre, Clinical Staff
Alan Barry, Clinical Staff
Susan L. Andersen, Research Staff

Four-week summer day camp for children ages 7-17 who have pervasive developmental disorders, Asperger's Syndrome, autism spectrum disorders and non-verbal learning disabilities. The camp is designed to help children develop social skills through fun activities including: communication games, swimming, field trips, drama, and arts and crafts. *$4500.00*

8752 Camp Meadowood Springs
Institute for Rehab., Research, & Recreation Inc
122 SE Court Ave
P.O. Box 1025
Pendleton, OR 97801
541-276-2752
Fax: 541-276-7227
info@meadowoodsprings.org
www.meadowoodsprings.com

8753 Camp Royall
250 Bill Ash Rd
Monure, NC 27559
919-542-1033
Fax: 919-542-6343
camproyall@autismsociety-nc.org
www.autismsociety-nc.org/camp-royall/

Lesley Fraser, Program Director, Camp Royall
Cindy Lodestro, Administrative Assistant
Sara Gage, Director, Social Recreation Services
Curtis Sobie, Fellow

A week-long overnight and day camp for children and adults with autism. Campers will participate in traditional camp activities in a structured environment that helps them develop confidence, independence, and a willingness to try new things.

8754 Camp Sisol
Jewish Community Center of Greater Rochester/JCC
1200 Edgewood Ave
Rochester, NY 14618
585-461-2000
Fax: 585-461-0805
www.jccrochester.org

Richard Gray, President
Daniel Goldstein, Vice President
Arnie Sohinki, Executive Director
Howard Cohen, Treasurer

Camp is located in Honeoye Falls, New York. Coed, ages 5-16. Camp Sisol accomodates children with special needs.

8755 Childrens Beach House
100 West 10th Street
Suite 411
Wilmington, DE 19801-1674
302-655-4288
Fax: 302-655-4216
www.cbhinc.org

Martha P. Tschantz, President
Mary Helms, Vice President
Richard T Garrett, Executive Director
Nicholas Imhoff, Business Manager

Camp is located in Lewes, Delaware. Four-week sessions June-August for Delaware children with hearing impairment or speech/communication impairment. Coed, ages 6-12.

8756   Easter Seals Oklahoma
701 NE 13th St
Oklahoma City, OK   73104   405-239-2525
info@eastersealsoklahoma.org
eastersealsok.org/

Keith McCombs, Chairman
Krista Massad, Chairman-Elect
Cassie Wilson, Secretary
Matt Vance, Treasurer
Offers an Adult Day Health Center, and Child Development Center. The Child Development Center offers developmentally appropriate learning activities and services to meet the unique needs of each child, and the adult center provides solutions to meet the physical, social and emotional needs of adults from the ages of 21 to 100+.

8757   New Horizons Summer Day Camp
YMCA
13821 Newport Avenue
Suite 200
Tustin, CA   92780   714-549-9622
Fax: 714-838-5976
www.ymcaoc.org

Robert Traut, Chair
Jeff Black, Vice Chair
Jeff McBride, President/CEO
Cara Owens, COO/VP,Operations
One-week sessions for children with ADD and speech/communication impairment. Coed, ages 5-14.

8758   Sequanota Lutheran Conference Center and Camp
P.O. Box 245
Jennerstown, PA   15547   814-629-6627
contact@sequanota.com
www.sequanota.com

Carol Custead, President
David Shoemaker, Vice President
Nathan Pile, Executive Director
Chris Brant, Treasurer
Runs Camp Bethesda, a summer camp for adults with developmental disabilities and speech/communication impairment. For ages 18 and up.

8759   Talisman Summer Camp
64 Gap Creek Rd
Zirconia, NC   28790   828-697-6313
info@talismancamps.com
www.talismancamps.com

Doug Smathers, Camp Director/Owner
Linda Tatsapaugh, Operations Director/Owner
Robiyn Mims, Admissions Coordinator
Lee Kisselburg, Facilities Manager
Talisman Summer Camp is located 40 miles south of Asheville, North Carolina. Offers a program of hiking, rafting, climbing, and caving for learning disabled ADD/ADHD and autistic young people. Coed, ages 9-18.

8760   Wendell Johnson Speech & Hearing Clinic
University Of Iowa
250 Hawkins Dr
Iowa City, IA   52242-1025   319-335-8736
Fax: 319-335-8851
kathy-miller@uiowa.edu
www.uiowa.edu

Chuck Wieland, President
Hans Hoerschelman, Vice President
Josh Smith, Budget Officer
Shannon Lizakowski, Secretary
The clinic offers assessment and remediation for communication disorders in adults and children. The clinic also offers a Intensive Summer Residential Clinic for school age children needing intervention services because of speech, language, hearing and/or reading problems.

8761   YMCA Camp Fitch
The YMCA's Camp Fitch on Lake Erie
12600 Abels Rd
North Springfield, PA   16430   814-922-3219
877-863-4824
Fax: 814-922-7000
hannahkight@campfitchymca.org
campfitchymca.org

Matt Pose, Executive Director
Tom Parker, Associate Executive Director
Hannah Kight, Office Manager
Jon Tully, Program Manager
Camp is located in North Springfield, Pennsylvania. Camping sessions for children and adults with diabetes or epilepsy. Ages 8-16, families and seniors.

Print: Books

8762   Autism 24/7: A Family Guide to Learning at Home & in the Community
Autism Society of North Carolina Bookstore
Ste 230
505 Oberlin Rd
Raleigh, NC   27605-1345   919-743-0204
800-442-2762
Fax: 919-743-0208
jchampion@autismsociety-nc.org
http://www.autismsociety-nc.org/

Sharon Jeffries-Jones, Chair
Elizabeth Phillippi, Vice Chair
Tracey Sheriff, Chief Executive Officer
Paul Wendler, Chief Financial Officer
Parents are encouraged to focus on skill sets and behaviors that most negatively affect family functioning, and replacing these behaviors with acceptable alternatives. *$19.95*

8763   Autism Handbook: Understanding & Treating Autism & Prevention Development
Oxford University Press
2001 Evans Road
Cary, NC   27513   919-677-0977
800-445-9714
Fax: 919-677-1303
custserv.us@oup.co
http://www.oup.com/us/

320 pages
ISBN 0-195076-67-2

8764   Autism and Learning
Taylor & Francis
37-41 Mortimer St
London, UK   W1T 3   http://www.informatandm.com
Stuart Powell, Author
Rita Jordan, Editor
This book is about how a cognitive perception on the way in which individuals with autism think and learn may be applied to particular curriculum areas.
160 pages Paperback
ISBN 1-853464-21-X

8765   Autism in Adolescents and Adults
Springer Publishing
233 Spring St
New York, NY   10013   877-283-3229
ainy@aveda.com
http://aveda.edu/new-york

Eric Schopler, Editor
Gary B. Mesibov, Editor
This book is a great history lesson in the development of understanding about autism spectrum disorders, and is a testament to how far research and services in the field have come. This book contains lots of information about what general thinking and ser-

vices used to be like, in an era when still little was understood about these disorders. *$63.00*
456 pages
ISBN 0-306410-57-5

8766   Autism...Nature, Diagnosis and Treatment
Autism Society of North Carolina Bookstore
Ste 230
505 Oberlin Rd
Raleigh, NC   27605-1345   919-743-0204
                                            800-442-2762
                                      Fax: 919-743-0208
                         jchampion@autismsociety-nc.com
                         http://www.autismsociety-nc.org/
Sharon Jeffries-Jones, Chair
Elizabeth Phillippi, Vice Chair
Paul Wendler, Chief Financial Officer
David Laxton, Director of Communications
Covers perspectives, issues, neurobiological issues and new directions in diagnosis and treatment. *$49.00*

8767   Autism: Explaining the Enigma
Wiley Publishers
111 River Street
Hoboken, NJ   07030-5774   201-748-6000
                                      Fax: 201-748-6088
                                           info@wiley.com
                                         http://as.wiley.com
Peter Booth Wiley, Chairman
Stephen M. Smith, President & CEO
John Kitzmacher, EVP, CFO
Ellis E. Cousens, Executive Vice President, COO
Explains the nature of autism. *$27.95*

8768   Autism: From Tragedy to Triumph
Branden Publishing Company
17 Station St
Brookline, MA   2445-7995   617-730-5757
                         http://www.yogainthevillage.com
Karen Wenc, Teaching Staff
Veronica Wolff, Teaching Staff
Annie Hoffman, Teaching Staff
Keith Beasley, Teaching Staff
A new book that deals with the Lovaas method and includes a foreward by Dr. Ivar Lovaas. The book is broken down into two parts — the long road to diagnosis and then treatment. *$12.95*

8769   Autism: Identification, Education and Treatment
Routledge (Taylor & Francis Group)
270 Madison Ave
New York, NY   10016-601   212-576-1411
              http://books.google.co.in/books/about/Autism.
Dianne Zager, Editor
Chapters include medical treatments, early intervention and communication development in autism. *$36.00*
ISBN 0-805820-44-7

8770   Autism: The Facts
Oxford University Press
2001 Evans Road
Cary, NC   27513   919-677-0977
                                            800-445-9714
                                      Fax: 919-677-1303
              http://www.oup.com/us/corporate/contact/?view
Simon Baron-Cohen, Co-Author
Patrick Bolton, Co-Author
   $22.50
128 pages
ISBN 0-192623-27-3

8771   Autistic Adults at Bittersweet Farms
Routledge (Taylor & Francis Group)
12660 Archbold-Whitehouse Rd.
Whitehouse, OH   43571   419-875-6986
                         http://www.bittersweetfarms.org/
Robert St. Clair, President
Matt Anderson, VP
Jan Toczynski, Secretary
Jon Ahlberg, Board Member
A touching view of an inspirational residential care program for autistic adolescents and adults. Also available in softcover. *$94.95*
Hardcover
ISBN 1-560240-42-3

8772   Beyond Baby Talk: From Sounds to Sentences, a Parent's Guide to Language Development
Prima Publishing
P.O.Box 1260
Rocklin, CA   95677-1260   916-787-7000
                                            800-632-8676
                                      Fax: 916-787-7001
Fernando Bueno, Editor in Chief
Julie Asbury, Managing Editor
Christopher Buffa, Sr. Editor
Andrea Hill, Community Manager
The authors discuss the best ways to help your child develop the all-important skill of communication and to recognize the signs of language development problems. *$15.95*
224 pages
ISBN 0-761526-47-1

8773   Breaking the Speech Barrier: Language Develpment Through Augmented Means
Brookes Publishing
P.O.Box 10624
Baltimore, MD   21285-0624   410-337-9580
                                            800-638-3775
                                      Fax: 410-337-8539
                         custserv@brookespublishing.com
                                           readplaylearn.com
Paul Brookes, Owner
This resource describes the creation of the System for Augmenting Language (SAL) for school-age youth with mental retardation and offers important insights into the language development of children who are not learning to communicate typically. *$39.95*
224 pages Paperback
ISBN 1-557663-90-0

8774   Breakthroughs: How to Reach Students with Autism
Aquarius Health Care Media
Ste 230
505 Oberlin Rd
Raleigh, NC   27605-1345   919-743-0204
                                            800-442-2762
                                      Fax: 919-743-0208
                         jchampion@autismsociety-nc.org
                         www.autismtreatmentcenter.org
Sharon Jeffries-Jones, Chair
Elizabeth Phillippi, Vice Chair
Tracey Sheriff, CEO
Paul Wendler, CFO
A hands-on, how-to program for reaching students with autism, featuring Karen Sewell, Autism Society of America's teacher of the year. Here Sewell demonstrates the successful techniques she's developed over a 20-year career. A separate 250 page manual ($59) is also available which covers math, reading, fine motor, self help, social adaptive, vocational and self help skills as well as providing numerous plan reproducibles and an exhaustive listing of equipment and materials resources. Video. *$99.00*

8775 Childhood Speech, Language & Listening Problems
Wiley Publishing
605 3rd Ave
New York, NY 10158-180   212-850-6000
                                       Fax: 212-850-6088
                    http://books.google.co.in/books/about/Childho
Patricia McAleer Hamaguchi
Language pathologist Hamaguchi employs her 15 years of experience to show parents how to recognize the most common speech, language, and listening problems. *$16.95*
224 pages Paperback
ISBN 0-471387-53-3

8776 Cognitive Behavioral Therapy for Adult Asperger Syndrome
Autism Society of North Carolina Bookstore
Ste 230
505 Oberlin Rd
Raleigh, NC 27605-1345   919-743-0204
                                            800-442-2762
                                       Fax: 919-743-0208
                    jchampion@autismsociety-nc.org
                    http://www.autismsociety-nc.org
Sharon Jeffries-Jones, Chair
Elizabeth Phillippi, Vice Chair
Tracey Sheriff, CEO
Paul Wendler, CFO
Text is prepared with case studies and examples from the author's own experiences working as a cognitive-behavioral therapist specializing in adults and adolescents with dual diagnosis, autism spectrum disorders, mood disorders, and anxiety disorders.

8777 Communication Development and Disorders in African American Children
Brookes Publishing
P.O.Box 10624
Baltimore, MD 21285-0624   410-337-9580
                                            800-638-3775
                                       Fax: 410-337-8539
                    custserv@brookespublishing.com
                    readplaylearn.com
Paul Brooks, Owner
Research, Assessment, and Intervention. This text presents research on communication disorders and language development in African American children. Also addresses multicultural aspects of service delivery and intervention and discusses issues in assessing, diagnosing, and treating communication disorders. *$39.00*
400 pages Paperback
ISBN 1-55766 -53-3

8778 Communication Development in Children with Down Syndrome
Brookes Publishing
P.O.Box 10624
Baltimore, MD 21285-0624   410-337-9580
                                            800-638-3775
                                       Fax: 410-337-8539
                    custserv@brookespublishing.com
                    readplaylearn.com
Paul Brooks, Owner
This book offers an extensive, detailed explanation of communication development in children with Down syndrome relative to their advancing cognitive skills. It introduces a critical framework for assessing and treating hearing, speech, and language problems and provides explicit intervention methods and tested clinical protocols.
Paperback
ISBN 1-55766 -50-5

8779 Coping for Kids Who Stutter
Speech Bin
P.O.Box 1579
Appleton, WI 54912   419-589-1425
                                            888-388-3224
                                       Fax: 888-388-6344
                                    info@speechbin.com
                                    www.speechbin.com
James R. Henderson, Chairman
Joseph M. Yorio, President & CEO
Rick Holden, EVP, Educators Publishing Service
Patrick T. Collins, EVP, Distribution
Informative book for children and adults about stuttering and how to manage it. *$15.95*
32 pages
ISBN 0-93785 -43-2

8780 Disorders of Motor Speech: Assessment, Treatment, and Clinical Characterization
Brookes Publishing
P.O.Box 10624
Baltimore, MD 21285-0624   410-337-9580
                                            800-638-3775
                                       Fax: 410-337-8539
                    custserv@brookespublishing.com
Paul Brooks, Owner
This book provides a probing examination of normal, dysarthric, and apraxic speech. Great for speech-language pathologists, neurologists, physical or occupational therapists, and physiatrists. *$47.00*
400 pages Hardcover
ISBN 1-55766 -23-1

8781 Employment for Individuals with Asperger Syndrome or Non-Verbal Learning Disability
Jessica Kingsley Publishers
400 Market Street
Suite 400
Philadelphia, PA 19106-2513   215-922-1161
                                            866-416-1078
                                       Fax: 215-922-1474
                                    orders@jkp.com
                                    www.jkp.com
Laurie Schlesinger, Vp Of Sales & Marketing
Yvona Fast, Author
Most people with Non-Verbal Learning Disorder (NLD) or Asperger Syndrome (AS) are underemployed. This book sets out to change this. With practical and technical advice on everything from job hunting to interview techniques, from 'fitting in' in the workplace to whether or not to disclose a diagnosis, this book guides people with NLD or AS successfully through the employment mine field. There is also information for employers, agencies and careers counsellors on AS and NLD as 'invisible' disabili *$22.95*
272 pages
ISBN 1-843107-66-X

8782 Encounters with Autistic States
Jason Aronson
400 Keystone Industrial Park
Dunmore, PA 18512-1507   800-782-0015
448 pages Hardcover
ISBN 0-765700-62-

8783 Kitten Who Couldn't Purr
William Morrow & Company
1350 Avenue of the Americas
New York, NY 10019-4702   212-261-6500
                                       Fax: 212-261-6925
                    http://www.goodreads.com/book/show/2319648.Th
Otis Chandler, CEO & Co-Founder
Eve Titus, Author
Jonathan the kitten doesn't know how to purr to say thank you, so he sets off to find someone to teach him. *$12.95*
32 pages

8784 Language Disabilities in Children and Adolescents
McGraw-Hill School Publishing
PO Box 182605
Columbus, OH 43218 800-338-3987
Fax: 609-308-4480
customer.service@mheducation.com
mcgraw-hill.com

David Levin, President and CEO
Patrick Milano, Chief Administrative Officer & CFO
Stephen Laster, Chief Digital Officer
David Stafford, SVP & General Counsel
A comprehensive review of research in language disabilities.

8785 Language and the Developing Child
International Dyslexia Association
40 York Rd.
4th Floor
Baltimore, MD 21204 410-296-0232
Fax: 410-321-5069
info@interdys.org
www.interdys.org

Rick Smith, Chief Executive Officer
Jennifer Topple, Chair
Elsa Cardenas-Hagan, Vice Chair
This collection of papers introduces a new generation of teachers, clinicians and parents to the work of one of the key figures in the search for the causes and treatment of dyslexia. *$15.00*

8786 Late Talker: What to Do If Your Child Isn't Talking Yet
St Martin's Griffin
175 5th Ave
New York, NY 10010-7703 646-307-5151
888-330-8477
Fax: 212-674-6132
customerservice@mpsvirginia.com

Marilyn C Agin, Author
This handbook offers advice on ways to identify the warning signs of a speech disorder, information on how to get the right kind of evaluations and therapy, ways to obtain appropriate services through the school system and health insurance, at-home activities that parents can do with their child to stimulate speech, benefits of nutritional supplementation, and advice from experienced parents who've been there on what to expect and what you can do to be your child's best advocate. *$13.95*
256 pages Paperback
ISBN 0-312309-24-4

8787 Let Community Employment be the Goal for Individuals with Autism
Indiana Resource Center For Autism
1905 North Range Road
Bloomington, IN 47408-9801 812-855-6508
800-825-4733
Fax: 812-855-9630
iidc@indiana.edu
www.iidc.indiana.edu/irca
Cathy Pratt, Director
Catherine Davies, Educational Consultant
Pamela Anderson, Outreach/Resource Specialist
Melissa Dubie, Research Associate
A guide designed for people who are responsible for preparing individuals with autism to enter the work force. *$7.00*

8788 Lollipop Lunch
Speech Bin-Abilitations
P.O.Box 1579
Appleton, WI 54912-1579 419-589-1425
888-388-3224
Fax: 888-388-6344
info@speechbin.com
www.speechbin.com

James R. Henderson, Chairman
Joseph M. Yorio, President & CEO
Rick Holden, EVP, Educators Publishing Service
Patrick T. Collins, EVP, Distribution

Cleverly illustrated stories and activities for phonological and language development. *$19.95*
128 pages
ISBN 0-937857-54-8

8789 Management of Autistic Behavior
Sage Publications
2455 Teller Road
Thousand Oaks, CA 91320 805-499-0721
800-818-7243
Fax: 805-499-0871
info@sagepub.com
www.sagepub.com

Sara Miller McCune, Founder, Publisher, Chairperson
Blaise R Simqu, President & CEO
Tracey A. Ozmina, Executive Vice President & Chief Operating Officer
Stephen Barr, Managing Director/SAGE London, President of SAGE Internation
This excellent reference is a comprehensive and practical book that tells what works best with specific problems. *$41.00*
450 pages

8790 Motor Speech Disorders
WB Saunders Company
14 Main Street
Southampton, NY 11968-2822 631-283-5050
800-523-1649
Fax: 631-283-2290
info@saunders.com
www.wbsaunders.com

Joseph R Duffy PhD, Author
Professional text on rehabilitation techniques for motor speech disorders. *$74.00*
592 pages
ISBN 0-323024-52-5

8791 Neurobiology of Autism
Johns Hopkins University Press
National Library of Medicine
Building 38A
Bethesda, MD 20894 410-516-6900
888-346-3656
888-FIN- NLM
Fax: 410-516-6998
info@ncbi.nlm.nih.gov
http://www.ncbi.nlm.nih.gov/pubmed/17919129
Pardo CA, Co-Author
Ebarhat CG, Co-Author
This book discusses recent advances in scientific research that point to a neurobiological basis for autism and examines the clinical implications of this research. *$28.00*
272 pages
ISBN 0-801880-47-5

8792 Nonverbal Learning Disabilities at Home: A Parent's Guide
Jessica Kingsley Publishers
400 Market Street
Suite 400
Philadelphia, PA 19106 215-922-1161
866-416-1078
Fax: 215-922-1474
hello.usa@jkp.com
www.jkp.com

Jessica Kingsley, Chairman & Managing Director
Jemima Kingsley, Director
Octavia Kingsley, Production Director
Lisa Clark, Sr. Commissioning Editor
Explores the variety of daily life problems children with NLD may face, and provides practical strategies for parents to help them cope and grow, from preschool age through their challenging adolescent years. *$19.95*
272 pages Paperback
ISBN 1-853029-40-0

8793   Parent Survival Manual
Springer Publishing Company
11 West 42nd Street
8th Floor
New York, NY   10036   212-355-1501
                                                         Fax: 212-355-7370
                                          christieseducation@christies.edu
                                          http://www.christieseducation.com
Craig Lickliter, Manager
A guide to crises resolution in autism and related developmental
disorders. *$39.95*

8794   Perspectives: Whole Language Folio
Gallaudet University Bookstore
PO Box 35009
Charlotte, NC   28235-5009   202-651-5750
                                                           800-995-0550
                                                         Fax: 202-651-5744
                                          www.cpcc.edu/disabilities
Edwin A. Dalrymple, Chairman
Judith N. Allison, Vice Chair
Tony Zeiss, President
Ellen Zaremba, Administrative Assistant to the President
The 19 articles in this collection offer practical help to teachers
seeking to emphasize whole language strategies in their class-
room. *$9.95*
64 pages

8795   Please Don't Say Hello
Human Sciences Press
233 Spring St
New York, NY   10013   877-283-3229
                                                         ainy@aveda.com
                                          http://aveda.edu/new-york
Phyllis Terri Gold, Author
Paul and his family moved into a new neighborhood. Paul's
brother was autistic. The children thought that Eddie was retarded until they learned that there were skills that he could do
better than they could. *$10.95*
47 pages Paperback
ISBN 0-89885-99-8

**8796   Promoting Communication in Infants and Young Children:
         500 Ways to Succeed**
Speech Bin-Abilitations
P.O.Box 1579
Appleton, WI   54912-1579   419-589-1425
                                                           888-388-3224
                                                         Fax: 888-388-6344
                                          info@speechbin.com
                                          www.speechbin.com
James R. Henderson, Chairman
Joseph M. Yorio, President & CEO
Rick Holden, EVP, Educators Publishing Service
Patrick T. Collins, EVP, Distribution
This practical reference for parents, caregivers and professional
service providers how to promote communication development
in infants and young children. Gives down-to-earth information
and activities to help your youngest children succeed. It provides
step-by-step suggestions for stimulationg children's speech and
language skills. Paperback. *$14.95*
ISBN 0-937857-72-6

8797   Reading, Writing and Speech Problems in Children
International Dyslexia Association
40 York Rd.
4th Floor
Baltimore, MD   21204   410-296-0232
                                                         Fax: 410-321-5069
                                          info@interdys.org
                                          www.interdys.org
Rick Smith, Chief Executive Officer
Jennifer Topple, Chair
Elsa Cardenas-Hagan, Vice Chair
This book provides reading, reading and speech execerises for
educating people with dyslexia. *$27.00*
ISBN 0-89079-79-1

**8798   Relationship Development Intervention with Young
         Children**
Taylor & Francis Group
73 Collier St.
London, N1 9BE   44- 0 -0 78
                                                         Fax: 44- 0 -0 78
                                          hello.usa@jkp.com
                                          http://www.jkp.com/jkp/distributors.php
Jessica Kingsley, Chairman
Jemima Kingsley, Director
Octavia Kingsley, Production Director
Lisa Clark, Sr. Commissioning Editor
Social and emotional development activities for Asperger Syndrome, Autism, PDD and NLD. Comprehensive set of activities
emphasizes foundation skills for younger children between the
ages of two and eight. Covers skills such as social referencing,
regulating behvior, conversational reciprocity, and synchronized
actions. For use in therapeutic settings as well as schools and parents. *$22.95*
256 pages
ISBN 1-843107-14-7

8799   Riddle of Autism: A Psychological Analysis
Jason Aronson
Ste 200
4501 Forbes Blvd
Lanham, MD   20706   301-459-3366
                                                           800-462-6420
                                                         Fax: 301-429-5746
                                          customercare@nbnbooks.com
                                          http://www.nbnbooks.com
Jason Brockwell, Sales Staff
Michael Sullivan, Sales
Mark Cozy, Sales Staff
Dennis Hayes, Director of Special Markets
Dr. Victor examines the myths that cloud an understanding of this
disorder and describes the meanings of its specific behavioral
symptoms. *$30.00*
356 pages Paperback
ISBN 1-568215-73-8

8800   Self-Therapy for the Stutterer
Stuttering Foundation of America
1805 Moriah Woods Blvd.
Suite 3
Memphis, TN   38117   901-761-0343
                                                           800-992-9392
                                                         Fax: 901-761-0484
                                          www.stutterhelp.org
Jane Fraser, President
Jean Gruss, Journalist
Robert M. Kurtz, Chairman & CEO
Malcolm Houg Fraser, Founder
A guide to help adults who stutter overcome the problem on their
own. *$3.00*
191 pages Paperback
ISBN 0-933388-32-2

8801   Sex Education: Issues for the Person with Autism
Indiana Resource Center For Autism
1905 North Range Road
Bloomington, IN   47408-9801   812-855-6508
                                                           800-825-4733
                                                         Fax: 812-855-9630
                                          iidc@indiana.edu
                                          www.iidc.indiana.edu/irca
Cathy Pratt, Director
Catherine Davies, Educational Consultant
Pamela Anderson, Outreach/Resource Specialist
Melissa Dubie, Research Associate
Discusses issues of sexuality and provides methods of instruction
for people with autism. *$4.00*

8802 Son-Rise: The Miracle Continues
2080 South Undermountain Road
Sheffield, MA 01257
413-229-2100
800-714-2779
sonrise@option.org
http://www.option.org
Samahria Lyt Kaufman, Co-Founder and Co-Director
Dane Griffith, Director of Administrative Services
Bears Kaufman, Co-Founder and Co-Director
Raun Kaufman, Director of Global Education
Part One is the astonishing record of Raun Kaufman's development from an autistic and retarded child into a loving, brilliant youngster who shows no traces of his former condition. Part Two follows Raun's development after the age of four, teaching the limitless possibilities of the Son-Rise Program. Part Three shares moving accounts of five other ordinary families who became extraordinary when they used the Son-Rise Program to reach their own unreachable children. *$12.95*
343 pages
ISBN 0-915811-53-7

8803 Sound Connections for the Adolescent
Speech Bin
P.O.Box 1579
Appleton, WI 54912-1579
419-589-1425
888-388-3224
Fax: 888-388-6344
info@speechbin.com
www.speechbin.com
James R. Henderson, Chairman
Joseph M. Yorio, President & CEO
Rick Holden, EVP, Educators Publishing Service
Patrick T. Collins, EVP, Distribution
A resource to help older elementary and secondary students understand their sound systems an how it functions. It targets skills critical for academic achievement: phonological awareness, phonemic relationships, phonemic processing, listening and memory and teaches linguistic rules they need to succeed. *$19.95*
Paperback

8804 Talkable Tales
Speech Bin-Abilitations
P.O.Box 1579
Appleton, WI 54912-1579
419-589-1425
888-388-3224
Fax: 888-388-6344
info@speechbin.com
www.speechbin.com
James R. Henderson, Chairman
Joseph M. Yorio, President & CEO
Rick Holden, EVP, Educators Publishing Service
Patrick T. Collins, EVP, Distribution
Read-a-rebus stories and pictures targeting most consonant phonemes for K-5 children. *$25.95*
128 pages
ISBN 0-93783-44-0

8805 Teaching Children with Autism: Strategies for Initiating Positive Interactions
Brookes Publishing
P.O.Box 10624
Baltimore, MD 21285-0624
410-337-9585
888-337-8808
Fax: 410-337-8539
custserv@healthpropress.com
http://www.healthpropress.com
Melissa A. Behm, President
Mary Magnus, Director
Stategies for initiating positive interactions and improving learning opportunities. This guide begins with an overview of characteristics and long-term strategies and proceeds through discussions that detail specific techniques for normalizing environments, reducing disruptive behavior, improving language and social skills, and enhancing generalization. *$32.95*
256 pages Paperback
ISBN 1-55766-80-4

8806 Teaching and Mainstreaming Autistic Children
Love Publishing Company
9101 East Kenyon Avenue
Suite 2200
Denver, CO 80237
303-221-7333
Fax: 303-221-7444
lpc@lovepublishing.com
http://www.lovepublishing.com/
Peter Knoblock, Author
Dr. Knoblock advocates a highly organized, structured environment for autistic children, with teachers and parents working together. His premise is that the learning and social needs of autistic children must be analyzed and a daily program designed with interventions that respond to this functional analysis of their behavior. *$24.95*
ISBN 0-89108-11-9

8807 Techniques for Aphasia Rehab: (TARGET) Generating Effective Treatment
Speech Bin
P.O.Box 1579
Appleton, WI 54912-1579
419-589-1425
888-388-3224
Fax: 888-388-6344
info@speechbin.com
www.speechbin.com
James R. Henderson, Chairman
Joseph M. Yorio, President & CEO
Rick Holden, EVP, Educators Publishing Service
Patrick T. Collins, EVP, Distribution
Practical treatment manual for use by aphasia clinicians. *$45.00*
384 pages
ISBN 0-93785-50-5

8808 Understanding & Controlling Stuttering: A Comprehensive New Approach Based on the Valsa Hyp
National Stuttering Association
119 West 40th Street
14th Floor
New York, NY 10018
212-944-4050
800-937-8888
Fax: 212-944-8244
info@westutter.org
www.nsastutter.org
Kenny Koroll, Chair
Tammy Flores, Executive Director
Stephanie Coopen, Family Programs Administrator
Mandy Finstad, Editor/Webmaster
Demonstrates how physical and psychological factors may interact to stimulate and perpetuate stuttering through a Valsalva-Stuttering cycle. *$25.00*
176 pages
ISBN 7-929773-01-3

8809 Verbal Behavior Approach: How to Teach Children with Autism & Related Disorders
Autism Society of North Carolina Bookstore
Ste 230
505 Oberlin Rd
Raleigh, NC 27605-1345
919-743-0204
800-442-2762
Fax: 919-743-0208
jchampion@autismsociety-nc.com
http://www.autismsociety-nc.org
Sharon Jeffries-Jones, Chair
Elizabeth Phillippi, Vice Chair
Tracey Sheriff, CEO
Paul Wendler, CFO
Provides full descriptions of how to teach the verbal operants that make up expressive languate which include: manding, tacting, echoing and intraverbal skills. *$19.95*

8810 **Without Reason: A Family Copes with two Generations of Autism**
Books on Special Children
721 W Abram St
Arlington, TX 76013-6995   817-277-0727
                                             800-489-0727
                                        Fax: 817-277-2270
                                        http://www.fhautism.com/
R. Wayne Gilpin, President
Jennifer Gilpin Yacio, Vice President and Editorial Director
David Reasor, CPA and Administrative Director
Teresa Corey, Conference Administrator
The author discovers his son has autism. He delves into problems of the autistic person and explains reasons for their actions.
$20.95
292 pages Hardcover

Print: Journals

8811 **American Journal of Speech-Language Pathology**
American Speech-Language-Hearing Association
2200 Research Boulevard
Rockville, MD 20850-3289   301-296-5700
                                             800-638-8255
                                        Fax: 301-296-8580
                                        nsslha@asha.org
                                        www.asha.org
Elizabeth S. McCrea, PhD, CCC-SLP, President
Barbara K. Cone, PhD, CCC-A, Vice President for Academic Affairs in Audiology
Carolyn W. Higdon, EdD, CCC-SLP, Vice President for Finance
Kaci Roger, Council Member
This is a quarterly journal of clinical practice for speech-language pathologists and language researchers. This journal will be online only beginning January 2010.

8812 **Journal of Speech, Language and Hearing Research**
American Speech-Language-Hearing Association
2200 Research Boulevard
Rockville, MD 20850-3289   301-296-5700
                                             800-638-8255
                                        Fax: 301-296-8580
                                        nsslha@asha.org
                                        www.asha.org
Elizabeth S. McCrea, PhD, CCC-SLP, President
Barbara K. Cone, PhD, CCC-A, Vice President for Academic Affairs in Audiology
Carolyn W. Higdon, EdD, CCC-SLP, Vice President for Finance
Kaci Roger, Council Member
This bimonthly journal contains basic, as well as applied research in normal and disordered communication processes. It will be available online only beginning January 2010.

8813 **Language, Speech, and Hearing Services in Schools**
International Fluency Association
Northern Illinois University
Dept. of Communicative Disorders
DeKalb, IL 60115-2899   www.theifa.org
David Shapiro, President
Norimune Kawat, Secretary
Rachel Everard, Treasurer
Shelley Brundage, Membership
This is a quarterly journal focusing on research appropriate to speech-language pathologists and audiologists in schools. The journal will only be available online beginning in January 2010.

Print: Magazines

8814 **Communication Outlook**
Artificial Language Laboratory
220 Trowbridge Road
East Lansing, MI 48824   517-353-8332
                                        Fax: 517-353-4766
                                        artling@msu.edu
                                        www.msu.edu
Lou Anna K. Simon, President
Satish Udpa, EVP for Administrative Services
Bill Beekman, VP & Secretary
Mark P. Haas, VP for Finance & Treasurer
Communication Outlook (CO) is an international quarterly magazine, which focuses on the techniques and technology of augmentative and alternative communication. CO provides information on technological developments for persons experiencing communication handicaps due to neurological, sensory or neuromuscular conditions. *$18.00*
32 pages Quarterly

Print: Newsletters

8815 **Access Audiology**
American Speech-Language-Hearing Association
2200 Research Boulevard
Rockville, MD 20850-3289   301-296-5700
                                             800-638-8255
                                        Fax: 301-296-8580
                                        nsslha@asha.org
                                        www.asha.org
Elizabeth S. McCrea, PhD, CCC-SLP, President
Barbara K. Cone, PhD, CCC-A, Vice President for Academic Affairs in Audiology
Carolyn W. Higdon, EdD, CCC-SLP, Vice President for Finance
Kaci Roger, Council Member
Dedicated to the specific needs of all professionals interested in hearing, balance, and the field of audiology. Each issue spotlights a specific topic of interest and relevance to audiologists.

8816 **Autism Research Review International**
Autism Research Institute
4182 Adams Avenue
San Diego, CA 92116-2599   619-281-7165
                                             866-366-3361
                                        Fax: 619-563-6840
                                        br@autismresearchinstitute.com
                                        autism.com
Stephen Edelson, Executive Director
Jane Johnson, Managing Director
Valerie Paradiz, Director
Anthony Morgali, Producer
Provides clearly written summaries of articles selected from computer searches. *$18.00*
8 pages Quarterly

8817 **Communicologist**
Texas Speech-Language-Hearing Association
Ste 200
918 Congress Ave
Austin, TX 78701-2342   512-494-1128
                                             888-729-8742
                                        Fax: 512-494-1129
Judith Keller, President
Larry Higdon, Director
Melanie McDonald, President Elect
Tori Gustafson, Vice President
A forum for distributing current information relevant to the practices of speech-language pathology and audiology across the state. Provides TSHA membership with the latest news from the Executive Board and Task Forces, as well as information about regional associations, distinguished service providers, the TSHA Annual Convention, and committee honors and nominations. Also contains advertisements of interest to the field.

8818   Connect
Hearing, Speech & Deafness Center (HSDC)
1625 19th Ave.
Seattle, WA   98122

206-323-5770
888-222-5036
Fax: 206-328-6871
seattle@hsdc.org
www.hsdc.org

Lindsay Klarman, Executive Director
Michelle Coleman, Operations Director
A newsletter that addresses concerns of those affected by speech
and language disorders. HSDC is a nonprofit for clients who are
deaf, hard of hearing, or who face other communication barriers
such as speech challenges.
8 pages Quarterly

8819   NSSLHA Now
Ntn'l Student Speech Language Hearing Association
2200 Research Boulevard
Rockville, MD   20850-3289

301-296-5700
800-638-8255
Fax: 301-296-8580
nsslha@asha.org
www.asha.org

Elizabeth S. McCrea, PhD, CCC-SLP, President
Barbara K. Cone, PhD, CCC-A, Vice President for Academic Af-
fairs in Audiology
Carolyn W. Higdon, EdD, CCC-SLP, Vice President for Finance
Kaci Roger, Council Member
Published three times per year.

8820   On Cue
National Cued Speech Association
1300 Pennsylvania Avenue, NW
Suite 190-713
Washington, DC 20004

301-915-8009
800-459-3529
www.cuedspeech.org

Shannon Howell, President
Penny Hakim, 1st Vice President
John Brubaker, VP Fundraising
Doug Dawson, Treasurer
Published several times a year and mailed to members of the As-
sociation.

8821   Stuttering & Your Child: Help For Parents
Stuttering Foundation of America
18005 Moriah Woods Blvd
PO Box 11749, Suite 3
Memphis, TN 38111-0749

901-761-0343
800-992-9392
Fax: 901-761-0484
info@stutteringhelp.org
www.StutteringHelp.org

Jane Fraser, President
Dennis Drayna, Director
Joseph R. G. Fulcher, Director
Frances Cook, Director
The Stuttering Foundation provides resources, services and support to those who stutter and their families, as well as support research into the cause of stuttering. The Stuttering Foundation
provides a referral list of speech-language pathologists and referrals to other information including research on stuttering, intensive workshops and camps. *$10.00*

8822   Stuttering Foundation Newsletter
Stuttering Foundation of America
P.O.Box 11749
Memphis, TN 38111-0749

901-761-0343
800-992-9392
Fax: 901-761-0484
info@stutteringhelp.org
www.stutteringhelp.org

Jane Fraser, President
Jean Gruss, Journalist
Robert M. Kurtz, Chairman & CEO
Malcolm Houg Fraser, Founder

8823   Voice
Providence Speech and Hearing Association
1301 Providence Avenue
Orange, CA   92868

714-923-1521
855-901-7742
Fax: 714-744-3841
pshc@pshc.org
www.pshc.org

Lewis Jaffe, President
Bret Rathwick, Vice President - Finance
Casey Immel, Treasurer
Marlene Woodworth, Secretary
People of all ages with speech and hearing problems by providing
specialized products and services.

Non Print: Newsletters

8824   Access Academics & Research
American Speech-Language-Hearing Association
2200 Research Boulevard
Rockville, MD   20850-3289

301-296-5700
800-638-8255
Fax: 301-296-8580
nsslha@asha.org
www.asha.org

Elizabeth S. McCrea, PhD, CCC-SLP, President
Barbara K. Cone, PhD, CCC-A, Vice President for Academic Af-
fairs in Audiology
Carolyn W. Higdon, EdD, CCC-SLP, Vice President for Finance
Kaci Roger, Council Member
Dedicated to the specific needs of academic and clinical faculty,
PhD students and researchers. The e-newsletter was developed as
part of the Focused Initiative on the PhD Shortage in Higher
Education.

8825   Access SLP Health Care
American Speech-Language-Hearing Association
2200 Research Boulevard
Rockville, MD   20850-3289

301-296-5700
800-638-8255
Fax: 301-296-8580
nsslha@asha.org
www.asha.org

Elizabeth S. McCrea, PhD, CCC-SLP, President
Barbara K. Cone, PhD, CCC-A, Vice President for Academic Af-
fairs in Audiology
Carolyn W. Higdon, EdD, CCC-SLP, Vice President for Finance
Kaci Roger, Council Member
An e-newsletter dedicated to the specific needs of speech-lan-
guage pathologists in healthcare settings. Each issue of Access
SLP Health Care features recent legislative activity impacting
SLPs and provides information on clinical issues, continuing ed-
ucation opportunities, and ASHA web-based resources.

8826   Access Schools
American Speech-Language-Hearing Association
2200 Research Boulevard
Rockville, MD   20850-3289

301-296-5700
800-638-8255
Fax: 301-296-8580
nsslha@asha.org
www.asha.org

Elizabeth S. McCrea, PhD, CCC-SLP, President
Barbara K. Cone, PhD, CCC-A, Vice President for Academic Af-
fairs in Audiology
Carolyn W. Higdon, EdD, CCC-SLP, Vice President for Finance
Kaci Roger, Council Member
Dedicated to the specific needs of school-based speech-language
pathologists. Each Access Schools e-newsletter features recent
legislative activity impacting school SLPs and provides informa-
tion on clinical issues, continuing education opportunities, and
ASHA web-based resources.

8827 Stuttering
Federal Government
31 Center Drive MSC 2320
Bethesda, MD 20892-2320
301-496-7243
800-241-1044
Fax: 301-402-0018
nidcdinfo@nidcd.nih.gov
www.nidcd.nih.gov

James F. Battey, Director
Judith A. Cooper, Deputy Director
Timothy J. Wheeles, Executive Officer
Tanya Brown, Executive Assistant
Describes how speech is produced, treatments for stuttering and research supported by the federal government.

Non Print: Video

8828 Autism: A World Apart
Fanlight Productions
c/o Icarus Films
32 Court Street, 21st Floor
Brooklyn, NY 11201
718-488-8900
800-876-1710
Fax: 718-488-8642
info@fanlight.com
www.fanlight.com

Ben Achtenberg, Owner, Founder
Nicole Johnson, Publicity Coordinator
Anthony Sweeney, Marketing Director
In this documentary, three families show us what the textbooks and studies cannot: what it's like to live with autism day after day; to raise and love children who may be withdrawn and violent and unable to make personal connections with their families. 29 minutes.
VHS/DVD
ISBN 1-572950-39-0

8829 Autism: the Unfolding Mystery
Aquarius Health Care Media
18 N Main St
Sherborn, MA 1770-1066
508-650-1616
Lesile Kussmann, Owner
Explore what it means to be autistic, how you can recognize the signs of autism in your child, and hear about new treatments and programs to help children learn to deal with the disorder. *$145.00*
DVD

8830 Getting Started with Facilitated Communication
Facilitated Communication Institute, Syracuse Univ
370 Huntington Hall
Syracuse, NY 13244-1
315-443-9657
Fax: 315-443-9218
fcstaff@syr.edu

Annegret Schubert, Producer
Describes in detail how to help individuals with autism and/or severe communication difficulties to get started with facilitated communication.
Video

8831 I Just Want My Little Boy Back
Autism Treatment Center Of America
2080 South Undermountain Road
Sheffield, MA 01257
413-229-2100
800-714-2779
happiness@option.org
http://www.option.org
Samahria Lyt Kaufman, Co-Founder and Co-Director
Dane Griffith, Director of Administrative Services
Bears Kaufman, Co-Founder and Co-Director
Raun Kaufman, Director of Global Education
A great video for parents and professionals caring for children with special needs. Join one British family and their autistic son before, during and after their journey to America to attend The Son-Rise Program at The Autism Treatment Center of America. This informative, inspirational and deeply moving story not only captures the joy, tears, challenges and triumps of this amazing lit-

tle boy and his family, but also serves as a powerful introduction to the attitude and principles of the program. *$25.00*

8832 Understanding Autism
Fanlight Productions
c/o Icarus Films
32 Court Street, 21st Floor
Brooklyn, NY 11201
718-488-8900
800-876-1710
Fax: 718-488-8642
info@fanlight.com
www.fanlight.com

Ben Achtenberg, Owner, Founder
Nicole Johnson, Publicity Coordinator
Anthony Sweeney, Marketing Director
Parents of children with autism discuss the nature and symptoms of this lifelong disability and outline a treatment program based on behavior modification principles. 19 minutes
VHS/DVD
ISBN 1-572951-00-1

Support Groups

8833 Autism Society of America
4340 East West Highway
Suite 350
Bethesda, MD 20814-3067
301-657-0881
800-328-8476
Fax: 301-657-0869
www.autism-society.org

Mary Beth Collins, Director of Programs
Tonia Ferguson, Senior Director of Content
Scott Badesch, President/Chief Executive Officer
John Dabrowski, Chief Financial Officer
ASA is the largest and oldest grassroots organization within the autism community, with a nationwide network of chapters and over 20,000 members and supporters nationwide. ASA is the leading source of education, information and referral about autism and has been the leader in advocacy and legislative initiatives for more than four decades.

8834 Cherab Foundation
P.O.Box 8524
Port St Lucie, FL 34985-8524
772-335-5135
Fax: 772-337-4812
help@cherab.org
www.cherab.org

Marilyn Agin, MD
Lisa Geng, Co Author
Helps to start, supports, and works together with other support groups and nonprofits (such as ECHO, VOICES, and Apraxia Network) that have mutual goals for helping children with apraxia and other speech disorders.

8835 Friends: National Association of Young People who Stutter
38 S Oyster Bay Rd
Syosset, NY 11791-5033
866-866-8335
lcaggiano@aol.com
www.friendswhostutter.org

Lee Caggiano, President
A national organization created to provide a network of love and support for children and teenagers who stutter, their families, and the professionals who work with them.

8836 National Health Information Center
US Department of Health
P.O.Box 1133
Washington, DC 20013-1133
301-565-4167
800-336-4797
301-468-7394
Fax: 301-984-4256
healthypeople@hhs.gov
http://www.healthypeople.gov

Jonathan Fielding, Chair
Shirika Kumanyika, Vice Chair

A health information referral service that puts health professionals and consumers who have health questions in touch with those organizations that are best able to provide answers.

8837   Speech Pathways
410 Meadow Creek Drive
Suite 206
Westminster, MD   21158   410-374-0555
                                            800-961-2724
                                      Fax: 410-374-8620
                               kim.bell@speechpathways.net
                                       speechpathways.net

Kimberly A. Bell, Owner
Karie Hadley, Therapist
Erica Hamilton, Therapist
Julie Kumpar, Therapist

We realize that parent and family support is critical to a child's success, in therapy as well as in life. We offer support at local and regional levels along with traditional speech and language services, and a wide variety of specialized pediatric programs. Our support groups/services are open to the larger community as well as to our clients.

Visual

Associations

8838 American Academy of Ophthalmology
655 Beach St
San Francisco, CA 94109
415-561-8540
866-561-8558
Fax: 415-561-8575
customer_service@aao.org
aao.org

Cynthia Ann Bradford, MD, President
David W Parke II, MD, CEO
Maria M Aaron, MD, Secretary for Annual Meeting
Lynn K Gordon, MD, PhD, Vice Chair, The Council
The American Academy of Ophthalmology is an association of doctors who provide comprehensive eye care, including medical, surgical and optical care. The academy is dedicated to advancing the profession of ophthalmology through programs, public education, courses and advocacy.

8839 American Action Fund for Blind Children and Adults
1800 Johnston St.
Baltimore, MD 21230-4914
410-659-9315
actionfund@actionfund.org
www.actionfund.org

Barbara Loos, President
Ramona Walhof, Vice President
Sandra Halverson, Second Vice President/Medical Transcriptionist
James Omvig, Treasurer
A service agency which specializes in providing to blind people help which is not readily available to them from government programs or other existing service systems. The services are planned especially to meet the needs of blind children, the elderly blind, and the deaf-blind.

8840 American Council of Blind Lions
148 Vernon Ave.
Louisville, KY 40206
502-897-1472
- - 66
carla40206@gmail.com
www.acb.org/affiliate-ACBL

Carla Ruschival, President
The American Council of Blind Lions (ACBL) works to educate members of local Lions Clubs about the needs and concerns of blind or visually impaired people. The ACBL is open to members from across the United States and encourages blind persons to join their local clubs and participate in civic projects.

8841 American Council of the Blind
1703 N. Beauregard St.
Suite 420
Alexandria, VA 22311
202-467-5081
800-424-8666
Fax: 703-465-5085
info@acb.org
www.acb.org

Eric Bridges, Executive Director
Anthony Stephens, Director, Advocacy & Governmental Affairs
The American Council of the Blind (ACB) is an association working to increase the independence, security, and opportunity for all blind or visually impaired individuals. The Council primarily focuses on developing and maintaining policies to implement the services needed for the blind or visually impaired.

8842 American Council of the Blind Radio Amateurs
19821 Vineyard Ln.
Saratoga, CA 95070
408-257-1034
acbra@acb.org
www.acbhams.org

John Glass, President
A special interest affiliate of the American Council of the Blind, the American Council of the Blind Radio Amateurs (ACBRA) promotes the interest of FCC licensed amaetur radio operators.

The ACBRA is made up of legally blind and fully sighted radio amateurs.

8843 American Foundation for the Blind
2 Penn Plaza
Suite 1102
New York, NY 10121
800-232-5463
www.afb.org

Kirk Adams, President & CEO
Darren M. Davis, Executive Administrator Executive Office
The American Foundation for the Blind (AFB) is a national non-profit that is dedicated to removing barriers, creating solutions, and expanding possibilities for the blind and visually impaired. The AFB is focused on spreading access to technology, elevating the quality of information and tools for professional who serve people with vision loss, and the promotion of independent living for those with vision loss.

8844 American Optometric Association
243 N Lindbergh Blvd
Floor 1
St. Louis, MO 63141-7881
800-365-2219
www.aoa.org

Christopher J. Quinn, O.D, President
Barbara L. Horn, O.D, Vice President
William T. Reynolds, O.D, Secretary-Treasurer
The American Optometric Association (AOA) advocates for improving the quality and availability of eye and vision care. The AOA represents more than 44,000 doctors of optometry, optometric professionals, and optometry students and works to set professional standards, lobby government and organizations on behalf of the profession, and provide research and education leadership.

8845 American Printing House for the Blind
American Printing House for the Blind, Inc.
1839 Frankfort Ave.
Louisville, KY 40206-0085
502-895-2405
800-223-1839
Fax: 502-899-2284
info@aph.org
www.aph.org

8846 Associated Services for the Blind and Visually Impaired
919 Walnut St.
Philadelphia, PA 19107
215-627-0600
Fax: 215-922-0692
asbinfo@asb.org
www.asb.org

Patricia C. Johnson, President & Chief Executive Officer
Kate Slattery Parghi, Director, Development
Associated Services for the Blind and Visually Impaired (ASB), is a private, nonprofit organization working to provide services, education, training, and resources to promote self-esteem, independence, and self determination in people who are blind or visually impaired. In addition, ASB advocates for the rights of blind and visually impaired persons through community actions and public education.

8847 Association for Education & Rehabilitationof the Blind & Visually Impaired
1703 N Beauregard St.
Suite 440
Alexandria, VA 22311- 1744
703-671-4500
Fax: 703-671-6391
aer@aerbvi.org
www.aerbvi.org

Jpe Catavero, President
Laura Bozeman, Secretary
Jennofer Wheeler, Treasurer
The Association for Education and Rehabilitation of the Blind and Visually Impaired (AER) is an international, nonprofit membership organization that supports professionals who provide education and rehabilitation services to people with visual impairments. The AER provides professional development and growth opportunities for its members and advocates to maintain specialized blind services.

8848 Association for Macular Diseases
The Association for Macular Diseases, Inc.
210 E 64th St
New York, NY 10065 212-605-3719
association@retinal-research.org
macula.org

Bernard Landou, President
The Association for Macular Diseases provides support and assistance to individuals with macular disease, their caregivers, and professional community.

8849 Association for Research in Vision and Ophthalmology
1801 Rockville Pike
Suite 400
Rockville, MD 20852-5622 240-221-2900
Fax: 240-221-0370
arvo@arvo.org
www.arvo.org

8850 Association for Vision Rehabilitation and Employment
174 Court St
Binghamton, NY 13901 607-724-2428
Fax: 607-771-8045
avreinfo@avreus.org
www.avreus.org

Ken Fernald, President & CEO
Jenn Small, Chief Operating Officer
Anthony Saccento, Chief Financial Officer
Teri Chamberlin, Director, Health & Rehabilitation Services
The Association for Vision Rehabilitation and Employment, Inc. (AVRE) is a private, nonprofit organization providing rehabilitation and employment services for people who are blind or visually impaired in the Twin Tiers of New York and Pennsylvania. Services include Low Vision, Early Intervention, Orientation and Mobility, Vision Rehabilitation Therapy, and employment preparation and placement.

8851 Association of Blind Citizens
PO Box 246
Holbrook, MA 02343 781-961-1023
Fax: 781-961-0004
president@blindcitizens.org
www.blindcitizens.org

8852 Blind Children's Center
4120 Marathon St
Los Angeles, CA 90029-3584 323-664-2153
info@blindchildrenscenter.org
www.blindchildrenscenter.org
Sarah E. Orth, MPA, Chief Executive Officer
Fernanda Armenta-Schmitt, PhD, Director, Education & Family Services
A nonprofit organization working to foster the development and education of children from birth to the 2nd grade who are blind or visually impaired. The Blind Children's Center serves about 100 children a year through a variety of family centered programs including the infant, preschool, and elementary.

8853 Blind Information Technology Specialists
8761 E Placita Bolivar
Tucson, AZ 85715-5650 520-232-2100
www.bits-acb.org

Tom L. Jones, President
Earlene Hughes, Vice President
David Tanner, Secretary
Richard Villa, Treasurer
The Blind Information Technology Specialists (BITS) is a nonprofit organization fostering the career development of computer professionals, promoting the use of computer technology and improved information access for people who are blind or visually impaired.

8854 Blinded Veterans Association
125 N West St
Suite 300
Alexandria, VA 22314 202-371-8880
800-669-7079
Fax: 202-371-8258
bva@bva.org
www.bva.org

Dale Stamper, National President
Joe Parker, National Vice President
Albert Avina, Executive Director
Stuart Nelson, Manager of Communications
The Blinded Veterans Association locates blinded veterans who need assistance, guides them through the rehabilitation process and acts as advocates for them before Congress and the Department of Veterans Affairs in securing the benefits they have earned through their service to the nation. The association also promotes access to technology, practical use of the latest research as well as offering programs for blinded veterans.

8855 Braille Institute of America
741 N Vermont Ave.
Los Angeles, CA 90029-3594 323-663-1111
800-272-4553
Fax: 323-663-0867
la@brailleinstitute.org
www.brailleinstitute.org

Peter A. Mindnich, President
Gloria Coulston, Vice President, Program Delivery
Nancy N. Neibrugge, Vice President, Program Content
The Braille Institute is a nonprofit organization providing assistance to blind and visually impaired individuals. The institute offers a variety of free programs, classes, and services at 5 regional centers in Southern California.

8856 California State Library Braille and Talking Book Library
PO Box 942837
Sacramento, CA 94237-0001 916-654-0640
800-952-5666
btbl@library.ca.gov
www.btbl.ca.gov

8857 Canine Helpers for the Handicapped
Canine Helpers for the Handicapped, Inc.
5699 Ridge Rd.
Lockport, NY 14094 716-433-4035
chhdogs@aol.com
www.caninehelpers.org

Beverly Underwood, Executive Director
Laura Gates, Trainer
Canine Helpers for the Handicapped is a nonprofit organization dedicated to training dogs in order to assist people with disabilities and promote independence.

8858 Caption Center
Media Access Group at WGBH
One Guest St.
Boston, MA 02135 617-300-3600
Fax: 617-300-1020
access@wgbh.org
www.wgbh.org/caption

Pat McDonald, Director
The Caption Center was the world's first captioning agency providing access to television for viewers who are visually impaired and/or hard of hearing. The Center develops new solutions and uses closed captioning and descriptive video to promote access to technology.

8859 Central Association for the Blind & Visually Impaired
507 Kent St.
Utica, NY 13501 315-797-2233
877-719-9996
www.cabvi.org

Edward P. Welsh, Chair
Kenneth C. Thayer, Vice Chair
Richard Evans, Treasurer
Marie Bord, Secretary

It assists people who are blind or visually impaired to achieve their highest levels of independence.

8860   Chicago Lighthouse for People who are Blind and Visually Impaired
1850 W Roosevelt Rd
Chicago, IL   60608-1298

312-666-1331
Fax: 312-243-8539
TTY:312-666-8874
www.chicagolighthouse.org

Bruce R. Hague, Chairman
Sandra C. Forsythe, Vice Chairman
Janet P. Szlyk, President
David Huber, Treasurer

A non profit agency committed to providing the highest quality educational, clinical, vocational, and rehabilitation services for children, youth and adults who are blind or visually impaired, including deaf blind and multi disabled. Also respects personal dignity and partners with individuals to enhance independent living and self sufficiency. This agency is a leader, innovator and advocate for people who are blind or visually impaired, enhancing the quality of life for all individuals.

8861   Clovernook Center for the Blind and Visually Impaired
7000 Hamilton Ave
Cincinnati, OH   45231-5240

513-522-3860
888-234-7156
Fax: 513-728-3946
TTY:513-522-3860
contact@clovernook.org
www.clovernook.org

Alfred J. Tuchfarber, Chair
Wilbert F. Schwartz, Vice Chair
Mark Jackson, Treasurer
Thomas R. Flottman, Secretary

Mission is to promote independence and foster the highest quality of life for people with visual impairments, including those with additional disabilities. We provide comprehensive program services including training and support for independent living, orientation and mobility instruction, vocational training, job placement, counseling, recreation, and youth services. Meaningful employment opportunities are also provided to individuals who are blind or visually impaired.

8862   Clovernook Printing House, The Clovernook Center for the Blind and Visually Impaired
7000 Hamilton Ave
Cincinnati, OH   45231-5240

513-522-3860
888-234-7156
Fax: 513-728-3946
contact@clovernook.org
www.clovernook.org

Alfred J. Tuchfarber, Chair
Wilbert F. Schwartz, Vice Chair
Mark Jackson, Treasurer
Thomas R. Flottman, Secretary

Clovernook also offers Braille Transcription Services including: Literary Books, Literary Magazines, Religious Materials, Instructional Manuals, ADA Conformance Materials, Literary Textbook Materials, Menus, Braille Alphabet Cards, and Forms. In addition, our Business Operations provide meaningful employment opportunities for individuals who are blind or visually impaired, while at the same time manufacturing high-quality products for customers across the country. *$145.00*
591 pages
ISBN 1-930956-48-7

8863   College of Optometrists in Vision Development
215 W Garfield Rd
Ste 200
Aurora, OH   44202-7884

330-995-0718
888-268-3770
Fax: 330-995-0719
info@covd.org
www.covd.org

David A. Damari, President
Kara Heying, Vice President
Christine Allison, Secretary-Treasurer
Pamela R. Happ, Executive Director

The College of Optometrists in Vision Development (COVD) is an international membership association of eye care professionals including optometrists, optometry students, and vision therapists. Members of COVD provide developmental vision care, vision therapy and vision rehabilitation services for children and adults.

8864   College of Syntonic Optometry
2052 W Morales Dr.
Pueblo West, CO   81007

719-547-8177
877-559-0541
Fax: 719-547-3750
Syntonics@q.com
www.collegeofsyntonicoptometry.com

Hans Lessmann, O.D, FCOVD, President
Robert Fox, O.D, FCOVD, FCSO, Vice President
Larry Wallace, O.D, Ph.D, Education Director

The College of Syntonic Optometry is an international organization dedicated to furthering Phototherapy in the treatment of the visual system. Members of the college include optometrists, and health care professionals.

8865   Columbia Lighthouse for the Blind
1825 K St NW
Suite 1103
Washington, DC   20006

202-454-6400
Fax: 202-955-6401
info@clb.org
www.clb.org

Tony Cancelosi, Chief Executive Officer
Kim Greenfield Alfonso, Chief Operating Officer
Cathy Miller, Director, Development

Columbia Lighthouse for the Blind (CLB) helps blind and visually impaired individuals in the greater Washington region. CLB provides lifestyle changing services including training and consultation in assistive technology, employment skills, career placement, low vision care, and counseling and rehabilitation services.

8866   Deaf-Blind Division of the National Federation of the Blind
200 East Wells Street
Baltimore, MD   21230-4914

410-659-9314
Fax: 410-685-5653
nfb@nfb.org
www.nfb.org

Marc Maurer, CEO

The nation's largest and most influential membership organization of blind persons, with a two-fold purpose: to help blind persons achieve self-confidence and self respect and to act as a vehicle for collective self-expression by the blind. The NFB improves blind people's lives through advocacy, education, research, technology, and programs encouraging independence and self-confidence. It is the leading force in the blindness field today and is the voice of the nations blind.

8867   Desert Blind & Handicapped Association
Desert Blind and Handicapped Association, Inc.
777 E Tahquitz Canyon Way
Suite 200
Palm Springs, CA 92262

760-969-5025
info@desertblind.org

Thomas Samulski, Executive Director
George Holliday, Treasurer

The Desert Blind & Handicapped Association provides free transportation for individuals who are blind or have a disability.

8868   Eye Bank Association of America
1101 17th St NW
Suite 400
Washington, DC 20036   202-775-4999
                                          Fax: 202-429-6036
                                          info@restoresight.org
                                          www.restoresight.org

Kevin P. Corcoran, CAE, President & CEO
Molly Georgakis, CAE, Vice President, Member Services
Stacey Gardner, Director, Education
The Eye Bank Association of America (EBAA) is a nonprofit organization advocating the restoration of sight by advancing donation, transplantation, and research. The EBAA is the oldest transplant association in the United States.

8869   Fidelco Guide Dog Foundation
103 Vision Way
Bloomfield, CT 06002   860-243-5200
                                          Fax: 860-769-0567
                                          admissions@fidelco.org
                                          www.fidelco.org

Karen C. Tripp, Chair
G. Kenneth Bernhard, Esq., Vice Chair
Gregg Barratt, Chief of Staff
Julie Unwin, Chief Operating Officer
The Fidelco Guide Dog Foundation creates increased freedom and independence for men and women who are blind by providing them with guide dogs.

8870   Fight for Sight
381 Park Ave S
Suite 809
New York, NY 10016   212-679-6060
                                          Fax: 212-679-4466
                                          Arthur@fightforsight.org
                                          www.fightforsight.org

Arthur Makar, Executive Director
Janice Benson, Associate Director
Fight for Sight is a nonprofit charity working to support eye and vision research through the providing of funds to scientists starting their careers.

8871   Foundation Fighting Blindness
7168 Columbia Gateway Dr.
Suite 100
Columbia, MD 21046   410-423-0600
                                          800-683-5555
                                          TTY:410363713951
                                          info@FightBlindness.org
                                          www.blindness.org

William T. Schmidt, Chief Executive Officer
Valerie Navy-Daniels, Chief Development Officer
Stephen M. Rose, PhD, Chief Research Officer
The Foundation Fighting Blindness (FFB) works to promote research in order to prevent, treat and restore vision. FFB is currently the world's leading private funder of retinal disease research, funding over 100 research grants and 150 researchers.

8872   Guide Dogs for the Blind
350 Los Ranchitos Rd.
PO Box 151200
San Rafael, CA 94915   information@guidedogs.com
                                          www.guidedogs.com

Christine Benninger, Cheif Executive Officer & President
Cathy Martin, Chief Financial Officer & Treasurer
Brent Ruppel, Vice President, Community Operations
Guide Dogs for the Blind (GDB) is a nonprofit organization working to provide safe mobility for those who are blind or visually impaired. GDB is the largest guide dog school in the United States offering training and follow up support for graduates of the school.

8873   Guiding Eyes for the Blind
611 Granite Springs Rd
Yorktown Heights, NY 10598-3499   914-245-4024
                                          800-942-0149
                                          Fax: 914-245-1609
                                          info@guidingeyes.org
                                          www.guidingeyes.org

Thomas Panek, President & Chief Executive Officer
Guiding Eyes for the Blind is a nonprofit organization providing guide dogs for individuals who are blind or visually impaired.

8874   Horizons for the Blind
125 Erick St.
A103
Crystal Lake, IL 60014   815-444-8800
                                          800-318-2000
                                          Fax: 815-444-8830
                                          mail@horizons-blind.org
                                          www.horizons-blind.org

Camille Caffarelli, Executive Director
Jeff T. Thorsen, First Vice President & Treasurer
Keith Myers, Second Vice President
Maryann Bartkowski, Secretary
Horizons for the Blind is a nonprofit organization working to improve the quality of life for people who are blind or visually impaired by increasing access to consumer products, services, culture, arts, education, and recreation.

8875   Independent Visually Impaired Entrepreneurs
                                          818-238-9321
                                          abazyn@bazyncommunications.com
                                          www.ivie-acb.org

Ardis Bazyn, President
The Independent Visually Impaired Entrepreneurs (IVIE) is a national organization for visually impaired business owners. The IVIE offers an annual convention, planning a program of interest for business owners.

8876   Institute for Families
1300 N Vermont Ave.
Suite 1004
Los Angeles, CA 90027   323-361-4649
                                          Fax: 323-665-7869
                                          info@instituteforfamilies.org
                                          instituteforfamilies.org

Gary Huffaker, Chairperson
Institute for Families is a nonprofit organization providing support and information for families of children with vision loss. The Institute provides guidance through a resource and referral network; referring families to organizations specializing in meeting the needs of children with specific vision loss problems.

8877   International Association of Audio Information Services
                                          800-280-5325
                                          lrk@ku.edu
                                          www.iaais.org

Lori Kesinger, Membership
The International Association of Audio Information Services (IAAIS) is a membership organization that works to turn text into speech and providing information through broadcast, telephone or internet. IAAIS connects and supports organizations that deliver equal access information for people with disabilities worldwide.

8878   Jewish Braille Institute International
JBI International
110 E 30th St
New York, NY 10016-7393   212-889-2525
                                          800-433-1531
                                          Fax: 212-689-3692
                                          admin@jbilibrary.org
                                          www.jbilibrary.org

Dr. Ellen Isler, President & Cheif Executive Officer
Israel A. Taub, Vice President & Cheif Financil Officer

The Jewish Braille Institute (JBI) International is a nonprofit organization working to meet the Jewish and general cultural needs of the blind and visually impaired.

8879 Keystone Blind Association
3056 East State St.
Hermitage, PA 16148
724-347-5501
Fax: 724-347-2204
info@keystoneblind.org
www.keystoneblind.org
Jonathan Fister, President/ CEO
Karen Anderson, Board Member
Sam Bellich, Board Member
Al Boland, Board Member
The Keystone Blind Association works to education, and employ individuals with vision loss. Headquartered in Hermitage, the Association has offices in Meadville and New Castle, Pennsylvania.

8880 Lighthouse Guild
250 W 64th St.
New York, NY 10023
800-284-4422
www.lighthouseguild.org
Alan R. Morse, JD, PhD, President & Cheif Executive Officer
The Lighthouse Guild is a nonprofit vision and healthcare organization working to address the needs of blind or visually impaired individuals.

8881 Lions Clubs International
300 W 22nd St
Oak Brook, IL 60523-8842
630-571-5466
Fax: 630-571-8890
TTY:630-571-6533
lions@lionsclubs.org
www.lionsclubs.org
Benedict Ancar, Director
Jui-Tai Chang, Director
Jaime Garcia Cepeda, Director
Kalle Elster, Director
Our 46,000 clubs and 1.35 million members make us the world's largest service club organization. We're also one of the most effective. Our members do whatever is needed to help their local communities. Everywhere we work, we make friends. With children who need eyeglasses, with seniors who don't have enough to eat and with people we may never meet.

8882 Macular Degeneration Foundation
PO Box 531313
Henderson, NV 89053-1313
702-450-2908
888-633-3937
liz@eyesight.org
www.eyesight.org
Liz Trauernicht, President/Director of Communications
Julie Zavala, VP/Asst Director of Operations
David Seftel, M.D., MBA, Executive Vice President/Director of Research Development
Ron Gallemore, Board Of Scientific Advisors
The Macular Degeneration Foundation is dedicated to those who have and will develop macular degeneration. We offer this growing community the latest information, news, hope and encouragement.

8883 National Alliance of Blind Students NABS Liaison
American Council of the Blind
1155 15th St NW
Ste 1004
Washington, DC 20005-2706
202-467-5081
800-424-8666
Fax: 202-467-5085
info@acb.org
www.acb.org
Jill Gaus, President
Lynn Jansen, Vice President
Debby Lieberman, Secretary
Mike Reese, Treasurer
A student affiliate of the American Council of the Blind which is a national organization of blind and visually impaired high school and college students who believe that every blind and visually impaired student has the right to an equal and accessible education.

Also encourages blind and visually impaired students to challenge their limits and reach their potential.

8884 National Association for Parents of Children with Visual Impairments (NAPVI)
PO Box 317
Watertown, MA 02471-317
617-972-7441
800-562-6265
Fax: 617-972-7444
spedex.com@gmail.com
www.spedex.com
Susan LaVenture, Executive Director
Julie Urban, President
Venetia Hayden, Vice President
Kim Alfonso, Treasurer
A non profit organization of, by and for parents committed to providing support to the parents of children who have visual impairments . Also a national organization that enables parents to find information and resources for their children who are blind or visually impaired including those with additional disabilities. NAPVI also provides leadership, support, and training to assist parents in helping children reach their potential.

8885 National Association for Visually Handicapped (NAVH)
111 E 59th S
Fl 6
New York, NY 10022-1202
212-889-3141
800-829-0500
Fax: 212-821-9707
TTY: 212-821-9713
info@lighthouse.org
www.lighthouse.org/navh
Mark G Ackerman, President & CEO
Barbara Gyde, Vice President
Ralph Caprio, Director
Karen Campbell, LCSW, Director of Social Services
NAVH is unique in the services it offers to the hard of seeing™ worldwide and is the only non-profit organization solely dedicated to providing assistance to this population. NAVH runs senior support groups, provides individual consultations, informational materials, training in the use of visual aids, and numerous other tools to ensure that the visually impaired can remain independent and lead fulfilling lives.

8886 National Association of Blind Educators
National Federation of the Blind
200 East Wells St
Baltimore, MD 21230-4914
410-659-9314
Fax: 410-685-5653
nfb@nfb.org
www.nfb.org
Marc Maurer, CEO
Membership organization of blind teachers, professors and instructors in all levels of education. Provides support and information regarding professional responsibilities, classroom techniques, national testing methods and career obstacles. Publishes The Blind Educator, national magazine specifically for blind educators.

8887 National Association of Blind Lawyers
National Federation of the Blind
1660 South Albion Street
Denver, CO 80222-4046
303-504-5979
Fax: 303-757-3640
slabarre@labarrelaw.com
www.nfb.org
Scott LaBarre, President
Membership organization of blind attorneys, law students, judges and others in the law field. Provides support and information regarding employment, techniques used by the blind, advocacy, laws affecting the blind, current information about the American Bar Association and other issues for blind lawyers.

8888 **National Association of Blind Merchants**
National Federation of the Blind
7450 Chapman Hwy #319
Knoxville, TN 37920 888-687-6226
www.blindmerchants.org

Nicky Gacos, President
Harold Wilson, First Vice President
Ed Birmingham, Second Vice President
Pam Schnurr, Treasurer
Membership organization of blind persons employed in either self-employment work or the Randolph-Sheppard vending program. Provides information regarding rehabilitation, social security, tax and other issues which directly affect blind merchants. Serves as advocacy and support group.

8889 **National Association of Blind Secretaries and Transcribers**
National Federation of the Blind
200 East Wells St
Baltimore, MD 21230-4914 410-659-9314
Fax: 410-685-5653
nfb@nfb.org
www.nfb.org

Marc Maurer, CEO
Membership organization of blind secretaries and transcribers at all levels, including medical and paralegal transcription, office workers, customer-service personnel and many other similar fields. Addresses issues such as technology, accomodation, career planning and job training.

8890 **National Association of Blind Students**
National Federation of the Blind
200 East Wells St
Baltimore, MD 21230-4914 410-659-9314
Fax: 410-685-5653
nfb@nfb.org
www.nfb.org

Marc Maurer, CEO
For over 30 years this national organization of blind students has provided support, information, and encouragement to blind college and university students. NABS leads the way in offering resources in issues such as national testing, accessible textbooks and materials, overcoming negative attitudes about blindness from school personnel, developing new techniques of accomplishing laboratory or field assignments, and many other college experiences.

8891 **National Association of Blind Teachers**
American Council of the Blind
1155 15th St NW
Ste 1004
Washington, DC 20005-2706 202-467-5081
800-424-8666
Fax: 202-467-5085
johnbuckley25@hotmail.com
www.blindteachers.net

Jill Gaus, President
Lynn Jansen, Vice President
Debby Lieberman, Secretary
Mike Reese, Treasurer
Works to advance the teaching profession for blind and visually impaired people, protects the interest of teachers, presents discussions and solutions for special problems encountered by blind teachers and publishes a directory of blind teachers in the US.

8892 **National Association of Blind Veterans**
PO Box 784957
Winter Garden, FL 34778 321-948-1466
president@nabv.org
www.nabv.org

Dwight Sayer, President
Gene Huggins, 1st Vice President
Larry Ball, 2nd Vice President
Patty Sayer, Secretary
A nationwide organization of blind and visually impaired veterans striving to serve fellow veterans who have lost their sight in the service of country or have lost their sight after serving country.

8893 **National Association of Guide Dog Users**
National Federation of the Blind
1003 Papaya Dr
Tampa, FL 33619-4629 813-626-2789
800-558-8261
888-624-3841
president@nagdu.org
www.nagdu.org

Marion Gwizdala, President
Provides information and support for guide dog users and works to secure high standards in guide dog training. Addresses issues of discrimination of guide dog users and offers public education about guide dog use. Biennial newsletter available: Harness Up!

8894 **National Association to Promote the Use of Braille**
National Federation of the Blind
39481 Gallaudet Dr
Apt 127
Fremont, CA 94538 510-248-0100
877-558-6524
Fax: 818-344-7930
mwillows@sbcglobal.net
www.nfbcal.org

Nadine Jacobson, President
Robert Jaquiss, Vice President
Linda Mentink, Second Vice President
Jennifer Dunnam, Secretary
Dedicated to securing improved Braille instruction, increasing the number of braille materials available to the blind and providing information of braille in securing independence, education and employment for the blind.

8895 **National Beep Baseball Association**
1501 41st NW
Apt G1
Rochester, MN 55901 866-400-4551
www.nbba.org

Stephen A. Guerra, Secretary
It facilitates and provides the adaptive version of America's favorite pastime for the blind, low vision and legally blind.

8896 **National Braille Association**
95 Allens Creek Rd
Bldg 1 Ste 202
Rochester, NY 14618- 3252 585-427-8260
Fax: 585-427-0263
nbaoffice@nationalbraille.org
www.nationalbraille.org

David Shaffar, Executive Director
Jan Carroll, President
Whitney Gregory-Williams, Vice President
Heidi Lehmann, Secretary
The only national organization dedicated to the professional development of individuals who prepare and produce braille materials.

8897 **National Braille Press**
88 Saint Stephen St
Boston, MA 02115-4312 617-266-6160
888-965-8965
888-965-8965
Fax: 617-437-0456
contact@nbp.org
www.nbp.org

Brian A. Mac Donald, President
Kimberley Ballard, Vice President
Tony Grima, Vice President of Braille Publications
Diane L. Croft, Publisher
The guiding purposes of National Braille Press are to promote the literacy of blind children through braille, and to provide access to information that empowers blind people to actively engage in work, family, and commuity affairs.

8898 National Center for Vision and Child Development
Lighthouse International
111 E 59th St
New York, NY 10022-1202 212-821-9200
800-829-0500
Fax: 212-821-9707
TTY: 212-821-9713
info@lighthouse.org
www.lighthouse.org

Mark G Ackerman, President/CEO
Barbara Gyde, Vice President
Ralph Caprio, Director
The worldwide leader in helping people of all ages who are blind
or partially sighted overcome the challenges of vision loss.

8899 National Diabetes Action Network for the Blind
National Federation of the Blind
1212 London Dr
Columbia, MO 65203-2012 573-875-8911
ebryant@socket.net
www.nfb.org

Ed Bryant, Manager
Leading support and information organization of persons losing
vision due to diabetes. Provides personal contact and resource information with other blind diabetics about non-visual techniques
of independently managing diabetes, monitoring glucose levels,
measuring insulin and other matters concerning diabetes. Publishes Voice of the Diabetic, the leading publication about
diabetes and blindness.

8900 National Eye Institute
31 Center Drive MSC 2510
Bethesda, MD 20892-2510 301-496-5248
Fax: 301-402-1065
2020@nei.nih.gov
www.nei.nih.gov

Paul A Sieving MD PhD, Director
To conduct and support research for blinding eye diseases, visual
disorders, mechanisms of visual function, and the preservation of
sight.

8901 National Federation of the Blind
200 E. Wells St.
at Jernigan Place
Baltimore, MD 21230- 4998 410-659-9314
Fax: 410-685-5653
nfb@nfb.org
nfb.org

John Berggren, Executive Director for Operation
John G. Paré Jr., Executive Director for Strategic Initiatives
Mark Riccobono, Executive Director, NFB Jernigan Institute
Joanne Wilson, Executive Director for Affiliate Action
The National Federation of the Blind (NFB) is the largest organization of the blind in the world. The Federation's purpose is to
help blind people achieve self-confidence, self-respect, and
self-determination. Their goal is the complete integration of the
blind into society on a basis of equality.

8902 National Industries for the Blind
1310 Braddock Pl
Alexandria, VA 22314-1691 703-310-0500
Fax: 703-998-8268
info@nib.org
www.nfb.org

Gary J. Krump, Chairperson
Ronald Tascarella, Vice Chairperson
Kristin Graham Koehler, Secretary
A nonprofit organization that represents over 100 associated industries serving people who are blind in thirty-six states. These
agencies serve people who are blind or visually impaired and help
them to reach their full potential. Services include job and family
counseling, job skills training, instruction in Braille and other
communication skills, children's programs and more.

**8903 National Library Service for the Blind and Physically
Handicapped**
Library of Congress
1291 Taylor St. NW
Washington, DC 20542-4962 202-707-5100
800-424-8567
Fax: 202-707-0712
TTY: 202-707-0744
nls@loc.gov
www.loc.gov/nls

**8904 National Library Services for the Blind& Physically
Handicapped**
Library of Congress
1291 Taylor Street North West
Washington, DC 20011 202-707-5100
Fax: 202-707-0712
TTY:202-707-0744
nls@loc.gov
www.loc.gov/nls

Karen Keninger, Director
NLS is responsible for the selection, copyright clearance, and
procurement of reading materials for blind and physically handicapped individuals. Distribution of the materials and relevant
biblographic information either directly or through cooperating
state and local network libraries. Design, development, and procurement of sound reproduction equipment and its distribution
either directly or through cooperating agencies.

8905 National Organization of Parents of Blind Children
National Federation of the Blind
200 East Wells St
Baltimore, MD 21230-4914 410-659-9314
Fax: 410-685-5653
www.nfb.org

Carlton Walker,, President
Barbara Cheadle,, President Emerita
Stephanie Kieszak-Holloway, First Vice-President
Andrea Beasley, Secretary
Support information and advocacy organization of parents of
blind or visually impaired children. Addresses issues ranging
from help to parents of a newborn blind infant, mobility and
braille instruction, education, social and community participation, development of self confidence and other vital factors
involved in growth of a blind child.

8906 New Eyes for the Needy
549 Millburn Avenue
PO Box 332
Short Hills, NJ 07078-332 973-376-4903
Fax: 973-376-3807
neweyesfortheneedy@verizon.net
www.neweyesfortheneedy.org

Susan Dyckman, Executive Director
Marianne Muench Busby, Vice President
Barbara Daney, Treasurer
Suzanne Escousee, Secretary
New Eyes provides new prescription glasses for poor children
and adults in the U.S. through a voucher system.

8907 Prevent Blindness America
211 W Wacker Drive
Suite 1700
Chicago, IL 60606 312-363-6001
800-331-2020
Fax: 312-363-6052
info@preventblindness.org
www.preventblindness.org

James E. Anderson, Chair
Kira Baldanado, Director
Arzu Bilazer, Creative Director
Mary Bregantini, Senior Director
The nation's leading volunteer eye health and safety organization
dedicated to fighting blindness and saving sight. Also touches the
lives of millions of people each year through public and professional education, advocacy, certified vision screening training,
community and patient service programs and research.

8908   Seeing Eye, The
10 Washington Valley Rd
PO Box 375
Morristown, NJ 07963-0375   973-539-4425
                                   Fax: 973-539-0922
                                   info@seeingeye.org
                                   www.seeingeye.org
Peggy Gibbon,, Director of Canine Development
James A Kutsch Jr, President/CEO
Dolores Holle, VMD,, Director of Canine Medicine & Surgery
Randall Ivens, Director of Human Resources
An organization that concentrates on its mission to enhance the independence, dignity, and self confidence of blind people through the use of seeing eye dogs. The Seeing Eye will be an organization that concentrates on its mission to enhance the independence, dignity, and self confidence of blind people through the use of Seeing Eye dogs, and on improving its ability to fulfill this mission. We will maintain and nuture the spirit of our founders and adhere to the highest standards of respect

8909   Services for the Visually Impaired
8720 Georgia Ave
Suite 210
Silver Spring, MD   20910-3614   301-589-0894
                                   Fax: 301-589-0884
                                   info@clb.org
                                   www.clb.org
Ann Cook, Executive Director
Anthony J. (Cancelosi, CEO
Provides skills and resources to DC area residents who are blind or experiencing vision loss, and are also committed to helping people regain their indepence and maintaining it.

8910   Society for the Blind
1238 S St.
Sacramento, CA   95811   916-452-8271
                                   Fax: 916-492-2483
                                   info@societyfortheblind.org
                                   societyfortheblind.org
Shari Roeseler, Executive Director
Shane Snyder, Director of Programs
Serving 26 counties in Northern California, Society for the Blind is a full service, nonprofit, agency providing services and programs for people who are blind or have low vision. services include the Low Vision Clinic, Braille Classes, computer training, support groups, living skills instruction, mobility training, and the Products for Independence Store.

8911   United States Association of Blind Athletes
1 Olympic Plaza
Colorado Springs, CO   80909-3508   719-866-3224
                                   Fax: 719-866-3400
                                   mlucas@usaba.org
                                   www.usaba.org
Mark A. Lucas, Executive Director
Ryan Ortiz, Assistant Executive Director
John Potts, Goalball High Performance Director
Lacey Markle, Public Relations and Events Coordinator
USABA is a Colorado-based 501(c) (3) organization that provides life-enriching sports opportunities for every individual with a visual impairment. A member of the U.S. Olympic Committee, USABA provides athletic opportunities in various sports including, but not limited to track and field, nordic and alpine skiing, biathlon, judo, wrestling, swimming, tandem cycling, powerlifting and goalball (a team sport for the blind and visually impaired).

8912   United States Blind Golfers Association
125 Gilberts Hill Rd
Lehighton, PA   18235   615-679-9629
                                   info@usblindgolf.com
                                   www.usblindgolf.com
Jim Baker, President
Diane Wilson, Vice President
Tony Schiros, Board Member
Alan Hooper, Board Member
It encourages and enhances opportunities of blind and visually impaired golfers to compete in golf.

8913   United States Braille Chess Association
1881 N. Nash St.
Unit 702
Arlington, VA   22209   516-223-8685
                                   www.americanblindchess.org
LA Pietrolungo, President
Alan Dicey, Vice President
Jay Leventhal, Secretary
Alan Schlank, Treasurer
It is dedicated to encourage and assist in the promotion and advancement of correspondence and over-the board chess among chess enthusiasts who are blind or visually impaired.

8914   Vermont Association for the Blind and Visually Impaired
60 Kimball Ave
South Burlington, VT   05403   802-863-1358
                                   800-639-5861
                                   Fax: 802-863-1481
                                   general@vabvi.org
                                   www.vabvi.org
James Mooney, President
Thomas Chase, Vice President
Debbie Balserus, Secretary
Patricia Henderson, Treasurer
The Vermont Association for the Blind and Visually Impaired (VABVI), a non-profit organization founded in 1926, is the only private agency to offer free training, services and support to visually impaired Vermonters. Each year we serve hundreds of children from birth to age 22 and adults age 55 and over.

8915   Vision Forward Association
912 N. Hawley Road
Milwaukee, WI   53213   414-615-0100
                                   855-878-6056
                                   Fax: 414-256-8748
                                   www.vision-forward.org
Terri Davis, Executive Director
Jacci Borchardt, Program Director
Jacque Cline, Human Resources Director
Dena Fellows, Marketing Director
Its mission is to empower, educate, and enhance the lives of individuals impacted by vision loss through all of life's transitions.

8916   Vision World Wide
Apt 302
5707 Brockton Dr
Indianapolis, IN   46220-5481   317-254-1332
                                   800-431-1739
                                   Fax: 317-251-6588
                                   www.visionww.org
Patricia L Prince, President
A non profit organization dedicated to improving the lives of the vision impaired through direct interaction and indirectly through the caregiving community. Also serve both the totally blind and those with various degrees and forms of vision loss.

8917   Visions Center on Blindness (VCB)
111 Summit Park Rd
Spring Valley, NY   10977-1221   212-625-1616
                                   888-245-8333
                                   Fax: 845-354-5130
                                   info@visionsvcb.org
                                   www.visionsvcb.org
Nancy T. Jones, President
Richard P. Simon, Vice President
Burton M. Strauss, Treasurer
Carol Spawn Desmond, Secretary
VISIONS VCB is a 35-acre year round residential rehabilitation and training center in Rockland County, New York, 35 miles north of New York City in the Village of New Hempstead. Since it's founding over 85 years ago, VCB has become one of the largest and most comprehensive overnight training and vision rehabilitation facilities in the United States. Year round on weekends and during summer sessions, VCB serves 600 people of all ages.

8918   Visually Impaired Veterans of America
American Council of the Blind
1155 15th St NW
Ste 1004
Washington, DC   20005-2706   202-467-5081
                                     800-424-8666
                                Fax: 202-467-5085
                                     www.acb.org

Jill Gaus, President
Lynn Jansen, Vice President
Debby Lieberman, Secretary
Mike Reese, Treasurer
Maintain, promote and foster the well bring and rehabilitation of all visually Impaired Veterans of the Armed Forces of the United States of America who are eligible to receive from the Veterans Administration; develops and encourages the practice of high standards of personal professional conduct among Visually Impaired Veterans; maintain, promote, and foster public confidence and awareness In Visually Impaired Veterans.

8919   Washington Ear
12061 Tech Rd
Ste B
Silver Spring, MD   20904-7826   301-681-6636
                                Fax: 301-625-1986
                                information@washear.org
                                     www.washear.org
George Long, Chairman
Neely Oplinger, Executive Director
Freddie L. Peaco, President
Paul D'Addario, President-Elect
A non profit organization providing reading and information services for blind, visually impaired and physically disabled people who cannot effectively read print, see plays, watch television programs and films, or view museum exhibits. Ear free services strive to substitute hearing for seeing, improving the lives of people with limited or no vision by enabling them to be well-informed, fully productive members of their families, their communities and the working world.

Camps

8920   Camp Barakel
P.O.Box 159
Fairview, MI   48621-0159   989-848-2279
                                Fax: 989-848-2280
                                info@campbarakel.org
                                     www.campbarakel.org
Paul Gardner, Camp Director
Hannah Gardner, Music Coordinator
Jon Ford, Head Lifeguard
Stacy Ford, Adult Program Staff
Five-day Christian camp experience in mid-August for campers ages 18-55 who are physically disabled, visually impaired, upper trainable mentally impaired or educable mentally impaired, bus transportation provided from locations in Lansing, Flint and Bay City, Michigan.

8921   Camp Challenge
8914 US Highway 50 East
Bedford, IN   47421   812-834-5159
                                info@gocampchallenge.com
                                     www.gocampchallenge.com
Maria , Director of Engagement
One and two-week sessions for campers with developmental and or physical disabilities, hearing impairment and the blind/visually impaired. Ages 6-99 and families.

8922   Camp Lawroweld
Northern New England Conference
228 West Side Road
Weld, ME   04285   207-585-2984
                                Fax: 207-585-2985
                                camplawroweld@gmail.com
                                     www.lawroweld.org

Harry Sabnani, Executive Director

Camp is located in Weld, Maine. Week sessions July for campers who are blind or visually impaired, all ages. Other camps coed, ages 9-16 and families, single adults, June - September.

8923   Camp Lou Henry Hoover
Girl Scouts of Washington Rock Council
201 East Grove Street
Westfield, NJ   07090   908-518-4400
                                Fax: 908-232-4508
                                girlscouts@gshnj.org
                                     www.gshnj.org
Samantha Basek, Field Executive
Susan Brooks, CEO
Camp is located in Middleville, New Jersey. Sessions for girls who are blind/visually impaired, ages 7-18.

8924   Camp Merrick
PO Box 56
Nanjemoy, MD   20662   301-870-5858
                                Fax: 301-246-9108
                                info@LionsCampMerrick.org
                                     lionscampmerrick.org
Wayne Magoon, President
Ray Shumaker, Vice President
Julie Andrew, Board Member
Frank Culhane, Treasurer
Programs offered April-January for children who are blind/visually impaired, hearing impaired or diabetic. Coed, ages 6-15.

8925   Camp Winnekeag
257 Ashby Road
Ashburnham, MA   01430   978-827-4455
                                Fax: 978-827-4551
                                sneconference@sneconline.org
                                     www.campwinnekeag.com
Frank Tochterman, Religious Leader
Camp is located in Ashburnham, Massachusetts. Camping sessions for blind/visually impaired children. Coed, ages 8-16.

8926   Columbia Lighthouse for the Blind Summer Camp
Columbia Lighthouse for the Blind
1825 K Street NorthWest
Suite 1103
Washington, DC   20006   202-454-6400
                                Fax: 877-595-9228
                                info@clb.org
                                     clb.org
Tony Cancelosi, President
Anthony Cancelosi, CEO
Helps enable the blind or visually impaired to obtain and maintain independence at home, school, work and in the community. Programs and services include early intervention services, training and consultation in assistive technology, career placement services, comprehensive low vision care and a wide range of rehabilitation services. Highly acclaimed summer camp, picnics and holiday activities encourage blind and visualy impaired children to make new friends and experience the joys of childhood.

8927   Easter Seals Oklahoma
701 NE 13th St
Oklahoma City, OK   73104   405-239-2525
                                info@eastersealsoklahoma.org
                                     eastersealsok.org/
Keith McCombs, Chairman
Krista Massad, Chairman-Elect
Cassie Wilson, Secretary
Matt Vance, Treasurer
Offers an Adult Day Health Center, and Child Development Center. The Child Development Center offers developmentally appropriate learning activities and services to meet the unique needs of each child, and the adult center provides solutions to meet the physical, social and emotional needs of adults from the ages of 21 to 100+.

8928   Enchanted Hills Camp for the Blind
Lighthouse for the Blind
214 Van Ness Avenue
San Francisco, CA   94102   415-431-1481
                                            888-400-8933
                                    Fax: 415-863-7568
                                    info@lighthouse-sf.org
                                    lighthouse-sf.org
Joshua A. Miele, President
Chris Downey, 1st Vice President
Gena Harper, Secretary
Joseph Chan, Treasurer
Camp is located in Napa, California. Half-week, one and
two-week sessions for blind, deaf/blind children and adults, ages
5 and up. This program offers a basic camping experience. Activi-
ties include music, art, dance, hiking and riding. Camperships are
available to California residents.

8929   Highbrook Lodge
Clevland Sight Center
1909 East 101st St
Cleveland, OH   44106   216-791-8118
                                            877-776-9563
                                    Fax: 216-791-1101
                                    TTY: 216-791-8119
                                    info@clevelandsightcenter.org
                                    www.clevelandsightcenter.org
Lawrence Benders, President/Executive Director
Kevin R. Krencisz, Chief Financial Officer
Karen Bain Hiller, Director of Development
Michael McManamon, Chief Information Officer
Camp is located in Chardon, Ohio. Summer sessions for children,
adults and families who are blind or have low vision. Sessopms
inclide a wide range of outdoor camp activities. Camp activities
focus on gaining independent skills, mobility, orientation and
self confidence in an accessable and traditional camp setting.

8930   Indian Creek Camp
Kentucky Tennessee Conference
150 Cabin Circle Drive
Liberty, TN   37095   615-548-4411
                                    Fax: 615-548-4029
                                    www.indiancreekcamp.com
Ken Wetmore, Director
Marty Sutton, Asst. Director
Toni Stephens, Program Director
Stephanie Rufo, Public Relations Director
Camp is located in Liberty, Tennessee. Summer sessions for chil-
dren and adults who are blind/visually impaired. Coed, ages 7-17,
families and seniors.

8931   Kamp A-Komp-Plish
9035 Ironsides Rd
Nanjemoy, MD   20662-3432   301-870-3226
                                            301-934-3590
                                    Fax: 301-870-2620
                                    recreation@melwood.org
                                    www.kampakomplish.org
Jonathan Rondeau, Chief Program Officer
Bekah Carmichael, Director
Doria Fleisher, Associate Director
Marisa Cucuzella, Assistant Director
Camp is located in Nanjemoy, Maryland. Half-week, one-week
and two-week sessions for blind/visually impaired children and
those with developmental disabilities and mobility limitation.
Coed, ages 8-16.

8932   Kamp Kaleo
46872 Willow Springs Road
Burwell, NE   68823   308-346-5083
                                    kampkaleo@gmail.com
                                    www.kampkaleo.com
Gaylene O'Brien, Administrator
Sandy Denton, Minister Of Faith Development
Kamp Kaleo provides summer sessions for campers who are
blind/visually impaired or have developmental disabilities.
Coed, ages 9-18 and families, seniors, single adults. In addition to

regular camp activities, there is a strong focus on religious
education.

8933   National Camp for Blind Children
Christian Record Services
P.O. Box 6097
Lincoln, NE   68506-0097   402-488-0981
                                    Fax: 402-488-7582
                                    www.christianrecord.org
Dan Jackson, Chair
Tom Lemon, Vice Chair
Larry Pitcher, President, Secretary
Al Burdick, Board Member
To enrich lives of those who are blind, visually impaired or physi-
cally challenged regardless of race, creed, economic status or
gender. Also encourages each camper to achieve greater self-es-
teem and self confidence while seeking to excel in the use of
his/her physical , mental, and spiritual capacities. Provides fee
Christian publications and programs for people with visual
impairments.
Monthly

8934   National Camps for Blind Children
Christian Record Services
5900 S 58th St
Suite M
Lincoln, NE   68516   402-488-0981
                                    Fax: 402-488-7582
                                    services@christianrecord.org
                                    www.christianrecord.org
Diane Thurber, President
Andrea Ahrens, Development Director
Jeri Lyn Rogge, Communication Director
Kalvin Follett, Studio & Library Services Director
Christian Record Services runs National Camps for Blind Chil-
dren, summer camps for people aged 9 to 65 who are considered
legally blind.

8935   Texas Lions Camp
Lions Club Of Texas
P.O.Box 290247
Kerrville, TX   78029   830-896-8500
                                    Fax: 830-896-3666
                                    www.lionscamp.com
Stephen Mabry, Executive Director
Steven King, Director of Operations
Patty Rodriguez, Program Supervisor
Bailey Carter, Program Supervisor
Texas Lions Camp is a camp dedicated to seving children in Texas
with physical diabilities, ages 7-16. While at camp, campers will
participate in a variety of acitivties and they will be encouraged to
become more independent and self-confident.

8936   VISIONS Vacation Camp for the Blind
VISIONS Center on Blindness
500 Greenwhich St
3rd Floor
Spring Valley, NY   10977-1354   212-625-1616
                                            888-245-8333
                                    Fax: 212-219-4078
                                    info@visionsvcb.org
                                    www.visionsvcb.org
Nancy T. Jones, President
Steve E. Kent, Vice President
Burton M. Strauss, Treasurer
Jasmine Campirides, Secretary
Is a non profit agency that promotes the independence of people
of all ages who are blind or visually impaired. Camp offers braille
classes, computers with large print and voice output, support
groups, discussions, mobility lessions, cooking classes, personal
and home management training, large print and Braille books.

8937 Wendell Johnson Speech And Hearing Clinic
University Of Iowa
250 Hawkins Dr
Iowa City, IA 52242-1025 319-335-8736
Fax: 319-335-8851
kathy-miller@uiowa.edu
www.uiowa.edu

Chuck Wieland, President
Hans Hoerschelman, Vice President
Josh Smith, Budget Officer
Shannon Lizakowski, Secretary
The clinic offers assessment and intervention for communication disorders in adults and children as well as an audiology clinic. The clinic also offers several summer programs for children with hearing, speech, language, autism and/or reading disorders, including a summer residential program for teens who stutter.

8938 YMCA Camp Chingachgook on Lake George
Capital District YMCA
1872 Pilot Knob Road
Kattskill Bay, NY 12844 518-656-9462
Fax: 518-656-9362
chingachgook@cdymca.org
camp.cdymca.org/

John Lefner, Executive Director
Carol Lewis, Office Manager
Jine Andreozzi, Summer Camp Program Director
Tricia Biles, Group Services Director
Sailing programs for people with disabilities. Coed, ages 7-16, families, seniors and single adults.

Print: Books

8939 A Christian Approach to Overcoming Disability: A Doctor's Story
Routledge (Taylor & Francis Group)
711 Third Ave.
New York, NY 10017 212-216-7800
Fax: 212-564-7854
orders@taylorandfrancis.com
www.routledge.com

Dr. Elaine Leong Eng, M.D.
A personal account of Dr. Elaine Leong Eng and her career move from obstetrician/gynecologist to full-time mom, as she faces the diagnosis of impending visual impairment. Dr. Eng offers personal experience and faith-based, psychological techniques for coping with disability.
142 pages Hardcover

8940 AFB Directory of Services for Blind and Visually Impaired Persons in the US and Canada
American Foundation for the Blind/AFB Press
2 Penn Plaza
Suite 1102
New York, NY 10121 212-502-7600
800-232-5463
Fax: 888-545-8331
afbinfo@afb.net
www.afb.org

Carl Augusto, President & Chief Executive Officer
Rick Bozeman, Finance Director, Chief Financial Officer
Kelly Bleach, Chief Administrative Officer
Stacy Rollins, Executive Administrative Assistant to the President
Comprehensive print resource containing more that 2,500 local, state, regional, and national services throughout the US and Canada for persons who are blind or visually impaired. *$79.95*
624 pages Paperback/onlin
ISBN 0-891288-05-3

8941 About Children's Eyes
National Association for Visually Handicapped
111 East 59th Street
New York, NY 10022-1202 212-821-9384
800-829-0500
Fax: 212-821-9707
info@lighthouse.org
lighthouse.org/navh

Mark G. Ackermann, President / CEO
How to identify the child with a visual problem. LightHouse acquired NAVH.

8942 About Children's Vision: A Guide for Parents
National Association for Visually Handicapped
111 East 59th Street
New York, NY 10022-1202 212-821-9384
800-829-0500
Fax: 212-821-9707
info@lighthouse.org
lighthouse.org/navh

Mark G. Ackermann, President / CEO
Offers a better understanding of the normal and possible abnormal development of a child's eyesight. LightHouse acquired NAVH. *$.50*

8943 Access to Art: A Museum Directory for Blind and Visually Impaired People
American Foundation for the Blind/AFB Press
2 Penn Plaza
Suite 1102
New York, NY 10121 212-502-7600
800-232-5463
Fax: 888-545-8331
afbinfo@afb.net
www.afb.org

Carl R. Augusto, President & Chief Executive Officer
Rick Bozeman, Finance Director, Chief Financial Officer
Kelly Bleach, Chief Administrative Officer
Stacy Rollins, Executive Administrative Assistant to the President
Details the access facilities of over 300 museums, galleries and exhibits in the United States. Also included are organizations offering art-related resources such as, art classes, competitions and traveling exhibits. *$19.95*
144 pages Large Print
ISBN 0-891281-56-8

8944 African Americans in the Profession of Blindness Services
Mississippi State University
P.O.Box 6189
Mississippi State, MS 39762 662-325-2001
Fax: 662-325-8989
TTY:662-325-2694
nrtc@colled.msstate.edu
www.blind.msstate.edu

Jacqui Bybee, Research Associate II
Douglas Bedsaul, Research and Training Coordinator
Anne Carter, Research and Training Coordinator
Brenda Cavenaugh, Ph.D., Research Professor
This study investigated the level of participation by African Americans in vocational rehab. (VR) services to persons who are visually impaired. Using surveys and interviews with all state VR directors, national census data and national RSA data, it was found nationally that African Americans are substantially under-represented in the service provider ranks, yet over-represented as clients. *$20.00*
61 pages Paperback

8945 Age-Related Macular Degeneration
National Association for Visually Handicapped
111 East 59th Street
New York, NY 10022-1202 212-821-9384
800-829-0500
Fax: 212-821-9707
info@lighthouse.org
lighthouse.org/navh

Mark G. Ackermann, President / CEO

A large booklet offering information and up-to-date research on Macular Degeneration. Also available in Russian. Revised in 2007. LightHouse acquired NAVH. *$5.00*

8946   American Anals of the Deaf Reference
800 Florida Ave NE
Washington, DC   20002-3600   202-651-5530
                                          Fax: 202-651-5489
                                      gupress@gallaudet.edu
                                  gupress.gallaudet.edu/annals
Stephanie Cawthon, Ph.D., Book Review Editor
Peter V. Paul, Ph.D., Editor, Literary Issues
Ye Wang, Ph.D., Senior Associate Editor
Feifei Ye, Ph.D., Associate Editor for Research Methodology
The controlled scope of GUPress operations allows the continuance of a highly focused commitment to individual titles that has contributed significantly to its 20 years of leadership in publishing on Deaf issues. Gallaudet University Press brings unmatched experience and knowledge to the marketplace for books on and for the Deaf community, its advocates, and scholars invested in the study of deaf society.

8947   Americans with Disabilities Act Guide for Places of Lodging: Serving Guests Who Are Blind
US Department of Justice
950 Pennsylvania Avenue NorthWest
Washington, DC   20530   202-307-0663
                                               800-574-0301
                                          Fax: 202-307-1197
                                          TTY: 800-514-0383
                                               www.ada.gov
Rebecca B. Bond, Chief
Zita Johnson Betts, Deputy Chief
Sally Conway, Deputy Chief
James Bostrom, Deputy Chief
A 12-page publication explaining what hotels, motels, and other places of transient lodging can do to accommodate guests who are blind or have low vision.

8948   Art and Science of Teaching Orientation and Mobility to Persons with Visual Impairments
American Foundation for the Blind/AFB Press
2 Penn Plaza
Suite 1102
New York, NY   10121   212-502-7600
                                               800-232-5463
                                          Fax: 888-545-8331
                                          afbinfo@afb.net
                                               www.afb.org
Carl R. Augusto, President & Chief Executive Officer
Rick Bozeman, Finance Director, Chief Financial Officer
Kelly Bleach, Chief Administrative Officer
Stacy Rollins, Executive Administrative Assistant to the President
Comprehensive decription of the techniques of teaching orientation and mobility, presented along with considerations and strategies for sensitive and effective teaching. Hardcover. Paperback also available. *$48.00*
200 pages
ISBN 0-891282-45-9

8949   Awareness Training
Landmark Media
3450 Slade Run Drive
Falls Church, VA   22042   703-241-2030
                                               800-342-4336
                                          Fax: 703-536-9540
                                      info@landmarkmedia.com
                                          landmarkmedia.com
Michael Hartogs, President
Peter Hartogs, VP New Business & Development
Richard Hartogs, VP Acquisitions
Beverly Weisenberg, Sales Representative
Covers disabilities of various types — vision, hearing, speech disorders, loss of limbs, loss of mobility, or mental/emotional limitations and how to integrate such individuals into various business and educational settings. It is a 4-part series designed to

identify and enable others to interact effectively with those suffering such disabilities. *$495.00*
Set of 4

8950   Babycare Assistive Technology
Through the Looking Glass
3075 Adeline Street
Suite 120
Berkeley, CA   94703   510-848-1112
                                               800-644-2666
                                          Fax: 510-848-4445
                                      tlg@lookingglass.org
                                          www.lookingglass.org
Maureen Block, J.D., President
Thomas Spalding, Treasurer
Alice Nemon, Secretary
Mega Kirshbaum, Author
Available in braille, large print or cassette. Provides an overview of the baby care assistive technology work at Through The Looking Glass including a discussion of TLG's intervention model, the impact of babycare equipment and guidelines for equipment development. *$2.00*
8 pages

8951   Babycare Assistive Technology for Parents with Physical Disabilties
Through the Looking Glass
3075 Adeline Street
Suite 120
Berkeley, CA   94703   510-848-1112
                                               800-644-2666
                                          Fax: 510-848-4445
                                      tlg@lookingglass.org
                                          www.lookingglass.org
Maureen Block, J.D., President
Thomas Spalding, Treasurer
Alice Nemon, Secretary
Mega Kirshbaum, Author
Examines the provision of babycare equipment through the lens of ithe infant/parent relationship, the lens of the family system, and through the lens of culture. Availiable in braille, large print or cassette. *$2.00*
7 pages

8952   Basic Course in American Sign Language
TJ Publishers
P.O. Box 702701
Dallas, TX   75370   972-416-0800
                                               800-999-1168
                                          Fax: 972-416-0944
                                          TTY: 301-585-4440
                                      TJPubinc@aol.com
                                          www.tjpublishers.com/
Tom Humphries, Author
Carol Padden, Co-Author
Terrance J O'Rourke, Co-Author
Accompanying videotapes and textbooks include voice translations. Hearing students can analyze sound for initial instruction, or opt to turn off the sound to sharpen visual acuity. Package includes the Basic Course in American Sign Language text, Student Study Guide, the original four 1-hour videotapes plus the ABCASI Vocabulary videotape. *$139.95*
280 pages

8953   Behavioral Vision Approaches for Persons with Physical Disabilities
Optometric Extension Program Foundation
7754 Braegger Road
Three Lakes, WI   54562   714-250-0176
                                      Info@depf.org
                                          www.depf.org
Kristin R. Jungbluth, President
Eric J. Lindberg, VP
Barbara Kuntz, Secretary
Patricia S. Lindberg, Treasurer

A discussion of the behavioral vision/neuro-motor approach to providing directions for prescriptive and therapeutic services for the visually handicapped child or adult. *$49.50*
197 pages

8954 Belonging
Dial Books
375 Hudson St
New York, NY 10014-3657   212-366-2000
                                         Fax: 212-414-3394
                                         www.penguin.com/

Deborah Kent, Author
Meg attended special schools for the blind until she was ready for high school. She decided that she wanted to go to a regular high school. She and her mother practiced her walks to school and studied the layout of the building prior to school starting, but Meg was unprepared for the trip when there were 1,500 students. She adjusted quickly to the crowds and the pace of the new school.
200 pages Hardcover
ISBN 0-80370 -30-1

8955 Berthold Lowenfeld on Blindness and Blind People
American Foundation for the Blind/AFB Press
2 Penn Plaza
Suite 1102
New York, NY 10121   212-502-7600
                                         800-232-5463
                                         Fax: 888-545-8331
                                         afbinfo@afb.net
                                         www.afb.org

Carl R. Augusto, President & Chief Executive Officer
Rick Bozeman, Finance Director, Chief Financial Officer
Kelly Bleach, Chief Administrative Officer
Stacy Rollins, Executive Administrative Assistant to the President
These writings of the pioneering educator, author and advocate range over a forty-year period include various ground-breaking papers for the blind educator, a remembrance of Helen Keller and other essays on education, sociology and history. *$21.95*
254 pages Paperback
ISBN 0-891281-01-0

8956 Blind and Vision-Impaired Individuals
Mainstream
Ste 830
3 Bethesda Metro Ctr
Bethesda, MD 20814-6301   301-961-9299
                                         800-247-1380
                                         Fax: 301-654-6714

Charles Moster
Mainstreaming blind individuals into the workplace. *$ 2.50*
12 pages

8957 Blindness and Early Childhood Development Second Edition
American Foundation for the Blind/AFB Press
2 Penn Plaza
Suite 1102
New York, NY 10121   212-502-7600
                                         800-232-5463
                                         Fax: 888-545-8331
                                         afbinfo@afb.net
                                         afb.org

Carl R. Augusto, President & Chief Executive Officer
Rick Bozeman, Finance Director, Chief Financial Officer
Kelly Bleach, Chief Administrative Officer
Stacy Rollins, Executive Administrative Assistant to the President
A review of current knowledge on motor and locomotor development, perceptual development, language and cognitive processes, and social, emotional and personality development. Paperback. *$34.95*
384 pages
ISBN 0-891281-23-8

8958 Blindness: What it is, What it Does and How to Live with it
American Foundation for the Blind/AFB Press
2 Penn Plaza
Suite 1102
New York, NY 10121   212-502-7600
                                         800-232-5463
                                         Fax: 888-545-8331
                                         afbinfo@afb.net
                                         www.afb.org

Carl R. Augusto, President & Chief Executive Officer
Rick Bozeman, Finance Director, Chief Financial Officer
Kelly Bleach, Chief Administrative Officer
Stacy Rollins, Executive Administrative Assistant to the President
A classic work on how blindness affects self-perception and social interaction and what can be done to restore basic skills, mobility, daily living and an appreciation of life's pleasures. *$15.95*
396 pages Paperback
ISBN 0-891282-05-

8959 Books are Fun for Everyone
Nat'l Lib Svc/Blind And Physically Handicapped
1291 Taylor Street North West
Washington, DC 20011   202-707-5100
                                         Fax: 202-707-0712
                                         TTY:202-707-0744
                                         nls@loc.gov
                                         www.loc.gov/nls

Karen Keninger, Director

8960 Books for Blind & Physically Handicapped Individuals
Nat'l Lib Svc/Blind And Physically Handicapped
1291 Taylor Street North West
Washington, DC 20011   202-707-5100
                                         Fax: 202-707-0712
                                         TTY:202-707-0744
                                         nls@loc.gov
                                         www.loc.gov/nls

Karen Keninger, Director
A free national library program of braille and recorded materials for blind and physically handicapped persons.

8961 Books for Blind and Physically Handicapped Individuals
Nat'l Lib Svc/Blind And Physically Handicapped
1291 Taylor Street North West
Washington, DC 20011   202-707-5100
                                         Fax: 202-707-0712
                                         TTY:202-707-0744
                                         nls@loc.gov
                                         www.loc.gov/nls

Karen Keninger, Director
A free national library program of braille and recorded materials for blind and physically handicapped persons is administered by the National Library Service for the Blind and Physically Handicapped Library of Congress.
Annual

8962 Braille Book Bank, Music Catalog
National Braille Association
95 Allens Creek Road
Building 1, Suite 202
Rochester, NY 14618   585-427-8260
                                         Fax: 585-427-0263
                                         nbaoffice@nationalbraille.org
                                         www.nationalbraille.org

Jan Carroll, President
Cindi Laurent, Vice President
David Shaffer, Executive Director
Heidi Lehmann, Secretary
Offers hundreds of musical titles in print form, braille and on cassette.
62 pages

8963   Braille: An Extraordinary Volunteer Opportunity
Nat'l Lib Svc/Blind And Physically Handicapped
1291 Taylor Street North West
Washington, DC   20011   202-707-5100
                                            Fax: 202-707-0712
                                          TTY:202-707-0744
                                               nls@loc.gov
                                             www.loc.gov/nls

Karen Keninger, Director

8964   Burns Braille Transcription Dictionary
American Foundation for the Blind/AFB Press
2 Penn Plaza
Suite 1102
New York, NY   10121   212-502-7600
                                               800-232-5463
                                          Fax: 888-545-8331
                                            afbinfo@afb.net
                                                    afb.org

Carl R. Augusto, President & Chief Executive Officer
Rick Bozeman, Finance Director, Chief Financial Officer
Kelly Bleach, Chief Administrative Officer
Stacy Rollins, Executive Administrative Assistant to the President
A handy, portable guide that is a quick reference for anyone who
needs to check print-to-braille and braille-to-print meanings and
symbols. Paperback. *$21.95*
96 pages 96 pages
ISBN 0-891282-32-7

**8965   Can't Your Child See? A Guide for Parents of Visually
         Impaired Children**
Sage Publications
2455 Teller Road
Thousand Oaks, CA   91320   805-499-0721
                                               800-818-7243
                                          Fax: 805-499-0871
                                           info@sagepub.com
                                             www.sagepub.com
Sara Miller McCune, Founder, Publisher, Executive Chairman
Blaise R Simqu, President & CEO
*Tracey A. Ozmina, Executive Vice President & Chief Operating Of-
ficer*
*Stephen Barr, Managing Director/SAGE London, President of
SAGE Internation*
This second edition offers parents optimistic, practical guide-
lines for helping visually impaired children reach their full poten-
tial. *$26.00*
279 pages Paperback

**8966   Career Perspectives: Interviews with Blindand Visually
         Impaired Professionals**
American Foundation for the Blind/AFB Press
2 Penn Plaza
Suite 1102
New York, NY   10121   212-502-7600
                                               800-232-5463
                                          Fax: 888-545-8331
                                            afbinfo@afb.net
                                                    afb.org
Carl R. Augusto, President & Chief Executive Officer
Rick Bozeman, Finance Director, Chief Financial Officer
Kelly Bleach, Chief Administrative Officer
Stacy Rollins, Executive Administrative Assistant to the President
Profiles of 20 successful archivers who describe in their own
words what it takes to pursue and attain professional success in a
sighted world. Available in large print, cassette and braille.
$19.95
96 pages
ISBN 0-891281-70-2

8967   Careers in Blindness Rehabilitation Services
Mississippi State University
P.O.Box 6189
Mississippi State, MS   39762   662-325-2001
                                          Fax: 662-325-8989
                                          TTY:662-325-2694
                                        nrtc@colled.msstate.edu
                                           www.blind.msstate.edu

Jacqui Bybee, Research Associate II
Douglas Bedsaul, Research and Training Coordinator
Anne Carter, Research and Training Coordinator
Brenda Cavenaugh, Ph.D., Research Professor
In a follow-up study in a series examining the substantial un-
der-representation of African Americans as professionals in
blindness services, researchers questioned college students
about their knowledge, opinions and interests in blindness services. *$15.00*
54 pages Paperback

8968   Cataracts
National Association for Visually Handicapped
111 East 59th Street
New York, NY   10022-1202   212-821-9384
                                               800-829-0500
                                          Fax: 212-821-9707
                                            info@lighthouse.org
                                           lighthouse.org/navh
Mark G. Ackermann, President / CEO
A booklet offering information about Cataracts, diagnosis and
treatment of this common condition. LightHouse acquired
NAVH. *$ 4.00*

**8969   Characteristics, Services, & Outcomes of Rehab. Consumers
         who are Blind/Visually Impaired**
Mississippi State University
P.O.Box 6189
Mississippi State, MS   39762   662-325-2001
                                          Fax: 662-325-8989
                                          TTY:662-325-2694
                                        nrtc@colled.msstate.edu
                                           www.blind.msstate.edu

Jacqui Bybee, Research Associate II
Douglas Bedsaul, Research and Training Coordinator
Anne Carter, Research and Training Coordinator
Brenda Cavenaugh, Ph.D., Research Professor
Issues regarding the efficacy of separate state agencies providing
specialized vocational rehabilitation (VR) services to consumers
who are blind have generated spirited discussions within the rehabilitation community throughout the history of the state-fed-
eral program. In this monograph, RRTC researches report results
of their investigation of services provided to blind consumers in
separate and general (combined) rehabilitation agencies. *$20.00*
45 pages Paperback

8970   Childhood Glaucoma: A Reference Guide for Families
NAPVI
1 North Lexington Avenue
White Plains, NY   10601   617-972-7441
                                               800-562-6265
                                          Fax: 617-972-7444
                                          napvi@guildhealth.org
                                               www.napvi.org

Julie Urban, President
Venetia Hayden, Vice President
Susan LaVenture, Executive Director
Randi Sher, Secretary
A vauluable tutorial and resource covering all aspects from genet-
ics through diagnosis, sibling relationships and more.
36 pages

8971   Children with Visual Impairments: A Guide For Parents
American Foundation for the Blind/AFB Press
105 East 22nd Street
New York, NY   10010   212-949-4800
                                           childrensaidsociety.org
William D. Weisberg, Ph.D., President & CEO
Drema Brown, VP of Education
Katherine Eckstein, Chief of Staff
Beverly Colon, VP for Health & Wellness
Written by parents and professional, this book presents a compre-
hensive overview of the issues that are crucial to the healthy de-
velopment of children with mild to severe visual impaiments. It
also offers insight from parents about coping with the emotional
aspects of raising a child with special needs. *$16.95*
416 pages
ISBN 0-933149-36-0

8972   Classification of Impaired Vision
National Association for Visually Handicapped
111 East 59th Street
New York, NY   10022-1202   212-821-9384
                                           800-829-0500
                                           Fax: 212-821-9707
                                           info@lighthouse.org
                                           lighthouse.org/navh
Mark G. Ackermann, President / CEO
Designed to provide a foundation for a better understanding of
teaching reading, writing, and listning skills to students with vi-
sual impairments from preschool age through adult levels. Light-
House acquired NAVH. *$57.95*
322 pages
ISBN 0-398066-93-2

8973   Communication Skills for Visually Impaired Learners
Charles C. Thomas
2600 S First St
Springfield, IL   62704-4730   217-789-8980
                                           800-258-8980
                                           Fax: 217-789-9130
                                           books@ccthomas.com
                                           www.ccthomas.com
Michael P. Thomas, President
Randall Harley, Author
Mila Truan, Author
LaRhea Sanford, Author
This book has been designed to provide a foundation for a better
understanding of teaching reading, writing, and listening skills to
students with visual impairments from preschool age through
adult levels. The plan of the book incorporates the latest research
findings with the practical experiences learned in the classroom.
$57.95
322 pages Paperback
ISBN 0-398066-93-2

**8974   Comprehensive Examination of Barriers to Employment
         Among Persons who are Blind or Impaire**
Mississippi State University
P.O.Box 6189
Mississippi State, MS   39762   662-325-2001
                                           Fax: 662-325-8989
                                           TTY:662-325-2694
                                           nrtc@colled.msstate.edu
                                           www.blind.msstate.edu
Jacqui Bybee, Research Associate II
Douglas Bedsaul, Research and Training Coordinator
Anne Carter, Research and Training Coordinator
Brenda Cavenaugh, Ph.D., Research Professor
A multi-phase research project designed to: identify barriers to
employment; identify and develop innovative successful strategies to overcome these barriers; develop methods for others to
utilize these strategies; disseminate this information to rehabilitation providers; replicate the use of selected strategies in other
settings. *$20.00*
90 pages Paperback

**8975   Contrasting Characteristics of Blind and Visually Impaired
         Clients**
Mississippi State University
P.O.Box 6189
Mississippi State, MS   39762   662-325-2001
                                           Fax: 662-325-8989
                                           TTY:662-325-2694
                                           nrtc@colled.msstate.edu
                                           www.blind.msstate.edu
Jacqui Bybee, Research Associate II
Douglas Bedsaul, Research and Training Coordinator
Anne Carter, Research and Training Coordinator
Brenda Cavenaugh, Ph.D., Research Professor
This report examines cases in the National Blindness and Low Vision Employment Database to identify and profile environmental
and personal characteristics of clients who are blind or visually
impaired and who were achieving successful and unsuccessful retention of competitive jobs. A total of 787 cases were analyzed.
$15.00
44 pages Paperback

8976   Dancing Cheek to Cheek
Blind Children's Center
4120 Marathon Street
Los Angeles, CA   90029-3584   323-664-2153
                                           800-222-3567
                                           Fax: 323-665-3828
                                           info@blindchildrenscenter.org
                                           www.blindchildrenscenter.org
Scott E. Schaldenbrand, President
Mark Correa, Board Member
Midge Horton, Executive Director
Pamela Lansky, Co-Author
Beginning social, play and language interactions. *$ 10.00*
23 pages

**8977   Development of Social Skills by Blind and Visually Impaired
         Students**
American Foundation for the Blind/AFB Press
2 Penn Plaza
Suite 1102
New York, NY   10121   212-502-7600
                                           800-232-5463
                                           Fax: 888-545-8331
                                           afbinfo@afb.net
                                           www.afb.org
Carl R. Augusto, President & Chief Executive Officer
Rick Bozeman, Finance Director, Chief Financial Officer
Kelly Bleach, Chief Administrative Officer
Stacy Rollins, Executive Administrative Assistant to the President
Offers an examination of the social interactions of blind and visu-
ally impaired children in mainstreamed settings and the commu-
nity that highlights the need to teach social interaction skills to
children and provide them with support. Paperback. *$45.95*
232 pages
ISBN 0-891282-17-4

8978   Diabetic Retinopathy
National Association for Visually Handicapped
111 East 59th Street
New York, NY   10022-1202   212-821-9384
                                           800-829-0500
                                           Fax: 212-821-9707
                                           info@lighthouse.org
                                           lighthouse.org/navh
Mark G. Ackermann, President / CEO
A booklet offering information about Diabetic Retinopathy.
LightHouse acquired NAVH.

8979 **Diversity and Visual Impairment: The Influence of Race, Gender, Religion and Ethnicity**
American Foundation for the Blind
2 Penn Plaza
Suite 1102
New York, NY 10121

212-502-7600
800-232-5463
Fax: 888-545-8331
afbinfo@afb.net
www.afb.org

Carl R. Augusto, President & Chief Executive Officer
Rick Bozeman, Finance Director, Chief Financial Officer
Kelly Bleach, Chief Administrative Officer
Stacy Rollins, Executive Administrative Assistant to the President
Cultural, social, ethnic, gender, and religious issues can influence the way an individual perceives and copes with a visual impairment. *$45.95*
480 pages
ISBN 0-891283-83-8

8980 **Do You Remember the Color Blue: The Questi Ons Children Ask About Blindness**
Viking Books
375 Hudson Street
New York, NY 10014-3657

212-366-2000
Fax: 212-366-2933
ecommerce@us.penguingroup.com
www.us.penguingroup.com

John Makinson, Chairman & CEO
The author answers thirteen thought-provoking questions that children have asked her over the years about being blind.
78 pages
ISBN 0-670880-43-4

8981 **Don't Lose Sight of Glaucoma**
National Eye Institute
2020 Vision Place
Building 31 Room 6a32
Bethesda, MD 20892-3655

301-496-5248
800-869-2020
Fax: 301-402-1065
2020@nei.nih.gov
www.nei.nih.gov

8982 **Early Focus: Working with Young Children Who Are Blind or Visually Impaired & Their Families**
American Foundation for the Blind/AFB Press
2 Penn Plaza
Suite 1102
New York, NY 10121

212-502-7600
800-232-5463
Fax: 888-545-8331
afbinfo@afb.net
www.afb.org

Carl R. Augusto, President & Chief Executive Officer
Rick Bozeman, Finance Director, Chief Financial Officer
Kelly Bleach, Chief Administrative Officer
Stacy Rollins, Executive Administrative Assistant to the President
Describes early intervention techniques used with blind and visually impaired children and stresses the benefits of family involvement and transdisciplinary teamwork. Paperback. *$32.95*
176 pages
ISBN 0-891282-15-7

8983 **Encyclopedia of Blindness and Vision Impairment Second Edition**
Facts on File
132 West 31st Street
17th Floor
New York, NY 10001

800-322-8755
Fax: 800-678-3633
CustServ@InfobaseLearning.com
www.factsonfile.com

Jill Sardenga, Author
Susan Shelly, Co-Author
Alan Shelly MD, Co-Author
Scott M Steidl MD, Co-Author

Designed to provide both laymen and professionals with concise, practical information on the second most common disability in the U.S. *$65.00*
340 pages Hardcover
ISBN 0-816042-80-2

8984 **Equals in Partnership: Basic Rights for Families of Children with Blindness**
NAPVI
1 North Lexington Avenue
White Plains, NY 10601

617-972-7441
800-562-6265
Fax: 617-972-7444
napvi@guildhealth.org
www.napvi.org

Julie Urban, President
Venetia Hayden, Vice President
Susan LaVenture, Executive Director
Randi Sher, Secretary
A comprehensive compilation of educational advocacy materials to help parents better understand the special needs of their children with visual impairments and to assist them in accessing appropriate services for their children.

8985 **Eye Research News**
Research to Prevent Blindness
645 Madison Avenue
Floor 21
New York, NY 10022-1010

212-752-4333
800-621-0026
Fax: 212-688-6231
www.rpbusa.org

Diane S. Swift, Chair
Brian F. Hofland, PhD, President
David H. Brenner, VP & Secretary
Richard E. Baker, Treasurer & Asst. Secretary
Yearly publication from Research to Prevent Blindness. Free.
4 pages Yearly

8986 **Eye and Your Vision**
National Association for Visually Handicapped
111 East 59th Street
New York, NY 10022-1202

212-821-9384
800-829-0500
Fax: 212-821-9707
info@lighthouse.org
lighthouse.org/navh

Mark G. Ackermann, President / CEO
A large booklet offering information, with illustrations, on the eye. Includes information on protection of eyesight, how the eye works and vision disorders. Available in Russian and Spanish also. LightHouse acquired NAVH. *$5.00*

8987 **Eye-Q Test**
National Association for Visually Handicapped
111 East 59th Street
New York, NY 10022-1202

212-821-9384
800-829-0500
Fax: 212-821-9707
info@lighthouse.org
lighthouse.org/navh

Mark G. Ackermann, President / CEO
Five questions and answers to assist in knowing more about vision. Also available in Spanish and Russian. LightHouse acquired NAVH.

8988 Family Context and Disability Culture Reframing: Through the Looking Glass
Through the Looking Glass
3075 Adeline Street
Suite 120
Berkeley, CA 94703

510-848-1112
800-644-2666
Fax: 510-848-4445
tlg@lookingglass.org
www.lookingglass.org

Maureen Block, J.D., President
Thomas Spalding, Treasurer
Alice Nemon, Secretary
Mega Kirshbaum, Author
This article provides an overview of the issues and guiding perspectives underlying 'Through the Lookinglass' eighteen years of work with families. Available in braille, large print or cassette. *$2.00*
5 pages

8989 Family Guide to Vision Care (FG1)
American Optometric Association
243 North Lindbergh Boulevard
Floor 1
Saint Louis, MO 63141-7881

800-365-2219
aoa.org

David A. Cockrell, OD, President
Andrea P. Thau, OD, Vice President
Barry Barresi, Executive Director
Christopher Quinn, OD, Secretary-Treasurer
Offers information on the early developmental years of your vision, finding a family optometrist and how to take care of your eyesight through the learning years, the working years and the mature years.

8990 Family Guide: Growth & Development of the Partially Seeing Child
National Association for Visually Handicapped
111 East 59th Street
New York, NY 10022-1202

212-821-9384
800-829-0500
Fax: 212-821-9707
info@lighthouse.org
lighthouse.org/navh

Mark G. Ackermann, President / CEO
Offers information for parents and guidelines in raising a partially seeing child. LightHouse acquired NAVH. *$.60*

8991 Fathers: A Common Ground
Blind Children's Center
4120 Marathon Street
Los Angeles, CA 90029-3584

323-664-2153
800-222-3567
Fax: 323-665-3828
info@blindchildrenscenter.org
www.blindchildrenscenter.org

Scott E. Schaldenbrand, President
Mark Correa, Board Member
Midge Horton, Executive Director
Fernanda Schmitt PhD, Co-Author
Exploring the concerns and roles of fathers of children with visual impairments. *$10.00*
50 pages

8992 Fighting Blindness News
Foundation Fighting Blindness
7168 Columbia Gateway Drive
Suite 100
Columbia, MD 21046

410-423-0600
800-683-5555
Fax: 410-363-2393
TTY: 800-683-5551
info@FightBlindness.org
www.blindness.org

Gordon Gund, Chair
David Brent, Vice Chair of Research
Edward H. Gollob, President
Steve Alper, Director

Offers information on medical updates, donor programs, assistive devices, resources and clinical trial information for persons with visual impariments, blindness and retinal degenerative diseases.
2x Year

8993 First Steps
Blind Children's Center
4120 Marathon Street
Los Angeles, CA 90029-3584

323-664-2153
800-222-3567
Fax: 323-665-3828
info@blindchildrenscenter.org
www.blindchildrenscenter.org

Scott E. Schaldenbrand, President
Mark Correa, Board Member
Midge Horton, Executive Director
Ferdinand Schmitt PhD, Co-Author
A handbook for teaching young children who are visually impaired. Designed to assist students, professionals and parents working with children who are visually impaired. Visit our website for many publications addressing training very young children who are blind or visually impaired. *$35.00*
203 pages

8994 Foundations of Orientation and Mobility
American Foundation for the Blind/AFB Press
2 Penn Plaza
Suite 1102
New York, NY 10121

212-502-7600
800-232-5463
Fax: 888-545-8331
afbinfo@afb.net
www.afb.org

Carl R. Augusto, President & Chief Executive Officer
Rick Bozeman, Finance Director, Chief Financial Officer
Kelly Bleach, Chief Administrative Officer
Stacy Rollins, Executive Administrative Assistant to the President
This text has been updated and revised and includes current research from a variety of disciplines, an international perspective, and expanded contents on low vision, aging, multiple disabilities, accessibility, program design and adaptive technology from more that 30 eminent subject experts. *$79.95*
775 pages
ISBN 0-891289-46-3

8995 Foundations of Rehabilitation Counseling with Persons Who Are Blind r Visually Impaired
American Foundation for the Blind/AFB Press
2 Penn Plaza
Suite 1102
New York, NY 10121

212-502-7600
800-232-5463
Fax: 888-545-8331
afbinfo@afb.net
www.afb.org

Carl R. Augusto, President & Chief Executive Officer
Rick Bozeman, Finance Director, Chief Financial Officer
Kelly Bleach, Chief Administrative Officer
Stacy Rollins, Executive Administrative Assistant to the President
Rehabilitation professionals have long recognized that the needs of people who are blind or visually impaired are unique and requie a special knowledge and expertise to provide and corrdinate rehabilitation services. *$59.95*
477 pages
ISBN 0-891289-45-3

8996 General Facts and Figures on Blindness
Prevent Blindness America
211 West Wacker Drive
Suite 1700
Chicago, IL 60606

800-331-2020
info@preventblindness.org
www.preventblindness.org

Paul G. Howes, Chairman
Hugh R. Parry, President & CEO,Prevent Blindness America
Jerome Desserich, Vice President & Chief Financial Officer
Danielle Disch, Development Manager

8997 Get a Wiggle On
American Alliance for Health, Phys. Ed. & Dance
1900 Association Drive
Reston, VA 20191-1598
703-476-3400
800-213-7193
Fax: 703-476-9527
aapar@aahperd.org
aahperd.org

Dolly D. Lambdin, President
E. Paul Roetert, CEO
Marybell Avery, Director
Frances E. Cleland, Director
Gives teachers and parents practical suggestions for helping blind and visually impaired infants grow and learn like other children. *$5.00*
80 pages
ISBN 0-88314-77-2

8998 Gift of Sight
RP Foundation Fighting Blindness
1401 W Mount Royal Ave
Baltimore, MD 21217-4245
410-225-9409
800-683-5555
Fax: 410-225-3936

8999 Glaucoma
Glaucoma Research Foundation
251 Post Street
Suite 600
San Francisco, CA 94108
415-986-3162
800-826-6693
Fax: 415-986-3763
question@glaucoma.org
glaucoma.org

Andrew L. Iwach, MD, Chair
Robert L. Stamper, MD, Vice Chair
Thomas M. Brunner, President and CEO
Bill Stewart, Secretary
Offers information on what glaucoma is, the causes, treatments, types of glaucoma, eye exams and prevention.

9000 Glaucoma: The Sneak Thief of Sight
National Association for Visually Handicapped
Fl 6
22 W 21st St
New York, NY 10010-6943
212-242-4438
800-3 C-NCOS
Fax: 631-736-0371
customerservice@cancos.com
cancos.com

Denise Green, Owner
A pamphlet describing the disease, treatment and medications. Also available in Russian and Spanish. Revised in 1999. *$3.50*

9001 Guidelines and Games for Teaching Efficient Braille Reading
American Foundation for the Blind/AFB Press
2 Penn Plaza
Suite 1102
New York, NY 10121
212-502-7600
800-232-5463
Fax: 888-545-8331
afbinfo@afb.net
www.afb.org

Carl R. Augusto, President & Chief Executive Officer
Rick Bozeman, Finance Director, Chief Financial Officer
Kelly Bleach, Chief Administrative Officer
Stacy Rollins, Executive Administrative Assistant to the President
Based on research in the areas of rapid reading and precision teaching, these guidelines represent a unique adaptation of a general reading program to the needs of braille readers. Paperback. *$24.95*
116 pages Paperback
ISBN 0-891281-05-4

9002 Guidelines for Comprehensive Low Vision Care
National Association for Visually Handicapped
111 East 59th Street
New York, NY 10022-1202
212-821-9384
800-829-0500
Fax: 212-821-9707
info@lighthouse.org
lighthouse.org/navh

Mark G. Ackermann, President / CEO
A description of the proper method to conduct a low vision evaluation.LightHouse acquired NAVH. *$.50*

9003 Handbook for Itinerant and Resource Teachers of Blind Students
National Federation of the Blind
200 East Wells St
Baltimore, MD 21230-4914
410-659-9314
nfb@iamdigex.net

Doris Willoughby, Author
Sharon L Monthei, Co-Author
The Handbook provides help to teachers, school administrators or other school personnel that have experience with blind or visually impaired students. The Handbook devotes 45 pages to Braille and how to teach Braille for parents and teachers. There are other chapters offering information on the law, physical education, fitting in socially, testing and evaluation, home economics, daily living skills and more. *$23.00*
533 pages Softcover
ISBN 0-962412-20-1

9004 Handbook of Information for Members of the Achromatopsia Network
P.O.Box 214
Berkeley, CA 94701-214
510-540-4700
Fax: 510-540-4767
futterman@achromat.org
www.achromat.org

9005 Health Care Professionals Who Are Blind or Visually Impaired
American Foundation for the Blind
2 Penn Plaza
Suite 1102
New York, NY 10121
212-502-7600
800-232-5463
Fax: 888-545-8331
afbinfo@afb.net
afb.org

Carl R. Augusto, President & Chief Executive Officer
Rick Bozeman, Finance Director, Chief Financial Officer
Kelly Bleach, Chief Administrative Officer
Stacy Rollins, Executive Administrative Assistant to the President
This resource is essential reading for older students and young adults who are blind or visually impaired, their families, and the professionals who work with them. *$21.95*
160 pages
ISBN 0-891283-88-9

9006 Heart to Heart
Blind Children's Center
4120 Marathon Street
Los Angeles, CA 90029-3584
323-664-2153
800-222-3567
Fax: 323-665-3828
info@blindchildrenscenter.org
www.blindchildrenscenter.org

Scott E. Schaldenbrand, President
Mark Correa, Board Member
Midge Horton, Executive Director
Dori Hayashi MA, Co-Author
Parents of children who are blind and partially sighted talk about their feelings. *$10.00*
12 pages

9007   Heartbreak of Being A Little Bit Blind
National Association for Visually Handicapped
111 East 59th Street
New York, NY   10022-1202

212-821-9384
800-829-0500
Fax: 212-821-9707
info@lighthouse.org
lighthouse.org/navh

Mark G. Ackermann, President / CEO
Summary of what it means to have impaired vision; includes illustrations. LightHouse acquired NAVH.

9008   Helen Keller National Center Newsletter
141 Middle Neck Road
Sands Point, NY   11050

516-944-8900
800-225-0411
Fax: 516-944-7302
hkncinfo@hknc.org
www.hknc.org

Joseph McNulty, Executive Director
The center provides evaluation and training in vocational skills, adaptive technology and computer skills, orientation and mobility, independent living, communication, speech-language skills, creative arts, fitness and leisure activities.

9009   Helping the Visually Impaired Child with Developmental Problems
Teachers College Press
1234 Amsterdam Avenue
New York, NY   10027

212-678-3929
800-575-6566
Fax: 212-678-4149
tcpress@tc.columbia.edu
www.teacherscollegepress.com

Mary Lynch, Manager
Brian Ellerbeck, Executive Acquisitions Editor
Marie Ellen Larcada, Senior Acquisitions Editor
Emily Spangler, Acquisitions Editor
This book aims to explore the human consequences of severe visual problems combined with other handicaps. The application of child development research to educational interventions, the need for educational and rehabilitative services that serve the human and the special needs of children and their families and the promise of technology in helping to expand communicative possibilities are also discussed. *$18.95*
216 pages Paperback
ISBN 0-807729-02-7

9010   History and Use of Braille
American Council of the Blind
2200 Wilson Boulevard
Suite 650
Arlington, VA   22201-3354

202-467-5081
800-424-8666
Fax: 703-465-5085
info@acb.org
acb.org

Kim Charlson, President
Jeff Thom, 1st Vice President
Melanie Brunson, Executive Director
A system of touch reading and writing for blind persons in which raised dots represent the letters of the alphabet.

9011   How to Thrive, Not Just Survive
American Foundation for the Blind/AFB Press
2 Penn Plaza
Suite 1102
New York, NY   10121

212-502-7600
800-232-5463
Fax: 888-545-8331
afbinfo@afb.net
www.afb.org

Carl R. Augusto, President & Chief Executive Officer
Rick Bozeman, Finance Director, Chief Financial Officer
Kelly Bleach, Chief Administrative Officer
Practical, hands-on guide for parents, teachers, and everyone involved in helping children develop the skills necessary for socialization, orientations and mobility, and leisure and recreational

activities. Some of the subjects covered are eating, dressing, personal hygiene, self-esteem and etiquette. *$24.95*
104 pages Paperback
ISBN 0-89128 -48-7

9012   Hub
SPOKES Unlimited
1006 Main Street
Klamath Fals, OR   97601

541-883-7547
Fax: 541-885-2469
spokesunlimited.org

Wendy Howard, Executive Director
Celeste Wolf, Clerical Support Specialist II
Newsletter on rehabilitation, peer counseling, blindness, visual impairments, information and referral.

9013   If Blindness Comes
National Federation of the Blind
200 East Wells St
Baltimore, MD   21230-4914

410-659-9314
Fax: 410-685-5653
nfb@iamdigex.net
www.nfb.org

Kenneth Jerrigan, Editor
An introduction to issues relating to vision loss and provides a positive, supportive philosophy about blindness. It is a general information book which includes answers to many common questions about blindness, information about services and programs for the blind and resource listings. Contact the Materials Center.

9014   If Blindness Strikes Don't Strike Out
2600 South 1st Street
Springfield, IL   62704

217-789-8980
800-258-8980
Fax: 217-789-9130
books@ccthomas.com
www.ccthomas.com

Bob Stork, Owner

9015   Imagining the Possibilities: Creative Approaches to Orientation and Mobility Instructio
American Foundation for the Blind
2 Penn Plaza
Suite 1102
New York, NY   10121

212-502-7600
800-232-5463
Fax: 888-545-8331
afbinfo@afb.net
afb.org

Carl R. Augusto, President & Chief Executive Officer
Rick Bozeman, Finance Director, Chief Financial Officer
Kelly Bleach, Chief Administrative Officer
Innovative and varied approaches to O&M techniques and teaching and dynamic suggestions on how to analyze learning styles are just some of the important topics included. *$49.95*
378 pages
ISBN 0-891283-82-X

9016   Increasing Literacy Levels: Final Report
Mississippi State University
P.O.Box 6189
Mississippi State, MS   39762

662-325-2001
Fax: 662-325-8989
TTY:662-325-2694
nrtc@colled.msstate.edu
www.blind.msstate.edu

Jacqui Bybee, Research Associate II
Douglas Bedsaul, Research and Training Coordinator
Anne Carter, Research and Training Coordinator
Brenda Cavenaugh, Ph.D., Research Professor
This study is composed of three research projects to identify and analyze the appropriate use of and instruction in Braille, optical devices and other technologies as they relate to literacy and employment of individuals who are blind or visually impaired. *$20.00*
148 pages Paperback

9017   Information Access Project
National Federation of the Blind
200 East Wells St
Baltimore, MD   21230-4914   410-659-9314
                                    Fax: 410-685-5653
                                         nfb@nfb.org
                                              nfb.org
Marc Maurer, President
Assists entities covered by the ADA in finding methods for converting visually displayed information, such as flyers, brochures and pamphlets, to formats accessible to individuals who are visually impaired.

9018   Information on Glaucoma
Glaucoma Research Foundation
251 Post Street
Suite 600
San Francisco, CA   94108   415-986-3162
                                          800-826-6693
                                    Fax: 415-986-3763
                                 question@glaucoma.org
                                    www.glaucoma.org
Andrew L. Iwach, MD, Chair
Robert L. Stamper, MD, Vice Chair
Thomas M. Brunner, President and CEO
Bill Stewart, Secretary

9019   Intervention Practices in the Retention of Competitive Employment
Mississippi State University
P.O.Box 6189
Mississippi State, MS   39762   662-325-2001
                                    Fax: 662-325-8989
                                    TTY:662-325-2694
                                 nrtc@colled.msstate.edu
                                  www.blind.msstate.edu
Jacqui Bybee, Research Associate II
Douglas Bedsaul, Research and Training Coordinator
Anne Carter, Research and Training Coordinator
Brenda Cavenaugh, Ph.D., Research Professor
This study investigated the methods by which an individual can retain competitive employment after the onset of a significant vision loss. Interviews were conducted with 89 rehabilitation counselors across the US Strategies that contribute to successful job retention were identified as well as best rehabilitation practices in job retention. *$15.00*
60 pages Paperback

9020   Know Your Eye
American Council of the Blind
2200 Wilson Boulevard
Suite 650
Arlington, VA   22201-3354   202-467-5081
                                          800-424-8666
                                    Fax: 703-465-5085
                                          info@acb.org
                                              acb.org
Kim Charlson, President
Jeff Thom, 1st Vice President
Melanie Brunson, Executive Director

9021   Large Print Loan Library
National Association for Visually Handicapped
111 East 59th Street
New York, NY   10022-1202   212-821-9384
                                          800-829-0500
                                    Fax: 212-821-9707
                                     info@lighthouse.org
                                    lighthouse.org/navh
Mark G. Ackermann, President / CEO
A huge large print catalog of all the publications, fiction and non-fiction, cassette tapes, books-on-tape and videos available for the visually impaired from the loan library of the National Association for the Visually Handicapped. LightHouse acquired NAVH.

9022   Large Print Loan Library Catalog
National Association for Visually Handicapped
111 East 59th Street
New York, NY   10022-1202   212-821-9384
                                          800-829-0500
                                    Fax: 212-821-9707
                                     info@lighthouse.org
                                    lighthouse.org/navh
Mark G. Ackermann, President / CEO
Listing of over 7,000 commercially published and NAVH large print books available through NAVH on a loan basis. Includes a limited selection of titles available for purchase. LightHouse acquired NAVH.

9023   Large Print Recipies for a Healthy Life
123601 Wilshire
Los Angeles, CA   90025   310-826-8280
                                          800-481-EYES
                                    Fax: 310-458-8179
Judith Caditz PhD, Author
   $21.95
   283 pages
   ISBN 0-962236-82-9

9024   Learning to Play
Blind Children's Center
4120 Marathon Street
Los Angeles, CA   90029-3584   323-664-2153
                                          800-222-3567
                                    Fax: 323-665-3828
                               info@blindchildrenscenter.org
                               www.blindchildrenscenter.org
Scott E. Schaldenbrand, President
Mark Correa, Board Member
Midge Horton, Executive Director
Presenting play activities to the pre-school child who is visually impaired. *$10.00*
12 pages

9025   Let's Eat
Blind Children's Center
4120 Marathon Street
Los Angeles, CA   90029-3584   323-664-2153
                                          800-222-3567
                                    Fax: 323-665-3828
                               info@blindchildrenscenter.org
                               www.blindchildrenscenter.org
Scott E. Schaldenbrand, President
Mark Correa, Board Member
Midge Horton, Executive Director
Feeding a child with visual impairment. *$10.00*
28 pages

9026   Library Services for the Blind
South Carolina State University
300 College Street NorthEast
P.O. Box 7491
Orangeburg, SC 29117   803-536-7045
                                    Fax: 803-536-8902
                                     reference@scsu.edu
                                       library.scsu.edu
Adrienne C. Webber, Dean, Library/Information Services
Ramona S. Evans, Administrative Specialist
Ruth A. Hodges, Reference & Information Specialist
Wanda L. Priester, Library Technical Asst.
News and information on developments in library services for readers who are blind and physically disabled.

9027 Lifestyles of Employed Legally Blind People
Mississippi State University
P.O.Box 6189
Mississippi State, MS   39762   662-325-2001
                                    Fax: 662-325-8989
                                    TTY:662-325-2694
                                    nrtc@colled.msstate.edu
                                    www.blind.msstate.edu

Jacqui Bybee, Research Associate II
Douglas Bedsaul, Research and Training Coordinator
Anne Carter, Research and Training Coordinator
Brenda Cavenaugh, Ph.D., Research Professor
Results from a telephone survey show that visually impaired respondents are involved in a wide variety of activities with little
restrictions on their range of activities. Sighted respondents
tended to spend more time in child care, obtaining goods and services, attending to self-care activities and engaging in social activities, while visually impaired respondents spent more time in
education and passive activities. This report is a study of expenditures and time use. *$ 10.00*
193 pages Paperback

9028 Lion
Lion's Clubs International
300 West 22nd Street
Oak Brook, IL   60523-8842   630-571-5466
                                    Fax: 630-571-8890
                                    TTY:630-571-6533
                                    www.lionsclubs.org/

Joseph Preston, International President
Jitsuhiro Yamada, 1st Vice President
Robert E. Corlew, 2nd Vice President
Peter Lynch, Executive Director
Publication for the blind.

9029 Living with Achromatopsia
P.O.Box 214
Berkeley, CA   94701-214   510-540-4700
                                    Fax: 510-540-4767
                                    www.achromat.org

Frances Futterman, Author
Consists entirely of comments from persons who know firsthand
about living with achromatopsia.

**9030 Low Vision Questions and Answers: Definitions, Devices,
Services**
American Foundation for the Blind/AFB Press
2 Penn Plaza
Suite 1102
New York, NY   10121   212-502-7600
                                    800-232-5463
                                    Fax: 888-545-8331
                                    afbinfo@afb.net
                                    afb.org

Carl R. Augusto, President & Chief Executive Officer
Rick Bozeman, Chief Financial Officer
Kelly Bleach, Chief Administrative Officer
Stacy Rollins, Executive Administrative Assistant to the President
What does low vision mean? What do low vision services cost?
What diseases cause low vision? Answers to these and other ques-
tions are presented in a comprehensive format with accompany-
ing photographs. $50.00/pack of 25.
21 pages Pamphlet
ISBN 0-891281-96-7

9031 Low Vision: Reflections of the Past, Issues for the Future
American Foundation for the Blind/AFB Press
2 Penn Plaza
Suite 1102
New York, NY   10121   212-502-7600
                                    800-232-5463
                                    Fax: 888-545-8331
                                    afbinfo@afb.net
                                    www.afb.org

Carl R. Augusto, President & Chief Executive Officer
Rick Bozeman, Chief Financial Officer
Kelly Bleach, Chief Administrative Officer
Stacy Rollins, Executive Administrative Assistant to the President

Background papers and a strategies section are used to identify
the shifting needs of visually impaired persons and the resources
that may be needed to address them. Paperback. *$34.95*
Paperback
ISBN 0-891282-18-1

9032 Mainstreaming and the American Dream
American Foundation for the Blind/AFB Press
2 Penn Plaza
Suite 1102
New York, NY   10121   212-502-7600
                                    800-232-5463
                                    Fax: 888-545-8331
                                    afbinfo@afb.net
                                    www.afb.org

Carl R. Augusto, President & Chief Executive Officer
Rick Bozeman, Chief Financial Officer
Kelly Bleach, Chief Administrative Officer
Stacy Rollins, Executive Administrative Assistant to the President
Based on in-depth interviews with parents and professionals, this
research monograph presents information on the needs and aspi-
rations of parents of blind and visually impaired children. Paper-
back. *$34.95*
256 pages Paperback
ISBN 0-891281-91-7

9033 Mainstreaming the Visually Impaired Child
NAPVI
1 North Lexington Avenue
White Plains, NY   10601   617-972-7441
                                    800-562-6265
                                    Fax: 617-972-7444
                                    napvi@guildhealth.org
                                    www.napvi.org

Julie Urban, President
Venetia Hayden, Vice President
Susan LaVenture, Executive Director
Randi Sher, Secretary
A unique, informative guide for teachers and educational profes-
sionals that work with the visually impaired. *$10.00*
121 pages Paper

9034 Making Life More Livable
American Foundation for the Blind
2 Penn Plaza
Suite 1102
New York, NY   10121   212-502-7600
                                    800-232-5463
                                    Fax: 888-545-8331
                                    afbinfo@afb.net
                                    www.afb.org

Carl R. Augusto, President & Chief Executive Officer
Rick Bozeman, Chief Financial Officer
Kelly Bleach, Chief Administrative Officer
Stacy Rollins, Executive Administrative Assistant to the President
Shows how simple adaptations in the home and environment can
make a big difference in the lives of blind and visually impaired
older persons. The suggestions offered are numerous and specific, ranging from how to mark food cans for greater visibility to
how to get out of the shower safley. Large print. *$24.95*
128 pages
ISBN 0-891283-87-0

**9035 Meeting the Needs of People with Vision Loss:
Multidisciplinary Perspective**
Resources for Rehabilitation
22 Bonad Road
Winchester, MA   01890   781-368-9080
                                    Fax: 781-368-9096
                                    orders@rfr.org
                                    www.rfr.org

Susan L Greenblatt, Editor
Written by rehabilitation professionals, physicians, and a sociologist, this book discusses how to provide appropriate information
and how to serve special populations. Chapters on the role of the

family, diabetes and vision loss, special needs of children and adolescents, adults with hearing and vision loss. *$29.95*
ISBN 0-929718-07-0

9036 Model Program Operation Manual: Business Enterprise Program Supervisors
Mississippi State University
P.O.Box 6189
Mississippi State, MS 39762 662-325-2001
Fax: 662-325-8989
TTY:662-325-2694
nrtc@colled.msstate.edu
www.blind.msstate.edu
Jacqui Bybee, Research Associate II
Douglas Bedsaul, Research and Training Coordinator
Anne Carter, Research and Training Coordinator
Brenda Cavenaugh, Ph.D., Research Professor
This monograph serves as a Model Program Operation Manual for Business Enterprise Program Supervisors who administer Randolph-Sheppard vending facilities under the Randolph-Sheppard Act. A wide variety of topics are covered including the role of the State Committee of Blind Venders, the role and responsibilities of the Vending Facility Operator, model qualification, for potential Facility Managers, guidelines for location of vending facilities and policies for closing vending facilities. *$20.00*
199 pages Paperback

9037 More Alike Than Different: Blind and Visually Impaired Children
American Foundation for the Blind/AFB Press
2 Penn Plaza
Suite 1102
New York, NY 10121 212-502-7600
800-232-5463
Fax: 888-545-8331
afborders@abdintl.com
www.afb.org
Carl R. Augusto, President & Chief Executive Officer
Rick Bozeman, Chief Financial Officer
Kelly Bleach, Chief Administrative Officer
Stacy Rollins, Executive Administrative Assistant to the President
Offers photographs of blind and visually impaired children around the world learning to read and write, travel independently and performing basic living skills. Covers the most recent technological advances and demonstrates the universality of educational needs and goals. Paperback. $100.00/pack of 25.
ISBN 0-891281-69-0

9038 Mothers with Visual Impairments who are Raising Young Children
American Foundation for the Blind/AFB Press
2 Penn Plaza
Suite 1102
New York, NY 10121 212-502-7600
800-232-5463
Fax: 888-545-8331
afbinfo@afb.net
www.afb.org
Carl R. Augusto, President & Chief Executive Officer
Rick Bozeman, Chief Financial Officer
Kelly Bleach, Chief Administrative Officer
Stacy Rollins, Executive Administrative Assistant to the President
Available in braille, large print or cassette. *$2.00*
16 pages

9039 Move With Me
Blind Children's Center
4120 Marathon Street
Los Angeles, CA 90029-3584 323-664-2153
800-222-3567
Fax: 323-665-3828
info@blindchildrenscenter.org
www.blindchildrenscenter.org
Scott E. Schaldenbrand, President
Mark Correa, Board Member
Midge Horton, Executive Director
Nancy Chernus-Mansfield MA, Co-Author

A parent's guide to movement development for babies who are visually impaired. *$10.00*
12 pages

9040 National Eye Institute
National Institute of Health
31 Center Drive MSC 2510
Bethesda, MD 20892-2510 301-496-5248
Fax: 301-402-1065
2020@nei.nih.gov
www.nei.nih.gov

9041 Orientation and Mobility Primer for Families and Young Children
American Foundation for the Blind/AFB Press
2 Penn Plaza
Suite 1102
New York, NY 10121 212-502-7600
800-232-5463
Fax: 888-545-8331
afbinfo@afb.net
www.afb.org
Carl R. Augusto, President & Chief Executive Officer
Rick Bozeman, Chief Financial Officer
Kelly Bleach, Chief Administrative Officer
Stacy Rollins, Executive Administrative Assistant to the President
Practical information for helping a child learn about his or her environment right from the start. Covers sensory training, concept development and orientation skills. Paperback. *$14.95*
48 pages
ISBN 0-891281-57-6

9042 Out of the Corner of My Eye: Living with Vision Loss in Later Life
American Foundation for the Blind/AFB Press
2 Penn Plaza
Suite 1102
New York, NY 10121 212-502-7600
800-232-5463
Fax: 888-545-8331
www.afb.org
Carl R. Augusto, President & Chief Executive Officer
Rick Bozeman, Chief Financial Officer
Kelly Bleach, Chief Administrative Officer
Stacy Rollins, Executive Administrative Assistant to the President
A personal account of students' vision loss and subsequent adjustment that is full of practical advice and cheerful encouragement, told by an 87 year old retired college teacher who has maintained her independence and zest for life. Available in paperback or on audio cassette. *$23.95*
120 pages
ISBN 0-891281-82-1

9043 Out of the Corner of My Eye: Living with Macular Degeneration
American Foundation for the Blind/AFB Press
2 Penn Plaza
Suite 1102
New York, NY 10121 212-502-7600
800-232-5463
Fax: 888-545-8331
afbinfo@afb.net
www.afb.org
Carl R. Augusto, President & Chief Executive Officer
Rick Bozeman, Chief Financial Officer
Kelly Bleach, Chief Administrative Officer
Stacy Rollins, Executive Administrative Assistant to the President
A personal account of students' vision loss and subsequent adjustment that is full of practical advice and cheerful encouragement, told by an 87 year old retired college teacher who has maintained her independence and zest for life. *$29.95*
168 pages Paperback
ISBN 0-891238-31-2

9044   Pain Erasure: the Bonnie Prudden Way
Ballantine Books
1540 Broadway
New York, NY   10036-4039   212-751-2600
                                        Fax: 212-572-4949

Bonnie Prudden, Author
Revolutionary breakthrough in pain relief involves trigger
points-tender areas where muscles have been damaged from falls,
childhood ailments, poor posture, and the stresses of daily life.

9045   Patient's Guide to Visual Aids and Illumination
National Association for Visually Handicapped
111 East 59th Street
New York, NY   10022-1202   212-821-9384
                                             800-829-0500
                                        Fax: 212-821-9707
                                        info@lighthouse.org
                                        lighthouse.org/navh

Mark G. Ackermann, President / CEO
A reference booklet offering information on aids for the visually
impaired. LightHouse acquired NAVH. *$.75*

9046   Pediatric Visual Diagnosis Fact Sheets
Blind Children's Center
4120 Marathon Street
Los Angeles, CA   90029-3584   323-664-2153
                                             800-222-3567
                                        Fax: 323-665-3828
                                     info@blindchildrenscenter.org
                                        blindchildrenscenter.org

Scott E. Schaldenbrand, President
Mark Correa, Board Member
Midge Horton, Executive Director
Collection of fact sheets addressing commonly encountered eye
conditions, diagnostic tests and materials. *$10.00*
10 pages

**9047   Perkins Activity and Resource Guide: A Handbook for
Teachers**
Perkins School for the Blind
175 North Beacon Street
Watertown, MA   02472   617-924-3434
                                        Fax: 617-972-7363
                                        info@perkins.org
                                        www.perkins.org

Frederic M. Clifford, Chair of the Board
Philip L. Ladd, Vice Chair of the Board
Leslie Nordon, Secretary
Charles C.J. Platt, Treasurer
This is a comprehensive, two volume guide with over 1,000 pages
of activities, resources and instructional strategies for teachers
and parents of students with visual and multiple disabilities.
$80.00

9048   Personal Reader Update
Personal Reader Department
9 Centennial Dr
Peabody, MA   01960-7906   978-977-2000
                                             800-343-0311
                                        Fax: 978-977-2409

**9049   Preschool Learning Activities for the Visually Impaired
Child**
NAPVI
1 North Lexington Avenue
White Plains, NY   10601   617-972-7441
                                             800-562-6265
                                        Fax: 617-972-7444
                                        napvi@guildhealth.org
                                        www.napvi.org

Julie Urban, President
Venetia Hayden, Vice President
Susan LaVenture, Executive Director
Randi Sher, Secretary
This guide for parents offers games and activities to keep visually
impaired children active during the preschool years. *$8.00*
91 pages Paperback

9050   Reaching, Crawling, Walking....Let's Get Moving
Blind Children's Center
4120 Marathon Street
Los Angeles, CA   90029-3584   323-664-2153
                                             800-222-3567
                                        Fax: 323-665-3828
                                     info@blindchildrenscenter.org
                                        www.blindchildrenscenter.org

Scott E. Schaldenbrand, President
Mark Correa, Board Member
Midge Horton, Executive Director
Orientation and mobility for preschool children who are visually
imapired. *$10.00*
24 pages

9051   Reading Is for Everyone
Nat'l Lib Svc/Blind And Physically Handicapped
1291 Taylor Street North West
Washington, DC   20011   202-707-5100
                                        Fax: 202-707-0712
                                        TTY:202-707-0744
                                        nls@loc.gov
                                        www.loc.gov/nls

Karen Keninger, Director

9052   Reading with Low Vision
Nat'l Lib Svc/Blind And Physically Handicapped
1291 Taylor Street North West
Washington, DC   20011   202-707-5100
                                        Fax: 202-707-0712
                                        TTY:202-707-0744
                                        nls@loc.gov
                                        www.loc.gov/nls

Karen Keninger, Director

9053   Recording for the Blind & Dyslexic
20 Roszel Road
Princeton, NJ   08540   800-221-4792
                                        Fax: 609-987-8116
                                     Custserv@LearningAlly.org
                                        www.learningally.org/

Brad Grob, Chairman
Harold J. Logan, Vice Chairman
Andrew Friedman, President & CEO
Jim Halliday, Executive Vice President
Provides recorded and computerized textbooks, library services
and other educational resources to people who cannot effectively
read standard print because of visual impairment, dyslexia or
other physical disability. RFB&D is now Learning Ally.

9054   Reference and Information Services From NLS
Nat'l Lib Svc/Blind And Physically Handicapped
1291 Taylor Street North West
Washington, DC   20011   202-707-5100
                                        Fax: 202-707-0712
                                        TTY:202-707-0744
                                        nls@loc.gov
                                        www.loc.gov/nls

Karen Keninger, Director

9055   Resource List for Persons with Low Vision
American Council of the Blind
2200 Wilson Boulevard
Suite 650
Arlington, VA   22201-3354   202-467-5081
                                             800-424-8666
                                        Fax: 703-465-5085
                                        info@acb.org
                                        acb.org

Kim Charlson, President
Jeff Thom, 1st Vice President
Melanie Brunson, Executive Director

9056 Rose-Colored Glasses
Human Sciences Press
233 Spring St
New York, NY 10013-1522
212-229-2859
800-221-9369
Fax: 212-463-0742

30 pages Hardcover
ISBN 0-87705 -08-8

9057 Say it with Sign
Harris Communications
15155 Technology Drive
Eden Prairie, MN 55344
952-388-2152
800-825-6758
Fax: 952-906-1099
info@harriscomm.com
harriscomm.com

Robert Harris, Owner
Contains both the serious and fun side of signing and provides the basic signs that might be needed in an emergency situation. *$299.50*
10-DVD set

9058 See A Bone
Facts on File
132 West 31st Street
14th Floor
New York, NY 10001
212-967-8800
800-683-5433
Fax: 212-760-0862
info@northernleasing.com
northernleasing.com

Mark Donnell, President
$65.00
352 pages
ISBN 0-816042-80-2

9059 See What I Feel
Britannica Film Company
345 4th Street
San Francisco, CA 94107
415-928-8466
Fax: 415-928-5027
Dave Bekowich, Owner
A blind child tells her friends about her trip to the zoo. Each experience was explained as a blind child would experience it. A teacher's guide comes with this video.
Film

9060 Selecting a Program
Blind Children's Center
4120 Marathon Street
Los Angeles, CA 90029-3584
323-664-2153
800-222-3567
Fax: 323-665-3828
info@blindchildrenscenter.org
www.blindchildrenscenter.org

Scott E. Schaldenbrand, President
Mark Correa, Board Member
Midge Horton, Executive Director
A guide for parents of infants and preschoolers with visual impairments. *$10.00*
28 pages

9061 Show Me How: A Manual for Parents of Preschool Blind Children
American Foundation for the Blind/AFB Press
2 Penn Plaza
Suite 1102
New York, NY 10121
212-502-7600
800-232-5463
Fax: 888-545-8331
afbinfo@afb.net
www.afb.org

Carl R. Augusto, President & Chief Executive Officer
Rick Bozeman, Chief Financial Officer
Kelly Bleach, Chief Administrative Officer
Stacy Rollins, Executive Administrative Assistant to the President

A practical guide for parents, teachers and others who help preschool children attain age-related goals. Covers issues on playing precautions, appropriate toys and facilitating relationships with playmates. Paperback. *$12.95*
56 pages
ISBN 0-891281-13-4

9062 Sign of the Times
Fanlight Productions
c/o Icarus Films
32 Court Street, 21st Floor
Brooklyn, NY 11201
718-488-8900
800-876-1710
Fax: 718-488-8642
info@fanlight.com
www.fanlight.com

Ben Achtenberg, Owner, Founder
Profiles a public school in the heart of Los Angeles - an American microcosm where over 300 languages are spoken, and where cultures and races collide. Fairfax High, publicized as the site of gang activity and murder, has long been a focus for bad press. But something very right is going on in this school. A Sign of the Times offers a positive example of how the American dream and American education are still alive

9063 Special Technologies Alternative Resources
210 McMorran Boulevard
Port Huron, MI 48060
810-987-7323
877-987-READ
star@sccl.lib.mi.us

Arnold H. Larson, Chairman
Kathleen J. Wheelihan, Vice Chairman
Arlene M. Marcetti, Board Member
Stan Arnetti, Director
Addresses the needs of a very unique diverse group of people by offering a full range of library services for people who cannot read standard print. Provides reading material in specialized formats that permit individuals with disabilities to have access to the written word, delivering to customer's mailboxes free of charge. Talking Book Machines, recorded books and magazines, descriptive videos, large print editions and braille books and magazines.

9064 Standing on My Own Two Feet
Blind Children's Center
4120 Marathon Street
Los Angeles, CA 90029-3584
323-664-2153
800-222-3567
Fax: 323-665-3828
info@blindchildrenscenter.org
www.blindchildrenscenter.org

Scott E. Schaldenbrand, President
Mark Correa, Board Member
Midge Horton, Executive Director
A guide to constructing mobility devices for children who are visually impaired. *$10.00*
38 pages

9065 Starting Points
Blind Children's Center
4120 Marathon Street
Los Angeles, CA 90029-3584
323-664-2153
800-222-3567
Fax: 323-665-3828
info@blindchildrenscenter.org
www.blindchildrenscenter.org

Scott E. Schaldenbrand, President
Mark Correa, Board Member
Midge Horton, Executive Director
Basic information for the classroom teacher of 3 to 8 year olds whose multiple disabilities include visual impairment. *$35.00*
157 pages
ISBN 0-891280-61-8

9066 **Step-By-Step Guide to Personal Management for Blind Persons**
American Foundation for the Blind/AFB Press
2 Penn Plaza
Suite 1102
New York, NY 10121
212-502-7600
800-232-5463
Fax: 888-545-8331
afbinfo@afb.net
www.afb.org

Carl R. Augusto, President & Chief Executive Officer
Rick Bozeman, Chief Financial Officer
Kelly Bleach, Chief Administrative Officer
Stacy Rollins, Executive Administrative Assistant to the President
A manual of techniques in the areas of hygiene, grooming, clothing, shopping and child care. *$19.95*
136 pages Spiralbound
ISBN 0-891280-61-8

9067 **Student Teaching Guide for Blind and Visually Impaired College Students**
American Foundation for the Blind/AFB Press
2 Penn Plaza
Suite 1102
New York, NY 10121
212-502-7600
800-232-5463
Fax: 888-545-8331
afbinfo@afb.net
www.afb.org

Carl R. Augusto, President & Chief Executive Officer
Rick Bozeman, Chief Financial Officer
Kelly Bleach, Chief Administrative Officer
Stacy Rollins, Executive Administrative Assistant to the President
A comprehensive resource designed to enable the student to enter the classroom of a university or college with confidence. Large print. *$14.95*
52 pages
ISBN 0-891281-42-8

9068 **Survey of Direct Labor Workers Who Are Blind & Employed by NIB**
Mississippi State University
P.O.Box 6189
Mississippi State, MS 39762
662-325-2001
Fax: 662-325-8989
TTY:662-325-2694
nrtc@colled.msstate.edu
www.blind.msstate.edu

Jacqui Bybee, Research Associate II
Douglas Bedsaul, Research and Training Coordinator
Anne Carter, Research and Training Coordinator
Brenda Cavenaugh, Ph.D., Research Professor
This report is a follow-up to surveys by National Industries for the Blind in 1983 and 1987 and summarizes the results of a national survey of approximately 500 legally blind direct labor workers. *$10.00*
101 pages Paperback

9069 **Talk to Me**
Blind Children's Center
4120 Marathon Street
Los Angeles, CA 90029-3584
323-664-2153
800-222-3567
Fax: 323-665-3828
info@blindchildrenscenter.org
www.blindchildrenscenter.org

Scott E. Schaldenbrand, President
Mark Correa, Board Member
Midge Horton, Executive Director
A language guide for parents of children who are visually impaired. *$10.00*
11 pages

9070 **Talk to Me II**
Blind Children's Center
4120 Marathon Street
Los Angeles, CA 90029-3584
323-664-2153
800-222-3567
Fax: 323-665-3828
info@blindchildrenscenter.org
www.blindchildrenscenter.org

Scott E. Schaldenbrand, President
Mark Correa, Board Member
Midge Horton, Executive Director
a sequel to Talk to Me *$10.00*
15 pages

9071 **Talking Books & Reading Disabilities**
Nat'l Lib Svc/Blind And Physically Handicapped
1291 Taylor Street North West
Washington, DC 20011
202-707-5100
Fax: 202-707-0712
TTY:202-707-0744
nls@loc.gov
www.loc.gov/nls

Karen Keninger, Director

9072 **Talking Books for People with Physical Disabilities**
Nat'l Lib Svc/Blind And Physically Handicapped
1291 Taylor Street North West
Washington, DC 20011
202-707-5100
Fax: 202-707-0712
TTY:202-707-0744
nls@loc.gov
www.loc.gov/nls

Karen Keninger, Director

9073 **Teaching Orientation and Mobility in the Schools: An Instructor's Companion**
American Foundation for the Blind
2 Penn Plaza
Suite 1102
New York, NY 10121
212-502-7600
800-232-5463
Fax: 888-545-8331
afbinfo@afb.net
www.afb.org

Carl R. Augusto, President & Chief Executive Officer
Rick Bozeman, Chief Financial Officer
Kelly Bleach, Chief Administrative Officer
Stacy Rollins, Executive Administrative Assistant to the President
This book, with its useful forms, checklists, and tips, will help O&M instructors and teachers of visually impaired students master the arts of planning schedules, organizing equipment and work routines, working with school personnel and educational team members, and effectively providing instruction to children with diverse needs. *$ 45.95*
176 pages
ISBN 0-891283-91-1

9074 **Teaching Visually Impaired Children**
Charles C. Thomas
2600 S First St
Springfield, IL 62704-4730
217-789-8980
800-258-8980
Fax: 217-789-9130
books@ccthomas.com
www.ccthomas.com

Michael P. Thomas, President
A comprehensive resource for the classroom teacher who is working with a visually impaired child for the first time, as well as a systematic overview of education for the specialist in visual disabilities. It approaches instructional challenges with clear explanations and practical suggestions, and it addresses common concerns of teachers in a reassuring and positive manner. Also available in cloth. *$49.95*
352 pages Paper 2004
ISBN 0-398074-77-7

9075 Textbook Catalog
National Braille Association
95 Allens Creek Road
Building 1, Suite 202
Rochester, NY 14618

585-427-8260
Fax: 585-427-0263
nbaoffice@nationalbraille.org
www.nationalbraille.org

Jan Carroll, President
Cindi Laurent, Vice President
David Shaffer, Executive Director
Heidi Lehmann, Secretary

Lists hundreds of scholarly, college and professional textbooks offered in large print, braille or on cassette for visually impaired readers.
80 pages

9076 Three Rivers News
Carnegie Library of Pitts. Library for the Blind
4724 Baum Boulevard
Pittsburgh, PA 15213

412-687-2440
800-242-0586
Fax: 412-687-2442
clbph@clpgh.org
www.clpgh.org

Kathleen Kappel, Executive Director

Loans recorded books/magazines and playback equipment, large print books and described videos to western PA residents unable to use standard printed materials due to a visual, physical, or physically-based reading disability.
12 pages Quarterly

9077 To Love this Life: Quotations by Helen Keller
American Foundation for the Blind/AFB Press
2 Penn Plaza
Suite 1102
New York, NY 10121

212-502-7600
800-232-5463
Fax: 888-545-8331
www.afb.org

Carl R. Augusto, President & Chief Executive Officer
Rick Bozeman, Chief Financial Officer
Kelly Bleach, Chief Administrative Officer
Stacy Rollins, Executive Administrative Assistant to the President

Inspirational work that offers the penetrating observations of Helen Keller, the beloved deaf-blind champion of the rights of people with disabilities. Also available on cassette at $21.95 (ISBN# 0-89128-348-X) *$21.95*
144 pages Hardcover
ISBN 0-891283-47-1

9078 Touch the Baby: Blind & Visually Impaired Children As Patients
American Foundation for the Blind/AFB Press
2 Penn Plaza
Suite 1102
New York, NY 10121

212-502-7600
800-232-5463
Fax: 888-545-8331
afbinfo@afb.net
www.afb.org

Carl R. Augusto, President & Chief Executive Officer
Rick Bozeman, Chief Financial Officer
Kelly Bleach, Chief Administrative Officer
Stacy Rollins, Executive Administrative Assistant to the President

A how-to manual for health care professionals working in hospitals, clinics and doctors' offices. Teaches the special communication and touch-related techniques needed to prevent blind and visually impaired patients from withdrawing from the healthcare workers and the outside world. $25.00/pack of 25.
13 pages
ISBN 0-891281-97-5

9079 Transition Activity Calendar for Students with Visual Impairments
Mississippi State University
P.O.Box 6189
Mississippi State, MS 39762

662-325-2001
Fax: 662-325-8989
TTY:662-325-2694
nrtc@colled.msstate.edu
www.blind.msstate.edu

Jacqui Bybee, Research Associate II
Douglas Bedsaul, Research and Training Coordinator
Anne Carter, Research and Training Coordinator
Brenda Cavenaugh, Ph.D., Research Professor

The Transition Activity Calendar guides the student with a visual disability through the maze of college preparation. Beginning in junior high school, clearly written steps are listed for each grade level. Students planning to enter college after high school graduation can check-off their accomplishments each step of the way. The calendar helps students focus on their goals while providing reminders of tasks yet to be completed. It can be used in a self-directed manner or in a group format. *$4.25*
16 pages Paperback

9080 Transition to College for Students with Visual Impairments: Report
Mississippi State University
P.O.Box 6189
Mississippi State, MS 39762

662-325-2001
Fax: 662-325-8989
TTY:662-325-2694
nrtc@colled.msstate.edu
www.blind.msstate.edu

Jacqui Bybee, Research Associate II
Douglas Bedsaul, Research and Training Coordinator
Anne Carter, Research and Training Coordinator
Brenda Cavenaugh, Ph.D., Research Professor

A report offering results from telephone interviews of college students with visual impairments and mail surveys of college officials which examines the transition experience of successful college students. General domains in the study include demographics, educational history, computers, specialized and adaptive equipment, resources, college preparation, problems adjusting to college and O&M skills. A literature review covers preparing for college, task timelines,and classroom, labs and tests. *$20.00*
151 pages Paperback

9081 Unseen Minority: A Social History of Blindness in the United States
American Foundation for the Blind/AFB Press
2 Penn Plaza
Suite 1102
New York, NY 10121

212-502-7600
800-232-5463
Fax: 888-545-8331
abfinfo@abf.org
www.afb.org

Carl R. Augusto, President & Chief Executive Officer
Rick Bozeman, Chief Financial Officer
Kelly Bleach, Chief Administrative Officer
Stacy Rollins, Executive Administrative Assistant to the President

A lively narrative, with anecdotes, that recounts how the blind overcame discrimination to gain full participation in the social, educational, economic and legislative spheres. Hardcover. *$59.95*
573 pages Paperback
ISBN 0-891288-96-1

9082 Vision Enhancement
UN Printing
122
1790 E 54th St
Indianapolis, IN 46220-3454

317-254-1332
800-431-1739
Fax: 317-251-6588
www.visionww.org

Patricia L Price, Managing Editor

Designed to encourage and support individuals with vision loss, family members, and caregivers. *$25.00*
72-78 pages Quarterly

9083 Visual Impairment: An Overview

American Foundation for the Blind/AFB Press
2 Penn Plaza
Suite 1102
New York, NY   10121

212-502-7600
800-232-5463
Fax: 888-545-8331
afbinfo@afb.net
www.afb.org

Carl R. Augusto, President & Chief Executive Officer
Rick Bozeman, Chief Financial Officer
Kelly Bleach, Chief Administrative Officer
Stacy Rollins, Executive Administrative Assistant to the President
An overall look at the most common forms of vision loss and their impact on the individual. Includes drawings as well as photographs that stimulate how people with vision loss see. Paperback. *$19.95*
56 pages
ISBN 0-891281-74-0

9084 Visual Impairments And Learning

Sage Publications
2455 Teller Road
Thousand Oaks, CA   91320

805-499-0721
800-818-7243
Fax: 805-499-0871
info@sagepub.com
www.sagepub.com

Sara Miller McCune, Founder, Publisher, Executive Chairman
Blaise R Simqu, President & CEO
Tracey A. Ozmina, Executive Vice President & Chief Operating Officer
Stephen Barr, Managing Director/SAGE London, President of SAGE Internation
The major focus of this new, third edition is to present a new way of thinking about individuals with visual impairment so that they are viewed as participating members of a seeing world despite their reduced visual functioning. *$40.00*
213 pages
ISBN 0-890798-68-3

9085 Walking Alone and Marching Together

National Federation of the Blind
200 East Wells St
Baltimore, MD   21230-4914

410-659-9314
Fax: 410-685-5653
www.nfb.org

Floyd Matson, Author
The history of the organized blind movement, this book spans more than 50 years of civil rights, social issues, attitudes and experiences of the blind. Published in 1990, it has been read by thousands of blind and sighted persons and is used in colleges, libraries and programs across the country as an important tool in understanding blindness and it's impact on both personal lives and the society at large. Braille $130, 2 track or 4 track cassette $40, Print $33.00. Contact Materials Center.

9086 What Do You Do When You See a Blind Person- and What Don't You Do?

American Foundation for the Blind/AFB Press
2 Penn Plaza
Suite 1102
New York, NY   10121

212-502-7600
800-232-5463
Fax: 888-545-8331
afbinfo@afb.net
afb.org

Carl R. Augusto, President & Chief Executive Officer
Rick Bozeman, Chief Financial Officer
Kelly Bleach, Chief Administrative Officer
Stacy Rollins, Executive Administrative Assistant to the President
Examples of real-life situations that teach sighted persons how to interact effectively with blind persons. Topics covered include

how to help someone across the street, how not to distract a guide dog and how to take leave of a blind person. *$25.00*
8 pages
ISBN 0-891281-95-5

9087 What Museum Guides Need to Know: Access for the Blind and Visually Impaired

American Foundation for the Blind/AFB Press
2 Penn Plaza
Suite 1102
New York, NY   10121

212-502-7600
800-232-5463
Fax: 888-545-8331
afbinfo@afb.net
www.afb.org

Carl R. Augusto, President & Chief Executive Officer
Rick Bozeman, Chief Financial Officer
Kelly Bleach, Chief Administrative Officer
Stacy Rollins, Executive Administrative Assistant to the President
Explains how blind and visually impaired museum-goers experience art and offers pointers on greeting people, asking if help is needed and teaching about a specific work of art. Contains information on access laws, resources, training guides and guidelines for preparing large print, cassette and braille materials. *$14.95*
64 pages Paperback
ISBN 0-891281-58-4

9088 Work Sight

Lighthouse International
111 East 59th Street
New York, NY   10022-1202

212-821-9384
800-829-0500
Fax: 212-821-9707
info@lighthouse.org
www.lighthouse.org

Mark G. Ackermann, President / CEO
Intended for employers and employees who have concerns about vision loss and job performance. *$25.00*

9089 World Through Their Eyes

Lighthouse International
111 East 59th Street
New York, NY   10022-1202

212-821-9384
800-829-0500
Fax: 212-821-9707
info@lighthouse.org
www.lighthouse.org

Mark G. Ackermann, President / CEO
Intended to help nursing home staff understand how residents with impaired vision perceive the world. Concrete suggestions help staff provide better care to visually impaired residents. *$25.00*

9090 You Seem Like a Regular Kid to Me

American Foundation for the Blind/AFB Press
2 Penn Plaza
Suite 1102
New York, NY   10121

212-502-7600
800-232-5463
Fax: 888-545-8331
afbinfo@afb.net
www.afb.org

Carl R. Augusto, President & Chief Executive Officer
Rick Bozeman, Chief Financial Officer
Kelly Bleach, Chief Administrative Officer
Stacy Rollins, Executive Administrative Assistant to the President
An interview with Jane, a blind child, tells other children what it's like to be blind. Jane explains how she gets around, takes care of herself, does her school work, spends her leisure time and even pays for things when she can't see money.
16 pages
ISBN 0-891289-21-6

Print: Journals

9091   Journal of Visual Impairment and Blindness
Sheridan Press,
450 Fame Ave
Hanover, PA   17331-1585   717-632-3535
                                            800-352-2210
                                    Fax: 717-633-8929
                                    pubsvc@tsp.sheridan.com
                                    www.sheridanreprints.com
Sharon Shively, Editor
Published in braille, regular print and on ASC II disk and cassette,
this journal contains a wide variety of subjects including rehabilitation, psychology, education, legislation, medicine, technology,
employment, sensory aids and childhood development as they relate to visual impairments. $130 annual individual subscription,
$180 annual institutional subscription.
64 pages Monthly
ISSN 0145-48 x

Print: Magazines

9092   Blind Educator
National Organization of Blind Educators
200 East Wells Street
Jernigan Place
Baltimore, MD   21230   410-659-9314
                                    Fax: 410-685-5653
                                    nfb@nfb.org
                                    www.nfb.org
Marc Mauer, President
Magazine specifically for blind educators.

9093   Braille Forum
American Council of the Blind
2200 Wilson Boulevard
Suite 650
Arlington, VA   22201-3354   202-467-5081
                                            800-424-8666
                                    Fax: 703-465-5085
                                    info@acb.org
                                    www.acb.org
Kim Charlson, President
Jeff Thom, 1st Vice President
Melanie Brunson, Executive Director
Offered in print, braille, cassette, IBM computer disk and e-mail.
$25 per format per year for companies and non-US residents.
48 pages Magazine

9094   Braille Monitor
Deaf-Blind Division of the Ntn'l Fed of the Blind
200 East Wells St
Baltimore, MD   21230-4914   410-659-9314
                                    Fax: 410-685-5653
                                    nfbpublications@nfb.org
                                    www.nfb.org
Marc Maurer, CEO
Barbara Pierce, Editor
The Braille Monitor is the leading publication of the National
Federation of the Blind. It covers the events and activities of the
NFB and addresses the many issues and concerns of the blind.

9095   Dialogue Magazine
Blindskills Inc.
P.O. Box 5181
Salem, OR   97304-0181   503-581-4224
                                            800-860-4224
                                    Fax: 503-581-0178
                                    info@blindskills.com
                                    www.blindskills.com
Marja Byers, Executive Director
B.T. Kimbrough, Editor
Publishes quarterly magazine in braille, large-type, cassette and
email of news items, technology and articles of special interest to

visually impaired youth and adults. Annual subscription cost $35
for braille, large print or cassette, $20 for email. *$35.00*
Quarterly

9096   Future Reflections
Deaf-Blind Division of the Ntn'l Fed of the Blind
200 East Wells Street
Baltimore, MD   21230-4914   410-659-9314
                                    Fax: 410-685-5653
                                    www.nfb.org
Marc Maurer, President
A magazine for parents and teachers of blind children.

9097   Guide Magazine
The Seeing Eye
P.O.Box 375
10 Washington Valley Road
Morristown, NJ 7963   973-539-4425
                                    Fax: 973-539-0922
                                    info@seeingeye.org
                                    seeingeye.org
James A. Kutsch, Jr., Ph.D., President & CEO
Robert Pudlak, CFO & Director of Administration & Finance
Glenn Cianci, Director of Facilities Management
Jean Thomas, Director of Donor & Public Relations
The Guide offers stories of inspiration from our graduates and
news of the latest program developments.

9098   JBI Voice
Jewish Braille Institute of America
110 Est 30th Street
New York, NY   10016   212-889-2525
                                            800-433-1531
                                    Fax: 212-689-3692
                                    admin@jbilibrary.org
                                    www.jbilibrary.org
Judy E. Tenney, Chairman
Thomas G. Kahn, Viec Chairman
Dr. Ellen Isler, President and CEO
Israel A Taub, Vice President and CFO
Monthly recorded magazine emphasizing Jewish current events
and culture.

9099   Jewish Braille Review
Jewish Braille Institute of America
110 Est 30th Street
New York, NY   10016   212-889-2525
                                            800-433-1531
                                    Fax: 212-689-3692
                                    admin@jbilibrary.org
                                    www.jbilibrary.org
Judy E. Tenney, Chairman
Thomas G. Kahn, Viec Chairman
Dr. Ellen Isler, President and CEO
Israel A Taub, Vice President and CFO
The JBI seeks the integration of Jews who are blind, visually im-
paired and reading disabled into the Jewish community and soci-
ety in general. More than 20,000 men, women and children in 50
countries receive a broad variety of JBI services.

9100   Musical Mainstream
Nat'l Lib Svc/Blind And Physically Handicapped
1291 Taylor Street North West
Washington, DC   20011   202-707-5100
                                    Fax: 202-707-0712
                                    TTY:202-707-0744
                                    nls@loc.gov
                                    www.loc.gov/nls
Karen Keninger, Director
Articles selected from print music magazines.
Quarterly

9101 **Opportunity**
National Industries for the Blind
1310 Braddock Place
Alexandria, VA 22314-1691   703-310-0500
                                          Fax: 703-998-8268
                                            services@nib.org
                                                www.nib.org

The Honorabl Krump, Esq., Chairman
Louis J. Jablonski, Jr., Vice Chairman
Kevin A. Lynch, President and Chief Executive Officer
James M Kesteloot, Director
Offers information and articles on the newest technology, equipment, services and programs for blind and visually impaired persons.
Quarterly

9102 **Providing Services for People with Vision Loss:**
Multidisciplinary Perspective
Resources for Rehabilitation
22 Bonad Road
Winchester, MA 01890-1302   781-368-9080
                                          Fax: 781-368-9096
                                            orders@rfr.org
                                                www.rfr.org

Susan L Greenblatt, Editor
A collection of articles by ophthalmologists and rehabilitation professionals, including chapters on operating a low vision service, starting self-help programs, mental health services, aids and techniques that help people with vision loss. *$19.95*
136 pages
ISBN 0-929718-02-0

Print: Newsletters

9103 **AFB News**
American Foundation for the Blind/AFB Press
2 Penn Plaza
Suite 1102
New York, NY 10121   212-502-7600
                                               800-232-5463
                                          Fax: 888-545-8331
                                            afbinfo@afb.net
                                                www.afb.org

Carl R. Augusto, President & Chief Executive Officer
Rick Bozeman, Chief Financial Officer
Kelly Bleach, Chief Administrative Officer
Stacy Rollins, Executive Administrative Assistant to the President
National newsletter for general readership about blindness and visual impairments featuring people, programs, services and activities.
12 pages Quarterly

9104 **ASB Visions Newsletter**
Associated Services for the Blind
919 Walnut Street
Philadelphia, PA 19107   215-627-0600
                                          Fax: 215-922-0692
                                            asbinfo@asb.org
                                                www.asb.org

Patricia C. Johnson, President and CEO
Tim McGovern, Human Relations
Brian Rusk, Public Relations Officer
Derby Ewing, Director, Human Services
Newsletter associated services for the blind and visually impaired.

9105 **Adaptive Services Division**
District of Columbia Public Library
901G St NW,
Rm 215
Washington, DC 20001-4531   202-727-2142
                                          Fax: 202-727-0322
                                          TTY:202-559-5368
                                            lbph.dcpl@dc.gov
                                                www.dclibrary.org

Venetia Demson, Chief, Adaptive Services

DC Regional Library for the blind, deaf and physically handicapped. Provides adaptive technology and training programs.
8 pages Quarterly

9106 **Alumni News**
Guide Dogs for the Blind
P.O.Box 151200
San Rafael, CA 94915-1200   415-499-4000
                                               800-295-4050
                                          Fax: 415-499-4035
                                                guidedogs.com

Bob Burke, Chairman
Stuart Odell, Vice Chairman
Chris Benninger, President and CEO
Jay Harris, Secretary
Restricted to graduates only.

9107 **Annual Report/Newsletter**
National Accreditation Council for Agencies/Blind
Rm 1004
15 E 40th St
New York, NY 10016-401   212-683-5068
                                          Fax: 212-683-4475

Ruth Westman, Executive Director
Provides standards and a program of accreditation for schools and organizations which serve children and adults who are blind or vision impaired.

9108 **Association for Macular Diseases Newsletter**
210 East 64th Street
New York, NY 10065   212-605-3719
                                          Fax: 212-605-3795
                                  association@retinal-research.org
                                                macula.org

Bernard Landou, President
Mary Fern Breheny, Board Member
Patricia Dahl, Board Member
Walter Ross, Editor-In-Chief
Not-for-profit organization promotes education and research in this scarcely explored field. Acts as a nationwide support group for individuals and their families endeavoring to adjust to the restrictions and changes brought about by macular disease. Offers hotline, educational materials, quarterly newsletter, support groups, referrals and seminars for persons and families affected by macular disease.

9109 **Awareness**
NAPVI
1 North Lexington Avenue
White Plains, NY 10601   617-972-7441
                                               800-562-6265
                                          Fax: 617-972-7444
                                            napvi@guildhealth.org
                                                www.napvi.org

Julie Urban, President
Venetia Hayden, Vice President
Susan LaVenture, Executive Director
Randi Sher, Secretary
Newsletter offering regional news, sports and activities, conferences, camps, legislative updates, book reviews, audio reviews, professional question and answer column and more for the visually impaired and their families.
Quarterly

9110 **BTBL News**
Braille and Talking Book Library
P.O. Box 942837
Sacramento, CA 94237-0001   916-654-0261
                                               800-952-5666
                                          Fax: 916-654-1119
                                            btbl@library.ca.gov
                                                www.btbl.ca.gov

Janet Coles, Editor
Christopher Berger, Senior Librarian
Olena Bilyk, Web Developer
Kim Brown, Communications Officer

BTBL News, the quarterly newsletter of the California Braille and Talking Book Library, features articles on topics of interest to library customers, including information about new services, existing services, events, staff and more.

9111 Canes and Trails
Guide Dogs for the Blind
P.O.Box 151200
San Rafael, CA 94915-1200   415-499-4000
                                          800-295-4050
                                     Fax: 415-499-4035
                                          guidedogs.com

Bob Burke, Chairman
Stuart Odell, Vice Chairman
Chris Benninger, President and CEO
Jay Harris, Secretary
A quarterly newsletter for orientation and mobility specialists, rehabilitation professionals, teachers, and service providers in the field of blindness and visual impairment.

9112 Community Connection
Guide Dogs for the Blind
P.O.Box 151200
San Rafael, CA 94915-1200   415-499-4000
                                          800-295-4050
                                     Fax: 415-499-4035
                                          guidedogs.com

Bob Burke, Chairman
Stuart Odell, Vice Chairman
Chris Benninger, President and CEO
Jay Harris, Secretary
A newsletter produced for our volunteers and other friends of Guide Dogs.

9113 DVH Quarterly
University of Arkansas at Little Rock
2801 S University Ave
Little Rock, AR 72204-1000   501-569-3000
Bob Brasher, Editor
Mary Boaz, Manager
Offers information on upcoming events, conferences and workshops on and for visual disabilities. Book reviews, information on the newest resources and technology, educational programs, want ads and more.
Quarterly

9114 Deaf-Blind Perspective
National Consortium on Deaf-Blindness
345 North Monmouth Avenue
Monmouth, OR 97361   503-838-8391
                                          800-438-9376
                                     Fax: 503-838-8150
                                     TTY: 800-854-7013
                                          www.tr.wou.edu

Ingrid Amerson, Child Development Center
Lyn Ayer, Center on Deaf & Blindness
Robert Ayres, Evaluation and Research
Cori Brownell, Center on Early Learning
A free publication with articles, essays, and announcements about topics related to people who are deaf-blind. Published two times a year (Spring and Fall) by the Teaching Research Institute of Western Oregon University, its purpose is to provide information and serve as a forum for discussion and sharing ideas.

9115 Fidelco
Fidelco Guide Dog Foundation
103 Vision Way
Bloomfield, CT 06002   860-243-5200
                                     Fax: 860-769-0567
                                          info@fidelco.org
                                          fidelco.org

Karen C. Tripp, Chairman
G. Kenneth Bernhard, Vice Chairman
Eliot D. Matheson, CEO
Diane R. Lindeland, VP, Finance
A newsletter published by Fidelco Guide Dog Foundation.

9116 Focus
Visually Impaired Center
1422 W Court St
Flint, MI 48503-5008   810-767-4014
                                     Fax: 810-767-0020

Charles Tommasulo, Executive Director
Newsletter offering information for the visually impaired person in the forms of legislative and law updates, ADA information, support groups, hotlines, and articles on the newest technology in the field.
Quarterly

9117 Gleams Newsletter
Glaucoma Research Foundation
2345 Yale Street
2nd Floor
Palo Alto, CA 94306   650-328-3388
                                          800-826-6693
                                     Fax: 415-986-3763
                                          info@glaucoma.org
                                          auorthodontics.com

Tom Brunner, CEO
Offers updated medical & research information on glaucoma. Included are glaucoma treatment and coping tips, legsilative information, professional articles and book reviews.
6 pages Quarterly

9118 Guide Dog News
Guide Dogs for the Blind
P.O.Box 151200
San Rafael, CA 94915-1200   415-499-4000
                                          800-295-4050
                                     Fax: 415-499-4035
                                          guidedogs.com

Bob Burke, Chairman
Stuart Odell, Vice Chairman
Chris Benninger, President and CEO
Jay Harris, Secretary
Read about changes to our teaching techniques, our new Adult Learning Program, vet tips, and find news about our graduates.

9119 Guideway
Guide Dog Foundation for the Blind
371 East Jericho Turnpike
Smithtown, NY 11787-2976   631-930-9000
                                          800-548-4337
                                     Fax: 631-930-9009
                                          info@guidedog.org
                                          www.guidedog.org

James C. Bingham, Chairman
Alphonce J. Brown, Jr., Vice Chairman
Wells B. Jones, CEO
Jack Sage, Secretary
Offers updates and information on the foundation's activities and guide dog programs. In print form but is also available on cassette.
Monthly

9120 Guild Briefs
Catholic Guild for The Blind
65 East Wacker Place
Suite 1010
Chicago, IL 60601   312-236-8569
                                     Fax: 312-236-8128
                                          info@guildfortheblind.org
                                          www.guildfortheblind.org

Brett Christenson, President
Laura Rounce, Vice President
David Tabak, Executive Director
Toria Emas, Secretary
Monthly publication for individuals who are blind or visually impaired. It contains articles on topics such as service programs, scholarships, education, seniors, research, and government.
12 pages monthly

9121 IAAIS Report
Int'l Association of Audio Information Services
3920 Willshire Dr
Lawrence, KS 66049-3673 412-434-6023
800-280-5325
www.iaais.org
Stuart Holland, President
Marjorie Williams, 1st Vice President
Linda Hynson, Secretary
Andrea Pasquale, Treasurer
Newsletter for persons interested in radio reading services. *$7.00*
Quarterly

9122 Insight
United States Association of Blind Athletes
1 Olympic Plaza
Colorado Springs, CO 80909 719-630-0422
Fax: 719-630-0616
media@usaba.org
www.usaba.org
Mark A. Lucas, MS, Executive Director
Ryan Ortiz, Assistant Executive Director
John Potts, Goalball High Performance director
Matt Simpson, Membership & Outreach Coordinator
Covers news, announcements and activities of the association.
20 pages Quarterly

9123 LampLighter
Columbia Lighthouse for the Blind
1825 K Street NorthWest
Suite 1103
Washington, DC 20006 202-454-6400
Fax: 877-595-9228
info@clb.org
clb.org
Tony Cancelosi, President
Anthony Cancelosi, CEO
Dedicated to helping the blind or visually impaired population.

9124 Library Users of America Newsletter
American Council of the Blind
2200 Wilson Boulevard
Suite 650
Arlington, VA 22201-3354 202-467-5081
800-424-8666
Fax: 703-465-5085
info@acb.org
www.acb.org
Kim Charlson, President
Jeff Thom, 1st Vice President
Melanie Brunson, Executive Director
Published twice yearly, the newsletter contains much information
about library services of particular interest to blind and visually
impaired patrons, and is available in the following formats:
Braille, audiocassette, large print and e-mail.

9125 Light the Way
Blind Children's Center
4120 Marathon Street
Los Angeles, CA 90029-3584 323-664-2153
800-222-3567
Fax: 323-665-3828
info@blindchildrenscenter.org
blindchildrenscenter.org
Scott E. Schaldenbrand, President
Mark Correa, Board Member
Midge Horton, Executive Director
Newsletter of the Blind Childrens Center, a family-centered
agency which serves young children with visual impairments.
The center-based and home-based services help the children to
acquire skills and build their independence. The center utilizes its
expertise and experience to serve families and professionals
worldwide through support services, education and research.

9126 Lighthouse Publication
Chicago Lighthouse
1850 West Roosevelt Road
Chicago, IL 60608-1298 312-666-1331
Fax: 312-243-8539
TTY:312-666-8874
publications@chicagolighthouse.org
www.thechicagolighthouse.org
Janet P. Szlyk, Ph.D., President & Chief Executive Officer
Mary Lynne Januszewski, Executive Vice President/CFO
Melanie M. Hennessy, SVP
Terrence J. longo, Executive Vice President/COO

9127 Lights On
Fight for Sight
Ste 809
391 Park Ave S
New York, NY 10016-8806 212-679-6060
Fax: 212-679-4466
www.fightforsight.com
Mary Prudden, Executive Director
A newsletter published by Fight for Sight.

9128 Long Cane News
American Foundation for the Blind/AFB Press
2 Penn Plaza
Suite 1102
New York, NY 10121 212-502-7600
800-232-5463
Fax: 888-545-8331
afbinfo@afb.net
www.afb.org
Carl R. Augusto, President & Chief Executive Officer
Rick Bozeman, Chief Financial Officer
Kelly Bleach, Chief Administrative Officer
Stacy Rollins, Executive Administrative Assistant to the President
SemiAnnual

9129 Magnifier
Macular Degeneration Foundation
P.O.Box 531313
Henderson, NV 89053 702-450-2908
888-633-3937
liz@eyesight.org
www.eyesight.org
Liz Trauernicht, President & Director of Communications
Julie Zavala, VP & Asst. Director of Operations
David Seftel, EVP & Dircetor, R & D
Ron Gallamore, Board of Scientific Advisors
The Magnifier is the distributed without charge via email and by
regular mail to those without access to the Internet. It features
breaking news, clinical trails, clarifies recent reports in the media, announces new Internet resources and informs the public of
important additions to the web site.

9130 NAVH Update
National Association of Visually Handicapped
111 East 59th Street
New York, NY 10022-1202 212-821-9384
800-829-0500
Fax: 212-821-9707
info@lighthouse.org
lighthouse.org/navh
Mark G. Ackermann, President / CEO
A newsletter published by the National Association of Visually
Impaired. LightHouse acquired NAVH.

9131 NBA Bulletin
National Braille Association
95 Allens Creek Road
Building 1, Suite 202
Rochester, NY 14618   585-427-8260
                              Fax: 585-427-0263
                       nbaoffice@nationalbraille.org
                          www.nationalbraille.org
Jan Carroll, President
Cindi Laurent, Vice President
David Shaffer, Executive Director
Heidi Lehmann, Secretary
Published quarterly and included int he price of the regular and
student NBA membership.

9132 NLS News
Nat'l Lib Svc/Blind And Physically Handicapped
1291 Taylor Street North West
Washington, DC 20011   202-707-5100
                              Fax: 202-707-0712
                              TTY:202-707-0744
                                    nls@loc.gov
                                www.loc.gov/nls
Karen Keninger, Director
Newsletter on current program developments.
Quarterly

9133 NLS Newsletter
Nat'l Lib Svc/Blind And Physically Handicapped
1291 Taylor Street North West
Washington, DC 20011   202-707-5100
                              Fax: 202-707-0712
                              TTY:202-707-0744
                                    nls@loc.gov
                                www.loc.gov/nls
Karen Keninger, Director
Newsletter on the service's volunteer activities.
Quarterly

9134 PBA News
Prevent Blindness America
211 West Wacker Drive
Suite 1700
Chicago, IL 60606   800-331-2020
                       info@preventblindness.org
                          www.preventblindness.org
Paul G. Howes, Chairman
Hugh R. Parry, President & CEO,Prevent Blindness America
Jerome Desserich, Vice President & Chief Financial Officer
Danielle Disch, Development Manager
Newsletter is filled with the information you need to protect your
eyes, preserve your sight, and educate yourself about your own
eye condition or that of a family member. Publication offered
three times yearly.
3 times yearly

9135 Planned Giving Department of Guide Dogs for the Blind
Guide Dogs for the Blind
P.O.Box 151200
San Rafael, CA 94915-1200   415-499-4000
                                       800-295-4050
                              Fax: 415-499-4035
                                    guidedogs.com
Bob Burke, Chairman
Stuart Odell, Vice Chairman
Chris Benninger, President and CEO
Jay Harris, Secretary
A newsletter published by Guide Dogs for the Blind.

9136 Playback
Recording for the Blind & Dyslexic
20 Roszel Road
Princeton, NJ 08540   800-221-4792
                              Fax: 609-987-8116
                        Custserv@LearningAlly.org
                          www.learningally.org/
Brad Grob, Chairman
Harold J. Logan, Vice Chairman
Andrew Friedman, President & CEO
Jim Halliday, Executive Vice President
A publication dedicated to our unit's family of members, volun-
teers, supporters and staff. RFB&D is now Learning Ally.
3x Year

9137 Quarterly Update
National Association for Visually Handicapped
111 East 59th Street
New York, NY 10022-1202   212-821-9384
                                       800-829-0500
                              Fax: 212-821-9707
                              info@lighthouse.org
                              lighthouse.org/navh
Mark G. Ackermann, President / CEO
Quarterly newsletter offering information on new products for
the visually impaired, advances in medical treatments, new books
available in the NAVH large print loan library and any new/up-
dated booklets. Free. LightHouse acquired NAVH.

9138 RP Messenger
Texas Association of Retinitis Pigmentosa
P.O.Box 8388
Corpus Christi, TX 78468-8388   361-852-8515
                              Fax: 361-852-8515
                              tarp@homebiz101.com
                                www.geocities.com
Dorothy Steifel, Executive Director
A bi-annual newsletter offering information on Retinitis
Pigmentosa. *$15.00*
BiAnnual

9139 SCENE
Braille Institute
527 North Dale Avenue
Anaheim, CA 92801   714-821-5000
                                       800-272-4553
                              Fax: 714-527-7621
                              oc@brailleinstitute.org
                              brailleinstitute.org
Lester M. Sussman, Chairman
Peter A. Mindnich, President
Jon K. Hayashida, OD, FAAO, Vice President, Programs & Ser-
vices
Rezaur Rehman, Vice President, Finance
Offers information on the organization, question and answer col-
umn, articles on the newest technology and more for visually im-
paired persons.

9140 STAR
Special Technologies Alternative Resources
210 McMorran Boulevard
Port Huron, MI 48060   810-987-7323
                                       877-987-READ
                              star@sccl.lib.mi.us
                                www.sccl.lib.mi.us
Arnold H. Larson, Chairman
Kathleen J. Wheelihan, Vice Chairman
Arlene M. Marcetti, Board Member
Stan Arnetti, Director
A newsletter published by Special Technologies Alternative Re-
sources.

9141   Seeing Eye Guide
The Seeing Eye
P.O.Box 375
10 Washington Valley Road
Morristown, NJ 07963   973-539-4425
                                                 Fax: 973-539-0922
                                          info@seeingeye.org
                                                seeingeye.org

James A. Kutsch, Jr., Ph.D., President & CEO
Randall Ivens, Director of Human Resources
Robert Pudlak, CFO & Director of Adninistration & Finance
David Johnson, Director of Instruction & Training
A quarterly publication from Seeing Eye.
Quarterly

9142   Shared Visions
Vista Center for the Blind & Visually Impaired
413 Laurel St
Santa Cruz, CA   95060-4904   831-458-9766
                                                 800-705-2970
                                                 Fax: 831-426-6233
                                       information@vistacenter.org
Pam Brandin, Executive Director
A quarterly publication for Blind and Visually Impaired individu-
als from Vista Center for the Blind and Visually Impaired.

9143   Sharing Solutions: A Newsletter for Support Groups
Lighthouse International
111 East 59th Street
New York, NY   10022-1202   212-821-9384
                                                 800-829-0500
                                                 Fax: 212-821-9707
                                             info@lighthouse.org
                                             www.lighthouse.org
Mark G. Ackermann, President / CEO
A newsletter for members and leaders of support groups for older
adults with impaired vision. The letter provides a forum for support groups members to network and share information, printed
in a very large type format.

9144   Sightings Newsletter
Schepens Eye Research Institute
20 Staniford Street
Boston, MA   02114   617-912-0100
                                                 Fax: 617-912-0110
                                          www.schepens.harvard.edu
Michael Gilmore, Director
Mary E. Leach, Director of Public Affairs
Frances Ng, Director of Human Resources
Ojas P. Mehta, Director, Intellectual Property & Commercial
Ventures
Publication of prominent center for research on eye, vision, and
blinding diseases; dedicated to research that improves the understanding, management, and prevention of eye diseases and visual
deficiencies; fosters collaboration among its faculty members;
trains young scientists and clinicians from around the world; promotes communication with scientists in allied fields; leader in the
worldwide dispersion of basic scientific knowledge of vision.

**9145   Smith Kettlewell Rehabilitation Engineering Research
Center**
2318 Fillmore Street
San Francisco, CA   94115   415-345-2000
                                                 Fax: 415-345-8455
                                                  rerc@ski.org
                                                  ski.org
John Brabyn, Ph.D., CEO/Executive Director
Ruth S. Poole, COO
Arthur Jampolsky, Director
Arthur Jampolsky,M.D., Founder
Reports on technology and devices for persons with visual im-
pairments.

9146   Student Advocate
National Alliance of Blind Students NABS Liaison
Ste 1004
1155 15th St NW
Washington, DC   20005-2706   202-467-5081
                                                 800-424-8666
                                                 Fax: 202-467-5085
                                             www.blindstudents.org
Melanie Brunson, Executive Director
A newsletter created by members of NABS and for any interested
parties.

9147   TBC Focus
Chicago Public Library Talking Books Center
400 South State Street
Chicago, IL   60605   312-747-4300
                                                 800-757-4654
                                                 Fax: 312-747-1609
                                             www.chipublib.org
Linda Johnson Rice, President
Christopher Valenti, VP
Christina Benitez, Secretary
Karim Adib, Director
Published quarterly by the Chicago Public Library Talking Book
Center. Free of charge.
4 pages Quarterly

9148   Talking Books Topics
Nat'l Lib Svc/Blind And Physically Handicapped
1291 Taylor Street North West
Washington, DC   20011   202-707-5100
                                                 Fax: 202-707-0712
                                                 TTY:202-707-0744
                                                  nls@loc.gov
                                             www.loc.gov/nls
Karen Keninger, Director
New recorded books and program news
Bi-monthly

9149   Upstate Update
New York State Talking Book & Braille Library
222 Madison Avenue
Albany, NY   12230-1   518-474-5935
                                                 800-342-3688
                                                 Fax: 514-474-5786
                                                 TTY: 518-474-7121
                                           nyslweb@mail.nysed.gov
                                             www.nysl.nysed.gov
Bernard A. Margolis, State Librarian & Asst. Commissioner for Li-
braries
Loretta Ebert, Research Library Director
Liza Duncan, Technical Services & Systmes
Books on audio cassette, cassette players, braille books, summer
reading programs, braille writer, magnifiers, closed-circuit T.V.,
large-print photocopier, cassette books and magazines, children's books on cassette, reference materials on blindness and
other handicaps.
4 pages Quarterly

9150   Visual Aids and Informational Material
National Association for Visually Handicapped
111 East 59th Street
New York, NY   10022-1202   212-821-9384
                                                 800-829-0500
                                                 Fax: 212-821-9707
                                             info@lighthouse.org
                                             lighthouse.org/navh
Mark G. Ackermann, President / CEO
A complete listing of the visual aids NAVH carries such as magnifiers, talking clocks, large print playing cards, etc. LightHouse
acquired NAVH. *$2.50*
65 pages

9151 Voice
Vermont Assn for the Blind & Visually Impaired
60 Kimball Avenue
South Burlington, VT 05403 802-863-1358
800-639-5861
Fax: 802-863-1481
General@vabvi.org
vabvi.org

Thomas Chase, President
Stephen Pouliot, Executive Director
Kathleen Quinlan, Director of Operations
Lori Newsome, Office Manager
The Voice is a newsletter published by Vermont Association for the Blind and Visually Impaired.

9152 Voice of Vision
GW Micro
725 Airport North Office Park
Fort Wayne, IN 46825 260-489-3671
Fax: 260-489-2608
www.gwmicro.com

Dan Weirich, Owner
Offers product reviews, product announcements, tips for making systems or applications more accessible, or explanations of concepts of interest to any computer user or would-be computer user. This association newsletter is available in braille, in large print, on audio cassette and on 3.5 or 5.25 IBM format diskette.
Quarterly

Non Print: Newsletters

9153 Insight
Eye Bank Association of America
Ste 1010
1015 18th Street NorthWest
Washington, DC 20036 202-775-4999
Fax: 202-429-6036
info@restoresight.org
www.restoresight.org

David Glasser, Chairman
Kevin Corcoran, President & Chief Executive Officer
Molly Georgakis, VP of Member Services
Patricia Hardy, Manager of Communications
An electronic newsletter.

9154 Listen Up
Recording for the Blind & Dyslexic
20 Roszel Rd
Princeton, NJ 8540-6206 609-452-0606
866-732-3585
Fax: 609-520-7990
www.learningally.org

John Kelly, CEO
RFB&D's bi-monthly electronic newsletter for members.

Non Print: Video

9155 Aging and Vision: Declarations of Independence
American Foundation for the Blind/AFB Press
2 Penn Plaza
Suite 1102
New York, NY 10121 212-502-7600
800-232-5463
Fax: 888-545-8331
afbinfo@afb.net
www.afb.org

Carl R. Augusto, President & Chief Executive Officer
Rick Bozeman, Chief Financial Officer
Kelly Bleach, Chief Administrative Officer
Stacy Rollins, Executive Administrative Assistant to the President
A very personal look at five older people who have successfully coped with visual impairmant and continue to lead active, satisfying lives. Their stories are not only inspirational, but also provide practical, down-to-earth suggestions for adapting to vision loss

later in life. 18 minute video tape. Also available in PAL, $52.95, 0-89128-276-9. *$42.95*
VHS
ISBN 0-891282-20-3

9156 Blindness, A Family Matter
American Foundation for the Blind/AFB Press
2 Penn Plaza
Suite 1102
New York, NY 10121 212-502-7600
800-232-5463
Fax: 888-545-8331
afbinfo@afb.net
www.afb.org

Carl R. Augusto, President & Chief Executive Officer
Rick Bozeman, Chief Financial Officer
Kelly Bleach, Chief Administrative Officer
Stacy Rollins, Executive Administrative Assistant to the President
A frank exploration of the effects of an individual's visual impairment on other members of the family and how those family members can play a positive role in the rehabilitation process. Features interviews with three families whose 'success stories' provide advice and encouragement, as well as interviews with newly blinded adults currently involved in a rehabilitation program. 23 minute video tape. Also available in PAL, $49.95, 0-89128-271-8. *$43.95*
VHS
ISBN 0-891282-22-X

9157 Building Blocks: Foundations for Learning for Young Blind and Visually Impaired Children
American Foundation for the Blind/AFB Press
2 Penn Plaza
Suite 1102
New York, NY 10121 212-502-7600
800-232-5463
Fax: 888-545-8331
afbinfo@afb.net
www.afb.org

Carl R. Augusto, President & Chief Executive Officer
Rick Bozeman, Chief Financial Officer
Kelly Bleach, Chief Administrative Officer
Stacy Rollins, Executive Administrative Assistant to the President
Presents the essential components of a successful early intervnetion program, including collaboration with family members, positive relationships between parents and professionals, public education, and attention to important programming components such as space exploration, braille readiness, orientation and mobility, play, cooking and music. Includes interviews with parents. Available in English or Spanish. 10 minute video tape. Also available in PAL, $33.95, 0-89128-268-8. *$26.95*
VHS
ISBN 0-891282-14-9

9158 Choice Magazine Listening
85 Channel Drive
Port Washington, NY 11050 516-883-8280
888-724-6423
888-724-6423
Fax: 516-944-5849
choicemag@aol.com
www.choicemagazinelistening.org

Pamela Loeser, Editor in Chief
Ann Schlegel-Kyrkostas, Associate Editor
David Graham Pade, Associate Editor
Michael Tedeschi, Webmaster
A free audio anthology is available bi-monthly to visually impaired/physically disabled or dislexic persons nationwide. Playable on the special free 4-track cassette playback equipment which is provided by the Library of Congress through the National Library Service. Each issue features eight hours of unabridged magazine articles, short stories, poetry and media selections from over 100 sources. College level and older. Bimonthly distribution.
Bi-Monthly

9159   Juggler
Beacon Press
24 Farnsworth Street
Boston, MA   02210   617-742-2110
                                            Fax: 617-723-3097
                                                   beacon.org
Helene Atwan, Executive Director
Andre was the young son of a wealthy, early Quebec fur trader.
Because he was almost totally blind, he was overly protected by
his family, and his movement outside his home was very limited.
Film

9160   Let's Eat Video
Blind Children's Center
4120 Marathon Street
Los Angeles, CA   90029-3584   323-664-2153
                                                  800-222-3567
                                            Fax: 323-665-3828
                                 info@blindchildrenscenter.org
                                      blindchildrenscenter.org
Scott E. Schaldenbrand, President
Mark Correa, Board Member
Midge Horton, Executive Director
Babies and toddlers with visual impairments lack one major ave-
nue of exploration, and this significantly infulences their aware-
ness, perceptions, and anticipation of the food which is presented
to them. *$35.00*
VHS/DVD

9161   Look Out for Annie
Lighthouse International
111 East 59th Street
New York, NY   10022-1202   212-821-9384
                                                  800-829-0500
                                            Fax: 212-821-9706
                                            info@lighthouse.org
                                            www.lighthouse.org
Mark G. Ackermann, President / CEO
Depicts an older woman coping with her vision loss. It focuses on
the emotional issues surrounding vision loss and conveys the idea
that both the person with the vision disorder and their family and
friends will need to make adjustments. *$25.00*
Video

9162   Not Without Sight
American Foundation for the Blind/AFB Press
PO Box 1020
Sewickley, PA   15143-920   412-741-1142
                                                  800-232-3044
                                            Fax: 412-741-0609
                                                   www.afb.org
Carl R Augusto, President/CEO
Tracy Charlovich, Css
This video describes the major types of visual impairment and
their causes and effects on vision, while camera simulations ap-
proximate what people with each impairment actually see. Also
demonstrates how people with low vision make the best use of the
vision they have. 20 minute video tape, $49.95. *$42.95*
VHS 17 min
ISBN 0-891282-27-3

9163   Out of Left Field
American Foundation for the Blind/AFB Press
2 Penn Plaza
Suite 1102
New York, NY   10121   212-502-7600
                                                  800-232-5463
                                            Fax: 888-545-8331
                                               afbinfo@afb.net
                                                      afb.org
Carl R. Augusto, President & Chief Executive Officer
Rick Bozeman, Chief Financial Officer
Kelly Bleach, Chief Administrative Officer
Stacy Rollins, Executive Administrative Assistant to the President
Illustrates how youngsters who are blind or visually impaired in-
tegrated with their sighted peers in a variety of recreational and

athletic activities. 17 minute video tape. Also available in PAL,
$33.95, 0-89128-270-X. *$29.95*
VHS 17 minutes
ISBN 0-891282-28-0

9164   See What I'm Saying
Fanlight Productions
c/o Icarus Films
32 Court Street, 21st Floor
Brooklyn, NY   11201   718-488-8900
                                                  800-876-1710
                                            Fax: 718-488-8642
                                             info@fanlight.com
                                               www.fanlight.com
Ben Achtenberg, Founder, Owner
The documentary follows Patricia, who is deaf and from a Span-
ish-speaking family, through her first year at the Kendall Demon-
stration Elementary School of Gallaudet University.
VHS/DVD

9165   See for Yourself
Lighthouse International
111 East 59th Street
New York, NY   10022-1202   212-821-9384
                                                  800-829-0500
                                            Fax: 212-821-9706
                                            info@lighthouse.org
                                            www.lighthouse.org
Mark G. Ackermann, President / CEO
This video features older adults with impaired vision who have
been helped by vision rehabilitation. *$50.00*

9166   Shape Up 'n Sign
Harris Communications
15155 Technology Dr
Eden Prairie, MN   55344-2273   952-906-1180
                                                  800-825-6758
                                            Fax: 952-906-1099
                                            info@harriscomm.com
Robert Harris, Owner
An aerobic exercise tape introducing the basic sign language for
deaf and hearing children ages six to ten. *$29.95*
30 Minutes DVD

9167   Sight by Touch
Landmark Media
3450 Slade Run Drive
Falls Church, VA   22042   703-241-2030
                                                  800-342-4336
                                            Fax: 703-536-9540
                                           info@landmarkmedia.com
                                               landmarkmedia.com
Michael Hartogs, President
Peter Hartogs, VP New Business & Development
Beverly Weisenberg, Sales Rep
Richard Hartogs, VP Acquisitions
This video features the life and importance of Louis Braille. Vi-
sion-impaired performers and teachers demonstrate how Braille
has benefitted their lives, and how improvements are constantly
being made. *$195.00*
Video

9168   Taping for the Blind
3935 Essex Lane
Houston, TX   77027   713-622-2767
                                            Fax: 713-622-2772
                                                   www.afb.org
Carl R. Augusto, President & Chief Executive Officer
Rick Bozeman, Chief Financial Officer
Robin Vogel, VP, Resource Development
Cynthia Fanzetti, Executive Director
An independent non profit educational organization funded by
corporations, listeners and individuals, with a mission to turn
sight into sound, enriching the lives of individuals with visual,
physical and learning disabilities. Founded in 1967 to read materials not availiable through other sources onto standard audio cassettes in our custom recording division. In 1978, Houston Taping

fFor The Blind signed on the air. Reading several dozen popular magazines and best selling books on the air.

9169   We Can Do it Together!
American Foundation for the Blind/AFB Press
2 Penn Plaza
Suite 1102
New York, NY   10121   212-502-7600
                                               800-232-5463
                                          Fax: 888-545-8331
                                              afbinfo@afb.net
                                                      afb.org
Carl R. Augusto, President & Chief Executive Officer
Rick Bozeman, Chief Financial Officer
Kelly Bleach, Chief Administrative Officer
Stacy Rollins, Executive Administrative Assistant to the President
This video illustrates a transdisciplinary team orientation and mobility program for students with severe visual and multiple impairments, covering both adapted communication systems used to teach mobility skills and basic indoor mobility in the school. For mobility instructors, administrators, teachers of the visually and severely handicapped, occupational, physical and speech therapists and parents. Discussion guide included. 10 minute video tape. Also available in PAL, $33.95, 0-89128-267-X. *$26.95*
VHS
ISBN 0-891282-13-0

Sports

9170   American Blind Bowling Association
1209 Somerset Road
Raleigh, NC   27610   919-755-0700
                                              www.abba1951.org
Thomas Lester, President
A.J. Inglesby, 1st Vice President
James Benton, 2nd Vice President
Judy Mandelkow, Tournament Director
Promotes blind bowling throughout the US and Canada by sanctioning blind bowling leagues and conducting a National Tournament. Current membership exceeds 2,000 people in the United States and Canada.

9171   Basketball: Beeping Foam
Maxi Aids
42 Executive Boulevard
Farmingdale, NY   11735   631-752-0521
                                               800-522-6294
                                          Fax: 631-752-0689
                                             TTY: 631-752-0738
                                            sales@maxiaids.com
                                              www.maxiaids.com
Elliot Zaretsky, President
This sound making basketball enables the visually impaired to play basketball or other games. *$29.95*

9172   Blind Outdoor Leisure Development
P.O.Box 6639
Snowmass Village, CO   81615   970-923-0578
                                          Fax: 970-923-7338
                               possibilities@challengeaspen.com
                                            challengeaspen.org
Jimmy Yeager, President
Jack Kennedy, VP
Grayson Stover, Secretary
Kevin Berg, Director
Outdoor recreation for the blind. Winter program of skiing with guides plus numerous summer programs for the visually impaired.

9173   Challenge Golf
 otivation Media
1245 Milwaukee Ave
Glenview, IL   60025-2400   847-827-9057
                                          Fax: 847-297-6829
Dorothy Bauer, Coordinator

A plain-language video, Challenge Golf is packed with information for beginners or veterans. Peter Longo covers 5 handicaps (one-arm, one-leg, in a seated position, blind, and arthritis) clearly and concisely, on how to play golf with a physical disability. In color, complete with special effects, graphs and real handicapped golfers at play. *$38.95*
Home Edition

9174   US Association of Blind Athletes
1 Olympic Plaza
Colorado Springs, CO   80909   719-630-0422
                                          Fax: 719-630-0616
                                                www.usaba.org
Mark A. Lucas, MS, Executive Director
Ryan Ortiz, Assistant Executive Director
John Potts, Goalball High Performance director
Matt Simpson, Membership & Outreach Coordinator
Provides athletic opportunities and training in competitive sports for visually impaired and blind individuals throughout the US Competitions indlcude local, regional and national events, internation events, and the Winter and Summer Paralympic Games.

9175   United States Blind Golf Association
3094 Shamrock St N
Tallahassee, FL   32309-2735   520-648-1088
                                          info@usblindgolf.com
                                             www.blindgolf.com
Dick Pomo, President
Provides blind and vision impaired gold tournaments to members.

Support Groups

9176   Braille Institute Orange County Center
527 North Dale Avenue
Anaheim, CA   92801   714-821-5000
                                               800-272-4553
                                          Fax: 714-527-7621
                                           oc@brailleinstitute.org
                                             brailleinstitute.org
Lester M. Sussman, Chairman
Peter A. Mindnich, President
Jon K. Hayashida, OD, FAAO, Vice President, Programs & Services
Rezaur Rehman, Vice President, Finance
Offers services, publications, information and programs free of charge to blind and visually impaired persons of all ages.

9177   Consumer and Patient Information Hotline
Prevent Blindness America
211 West Wacker Drive
Suite 1700
Chicago, IL   60606   800-331-2020
                                        info@preventblindness.org
                                         www.preventblindness.org/
Paul G. Howes, Chairman
Hugh R. Parry, President & CEO,Prevent Blindness America
Jerome Desserich, Vice President & Chief Financial Officer
Danielle Disch, Development Manager
A toll-free line offering free information on a broad range of vision, eye health and safety topics including sports eye safety, diabetic retinopathy, glaucoma, cataracts, children's eye disorders and more.

9178   Department of Ophthalmology Information Line
Eye & Ear Infirmary
1855 W Taylor St
Chicago, IL   60612-7242   312-996-6590
                                          Fax: 312-996-7770
                                                eyeweb@uic.edu
                                                    www.uic.edu
Jospeh White, President
Offers eye clinic and physician referrals to persons suffering from vision disorders as well as offers emergency information.

9179 Lighthouse International Information and Resource Service
111 East 59th Street
New York, NY 10022-1202
212-821-9384
800-829-0500
Fax: 212-821-9707
info@lighthouse.org
lighthouse.org

Mark G. Ackermann, President / CEO

Provides information about eye diseases, low vision, age-related vision loss, adaptive technology, optical devices, large print and braille publishers, helps people find low vision services, vision rehabilitation services, and support groups across the U.S.; offers large selection of consumer products.

9180 National Association for Parents of Children with Visual Impairments (NAPVI)
1 North Lexington Avenue
White Plains, NY 10601
617-972-7441
800-562-6265
Fax: 617-972-7444
napvi@guildhealth.org
www.napvi.org

Julie Urban, President
Venetia Hayden, Vice President
Susan LaVenture, Executive Director
Randi Sher, Secretary

In 1979, a group of parents responding to their own needs founded NAPVI, the National Association for Parents of the Visually Impaired, Inc. Never before was there a self-help organization specific to the needs of families of children with visual impairments. Since that time, NAPVI has grown and helped families across the US and in other countries.

9181 VUE: Vision Use in Employment
Carroll Center for the Blind
770 Centre Street
Newton, MA 02458-2597
617-969-6200
800-852-3131
Fax: 617-969-6204
www.carroll.org

Joseph Abely, President
Brian Charlson, Director of Technology
Diane M. Newark, Chief Development Officer
Janet Perry, Human Resources Director

Provides engineering solutions plus training to help people keep jobs despite their vision loss.

9182 Washington Connection
American Council of the Blind
1703 N. Beauregard St
Ste 420
Alexandria, VA 22311
202-467-5081
800-424-8666
Fax: 703-465-5085
info@acb.org
www.acb.org/wc

Kim Charlson, President
Jeff Thom, 1st Vice President
Eric Bridges, Executive Director

Coverage of issues affecting blind people via legislative information, participates in law-making, legislative training seminars and networking of support resources across the US.

A

A-Solution, 538
AACRAO, 2236
AACRC Annual Meeting, 1884
AADB E-News, 7640
AADB National Conference, 1885
AAIDD Annual Meeting, 1886
AAMHL, Inc., 7955
AAN's Toll-Free Hotline, 8694
AAO Annual Meeting, 1887
AAPD Newsletter, 8129
AARP, 2250, 7492
AARP Fulfillment, 5149, 5181, 5268, 7551
AARP Magazine, 7575
ABA Commission on Mental & Physical Disability Law, 4650, 4678
ABA Commission on Mental and Physical Disability, 2519
Abacus, 1664
Abbot and Dorothy H Stevens Foundation, 2996
ABC Mark of Merit Newsletter, 7942
ABC of Asthma, Allergies & Lupus, 8475
ABC Union, ACE, ANLV, Vegas Western Cab, 5592
ABC-CLIO, 2482
ABD Winter Conference, 1888
ABDA/ABMPP Annual Conference, 4632
Abell-Hangar Foundation, 3243
ABI Professional Publications, 8567
Abilitations, 2050
Abilitations - Speech Bin, 8115
Abilities Center of New Jersey, 6147
Abilities Expo, 1897
Abilities in Motion, 4469
Abilities of Florida: An Affiliate of Service Source, 5968
Abilities of Northwest New Jersey, 6148
Abilities Without Boundaries, 5943
Abilities!, 757
Abilitree, 4461
Ability 1st, 4053
Ability Center, 71, 4383
Ability Center of Greater Toledo, 1665, 4444
Ability Center of Greater Toledo: Defiance, 4445
Ability Center of Greater Toledo: Port Cli nton, 4446
Ability Jobs, 5435
Ability Magazine, 5351, 5435
Ability Research, 1560
Ability Resources, 4457
Ability Works Incorporated, 6121
AbilityFirst, 5885, 6597
Abingdon Press, 5320
ABLE Center for Independent Living, 4521
ABLE Industries, 5883
ABLE Program MCC-Longview, 2712
Able to Laugh, 5361
Able Trek Tours, 5567
Able Trust, 2889
Able Trust, The, 5969
AbleApparel - Affordable Adaptive Clothing and Accessories, 5436
AbleArts, 1
AbleData, 1611, 5437
AbleNet, 196, 220, 224, 292, 320, 341, 358, 361, 502, 503, 508, 528, 533, 1567, 1576, 1586, 1596, 1691, 1993, 2372, 5532
Ablenet, 227
AbleNet, Inc., 5509
Ablex Publishing Corporation, 2613
About Children's Eyes, 8941
About Children's Vision: A Guide for Parents, 8942
About Special Kids, 6364
ABS Newsletter, 8249
ACA Annual Conference, 1889
Academic Language Therapy Association, 8719
Academic Press, Journals Division, 2268
Academic Software, 1563, 1584, 1597, 1738, 1751, 1772
Academic Software Inc, 1561
Academic Therapy Publications, 2125, 2376

Academic Therapy Publications / High Noon Books, 2125, 2142
Academy Eye Associates, 7121
Academy for Guided Imagery, 2713
Academy of Cognitive Therapy, 7653
Academy of Rehabilitative Audiology, 2071, 8121, 8146
Academy of Spinal Cord Injury Professionals, 8165
Academy of Spinal Cord Injury Professional s: Psychologists, Social Workers & Counselors, 8166
Academy of Spinal Cord Injury Professionals, 8166
Acc-u-trol, 72
Accent Books & Products, 1952, 5147, 5148, 5150, 5176, 5192, 5212, 5224, 5280, 5543
Accent on Living Magazine, 5059
Accent Special Publications, 1943
Accentcare, 6598
Access Academics & Research, 8824
Access Alaska: ADA Partners Project, 3928
Access Alaska: Fairbanks, 3929
Access Alaska: Mat-Su, 3930
Access America, 5550
Access Audiology, 8815
Access Center for Independent Living, 4447
Access Center of San Diego, 3955
Access Control Systems: NHX Nurse Call System, 188
Access Currents, 1940
Access Design Services: CILs as Experts, 5060
Access Equals Opportunity, 1941
Access for 911 and Telephone Emergency Services, 5062
Access for All, 1942
Access for All: Integrating Deaf, Hard of Hearing and Hearing Preschoolers, 8039
Access for Disabled Americans, 5537
Access II Independent Living Center, 4326
Access II Independent Living Centers, 7579
Access Independence, 4559
Access Living of Metropolitan Chicago, 4112
Access Mobility Systems, 115
Access Schools, 8826
Access Services, 4974
Access SLP Health Care, 8825
Access Store Products for Barrier Free Environments, 430
Access Store.Com, 430
Access to Art: A Museum Directory for Blind and Visually Impaired People, 8943
Access to Health Care: Number 3&4, 2334
Access to Independence, 3956, 5061
Access To Independence Inc., 5061
Access to Independence of Cortland County , Inc., 4395
Access to Independence of Imperial Valley, 3957
Access to Independence of North County, 3958
Access To Recreation, 640, 681
Access to Recreation, 431, 223, 412
Access to Sailing, 8267
Access Travel: Airports, 5539
Access Unlimited, 5438
Access Utah Network, 3851
Access with Ease, 339
Access Yosemite National Park, 5551
Access-USA, 491, 600
Access-USA: Transcription Services, 492
Accessibility Lift, 368
Accessible Home of Your Own, 1943
Accessible Journeys, 5569, 5568
Accessible Space, Inc., 4298
Accessible Vans Of America, 5593
Accessnorth CIL of Northeastern MN: Aitkin, 4299
Accessnorth CIL of Northeastern MN: Duluth, 4300
AccessText Network, 2126
AccessToThePlanet, 5568
Ace Mobility, LLC, 72, 77, 80, 87, 103, 106, 117, 119, 120, 124, 129, 141
Ace Mobility, LLc, 88
Aces Adventure Weekend, 1370
ACES/ACCESS Inclusion Program, 6742
Achieva, 1371
Achievement Centers For Children, 1321, 8378

Achievement Centers for Children, 1337
Achievement House & NCI Affiliates, 5886
Achievement Products, 432
Achieving Diversity and Independence, 5063
Achilles Track Club, 8268
Acid Maltase Deficiency Association, 8167
ACLD/An Association for Children and Adult s with Learning Disabilities: Greater Pittsburgh, 6216
ACM Lifting Lives Music Camp, 1414
ACPOC News, 8661
Acrontech International, 1816
ACS Federal Healthcare, 752
ACT Assessment Test Preparation Reference Manual, 6060
Acting Blind, 5362
Action Camp, 1455
Action Products, 259
Action Toward Independence: Middletown, 4396
Action Toward Independence: Monticello, 4397
Active Citizenship and Disability: Impleme nting the Personalization of Support, 5029
Active Living Magazine, 7943
Active Re-Entry, 4544
Active Re-Entry: Vernal, 4545
Activities in Action, 7541
Activities with Developmentally Disabled Elderly and Older Adults, 7542
Activity-Based Approach to Early Intervention, 2nd Edition, 2335
Activity-Based Intervention: 2nd Edition, 5064
Ad Lib Drop-In Center: Consumer Management, Ownership and Empowerment, 5065
AD/HD and the College Student: The Everyth ing Guide to Your Most Urgent Questions, 2328
ADA and City Governments: Common Problems, 5054
ADA Annual Scientific Sessions, 1890
ADA Camp Aspire, 1269
ADA Camp for Kids, 8360
ADA Camp GrenADA, 1105
ADA Camp Grenada, 8358
ADA Camp Needlepoint, 8359
ADA Guide for Small Businesses, 5049
ADA Hotel Built-In Alerting System, 187
ADA In Details: Interpreting the 2010 Amer icans with Disabilities Act Stands, 4610
ADA Information Services, 5050
ADA Pipeline, 5051
ADA Questions and Answers, 5052, 5434
Ada S McKinley Vocational Services, 6014
ADA Tax Incentive Packet for Business, 5053
ADA Technical Assistance Program, 3472
ADA Teen Adventure Camp, 1106, 8361
ADA Triangle D Camp, 1107, 8362
ADA-TA: A Technical Assistance Update from the Department of Justice, 5055
Adam's Camp, 1039, 1040, 1177, 1242, 1428
Adam's Camp: Alaska, 976
Adam's Camp: Colorado, 1040
Adam's Camp: Nantucket, 1177
Adam's Camp: New Hampshire, 1242
Adam's Camp: Texas, 1428
Adams Media, 5012
Adaptable Housing: A Technical Manual for Implementing Adaptable Dwelling, 1944
Adaptations by Adrian, 1516
Adapted Physical Activity, 5248
Adapted Physical Activity Programs, 2227
Adapted Physical Education and Sport, 8213
Adapted Physical Education for Students with Autism, 2336
Adaptek Systems, 189
Adapting Early Childhood Curricula for Children with Special Needs (9th Edition), 2337
Adapting Instruction for the Mainstream: A Sequential Approach to Teaching, 2338
Adaptivation, 1562
Adaptive Baby Care, 5363
Adaptive Baby Care Equipment Video and Book Through the Looking Glass, 5364
Adaptive Clothing: Adults, 433, 1517
Adaptive Education Strategies Building on Diversity, 2339
Adaptive Environments Center, 1931, 1945

Adaptive Mainstreaming: A Primer for Teachers and Principals, 3rd Edition, 2643
Adaptive Services Division, 9105
Adaptive Sports Center, 8269, 8664
The Adaptive Sports Foundation, 3143
Adaptive Technology Catalog, 434
Adaptive Tracks, 8664
Adaptivemall.com, 1961
ADARA, 8117
ADD Challenge: A Practical Guide for Teachers, 2329
ADD Warehouse, 7796, 7911, 7920
ADD, Stepping Out of the Dark, 7900
ADD-SOI Center, The, 2636
ADD: Helping Your Child, 7762
Addictive & Mental Disorders Division, 3629
Addie McBryde Rehabilitation Center for the Blind, 7063
Addison Point Specialized Services, 6085
Addison-Wesley Publishing Company, 5100
ADDitude Directory, 2102
Address Book, 601
ADEC Resources for Independence, 6038
Adelante Development Center, 6176
ADHD Book of Lists: A Practical Guide for Helping Children and Teens with ADDs, 7763
ADHD Coaching: A Guide for Mental Health P rofessionals, 2330
ADHD in Adults, 7901
ADHD in the Classroom: Strategies for Teachers, 2331
ADHD in the Schools: Assessment and Intervention Strategies, 2332, 7764
ADHD Report, 7880
ADHD with Comorbid Disorders: Clinical Assessment and Management, 7765
ADHD: What Can We Do?, 7902
ADHD: What Do We Know?, 7903
Adjustable Bath Seat, 142
Adjustable Bed, 173
Adjustable Chair, 238
Adjustable Clear Acrylic Tray, 239
Adjustable Incline Board, 369
Adjustable Raised Toilet Seat & Guard, 143
Adjustable Rigid Chair, 240
Adjustable Tee Stool, 241
Adjustable Wedge, 260
Adjustment Training Center, 4506
Adlib, 4250
Administration Building D HS S Campus, 3438
Administration for Community Living, 2167
Administration on Aging, 3341
Administration on Children, Youth and Families, 3342
Administration on Developmental Disabilities, 3343
Administrative Office, 1375, 1433, 8375
Adobe News, 5066
Adolescents and Adults with Learning Disab ilities and ADHD, 2340
Adolescents with Down Syndrome: Toward a More Fulfilling Life, 7766
Adolph Coors Foundation, 2854
ADRS Lakeshore, 5842
Adult Absorbent Briefs, 1551
Adult ADD: The Complete Handbook: Everyt hing You Need to Know About How to Cope with ADD, 7767
Adult Day Training, 4054
Adult Lap Shoulder Bodysuit, 1552
Adult Leukemia: A Comprehensive Guide for Patients and Families, 8479
Adult Long Jumpsuit with Feet, 435
Adult Short Jumpsuit, 436, 1518
Adult Sleeveless Bodysuit, 1553
Adult Swim Diaper, 1554
Adult Tee Shoulder Bodysuit, 1555
Adult Waterproof Overpant, 1556
Advance for Providers of Post-Acute Care, 2228
Advanced Breast Cancer: A Guide to Living with Metastic Disease, 8480
Advanced Language Tool Kit, 1962
Advanced Sign Language Vocabulary: A Resource Text for Educators, 8040

Advanced Sign Language Vocabulary: A Resource Text for Educators, 2341
Advances in Cardiac and Pulmonary Rehabilitation, 2342
Advantage Wheelchair & Walker Bags, 661
Adventist HealthCare, 2714
Adventist Hinsdale Hospital, 8712
Adventure Day Camp, 8364
Adventure Learning Center at Eagle Village, 7710
Adventures in Musicland, 1719
Adventures Without Limits, 1355
Advocacy, 3845
Advocacy Center, 758, 3549
Advocacy Center for Persons with Disabilities, 3456
Advocacy Center of Louisiana, 759
The Advocacy Centre, 946
Advocacy Centre for the Elderly, 760
Advocacy Pulse, 7946
Advocacy Services of Alaska, 3386
Advocado Press, 4674
The Advocado Press, 5042
Advocate, 5067
Advocate Christ Hospital and Medical Center, 6857
Advocate Christ Medical Center & Advocate Hope Children's Hospital, 6858
Advocate Illinois Masonic Medical Center, 6859
Advocates for Better Living For Everyone (A.B.L.E.), 4172
Advocates for Children of New York, 761
Advocates for Developmental Disabilities, 762
AEPS Child Progress Record: For Children Ages Three to Six, 1957
AEPS Child Progress Report: For Children Ages Birth to Three, 2637
AEPS Curriculum for Birth to Three Years, 2333
AEPS Curriculum for Three to Six Years, 1958
AEPS Data Recording Forms: For Children Ages Birth to Three, 2638
AEPS Data Recording Forms: For Children Ages Three to Six, 1959
AEPS Family Interest Survey, 1960
AEPS Family Report: Birth to Three Years, 5246
AEPS Family Report: For Children Ages Birth to Three, 5056
AEPS Family Report: For Children Ages Three to Six, 5247
AEPS Measurement for Birth to Three Years, 2639
AEPS Measurement for Three to Six Years, 2640
AER Annual International Conference, 1891
Aerie Experiences, 1085
Aerospace America, 560
Aerospace Compadre, 560
Aetna Foundation, 2861
AFB Center on Vision Loss, 3080
AFB Directory of Services for Blind and Visually Impaired Persons in the US and Canada, 8940
AFB News, 9103
AFB Press, 2124, 8076
A4 Tech (USA) Corporation, 1663
African Americans in the Profession of Blindness Services, 8944
The AG Academy for Listening and Spoken Language, 2100
AG Bell Convention, 1892
Agassiz Village, 8365
Age Appropriate Puzzles, 5508
Age-Related Macular Degeneration, 8945
Agency for Healthcare Research and Quality, 2183
Agency of Human Services, 1662, 6249
Agency of Human Svcs Dept Disabilities, Aging & IL, 3872
Ages & Stages Questionnaires, 2644
Aging & Disability Services, 3875
Aging & Vision News, 7576
Aging and Developmental Disability: Current Research, Programming, and Practice, 7543
Aging and Disabilities, 3869
Aging and Disability Services, 3876, 7487
Aging and Disability Services Division, 3648
Aging and Disability: Crossing Network Lin es, 2344

Aging and Family Therapy: Practitioner Perspectives on Golden Pond, 7544
Aging and Rehabilitation II: The State of the Practice, 2345
Aging and Vision News, 7578
Aging and Vision: Declarations of Independence, 9155
Aging Brain, 2343
Aging in America, 7488
Aging in Stride, 7545
Aging in the Designed Environment, 7546
Aging Life Care Association, 7483
Aging News Alert, 7577, 7583
Aging Services of Michigan, 7484
Aging Services of South Carolina, 7485
Aging Services of Washington, 7486
Aging with a Disability, 7547
Agnes M Lindsay Trust, 3060
AGRAM, 7582
AGS, 1980, 2006, 2032, 2048, 2063, 2667, 2668, 2669, 2671, 2679, 2681, 2682, 2683, 2699
AHC Media LLC, 8663
AHEAD, 2263, 5104
AHEAD Association, 753
Ahmanson Foundation, 2791
AHRC New York, 1275, 1296
A I Squared, 1685
AI Squared, 1683
Ai Squared, 1720, 5439
AID Bulletin, 8662
AIDS Alert, 8663
AIDS and Other Manifestations of HIV Infec tion, 8477
AIDS Healthcare Foundation, 754
AIDS in the Twenty-First Century: Disease and Globalization, 8478
AIDS Legal Council of Chicago, 4611
AIDS Sourcebook, 8476
AIDS Treatment Data Network, 2321
AIDS United, 8292
AIDS Vancouver, 755
AIDS: The Official Journal of the Internat ional AIDS Society, 8645
AIDSLAW of Louisiana, 4612
AIM Independent Living Center: Corning, 4389
AIM Independent Living Center: Elmira, 4390
AIMS Multimedia, 1697
Aiphone Corporation, 188
Air Lift Oxygen Carriers, 631
Air Lift Unlimited, 631
Air Products Foundation, 3193
AIR: Assessment of Interpersonal Relations, 2641
AJ Pappanikou Center, 2314, 2315
Akron Community Foundation, 3160
Akron Resources, 190
AL Baptist State Board of Missions, 8019
Alabama Council For Developmental Disabilities, 3365
Alabama Department of Education: Division of Special Education Services, 2159
Alabama Department of Labor, 5848
Alabama Department of Public Health, 3366
Alabama Department of Rehabilitation Services, 3367, 6537
Alabama Department Of Rehabilitation Services, 5842, 5851
Alabama Department of Rehabilitation Services, 5849, 5850, 5854, 5855, 5856, 5857, 5858, 5859, 5860, 5861, 5862, 5863, 5864, 5865, 5866, 6542
Alabama Department of Senior Services, 3368
Alabama Disabilities Advocacy Program, 3369
Alabama Division of Rehabilitation and Crippled Children, 3370
Alabama Easter Seal Society, 8363
Alabama Goodwill Industries, 5843
Alabama Governor's Committee on Employment of Persons with Disabilities, 3371
Alabama Institute for Deaf & Blind, 8002
Alabama Institute for Deaf and Blind, 7650
Alabama Institute for Deaf and Blind Library and Resource Center, 4700
Alabama Power Foundation, 2779
Alabama Public Library Service, 4702

Arc of Alaska, 2782
The Arc of Allen County, 2209
The Arc of Anchorage, 2782
Arc of Anderson County, 3231
Arc of Arizona, 7889
The Arc of Arizona, 2785
Arc of Arkansas, 2789
Arc of Bergen and Passaic Counties, 6151
Arc of Blackstone, 4495
Arc of Blackstone Valley, 3218
Arc of California, 2794
Arc of Cape Cod, 4251
Arc of Colorado, 2855
Arc of Connecticut, 2862
Arc of Davidson County, 3232
Arc of Delaware, 2875, 3442
Arc of Dunn County, 3299
Arc of Eau Claire, 3300
Arc of Florida, 2890
Arc of Fox Cities, 3301
Arc Of Georgia, 2904
ARC of Gloucester, 1258
ARC of Gloucester County, 6143
Arc of Hamilton County, 3233
Arc of Hawaii, 2915
ARC of Hunterdon County, The, 6144
Arc of Illinois, 2924
Arc of Indiana, 2959
Arc of Iowa, 2963
Arc of Jefferson County, 5844
Arc of Kansas, 2968
Arc of Kentucky, 2971
Arc of Louisiana, 2972
Arc of Maryland, 2979
Arc of Massachusetts, The, 2997
ARC of Mercer County, 6145
Arc Of Meriden-Wallingford, Inc., 6744
Arc of Michigan, 3013
Arc of Minnesota, 3031
Arc of Mississippi, 3041
ARC of Monmouth, 6146
Arc of Natrona County, 3313
Arc of Nebraska, 3052
Arc of New Jersey, 3062
The Arc of New Jersey, 2204
Arc of New London County, 8390
Arc of New Mexico, 3076
Arc of North Carolina, 3149
The Arc of North Carolina, 7705
Arc of North Dakota, 3158
Arc of Northern Bristol County, 2998
Arc of Northern Rhode Island, 3219
Arc of Ohio, 3162
Arc of Oregon, 3189
Arc of Pennsylvania, 3194
Arc of Racine County, 3302
Arc of San Diego, 7726
The Arc of San Diego, 1026
ARC Of San Diego-ARROW Center, The, 6590
ARC Of San Diego-East County Training Center,
The, 6591
ARC Of San Diego-Rex Industries, The, 6592
ARC Of San-Diego-South Bay, 6593
ARC of Somerset County, 1253
Arc of South Carolina, 3228
ARC Of Southeast Los Angeles-Southeast
Industries, 6594
Arc of Tennessee, 3234, 5074, 7881
Arc of Texas, The, 3246
Arc of the District of Columbia, 2878, 5057
Arc of the Farmington Valley, 6745
Arc of the United States, 5450
The Arc of the United States, 7706
Arc of the US Missouri Chapter, 3044
Arc of Utah, 3276
Arc of Virginia, 3280
Arc of Washington County, 3235
Arc of Washington State, 3287
Arc Of West Virginia, The, 3297
Arc of Williamson County, 3236
Arc of Wisconsin Disability Association, 3303
Arc South County Chapter, 3217
ARC's Government Report, 5057
ARC-Adult Vocational Program, 5884
Arc-Dane County, 3304

Arc-Diversified, 3237
Arc/Muskegon, 4270
ARC: VC Community Connections West, 6595
ARC: VC Ventura, 6596
ARCA - Dakota County Technical College, 5058
ARCA Newsletter, 5058
Arcadia Foundation, 3195
Arcadia University, 2753
Architectural Barriers Action League, 5540
Archives of Neurology, 8648
Arcoa Travel Chair, 684
Arcola Mobility, 73, 112, 114
Arctic Access, 3932
Arden Rehabilitation And Healthcare Center, 7241
Arden Rehabilitation and Healthcare Center, 7456
Ardence, 6430
Ardmore Developmental Center, 6093
Area Access, 371
Area Agency on Aging of Southwest Arkansas,
7597
Area Agency on Aging: Region One, 7598
Area Cooperative Educational Services (ACES),
5945
Arena Stage, 6, 7613
ARISE, 4391
ARISE: Oneida, 4392
ARISE: Oswego, 4393
ARISE: Pulaski, 4394
Arista Surgical Supply Company, 632
Arista Surgical Supply Company/AliMed, 169,
639, 649, 720
Arizona State Department of Health Services,
2326
Arizona Autism Resources, 2785
Arizona Braille and Talking Book Library, 4708
Arizona Bridge to Independent Living, 3941, 5090
Arizona Bridge to Independent Living: Phoenix,
3942
Arizona Bridge to Independent Living: Mesa, 3943
Arizona Camp Sunrise, 8366
Arizona Camp Sunrise & Sidekicks, 979
Arizona Center for Disability Law, 3395
Arizona Center for the Blind and Visually
Impaired, 6560
Arizona Civil Rights Division, 5873
Arizona Community Foundation, 2786
Arizona Department of Economic Security, 3388
Arizona Department of Health Services, 3389,
2327, 2453
Arizona Division of Aging and Adult Services,
3390
Arizona Hemophilia Association, 8308, 984, 985,
8395
Arizona Industries for the Blind, 6561
Arizona Instructional Resource Center for
Students who are Blind or Visually Impaired,
The, 2787
Arizona Rehabilitation State Services for the Blind
and Visually Impaired, 3391
Arizona State Library, 4708
Arjo Inc, 163, 244, 245, 404, 409, 410
ArjoHuntleigh, 144, 157
Arkansas Assistive Technology Projects, 3398
Arkansas Children's Neuroscience Center, 991
Arkansas Department of Human Services, 5882
Arkansas Department of Special Education, 2161
Arkansas Division of Aging & Adult Services,
3399
Arkansas Division of Developmental Disabilities
Services, 3400
Arkansas Division of Services for the Blind, 3401
Arkansas Employment Security Department, 5878
Arkansas Employment Service Agency and Job
Training Program, 5878
Arkansas Governor's Developmental Disabilities
Council, 3402
Arkansas Independent Living Council, 3949
Arkansas Lighthouse for the Blind, 6582
Arkansas Regional Library for the Blind and
Physically Handicapped, 4716
Arkansas School for the Blind, 4717
Arkasas Rehab Services, 5880
Arkenstone: The Benetech Initiative, 1564
Arlington County Department of Libraries, 4976
Arlington County Library, 4976

Arms Wide Open, 4082
Armstrong Medical, 440
Army and Air Force Exchange Services, 2750
Arnold A Schwartz Foundation, 3063
Aromatherapy Book: Applications and Inhalations,
5075
Aromatherapy for Common Ailments, 5076
Around the Clock: Parenting the Delayed AD HD
Child, 7904
Arrowhead West, 6952
Art and Disabilities, 8
Art and Healing: Using Expressive Art to Heal
Your Body, Mind, and Soul, 9
Art and Science of Teaching Orientation and
Mobility to Persons with Visual Impairments,
8948
Art for All the Children: Approaches to Art
Therapy for Children with Disabilities, 10
Art Therapy, 5330
Art Therapy SourceBook, 7
Art-Centered Education and Therapy for Children
with Disabilities, 2352
Arthritis Bible, 8214
Arthritis Foundation, 8174, 5184, 5185, 7939,
8223, 8229, 8232, 8234, 8242, 8243, 8244,
8245, 8611
Arthritis Foundation Distribution Center, 5410
Arthritis Foundation Great West Region, 8242
Arthritis Foundation, Southeast Region Inc, 8290
Arthritis Helpbook: A Tested Self Manageme nt
Program for Coping with Arthritis, 8215
Arthritis Self-Management, 8665
Arthritis Sourcebook, 8216
Arthritis Sourcebook., 8487
Arthritis Today, 8234
Arthritis Update, 8243
Arthritis, What Exercises Work: Breakthrou gh
Relief for the Rest of Your Life, 8217
Arthritis: A Take Care of Yourself Health Guide,
8218
Arthur C. Luf Children's Burn Camp, 1058
Arthur Ross Foundation, 3086
Artic Business Vision (for DOS) and Artic
WinVision (for Windows 95), 1686
Artic Technologies, 1686
Artificial Language Laboratory, 4864, 8814
Artificial Larynx, 194
Artists Fellowship, 3087
The Arts of Life, 66
Arts Unbound, 11
As I Am, 5077
ASB Visions Newsletter, 9104
ASCCA, 8363
Ascension Health, 6409
ASD Athletics, 7650
ASD Summer Camp, 8002
ASHA Convention, 1894
ASHA Leader, The, 8130
Asheville VA Medical Center, 5761
Ashton Memorial Nursing Home and Chemical
Dependency Center, 6853
ASIA Annual Scientific Meeting, 1895
Aspen Camp, 1041
Aspen Camp of the Deaf & Hard of Hearing, 8004
Aspen Camp School for the Deaf earing, 8003
Aspen Publishers, 5070, 5231
Aspire of Western New York, 7101
Assemblies of God Center for the Blind, 4892
Assessing Students with Special Needs, 2646
Assessing the Handicaps/Needs of Children, 2353
Assessment & Management of Mainstreamed
Hearing-Impaired Children, 2354
Assessment and Remediation of Articulatory and
Phonological Disorders, 2356
Assessment in Mental Handicap: A Guide to
Assessment Practices & Tests, 2357
Assessment Log & Developmental Progress Charts
for the CCPSN, 2355, 2647
Assessment of Children and Youth, 2358
Assessment of Individuals with Severe
Disabilities, 2359
Assessment of Learners with Special Needs, 2648
Assessment of the Feasibility of Contracting with
a Nominee Agency, 4636

David Fulton Publishers (Routledge), 2618
David J Green Foundation, 3099
Davidson College, 2756
Davidson College, Office of Study Abroad, 2756
Davis Center, 198, 7962, 8728
The Davis Center, 948, 1613
Davis Center for Rehabilitation Baptist Hospital of Miami, 6781
DAWN Center for Independent Living, 4371
Dawn Enterprises, 4099
DawnSign Press, 8047, 8087, 8158
Dayle McIntosh Center: Laguna Niguel, 3987
DAYS: Depression and Anxiety in Youth Scale, 2659
Dayspring Associates, 451
Dayton VA Medical Center, 5772
Dazor Manufacturing Corporation, 505, 619, 628
DB-Link, 834
DBTAC-Great Lakes ADA Center, 6358
DD Center/St Lukes: Roosevelt Hospital Center, 4406
DDDS/Georgetown Center, 6759
DE French Foundation, 3097
Deaf Action Center Of Greater New Orleans, 6975
Deaf Camps, 1174
Deaf Catholic, 8134
Deaf Centers of Nevada, 1239
Deaf Children Signers, 5378
Deaf Culture Series, 5379
Deaf Empowerment: Emergence, Struggle and Rhetoric, 8058
Deaf History Unveiled: Interpretations from the New Scholarship, 8059
Deaf in America: Voices from a Culture, 8062
Deaf Kid's Kamp, 8022
Deaf Like Me, 8060
Deaf Mosaic, 5380
Deaf Parents and Their Hearing Children, 8061
Deaf REACH, 7963
Deaf West Theatre, 21
Deaf Women United, 7964
Deaf-Blind American, 7634
Deaf-Blind Division of the National Federa tion of the Blind, 8866
Deaf-Blind Division of the Ntn'l Fed of the Blind, 9094, 9096
Deaf-Blind Perspective, 7637, 9114
Deafness and Communicative Disorders Branch of Rehab Services Administration Office, 8729
Deafness Research Foundation, 7965, 8126
Dean A McGee Eye Institute, 7166
Deciphering the System: A Guide for Families of Young Disabled Children, 2412
DecisionHealth, 7580
Defining Rehabilitation Agency Types, 2413
Delano Regional Medical Center, 6634
Delaware Assistive Technology Initiative (DATI), 4747
Delaware Assistive Technology Initiative (DATI), 3436
Delaware Association for the Blind, 6760
Delaware Client Assistance Program, 3437
Delaware Department of Health and Social Services, 3438
Delaware Department of Labor, 5957
Delaware Department of Public Instructing, 3439
Delaware Developmental Disability Council, 3440
Delaware Division for the Visually Impaire d, 3441
Delaware Division of Vocational Rehabilita tion, 5957
Delaware Job Training Program Liaison, 5958
Delaware Library for the Blind and Physically Handicapped, 4748
Delaware Protection & Advocacy for Persons with Disabilities, 3442
Delaware VA Regional Office, 5646
Delaware Veterans Center, 6761
Delaware Workers Compensation Board, 3443
Dell Rapids Sportsmens Club, 5573
Delmar Cengage Learning, 8559
Delta Center, 6877
Delta Center for Independent Living, 4329
Delta Resource Center for Independent Living, 3950

Delta Society National Service Dog Center, 521
Deluxe Bath Bench with Adjustable Legs, 155
Deluxe Convertible Exercise Staircase, 381
Deluxe Corporation, 3032
Deluxe Corporation Foundation, 3032
Deluxe Long Ring Low Vision Timer, 342
Deluxe Nova Wheeled Walker & Avant Wheeled Walker, 638
Deluxe Roller Knife, 343
Deluxe Signature Guide, 608
Deluxe Sock and Stocking Aid, 288
Deluxe Standard Wood Cane, 639
Demand Response Transportation Through a Rural ILC, 5112
Dementia Society of America, 7678
Demos Health Publishing, 5082
Demos Medical Publishing, 5159, 7941, 8486, 8511, 8522, 8523, 8527, 8545, 8572, 8573, 8574, 8575, 8577
Demystifying Job Development: Field-Based Approaches to Job Development for the Disabled, 5353
Den-Mar Rehabilitation and Nursing Center, 7352
Dennis Developmental Center, 2661
Dental Amalgam Syndrome (DAMS) Newsletter, 4727
Denver CIL, 4028
Denver Foundation, 2858
Denver VA Medical Center, 5640
Department Human Services, 3676
Department of Heath Education, 3700
Department of Aging and Independent Living, 4555
Department of Blind Rehabilitation, 3583
Department of Education, 2166, 3647, 3660, 4887, 6142
Department of Employment Security, 6021
Department of Health, 3488
Department of Health & Rehabilitative Services, 3459
Department Of Health & Social Services - Division Of Behaviorial Health, 3382
Department Of Health and Human Services, 3401
Department of Health and Human Services, 3645, 3661, 6190
Department of Housing & Urban Development (HUD), 5155
Department of Human Rights, 3526
Department Of Human Services, 6110
Department of Human Services, 3399, 4115, 4118, 6164, 6234
Department of Justice ADA Mediation Program, 4647
Department of Labor, 3755, 3874, 6132, 6165
Department of Labor & Workforce Development, 3387, 5869
Department of Labor and Employment, 5931
Department of Labor and Industrial Realtions, 3628
Department of Medicine and Surgery Veterans Administration, 5605
Department of Mental Health, Retardation and Hospitals of Rhode Island, 3783
Department Of Ophthalmalogy, 4769
Department of Ophthalmology and Visual Science, 4792
Department of Ophthalmology Information Line, 9178
Department of Pennsylvania, 3775
Department of Physical Medicine & Rehabilitation at Sinai Hospital, 835
Department of Physical Medicine and Rehabilitation, 7079
Department of Physical Medicine and Rehabilitation, 6773
Department of Public Health Human Services, 2195
Department of Public Instruction: Exceptional Children & Special Programs Division, 2166
Department of Rehabilitation Services & Bureau of Education And Services for the Blind, 2165
Department Of Rehabilitative Services, 6253
Department of Services for the Blind, 6262
Department of Services for the Blind National Business & Disability Council, 6262

Department of Social and Health, 6266
Department of Social Services, 3556, 5956
Department of Veteran s Affairs, 5631
Department of Veterans Affairs, 5689, 5808
Department of Veterans Affairs Vet Center #418, 6929
Department of Veterans Affairs of Washington DC, 6587
Department of Veterans Affairs Regional Office - Vocational Rehab Division, 5606
Department of Veterans Benefits, 5607
Department Of Workforce Development, 6103
Depression and Bipolar Support Alliance, 7679
Dept of Labor & Workforce Development, 3822
Des Moines Division-VA Central Iowa Health Care System, 6936
Des Moines VA Medical Center, 5677
Des Moines VA Regional Office, 5678
Desert Area Resources and Training, 6639
Desert Blind & Handicapped Association, 8867
Desert Blind and Handicapped Association, Inc., 8867
Desert Haven Enterprises, 5893
Desert Life Rehabilitation & Care Center, 6565, 7266
Desert Regional Medical Center, 6635
Design for Acessibility, 1946
Designing and Using Assistive Technology: The Human Perspective, 2414
Designs for Comfort, 1523
Detroit Center for Independent Living, 4278
DEUCE Environmental Control Unit, 504
Deutsch Foundation, 2809
Developing Cross-Cultural Competence:Guide to Working with Young Children & Their Families, 2415
Developing Individualized Family Support Plans: A Training Manual, 2416
Developing Organized Coalitions and Strategic Plans, 5113
Developing Personal Safety Skills in Children with Disabilities, 5258
Developing Staff Competencies for Supporting People with Disabilities, 2417
Development of Language, 2418
Development of Social Skills by Blind and Visually Impaired Students, 8977
Developmental Disabilities Council, 1629
Developmental Disabilities in Infancy and Childhood, 5259
Developmental Disabilities of Learning, 2419
Developmental Disabilities Planning Council, 6366
Developmental Disabilities: A Handbook for Occupational Therapists, 2420
Developmental Disabilities: A Handbook for Interdisciplinary Practice, 2421
Developmental Disability Council: Arizona, 3392
Developmental Disability Services Section, 3724
Developmental Evaluation and Adjustment Fa cilities, 4257
Developmental Services Center, 2662
Developmental Services of Northwest Kansas, 6954
Developmental Training Services, 5932
Developmental Variation and Learning Disorders, 2422
Devereax Foundation, 7221
Devereux Advanced Behavioral Health - Texas Victoria Campus, 7212
Devereux Advanced Behavioral Health Arizona - Scottsdale, 6566
Devereux Advanced Behavioral Health California, 6636
Devereux Advanced Behavioral Health Colorado, 6729
Devereux Advanced Behavioral Health Florida - Titusville Campus, 6782
Devereux Advanced Behavioral Health Georgia, 6841
Devereux Advanced Behavioral Health Massachusetts & Rhode Island, 7017
Devereux Advanced Behavioral Health - Florida, 6783

Devereux Advanced Behavioral Health - National Office, 7183
Devereux Advanced Behavioral Health Connecticut, 2740
Devereux Advanced Behavioral Health New Jersey, 7089
Devereux Advanced Behavioral Health New York, 7106
Devereux Advanced Behavioral Health Texas - League City Campus, 7213
Devereux Arizona - Tucson, 6567
Devereux Florida - Orlando Campus, 6784
Devereux Florida - Viera Campus, 6785
Devereux Florida Corporate Office, 6783
Devereux Foundation, 7205, 7207, 7211
Devereux Georgia Treatment Network, 6841
Devereux New Jersey, 7089
Devereux New York, 7106
Devereux Orlando Campus, 6784
Devereux Pennsylvania, 7184
Devereux School, 7017
Devereux Threshold Center for Autism, 6786
Devereux Viera Campus, 6785
Diabetes Camp, 8430
Diabetes Camping And Educational Services, Inc., 999
Diabetes Dayton, 1329, 8401
Diabetes Network of East Hawaii, 3485
Diabetes Self-Management, 8668
Diabetes Society, 8427
Diabetes Solutions of Oklahoma, Inc., 1351
Diabetes Sourcebook., 8516
Diabetic Cruise Desk, 5574
Diabetic Retinopathy, 8978
Diabetic Youth Families, 995
Diabetic Youth Foundation, 8367
Diabetic Youth Services, 8381
Diagnostic Report Writer, 1818
Dial Books, 8954
Dial-a-Hearing Screening Test, 8164
Dial: Disabled Information Awareness & Liv ing, 4372
Dialog Corporation, 1638
Dialogue Magazine, 9095
Dialysis at Sea Cruises, 5575
Dialysis Clinic, Inc., 1423
DiaMedica Inc., 5303
Dice: Jumbo Size, 5523
Dictionary of Congenital Malformations & Disorders, 5114
Dictionary of Developmental Disabilities Terminology, 5115, 5260
Didlake, 6254
Diestco Manufacturing Company, 678
Different Dream Parenting: A Practical Guide to Raising a Child with Special Needs, 5304
Different Roads to Learning, 1983
Difficult Child, 7801
Digest of Neurology and Psychiatry, 2423
Digestive Diseases & Disorders Sourcebook, 8517
Digi-Flex, 506
Digital Hearing Aids, 322
Dilemma, 1737
Dimensions of State Mental Health Policy, 4648
Dino-Games, 1738
Diocese of Maine Episcopal, 8007
Dionysus Theatre, 22
DIRECT Center for Independence, 3945
Directions, 8669
Directions Unlimited Acccessible Tours, 5576
Directions: Technology in Special Education, 1739
Directory for Exceptional Children, 2110
Directory of Accessible Building Products, 1947
Directory of Financial Aids for Women, 3317
Directory of Members, 5116
Directory Of Services For People With Disa bilities, 2109
Directory of Travel Agencies for the Disabled, 5541
DIRLINE, 1628
Disabilities Network of Eastern Connecticu t, 4041
Disabilities Rights Center, Inc, 3668
Disabilities Sourcebook, 452
Disability & Rehabilitation Journal, 5336
Disability & Society, 2241

Disability Action Center, 4502
Disability Action Center NW, 4100
Disability Action Center NW: Coeur D'Alene, 4101
Disability Action Center NW: Lewiston, 4102
Disability Advocates of Kent County, 4279
Disability Analysis Handbook: Tools for Independent Practice, 5337
Disability Analyst, 1900
Disability and Communication Access Board, 3486
Disability and Health Journal, 2243
Disability and Health: National Center for Birth Defects and Developmental Disabilities, 8701
Disability and Rehabilitation, 2426
Disability and Social Performance: Using Drama to Achieve Successful Acts, 23
Disability and Sport, 8219
Disability Awareness Guide, 5117
Disability Awareness Network, 4431
Disability Bookshop Catalog, 453
Disability Center for Independent Living, 4029
Disability Coalition of Northern Kentucky, 4223
Disability Compliance for Higher Education, 2287, 4649
Disability Connection, 4280
Disability Connections, 4084
disAbility Connections, 4297
Disability Culture Perspective on Early Intervention, 7802
Disability Determination Section, 3897
Disability Determination Service: Birmingham, 3374
Disability Determination Services, 3813
Disability Discrimination Law, Evidence an d Testimony, 4650
Disability Funders Network, 837
Disability Funding News, 2424, 3318
DisAbility Information and Resources, 5459
Disability Law Center, 3861
Disability Law Center of Alaska, 3385
Disability Law Colorado, 4616
Disability Law in the United States, 4651
Disability Law Project, 3862
DisAbility LINK, 836
disABILITY LINK: Rome, 4092
Disability Matters, 1912
Disability Ministries at St. Augustine Parish, 1346
Disability Network, 8700
Disability Network of Mid-Michigan, 4282
Disability Network of Oakland & Macomb, 4283
Disability Network Southwest Michigan, 4281
Disability Network/Lakeshore, 4284
Disability Policy Consortium, 3823
Disability Pride Newsletter, 2288
Disability Resource Agency for Independent Living: Modesto, 3988
Disability Resource Association, 4330
Disability Resource Center, 4071, 4565
Disability Resource Center of Fairfield County, 4042
DisAbility Resource Center: Knoxville, 4516
DisAbility Resource Connection: Everett, 4584
Disability Resource Initiative, 4224
Disability Resources, 2289
Disability Resources Monthly, 2289
Disability Rights & Resources, 4432
Disability Rights Activist, 5460
Disability Rights Advocates, 4617
Disability Rights Bar Association, 838
Disability Rights Center of Kansas, 3540
Disability Rights Education and Defense Fund, 4618
Disability Rights Education and Defense Fn, 4637
Disability Rights Education and Defense Fund, 4652, 5404
Disability Rights Florida, 839
Disability Rights Montana, 3630
Disability Rights Movement, 5118
Disability Rights New Jersey, 4373
Disability Rights Now, 4652
Disability Rights of Pennsylvania (DRP), 3771
Disability Rights Texas, 4619
Disability Rights Vermont, 3863
Disability Rights Wisconsin: Milwaukee Office, 3906

Disability Rights: Washington, 3886
Disability Services & Legal Center, 3989
Disability Services Division of Montana, 7076
disAbility Solutions for Independent Livin g, 4081
Disability Studies and the Inclusive Class room, 2425
Disability Studies Quarterly, 2242
Disability Under the Fair Employment & Housing Act: What You Should Know About the Law, 4653
Disability, Sport and Society, 2427
DisabilityAdvisor.com, 2134, 5461
DisabilityResources.org, 5462
Disabled & Alone/Life Services for the Handicapped, 5170, 5269
Disabled American Veterans, 5649
Disabled American Veterans Headquarters, 5608
Disabled American Veterans: Ocean County, 5739
Disabled and Alone: Life Services for the Handicapped, Inc., 844
Disabled Athlete Sports Association, 840
Disabled Businesspersons Association, 841
Disabled Children's Fund, 842
Disabled Drummers Association, 843
Disabled God: Toward a Liberatory Theology of Disability, 5320
Disabled People's International Fifth World Assembly as Reported by Two US Participants, 5119
Disabled Resource Services, 4030, 5111
Disabled Resources Center, 3990
Disabled Rights: American Disability Polic y and the Fight for Equality, 2428
Disabled Sports Program Center, 8272
Disabled Sports USA, 8273
Disabled Sports USA Far West, 8272
Disabled Watersports Program, 8274
Disabled We Stand, 5120
Disabled, the Media, and the Information Age, 5121
Disbled Resource Services, 4031
Discount School Supply, 1984
Discover Technology, 5463
Discovery Camps, 1463
Discovery Day Camp, 1241
Discovery Education, 1697
Discovery House Publishers, 5304
Discovery Newsletter, 5122
Discrimination is Against the Law, 4654
Discriptive Language Arts Development, 1819
Disorders of Motor Speech: Assessment, Treatment, and Clinical Characterization, 8780
District of Columbia Center for Independen t Living, 4051
District of Columbia Department of Employment Services, 5960
District of Columbia Department of Handicapped Children, 3446
District of Columbia Dept. of Employment Services: Office of Workforce Development, 5961
District of Columbia Fair Employment Practice Agencies, 5962
District of Columbia General Hospital Physical Medicine & Rehab Services, 6768
District of Columbia Office on Aging, 3447
District of Columbia Public Library, 4750, 9105
District of Columbia Public Library: Services for the Deaf Community, 4750
District of Columbia Public Schools: Special Education Division, 2168
District of Columbia Regional Library for the Blind and Physically Handicapped, 4751
Diversified Opportunities, 7122
Diversity and Visual Impairment: The Influ ence of Race, Gender, Religion and Ethnicity, 8979
Divided Legacy: A History of the Schism in Medical Thought, The Bacteriological Era, 2429
Division for Early Childhood of the Counci l for Exceptional Children, 2079
Division for Physical, Health & Multiple Disabilities, 2080, 8315
Division for the Blind and Visually Impaired, 6092
The Division for the Visually Impaired, 3445

F

Katy Isaacson Elaine Gordon Lodge, 1296
Kauai Center for Independent Living, 4097
Kaufman Test of Educational Achievement (K-TEA), 2671
Kay Elemetrics Corporation, 1687, 1825
Kayelemetrics Corporation, 1830
Keats Publishing, 5196
Keep the Promise: Managed Care and People with Disabilities, 5167
Keeping Ahead in School, 2005
Keeping Our Families Together, 5168
Kelley Diversified, 6001
Kelly Services Foundation, 3025
Ken McRight Supplies, 174, 262
Kenai Peninsula Independent Living Center, 3934
Kenai Peninsula Independent Living Center: Seward, 3935
Kendall Demonstration Elementary School Curriculum Guides, 2500
Keni Peninsula Independent Living Center: Central Peninsula, 3936
Kennebunk Nursing & Rehabilitation Center, 7354
Kennedy Center, 5952
Kennedy Job Training Center, 6024
Kennedy Krieger Institute, 2726, 2991
Kennedy Park Medical Rehabilitation Center, 7472
Kenneth & Evelyn Lipper Foundation, 3119
Kenneth T and Eileen L Norris Foundation, 2824
Kenny Foundation, 5556
Kensington Publishing, 5301
Kent County Arc, 3026
Kent District Library for the Blind and Physically Handicapped, 4869
Kentfield Rehabilitation Hospital & Outpatient Center, 6298
Kentucky Assistive Technology Service Network, 1636
Kentucky Committee on Employment of People with Disabilities, 6073
Kentucky Council on Developmental Disability, 3541
Kentucky Department for Employment Service and Job Training Program Liaison, 6074
Kentucky Department for Mental Health and Mental Retardation Services, 3542
Kentucky Department for Mental Health:, 3543
Kentucky Department of Education: Division of Exceptional Children's Services, 2179
Kentucky Office for the Blind, 3544, 6075
Kentucky Office of Aging Services, 3545
Kentucky Protection & Advocacy, 3546
Kentucky Talking Book Library - Kentucky Dept. for Libraries and Archives, 4827
Kentucky Tennessee Conference, 8930
Kentucky Vocational Rehabilitation Agency, 6076
Keshet Dance and Center for the Arts, 35
Kessler Institute for Rehabilitation, 104
Kessler Institute for Rehabilitation, Welkind Facility, 6426
Kessler Rehabilitation Corporation, 2727
Ketch Industries, 6959
Ketogenic Diet: A Treatment for Children and Others with Epilepsy, 8545
Key Changes: A Portrait of Lisa Thorson, 8263
Key Holders, Ignition & Door Keys, 105
Key Tronic KB 5153 Touch Pad Keyboard, 1673
Keyboard Tutor, Music Software, 1760
Keyboarding by Ability, 1761
Keyboarding for the Physically Handicapped, 1762
Keyboarding with One Hand, 1763
KeyMath Teach and Practice, 2006
Keys to Parenting a Child with Attention Deficit Disorder, 7831
Keys to Parenting a Child with Downs Syndrome, 7832
Keys to Parenting the Child with Autism, 7833
Keystone Blind Association, 8879
The Keystone Group, 3221
KeyTronic, 1673
Keywi, 1690
KG Saur/Division of RR Bowker, 5160
Kid's Custom, 725
Kid's Edge, 726
Kid's Liberty, 727
Kid-Friendly Chairs, 728

Kid-Friendly Parenting with Deaf and Hard of Hearing Children, 8083
KIDS (Keyboard Introductory Development Series), 1759
Kids Cancer Alliance, 1150
KiDS NEED MoRE, 1274
Kids on the Block Programs, 8291
Kindered Health Care, 7429
Kindred, 6727, 7270, 7473
Kindred Health Care, 7252, 7273, 7334, 7440, 7447, 7460, 7482
Kindred Health Care Center, 7271
Kindred Health Care Publications, 7448
Kindred Healthcare, 7015, 7266, 7317, 7344, 7421, 7428, 7450, 7459, 7472, 7481
Kindred Healthcare, Inc., 6722
Kindred Heights Nursing & Rehabilitation Center, 7428
Kindred Hospital-La Mirada, 6661
Kindred Transitional Care and Rehabilitation, 7315
King's Daughter's Medical Center's Rehab Unit/Work Hardening Program, 6965
King's Rehabilitation Center, 5902
King's Rule, 1703
King's View Work Experience Center- Atwater, 6662
Kings Harbor Multicare Center, 7392
Kiplinger Foundation, 2885
Kitsap Community Resources, 4585
Kitten Who Couldn't Purr, 8783
Kiwanis Camp Wyman, 8444
Kiwanis Club of Montavilla, 1366
Kleinert's, 470
KLST-2: Kindergarten Language Screening Test Edition, 2nd Edition, 2670
Kluge Children's Rehabilitation Center, 6525
Knee Socks, 1524
Knock Light, 515
Know Your Eye, 9020
Knowing Your Rights, 4667
Knox County Council for Developmental Disabilities, 6025
Knoxville VA Medical Center, 5680
Koala Miniflex, 729
Koicheff Health Care Center, 7114
Kokomo Rehabilitation Hospital, 6371
Koret Foundation, 2825
Kostopulos Dream Foundation, 1459
Kota Camp, 994
Kreider Services, 6026
Kresge Foundation, 3027
Krieger Publishing Company, 2388, 2594, 8222
Kris' Camp, 1083
Kris' Camp/Therapy Intensive Programs, Inc., 1083
Kroepke Kontrols, 83, 92, 95, 97, 100, 102, 108
Kuhn Employment Oppurtunities, 6752
Kuschall North America, 240
Kuschall of America, 687, 688, 689, 697
Kuzell Institute for Arthritis and Infectious Diseases, 4731

L

La Frontera Center, 6572
La-Z-Boy, 399
LA84 Foundation, 2826
Lab School of Washington, 2170, 7738
LaBac Systems, 743
Labeling the Mentally Retarded, 7835
Laboure College Library, 4860
Ladacain Network, 7090
Ladybug Corner Chair, 250
Lafayette Nursing and Rehabilitation Center, 7307
LaFayette-Walker Public Library, 4782
Lake County Center for Independent Living, 4126
Lake County Health Department, 6892
Lake County Public Library Talking Books Service, 4810
Lake Erie College, 2762
Lake Michigan Academy, 2728
Lakeland Adult Day Training, 4072
Lakeland Center, 7047

Lakemary Center, 6960
LakeMed Nursing and Rehabilitation Center, 7417
Lakeshore Camp & Retreat Center, 1417, 1420
Lakeshore Foundation, 8278
Lakeshore Learning Materials, 2007
Lakeside Milam Recovery Centers (LMRC), 7247
Lakeview NeuroRehabilitation Center, 6419
Lakeview Rehabilitation Hospital, 6388
Lakeview Subacute Care Center, 7380
Lakewood Health Care Center, 7248
Lambs Farm, 6027
Lambton County Developmental Services, 888
LampLighter, 9123
Lamplighter's Work Center, 6111
Lanakila Rehabilitation Center, 6006
Land of Lincoln Goodwill Industries, 6028
Land-of-Sky Regional Council Area Agency on Aging, 7601
Landmark Media, 5369, 5394, 5422, 7649, 8949, 9167
Lane Community College, 2763
Language and Communication Disorders in Children, 2503
Language and the Developing Child, 8785
Language Arts: Detecting Special Needs, 2501
Language Disabilities in Children and Adolescents, 8784
Language Learning Practices with Deaf Children, 2502
Language Parts Catalog, 2008
Language Tool Kit, 2009
Language, Learning & Living, 204
Language, Speech and Hearing Services in School, 2010
Language, Speech, and Hearing Services in Schools, 8813
Lanting Foundation, 3028
LaPalma Intercommunity Hospital, 6663
Lapeer: Blue Water Center for Independent Living, 4288
LaRabida Children's Hospital and Research Center, 6360
Laradon Hall Society for Exceptional Children and Adults, 6730
Large Button Speaker Phone, 205
Large Print DOS, 1765
Large Print Keyboard Labels, 1577
Large Print Loan Library, 9021
Large Print Loan Library Catalog, 9022
Large Print Recipies for a Healthy Life, 9023
Large Print Telephone Dial, 206
Large Print Touch-Telephone Overlays, 207
Large Type, 1880
Las Animas County Rehabilitation Center, 5937
Las Vegas Healthcare And Rehabilitation Center, 7077
Las Vegas Healthcare and Rehabilitation Center, 7375
Las Vegas Veterans Center, 5732
Las Vegas-Clark County Library District, 4902
Lash & Associates Publishing/Training, 7827
Latchloc Automatic Wheelchair Tiedown, 106
Late Talker: What to Do If Your Child Isn't Talking Yet, 8786
Latex Allergy in Spina Bifida Patients, 8546
Laureate Learning Systems, 1766
Laurel Designs, 661, 5135
Laurel Grove Hospital: Rehab Care Unit, 6299
Laurel Hill Center, 4465
Laurent Clerc: The Story of His Early Years, 8084
Law Center Newsletter, 4668
LC Technologies Inc, 1572
LD Child and the ADHD Child: Ways Parents & Professionals Can Help, 7834
LD Monthly Report, 2303
LD Online, 2087
LD OnLine - WETA Public Television, 5478
LDS Hospital Rehabilitation Center, 6518
LeadingAge, 7504
LeadingAge Arizona, 7505
LeadingAge California, 7506
LeadingAge Connecticut, 7507
LeadingAge Gulf States, 7508
LeadingAge Illinois, 7509
LeadingAge Indiana, 7510

Lions Camp Crescendo, Inc., 8025
Lions Camp Kirby, 1393, 8026
Lions Camp Merrick, 1176, 8027
Lions Camp Tatiyee, 988
Lions Club Industries for the Blind, 7128
Lions Club of Oregon and Washington, 8020
Lions Club Of Texas, 8461, 8935
Lions Club of Texas, 1454, 8032
Lions Clubs International, 2764, 8881
Lions Clubs of District 22-C, 8027
Lions Clubs of California and Nevada, 8028
Lions Den Outdoor Learning Center, 7739
Lions of Multiple District 35, 7625
Lions Services Inc., 7129
Lions Wilderness Camp for Deaf Children, Inc., 1033, 9028
Lions Wilderness Camp Headquarters, 1033
Lions World Services for the Blind, 6586
Lipomas & Lipomyelomeningocele, 8552
Lippincott Williams And Wilkins, 2532
Lippincott Williams & Wilkins, 8515, 8645
Lippincott, Williams & Wilkins, 2383, 2517, 2520, 2521, 2552, 5327, 5335, 7559, 8530, 8650, 8660
Lisa Beth Gerstman Camp, 1297
Lisle, 2765
Listen Up, 9154
Listner, 8144
Literacy & Your Deaf Child: What Every Pa rent Should Know, 8086
Literacy Program, 2014
Literature Based Reading, 2015
Literature Journal, The, 8122
Little City Foundation, 2941
Little Friends, Inc., 6893
Little Heroes Preschool Burn Camp, 1034
Little Mack Communicator, 1691
Little People of America, 8329
Little Red Door Cancer Agency, 1128
Little Red Hen, 1768
Little Rock Vet Center #0713, 6587
Live Independently Networking Center, 4434
Live Independently Networking Center: Hickory, 4435
Live Oaks Career Development Campus, 7152
Liver Disorders Sourcebook, 8553
Livin', 5172
Living an Idea: Empowerment and the Evolution of an Alternative School, 2016
Living Beyond Multiple Sclerosis: A Woman 's Guide, 8554
Living in a State of Stuck, 5173
Living in the Community, 5174
Living Independence for Everyone (LIFE), 4086
Living Independence Network Corporation, 4105
Living Independence Network Corporation: Twin Falls, 4106
Living Independence Network Corporation: C aldwell, 4107
Living Independent for Everyone (LIFE): Pocatello Office, 4108
Living Independently for Everyone (LIFE): Blackfoot Office, 4109
Living Independently for Everyone (LIFE): Pocate, 4109
Living Independently for Everyone: Burley, 4110
Living Independently for Today and Tomorro w, 4347
Living Independently in Northwest Kansas: Hays, 4186
Living Independently Now Center (LINC), 4128
Living Independently Now Center: Sparta, 4129
Living Independently Now Center: Waterloo, 4130
Living Skills Center for the Visually Impaired, 6670
Living Well with Asthma, 8555
Living Well with Chronic Fatigue Syndrome and Fibromyalgia, 8556
Living Well with HIV and AIDS, 8557
Living with a Brother or Sister with Speci al Needs: A Book for Sibs, 5270
Living with Achromatopsia, 9029
Living with Brain Injury: A Guide for Fami lies, 8559
Living with Spina Bifida: A Guide for Fami lies and Professionals, 8560

Living With Spinal Cord Injury Series, 8558
Livingston Center for Independent Living, 4289
LJ Skaggs and Mary C Skaggs Foundation, 2827
Lloyd Hearing Aid Corporation, 321, 322, 325, 332
Lodi Memorial Hospital, 6300
Lodi Memorial Hospital West, 6300
Lola Wright Foundation, 3266
Lollipop Lunch, 8788
Loma Linda University Orthopedic and Rehabilitation Institute, 6671
Long Beach Department of Health and Human Services, 3415
Long Beach Memorial Medical Center Memorial Rehabilitation Hospital, 6301, 7275
Long Beach VA Medical Center, 5627
Long Cane News, 9128
Long Handled Bath Sponges, 159
Long Island Alzheimer's Foundation, 3120
Long Island Center for Independent Living, 4410
Long Island Talking Book Library System, 4928
Long Oven Mitts, 353
Long-Term Care: How to Plan and Pay for It, 7561
Longman Education/Addison Wesley, 2358, 2491
Longman Group, 2588
Longman Publishing Group, 2444, 2556, 2643, 2646
Longreach Reacher, 518
Longwood Foundation, 2876
Look Out for Annie, 9161
Look Who's Laughing, 5399
Looking Good: Learning to Improve Your Appearance, 1769
Loop Scissors, 519
Los Angeles County Department of Health Services, 3416
Los Angeles Regional Office, 5628
LoSeCa Foundation, 892
A Loss for Words, 8038
Lost Tree Village Charitable Foundation, 2899
Lotus Press, 8498
Loud, Proud and Passionate, 5175
Loudoun County Adaptive Recreation Camps, 1477
Loudoun County Local Government, 1477
Louis A Johnson VA Medical Center, 5831
Louis and Anne Abrons Foundation, 3121
Louis de la Parte Florida Mental Health Institute Research Library, 4762
Louis R Lurie Foundation, 2830
Louis Stokes VA Medical Center - Wade Park Campus, 5773
Louisiana Assistive Technology Access Network, 3550
Louisiana Center for Dyslexia and Related Learning Disorders, 3551
Louisiana Center for the Blind, 6983
Louisiana Department of Aging, 3552
Louisiana Department of Education, 2180
Louisiana Department of Education: Office of Special Education Services, 2180
Louisiana Department of Health - Mental Health Services, 3553
Louisiana Developmental Disability Council, 3554
Louisiana Employment Service and Job Training Program Liaison, 6081
Louisiana Learning Resources System, 3555
Louisiana Lions Camp, 1158, 8411
Louisiana State Library, 4830
Louisiana State University Eye Center, 6984
Louisiana State University Genetics Sectio n of Pediatrics, 4831
Louisiana Vocational Rehabilitation Agency, 6082
Louisville Free Public Library, 4828
Louisville VA Medical Center, 5687
Louisville VA Regional Office, 5688
Lourdes Regional Rehabilitation Center, 7091
Lousiana State University, 6984
Love Publishing Company, 2248, 2370, 2398, 2605, 2614, 4662, 7865, 8806
Love: Where to Find It, How to Keep It, 5176
Loving & Letting Go, 5271
Loving Justice, 4673
A Loving Spoonful, 751
Low Effort and No Effort Steering, 111

Low Tech Assistive Devices: A Handbook for the School Setting, 2017
Low Vision Questions and Answers: Definitions, Devices, Services, 9030
Low Vision Services of Kentucky, 6967
Low Vision Telephones, 621
Low Vision: Reflections of the Past, Issues for the Future, 9031
Lowe Syndrome Association, 1916
Lowe Syndrome Conference, 1916
Loyola Press, 5324
LPB Communications, 203
LPDOS Deluxe, 1764
LRP Publications, 2287, 2292, 2317, 3320, 3327, 4649, 4671, 5021, 6345
LS&S, 471, 483
Lucy Lee Hospital, 7070
Luke B Hancock Foundation, 2831
Lumber River Council of Governments Area A gency on Aging, 7602
Lumex Cushions and Mattresses, 273
Lumex Recliner, 251
Luminaud, 473, 464, 1689
Lung Cancer: Making Sense of Diagnosis, Treatment, and Options, 8561
Lung Disorders Sourcebook, 8562
Lung Line Information Service, 8707
Lupus: Alternative Therapies That Work, 8563
Lutheran Blind Mission, 4895
Lutheran Charities Foundation of St Louis, 3049
Lutherans Outdoors in South Dakota, 1413, 8451
Lutherdale Bible Camp, 1494
Lutherdale Ministries, 1494
Lyme Disease Foundation, 5479
Lymphoma Canada, 8330
Lynchburg Area Center for Independent Living, 4573
Lynde and Harry Bradley Foundation, 3308
Lynne Rienner Publishers, 2144
Lyons Campus of the VA New Jersey Healthcare System, 5741

M

M ER S Goodwill, 7068
M Evans and Company, 5277
M&M Health Care Apparel Company, 1525
MA Report, 2305
Mac's Lift Gate, 403
MacDonald Training Center, 6807
MAClown Vocational Rehabilitation Workshop, 5985
MacMillan - St. Martin's Press, 8217
Macomb Library for the Blind & Physically Handicapped, 4870
Macon Library for the Blind and Physically Handicapped, 4780
Macon Resources, 6895
Macular Degeneration Foundation, 8882, 9129
Mad Hatters: Theatre That Makes a World of Difference, 2730
Mada Medical Products, 148, 299, 306, 309, 313, 317, 635, 641, 642, 645, 646, 647, 650, 655, 709, 717
MADAMIST 50/50 PSI Air Compressor, 309
Maddak Inc., 475
Madison County Hospital, 7341
Madison County Rehab Services, 7341
Madison Healthcare and Rehabilitation Cent er, 7437
Madonna Rehabilitation Hospital, 6416, 7373
Magee Rehabilitation Hospital, 6470
MAGIC Foundation for Children's Growth, 2942, 8564
MAGIC Touch, 8564
Magic Wand Keyboard, 1674
Magnetic Card Reader, 354
Magni-Cam & Primer, 622
Magnifier, 9129
Magnifier Bookweight, 623
Magnolia Health Systems, 7330
Main Office & Developmental Training Center, 6883
Maine Assistive Technology Projects, 3558

Maine Association of Non Profits, 2976
Maine Bureau of Elder and Adult Services, 3559
Maine CITE, 1639
Maine Department of Health and Human Services, 3560
Maine Department Of Labor, 6088
Maine Developmental Disabilities Council, 3561
Maine Division for the Blind and Visually Impaired, 3562
Maine Governor's Committee on Employment of the Disabled, 6089
Maine Human Rights Commission, 6090, 6090
Maine Office of Elder Services, 3563
Maine State, 4836
Maine State Library, 4836
Maine VA Regional Office, 5692
Maine Workers' Compensation Board, 3564
Mainland Center Hospital RehabCare Unit, 7223
Mainstay Life Services, 1394
Mainstay Life Services Summer Program, 1394
Mainstream, 893, 3951, 6095, 2522, 5377, 6101, 8956
Mainstream Living, 5480
Mainstream Magazine, 5178
Mainstream Online Magazine of the Able-Disabled, 5481
Mainstreaming and the American Dream, 9032
Mainstreaming Deaf and Hard of Hearing Students: Questions and Answers, 2513
Mainstreaming Exceptional Students: A Guide for Classroom Teachers, 2514
Mainstreaming the Visually Impaired Child, 9033
Mainstreaming: A Practical Approach for Teachers, 2515
Majors Medical Equipment, 707
Makemie Woods Camp, 8445
Makemie Woods Camp/Conference Retreat, 8446
Making a Difference, 5182
Making a Difference: A Wise Approach, 5183
Making Changes: Family Voices on Living Disabilities, 5179
Making Choices for Independent Living, 4247
Making Informed Medical Decisions: Where to Look and How to Use What You Find, 5180
Making Life More Livable, 9034
Making News: How to Get News Coverage of Disability Rights Issues, 4674, 5042
Making School Inclusion Work: A Guide to Everyday Practice, 2019
Making Self-Employment Work for People wit h Disabilities, 5043
Making the Writing Process Work, 7837
Making the Writing Process Work: Strategie s for Composition and Self-Regulation, 2020
Making Wise Decisions for Long-Term Care, 5181
Man's Low-Vision Quartz Watches, 624
Management of Autistic Behavior, 7838, 8565, 8789
Management of Children and Adolescents with ADHD, 7839
Management of Genetic Syndromes, 8566
Managing Attention Deficit Hyperactivity in Children: A Guide for Practitioners, 7840
Managing Diagnostic Tool of Visual Perception, 2516
Managing Post Polio: A Guide to Living Well with Post Polio, 8567
Managing Your Activities, 5184
Managing Your Health Care, 5185
Managing Your Symptoms, 8161
Manatee Springs Care & Rehabilitation Center, 6333
Manchester Regional Office, 5736
Manchester VA Medical Center, 5737
Mane Stream, 1262
Manhattan Public Library, 4819
Manor Care Health Services- Citrus Heights, 6672
Manor Care Health Services- Palm Desert, 6673
Manor Care Health Services-Fountain Valley, 6674
Manor Care Health Services-Hemet, 6675
Manor Care Health Services-Sunnyvale, 6676
Manor Care Health Services-Tacoma, 7249
Manor Care Health Services-Walnut Creek, 6677

Manor Care Nursing and Rehab Center: Tucson, 6573
Manor Care Nursing and Rehabilitation Center: Boulder, 6733
Manor Care Nursing: Denver, 6734
Manor Care Ohio, 6733
ManorCare Health Services-Arlington, 7236
ManorCare Health Services-Lynnwood, 7250
ManorCare Health Services-Spokane, 7251
Manual Alphabet Poster, 2021
Manual of Sequential Art Activities for Classified Children and Adolescents, 37
Many Faces of Dyslexia, 2022
MAP Training Center, 6894
MAPCON Technologies, 2145
Maplebrook School, 1298, 7740
Mapleton Center, 6323
MarbleSoft, 5524, 5531
March of Dimes Birth Defects Foundation, 894
Margaret L Wendt Foundation, 3122
Margaret T Morris Foundation, 2788
Marianjoy Rehabilitation Hospital and Clinics, 6361
Marin Center for Independent Living, 4008
Marin Community Foundation, 2832
Mariner Health Care: Connecticut, 6325
Mariner Health of Nashville, 7438
Mariner Shower and Commode Chair, 160
Marion VA Medical Center, 5670
Marist Brothers Mid-Hudson Valley Camp, 1299, 8447
Mark Elmore Associates Architects, 1934
Mark Seven Deaf Foundation, 1282, 8016
Marmon Valley, 1340
Marriner S Eccles Foundation, 3277
Marshall & Ilsley Trust Company, 3312
Marshall & Ilsley Trust of Florida, 2970
Marshall University College Of Educational & Human, 4998
Martin Luther Homes of Indiana, 4159
Martin Luther Homes of Iowa, 4169
Martin Technology, 653
Martinez Outpatient Clinic, 5629
Martinsburg VA Medical Center, 5832
Marvelwood School, 7741
Marvelwood Summer, 7741
Mary A Crocker Trust, 2833
Mary Bryant Home for the Blind, 6896
Mary Free Bed Rehabilitation Hospital, 7048
Mary Lanning Memorial Hospital, 7374
Mary Reynolds Babcock Foundation, 3155
Maryland Client Assistance Program Division of Rehabilitation Services, 3568
Maryland Department of Aging, 3569
Maryland Department of Disabilities, 1640
Maryland Department of Handicapped Children, 3570
Maryland Developmental Disabilities Council, 3571
Maryland Division of Mental Health, 3572
Maryland Employment Services and Job Training Program Liaison, 6096
Maryland Fair Employment Practice Agency, 6097
Maryland State Department of Education, 6098, 4842
Maryland State Department of Education: Division of Special Education, 2186
Maryland State Library for the Blind and Physically Handicapped, 4842
Maryland Technology Assistance Program, 1640
Maryland Veterans Centers, 5697
Mask of Benevolence: Disabling the Deaf Community, The, 8087
Masonic Healthcare Center, 7287
MasoniCare Corporation, 7287
Massachusetts Assistive Technology Partnership, 3577
Massachusetts Client Assistance Program, 3578
Massachusetts Department of Education, 2182
Massachusetts Department of Education: Program Quality Assurance, 2182
Massachusetts Department of Mental Health, 3579
Massachusetts Developmental Disabilities Council, 3580

Massachusetts Eye & Ear Infirmary, 4859
Massachusetts Eye and Ear Infirmary & Vision Rehabilitation Center, 7027
Massachusetts Fair Employment Practice Agency, 6105
Massachusetts Governor's Commission on Employment of Disabled Persons, 6106
Massachusetts Office on Disability, 3578
Massachusetts Rehabilitation Commission, 4861
Massena Independent Living Center, 4411
Mat Factory, 670, 673, 675
Match-Sort-Assemble Job Cards, 2023
Match-Sort-Assemble Pictures, 2024
Match-Sort-Assemble SCHEMATICS, 2025
Match-Sort-Assemble TOOLS, 2026
Math for Everyday Living, 1706
Math for Successful Living, 1707
Math Rabbit, 1705
Maumee Valley Girl Scout Center, 8405
Maxi Aids, 476, 99, 154, 155, 158, 160, 168, 170, 176, 206, 207, 287, 289, 294, 295, 315, 316, 336, 337, 340, 342, 345, 346, 348, 350, 351, 354, 355, 362, 382, 497, 513, 547, 549, 551, 552, 555, 556, 559, 571, 579, 602, 604, 605, 608, 612, 616, 617, 625, 626, , 627, 633, 634, 636, 637, 643, 657, 659, 684, 718, 738, 739, 748, 1601, 5511, 5512, 5513, 5514, 5515, 5516, 5517, 5518, 5520, 5521, 5522, 5527, 5535, 5536, 9171
Maxi Marks, 547
Maxi Superior Cane, 643
Maxi-Aids Braille Timer, 355
Maxi-Aids, 494
MaximEyes, 7647
Maynord's Chemical Dependency Recovery Centers, 6678
Maynord's Ranch for Men, 6679
Mayo Clinic Scottsdale, 7269
Mayor of the West Side, 5015
Mc Graw- Hill, School Publishing, 2598
McAlester Regional Health Center RehabCare Unit, 7168
McCune Charitable Foundation, 3078
McDonald's Corporation Contributions Program, 2943
McFarland & Company, 1748, 2511
McGraw-Hill, 8495
McGraw-Hill Company, 2146, 7, 2540, 5138, 8632
McGraw-Hill Professional, 8216
McGraw-Hill School Publishing, 2003, 2338, 2356, 2445, 2449, 2498, 2505, 2515, 2539, 2582, 2585, 2607, 8784
McGraw-Hill School Publishn, 2503
McGraw-Hill, School Publishing, 2058, 2418, 7841
McInerny Foundation Bank Of Hawaii, Corporate Trustee, 2919
McKey Mouse, 1675
McKinnon Body Therapy Center, 895
Mclean Hospital Child/Adolescent Program, 7711, 8751
MDA Newsmagazine, 2272
MDA Summer Camp, 1118
The Mead Center for American Theater, 6
Meadowbrook Manor, 6680
Meadows Foundation, 3267
Meadowvale Health and Rehabilitation Cente r, 7334
Meadowview Manor, 6681
Measure of Cognitive-Linguistic Abilities (MCLA), 2675
Measurement and Evaluation in Counseling, 2273
Mecalift Sling Lifter, 404
Med Covers, 680
Med-Camps of Louisiana, 8448
MedCamps of Louisiana, 1159
MedDev Corporation, 310
MedEscort International, 5557
Medford Rehabilitation and Healthcare Cent er, 7421
Medi-Grip, 311
Media Access Group at WGBH, 4857, 8858
Media America, 8651
Media Projects Inc, 7919

Nat'l Lib Svc/Blind And Physically Handicapped, 8959, 8960, 8961, 8963, 9051, 9052, 9054, 9071, 9072, 9100, 9132, 9133, 9148
NAT-CENT, 7645
National 4-H Council, 2766
National Ability Center, 1455
National Accreditation Council for Agencies/Blind, 9107
National AIDS Hotline, 8708
National Allergy and Asthma Network, 2305
National Alliance of Black Interpreters, 7982
National Alliance of Blind Students NABS Liaison, 8883
National Alliance of Blind Students NABS Liaison, 9146
National Alliance of the Disabled (NAOTD), 5485
National Alliance on Mental Illness, 7895
National Alliance on Mental Illness (NAMI), 7690
National Alliance on Mental Illness of New York State, 3697
National Amputation Foundation, 7934
National Aphasia Association, 8736
National Arts and Disability Center (NADC), 48
National Assoc of State Directors of DD Services, 5211
National Association for Adults with Speci al Learning Needs, 2090
National Association for Children of Alcoholics, 8333
National Association for Continence, 8191, 8679
National Association for Developmental Disabilities (NADD), 7691
National Association for Down Syndrome, 7692
National Association for Drama Therapy, 49
National Association for Holistic Aromatherapy, 899
National Association for Home Care & Hospice, 8334
National Association for Home Care and Hospice, 7529
National Association for Medical Direction of Respiratory Care, 8335
National Association for Parents of Children with Visual Impairments (NAPVI), 8884, 9180
National Association for Proton Therapy, 8336
National Association for the Dually Diagnosed, 1918
National Association for Visually Handicapped (NAVH), 8885
National Association for Visually Handicap ped Lighthouse International, 5486
National Association for Visually Handicapped, 7628, 8941, 8942, 8945, 8968, 8972, 8978, 8986, 8987, 8990, 9000, 9002, 9007, 9021, 9022, 9045, 9137, 9150
National Association of Anorexia Nervosa and Associated Disorders, 8337
National Association of Area Agencies on Aging, 7530
National Association of Blind Educators, 8886
National Association of Blind Lawyers, 8887
National Association of Blind Merchants, 900, 8888
National Association of Blind Secretaries and Transcribers, 8889
National Association of Blind Students, 8890
National Association of Blind Teachers, 8891
National Association of Blind Veterans, 8892
National Association of Chronic Disease Directors, 8338
National Association of Cognitive- Behavioral Therapists, 7693
National Association of Colleges and Employers, 2091
National Association of Councils on Develo pmental Disabilities, 901
National Association of Counties, 7531
National Association of Disability Represe ntatives, 902
National Association of Disability Representatives, 1919
National Association of Epilepsy Centers, 7694
National Association of Guide Dog Users, 8893
National Association of Hearing Officials, 7983, 8137

National Association of Nutrition and Aging Services Programs (NANASP), 7532
National Association of Parents with Child ren in Special Education, 2092, 7984
National Association of School Psychologists, 2147
National Association of School Psychologists, 2347, 2387, 2507, 2690
National Association of Special Education Teachers, 7985, 8737
National Association of State Directors of Developmental Disabilities Services (NASDDDS), 903
National Association of State Directors of Special Education, 2093
National Association of State Units on Aging, 7591
National Association of States United for Aging and Disabilities, 7533
National Association of the Deaf, 7986, 4670, 4683, 8034, 8145
National Association of Visually Handicapped, 9130
National Association to Advance Fat Acceptance, 8339
National Association to Promote the Use of Braille, 8894
National Ataxia Foundation, 7695
National Autism Association, 7696
National Autism Hotline, 7922
National Autism Resources, 2031
National Beep Baseball Association, 8895
National Black Association for Speech Language and Hearing, 7987
National Black Association for Speech-Lang uage and Hearing, 8738
National Black Deaf Advocates, 7988
National Braille Association, 4923, 8896, 8962, 9075, 9131
National Braille Press, 8897
National Brain Tumor Foundation - National Brain Tumor Society, 5487
National Business & Disability Council, 904, 5488
National Camp for Blind Children, 8933
National Camps for Blind Children, 1236, 8934
National Cancer Institute, 8340, 8696
National Car Rental System, 5597
National Care Planning Council, 3350
National Catholic Office for the Deaf, 8066
National Catholic Office of the Deaf, 7989, 8147
National Center for Education in Maternal and Child Health, 905
National Center for Homeopathy, 2094
National Center for Learning Disabilities, 2148
National Center for PTSD, 4971
National Center for Vision and Child Development, 8898
National Center on Birth Defects and Developmental Disabilities, 4781
National Center on Caregiving at Family Caregiver Alliance (FCA), 2835
National Center on Deaf-Blindness, 7622
National Cerebral Palsy of American, 3850
National Clearinghouse on Disability and Exchange, 5189
National Clearinghouse on Family Support and Children's Mental Health, 2171
National Clearinghouse on Postsecondary Education, 2143
National Coalition for Assistive and Rehab Technology, 8192
National Coalition of Federal Aviation Employees with Disabilities, 3351
National Commission on Orthotic and Prosth etic Education, 7935
National Conference on Building Codes and Standards, 1935
National Consortium on Deaf-Blindness, 834, 7637, 9114
National Council of Architectural Registration Boards (NCARB), 1936
National Council on Aging, 7534, 7590, 7592, 7596
National Council on Disability, 906, 3352, 4693, 5188

National Council on Independent Living, 907, 4052, 8193
National Council on Multifamily Housing Industry, 1951
National Council on Rehabilitation Education (NCRE), 2095
National Council on the Aging, 7573
National Council on the Aging Conference, 1921
National Cued Speech Association, 7990, 8739, 8820
National Deaf Education Network and Clearinghouse, 908
National Deaf Women's Bowling Association, 7991
National Diabetes Action Network for the Blind, 8899
National Diabetes Information Clearinghouse, 8341
National Digestive Diseases Information Clearinghouse, 8342
National Directory of Corporate Giving, 3338
National Disability Rights Network, 909
National Disability Sports Alliance, 8279
National Division of the Blind and Visually Impaired, 3353
National Down Syndrome Congress, 7697, 7884
National Down Syndrome Society, 7698
National Early Childhood Technical Assistance Center, 910
National Easter Seals Chicago, 7141
National Education Association of the United States, 2096
National Endowment for the Arts Office, 1946
National Endowment for the Arts: Office for AccessAbility, 50
National Epilepsy Library (NEL), 4844
National Eye Institute, 8900, 9040, 8981
National Eye Research Foundation, 2945
National Eye Research Foundation (NERF), 4799
National Family Association for Deaf-Blind, 7623, 7639
National Federation of the Blind, 2993, 7624, 8901, 900, 6094, 8706, 8886, 8887, 8888, 8889, 8890, 8893, 8894, 8899, 8905, 9003, 9013, 9017, 9085
National Federation of the Blind Jernigan Institute, 4845
National Federation of the Blind Senior Division, 7633
National Fibromyalgia Association, 8194, 8343, 7878, 8235, 8253
National Foundation for Ectodermal Dysplasias, 2946
National Foundation for Facial Reconstruction, 3127
National Foundation of Wheelchair Tennis, 2836
National Fragile X Foundation, 8740
National Gerontological Nursing Association, 7535
National Guild of Hypnotists, 911
National Headache Foundation, 2947
National Headquarters, 7183
National Health Information Center, 7923, 8836
National Health Law Program (NHeLP), 4627
National Hearing Conservation Association, 7992
National Hemophilia Foundation, 3128, 8344
National Hemophilia Foundation: Lone Star Chapter, 1429
National Hispanic Council on Aging, 7536
National Hookup, 5191
National Human Genome Research Institute, 2187
National Hydrocephalus Foundation, 7699, 8551
National Indian Council on Aging, 7589
National Indian Council on Aging, Inc., 7537
National Industries for the Blind, 8902, 9101
National Institue Health, 4850
National Institute of Environmental Health Sciences, 2196
National Institute of General Medical Scie nces, 2188
National Institute of Health, 9040
National Institute of Neurological Disorde Disorders & Stroke, 7936
National Institute on Aging, 3354, 4846

New Jersey Speech-Language-Hearing Association, 2203
New Jersey YMHA/YWHA, 1264
New Jersey YMHA/YWHA Camps Milford, 7743
New Language of Toys: Teaching Communicati on Skills to Children with Special Needs, 5274, 5529
New Medico Community Re-Entry Service, 7052
New Medico Rehabilitation and Skilled Nursing Center at Lewis Bay, 7030
New Medico, Highwatch Rehabilitation Center, 7084
New Mexico Aging and Long-Term Services Department, 3681
New Mexico Client Assistance Program, 3682
New Mexico Commission for the Blind, 3683
New Mexico Department of Health: Children's Medical Services, 3684
New Mexico Employment Services and Job Training Liaison, 6178
New Mexico Governor's Committee on Concerns of the Handicapped, 3685
New Mexico Protection & Advocacy for Persons with Disabilities, 3686
New Mexico State Department of Education, 2205
New Mexico State Library for the Blind and Physically Handicapped, 4911
New Mexico State Veterans' Home, 5743
New Mexico Technology Assistance Program, 1645, 3687, 4386
New Mexico VA Healthcare System, 5744
New Mexico Workers Compensation Administration, 3688
New Mobility, 8236
New Music Therapist's Handbook, 2nd Ed. Berklee School of Music, 54
New Orleans Resources for Independent Living, 4231
New Orleans Speech and Hearing Center, 6985
New Orleans VA Medical Center, 5690
New State Office of Mental Health Agency, 3698
New Ventures, 6002
New Vision Enterprises, 6969
New Vision Store, 477, 5523
New Vistas, 4387
New Voices: Self Advocacy By People with Disabilities, 5193
New World Library, 8532, 8620, 8627
New York Arthritis Reporter, 8256
New York Branch International Dyslexia Association, 1901
New York Chapter of the Arthritis Foundation, 8256
New York City Bar, 4646
New York City Campus of the VA NY Harbor Healthcare System, 5753
New York Client Assistance Program, 3699
New York Community Trust, 3130
New York Department of Handicapped Children, 3700
New York District Kiwanis Foundation, 1295
New York Families For Autistic Children, 7869
New York Foundation, 3131
New York Public Library, 4912
New York Regional Office, 5754
New York Service for the Handicapped, 1256, 8208
New York State Commisionon Qualityof Careand Advoc, 3706
New York State Commission for the Blind, 3701
New York State Commission on Quality of Care, 3702
New York State Congress of Parents and Teachers, 3703
New York State Department of Labor, 6185
New York State Education Department, 2207, 3720
New York State Library and Education, 4924
New York State Office of Advocates for Persons with Disabilities, 3704
New York State Office of Mental Health, 3705
New York State Talking Book & Braille Library, 4924
New York State Talking Book & Braille Library, 9149

New York State Talking Book and Braille Library, 5022
New York State TRAID Project, 3706
New York Therapeutic Riding Center-Equestr ia, 920
New York University Medical Center, 4915
New York-Presbyterian Hospital, 7115
Newark Healthcare Center, 7156
Newark Regional Office, 5742
Newport County Chapter of Retarded Citizens, 6226
Newport Hospital, 7194
Newport News Public Library System, 4981
News from Advocates for Deaf-Blind, 7639
Newsletter of PA's AT Lending Library, 5492
NewsLine, 5275
Nexus Health Systems, 6515
NEXUS Wheelchair Cushioning System, 277
NFB Diabetes Action Network, 8686
NIAD Art Center (Nurturing Independence through Artistic Development), 47
Nick & Kelly Children's Fund, 989
Nick & Kelly's Heart Camp, 989
Nick Joins In, 8581
Nicklaus Children's Hospital, 1077
Nightshirts, 1538
NINDS Notes, 7945
Nintendo, 5526
NISH, 6256
Nishna Productions-Shenandoah Work Center, 6945
NLP Comprehensive, 7688, 7896
NLP News, 7896
NLP University, 7689
NLP University - Dynamic Learning Center, 7689
NLS News, 9132
NLS Newsletter, 9133
NNEAHSA, 7593
No Barriers, 5402
No Boundaries, 569, 574
No Limits, 55
No Limits Communications & New Mobility, 531
No Limits Foundation, 1004, 1062, 1074, 1103, 1162, 1163, 1166, 1171, 1222, 1442
No Longer Disabled: the Federal Courts & the Politics of Social Security Disability, 4684
No Longer Immune: A Counselor's Guide to AIDS, 2527
No More Allergies, 8582
No Time for Jello: One Family's Experience, 8583
Noble Of Indiana, 6053
Noble, Inc., 6053
Nocturnal Asthma, 8584
NOD E-Newsletter, 5190
NOLO, 4685, 5094, 7561, 7567
NOLO (Internet Brands), 5010, 5314
Nolo's Guide to Social Security Disability Getting and Keeping Your Benefits, 4685
Non-Traditional Casting Project, 56
Nonverbal Learning Disabilities at Home: A Parent's Guide, 8792
NorCal Services For Deaf & Hard Of Hearing, 1000
NorCal Services For Deaf & Hard Of Hearing, Inc., 8012
Norcliffe Foundation, 3294
Nordson Corporate Giving Program, 3177
NORESCO Workshop, 5938
Norfolk Foundation, 3284
Norman Marcus Pain Institute, 7116
North America Riding for the Handicapped Association, 921
North American Riding for the Handicapped Association, 8283
North American Riding for the Handicapped Assoc, 8240
North Atlantic Books, 2429
North Auburn Rehabilitation And Health Center, 7461
North Broward Medical Center, 7298, 6813
North Broward Rehab Unit, 6813
North Carolina Workers Compensation Board, 3726
North Carolina Accessibility Code, 1953

North Carolina Assistive Technology Project, 3727
North Carolina Children & Youth Branch, 3728
North Carolina Client Assistance Program, 3729
North Carolina Department of Insurance, 1953
North Carolina Department of Public Instruction: Exceptional Children Division, 2197
North Carolina Developmental Disabilities, 3730
North Carolina Division of Aging, 3731
North Carolina Division of Services for the Blind, 6190
North Carolina Industrial Commission, 3732
North Carolina Library for the Blind and Physically Handicapped, 4933
North Carolina Publc of Health, 3728
North Central Independent Living Services, 4349
North Chicago VA Medical Center, 5671
North Coast Rehabilitation Center, 6302
North Country Center for Independent Livin g, 4414
North Country Independent Living, 4599
North Country Independent Living: Ashland, 4600
North Dakota Workers Compensation Board, 3735
North Dakota Client Assistance Program, 3736
North Dakota Community Foundation, 3159
North Dakota Department of Education: Special Education, 2198
North Dakota Department of Human Resources, 3737
North Dakota Department of Human Services, 3738
North Dakota Department of Labor, and Human Rights, 6198
North Dakota Employment Service and Job Training Program Liaison, 6199
North Dakota State Library Talking Book Services, 4936
North Dakota State Library Talking Book Services, 5122
North Dakota VA Regional Office - Fargo Regional Office, 5768
North Dakota Vocational Rehabilitation Agency, 6200
North District Independent Living Program, 4088
North Georgia Talking Book Center, 4782
North Hastings Community Integration Assoc iation, 922
North Hills Hospital, 7444
North Little Rock Regional Office, 5625
North Ridge Medical and Rehabilitation Cen ter, 7476
North Star Community Services, 5194
North Texas Rehabilitation Center, 7224
North Valley Services, 6686
Northampton VA Medical Center, 5702
Northeast Independent Living Program, 4264
Northeast Independent Living Services, 4334
Northeast Occupational Exchange, 6091
Northeast Rehabilitation Clinic, 7377
Northeast Rehabilitation Hospital, 6420
Northeast Wisconsin Directory of Services for Older Adults, 2117
Northeastern Pennsylvania Center for Independent Living, 4488
Northern Arizona University, 6570
Northern Arizona VA Health Care System, 5620
Northern Cartographic, 5550
Northern Illinois Center for Adaptive Technology, 1646
Northern Illinois Special Recreation Association (NISRA), 6897
Northern Nevada Center for Independent Liv ing: Fallon, 4362
Northern Nevada Center for Independent Living, 5108
Northern New England Conference, 8922
Northern New Hampshire Mental Health and Developmental Services, 7085
Northern New York Community Foundation, 3132
Northern Regional Center for Independent Living: Watertown, 4415
Northern Regional Center for Independent L iving: Lowville, 4416
Northern Utah Center for Independent Living, 4547

Q

X

Y

Alabama

ADRS Lakeshore, 5842
Alabama Goodwill Industries, 5843
Alabama Institute for Deaf and Blind Library and Resource Center, 4700
Alabama Power Foundation, 2779
Alabama Radio Reading Service Network (ARRS), 4701
Alabama Regional Library for the Blind and Physically Handicapped, 4702
Alabama VA Benefits Regional Office - Montgomery, 5612
Alabama VA Medical Center - Birmingham, 5613
Andalusia Health Services, 2780
Arc Of Alabama, The, 2781
Arc of Jefferson County, 5844
Birdie Thornton Center, 3922
Camp Evoked Potential, 961
Camp Rap-A-Hope, 962
Camp Seale Harris, 963
Camp Shocco for the Deaf, 964
Camp Smile-A-Mile, 965
Camp Smile-A-Mile: Jr./Sr. Weekend Camp, 966
Camp Smile-A-Mile: Off Therapy Family Camp, 967
Camp Smile-A-Mile: On Therapy Family Camp, 968
Camp Smile-A-Mile: Sibling Camp, 969
Camp Smile-A-Mile: Teen Camp, 970
Camp Smile-A-Mile: Young Adult Retreat, 971
Camp Smile-A-Mile: Youth Weeklong Camp, 972
Camp WheezeAway, 973
Central Alabama Veterans Healthcare System, 5614
Coffee County Training Center, 5845
Dothan Houston County Library System, 4703
Easter Seals Camp ASCCA, 974
Easter Seals: Achievement Center, 5846
Easter Seals: Opportunity Center, 5847
Happy Camp, 975
Huntsville Subregional Library for the Blind & Physically Handicapped, 4704
Independent Living Center of Mobile, 3923
Independent Living Resources Of Greater Birmingham: Alabaster, 3924
Independent Living Resources of Greater Birmingham: Jasper, 3925
Independent Living Resources of Greater Birmingham, 3926
Montgomery Career Center: Alabama Employment Services Division, 5848
Montgomery Center for Independent Living, 3927
Public Library Of Anniston-Calhoun County, 4705
Technology Assistance for Special Consumers, 4706
Tuscaloosa VA Medical Center, 5615
Vocational Rehabilitation Service - Opelika, 5849
Vocational Rehabilitation Service - Dothan, 5850
Vocational Rehabilitation Service - Homewood, 5851
Vocational Rehabilitation Service - Huntsville, 5852
Vocational Rehabilitation Service - Jackson, 5853
Vocational Rehabilitation Service - Jasper, 5854
Vocational Rehabilitation Service - Mobile, 5855
Vocational Rehabilitation Service - Muscle Shoals, 5856
Vocational Rehabilitation Service - Selma, 5857
Vocational Rehabilitation Service - Tallad ega, 5858
Vocational Rehabilitation Service - Troy, 5859
Vocational Rehabilitation Service - Tuscal oosa, 5860
Vocational Rehabilitation Service- Gadsden, 5861
Vocational Rehabilitation Service: Scottsboro, 5862
Vocational Rehabilitation Services - Andalusia, 5863
Vocational Rehabilitation Services - Anniston, 5864
Vocational and Rehabilitation Service - Decatur, 5865

Vocational and Rehabilitation Services - Montgomery, 5866
Wiregrass Rehabilitation Center, Inc., 5867
Workshops, Inc., 5868

Alaska

Access Alaska: ADA Partners Project, 3928
Access Alaska: Fairbanks, 3929
Access Alaska: Mat-Su, 3930
Adam's Camp: Alaska, 976
Alaska Division of Vocational Rehabilitati on, 5869
Alaska Fair Employment Practice Agency, 5870
Alaska Job Center Network, 5871
Alaska SILC, 3931
Alaska State Library Talking Book Center, 4707
Alaska VA Healthcare System - Anchorage, 5616
Arc of Alaska, 2782
Arctic Access, 3932
Camp Abilities, 977
Camp Alpine, 978
DAV Department of Alaska, 5617
Hope Community Resources, 3933
Kenai Peninsula Independent Living Center, 3934
Kenai Peninsula Independent Living Center: Seward, 3935
Keni Peninsula Independent Living Center: Central Peninsula, 3936
Rasmuson Foundation, 2783
Southeast Alaska Independent Living, 3937
Southeast Alaska Independent Living: Ketch ikan, 3938
Southeast Alaska Independent Living: Sitka, 3939
Veteran Benefits Administration - Anchorage Regional Office, 5618

Arizona

ASSIST! to Independence, 3940
American Foundation Corporation, 2784
Arizona Autism Resources, 2785
Arizona Braille and Talking Book Library, 4708
Arizona Bridge to Independent Living, 3941
Arizona Bridge to Independent Living: Phoenix, 3942
Arizona Bridge to Independent Living: Mesa, 3943
Arizona Camp Sunrise & Sidekicks, 979
Arizona Community Foundation, 2786
Arizona Instructional Resource Center for Students who are Blind or Visually Impaired, The, 2787
Bonnie Prudden Myotherapy, 808
Books for the Blind of Arizona, 4709
CARF Rehabilitation Accreditation Commission, 812
Camp AZDA, 980
Camp Abilities Tucson, 981
Camp Candlelight, 982
Camp Civitan, 983
Camp H.U.G, 984
Camp Honor, 985
Camp Not-A-Wheeze, 986
Carl T Hayden VA Medical Center, 5619
Children's Center for Neurodevelopmental Studies, 4710
Community Outreach Program for the Deaf, 3944
DIRECT Center for Independence, 3945
Downtown Neighborhood Learning Center, 5872
Fair Employment Practice Agency: Arizona, 5873
Flagstaff City-Coconino County Public Library, 4711
Fountain Hills Lioness Braille Service, 4712
International Association of Yoga Therapists, 876
International Child Amputee Network, 877
JOBS Administration Job Opportunities & Basic Skills, 5874
Lions Camp Tatiyee, 988
Margaret T Morris Foundation, 2788
New Horizons Independent Living Center: Prescott Valley, 3946
Nick & Kelly's Heart Camp, 989
Northern Arizona VA Health Care System, 5620
Prescott Public Library, 4713

Services Maximizing Independent Living and Empowerment (SMILE), 3947
Southern Arizona VA Healthcare System, 5621
Special Needs Center/Phoenix Public Library, 4714
Sterling Ranch: Residence for Special Women, 3948
TETRA Services, 5875
Vocational and Rehabilitation Agency Rehabilitation Services Administrations, 5876
Wheelers - Marauatha Baptist Church, 5603
Wheelers Handicapped Accessible Van Rental s, 5604
World Research Foundation, 4715
Yavapai Regional Medical Center-West, 5877

Arkansas

Arc of Arkansas, 2789
Arkansas Employment Service Agency and Job Training Program, 5878
Arkansas Independent Living Council, 3949
Arkansas Regional Library for the Blind and Physically Handicapped, 4716
Arkansas School for the Blind, 4717
Camp Aldersgate, 990
Camp Laughter, 991
Camp Quality Arkansas, 992
Case Management Society of America, 818
Delta Resource Center for Independent Living, 3950
Easter Seal Work Center, 5879
Educational Services for the Visually Impaired, 4718
Eugene J Towbin Healthcare Center, 5622
John L McClellan Memorial Hospital, 5624
Kota Camp, 994
Library for the Blind and Physically Handi capped SW Region of Arkansas, 4719
North Little Rock Regional Office, 5625
Northwest Ozarks Regional Library for the Blind and Handicapped, 4720
Sources for Community IL Services, 3953
Spa Area Independent Living Services, 3954
VCT/A Job Retention Skill Training Program, 5880
Vocational and Rehabilitation Agency Division of Services for the Blind, 5881
Vocational and Rehabilitation Agency for Persons Who Are Visually Impaired, 5882
Winthrop Rockefeller Foundation, 2790

California

AAO Annual Meeting, 1887
ABLE Industries, 5883
AIDS Healthcare Foundation, 754
ARC-Adult Vocational Program, 5884
Abilities Expo, 1897
Ability 1st, 4053
AbilityFirst, 5885
Access Center of San Diego, 3955
Access to Independence, 3956
Access to Independence of Imperial Valley, 3957
Access to Independence of North County, 3958
Achievement House & NCI Affiliates, 5886
Ahmanson Foundation, 2791
Alice Tweed Touhy Foundation, 2792
American Holistic Medical Association, 783
Anglo California Travel Service, 5571
Arc of California, 2794
Atkinson Foundation, 2795
Baker Commodities Corporate Giving Program, 2796
Bakersfield ARC, 5887
Balance Centers of America, 6041
Bank of America Foundation, 2797
Bearskin Meadow Camp, 995
Beaumont Senior Center: Community Access Center, 3959
Blind Babies Foundation, 2798
Blind Children's Center Annual Meeting, 1906
Bothin Foundation, 2799
Braille Institute Library, 4721

West Palm Beach VA Medical Center, 5658
Work Exploration Center, 5996
Young Onset Parkinson Conference, 1930
disAbility Solutions for Independent Livin g, 4081

Georgia

AADB National Conference, 1885
Aerie Experiences, 1085
Arc Of Georgia, 2904
Arms Wide Open, 4082
Athens Talking Book Center-Athens-Clarke
    County Regional Library, 4772
Atlanta Regional Office, 5659
Atlanta VA Medical Center, 5660
Augusta Talking Book Center, 4773
Augusta VA Medical Center, 5661
Bain, Inc. Center For Independent Living, 4083
Bainbridge Subregional Library for the Blind &
    Physically Handicapped, 4774
Camp Breathe Easy, 1086
Camp Caglewood, 1087
Camp Dream, 1088
Camp Hawkins, 1090
Camp Independence, 1091
Camp Juliena, 1092
Camp Kudzu, 1093
Camp Twin Lakes, 1095
Camp Twin Lakes: Camp Dream, 1096
Camp Twin Lakes: Rutledge, 1097
Camp Twin Lakes: Will-A-Way, 1098
Carl Vinson VA Medical Center, 5662
Center for Assistive Technology and
    Environmental Access, 819
Columbus Subregional Library For The Blind And
    Physically Handicapped, 4775
Community Foundation for Greater Atlanta, 2905
DisAbility LINK, 836
Disability Connections, 4084
Emory Autism Resource Center, 4776
Emory University Laboratory for Ophthalmic
    Research, 4777
Employment and Training Division, Region B,
    5997
Fair Housing and Equal Employment, 5998
Florence C and Harry L English Memorial Fund,
    2906
Georgia Library for the Blind and Physically
    Handicapped, 4778
Georgia Power, 2907
Griffin Area Resource Center Griffin Community
    Workshop Division, 5999
Hall County Library: East Hall Branch and Special
    Needs Library, 4779
Harriet McDaniel Marshall Trust in Memory of
    Sanders McDaniel, 2909
Human Ecology Action League (HEAL), 873
IBM National Support Center, 6000
John H and Wilhelmina D Harland Charitable
    Foundation, 2911
Kelley Diversified, 6001
Lettie Pate Whitehead Foundation, 2912
Living Independence for Everyone (LIFE), 4086
Macon Library for the Blind and Physically
    Handicapped, 4780
Multiple Choices Center for Independent Living,
    4087
National Center on Birth Defects and
    Developmental Disabilities, 4781
New Ventures, 6002
North District Independent Living Program, 4088
North Georgia Talking Book Center, 4782
Oconee Regional Library, 4783
Rome Subregional Library for the Blind and
    Physically Handicapped, 4784
South Georgia Regional Library-Valdosta Talking
    Book Center, 4785
Southeastern Paralyzed Veterans of America
    (PVA), 5663
Southwest District Independent Living Program,
    4089
Squirrel Hollow Summer Camp, 1099
Statewide Independent Living Council of Ge orgia,
    4090

SunTrust Bank, Atlanta Foundation, 2914
Talking Book Center Brunswick-Glynn County
    Regional Library, 4786
Walton Options for Independent Living, 4091
disABILITY LINK: Rome, 4092

Hawaii

Arc of Hawaii, 2915
Assets School, 6003
Assistive Technology Resource Centers of Hawaii
    (ATRC), 4787
Atherton Family Foundation, 2916
Camp Anuenue, 1100
Camp Taylor: Family Camp, 1019, 1101
Center For Independent Living- Kauai, 4093
GN Wilcox Trust, 2917
Hawaii Center for Independent Living, 4094
Hawaii Center for Independent Living-Maui, 4095
Hawaii Centers for Independent Living, 4096
Hawaii Community Foundation, 2918
Hawaii Fair Employment Practice Agency, 6004
Hawaii State Library for the Blind and Physically
    Handicapped, 4788
Hawaii Vocational Rehabilitation Division, 6005
Hilo Vet Center, 5664
Honolulu VBA Regional Office, 5665
Kauai Center for Independent Living, 4097
Lanakila Rehabilitation Center, 6006
McInerny Foundation Bank Of Hawaii, Corporate
    Trustee, 2919
Over the Rainbow Disabled Travel Services &
    Wheelers Accessible Van Rentals, 5599
Pacific Islands Health Care System, 5666
Pacific Rim International Conference on Disability
    And Diversity, 1924
Sophie Russell Testamentary Trust Bank Of
    Hawaii, 2920
Wahiawa Family, 6008

Idaho

American Falls Office: Living Independently for
    Everyone (LIFE), 4098
Boise Regional Office, 5667
Boise VA Medical Center, 5668
Camp Hodia, 1102
Camp No Limits Idaho, 1103
Camp Rainbow Gold, 1104
Dawn Enterprises, 4099
Disability Action Center NW, 4100
Disability Action Center NW: Coeur D'Alene,
    4101
Disability Action Center NW: Lewiston, 4102
Idaho Assistive Technology Project, 4789
Idaho Commission for Libraries: Talking Book
    Service, 4790
Idaho Employment Service and Job Training
    Program Liaison, 6009
Idaho Fair Employment Practice Agency, 6010
Idaho Falls Office: Living Independently for
    Everyone (LIFE), 4103
Idaho Governor's Committee on Employment of
    People with Disabilities, 6011
Idaho Vocational Rehabilitation Agency, 6012
Living Independence Network Corporation, 4105
Living Independence Network Corporation: Twin
    Falls, 4106
Living Independence Network Corporation: C
    aldwell, 4107
Living Independent for Everyone (LIFE): Pocatello
    Office, 4108
Living Independently for Everyone (LIFE):
    Blackfoot Office, 4109
Living Independently for Everyone: Burley, 4110
ROW Adventures, 5586
Southwestern Idaho Housing Authority, 4111

Illinois

ADA Camp GrenADA, 1105
ADA Teen Adventure Camp, 1106
ADA Triangle D Camp, 1107

ATIA Conference, 1896
Access Living of Metropolitan Chicago, 4112
Ada S McKinley Vocational Services, 6014
Alzheimer's Association, 2921
American Academy of Pain Medicine, 766
American Academy of Pain Medicine Foundati on,
    767
American Academy of Pediatrics, 768
American Massage Therapy Association, 784
American Pain Society, 787
American Society of Clinical Hypnosis, 792
Amerock Corporation, 2923
Anixter Center, 6015
Arc of Illinois, 2924
Association of Assistive Technology Act Pr
    ograms, 799
Benjamin Benedict Green-Field Foundation, 2925
Blowitz-Ridgeway Foundation, 2926
C-4 Work Center, 6016
Camp "I Am Me", 1108
Camp Callahan, 1109
Camp Discovery, 1059, 1110, 1206, 1206, 1377,
    1419, 1437
Camp FRIENDship, 1111
Camp Little Giant, 1112
Camp One Step, 1114
Camp Quality Illinois, 1115
Camp Red Leaf, 1116
Center for Creative Arts Therapy, 820
Center on Deafness, 4113
Chaddick Institute for Metropolitan Development,
    2927
Chicago Community Trust, 2928
Chicago Community Trust and Affiliates, 2929
Chicago Public Library Talking Book Center, 4791
Clearbrook, 6017
Community Foundation of Champaign County,
    2930
Community Residential Alternative, 4114
Cornerstone Services, 6018
Department of Ophthalmology and Visual Science,
    4792
Division of Rehabilitation Services, 4085, 4115
Dr Scholl Foundation, 2931
DuPage Center for Independent Living, 4116
Duchossois Foundation, 2932
Easterseal, 845
Easterseals, 846
Edward Hines Jr Hospital, 5669
Evenston Community Foundation, 2933
Family Resource Center on Disabilities, 852
Field Foundation of Illinois, 2934
Fite Center for Independent Living, 4117
Francis Beidler Charitable Trust, 2935
Fred J Brunner Foundation, 2936
Fulton County Rehab Center, 6019
George M Eisenberg Foundation for Charities,
    2937
Glenkirk, 6020
Grover Hermann Foundation, 2938
Guild for the Blind, 4793
Horizons for the Blind, 4794
Illinois Department of Rehab Services, 4118
Illinois Early Childhood Intervention
    Clearinghouse, 4795
Illinois Employment Service, 6021
Illinois Machine Sub-Lending Agency, 4796
Illinois Regional Library for the Blind and
    Physically Handicapped, 4797
Illinois Valley Center for Independent Living, 4119
Illinois Wheelchair Sport Camps, 1117
Illinois and Iowa Center for Independent L iving,
    4120
Impact Center for Independent Living, 4121
International Academy of Independent Medical
    Evaluators, 875
Jacksonville Area CIL: Havana, 4122
Jacksonville Area Center for Independent Living,
    4123
Jewish Vocational Services, 6022
JoDavies Workshop, 6023
John D and Catherine T MacArthur Foundation,
    2939
Kennedy Job Training Center, 6024

Indiana

Iowa

Kansas

Central Kansas Library Systems Headquarter s (CSLS), 4818
Coalition for Independence, 4176
Colmery-O'Neil VA Medical Center, 5682
Cowley County Developmental Services, 4177
Dwight D Eisenhower VA Medical Center, 5683
Hutchinson Community Foundation, 2969
Independence, 4178
Independent Connection, 4179
Independent Connection: Abilene, 4180
Independent Connection: Beloit, 4181
Independent Connection: Concordia, 4182
Independent Living Resource Center, 3996, 4183
Kansas Fair Employment Practice Agency, 6071
Kansas Services for the Blind & Visually Impaired, 4184
Kansas VA Regional Office, 5684
Kansas Vocational Rehabilitation Agency, 6072
LINK: Colby, 4185
Living Independently in Northwest Kansas: Hays, 4186
Manhattan Public Library, 4819
Northwest Kansas Library System Talking Books, 4820
Prairie IL Resource Center, 4187
Prairie Independent Living Resource Center, 4188
Resource Center for Independent Living: Emporia, 4191
Resource Center for Independent Living: Ar kansas City, 4192
Resource Center for Independent Living: Bu rlington, 4193
Resource Center for Independent Living: Co ffeyville, 4194
Resource Center for Independent Living: El Dorado, 4195
Resource Center for Independent Living: Ft Scott, 4196
Resource Center for Independent Living: Ot tawa, 4197
Resource Center for Independent Living: Ov erland Park, 4198
Resource Center for Independent Living: To peka, 4199
Richard W Higgins Charitable Foundation, 2970
Robert J Dole VA Medical Center, 5685
South Central Kansas Library System, 4821
Southeast Kansas Independent Living (SKIL), 4200
Southeast Kansas Independent Living: Independence, 4201
Southeast Kansas Independent Living: Chanu te, 4202
Southeast Kansas Independent Living: Colum bus, 4203
Southeast Kansas Independent Living: Fredo nia, 4204
Southeast Kansas Independent Living: Hays, 4205
Southeast Kansas Independent Living: Pitts burg, 4206
Southeast Kansas Independent Living: Sedan, 4207
Southeast Kansas Independent Living: Yates Center, 4208
State Library of Kansas, 4822
Three Rivers Independent Living Center, 4209
Three Rivers Independent Living Center: Clay, 4210
Three Rivers Independent Living Center: Ma nhattan, 4211
Three Rivers Independent Living Center: Se neca, 4212
Three Rivers Independent Living Center: To peka, 4213
Topeka & Shawnee County Public Library Talking Books Service, 4823
Topeka Independent Living Resource Center, 4214
Whole Person: Nortonville, 4215
Whole Person: Nortonville, The, 4216
Whole Person: Prairie Village, 4217
Whole Person: Prairie Village, The, 4218
Whole Person: Tonganoxie, 4219
Wichita Public Library/Talking Book Service, 4824

Wichita Public Library/Talking Book Servic e, 4825

Kentucky

Arc of Kentucky, 2971
Camp Quality Kentuckiana, 1131, 1149
Center for Accessible Living, 4220
Center for Accessible Living: Murray, 4221
Center for Independent Living: Kentucky Department for the Blind, 4222
Children's Alliance, 828
Disability Coalition of Northern Kentucky, 4223
Disability Resource Initiative, 4224
Disabled American Veterans Headquarters, 5608
EnTech: Enabling Technologies of Kentuckiana, 4826
Independence Place, 4225
Kentucky Committee on Employment of People with Disabilities, 6073
Kentucky Department for Employment Service and Job Training Program Liaison, 6074
Kentucky Office for the Blind, 6075
Kentucky Talking Book Library - Kentucky Dept. for Libraries and Archives, 4827
Kentucky Vocational Rehabilitation Agency, 6076
Kids Cancer Alliance, 1150
Lexington VA Medical Center, 5686
Lions Camp Crescendo, 1151
Louisville Free Public Library, 4828
Louisville VA Medical Center, 5687
Louisville VA Regional Office, 5688
Office for the Blind, 6077
Pathfinders for Independent Living, 4226
Pioneer Vocational/Industrial Services, 6078
SILC Department of Vocational Rehabilitation, 4227
The Center for Courageous Kids, 1152
Work Enhancement Center of Western Kentucky, 6079

Louisiana

Advocacy Center of Louisiana, 759
Alexandria VA Medical Center, 5689
Arc of Louisiana, 2972
Baton Rouge Area Foundation, 2973
Camp Bon Coeur, 1153
Camp Challenge, 1154
Camp Pelican, 1155
Camp Quality Louisiana, 1156
Central Louisiana State Hospital Medical and Professional Library, 4829
Community Foundation of Shreveport-Bossier, 2974
Community Opportunities of East Ascension, 6080
Dynamic Dimensions, 5933
Louisiana Employment Service and Job Training Program Liaison, 6081
Louisiana Lions Camp, 1158
Louisiana State Library, 4830
Louisiana State University Genetics Sectio n of Pediatrics, 4831
Louisiana Vocational Rehabilitation Agency, 6082
MedCamps of Louisiana, 1159
New Horizons: Central Louisiana, 4228
New Horizons: Northeast Louisiana, 4229
New Horizons: Northwest Louisiana, 4230
New Orleans VA Medical Center, 5690
Resources for Independent Living: Baton Rouge, 4231
Resources for Independent Living: Metairie, 4232
Shreveport VA Medical Center, 5691
Southwest Louisiana Independence Center: L ake Charles, 4233
Southwest Louisians Independence Center: Lafayette, 4234
St. James Association for Retarded Citizens, 6083
State Library of Louisiana: Services for the Blind and Physically Handicapped, 4832
Volunteers of America of Greater New Orlea ns, 4235
W Troy Cole Independent Living Specialist, 4236

Westbank Sheltered Workshop, 6084

Maine

Addison Point Specialized Services, 6085
Alpha One: South Portland, 4238
BCR Foundation, 2975
Bangor Public Library, 4833
Bangor Veteran Center: Veterans Outreach Center, 6086
Camp CaPella, 1160
Camp Lawroweld, 1161
Camp No Limits Maine, 1162
Camp Snow Maine, 1163
Camp Sunshine, 993, 1094, 1164, 1164
Camp sNOw Maine, 1166
Cary Library, 4834
Creative Work Systems, 6087
High School Students Guide to Study, Travel, and Adventure Abroad, 2757
Lewiston Public Library, 4835
Maine Department Of Labor, 6088
Maine Governor's Committee on Employment of the Disabled, 6089
Maine Human Rights Commission, 6090
Maine State Library, 4836
Maine VA Regional Office, 5692
Motivational Services, 4239
Northeast Occupational Exchange, 6091
Pine Tree Camp, 1167
Portland Public Library, 4838
Shalom House, 4240
Togus VA Medical Center, 5693
UNUM Charitable Foundation, 2976
Waban Projects, 956
Waterville Public Library, 4839
Women to Women, 957

Maryland

APSE, 756
APSE National Conference, 1893
ASHA Convention, 1894
American Association on Health and Disabil ity, 771
American College of Nurse Midwives, 777
American Health Assistance Foundation, 2977
American Occupational Therapy Association, 785
American Occupational Therapy Foundation, 2978
Anxiety and Depression Association of Amer ica, 795
Arc of Maryland, 2979
Ardmore Developmental Center, 6093
Association for International Practical Training, 2751
Association for Persons in Supported Employment, 797
Association of University Centers on Disabilities, 803
Baltimore Community Foundation, 2980
Baltimore Regional Office, 5694
Baltimore VA Medical Center, 5695
Broadmead, 4241
CASA Inc., 4384
CQL Accreditation, 1908
Camp Great Rock, 1169
Camp Littlefoot, 1170
Camp No Limits Maryland, 1171
Camp Sunrise, 1172
Camp Superkids, 1173
Candlelighters Childhood Cancer Foundation, 2981
Children's Fresh Air Society Fund, 2982
Clark-Winchcole Foundation, 2983
Columbia Foundation, 2984
Community Health Funding Report, 3316
Corporate Giving Program, 2985
Cystic Fibrosis Foundation, 2986
Deaf Camps, 1174
Department of Physical Medicine & Rehabilitation at Sinai Hospital, 835
Disability Funding News, 3318
Disabled Children's Fund, 842
Eastern Shore Center for Independent Living, 4242

Montana Governor's Committee on Employment of Disabled People, 6131
Montana Independent Living Project, Inc., 4348
Montana State Library-Talking Book Library, 4899
Montana VA Regional Office, 5724
North Central Independent Living Services, 4349
Summit Independent Living Center: Kalipsell, 4350
Summit Independent Living Center: Hamilton, 4351
Summit Independent Living Center: Missoula, 4352
Summit Independent Living Center: Ronan, 4353
V A Montana Healthcare System, 5725
VA Montana Healthcare System, 5726
Vet Center, 5716, 5727

Nebraska

Arc of Nebraska, 3052
Camp Floyd Rogers, 1232
Camp Kindle, 1002, 1233
Center for Independent Living of Central Nebraska, 4354
Cooper Foundation, 3053
Easter Seals Nebraska, 1234
Grand Island VA Medical System, 5728
Kamp Kaleo, 1235
League of Human Dignity: Lincoln, 4355
League of Human Dignity: Norfolk, 4356
League of Human Dignity: Omaha, 4357
Lincoln Regional Office, 5729
Lincoln VA Medical Center, 5730
Mosaic, 3054
Mosaic Of De, 4050
Mosaic of Axtell Bethpage Village, 4358
Mosaic of Beatrice, 4359
Mosaic: Pontiac, 4131
Mosiac: York, 4360
National Camps for Blind Children, 1236
Nebraska Assistive Technology Partnership Nebraska Department of Education, 4900
Nebraska Employment Services, 6132
Nebraska Fair Employment Practice Agency, 6133
Nebraska Library Commission: Talking Book and Braille Service, 4901
Nebraska Vocational Rehabilitation Agency, 6134
Slosburg Family Charitable Trust, 3055
Union Pacific Foundation, 3056
VA Nebraska-Western Iowa Health Care System, 5731

Nevada

ABC Union, ACE, ANLV, Vegas Western Cab, 5592
Camp Buck, 1237
Camp Lotsafun, 1238
Camp SignShine, 1239
CampCare, 1240
Carson City Center for Independent Living, 4361
Discovery Day Camp, 1241
EL Wiegand Foundation, 3057
Las Vegas Veterans Center, 5732
Las Vegas-Clark County Library District, 4902
Nell J Redfield Foundation, 3058
Nevada Equal Rights Commission - Dept. of Employment, Training & Rehabilitation, 6135
Nevada Governor's Committee on Employment of Persons with Disabilities, 6136
Nevada State Library and Archives, 4903
Northern Nevada Center for Independent Living: Fallon, 4362
Reno Regional Office, 5733
Rural Center for Independent Living, 4363
Southern Nevada Center for Independent Living: North Las Vegas, 4364
Southern Nevada Center for Independent Living: Las Vegas, 4365
VA Sierra Nevada Healthcare System, 5734
VA Southern Nevada Healthcare System, 5735
William N Pennington Foundation, 3059

New Hampshire

Adam's Camp: New Hampshire, 1242
Agnes M Lindsay Trust, 3060
Camp Allen, 1243
Camp Connect, 1244
Camp Inter-Actions, 1245
Camp Sno Mo, 1246
Camp Yavneh: Yedidut Program, 1247
Fit for Work at Exeter Hospital, 6138
Foundation for Seacoast Health, 3061
Granite State Independent Living Foundation, 4366
Manchester Regional Office, 5736
Manchester VA Medical Center, 5737
National Guild of Hypnotists, 911
New Hampshire Employment Security, 6139
New Hampshire Fair Employment Practice Agency, 6140
New Hampshire Job Training Program Liaison, 6141
New Hampshire State Library: Talking Book Services, 4904
New Hampshire Veterans Centers, 5738
Wediko Summer Program, 1248

New Jersey

ARC of Gloucester County, 6143
ARC of Hunterdon County, The, 6144
ARC of Mercer County, 6145
ARC of Monmouth, 6146
Abilities Center of New Jersey, 6147
Abilities of Northwest New Jersey, 6148
Alliance Center for Independence, 4367
Alliance Center for Independence (ACI), 6149
Alternatives for Growth: New Jersey, 6150
American Organization for Bodywork Therapies of Asia, 786
Arc of Bergen and Passaic Counties, 6151
Arc of New Jersey, 3062
Arnold A Schwartz Foundation, 3063
Autism New Jersey, 4905
Avis Rent A Car, 5594
Camden City Independent Living Center, 4368
Camp Chatterbox, 1250
Camp Deeny Riback, 1251
Camp Dream Street, 1217, 1252
Camp Jotoni, 1253
Camp Merry Heart, 1254
Camp Nejeda, 1255
Camp Oakhurst, 1256
Camp Quality New Jersey, 1257
Camp Sun'N Fun, 1258
Campbell Soup Foundation, 3064
Career Opportunity Development of New Jersey, 6152
Center for Educational Advancement New Jersey, 6153
Center for Independent Living: Long Branch, 4369
Center for Independent Living: South Jersey, 4370
Cerebral Palsy Association of Middlesex County, 6154
Children's Hopes & Dreams Wish Fulfillment Foundation, 3065
Children's Specialized Hospital Medical Library - Parent Resource Center, 4906
Christopher & Dana Reeve Foundation, 4907
Community Foundation of New Jersey, 3066
DAWN Center for Independent Living, 4371
Dial: Disabled Information Awareness & Living, 4372
Disability Matters, 1912
Disability Rights New Jersey, 4373
Disabled American Veterans: Ocean County, 5739
East Orange Campus of the VA New Jersey Healthcare System, 5740
Easter Seal Society of New Jersey Highlands Workshop, 6155
Easter Seal of Ocean County, 6156
Easter Seals New Jersey, 6157
Eden Acres Administrative Services, 6158
Edison Sheltered Workshop, 6159
Explorer's Club Camp, 1259
Eye Institute of New Jersey, 4908

FM Kirby Foundation, 3067
Family Resource Associates, 4374
Fannie E Rippel Foundation, 3068
First Occupational Center of New Jersey, 6160
Fund for New Jersey, 3069
Goodwill Industries of Southern New Jersey, 6161
Happiness Is Camping, 1260
Harbor Haven Summer Program, 1261
Hausmann Industries, 6162
Heightened Independence and Progress: Hackensack, 4375
Heightened Independence and Progress: Jersey City, 4376
Jersey Cape Diagnostic Training & Opportunity Center, 6163
Lyons Campus of the VA New Jersey Healthcare System, 5741
Mane Stream, 1262
Martin Luther Homes of Iowa, 4169
Merck Company Foundation, 3070
Mycoclonus Research Foundation, 4909
Nabisco Foundation, 3071
New Jersey Camp Jaycee, 1263
New Jersey Commission for the Blind and Visually Impaired, 6164
New Jersey Employment Service and Job Training Program Services, 6165
New Jersey Library for the Blind and Handicapped, 4910
Newark Regional Office, 5742
Occupational Center of Hudson County, 6166
Occupational Center of Union County, 6167
Occupational Training Center of Burlington County, 6168
Occupational Training Center of Camden County, New Jersey, 6169
Ostberg Foundation, 3072
Pathways to Independence, Inc., 6170
Progressive Center for Independent Living, 4377
Progressive Center for Independent Living: Flemington, 4378
Project Freedom, 4379
Project Freedom: Hamilton, 4380
Project Freedom: Lawrence, 4381
Prudential Foundation, 3073
Robert Wood Johnson Foundation, 3074
Round Lake Camp, 1264
Somerset Training and Employment Program, 6171
St. John of God Community Services Vocational Rehabilitation, 6172
Summit Camp, 1265
The Davis Center, 948
Total Living Center, 4382
United Cerebral Palsy Associations of New Jersey, 6173
Verizon Foundation, 3146
Victoria Foundation, 3075
West Essex Rehab Center, 6175

New Mexico

Ability Center, 4383
Adelante Development Center, 6176
Arc of New Mexico, 3076
CHOICES Center for Independent Living, 4385
Camp Enchantment, 1266
Camp Rising Sun, 1267
Camp for Kids With Diabetes: Camp 180, 1268
Dental Amalgam Syndrome (DAMS) Newsletter, 4727
Family Voices, 853
Frost Foundation, 3077
Goodwill Industries of New Mexico, 6177
JoanBorysenko.Com, 884
McCune Charitable Foundation, 3078
Native American Disability Law Center, 919
New Mexico Employment Services and Job Training Liaison, 6178
New Mexico State Library for the Blind and Physically Handicapped, 4911
New Mexico State Veterans' Home, 5743
New Mexico Technology Assistance Program, 4386
New Mexico VA Healthcare System, 5744

Special Education and Vocational Rehabilitation Agency: New York, 6187
St George's Society of New York, 3139
Stanley W Metcalf Foundation, 3140
State University of New York, 2772
State University of New York Health Sciences Center, 4927
Staten Island Center for Independent Living, Inc., 4426
Stonewall Community Foundation, 3141
Suffolk Cooperative Library System: Long Island Talking Book Library, 4928
Suffolk Independent Living Organization (SILO), 4427
Sunshine Campus, 1303
Surdna Foundation, 3142
Syracuse VA Medical Center, 5756
TSA National Conference, 1929
Taconic Resources for Independence, 4428
The Adaptive Sports Foundation, 3143
Tisch Foundation, 3144
Torah Alliance of Families of Kids with Disabilities, 5757
United Spinal Association, 4929
VA Hudson Valley Health Care System, 5758
VA Western NY Healthcare System, Batavia, 5759
VA Western NY Healthcare System, Buffalo, 5760
VISIONS Vacation Camp for the Blind, 1304
Van Ameringen Foundation, 3145
Wabash/Employability Center, 6059
Wagon Road Camp, 1305
Wallace Memorial Library, 4930
West Hills Day Camp: Gersh Academy, 1306
Westchester Disabled on the Move, 4429
Westchester Independent Living Center, 4430
Western New York Foundation, 3147
William T Grant Foundation, 3148
Xavier Society for the Blind, 4931
YAI: National Institute for People with Disabilities, 960
YMCA Camp Chingachgook on Lake George, 1307

North Carolina

AHEAD Association, 753
American Herbalists Guild, 782
Arc of North Carolina, 3149
Asheville VA Medical Center, 5761
Association on Higher Education and Disability, 1904
Bob & Kay Timberlake Foundation, 3150
Camp Carefree, 1249, 1308
Camp Carolina Trails, 1309
Camp Dogwood, 1310
Camp New Hope, 1113, 1311
Camp Royall, 1312
Camp Sertoma, 1313
Camp Tekoa UMC, 1314
Center for Universal Design, 823
Charlotte Vet Center, 5762
Davidson College, Office of Study Abroad, 2756
Disability Awareness Network, 4431
Disability Rights & Resources, 4432
Division Of Workforce Development, 6188
Duke Endowment, 3151
Durham VA Medical Center, 5763
Fayetteville VA Medical Center, 5623, 5764
First Union Foundation, 3152
Foundation for the Carolinas, 3153
Genova Diagnostics, 4932
Grayson Foundation, 2908
Iredell Vocational Workshop, 6189
Joy: A Shabazz Center for Independent Living, 4433
Kate B Reynolds Charitable Trust, 3154
Live Independently Networking Center, 4434
Live Independently Networking Center: Hickory, 4435
Mary Reynolds Babcock Foundation, 3155
Metametrix Clinical Laboratory, 897
National Association for Holistic Aromatherapy, 899

National Early Childhood Technical Assistance Center, 910
North Carolina Division of Services for the Blind, 6190
North Carolina Library for the Blind and Physically Handicapped, 4933
Older Americans Report, 3339
Pathways for the Future Center for Independent Living, 4436
Pediatric Rheumatology Clinic, 4934
Rowan County Vocational Workshop, 6191
Rutherford Vocational Workshop, 6192
SOAR Summer Adventures, 1315
Talisman Summer Camp, 1316
Transylvania Vocational Services, 6193
Triangle Community Foundation, 3156
United States Disabled Golf Association, 952
University of North Carolina at Chapel Hill: Neuroscience Research Building, 4935
Victory Junction Gang Camp, 1317
WG Hefner VA Medical Center - Salisbury, 5765
Webster Enterprises Inc., 6196
Western Alliance Center for Independent Living, 4437
Western Alliance for Independent Living, 4438
Western Regional Vocational Rehabilitation Facility Clifford File, Jr., 6197
Winston-Salem Regional Office, 5766

North Dakota

Alex Stern Family Foundation, 3157
Arc of North Dakota, 3158
Camp Sioux, 1318
Dakota Center for Independent Living: Dickinson, 4439
Dakota Center for Independent Living: Bism arck, 4440
Fargo VA Medical Center, 5767
Fraser, 4441
Freedom Resource Center for Independent Li ving: Fargo, 4442
North Dakota Community Foundation, 3159
North Dakota Department of Labor, and Human Rights, 6198
North Dakota Employment Service and Job Training Program Liaison, 6199
North Dakota State Library Talking Book Services, 4936
North Dakota VA Regional Office - Fargo Regional Office, 5768
North Dakota Vocational Rehabilitation Agency, 6200
Resource Center for Independent Living: Minot, 4443

Ohio

Ability Center of Greater Toledo, 4444
Ability Center of Greater Toledo: Defiance, 4445
Ability Center of Greater Toledo: Port Cli nton, 4446
Access Center for Independent Living, 4447
Akron Community Foundation, 3160
Albert G and Olive H Schlink Foundation, 3161
American Society for the Alexander Technique, 790
Antioch College, 2749
Arc of Ohio, 3162
Bahmann Foundation, 3163
CYO Camp Happiness Day Camp, 1319
Camp Arye, 1320
Camp Cheerful, 1321
Camp Christopher: SumFun Day Camp, 1322
Camp Courageous, 1323
Camp Echoing Hills, 1324
Camp Emanuel, 1325
Camp Hamwi, 1326
Camp Ho Mita Koda, 1327
Camp Ko-Man-She, 1329
Camp Korelitz, 1330
Camp Nuhop, 1331
Camp Oty'Okwa, 1332

Camp Paradise, 1333
Camp Quality Ohio, 1334
Camp Stepping Stone, 1335
Camp Tiponi, 1336
Case Western Reserve University, 4937
Case Western Reserve University Northeast Ohio Multipurpose Arthritis Center, 4938
Center for Independent Living Options, 4448
Champ Camp, 1047, 1337
Chillicothe VA Medical Center, 5769
Cincinnati Children's Hospital Medical Center, 4939
Cincinnati VA Medical Center, 5770
Cleveland FES Center, 4940
Cleveland Foundation, 3164
Cleveland Public Library, 4941
Cleveland Regional Office, 5771
Columbus Foundation and Affiliated Organizations, 3165
Cornucopia, 6201
Dayton VA Medical Center, 5772
Eleanora CU Alms Trust, 3166
Eva L And Joseph M Bruening Foundation, 3167
Fairfield Center for Disabilities and Cerebral Palsy, 4449
Flying Horse Farms, 1338
Fred & Lillian Deeks Memorial Foundation, 3168
GAR Foundation, 3169
George Gund Foundation, 3170
Great Oaks Joint Vocational School, 6202
Greater Cincinnati Foundation, 3171
HCR Manor Care Foundation, 3172
HWH Foundation, 3173
Harry C Moores Foundation, 3174
Hearth Day Treatment and Vocational Services, 6203
Helen Steiner Rice Foundation, 3175
Highbrook Lodge, 1339
Highland Unlimited Business Enterprises of CRI, 6204
Innovative Industries, 6062
Insight Horse Camp, 1340
Lake Erie College, 2762
Linking Employment, Abilities and Potentia l, 4450
Louis Stokes VA Medical Center - Wade Park Campus, 5773
Mid-Ohio Board for an Independent Living Environment (MOBILE), 4451
Nationwide Foundation, 3176
Nordson Corporate Giving Program, 3177
Ohio Civil Rights Commission, 6205
Ohio Commission On Minority Health, 6206
Ohio Regional Library for the Blind and Physically Handicapped, 4942
Ohio Statewide Independent Living Council, 4452
Parker-Hannifin Foundation, 3178
Recreation Unlimited: Day Camp, 1341
Recreation Unlimited: Residential Camp, 1342
Recreation Unlimited: Respite Weekend Camp, 1343
Recreation Unlimited: Specialty Camp, 1344
Rehabilitation Service of North Central Oh io, 4453
Reinberger Foundation, 3179
Robert Campeau Family Foundation, 3180
Rotary Camp, 1345
Samuel W Bell Home for Sightless, 4454
Services for Independent Living, 4341, 4455
Sisler McFawn Foundation, 3181
Society for Equal Access: Independent Living Center, 4456
St. Augustine Rainbow Camp, 1346
Stark Community Foundation, 3182
State Library of Ohio: Talking Book Program, 4943
Stepping Stones: Camp Allyn, 1347
Stocker Foundation, 3183
Toledo Community Foundation, 3184
United States Trager Association, 953
William J and Dorothy K O'Neill Foundation, 3185
YMCA Outdoor Center Campbell Gard, 1348
Youngstown Foundation, 3186

Oklahoma

Ability Resources, 4457
Anne and Henry Zarrow Foundation, 3187
Camp CANOE, 1349
Camp ClapHans, 1350
Camp Endres, 1351
Camp Loughridge, 1352
Camp Perfect Wings, 1353
Easter Seals Oklahoma, 1354
Green County Independent Living Resource
  Center, 4458
Jack C. Montgomery VA Medical Center, 5774
Jack C. Montomery VA Medical Center, 5775
Oklahoma City VA Medical Center, 5776
Oklahoma Department of Rehabilitation Services,
  6208
Oklahoma Employment Services and Job Training
  Program Liaison, 6209
Oklahoma Governor's Committee on Employment
  of People with Disabilities, 6210
Oklahoma Library for the Blind & Physically
  Handicapped, 4944
Oklahoma Medical Research Foundation, 4945
Oklahoma Veterans Centers Vet Center, 5777
Oklahomans for Independent Living, 4459
Progressive Independence, 4460
Sarkeys Foundation, 3188
Tulsa City-County Library System: Outreach
  Services, 4946

Oregon

A Guide to International Educational Excha nge,
  2745
Abilitree, 4461
Adventures Without Limits, 1355
American Tinnitus Association, 793
Arc of Oregon, 3189
B'nai B'rith Camp: Kehila Program, 1356
Bend Work Activity Center, 6211
Building Bridges: Including People with
  Disabilities in International Programs, 2755
Cambia Health Foundation, 813
Camp Magruder, 1357
Camp Meadowood Springs, 1358
Camp Millennium, 1359
Camp Starlight, 1360
Camp Taloali, 1361
Camp Ukandu, 1362
Creating Memories, 1363
DB-Link, 834
Eastern Oregon Center for Independent Living,
  4462
Gales Creek Diabetes Camp, 1364
HASL Independent Abilities Center, 4463
Hull Park, 1365
Independent Living Resources, 4464
International Partnership for Service-Learning and
  Leadership, 2759
Jackson Foundation, 3191
Lane Community College, 2763
Laurel Hill Center, 4465
Leslie G Ehmann Trust, 3192
Mt Hood Kiwanis Camp, 1366
National University of Natural Medicine, 916
Oregon Fair Employment Practice Agency, 6212
Oregon Health Sciences University, 5778
Oregon Health Sciences University, Elks'
  Children's Eye Clinic, 4947
Oregon Talking Book & Braille Services, 4948
Portland Regional Office, 5779
Portland VA Medical Center, 5780
Postpartum Support International, 932
Progressive Options, 4466
Roseburg VA Medical Center, 5781
SPOKES Unlimited, 4467
Southern Oregon Rehabilitation Center & Cl inics,
  5782
State of Oregon Office of Vocational
  Rehabilitation Service, 6213
Strength for the Journey, 1367
Sundial Special Vacations, 5587
Suttle Lake Camp, 1368

Swindells Charitable Foundation Trust, 2874
Talking Book & Braille Services Oregon State
  Library, 4949
Trips Inc., 5588
Umpqua Valley Disabilities Network, 4468
University of Oregon, 2774
Upward Bound Camp, 1369
Vocational and Rehabilitation Agency: Oregon
  Commission for the Blind, 6215
World of Options, 2777

Pennsylvania

ACLD/An Association for Children and Adult s
  with Learning Disabilities: Greater Pittsburgh,
  6216
Abilities in Motion, 4469
AccessToThePlanet, 5568
Accessible Journeys, 5569
Aces Adventure Weekend, 1370
Achieva, 1371
Air Products Foundation, 3193
Anthracite Region Center for Independent Living,
  4470
Arc of Pennsylvania, 3194
Arcadia Foundation, 3195
Associated Services for the Blind and Visu ally
  Impaired, 4950
Beaver College, 2753
Brachial Plexus Palsy Foundation, 3196
Brian's House, 4471
Butler VA Medical Center, 5783
Camp AIM, 1372
Camp Akeela, 1373
Camp Amp, 1374
Camp Can Do, 1375
Camp Freedom, 1378
Camp Hot-to-Clot, 1379
Camp Lee Mar, 1380
Camp Lily Lehigh Valley, 1381
Camp Orchard Hill, 1382
Camp Ramah in the Poconos Education, Inc., 1383
Camp STAR, 1384
Camp Setebaid, 1385
Camp Spencer Superstars, 1386
Camp Victory, 1157, 1387
Camp Wesley Woods: Exceptional Persons Camp,
  1388
Camp Woodlands, 1389
Carnegie Library of Pittsburgh Library for the
  Blind & Physically Handicapped, 4951
Coatesville VA Medical Center, 5784
Columbia Gas of Pennsylvania Corporate Giv ing,
  3197
Community Resources for Independence, 4472
Community Resources for Independence, Inc.,
  Bradford, 4473
Community Resources for Independence:
  Lewistown, 4474
Community Resources for Independence: Alto ona,
  4475
Community Resources for Independence: Clar ion,
  4476
Community Resources for Independence: Clea
  rfield, 4477
Community Resources for Independence: Herm
  itage, 4478
Community Resources for Independence: Lewi
  sburg, 4479
Community Resources for Independence: Oil City,
  4480
Community Resources for Independence: Warr en,
  4481
Community Resources for Independence: Well
  sboro, 4482
Connelly Foundation, 3198
Dolfinger-McMahon Foundation, 3199
Dragonfly Forest Summer Camp, 1390
Elwyn, 848
Elwyn Delaware, 4749
Erie VA Medical Center, 5785
Free Library of Philadelphia: Library for the Blind
  and Physically Handicapped, 4952
Freedom Valley Disability Center, 4483

Guided Tour for Persons 17 & Over with
  Developmental and Physical Challenges, 5581
Handi Camp, 1391
Heinz Endowments, 3200
Henry L Hillman Foundation, 3201
Innabah Camps, 1392
Institute on Disabilities At Temple Univ., 4484
International University Partnerships, 2761
James E Van Zandt VA Medical Center, 5786
Jewish Healthcare Foundation of Pittsburgh, 3202
Juliet L Hillman Simonds Foundation, 3203
Learning Disabilities Association of Ameri ca, 889
Lebanon VA Medical Center, 5787
Lehigh Valley Center for Independent Living, 4485
Liberty Resources, 4486
Life and Independence for Today, 4487
Lions Camp Kirby, 1393
Mainstay Life Services Summer Program, 1394
Northeastern Pennsylvania Center for Independent
  Living, 4488
Oberkotter Foundation, 3204
Office of Vocational Rehabilitation, 6217
Outside In School Of Experiential Education, Inc.,
  1395
PECO Energy Company Contributions Program,
  3205
PNC Bank Foundation, 3206
Pennsylvania College of Optometry Eye Institute,
  4953
Pennsylvania Employment Services and Job
  Training, 6218
Pennsylvania Governor's Committee on
  Employment of Disabled Persons, 6219
Pennsylvania Human Relations Commission
  Agency, 6220
Pennsylvania Veterans Centers, 5788
Phelps School Academic Support Program, 1396
Philadelphia Foundation, 3207
Philadelphia Regional Office and Insurance Center,
  5789
Philadelphia VA Medical Center, 5790
Pittsburgh Foundation, 3208
Pittsburgh Regional Office, 5791
Raising Deaf Kids, 934
Reading Rehabilitation Hospital, 4954
Sequanota Lutheran Conference Center and Camp,
  1397
Shenango Valley Foundation, 3209
South Central Pennsylvania Center for Inde
  pendence Living, 4489
Staunton Farm Foundation, 3210
Stewart Huston Charitable Trust, 3211
Stuttering Center of Western Pennsylvania, 944
Teleflex Foundation, 3212
Three Rivers Center for Independent Living: New
  Castle, 4490
Three Rivers Center for Independent Livi ng:
  Washington, 4491
Three.Rivers Center for Independent Living, 4171,
  4492
Tri-County Patriots for Independent Living, 4493
USX Foundation, 3213
VA Pittsburgh Healthcare System, University
  Drive Division, 5792
VA Pittsburgh Healthcare System, Highland Drive
  Division, 5793
Variety Club Camp & Development Center, 1398
Vocational and Rehabilitation Agency, 5941, 5955,
  6007, 6013, 6035, 6058, 6092, 6120,
  6137, 6142, 6174, 6182, 6194, 6207, 6214, 6222
Voices for Independence, 4494
West Penn Burn Camp, 1399
Wilkes-Barre VA Medical Center, 5794
William B Dietrich Foundation, 3214
William Talbott Hillman Foundation, 3215
William V and Catherine A McKinney Charitable
  Foundation, 3216
YMCA Camp Fitch, 1400

Rhode Island

Arc South County Chapter, 3217
Arc of Blackstone, 4495
Arc of Blackstone Valley, 3218

LIFE: Fort Hall, 4104
Lisle, 2765
Lola Wright Foundation, 3266
Meadows Foundation, 3267
Michael E. Debakey VA Medical Center, 5811
Moody Foundation, 3268
NADR Conference, 1919
National Association of Disability Repre se
ntatives, 902
Office for Students with Disabilities, University of
Texas at Arlington, 4532
Palestine Resource Center for Independent Living,
4533
Panhandle Action Center for Independent Living
Skills, 4534
Pearle Vision Foundation, 3269
REACH of Dallas Resource Center on Independent
Living, 4535
REACH of Denton Resource Center on
Independent Living, 4536
REACH of Fort Worth Resource Center on Ind
ependent Living, 4537
RISE-Resource: Information, Support and
Empowerment, 4538
SAILS, 4539
San Antonio Area Foundation, 3270
Shell Oil Company Foundation, 3271
South Texas Charitable Foundation, 3272
South Texas Veterans Healthcare System, 5812
Sterling-Turner Foundation, 3273
TLL Temple Foundation, 3274
Talking Book Program/Texas State Library, 4967
Texas Department of Assistive and Rehabili tative
Services, 4540
Texas Employment Services and Job Training
Program Liaison, 6242
Texas Lions Camp, 1454
University of Texas Southwestern Medical
Center/Allergy & Immunology, 4968
University of Texas at Austin Library, 4969
VA North Texas Health Veterans Affairs Car e
System: Dallas VA Medical Center, 5813
VOLAR Center for Independent Living, 4541
Valley Association for Independent Living (VAIL),
4542
Valley Association for Independent Living:
Harlingen, 4543
Vocational and Rehabilitation Agency: State
Rehabilitation Commission, 5956, 6243
Waco Regional Office, 5814
West Texas VA Healthcare System, 5815
William Stamps Farish Fund, 3275

Utah

Action Camp, 1455
Active Re-Entry, 4544
Active Re-Entry: Vernal, 4545
Camp Giddy-Up, 1456
Camp Hobe, 1457
Camp ICANDO, 1458
Camp Kostopulos, 1459
Camp Nah-Nah-Mah, 1460
Camp Vision, 1461
Camp X-Treme, 1462
Central Utah Independent Living Center, 4546
Discovery Camps, 1463
FCYD Camp Utada, 1464
Marriner S Eccles Foundation, 3277
OPTIONS for Independence, 4547
OPTIONS for Independence: Brigham Satellit e,
4548
Overnight Camps, 1465
Questar Corporation Contributions Program, 3278
Red Rock Center for Independence, 4549
Utah Assistive Technology Program (UTAP) Utah
State University, 4551
Utah Division of Veterans Affairs, 5816
Utah Employment Services, 6244
Utah Governor's Committee on Employment of the
Handicapped, 6245
Utah Independent Living Center, 4552
Utah Independent Living Center: Minersville, 4553
Utah Independent Living Center: Tooele, 4554

Utah State Library Division: Program for the Blind
and Disabled, 4970
Utah Veterans Centers, 6246
VA Salt Lake City Healthcare System, 5817

Vermont

Camp Thorpe, 1466
National Center for PTSD, 4971
Silver Towers Camp, 1467
State of Vermont Department of Disabilitie s,
Aging and Independent Living, 6249
Vermont Assistive Technology Program, 4555
Vermont Center for Independent Living: Ben
nington, 4556
Vermont Center for Independent Living: Chi
ttenden, 4557
Vermont Center for Independent Living: Mon
tpelier, 4558
Vermont Community Foundation, 3279
Vermont Department of Libraries - Special
Services Unit, 4972
Vermont Department of Libraries -Special Services
Unit, 4973
Vermont Employment Services and Job Training,
6250
Vermont Governor's Committee on Employment of
People with Disabilities, 6251
Vermont VA Regional Office Center, 5818
Vermont Veterans Centers, 5819

Virginia

ACA Annual Conference, 1889
ACS Federal Healthcare, 752
ADA Annual Scientific Sessions, 1890
AER Annual International Conference, 1891
ASIA Annual Scientific Meeting, 1895
Access Independence, 4559
Access Services, 4974
Alexandria Community Y Head Start, 6252
Alexandria Library Talking Book Service, 4975
American Academy of Audiology, 764
American Chiropractic Association, 775
American Counseling Association, 778
American National Bank and Trust Company, 2922
Amputee Coalition, 794
Appalachian Independence Center, 4560
Arc of Virginia, 3280
Arlington County Department of Libraries, 4976
Association of Medical Professionals with Hearing
Losses (Amphl), 802
Beacon Tree, 806
Blinded Veterans Association National
Convention, 1907
Blue Ridge Independent Living Center, 4561
Blue Ridge Independent Living Center:
Christianburg, 4562
Blue Ridge Independent Living Center: Low Moor,
4563
Braille Circulating Library for the Blind, 4977
Brain Injury Association of America, 810
Camp Dickenson, 1469
Camp Easter Seals Virginia, 1470
Camp Foundation, 3281
Camp Holiday Trails, 1471
Camp Jordan, 1472
Camp Loud And Clear, 1473
Camp Virginia Jaycee, 1474
Camps for Children & Teens with Diabetes, 1475
Central Rappahannock Regional Library, 4978
Civitan Acres for the Disabled, 1476
Clinch Independent Living Services, 4564
Community Foundation of Richmond & Central
Virginia, 3282
Council For Exceptional Children, 833
Council for Exceptional Children, 4979
Council for Exceptional Children Annual
Convention and Expo, 1911
Department Of Rehabilitative Services, 6253
Developmental Training Services, 5932
Didlake, 6254
Disability Funders Network, 837

Disability Resource Center, 4071, 4565
ENDependence Center of Northern Virginia, 4566
Equal Access Center for Independence, 4567
From the State Capitals: Public Health, 3331
Hampton VA Medical Center, 5820
Hunter Holmes McGuire VA Medical Center, 5821
Independence Empowerment Center, 4568
Independence Resource Center, 4569
Independent Living Center Network: Department
of the Visually Handicapped, 4570
International Chiropractors Association, 878
International Student Exchange Programs (I SEP),
2760
James Branch Cabell Library, 4980
John Randolph Foundation, 3283
Junction Center for Independent Living, 4571
Junction Center for Independent Living: Du ffield,
4572
Learning Services: Shenandoah, 6255
Loudoun County Adaptive Recreation Camps,
1477
Lynchburg Area Center for Independent Living,
4573
Mental Health America, 896
NISH, 6256
National Association of State Directors of
Developmental Disabilities Services
(NASDDDS), 903
National Council on the Aging Conference, 1921
National Rehabilitation Association (NRA), 914
National Vaccine Information Center, 917
Newport News Public Library System, 4981
Norfolk Foundation, 3284
Northern Virginia Resource Center for Deaf and
Hard of Hearing Persons, 4982
Oakland School & Camp, 1478
Peidmont Independent Living Center, 4574
Peninsula Center for Independent Living, 4575
Piedmont Independent Living Center, 4576
RESNA Annual Conference, 1925
Rehabiliation Engineering Center for Personal
Licensed Transportation, 5601
Resources for Independent Living, 4011, 4577
Richmond Research Training Center, 6257
Roanoke City Public Library System, 4983
Roanoke Regional Office, 5822
Robey W Estes Family Foundation, 3285
Salem VA Medical Center, 5823
ServiceSource, 6258
Sheltered Occupational Center of Virginia, 6259
Source-APTA Audio Conference, 1927
Staunton Public Library Talking Book Center,
4984
Technology and Media Division, 945
University of Virginia Health System General
Clinical Research Group, 4985
Valley Associates for Independent Living (VAIL),
4578
Valley Associates for Independent Living:
Lexington, 4579
Virginia Autism Resource Center, 4986
Virginia Beach Foundation, 3286
Virginia Beach Public Library Special Services
Library, 4987
Virginia Chapter of the Arthtitis Foundation, 4988
Virginia Department of Veterans Services, 5824
Virginia State Library for the Visually and
Physically Handicapped, 4989
Vocational and Rehabilitation Agency: Department
for the Blind/Visually Impaired, 6195, 6223,
6228, 6228, 6260
Volunteers of America, 750
Woodrow Wilson Rehabilitation Center Training
Program, 4580
World Federation for Mental Health, 958

Washington

Alliance for People with Disabilities: Sea ttle, 4581
Alliance of People with Disabilities: Redmond,
4582
American Disability Association, 779
Arc of Washington State, 3287
Bastyr University Natural Health Clinic, 804

Ben B Cheney Foundation, 3288
Camp Goodtimes, 1479
Camp Killoqua, 1480
Camp Korey, 1481
Camp Prime Time, 1482
Camp Sealth, 1483
Camp Stix, 1484
Community Foundation of North Central
    Washington, 3289
Community Services for the Blind and Parti ally
    Sighted Store: Sight Connection, 4583
Department of Services for the Blind National
    Business & Disability Council, 6262
DisAbility Resource Connection: Everett, 4584
Division of Developmental Disabilities: De
    partment of Social & Health Services, 6263
Easter Seals Camp Stand by Me, 1485
Glaser Progress Foundation, 3290
Greater Tacoma Community Foundation, 3291
Inland Northwest Community Foundation, 3292
Jonathan M Wainwright Memorial VA Medical
    Center, 5825
Kitsap Community Resources, 4585
Medina Foundation, 3293
Meridian Valley Clinical Laboratory, 4990
Norcliffe Foundation, 3294
Northwest Kiwanis Camp, 1486
Ophthalmic Research Laboratory Eye Institute/First
    Hill Campus, 4991
SL Start and Associates, 6264
School of Piano Technology for the Blind, 6265
Seattle Regional Office, 5826
Spokane Center for Independent Living, 4586
Spokane VA Medical Center, 5827
Stewardship Foundation, 3295
Tacoma Area Coalition of Individuals with
    Disabilities, 4587
VA Puget Sound Health Care System, 5828
Vocational and Rehabilitation Agency: Division of
    Vocational Rehabilitation, 5995, 6248, 6266,
    6266
Washington Talking Book and Braille Library,
    4992
Western Washington University, 2775
Westside Parents Work Activity Center, 6037
Weyerhaeuser Company Foundation, 3296
Wheelchair Getaways, 5590
Wheelchair Getaways Wheelchair/Scooter
    Accessible Van Rentals, 5602

West Virginia

Appalachian Center for Independent Living, 4588
Appalachian Center for Independent Living:
    Spencer, 4589
Arc Of West Virginia, The, 3297
Bernard McDonough Foundation, 3298
Cabell County Public Library/Talking Book
    Department/Subregional Library for the Blind,
    4993
Division of Rehabilitation Services: Staff Library,
    4994

High Technology Foundation, 869
Huntington Regional Office, 5829
Huntington VA Medical Center, 5830
Kanawha County Public Library, 4995
Louis A Johnson VA Medical Center, 5831
Martinsburg VA Medical Center, 5832
Mountain State Center for Independent Living,
    4590
Mountain State Center for Independent Living,
    4591
Mountaineer Spina Bifida Camp, 1487
Northern West Virginia Center for Independent
    Living, 4592
Ohio County Public Library Services for the Blind
    and Physically Handicapped, 4996
Ronald McDonald House, 937
Talking Book Department, Parkersburg and Wood
    County Public Library, 4997
US Department Veterans Affairs Beckley Vet
    Center, 5833
West Virginia Autism Training Center, 4998
West Virginia Division of Rehabilitation Services,
    6267
West Virginia Employment Services and Job
    Training Programs Liaison, 6268
West Virginia Library Commission, 4999
West Virginia School for the Blind Library, 5000
West Virginia Vocational Rehabilitation, 6269

Wisconsin

AACRC Annual Meeting, 1884
Able Trek Tours, 5567
American Academy for Cerebral Palsy and
    Developmental Medicine Annual Conference,
    1898
Arc of Dunn County, 3299
Arc of Eau Claire, 3300
Arc of Fox Cities, 3301
Arc of Racine County, 3302
Arc of Wisconsin Disability Association, 3303
Arc-Dane County, 3304
Association of Children's Residential Centers, 800
Association of Educational Therapists, 801
Brown County Library, 5001
Camp Daypoint, 1488
Camp Kee-B-Waw, 1489
Camp Klotty Pine, 1490
Camp Lakota, 1491
Camp Needlepoint, 1492
Center for Independent Living of Western
    Wisconsin, 4593
Clement J Zablocki VA Medical Center, 5834
Easter Seal Camp Wawbeek, 1493
Eye Institute of the Medical College of Wisconsin
    and Froedtert Clinic, 5002
Faye McBeath Foundation, 3305
Helen Bader Foundation, 3306
Independence First, 4594
Independence First: West Bend, 4595
Inspiration Ministries, 4596
Johnson Controls Foundation, 3307

Lutherdale Bible Camp, 1494
Lynde and Harry Bradley Foundation, 3308
Mid-State Independent Living Consultants:
    Wausau, 4597
Mid-state Independent Living Consultants: Stevens
    Point, 4598
Milwaukee Foundation, 3309
North Country Independent Living, 4599
North Country Independent Living: Ashland, 4600
Northwestern Mutual Life Foundation, 3310
Options for Independent Living, 4601
Options for Independent Living: Fox Valley, 4602
Phantom Lake YMCA Camp, 1495
SB Waterman & E Blade Charitable Foundation,
    3312
Society's Assets: Elkhorn, 4603
Society's Assets: Kenosha, 4604
Society's Assets: Racine, 4605
Timbertop Nature Adventure Camp, 1496
Tomah VA Medical Center, 5835
Trace Research and Development Center, 5003
Vocational and Rehabilitation: State of Wisconsin,
    6270
William S Middleton Memorial VA Hospital
    Center, 5836
Wisconsin Badger Camp, 1497
Wisconsin Elks/Easter Seals Respite Camp, 1498
Wisconsin Lions Camp, 1499
Wisconsin Regional Library for the Blind &
    Physically Handicapped, 5004
Wisconsin VA Regional Office, 5837

Wyoming

Arc of Natrona County, 3313
Camp Hope, 1500
Casper Vet Center, 5838
Cheyenne VA Medical Center, 5839
Division of Vocational Rehabilitation of Wyoming,
    6271
Eagle View Ranch, 1501
RENEW: Gillette, 4606
RENEW: Rehabilitation Enterprises of North
    Eastern Wyoming, 4607
Rehabilitation Enterprises of North Easter n
    Wyoming: Newcastle, 4608
Sheridan VA Medical Center, 5840
Vocational Rehabilitation, Division of Department
    of Workforce Services, 6272
Wyoming Department of Employment
    Unemployment Insurance, 6273
Wyoming Governor's Committee on Employment
    of the Handicapped, 6274
Wyoming Services for Independent Living, 4609
Wyoming Services for the Visually Impaired, 5005
Wyoming's New Options in Technology
    (WYNOT) - University of Wyoming, 5006

AIDS

AIDS Alert, 8663
AIDS and Other Manifestations of HIV Infection, 8477
AIDS Healthcare Foundation, 754
AIDS in the Twenty-First Century: Disease and Globalization, 8478
AIDS Legal Council of Chicago, 4611
AIDS Sourcebook, 8476
AIDS United, 8292
AIDS Vancouver, 755
AIDS: The Official Journal of the International AIDS Society, 8645
AIDSLAW of Louisiana, 4612
Camp Heartland, 1207
Camp Hollywood HEART, 1001
Camp Kindle, 1002, 1233
Camp Starlight, 1360
Camp Sunburst, 1016
Caremark Healthcare Services, 6869
Children with Disabilities, 5255
FC Search, 3319
Glaser Progress Foundation, 3290
Guide to Living with HIV Infection: Developed at the Johns Hopkins AIDS Clinic, 8528
Harborview Medical Center, Low Vision Aid Clinic, 7245
HEAL: Health Education AIDS Liaison, 2082
HIV Infection and Developmental Disabilities, 2463
Legal Action Center, 4625
Legislative Network for Nurses, 4672
Levi Strauss Foundation, 2829
Living Well with Chronic Fatigue Syndrome and Fibromyalgia, 8556
Living Well with HIV and AIDS, 8557
A Loving Spoonful, 751
Miami VA Medical Center, 5656
Michigan Association for Deaf, and Hard of Hearing, 3585
Michigan Protection & Advocacy Service, 3598
National AIDS Hotline, 8708
No Longer Immune: A Counselor's Guide to AIDS, 2527
Penitent, with Roses: An HIV+ Mother Reflects, 8603
Project Inform, 933
Questions and Answers: The ADA and Personswith HIV/AIDS, 8610
Ryan White & Global HIV/AIDS Program, 938
Sight by Touch, 9167
Strength for the Journey, 1367, 8456
Sunburst Projects, 8354
Suttle Lake Camp, 1368, 8459
Vinfen Corporation, 7035
Visiting Nurse Association of North Shore, 7036

Aging

Activities in Action, 7541
ADHD: What Can We Do?, 7902
Administration on Aging, 3341
Advocacy Center of Louisiana, 759
Advocacy Centre for the Elderly, 760
Aging & Vision News, 7576
Aging and Disability Services, 3876, 7487
Aging and Disability Services Division, 3648
Aging and Disability: Crossing Network Lines, 2344
Aging and Family Therapy: Practitioner Perspectives on Golden Pond, 7544
Aging and Rehabilitation II: The State ofthe Practice, 2345
Aging and Vision News, 7578
Aging and Vision: Declarations of Independence, 9155
Aging Brain, 2343
Aging in America, 7488
Aging in Stride, 7545
Aging in the Designed Environment, 7546
Aging Life Care Association, 7483
Aging News Alert, 7577, 7583
Aging Services of Michigan, 7484

Aging Services of South Carolina, 7485
Aging Services of Washington, 7486
Aging with a Disability, 7547
Alabama Department of Senior Services, 3368
Alabama VA Benefits Regional Office - Montgomery, 5612
Alaska Commission on Aging, 3378
Albany County Department for Aging and Albany Social Services, 3692
Albany VA Medical Center: Samuel S Stratton, 5745
Aleda E Lutz VA Medical Center, 5706
Alexandria VA Medical Center, 5689
Alliance for Aging Research, 7489
Alliance for Retired Americans, 7490
Alvin C York VA Medical Center, 5802
Amarillo VA Healthcare System, 5807
American Aging Association, 7491
American Association of Retired Persons, 7492
American Geriatrics Society, 7493
American Planning Association, 7494
American Society on Aging, 7495
American Wheelchair Bowling Association, 8270
Amyotrophic Lateral Sclerosis: A Guide for Patients and Families, 8486
ARC Of Southeast Los Angeles-Southeast Industries, 6594
Area Agency on Aging of Southwest Arkansas, 7597
Area Agency on Aging: Region One, 7598
Arizona Division of Aging and Adult Services, 3390
Arkansas Division of Aging & Adult Services, 3399
Asheville VA Medical Center, 5761
Association for Gerontology in Higher Education, 7496
Association for International Practical Training, 2751
Association of Jewish Aging Services, 7497
Association on Aging with Developmental Disabilities, 7498
Atlanta Regional Office, 5659
Atlanta VA Medical Center, 5660
Attention Getter, 1724
Attention Teens, 1725
Augusta VA Medical Center, 5661
Baltimore Regional Office, 5694
Baltimore VA Medical Center, 5695
Bath VA Medical Center, 5747
Battle Creek VA Medical Center, 5707
Bay Pines VA Medical Center, 5653
Biloxi/Gulfport VA Medical Center, 5717
Blindness, A Family Matter, 9156
Boise Regional Office, 5667
Boise VA Medical Center, 5668
Boston VA Regional Office, 5700
Bronx VA Medical Center, 5748
Brooklyn Campus of the VA NY Harbor Healthcare System, 5749
Buffalo Regional Office - Department of Veterans Affairs, 5750
Building Blocks: Foundations for Learning for Young Blind and Visually Impaired Children, 9157
Butler VA Medical Center, 5783
California Department of Aging, 3407
Canandaigua VA Medical Center, 5751
CARF International (Commission on Accreditation of Rehabilitation Facilities), 2077
CARF Rehabilitation Accreditation Commission, 812
Caring for Those You Love: A Guide to Compassionate Care for the Aged, 7549
Carl T Hayden VA Medical Center, 5619
Carl Vinson VA Medical Center, 5662
Castle Point Campus of the VA Hudson Valley Healthcare System, 5752
Center for Disability and Elder Law, Inc., 4613
Center for Positive Aging, 7499
Change Your Brain, Change Your Life: The Breakthrough Program for Conquering Depression, 7791

Cheyenne VA Medical Center, 5839
Children of Aging Parents, 7500
Chillicothe VA Medical Center, 5769
Cincinnati VA Medical Center, 5770
Clement J Zablocki VA Medical Center, 5834
Cleveland Regional Office, 5771
Coatesville VA Medical Center, 5784
Colmery-O'Neil VA Medical Center, 5682
Colorado Association of Homes and Services for the Aging, 7501
Colorado Department of Aging & Adult Services, 3422
Colorado Springs Independence Center, 4026
Colorado/Wyoming VA Medical Center, 5639
Columbia Foundation, 2984
Columbia Regional Office, 5797
Communication Skills for Working with Elders, 2400
Complementary Alternative Medicine and Multiple Sclerosis, 8511
Connecticut Commission on Aging, 3431
Coping and Caring: Living with Alzheimer's Disease, 7551
Court-Related Needs of the Elderly and Persons with Disabilities, 4645
CurePSP Magazine, 8652
Dayton VA Medical Center, 5772
Deaf-Blind Division of the National Federation of the Blind, 8866
Delaware Department of Health and Social Services, 3438
Delaware VA Regional Office, 5646
Denver VA Medical Center, 5640
Des Moines VA Medical Center, 5677
Des Moines VA Regional Office, 5678
District of Columbia Office on Aging, 3447
DSHS/Aging & Adult Disability Services Administration, 3885
Duchenne Muscular Dystrophy, 8518
Durham VA Medical Center, 5763
Dwight D Eisenhower VA Medical Center, 5683
East Orange Campus of the VA New Jersey Healthcare System, 5740
Edith Nourse Rogers Memorial Veterans Hospital, 5701
Edward Hines Jr Hospital, 5669
Ehrman Medical Library, 4915
El Paso VA Healthcare Center, 5809
Elder Abuse and Mistreatment, 7552
Elder Visions Newsletter, 7589
ElderLawAnswers.com, 4656
Elgin Training Center, 6884
Employment for Individuals with Asperger Syndrome or Non-Verbal Learning Disability, 8781
Enabling News, 7579
Erie VA Medical Center, 5785
Eugene J Towbin Healthcare Center, 5622
Explore Your Options, 7553
Facilitating Self-Care Practices in the Elderly, 2451
Falling in Old Age, 7554
Family Intervention Guide to Mental Illness, 7555
Family-Guided Activity-Based Intervention for Toddlers & Infants, 5385
Fanlight Productions, 25
Fargo VA Medical Center, 5767
Fayetteville VA Medical Center, 5623, 5764
Federation for Children with Special Needs, 856
Films & Videos on Aging and Sensory Change, 5388
Florida Adult Services, 3461
Fort Howard VA Medical Center, 5696
Foundations of Orientation and Mobility, 8994
Gainesville Division, North Florida/South Georgia Veterans Healthcare System, 5654
Georgia Department of Aging, 3477
The Gerontological Society of America, 7540
Gerontology: Abstracts in Social Gerontology, 7573
Getting Better, 8159
Golf Xpress, 7494
Goodwill Industries of Central Indiana, 6047
Grand Island VA Medical System, 5728
Grand Junction VA Medical Center, 5641

Southern Oregon Rehabilitation Center & Clinics, 5782

Spokane VA Medical Center, 5827

St. Cloud VA Medical Center, 5714

St. Louis Regional Office, 5722

St. Louis VA Medical Center, 5723

St. Paul Regional Office, 5715

St. Petersburg Regional Office, 5657

Start-to-Finish Library, 1857

State of Vermont Department of Disabilities, Aging and Independent Living, 6249

Stickybear Typing, 1874

Storybook Maker Deluxe, 1793

Strategies for Teaching Students with Learning and Behavior Problems, 2586

Strides Magazine, 8240

Successful Models of Community Long Term Care Services for the Elderly, 7568

Syracuse VA Medical Center, 5756

Teaching Special Students in Mainstream, 2123

Tennessee Commission on Aging and Disability, 3817

Tennessee Hospital Association, 7539

Texas Department on Aging, 3842

Therapeutic Activities with Persons Disabled by Alzheimer's Disease, 7569

Togus VA Medical Center, 5693

Tomah VA Medical Center, 5835

Tomorrow's Promise: Language Arts, 1863

Tomorrow's Promise: Spelling, 1865

Tompkins County Office for the Aging, 7607

Tourette Syndrome: The Facts, 8629

Triangle J Council of Governments Area Agency on Aging, 7608

University of California Memory and Aging Center, 7609

US Department of Veterans Affairs National Headquarters, 5610

US Servas, 5563

Utah Department of Aging, 3855

Utah Division of Veterans Affairs, 5816

V A Montana Healthcare System, 5725

VA Ann Arbor Healthcare System, 5711

VA Boston Healthcare System: Brockton Division, 5703

VA Boston Healthcare System: Jamaica Plain Campus, 5704

VA Boston Healthcare System: West Roxbury Division, 5705

VA Central California Health Care System, 5634

VA Connecticut Healthcare System: Newington Division, 5644

VA Connecticut Healthcare System: West Haven, 5645

VA Greater Los Angeles Healthcare System, 5635

VA Illiana Health Care System, 5672

VA Montana Healthcare System, 5726

VA Nebraska-Western Iowa Health Care System, 5731

VA North Indiana Health Care System: Fort Wayne Campus, 5675

VA Northern California Healthcare System, 5636

VA Northern Indiana Health Care System: Marion Campus, 5676

VA Pittsburgh Healthcare System, Highland Drive Division, 5793

VA Pittsburgh Healthcare System, University Drive Division, 5792

VA Puget Sound Health Care System, 5828

VA Salt Lake City Healthcare System, 5817

VA San Diego Healthcare System, 5637

VA Sierra Nevada Healthcare System, 5734

VA Southern Nevada Healthcare System, 5735

VA Western NY Healthcare System, Batavia, 5759

VA Western NY Healthcare System, Buffalo, 5760

Vermont Department of Aging, 3867

Vermont Department of Disabilities, Aging and Independent Living, 3869

Vermont Division of Disability & Aging Services, 3873

Vermont VA Regional Office Center, 5818

Veteran Benefits Administration - Anchorage Regional Office, 5618

Visiting Nurse Association of America, 8718

Visually Impaired Seniors as Senior Companions: A Reference Guide, 7570

Waco Regional Office, 5814

Washington County Disability, Aging and Veteran Services, 3770

Washington DC VA Medical Center, 5652

We Can Do it Together!, 9169

West Palm Beach VA Medical Center, 5658

West Texas VA Healthcare System, 5815

West Virginia Department of Aging, 3901

WG Hefner VA Medical Center - Salisbury, 5765

Wilkes-Barre VA Medical Center, 5794

William Jennings Bryan Dorn VA Medical Center, 5799

William S Middleton Memorial VA Hospital Center, 5836

Wilmington VA Medical Center, 5647

Winston-Salem Regional Office, 5766

Wisconsin Bureau of Aging, 3911

Wisconsin VA Regional Office, 5837

Work Exploration Center, 5996

Work, Health and Income Among the Elderly, 7571

Wyoming Department of Aging, 3919

Wyoming/Colorado VA Regional Office, 5841

Yoga for Fibromyalgia: Move, Breathe, and Relax to Improve Your Quality of Life, 8233

Young Person's Guide to Spina Bifida, 8641

Alternative Therapies

Academy for Guided Imagery, 2713

American Academy of Environmental Medicine: Annual Conference, 1899

American Academy of Osteopathy, 8168

American Association of Neuromuscular & Electrodiagnostic Medicine, 8169

American Association of Oriental Medicine, 769

American College of Advancement in Medicine, 776

American College of Nurse Midwives, 777

American Council for Headache Education(ACHE), 2073

American Herb Association Newsletter, 5068

American Holistic Medical Association, 783

American Sexual Health Association, 8304

American Society for the Alexander Technique, 790

American Society of Clinical Hypnosis, 792

Aromatherapy Book: Applications and Inhalations, 5075

Aromatherapy for Common Ailments, 5076

Association for Applied Psychophysiology and Biofeedback, 796

Ayurvedic Institute, 2718

Bach Flower Therapy: Theory and Practice, 5081

Bastyr University Natural Health Clinic, 804

Beliefs, Values, and Principles of Self Advocacy, 5083

Brain Allergies: The Psychonutrient and Magnetic Connections, 8495

Center for Mind-Body Studies, 822

Chinese Herbal Medicine, 5101

Chronic Fatigue Syndrome: Your Natural Gu ide to Healing with Diet, Herbs and Other Methods, 8507

Colon Health: Key to a Vibrant Life, 8510

Creating Wholeness: Self-Healing Workbook Using Dynamic Relaxation, Images and Thoughts, 5110

Curing MS: How Science is Solving the Mysteries of Multiple Sclerosis, 8514

Department of Physical Medicine & Rehabilitation at Sinai Hospital, 835

Designing and Using Assistive Technology: The Human Perspective, 2414

Divided Legacy: A History of the Schism in Medical Thought, The Bacteriological Era, 2429

Environmental Health Center: Dallas, 8317

Esalen Institute, 850

Everybody's Guide to Homeopathic Medicines, 5129

Feldenkrais Guild of North America (FGNA), 859

Handbook of Chronic Fatigue Syndrome, 8529

Healing Herbs, 5143

Health Action, 867

Heart of the Mind, 8532

Herb Research Foundation, 5473

Homeopathic Educational Services, 871

Human Ecology Action League (HEAL), 873

Imagery in Healing Shamanism and Modern Medicine, 5151

Informed Touch; A Clinician's Guide To The Evaluation Of Myofascial Disorders, 8538

International Association of Hygienic Physicians, 8325

International Association of Yoga Therapists, 876

International Childbirth Education Association, 2084

International Clinic of Biological Regeneration, 879

It's All in Your Head: The Link Between Mercury Amalgams and Illness, 8542

JoanBorysenko.Com, 884

Living an Idea: Empowerment and the Evolution of an Alternative School, 2016

Living Beyond Multiple Sclerosis: A Woman's Guide, 8554

Long Beach Department of Health and Human Services, 3415

Los Angeles County Department of Health Services, 3416

Lupus: Alternative Therapies That Work, 8563

McKinnon Body Therapy Center, 895

National Association for Holistic Aromatherapy, 899

National Association to Advance Fat Acceptance, 8339

National Center for Homeopathy, 2094

National Guild of Hypnotists, 911

National Headache Foundation, 2947

National University of Natural Medicine, 916

National Vaccine Information Center, 917

New York Therapeutic Riding Center-Equestria, 920

Nothing is Impossible: Reflections on a New Life, 5195

Nurse Healers: Professional Associates International, 923

Nutritional Desk Reference, 5196

Nutritional Influences on Illness:, 5197

Optometric Extension Program Foundation, 2994

Our Own Road, 5406

PACER Center (Parent Advocacy Coalition for Educational Rights), 924

Pacific Institute of Aromatherapy, 926

Pain Erasure, 5277

Pain Erasure: the Bonnie Prudden Way, 9044

Rolf Institute, 936

Small Wonder, 2048

Sofia University, 941

Solving the Puzzle of Chronic Fatigue, 8619

Tourette's Syndrome: Tics, Obsessions, Compulsions: Developmental Psychopathology, 8631

United States Trager Association, 953

Upledger Institute Clinic, 955

Weiner's Herbal, 5242

Amputation

American Amputee Foundation, 7924

Amputee Coalition, 794

Baylor Institute for Rehabilitation, 7206

Botsford Center For Rehabilitation & Health Improvement-Redford, 7039

Breaking New Ground Resource Center, 8695

Camp No Limits California, 1004

Camp No Limits Connecticut, 1062

Camp No Limits Florida, 1074

Camp No Limits Idaho, 1103

Camp No Limits Maine, 1162

Camp No Limits Maryland, 1171

Camp No Limits Missouri, 1222

Camp No Limits Texas, 1442

Camp Snow Maine, 1163

Camp sNOw Maine, 1166

Camp STAR, 1384

Amythrophic Lateral Sclerosis

Art & Music Therapies

Arthritis

Asthma

Attention Deficit Disorder

Autism

Helping People with Autism Manage Their Behavior, 7819
Hidden Child: The Linwood Method for Reaching the Autistic Child, 7821
Hillcroft Services, 1135
Illinois Center for Autism, 6890
Imagery Procedures for People with Special Needs, 5395
Imagine: Innovative Resources for Cognitive & Physical Challenges, 5936
Indiana Resource Center for Autism, 4808
Judevine Center for Autism, 4894
Keys to Parenting the Child with Autism, 7833
Kris' Camp, 1083
Let Community Employment be the Goal for Individuals with Autism, 7836, 8787
Little City Foundation, 2941
Little Friends, Inc., 6893
Living with Spina Bifida: A Guide for Families and Professionals, 8560
Louis de la Parte Florida Mental Health Institute Research Library, 4762
Management of Autistic Behavior, 7838, 8565, 8789
Mount Sinai Medical Center, 2901
Music Therapy, 39
National Autism Association, 7696
National Autism Hotline, 7922
Neurobiology of Autism, 7843, 8791
New England Center for Children, 7028
New Jersey Camp Jaycee, 1263
Parent Survival Manual, 7846, 8793
Please Don't Say Hello, 7850, 8795
Prufrock Press, 2152
Reaching the Autistic Child: A Parent Training Program, 8612
Reaching the Child with Autism Through Art, 62
Riddle of Autism: A Psychological Analysis, 7857, 8799
Rimland Services for Autistic Citizens, 1120, 7749
Schools And Services For Children With Autism Spectrum Disorders., 3710
Sex Education: Issues for the Person with Autism, 7859, 8801
Sometimes You Just Want to Feel Like a Human Being, 5228
Son Rise: The Miracle Continues, 8620
Son-Rise Program, 8714
Son-Rise: The Miracle Continues, 7860, 8802
Soon Will Come the Light, 7861
Special Needs Advocacy Resource Book, 2696
Special Needs Project, 2156
Spokane Center for Independent Living, 4586
Sunnyhill Adventure Center, 7756
TEACCH Autism Program, 7704
Teaching and Mainstreaming Autistic Children, 7865, 8806
Teaching Asperger's Students Social Skills Through Acting, 64
Teaching Children With Autism in the General Classroom, 2595
Teaching Children with Autism: Strategies for Initiating Positive Interactions, 7864, 8805
Teaching Students with Moderate/Severe Disabilities, Including Autism, 2610
Treating Disordered Speech Motor Control, 2625
Treatment and Learning Centers (TLC), 6102
Uncommon Fathers, 5298
Understanding Autism, 7918, 8832
Valley News Dispatch, 7869
Vanguard School, The, 2743
Virginia Autism Resource Center, 4986
Wendell Johnson Speech And Hearing Clinic, 7652, 7760, 8750, 8937
West Hills Day Camp: Gersh Academy, 1306
West Virginia Autism Training Center, 4998
Without Reason: A Family Copes with two Generations of Autism, 7871, 8810

Behavioral Disorders

AACRC Annual Meeting, 1884
Alternative Teaching Strategies, 2348
American Group Psychotherapy Association, 8300

Association for Contextual Behavioral Science, 7659
Behavior Analysis in Education: Focus on Measurably Superior Instruction, 2367
Behavior Modification, 2368
Behavioral Disorders, 2369
Camp Ruggles, 1402, 7723
Center for Neuro Skills, 6619
Childhood Behavior Disorders: Applied Research & Educational Practice, 2384
Creating Positive Classroom Environments: Strategies for Behavior Management, 2407
Devereux Advanced Behavioral Health - National Office, 7183
Devereux Advanced Behavioral Health - Texas Victoria Campus, 7212
Devereux Advanced Behavioral Health Arizona - Scottsdale, 6566
Devereux Advanced Behavioral Health Georgia, 6841
Devereux Advanced Behavioral Health Massachusetts & Rhode Island, 7017
Devereux Advanced Behavioral Health New Jersey, 7089
Devereux Advanced Behavioral Health New York, 7106
Devereux Advanced Behavioral Health Texas - League City Campus, 7213
Devereux Arizona - Tucson, 6567
Devereux Florida - Orlando Campus, 6784
Devereux Florida - Viera Campus, 6785
Devereux Pennsylvania, 7184
Explorer's Club Camp, 1259
Getting Around Town, 2459
Groden Center, 6225
Journal of Emotional and Behavioral Disorders, 2258
Journal of Motor Behavior, 2260
Journal of Vocational Behavior, 2268
Lakeview NeuroRehabilitation Center, 6419
Progress Without Punishment: Approaches for Learners with Behavior Problems, 2550
RCI, 6179
Social Skills for Students With Autism Spectrum Disorders and Other Dev Disabilities, 2576
Teaching Students with Learning and Behavior Problems, 2608
ValueOptions, 5501
Volunteers of America, 750
What School Counselors Need to Know, 2631
Working Bibliography on Behavioral and Emotional Disorders, 2633

Birth Defects

Baylor College of Medicine Birth Defects Center, 4961
BDRC Newsletter, 5454
Birth Defect Research for Children, 807
Camp Bon Coeur, 1153, 8373
Camp Del Corazon, 8383
Camp del Corazon, 1025
Camp Odayin, 1209
Camp Odayin Day Camp, 1210
Camp Odayin Summer Camp, 1211
Camp Odayin Winter Camp, 1212
Camp Odayin Young Adult Retreat, 1213
Camp Taylor, 1018
Camp Taylor: Family Camp, 1019, 1101
Camp Taylor: Leadership Camp, 1020
Camp Taylor: Teen Camp, 1021
Camp Taylor: Young Adult Program, 1022
Camp Taylor: Youth Camp, 1023
Cornelia de Lange Syndrome Foundation, 2865
Dictionary of Congenital Malformations& Disorders, 5114
Division of Birth Defects and Developmental Disabilities, 3473
Edward J Madden Open Hearts Camp, 8434
Management of Genetic Syndromes, 8566
March of Dimes Birth Defects Foundation, 894
National Center on Birth Defects and Developmental Disabilities, 4781
National Fragile X Foundation, 8740

National Organization for Albinism and Hypopigmentation, 8346
National Organization on Fetal Alcohol Syndrome, 8348
Nick & Kelly's Heart Camp, 989
Open Hearts Camp, 1183
University of Miami: Mailman Center for Child Development, 4770
Why My Child, 5433

Blind/Deaf

AADB National Conference, 1885
ABD Winter Conference, 1888
Alaska Center for the Blind and Visually Impaired, 6559
American Association of the Deaf-Blind, 7611
American Board of Disability Analysts Annual Conference, 1900
Arena Stage, 6, 7613
ASD Athletics, 7650
Camp Abilities Brockport, 1273
Canadian Deafblind Association, 7615
Communicating with People Who Have Trouble Hearing & Seeing: A Primer, 7628
Deaf-Blind Perspective, 7637, 9114
Florida School for the Deaf and Blind, 7626
A Handbook for Writing Effective Psychoeducational Reports (2nd Edition), 7627
Hearing Loss Association of America, 7617, 7972
Helen Keller National Center for Deaf- Blind Youths and Adults, 7618
InFocus, 7638
National Center on Deaf-Blindness, 7622
National Family Association for Deaf-Blind, 7623

Brain Injuries

Bancroft, 7087
Before and After Zachariah, 5318
Brain Injury Alliance of Texas, 7667
Brain Injury Association of America, 810, 7668
Brain Injury Association of New York State, 7669
Camp Barefoot, 1192
Center for Comprehensive Services, 6871
Center for Neuro-Rehabilitation, 6997
Communitas Supportive Care Society, 831
Easter Seals Superior California, 6642
The Education of Children with Acquired Brain Injury, 2618
The Essential Brain Injury Guide (5th Edition), 5347
Hope Network Neuro Rehabilitation, 872, 7046
Hospital For Special Care (HSC), 7286
Living with Brain Injury: A Guide for Families, 8559
Measure of Cognitive-Linguistic Abilities(MCLA), 2675
National Hydrocephalus Foundation, 7699
Neurobehavioral Medicine Center, 6812
North Broward Rehab Unit, 6813
Occupational Therapy Approaches to Traumatic Brain Injury, 2529
Preventable Brain Damage, 7851
Rasmussen's Syndrome and Hemispherectomy Support Network Newsletter, 8680
Students with Acquired Brain Injury: The School's Response, 2587
Universal Institute Rehabilitation & Fitness Center, 6428
When Billy Broke His Head...and Other, 5429

Cancer

Adult Leukemia: A Comprehensive Guide for Patients and Families, 8479
Advanced Breast Cancer: A Guide to Living with Metastic Disease, 8480
Adventure Day Camp, 8364
Alexander and Margaret Stewart Trust, 2877
AMC Cancer Research Center, 4737
American Public Health Association, 788

Diabetes

Diet & Nutrition

Down Syndrome

Dyslexia

Education & Counseling

Emergency Alert

Environmental Disorders

Epilepsy

Head & Neck Injuries

Hemophilia

Herbal Medicine

Human Interaction Disabilities

Immune Deficiencies

Incontinence

Lowe's Syndrome

Lung Disorders

Massage Therapy

Mental Disabilities

Mental Retardation

Multiple Disabilities

Multiple Sclerosis

Muscular Dystrophy

Neurological Impairments

Obesity

Obsessive Compulsive Disorders

Orthopedical Disabilities

Pain Management

Parkinson Disease

Pediatric Issues

Phenylketonuria

Physical Disabilities

Women

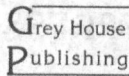
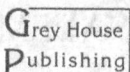

2017 Title List

Visit www.GreyHouse.com for Product Information, Table of Contents, and Sample Pages.

General Reference

An African Biographical Dictionary
America's College Museums
American Environmental Leaders: From Colonial Times to the Present
Encyclopedia of African-American Writing
Encyclopedia of Constitutional Amendments
An Encyclopedia of Human Rights in the United States
Encyclopedia of Invasions & Conquests
Encyclopedia of Prisoners of War & Internment
Encyclopedia of Religion & Law in America
Encyclopedia of Rural America
Encyclopedia of the Continental Congress
Encyclopedia of the United States Cabinet, 1789-2010
Encyclopedia of War Journalism
Encyclopedia of Warrior Peoples & Fighting Groups
The Environmental Debate: A Documentary History
The Evolution Wars: A Guide to the Debates
From Suffrage to the Senate: America's Political Women
Gun Debate: An Encyclopedia of Gun Control & Gun Rights
Political Corruption in America
Privacy Rights in the Digital Era
The Religious Right: A Reference Handbook
Speakers of the House of Representatives, 1789-2009
This is Who We Were: 1880-1900
This is Who We Were: A Companion to the 1940 Census
This is Who We Were: In the 1900s
This is Who We Were: In the 1910s
This is Who We Were: In the 1920s
This is Who We Were: In the 1940s
This is Who We Were: In the 1950s
This is Who We Were: In the 1960s
This is Who We Were: In the 1970s
This is Who We Were: In the 1980s
This is Who We Were: In the 1990s
U.S. Land & Natural Resource Policy
The Value of a Dollar 1600-1865: Colonial Era to the Civil War
The Value of a Dollar: 1860-2014
Working Americans 1770-1869 Vol. IX: Revolutionary War to the Civil War
Working Americans 1880-1999 Vol. I: The Working Class
Working Americans 1880-1999 Vol. II: The Middle Class
Working Americans 1880-1999 Vol. III: The Upper Class
Working Americans 1880-1999 Vol. IV: Their Children
Working Americans 1880-2015 Vol. V: Americans At War
Working Americans 1880-2005 Vol. VI: Women at Work
Working Americans 1880-2006 Vol. VII: Social Movements
Working Americans 1880-2007 Vol. VIII: Immigrants
Working Americans 1880-2009 Vol. X: Sports & Recreation
Working Americans 1880-2010 Vol. XI: Inventors & Entrepreneurs
Working Americans 1880-2011 Vol. XII: Our History through Music
Working Americans 1880-2012 Vol. XIII: Education & Educators
Working Americans 1880-2016 Vol. XIV: Industry Through the Ages
World Cultural Leaders of the 20th & 21st Centuries

Education Information

Charter School Movement
Comparative Guide to American Elementary & Secondary Schools
Complete Learning Disabilities Directory
Educators Resource Directory
Special Education: Policy and Curriculum Development

Health Information

Comparative Guide to American Hospitals
Complete Directory for Pediatric Disorders
Complete Directory for People with Chronic Illness
Complete Directory for People with Disabilities
Complete Mental Health Directory
Diabetes in America: Analysis of an Epidemic
Directory of Health Care Group Purchasing Organizations
HMO/PPO Directory
Medical Device Market Place
Older Americans Information Directory

Business Information

Complete Television, Radio & Cable Industry Directory
Directory of Business Information Resources
Directory of Mail Order Catalogs

Directory of Venture Capital & Private Equity Firms
Environmental Resource Handbook
Food & Beverage Market Place
Grey House Homeland Security Directory
Grey House Performing Arts Directory
Grey House Safety & Security Directory
Hudson's Washington News Media Contacts Directory
New York State Directory
Sports Market Place Directory

Statistics & Demographics

American Tally
America's Top-Rated Cities
America's Top-Rated Smaller Cities
Ancestry & Ethnicity in America
The Asian Databook
Comparative Guide to American Suburbs
The Hispanic Databook
Profiles of America
"Profiles of" Series – State Handbooks
Weather America

Financial Ratings Series

TheStreet Ratings' Guide to Bond & Money Market Mutual Funds
TheStreet Ratings' Guide to Common Stocks
TheStreet Ratings' Guide to Exchange-Traded Funds
TheStreet Ratings' Guide to Stock Mutual Funds
TheStreet Ratings' Ultimate Guided Tour of Stock Investing
Weiss Ratings' Consumer Guides
Weiss Ratings' Financial Literary Basic Guides
Weiss Ratings' Guide to Banks
Weiss Ratings' Guide to Credit Unions
Weiss Ratings' Guide to Health Insurers
Weiss Ratings' Guide to Life & Annuity Insurers
Weiss Ratings' Guide to Property & Casualty Insurers

Bowker's Books In Print® Titles

American Book Publishing Record® Annual
American Book Publishing Record® Monthly
Books In Print®
Books In Print® Supplement
Books Out Loud™
Bowker's Complete Video Directory™
Children's Books In Print®
El-Hi Textbooks & Serials In Print®
Forthcoming Books®
Law Books & Serials In Print™
Medical & Health Care Books In Print™
Publishers, Distributors & Wholesalers of the US™
Subject Guide to Books In Print®
Subject Guide to Children's Books In Print®

Canadian General Reference

Associations Canada
Canadian Almanac & Directory
Canadian Environmental Resource Guide
Canadian Parliamentary Guide
Canadian Venture Capital & Private Equity Firms
Financial Post Directory of Directors
Financial Services Canada
Governments Canada
Health Guide Canada
The History of Canada
Libraries Canada
Major Canadian Cities

Grey House Publishing | Salem Press | H.W. Wilson | 4919 Route, 22 PO Box 56, Amenia NY 12501-0056

2017 Title List
Visit **www.SalemPress.com** for Product Information, Table of Contents, and Sample Pages.

Science, Careers & Mathematics
Ancient Creatures
Applied Science
Applied Science: Engineering & Mathematics
Applied Science: Science & Medicine
Applied Science: Technology
Biomes and Ecosystems
Careers in The Arts: Fine, Performing & Visual
Careers in Building Construction
Careers in Business
Careers in Chemistry
Careers in Communications & Media
Careers in Environment & Conservation
Careers in Financial Services
Careers in Healthcare
Careers in Hospitality & Tourism
Careers in Human Services
Careers in Law, Criminal Justice & Emergency Services
Careers in Manufacturing
Careers in Overseas Jobs
Careers in Physics
Careers in Sales, Insurance & Real Estate
Careers in Science & Engineering
Careers in Sports & Fitness
Careers in Technology Services & Repair
Computer Technology Innovators
Contemporary Biographies in Business
Contemporary Biographies in Chemistry
Contemporary Biographies in Communications & Media
Contemporary Biographies in Environment & Conservation
Contemporary Biographies in Healthcare
Contemporary Biographies in Hospitality & Tourism
Contemporary Biographies in Law & Criminal Justice
Contemporary Biographies in Physics
Earth Science
Earth Science: Earth Materials & Resources
Earth Science: Earth's Surface and History
Earth Science: Physics & Chemistry of the Earth
Earth Science: Weather, Water & Atmosphere
Encyclopedia of Energy
Encyclopedia of Environmental Issues
Encyclopedia of Environmental Issues: Atmosphere and Air Pollution
Encyclopedia of Environmental Issues: Ecology and Ecosystems
Encyclopedia of Environmental Issues: Energy and Energy Use
Encyclopedia of Environmental Issues: Policy and Activism
Encyclopedia of Environmental Issues: Preservation/Wilderness Issues
Encyclopedia of Environmental Issues: Water and Water Pollution
Encyclopedia of Global Resources
Encyclopedia of Global Warming
Encyclopedia of Mathematics & Society
Encyclopedia of Mathematics & Society: Engineering, Tech, Medicine
Encyclopedia of Mathematics & Society: Great Mathematicians
Encyclopedia of Mathematics & Society: Math & Social Sciences
Encyclopedia of Mathematics & Society: Math Development/Concepts
Encyclopedia of Mathematics & Society: Math in Culture & Society
Encyclopedia of Mathematics & Society: Space, Science, Environment
Encyclopedia of the Ancient World
Forensic Science
Geography Basics
Internet Innovators
Inventions and Inventors
Magill's Encyclopedia of Science: Animal Life
Magill's Encyclopedia of Science: Plant life
Notable Natural Disasters
Principles of Astronomy
Principles of Biology
Principles of Chemistry
Principles of Physical Science
Principles of Physics
Principles of Research Methods
Principles of Sustainability
Science and Scientists
Solar System
Solar System: Great Astronomers
Solar System: Study of the Universe
Solar System: The Inner Planets
Solar System: The Moon and Other Small Bodies

Solar System: The Outer Planets
Solar System: The Sun and Other Stars
World Geography

Literature
American Ethnic Writers
Classics of Science Fiction & Fantasy Literature
Critical Approaches: Feminist
Critical Approaches: Multicultural
Critical Approaches: Moral
Critical Approaches: Psychological
Critical Insights: Authors
Critical Insights: Film
Critical Insights: Literary Collection Bundles
Critical Insights: Themes
Critical Insights: Works
Critical Survey of Drama
Critical Survey of Graphic Novels: Heroes & Super Heroes
Critical Survey of Graphic Novels: History, Theme & Technique
Critical Survey of Graphic Novels: Independents/Underground Classics
Critical Survey of Graphic Novels: Manga
Critical Survey of Long Fiction
Critical Survey of Mystery & Detective Fiction
Critical Survey of Mythology and Folklore: Heroes and Heroines
Critical Survey of Mythology and Folklore: Love, Sexuality & Desire
Critical Survey of Mythology and Folklore: World Mythology
Critical Survey of Poetry
Critical Survey of Poetry: American Poets
Critical Survey of Poetry: British, Irish & Commonwealth Poets
Critical Survey of Poetry: Cumulative Index
Critical Survey of Poetry: European Poets
Critical Survey of Poetry: Topical Essays
Critical Survey of Poetry: World Poets
Critical Survey of Science Fiction & Fantasy
Critical Survey of Shakespeare's Plays
Critical Survey of Shakespeare's Sonnets
Critical Survey of Short Fiction
Critical Survey of Short Fiction: American Writers
Critical Survey of Short Fiction: British, Irish, Commonwealth Writers
Critical Survey of Short Fiction: Cumulative Index
Critical Survey of Short Fiction: European Writers
Critical Survey of Short Fiction: Topical Essays
Critical Survey of Short Fiction: World Writers
Critical Survey of World Literature
Critical Survey of Young Adult Literature
Cyclopedia of Literary Characters
Cyclopedia of Literary Places
Holocaust Literature
Introduction to Literary Context: American Poetry of the 20th Century
Introduction to Literary Context: American Post-Modernist Novels
Introduction to Literary Context: American Short Fiction
Introduction to Literary Context: English Literature
Introduction to Literary Context: Plays
Introduction to Literary Context: World Literature
Magill's Literary Annual 2015
Magill's Survey of American Literature
Magill's Survey of World Literature
Masterplots
Masterplots II: African American Literature
Masterplots II: American Fiction Series
Masterplots II: British & Commonwealth Fiction Series
Masterplots II: Christian Literature
Masterplots II: Drama Series
Masterplots II: Juvenile & Young Adult Literature, Supplement
Masterplots II: Nonfiction Series
Masterplots II: Poetry Series
Masterplots II: Short Story Series
Masterplots II: Women's Literature Series
Notable African American Writers
Notable American Novelists
Notable Playwrights
Notable Poets
Recommended Reading: 600 Classics Reviewed
Short Story Writers

Grey House Publishing | Salem Press | H.W. Wilson | 4919 Route, 22 PO Box 56, Amenia NY 12501-0056

2017 Title List

Visit **www.SalemPress.com** for Product Information, Table of Contents, and Sample Pages.

History and Social Science

The 2000s in America
50 States
African American History
Agriculture in History
American First Ladies
American Heroes
American Indian Culture
American Indian History
American Indian Tribes
American Presidents
American Villains
America's Historic Sites
Ancient Greece
The Bill of Rights
The Civil Rights Movement
The Cold War
Countries, Peoples & Cultures
Countries, Peoples & Cultures: Central & South America
Countries, Peoples & Cultures: Central, South & Southeast Asia
Countries, Peoples & Cultures: East & South Africa
Countries, Peoples & Cultures: East Asia & the Pacific
Countries, Peoples & Cultures: Eastern Europe
Countries, Peoples & Cultures: Middle East & North Africa
Countries, Peoples & Cultures: North America & the Caribbean
Countries, Peoples & Cultures: West & Central Africa
Countries, Peoples & Cultures: Western Europe
Defining Documents: American Revolution
Defining Documents: American West
Defining Documents: Ancient World
Defining Documents: Civil Rights
Defining Documents: Civil War
Defining Documents: Court Cases
Defining Documents: Dissent & Protest
Defining Documents: Emergence of Modern America
Defining Documents: Exploration & Colonial America
Defining Documents: Immigration & Immigrant Communities
Defining Documents: Manifest Destiny
Defining Documents: Middle Ages
Defining Documents: Nationalism & Populism
Defining Documents: Native Americans
Defining Documents: Postwar 1940s
Defining Documents: Reconstruction
Defining Documents: Renaissance & Early Modern Era
Defining Documents: 1920s
Defining Documents: 1930s
Defining Documents: 1950s
Defining Documents: 1960s
Defining Documents: 1970s
Defining Documents: The 17th Century
Defining Documents: The 18th Century
Defining Documents: Vietnam War
Defining Documents: Women
Defining Documents: World War I
Defining Documents: World War II
The Eighties in America
Encyclopedia of American Immigration
Encyclopedia of Flight
Encyclopedia of the Ancient World
Fashion Innovators
The Fifties in America
The Forties in America
Great Athletes
Great Athletes: Baseball
Great Athletes: Basketball
Great Athletes: Boxing & Soccer
Great Athletes: Cumulative Index
Great Athletes: Football
Great Athletes: Golf & Tennis
Great Athletes: Olympics
Great Athletes: Racing & Individual Sports
Great Events from History: 17th Century
Great Events from History: 18th Century
Great Events from History: 19th Century
Great Events from History: 20th Century (1901-1940)
Great Events from History: 20th Century (1941-1970)

Great Events from History: 20th Century (1971-2000)
Great Events from History: 21st Century (2000-2016)
Great Events from History: African American History
Great Events from History: Cumulative Indexes
Great Events from History: LGBTG
Great Events from History: Middle Ages
Great Events from History: Modern Scandals
Great Events from History: Renaissance & Early Modern Era
Great Lives from History: 17th Century
Great Lives from History: 18th Century
Great Lives from History: 19th Century
Great Lives from History: 20th Century
Great Lives from History: 21st Century (2000-2016)
Great Lives from History: American Women
Great Lives from History: Ancient World
Great Lives from History: Asian & Pacific Islander Americans
Great Lives from History: Cumulative Indexes
Great Lives from History: Incredibly Wealthy
Great Lives from History: Inventors & Inventions
Great Lives from History: Jewish Americans
Great Lives from History: Latinos
Great Lives from History: Notorious Lives
Great Lives from History: Renaissance & Early Modern Era
Great Lives from History: Scientists & Science
Historical Encyclopedia of American Business
Issues in U.S. Immigration
Magill's Guide to Military History
Milestone Documents in African American History
Milestone Documents in American History
Milestone Documents in World History
Milestone Documents of American Leaders
Milestone Documents of World Religions
Music Innovators
Musicians & Composers 20th Century
The Nineties in America
The Seventies in America
The Sixties in America
Survey of American Industry and Careers
The Thirties in America
The Twenties in America
United States at War
U.S. Court Cases
U.S. Government Leaders
U.S. Laws, Acts, and Treaties
U.S. Legal System
U.S. Supreme Court
Weapons and Warfare
World Conflicts: Asia and the Middle East

Health

Addictions & Substance Abuse
Adolescent Health & Wellness
Cancer
Complementary & Alternative Medicine
Community & Family Health
Genetics & Inherited Conditions
Health Issues
Infectious Diseases & Conditions
Magill's Medical Guide
Nutrition
Nursing
Psychology & Behavioral Health
Psychology Basics

Grey House Publishing | Salem Press | H.W. Wilson | 4919 Route, 22 PO Box 56, Amenia NY 12501-0056

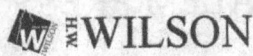
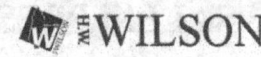
Current Biography
Current Biography Cumulative Index 1946-2013
Current Biography Monthly Magazine
Current Biography Yearbook: 2003
Current Biography Yearbook: 2004
Current Biography Yearbook: 2005
Current Biography Yearbook: 2006
Current Biography Yearbook: 2007
Current Biography Yearbook: 2008
Current Biography Yearbook: 2009
Current Biography Yearbook: 2010
Current Biography Yearbook: 2011
Current Biography Yearbook: 2012
Current Biography Yearbook: 2013
Current Biography Yearbook: 2014
Current Biography Yearbook: 2015
Current Biography Yearbook: 2016

Core Collections
Children's Core Collection
Fiction Core Collection
Graphic Novels Core Collection
Middle & Junior High School Core
Public Library Core Collection: Nonfiction
Senior High Core Collection
Young Adult Fiction Core Collection

The Reference Shelf
Aging in America
American Military Presence Overseas
The Arab Spring
The Brain
The Business of Food
Campaign Trends & Election Law
Conspiracy Theories
The Digital Age
Dinosaurs
Embracing New Paradigms in Education
Faith & Science
Families: Traditional and New Structures
The Future of U.S. Economic Relations: Mexico, Cuba, and Venezuela
Global Climate Change
Graphic Novels and Comic Books
Guns in America
Immigration
Immigration in the U.S.
Internet Abuses & Privacy Rights
Internet Safety
LGBTQ in the 21st Century
Marijuana Reform
The News and its Future
The Paranormal
Politics of the Ocean
Prescription Drug Abuse
Racial Tension in a "Postracial" Age
Reality Television
Representative American Speeches: 2008-2009
Representative American Speeches: 2009-2010
Representative American Speeches: 2010-2011
Representative American Speeches: 2011-2012
Representative American Speeches: 2012-2013
Representative American Speeches: 2013-2014
Representative American Speeches: 2014-2015
Representative American Speeches: 2015-2016
Representative American Speeches: 2016-2017
Rethinking Work
Revisiting Gender
Robotics
Russia
Social Networking
Social Services for the Poor
Space Exploration & Development
Sports in America

The Supreme Court
The Transformation of American Cities
U.S. Infrastructure
U.S. National Debate Topic: Educational Reform
U.S. National Debate Topic: Surveillance
U.S. National Debate Topic: The Ocean
U.S. National Debate Topic: Transportation Infrastructure
Whistleblowers

Readers' Guide
Abridged Readers' Guide to Periodical Literature
Readers' Guide to Periodical Literature

Indexes
Index to Legal Periodicals & Books
Short Story Index
Book Review Digest

Sears List
Sears List of Subject Headings
Sears: Lista de Encabezamientos de Materia

Facts About Series
Facts About American Immigration
Facts About China
Facts About the 20th Century
Facts About the Presidents
Facts About the World's Languages

Nobel Prize Winners
Nobel Prize Winners: 1901-1986
Nobel Prize Winners: 1987-1991
Nobel Prize Winners: 1992-1996
Nobel Prize Winners: 1997-2001

World Authors
World Authors: 1995-2000
World Authors: 2000-2005

Famous First Facts
Famous First Facts
Famous First Facts About American Politics
Famous First Facts About Sports
Famous First Facts About the Environment
Famous First Facts: International Edition

American Book of Days
The American Book of Days
The International Book of Days

Monographs
American Reformers
The Barnhart Dictionary of Etymology
Celebrate the World
Guide to the Ancient World
Indexing from A to Z
The Poetry Break
Radical Change: Books for Youth in a Digital Age

Wilson Chronology
Wilson Chronology of Asia and the Pacific
Wilson Chronology of Human Rights
Wilson Chronology of Ideas
Wilson Chronology of the Arts
Wilson Chronology of the World's Religions
Wilson Chronology of Women's Achievements